The American Psychiatric Publishing

Textbook of Psychosomatic Medicine

Editorial Board

The American Psychiatric Publishing

Textbook of Psychosomatic Medicine

Edited by

James L. Levenson, M.D.

Chair, Consultation-Liaison Psychiatry, and Vice-Chair, Psychiatry
Professor of Psychiatry, Medicine, and Surgery
Virginia Commonwealth University
Richmond, Virginia

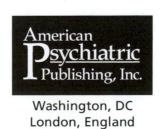

American Psychiatric Publishing, Inc.

Washington, DC
London, England

Note: The authors have worked to ensure that all information in this book is accurate at the time of publication and consistent with general psychiatric and medical standards, and that information concerning drug dosages, schedules, and routes of administration is accurate at the time of publication and consistent with standards set by the U.S. Food and Drug Administration and the general medical community. As medical research and practice continue to advance, however, therapeutic standards may change. Moreover, specific situations may require a specific therapeutic response not included in this book. For these reasons and because human and mechanical errors sometimes occur, we recommend that readers follow the advice of physicians directly involved in their care or the care of a member of their family.

Books published by American Psychiatric Publishing, Inc., represent the views and opinions of the individual authors and do not necessarily represent the policies and opinions of APPI or the American Psychiatric Association.

Manufactured in the United States of America on acid-free paper
09 08 07 06 05   5 4 3 2 1
First Edition

Typeset in Adobe's Janson Text and Frutiger 55 Roman

American Psychiatric Publishing, Inc.
1000 Wilson Boulevard
Arlington, VA 22209-3901
www.appi.org

Library of Congress Cataloging-in-Publication Data
The American Psychiatric Publishing textbook of psychosomatic medicine / edited by James L. Levenson.—1st ed.
    p. ; cm.
  Includes bibliographical references and index.
  ISBN 1-58562-127-7 (hardcover : alk. paper)
  1. Medicine, Psychosomatic. I. Title: Textbook of psychosomatic medicine. II. Levenson, James L.
  III. American Psychiatric Publishing.
  [DNLM: 1. Psychophysiologic Disorders. 2. Psychosomatic Medicine—methods. WM 90 A512 2005]
  RC49.A417 2005
  616.08—dc22

                                         2004050259

British Library Cataloguing in Publication Data
A CIP record is available from the British Library.

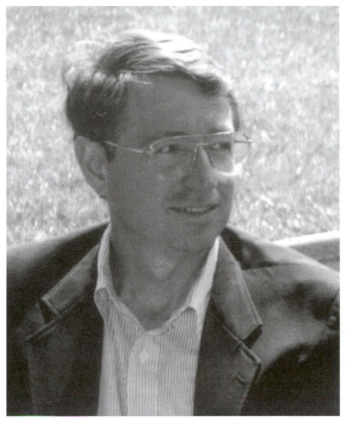

Alan Stoudemire, M.D.
Professor of Psychiatry and Behavioral Sciences
Director of Medical Student Education in Psychiatry
Emory University School of Medicine

This book is dedicated to the memory of Alan Stoudemire (1951–2000), a brilliant clinician, true scholar, prolific writer, and dedicated teacher and mentor. His contributions profoundly transformed our field. He was and remains an inspiration to others, in and outside our profession, for he lived life fully with passion and principle. He transcended his own illnesses with rare strength of spirit, deepening his compassion for and commitment to the medically ill, even while his own life was tragically abbreviated. Those of us who knew him well will forever miss his warmth, wit, and heartfelt friendship.[1]

---

[1]See also Thompson T: "A Tribute to Alan Stoudemire, M.D.: 1951–2000." *Psychosomatics* 42:1–4, 2001.

Contents

PART I
General Principles in Evaluation and Management

PART II
Symptoms and Disorders

PART III
Specialties and Subspecialties

PART IV
Treatment

Contributors

Susan E. Abbey, M.D., F.R.C.P.C.
Director, Program in Medical Psychiatry, and Director, Psychosocial Team, Multi-Organ Transplant Program, University Health Network; Associate Professor, Department of Psychiatry, Faculty of Medicine, University of Toronto, Toronto, Ontario, Canada

Lesley M. Arnold, M.D.
Associate Professor of Psychiatry and Director, Women's Health Research Program, Department of Psychiatry, University of Cincinnati College of Medicine, Cincinnati, Ohio

Roxann D. Barnes, M.D.
Assistant Professor of Anesthesiology, Department of Anesthesiology, Mayo Clinic College of Medicine, Rochester, Minnesota

Charles H. Bombardier, Ph.D.
Associate Professor, Department of Rehabilitation Medicine, University of Washington, Seattle, Washington

John Michael Bostwick, M.D.
Associate Professor of Psychiatry, Mayo Clinic College of Medicine, Rochester, Minnesota

William Breitbart, M.D.
Chief, Psychiatry Service, Department of Psychiatry and Behavioral Sciences, and Attending Psychiatrist, Pain and Palliative Care Service, Department of Neurology, Memorial Sloan-Kettering Cancer Center; Professor of Psychiatry, Department of Psychiatry, Weill Medical College of Cornell University, New York, New York

George R. Brown, M.D.
Professor and Associate Chair, Department of Psychiatry, East Tennessee State University; Chief of Psychiatry, Mountain Home VAMC, Johnson City, Tennessee

Brenda Bursch, Ph.D.
Associate Professor of Psychiatry and Biobehavioral Sciences, and Pediatrics, David Geffen School of Medicine at UCLA, Los Angeles, California

Alan J. Carson, M.Phil., M.D., M.R.C.Psych.
Consultant Neuropsychiatrist and part-time Senior Lecturer, Department of Clinical Neurosciences, Western General Hospital, University of Edinburgh, Edinburgh, United Kingdom

Harvey Max Chochinov, M.D., Ph.D., F.R.C.P.C.
Director and Canada Research Chair in Palliative Medicine, Manitoba Palliative Care Research Unit, CancerCare Manitoba; Professor of Psychiatry and Family Medicine, Departments of Psychiatry and Family Medicine, University of Manitoba, Winnipeg, Manitoba, Canada

Maciej P. Chodynicki, M.D.
Senior Clinical Fellow, Department of Psychiatry and Behavioral Sciences, The Johns Hopkins University School of Medicine, Baltimore, Maryland

Eric J. Christopher, M.D.
Director, Consultation-Liaison Psychiatry, and Clinical Associate Professor, Departments of Internal Medicine and Psychiatry, Duke University Medical Center, Durham, North Carolina

Michael R. Clark, M.D., M.P.H.
Associate Professor and Director, Adolf Meyer Chronic Pain Treatment Programs, Department of Psychiatry and Behavioral Sciences, Johns Hopkins Medical Institutions, Baltimore, Maryland

Greg L. Clary, M.D.
Consulting Assistant Clinical Professor, Duke University Medical Center, Durham, North Carolina

Kathy Coffman, M.D.
Attending Psychiatrist, Cedars–Sinai Medical Center, Los Angeles, California

Lewis M. Cohen, M.D.
Associate Professor of Psychiatry, Tufts University School of Medicine, Boston, Massachusetts; Director of Renal Palliative Care Initiative, Baystate Medical Center, Springfield, Massachusetts

Wendy Cohen, M.D.
Clinical Assistant Professor of Psychiatry, Virginia Commonwealth University, Richmond, Virginia

Francis Creed, M.D., F.R.C.P.C., F.R.C.Psych., F.Med.Sci.
Professor of Psychological Medicine, School of Psychiatry and Behavioural Sciences, University of Manchester, United Kingdom

Niccolo D. Della Penna, M.D.
Fellow, Department of Psychiatry and Behavioral Sciences, The Johns Hopkins School of Medicine, Baltimore, Maryland

Michael J. Devlin, M.D.
Associate Professor of Clinical Psychiatry, Columbia University College of Physicians and Surgeons; Clinical Co-Director, Eating Disorders Research Unit, New York State Psychiatric Institute, New York, New York

Mary Amanda Dew, Ph.D.
Professor of Psychiatry, Psychology, and Epidemiology; Director of Quality of Life Research, Artificial Heart Program, Western Psychiatric Institute and Clinics, University of Pittsburgh Medical Center, Pittsburgh, Pennsylvania

Chris Dickens, M.B.B.S., Ph.D.
Senior Lecturer in Psychological Medicine, Department of Psychiatry, Manchester Royal Infirmary, Manchester, United Kingdom

Andrea F. DiMartini, M.D.
Associate Professor of Psychiatry and Surgery, and Liaison to the Starzl Transplant Institute, Western Psychiatric Institute and Clinics, University of Pittsburgh Medical Center, Pittsburgh, Pennsylvania

Ilyse J. Dobrow, B.A.
Research Assistant, Eating Disorders Research Unit, New York State Psychiatric Institute, New York, New York

Steven A. Epstein, M.D.
Professor and Chair, Department of Psychiatry, Georgetown University Medical Center, Washington, D.C.

Jesse R. Fann, M.D., M.P.H.
Assistant Professor, Department of Psychiatry and Behavioral Sciences, and Adjunct Assistant Professor, Department of Rehabilitation Medicine, University of Washington, Seattle; Associate in Clinical Research, Fred Hutchinson Cancer Research Center; Director, Psychiatry and Psychology Consultation Service, Seattle Cancer Care Alliance, Seattle, Washington

Charles V. Ford, M.D.
Professor of Psychiatry, School of Medicine, University of Alabama at Birmingham, Birmingham, Alabama

John E. Franklin Jr., M.D., M.Sc.
Associate Dean, Minority and Cultural Affairs, and Associate Professor of Psychiatry, Northwestern University Medical School, Chicago, Illinois

Michael J. Germain, M.D.
Associate Professor of Medicine, Tufts University School of Medicine, Boston, Massachusetts; Medical Director, Renal Transplantation Service, Baystate Medical Center, Springfield, Massachusetts

Christopher Gibson, Ph.D.
Research Associate, Psychiatry Service, Department of Psychiatry and Behavioral Sciences, Memorial Sloan-Kettering Cancer Center, New York, New York

Ann Goebel-Fabbri, Ph.D.
Instructor in Psychology, Department of Psychiatry, Harvard Medical School; Psychologist, Behavioral and Mental Health Research Section, Joslin Diabetes Center, Harvard Medical School, Boston, Massachusetts

Donna B. Greenberg, M.D.
Psychiatrist, Massachusetts General Hospital; Associate Professor of Psychiatry, Harvard Medical School, Boston, Massachusetts

Judy A. Greene, M.D.
Clinical Fellow in Psychiatry, Department of Psychiatry, Beth Israel Deaconess Medical Center, Boston, Massachusetts

Mark S. Groves, M.D.
Attending Psychiatrist, Departments of Psychiatry and Neurology, Beth Israel Medical Center, New York, New York

Richard C. Haaser, M.D.
Assistant Professor, Department of Psychiatry, East Tennessee State University; Director, Consultation-Liaison Psychiatry, Mountain Home VAMC, Johnson City, Tennessee

Daniel Hicks, M.D.
Associate Professor and Director, Consultation-Liaison Psychiatry, Georgetown University Medical Center, Washington, D.C.

Alan M. Jacobson, M.D.
Senior Vice President, Strategic Initiatives Division, Joslin Diabetes Center, Harvard Medical School; and Professor of Psychiatry, Harvard Medical School, Boston, Massachusetts

Joel P. Jahraus, M.D.
Medical Director of Remuda Life Programs, Remuda Treatment Centers, Wickenberg, Arizona

Mark R. Katz, M.D., F.R.C.P.C.
Staff Psychiatrist, Departments of Psychiatry and Psychosocial Oncology and Palliative Care, Toronto General Hospital and Princess Margaret Hospital, University Health Network; Assistant Professor of Psychiatry, University of Toronto, Toronto, Ontario, Canada

Jennifer W. Kaupp, Ph.D.
Private practice, Santa Cruz, California; Lecturer, Department of Psychology, University of California at Santa Cruz, Santa Cruz, California

Gary G. Kay, Ph.D.
Associate Professor of Neurology, Georgetown University School of Medicine, Washington, D.C.

Richard Kennedy, M.D.
Assistant Professor, Department of Psychiatry and Department of Physical Medicine and Rehabilitation, Virginia Commonwealth University, Richmond, Virginia

Lois E. Krahn, M.D.
Associate Professor of Psychiatry, Mayo Clinic College of Medicine; Chair, Department of Psychiatry and Psychology, Mayo Clinic, Scottsdale, Arizona

Wendy A. Law, Ph.D.
Assistant Professor of Medical and Clinical Psychology and Psychiatry, Uniformed Services University of the Health Sciences, Bethesda, Maryland

James L. Levenson, M.D.
Chair, Consultation-Liaison Psychiatry, and Vice-Chair, Psychiatry; Professor of Psychiatry, Medicine, and Surgery; Virginia Commonwealth University, Richmond, Virginia

Norman B. Levy, M.D.
Clinical Professor of Psychiatry, State University of New York Downstate Medical Center; Director of Psychiatry, Kingsboro Psychiatric Center, Brooklyn, New York

Antonio Lobo, M.D., Ph.D.
Professor and Chairman, Department of Medicine and Psychiatry, Universidad de Zaragoza; and Chief, Psychosomatics and Consultation-Liaison Psychiatry Service, Hospital Clínico Universitario, Zaragoza, Spain

Constantine G. Lyketsos, M.D., M.H.S.
Professor of Psychiatry and Behavioral Sciences and Director, Division of Geriatric Psychiatry and Neuropsychiatry, The Johns Hopkins Hospital, Baltimore, Maryland

Rajnish Mago, M.D.
Assistant Professor of Psychiatry and Human Behavior and Associate Director of Consultation-Liaison Psychiatry, Thomas Jefferson University, Philadelphia, Pennsylvania

Robert L. Mapou, Ph.D.
Research Associate Professor of Psychiatry and Research Assistant Professor of Neurology, Uniformed Services University of the Health Sciences, Bethesda, Maryland; Clinical Associate Professor of Neurology (Psychology), Georgetown University School of Medicine, Washington, D.C.

Prakash S. Masand, M.D.
Consulting Professor of Psychiatry, Department of Psychiatry, Duke University Medical Center, Durham, North Carolina

Mary Jane Massie, M.D.
Attending Psychiatrist, Memorial Sloan-Kettering Cancer Center; Professor of Clinical Psychiatry, Weill Medical College of Cornell University, New York, New York

Elinore F. McCance-Katz, M.D., Ph.D.
Professor of Psychiatry and Chair, Division of Addiction, Virginia Commonwealth University, Richmond, Virginia

David J. Meagher, M.D., M.R.C.Psych., M.Sc.
Consultant Psychiatrist and Clinical Research Tutor, Limerick Mental Health Services, Midwestern Regional Hospital, Dooradoyle, Limerick, Ireland

Franklin G. Miller, Ph.D.
Bioethicist, Clinical Bioethics Department, Warren Grant Magnuson Clinical Center, Bethesda, Maryland

Sarah E. Munce, B.Sc.
Graduate student, University of Toronto, University Health Network Women's Health Program, Toronto, Ontario, Canada

Gail Musen, Ph.D.
Assistant Investigator, Behavioral and Mental Health Research Section, Joslin Diabetes Center; Instructor in Psychiatry, Department of Psychiatry, Harvard Medical School, Boston, Massachusetts

Philip R. Muskin, M.D.
Chief, Consultation-Liaison Psychiatry, Columbia University Medical Center; Professor of Clinical Psychiatry, Columbia University College of Physicians and Surgeons; Faculty, Columbia University Psychoanalytic Center for Training and Research, New York, New York

Lynn Myles, B.Sc., M.D., F.R.C.S.Ed.
Consultant Neurosurgeon, Department of Clinical Neurosciences, Western General Hospital, University of Edinburgh, Edinburgh, United Kingdom

Robert P. Nolan, Ph.D., R.Psych.
Director, Behavioural Cardiology Research Unit, Cardiac Program, University Health Network; Assistant Professor, Faculty of Medicine, University of Toronto, Toronto, Ontario, Canada

Kevin W. Olden, M.D.
Professor of Medicine and Psychiatry, Division of Gastroenterology, University of South Alabama School of Medicine, Mobile, Alabama

Patrick G. O'Malley, M.D., M.P.H.
Associate Professor of Medicine, Uniformed Services University of the Health Sciences, Bethesda, Maryland

Chiadi U. Onyike, M.D., M.H.S.
Assistant Professor of Psychiatry and Behavioral Sciences; Faculty, Division of Geriatric Psychiatry and Neuropsychiatry; Director, Psychiatry Emergency Services, The Johns Hopkins University and Hospital, Baltimore, Maryland

James A. Owen, Ph.D.
Associate Professor, Department of Psychiatry and Department of Pharmacology and Toxicology, Queen's University; Director, Psychopharmacology Lab, Providence Continuing Care Center Mental Health Services, Kingston, Ontario, Canada

Ashwin A. Patkar, M.D.
Associate Professor of Psychiatry and Human Behavior, Department of Psychiatry, Thomas Jefferson University, Philadelphia, Pennsylvania

Pauline S. Powers, M.D.
Professor of Psychiatry and Behavioral Medicine, Department of Psychiatry and Behavioral Medicine, College of Medicine, University of South Florida, Tampa, Florida

John Querques, M.D.
Associate Director, Psychiatry Consultation Service, Beth Israel Deaconess Medical Center; Instructor in Psychiatry, Harvard Medical School, Boston, Massachusetts

Nathalie Rapoport-Hubschman, M.D.
Rabin Medical Center, Beilinson Campus, Petah-Tikva, Israel

Keith G. Rasmussen, M.D.
Assistant Professor of Psychiatry, Department of Psychiatry and Psychology, Mayo Clinic College of Medicine, Rochester, Minnesota

Jarrett W. Richardson, M.D.
Associate Professor of Psychiatry, Mayo Clinic College of Medicine; Consultant, Department of Psychiatry and Psychology, Mayo Clinic, Rochester, Minnesota

Michael J. Robinson, M.D., F.R.C.P.C.
Adjunct Assistant Professor, Department of Psychiatry, Queens University, Kingston, Ontario, Canada; Clinical Research Physician, Eli Lilly and Company, U.S. Affiliate Medical Division, Indianapolis, Indiana

Gary M. Rodin, M.D., F.R.C.P.C.
Head, Behavioural Sciences and Health Research Division, Toronto General Hospital, University Health Network; Head, Psychosocial Oncology and Palliative Care Program, Princess Margaret Hospital, University Health Network; Professor, Department of Psychiatry, University of Toronto, Toronto, Ontario, Canada

Danielle E. Rolfe, B.P.H.E.
Graduate student, University of Toronto, University Health Network Women's Health Program, Toronto, Ontario, Canada

Donald L. Rosenstein, M.D.
Chief, Psychiatry Consultation-Liaison Service, and Deputy Clinical Director, National Institute of Mental Health, Bethesda, Maryland

Teresa A. Rummans, M.D.
Professor of Psychiatry, Department of Psychiatry and Psychology, Mayo Clinic College of Medicine, Rochester, Minnesota

Carlos A. Santana, M.D.
Associate Professor, Department of Psychiatry and Behavioral Medicine, College of Medicine, University of South Florida, Tampa, Florida

Pedro Saz, M.D., Ph.D.
Professor, Department of Medicine and Psychiatry, Universidad de Zaragoza, Zaragoza, Spain

Stephen C. Scheiber, M.D.
Clinical Professor of Psychiatry, Northwestern University Medical School, Evanston, Illinois; Clinical Professor of Psychiatry, Medical College of Wisconsin, Milwaukee, Wisconsin; Executive Vice President, American Board of Psychiatry and Neurology, Inc., Deerfield, Illinois

Barbara A. Schindler, M.D.
Vice Dean for Educational and Academic Affairs and Professor of Psychiatry, Drexel University College of Medicine, Philadelphia, Pennsylvania

Robert K. Schneider, M.D.
Associate Professor of Psychiatry, Internal Medicine, and Family Practice; Chair, Division of Ambulatory Psychiatry: Virginia Commonwealth University, Richmond, Virginia

Peter A. Shapiro, M.D.
Associate Professor of Clinical Psychiatry, Columbia University College of Physicians and Surgeons; Associate Director, Consultation-Liaison Psychiatry Service; Director, Transplantation Psychiatry Service, Columbia University Medical Center, New York–Presbyterian Hospital, New York, New York

Michael C. Sharpe, M.A., M.D., F.R.C.P., M.R.C.Psych.
Professor of Psychological Medicine and Symptoms Research, School of Molecular and Clinical Medicine, University of Edinburgh, Edinburgh, United Kingdom

Robert I. Simon, M.D.
Clinical Professor of Psychiatry and Director, Program in Psychiatry and Law, Georgetown University School of Medicine, Washington, D.C.; Chairman, Department of Psychiatry, Suburban Hospital, Bethesda, Maryland

Felicia A. Smith, M.D.
Postgraduate Fellow, Psychiatric Consultation-Liaison Service, Massachusetts General Hospital, Boston, Massachusetts

Caitlin R. Sparks, B.A.
Senior Research Assistant, Behavioral and Mental Health Research Section, Joslin Diabetes Center, Harvard Medical School, Boston, Massachusetts

Jack Spector, Ph.D.
Clinical Neuropsychologist, private practice, Baltimore and Chevy Chase, Maryland

David Spiegel, M.D.
Jack, Lulu and Sam Willson Professor, School of Medicine; Associate Chair, Psychiatry and Behavioral Sciences; Medical Director, Center for Integrative Medicine, Stanford University Medical Center, Stanford, California

Theodore A. Stern, M.D.
Chief, Psychiatric Consultation Service, Massachusetts General Hospital; Professor of Psychiatry, Harvard Medical School, Boston, Massachusetts

Donna E. Stewart, M.D., F.R.C.P.C.
Professor and Chair of Women's Health, University of Toronto, University Health Network Women's Health Program, Toronto, Ontario, Canada

Nada L. Stotland, M.D., M.P.H.
Professor of Psychiatry and Obstetrics/Gynecology, Rush Medical College, Chicago, Illinois

Margaret Stuber, M.D.
Professor of Psychiatry and Biobehavioral Sciences, David Geffen School of Medicine at UCLA, Los Angeles, California

Edward G. Tessier, Pharm.D., M.P.H.
Lecturer, School of Nursing, University of Massachusetts Amherst, Amherst, Massachusetts

Glenn J. Treisman, M.D., Ph.D.
Associate Professor, Department of Psychiatry and Behavioral Sciences and Department of Medicine, The Johns Hopkins School of Medicine, Baltimore, Maryland

Paula T. Trzepacz, M.D.
Medical Director, U.S. Neurosciences, Lilly Research Laboratories; Clinical Professor of Psychiatry, University of Mississippi Medical School, Jackson, Mississippi; Adjunct Professor of Psychiatry, Tufts University School of Medicine, Boston, Massachusetts

Teresa S.M. Tsang, M.D.
Associate Professor of Medicine, Department of Internal Medicine, Division of Cardiovascular Disease, Mayo Clinic, Rochester, Minnesota

Adam Zeman, M.A., D.M., M.R.C.P.
Consultant Neurologist and part-time Senior Lecturer, Department of Clinical Neurosciences, Western General Hospital, University of Edinburgh, Edinburgh, United Kingdom

Foreword

Stephen C. Scheiber, M.D.

JIM LEVENSON HAS done superb work in organizing and editing this excellent textbook, which presents the current knowledge base of Psychosomatic Medicine for physicians in all specialties. Dr. Levenson has brought together a superb editorial board, including members from the United States, Canada, United Kingdom, Australia, Spain, Italy, and Mexico. The authors' contributions reflect the breadth and depth of this psychiatric subspecialty, which gained official recognition by the American Board of Psychiatry and Neurology in 2003 through the American Board of Medical Specialties.

The text is neatly divided into sections, including general principles, symptoms and disorders, and different organ systems, which are reflected in the specialties and subspecialties of medicine. It concludes with a detailed discussion of the different treatments and management approaches.

At the interface between psychiatry and other medical specialties, Psychosomatic Medicine is the newest psychiatric subspecialty recognized by the American Board of Medical Specialties. The American Board of Psychiatry and Neurology is developing the competencies and certification examination for this field, with the first examination to be held in June 2005. The Accreditation Council of Graduate Medical Education and the Psychiatry Residency Review Committee have begun the process of accrediting fellowship programs in Psychosomatic Medicine.

While research, clinical treatment, and teaching in Psychosomatic Medicine have been growing rapidly in the past decade, this field has evolved and matured over many years, with contributions from many great psychiatrists and other physicians such as Flanders Dunbar, Felix Deutsch, Franz Alexander, Harold Wolff, and Roy Grinker in the development of Psychosomatic Medicine in the first half of the twentieth century. In the 1930s, the American Psychosomatic Society was founded, and the first issue of the journal *Psychosomatic Medicine* was published, followed in the 1950s by the founding of the Academy of Psychosomatic Medicine and the first issue of *Psychosomatics*.

Another growth spurt of Psychosomatic Medicine occurred in the 1970s, with the appearance of a plethora of major texts, including those by Oscar Hill; Allister Munro; Wittkower and Warnes; Herbert Weiner; Lipowski, Lipsitt, and Whybrow; and a number of others. George Engel, an internist and psychoanalyst, brought psychiatry and medicine closer together and refocused the conceptual basis of the field through the biopsychosocial model. In the 1970s and 1980s, consultation-liaison psychiatry blossomed as the clinical application of psychosomatic principles over many years, with leaders such as Bish Lipowski, John Schwab, Tom Hackett, Jim Strain, Bob Pasnau, and Jimmie Holland.

Today, Psychosomatic Medicine is a vibrant clinical field informed by a rapidly expanding research base, growing not only in North America and Europe but also in Japan, Australia, New Zealand, and many other nations. This fine work demonstrates the acceleration of advances in the field of Psychosomatic Medicine. The increasing complexity and subspecialization in the rest of medicine requires that the expert in Psychosomatic Medicine keep abreast of the latest advances in diagnosis and treatment in the other medical specialties. The contributors to this latest and most advanced textbook of Psychosomatic Medicine are widely recognized experts who comprehensively cover all of the major psychiatric symptoms and disorders in the medically ill. For each major psychiatric disorder and each major medical disorder, they review epidemiology and risk factors; the effects of the psychiatric disorder on medical disorders and, conversely, the effects of medical diseases on the psyche; clinical features; diagnosis and assessment; differential diagnosis; management; and treatment. This textbook is very up-to-date, scholarly, and encyclopedic but also reflects an understanding that one must approach each patient as a unique, suffering individual.

Introduction

James L. Levenson, M.D.

WHAT IS PSYCHOSOMATIC Medicine? In the past, Psychosomatic Medicine has had ambiguous connotations, alternatively "psychogenic" or "holistic," but it is the latter meaning that has characterized its emergence as a contemporary scientific and clinical discipline (Lipowski 1984). In this book, it refers to a specialized area of psychiatry whose practitioners have particular expertise in the diagnosis and treatment of psychiatric disorders and difficulties in complex medically ill patients (Gitlin et al. 2004).

We treat and study three general groups of patients: those with comorbid psychiatric and general medical illnesses complicating each other's management, those with somatoform and functional disorders, and those with psychiatric disorders that are the direct consequence of a primary medical condition or its treatment. Psychosomatic Medicine practitioners work as hospital-based consultation-liaison psychiatrists (Kornfeld 1996), on medical-psychiatric inpatient units (Kathol and Stoudemire 2002), and in settings in which mental health services are integrated into primary care (Unutzer et al. 2002). Thus the field's name reflects the fact that it exists at the interface of psychiatry and medicine.

Psychosomatic Medicine is the newest psychiatric subspecialty formally approved by the American Board of Medical Specialties. There have been many other names for this specialized field, including consultation-liaison psychiatry, medical-surgical psychiatry, psychological medicine, and psychiatric care of the complex medically ill,

among others. In 2001, the Academy of Psychosomatic Medicine applied to the American Board of Psychiatry and Neurology (ABPN) for the recognition of "Psychosomatic Medicine" as a subspecialty field of psychiatry, choosing to return to the name for the field embedded in our history, our journals, and our national organizations (for a detailed account of the field, see Lyketsos et al. 2001). Subsequent formal approval was received from the American Psychiatric Association, ABPN, the Residency Review Committee (RRC) of the Accreditation Council for Graduate Medical Education (ACGME), and the American Board of Medical Specialties (ABMS). The first certifying examination is scheduled for June 2005.

Psychosomatic Medicine has a rich history. The term *psychosomatic* was introduced by Johann Heinroth in 1818, and Felix Deutsch introduced the term *psychosomatic medicine* around 1922 (Lipsitt 2001). Psychoanalysts and psychophysiologists pioneered the study of mind-body interactions from very different vantage points, each contributing to the growth of Psychosomatic Medicine as a clinical and scholarly field. The modern history of the field (see Table 1) perhaps starts with the Rockefeller Foundation's funding of psychosomatic medicine units in several U.S. teaching hospitals in 1935. The National Institute of Mental Health made it a priority to foster the growth of consultation-liaison psychiatry, through training grants (circa 1975) and a research development program (circa 1985).

Table 1: Key dates in the modern history of psychosomatic medicine	
1935	Rockefeller Foundation opens first Consultation-Liaison (C/L)–Psychosomatic Units at Massachusetts General, Duke, and Colorado
1936	American Psychosomatic Society founded
1939	First issue of *Psychosomatic Medicine*
1953	First issue of *Psychosomatics*
1954	Academy of Psychosomatic Medicine (APM) founded
1975	National Institute of Mental Health (NIMH) Training Grants for C/L Psychiatry
1985	NIMH Research Development Program for C/L Psychiatry
1991	APM-recognized fellowships number 55
2001	Subspecialty application for Psychosomatic Medicine
2003	Approval as subspecialty by American Board of Medical Specialties

Table 2: Selected classic texts in psychosomatic medicine

1935	*Emotions and Body Change* (Dunbar)
1943	*Psychosomatic Medicine* (Weiss and English)
1950	*Psychosomatic Medicine* (Alexander)
1968	*Handbook of Psychiatric Consultation* (Schwab)
1978	*Organic Psychiatry* (Lishman)
1978	*Massachusetts General Hospital Handbook of General Hospital Psychiatry* (Hackett and Cassem)
1993	*Psychiatric Care of the Medical Patient* (Stoudemire and Fogel)

Psychosomatic Medicine is a scholarly discipline, with classic influential texts (Table 2), many devoted journals (Table 3), and both national (Table 4) and international (Table 5) professional/scientific societies. The Academy of Psychosomatic Medicine is the only U.S. national organization primarily dedicated to Psychosomatic Medicine as a psychiatric subspecialty. The American Psychosomatic Society, an older cousin, is primarily devoted to psychosomatic research, and its members come from many disciplines (Wise 1995). While consultation-liaison psychiatry and psychosomatic medicine flourished first in the United States, exciting work now comes from around the world. This is reflected in the membership of the Editorial Board and the contributors to this text, who include psychiatrists from the United States, Canada, United Kingdom, Australia, Spain, Italy, and Mexico.

This book is organized into four sections. The first five chapters cover general principles in evaluation and management. Chapters 6–18 are devoted to psychiatric symptoms and disorders in the medically ill. Chapters 19–36 address issues within each of the medical specialties and subspecialties. The final four chapters are summaries of psychiatric treatment in the medically ill. This book has attempted to capture the diversity of our field, whose practitioners do not place equal emphasis on the syllables of "bio-psycho-social." There is not unanimity among us on some questions, and diverse opinions will be found in this book. Psychosomatic Medicine has evolved, since its start, from a field based on clinical experience, conjecture, and theorizing into a discipline grounded in empirical research that is growing and spreading its findings into many areas of medical care (Levenson 1997).

Acknowledgments

This book has benefited from those who have gone before in creating comprehensive textbooks for our field, especially Stoudemire, Fogel, and Greenberg's *Psychiatric Care of the Medical Patient* (2000) and Wise and Rundell's *The American Psychiatric Publishing Textbook of Consultation-Liaison Psychiatry* (2002).

Table 3: Selected journals in pychosomatic medicine

Journal name	Date of initial publication
Psychosomatic Medicine	1939
Psychosomatics	1953
Psychotherapy and Psychosomatics	1953
Psychophysiology	1954
Journal of Psychosomatic Research	1956
Advances in Psychosomatic Medicine	1960
International Journal of Psychiatry in Medicine	1970
General Hospital Psychiatry	1979
Journal of Psychosomatic Obstetrics and Gynecology	1982
Journal of Psychosocial Oncology	1983
Stress Medicine	1985
Psycho-oncology	1986

Table 4: National organizations

Academy of Psychosomatic Medicine
Association for Medicine and Psychiatry
American Psychosomatic Society
American Association for General Hospital Psychiatry
Society for Liaison Psychiatry
Association for Academic Psychiatry—Consultation-Liaison Section
American Neuropsychiatric Association
American Psychosocial Oncology Society
North American Society for Psychosomatic Obstetrics and Gynecology

Table 5: International organizations

European Association for Consultation-Liaison Psychiatry and Psychosomatics
International Organization for Consultation-Liaison Psychiatry
World Psychiatric Association—Section of General Hospital Psychiatry
International College of Psychosomatic Medicine
International Neuropsychiatric Association
International Psychooncology Society

I owe an enormous debt of gratitude to the many people who made this book possible. First, to Bob Hales, Editor-in-Chief, and Tom Wise, Chair of the Editorial Board at American Psychiatric Publishing, Inc. (APPI), whose faith in me and encouragement were inspirational. This book would not have been conceived if Psychosomatic Medicine had not become an official subspecialty of American psychiatry, and for that we all owe a great deal to Kostas Lyketsos, leader and comrade-in-arms in the long campaign, along with many others from the Academy of Psychosomatic Medicine who worked to make it a reality, including Dan Winstead, whose wise counsel has been invaluable. The value of this text comes from the untiring labors of the contributors, who were patient under repeated onslaughts of red ink from me. An assertive Editorial Board pushed us all toward the highest standards.

Every chapter in this book has been critically reviewed by at least one member of the Editorial Board, and most have been externally reviewed as well. Chapters 19–36 have also been reviewed by one or more nonpsychiatric physician experts of the relevant specialty or subspecialty. I am particularly grateful to my nonpsychiatric colleagues at Virginia Commonwealth University (VCU) who generously gave their time to critique chapters in their respective disciplines, including David Gardner, Mike Edmond, Laurie Lyckholm, Lex Tartaglia, Paul Fairman, Lenore Buckley, Sara Monroe, Brian Kaplan, Michael King, Bob Perry, Ken Ellenbogen, and Marjolein de Wit. Psychiatric colleagues at VCU, including Susan Kornstein, Alison Lynch, Anand Pandurangi, Jim Wade, and Neil Sonenklar, did the same in their areas of expertise. UCLA child psychiatrists Brenda Bursch and Margaret Stuber (authors of Chapter 34) provided expert reviews of several other chapters' coverage of topics involving children and adolescents.

Tina Coltri-Marshall provided invaluable service, keeping everyone organized and on schedule. APPI's John McDuffie and Bob Pursell gave expert advice and encouragement from start to finish, and I am grateful to all of the APPI staff, including Robin Simpson, Pam Harley, Greg Kuny, Katie Duffy, Abdul Kargbo, Julia Bozzolo, Rebecca Richters, and Judy Castagna.

Finally, this book would not have been possible without the most enthusiastic support from my chair, Joel Silverman; the help of my secretary, Pam Copeland; and the patience and tolerance of my family.

References

Gitlin DF, Levenson JL, Lyketsos CG: Psychosomatic medicine: a new psychiatric subspecialty. Acad Psychiatry 28:4–11, 2004

Kathol RG, Stoudemire A: Strategic integration of inpatient and outpatient medical-psychiatry services, in The American Psychiatric Publishing Textbook of Consultation-Liaison Psychiatry. Edited by Wise MG, Rundell JR. Washington, DC, American Psychiatric Publishing, 2002, pp 871–888

Kornfeld DS: Consultation-liaison psychiatry and the practice of medicine. The Thomas P. Hackett Award lecture given at the 42nd annual meeting of the Academy of Psychosomatic Medicine, 1995. Psychosomatics 37:236–248, 1996

Levenson JL: Consultation-liaison psychiatry research: more like a ground cover than a hedgerow. Psychosom Med 59:563–564, 1997

Lipowski ZJ: What does the word "psychosomatic" really mean? A historical and semantic inquiry. Psychosom Med. 46:153–71, 1984

Lipsitt DR: Consultation-liaison psychiatry and psychosomatic medicine: the company they keep. Psychosom Med 63:896–909, 2001

Lyketsos CG, Levenson JL, Academy of Psychosomatic Medicine (APM) Task Force for Subspecialization: Proposal for recognition of "PSYCHOSOMATIC MEDICINE" as a psychiatric subspecialty. Academy of Psychosomatic Medicine, July 2001

Unutzer J, Katon W, Callahan CM, et al: Collaborative care management of late-life depression in the primary care setting: a randomized controlled trial. JAMA 288:2836–2845, 2002

Wise TN: A tale of two societies. Psychosom Med 57:303–309, 1995

PART I

General Principles in Evaluation and Management

1

Psychiatric Assessment and Consultation

Felicia A. Smith, M.D.

John Querques, M.D.

James L. Levenson, M.D.

Theodore A. Stern, M.D.

PSYCHOSOMATIC MEDICINE IS clinically rooted in consultation-liaison psychiatry, expanding from its beginnings on a few general medical wards of large hospitals in the 1930s to specialized medical units throughout various parts of the health care delivery system. Practitioners in this discipline assist with the care of a variety of patients, especially those with complex illnesses such as cancer, organ transplantation, and HIV infection (Gitlin et al. 2004; Hackett et al. 2004). In the medical setting, prompt recognition and evaluation of psychiatric problems are essential because psychiatric comorbidity often exacerbates the course of medical illness, causes significant distress in the patient, prolongs hospital length of stay, and increases costs of care. Psychiatrists in medical settings may be asked to evaluate a wide variety of conditions. These can include dementia, delirium, agitation, psychosis, substance abuse or withdrawal, somatoform disorders, personality disorders, and mood and anxiety disorders, as well as suicidal ideation, noncompliance, and aggressive and other behavioral problems. In addition, ethical and legal considerations are often critical elements of the psychiatric consultation.

In this introductory chapter, we present a detailed approach to psychiatric assessment and consultation in a medical setting. Flexibility is essential for psychiatric consultants to be successful in the evaluation of affective, behavioral, and cognitive disturbances in medically ill patients. In the final section of the chapter, we briefly outline the benefits of psychiatric consultation for patients as well as for the greater hospital and medical communities.

Psychiatric Consultation in the General Hospital

Psychiatrists who work in medical settings are charged with providing expert consultation to medical and surgical patients. In many respects, psychiatric care of such patients is no different from the treatment of patients in a psychiatric clinic or in a private office. However, the constraints of the modern hospital environment demand a high degree of adaptability. Comfort, quiet, and privacy are scarce commodities in medical and surgical units. Interruptions by medical or nursing staff, visitors, and roommates erode the privacy that the psychiatrist usually expects. Patients who are sick, preoccupied with their physical condition, and in pain are ill-disposed to engage in the exploratory interviews that often typify psychiatric evaluations in other settings. Monitoring devices replace the plants, pictures, and other accoutrements of a typical office. Nightstands and tray tables are littered with medical paraphernalia commingled with personal effects.

The consultant must be adept at gathering the requisite diagnostic information efficiently from the data permitted by the patient's clinical condition and must be able to tolerate the sights, sounds, and smells of the sickroom. Additional visits for more history are often inevitable. In the end, the diagnosis will likely fall into one (or more) of the categories outlined in Lipowski's (1967) classification, which is still relevant today (Table 1–1).

TABLE 1–1. Categories of psychiatric differential diagnoses in the general hospital

- Psychiatric presentations of medical conditions
- Psychiatric complications of medical conditions or treatments
- Psychological reactions to medical conditions or treatments
- Medical presentations of psychiatric conditions
- Medical complications of psychiatric conditions or treatments
- Comorbid medical and psychiatric conditions

Source. Adapted from Lipowski 1967.

Although the consultant is summoned by the patient's physician, in most cases the visit is unannounced and is not requested by the patient, from whom cooperation is expected. Explicitly acknowledging this reality and apologizing if the patient was not informed are often sufficient to gain the patient's cooperation. Cooperation is enhanced if the psychiatrist sits down and operates at eye level with the patient. By offering to help the patient get comfortable (e.g., by adjusting the head of the bed, bringing the patient a drink or a blanket, or adjusting the television) before and after the encounter, the consultant can increase the chances of being welcomed then and for follow-up evaluations.

When psychiatrists are consulted for unexplained physical symptoms or for pain management, it is useful to empathize with the distress that the patient is experiencing. This avoids conveying any judgment on the etiology of the pain except that the suffering is real. After introductions, if the patient is in pain, the consultant's first questions should address this issue. Failing to do so conveys a lack of appreciation for the patient's suffering and may be taken by the patient as disbelief in his or her symptoms. Starting with empathic questions about the patient's suffering establishes rapport and also guides the psychiatrist in setting the proper pace of the interview. Finally, because a psychiatric consultation will cause many patients to fear that their physician thinks they are "crazy," the psychiatrist may first need to address this fear.

The Process of the Consultation

Although it is rarely as straightforward as the following primer suggests, the process of psychiatric consultation should, in the end, include all the components explained below and summarized in Table 1–2.

Speak Directly With the Referring Clinician

Requests for psychiatric consultation are notorious for being vague and imprecise (e.g., "rule out depression" or

TABLE 1–2. Procedural approach to psychiatric consultation

- Speak directly with the referring clinician.
- Review the current records and pertinent past records.
- Review the patient's medications.
- Gather collateral data.
- Interview and examine the patient.
- Formulate diagnostic and therapeutic strategies.
- Write a note.
- Speak directly with the referring clinician.
- Provide periodic follow-up.

"patient with schizophrenia"). They sometimes signify only that the team recognizes that a problem exists; such problems may range from an untreated psychiatric disorder to the experience of countertransferential feelings. In speaking with a member of the team that has requested the consultation, the consultant employs some of the same techniques that will be used later in examining the patient; that is, he or she listens to the implicit as well as the explicit messages from the other physician (Murray 2004). Is the physician angry with the patient? Is the patient not doing what the team wants him or her to do? Is the fact that the patient is young and dying leading to the team's overidentification with him or her? Is the team frustrated by an elusive diagnosis? All of these situations generate emotions that are difficult to reduce to a few words conveyed in a consultation request; moreover, the feelings often remain out of the team's conscious awareness. This brief interaction may give the consultant invaluable information about how the consultation may be useful to the team and to the patient.

Review the Current Records and Pertinent Past Records

When it is done with the unfailing curiosity of a detective hot on the trail of hidden clues, reading a chart can be an exciting and self-affirming part of the consultation process. Although it does not supplant the consultant's independent history taking or examination, the chart review provides a general orientation to the case. Moreover, the consultant is in a unique position to focus on details that may have been previously overlooked. For example, nurses often document salient neurobehavioral data (e.g., the level of awareness and the presence of confusion or agitation); physical and occupational therapists estimate functional abilities crucial to the diagnosis of cognitive disorders and to the choice of an appropriate level of care (e.g., nursing home or assisted-living facility); and speech pathologists note alterations in articulation, swallowing, and language, all of which may indicate an organic brain disease. All of them may have written progress notes about adherence to treatment regimens, unusual behavior, interpersonal difficulties, or family issues encountered in their care of the patient. These notes may also provide unique clues to the presence of problems such as domestic violence, factitious illness, or personality disorders. In hospitals or clinics where nurses' notes are kept separate from the physician's progress notes, it is essential for the consultant to review those sections.

Review the Patient's Medications

Construction of a medication list at various time points (e.g., at home, on admission, on transfer within the hospital, and at present) is always good, if not essential, practice. Special attention should be paid to medications with psychoactive effects and to those associated with withdrawal syndromes (both obvious ones like benzodiazepines and opiates, and less obvious ones like antidepressants, anticonvulsants, and beta-blockers). Review of order sheets or computerized order entries is not always sufficient, because—for a variety of reasons—patients may not always receive prescribed medications; therefore, medication administration records should also be reviewed. Such records are particularly important for determining the frequency of administration of medicines ordered on an as-needed basis. For example, an order for lorazepam 1–2 mg every 4–6 hours as needed may result in a patient receiving anywhere from 0 mg to 12 mg in a day, which can be critical in cases of withdrawal or oversedation.

Gather Collateral Data

Histories from hospitalized medically ill patients may be especially spotty and unreliable, if not nonexistent (e.g., with a patient who is somnolent, delirious, or comatose). Data from collateral sources (e.g., family members; friends; current and outpatient health care providers; case managers; and, in some cases, police and probation officers) may be of critical importance. However, psychiatric consultants must guard against prizing any single party's version of historical events over another's; family members and others may lack objectivity, be in denial, be overinvolved, or have a personal agenda to advance. For example, family members tend to minimize early signs of dementia and to overreport depression in patients with dementia. Confidentiality must be valued when obtaining collateral information. Ideally, one obtains the patient's consent first; however, this may not be possible if the patient lacks capacity or if a dire emergency is in progress (see Chapter 3, "Le-

gal Issues," and Chapter 4, "Ethical Issues"). Moreover, in certain situations there may be contraindications to contacting some sources of information (e.g., an employer of a patient with substance abuse or the partner of a woman who is experiencing abuse). Like any astute physician, the psychiatrist collates and synthesizes all available data and weighs each bit of information according to the reliability of its source.

Interview and Examine the Patient

Armed with information gleaned and elicited from other sources, the psychiatric consultant now makes independent observations of the patient and collects information that may be the most reliable of all because it comes from direct observations. For non-English-speaking patients, a translator is often needed. Although using family members may be expedient, their presence often compromises the questions asked and the translations offered because of embarrassment or other factors. It is therefore important to utilize hospital translators or, for less common languages, services via telephone. This can be difficult, but it may be necessary in obtaining a full and accurate history.

Mental Status Examination

A thorough mental status examination is central to the psychiatric evaluation of the medically ill patient. Because the examination is hierarchical in nature, care must be taken to complete it in a systematic fashion (Hyman and Tesar 1994). The astute consultant will glean invaluable diagnostic clues from a combination of observation and questioning.

Level of consciousness.   Level of consciousness depends on normal cerebral arousal by the reticular activating system. A patient whose level of consciousness is impaired will inevitably perform poorly on cognitive testing. The finding of *disorientation* implies cognitive failure in one or several domains, and it is helpful to test orientation near the start of the mental status examination.

Attention.   The form of attention most relevant to the clinical mental status examination is the sustained attention that allows one to concentrate on cognitive tasks. Disruption of attention—often by factors that diffusely disturb brain function, such as drugs, infection, or organ failure—is a hallmark of delirium. Sustained attention is best tested with moderately demanding, nonautomatic tasks such as reciting the months backward or, as in the Mini-Mental State Examination (MMSE; Folstein et al. 1975), spelling *world* backward or subtracting 7 serially from 100. Serial subtraction is intended to be a test of attention, not arithmetic ability, so the task should be adjusted to the patient's native ability and educational level (serial *3*s from 50, serial *1*s from 20). An inattentive patient's performance on other parts of the mental status examination may be affected on any task requiring sustained focus.

Memory.   *Working memory* is tested by asking the patient to *register* some information (e.g., three words) and to *recall* that information after an interval of at least 3 minutes during which other testing prevents rehearsal. This task can also be considered a test of *recent memory*. Semantic memory is tapped by asking general-knowledge questions (e.g., "Who is the President?") and by naming and visual recognition tasks. The patient's ability to remember aspects of his or her history serves as an elegant test of *episodic memory* (as well as of *remote memory*). Because semantic and episodic memories can be articulated, they constitute *declarative memory*. In contrast, *procedural memory* is implicit in learned action (e.g., riding a bicycle) and cannot be described in words. Deficits in procedural memory can be observed in a patient's behavior during the clinical evaluation.

Executive function.   *Executive function* refers to the abilities that allow one to plan, initiate, organize, and monitor thought and behavior. These abilities, which localize broadly to the frontal lobes, are essential for normal social and professional performance but are difficult to test. Frontal lobe disorders often make themselves apparent in social interaction with a patient and are suspected when one observes disinhibition, impulsivity, disorganization, abulia, or amotivation. Tasks that can be used to gain some insight into frontal lobe function include verbal fluency, such as listing as many animals as possible in 1 minute; motor sequencing, such as asking the patient to replicate a sequence of three hand positions; the go/no-go task, which requires the patient to tap the desk once if the examiner taps once, but not to tap if the examiner taps twice; and tests of abstraction, including questions like "What do a tree and a fly have in common?"

Language.   *Language disorders* result from lesions of the dominant hemisphere. In assessing language, one should first note characteristics of the patient's speech (e.g., non-fluency or paraphasic errors) and then assess comprehension. Naming is impaired in both major varieties of aphasia, and anomia can be a clue to mild dysphasia. Reading and writing should also be assessed. Expressive (Broca's or motor) aphasia is characterized by effortful, nonfluent speech with use of phonemic paraphasias (incorrect words that approximate the correct ones in sound), reduced use of function words (e.g., prepositions and articles), and well-preserved comprehension. Receptive (Wernicke's or sensory) aphasia is characterized by fluent speech with both phonemic and semantic paraphasias (incorrect words that approximate the correct ones in meaning) and poor comprehension. The stream of incoherent speech and the lack of insight in patients with Wernicke's aphasia sometimes lead to misdiagnosis of a primary thought disorder and psychiatric referral; the clue to the diagnosis of a language disorder is the severity of the comprehension deficit. Global dysphasia combines features of Broca's and Wernicke's aphasias. Selective impairment of repetition characterizes conduction aphasia. The nondominant hemisphere plays a part in the appreciation and production of the emotional overtones of language.

Praxis.   *Apraxia* refers to an inability to perform skilled actions (e.g., using a screwdriver, brushing one's teeth) despite intact basic motor and sensory abilities. These abilities can be tested by asking a patient to mime such actions or by asking the patient to copy unfamiliar hand positions. *Constructional apraxia* is usually tested with the Clock Drawing Test. *Gait apraxia* involves difficulty in initiating and maintaining gait despite intact basic motor function in the legs. *Dressing apraxia* is difficulty in dressing caused by an inability to coordinate the spatial arrangement of clothes with the body.

Mood and affect.   Mood and affect both refer to the patient's emotional state, mood being the patient's perception and affect being the interviewer's perception. The interviewer must interpret both carefully, taking into account the patient's medical illness. Normal but intense expressions of emotion (e.g., grief, fear, or irritation) are common in patients with serious medical illness but may be misperceived by nonpsychiatric physicians as evidence of psychiatric disturbance. Disturbances in mood and affect may also be the result of brain dysfunction or injury. Irritability may be the first sign of many illnesses, ranging from alcohol withdrawal to rabies. Blunted affective expression may be a sign of Parkinson's disease. Intense affective lability (e.g., pathological crying or laughing) with relatively normal mood occurs with some diseases or injuries of the frontal lobes.

Perception.   Perception in the mental status examination is primarily concerned with hallucinations and illusions. However, before beginning any part of the clinical interview and the mental status examination, the interviewer should establish whether the patient has any impairment in vision or hearing that could interfere with communication. Unrecognized impairments have led to erroneous impressions that patients were demented, delirious, or psychotic. Although hallucinations in any modality may occur in primary psychotic disorders (e.g., schizophrenia or affective psychosis), prominent visual, olfactory, gustatory, or tactile hallucinations suggest a secondary medical etiology. Olfactory and gustatory hallucinations may be manifestations of seizures, and tactile hallucinations are often seen with substance abuse.

Judgment and insight. The traditional question for the assessment of *judgment* (i.e., "What would you do if you found a letter on the sidewalk?") is much less informative than questions tailored to the problems faced by the patient being evaluated; for example, "If you couldn't stop a nosebleed, what would you do?" "If you run out of medicine and you can't reach your doctor, what would you do?" Similarly, questions to assess *insight* should focus on the patient's understanding of his or her illness, treatment, and life circumstances.

Further guidance on mental status examination. An outline of the essential elements of a comprehensive mental status examination is presented in Table 1–3. Particular cognitive mental status testing maneuvers are described in more detail in Table 1–4. More detailed consideration of the mental status examination can be found elsewhere (Strub and Black 2000; Trzepacz and Baker 1993).

Physical Examination

Although the interview and mental status examination as outlined above are generally thought to be the primary diagnostic tools of the psychiatrist, the importance of the physical examination should not be forgotten, especially in the medical setting. Most psychiatrists do not perform physical examinations on their patients. The consultation psychiatrist, however, should be familiar with and comfortable performing neurological examinations and other selected features of the physical examination that may uncover the common comorbidities in psychiatric patients (Granacher 1981; Summers et al. 1981a, 1981b). At an absolute minimum, the consultant should review the physical examinations performed by other physicians. However, the psychiatrist's examination of the patient, especially of central nervous system functions relevant to the differential diagnosis, is often essential. A fuller physical examination is appropriate on medical-psychiatric units or whenever the psychiatrist has assumed responsibility for the care of a patient's medical problems. Even with a sedated or comatose patient, simple observation and a few maneuvers that involve a laying on of hands may potentially yield a bounty of findings. Although it is beyond the scope of this chapter to discuss a comprehensive physical examination, Table 1–5

TABLE 1–3. The mental status examination

Level of consciousness
- Alert, drowsy, somnolent, stuporous, comatose; fluctuations suggest delirium

Appearance and behavior
- Overall appearance, grooming, hygiene
- Cooperation, eye contact, psychomotor agitation or retardation
- Abnormal movements: tics, tremors, chorea, posturing

Attention
- Vigilance, concentration, ability to focus, sensory neglect

Orientation and memory
- Orientation to person, place, time, situation
- Recent, remote, and immediate recall

Language
- Speech: rate, volume, fluency, prosody
- Comprehension and naming ability
- Abnormalities include aphasia, dysarthria, agraphia, alexia, clanging, neologisms, echolalia

Constructional ability
- Clock drawing to assess neglect, executive function, and planning
- Drawing of a cube or intersecting pentagons to assess parietal function

Mood and affect
- Mood: subjective sustained emotion
- Affect: observed emotion—quality, range, appropriateness

Form and content of thought
- Form: linear, circumstantial, tangential, disorganized, blocked
- Content: delusions, paranoia, ideas of reference, suicidal or homicidal ideation

Perception
- Auditory, visual, gustatory, tactile, olfactory hallucinations

Judgment and insight
- Understanding of illness and consequences of specific treatments offered

Reasoning
- Illogical versus logical; ability to make consistent decisions

Source. Adapted from Hyman and Tesar 1994.

---

provides a broad outline of selected findings of the physical examination and their relevance to the psychiatric consultation.

Formulate Diagnostic and Therapeutic Strategies

By the time the consultant arrives on the scene, routine chemical and hematological tests and urinalyses are almost

TABLE 1–4.   Detailed assessment of cognitive domains

Cognitive domain	Assessment
Level of consciousness and arousal	Inspect the patient
Orientation to place and time	Ask direct questions about both of these
Registration (recent memory)	Have the patient repeat three words immediately
Recall (working memory)	Have the patient recall the same three words after performing another task for at least 3 minutes
Remote memory	Ask about the patient's age, date of birth, milestones, or significant life or historical events (e.g., names of presidents, dates of wars)
Attention and concentration	Subtract serial 7s (adapt to the patient's level of education; subtract serial 3s if less educated). Spell *world* backward (this may be difficult for non-English speakers). Test digit span forward and backward. Have the patient recite the months of the year (or the days of the week) in reverse order.
Language	
• *Comprehension*	(Adapt the degree of difficulty to the patient's educational level)
	Inspect the patient while he or she answers questions
	Ask the patient to point to different objects
	Ask yes or no questions
	Ask the patient to write a phrase (paragraph)
• *Naming*	Show a watch, pen, or less familiar objects, if needed
• *Fluency*	Assess the patient's speech
	Have the patient name as many animals as he or she can in 1 minute
• *Articulation*	Listen to the patient's speech
	Have the patient repeat a phrase
• *Reading*	Have the patient read a sentence (or a longer paragraph if needed)
Executive function	Determine if the patient requires constant cueing and prompting
• *Commands*	Have the patient follow a three-step command
• *Construction tasks*	Have the patient draw interlocked pentagons
	Have the patient draw a clock
• *Motor programming tasks*	Have the patient perform serial hand sequences
	Have the patient perform reciprocal programs of raising fingers
Judgment and reasoning	Listen to the patient's account of his or her history and reason for hospitalization
	Assess abstraction (similarities: dog/cat; red/green)
	Ask about the patient's judgment about simple events or problems: "A construction worker fell to the ground from the seventh floor of the building and broke his two legs; he then ran to the nearby hospital to ask for medical help. Do you have any comment on this?"

TABLE 1–5. Selected elements of the physical examination and significance of findings

Elements	Examples of possible diagnoses
General	
General appearance healthier than expected	Somatoform disorder
Fever	Infection or NMS
Blood pressure or pulse abnormalities	Withdrawal, thyroid or cardiovascular disease
Body habitus	Eating disorders, polycystic ovaries, or Cushing syndrome
Skin	
Diaphoresis	Fever, withdrawal, NMS
Dry, flushed	Anticholinergic toxicity, heat stroke
Pallor	Anemia
Changes in hair, nails, skin	Malnutrition, thyroid or adrenal disease
Jaundice	Liver disease
Characteristic stigmata	Syphilis, cirrhosis, or self-mutilation
Bruises	Physical abuse, ataxia, traumatic brain injury
Eyes	
Mydriasis	Opiate withdrawal, anticholinergic toxicity
Miosis	Opiate intoxication, cholinergic toxicity
Kayser-Fleischer pupillary rings	Wilson's disease
Neurological	
Tremors	Delirium, withdrawal syndromes, parkinsonism
Primitive reflexes present (e.g., snout, glabellar, and grasp)	Dementia, frontal lobe dysfunction
Hyperactive deep-tendon reflexes	Withdrawal, hyperthyroidism
Ophthalmoplegia	Wernicke's encephalopathy, brain stem dysfunction, dystonic reaction
Papilledema	Increased intracranial pressure
Hypertonia, rigidity, catatonia, parkinsonism	EPS, NMS
Abnormal movements	Parkinson's disease, Huntington's disease, EPS
Abnormal gait	Normal pressure hydrocephalus, Parkinson's disease, Wernicke's encephalopathy
Loss of position and vibratory sense	Vitamin B_{12} deficiency

Note. EPS = extrapyramidal side effects; NMS = neuroleptic malignant syndrome.

always available and should be reviewed along with any other laboratory, imaging, and electrophysiological tests. The consultant then considers what additional tests are needed to arrive at a diagnosis. Attempts have been made in the past to correlate biological tests, such as the dexamethasone suppression test, with psychiatric illness; despite extensive research, however, no definitive biological tests are available to identify psychiatric disorders. Before ordering a test, the consultant must consider the likelihood that the test will contribute to making a diagnosis.

There is an extensive list of studies that could be relevant to psychiatric presentations; the most common screening tests in clinical practice are listed in Table 1–6. It was once common practice for the psychiatrist to order routine batteries of tests, especially in cognitively impaired patients, in a stereotypical diagnostic approach to the evaluation of dementia or delirium. In modern practice, tests should be ordered selectively, with consider-

TABLE 1–6. Common tests in psychiatric consultation

Complete blood cell count
Serum chemistry panel
Thyroid-stimulating hormone (thyrotropin) concentration
Vitamin B_{12} (cyanocobalamin) concentration
Folic acid (folate) concentration
Human chorionic gonadotropin (pregnancy) test
Toxicology
  Serum
  Urine
Serological tests for syphilis
HIV tests
Urinalysis
Chest X ray
Electrocardiogram

ation paid to sensitivity, specificity, and cost-effectiveness. Perhaps most importantly, careful thought should be given to whether the results of each test will affect the patient's management. Finally, further studies may be beneficial in certain clinical situations as described throughout this book.

Routine Tests

As far as screening is concerned, a complete blood cell count may reveal anemia that contributes to depression or infection that causes psychosis. Leukocytosis is seen with infection and other acute inflammatory conditions, lithium therapy, and neuroleptic malignant syndrome, whereas leukopenia and agranulocytosis may be caused by certain psychotropic medications. A serum chemistry panel may point to diagnoses as varied as liver disease, eating disorders, renal disease, malnutrition, and hypoglycemia—all of which may have psychiatric manifestations (Alpay and Park 2004). Serum and urine toxicological screens are helpful in cases of altered sensorium and obviously whenever substance abuse, intoxication, or overdose is suspected. Because blood tests for syphilis, thyroid disease, and deficiencies of vitamin B_{12} and folic acid (conditions that are curable) are readily available, they warrant a low threshold for their use. In patients with a history of exposures, HIV infection should not be overlooked. Obtaining a pregnancy test is often wise in women of childbearing age to inform diagnostically as well as to guide treatment options. Urinalysis, chest radiography, and electrocardiography are particularly important screening tools in the geriatric population. Although it is not a first-line test, cerebrospinal fluid analysis should be considered in cases of mental status changes associated with fever, leukocytosis, meningismus, or unknown etiology. Increased intracranial pressure should be ruled out before a lumbar puncture is performed, however. More detailed discussion of specific tests is provided in relevant chapters throughout this text.

Neuroimaging

The psychiatric consultant must also be familiar with neuroimaging studies. Neuroimaging may aid in fleshing out the differential diagnosis of neuropsychiatric conditions, although it rarely establishes the diagnosis by itself (Dougherty and Rauch 2004). In most situations, magnetic resonance imaging (MRI) is preferred over computed tomography (CT). MRI provides greater resolution of subcortical structures (e.g., basal ganglia, amygdala, and other limbic structures) of particular interest to psychiatrists. It is also superior for detection of abnormalities of the brain stem and posterior fossa. Furthermore, MRI is better able to distinguish between gray-matter and white-matter lesions. CT is most useful in cases of suspected acute intracranial hemorrhage (having occurred within the past 72 hours) and when MRI is contraindicated (in patients with metallic implants). Dougherty and Rauch (2004) suggest that the following conditions and situations merit consideration of neuroimaging: new-onset psychosis, new-onset dementia, delirium of unknown cause, prior to an initial course of electroconvulsive therapy, and an acute mental status change with an abnormal neurological examination in a patient with either a history of head trauma or an age of 50 years or older. Regardless of the modality, the consultant should read the radiologist's report, because other physicians tend to dismiss all but acute focal findings or changes and as a result misleadingly record the results of the study as normal in the chart. Psychiatrists recognize, however, that even small abnormalities (e.g., periventricular white-matter changes) or chronic changes (e.g., cortical atrophy) have diagnostic and therapeutic implications (see Chapter 7, "Dementia," Chapter 9, "Depression," and Chapter 32, "Neurology and Neurosurgery").

Electrophysiological Tests

The electroencephalogram (EEG) is the most widely available test that can assess brain activity. The EEG is most often indicated in patients with paroxysmal or other symptoms suggestive of a seizure disorder, especially complex partial seizures, or pseudoseizures (see Chapter 32, "Neurology and Neurosurgery"). An EEG may also be helpful in distinguishing between neurological and psychiatric etiologies for a mute, uncommunicative patient. An EEG may be helpful in documenting the presence of generalized slowing in a delirious patient, but it rarely indicates a specific etiology of delirium and it is not indicated in every delirious patient. However, when the diagnosis of delirium is uncertain, electroencephalographic evidence of dysrhythmia may prove useful. For example, when the primary treatment team insists that a patient should be transferred to a psychiatric inpatient service because of a mistaken belief that the symptoms of delirium represent schizophrenia or depression, an EEG may provide concrete data to support the correct diagnosis. EEGs may also facilitate the evaluation of rapidly progressive dementia or profound coma; but because findings are neither sensitive nor specific, they are not often helpful in the evaluation of space-occupying lesions, cerebral infarctions, or head injury (Bostwick and Philbrick 2002). Continuous electroencephalographic recordings with video monitoring or ambulatory electroencephalographic monitoring may be necessary in order to document abnormal electrical activity in cases of complex partial sei- zures or when factitious seizures are suspected. As with neuroimaging reports, the psychiatric consultant must read the electroencephalographic report, because non- psychiatrists often misinterpret the absence of dramatic focal abnormalities (e.g., spikes) as indicative of normal- ity, even though psychiatrically significant brain dysfunc- tion may manifest as focal or generalized slowing or as sharp waves. Other electrophysiological tests may be helpful in specific situations; for example, sensory evoked potentials to distinguish multiple sclerosis from conver- sion disorder, or electromyography with nerve conduc- tion velocities to differentiate neuropathy from malingering.

Other Tests

Other diagnostic tools may also prove useful as adjuncts. Neuropsychological testing may be helpful in diagnosis, prognosis, and treatment planning in patients with neu- ropsychiatric disorders. Psychological testing can help the consultant better understand a patient's emotional functioning and personality style. For example, elevations on the Hypochondriasis and Hysteria scales of the Min- nesota Multiphasic Personality Inventory and a normal or minimally elevated result on the Depression scale consti- tute the so-called conversion V or psychosomatic V pat- tern, classically regarded as indicative of a significant psy- chological contribution to the etiology of somatic symptoms but now recognized as confounded by medical illness. (See Chapter 2, "Neuropsychological and Psycho- logical Evaluation," for a full description of neuropsycho- logical and psychological testing.)

The amobarbital interview has been used as a tool in the diagnosis and treatment of a variety of psychiatric conditions (e.g., conversion disorder, posttraumatic stress disorder, factitious disorder, psychogenic amnesia, neuro- sis, and catatonia) for the past 70 years (Kavarirajan 1999). The psychiatric literature has been mixed, however, on the utility of the amobarbital interview, and intravenous lorazepam is now generally regarded as a safer alternative. However, the diagnostic validity of amobarbital and lorazepam interviews has not been systematically assessed.

Write a Note

The consultation note should be clear, concise, and free of jargon and should focus on specific diagnostic and therapeutic recommendations. Although an understand- ing of the patient's psychodynamics may be helpful, the consultant should usually avoid speculations in the chart regarding unconscious motivations. Consultees funda- mentally want to know what is going on with the patient and what they should and can do about it; these themes should dominate the note. Mental health professionals are trained to construct full developmental and psychoso- cial formulations, but these do not belong in a consulta- tion note (although they may inform key elements of the assessment and recommendations). Finger-pointing and criticism of the primary team or other providers should be avoided. The consultant should also avoid rigid insistence on a preferred mode of management if there is an equally suitable alternative (Kontos et al. 2003).

The consultation note should include a condensed version of all the elements of a general psychiatric note with a few additions (Querques et al. 2004). The consult- ant should begin the note with a summary of the patient's medical and psychiatric history, the reason for the current admission, and the reason for the consultation. Next should be a brief summary of the present medical illness with pertinent findings and hospital course; this summary is meant to demonstrate an appreciation for the current medical issues rather than to repeat what has already been documented in the chart. It is often helpful for the con- sultant to include a description of the patient's typical pat- terns of response to stress and illness, if known. Physical and neurological examinations, as well as germane labo- ratory results or imaging studies, should also be summa- rized. The consultant should then list the differential di- agnosis in order of decreasing likelihood, making clear which is the working diagnosis or diagnoses. If the pa- tient's symptoms are not likely to be due to a psychiatric disorder, this should be explicitly stated. Finally, the con- sultant should make recommendations or clearly describe plans in order of decreasing importance. Recommenda- tions include ways to further elucidate the diagnosis as well as therapeutic suggestions. It is especially important to anticipate and address problems that may appear at a later time (e.g., offering a medication recommendation for treatment of agitation in a delirious patient who is cur- rently calm). For medication recommendations, brief no- tation of side effects and their management is useful. The inclusion of a statement indicating that the consultant will provide follow-up will reassure the consulting team, and the consultant should include contact information in the event that they have further questions.

Speak Directly With the Referring Clinician

The consultation ends in the same way that it began— with a conversation with the referring clinician. Personal contact is especially crucial if diagnostic or therapeutic suggestions are time sensitive. Some information or rec- ommendations may be especially sensitive, whether for reasons of confidentiality or risk management, and are bet- ter conveyed verbally than fully documented in the chart.

The medical chart is read by a variety of individuals, including the patient at times, and, thus, discretion is warranted.

Provide Periodic Follow-Up

Many consultations cannot be completed in a single visit. Rather, several encounters may be required before the problems identified by both the consultee and the consultant are resolved. Moreover, new issues commonly arise during the course of the consultative process, and a single consultation request often necessitates frequent visits, disciplined follow-up, and easy accessibility. All follow-up visits should be documented in the chart. Finally, it may be appropriate to sign off of a case when the patient stabilizes or when the consultant's opinion and recommendations are being disregarded (Kontos et al. 2003).

Role of Other Providers

Although the emphasis of this chapter is on the psychiatrist as consultant, the value of members of other professions, working together as a team, should not be overlooked. Psychologists play an essential role in performing neuropsychological and psychological testing and providing psychotherapeutic and behavioral interventions. Psychiatric clinical nurse specialists provide services to the nursing staff that parallel those that the psychiatrist provides to the medical team. They are especially helpful in organizing interdisciplinary care conferences and nursing behavioral treatment plans that include behavioral contracts with patients. Case managers facilitate transfers and set up aftercare. Chaplains address the spiritual needs of patients in distress. Finally, communication with primary care physicians remains of utmost importance, since the primary care physician is well positioned to oversee and coordinate ongoing care after discharge.

Screening

Screening tools may also be helpful in specific situations. Although a comprehensive survey of cognitive function is not required for every patient, even a slim suspicion of the possibility of a cognitive deficit should prompt performance of cognitive screening. Although individualized mental status examinations performed as part of a psychiatrist's clinical interview are much preferred to standardized tests, screening tests have been useful in case finding and research.

Tests such as the MMSE or the Mini-Cog (Borson et al. 2000) are helpful adjuncts in the hands of nonpsychiatrists to quickly identify potential cognitive disorders. The MMSE is a 19-question test that provides an overview of a patient's cognitive function at a moment in time; it includes assessment of orientation, attention, and memory. It is of limited use without modification, however, in patients who are deaf or blind, are intubated, or do not speak English. The MMSE is also particularly insensitive in measuring cognitive decline in very intelligent patients, who may appear less impaired than they really are. The Mini-Cog, on the other hand, combines a portion of the MMSE (3-minute recall) with the Clock Drawing Test, as described by Critchley in 1953 (Scanlan and Borson 2001). In screening for dementia, the MMSE and the Mini-Cog have been shown to have similar sensitivity (76%–79%) and specificity rates (88%–89%) (Borson et al. 2003). However, the Mini-Cog is significantly shorter and enables screening temporoparietal and frontal cortical areas via the Clock Drawing Test—areas that are not fully assessed by the MMSE.

In addition, these tests may be supplemented with others—including Luria maneuvers and cognitive estimations (e.g., How many slices are there in an average loaf of white bread? How long is the human spinal cord?)—that further assess the functioning of frontal-subcortical networks. A formal neuropsychological battery may be useful if these bedside tests produce abnormal results (see Chapter 2, "Neuropsychological and Psychological Evaluation"). In a patient with an altered level of awareness or attention, formal cognitive tests should be deferred until the sensorium clears, because clouding of consciousness will produce uninterpretable results.

Other screening instruments may also prove beneficial, especially in research, for identifying patients in medical settings who could benefit from a comprehensive psychiatric interview. The Primary Care Evaluation of Mental Disorders (PRIME-MD) is a two-stage evaluation tool developed for primary care physicians to screen for five of the most common psychiatric disorders seen in the primary care setting: major depression, substance use disorders, anxiety, somatoform disorders, and eating disorders (Spitzer et al. 1999). The first stage involves a patient questionnaire, and the second stage consists of a clinician-guided evaluation that takes roughly 8 minutes to administer. The PRIME-MD Patient Health Questionnaire (PHQ), an abbreviated form of the PRIME-MD, consists of a shorter three-page questionnaire that can be entirely self-administered by the patient (Spitzer et al. 1999). In addition to the assessment of mood, anxiety, eating, alcohol, and somatoform disorders (as in the original PRIME-MD), the PHQ screens for posttraumatic stress disorder and common psychosocial stressors and also provides a pregnancy history. Although it has also been shown to be a valid screening tool, the PHQ is more efficient, given that the amount of the physician's time required to administer the tool is diminished. Both the PRIME-MD and the PHQ have improved the diagnosis of psychiatric conditions in primary care settings (Spitzer et al. 1999) and may find a role at the bedside as well.

The General Health Questionnaire is another screening instrument originally developed in the 1970s to help identify the possibility that a medical outpatient has symptoms suggestive of a psychiatric disorder (Goldberg and Blackwell 1970). The original 60-item version has been replaced with well-validated 28- and 12-item versions, and it has been translated into numerous languages worldwide and been cross-culturally validated (Tait et al. 2003). Because of its emphasis on identifying *new* symptoms, the General Health Questionnaire examines state rather than trait conditions (Tait et al. 2003).

The CAGE is a well-known screening device developed by Ewing (1984) to identify alcohol abuse. A total of two or more positive responses on the four-question screen correlates with an 89% chance of alcohol abuse (Mayfield et al. 1974) (see Chapter 18, "Substance-Related Disorders").

Benefits of Psychiatric Services

The benefits of psychiatric services in health care delivery are significant. A growing body of evidence suggests a link between comorbid psychopathology and increased length of hospital stay and, consequently, increased inpatient costs. Levenson et al. (1990) described a longer median length of hospital stay (a 40% increase) and hospital costs that were 35% higher in a group of medical inpatients with depression, anxiety, cognitive dysfunction, or high levels of pain (independent of severity of medical illness). Cognitively impaired geriatric patients were shown to have an increased length of stay compared with those without cognitive impairment (Fulop et al. 1998), whereas depressed elderly patients in another sample had more hospitalizations and longer hospital stays (Koenig and Kuchibhatla 1998). Although some have suggested that psychiatric consultation might decrease length of stay and inpatient costs (Levitan and Kornfeld 1981; Strain et al. 1991), that is not where its primary value lies. Patients benefit from reductions in mental suffering and improvements in psychological well-being, from more accurate diagnosis, and from more appropriate treatment. Providers of health care profit from the added diagnostic and therapeutic expertise of the psychiatric consultant as well as from a better understanding of health behaviors. The hospital milieu benefits from assistance with disruptive and dangerous patients and is enriched by a safer and more pleasant work environment and better risk management.

Conclusion

Psychiatric assessment and consultation can be crucial to seriously ill medical patients. The psychosomatic medicine psychiatrist is an expert in the diagnosis and care of psychopathology in the medically ill. Psychiatric consultation affords a unique ability to offer a panoramic view of the patient, the illness, and the relationship between the two. The psychiatric consultant will be called on to help diagnose, understand, and manage a wide array of conditions; when effective, the consultant addresses the needs of both the patient and the medical-surgical team. In this manner, psychiatric consultation is essential to the provision of comprehensive care in the medical setting.

References

Alpay M, Park L: Laboratory tests and diagnostic procedures, in Massachusetts General Hospital Psychiatry Update and Board Preparation, 2nd Edition. Edited by Stern TA, Herman JB. New York, McGraw-Hill, 2004, pp 251–265

Borson S, Scanlan J, Brush M, et al: The Mini-Cog: a cognitive "vital signs" measure for dementia screening in multi-lingual elderly. Int J Geriatr Psychiatry 15:1021–1027, 2000

Borson S, Scanlan JM, Chen P, et al: The Mini-Cog as a screen for dementia: validation in a population-based sample. J Am Geriatr Soc 51:1451–1454, 2003

Bostwick JM, Philbrick KL: The use of electroencephalography in psychiatry of the medically ill. Psychiatr Clin North Am 25:17–25, 2002

Critchley M: The Parietal Lobes. New York, NY, Hafner, 1953

Dougherty DD, Rauch SL: Neuroimaging in psychiatry, in Massachusetts General Hospital Psychiatry Update and Board Preparation, 2nd Edition. Edited by Stern TA, Herman JB. New York, McGraw-Hill, 2004, pp 227–232

Ewing JA: Detecting alcoholism. The CAGE questionnaire. JAMA 252:1905–1907, 1984

Folstein MF, Folstein SE, McHugh PR: "Mini-Mental State": a practical method for grading the cognitive state of patients for the clinician. J Psychiatr Res 12:189–198, 1975

Fulop G, Strain JJ, Fahs MC, et al: A prospective study of the impact of psychiatric comorbidity on length of hospital stays of elderly medical surgical inpatients. Psychosomatics 39:273–280, 1998

Gitlin DF, Levenson JL, Lyketsos CG: Psychosomatic medicine: a new psychiatric subspecialty. Acad Psychiatry 28:4–11, 2004

Goldberg DP, Blackwell B: Psychiatric illness in general practice: a detailed study using a new method of case identification. BMJ 1(707):439–443, 1970

Granacher RP: The neurologic examination in geriatric psychiatry. Psychosomatics 22:485–499, 1981

Hackett TP, Cassem NH, Stern TA, et al: Beginnings: psychosomatic medicine and consultation psychiatry in the general hospital, in Massachusetts General Hospital Handbook of General Hospital Psychiatry, 5th Edition. Edited by Stern TA, Fricchione GL, Cassem NH, et al. St Louis, MO, Mosby, 2004, pp 1–7

Hyman SE, Tesar GE: The emergency psychiatric evaluation, including the mental status examination, in Manual of Psychiatric Emergencies, 3rd Edition. Edited by Hyman SE, Tesar GE. Boston, MA, Little, Brown, 1994, pp 3–11

Kavarirajan H: The amobarbital interview revisited: a review of the literature since 1966. Harv Rev Psychiatry 3:153–165, 1999

Koenig HG, Kuchibhatla M: Use of health services by hospitalized medically ill depressed elderly patients. Am J Psychiatry 155:871–877, 1998

Kontos N, Freudenreich O, Querques J, et al: The consultation psychiatrist as effective physician. Gen Hosp Psychiatry 25:20–23, 2003

Levenson JL, Hamer RM, Rossiter LF: Relation of psychopathology in general medical inpatients to use and cost of services. Am J Psychiatry 147:1498–1503, 1990

Levitan SJ, Kornfeld DS: Clinical and cost benefits of liaison psychiatry. Am J Psychiatry 138:790–793, 1981

Lipowski ZJ: Review of consultation psychiatry and psychosomatic medicine, II: clinical aspects. Psychosom Med 29:201–224, 1967

Mayfield D, McLeod G, Hall P: The CAGE questionnaire: validation of a new alcoholism screening instrument. Am J Psychiatry 131:1121–1124, 1974

Murray GB: Limbic music, in Massachusetts General Hospital Handbook of General Hospital Psychiatry, 5th Edition. Edited by Stern TA, Fricchione GF, Cassem NH, et al. St Louis, MO, Mosby, 2004, pp 21–28

Querques J, Stern TA, Cassem NH: Psychiatric consultation to medical and surgical patients, in Massachusetts General Hospital Psychiatry Update and Board Preparation, 2nd Edition. Edited by Stern TA, Herman JB. New York, McGraw-Hill, 2004, pp 507–510

Scanlan JM, Borson S: The Mini-Cog: receiver operation characteristics with expert and naïve raters. Int J Geriatr Psychiatry 16:216–222, 2001

Spitzer RL, Kroenke K, Williams JB: Validation and utility of a self-report version of PRIME-MD: the PHQ Primary Care Study. Primary Care Evaluation of Mental Disorders. Patient Health Questionnaire. JAMA 282:1737–1744, 1999

Strain JJ, Lyons JS, Hammer JS, et al: Cost offset from a psychiatric consultation-liaison intervention with elderly hip fracture patients. Am J Psychiatry 148:1044–1049, 1991

Strub RL, Black FW: Mental Status Examination in Neurology, 4th Edition. Philadelphia, PA, FA Davis, 2000

Summers WK, Munoz RA, Read MR: The psychiatric physical examination, part I: methodology. J Clin Psychiatry 42:95–98, 1981a

Summers WK, Munoz RA, Read MR, et al: The psychiatric physical examination, part II: findings in 75 unselected psychiatric patients. J Clin Psychiatry 42:99–102, 1981b

Tait RJ, French DJ, Hulse GK: Validity and psychometric properties of the General Health Questionnaire—12 in young Australian adolescents. Aust N Z J Psychiatry 37:374–381, 2003

Trzepacz PT, Baker RW: The Psychiatric Mental Status Examination. New York, Oxford University Press, 1993

2 Neuropsychological and Psychological Evaluation

Wendy A. Law, Ph.D.

Robert L. Mapou, Ph.D.

Jack Spector, Ph.D.

Gary G. Kay, Ph.D.

TWO SPECIALIZED AREAS within the field of psychology specifically address the interrelationships between mental and physical health. These specialties are represented by the divisions of Health Psychology (behavioral medicine) (Division 38, http://www.health-psych.org) and Clinical Neuropsychology (Division 40, http://www.div40.org) of the American Psychological Association (http://www.apa.org). Although some practitioners specialize in these areas, many general clinical psychologists make them part of their practice as well.

Clinical neuropsychology provides methods for diagnosis, assessment, and intervention of known or suspected brain dysfunction resulting from illness, trauma, or developmental abnormality (Eubanks 1997). Initially, neuropsychological assessment was most often used for diagnosis, but recently developed neuroimaging techniques have proved more efficient for detecting or localizing brain dysfunction (Mapou 1988). Nevertheless, neuropsychological assessment remains valuable in answering questions about the likely etiology in patients with symptoms suggestive of central nervous system (CNS) injury or disease that cannot be resolved by bedside mental status, physical, and neuroradiological examinations. This in-

cludes the legal arena, where neuropsychological assessment can be relied on, for example, to help distinguish between mild traumatic brain injury, posttraumatic stress disorder, and malingering. For individuals with known CNS-related impairments, neuropsychological assessment can inform prognosis and guide treatment and rehabilitation. For example, a patient who presents with significant problems remembering new information may be found to have either a lack of consolidation (i.e., the new information never gets into memory) or difficulty recalling what was learned (i.e., the information was stored in memory but cannot be retrieved efficiently), each of which requires differentiated treatment.

Finally, with repeated testing, neuropsychological evaluations can provide an objective means to monitor a patient's progress (or decline). These contributions appear to be the most significant goals of neuropsychological evaluation at present, with diagnosis more often being a secondary component (Mapou 1995). Although a full neuropsychological evaluation can be costly, use of repeated measures can be accomplished with a more limited, targeted test battery that evaluates the specific areas of interest.

The views and opinions expressed herein are the private views of the authors and are not to be considered as official or as reflecting the views of the U.S. Department of Defense. The authors would like to thank Su-Jong Kim for technical assistance in preparation of this chapter.

This chapter is a revision and update of a previous publication (Mapou et al. 2002).

In addition to neuropsychological evaluation, psychological assessment provides a complementary methodology for understanding a patient's emotional functioning and personality style. In some clinical situations, the use of both together is synergistically informative. For example, combined psychological and neuropsychological assessment can better detect patients who intentionally or unintentionally exaggerate their difficulties.

In this chapter, we review neuropsychological and psychological assessments in the medically ill or injured. We review the most often used neuropsychological techniques and discuss their application for differential diagnosis. An overview of psychological assessment techniques follows, with illustrations in both neurological and psychiatric disorders. We close the chapter by discussing special issues in assessment and conclude with some guidelines for selecting a neuropsychologist.

Neuropsychological Evaluation

The neuropsychological evaluation represents an integration of clinical information and empirical findings from neuropsychological testing. Although the different schools of neuropsychology differ somewhat in their approaches to the evaluation of a patient who has or is suspected of having brain dysfunction, all aim to describe cognitive, motor, and affective functioning; contribute to final diagnosis; and summarize how identified difficulties affect everyday functioning.

Each of the approaches to neuropsychological evaluation has advantages and disadvantages (Table 2–1). However, all approaches have been applied to a range of medical-surgical patients (see, for example, Tarter et al. 1988), and each has value for use in the medical setting; the best choice depends on the specific clinical situation and should be individualized.

Patient-Centered and Process-Oriented Approaches

In patient-centered, process-oriented approaches, neuropsychological assessment is organized around the referral question. Although a consistent core set of measures is typically administered, additional supplementary measures are selectively added. In addition, some of the testing procedures are modified to test the limits of cognitive and behavioral ability, and qualitative data are used to supplement actuarial test scores. The advantage of this approach is that assessment can be limited to the measures that are likely to be most effective for answering the referral question. The disadvantage is that some scores (e.g., IQ, im-

pairment index) cannot be determined with more limited sets of measures, and these scores are sometimes required by the referral source. In addition, although individual measures in patient-centered approaches have established reliability, validity, and sensitivity to brain dysfunction, these characteristics have not been evaluated when all the measures are administered together in combination as a finite battery of tests. Nonetheless, this approach is highly useful when the referring practitioner is primarily interested in understanding limitations in the patient's daily functioning and for considerations of rehabilitation. Additional information on this approach to neuropsychological evaluation can be found elsewhere (Christensen 1979; Jørgensen and Christensen 1995; E. Kaplan 1988, 1990, 1993; Lezak 1983, 1995; Luria 1973, 1980).

Battery-Based Approaches

In contrast to a more patient-centered approach, battery-based approaches consist of always administering a group of tests that have been standardized and validated together with a well-defined standardization sample. Specific subtests are combined in different fixed batteries, with a primary shared feature among batteries being their empirically established sensitivity to brain dysfunction overall. Interpretation of results from a fixed battery is based on the level and pattern of subtest performance of the individuals in comparison with the group findings from the standardization sample.

Relative to patient-oriented, flexible-battery approaches, battery-based approaches are generally more time-consuming and limited for understanding the unique features of an individual patient. In practice, however, most clinicians use standardized test batteries in a flexible manner. Because most batteries do not provide a comprehensive assessment of cognitive function, additional measures are generally used (Heaton et al. 1991). Clinicians are also likely to use subtests selectively based on observed qualitative aspects of performance, which technically alters the battery's standardized comparison of the individual results with a group. Nonetheless, because practitioners are likely to encounter such batteries, particularly in forensic contexts, we briefly describe the most common of them, noting their strengths and limits.

Halstead-Reitan Neuropsychological Test Battery

The Halstead-Reitan Neuropsychological Test Battery (HRNTB) (Reitan and Wolfson 1985) is arguably the most frequently used neuropsychological battery in clinical practice. Since its initial development by Halstead in the 1940s, the battery has been refined and has been administered to thousands of patients with different neurologi-

TABLE 2–1. Advantages and disadvantages of neuropsychological assessment approaches in psychosomatic medicine consultation

Method	Advantages	Disadvantages
Patient-centered and process-oriented approaches	Comprehensive assessment Can be tailored to answer the referral question	Methods not validated together Can be time-consuming if not applied selectively
Battery-based approaches	Highly standardized and quantified Very sensitive to neurological dysfunction	Require special equipment May not answer specific referral questions Provide limited assessment of certain cognitive realms
Halstead-Reitan Neuropsychological Test Battery (Reitan and Wolfson 1985)	Large body of supporting research	Always time-consuming Difficult for bedside evaluation
Luria-Nebraska Neuropsychological Battery (Golden et al. 1985)	Relatively brief	Criticized for problems with design and validity
Mental status assessment and screening instruments (e.g., Mini-Mental State Examination [Folstein et al. 2001])	Brief, easily learned Can be done anywhere Familiar in medical settings	Not comprehensive Limited sensitivity and specificity

cal and psychiatric disorders, generating extensive normative data. The battery consists of five types of measures: "1) input measures; 2) tests of verbal abilities; 3) measures of spatial, sequential, and manipulatory abilities; 4) tests of abstraction, reasoning, logical analysis, and concept formation; and 5) output measures" (Reitan and Wolfson 1986, p. 136). Strict interpretation emphasizes the pattern and level of performance on individual measures and on computed summary indices, including a measure of overall impairment (see Reitan and Wolfson 1985).

Normative data stratified by age, education, and gender are available (Heaton et al. 1991). When strictly standardized testing procedures are necessary (e.g., in forensic settings), the HRNTB is most often recommended. However, when time is limited (the full battery requires 6–7 hours), as in inpatient medical consultation, or when more in-depth assessment of particular cognitive functions is necessary, the complete HRNTB is less useful. Many clinicians use portions of the HRNTB, to take advantage of its standardization, and supplement the selected measures with other tests and procedures as time permits. However, as indicated, when the battery is not administered in its entirety, it is more comparable to a flexible-battery approach and should be interpreted more cautiously in comparison with the standardization sample for the battery as a whole.

Luria-Nebraska Neuropsychological Battery

The Luria-Nebraska Neuropsychological Battery (LNNB) (Golden et al. 1985) was developed based on procedures described by Christensen (1979), in an effort to standard-

ize the administration and interpretation of procedures associated with Luria's (1973, 1980) functional systems approach. There are two different forms of the battery (Forms I and II), and a short screening test version has also been published (Golden 1988) to determine whether or not the full battery should be completed. The LNNB has been administered to patients with different neurological and psychiatric disorders, and data from these groups have been compared with those from control subjects (Golden and Maruish 1986). The LNNB is as sensitive to the presence of brain dysfunction as the HRNTB (Kane et al. 1985), but it samples a wider range of cognitive skills and requires considerably less administration time.

A variety of concerns have been raised about the statistical characteristics of the LNNB (Adams 1980, 1984; Stambrook 1983) and the content validity of its clinical scales (Delis and Kaplan 1983; Klein 1993; Spiers 1984). Although the LNNB has utility as an instrument for determining likely cognitive dysfunction, it is limited as an in-depth measure of specific cognitive and motor functions. Because of these difficulties, the LNNB must be used with caution and should always be supplemented with other measures. However, this again changes the standardized nature of the battery as a single entity.

Bedside Screening and Extended Cognitive Examinations

The mental status examination has a long history in psychiatry and neurology and should always be included in a standard psychiatric or neurological examination (see also Chapter 1, "Psychiatric Assessment and Consultation"). Physicians perform cognitive screening to determine whether cognitive impairment is present and to develop initial hypotheses about diagnosis. Hodges (1994) outlined an approach to cognitive screening and summarized available measures. Mental status tests run the gamut from informal and idiosyncratic measures of cognitive and motor function, to the brief but standardized Mini-Mental State Examination (MMSE) (Folstein et al. 1975, 2001), to more comprehensive screening tests such as the Dementia Rating Scale (Mattis 1988) and the Neurobehavioral Cognitive Status Examination (Schwamm et al. 1987), now known as COGNISTAT (Northern California Neurobehavioral Group 1995). All such screening measures require little time for administration (5–45 minutes), do not require the use of specialized equipment (although some measures use stimuli presented on printed cards), and are easily administered in the clinic or at the bedside. Therefore, in contrast to more extensive neuropsychological testing, extended cognitive mental status examinations have the advantages of brevity and flexibility of administration.

Most mental status examinations assess the following areas of function: orientation, simple attention, short-term memory, comprehension, repetition, naming, construction, and abstraction skills. Within each area, however, the assessment is necessarily brief. Thus, what is gained in time and flexibility is lost in sensitivity and specificity. Although brief examinations, such as the MMSE, can detect gross changes in cognitive function and provide a baseline for follow-up assessment, they are likely to miss subtle cognitive deficits (Stokes et al. 1991). A. Nelson et al. (1986) reviewed five frequently used bedside screening examinations: the MMSE, Dementia Rating Scale, Cognitive Capacity Screening Examination (Jacobs et al. 1977), Mental Status Questionnaire (Montgomery and Costa 1983), and Short Portable Mental Status Questionnaire (Omer et al. 1983). The researchers found all the tests to be useful in diagnosing dementia and delirium but expressed concern that these measures were likely to miss subtle cognitive deficits.

A new measure, the Repeatable Battery for the Assessment of Neuropsychological Status (RBANS) (Randolph 1998), was designed to address shortcomings of past measures but retain brevity of testing time. This measure has 12 subtests that evaluate immediate memory, visuospatial and constructional skills, attention, language, and delayed memory. It takes 30 minutes to administer; has two parallel forms specifically designed to permit repeated testing, with an emphasis on detection of dementia; and has normative data for individuals ages 20–89 years. The RBANS has shown reasonable sensitivity and specificity for identifying neurological dysfunction and the nature of the dysfunction in different cognitive domains (Randolph 1998).

Bedside screening and extended mental status examinations are often important for initial evaluation but may be inadequate for a full assessment of a complex medical/psychiatric case. An examination that is too brief and too restricted in scope will assess a limited range of functions and is unlikely to be sensitive to subtle deficits. However, a full neuropsychological evaluation that provides more specific data is likely to be lengthy (a problem in the inpatient setting) and more difficult (a problem for patients with limited cognitive or physical abilities). Therefore, the specific purpose of the evaluation should guide the choice of assessment procedures. A careful cognitive screening examination clarifies whether there is a need for more detailed, formal neuropsychological evaluation.

Applications in Psychosomatic Medicine

In medical settings, neuropsychologists are most frequently consulted to help with differential diagnosis or prognosis of neuropsychiatric disorders and to guide treatment and rehabilitation. Table 2–2 provides examples of typical outcomes that may be gained from neuropsychological evaluation, depending on the referral question. It should be emphasized that no individual neuropsychological test score can be considered pathognomonic for determining or localizing CNS disruption. Nevertheless, individual tests can be informative. For example, a patient with mild hypoactive delirium due to hepatic encephalopathy who completes a basic visuomotor tracking task (e.g., Part A of the Trail Making Test) in the expected amount of time but completes the complex visuomotor tracking task (e.g., Part B of the Trail Making Test) in twice the normal expected time provides objective evidence of slowed processing that is not likely to be solely related to nonspecific illness-related fatigue. In the following sections, case examples are presented to describe some common applications of neuropsychological evaluation.

Dementia

In patients suspected of having dementing conditions, neuropsychological assessment is most valuable in the very earliest stages, during which bedside examination and neuroradiological findings are often equivocal (see also Chapter 7, "Dementia"). Neuropsychological evaluation can also help differentiate degenerative dementias from static and metabolic cognitive disorders, and cortical from subcortical dementias. Cortical dementias, such as Alzheimer's disease, are characterized by memory deficits, language dysfunction or visuospatial impairment, execu-

---

TABLE 2–2. Applications of neuropsychological assessment

- Differential diagnosis of degenerative and static neurological conditions contributing to cognitive and behavioral dysfunction
- Differentiation of symptoms due to neurological conditions versus psychiatric disorders
- Selection of candidates for surgery for intractable epilepsy
- Documentation of sequelae of acute brain insults and application to prognosis and treatment
- Assessment of neurocognitive function in patients with cardiac, pulmonary, hepatic, or renal insufficiency
- Assessment of benefits and adverse effects of new treatments
- Evaluation for a specific learning disability or attention-deficit/hyperactivity disorder
- Assessment of ability of an impaired individual to return to work or school or to perform independent living skills
- Assessment of competence to make medical, legal, or financial decisions
- Longitudinal evaluation to assess level of functioning and treatment responsiveness

---

tive function deficits, and diminished self-awareness, typically observed in the context of normal psychomotor abilities and near-normal attention (Cummings 1985). In contrast, subcortical dementias, such as those associated with Parkinson's disease, are marked by psychomotor retardation, attentional impairment, and emotional lability, typically in the context of intact language and visuospatial skills and recognition memory (Cummings 1985, 1990) (see Chapter 7, "Dementia"). Repeated neuropsychological evaluation can also be useful for periodic objective assessment of the nature of the deficits and evaluation of competence and response to treatment.

Case Example 1

Ms. A, a 77-year-old widow of 20 years with a 2-year history of memory problems and depression, was referred by her physician for neuropsychological evaluation to help determine the nature of her memory difficulties. She acknowledged feeling lonely and had experienced some loss of interest in her usual activities, although she continued to play bridge on a monthly basis with old friends. Ms. A lived independently and had experienced a fall the preceding month associated with slippery conditions during her daily walk. She did not seek medical attention, and her adult son initiated contact with her physician after his mother informed him of her fall. Her son reported that she seemed to have some difficulties with short-term memory and frequently repeated things she had already told him. He also reported that she continued to play a very strong game of bridge, which he also enjoyed.

Initial screening conducted by the referring physician revealed an MMSE score of 25, with difficulty reporting the day of the week and the specific date of the month and failure to recall three words. She acknowledged that she was not as sharp as she used to be and that she did not remember things as well. She also had started to let her household finances lapse, forgetting to pay bills on time. A computed tomographic scan of the head showed "mild age-related cortical atrophy." Ms. A's medical history included hypercholesterolemia and hypertension controlled with medication. Her additional medical history was believed to be noncontributory.

Results of the initial evaluation indicated some problems with depression (Geriatric Depression Scale score of 18). The primary care physician prescribed fluoxetine and referred her for neuropsychological assessment. At the time of the evaluation 1 month later, Ms. A felt that her mood had improved, although she still felt lonely. Her Geriatric Depression Scale score at the time of the evaluation was 5. Results from the neuropsychological evaluation indicated that she was a highly intelligent woman with very strong verbally based communication skills. However, test results also showed severe memory encoding and retrieval problems, inability to perform simple mathematical calculations, problems copying a complex figure, impaired simple object naming, and weaknesses in simple auditory attention. On the basis of the findings from the evaluation, Ms. A was given a tentative diagnosis of dementia (probable Alzheimer's disease) and was prescribed donepezil. Follow-up evaluation 1 year later showed continued decline in short-term memory and memory retrieval, but notable improvement in simple auditory attention as well as stability of the remaining affected domains, suggesting that donepezil had been beneficial.

Although it is generally rare, a specific amnestic disorder can occur as a result of several different neuropathological processes (see Chapter 32, "Neurology and Neurosurgery"). Neuropsychological assessment can help differentiate amnestic disorders from degenerative dementias, providing reassurance to patients and families, and informing treatment decisions (e.g., whether to prescribe a cholinesterase inhibitor for the patient). Amnestic difficulties following neurosurgery (e.g., for intractable epilepsy) have been lessened substantially through preoperative neuropsychological assessment (Kapur and Pravett 2003). In other instances, neuropsychological testing can contribute to decision making regarding whether invasive preoperative assessment procedures would be useful in relation to the risks and benefits expected for surgical intervention (M.D. Holmes et al. 2003).

Cerebrovascular Accident

Neuropsychological evaluation has been described as an essential component of the treatment planning process for many survivors of cerebrovascular accident (CVA)

(Tupper 1991) (see also Chapter 32, "Neurology and Neurosurgery"). Patients with severe dominant-hemisphere lesions will often be served best through consultation with speech pathologists, particularly during the initial phases of recovery. When language is not severely disrupted (or after improvement in language-impaired patients), a comprehensive neuropsychological evaluation can identify subtle deficits in memory, attention, or judgment (Brown et al. 1996; Lishman 1998). Disruption of any of these cognitive domains has implications for continued functional recovery and for rehabilitation. This may be particularly relevant when the patient also has psychiatric sequelae, such as depression or personality change. Patients with right parietal or frontal lobe CVA may not acknowledge their deficits or even notice obvious motor or sensory disabilities (neglect and denial syndromes) (McGlynn and Schacter 1989). They often want to drive or return to work, unaware of potential risk to themselves or others. Neuropsychological assessment can objectively document such deficits, and the results of such an assessment can aid interventions by primary clinicians and families (e.g., taking away driving privileges).

Like most acute neurological disorders, CVA syndromes can change rapidly in the weeks immediately following occurrence (Meier and Strauman 1991). Therefore, during acute recovery, a relatively brief cognitive evaluation should be administered periodically to annotate changes associated with resolution of nonspecific inflammation and injury effects (DeGraba 1998). Residual difficulties, including neuropsychiatric sequelae, are more likely to become apparent after the patient is medically stabilized. At this point, referral for neuropsychological evaluation may be useful to help differentiate psychological reactions to the stroke from more CNS-based causes of cognitive, behavioral, and affective symptoms.

Case Example 2

Ms. B—a 45-year-old previously successful independent Web site designer—experienced a subarachnoid hemorrhage due to rupture of an anterior communicating artery aneurysm. She was referred for a neuropsychological evaluation 6 months after hospital discharge because of her husband's concerns regarding her changed personality and problems with memory. Specifically, since her CVA she was doggedly insistent on rehashing problems with members of her extended family that the couple had resolved years earlier. When her husband returned from work each night, she would begin talking to him as soon as the door opened with complaints of past family interferences and emphatic vehemence that none of their family members were going to be allowed to visit over the summer. She also became despondent nightly, worrying that she would have a second aneurysm and not survive.

The purpose of neuropsychological evaluation was to better characterize Ms. B's deficits and abilities and to shed light on the cause of her difficulties (brain injury vs. emotional adjustment vs. preexisting limitations). Results of the evaluation indicated that she was at least of average general intellectual ability, based on a composite measure from the Wechsler Adult Intelligence Scale—3rd Edition (WAIS-III; Wechsler 1997). However, marked variability among the subtest scores included below-average retrieval of old knowledge, well-above-average vocabulary, above-average abstract reasoning, and low-average ability on some of the visual tasks. Additional findings on tests of memory included impaired encoding for learning unstructured (word list) material and deficient retrieval in a more highly structured task (paragraph memory). Ms. B also "remembered" incorrect information on the paragraph recall task that never was a part of the initial information (confabulation). On other tasks, Ms. B demonstrated marked repetition of responses, whether the response was correct or incorrect (perseveration). The results of the evaluation indicated that she was experiencing cognitive dysfunction attributable to the subarachnoid hemorrhage. She and her husband were informed of the findings and the relation to the behaviors she was exhibiting at home. Although she did not freely recall this explanation on a daily basis, when reminded by her husband of the results from the evaluation, she was able to remember the gist of the feedback and could then alter her behavior, redirecting her attention to less aggravating topics.

Traumatic Brain Injury

Neuropsychological evaluation is generally of limited use in moderate to severe traumatic brain injury (TBI) during the acute postinjury period because most patients are still experiencing acute posttraumatic confusion and altered consciousness (see also Chapter 35, "Physical Medicine and Rehabilitation"). The duration of impaired consciousness and the rate of improvement in cognitive functions are both predictive of cognitive function outcome after rehabilitation (Zafonte et al. 1997). The Galveston Orientation and Amnesia Test (Levin et al. 1979) is a 100-point, 16-item questionnaire that evaluates orientation and memory for events occurring before and after moderate to severe injuries. This brief measure is particularly useful because it can be administered in a very short time and can be given repeatedly, even multiple times within the same day if there is a rapid change in the patient's status. If the patient achieves a stable score of at least 75 of the 100 points, it is appropriate to administer a neuropsychological evaluation to assess the presence, extent, and impact of brain injury–related difficulties. Most moderate to severe closed-head injuries produce deficits in attention, memory, and executive skills (Brooks 1984; Levin et al. 1982, 1987). Judgment and reasoning may also be impaired and can affect willingness to participate in treatment. Although subtle naming and perceptual deficits can be identified, more severe impairment in these areas is rare in the absence of focal damage to the relevant areas.

Preexisting learning disabilities, attention-deficit/hyperactivity disorder (ADHD), substance abuse, and prior head injuries are frequent in TBI; their contributions to the patient's postinjury status must always be carefully considered (Dikmen and Levin 1993), and careful assessment of the patient's emotional status and personality structure before and after injury is essential for evaluation of functional deficit and prediction of outcome (Prigatano 1991; Prigatano et al. 1986) (see also Chapter 35, "Physical Medicine and Rehabilitation").

Case Example 3

Ms. C, a 20-year-old client at a TBI day treatment program, was referred for neuropsychological evaluation to assist with treatment and college planning. Specifically, the referral requested an evaluation to determine her residual cognitive strengths and weaknesses and the likelihood that she would be able to pursue further education, either with or without accommodations. Ms. C had experienced a severe TBI 1 year earlier, with coma for about 11 weeks. She described some improvement in memory over the 6 months after the injury, but she still had 6-month retrograde amnesia for events preceding the date of injury. Ms. C had been forced to switch from her dominant left to her nondominant right hand because of tremor and ataxia. During testing, she expressed frustration with her rehabilitation, complaining that not enough was being done to help her left hand. She indicated that she preferred to focus on physical rather than on cognitive or functional issues. However, she did report word-finding difficulties, distractibility, and problems with vision when reading.

Ms. C's estimated verbal IQ was in the low-average range, whereas her estimated performance IQ was moderately impaired, judged to be a decline from estimated preinjury functioning in the average range. Impairments were evident in attention, marked by very low processing speed and susceptibility to interference. Difficulties in executive functioning were marked by poor planning and impulsivity, weak organizational skills when learning new information, and deficits in visually based reasoning. Learning and memory were best for organized verbal information and were far poorer for a word list and complex visual design. Naming, timed word retrieval, and visuospatial constructional skills were impaired. Access to school-based knowledge, span for verbal information, and mental manipulation skills were relatively spared, and strength was evident in flexibility of thinking and use of feedback. A comprehensive academic evaluation, accommodations in college, a light class load, and tutoring were recommended. A neuro-ophthalmological evaluation, to determine the cause of her complaints of visual problems that also were revealed by testing, was recommended as well. On the basis of the reported findings, Ms. C was able to obtain accommoda-

tions in school and continue her academic pursuits, albeit at a slower rate. She also continued to improve cognitively and successfully completed classes at the local community college.

Depression Versus Dementia

Knowledgeable older patients who note difficulties with attention, memory, and word finding may worry that they are in the early stages of dementia (see also Chapter 7, "Dementia," and Chapter 9, "Depression"). In addition to early dementia, the differential diagnosis includes normal age-related memory decline, depression, medication side effects, and metabolic derangements.

Major depression is often accompanied by impairment in attention and in the ability to actively encode information, with associated reduction in learning and memory (Burt et al. 1995; Cassens et al. 1990; Sweeney et al. 1989; Veiel 1997). Psychomotor slowing and reductions in performance IQ (nonverbal intelligence) and in visuospatial skills may be observed. In contrast, focal language deficits are unlikely in depressed patients, and difficulties with memory from depression tend to reflect inadequate encoding rather than the forgetting that is more typical of dementia. In fact, despite the frequency of word-finding complaints, formal tests of naming often help differentiate depression from dementia; naming deficits are much less common in depressed individuals (Hill et al. 1992). However, recent studies have demonstrated that it is not uncommon for depression to be the first manifestation of Alzheimer's disease or another dementia. Although some depressed individuals show no cognitive deficits on formal testing, others manifest a neuropsychological pattern similar to that associated with subcortical dementia (Massman et al. 1992). In the latter case, in elderly patients in whom there is no other explanation for subcortical dementia (e.g., Parkinson's disease, acquired immune deficiency syndrome), recent studies have suggested a vascular etiology for both the depressive and the cognitive symptoms, correlated with subcortical lesions that are seen on magnetic resonance imaging (see Chapter 7, "Dementia").

Case Example 4

Ms. D, a 65-year-old woman, was referred by her psychotherapist because of a 20-year history of forgetfulness. Previous evaluations, including a recent magnetic resonance imaging (MRI) scan, had revealed no evidence of dementia despite the fact that Ms. D believed her problems were worsening. Ms. D had a history of diabetes mellitus, hypothyroidism, migraine, and hypertension (all controlled with medication) and a lifelong history of depression, for which she had received antidepressants and psychotherapy without a lasting remission. She commented that each time her memory problems worsened, she became more depressed.

Ms. D's skills on neuropsychological testing were largely in the superior range and were consistent with expectations based on her background. Although she had some problems retrieving learned information on measures of learning and memory, she retained information without difficulty over a delay. There was some evidence of weakness in attention and overall cognitive efficiency. Sometimes, when she perceived a task as difficult, she became frustrated and continued to ruminate into the next task, even when her performance was fine. Ms. D later acknowledged that she often "beat up" herself when she had cognitive difficulty. Psychological testing indicated a coping style in which Ms. D appeared more comfortable with a physical explanation for her difficulties. It was concluded that Ms. D did not have dementia. Her depression, and perhaps personality style, appeared to account for her cognitive inefficiency. Her other medical conditions were well controlled and were unlikely to be contributing. Expectations of cognitive failure occupied her thoughts and became a self-fulfilling prophecy. It was believed that if she were able to focus her thoughts on her cognitive successes rather than her failures, it was likely that her everyday skills could improve. Cognitive-behavioral psychotherapy and compensatory strategies designed to improve her attention and memory skills were recommended.

Psychological Assessment

A psychological evaluation represents a comprehensive integration of psychological assessment results (objective and projective test results, behavioral observations, and a patient's self-report) with professional knowledge and expertise for the purpose of identifying a patient's emotional status, personality structure, psychological symptoms, and motivational state. Psychological assessment can supplement the standard clinical interview both because clinicians tend to miss what they do not anticipate and because some states and traits may be hard to confirm through interviewing even when they are suspected (e.g., malingering, occult psychosis). Psychological assessment typically involves combining information obtained through psychological tests, interviews, and other clinical evaluations. A wide range of tests and approaches to testing are available, and most instruments have established standardization, reliability, and validity (Anastasi and Urbina 1997).

In medical settings, psychological evaluation can help clarify differential diagnosis; assess a patient's resistance to specific treatment approaches; evaluate the role of psychological factors in a patient's medical condition; determine the need for psychosocial interventions (e.g., stress management in anxious individuals before a medical procedure); and predict outcomes of surgical, medical, or psychiatric treatments. In addition, psychological assessment is a requisite portion of any neuropsychological evaluation.

Objective Personality Measures

In this section, we discuss the most frequently used clinical instruments having well-established reliability and validity. These personality instruments are self-report measures, in which the patient responds to a series of statements or questions relating to attitudes, beliefs, symptoms, and experiences and for which the scoring of the individual's response is based solely on an objective format in which all raters would agree (e.g., Likert scale items in which a response of "1" has the same meaning to all raters). On some tests, patients simply agree or disagree with target statements; on other tests, they report a degree of endorsement on a scale. Typically, the patient's responses are aggregated, scaled, and compared with data from normative groups.

There are some general cautions when using self-report instruments with medically ill patients. Instruments that are reliable and valid for identification of psychopathology in psychiatric patients may be inappropriate for use with medical patients, among other reasons because somatic items on these instruments will be endorsed by medical patients on the basis of symptoms of their illness. Because psychological evaluation represents an integration of multiple sources of information, idiographic features of the individual patient also must be considered in relation to standardized psychological assessment results. In the following sections, we discuss the use of specific psychological assessment instruments in medical settings, with the caveat that specific features of the individual patient may alter the interpretation of even these well-standardized and highly reliable measures.

Minnesota Multiphasic Personality Inventory

The Minnesota Multiphasic Personality Inventory (MMPI), developed by Hathaway and McKinley (1967) in the early 1940s, is the most widely used and researched objective personality measure. It has demonstrated sensitivity to many psychiatric disorders. The MMPI was restandardized (MMPI-2) (Butcher et al. 1989), and debate continues regarding the comparability of the two forms (see Helmes and Reddon 1993). The MMPI-2 consists of 567 true–false items. It yields scores on 3 major validity indices and 10 major clinical scales. In addition to these scales, many specific content scales are sensitive to health concerns, neurological disorders, affective symptoms, thought disturbance, and ego strength, among other factors. Other scales also permit assessment of response bias and potential symptom embellishment. Test results are interpreted relative to census-based normative data. Additional information is learned by reviewing a patient's responses to critical items. A vast body of literature exists on the interpretation of MMPI results in mental health settings, and a similar research literature is developing for the updated MMPI-2. For the purposes of this chapter, unless specifically indicated, we use MMPI to refer to the general test, without differentiating the original form of the test from the more recent update.

Despite the significant empirical basis of the MMPI, it may be inappropriate to apply these interpretations to general medical patients, given the sensitivity of the MMPI to the "normal" experiences and symptoms of patients with well-defined medical conditions (Cripe 1989). Pincus and Callahan (1993), for example, studied the MMPI in patients with rheumatoid arthritis. The researchers asked rheumatologists to identify the test items that were expected to differ between patients with rheumatoid arthritis and matched individuals without arthritis, based on rheumatoid arthritis symptoms and not psychological state. The researchers also compared MMPI results from rheumatoid arthritis patients with those from control subjects without medical or psychiatric illness. Using these criteria, the authors identified five items from the original MMPI that were clearly related to rheumatoid arthritis. These items appeared to account for the higher scores of rheumatoid arthritis patients on scales 1 (Hypochondriasis), 2 (Depression), and 3 (Hysteria).

Other MMPI items are frequently endorsed by patients with neuropsychiatric disorders. Specifically, patients with seizure disorders, TBI, and CVA often have clinically elevated scores on scales that were primarily designed to measure somatic preoccupation (scale 1, Hypochondriasis), conversion (scale 3, Hysteria), depression (scale 2, Depression), and thought disorder (scale 8, Schizophrenia, Sc) (Alfano et al. 1992; Bornstein and Kozora 1990; Gass and Russell 1986; Wooten 1983). For this reason, Alfano and colleagues (1992) and Gass and Russell (1986) recommended computing "neurocorrected" scores on these scales by eliminating specific items when determining the total scale score, to separate the effects of neurological disorder. The resulting MMPI profile would then presumably reflect only the "pure" psychiatric symptoms experienced by the patient. A competing view, however, is that a neuropsychiatric patient's report of atypical experiences is due to the actual cognitive deficits, affective reactions, and personality changes associated with these disorders. Therefore, increased scores on scales that assess these symptoms may accurately reflect a patient's experience of his or her

disorder, but results for patients with neuropsychiatric disorders still should be interpreted differently from results from psychiatric patients (Mack 1979).

In general, because somatic items are prevalent in MMPI scales used to identify depression, conversion, somatization, and somatoform disorders, scores on these scales often may be increased among medically ill patients. For example, Mayo Clinic data on the MMPI for general medical outpatients showed that 32.4% of females and 24.5% of males had significantly increased scores on scale 1 (Hypochondriasis) and scale 3 (Hysteria) compared with the original MMPI normative data (Osborne et al. 1983). In a parallel study, new MMPI normative data were collected. These data were considered more comparable to MMPI-2 normative data than the original MMPI data (Colligan et al. 1983). Investigators who used these normative data found that 37.8% of females and 30.6% of males in a general medical outpatient sample had elevated scores on the same two scales (Osborne et al. 1983). Some of these elevations may be explained by the increased prevalence of psychiatric disorders in medical inpatients and outpatients, but it is clear that caution is still warranted when interpreting MMPI scores of medical patients on these somatically loaded scales.

Finally, an elevation in scores on scales 1 (Hypochondriasis) and 3 (Hysteria), with a significantly lower score on scale 2 (Depression), is often referred to as the classic "conversion V" configuration. In psychiatric patients, this pattern is interpreted as showing that the "client is using somatic symptoms to avoid thinking about or dealing with psychological problems...[and is] converting personally distressing troubles into more rational or socially acceptable problems" (Greene 1991, p. 148). Patients with this profile are described as lacking insight, being very resistant to psychological interpretations of their problems, and presenting bizarre somatic complaints. However, these interpretations may not apply to medical patients, whose scores on these scales may be elevated to a level approximately equivalent to that among patients with conversion disorders (Fricke 1956; Lair and Trapp 1962). As noted, studies have shown significant overlap between symptoms of physical diseases (e.g., multiple sclerosis, pulmonary disease) and MMPI items that lead to clinically significant increases in scale scores (Labott et al. 1996; Meyerink et al. 1988; Mueller and Girace 1988). Even in the absence of a medical explanation for the symptoms, the presence of a conversion V does not itself prove diagnosis of a somatoform disorder. Furthermore, in some patients "unexplained" somatic complaints cannot be clearly attributed to medical or psychiatric causes and are best regarded as functional disorders. Thus, the presence of a conversion V in patients with physical symptoms in medical settings should not be interpreted as indicating a conversion disorder without careful consideration of and integration with the patient's history, physical examination, review of specific MMPI items endorsed, and any other diagnostic tests.

In summary, the MMPI-2 and its predecessor are powerful tools, but they must be interpreted in light of the patient's medical condition and other information, particularly if positive test results occur in the absence of other findings of psychiatric illness. When included as one component of a comprehensive psychological assessment, MMPI results can help the clinician understand medical patients' experience of their disorder. In the past the MMPI was used to help predict outcome and identify treatment modalities for some specific medical conditions (e.g., headache [Kudrow and Sutkers 1979] and impotence [Beutler et al. 1975]) and for some surgical procedures (e.g., candidates for cardiac surgery [Henrichs and Waters 1972] or laminectomy [Long 1981] and patients with intractable seizures who are candidates for surgery [Dodrill et al. 1986]). However, because of the frequent misuse of MMPI results in patients with medical conditions, others have cautioned about use of the MMPI in evaluation of medical patients when psychiatric disorder is not present (Green 1982).

Millon Clinical Multiaxial Inventory

The Millon Clinical Multiaxial Inventory–II (MCMI-II) (Goncalves and Woodward 1994; Groth-Marnat 1997; Millon 1987) addresses psychopathology according to DSM-III-R diagnostic categories (American Psychiatric Association 1987). The MCMI-III (Davis et al. 1999; Groth-Marnat 1997; Millon 1994) is an updated version using DSM-IV categories (American Psychiatric Association 1994, 2000). The MCMI-III consists of 175 true–false questions about basic personality patterns, severe personality disorders, and clinical syndromes. The test is scored by computer; specific normative data, such as the distribution of scores on specific scales, are treated as proprietary and generally are not available to the user. Thus, it is difficult to evaluate individual differences in factors associated with a specific patient that might contribute to elevations for reasons other than the test's expressed purpose.

The MCMI-III generates a narrative report and a score profile. The test is designed for use in mental health settings and assumes that the examinee is seeking assistance. The explicit purpose of the MCMI-III is to determine personality and characterological contributions to behavioral difficulties in individuals with confirmed Axis I psychopathology. As of January 7, 2004, 14 studies of any MCMI were identified through a MEDLINE search as

having direct reference to medical populations. However, for most of these studies, the profiles of the target medical samples were established on the basis of the existing MCMI standardization sample rather than by comparing performance of the research study samples with that of a nonpsychiatric sample. Therefore, published findings of studies evaluating MCMI/MCMI-II/MCMI-III profiles and score elevations in medical and surgical populations must be interpreted with caution.

Personality Assessment Inventory

The Personality Assessment Inventory (PAI) (Morey 1991) is an instrument with psychometric properties that is intended to be an advance over the MMPI. The PAI consists of 344 items, yielding standard scores on 4 validity scales, 11 clinical scales, 5 treatment scales, and 2 interpersonal scales. The test can be completed by persons who are able to read at the fourth-grade level, requires approximately 45 minutes to complete, and is easily scored by hand or by computer. The patient's responses are plotted and compared with data from a large, census-based, psychiatrically healthy population and from a large, community-based sample of psychiatric patients. In addition to measures of type and severity of psychopathology, the test yields measures of suicidality, aggression, perception of social support, level of recent stress, and resistance to psychological treatment.

As with the MMPI tests, one must be careful interpreting PAI findings obtained from medically ill patients. Medical symptoms elevate scores on clinical scales, leading to a risk of overdiagnosis of conversion or other somatoform disorders. Therefore, the same caveats mentioned regarding the MMPI and MCMI tests must also be considered when the PAI is used in clinical settings.

Millon Behavioral Health Inventory

The Millon Behavioral Health Inventory (MBHI) (Millon et al. 1982) was designed specifically to assess personality traits, interpersonal style, impact of stress, motivation for change, and compliance with care in medical settings. The test provides specific predictions for patients with cardiac, gastrointestinal, genitourinary, or orthopedic disease, as well as predictions about compliance with treatment. Our experience with the test, however, suggests that it is somewhat lacking in terms of assessment of personality traits and that its content is too obvious to many patients.

Millon Behavioral Medicine Diagnostic

The Millon Behavioral Medicine Diagnostic (MBMD) (Millon et al. 2001) was developed to provide a self-report measure of psychosocial factors that can affect health outcome in the medically ill. Standardized on a wider-based sample of the medically ill than the MBHI, the MBMD provides summary information on seven scales (Response Patterns, Negative Health Habits, Psychiatric Indicators, Coping Styles, Stress Moderators, Treatment Prognostics, and Management Guide) based on patient responses to 165 true–false questions. Although this more recent assessment tool has improved some of the weaknesses associated with the MBHI, because of its recency there has been little empirical research demonstrating its application effectiveness. Thus, the utility of the MBMD in the context of psychosomatic medicine has not yet been established.

Projective Personality Measures

Among the best-known and least-understood psychological tests are the projective measures (e.g., Rorschach inkblot test, Thematic Apperception Test). These tests employ less structure with more ambiguous stimuli and have greater task demands in comparison with the aforementioned objective personality measures. In addition, a primary goal of projective assessment is to elicit responses rich enough to permit psychodiagnostic inference and detect disorders of reality testing and thought processes (Anastasi and Urbina 1997). Although many clinicians rely on qualitative analysis of patient responses, quantitative summaries from some of these measures are as reliable, valid, and objective as results from the personality inventories described earlier in this chapter. However, data on medically ill populations are available for few of the projective test measures, and caution must be exercised when using these instruments with cognitively impaired patients. Deficits in attention, executive function, language, and visuospatial skills can render a patient's responses on these instruments unsuitable for measuring psychopathology.

When applied appropriately, projective tests such as the Rorschach inkblot test (Exner 1993; Rorschach 1921) may provide extensive information on how the individual's medical condition affects his or her perceptual processing and may be useful for treatment planning. However, it is even more important for the referring physician to be aware of and recognize the potential misuse of the results from such tests, so that medical conditions that may produce perceptual distortion are not inaccurately characterized as psychiatric disorders. Because these tests are less frequently used or are less appropriate for medical-illness samples, specific information or discussion of the various projective measures is not included in this chapter.

Self-Rating Scales

In addition to the objective and projective personality measures, which are most commonly administered and interpreted by qualified professionals, there are a variety of self-rating scales that have been developed to measure anxiety, depression, life-event stress, and other behavioral and affective symptoms. Newer instruments have been designed to measure health-related quality of life and well-being in medical patients, with less emphasis placed on diagnosing psychiatric disorders. Self-rating scales have the advantage of permitting a relatively brief assessment of current emotional functioning and are sensitive to factors that can affect neuropsychological functioning. Because their purpose is usually obvious, however, patients are prone to underreport or overreport difficulties. Furthermore, by definition of their targeted focus on current state, these measures provide little information about personality structure or typical coping style. If more extensive information is needed, more-detailed, objective measures should be used. For self-rating instruments that include somatic items but that have not been validated in the medically ill, results should be interpreted with caution in patients with medical illness.

Because of the ease of use, brevity of administration, and wealth of information that can be obtained from self-report instruments, the number of tests that have been developed is almost innumerable. Common examples of self-report measures with well-established reliability, validity, and standardization are described in the following subsections. A more complete description of currently available self-report measures is contained in the *Handbook of Psychiatric Measures* (American Psychiatric Association 2002).

Depression Scales

Among the best-known scales for measuring depression are the Beck Depression Inventory (BDI) (Beck and Steer 1987) and its revision, the BDI-II (Beck et al. 1996), a 21-item scale on which a patient rates the severity of current affective and somatic symptoms (see Chapter 9, "Depression"). Although the BDI is sensitive to depressive symptoms, its use among patients with medical illness has been criticized because of the scale's somatic content (Cavanaugh et al. 1983; Emmons et al. 1987; Schulberg et al. 1985). For this reason, Cavanaugh and colleagues (1983) recommended using only affective items on the BDI when evaluating general medical patients. Similarly, Pincus and Callahan (1993), in the study described earlier in the subsection "Minnesota Multiphasic Personality Inventory," found that six BDI items were likely to be endorsed by rheumatoid arthritis patients. Thus, clinicians using the BDI or the newer BDI-II (Beck et al. 1996) with medical and surgical patients should examine the pattern and level of item endorsement before interpreting a total score that is in the clinical range.

The Zung Self-Rating Depression Scale (Zung 1965), also known as the Zung Depression Scale, is frequently used in medical settings. It is a 20-item scale that measures severity of affective and physiological symptoms of depression. The Zung Depression Scale is less highly standardized than the BDI (Green 1982). As with the BDI, the total score must be interpreted judiciously in patients with medical illness. Another popular depression inventory is the Geriatric Depression Scale (Gallagher 1986; Yesavage et al. 1983), but the validity of this scale in patients with dementia is questionable (Feher et al. 1992).

In general, self-report measures of depression are less sensitive to changes due to treatment compared with assessment scales requiring professional expertise (e.g., the Hamilton Rating Scale for Depression [Hamilton 1960]). In general, specific symptom items included in these scales are less sensitive to change in response to treatment in comparison with overall summary scores (Lambert and Lambert 1999).

The Chicago Multiscale Depression Inventory (CMDI) (Nyenhuis et al. 1998) was developed for differentiating self-report symptoms of depression associated with mood, negative evaluation, and vegetative features. The CMDI is a one-page, 50-item self-report measure in which target items are presented as either a single word or a simple phrase and patients rate the relevance of each item to themselves with a Likert rating scale, ranging from 1 to 5. The CMDI has been used in patients with multiple sclerosis, and separating the participants with multiple sclerosis into groups based on the subscale scores was found to be useful in differentiating cognitive changes associated with mood state rather than medical illness symptoms (Nyenhuis et al. 1995). Similarly, depression rates in patients with myasthenia gravis were elevated only for the Vegetative Features scale of the CMDI, validating the importance of separating depression symptoms into distinct components when evaluating patients with medical disorders (Paul et al. 2000). Thus, the CMDI may be useful for differentiating the types of symptoms endorsed by various medically ill samples and for separating symptoms of depression from illness-related symptoms.

Anxiety Scales

The best-known anxiety scale is the State-Trait Anxiety Inventory (STAI) (Spielberger et al. 1983) (see also Chapter 12, "Anxiety Disorders"). It consists of two sections: 20 items that assess the patient's anxiety at the time of evaluation (state) and 20 items that evaluate the pa-

tient's long-standing, characteristic level of anxiety (trait). Unfortunately, if patients do not read the instructions for each section carefully, the distinction between state and trait measures can be minimal. The STAI was designed as a research instrument, and normative data are limited (Spielberger et al. 1983). However, this instrument has been successfully applied in repeated assessments of patient anxiety in research involving medically ill samples (e.g., patients undergoing coronary artery bypass surgery [Phillips et al. 2003]). In addition, the STAI successfully discriminated medical care factors that could affect patients' experienced anxiety after receiving adverse health information from test findings (e.g., Bekkers et al. 2002). Thus, the STAI may have utility for evaluating and assessing changes in experienced anxiety. Of particular relevance, several studies show that heightened anxiety is predictive of reduced treatment compliance across different medical conditions (e.g., cardiac rehabilitation [Whitmarsh et al. 2003]; medication regimen adherence in HIV infection [Escobar et al. 2003]; and cancer assessment follow-up [Yassin et al. 2002]).

The Beck Anxiety Inventory (Beck 1993) is an alternative to the STAI and is reportedly more effective in differentiating individuals with anxiety from those with depression. However, the extensive overlap between these two disorders complicates differential diagnosis, and reliance should not be placed solely on summary scores of self-report measures (Wilson et al. 1999).

General Distress and Life-Event Scales

A more general instrument that surveys psychiatric and medical symptoms as well as general level of distress is the Hopkins Symptom Checklist–90—Revised (SCL-90-R) (Derogatis 1994); the abbreviated version of this measure is the Brief Symptom Inventory (Derogatis 1993). The SCL-90-R includes 90 items, which patients are asked to rate in terms of severity, and provides results on several psychiatric symptom scales. Its utility for both psychiatric and medical populations has been criticized (Green 1982), but it has been used extensively in research with diverse medical and psychiatric patients. When this type of self-report measure is included as part of a comprehensive assessment, it can provide useful information about specific symptoms experienced by the patient (Anastasi and Urbina 1997).

The General Health Questionnaire (GHQ) (Goldberg and Blackwell 1970; Goldberg and Williams 1988) is another widely used and multidimensional scale that assesses self-reported symptoms. Available in the original 60-item version as well as several shortened versions (e.g., GHQ-12), this measure evaluates patients' reports of mental health concerns associated with somatic, affective, and social functioning and disturbances. Shortened versions have also been validated as mental health screening measures across diverse cultures in a World Health Organization study (Goldberg et al. 1997). Another popular measure relevant to psychosomatic medicine is the Profile of Mood States (McNair et al. 1981). Patients rate a series of words that are specific to affective state, and results are reported on several different scales. Because this measure includes few somatic items, it can be used for the assessment of medically ill patients. For measurement of life-event stress, the Schedule of Recent Experience (Casey et al. 1967) and the Social Readjustment Rating Scale (T.H. Holmes and Rahe 1967) are particularly well established.

Health-Related Quality-of-Life and Well-Being Scales

Self-report questionnaires addressing quality of life have been developed with medical patients in mind. These scales evaluate well-being, distress, and life events that can affect coping and psychological response to medical conditions. They either target behavioral characteristics and complaints associated with an illness or survey multiple attributes that are prevalent features of an illness. Well-being and quality of life are subjective individual characteristics that are measured best by self-report. Effective treatment of symptoms (psychological or medical) does not always result in improved subjective satisfaction or perceived quality of life. Conversely, quality of life can sometimes be improved with treatment without a corresponding change in medical symptoms (Frisch 1999). The importance of measuring quality of life through patient self-report, rather than through physician observation, has been emphasized (Gill and Feinstein 1994). Some have even argued that behavioral outcomes are even more important measures of health outcomes than are indices of symptoms (R.M. Kaplan 1990). Consequently, these measures can be useful supplements to more traditional measures of psychiatric (and medical) symptoms.

The Quality of Life Inventory (Frisch 1994) is a brief self-report measure that assesses satisfaction and perceived importance of basic life pursuits in 16 domains (e.g., personal health, relationship status). The measure's psychometric properties have been well established and have contributed to its frequent description as one of the best of the available measures of health-related quality of life (Frisch 1999). Another well-known measure was developed by the RAND Corporation for the Medical Outcomes Study (Tarlov et al. 1989). This instrument has also been used frequently in research, particularly an abbreviated version (36-item short form, or SF-36) (Hays 1998; Ware and Sherbourne 1992) and its updated version (SF-36v2) (Ware and Kosinski 1996). The SF-36 has been widely used as a measure of health-related quality-of-life outcome across the eight domains that are the most significantly affected by medical illness and also provides summary outcome scores for physical, mental, and overall health (Ware 1999). The Functional Assessment of Cancer Therapy Scale (Cella et al. 1993) was designed to measure quality of life in cancer patients. The scale contains questions for all cancer patients, and additional scales have been designed to measure symptoms of specific cancers and of HIV infection (Cella 1994). All these measures of patients' subjective status can provide useful indications of the need for psychological intervention or the effectiveness of a medical treatment regimen, independent of changes in primary symptoms. With any of these measures, however, the selection of the appropriate normative comparison group is still critical in making a diagnosis and planning treatment for medically ill patients with psychiatric symptoms (Derogatis et al. 1995).

The Stress Profile (Nowack 1999) is a 123-item, Likert-type self-report measure of seven major categories of individual functioning and coping (Stress Domains, Health Habits, Social Support Network, Type A Behavior, Cognitive Hardiness, Coping Style, and Psychological Well-Being) that are reported in terms of 15 subscales found to moderate the impact of perceived and experienced stress on health and well-being. The questionnaire also includes two measures of response validity (response bias and response inconsistency) and yields standard scores represented as Health Risk Alerts and Health Protection Resources. The questionnaire was standardized on a nonclinical sample. Administration of this measure typically requires 20–25 minutes. Results from this comprehensive health risk appraisal provide targeted information on lifestyle and health behaviors that contribute to illness, and it has been shown to have adequate psychometric characteristics. The Stress Profile has been found to effectively categorize stress effects on health outcomes, work absenteeism, and job burnout in both retrospective and prospective analysis studies (Nowack 1999).

Summary of Psychological Assessment and Self-Report Instruments

Advantages and disadvantages of the different types of psychological assessment measures are listed in Table 2–3. As noted, caution must always be exercised when interpreting scores of patients with medical illness because normative data established for normal samples or psychiatric patients are not directly applicable. This is especially true when using computer-generated interpretations of

TABLE 2–3.   Advantages and disadvantages of psychological assessment methods

Method	Advantages	Disadvantages
Objective personality measures	Standardized, reliable, and valid for psychiatric diagnosis Large body of supporting data Quantitative indices of distress, coping, and personality style	Time-consuming (30–45 minutes) Results must be interpreted with caution in patients with medical illness Can be difficult for patients with cognitive deficits to complete
Projective personality measures	Qualitative information on personality structure Sensitive to thought disorder Rich psychodiagnostic information Less vulnerable to self-report bias	Time-consuming (45–60 minutes) Few data on profiles of medical patients Results are difficult to interpret when cognitive dysfunction is present
Self-rating symptom scales	Standardized, reliable, and valid for psychiatric diagnosis Brief (5–15 minutes) Easily administered at bedside	Results must be interpreted with caution in patients with medical illness Prone to underreporting or overreporting of symptoms Do not provide comprehensive assessment of psychopathology
Health-related quality-of-life scales	Standardized, reliable, and valid Brief (5–15 minutes) Easily administered at bedside Supplement traditional measures of psychopathology Evaluate issues important to recovery from illness	Must be selected with reference to a specific medical condition Prone to underreporting or overreporting of symptoms Do not assess psychopathology

measures such as the MMPI, which do not take any individual factors into account. In addition, cognitive disorders can make it difficult for a patient to complete a measure and can render results invalid. However, when results from these instruments are interpreted in the context of the patient's history, clinical interview, and other diagnostic information, they can provide information on current coping style, emotional state, reactions to illness, quality of life, and general well-being. For a classic review regarding factors that must be considered when administering psychological tests to general medical patients, the reader is referred to Green 1982.

Applications to Psychosomatic Medicine

Psychological evaluation and self-report measures can be useful in a variety of circumstances in psychosomatic medicine. In the following subsections, we provide several examples of relevant applications.

Emotional Factors and Physical Symptoms

Psychological tests can help to determine how emotional factors contribute to a patient's physical symptoms. A patient's current and chronic levels of stress can be evaluated with instruments such as the PAI, STAI, and specific Ror-schach indices. These instruments assess tendencies toward repression and denial, coping resources, and personal reaction to illness, among other factors. These factors affect the development, maintenance, and progression of a disorder, as well as success or failure of treatment programs. The MMPI and PAI provide measures of guardedness, willingness to address psychological conflicts, and ability to admit directly to experiencing distress.

Case Example 5

E, an adolescent male, was admitted to a neurology unit for evaluation of atypical dystonia and intermittent seizures. While hospitalized, he experienced prolonged periods of tonic-clonic movements, marked by head thrashing, pelvic thrusting, and bilateral cycling motions with his legs. These events almost always occurred during clinician visits and were unaccompanied by incontinence, postevent confusion, or baseline cognitive deficit. Electroencephalographic recordings during the patient's spells were normal. E's approach to the MMPI-2 was guarded and defensive. He denied common shortcomings and presented himself in an unusually positive light. He expressed no psychological concerns. The clinical scale profile revealed a tendency to emphasize physical symptoms as a defense against emotional discomfort. Similar patients are described as naive, immature, and demanding and are prone to employ repression and denial as defenses against psychological stress or conflict. The psychiatric consultant was able to alternately provoke and terminate the patient's attacks during an amobarbital interview. Eventually, suggestion-based intervention resulted in remission of the events, and the dystonic posturing resolved. However, the patient's spells returned shortly after he was discharged to his home. At that point, hypnotic suggestion–based intervention with the patient was combined with family therapy and parent training to minimize the contingencies that appeared to be maintaining the patient's symptoms.

Although findings of psychological contributions to physical symptoms can often be made in the absence of psychological test data, the addition of such data can provide important support for a diagnosis of a somatoform disorder (as in Case Example 5 above), which should not be made solely on the basis of a normal medical evaluation. Psychological test data that strongly support a diagnosis of conversion disorder can help avoid multiple unnecessary neurological diagnostic tests. Psychological assessment may be especially helpful when the questionable symptoms appear in a patient with a known neurological disorder (L. D. Nelson et al. 2003).

Adjustment to Medical Illness

Interpersonal style, psychosocial competencies, and character structure can interact with physical illness and can determine a patient's ability to cope with illness, deal with health care providers, and respond to intervention. Psychological and personality testing can be valuable components of the psychiatric assessment of patients whose physical conditions force them into intense regressed relationships with their care providers. In some patients, severe character pathology may manifest as unusual physical symptoms or as pathological interactions with the treatment team. Careful assessment of personality variables can protect both patient and provider from maladaptive or destructive interactions.

Case Example 6

Ms. F, a 35-year-old licensed practical nurse, was referred for testing by a defense law firm; she presented with severe cognitive and emotional difficulties after a very mild head injury sustained in a fall from a chair. Clinical interview, projective testing, and responses on personality inventories revealed chronic impairment in emotionality, judgment, impulse control, and interpersonal relationships. Her interpersonal boundaries were weak, with marked evidence of chronic overidealization and undervaluation of those close to her. Symptom inventories and a review of records revealed impulsive behaviors, including buying sprees, bingeing-purging, sexual improprieties, and substance abuse. Her relationships were typically intense and short-lived. On self-report checklists and on structured interviews, Ms. F re-

ported many inconsistent and incompatible symptoms and could be led to endorse vague, unusual, and nonphysiological complaints. A review of the patient's record revealed marked inconsistencies and outright fabrications in her medical and psychosocial history. Evidence suggested that she may have misrepresented her symptoms in the past, which caused her to undergo a number of painful and invasive diagnostic and operative procedures. Projective and personality testing supported the diagnosis of borderline personality disorder and a probable factitious disorder with physical symptoms. It was later discovered that the patient had been pursuing treatment elsewhere, having attended nearly 140 diagnostic and treatment appointments in the 90 days before her psychological evaluation.

Emotional Sequelae of Neurological Disorders

A number of neurological and medical disorders are associated with cognitive and emotional sequelae. At times, CNS manifestations of a patient's disorder are difficult to discriminate from emotional reactions to the disorder. Psychological testing can help to determine how the psychomotor retardation, agitation, cognitive inefficiency, or emotional lability of patients with brain disease is related to illness.

Competence and Other Medical–Legal Issues

Neuropsychological and psychological testing can provide objective data on cognitive or emotional factors that affect patients' ability to appreciate their circumstances and the consequences of their decisions and to respond to environmental demands in an appropriate manner. Such evaluations can be very helpful in complex competency determinations, especially when competency is being contested (see Chapter 3, "Legal Issues"), as well as in determining the extent of injuries (especially brain injuries) in personal injury and workers' compensation litigation.

Case Example 7

Mr. H, a 67-year-old resident of a senior citizen apartment complex, sustained a left middle cerebral artery infarction, which initially left him globally aphasic, emotionally labile, and right hemiparetic. Immediately after the CVA, he was not believed to be competent to make decisions on his own behalf, and plans were made to have him transferred from the hospital to a nursing home near his eldest daughter, hundreds of miles from his home and friends. Mr. H grew increasingly alert, oriented, and engaged as he recovered from his CVA and was markedly upset by the decision to move him to a nursing facility so far away from his home. Neuropsychological testing revealed that Mr. H had relatively intact intellectual resources. Despite language difficulties, his nonverbal processing skills, memory, and reasoning abilities were nearly normal for his age and education. He became facile at using gesture and other forms of nonverbal communication to overcome his expressive language deficits and was able to communicate an understanding of most of what he heard. Mr. H expressed his desire to remain in his home and to receive outpatient rehabilitation services and home health care. He formulated a plan to receive these services and demonstrated the skills necessary to manage the social and financial resources needed to remain in his home. The family's initial reticence was overcome as Mr. H demonstrated his competencies.

Malingering

A patient may intentionally misrepresent or exaggerate his or her symptoms. Even the most experienced clinicians may be less capable than they suspect of determining when patients are feigning psychological or cognitive deficits (Bernard 1990; Faust et al. 1988; Heaton et al. 1978). Psychological testing can help clinicians detect feigning of symptoms. The MMPI and PAI both contain scales sensitive to intentional efforts to misrepresent symptoms (Bagby et al. 2002; Rothke et al. 2000). The Structured Interview of Reported Symptoms (Rogers et al. 1992) is a "rare symptom" inventory that is sensitive to inconsistent or unusual complaints not associated with known clinical entities. Careful analysis of neuropsychological test performance also helps to identify patients whose complaints are highly inconsistent with or disproportionate to their objective deficits (Ruff et al. 1993; Trueblood and Schmidt 1993).

Symptom validity testing refers to the process of repeatedly administering a simple binary forced-choice task to assess possible malingering (Bianchini et al. 2001; Pankrantz 1979, 1983). Trials with longer interresponse intervals and more complex interresponse tasks are described to the patient as "harder," and a large number of such trials are used. Malingering patients frequently deviate from the standard normal distribution, perform significantly worse than chance (a patient responding randomly is expected to respond correctly 50% of the time), and often perform far worse than patients with genuine brain injuries (Binder 1993). One can generate statistical probabilities that a patient's performance on this deceptively easy procedure reflects a conscious effort to perform poorly. The Portland Digit Recognition Test (PDRT) (Binder 1993; Binder and Willis 1991) is a frequently used version of this procedure. Computerized versions of the PDRT

and other forced-choice procedures have been developed and are seeing increased clinical use (Bianchini et al. 2001; Gutierrez and Gur 1998).

Case Example 8

Mr. I is a 32-year-old right-handed cab driver who was referred for an independent medical examination about 20 months after he sustained blunt chest trauma, a fractured ankle, and an apparent mild head injury in a motor vehicle accident. Mr. I's reports of coma and posttraumatic amnesia expanded over time, such that by the time of his neuropsychological evaluation he reported that he had lost consciousness for several days and reported nearly 1 year's retrograde memory loss and nearly 6 months' postconcussive amnesia. In the ensuing months Mr. I complained of changes in personality and behavior and reported severe difficulties in memory and concentration affecting all elements of personal and vocational functioning. He consistently misrepresented his premorbid abilities and accident-related disabilities.

Neuropsychological evaluation found Mr. I to be of borderline impaired intelligence with markedly impaired spatial, psychomotor, and attention-related intellectual abilities. These latter IQ scores were below levels expected from Mr. I's past academic attainment and vocational functioning and seemed to have been suppressed by an apparent motivation to perform poorly during testing. Performance on the remainder of this evaluation revealed uniformly severe cognitive impairment, in most cases much worse than is typically observed in more obviously severely injured patients. The pattern, extent, and progress of deficits were judged to be inconsistent with what is seen after much more severe, objectively demonstrable CNS insults. Mr. I performed below chance levels on procedures demonstrated to be sensitive to the effects of embellished or feigned deficit. His performance on objective indicators of dissimulation and pattern of performance on other standardized procedures very strongly suggested that Mr. I was intentionally spoiling his test performance. The ongoing litigation, the discrepancy between his subjective report and objective findings, his lack of normal effort during assessment, his complaints of remote memory loss, his exaggeration and fabrication of elements of personal history, and the improbable mechanism of injury relative to the nature and extent of his deficits were all consistent with the conclusion that the patient was malingering.

Computerized Testing

Several familiar neuropsychological measures have been adapted for computerized administration, and new computerized neuropsychological tests have also been developed.

Computerized cognitive screening tests represent some of the recent innovations in computerized testing. Computers offer a way to administer brief cognitive function tests; laptop computers enable bedside administration. Two batteries have been available for several years. CogScreen (Kay 1995), a group of 11 tests, requires approximately 30 minutes for administration. CogScreen was designed to detect subtle cognitive deficits that could affect aviation performance and is sensitive to mild neurocognitive disorder in general. MicroCog (Powell et al. 1996) was designed to assess mild cognitive decline in physicians, but it has been applied to cognitive screening of a wide range of patients, particularly older adults. The Cambridge Neuropsychological Test Automated Battery (Sahakian and Owen 1992) includes computerized versions of several common neuropsychological tasks accompanied by novel measures of reaction time and executive problem solving; it has been used extensively in research. Although to date these computerized batteries have not seen widespread clinical use, it is likely they and others will become more prevalent.

Computerized continuous performance tests (CPTs) have been increasingly used as part of a more comprehensive neuropsychological battery. These measures of sustained attention require a client to respond to a specific but infrequent stimulus (e.g., the number 1 presented among many 2s, an X presented among many different letters) for a lengthy period (Rosvold et al. 1956). Examples of these instruments include the Test of Variables of Attention (Leark et al. 1996), Integrated Auditory and Visual Continuous Performance Test (Sandford and Turner 1999), and Conners Continuous Performance Test (Conners 1994). The most common application of these measures has been in diagnosing ADHD. Unfortunately, because of their ease of administration, they have been used in isolation, with some professionals making a diagnosis of ADHD solely on the basis of an abnormal CPT result. This is inappropriate because it has been well established that there is no single cognitive test, the CPT included, that is sufficiently sensitive to and specific for diagnosing ADHD (Barkley 1998).

Selecting a Neuropsychologist

Clinical neuropsychology is a specialized area of practice within clinical psychology. It is unfortunate that no formal regulations exist regarding use of the title of neuropsychologist. Although guidelines for training and continuing education in neuropsychology have been published (Bornstein 1988; Hannay et al. 1998; Reports of the INS–Division 40 Task Force 1987), adherence to these guidelines is not yet required. Neuropsychology has now been recognized as a specialty by the American Psychological Association, which is responsible for credentialing psychological training programs in the United States, but it will be several years before graduates begin emerging from accredited programs. One indicator of competence is board certification in Clinical Neuropsychology by either the American Board of Professional Neuropsychology or the American Board of Professional Psychology, recognized as the "clearest evidence of competence as a Clinical Neuropsychologist" by the Clinical Neuropsychology Division of the American Psychological Association ("Definition of a Clinical Neuropsychologist" 1989, p. 22).[1] However, there are no legal requirements for certification, and some excellent neuropsychologists are not board certified.

References

Adams KM: In search of Luria's battery: a false start. J Consult Clin Psychol 48:511–516, 1980

Adams KM: Luria left in the lurch: unfulfilled promises are not valid tests. J Clin Neuropsychol 6:455–458, 1984

Alfano DP, Neilson PM, Paniak CE: The MMPI and closed-head injury. Clin Neuropsychol 6:134–142, 1992

American Psychiatric Association: Diagnostic and Statistical Manual of Mental Disorders, 3rd Edition, Revised. Washington, DC, American Psychiatric Association, 1987

American Psychiatric Association: Diagnostic and Statistical Manual of Mental Disorders, 4th Edition. Washington, DC, American Psychiatric Association, 1994

American Psychiatric Association: Handbook of Psychiatric Measures. Washington, DC, American Psychiatric Publishing, 2002

Anastasi A, Urbina S: Psychological Testing, 7th Edition. Englewood Cliffs, NJ, Prentice Hall, 1997

Bagby RM, Nicholson RA, Bacchiochi JR, et al: The predictive capacity of the MMPI-2 and PAI validity scales and indexes to detect coached and uncoached feigning. J Pers Assess 78:69–96, 2002

Barkley RA: Attention-Deficit Hyperactivity Disorder: A Handbook for Diagnosis and Treatment, 2nd Edition. New York, Guilford, 1998

Beck AT: Beck Anxiety Inventory. San Antonio, TX, Psychological Corporation, 1993

---

[1]A directory of diplomates in clinical neuropsychology, listed alphabetically and geographically, is available from the American Academy of Clinical Neuropsychology, Department of Psychiatry (B2954, CFOB), University of Michigan Health Systems, 1500 East Medical Center Drive, Ann Arbor, MI 48109-0704.

Beck AT, Steer RA: Beck Depression Inventory Manual. San Antonio, TX, Psychological Corporation, 1987

Beck AT, Steer RA, Brown GK: Beck Depression Inventory–II. San Antonio, TX, Psychological Corporation, 1996

Bekkers RL, van der Donck M, Klaver FM, et al: Variables influencing anxiety of patients with abnormal cervical smears referred for colposcopy. J Psychosom Obstet Gynaecol 23: 257–261, 2002

Bernard L: Prospects for faking believable memory deficits on neuropsychological tests and the use of incentives in simulation research. J Clin Exp Neuropsychol 12:715–728, 1990

Beutler LE, Karacan I, Anch AM, et al: MMPI and MIT discriminators of biogenic and psychogenic impotence. J Consult Clin Psychol 43:899–903, 1975

Bianchini KJ, Mathias CW, Greve KW: Symptom validity testing: a critical review. Clin Neuropsychol 15:19–45, 2001

Binder LM: Assessment of malingering after mild head trauma with the Portland Digit Recognition Test. J Clin Exp Neuropsychol 15:170–182, 1993

Binder LM, Willis SC: Assessment of motivation after financially compensable minor head trauma. Psychol Assess 3:175–181, 1991

Bornstein RA: Guidelines for continuing education in clinical neuropsychology. Clin Neuropsychol 2:25–29, 1988

Bornstein RA, Kozora E: Content bias of the MMPI Sc scale in neurological patients. Neuropsychiatry Neuropsychol Behav Neurol 3:200–205, 1990

Brooks N (ed): Closed Head Injury: Psychological, Social, and Family Consequences. New York, Oxford University Press, 1984

Brown GG, Baird AD, Shatz MW, et al: The effects of cerebrovascular disease on neuropsychological functioning, in Neuropsychological Assessment of Neuropsychiatric Disorders, 2nd Edition. Edited by Grant I, Adams KM. New York, Oxford University Press, 1996, pp 342–378

Burt DB, Zembar MJ, Niederehe G: Depression and memory impairment: a meta-analysis of the association, its pattern, and specificity. Psychol Bull 117:285–305, 1995

Butcher JN, Dahlstrom WG, Graham JR, et al: Minnesota Multiphasic Personality Inventory–2 (MMPI-2): Manual for Administration and Scoring. Minneapolis, University of Minnesota Press, 1989

Casey RL, Masuda M, Holmes TH: Quantitative study of recall of life events. J Psychosom Res 11:239–247, 1967

Cassens G, Wolfe L, Zola M: The neuropsychology of depressions. J Neuropsychiatry Clin Neurosci 2:202–213, 1990

Cavanaugh S, Clark DC, Gibbons RD: Diagnosing depression in the hospitalized medically ill. Psychosomatics 24:809–815, 1983

Cella D: Manual: Functional Assessment of Cancer Therapy (FACT) Scales and the Functional Assessment of HIV Infection (FAHI) Scale (Version 3). Chicago, IL, D Cella, 1994

Cella DF, Tulsky DS, Gray G, et al: The Functional Assessment of Cancer Therapy Scale: development and validation of the general measure. J Clin Oncol 11:570–579, 1993

Christensen A-L: Luria's Neuropsychological Investigation, 2nd Edition. Copenhagen, Munksgaard, 1979

Colligan RC, Osborne D, Swensen WM, et al: The MMPI: a contemporary normative study. Paper presented at the 91st annual convention of the American Psychological Association, Anaheim, CA, August 26–30, 1983

Conners CK: Conners' Continuous Performance Test Computer Program. Orlando, FL, Psychological Assessment Resources, 1994

Cripe LI: Neuropsychological and psychosocial assessment of the brain-injured person: clinical concepts and guidelines. Rehabil Psychol 34:93–100, 1989

Cummings JL: Clinical Neuropsychiatry. Boston, MA, Allyn & Bacon, 1985

Cummings JL (ed): Subcortical Dementia. New York, Oxford University Press, 1990

Davis RD, Meagher SE, Goncalves A, et al: Treatment planning and outcome in adults: the Millon Clinical Multiaxial Inventory–III, in The Use of Psychological Testing for Treatment Planning and Outcome Assessment, 2nd Edition. Edited by Maruish M. Mahwah, NJ, Erlbaum, 1999, pp 1051–1081

DeGraba TJ: The role of inflammation after acute stroke: utility of pursuing anti-adhesion molecule therapy. Neurology 51 (3, suppl 3):S62–S68, 1998

APA Division 40 Executive Committee: Definition of a clinical neuropsychologist (executive statement). Clin Neuropsychol 3:22, 1989

Delis DC, Kaplan E: Hazards of a standardized neuropsychological test with low content validity: comment on the Luria-Nebraska Neuropsychological Battery. J Consult Clin Psychol 51:396–398, 1983

Derogatis LR: BSI: Administration, Scoring, and Procedures Manual, 3rd Edition. Minneapolis, MN, National Computer Systems, 1993

Derogatis LR: SCL-90-R: Administration, Scoring, and Procedures Manual. Minneapolis, MN, National Computer Systems, 1994

Derogatis LR, Fleming MP, Sudler NC, et al: Psychological assessment, in Managing Chronic Illness: A Biopsychosocial Perspective. Edited by Nicasio PM, Smith TW. Washington DC, American Psychological Association, 1995, pp 59–116

Dikmen SS, Levin HS: Methodological issues in the study of mild head injury. J Head Trauma Rehabil 8:30–37, 1993

Dodrill CB, Wilkus RJ, Ojemann GA, et al: Multidisciplinary prediction of seizure relief from cortical resection surgery. Ann Neurol 20:2–12, 1986

Emmons CA, Fetting JH, Zonderman AB: A comparison of the symptoms of medical and psychiatric patients matched on the Beck Depression Inventory. Gen Hosp Psychiatry 9:398–404, 1987

Escobar I, Campo M, Martin J, et al: Factors affecting patient adherence to highly active antiretroviral therapy. Ann Pharmacother 37:775–781, 2003

Eubanks JD: Division 40 Report: clinical neuropsychology summary information prepared by Division 40, Clinical Neuropsychology, American Psychological Association. Clin Neuropsychol 11:77–80, 1997

Exner JE: The Rorschach: A Comprehensive System, 3rd Edition. Vol 1: Basic Foundations. New York, Wiley, 1993

Faust D, Hart K, Guilmette TJ: Pediatric malingering: the capacity of children to fake believable deficits on neuropsychological testing. J Consult Clin Psychol 56:578–582, 1988

Feher EP, Larrabee GJ, Crook TH: Factors attenuating the validity of the Geriatric Depression Scale in a dementia population. J Am Geriatr Soc 40:906–909, 1992

Folstein MF, Folstein SE, McHugh PR: "Mini-Mental State": a practical method for grading the cognitive state of patients for the clinician. J Psychiatr Res 12:189–198, 1975

Folstein MF, Folstein SE, McHugh R: Mini-Mental State Examination. Odessa, FL, Psychological Assessment Resources, 2001

Fricke BG: Conversion hysterics and the MMPI. J Clin Psychol 12:322–326, 1956

Frisch MB: Quality of Life Inventory (QOLI). Minneapolis, MN, National Computer Systems, 1994

Frisch MB: Quality of life assessment/intervention and the Quality of Life Inventory (QOLI), in The Use of Psychological Testing for Treatment Planning and Outcome Assessment, 2nd Edition. Edited by Maruish M. Mahwah, NJ, Erlbaum, 1999, pp 1277–1331

Gallagher D: Assessment of depression by interview methods and psychiatric rating scales, in Handbook for Clinical Memory Assessment of Older Adults. Edited by Poon LW. Washington, DC, American Psychological Association, 1986, pp 202–212

Gass CS, Russell EW: Minnesota Multiphasic Personality Inventory correlates of lateralized cerebral lesions and aphasic deficits. J Consult Clin Psychol 54:359–363, 1986

Gill TM, Feinstein AR: A critical appraisal of the quality of quality-of-life measurements. JAMA 272:619–626, 1994

Goldberg DP, Blackwell B: Psychiatric illness in general practice. A detailed study using a new method of case identification. Br Med J 1:439–443, 1970

Goldberg DP, Williams P: A User's Guide to the GHQ. Windsor, England, NFER-Nelson, 1988

Goldberg DP, Gater R, Sartorius N, et al: The validity of two versions of the GHQ in the WHO study of mental illness in general health care. Psychol Med 27:191–197, 1997

Golden CJ: Screening Test for the Luria-Nebraska Neuropsychological Battery. Los Angeles, CA, Western Psychological Services, 1988

Golden CJ, Maruish M: The Luria-Nebraska Neuropsychological Battery, in The Neuropsychology Handbook. Edited by Wedding DJ, Horton AM, Webster J. New York, Springer, 1986, pp 161–193

Golden CJ, Hammeke TA, Purisch AD: Luria-Nebraska Neuropsychological Battery. Los Angeles, CA, Western Psychological Services, 1985

Goncalves AA, Woodward MJ: Millon Clinical Multiaxial Inventory–II, in The Use of Psychological Testing for Treatment Planning and Outcome Assessment. Edited by Maruish M. Hillsdale, NJ, Erlbaum, 1994, pp 161–184

Green CJ: Psychological assessments in medical settings, in Handbook of Clinical Health Psychology. Edited by Millon T, Meagher R. New York, Plenum, 1982, pp 339–375

Greene RL: The MMPI-2/MMPI: An Interpretive Manual. Boston, MA, Allyn & Bacon, 1991

Groth-Marnat G: Handbook of Psychological Assessment, 3rd Edition. New York, Wiley, 1997

Gutierrez JM, Gur RC: Detection of malingering using forced choice techniques, in Detection of Malingering During Head Injury Litigation. Edited by Reynolds CR. New York, Plenum, 1998, pp 81–104

Hamilton M: A rating scale for depression. J Neurol Neurosurg Psychiatry 23:56–62, 1960

Hannay HJ, Bieliauskas LA, Crosson BA, et al: Proceedings of the Houston Conference on Specialty Education Training in Clinical Neuropsychology. Arch Clin Neuropsychol 13:157–250, 1998

Hathaway SR, McKinley JC: Minnesota Multiphasic Personality Inventory, Revised Edition. New York, Psychological Corporation, 1967

Hays RD: RAND-36 Health Status Inventory. San Antonio, TX, Psychological Corporation, 1998

Heaton RK, Smith HH, Lehman RAW, et al: Prospects for faking believable deficits on neuropsychological testing. J Consult Clin Psychol 46:892–900, 1978

Heaton RK, Grant I, Matthews CG: Comprehensive Norms for an Expanded Halstead-Reitan Battery. Orlando, FL, Psychological Assessment Resources, 1991

Helmes E, Reddon JR: A perspective on developments in assessing psychopathology: a critical review of the MMPI and MMPI-2. Psychol Bull 113:453–471, 1993

Henrichs TF, Waters WF: Psychological adjustment and response to open-heart surgery: some methodological considerations. Br J Psychiatry 120:491–496, 1972

Hill CD, Stoudemire A, Morris R, et al: Dysnomia in the differential diagnosis of major depression, depression-related cognitive dysfunction, and dementia. J Neuropsychiatry Clin Neurosci 4:64–69, 1992

Hodges JR: Cognitive Assessment for Clinicians. New York, Oxford University Press, 1994

Holmes MD, Miles AN, Dodrill CB, et al: Identifying potential surgical candidates in patients with evidence of bitemporal epilepsy. Epilepsia 44:1075–1079, 2003

Holmes TH, Rahe RH: The Social Readjustment Rating Scale. J Psychosom Res 11:213–218, 1967

Jacobs JW, Bernhard MR, Delgado A, et al: Screening for organic mental syndromes in the medically ill. Ann Intern Med 86:40–46, 1977

Jørgensen K, Christensen A-L: The approach of A.R. Luria to neuropsychological assessment, in Clinical Neuropsychological Assessment: A Cognitive Approach. Edited by Mapou RL, Spector J. New York, Plenum, 1995, pp 217–236

Kane RL, Parsons OA, Goldstein G: Statistical relationships and discriminative accuracy of the Halstead-Reitan, Luria-Nebraska, and Wechsler IQ scores in the identification of brain damage. J Clin Exp Neuropsychol 7:211–223, 1985

Kaplan E: A process approach to neuropsychological assessment, in Clinical Neuropsychology and Brain Function: Research, Measurement, and Practice. Edited by Boll T, Bryant BK. Washington, DC, American Psychological Association, 1988, pp 129–167

Kaplan E: The process approach to neuropsychological assessment of psychiatric patients. J Neuropsychiatry Clin Neurosci 2:72–87, 1990

Kaplan E: The Boston Process Approach to neuropsychological assessment. Workshop presented at Walter Reed Army Medical Center, Washington, DC, March 1993

Kaplan RM: Behavior as the central outcome in health care. Am Psychol 45:1211–1220, 1990

Kapur N, Prevett M: Unexpected amnesia: are there lessons to be learned from cases of amnesia following unilateral temporal lobe surgery? Brain 126(Pt 12):2573–2585, 2003

Kay GG: CogScreen—Aeromedical Edition: Professional Manual. Odessa, FL, Psychological Assessment Resources, 1995

Klein SH: Misuse of the Luria-Nebraska localization scales—comments on a criminal case study. Clin Neuropsychol 7:297–299, 1993

Kudrow L, Sutkers BJ: MMPI pattern specificity in primary headache disorders. Headache 19:18–24, 1979

Labott SM, Preisman RC, Torosian T, et al: Screening for somatizing patients in the pulmonary subspecialty clinic. Psychosomatics 37:327–338, 1996

Lair CV, Trapp EP: The differential diagnostic value of MMPI with somatically disturbed patients. J Clin Psychol 37:744–749, 1962

Lambert MJ, Lambert JM: Use of psychological tests for assessing treatment outcome, in The Use of Psychological Testing for Treatment Planning and Outcomes Assessment, 2nd Edition. Edited by Maruish M. Mahwah, NJ, Erlbaum, 1999, pp 115–151

Leark RA, Dupuy TR, Greenberg LM, et al: Test of Variables of Attention Professional Manual, Version 7.0. Los Alamitos, CA, Universal Attention Disorders, 1996

Levin HS, O'Donnell VM, Grossman RG: The Galveston Orientation and Amnesia Test: a practical scale to assess cognition after head injury. J Nerv Ment Dis 167:675–684, 1979

Levin HS, Benton AL, Grossman RG: Neurobehavioral Consequences of Closed Head Injury. New York, Oxford University Press, 1982

Levin HS, Grafman J, Eisenberg HM (eds): Neurobehavioral Recovery From Head Injury. New York, Oxford University Press, 1987

Lezak MD: Neuropsychological Assessment, 2nd Edition. New York, Oxford University Press, 1983

Lezak MD: Neuropsychological Assessment, 3rd Edition. New York, Oxford University Press, 1995

Lishman WA: Organic Psychiatry: The Psychological Consequences of Cerebral Disorder, 3rd Edition. Malden, MA, Blackwell Science, 1998

Long CJ: The relationship between surgical outcome and MMPI in chronic pain patients. J Clin Psychol 37:744–749, 1981

Luria AR: The Working Brain: An Introduction to Neuropsychology. New York, Basic Books, 1973

Luria AR: Higher Cortical Functions in Man, 2nd Edition. New York, Basic Books, 1980

Mack JL: The MMPI and neurological dysfunction, in MMPI: Clinical and Research Trends. Edited by Newmark CS. New York, Praeger, 1979, pp 53–79

Mapou RL: Testing to detect brain damage: an alternative to what may no longer be useful. J Clin Exp Neuropsychol 10:271–278, 1988

Mapou RL: Introduction, in Clinical Neuropsychological Assessment: A Cognitive Approach. Edited by Mapou RL, Spector J. New York, Plenum, 1995, pp 1–13

Mapou RL, Law WA, Spector J, et al: Neuropsychological and psychological assessment, in The American Psychiatric Publishing Textbook of Consultation-Liaison Psychiatry: Psychiatry in the Medically Ill, 2nd Edition. Edited by Wise MG, Rundell JR. Washington, DC, American Psychiatric Publishing, 2002, pp 77–106

Massman PJ, Delis DC, Butters N, et al: The subcortical dysfunction hypothesis of memory deficits in depression: neuropsychological validation in a subgroup of patients. J Clin Exp Neuropsychol 14:687–706, 1992

Mattis S: Dementia Rating Scale. Odessa, FL, Psychological Assessment Resources, 1988

McGlynn SM, Schacter DL: Unawareness of deficits in neuropsychological syndromes. J Clin Exp Neuropsychol 11:143–205, 1989

McNair DM, Lorr M, Droppelman LS: Profile of Mood States Manual. San Diego, CA, Educational and Industrial Testing Service, 1981

Meier M, Strauman SE: Neuropsychological recovery after cerebral infarction, in Neurobehavioral Aspects of Cerebrovascular Disease. Edited by Bornstein RA, Brown G. New York, Oxford University Press, 1991, pp 273–296

Meyerink LH, Reitan RM, Selz M: The validity of the MMPI with multiple sclerosis patients. J Clin Psychol 44:764–769, 1988

Millon T: Millon Clinical Multiaxial Inventory–II Manual. Minneapolis, MN, National Computer Systems, 1987

Millon T: MCMI-III Test Manual. Minneapolis, MN, National Computer Systems, 1994

Millon T, Green CJ, Meagher RB: Millon Behavioral Health Inventory Manual, 3rd Edition. Minneapolis, MN, National Computer Systems, 1982

Millon T, Antoni MH, Millon C, et al: Test Manual for the Millon Behavioral Medicine Diagnostic (MBMD). Minneapolis, MN, National Computer Services, 2001

Montgomery K, Costa L: Neuropsychological test performance of a normal elderly sample. Paper presented at the 6th European conference of the International Neuropsychological Society, Lisbon, Portugal, June 1983

Morey LC: The Personality Assessment Inventory Manual. Odessa, FL, Psychological Assessment Resources, 1991

Mueller SR, Girace M: Use and misuse of the MMPI: a reconsideration. Psychol Rep 63:483–491, 1988

Nelson A, Fogel BS, Faust D: Bedside cognitive screening instruments: a critical assessment. J Nerv Ment Dis 174:73–83, 1986

Nelson LD, Elder JT, Tehrani P, et al: Measuring personality and emotional functioning in multiple sclerosis: a cautionary note. Arch Clin Neuropsychol 18:419–429, 2003

Northern California Neurobehavioral Group: Manual for COGNISTAT (The Neurobehavioral Cognitive Status Examination). Fairfax, CA, Northern California Neurobehavioral Group, 1995

Nowack KM: Stress Profile: Manual. Los Angeles, CA, Western Psychological Services, 1999

Nyenhuis DL, Rao SM, Zajecka JM, et al: Mood disturbance versus other symptoms of depression in multiple sclerosis. J Int Neuropsychol Soc 1:291–296, 1995

Nyenhuis DL, Luchetta T, Yamamoto C, et al: The development, standardization, and initial validation of the Chicago Multiscale Depression Inventory. J Pers Assess 70:386–401, 1998

Omer H, Foldes J, Toby M, et al: Screening for cognitive deficits in a sample of hospitalized geriatric patients: a re-evaluation of a brief mental status questionnaire. J Am Geriatr Soc 31:266–268, 1983

Osborne D, Colligan RC, Swensen WM, et al: Use of contemporary MMPI norms in a medical population. Paper presented at the 91st annual convention of the American Psychological Association, Anaheim, CA, August 26–30, 1983

Pankrantz L: Symptom validity testing and symptom retraining: procedures for the assessment and treatment of functional sensory deficits. J Consult Clin Psychol 47:409–410, 1979

Pankrantz L: A new technique for the assessment and modification of feigned memory deficit. Percept Mot Skills 57:367–372, 1983

Paul RH, Cohen RA, Goldstein JM, et al: Severity of mood, self-evaluative, and vegetative symptoms of depression in myasthenia gravis. J Neuropsychiatry Clin Neurosci 12:499–501, 2000

Phillips Bute B, Mathew J, Blumenthal JA, et al: Female gender is associated with impaired quality of life 1 year after coronary artery bypass surgery. Psychosom Med 65:944–951, 2003

Pincus T, Callahan LF: Depression scales in rheumatoid arthritis: criterion contamination in interpretation of patient responses. Patient Educ Couns 20:133–143, 1993

Powell D, Kaplan E, Whitla D, et al: MicroCog: Assessment of Cognitive Functioning, Version 2.4. San Antonio, TX, Psychological Corporation, 1996

Prigatano GP: Disordered mind, wounded soul: the emerging role of psychotherapy in rehabilitation after brain injury. J Head Trauma Rehabil 6:1–10, 1991

Prigatano GP, Fordyce DJ, Zeiwer HK, et al: Neuropsychological Rehabilitation After Brain Injury. Baltimore, MD, Johns Hopkins University Press, 1986

Randolph C: Repeatable Battery for the Assessment of Neuropsychological Status (RBANS). San Antonio, TX, Psychological Corporation, 1998

Reitan RM, Wolfson D: The Halstead-Reitan Neuropsychological Test Battery: Theory and Clinical Interpretation. Tucson, AZ, Neuropsychology Press, 1985

Reitan RM, Wolfson D: The Halstead-Reitan Neuropsychological Test Battery, in The Neuropsychology Handbook. Edited by Wedding DJ, Horton AM, Webster J. New York, Springer, 1986, pp 134–160

Reports of the INS–Division 40 Task Force on Education, Accreditation, and Credentialing. Clin Neuropsychol 1:29–34, 1987

Rogers R, Bagby RM, Dickens SE: SIRS—Structured Interview of Reported Symptoms: Professional Manual. Odessa, FL, Psychological Assessment Resources, 1992

Rorschach H: Psychodiagnostics. Bern, Switzerland, Bircher, 1921

Rosvold HE, Mirksy AF, Sarason I, et al: A continuous performance test of brain damage. J Consult Psychol 20:343–350, 1956

Rothke SE, Friedman AF, Jaffe AM, et al: Normative data for the F(p) scale of the MMPI-2: Implications for clinical and forensic assessment of malingering. Psychol Assess 12:335–340, 2000

Ruff RM, Wylie T, Tennant W: Malingering and malingering-like aspects of mild closed head injury. J Head Trauma Rehabil 8:60–73, 1993

Sahakian BJ, Owen AM: Computerized assessment in neuropsychiatry using CANTAB. Journal of Research in Social Medicine 85:399–402, 1992

Sandford JA, Turner A: Integrated Auditory and Visual Continuous Performance Test Manual. Richmond, VA, Braintrain, 1999

Schulberg HC, Saul M, McClelland M, et al: Assessing depression in primary medical and psychiatric practices. Arch Gen Psychiatry 42:1164–1170, 1985

Schwamm LH, Van Dyke C, Kiernan RJ: The Neurobehavioral Cognitive Status Examination: comparison with the Cognitive Capacity Screening Examination and the Mini-Mental State Examination in a neurosurgical population. Ann Intern Med 107:486–491, 1987

Spielberger CD, Gorsuch RL, Lushene R, et al: Manual for the State-Trait Anxiety Inventory (Form Y). Palo Alto, CA, Consulting Psychologists Press, 1983

Spiers PA: Have they come to praise Luria or to bury him? The Luria-Nebraska Battery controversy. J Consult Clin Psychol 49:331–341, 1984

Stambrook M: The Luria-Nebraska Neuropsychological Battery: a promise that may be partly fulfilled. J Clin Neuropsychol 5:247–269, 1983

Stokes AF, Banich MT, Elledge VC: Testing the tests—an empirical evaluation of screening tests for the detection of cognitive impairment in aviators. Aviat Space Environ Med 62:783–788, 1991

Sweeney JA, Wetzler S, Stokes P, et al: Cognitive functioning in depression. J Clin Psychol 45:836–842, 1989

Tarlov AR, Ware JE, Greenfield S, et al: The Medical Outcomes Study: an application of methods for monitoring the results of medical care. JAMA 262:925–930, 1989

Tarter RE, van Thiel DH, Edwards KL (eds): Medical Neuropsychology. New York, Plenum, 1988

Trueblood W, Schmidt M: Malingering and other validity considerations in the neuropsychological evaluation of mild head injury. J Clin Exp Neuropsychol 15:578–590, 1993

Tupper D: Rehabilitation of cognitive and neuropsychological deficit following stroke, in Neurobehavioral Aspects of Cerebrovascular Disease. Edited by Bornstein RA, Brown G. New York, Oxford University Press, 1991, pp 273–296

Veiel HOF: A preliminary profile of neuropsychological deficits associated with major depression. J Clin Exp Neuropsychol 19:587–603, 1997

Ware JE: SF-36 Health Survey, in The Use of Psychological Testing for Treatment Planning and Outcomes Assessment, 2nd Edition. Edited by Maruish ME. Mahwah, NJ, Erlbaum, 1999, pp 1227–1246

Ware JE, Kosinski M: The SF-36 Health Survey (Version 2.0) Technical Note. Boston: Health Assessment Lab, 1996

Ware JE, Sherbourne CD: The MOS 36-item short-form health survey (SF-36), I: conceptual framework and item selection. Med Care 30:473–483, 1992

Wechsler D: Wechsler Adult Intelligence Scale—3rd Edition. San Antonio, TX, Psychological Corporation, 1997

Whitmarsh A, Koutantji M, Sidell K: Illness perceptions, mood and coping in predicting attendance at cardiac rehabilitation. Br J Health Psychol 8 (pt 2):209–221, 2003

Wilson KA, de Beurs E, Palmer CA, et al: Beck Anxiety Inventory, in The Use of Psychological Testing for Treatment Planning and Outcomes Assessment, 2nd Edition. Edited by Maruish M. Mahwah, NJ, Erlbaum, 1999, pp 971–992

Wooten A: MMPI profiles among neuropsychology patients. J Clin Psychol 39:392–406, 1983

Yassin AS, Howell RJ, Nysenbaum AM: Investigating nonattendance at colposcopy clinic. J Obstet Gynaecol 22:79–80, 2002

Yesavage J, Brink T, Rose T, et al: Development and validation of a geriatric depression screening scale: a preliminary report. J Psychiatr Res 17:37–49, 1983

Zafonte R, Mann NR, Millis S, et al: Posttraumatic amnesia: its relation to functional outcome. Arch Phys Med Rehabil 78:1103–1106, 1997

Zung WK: A self-rating depression scale. Arch Gen Psychiatry 12:63–70, 1965

3 Legal Issues

Robert I. Simon, M.D.

Barbara A. Schindler, M.D.

James L. Levenson, M.D.

PSYCHIATRISTS WORKING IN medical settings regularly encounter a number of difficult ethical and legal issues. Although these issues are not unique, there are special challenges in caring for patients with multiple comorbid medical and psychiatric illnesses in settings in which multiple disciplines are involved. In this chapter, we discuss confidentiality, the Health Insurance Portability and Accountability Act (HIPAA), informed consent, competency, guardianship, substituted judgment, end-of-life decisions, advance directives, voluntary and involuntary treatment, discharges against medical advice (AMA), the use of physical restraints, the Emergency Medical Treatment and Active Labor Act (EMTALA), collaborative care, managed care, and risk management. Although there can be clinically significant overlap, this chapter focuses primarily on legal issues; corresponding ethical issues are covered in Chapter 4, "Ethical Issues." It should be noted that this chapter refers to the laws of the United States. Similar principles are applicable to other nations whose jurisprudence has English origins.

Confidentiality and Testimonial Privilege

Confidentiality

Confidentiality refers to the right of a patient to have confidential communications withheld from outside parties without implied or expressed authorization. Once the doctor–patient relationship is created, the physician assumes an automatic duty to safeguard a patient's disclosures. This duty is not absolute, and in some circumstances breaching confidentiality is both ethical and legal (Table 3–1) (American Psychiatric Association 1987).

TABLE 3–1.   Common statutory exceptions to confidentiality between physician and patient

Child abuse
Competency proceedings
Court-ordered examination
Posing a danger to self or others
Patient–litigant exception
Intent to commit a crime or harmful act
Civil commitment proceedings
Communication with other treatment providers

Consultation psychiatrists are faced with a unique challenge of balancing patient confidentiality with the need to provide adequate information to the medical staff requesting the consultation. Sensitive clinical information flows between the patient and consulting psychiatrist, the patient's nonpsychiatric physicians, and the team of health care providers, as well as to family members and other personnel and agencies outside the acute health care setting (e.g., nursing home, boarding home, or rehabilitation center). Documentation in the medical record and verbal communication to the staff providing patient care require careful consideration of what to communicate and what to keep confidential. The medical record is widely available to all who provide care to the patient as well as a very large number of nonclinical personnel inside and outside the hospital (Siegler 1982). To further complicate the issue of confidentiality, the involvement of the consulting psychiatrist is most often initiated at the request of the attending physician, not the patient. The psychiatrist's working relationship with the attending physician is as key to the consultative process as the relationship with the patient. In addition, in complicated clinical situations a large number of health care providers and family members must be involved, increasing the burden of maintaining confidentiality. In most circumstances the consulting psychiatrist should obtain the competent patient's verbal permission before speaking to the patient's family or other third parties and if possible should have the patient confirm what sensitive data may be shared in the medical record and with the attending physician. Most patients are either agreeable to sharing pertinent data or quite specific about what data cannot be disclosed. There is less need for consent when seeking information from family members than when sharing information obtained from the patient.

In general, psychiatrists should not assume that they possess carte blanche authorization when speaking to hospital staff members about all matters revealed by the patient. Information should be provided that would enable the staff to function effectively in caring for the patient. It is often unnecessary to disclose intimate details of the patient's history or current mental life.

Recent federal legislation addresses confidentiality issues in the health care environment. The Health Insurance Portability and Accountability Act (HIPAA) of 1996 established standards for the protection of patient privacy that were implemented in 2003. The U.S. Department of Health and Human Services has developed regulations for maintaining the confidentiality and transmission of personal health information. Health care organizations, providers, and insurers are mandated to comply with both the "Transactions" and "Privacy" rules of the HIPAA legislation. The two HIPAA guidelines that are most relevant to consulting psychiatrists are that 1) treating health care providers are explicitly exempted from requiring patient consent for sharing information with each other, and 2) psychotherapy notes receive extra confidentiality protection when they are kept separate from the rest of the medical record. The psychiatric consultant's note on the medical chart would not be considered a psychotherapy note even if it documented psychotherapy (American Psychiatric Association 1987; Appelbaum 2002).

Testimonial Privilege

Testimonial privilege is the privilege to withhold information that applies only to the judicial setting. The patient, not the psychiatrist, holds the testimonial privilege that controls the release of confidential information. In other words, if a competent patient waives the right to confidentiality about his or her treatment, a psychiatrist cannot claim doctor–patient privilege and must testify. Privilege statutes represent the most common recogni-

tion by the state of the importance of protecting information provided by a patient to a psychotherapist. This recognition moves away from the essential purpose of the American system of justice (e.g., "truth finding") by insulating certain information from disclosure in court. The rationale for this protection is that the special need for privacy in the doctor–patient relationship outweighs the unbridled quest for an accurate outcome in court.

There are specific exceptions to testimonial privilege. Although exceptions vary, the most common include child abuse reporting, civil commitment proceedings, court-ordered evaluations, criminal proceedings, and cases in which a patient's mental state is part of the litigation. This last exception, known as the *patient–litigant exception*, commonly occurs in will contests, workers' compensation cases, child custody disputes, personal injury actions, and malpractice actions. The extent of testimonial privilege and its exceptions varies among jurisdictions.

Informed Consent and the Right to Refuse Treatment

> Mr. J, a 73-year-old retired mechanic with known peripheral vascular disease and chronic atrial fibrillation, is brought to the emergency room with severe acute right leg pain. His peripheral pulses are absent, and he is diagnosed with an embolus to the right femoral artery. He refuses embolectomy, a potentially limb-saving and life-saving procedure. A psychiatric consultation is called to evaluate competency. His decisional capacity is judged to be sufficiently intact to refuse treatment.

Although the process of informed consent is highly integrated in modern health care settings, many legal issues remain regarding informed consent in seriously medically compromised patients, especially those with neuropsychiatric impairment. Medical staff members routinely overestimate patients' capacity to fully understand the informed consent forms they are signing, basing their views on a gestalt impression rather than explicit assessment. It is most often when patients refuse treatment that their understanding of the consent process is called into question, resulting in a psychiatric consultation to evaluate competency. Consultations are rarely called to evaluate patients who willingly sign a consent form (Lippert and Stewart 1988).

The right to refuse treatment is intimately connected with the doctrine of informed consent (Simon 1989). By withholding consent, patients such as Mr. J express their right to refuse treatment except under certain circumstances. The right to refuse treatment also reflects the exercise of basic constitutional rights. As Stone (1981) pointed out, the right to refuse psychiatric medication is not an isolated issue. Protection of individual autonomy includes the right to refuse emergency life-saving treatment, the right to establish advance directives, and the so-called right to die.

Informed Consent

Informed consent provides patients with a legal cause of action if they are not adequately informed about the nature and consequences of a particular medical treatment or procedure. The legal theory of informed consent is based on two distinct principles. First, every patient has the right to determine what is or is not done to his or her body (also referred to as the right of self-determination) (*Schloendorff v. Society of New York Hospital* 1914). The second principle emanates from the fiduciary nature of the doctor–patient relationship (Simon 1987). Inherent in a physician's fiduciary duty is the responsibility to disclose honestly and in good faith all requisite facts about a patient's condition. The primary purpose of the doctrine of informed consent is to promote individual autonomy; a secondary purpose is to facilitate rational decision making (Appelbaum et al. 1987).

Informed consent has three essential ingredients:

1. *Competency.* Clinicians provide the first level of screening to establish patient competency and to determine whether to accept a patient's treatment decision. The risk–benefit ratio in any given medical intervention should influence the amount of scrutiny that physicians apply to the patient's decisional capacity, as discussed later in this chapter.
2. *Information.* The patient or a bona fide representative must be given adequate information.
3. *Voluntariness.* The patient must voluntarily consent to or refuse the proposed treatment or procedure.

Exceptions and Liability

Table 3–2 shows the four basic exceptions to the requirement for obtaining informed consent. When emergency treatment is necessary to save a life or prevent imminent serious harm, and it is impossible to obtain either the patient's consent or that of someone authorized to provide consent for the patient, the law will typically "presume" that consent is granted. Inability to obtain the patient's consent may be related to clear lack of decisional capacity, to indeterminate capacity, to inability to communicate (e.g., intubation), or, in extreme emergencies, to insufficient time to evaluate capacity. Two qualifications are

---

TABLE 3–2.   Basic exceptions to obtaining informed consent

Emergencies
Incompetence
Therapeutic privilege
Waiver

---

necessary to apply this exception. First, the emergency must be serious and imminent, and second, the patient's condition, and not other circumstances (e.g., availability of the surgeon), must determine that an emergency exists. This exception does not apply if the patient is competent and is refusing treatment, even if the intervention is life-saving (e.g., transfusion in a Jehovah's Witness). Such emergency interventions should be guided by patients' advance directives, if they are clearly known. This was not the case with Mr. J.

The second exception to informed consent exists when a patient lacks sufficient mental capacity to give consent (e.g., a patient with delirium) or is legally incompetent. Someone who is incompetent is incapable of giving informed consent. Under these circumstances, consent is obtained from a substitute decision maker.

The third exception, therapeutic privilege, is the most difficult to apply. Informed consent may not be required if a psychiatrist determines that a complete disclosure of possible risks and alternatives might have a deleterious effect on the patient's health and welfare. Jurisdictions vary in their application of this exception. When specific case law or statutes outlining the factors relevant to such a decision are absent, a doctor must substantiate a patient's inability to psychologically withstand being informed of the proposed treatment. Some courts have held that therapeutic privilege may be invoked only if informing the patient will worsen his or her condition or will so frighten the patient that rational decision making is precluded (*Canterbury v. Spence* 1972; *Natanson v. Kline* 1960). Therapeutic privilege is not a means of circumventing the legal requirement for obtaining informed consent from the patient before initiating treatment. It should be very rarely necessary to invoke therapeutic privilege in the medical setting, because a skilled clinician should be able to explain the diagnosis and proposed treatment in language the patient can cognitively and emotionally handle, aided by the consulting psychiatrist.

Finally, a physician need not disclose risks of treatment when the patient has competently, knowingly, and voluntarily waived his or her right for information (e.g., when the patient refuses information on drug side effects). However, the physician should then consider whether the patient's lack of information could adversely affect treatment outcome, in which case it may be more appropriate not to proceed with treatment.

Aside from these four exceptions, a physician who treats a patient without obtaining informed consent is subject to legal liability. In some jurisdictions, however, case law or statutes specify that informed consent is unnecessary if a reasonable person under the given circumstances would have consented to treatment. As a rule, treatment without any consent or against a patient's wishes may constitute battery (intentional tort), whereas treatment commenced with inadequate consent is treated as an act of medical negligence. On rare (usually emergent) occasions, the physician may decide to treat a patient without fully disclosing the risks, benefits, and alternatives, understanding that it is better to be at risk for battery than for medical negligence.

Infrequently, courts have authorized treatment against the wishes of a competent patient. Generally, these cases involve situations in which the life of a fetus is at risk, a patient is encumbered with or is responsible for the care of dependent children and can be restored to full health through the intervention in question (e.g., blood transfusions), or a patient has attempted suicide.

Patient Competency in Health Care Decision Making

Ms. L—a 73-year-old single, retired librarian with diabetes mellitus and multiple complications, including retinopathy and poorly healing leg ulcers—is admitted to the hospital for the third time in 6 months in a state of ketoacidosis. She lives alone in the house in which she was born, has minimal family support, and has consistently refused home health aides or nursing home placement. She insists that she can care for herself and that she wants to die in the house she was born in. A psychiatric consultation is requested to evaluate the patient's competency to care for herself at home and to make medical treatment decisions.

Consulting psychiatrists are frequently asked to assess a patient's competency. The case of Ms. L is a common example of a complex clinical situation that precipitates such a consultation.

Competency can be defined as "having sufficient capacity, ability...(or) possessing the requisite physical, mental, natural, or legal qualifications" (Black 1990, p. 284). This definition is deliberately vague and ambiguous because the term *competency* is a broad concept encompassing many different legal issues and contexts. As a result, its definition, requirements, and application can vary widely depending on the circumstances (e.g., making health care decisions, executing a will, or confessing to a crime).

In general, *competency* refers to some minimal mental, cognitive, or behavioral ability, trait, or capability that is required for a person to perform a particular legally recognized act or to assume a legal role. The determination of impaired competency requires a judicial decision. Although the term *competency* is widely used in the clinical setting, health care providers cannot declare an individual incompetent. In this regard, it is clinically useful to distinguish the terms *incompetence* and *lack of decisional capacity*. *Incompetence* refers to a court decision, whereas *lack of decisional capacity* refers to a determination made by a clinician (Mishkin 1989). Legally, only competent persons may give informed consent. An adult patient is considered legally competent unless he or she has been adjudicated incompetent or temporarily incapacitated because of a medical condition. Incapacity does not prevent treatment. It merely means that the clinician must obtain substitute consent, usually from a designated family member. Legal competence is very narrowly defined in terms of cognitive capacity. This definition derives largely from the laws governing transactions. Important clinical concepts such as incompetence due to a psychiatric illness may not be recognized by the law unless the disorder significantly diminishes cognitive capacity. Psychiatric treatment may be refused by severely depressed patients because of hopelessness, by manic patients because of grandiosity, and by schizophrenic patients because of paranoia. The challenge becomes more complex in the medical setting, where serious mental illness causes a patient to reject needed medical as well as psychiatric treatment. Denial of illness often interferes with insight and the ability to appreciate the significance of information provided to the patient. In the case *In the Guardianship of John Roe* (1992), the Massachusetts Supreme Judicial Court recognized that denial of illness can render a patient incompetent to make treatment decisions.

Under the Anglo-American system of law, an individual is presumed to be competent unless adjudicated incompetent. Thus, incompetence is a legal determination made by a judge based on evidence from health care providers and others that the individual's functional mental capacity is significantly impaired. The Uniform Guardianship and Protective Proceedings Act (UGPPA) or the Uniform Probate Code (UPC) is used as a basis for laws governing competency in many states (Mishkin 1989). The Uniform Acts were drafted by legal scholars and practicing attorneys to achieve uniformity among states by enactment of model laws (Uniform Guardianship and Protective Proceedings Act, sec. 5-101).

Competency is not a scientifically determinable state; it is situation specific. Although there are no hard-and-fast rules, germane to determining competency is the patient's ability to 1) understand the particular treatment choice being proposed, 2) make a treatment choice, and 3) be able to verbally or nonverbally communicate that choice. The above standard, however, obtains only a simple consent from the patient rather than an informed consent because alternative treatment choices are not provided.

A review of case law and scholarly literature reveals four standards for determining mental incapacity in decision making (Appelbaum et al. 1987; Appelbaum and Grisso 1997). In the order of levels of mental capacity required, these standards include 1) communication of choice, 2) understanding of information provided, 3) appreciation of options available, and 4) rational decision making. Cognitive disorders can reduce all four of these capacities, while noncognitive psychiatric disorders primarily affect the third and fourth capacities.

Psychiatrists are generally most comfortable with a rational decision-making standard in determining mental incapacity. Most courts, however, prefer the first two standards. A truly informed consent that considers the patient's autonomy, personal needs, and values occurs when rational decision making is applied by the patient to the risks and benefits of appropriate treatment options provided by the clinician. Grisso and Applebaum (1995; Grisso et al. 1997) found that the choice of standards determining competence affected the type and proportion of patients classified as impaired. When compound standards were used, the proportion of patients identified as impaired increased. They advise that clinicians should be aware of the applicable standards in their jurisdictions.

Assessing the risk–benefit ratio of each medical intervention should dictate the level of understanding required of each patient in the decision-making process. While a lumbar puncture is a low-risk, highly beneficial procedure in a patient with a high fever and stiff neck, heart transplantation is a high-risk, potentially highly beneficial procedure in the patient with end-stage cardiac disease. While both may be life-saving procedures, a different level of understanding of the risks and benefits is usually expected from each patient. Table 3–3 provides a useful

tool in conceptualizing the level of scrutiny needed in different risk–benefit ratios.

Scrutiny of capacity should always be high for high-benefit, high-risk interventions. Scrutiny should be high for patients who refuse high-benefit, low-risk interventions. On the other hand, less scrutiny is warranted for patients *refusing* low-benefit, high-risk treatment. Careful attention should be directed at patients who readily agree to such treatment. Finally, it is less important to scrutinize capacity when both the benefits and risks of treatment are low, for there is little at stake for the patient.

States vary with regard to the extent of their reliance on psychiatric assessments. Nonmedical personnel, such as social workers, psychologists, family members, friends, colleagues, and even the individual who is the subject of the proceeding, may testify.

Because severely mentally disordered patients frequently lack adequate understanding of or deny their illness, they may communicate a choice and appear to understand the information provided but lack the insight or ability to truly appreciate the information. Rational decision making is impaired as well. For example, a schizophrenic patient with end-stage renal disease may understand that his kidneys are not working and may clearly communicate whether he will agree to dialysis without fully understanding the dialysis process, its complications, or the long-term commitment to treatment. Furthermore, his decision may be driven by irrational thoughts (e.g., "the machine will control me").

A valid consent is either expressed (orally or in writing) or implied from the patient's actions. The issue of competency, whether in a civil or criminal context, is commonly raised in two situations: when the person is a minor and when he or she is mentally disabled and lacks the requisite cognitive capacity for health care decision making. In many situations, minors are not considered legally competent; therefore the consent of a parent or designated guardian is required. However, there are exceptions to this general rule, such as minors who are considered emancipated (Smith 1986) or mature (*Gulf S I R Co. v. Sullivan* 1928), or in some cases of medical need, such as abortion (*Planned Parenthood v. Danforth* 1976) or mental health counseling (*Jehovah's Witnesses v. King County Hospital* 1968).

TABLE 3–3.	**Level of scrutiny needed in different risk–benefit ratios**	
	High benefit	**Low benefit**
High risk	Scrutinize capacity closely (e.g., cardiac transplantation)	Scrutinize accepters > refusers (e.g., chemotherapy for metastatic large-cell lung cancer)
Low risk	Scrutinize refusers > accepters (e.g., intravenous penicillin for endocarditis)	Close scrutiny not necessary (e.g., cholinesterase inhibitors in dementia)

Mentally disabled patients, including mentally impaired psychiatric patients and psychiatrically impaired medically ill patients, present a slightly different problem in evaluating competency. Lack of capacity or competency *cannot* be presumed from either treatment for mental illness (*Wilson v. Lehman* 1964) or institutionalization (*Rennie v. Klein* 1978). Mental disability or illness does *not* in itself render a person incompetent in all areas of functioning. Instead, the patient must be examined to determine whether specific functional incapacities render a person incapable of making a particular kind of decision or performing a particular type of task. Generally, the law will recognize only those decisions or choices that are made by a competent individual. The law seeks to protect incompetent individuals from the harmful consequences of their acts. Persons older than 18 years (U.S. Department of Health and Human Services 1981) are presumed to be competent (*Meek v. City of Loveland* 1929). This presumption, however, is rebuttable by evidence of an individual's incapacity (*Scaria v. St. Paul Fire and Marine Ins Co* 1975). Perception, short- and long-term memory, judgment, language comprehension, verbal fluency, and reality orientation are mental functions that a court will scrutinize regarding mental capacity and competency.

Medically ill patients who are found to lack the requisite functional mental capacity to make a treatment decision, except in cases of an emergency (*Frasier v. Department of Health and Human Resources* 1986), must have a surrogate (usually next of kin) or appointed guardian to make health care decisions on their behalf (*Aponte v. United States* 1984). Several consent options are available for patients who lack the mental capacity for health care decisions, depending on the jurisdiction. In most states, proxy consent for the evaluation and treatment of a medical condition is available for the patient lacking health care decision-making capacity, without the need to involve the courts. However, in many states, proxy consent in the patient lacking health care decision-making capacity is prohibited for specific types of treatment (e.g., psychiatric treatment, abortion, sterilization, psychosurgery).

Guardianship

Historically, the state or sovereign possessed the power and authority to safeguard the estate of incompetent persons (Regan 1972). In modern times, guardianship is a method of substitute decision making for individuals who are judicially determined to be unable to act for themselves (Parry 1985). In some states, there are separate provisions for the appointment of a "guardian of one's person" (e.g., health care decision making) and for a "guardian of one's estate" (e.g., authority to make contracts to sell one's property) (Sales et al. 1982, p. 461). The latter guardian is frequently referred to as a *conservator*, although this designation is not uniformly used throughout the United States. Two further distinctions—*general (plenary)* and *specific* guardianship—are made in some jurisdictions (Sales et al. 1982). As the name implies, a specific guardian is restricted to making decisions about a particular subject area. For instance, the specific guardian is authorized to make decisions about major or emergency medical procedures, and the disabled person retains the freedom to make decisions about all other medical matters. The general guardian, by contrast, has total control over the disabled individual's person, estate, or both (Sales et al. 1982).

Guardianship arrangements are increasingly used with patients who have dementia, particularly AIDS-related dementia and Alzheimer's disease (Overman and Stoudemire 1988). Under the Anglo-American system of law, an individual is presumed to be competent unless adjudicated incompetent. Thus, incompetence is a legal determination made by a court of law based on evidence from health care providers and others that the individual's functional mental capacity is significantly impaired. In many states either the UGPPA (sec. 5-101) or the UPC is used as a basis for laws governing competency (Mishkin 1989). The Uniform Acts were drafted by legal scholars and practicing attorneys to achieve uniformity among states by enactment of model laws.

General incompetency is defined in the UGPPA as meaning impaired by reason of mental illness, mental deficiency, physical illness or disability, advanced age, chronic use of drugs, chronic intoxication, or other cause (except minority) to the extent of lacking sufficient understanding or capacity to make or communicate reasonable decisions (Uniform Guardianship and Protective Proceedings Act, sec. 1-101[7]; see also Uniform Probate Code, sec. 5-101).

A significant number of patients with severe medical or psychiatric disorders meet the above definition. Generally, the appointment of a guardian is limited to situations in which the individual's decision-making capacity is so impaired that he or she is unable to care for personal safety or provide necessities such as food, shelter, clothing, and medical care (*In re Boyer* 1981).

The standard of proof required for a judicial determination of incompetency is clear and convincing evidence. Although the law does not assign percentages to proof, Simon (1992) has suggested that clear and convincing evidence should be in the range of 75% certainty.

Substituted Judgment

Psychiatrists often find that the process required to obtain an adjudication of incompetence is unduly burdensome, is costly, and frequently interferes with the provision of quality treatment. Moreover, families may be reluctant to face the formal court proceedings necessary to declare their family member incompetent, particularly when sensitive family matters are disclosed. Common consent options for patients lacking health care decision-making capacity are listed in Table 3–4.

Clear advantages are associated with having the family serve as decision makers (Perr 1984). First, the use of responsible family members as surrogate decision makers maintains the integrity of the family unit and relies on the sources who are most likely to know the patient's wishes. Second, it is more efficient and less costly. The President's Commission for the Study of Ethical Problems in Medicine and Biomedical and Behavioral Research (1982) recommended that the relatives of incompetent patients be selected as proxy decision makers for the following reasons:

1. The family is generally most concerned about the good of the patient.
2. The family is usually most knowledgeable about the patient's goals, preferences, and values.
3. The family deserves recognition as an important social unit to be treated, within limits, as a single decision maker in matters that intimately affect its members.

There are some disadvantages, however. Proxy decision making requires synthesizing the diverse values, beliefs, practices, and prior statements of the patient for a specific circumstance (Emanuel and Emanuel 1992). As one judge characterized the problem, any proxy decision made in the absence of specific directions is at best only an optimistic approximation (*In re Jobes* 1987). Ambivalent feelings, conflicts within the family and with the patient, and conflicting economic interests may make certain family members suspect as guardians (Gutheil and Appelbaum 1980). Some family members are more impaired than the patient for whom proxy consent is being sought. In addition, relatives may not be available or may not want to get involved.

Some states permit proxy decision making by statute, mainly through their informed consent statute (Solnick 1985). Some state statutes specify that another person (e.g., specific relatives) may authorize consent on behalf of the incompetent patient. As noted earlier in this chap-

TABLE 3–4. Common consent options for patients who lack the mental capacity for health care decisions

Proxy consent of next of kin

Adjudication of incompetence; appointment of a guardian

Institutional administrators or committees

Treatment review panels

Substituted consent of the court

Advance directives (living will, durable power of attorney, health care proxy)

Statutory surrogates (spouse or court-appointed guardian)[a]

[a]Medical statutory surrogate laws (when treatment wishes of the patient are unstated).

ter, a number of states permit proxy consent by next of kin only for patients with medical conditions. Proxy consent is not available in many states for individuals with psychiatric conditions (Simon 2001).

As noted above, in most jurisdictions, a durable power of attorney or health care proxy permits the next of kin to consent (Solnick 1985). When proxy consent by a relative is not provided by statute or by case law authority within the state, physicians should be cautious about relying on the good-faith consent by next of kin in treating a patient believed to be incompetent (Macbeth 1994). The legally conservative procedure is to seek judicial recognition of the family member as the substitute decision maker. This approach can be impractical medically because of unacceptable delays in treatment and can be impractical legally because courts are not capable of handling the potential volume of such cases.

Some patients recover competency within a few days (e.g., those with delirium). As soon as the patient recovers sufficient mental capacity, consent for further treatment should be obtained directly from the patient. For the patient who continues to lack mental capacity for health care decisions, an increasing number of states have statutes that permit involuntary treatment of incompetent medically ill patients who refuse treatment, even if the patient does not meet current standards for involuntary civil commitment (Hassenfeld and Grumet 1984; Zito et al. 1984).

End-of-Life Decisions

Psychiatric consultations are often requested regarding the termination of medical treatment, especially in terminally ill patients with chronic, progressively debilitating illnesses (Cohen 2000). Although many of these consultations are called ostensibly to assess the patient's competency, a covert reason for the consultation may be the physician's and staff's anxiety or conflict surrounding end-of-life decisions (Umapathy et al. 1999). Withholding or withdrawing life support may trigger an emotional response from the health care team that can cloud established legal mandates. In addition to the overt request to evaluate competency, the consulting psychiatrist needs to carefully evaluate any contributing factors to the patient's and the health care team's decision. Both untreated depression and inadequate pain management can contribute significantly to a premature decision to terminate treatment (Leeman 1999; Leeman et al. 2001). Full evaluation and provision of adequate treatment make it rarely necessary for the courts to become involved. In addition, a clear understanding of family and team support of the decision to terminate treatment and the family dynamics is a necessary part of the consultative process, especially when there is a disagreement between the patient and the family. For example, with a uremic patient who is refusing dialysis, if the family is having difficulty letting go of their loved one, they might wait until the patient becomes delirious and then insist on beginning dialysis.

Right to Die

Legal decisions addressing the issue of a patient's right to die involve one of two categories of patients: 1) patients who are incompetent (i.e., removal of life-support systems) (*In re Conroy* 1985; *In re Quinlan* 1976) or 2) patients who are competent.

Incompetent Patients

On the very difficult and personal question of patient autonomy, the United States Supreme Court ruled in *Cruzan v. Director, Missouri Department of Health* (1990) that the state of Missouri could prohibit the removal of a feeding tube surgically implanted in the stomach of Nancy Cruzan without clear and convincing evidence of her wishes. The patient had been in a persistent vegetative state for 7 years. Without clear and convincing evidence of a patient's decision to have life-sustaining measures withheld in a particular circumstance, the state has an interest in maintaining that individual's life, even to the exclusion of the family's wishes.

The importance of the *Cruzan* decision for physicians treating severely or terminally impaired patients is that they must seek clear and competent instructions from the patient regarding foreseeable treatment decisions. For example, physicians treating patients with progressive degenerative brain diseases should attempt to obtain the patient's wishes regarding the use of life-sustaining measures while that patient can still competently articulate

those wishes. This information is best provided in the form of a living will, durable power of attorney agreement, or health care proxy. However, any written document that clearly and convincingly sets forth the patient's wishes—including contemporaneous documentation by the physician in the patient's chart—could serve the same purpose. Most states have enacted legislation since *Cruzan* that allows surrogate decision makers to make critical end-of-life decisions in the absence of written evidence of the patient's wishes.

Although physicians fear civil or criminal liability for stopping life-sustaining treatment, liability may in theory also arise from overtreating critically or terminally ill patients (Weir and Gostin 1990), although such suits are rare. Legal liability may occur for providing unwanted treatment to a competent patient or treatment that is against the best interests of an incompetent patient.

Competent Patients

A small but growing body of cases has emerged involving competent patients who usually have excruciating pain, severe chronic debilitating illness, and terminal diseases and seek to stop further medical treatment (e.g., dialysis). The single most significant influence in the development of this body of law is the doctrine of *informed consent*. Beginning with the fundamental tenet that "no right is held more sacred…than the right of every individual to the possession and control of his own person" (*Schloendorff v. Society of New York Hospital* 1914, pp. 92–93; see also *Union Pacific Ry Co v. Botsford* 1891, pp. 250–251), courts have fashioned the present-day informed consent doctrine and have applied it to right-to-die cases.

Notwithstanding these principles, the right to decline life-sustaining medical intervention, even for a competent person, is not absolute. As noted in *In re Conroy* (1985), four countervailing interests may limit the exercise of that right: 1) preservation of life, 2) prevention of suicide, 3) safeguarding the integrity of the medical profession, and 4) protection of innocent third parties. In each of these situations, and depending on the surrounding circumstances, the trend is to support a competent patient's right to have artificial life-support systems discontinued (*Bartling v. Superior Court* 1984; *Bouvia v. Superior Court* 1986; *In re Farrell* 1987; *In re Jobes* 1987; *In re Peter* 1987; *Tune v. Walter Reed Army Medical Hosp* 1985).

As a result of the *Cruzan* decision, courts will focus primarily on the reliability of the evidence presented to establish the patient's competence—specifically, the clarity and certainty with which a decision to withhold medical treatment was made. Assuming that a terminally ill patient chose to forgo any further medical intervention *and* the patient was competent at the time of the decision, courts are unlikely to overrule or subvert the patient's right to privacy and autonomy

Do-Not-Resuscitate Orders

Cardiopulmonary resuscitation (CPR) is a medical life-saving intervention. Immediate initiation of CPR at the time of cardiac arrest leaves no time to think about the consequences of reviving a patient. Most patients requiring CPR have not thought about or expressed a preference for or against its use. Physicians and their patients can have significant anxiety discussing do-not-resuscitate (DNR) orders despite clear clinical indications and established hospital policies grounded in legal guidelines. Failure of adequate and appropriate doctor–patient communication can result in significant misunderstanding of the purpose of DNR orders. Patients can feel overwhelmed and paralyzed by the decision or railroaded by their physician into making a decision that might not reflect their true intentions. The consulting psychiatrist can help facilitate this difficult conversation between the patient and his or her primary physician.

The ethical principle of patient autonomy justifies the position that the patient or substitute decision maker should make the decision about the use of CPR. A seriously ill, competent patient's request not to be resuscitated should be respected, and a DNR order should be documented in the clinical record.

Schwartz (1987) noted that two key principles have emerged concerning DNR decisions:

1. DNR decisions are reached consensually by the attending physician and the patient or substitute decision maker.
2. DNR orders, including date and time, are written on the doctor's order sheet, and the reasons for the DNR order are documented in the chart.

The laws regarding DNR orders may vary among states, and hospital policies may vary as well (Luce 1990). In some jurisdictions a physician may enter a DNR order, even without the consent of the patient or family, when CPR is judged utterly futile (e.g., sepsis with advanced multi-organ failure). Ethical and legal guidance for CPR and emergency cardiac care is available (Council on Ethical and Judicial Affairs 1991).

Physician-Assisted Suicide

With the increasing legal recognition of physician-assisted suicide, psychiatrists are likely to be called on to become gatekeepers as part of their practice in medical settings (see also Chapter 10, "Suicidality," and Chapter 40, "Palliative Care"). Such a role would be a radical departure from the physician's code of ethics, which prohibits participation by an ethical doctor in any intervention that hastens death. Previously, the Supreme Court ruled in *Cruzan* that terminally ill persons could refuse life-sustaining medical treatment. Courts and legislatures will determine whether hastening death is an unwarranted extension of the right to refuse treatment. Almost every proposal for physician-assisted suicide requires a psychiatric screening or consultation to determine the terminally ill person's competence to terminate his or her life, although the state of Oregon does not require it. The presence of psychiatric disorders associated with suicide, particularly depression, will have to be ruled out as the driving factor behind physician-assisted suicide. Much controversy rages over the ethics of this gatekeeping function (Council on Ethical and Judicial Affairs 1994). Currently, the only jurisdictions that legally sanction physician-assisted suicide are Oregon in the United States and the Netherlands in Europe (Batlle 2003; Hedberg et al. 2003).

Advance Directives

Advance directives such as a living will, health care proxy, or durable medical power of attorney are recommended so that a patient's preferences can guide the health care team and family and to avoid ethical and legal complications, particularly in withholding or withdrawing life-sustaining treatment (Simon 1992; Solnick 1985). The Patient Self-Determination Act (Omnibus Budget Reconciliation Act of 1990), which became effective on December 1, 1991, requires all hospitals, nursing homes, hospices, managed care organizations, and home health care agencies to advise patients or family members of their right to accept or refuse medical care in the form of an advance directive and to inquire if the patient has made an advance directive (LaPuma et al. 1991). If possible, copies of an advance directive should be included as part of the patient's medical record.

Federal law does not specify the right to formulate advance directives; therefore, state law applies. State legislators have recognized that individuals may want to stipulate who should make important health care decisions if they become incapacitated and unable to act in their own behalf. All 50 states and the District of Columbia permit individuals to create a durable power of attorney (i.e., one that endures even if the competence of the creator does not) (*Cruzan v. Director, Missouri Department of Health* 1990). Several states and the District of Columbia have durable power of attorney statutes that expressly authorize the appointment of proxies for making health care decisions (see, e.g., *Cruzan v. Director, Missouri Department of Health* 1990).

Generally, durable power of attorney is construed to empower an agent to make health care decisions. Such a document is much broader and more flexible than a living will, which covers just the period of a diagnosed terminal illness and usually specifies only that no "extraordinary treatments" be used to prolong the act of dying (Mishkin 1985). To clarify the uncertain status of the durable power of attorney for health care decisions, several states have passed health care proxy laws. The health care proxy is a legal instrument akin to the durable power of attorney but is specifically created for the delegation of health care decisions. It provides a mechanism for a patient to designate a decision maker other than next of kin (e.g., an unmarried partner instead of a parent).

In a durable power of attorney or health care proxy, general or specific directions can be set forth about how future decisions are to be made in the event that one becomes unable to make these decisions. The determination of a patient's competence, however, is not specified in most durable power of attorney and health care proxy statutes. When this becomes a clinical issue, an examination by two physicians to determine the patient's ability to understand the nature and consequences of the proposed treatment or procedure, ability to make a choice, and ability to communicate that choice usually is sufficient. This information, like all significant medical observations, should be clearly documented in the patient's chart. If the determination is disputed, an independent examination by another physician should be obtained.

Despite the growing use of advance directives, increasing evidence suggests that physician values rather than patient values are more decisive in end-of-life decisions (Orentlicher 1992).

The application of advance directives to patients with serious psychiatric illness may present difficulties. For example, a patient with an intermittent thought disorder may draw up an advance directive during a period of mental stability and then disavow it when psychotic. Because durable power of attorney agreements or health care proxies are easily revoked, the treating clinician or institution may have to honor the patient's refusal, even if there is reasonable evidence that the patient lacks decisional capacity. If this situation occurs, legal consultation should be considered. When the patient is grossly confused and is an immediate danger to self and others, the physician or hospital is on firmer ground, both medically and legally, to consult with the previously disregarded proxy and to temporarily override the patient's treatment refusal. Otherwise, it is generally better to seek a court order for treatment. Typically, unless there are compelling medical reasons to do otherwise, courts will generally honor the patient's original treatment directions.

Maternal Competency

Ms. N, a 32-year-old woman with a 5-year history of almost daily crack cocaine abuse, is admitted to the maternity service at 36 weeks' gestation in active labor with premature rupture of the membranes. The newborn male infant is small for gestational age and has a positive toxicology screen for cocaine but is otherwise healthy. A psychiatric consultation is called to determine Ms. N's maternal competency to care for the newborn infant, as well for her other three children (all under age 10), at home.

Psychiatric consultations are increasingly being requested for evaluations of maternal (or, more rarely, paternal) competency (i.e., capacity to care for a child) when it is thought that a vulnerable infant or child in the pediatric ward, clinic, or newborn nursery will be at risk if the parent is allowed to take the child home (Nair and Morrison 2000). This most commonly occurs in situations of maternal substance abuse, maternal psychiatric illness, or child abuse or neglect or when there is question of Munchausen syndrome by proxy. Child protective services frequently become involved. Courts can be asked to temporarily or even permanently terminate parental rights given the clinical situation. The determination to sever parental rights even temporarily is extremely stressful and painful for all involved in the decision. This is not a competency evaluation in the legal sense described above; rather, it is an assessment of maternal capacity to care for the child and of potential threats to the child's safety. The consulting psychiatrist will require significant input from a variety of sources—including family members, pediatricians, social workers, and nursing staff—to determine maternal capacity to care for the child. Those individuals may have very polarized opinions about what is needed to protect the child, and in the case of maternal substance abuse, strong negative countertransference may be involved. Awareness of local laws pertaining to parental rights, physician reporting of suspected abuse and neglect, and guardianship is necessary.

Whether maternal substance abuse during pregnancy should be legally considered child abuse is controversial in both the medical and legal fields. Two relevant recent legal cases in South Carolina, both of which threatened the doctor–patient relationship and confidentiality, have received national attention. In *Ferguson v. City of Charles-*

ton (2001), medical personnel in a Charleston hospital reported to police positive urine toxicology screenings from pregnant women and postpartum mothers that were obtained without a warrant or consent. These women were arrested in the hospital without appropriate medical or psychiatric referral and treatment for their addictions. In 2001, the United States Supreme Court ruled that the hospital's policy of searching for evidence of substance abuse violated the Fourth Amendment's prohibition of unlawful searches. More recently, in *McKnight v. South Carolina* (2003), a woman who used cocaine during pregnancy and delivered a stillborn child was convicted of homicide by child abuse and is serving a 12-year prison sentence. The conviction was upheld after one mistrial by the South Carolina Supreme Court. This case is being appealed to the United States Supreme Court.

Voluntary and Involuntary Psychiatric Treatment in the Medical Setting

Psychiatrists frequently become involved when medical inpatients with psychiatric disorders refuse treatment or a psychiatric disorder interferes significantly in the medical decision-making process or compliance with treatment. The needs of these patients are often inadequately evaluated and undertreated (Lamden 1997). In addition, confusion exists about the legal power of temporary psychiatric detention and psychiatric commitment. Involuntary psychiatric detention or commitments specifically allow only acute psychiatric evaluation, not other involuntary medical evaluations or treatments (Wise 1987). Psychiatric treatment may occur only when further judicial authorization is obtained or a second psychiatric opinion is documented, depending on the jurisdiction. The mental health laws of each state determine the criteria for involuntary psychiatric treatment, typically based on dangerousness to self or others in the presence of a psychiatric illness. The laws that specifically allow nonpsychiatric medical treatment without patient consent are based on competency criteria. In other words, judicial authorization for involuntary medical treatment depends on demonstrating that the patient does not have sufficient capacity to refuse treatment; it does not require that the patient's medical condition be life- or limb-threatening.

When a medical patient is so psychiatrically ill as to require court-ordered treatment, there is often pressure from nonpsychiatric physicians, nurses, hospital administrators, and even the legal process to transfer the patient to a psychiatric unit. Decisions on whether or not to do so should be based primarily on what is in the patient's best interest and the need to protect other patients' welfare. It is the consulting psychiatrist's responsibility to independently assess whether the patient is sufficiently medically stable for transfer and to advocate for the patient. When available, medical-psychiatric units may be an ideal solution for some patients. Other patients can be best managed on secure medical units with one-to-one nursing supervision until they are stable enough for transfer. Concomitant psychiatric treatment should be provided while the patient is being medically treated.

Although an expressed or implied contract may be lacking, it is well established legally that a doctor is not obligated to accept a patient who simply seeks medical or psychiatric treatment (*Salas v. Gamboa* 1988). In some situations, however, an implied contractual arrangement does exist, even between a physician and a patient who have had no contact. The most common situation is a hospital's emergency room, where it is expected that emergency medical services will be provided to all who need them. This principle may extend to include physicians and psychiatrists who are on call for patient admissions or who consult with the emergency room staff (*Dillon v. Silver* 1987). Once a patient is admitted to a hospital, whether through voluntary or involuntary admission, the hospital is responsible to provide reasonable care.

Depending on the circumstances, liability associated with patient admission may arise involving the psychiatrist's failure to comply with civil commitment requirements, giving rise to a lawsuit based on the theories of false imprisonment (*Gonzalez v. New York* 1983), malicious prosecution, or assault (*St. Vincent's Medical Center v. Oakley* 1979).

Medical-surgical patients who are transferred to a psychiatric unit may want to leave. Because these patients were originally admitted for a medical or surgical problem, transfer to a psychiatric unit can be a bewildering, frightening experience. On encountering disturbed, noisy, or threatening patients, the medical-surgical patient may become terrified and demand immediate release. Grounds for a lawsuit may exist when a voluntary patient seeks to leave a hospital and is then coerced to remain in the hospital by threat of civil commitment. A patient should not be told that he or she will be involuntarily hospitalized unless that is the psychiatrist's actual intention (*Marcus v. Liebman* 1978).

In addition, a lawsuit can result when actual commitment proceedings are initiated without appropriate evidence for such an action (*Plumadore v. State* 1980). Liability may also arise if a patient represents a foreseeable risk of danger to self or others and the hospital does not hospitalize such a patient (*Clark v. State* 1985).

To protect a patient's civil rights, the consultant should inform the patient about the types of voluntary admission. Pure or informal voluntary admission permits the patient to leave the hospital at any time. Only persuasion is available to encourage the patient to stay. Conditional or formal voluntary admissions contain provisions that may require the patient to stay for a period of time after giving written notice of intention to leave. The latter provision is used when the patient is judged to be a danger to self or others. In reality, the distinction between voluntary and involuntary admissions is not always clear. Patients are often induced or pressured into accepting voluntary admissions. If voluntary admission were maintained as truly voluntary, involuntary admissions would likely increase. In addition to voluntary admissions procedures, an increasing number of states permit nonjudicial hospitalization of nonprotesting persons. For example, the District of Columbia statute provides a simple, nontraumatic admission process for individuals who either do not recognize their need for hospitalization or are unwilling to seek admission but nevertheless sign a "no objection" statement when others initiate the admission process (DC CODE ANN 1981/1984).

Discharges Against Medical Advice

Voluntary patients may demand to leave the hospital against medical advice (AMA). This commonly occurs with patients who have experienced failures in physician–patient communication, who have external family or other pressures to leave the hospital, or who have an addictive disorder that has not been adequately diagnosed or treated in the hospital (e.g., heroin or nicotine withdrawal) (Schindler et al. 1988). The consulting psychiatrist must determine if the patient is a danger to self or others and if the patient has decisional capacity. In addition, the psychiatrist plays a key role in determining the reason the patient wants to leave the hospital AMA and in offering appropriate interventions. Regardless of whether the patient signs an AMA form, clear and complete documentation should be made in the medical record detailing the recommendations made to the patient about the need for further treatment as well as the possible risks of premature discharge (Gerbasi and Simon 2003). Voluntary patients who lack decisional capacity but are not dangerous or gravely disabled can be kept in the hospital against their will if they have been adjudicated incompetent and a guardian gives consent for continued hospitalization. This authority also exists for individuals vested with durable power of attorney for health care decisions. For other cases, an emergency judicial order should be sought to restrain the incompetent patient who wishes to leave

AMA. In contrast to involuntary hospitalization for psychiatric treatment, a judicial order to permit continued treatment of an objecting incompetent medical patient does not require demonstration of dangerousness. From a clinical perspective, family or other responsible parties should be involved if possible to prevent a premature discharge.

Although competent patients can leave the hospital AMA, the consulting psychiatrist can provide significant input and intervention in preventing such a discharge (Schindler et al. 1988).

> Mr. T, a 36-year-old male intravenous heroin user admitted with bacterial endocarditis, demanded to leave the hospital AMA after only 3 days of intravenous antibiotics. He refused to stay until home treatment could be arranged. He was able to describe his illness, his need for treatment, and the consequences of terminating treatment. He appeared restless and uncomfortable. His decisional capacity was determined to be intact. On further investigation, it was discovered that the medical staff had decided to give him clonidine instead of methadone to manage his withdrawal symptoms, that the patient in the next bed had had cardiac arrest during the previous night and died, and that the patient's wife was to be discharged from the psychiatric unit that day after a suicide attempt.

This case illustrates some of the areas in which psychiatric consultation can play a key role in preventing potentially life-threatening AMA discharges. First, the consultant should develop a differential diagnosis of the patient's reasons to leave AMA and should attempt to address one or all of them with the patient, family, and medical staff. In the case of Mr. T, an initial priority is better control of withdrawal symptoms by the addition of methadone. For other patients, analogous interventions include nicotine patches and adequate pain control. A second priority in the case of Mr. T is to address his anxiety about his roommate's death and his fear of his wife being home alone. A combination of supportive psychotherapy, anxiolytics, and environmental changes (e.g., having his wife spend the rest of the day and night in the patient's hospital room) may result in a marked decrease in the patient's anxiety and an increase in his trust in the health care team. Discussions with staff about the patient's current emotional state and the determinants of his wish to leave AMA helped decrease the staff's countertransference, resulting in more supportive patient–staff interactions and improved staff–patient communication.

When such efforts fail, anger directed at the patient by any member of the health care team is not clinically constructive and may contribute to legal liability. Such angry responses are understandable when physicians and nurses have worked hard to help the patient. The consulting psychiatrist can help the team members modulate their feelings. The patient should be told that he is welcome to return to the hospital if he changes his mind or his symptoms get worse. The key goals in such interventions are to ensure the patient is making an informed, competent decision to leave and to encourage the patient to return if further care is needed. All too often, a power struggle ensues and the physicians or nurses become fixated on getting the patient to sign the AMA form, a step that is neither necessary nor sufficient for proper documentation.

Involuntary Hospitalization

The consulting psychiatrist must often consider involuntary hospitalization for patients on medical units who have made suicide attempts requiring acute medical care or who have complex comorbid medical and acute psychiatric symptoms. The criteria are identical to those governing all psychiatric commitments (Simon 1998a, 2001; Tardiff 1996). The individual must be 1) mentally ill, 2) dangerous to self or others, and/or 3) unable to provide for basic needs. Generally, each state determines which criteria are required and defines each criterion. Because terms such as mentally ill are often loosely described, the proper definition relies on the clinician's judgment and a clear understanding of the local commitment laws.

Clinicians cannot themselves legally commit patients. This process is solely under the court's jurisdiction. Psychiatrists who use reasonable professional judgment and act in good faith when requesting involuntary hospitalization are granted immunity from liability in many states. It is helpful to keep this in mind, especially when the non-psychiatric health care professional may not understand and even oppose psychiatric commitment and transfer of patients (e.g., a superficially rational patient with anorexia nervosa and a dangerously low weight) (Appelbaum and Rumpf 1998).

Commitment statutes do not mandate involuntary hospitalization (Appelbaum et al. 1987). The statutes are permissive and enable mental health professionals and others to seek involuntary hospitalization for persons who meet certain criteria. On the other hand, the duty to seek involuntary hospitalization is a standard-of-care issue. That is, patients who are mentally ill and pose an imminent, serious threat to themselves or others may require involuntary hospitalization as a primary psychiatric intervention. This is equally true of the patient who starts out as a medical-surgical patient.

Physical Restraints

The psychiatric-legal issues surrounding physical restraints are complex (Tardiff 1984). What the general psychiatrist may regard as contraindications to the use of restraints on psychiatric units are often viewed as indications by consulting psychiatrists on medical units. Physical restraint may be required in confused, medically unstable patients, especially when chemical restraint is ineffective or contraindicated. If restraints are not used in some delirious patients or patients with dementia, the patients may pull out their intravenous lines, endotracheal tubes, arterial lines, or other vital lines or tubes. Furthermore, confused medically ill patients often climb over bed rails, risking falls, which may result in fractures and subdural hematomas. Physical restraint is sometimes the most humane alternative.

Stringent legal regulation of physical restraints has increased during the past decade, as have legal challenges to their use. Generally, courts hold that restraints and seclusion are appropriate only when a patient presents a risk of harm to self or others and a less restrictive alternative is not available. Some health care professionals have overused restraints, whereas others are uncomfortable with their use, viewing it as an assault on the patient. Psychiatrists can help explore the various options for managing the patient and address the discomfort of the staff while keeping in mind that there are clinical and legal risks both in using and in forgoing restraints.

Emergency Medical Treatment and Active Labor Act

The Emergency Medical Treatment and Active Labor Act (EMTALA), a United States federal law enacted in 1986, obligates emergency departments of all hospitals that participate in Medicare to examine patients who seek emergency care and to either stabilize them before discharge or transfer to another facility or admit them if medically indicated (Quinn et al. 2002). In this situation, health care providers cannot discriminate against patients because of their inability to pay for medical care. The law has been interpreted by the courts to require nondiscrimination in medical care rather than the establishment of standard-of-care quality (Rosenbaum 2003). In the infamous Baby K case (*In re Baby K* 1993), the United States Supreme Court went further and ruled that EMTALA requires the provision of "stabilizing treatment" even if such treatment is outside the prevailing standard of care and is considered clinically and ethically inappropriate. Difficult EMTALA problems may arise with patients presenting to emergency rooms with unstable medical and psychiatric illness who may be uncooperative with treatment.

Conflicts between hospitals and between physicians occur when the patient appears too psychiatrically unstable to be treated in a medical facility and too medically unstable to transfer to a psychiatric facility. The potential penalties for violations of the law are so severe that it has led to "EMTALA-phobic" behaviors in which emergency physicians have admitted patients against the advice of psychiatric consultants, or psychiatrists have admitted patients they regard as clinically inappropriate. EMTALA does not apply to discharges from medical or psychiatric inpatient units of previously stabilized patients, although this is a commonly expressed fear. New rules (issued in September 2003) clarified that the EMTALA obligation ends once a patient has been admitted. Issues regarding the transfer of psychiatric patients were not addressed in the new rules.

Legal Issues in Collaborative Care in the Medical Hospital

Psychiatrists in the medical setting work in a complex environment with a variety of health care and administrative professionals, requiring a sound understanding of the boundaries of their role in the health care setting and in the care of each patient (Appelbaum 1991; Kleinman 1991). In the medical inpatient setting, the psychiatric consultant is called to the bedside by the primary physician to evaluate and at times co-manage the patient with psychiatric symptoms. The consulting psychiatrist is not the patient's primary physician. The consultant's relationship is with the physician who called for the consultation, not the patient. The primary physician is free to accept or reject the findings and recommendations of the psychiatric consultant. Although psychiatrists are not likely to be found ultimately liable for adverse outcomes when their suggestions are not acted on, ironically they may be sued along with the primary physician. Whereas primary responsibility for the patient remains with the consultee, who normally relies on the consultant's recommendations and writes the orders in the chart, both parties can be held liable for negative patient outcomes (Beran 1997; Garrick and Weinstock 1994). For example, both the nonpsychiatric physician and the consulting psychiatrist may be sued when a patient given haloperidol on the psychiatrist's advice develops neuroleptic malignant syndrome, even when there is no negligence. In addition, psychiatrists need to be aware of their supervisory role and re-

sponsibilities with psychiatric nurse practitioners, social workers, and trainees in the hospital setting (see American Psychiatric Association 1980)

A number of nonclinical roles that psychiatrists may play in the medical setting can raise both legal and ethical concerns. Frequent interactions with the medical health care team around patient care issues lead to involvement on hospital committees (e.g., impaired physician, ethics, pharmacy and therapeutics) and often to leadership roles in the hospital system. Psychiatrists in the medical setting are also sought out for curbside consultations and referrals for staff members and their families. The consultant may also be privy to information about other health care providers (attending physicians, house staff, medical students, nurses, and other staff)—ranging from minor complaints to allegations of impairment, incompetence, or unprofessional behavior—and may become aware of health professionals who are struggling with mental health or addiction problems. Patients, families, or staff may ventilate to the psychiatrist about quality-of-care concerns. Psychiatrists should maintain awareness of the conflicts of interest that may arise and at the same time assess the likely accuracy and validity of the information. They then must balance competing legal as well as ethical obligations (e.g., the information may have been obtained confidentially from a patient, but there may be a legal mandate requiring reporting of impaired health care professionals). When in doubt, psychiatrists should seek consultation with legal services or the chief of staff of the hospital.

Managed Care: Impact on Psychiatric Care in the Medical Setting

A number of managed care issues have been particularly problematic in providing psychiatric care in the medical setting. These include conflicts over responsibility for payment for psychiatric consultations, limited formularies, and restrictive determinations by insurance companies of availability and sites for posthospital psychiatric treatment (Alter et al. 1997). There may be limited or no provisions for psychiatric consultation and treatment during medical hospitalization, which has fallen between the cracks of the medical insurer and the psychiatric "carve out." Regardless of insurance coverage, psychiatrists should strive to ensure that the medical patient receives any urgently needed psychiatric intervention. If another staff psychiatrist is a part of the patient's insurer's panel, he or she should provide the service. If not, then the psychiatrist should provide the clinical service and is normally entitled to bill the insurer full charges. Psychiatrists' primary responsibility is always to the patient first; they must use their best clinical judgment in providing competent care to patients regardless of what the managed care company states it will allow (Simon 1998b). Psychiatrists must not suspend their judgment in making competent dispositions and referrals for patients, because they are more likely to be held responsible for making a negligent choice than the insurer.

Risk Management and Risk Reduction

Dr. P, a 73-year-old recently retired physician, is admitted to the orthopedic service with a right hip fracture. On his fifth postoperative day, he is noted to be missing from his room, only to be found 30 minutes later in the hospital stairwell with new pelvic and ulnar fractures. A psychiatric consultation is called 2 days later when the patient becomes agitated and repeatedly removes his intravenous line. Review of the medical record by the consultant reveals several physician and nursing notes documenting the patient's confusion and irritability on initial admission to the hospital and worsening on subsequent hospital days. The patient's daughter confirms that the patient had retired because of cognitive impairment and had occasionally wandered away from home since his wife's death 6 months ago. Soon after Dr. P's discharge to a nursing home, the family files a malpractice suit against the hospital.

Psychiatrists and other mental health professionals contribute to risk reduction in the hospital through their assistance with patients who are angry, suicidal, disruptive, confused, noncompliant, or otherwise difficult and in decisions about restraint, level of observation, AMA discharges, and determination of decisional capacity. In the case of Dr. P described above, earlier psychiatric consultation could have recognized the likely preexisting dementia and the high risk of postoperative delirium and could have facilitated appropriate precautions and management.

It is widely believed that poor doctor–patient communication is a frequent underlying stimulus for avoidable malpractice suits, and there are data to support this belief (Moore et al. 2000). Psychosomatic medicine specialists have considerable expertise on the doctor–patient relationship and can assist other physicians and other health care professionals in preventing breakdown of the relationship, improving communications, and repairing damaged relationships. Primary prevention of malpractice suits through physician continuing medical education about the psychodynamics of the doctor–patient relationship has been considered helpful (Virshup et al. 1999).

References

Alter CL, Schindler BA, Hails KC, et al: Funding for consultation-liaison services in public sector managed care plan: the experience of the Consultation-Liaison Association of Philadelphia. Psychosomatics 38:93–97, 1997

American Psychiatric Association: Official actions: guidelines for psychiatrists in consultative, supervisory, or collaborative relationships with nonmedical therapists. Am J Psychiatry 137:1489–1491, 1980

American Psychiatric Association: Guidelines on confidentiality. Am J Psychiatry 144:1522–1526, 1987

Appelbaum PS: General guidelines for psychiatrists who prescribe medication for patients treated by nonmedical therapists. Hosp Community Psychiatry 42:281–282, 1991

Appelbaum PS: Privacy in psychiatric treatment: threats and responses. Am J Psychiatry 159:1809–1818, 2002

Appelbaum PS, Grisso T: Capacities of hospitalized, medically ill patients to consent to treatment. Psychosomatics 38:119–125, 1997

Appelbaum PS, Rumpf T: Civil commitment of the anorexic patient. Gen Hosp Psychiatry 20:225–230, 1998

Appelbaum PS, Lidz CW, Meisel A: Informed Consent: Legal Theory and Clinical Practice. New York, Oxford University Press, 1987

Batlle JC: Legal status of physician-assisted suicide. JAMA 289:2279–2281, 2003

Beran RG: Shared care-responsibilities of the doctors. Med Law 16:235–243, 1997

Black HC: Black's Law Dictionary, 6th Edition. St Paul, MN, West Publishing, 1990

Cohen LM, Steinberg MD, Hails KC, et al: Psychiatric evaluation of death-hastening requests. Lessons from dialysis discontinuation. Psychosomatics 41:195–203, 2000

Council on Ethical and Judicial Affairs, American Medical Association: Guidelines for the appropriate use of do-not-resuscitate orders. JAMA 265:1868–1871, 1991

Council on Ethical and Judicial Affairs, American Medical Association: Physician-assisted suicide, in Code of Medical Ethics. Reports of the Council on Ethical and Judicial Affairs of the American Medical Association, Vol 5, No 2. Chicago, IL, American Medical Association, 1994, pp 269–275

Emanuel EJ, Emanuel LL: Proxy decision making for incompetent patients—an ethical and empirical analysis. JAMA 267:2067–2071, 1992

Garrick TR, Weinstock R: Liability of psychiatric consultants. Psychosomatics 35:474–484, 1994

Gerbasi JB, Simon RI: Patients' rights and psychiatrists' duties: discharging patients against medical advice. Harv Rev Psychiatry 11:333–343, 2003

Grisso T, Appelbaum PS: Comparison of standards for assessing patients: capacities to make treatment decisions. Am J Psychiatry 152:1033–1037, 1995

Grisso T, Appelbaum PS, Hill-Fotouhi C: The MacCAT-T: a clinical tool to assess patients' capacities to make treatment decisions Psychiatr Serv 48:1415–1419, 1997

Gutheil TG, Appelbaum PS: Substituted judgment and the physician's ethical dilemma: with special reference to the problem of the psychiatric patient. J Clin Psychiatry 41:303–305, 1980

Hassenfeld IN, Grumet B: A study of the right to refuse treatment. Bull Am Acad Psychiatry Law 12:65–74, 1984

Hedberg K, Hopkins D, Kohn M: Five years of legal physician-assisted suicide in Oregon. N Engl J Med 348:961–964, 2003

Kleinman CC: Psychiatrists' relationships with nonmedical professionals, in American Psychiatric Press Review of Clinical Psychiatry and the Law, Vol 2. Edited by Simon RI. Washington, DC, American Psychiatric Press, 1991, pp 241–257

Lamden RM, Ramchandani D, Schindler BA: The chronic mentally ill in the general hospital consultation-liaison service: their needs and management. Psychosomatics 38:472–477, 1997

LaPuma J, Orentlicher D, Moss RJ: Advance directives on admission: clinical implications and analysis of the Patient Self-Determination Act of 1990. JAMA 266:402–405, 1991

Leeman CP: Depression and the right to die. Gen Hosp Psychiatry 21:112–115, 1999

Leeman CP, Blum J, Lederberg MS: A Combined ethics and psychiatric consultation. Gen Hosp Psychiatry 23:73–76, 2001

Lippert GP, Stewart DE: The psychiatrist's role in determining competency to consent in the general hospital. Can J Psychiatry 33:250–253, 1988

Luce JM: Ethical principles in critical care. JAMA 263:696–700, 1990

Macbeth JE, Wheeler AM, Sither JW, et al: Legal and Risk Management Issues in the Practice of Psychiatry. Washington, DC, Psychiatrists Purchasing Group, 1994

Mishkin B: Decisions in Hospice. Arlington, VA, The National Hospice Organization, 1985

Mishkin B: Determining the capacity for making health care decisions, in Issues in Geriatric Psychiatry (Advances in Psychosomatic Medicine Series, Vol 19). Edited by Billig N, Rabins PV. Basel, Switzerland, Karger, 1989, pp 151–166

Moore PJ, Adler NE, Robertson PA: Medical malpractice: the effect of doctor-patient relations on medical patient perceptions and malpractice intentions. West J Med 173:244–250, 2000

Nair S, Morrison M: The evaluation of maternal competency. Psychosomatics 41:523–530, 2000

Orentlicher D: The illusion of patient choice in end-of-life decisions. JAMA 267:2101–2104, 1992

Overman W, Stoudemire A: Guidelines for legal and financial counseling of Alzheimer's disease patients and their families. Am J Psychiatry 145:1495–1500, 1988

Parry J: Incompetency, guardianship, and restoration, in The Mentally Disabled and the Law, 3rd Edition. Edited by Brakel SJ, Parry J, Weiner BA. Chicago, IL, American Bar Foundation, 1985, pp 370–371

Perr IN: The clinical considerations of medication refusal. Legal Aspects of Psychiatric Practice 1:5–8, 1984

President's Commission for the Study of Ethical Problems in Medicine and Biomedical and Behavioral Research: Making Health Care Decisions: A Report on the Ethical and Legal Implications of Informed Consent in the Patient Practitioner Relationship, Vol 1: Report. Washington, DC, U.S. Government Printing Office, 1982

Quinn DK, Geppert CM, Maggiore WA: The Emergency Medical Treatment and Active Labor Act of 1985 and the practice of psychiatry. Psychiatr Serv 53(10):1301–1307, 2002

Regan M: Protective services for the elderly: commitment, guardianship, and alternatives. William Mary Law Rev 13:569–573, 1972

Rosenbaum S: The impact of United States law on medicine as a profession. JAMA 289:1546–1556, 2003

Sales BD, Powell DM, Van Duizend R: Disabled Persons and the Law: Law, Society, and Policy Services, Vol 1. New York, Plenum, 1982

Schindler BA, Blum D, Malone R: Non-compliance in the treatment of endocarditis: the medical staff as co-conspirators Gen Hosp Psychiatry 10:197–201, 1988

Schwartz HR: Do not resuscitate orders: the impact of guidelines on clinical practice, in Geriatric Psychiatry and the Law. Edited by Rosner R, Schwartz HR. New York, Plenum, 1987, pp 91–100

Siegler M: Sounding Board. Confidentiality in medicine—a decrepit concept. N Engl J Med 307:1518–1521, 1982

Simon RI: The psychiatrist as a fiduciary: avoiding the double agent role. Psychiatric Annals 17:622–626, 1987

Simon RI: Beyond the doctrine of informed consent—a clinician's perspective. Journal for the Expert Witness, the Trial Attorney, the Trial Judge 4:23–25, 1989

Simon RI: Clinical Psychiatry and the Law, 2nd Edition. Washington, DC, American Psychiatric Press, 1992

Simon RI: Psychiatrists awake! Suicide risk assessments are all about a good night's sleep. Psychiatr Ann 28:479–485, 1998a

Simon RI: Psychiatrists' duties in discharging sicker and potentially violent inpatients in the managed care era. Psychiatr Serv 49:62–67, 1998b

Simon RI: Concise Guide to Psychiatry and Law for Clinicians, 3rd Edition. Washington, DC, American Psychiatric Press, 2001

Smith JT: Medical Malpractice: Psychiatric Care. Colorado Springs, CO, Shepard's/McGraw-Hill, 1986

Solnick PB: Proxy consent for incompetent non-terminally ill adult patients. J Leg Med 6:1–49, 1985

Stone AA: The right to refuse treatment. Arch Gen Psychiatry 38:358–362, 1981

Tardiff K (ed): The Psychiatric Uses of Seclusion and Restraint. Washington, DC, American Psychiatric Press, 1984

Tardiff K: Assessment and Management of Violent Patients, 2nd Edition. Washington, DC, American Psychiatric Press, 1996

Umapathy C, Ramchandani D, Lamden R, et al: Competency evaluations on the consultation-liaison service: some overt and covert aspects. Psychosomatics 40:28–33, 1999

U.S. Department of Health and Human Services: The Legal Status of Adolescents 1980. Rockville, MD, U.S. Department of Health and Human Services, 1981

Virshup BB, Oppenberg AA, Coleman MM: Strategic risk management: reducing malpractice claims through more effective patient-doctor communication. Am J Med Qual 14:153–159, 1999

Weir RF, Gostin L: Decisions to abate life-sustaining treatment for nonautonomous patients: ethical standards and legal liability for physicians after Cruzan. JAMA 264:1846–1853, 1990

Wise TN, Berlin R: Involuntary hospitalization: an issue for the consultation-liaison psychiatrist. Gen Hosp Psychiatry 9:40–44, 1987

Zito JM, Lentz SL, Routt WW, et al: The treatment review panel: a solution to treatment refusal? Bull Am Acad Psychiatry Law 12:349–358, 1984

Legal Citations

Aponte v United States, 582 F Supp 555, 566–569 (D PR 1984)

Bartling v Superior Court, 163 Cal App 3d 186, 209 Cal Rptr 220 (1984)

Bouvia v Superior Court, 179 Cal App 3d 1127, 225 Cal Rptr 297 (1986)

Canterbury v Spence, 464 F2d 772 (DC Cir), cert denied, Spence v Canterbury, 409 US 1064 (1972)

Clark v State, No 62962 Albany Court of Claims (NY 1985)

Cruzan v Director, Missouri Department of Health, 110 S Ct 284 (1990)

Dillon v. Silver, 520 NYS2d 751, 134 AD2d 159 (NY App Div 1987)

Ferguson v City of Charleston, 532 US 67, 121 S Ct 1281, 149, L Ed 2d 2095 (2001)

Frasier v Department of Health and Human Resources, 500 So 2d 858, 864, La Ct App (1986)

Gonzalez v New York, 121 Misc 2d 410, 467 NYS2d 538 (1983), rev'd on other grounds, 110 AD 2d 810 488 NYS 2d 231

Gulf S I R Co v Sullivan, 155 Miss 1, 119 So 501 (1928)

In re Baby K, 832 F Supp 1022, 1031 (ED Va 1993)

In re Boyer, 636 P 2d 1085, 1089, Utah (1981)

In re Conroy, 98 NJ 321, 486 A2d 1209, 1222–1223 (1985)

In re Farrell, 108 NJ 335, 529 A2d 404 (1987)

In re Jobes, 108 NJ 365, 529 A2d 434 (1987)

In re Peter, 108 NJ 365, 529 A2d 419 (1987)

In re Quinlan, 70 NJ 10, 355 A2d 647, cert denied, 429 US 922 (1976)

In the Guardianship of John Roe, 411 MA 666 (1992)

Jehovah's Witnesses v King County Hospital, 278 F Supp 488 (WD Wash 1967), aff'd, 390 US 598 (1968)

Marcus v Liebman, 59 Ill App 3d 337, 375 NE2d 486 (Ill App Ct 1978)

McKnight v South Carolina, 576 SE2d 168, 352 SC 635 (2003)

Meek v City of Loveland, 85 Colo 346, 276 P 30 (1929)

Natanson v Kline, 186 Kan 393, 350 P2d 1093 (1960)

Planned Parenthood v Danforth, 428 US 52, 74 (1976)

Plumadore v State, 75 AD2d 691, 427 NYS2d 90 (1980)

Rennie v Klein, 462 F Supp 1131 (D NJ 1978), remanded, 476 F Supp 1294 (D NJ 1979) aff'd in part, modified in part and remanded, 653 F2d 836, 3rd Cir (1980), vacated and remanded, 458 US 1119 (1982), 720 F2d 266, 3rd Cir (1983)

Salas v Gamboa, 760 SW2d 838, Tex App (1988)

Scaria v St. Paul Fire and Marine Ins Co, 68 Wis 2d 1, 227 NW2d 647 (1975)

Schloendorff v Society of New York Hospital, 211 NY 125, 105 NE 92 (1914), overruled, Bing v Thunig, 2 NY2d 656, 143 NE2d 3, 163 NYS2d 3 (1957)

St. Vincent's Medical Center v Oakley, 371 So 2d 590, Fla App (1979)

Tune v Walter Reed Army Medical Hosp, 602 F Supp 1452, DDC (1985)

Union Pacific Ry Co v Botsford, 141 US 250, 251 (1891)

Wilson v Lehman, 379 SW2d 478, 479, Ky (1964)

Civil Statutes

DC CODE ANN, sec. 21-513 (1981 and 1984 Supp)

Emergency Medical Treatment and Active Labor Act (42 USC sec. 1395dd), Centers for Medicare and Medicaid Services, 68 FR 53222–53264 (September 9, 2003)

Health Insurance Portability and Accountability Act of 1996, U.S. Department of Health and Human Services, Office of the Secretary, 45 CFR Parts 160, 162, 164 (February 20, 2003)

Omnibus Budget Reconciliation Act of 1990, Pub. L. No. 101-508 (Nov. 5, 1990), sec. 4206, 4751 (42 USC, scattered sections)

Uniform Guardianship and Protective Proceedings Act, sec. 5-101

Uniform Probate Code, sec. 1-101[7]

4 Ethical Issues

Donald L. Rosenstein, M.D.
Franklin G. Miller, Ph.D.

ETHICAL ISSUES PERMEATE the practice of psychosomatic medicine. Psychiatrists who work in medical and surgical settings routinely perform clinical evaluations and make treatment recommendations with deep moral significance. For example, psychiatrists render opinions about the decision-making capacity of medically ill patients, whether they pose a danger to themselves or others, or if they are appropriate candidates for organ transplantation. These clinical assessments bear directly on patients' autonomy and the medical care they receive. Similarly, psychiatrists who provide end-of-life care frequently confront the possibility that medical interventions provided to their patients delay death rather than prolong life. The fact that there are no clear lines of demarcation between these types of clinical considerations and their ethical ramifications makes the practice of clinical ethics in psychosomatic medicine both compelling and challenging. All consulting psychiatrists should be adept at identifying ethical issues relating to the practice of psychosomatic medicine and need to be familiar with ethical rules, principles, and standards that should guide solving moral problems in patient care.

Historically, practitioners of psychosomatic medicine and consultation-liaison psychiatry have been active and influential participants in the ethical life of hospitals, hospice settings, and nursing homes. Many serve as members or chairs of ethics committees, institutional review boards, and ethics consultation services. Even for clinical or research psychiatrists who do not participate in these formal ethics activities, the practice of psychosomatic medicine requires familiarity with the principles of biomedical ethics.

The routine care of medically ill patients usually requires neither psychiatric consultation nor explicit ethical deliberation. However, when difficulties arise in the provision of clinical care, ethical and psychiatric concerns are often packaged together in partially formulated and emotionally charged requests for help (Lederberg 1997). In some cases, a psychiatric disorder may be inaccurately perceived as an ethical problem. For example, a patient's missed dialysis appointments might be interpreted as refusal of treatment when the patient's absences are actually due to panic attacks. In this case, the proper psychiatric diagnosis and clinical intervention may obviate misplaced ethical concerns. Conversely, a legitimate ethical dilemma (i.e., an impasse in the clinical care of a patient due to conflicting moral values) can prompt a misguided request for a psychiatric evaluation (e.g., disagreement between family members and the medical team about the value of continued aggressive medical interventions for a severely ill and clearly incapacitated patient). This second example requires careful moral deliberation among the relevant decision makers rather than a specialist's assessment of the patient's decision-making capacity. Such cases often require the help of an ethics consultant or committee. Nonetheless, the successful resolution of the ethical issues may not be possible until the presence of psychopathology in the patient, or a systems problem involving the health care team, has been identified and addressed by the psychiatric consultant.

Psychiatrists and ethicists are frequently consulted on the same complicated patients at the same urgent moment. Just as the psychiatrist has been trained to enter carefully into a dynamic system, gather information, and formulate the proper questions in the proper sequence, so too must the ethicist. Either consultant may call for a multidisciplinary team meeting to get the critical decision makers talking with each other in the same room rather than through notes in the patient's chart.

Despite the fact that many of the core skills needed for effective psychiatric intervention are also required for the resolution of ethical dilemmas that arise in the care of medically ill patients, there are important distinctions between the tasks and methods of these two consultative activities. Psychiatric consultation follows the medical model of providing expert advice on diagnosis and therapy. Physicians who ask for psychiatric consultations want specific answers to specific questions. They want to be told precisely how to manage a certain aspect of their patient's care. Health care professionals often desire the same type of direction from an ethics consultant. However, within the bioethics community the traditional medical model is one of the least favored approaches to ethics consultation. Instead, most ethics committees and consultation services seek to facilitate discussion and conflict resolution between the stakeholders in the case. The purpose of this process-oriented approach is to identify the range of ethically permissible options rather than to provide the "right answer" or stipulate a specific course of action. The consulting psychiatrist should be able to identify ethical issues that fall outside the scope of psychiatric expertise and encourage wider moral deliberation. Similarly, the ethics consultant who can identify unaddressed clinical questions (e.g., Is the patient depressed, anxious, or confused?) can help resolve an apparent ethical problem by bringing the prior clinical questions to the attention of the medical team or psychiatrist.

The purpose of this chapter is to provide a framework for integrating ethical considerations into the practice of psychosomatic medicine. The chapter is organized into two sections. The first section provides a brief overview of the discipline of ethics and the rules governing the behavior of physicians. The second section presents a case vignette to illustrate the complex interplay between several key clinical and ethical issues encountered in psychosomatic medicine and the process of moral problem solving. The case is interrupted at critical junctures in order to facilitate a discussion of specific ethical issues as they might unfold in actual practice (e.g., decision-making capacity and treatment refusal; involuntary medication; withdrawal of care). Although the primary focus of the case is on ethical issues related to the provision of clinical care, we also discuss the relevant differences between the ethics of clinical medicine and the ethics of clinical research.

This chapter does not cover all ethical issues in psychosomatic medicine. Relevant legal considerations are discussed in Chapter 3 ("Legal Issues"). Specific ethical topics covered elsewhere in this book include physician-assisted suicide in Chapter 10 ("Suicidality"), terminal weaning in Chapter 20 ("Lung Disease"), dialysis decisions in Chapter 22 ("Renal Disease"), transplant candi-date and donor issues in Chapter 31 ("Organ Transplantation"), sterilization in Chapter 33 ("Obstetrics and Gynecology"), placebos in Chapter 36 ("Pain"), and palliative care in Chapter 40 ("Palliative Care"). Readers are referred to other sources for ethics topics not covered, including confidentiality (Kimball and Silverman 1979), truth-telling (Horikawa et al. 1999, 2000), and the scope of the psychiatric consultant's role in medical settings (Agich 1985).

Overview of the Discipline of Ethics

The discipline of ethics consists of systematic investigation and analysis of moral issues, including judgments concerning deliberation and conduct in specific situations, the identification and application of appropriate moral rules or principles, methods of justifying actions and practices, and the development of moral character. In the field of medical ethics, the focus of inquiry is often morally problematic cases involving complex interactions between health care professionals and patients (or research subjects) in which competing moral considerations are relevant.

Ethical inquiry aimed at resolving a problem in patient care or clinical research proceeds in accordance with a series of connected steps (Fins et al. 1997). First, the factual contours of the case, including pertinent medical facts, patient needs and preferences, institutional contexts, and attitudes and actions of involved professionals, should be investigated. Second, the moral considerations relevant to the case are identified and assessed. This calls for discerning the bearing of specific moral rules and principles on the case and their relative weight in determining what to do when such moral considerations conflict. Third, a decision is made on a plan of action to resolve the moral problem. Finally, the plan is implemented and its results are evaluated. Typically, all these stages of ethical inquiry take place within a process of discussion among the individuals with a stake in the outcome of the case, which may also include ethics consultation with an ethicist or ethics committee in especially difficult situations.

The most general moral considerations guiding ethical inquiry in medical contexts are the principles of biomedical ethics. The leading conception identifies four such principles (Beauchamp and Childress 2001). *Respect for patient autonomy* requires that professionals recognize the right of competent adult individuals to make their own decisions about health care or participation in research. This includes the obligation to obtain informed consent and the right of competent patients to refuse recommended diagnostic interventions or therapy or to decline an invitation to enroll in research. In the therapeutic context, *beneficence* directs professionals to promote the health and well-being of particular patients by offering and providing competent medical care; in research it directs investigators to produce valuable knowledge with the aim of improving medical care for future patients. *Nonmaleficence* enjoins professionals to avoid harming patients or research subjects. Taken together, beneficence and nonmaleficence underlie the obligation of clinicians to assess the risk–benefit ratios of patient care and research interventions. The principle of *justice* requires that medical care and research be performed in a way that is fair and equitable.

Complex moral problems in medicine are rarely resolved by simple application of one of these principles. The specific relevance and weight of principles and subsidiary moral considerations are assessed in the deliberative process of ethical inquiry. An extensive and instructive account of the meaning and application of these principles is presented in *Principles of Biomedical Ethics* by Beauchamp and Childress (2001).

Ethical considerations relevant to the ethical practice of medicine and research are incorporated in various medical oaths (Hippocratic Oath) and codes (Nuremberg Code, American Medical Association Code of Ethics); declarations (Helsinki Declaration) (World Medical Association Declaration of Helsinki 2000); and reports, guidelines, policies, and laws regarding the behavior of physicians. Some of these documents conflict with each other, and some are even internally inconsistent with respect to permissible activities (Miller and Shorr 2002). Indeed, many physicians find their own beliefs at odds with existing laws and policies concerning specific medical practices (e.g., abortion, physician-assisted suicide, use of medical marijuana).

There is no specific code of ethics for psychosomatic medicine. The most relevant professional documents are the Principles of Medical Ethics of the American Medical Association (2001) and the annotation of this code by the American Psychiatric Association (2001). The American Psychiatric Association's annotation goes into substantial detail regarding specific behaviors (e.g., sexual boundary violations, breaches of confidentiality, fee splitting, abandonment of patients) and is directly relevant to all psychiatric practice, including subspecialties. However, certain aspects of the practice of psychosomatic medicine pose ethical challenges that are not specifically addressed by these codes. The case presented through the remainder of the chapter illustrates several of these difficult issues and suggests a clinically oriented approach to their resolution.

Assessment of Decision-Making Capacity

Mr. P, a 74-year-old man who was separated from his wife, was hospitalized for a recurrence of prostate cancer. He was first diagnosed with cancer in his early 60s and had been free of disease for 10 years following prostatectomy and hormonal therapy. Other than his prostate cancer, his health was excellent. He had not been taking any medications and reported drinking 2–4 beers per night. On the day before admission, he went to see his primary care physician because of low back pain. Diagnostic imaging revealed multiple lesions in his lumbar spine consistent with metastatic prostate cancer. His physician recommended hospitalization for a course of standard chemotherapy.

The morning after his admission, the patient appeared demoralized and withdrawn but was cooperative with the start of chemotherapy. He received intravenous lorazepam and oral prochlorperazine as part of his chemotherapy regimen. On the fourth day after admission, his nurse attempted to insert a new intravenous catheter for the continued administration of chemotherapy. The patient reacted with irritability and pulled his arm away from the nurse. Repeated attempts by the nurse to persuade Mr. P to allow the intravenous line to be restarted resulted in an escalation of his anger, and he demanded that he be "unhooked from all these tubes" so that he could go home. Psychiatric consultation was requested to determine if the patient was competent to refuse treatment.

Consultation requests concerning a patient's ability to make his or her own medical decisions pose two related questions. The first requires a *clinical judgment*: Does this patient have a medical, neurological, or psychiatric disorder that compromises his or her capacity to understand, appreciate, and reason with respect to the details of a given diagnostic or therapeutic procedure? The second question requires a *moral judgment*: Based on the clinical assessment described above, ought this person be allowed to give or refuse permission for medical care? Capacitated adults are entitled to refuse medical care or demand the withdrawal of life-saving treatments if they so desire. Consequently, the assessment of Mr. P's decision-making capacity (DMC) is a critical task in his hospitalization and exemplifies the importance of addressing the clinical issue before the ethical one.

The domains of legal competence, the capacity to make autonomous decisions, and the ability to provide informed consent are closely related but distinct from each other (Berg and Appelbaum 2001; Faden et al. 1986). In our society, there is a presumption that adults are legally competent to make their own decisions. A judgment that someone is incompetent is made by judicial ruling and is typically based on the ability to make specific decisions (e.g., choices concerning medical care, management of finances, designation of a substitute decision maker, execution of a will) at a given point in time. Standards for determining competence vary by jurisdiction but are based in large part on clinical assessments of an individual's cognitive state and DMC. From a legal perspective, a person is either competent to make decisions for himself or herself or incompetent to do so, in which case someone else makes decisions on his or her behalf (see also discussion of DMC in Chapter 3, "Legal Issues").

In contrast to the dichotomous nature of competency determinations, DMC varies along a continuum from incapacitated to fully capacitated (Figure 4–1). In the medical setting, it is common for patients to manifest diminished DMC in some domains but retain the ability to make decisions in other domains. For example, although a patient may have impaired DMC such that she does not understand the procedures, risks, and benefits of a complicated medical intervention, she may still be quite capable of designating her spouse or other loved one to make medical decisions for her. Furthermore, the nature of comorbid medical and psychiatric illnesses and their treatments is such that DMC often changes over time. Patients with secondary mania, traumatic brain injury, and delirium characteristically manifest fluctuating DMC. Despite the greater prevalence in hospital settings of delirium or comorbid delirium and dementia (Trzepacz et al. 1998) compared with uncomplicated dementia, the vast majority of published literature on clinical and ethical aspects of impaired DMC has focused on individuals with either stable or progressive cognitive impairment.

The assessment of DMC is particularly challenging in the setting of physical or behavioral communication barriers. Clinical decisions must also be made regarding patients who are either unable to speak (e.g., due to mechanical ventilation) or unwilling to be interviewed (e.g., due to a personality disorder). The use of written notes or communication boards (often of limited utility because of the patient's fatigue or weakness) and behavioral indicators may allow only tentative conclusions about the patient's DMC. These cases require frequent assessment, patience, and clinical creativity. Because medically ill patients rarely undergo formal competency evaluations and judicial proceedings, the clinical assessment of DMC carries an extra burden in health care settings to ensure that medical decisions are made by capacitated patients or appropriate substitute decision makers for those who are incapacitated.

Few human activities are as complex and individually determined as how we make decisions. Basic components of DMC include intellectual ability; memory; attention; concentration; conceptual organization; and aspects of executive function such as the ability to plan, solve problems, and make probability determinations. Most of the psychiatric literature on DMC has focused on these cognitive functions and has employed psychometric approaches to the study of subjects with neuropsychiatric illnesses such as dementia, psychosis, major depression, and bipolar disorder (Chen et al. 2002). In contrast, the contributions of mood, motivation, and other influences on risk assessment and decision making have received less

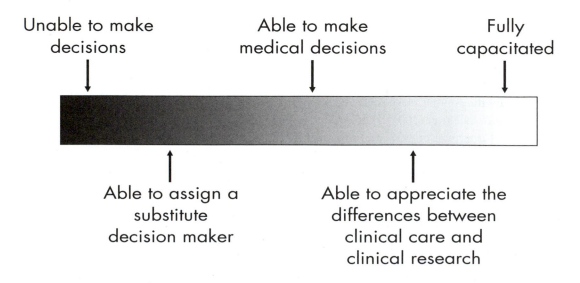

FIGURE 4–1.   **Continuum of decision-making capacity.**

attention but have clear implications for the process and quality of informed consent for both clinical procedures and research participation. The extent to which these factors (and less discrete concepts such as intuition, trust, and ambivalence) affect the decision-making process is not known. Although much work remains to be done to better understand the determinants of decision making, it is clear that focusing exclusively on measures of cognitive impairment is short-sighted.

A frequently observed but unfortunate phenomenon on medical and surgical wards is the differential threshold for concern about DMC depending on the degree to which the patient is compliant with medical care. Patients who refuse a diagnostic or therapeutic procedure are often suspected of having impaired DMC and are referred for psychiatric or neurological evaluation. In contrast, decisionally impaired patients who are passive and agreeable with requests from their nurses and doctors rarely engender these same concerns. The diagnosis of delirium, particularly the hypoactive subtype, is often missed in hospital settings (see Chapter 6, "Delirium") and can be very distressing to patients, family members, and health care professionals (Breitbart et al. 2002a). One of several reasons to diagnose and aggressively treat delirium (with or without agitation) is that its resolution may restore DMC and thus allow patients to make important medical decisions for themselves (Bostwick and Masterson 1998).

Medically ill patients are at risk for impaired DMC for multiple reasons. The most common causes for concern are related to the patient's underlying medical problems (e.g., respiratory compromise, hepatic failure, cerebrovascular event, severe pain) or their treatment (e.g., excessive narcotics, high-dose glucocorticoid or cytokine therapy) rather than due to a primary psychiatric disorder. In Mr. P's case, there are several potential medical causes for his treatment-refusing behavior (e.g., delirium due to alcohol withdrawal, inadequate pain control, akathisia). A judgment that Mr. P is or is not capacitated to refuse treatment would be premature without a careful clinical evaluation of his mental state.

Physical Restraint and Involuntary Medical Treatment

Dr. M, a psychiatrist specializing in psychosomatic medicine, visited Mr. P for a psychiatric examination. She observed that Mr. P was an elderly man who was unshaven and poorly groomed. His temperature was 38.4°C, and his pulse and blood pressure were slightly elevated. When asked if he understood the purpose of the psychiatric evaluation, he replied, "I'm not inter-

ested in talking to you. I'm not crazy. I just want to go home." The patient was irritable and uncooperative with the interview, and after a few minutes of complaining about his nursing care, he insisted that the psychiatrist leave his room. The nursing report and the description from his daughter revealed that the patient had been increasingly irritable over the past few days and was briefly disoriented the previous evening. His daughter was unsure of the patient's typical alcohol consumption but suspected that he drank more than he had reported to his physicians.

Suspecting that Mr. P was experiencing delirium, possibly due to alcohol withdrawal, Dr. M recommended treatment with benzodiazepines, a multivitamin, and folate and a workup for other metabolic, infectious, or structural causes of delirium (including blood tests, a lumbar puncture, and a magnetic resonance imaging scan). However, before completion of this workup, the patient struck a nurse and was placed in a harness and wrist restraints.

Physical restraint of patients should be used only when no less restrictive method is available to protect them and the staff from harm. The Centers for Medicare and Medicaid Services (U.S. Department of Health and Human Services 2003) and the Joint Commission on Accreditation of Healthcare Organizations (2003) require that hospitals have policies on physical restraint and seclusion. In cases of extreme agitation and violence, nuanced mental status examinations are unnecessary and often impossible, and most physicians and nurses are comfortable deciding whether and when a patient's behavior warrants physical restraint. However, when the underlying neuropsychiatric disorder is not well characterized, the consulting psychiatrist can provide critical information regarding the justification for restraint and steps to improve the patient's condition. The medical team is looking for an expert opinion as to the patient's degree of self-control and dangerousness. Is there an imminent risk of harm to the patient or staff, and how can that risk be reduced? If the patient is capacitated and not dangerous, then forcible restraint violates his dignity, privacy, and autonomy. On the other hand, if an incapacitated and dangerous patient is not restrained, the rights of staff and other patients, and the patient's safety, have been compromised.

It appears that Mr. P has temporarily lost DMC, and the principal concern at this point is his safety and that of his caregivers. Occasionally health care providers question whether it is ethically and legally permissible to physically restrain patients under these circumstances (see Chapter 3, "Legal Issues"). There should be no confusion in this regard: standard of care, as well as legal precedent, for acutely agitated and confused patients is to immediately ensure their safety even if it requires physical restraint. Compassionate care requires that the patient be treated with dignity and respect under such circumstances and that restraint be continued only for as long as necessary. The critical distinction to be made at this juncture is between capacitated, informed refusal of care that warrants respect and refusal behavior due to compromised DMC.

A comprehensive workup for delirium often involves invasive diagnostic procedures and may necessitate the use of force to overcome the patient's resistance. Under what circumstances is it permissible to hold a confused patient down for blood tests (e.g., electrolyte concentrations, serum drug levels, or blood cultures), a bladder catheterization, or a lumbar puncture? The clinical presentations that prompt such diagnostic interventions range from true medical emergencies to subacute and self-limiting syndromes. There is no simple solution to this problem. Such decisions require clinical judgments about the necessity of each diagnostic test, its associated risks, and the degree to which the patient's condition is deemed to threaten life or risk permanent serious injury. For minimally invasive testing that is judged to be of urgent and critical importance, physicians have an obligation to act in the best medical interests of their patients even if this entails the use of force. At the other end of the spectrum, a relatively high-risk, low-yield diagnostic test in a stable but incapacitated patient is substantially more difficult to justify.

Durable Power of Attorney and Advance Directives for Health Care

> Mr. P is separated but not legally divorced. He has lived alone for 5 years and has one adult daughter with whom he is very close. Mr. P's daughter thought that her father had a living will but did not know where it was or if his estranged wife was still the holder of a durable power of attorney.

At this point in his hospitalization, attempts should be made by the health care team to identify the most appropriate substitute decision maker for Mr. P. Involving a spouse, close relative, or friend in medical decision making for incapacitated patients demonstrates respect for them. As with competency standards, laws regarding substitute decision makers vary by jurisdiction. The Patient Self-Determination Act of 1991 (Omnibus Budget Reconciliation Act of 1990) was intended to inform patients of their right to direct their own medical care should they become incapacitated or otherwise lose the ability to communicate their preferences. These rights include designating a holder of a durable power of attorney (DPA) for health care decisions. The completion of a living will

or an advance directive for health care allows patients to specify in writing the medical care they wish to receive under different catastrophic medical circumstances (e.g., brain death, persistent vegetative state).

Clinicians and caregivers often make false assumptions about the legal status of family members and significant others when it comes to surrogate decision making. Parents of disabled adults (e.g., patients with mental retardation, autism, or psychotic disorders) may erroneously conclude that they automatically remain the patient's legal guardian even after their child's eighteenth birthday. In most of these cases, the parents are the logical and most appropriate choices as legal guardians or surrogate decision makers. However, not all parents of incapacitated adult patients have the best interests of their children in mind. Similarly, when an unmarried incapacitated patient has more than one adult child, differences of opinion among the children about what is best for that sick or dying parent are common. Consequently, clinicians should clarify the legal status of their patients' substitute decision makers whenever possible to avoid compromised medical care and its legal ramifications.

Research on the use of advance directives and the behavior of substitute decision makers suggests two important conclusions. First, most individuals are reluctant to put in writing the kind of medical care they would like to receive if they should become gravely ill and incapacitated. Several studies found that only 15%–20% of patients fill out an advance directive for health care or research when given an opportunity to do so (Gross 1998; SUPPORT Principal Investigators 1995; Wendler et al. 2002). Second, regardless of the expressed wishes of patients, substitute decision makers tend to make decisions based on what they would want to have happen to themselves or, alternatively, what they consider to be in the best interests of the patient, rather than employing a substituted judgment standard (i.e., what the patient would have wanted) when making decisions for someone else.

Depression in the Medically Ill

> The clinician in charge of Mr. P's care obtained verbal permission from the patient's daughter to continue the physical restraints and complete the diagnostic testing. The medical workup suggested delirium secondary to alcohol withdrawal and hypomagnesemia. The patient was treated with intravenous magnesium sulfate, lorazepam, and a low dosage of an antipsychotic to treat his confusion, conceptual disorganization, and agitation.
> Two days after initiation of treatment with magnesium, lorazepam, and haloperidol, Mr. P had a markedly improved sensorium. He was considerably less irritable

and was able to complete a detailed psychiatric interview. He was relieved to be able to "think clearly again," and over the course of several sessions he developed a trusting relationship with Dr. M. However, as his delirium resolved, Mr. P expressed a deepening sadness and sense of hopelessness about his medical condition. He expressed skepticism about the value of more chemotherapy and wished to avoid a painful death.

In Mr. P's case, the aggressive treatment of his delirium had the value of restoring his decision-making capacity but left him painfully aware of his progressive cancer and feeling depressed as a consequence. The clinicians caring for Mr. P are again faced with a complex clinical problem that raises ethical issues. Mr. P is contemplating stopping chemotherapy but is manifesting symptoms of depression. Is his depression influencing his decision making, and if so, what is the proper response from his health care providers? As discussed earlier, clinical considerations should be explored first in the service of an ethically desirable outcome for Mr. P.

It is important to recognize that major depression in the medically ill usually does not make the patient decisionally incapacitated. To be sure, the presence of depression may well influence patients' ability to tolerate uncomfortable symptoms, maintain hope, or assess a treatment's risk–benefit ratio but does not necessarily render them unable to make medical decisions for themselves (Elliott 1997). Untreated depression has been linked to poor compliance with medical care, increased pain and disability (Spiegel et al. 1994), and a greater likelihood of considering euthanasia and physician-assisted suicide (Emanuel et al. 1996). Depression produces more subtle distortions of decision making than delirium or psychosis, but refusal of even life-saving treatment by a depressed patient cannot be assumed to constitute suicidality or lack of capacity (Katz et al. 1995; Sullivan and Youngner 1994). Consequently, depressed patients should be strongly encouraged to accept treatment of depression, but decisions regarding overriding a refusal of medical treatment should be based on whether they lack DMC.

Differentiating the Ethics of Clinical Research From the Ethics of Medical Care

Mr. P was moderately depressed and declined the recommended trial of an antidepressant because he was not interested in "taking any more drugs." Although he was ambivalent about proceeding with chemotherapy, he agreed to resume the standard chemotherapy regimen and received another full cycle. When, after 4 weeks of chemotherapy, he complained of new chest pain, it was discovered that he had new metastatic bone lesions in his ribs.

At this point, he told his daughter he wanted to stop treatment and go home to die. He asked his oncologist to discharge him to his home or hospice. His oncologist responded that Mr. P could go home but recommended that he consider enrolling in a Phase I clinical trial of a new chemotherapeutic agent. Mr. P's daughter also encouraged him to enroll in the clinical trial and to "keep fighting."

In some respects, the option of enrolling in a clinical trial is a logical consideration following the failure of standard medical treatment. However, this decision point in Mr. P's clinical course warrants a thoughtful exploration of the differences between the practice of medicine and clinical research. Clinical medicine aims at providing optimal medical care for particular patients. The risks of diagnostic tests and treatments are justified by the prospect of compensating medical benefits for the patient. By contrast, clinical research is devoted to answering scientific questions to produce generalizable knowledge. Physician-investigators conduct clinical trials to evaluate experimental treatments in *groups* of patient-subjects, with the ultimate goal of benefiting future patients by improving medical care. To be sure, the contrast between the group focus of research trials and the individual focus of medical care should not be overstated. Physicians are obligated to practice medicine in the context of a professional standard of care rather than by idiosyncratic judgments about what is best for individual patients. Nonetheless, they are expected to make competent treatment recommendations tailored to the characteristics of their individual patients.

Many patients receive therapeutic benefits from participating in clinical trials, which may even surpass the benefits from standard medical care (Braunholtz et al. 2001). However, the randomized clinical trial differs fundamentally from patient care in its purpose, characteristic methods, and justification of risks. Interventions evaluated in these trials are allocated by chance. Double-blind conditions and often placebo controls are employed. For scientific reasons, protocols governing clinical trials typically restrict flexibility in dosing of study drugs and use of concomitant medications. Trials often include drug washouts before randomization to establish a drug-free baseline to assess treatment efficacy. Research interventions such as blood draws, imaging procedures, and biopsies are often administered to measure trial outcomes. These strictly research interventions pose risks to participants that are not compensated by medical benefits to them but are justified by the potential value of the knowledge to be gained from the trial. Although the differences between research trials and medical care have been frequently noted (Appelbaum et al. 1987; Beecher 1970; Levine 1986; Miller et al. 1998), their ethical significance has not been sufficiently appreciated. Accordingly, clinical trials continue to be conceived from a therapeutic perspective oriented around the physician–patient relationship (Miller and Rosenstein 2003).

Clinical research has changed dramatically in recent years. Two decades ago, the majority of clinical trials were conducted in academic medical centers. Today, they are more likely to be conducted in private practice settings under the direction of clinicians rather than full-time investigators. Increasingly, psychiatrists are being consulted on patients who either are enrolled in or are considering enrolling in a clinical trial. Practitioners of psychosomatic medicine can make several contributions in this context. They may be asked to render an opinion about the psychiatric appropriateness of a patient for a clinical trial. Their patients may ask for advice about enrolling in a study. There may be an opportunity to modify the existing study or design a new one that addresses psychiatric aspects of the medical illness or its treatment.

In each of these activities, the consulting psychiatrist is well served by possessing an understanding of the critical aspects of clinical research and how they differ from those related to standard medical care (Emanuel et al. 2000; Miller and Rosenstein 2003). For example, many patients and physicians do not appreciate that the primary purpose of a Phase I trial (what was offered to Mr. P) is to assess the tolerability and toxicity of a drug rather than to obtain preliminary data on the effectiveness of the drug (Phase II).

Another aspect of research ethics directly relevant to Mr. P's case is the issue of research involving subjects considered "mentally disabled." The regulations governing federally funded human-subjects research were written more than 20 years ago and mandated additional safeguards for research subjects considered "vulnerable to coercion or undue influence" (U.S. Department of Health and Human Services 1991). Included in this category of vulnerable subjects are the mentally disabled. These regulations, known as the Common Rule, were clearly intended to prevent the exploitation of individuals for the sake of scientific progress. Unfortunately, the Common Rule does not include a definition of mental disability, nor does it specify what would constitute either the degree or the likelihood of mood, cognitive, or behavioral impairment that would render someone vulnerable in this respect. In practice, a psychiatric consultation often serves as an important additional safeguard by virtue of eliciting an expert opinion about a prospective research subject's DMC and ability to provide informed consent.

The nature of the research protocol, rather than the disorder being studied, might also place research subjects at risk for impaired DMC. Oncology trials in which subjects receive interleukin-2 or interferon-alpha, cytokines that are associated with central nervous system toxicity, provide examples of protocols that place otherwise capacitated subjects at risk of losing DMC. In these cases, the concern is less about adequate informed consent on the "front end" of the study than it is on subjects losing their ability to provide adequate consent for continuing participation. For such studies, institutional review boards (IRBs) can require subjects to appoint a holder of a DPA as a condition of enrollment. This approach has the advantages of highlighting an important risk of the study (i.e., loss of DMC) and ensuring appropriate initial and ongoing research authorization.

Research Ethics in Psychosomatic Medicine

Guidance on ethical issues raised specifically by research in psychosomatic medicine is needed. For example, obtaining proper authorization for research with individuals who lack DMC is relevant to both research on delirium and research on other conditions in which delirium might develop as a complicating factor. In the case of delirium research, current publication standards for informed consent are highly variable. Investigators have described research authorization from subjects who provided prospective informed consent (Breitbart et al. 1996). Other manuscripts state that informed consent was obtained from the subjects or their surrogates (often without detailing the circumstances of surrogate consent) (Bogardus et al. 2003; Cole et al. 2002; Inouye et al. 1999; Laurila et al. 2002). It has also been argued that prospective IRB review and informed consent are not necessary for studies that involve very little deviation from (standard) clinical practice (Breitbart et al. 2002a, 2002b; Lawlor et al. 2000). We contend that this view confuses research with medical care and is inconsistent with the principle of respect for persons and federal regulations for human-subjects research (Davis and Walsh 2001; U.S. Department of Health and Human Services 1991). Some reports of delirium research are silent on the issue of IRB review (Lawlor et al. 2000). Finally, we have suggested that published reports of medical and psychiatric research should address ethical issues in a more comprehensive fashion (i.e., providing more detail than the standard sentence that the study was approved by a local IRB and informed consent was obtained from subjects) (Miller et al. 1999; Tanaka 1999).

When Patients Express a Wish to Die

After considering the pros and cons of enrolling in the Phase I clinical trial, Mr. P decided to "stop poisoning myself and let this thing run its course." He told his oncologist that he was ready to go home but that he was very afraid the cancer would spread to more of his bones. When he told his oncologist that he would rather end his life than suffer through a painful death, his oncologist responded that he would not do anything to "bring on" Mr. P's death and again requested a consult with Dr. M.

On psychiatric examination, Mr. P was judged to be capacitated and not depressed. He confided that he had cared for his father during a "prolonged, excruciating, and undignified" death. He had accepted the inevitability of his own death but wished to avoid the kind of experience his father had endured. Dr. M then facilitated a discussion between the oncologist and Mr. P about available options. Mr. P decided to stop eating and drinking and was discharged to hospice with assurances that he would be kept comfortable while awaiting death. Dr. M was also able to help Mr. P's daughter understand her father's decision. Mr. P died from terminal dehydration 12 days after his transfer to hospice.

Few clinical scenarios generate requests for psychiatric consultation more predictably than when a patient expresses a wish to die. The range of possible meanings underlying this communication is immense, and a comprehensive discussion of this area is beyond the scope of this chapter (see Chapter 3, "Legal Issues," Chapter 10, "Suicidality," and Chapter 40, "Palliative Care"). Is the patient expressing a passive wish to die, planning to commit suicide, rejecting life-sustaining treatments (withdrawal of care), eliciting help in ending his or her life (physician-assisted suicide), or asking to be killed (euthanasia)? Under any circumstances, an expression of suicidal ideation or a request for help with an intentionally arranged death is a complex message that warrants careful clinical assessment.

Muskin (1998) observed that physicians respond to requests to die by focusing predominantly on determinations of the patient's DMC. He argued persuasively that too often there is inadequate attention to the underlying meaning and importance of these requests. Although it is true that capacitated subjects have the right to refuse life-sustaining treatments (and in Oregon, to request physician-assisted suicide), a compassionate and comprehensive evaluation by the consulting psychiatrist can help frame both the clinical questions and the ethically permissible medical options.

Just as the clinical issues raised by requests to die are frequently reduced to questions of decision-making ca-

pacity, the ethical analysis of physician-assisted suicide is often characterized as a simple matter of autonomy versus nonmaleficence. Miller and Brody (1995) articulated an important distinction in the debate on physician-assisted suicide. In considering whether physician-assisted suicide was morally justifiable, they explored whether the practice of physician-assisted suicide as a last resort could be compatible with the professional integrity of physicians.

Ultimately, Mr. P made a capacitated and deliberate request for a comfortable and dignified death. His choice of terminal dehydration was a legal option that did not compromise the professional integrity of his caretakers (Ganzini et al. 2003; Miller and Meier 1998). In this case, the psychiatrist was able to successfully treat his delirium, manage his depression despite refusal of pharmacotherapy, and help resolve a potential impasse between Mr. P and his oncologist.

Ethics Training in Psychosomatic Medicine

Training in ethics is considered a key component of the educational programs in psychosomatic medicine/consultation-liaison psychiatry fellowships (Academy of Psychosomatic Medicine 2003). Recognizing the importance of the interface between psychosomatic medicine and clinical ethics, a task force of the Academy of Psychosomatic Medicine recently published an annotated bibliography for ethics training (Preisman et al. 1999). Curricula for teaching research ethics in psychiatry have also been developed in recent years (Beresin et al. 2003; Rosenstein et al. 2001). Ethics education should be oriented to developing basic competence in identification of ethical issues in the practice of psychosomatic medicine and in deliberation aimed at satisfactory resolution of moral problems in patient care or research.

Conclusion

The relationship between psychosomatic medicine and bioethics is rich and unique for both historical and conceptual reasons. The ethical issues considered in this chapter are often discussed in purely theoretical terms. We have attempted to illustrate some of the ways in which clinical considerations can color the expression and resolution of these issues as they are encountered at the bedside. All too often optimal patient care is hampered by the presence of psychiatric symptoms in the patient or systems problems among the health care team or family members. Practitioners of psychosomatic medicine are ideally positioned to facilitate the resolution of both clinical problems and ethical dilemmas as they arise in an increasingly complex health care environment.

References

Academy of Psychosomatic Medicine: Standards for Fellowship Training in Consultation-Liaison Psychiatry. Chicago, IL, Academy of Psychosomatic Medicine, 2003. Available at: http://www.apm.org/fellow.html. Accessed April 11, 2004.

Agich GJ: Roles and responsibilities: theoretical issues in the definition of consultation liaison psychiatry. J Med Philos 10:105–126, 1985

American Medical Association: Principles of Medical Ethics, June 2001. Chicago, IL, American Medical Association, 2001. Available at: http://www.ama-assn.org/ama/pub/category/2512.html. Accessed April 1, 2004.

American Psychiatric Association: The Principles of Medical Ethics: With Annotations Especially Applicable to Psychiatry, 2001 Edition. Arlington, VA, APA, 2001. Available at: http://www.psych.org/psych_pract/ethics/medicalethics2001_42001.cfm. Accessed April 11, 2004.

Appelbaum PS, Lidz CW, Meisel JD: Fulfilling the underlying purpose of informed consent, in Informed Consent: Legal Theory and Clinical Practice. New York, Oxford University Press, 1987, pp 237–260

Beauchamp TL, Childress JF: Principles of Biomedical Ethics, 5th Edition. New York, Oxford University Press, 2001

Beecher HK: Research and the Individual; Human Studies. Boston, MA, Little, Brown, 1970

Beresin EV, Baldessarini RJ, Alpert J, et al: Teaching ethics of psychopharmacology research in psychiatric residency training programs. Psychopharmacology (Berl) 171:105–111, 2003

Berg JW, Appelbaum PS: Informed Consent: Legal Theory and Clinical Practice, 2nd Edition. New York, Oxford University Press, 2001

Bogardus ST Jr, Desai MM, Williams CS, et al: The effects of a targeted multicomponent delirium intervention on postdischarge outcomes for hospitalized older adults. Am J Med 114:383–390, 2003

Bostwick JM, Masterson BJ: Psychopharmacological treatment of delirium to restore mental capacity. Psychosomatics 39:112–117, 1998

Braunholtz DA, Edwards SJL, Lilford RJ: Are randomized clinical trials good for us (in the short term)? Evidence for a "trial effect." J Clin Epidemiol 54:217–224, 2001

Breitbart W, Marotta R, Platt MM, et al: A double-blind trial of haloperidol, chlorpromazine, and lorazepam in the treatment of delirium in hospitalized AIDS patients. Am J Psychiatry 153:231–237, 1996

Breitbart W, Gibson C, Tremblay A: The delirium experience: delirium recall and delirium-related distress in hospitalized patients with cancer, their spouses/caregivers, and their nurses. Psychosomatics 43:183–194, 2002a

Breitbart W, Tremblay A, Gibson C: An open trial of olanzapine for the treatment of delirium in hospitalized cancer patients. Psychosomatics 43:175–182, 2002b

Chen DT, Miller FG, Rosenstein DL: Enrolling decisionally impaired adults in clinical research. Med Care 40 (9 suppl): V20–V29, 2002

Cole MG, McCusker J, Bellavance F, et al: Systematic detection and multidisciplinary care of delirium in older medical inpatients: a randomized trial. Can Med Assoc J 167:753–759, 2002

Davis MP, Walsh D: Methadone for relief of cancer pain: a review of pharmacokinetics, pharmacodynamics, drug interactions and protocols of administration. Support Care Cancer 9:73–83, 2001

Elliott C: Caring about risks: are severely depressed patients competent to consent to research? Arch Gen Psychiatry 54:113–116, 1997

Emanuel EJ, Fairclough DL, Daniels ER, et al: Euthanasia and physician-assisted suicide: attitudes and experiences of oncology patients, oncologists, and the public. Lancet 347:1805–1810, 1996

Emanuel EJ, Wendler D, Grady C: What makes clinical research ethical? JAMA 283:2701–2711, 2000

Faden RR, Beauchamp TL, King NMP: A History and Theory of Informed Consent. New York, Oxford University Press, 1986

Fins JJ, Bacchetta MD, Miller FG: Clinical pragmatism: a method of moral problem solving. Kennedy Inst Ethics J 7:129–145, 1997

Ganzini L, Goy ER, Miller LL, et al: Nurses' experiences with hospice patients who refuse food and fluids to hasten death. N Engl J Med 349:359–365, 2003

Gross MD: What do patients express as their preferences in advance directives? Arch Intern Med 158:363–365, 1998

Horikawa N, Yamazaki T, Sagawa M, et al: The disclosure of information to cancer patients and its relationship to their mental state in a consultation-liaison psychiatry setting in Japan. Gen Hosp Psychiatry 21:368–373, 1999

Horikawa N, Yamazaki T, Sagawa M, et al: Changes in disclosure of information to cancer patients in a general hospital in Japan. Gen Hosp Psychiatry 22:37–42, 2000

Inouye SK, Bogardus ST Jr, Charpentier PA, et al: A multicomponent intervention to prevent delirium in hospitalized older patients. N Engl J Med 340:669–676, 1999

Joint Commission on Accreditation of Healthcare Organizations: Available at: http://www.jcaho.org. Accessed June 29, 2004.

Katz M, Abbey S, Rydall A, et al: Psychiatric consultation for competency to refuse medical treatment: a retrospective study of patient characteristics and outcome. Psychosomatics 36:33–41, 1995

Kimball CP, Silverman AJ: The issue of confidentiality in the consultation-liaison process. Bibl Psychiatr 159:82–92, 1979

Laurila JV, Pitkala KH, Strandberg TE, et al: Confusion assessment method in the diagnostics of delirium among aged hospital patients: would it serve better in screening than as a diagnostic instrument? Int J Geriatr Psychiatry 17:1112–1119, 2002

Lawlor PG, Gagnon B, Mancini IL, et al: Occurrence, causes, and outcome of delirium in patients with advanced cancer: a prospective study. Arch Intern Med 160:786–794, 2000

Lederberg MS: Making a situational diagnosis: psychiatrists at the interface of psychiatry and ethics in the consultation-liaison setting. Psychosomatics 38:327–338, 1997

Levine RJ: Ethics and Regulation of Clinical Research. Baltimore, MD, Urban & Schwarzenberg, 1986

Miller FG, Brody H: Professional integrity and physician-assisted death. Hastings Cent Rep 25:8–17, 1995

Miller FG, Meier DE: Voluntary death: a comparison of terminal dehydration and physician-assisted suicide. Ann Intern Med 128:559–562, 1998

Miller FG, Rosenstein DL: The therapeutic orientation to clinical trials. N Engl J Med 348:1383–1386, 2003

Miller FG, Shorr AF: Unnecessary use of placebo controls: the case of asthma clinical trials. Arch Intern Med 162:1673–1677, 2002

Miller FG, Rosenstein DL, DeRenzo EG: Professional integrity in clinical research. JAMA 280:1449–1454, 1998

Miller FG, Pickar D, Rosenstein DL: Addressing ethical issues in the psychiatric research literature (letter). Arch Gen Psychiatry 56:763–764, 1999

Muskin PR: The request to die. Role for a psychodynamic perspective on physician-assisted suicide. JAMA 279:323–328, 1998

Omnibus Budget Reconciliation Act of 1990, Pub. L. No. 101-508 (Nov. 5, 1990), sec. 4206, 4751 (42 USC, scattered sections)

Preisman RC, Steinberg MD, Rummans TA, et al: An annotated bibliography for ethics training in consultation-liaison psychiatry. Psychosomatics 40:369–379, 1999

Rosenstein DL, Miller FG, Rubinow DR: A curriculum for teaching psychiatric research bioethics. Biol Psychiatry 50:802–808, 2001

Spiegel D, Sands S, Koopman C: Pain and depression in patients with cancer. Cancer 74:2570–2578, 1994

Sullivan MD, Youngner SJ: Depression, competence, and the right to refuse lifesaving medical treatment. Am J Psychiatry 151:971–978, 1994

SUPPORT Principal Investigators: A controlled trial to improve care for seriously ill hospitalized patients. The Study to Understand Prognoses and Preferences for Outcomes and Risks of Treatments (SUPPORT). JAMA 274:1591–1598, 1995

Tanaka E: Gender-related differences in pharmacokinetics and their clinical significance. J Clin Pharm Ther 24:339–346, 1999

Trzepacz PT, Mulsant BH, Dew MA, et al: Is delirium different when it occurs in dementia? A study using the delirium rating scale. J Neuropsychiatry Clin Neurosci 10:199–204, 1998

U.S. Department of Health and Human Services: Available at: http://www.hhs.gov. Accessed June 29, 2004.

Wendler D, Martinez RA, Fairclough D, et al: Views of potential subjects toward proposed regulations for clinical research with adults unable to consent. Am J Psychiatry 159:585–591, 2002

World Medical Association Declaration of Helsinki: Ethical principles for medical research involving human subjects. JAMA 284:3043–3045, 2000

5 Psychological Responses to Illness

Mark S. Groves, M.D.

Philip R. Muskin, M.D.

A CENTRAL TASK of the psychiatrist working with the medically ill is to understand patients' subjective experiences of illness in order to design therapeutic interventions that modulate the patients' behavioral or emotional responses, decrease their distress, and improve their medical outcomes. In outpatient practice or in the general hospital, physicians witness tremendous diversity of emotional and behavioral responses to illness. Some individuals seem able to face devastating illnesses for which no cure is currently available with courage and a sense of humor (Cousins 1983; Druss 1995; Druss and Douglas 1988). Others, facing easily treatable illnesses, have difficulty overcoming intense emotions such as anger, fear, or hopelessness. Clinical experience and research demonstrate that illness variables such as severity, chronicity, or organ system involvement cannot predict an individual's response to any given medical illness (Lipowski 1975; Lloyd 1977; Sensky 1997; Westbrook and Viney 1982). Rather, it is in the realm of the individual's subjective experience of an illness that one can begin to understand his or her emotional and behavioral responses (Lipowski 1970; Lloyd 1977).

During the past few decades, there has been considerable work in the fields of health psychology and psychiatry attempting to explain the tremendous variety of individual responses to the stresses of illness and to account for these interindividual differences (see, e.g., Druss 1995; Geringer and Stern 1986; Kahana and Bibring 1964; Lazarus 1999; Perry and Viederman 1981; Peterson 1974; Strain and Grossman 1975; Verwoerdt 1972). In this chapter, we provide a general overview of the stresses that accompany medical illness and hospitalization and review some of the psychological, emotional, and behavioral responses that these stresses frequently elicit.

The concepts of stress, personality types, coping strategies, and defense mechanisms can be integrated into a framework that illustrates the complexity of an individual's behavioral or emotional responses to illness (Figure 5–1). This framework, adapted from the work of Lazarus and Folkman (Lazarus 1999; Lazarus and Folkman 1984), attempts to integrate the psychodynamic concepts of character style and intrapsychic defenses with other psychological concepts such as stress and coping. The importance of individual subjectivity is emphasized in this model through the placement of coping styles, defense mechanisms, personality types, and the appraised meaning of illness as central mediators of the behavioral and emotional responses to the stresses of medical illness.

This chapter does not focus solely on maladaptive responses to illness or psychopathology. A coping strategy or defense mechanism may be relatively maladaptive or ineffective in one context, but adaptive and effective in another (Penley et al. 2002). For example, the maladaptive use of denial by a patient just diagnosed with early breast cancer might lead to a long delay in seeking treatment (Zervas et al. 1993). In contrast, the adaptive use of denial by a man diagnosed with untreatable metastatic pancreatic cancer might enable him to maximize his quality of life in the months before his death (Druss 1995).

Psychiatrists do not see most people who become ill, nor will most patients' responses to their illnesses concern their physicians (Patterson et al. 1993; Perry and Viederman 1981). That does not mean, of course, that there is no psychological response to the illness. An overt display

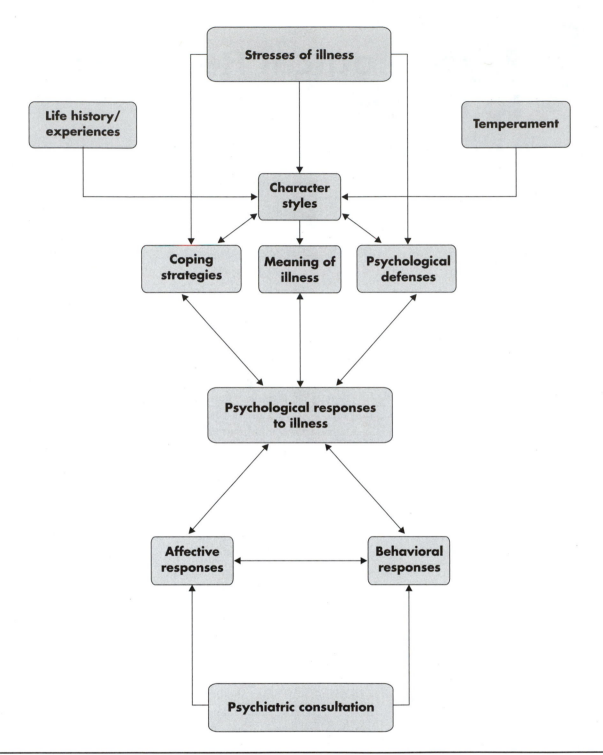

FIGURE 5–1. Framework illustrating the complexity of an individual's behavioral or emotional responses to illness.

Source. Adapted from Lazarus 1999; Lazarus and Folkman 1984.

of emotion may or may not be appropriate for a patient's racial and cultural background. In addition, patients may feel discouraged from expressing their thoughts and feelings about their illness to family members or physicians. The determination that a psychological response to illness is problematic must be based on the impact the response has on the patient, the patient's adherence to therapeutic plans, and the patient's social functioning.

There is no one correct way to characterize psychological responses to illness. Psychodynamic formulations, coping styles, and personality types offer different perspectives that may or may not be useful in understanding the response of a particular patient. Therefore, in this chapter, we provide an overview of the following topics without subscribing exclusively to any single theoretical framework: 1) the stresses of medical illness and hospitalization; 2) the influences of personality types, coping styles, and defense mechanisms on patients' subjective experiences of illness; 3) denial; 4) emotional responses to illness; and 5) behavioral responses to illness.

Stresses of Medical Illness and Hospitalization

The stresses of medical illness and hospitalization are both very significant and numerous (Strain and Grossman 1975). In their frequently cited study from 1967, Holmes and Rahe surveyed many individuals from a number of countries, asking them to rate the impact of various events on their lives. These ratings generated a ranked list of life events based on relative impact, which was used to create the Social Readjustment Rating Scale (Lazarus 1999). In this list of stressors, "personal injury or illness" ranked sixth (after death of spouse, divorce, marital separation, death of close family member, and jail term). Some of the stresses accompanying illness are nearly universal, whereas others vary by illness and are more specific (Druss 1995). In this section, we discuss some of the most common stresses experienced by patients in medical settings.

Apart from medical illness, the hospital environment itself can be stressful (Gazzola and Muskin 2003; Kornfeld 1972). To many, the hospital is a frightening place associated with painful personal or family memories. Hospitalization separates patients from their usual environments and social supports; it is by its very nature isolating. The inpatient is asked to wear a hospital gown, which results in de-individualization, loss of control, and loss of privacy (Gazzola and Muskin 2003). The machines, intravenous lines, blood withdrawals, interactions with strangers, and neighboring ill patients all contribute to the stress of hospitalization regardless of the patient's specific illness. In addition, the hospital demands that the patient be largely dependent on others for the most basic tasks—a change that in itself can be very stressful for many individuals (Kornfeld 1972; Muskin 1995; Perry and Viederman 1981). Perry and Viederman (1981) described three successive (though at times overlapping) tasks that patients facing medical illness must go through: 1) acknowledgment to themselves and others that they

are ill; 2) regressive dependency on others for care; and 3) resumption of normal functioning after recovery. Perry and Viederman proposed that all three tasks bring their own stresses and must be confronted for the patient to successfully cope with the illness and the hospitalization (Perry and Viederman 1981).

On a nearly universal level, medical illness results in narcissistic injury, that is, it demands that patients reexamine their views of themselves (Strain and Grossman 1975). Although most people would not overtly claim that they are invulnerable to serious medical illness, they may hold such a belief consciously. Unconscious fantasies of invulnerability may be unknown until the person is injured or becomes ill. The development of a medical illness shatters any such conscious or unconscious beliefs. The sick patient may feel "defective," "weak," or less desirable to others. Strain and Grossman (1975) have described the effects of illness on the sense of self:

> Sudden illness, hospitalization, and the threat of death undermine the universal, albeit irrational, beliefs that we are always capable, independent, and self-sufficient; that our bodies are indestructible; that we can control the world around us and we are the masters of our own destiny. These events challenge the infantile fantasy on which these beliefs are based—the fantasy that our omnipotent parents (and later, the doctor) can ensure our pain-free, pleasurable, and protected existence.... Similarly, the patient's belief in his autonomy and his conviction that he is "in control" of the world around him are challenged and reversed. (p. 25)

One determinant of the impact of an illness is whether it is acute or chronic (Verwoerdt 1972). Although an acute, non-life-threatening illness gives the individual little time to adapt, its effects are short term. Chronic illnesses, however, require the individual to more permanently change his or her self-view. The challenges of chronic illness are ongoing and become a part of daily life for the individual. A change in identity or body image is disorienting and often anxiety producing; the patient's previously held self-conception is disturbed, shaken up, or shattered.

Separation from family or friends in the hospital or at home when one is ill produces isolation, disconnection, and stress (Heiskell and Pasnau 1991; Strain and Grossman 1975). This can precipitate conscious or unconscious fears of abandonment. The stress of separation and fear of abandonment are not only experienced by children. Newly diagnosed with AIDS, a 30-year-old Latina mother of three may fear rejection by her community and abandonment by her parents. Or, after many years of chemotherapy for metastatic thyroid cancer, a 55-year-old bank executive may elect to undergo another course of chemotherapy despite the low likelihood of success rather than seek hospice care because the latter would signify giving up. Although not desirous of more treatment, the patient might fear that his oncologist who had worked with him for a decade would abandon him.

The lack of privacy in the hospital environment or clinic places additional stresses on the patient (Kornfeld 1972). Bodily exposure evokes discomfort. Given only a thin gown to wear, patients may be subjected to repeated examinations by doctors, nurses, and medical students. Exposure of the most private aspects of life can occur (Perry and Viederman 1981). A woman presenting with symptoms of a sexually transmitted disease must give a detailed account of her sexual history, and a young patient brought in with acute chest pain and hypertension is asked about use of cocaine, an illegal drug. For the vulnerable individual, such experiences of exposure can evoke feelings of shame and thus require the clinician to be tactful and empathic to put the patient at ease and maintain a therapeutic alliance.

Beyond simple exposure, the medical environment often involves experiences of bodily invasion that are very stressful for the patient (Gazzola and Muskin 2003). From the more invasive experiences of a colonoscopy, the placement of a nasogastric tube, or tracheal intubation to ostensibly more benign procedures such as a fine-needle biopsy of a breast lump or a rectal examination, the fear and discomfort of such interventions are often not fully recognized by the physician for whom such procedures have become routine. Individuals certainly vary in their fears; for example, the victim of repeated physical or sexual abuse might be especially fearful of such experiences and require the doctor to use greater care and psychological preparation than usual.

Pain should not be overlooked as a profound stressor that should be dealt with aggressively (Heiskell and Pasnau 1991). Even the most highly adapted patient with effective coping skills and strong social support can be taxed to the limit by extreme pain. Psychiatrists are frequently asked to evaluate patients for depression and hopelessness. On discovering inadequately treated pain, the consultant can facilitate increased pain control, sometimes leading to full remission of hopelessness and depression without any additional intervention. Like pain, sleep disturbances are extremely common in the medically ill, with significant psychological impact. A patient's outlook, emotional expression, and ability to cope may shift dramatically when insomnia is remedied.

When illness leads to disability—whether due to pain, physical limitations, or psychological effects—the disability is an additional stressor that can have a profound impact on the patient's regular activities of daily life (West-

brook and Viney 1982). What was previously routine and required no conscious planning can become tremendously challenging, both psychologically and practically. For example, on the acute rehabilitation unit, patients are assisted in their efforts to learn to walk again. What was previously automatic has become incredibly difficult and requires new techniques, assistive devices, and the help of others. Disabilities frequently preclude the possibility of an immediate return to work. For many this is a significant loss because it removes the natural opportunities to feel productive, which had provided a sense of accomplishment. For many people, feelings of accomplishment, productivity, and usefulness are important for their self-image. Thus, self-esteem is damaged when they lose this important source of gratification.

Although only a small proportion of medical illnesses signify the imminent or near approach of death and force affected individuals to directly confront their mortality, even minor illnesses can evoke a sense of the fragility and impermanence of life (Perry and Viederman 1981). Psychiatrists for the medically ill are often called to consult on patients who are experiencing anxiety or conflicts facing death (or patients whose illnesses evoke these difficulties in caregivers). Patients may refuse to give do-not-resuscitate orders despite clear evidence that resuscitation would be futile, because they equate do-not-resuscitate orders with suicide, which is morally unacceptable to them (Sullivan and Youngner 1993). Facing mortality—whether in the near future or later—can force a person to deeply reflect on life and can shatter previously held dreams of the future. This can stir up regrets and evoke numerous emotions, as described in the work of Elisabeth Kubler-Ross (1969). The various emotions evoked by medical illness are discussed later in this chapter.

Personality Types, Coping Styles, and Defense Mechanisms

There is great individual variation in responses to an environmental stressor such as receiving a diagnosis of cancer (Heim et al. 1993). Models of human behavior that only involve environmental stress and reflexive behavioral responses cannot account for this variation in responses and are therefore considered to have limited utility and explanatory power. Richard Lazarus has reviewed the historical transition in health psychology and other disciplines from the traditional stimulus → response model to the more contemporary stimulus → organism → response model, which emphasizes the importance of understanding individuals' *subjective* experiences (Lazarus 1999). It is only through understanding individuals' subjective experiences that the interindividual differences in reactions to a stressor can be accounted for.

Although the stressors of a situation and the behavioral responses of the patient may be readily identified by the medical team, the subjective experiences of the patient by their very nature are more elusive and require inquiry. Psychiatrists are often asked to evaluate patients with problematic behavioral or emotional reactions to the hospital setting or to their illnesses. Medical doctors can usually identify the stressors involved—for example, the need for emergent amputation in a 55-year-old diabetic patient with a gangrenous toe. The stated reason for consultation often also identifies the behavioral or emotional responses judged to be problematic, such as displaying anger and threatening to sign out against medical advice. Consulting psychiatrists seek to understand patients' subjective experiences of illness to explain their emotional and behavioral responses and to design interventions to help patients (and their caregivers).

Research investigating subjective variables that influence an individual's response to a given stressor has generally focused on three main areas: personality types, coping styles, and defense mechanisms. These areas are addressed separately in this section.

Personality Types

It is important to distinguish between the concepts of personality type or character style and personality disorder. As noted at the outset, this chapter is not concerned with psychopathology. Personality types may be understood as existing on a continuum with respective personality disorders (Oldham and Skodol 2000). In addition, most patients do not fit exclusively into one type but may exhibit characteristics of a number of personality types. Although the most accurate and complete understanding of personality may be achieved through a dimensional model, the characterization of discrete personality types is useful in highlighting differences and providing vivid prototypical examples. Much of the literature on personality types has been contributed by psychodynamic psychiatry. Although this rich literature continues to be tremendously useful for psychiatrists working in the medical setting, it is unfortunately often ignored because of the current emphasis on biological and descriptive psychiatry. In recognition of Kahana and Bibring's (1964) classic and still relevant paper "Personality Types in Medical Management," we have organized our discussion around the seven personality types they described (altering their terms to fit with more commonly used modern descriptions): 1) dependent, 2) obsessional, 3) histrionic, 4) masochistic, 5) paranoid, 6) narcis-

sistic, and 7) schizoid. What makes Kahana and Bibring's paper so valuable is its rich descriptions of these various personality types and the manner in which each type determines the individuals' subjective experiences of the meaning of illness.

Under conditions of stress, an individual's characteristic means of adapting to situations are heightened (Heiskell and Pasnau 1991; Kiely 1972). When confronted with the stress of a medical illness requiring hospitalization, the mildly obsessional patient might appear overly rigid or controlling. Similarly, a moderately dependent individual may appear "clingy" or excessively needy amid the acute stresses of hospitalization. Patients exhibiting extreme forms of these personality types can frustrate caregivers, often evoking intense negative emotions. It is important to recognize these countertransference responses, because they can be diagnostically useful tools. The negative emotions that patients with these extreme personality types evoke in the doctors and nurses may result in responses from the caregivers that aggravate the situation.

In another classic paper, "Taking Care of the Hateful Patient," Groves (1978) characterized four types of patients who most challenge physicians: dependent clingers, entitled demanders, manipulative help-rejecters, and self-destructive deniers. Groves also described the typical countertransference responses to each type and provided helpful tips on the management of these challenging patients. In this subsection, we integrate Groves's astute observations and descriptions of these four types with the seven personality types described by Kahana and Bibring.

Table 5–1 summarizes each of the seven personality types described in detail below—their characteristics, the meaning of illness to each type, frequent countertransference responses evoked among caregivers, and tips on management—drawing on the contributions of Geringer and Stern (1986), Groves (1978), Kahana and Bibring (1964), Muskin and Haase (2001), and others.

Dependent

The dependent patient is needy and demanding, is seemingly unable to independently solve problems or self-soothe, and continually asks for help from others. Patients with a dependent personality may initially evoke positive feelings from their physicians and are more likely to adhere to treatment recommendations (Bornstein 1994). The physician may enjoy feeling needed or powerful, much as a parent might feel toward a child. The dependent patient, however, can feel "sticky" or seem to have insatiable needs (Miller 2001), making it difficult for the caregiver to leave the room or end an interview. Such patients typically have limited frustration tolerance. His-

TABLE 5–1. Personality types

Type	Characteristics	Meaning of illness	Countertransference responses	Tips on management
Dependent	Needy, demanding, clingy Unable to reassure self Seeks reassurance from others	Threat of abandonment	Positive: doctor feels powerful and needed Negative: doctor feels overwhelmed and annoyed; may try to avoid patient	Reassure within limits Schedule visits Mobilize other supports Reward efforts toward independence Avoid tendency to withdraw from patient
Obsessional	Meticulous, orderly Likes to feel in control Very concerned with right/wrong	Loss of control over body/emotions/impulses	May admire When extreme: anger—a "battle of wills"	Try to set routine Give patient choices to increase sense of control Provide detailed information and "homework" Foster collaborative approach/avoid battle of wills
Histrionic	Entertaining Melodramatic Seductive, flirtatious	Loss of love or loss of attractiveness	Anxiety, impatience, off-putting Erotic; finds patient attractive	Strike a balance between warmth and formality Maintain clear boundaries Encourage patient to discuss fears Do not confront head-on
Masochistic	"Perpetual victim" Self-sacrificing martyr	Ego-syntonic Conscious or unconscious punishment	Anger, hate, frustration Helplessness, self-doubt	Avoid excessive encouragement Share patient's pessimism Deemphasize connection between symptoms and frequent visits Suggest that patient consider treatment as another burden to endure, or emphasize treatment's positive effect on loved ones
Paranoid	Guarded, distrustful Quick to blame or counterattack Sensitive to slights	Proof that world is against patient Medical care is invasive and exploitative	Anger, feeling attacked or accused May become defensive	Avoid defensive stance Acknowledge patient's feelings without disputing them Maintain interpersonal distance; avoid excessive warmth Do not confront irrational fears
Narcissistic	Arrogant, devaluing Vain, demanding	Threat to self-concept of perfection and invulnerability Shame evoking	Anger, desire to counterattack Activation of feelings of inferiority, or enjoyment of feeling of status of working with an important patient	Resist the desire to challenge patient's entitlement Reframe entitlement to foster treatment adherence Take a humble stance, provide opportunities for patient to show off, offer consultations if appropriate
Schizoid	Aloof, remote Socially awkward Inhibited	Fear of intrusion	Little connection to patient Difficult to engage	Respect patient's privacy Prevent patient from completely withdrawing Maintain gentle, quiet interest in patient Encourage routine and regularity

Source. Derived in large part from Geringer and Stern 1986; Kahana and Bibring 1964; Perry and Viederman 1981.

torically described as "oral" personalities, the extreme of this personality type corresponds to a DSM-IV-TR diagnosis of dependent personality disorder and sometimes borderline personality disorder (American Psychiatric Association 2000; Geringer and Stern 1986).

For the patient with a dependent personality, illness evokes an increased desire for care from others. Illness stimulates the patient's fear of abandonment (Perry and Viederman 1981). The person may feel that no one cares about him or her or may frantically cling to caregivers. Extremes of this personality style fit Groves's (1978) description of dependent clingers. These patients evoke aversion in their caregivers. The caregiver becomes overwhelmed by the patient's neediness, may feel manipulated, and may wish to avoid the patient, thus confirming the patient's fear of abandonment (Groves 1978). Tips on managing patients with this personality style, whether in a mild form or at the extreme, include appropriate reassurance that they will be taken care of, setting firm limits regarding what needs will be met, and setting a specific schedule of visits (e.g., 20 minutes three times a week) to set clear expectations regarding the doctor's time and availability (Miller 2001; Perry and Viederman 1981). For the overdemanding patient, it can be helpful to tactfully convey that behaviors such as incessantly ringing the call bell may have an opposite effect than what is intended and can lead caregivers to avoid the patient (Perry and Viederman 1981).

Obsessional

Individuals with an obsessional personality style are meticulous and orderly and like to feel in control. They place a strong emphasis on rationality, can be self-righteous at times, and are concerned with issues of right and wrong. These patients may be emotionally reserved and focus on details, sometimes to such an extent as to miss the broader picture. Ritual and regularity of schedule are important to them (Miller 2001). They are easily frustrated by the unpredictability of the hospital environment. Patients at the extreme end of the spectrum with this personality style might meet DSM-IV-TR criteria for obsessive-compulsive personality disorder.

Patients with an obsessional personality style will generally want a lot of information from their physicians regarding their medications, diagnoses, tests, etc. The physician may be pleased by the patient's desire to learn about his or her illness and its treatments. Under extreme stress, however, the patient may become increasingly rigid and inflexible, and at times the obsessional patient's only way to feel a sense of control is by refusing treatment or procedures (Kahana and Bibring 1964). A defiant refusal of procedures frequently leads to psychiatric consultation.

For example, the obsessional patient who is frustrated by the unpredictability of his hospital care and is angry after hours of fasting for an endoscopy that is subsequently canceled may refuse to allow a phlebotomist to draw his blood the following morning or refuse the second attempt to send him to the endoscopy suite. Conflicts between the extremes of compliance and defiance are common for these individuals.

Illness is experienced by the obsessional patient as a loss of control over the body, and it evokes a fear of loss of control over emotions or impulses (Heiskell and Pasnau 1991; Kahana and Bibring 1964; Miller 2001). When an inflexible or obstinate patient with this personality style confronts the physician, the physician may be tempted to engage in a battle of wills or try to exert greater control over the patient's treatment. Such a response, however, becomes counterproductive and often provokes the patient to resist even harder as in a tug-of-war. Instead, it may be helpful to offer detailed explanations of the procedures and tests and the reasons they are necessary. This emphasizes a collaborative approach, encouraging patients to actively participate in their care. Wherever possible, it is helpful to give patients choices and input in their care. This makes the patient a partner, not an opponent (Gazzola and Muskin 2003). Giving patients information, assigning them "homework," and providing opportunities for their input on decisions, where appropriate, will enable them to feel more in control of their care and will decrease anxiety and interpersonal friction (Muskin and Haase 2001).

Histrionic

Patients with a histrionic personality style can be entertaining, engaging, and at times seductive. This can be charming at times, or it can be uncomfortable or embarrassing for physicians (Miller 2001). Histrionic patients crave attention, approval, and admiration and tend to avoid anxiety-provoking situations through the use of denial. Illness in the patient with a histrionic personality style is experienced as a threat to the patient's masculinity or femininity (Geringer and Stern 1986). Illness activates such patients' fear of loss of love or attractiveness (Kahana and Bibring 1964; Strain and Grossman 1975).

The physician treating the histrionic patient should try to strike a balance between warmth and formality. Maintaining clear boundaries is essential, but an overly formal style will activate the patient's fear of loss of attractiveness or lovability (Heiskell and Pasnau 1991; Miller 2001). Encouraging the patient to discuss his or her fears will help bring to consciousness the anxiety that the patient is attempting to avoid. It is important, however, not to push patients too hard—a supportive and patient stance that gently encourages patients to voice fears when ready will be most helpful. "Confronting denial" head-on usually is counterproductive, as discussed in greater detail later in this chapter.

Masochistic

Patients with a masochistic personality style seem to be perpetual victims and readily recount their woes, experiencing themselves as self-sacrificing martyrs. One typically finds that such patients had miserable, abusive childhoods in which the experiences of physical illness paradoxically may have been bright spots, the only times they may have felt truly loved or cared for by parents or others (Heiskell and Pasnau 1991). The experience of illness, in part, provides reassurance to these patients that they will be able to maintain the attention and care of their physicians. Kahana and Bibring (1964) concretize this wish in the unspoken statement "You have to love me because I suffer so terribly." The patient may feel that the illness (consciously or unconsciously) is punishment for real or fantasized wrongdoings. Other patients may hold an unconscious wish to defeat their physicians (Douglas and Druss 1987; Heiskell and Pasnau 1991). The masochistic personality style can be particularly resistant to change.

Patients with the masochistic personality style may present with somatoform or factitious disorders. When the masochistic patient has no response (or a negative response) to treatment, or the physician's attempts to offer reassurance have no impact, the physician may become extremely frustrated. Encouragement and reassurance may actually have a paradoxical effect, provoking the patient to feel more pessimistic and leading to a worsening of symptoms. Those with an extreme version of this personality style have been described as "help-rejecters" (Groves 1978). They evoke feelings of irritation, depression, self-doubt, and hopelessness in their caregivers, who themselves may believe that such patients engineer their own misfortunes. The idea that someone could obtain psychological benefit from suffering is a concept that is difficult to understand, especially for physicians and other health care professionals.

Managing the patient with a masochistic personality should involve regularly scheduled follow-up visits irrespective of symptoms. It is important to deemphasize the connection between severity of symptoms and frequency of physician contact (Perry and Viederman 1981). Rather than encourage and reassure these patients, it is useful to acknowledge the patients' suffering and to "share their pessimism" (Groves 1978). It is sometimes of benefit for the physician to express to the patient an understanding that the illness and medical treatments are yet another burden for the patient to endure (Gazzola and Muskin

2003). It can also be helpful to emphasize the treatment's potential positive effect on others dear to the patient. This may reframe the treatment as another opportunity for the patient to suffer for the benefit of others (Heiskell and Pasnau 1991).

Paranoid

The paranoid patient is not generally a favorite of the physician. This patient maintains a guarded, distrustful stance; is quick to blame; and readily feels attacked (Heiskell and Pasnau 1991). Patients with a paranoid style do not forgive easily and may maintain lists of grievances. When these patients feel slighted, they tend to counterattack. It may not take much to provoke them, because they are extremely sensitive to anything experienced as a slight. When ill, patients with a paranoid personality style may blame others, and they may conceive of the illness as proof that the world is against them. They are prone to feeling hurt, invaded, or exploited by seemingly innocuous medical procedures (Miller 2001). Stress increases such patients' tendency to be suspicious, guarded, or controlling. This results in a request for psychiatric consultation because these patients evoke feelings of anger in their caregivers. They refuse procedures or tests, threaten to sign out against medical advice, and accuse the staff of doing things against them.

The physician assigned the task of treating a patient with this personality style often feels accused. If the physician is not aware of this, it can lead to defensive countertransference (Kahana and Bibring 1964). This may appear as a temptation to argue with the patient or as an attempt to prove the patient wrong. Taking a defensive stance will be counterproductive and can in essence prove the paranoid patient right; a defensive response will only increase the patient's paranoia. A more helpful approach is to acknowledge the patient's feelings without dispute or agreement, explaining in detail the justification for the treatments. Irrational fears often should not be confronted head-on or challenged; the patient will judge caregivers more on their actions and predominant emotional stance than on their words. Avoiding excessive warmth is helpful, as is maintaining sufficient interpersonal distance (Heiskell and Pasnau 1991). A calm, firm, direct stance is preferable to an angry, defensive stance or an intrusive, overly warm stance.

Narcissistic

Patients with a narcissistic personality style are typically easily recognized. Arrogant, devaluing, vain, and demanding, these patients can often be identified by one's immediate reaction. The narcissistic patient frequently begins the interview inquiring about the physician's title and rank. The patient may refuse to be examined by medical students, residents, or junior faculty members. These patients will devalue those believed to be inferior to them and will idealize the few people perceived to be highest in status. At the extreme, some patients will meet the criteria for narcissistic personality disorder. The patient's self-experience is frequently not validated by actual status in the world.

Narcissistic patients will experience an illness as a threat to their self-concept of perfection and invulnerability (Heiskell and Pasnau 1991; Kahana and Bibring 1964). Under such a threat, the patient's characteristic defense of grandiosity will be heightened. The physician or caregiver who is angered by the patient's devaluations and entitlement will be strongly tempted to put the patient in his or her place (Miller 2001). The psychiatric consultant who is called to assist in the management of a narcissistic patient may hear angry staff members say, "Who does he think he is? He's no better than anyone else!" and hear them put down the patient. Groves (1978) described patients at the extreme of this style as "entitled demanders," noting the intense feelings of anger and the desire to counterattack that these patients can evoke in their caregivers. The narcissistic patient can activate the physician's own feelings of inferiority, adding to the desire to avoid or attack the patient. The "power" of narcissistic V.I.P. patients can be very seductive to physicians, who may be tempted to cater to the unreasonable demands with the fantasy of some special status.

Managing patients with a narcissistic personality can be challenging. Resisting the desire to challenge the patient's entitlement is crucial in forming a therapeutic alliance. According to Groves (1978), "Entitlement is the patient's religion and should not be blasphemed." Although it is counterintuitive, the physician should not reflexively support the patient's entitlement but should reframe it in such a way as to foster the patient's adherence to the treatment regimen and working with the team. Frequent use of phrases such as "You deserve the best" can be very helpful (Muskin and Haase 2001). Taking a humble stance can be effective: "Understandably, Mr. Jones, you want the best care and certainly deserve no less—unfortunately, although we strive to provide you with the best care possible, we aren't perfect. We ask your indulgence to work with us so that we can give you the care that you deserve." Such statements can at times have a dramatic effect if delivered genuinely. Judicious use of "narcissistic strokes"— that is, providing opportunities for the patient to brag or show off—can assist in building rapport. Appropriate acknowledgment of mistakes made by the team and offering consultation by specialists can also assist in the management of these challenging patients. If the patient feels rec-

ognized as someone unique and special, he or she will feel reassured and will have less need to make demands (Heiskell and Pasnau 1991). The psychiatric consultant can assist members of the team not to take the patient's devaluations personally, but to understand them as the patient's frantic efforts to maintain self-esteem. If the caregivers can avoid feeling personally attacked, they will find it easier to work with these patients and will be less likely to engage in a counterattack.

Schizoid

Patients with a schizoid personality are seen as aloof, remote, and socially awkward or inhibited; they frequently avoid obtaining medical care until it is absolutely necessary (Kahana and Bibring 1964; Miller 2001). The physician charged with the care of the schizoid patient will find it difficult to build rapport or engage the patient in treatment.

At one end of the spectrum of this personality style are schizoid and avoidant personality disorders (Geringer and Stern 1986). These two personality disorders are distinguished in part by the apparent interest in social contact. The patient with schizoid personality disorder seems uninterested in social contact, whereas the patient with avoidant personality disorder desires social contact but avoids it out of fear of rejection. In the consultation setting, similar management tips apply to either of these two personality disorders and to patients who fall within this spectrum. In general, illness and hospitalization evoke a fear of intrusion and intense anxiety (Geringer and Stern 1986; Heiskell and Pasnau 1991). The physician should respect the patient's need for privacy but should prevent the patient from withdrawing completely (Gazzola and Muskin 2003). Maintaining a quiet, gentle interest in the patient and encouraging a regular, expectable routine can reassure the patient that he or she is safe and will not be intruded on (Miller 2001). Typically such patients have a fragile sense of self and therefore warrant gentle care, but care at a distance.

Summary of Personality Types

These seven prototypical personality styles cannot claim to capture every patient, and many patients fit into multiple categories. Understanding the common features of each style can aid the consulting psychiatrist. Knowing how each personality style experiences illness will inform interactions with such patients. Close monitoring of one's countertransference can also assist in identifying the patient's predominant personality style (e.g., feeling inferior with narcissistic patients or feeling attacked by paranoid patients). Knowledge of these personality types can assist the psychiatric consultant in educating the medical team about the proper management of these challenging patients and in assisting them not to react in counterproductive ways. At times, through understanding of the patient's personality style, the consulting psychiatrist is able to achieve rapid and remarkable therapeutic effects by choosing an appropriate intervention. Such effective interventions are impressive to nonpsychiatric physicians and staff members and demonstrate the utility of psychodynamic understanding in the psychiatric care of the medically ill.

Coping Styles

In the previous subsection, we illustrated how taking into account personality types can account for some of the interindividual variation in response to the stressors of illness. How individuals cope is another rich area of investigation (Jensen et al. 1991; Lazarus 1999; Penley et al. 2002), and problems in coping with illness have been shown to be a frequent reason for psychiatric consultation (Strain et al. 1993). Health psychologists have developed the concepts of appraisal (the assignment of meaning or value to a particular thing or event) and coping (Lazarus and Folkman 1984). An extensive body of literature developed over the past few decades has examined these processes among patients in health care settings. This psychological literature is often underrecognized by the psychiatric and medical communities but is extremely useful and can complement psychodynamic perspectives.

Coping can be defined as "thoughts and behaviors that the person uses to manage or alter the problem that is causing distress (problem-focused coping) and regulate the emotional response to the problem (emotion-focused coping)" (Folkman et al. 1993, pp. 409–410). A comprehensive review of the literature on the many defined coping strategies in medical illness is beyond the scope of this chapter. The reader is referred to the excellent reviews by Lazarus (1999) and Penley et al. (2002). Some important empirical generalizations that have emerged from decades of research on coping are discussed in this section (Lazarus 1999).

Use of Multiple Coping Styles in Stressful Situations

Folkman and colleagues (1986) identified eight categories of coping styles in a factor analysis of the Ways of Coping Questionnaire–Revised: 1) confrontative coping (hostile or aggressive efforts to alter a situation), 2) distancing (attempts to detach oneself mentally from a situation), 3) self-controlling (attempts to regulate one's feelings or actions), 4) seeking social support (efforts to seek emotional support or information from others), 5) accepting responsibility (acknowledgment of a personal role in the problem), 6) using escape-avoidance (cognitive or behavioral efforts to escape or avoid the problem or situation), 7) planful problem solving (deliberate and carefully thought-out efforts to alter the situation), and 8) conducting positive reappraisal (efforts to reframe the situation in a positive light) (Folkman et al. 1986; Penley et al. 2002). Research has shown that patients use multiple coping strategies in any given situation (Lazarus 1999). Individuals often prefer or habitually use certain strategies over others, but generally multiple strategies are used for a complex stressful situation such as a medical illness or hospitalization. People employ some trial and error in the selection of coping style (Lazarus 1999).

Coping as a Trait and a Process

Preferred coping styles are often tied to personality variables; sometimes they can be viewed as traits as well as processes (Heim et al. 1997; Lazarus 1999). Therefore, it is useful to ask patients how they previously dealt with very stressful situations. This can provide useful information for the physician, because patients are likely to use strategies in the present that are similar to those they used in the past, whether they were effective or not.

Research on women with breast cancer at various stages of illness has demonstrated that coping strategies may change as the nature of the stressor changes (Heim et al. 1993, 1997). For example, on initial detection of breast cancer, a woman may seek social support from her friends and spouse to cope with the uncertainties of her situation. Later, after lumpectomy and staging, she might shift her primary coping strategy to planful problem solving—a plan to follow up regularly for chemotherapy and to fully adhere to her oncologist's prescription of tamoxifen.

Problem-Focused Coping Versus Emotion-Focused Coping

One way in which various coping styles can be organized is whether they are problem focused or emotion focused. Research has shown that patients will tend to choose problem-focused coping strategies when they appraise the situation as being changeable or within their control (Folkman et al. 1993; Schussler 1992). In conditions considered out of their control, patients may choose emotion-focused coping styles (Folkman et al. 1993; Schussler 1992). In the medical setting, consulting psychiatrists can help change the patient's appraisal of the situation and encourage the patient to choose more adaptive coping styles. For example, if a patient newly diagnosed with diabetes mellitus misperceives high blood glucose as being unchangeable or out of his control, he might choose an emotion-focused coping strategy such as avoidance or denial. In educating this patient about how treatable hyperglycemia can be, the physician could encourage the patient to change his coping strategy to a problem-focused strategy such as making dietary changes or increasing exercise.

Variations in Usefulness of Coping Strategies Over Time

Coping is a powerful mediator of how a patient responds emotionally to a given stressor (Folkman and Lazarus 1988; Lipowski 1970). Coping strategies have also been demonstrated to have different effects on health outcomes—some positive, others negative (see Penley et al. 2002 for a meta-analysis on this research). Although some coping strategies may be considered more effective than others, they vary in usefulness depending on the situation. A strategy that is initially effective in dealing with a stressor may no longer be effective when the nature of the stressor changes (Penley et al. 2002). The discussion of maladaptive versus adaptive denial under "Denial" below illustrates this point.

Relationship Between Coping Styles and the Meaning of Illness

Lipowski (1970) described eight "illness concepts": 1) illness as challenge, 2) illness as enemy, 3) illness as punishment, 4) illness as weakness, 5) illness as relief, 6) illness as strategy, 7) illness as irreparable loss or damage, and 8) illness as value (Lipowski 1970). Lipowski proposed that a patient's choice of coping strategy is partially dependent on the underlying illness concept. In a study of 205 patients with chronic physical illness, the descriptors "illness as challenge/acceptance" and "illness as value" were found to be related to "adaptive coping and mental well-being." Conversely, "illness as enemy," "illness as punishment," and "illness as relief" were associated with psychological symptoms and maladaptive coping (Schussler 1992).

Defense Mechanisms

The psychoanalytic term *defense mechanism* was first described in the literature by Anna Freud in *The Ego and the Mechanisms of Defense* (Freud 1948). Defense mechanisms are automatic psychological processes by which the mind confronts a psychological threat (e.g., the fear of death or deformity) or conflict between a wish and the demands of reality or the dictates of conscience. There is

a rich history of this psychoanalytic concept that is beyond the scope of this chapter. Although there is some overlap of the concept of coping with that of defenses, the psychological concept of coping is more behavioral; it involves action (e.g., seeking social support, or productive problem solving) and is generally a conscious experience. Defenses are usually conceptualized as intrapsychic processes that are largely out of the individual's awareness. In *The Wisdom of the Ego*, George Vaillant (1993) emphasized the usefulness of the concept of defenses:

> Our lives are at times intolerable. At times we cannot bear reality. At such times our minds play tricks on us. Our minds distort inner and outer reality so that an observer might accuse us of denial, self-deception, even dishonesty. But such mental defenses creatively rearrange the sources of our conflict so that they become manageable and we may survive. The mind's defenses—like the body's immune mechanisms—protect us by providing a variety of illusions to filter pain and allow self-soothing. (p. 1)

He further noted that

> [a] clearly understood nomenclature of defenses not only enables us to understand adaptation to stress; it also offers us a means of uncoding, of translating if you will, much of what seems irrational in human behavior. (p. 28)

A basic understanding of the concept of defense and various defense mechanisms can provide the psychiatrist in the medical setting with another lens through which to examine a patient and to predict or explain the patient's emotional or behavioral responses to medical illness.

Vaillant (1993) identified a number of aspects of defenses:

1. *Defenses are generally outside of awareness of the individual or unconscious*—They enable the mind to "play tricks on" the individual to lessen distress or conflict.
2. *Defenses by nature distort inner and outer reality*—As is emphasized below, the degree of this distortion varies among various defense mechanisms, as does the focus of the distortion: some defenses distort a warded-off internal drive or desire, whereas others distort the external reality or interpersonal situation.
3. *Defenses can appear strange or overt to the observer while going unnoticed by the subject*—The psychiatrist must decide whether directing the patient's awareness to his or her use of certain defenses is indicated.
4. *Defenses are creative*—The mind creates a new perception distinct from reality.

5. *Defenses involve psychological conflict*—Through them the mind attempts to manage the often conflicting demands of inner wishes, conscience, other people, and reality.

6. *Defenses are adaptive and are not all pathological*—Some defenses are more adaptive than others, and the use of defenses is an inherent property of the mind.

Vaillant proposed a hierarchy of defense mechanisms ranked in four levels of adaptivity: psychotic, immature (or borderline), neurotic, and mature (Vaillant 1993). This hierarchy is based on the degree to which each defense distorts reality and how effectively it enables the expression of wishes or needs without untoward external consequences. Patients often employ many different defense mechanisms in different situations or under varying levels of stress. When a patient inflexibly and consistently uses lower-level defenses, this is often consistent with a personality disorder. Table 5–2 lists major defense mechanisms grouped into four levels.

The *psychotic defenses* are characterized by the extreme degree to which they distort external reality. Patients in psychotic states usually employ these defenses; psychotherapy is generally ineffective in altering them, and antipsychotic medication may be indicated.

The *immature defenses* are characteristic of patients with personality disorders, especially the cluster B personality disorders such as borderline personality disorder. Vaillant (1993) emphasized how many of these defenses are irritating to others and get under other people's skin. "Those afflicted with immature defenses often transmit their shame, impulses and anxiety to those around them" (p. 58).

In contrast to the immature defenses, the *neurotic defenses* do not typically irritate others and are more privately experienced—they are less interpersonal and often involve mental inhibitions. They distort reality less than immature or psychotic defenses and may go unnoticed by the observer. With appropriate tact and timing, neurotic defenses can be effectively interpreted in exploratory psychotherapy when it is considered appropriate by the treating psychiatrist. "Over the short haul, neurotic defenses make the user suffer; immature defenses make the observer suffer" (Vaillant 1993, p. 66).

The *mature defenses* "integrate sources of conflict... and thus require no interpretation" (Vaillant 1993, p. 67). The use of mature defenses such as humor or altruism in the confrontation of a stressor such as medical illness often earns admiration from others and can be inspirational. Such mature defenses are not interpreted by the psychiatrist but are praised. These defenses maximize expression of drives or wishes without negative consequences or distortion of reality.

Denial

Denial is an important and complex concept and a common reason that physicians request psychiatric consultation. Weisman and Hackett (1961) defined denial as "the conscious or unconscious repudiation of part or all of the total available meanings of an event to allay fear, anxiety, or other unpleasant affects" (p. 232). It is to be distinguished from a lack of awareness due to a cognitive deficit such as anosognosia or from the limited insight of a patient with chronic schizophrenia. Psychiatrists are often called to see a patient "in denial" about a newly diagnosed illness and may be asked to assess the patient's capacity to consent to or refuse certain treatments. As discussed below, denial can be adaptive, protecting the patient from being emotionally overwhelmed by an illness, or maladaptive, preventing or delaying diagnosis, treatment, and lifestyle changes.

Denial seems to be a very personal response that is prone to a double standard: we are often capable of—even comfortable with—ignoring our own denial but consider other people's denial abnormal. A smoker may minimize his risk of lung cancer, noting that only a small percentage of smokers get the disease, yet simultaneously criticize his son's obesity as a risk factor for diabetes. Physicians urge their patients to adopt healthy lifestyles yet may routinely overwork and get too little sleep (see Gaba and Howard 2002).

Psychiatrists are most likely to be called on when the patient's denial makes the physician uncomfortable, but health care providers use the term *denial* too often in a loose and inaccurate way (Goldbeck 1997; Havik and Maeland 1988; Jacobsen and Lowery 1992). A physician's statement that a patient is "in denial" may refer to a number of different situations: 1) the patient rejects the diagnosis, 2) the patient minimizes symptoms of the illness or does not seem to appreciate its implications, 3) the patient avoids or delays medical treatment, or 4) the patient appears to have no emotional reaction to the diagnosis or illness (Goldbeck 1997). The first task of the psychiatric consultant is to determine more specifically what the referring physician means by "denial."

The severity of denial varies by the nature of what is denied, by the predominant defense mechanisms at work (e.g., suppression, repression, psychotic denial), and by the degree of accessibility to consciousness (Goldbeck 1997). Patients using the mature defense of *suppression* in confronting an illness are not truly in denial. Rather, they have chosen to put aside their fears about illness and treatment until a later time. Their fears are not deeply unconscious but are easily accessible if patients choose to access them. These patients typically accept treatment,

TABLE 5–2.	Defense mechanisms
Mature defenses	
Suppression	Consciously putting a disturbing experience out of mind
Altruism	Vicarious but instinctively gratifying service to others
Humor	Overt expression of normally unacceptable feelings without unpleasant effect
Sublimation	Attenuated expression of drives in alternative fields without adverse consequences
Anticipation	Realistic planning for inevitable discomfort
Neurotic defenses	
Repression	Involuntary forgetting of a painful feeling or experience
Control	Manipulation of external events to avoid unconscious anxiety
Displacement	Transfer of an experienced feeling from one person to another or to something else
Reaction formation	Expression of unacceptable impulses as directly opposite attitudes and behaviors
Intellectualization	Replacing of feelings with facts/details
Rationalization	Inventing a convincing, but usually false, reason why one is not bothered
Isolation of affect	Separating a painful idea or event from feelings associated with it
Undoing	Ritualistic "removal" of an offensive act, sometimes by atoning for it
Immature defenses	
Splitting	Experiencing oneself and others as all good or all bad
Idealization	Seeing oneself or others as all-powerful, ideal, or godlike
Devaluation	Depreciating others
Projection	Attributing unacceptable impulses or ideas to others
Projective identification	Causing others to experience one's unacceptable feelings; one then fears or tries to control the unacceptable behavior in the other person
Acting out	Direct expression of an unconscious wish or impulse to avoid being conscious of the affect, and thoughts that accompany it
Passive aggression	Expressing anger indirectly and passively
Intermediate denial	Refusal to acknowledge painful realities

TABLE 5–2.	Defense mechanisms *(continued)*
Psychotic defenses	
Psychotic denial	Obliteration of external reality
Delusional projection	Externalization of inner conflicts and giving them tangible reality—minimal reality testing
Schizoid fantasy	Withdrawal from conflict into social isolation and fantasizing

Source.   Carlat 1999; Muskin and Haase 2001; Vaillant 1993.

face their illnesses with courage, and do not let their emotions overtake them. Such "denial" is considered adaptive (Druss and Douglas 1988). Many authors have proposed that some denial is perhaps necessary for very effective coping with an overwhelming illness (see discussions in Druss 1995; Ness and Ende 1994; Schussler 1992; Wool 1988).

In contrast to suppression, the patient using *repression* as a defense is generally unaware of the internal experience (fear, thought, wish, etc.) being warded off. Repressed thoughts or feelings are not easily accessible to consciousness. Such a patient may feel very anxious without understanding why. For example, a 39-year-old man whose father died of a myocardial infarction at age 41 may become increasingly anxious as his 40th birthday approaches without being aware of the connection.

When it is more severe and pervasive, denial can cause patients to flatly deny they are ill and to never seek health care. If they are already in care, they decline treatment or are nonadherent. Repeated attempts by the medical team to educate them about their illness have no impact. Extreme denial may be severe enough to distort the perception of reality, sometimes described as *psychotic denial*. Most patients with pervasive denial of illness are not psychotic in the usual sense of the word and should be distinguished from those who are. The latter usually have a psychotic illness such as schizophrenia and may pay no attention to signs or symptoms of illness or may incorporate them into somatic delusions. Psychotic patients who deny illness usually do not conceal its signs; others often readily recognize they are ill. In contrast, nonpsychotic patients with pervasive denial often conceal signs of their illness from themselves and others. For example, a nonpsychotic woman with pervasive denial of a growing breast mass avoided medical care and undressing in front of others and kept a bandage over what she regarded as a bruise. Although pregnancy is not a medical illness, a dramatic example of pervasive (sometimes psychotic) denial is the denial of pregnancy (see Chapter 33, "Obstetrics and Gynecology").

Strauss et al. (1990) proposed a new DSM diagnosis, maladaptive denial of physical illness, to describe patients whose denial of illness is maladaptive. How does one determine whether denial is adaptive or maladaptive? For the woman with a growing breast tumor, denial is clearly maladaptive because it has prevented her from receiving potentially life-saving treatment. In other situations denial may be quite adaptive. In determining the adaptivity of a patient's denial, it is important to answer the following questions (Goldbeck 1997):

1. Does the patient's denial impair or prevent the patient from receiving necessary treatment or lead to actions that endanger the patient's health? If so, then the denial is deemed maladaptive. In cases in which no effective treatment is available, the denial might be judged as adaptive to the extent that it decreases distress and improves quality of life, or it may be maladaptive if it prevents critical life planning (e.g., a single parent with little support and a terminal illness who has made no plans for his or her young children).

2. Which component of denial—denial of the facts of illness, denial of the implications of the illness, or denial of the emotional reaction to illness—does the patient exhibit? The latter two components of denial are not as maladaptive as the first component and may be adaptive in some situations. Denying the full implications of a disease, such as inevitable death, might be adaptive because it facilitates hope and improved quality of life. Likewise, denial of certain emotional reactions to the illness such as fear or hopelessness might enable a patient to stay motivated through a completed course of treatment.

3. Is the denial a temporary means of "buying time" to gradually accept a diagnosis so that the immediate impact is not so overwhelming, or has the denial been so protracted that it has prevented adaptive action? Many patients are unable to immediately accept a diagnosis, and denial may be a way for them to slowly adjust their emotional distress during a period of gradual acceptance. In many situations this would be considered adaptive.

Even when denial is adaptive for the patient, it may bother physicians or other caregivers. The following case example illustrates this point.

A psychiatric consultation was requested for a 24-year-old man who was quadriplegic after a gunshot wound to the spine. The physician was insistent that the patient's denial be "broken through" because the patient was convinced he would walk again. The patient demonstrated a thorough understanding of his condition and maintained that his hard work and faith would restore his physical abilities. The physician was concerned that the patient might commit suicide when he realized that there was no chance of recovery of function. Instead of forcing the patient to face the prognosis, the consultant recommended that the physician offer the patient training in the skills necessary to maintain himself in his current state, because recovery, in whatever form it took, would take a considerable amount of time. The patient continued to cooperate with physical therapy, learned how to use a motorized wheelchair, and discussed the plans for his living arrangements. The physician felt comfortable with this approach because it was "realistic."

All too often, physicians misjudge patients as being in denial. This tends to occur with three types of patients: 1) patients without an overt emotional reaction to an illness or diagnosis, 2) patients whose reactions differ from those expected by their caregivers, and 3) patients who have been inadequately informed about their illness. The absence of an overt reaction to medical illness is a style of psychological response. Although it is not evident to an observer, individuals may actually be aware of their emotions and thoughts about their illness. Some physicians have a tendency to misjudge patients as being in denial who do not express an expected emotional response or who seek alternative treatments than those recommended by the physician (Cousins 1982). An obsessional middle-aged accountant in the coronary care unit, for example, may be acutely aware of his condition and may be quite concerned about it, yet he may not express any of the fears or anxiety that his caregivers would expect, appearing calm and hopeful. This patient is not denying his illness but may be considered to be doing so by caregivers because he "looks too relaxed and in too good a mood."

One must ensure that patients are fully informed about their illness and treatment before assessing patients as being in denial. Gattelari et al. (1999) demonstrated that a portion of patients judged by their caregivers to be using denial were in fact relatively uninformed about the details of their illness or its prognosis. On the other hand, some patients who say they have not been informed have in fact been repeatedly educated by their health care professionals and are really in denial.

Studies of the impact of denial on medical outcomes have found both beneficial and adverse effects. It is a literature with several methodological limitations, including sometimes failing to clearly define how denial was measured, treating denial as an all-or-nothing phenomenon, and using a lack of observable negative affect as a primary indicator of denial (problematic for the reasons discussed above). The use of different measures of denial and distinct patient populations makes comparisons across studies very difficult (Goldbeck 1997).

A number of studies have demonstrated positive effects of denial of physical illness on outcome. Hackett and Cassem (1974) found that "major deniers" in coronary care units after myocardial infarction had a better outcome than "minor deniers." Levenson et al. (1989) demonstrated that among patients with unstable angina, "high deniers" had fewer episodes of angina and more favorable outcomes than "low deniers." Other studies suggest that denial is useful for specific clinical situations such as elective surgery (Cohen and Lazarus 1973) and wound healing (Marucha et al. 1998). Denial was associated with better survival rates in a small study of patients awaiting heart transplantation (Young et al. 1991).

Other research studies have found a mixed or negative impact of denial on medical outcome. "Major deniers" have shorter stays in the intensive care unit but are more likely to be noncompliant after discharge (Levine et al. 1987). Greater denial was associated with a worse medical outcome but was associated with decreased mood symptoms and sleep problems in patients with end-stage renal disease (Fricchione et al. 1992). Denial may be counterproductive in asthma patients (Staudenmeyer et al. 1979). Croog et al. (1971) noted lower treatment adherence among deniers in their large sample of myocardial infarct patients. In a study of women scheduled for breast biopsy, those with a history of habitual use of denial were observed to have been more likely to delay medical evaluation (Greer 1974).

When denial is present and is assessed as maladaptive, interventions should usually be directed toward the underlying emotions provoking the denial (e.g., fear). Direct confrontation of denial should be generally avoided because it is counterproductive (Ness and Ende 1994; Perry and Viederman 1981). For example, a 17-year-old adolescent who is newly diagnosed with diabetes mellitus may not want to accept this diagnosis and the need for changes in his lifestyle because of his painful memories of seeing other family members suffer through complications of diabetes. The physician may be tempted to frighten the patient into compliance with a statement such as, "If you don't change your diet, measure your blood sugar, and take insulin regularly, you will wind up with complications just like your mother's." Such statements are usually counterproductive because they increase anxiety, which is driving the patient's use of denial in the first place. Instead, a gentle, empathic, and nonjudgmental stance is more effective (Ness and Ende 1994). Diminishing the intensity of negative affects such as anxiety through psychopharmacological or psychotherapeutic interventions can also be helpful because these affects may be driving the patient's need for denial.

In addition, the consulting psychiatrist should consider whether a patient's maladaptive denial is fostered by particular interpersonal relationships, such as those with family members, friends, a religious community, physicians, or other caregivers (Goldbeck 1997). In such cases, interventions aimed solely at the individual patient's denial without addressing the reinforcing interpersonal relationships are likely to be unsuccessful.

Emotional Responses to Medical Illness

Psychiatrists in the medical setting are frequently called on to help a patient manage emotional responses to illness and hospitalization (e.g., anger, fear, grief, shame). Usually the patient's emotional response is identified in the consultation request. For example, "Please come see this 25-year-old man just diagnosed with testicular cancer who is angry and refusing treatment." The 25-year-old man's internist cannot understand why he would refuse the very treatment needed to treat (and possibly cure) his testicular cancer. With an understanding of the patient's subjective experience of his illness, his predominant coping styles, and his prominent defense mechanisms, the consulting psychiatrist can help the patient and his internist to understand his anger, facilitating an alliance with which treatment is more likely to be accepted.

Because every patient is unique, empathic listening to a patient's story of his or her illness will reveal the predominant emotional response, which is a potential clue to the subjective meaning of illness for that patient (Lazarus 1999). Core relational themes for the most common emotions (Lazarus 1999) can serve as hypotheses about the meaning of the illness for the patient (Table 5–3). An illness can evoke multiple emotional responses simultaneously or sequentially. The illness may have multiple meanings, and the meanings may change over the course of the illness. The predominant emotional response should not be the sole focus of the psychiatrist's attention (although it may demand the most attention). For example, the 25-year-old man just diagnosed with testicular cancer is markedly angry and refuses treatment. One can hypothesize that it might be because he feels frightened, weakened, or emasculated or that he fears castration. In viewing the physician as the bearer of bad news, the patient is not only angry at having been diagnosed with cancer but also angry at his physician. Accepting and attempting to understand the patient's anger aids the psychiatrist in giving this man permission to express his feelings while tactfully helping him to see that he can do so without forgoing his own treatment. The patient's refusal of treatment may be also determined by fear of what the treatment will involve. The psychiatrist might also

TABLE 5–3.   Core relational themes underlying affective responses

Anger	A demeaning offense against me and mine
Anxiety	Facing uncertain, existential threat
Fright	An immediate, concrete, and overwhelming danger
Guilt	Having transgressed a moral imperative
Shame	Failing to live up to an ego ideal
Sadness	Having experienced an irrevocable loss
Happiness	Making reasonable progress toward the realization of a goal
Envy	Wanting what someone else has
Relief	A distressing goal-incongruent condition that has changed for the better or gone away
Hope	Fearing the worst but yearning for better

Source.   Reprinted from *Emotion and Adaptation* by Richard S. Lazarus, copyright © 1991 by Oxford University Press, Inc. Used by permission of Oxford University Press, Inc.

work with the oncologist and his or her response to the patient's anger. Education by the physicians about the treatment options and the high likelihood of cure could dramatically shift the patient's emotional and behavioral responses and evoke relief and hope. Assisting the patient in naming his emotional responses and understanding *why* they are present can help the patient feel understood. This can facilitate the acceptance of an individualized treatment plan that appropriately involves medication, psychotherapy, psychoeducation, or other interventions.

Anger

Anger is a common emotional response to medical illness and may be the most difficult emotional response for physicians to confront. This is particularly true when the anger is directed toward them or is expressed as treatment refusal. Patients with paranoid, narcissistic, borderline, or antisocial personality styles or disorders are particularly likely to express anger in the face of medical illness (Muskin and Haase 2001). Common reflexive reactions include counterattacking or distancing oneself from the patient. The psychiatrist who is skilled in psychosomatic medicine will convey appropriate empathy along with necessary limit setting for the angry patient. Many maneuvers are possible, such as a tactful redirection of the patient's anger toward more productive targets (e.g., away from refusal of treatment and toward planning with the oncologist to attack the illness through potentially curative chemotherapy). Helping the team respond appropriately to the patient is just as important. Viewing expressed

anger as natural and diffusing the intensity of affect can help to reestablish collaborative relationships with the patient.

Anxiety and Fear

Some degree of anxiety is likely to be experienced universally by patients in the medical setting (Lloyd 1977). The degree of anxiety varies tremendously by individual and by situation. Patients with premorbid anxiety disorders are more likely to experience severe anxiety when confronted with medical illness. The patient with a dependent personality style may experience acute anxiety on hospitalization when faced with separation from his or her support system. The obsessional patient is likely to become anxious if the treatment plan or diagnosis remains unclear. The intrusiveness of the medical setting may evoke anxiety in the schizoid patient.

Psychotherapies, education regarding the illness and treatments, and judicious use of medication can greatly diminish the patient's anxiety (Perry and Viederman 1981). Although fear (usually involving a specific threat or danger) and anxiety (the feeling of nervousness or apprehension experienced on facing uncertain threats) are distinct emotions, they are often managed similarly. It is important to specifically elicit what the patient fears—pain, death, abandonment, disfigurement, dependence, disability, etc. Blanket reassurance is usually ineffective and may actually be detrimental because the patient may perceive it as unempathic, superficial, false, or patronizing. Empathy and reassurance tailored to the patient's specific fears can offer significant relief (Perry and Viederman 1981).

Sadness

Sadness is evoked in situations where there is a loss (Lloyd 1977). Medical illness can lead to multiple types of loss: loss of physical function or social role, loss of ability to work, loss of the pursuit of a goal or dream, or loss of a part of one's body. Internal losses of organs or organ functions can be as significant as external losses such as amputation of a limb. Patients with untreated mood disorders may be more likely to develop clinically significant depression in the face of medical illness. Sadness may be the primary manifestation of an adjustment disorder, which is common in medically ill patients (Strain et al. 1998). Drawing an analogy to the process of mourning is often appropriate and helps to normalize the patient's sadness (Fitzpatrick 1999). Mourning a loss takes time, a fact that is often neglected in medical settings. It is important for the physician to convey a sense of appropriate hope. Describing true examples of other patients' positive outcomes in similar situations can often be helpful. Even when the patient's sadness represents a normal grieflike reaction, physicians are often tempted to prescribe antidepressant medication, desiring to make the patient feel better. In such cases, the psychosomatic medicine specialist can redirect the treatment plan to interventions that are more likely to be helpful, such as psychotherapy, pastoral care, and—often most important—more time speaking with the primary treating physician.

Guilt

Some patients experience illness as a punishment for real or imagined sins. Clarifying that illness is not the patient's fault—and thereby confronting the guilt—is a helpful technique. Patients may also experience guilt related to earlier or current illness-promoting behaviors such as smoking cigarettes, nonadherence to medication regimens, or risky sexual practices. Education of family members can be critical if they blame the patient inappropriately for the illness. If the patient is religious, counseling from a hospital chaplain or the appropriate clergy member should be considered.

Shame

Illness is universally experienced as narcissistic injury to some degree. Narcissistic patients are more susceptible to experiencing shame in the face of medical illness. Patients who view their illness as a result of earlier behaviors—such as contracting HIV through impulsive sexual liaisons, or developing lung cancer after a long history of smoking—may experience shame in the medical setting. It is important for physicians to take a nonjudgmental stance and avoid blaming patients for their illnesses. Critical, disapproving responses are counterproductive, heighten patients' shame, and frequently lead to treatment avoidance. For example, the noncompliant diabetic patient who is repeatedly admitted to the hospital for diabetic ketoacidosis frustrates her doctors and nurses. They are often tempted to scold the patient, thinking that this is necessary to avoid colluding with her acting-out and failure to take her disease seriously. Such responses are typically humiliating for the patient, are ineffective in motivating behavior change, and often worsen the vicious cycle of noncompliance.

Behavioral Responses to Illness

Patients' behavioral responses to illness vary tremendously within a spectrum ranging from maladaptive to adaptive. Adaptive responses may simply warrant encour-

agement or praise. Psychiatrists in the medical setting are often asked to see patients whose behavioral responses to illness or hospitalization are maladaptive and are interfering with their treatment. In understanding the patient's subjective experience, personality style, defense mechanisms, and coping strategies, one can design therapeutic interventions to help change the patient's responses to more adaptive behaviors. This section highlights a few of the common behavioral responses to illness.

Adaptive Responses

Support Seeking

Facing a new medical illness or hospitalization can be highly taxing for even the most well-adapted individual. Patients who are fortunate to have well-developed social support networks can benefit greatly from support from friends and family. Patients with conflicts about dependency might have more difficulty with this task, and psychotherapy can normalize this need and assist patients in reaching out to others. Referral to patient support groups can also be helpful for many patients; they can learn from the experiences of others facing the same illness and can feel less alone or alienated from other people. Information about self-help organizations can be obtained from various sources on the Internet, such as Dr. John Grohl's "Psych Central" Web site (http://psychcentral.com) and the "Self-Help Group Sourcebook Online" of the American Self-Help Group Clearinghouse (http://mentalhelp.net/selfhelp).

Altruism

Altruistic behavior such as volunteering to raise money for breast cancer, becoming a transplant advocate who meets with preoperative patients and shares experiences with them, or participating in an AIDS walkathon can represent a highly adaptive response to illness. One of the common stresses of illness is the impact on an individual's self-esteem and sense of productivity. Through helping others, patients feel a sense of purpose and gratification that can help improve their mood. Generally, the consulting psychiatrist needs only to support and encourage such behaviors. For many patients with severe illnesses, voluntary participation in research can have the same effect. Particularly for those with terminal illness, participation in research can provide a sense of purpose and hope by contributing to the potential for new treatment options in the future.

Epiphany Regarding Life Priorities

Although no one would generally claim that a medical illness is beneficial for the affected individual, it often helps patients regain perspective on what is most important to them in life. Normal daily hassles of living may no longer seem as stressful, and some patients facing a serious illness experience an epiphany and dramatically change their lives for the better. Patient narratives of the life-affirming effects of illness and stories of personal growth abound in literature (Druss 1995). At times, the consultation psychiatrist can witness and support a patient through a personal transformation. A 47-year-old male executive recently diagnosed with a myocardial infarction may dramatically change his diet, embark on a new exercise regimen, and reconfigure his role at work to reduce emotional stress. Similarly, a woman newly diagnosed with HIV who commits herself to taking her medications regularly, seeks treatment for substance use, and rejoins her church also exemplifies this phenomenon.

There can be great opportunities for effective psychotherapy in the medically ill, because patients are under tremendous stress when faced with serious medical illness, and the usual distractions of their daily lives no longer dominate their thoughts. Sometimes a therapeutic alliance can form and work can progress more rapidly than is typical in other settings (Muskin 1990).

Becoming an Expert in One's Illness

For the obsessional patient in particular, learning as much as possible about the illness can be adaptive and can give the individual a greater sense of control. Although the information itself may not be positive, patients often find that reality can seem more manageable than their imagined fears. However, this response to illness is not appealing to all patients. Some will prefer to put their trust in their physicians and to not know everything. The psychiatrist armed with an understanding of the patient's personality style and characteristic coping styles and defense mechanisms will be able to know whether or not increased information and knowledge might reduce the patient's distress and augment a sense of control.

Maladaptive Responses: Nonadherence to Treatment Regimens

Treatment nonadherence is more common than most physicians recognize. It has been estimated that up to 50% of patients fail to adhere to their prescribed medication regimens (Sackett and Haynes 1976). Patients typically overestimate their own adherence to the treatment, and physicians are often unaware of their patients' lack of adherence (Levenson 1998). Physicians working in all medical settings witness the negative effects of nonadherence, and psychiatrists are frequently called on to see

problem patients who are repetitively noncompliant. For such cases the consulting psychiatrist is often cast in the role of disciplinarian, detective, or magician; medical colleagues may expect the psychiatrist's interventions to bring rapid change to the patient's adherence patterns. Although it is possible in some cases, this scenario is typically unrealistic. It is possible to undertake interventions that improve patient adherence when the underlying factors accounting for nonadherence are correctly identified and addressed.

There are numerous reasons why patients do not fully adhere with treatment regimens. Psychiatric disorders and psychological motivations are not the only factors that may be involved. Other factors, such as cost, side effects, and treatment complexity, may play a role. It is important to determine the degree of a patient's nonadherence and its context. Is the patient occasionally or consistently nonadherent? Is the nonadherence specific to a certain medication or type of recommendation (e.g., dieting), or is it more generalized across different treatments and different physicians? Identifying the context of nonadherence can provide clues to the underlying factors involved when the patient cannot directly give the reasons for nonadherence. In this section we identify some of the most common reasons for treatment nonadherence and offer 11 general principles for management of this common clinical problem.

Psychologically Motivated Factors for Nonadherence

Perry and Viederman (1981) outlined a number of distinct psychological reasons why patients do not adhere with treatment recommendations. One reason they discuss is nonadherence to defend against humiliation (Perry and Viederman 1981). Rather than accept the stigma of his illness, a patient with HIV might stop his medications, which remind him daily of his illness. Active empathic work to counteract the illness concepts that cause shame can diminish this motivation for treatment nonadherence.

Another psychological motivation for nonadherence is to counteract a feeling of helplessness (Perry and Viederman 1981). An adolescent with newly diagnosed diabetes mellitus who is struggling with a developmentally appropriate desire to gain autonomy may believe that the only way to feel autonomous and in control is to rebel against her parents and caregivers by not taking insulin. Such nonadherence may also be motivated by the wish to be healthy like her peers.

Anger toward the treating physician or toward the illness or diagnosis itself may be another psychological motivator for treatment nonadherence, whether the anger is appropriate to the situation or is a product of character pathology. Varying degrees of denial may also be involved. Specific interventions for clinical situations in which anger and denial are primary motivators for nonadherence were discussed earlier in this chapter in the section "Denial" and in the subsection "Anger" under "Emotional Responses to Medical Illness."

Patients' trust in the physicians recommending their treatment is an important determinant of their likelihood of complying with the treatment regimen. Physicians must earn their patients' trust through building rapport and direct, honest communication. Patients with psychotic disorders or significant character pathology might have particular difficulty placing trust in their caregivers. Mistrust and paranoia may play a role in these patients' compliance with treatment regimens.

Comorbid Psychiatric Disorders and Nonadherence

Comorbid psychiatric disorders may also lead to treatment nonadherence. Affective disorders are particularly common. Depressed patients may not have the motivation, concentration, or energy required to fully comply with treatment recommendations. They might even stop treatment as an indirect means of attempting suicide. Manic patients may believe they no longer need treatment, may abuse substances, or may become disorganized or psychotic. Psychotic disorders, anxiety disorders, substance use disorders, and cognitive disorders are other psychiatric conditions that often play a role in treatment nonadherence. Therefore, a thorough psychiatric history and comprehensive review of symptoms are essential parts of the evaluation of the noncompliant patient.

Other Factors in Nonadherence

Nonadherence may be due to reality factors rather than psychological motivations. Cost of treatment, side effects (whether feared or experienced), and complicated or inconvenient medication dosing schedules are treatment-specific factors that should be considered. Other practical barriers, such as difficulties with transportation, inflexible and lengthy work schedules, or child-care responsibilities, may preclude consistent keeping of appointments (Levenson 1998).

A lack of information about the illness or its treatment should always be ruled out as a factor in nonadherence. Patients should understand their illness, their treatment options, and the reasons that treatment is necessary. Patient education should always be provided in the patient's primary language to ensure full understanding. To assess patient understanding, physicians should ask patients to repeat and to explain in their own words what they have been told about their illness. If possible, family members should be involved in the education. Written materials or visual materials may be helpful tools in patient education.

Incongruities between the health beliefs of patients and their physicians can also account for nonadherence and should be identified (Gaw 2001). Physicians of all disciplines must make an effort to understand their patients' cultural and religious backgrounds, paying particular attention to patients' beliefs and values about health and illness. Physicians should attempt to elicit their patients' explanatory models about diseases and the effects of treatments. When possible, attempts can be made to explain treatment plans within patients' explanatory models for illness and treatment. Or, at the least, mutual acknowledgment and acceptance of the differences between the explanatory models of the physician and the patient may facilitate treatment adherence and build doctor–patient rapport. When they feel that their caregivers accept and understand their cultural or religious beliefs, patients will also be more likely to voluntarily report their concomitant use of alternative or herbal treatments.

Interventions to Increase Treatment Adherence

The following general principles may assist the physician in facilitating greater patient adherence with treatment regimens (Becker and Maiman 1980; Chen 1991; Gaw 2001; Levenson 1998):

1. Ask patients directly about their adherence, maintaining a nonjudgmental stance. Design a collaborative plan to increase adherence. Normalizing statements and questions—such as "Many patients find it difficult to take their medications on a regular basis. Have you had this experience?"—are more effective in eliciting information about treatment adherence than questions such as "You've been taking your medication regularly, right?"
2. Ensure that patients are fully informed about their illness and treatments.
3. Rule out cognitive deficits (e.g., mental retardation or dementia), because they may play a role in nonadherence.
4. Uncover any underlying psychological motivating factors for nonadherence and address them specifically.
5. Diagnose and treat any comorbid psychiatric disorders.
6. Minimize treatment-related factors for nonadherence, such as side effects and cost and complexity of treatment regimens, when possible.

7. Identify, acknowledge, and contend with any cultural reasons for nonadherence.

8. Avoid shaming, scolding, or frightening the patient. Scolding patients or scaring them with statements such as "If you don't take your medications, you could have a heart attack and die!" is almost always counterproductive (Heiskell and Pasnau 1991). Such statements may shame patients or inflate their fears and can increase the likelihood that they will not return for treatment.

9. Use positive reinforcement as a motivator when possible, because it is generally more effective than negative reinforcement at facilitating behavior change.

10. Involve family members in facilitating patient treatment adherence when they are "on board" with the treatment plan.

11. Attend to doctor–patient rapport and build an effective treatment alliance.

Maladaptive Responses: Signing Out Against Medical Advice

A common reason for urgent psychiatric consultation in the medical hospital is a patient threatening to sign out against medical advice. Of all hospital discharges in the United States, 0.8%–2% are against medical advice (Hwang et al. 2003; Jeremiah et al. 1995; Weingart et al. 1998). Often the psychiatrist is asked to assess the decisional capacity of a patient who wants to sign out against medical advice. Legal aspects of this important assessment are discussed in Chapter 3, "Legal Issues." The patient's threat to sign out is usually not truly motivated by a primary desire to leave but more often reflects another agenda, intense affect, or interpersonal friction with physicians or nursing staff. In some cases, it is a means of expressing anger or frustration toward caregivers (Albert and Kornfeld 1973).

The motivations for signing out against medical advice vary significantly and are similar to those motivating treatment nonadherence. Among the more common motivations are 1) anger at caregivers or dissatisfaction with the treatment received (whether legitimate or partly due to character pathology); 2) overwhelming fear or anxiety; 3) substance craving or withdrawal (sometimes due to the medical team's inadequate use of prophylactic medications such as benzodiazepines or nicotine patches); 4) delirium or dementia; 5) psychosis or paranoia; 6) desire to leave the hospital to attend to outside responsibilities (e.g., child care, work, court dates, or a pet at home alone); and 7) impatience with discharge planning or feeling well enough to leave. In a classic study of patients threatening to sign out against medical advice, the most common underlying motivations were overwhelming fear, anger, and psychosis or confusion (Albert and Kornfeld 1973). In most cases there had been a progressive increase in the patient's distress for days before the threat to sign out that had not been recognized or addressed adequately (Albert and Kornfeld 1973).

Among interventions, *empathic listening* to the patient's frustrations is critical, in that it provides an opportunity for the patient to ventilate frustrations and to feel understood. Empathic listening will often have a dramatic de-escalating effect and will enable the team to re-engage the patient in treatment. The psychiatrist can also intervene in assisting the team to better understand a patient's behavior so as to diminish the patient's feelings of anger and frustration. Other guidelines for intervention are the following:

1. Understand the threat as a communication—Does the patient really want to leave, or is he or she expressing frustration, anger, anxiety, or another affect?

2. If the patient is justifiably angry, apologize on behalf of the system or hospital.

3. Avoid scare tactics or direct confrontation of denial, because these techniques are generally counterproductive.

4. Design interventions using an understanding of the patient's personality type.

5. Diagnose and treat any comorbid psychiatric disorders.

6. Involve social supports (if they are allied with the treatment plan).

7. Ensure that the patient is adequately informed about the illness and its need for treatment.

8. Assess the patient's capacity to sign out, if indicated (discussed further in Chapter 3, "Legal Issues").

9. When patients still sign out against medical advice, encourage them to return for treatment if they change their mind.

Conclusion

How does one integrate these various theoretical concepts into the consultation process? How do the psychological responses to illness guide the consultant to efficiently use his or her time to understand the situation and make useful suggestions? We are aware of no magic formula, but we believe that experienced consultants use their knowledge of human behavior and concepts such as personality types, coping styles, and defense mechanisms to understand their patients and to intervene. Opportunities abound in the medical setting for psychiatric interventions, which can dramatically modify patients' psychological responses to illness. The key to these interventions lies in the development of an understanding of the patient's subjective experience of illness. A curious inquiry into the internal experience of a patient facing medical illness and the appropriate conveyance of empathy will generally be rewarded. We hope the framework, concepts, and guidelines presented in this chapter will prove useful in assisting psychiatrists who have chosen to work with patients in medical settings.

References

Albert HD, Kornfeld DS: The threat to sign out against medical advice. Ann Intern Med 79:888–891, 1973

American Psychiatric Association: Diagnostic and Statistical Manual of Mental Disorders, 4th Edition, Text Revision. Washington, DC, American Psychiatric Association, 2000

Becker MH, Maiman LA: Strategies for enhancing patient compliance. J Community Health 6:113–135, 1980

Bornstein RF: Adaptive and maladaptive aspects of dependency: an integrative review. Am J Orthopsychiatry 64:622–634, 1994

Carlat DJ: The Psychiatric Interview: A Practical Guide. Philadelphia, PA, Lippincott Williams & Wilkins, 1999

Chen A: Noncompliance in community psychiatry: a review of clinical interventions. Hosp Community Psychiatry 42:282–286, 1991

Cohen F, Lazarus RS: Active coping processes, coping dispositions, and recovery from surgery. Psychosom Med 35:375–398, 1973

Cousins N: Denial: are sharper definitions needed? JAMA 248:210–212, 1982

Cousins N: The Healing Heart. New York, WW Norton, 1983

Croog SH, Shapiro DS, Levine S: Denial among male heart patients: an empirical study. Psychosom Med 33:385–397, 1971

Douglas CJ, Druss RG: Denial of illness: a reappraisal. Gen Hosp Psychiatry 9:53–57, 1987

Druss RG: The Psychology of Illness: In Sickness and in Health. Washington, DC, American Psychiatric Press, 1995

Druss RG, Douglas C: Adaptive responses to illness and disability. Gen Hosp Psychiatry 10:163–168, 1988

Fitzpatrick MC: The psychologic assessment and psychosocial recovery of the patient with an amputation. Clin Orthop 361:98–107, 1999

Folkman S, Lazarus R: The relationship between coping and emotion: implications for theory and research. Soc Sci Med 26:309–317, 1988

Folkman S, Lazarus R, Dunkel-Schetter C, et al: The dynamics of a stressful encounter: cognitive appraisal, coping and encounter outcomes. J Pers Soc Psychol 50:992–1003, 1986

Folkman S, Chesney M, Pollack L, et al: Stress, control, coping and depressive mood in human immunodeficiency virus–positive and –negative gay men in San Francisco. J Nerv Ment Dis 181:409–416, 1993

Freud A: The Ego and the Mechanisms of Defence. London, Hogarth Press, 1948

Fricchione GL, Howanitz E, Jandorf L, et al: Psychological adjustment to end-stage renal disease and the implications of denial. Psychosomatics 33:85–91, 1992

Gaba DM, Howard SK: Fatigue among clinicians and the safety of patients. N Engl J Med 347:1249–1255, 2002

Gattelari M, Butow PN, Tattersall HN, et al: Misunderstanding in cancer patients: why shoot the messenger? Ann Oncol 10:39–46, 1999

Gaw AC: Concise Guide to Cross-Cultural Psychiatry. Washington, DC, American Psychiatric Publishing, 2001

Gazzola L, Muskin PR: The impact of stress and the objectives of psychosocial interventions, in Psychosocial Treatment for Medical Conditions: Principles and Techniques. Edited by Schein LA, Bernard HS, Spitz HI, Muskin PR. New York, Brunner-Routledge, 2003, pp 373–406

Geringer ES, Stern T: Coping with medical illness: the impact of personality types. Psychosomatics 27:251–261, 1986

Goldbeck R: Denial in physical illness. J Psychosom Res 43:575–593, 1997

Greer S: Delay in the treatment of breast cancer. Proc R Soc Med 6:470–473, 1974

Groves JE: Taking care of the hateful patient. N Engl J Med 298:883–888, 1978

Hackett TP, Cassem NH: Development of a quantitative rating scale to assess denial. J Psychosom Res 18:93–100, 1974

Havik OE, Maeland J: Verbal denial and outcome in myocardial infarction patients. J Psychosom Res 32:145–157, 1988

Heim E, Augustiny KF, Schaffner L, et al: Coping with breast cancer over time and situation. J Psychosom Res 37:523–542, 1993

Heim E, Valach L, Schaffner L: Coping and psychological adaptation: longitudinal effects over time and stage in breast cancer. Psychosom Med 59:408–418, 1997

Heiskell LE, Pasnau RO: Psychological reaction to hospitalization and illness in the emergency department. Emerg Med Clin North Am 9:207–218, 1991

Holmes TH, Rahe RH: The social readjustment rating scale. J Psychosom Res 11:213–218, 1967

Hwang SW, Li J, Gupta R, et al: What happens to patients who leave hospital against medical advice? CMAJ 168:417–420, 2003

Jacobsen BS, Lowery BJ: Further analysis of the psychometric properties of the Levine Denial of Illness Scale. Psychosom Med 54:372–381, 1992

Jensen MP, Turner JA, Romano, KM, et al: Coping with chronic pain: a critical review of the literature. Pain 47:249–283, 1991

Jeremiah J, O'Sullivan P, Stein MD: Who leaves against medical advice?

Kahana RJ, Bibring G: Personality types in medical management, in Psychiatry and Medical Practice in a General Hospital. Edited by Zinberg NE. New York, International Universities Press, 1964, pp 108–123

Kiely WF: Coping with severe illness. Adv Psychosom Med 8:105–118, 1972

Kornfeld DS: The hospital environment: its impact on the patient. Adv Psychosom Med 8:252–270, 1972

Kubler-Ross E: On Death and Dying. New York, Macmillan, 1969

Lazarus RS: Stress and Emotion: A New Synthesis. New York, Springer, 1999

Lazarus RS, Folkman S: Stress, Appraisal and Coping. New York, Springer, 1984

Levenson JL: Psychiatric aspects of medical practice, in Clinical Psychiatry for Medical Students, 3rd Edition. Edited by Stoudemire A. Philadelphia, PA, Lippincott-Raven, 1998, pp 727–763

Levenson JL, Mishra A, Hamer RM, et al: Denial and medical outcome in unstable angina. Psychosom Med 51:27–35, 1989

Levine J, Warrenberg S, Kerns R, et al: The role of denial in recovery from coronary heart disease. Psychosom Med 49:109–117, 1987

Lipowski ZJ: Physical illness, the individual and the coping process. Psychiatry Med 1:91–102, 1970

Lipowski ZJ: Psychiatry of somatic diseases: epidemiology, pathogenesis, classification. Compr Psychiatry 16:105–124, 1975

Lloyd G: Psychological reactions to physical illness. Br J Hosp Med 18:352–358, 1977

Marucha PT, Kiecolt-Glaser JK, Favagehi M: Mucosal wound healing is impaired by examination stress. Psychosom Med 60:362–365, 1998

Miller MC: Personality disorders. Med Clin North Am 85:819–837, 2001

Muskin PR: The combined use of psychotherapy and pharmacotherapy in the medical setting. Psychiatr Clin North Am 13:341–353, 1990

Muskin PR: The medical hospital, in Psychodynamic Concepts in General Psychiatry. Edited by Schwartz HJ, Bleiberg E, Weissman SH. Washington, DC, American Psychiatric Press, 1995

Muskin PR, Haase EK: Difficult patients and patients with personality disorders, in Textbook of Primary Care Medicine, 3rd Edition. Edited by Noble J et al. St Louis, MO, Mosby, 2001, pp 458–464

Ness DE, Ende J: Denial in the medical interview. JAMA 272:1777–1781, 1994

Oldham JM, Skodol AE: Charting the future of Axis II. J Personal Disord 14:17–29, 2000

Patterson DR, Everett JJ, Bombardier CH, et al: Psychological effects of severe burn injuries. Psychol Bull 113:362–378, 1993

Penley JA, Tomaka J, Wiebe JS: The association of coping to physical and psychological health outcomes: a meta-analytic review. J Behav Med 25:551–603, 2002

Perry S, Viederman M: Management of emotional reactions to acute medical illness. Med Clin North Am 65:3–14, 1981

Peterson BH: Psychological reactions to acute physical illness in adults. Med J Aust 1(9):311–316, 1974

Sackett DL, Haynes RB (eds): Compliance With Therapeutic Regimens. Baltimore, MD, Johns Hopkins University Press, 1976

Schussler G: Coping strategies and individual meanings of illness. Soc Sci Med 34:427–432, 1992

Sensky T: Causal attributions in physical illness. J Psychosom Res 43:565–573, 1997

Staudenmeyer H, Kinsman RS, Dirks JF, et al: Medical outcome in asthmatic patients: effects of airways hyperactivity and symptom-focused anxiety. Psychosom Med 41:109–118, 1979

Strain JJ, Grossman S: Psychological reactions to medical illness and hospitalization, in Psychological Care of the Medically Ill: A Primer in Liaison Psychiatry. New York, Appleton-Century-Crofts, 1975, pp 23–36

Strain J, Hammer JS, Huertas D, et al: The problem of coping as a reason for psychiatric consultation. Gen Hosp Psychiatry 15:1–8, 1993

Strain JJ, Smith GC, Hammer JS, et al: Adjustment disorder: a multisite study of its utilization and interventions in the consultation-liaison psychiatry setting. Gen Hosp Psychiatry 20:139–149, 1998

Strauss DH, Spitzer R, Muskin PR: Maladaptive denial of physical illness: a proposal for DSM-IV. Am J Psychiatry 147:1168–1172, 1990

Sullivan MD, Youngner SJ: Depression, competence and the right to refuse lifesaving medical treatment. Am J Psychiatry 151:971–978, 1993

Vaillant GE: The Wisdom of the Ego. Cambridge, MA, Harvard University Press, 1993

Verwoerdt A: Psychopathological responses to the stress of physical illness. Adv Psychosom Med 8:119–141, 1972

Weingart SN, Davis RB, Phillips RS: Patients discharged against medical advice from a general medicine service. J Gen Intern Med 13:568–571, 1998

Weisman AD, Hackett TP: Predilection to death: death and dying as a psychiatric problem. Psychosom Med 23:232, 1961

Westbrook M, Viney LL: Psychological reactions to the onset of chronic illness. Soc Sci Med 16:899–905, 1982

Wool MS: Understanding denial in cancer patients. Adv Psychosom Med 18:37–53, 1988

Young LD, Schweiger J, Beitzinger J, et al: Denial in heart transplant candidates. Psychother Psychosom 55:141–144, 1991

Zervas IM, Augustine A, Fricchione GL: Patient delay in cancer: a view from the crisis model. Gen Hosp Psychiatry 15:9–13, 1993

PART II

Symptoms and Disorders

6 Delirium

Paula T. Trzepacz, M.D.

David J. Meagher, M.D., M.R.C.Psych., M.Sc.

DELIRIUM IS A complex neuropsychiatric disorder that occurs commonly among patients in all health care settings, especially among the elderly and those with preexisting brain lesions or cognitive impairment. It is primarily characterized by generalized impairment of cognition, especially orientation and attention, but also involves a range of noncognitive symptoms, including motor behavior, sleep–wake cycle, thinking, language, perception, and affect. It characteristically has an acute onset (hours to days) and a fluctuating course (waxing and waning symptom severity over a 24-hour period), often worsening at night. It may be preceded by a prodromal phase of 2–3 days of malaise, restlessness, poor concentration, anxiety, irritability, sleep disturbances, and nightmares. It has been called *acute organic brain syndrome* and *acute brain failure* because of its breadth of cognitive and behavioral symptoms. Table 6–1 highlights delirium's characteristic features.

Delirium is an abnormal state of consciousness along a continuum between normal alertness and awareness at one extreme and the reduced wakefulness associated with stupor or coma at the other extreme. Consciousness has two main components—level of wakefulness (alertness) and content of higher mental functions (awareness). Because delirium alters both of these components of consciousness, it impairs the person more broadly than most other psychiatric disorders do. Precise delineation between severe hypoactive delirium and stupor can be difficult. Emergence from coma usually involves a period of delirium before normal consciousness is achieved. A prospective study of intensive care unit (ICU) patients found that 89% of survivors of stupor or coma progressed to delirium (McNicoll et al. 2003), whereas the small number who progressed directly to normal consciousness without delirium tended to have had drug-induced comatose states (Ely et al. 2004a).

Although delirium is usually characterized by an acute onset replete with many symptoms, it may be preceded by a subclinical delirium with more insidious changes in sleep pattern or cognition (Harrell and Othmer 1987). Matsushima et al. (1997) prospectively studied 10 critical care unit patients with delirium and 10 nondelirious control subjects with electroencephalography. They found prodromal changes of background slowing on the electroencephalogram (EEG) and sleep disturbance associated with changing consciousness. Cole et al. (2003b) prospectively studied "subsyndromal delirium," defined as the presence of one or more of four core symptoms (clouding of consciousness, inattention, disorientation, and/or perceptual disturbances) but not meeting DSM-III-R (American Psychiatric Association 1987) criteria, in 164 elderly medical patients. The more symptoms present, especially on admission, the worse the prognosis, suggesting that even subclinical manifestations of delirium are significant.

Delirium also may be a transient state, as when a patient emerges from general anesthesia, during concussion following a head injury, or postictally. Football players who sustain a head injury during a game are removed to the sidelines until the disorienting effects of concussion resolve sufficiently. Most deliria are considered reversible, but in the terminally ill, delirium may be progressive and intractable despite measures to treat it. On the other hand, delirium occurring in patients with serious illness frequently resolves, as evidenced in the study by Breitbart et al. (2002b), in which two-thirds of the cases of delirium occurring in hospitalized patients with cancer resolved completely with treatment. Similarly, Ljubisavljevic and Kelly (2003) found that 85% of the patients admitted with cancer who developed delirium experienced successful symptom reversal.

TABLE 6–1.   Signs and symptoms of delirium

Diffuse cognitive deficits
  Attention
  Orientation (time, place, person)
  Memory (short- and long-term; verbal and visual)
  Visuoconstructional ability
  Executive functions

Temporal course
  Acute or abrupt onset
  Fluctuating severity of symptoms over 24-hour period
  Usually reversible
  Subclinical syndrome may precede and/or follow

Psychosis
  Perceptual disturbances (especially visual), including
    illusions, hallucinations, metamorphoses
  Delusions (usually paranoid and poorly formed)
  Thought disorder (tangentiality, circumstantiality, loose
    associations)

Sleep–wake disturbance
  Fragmented throughout 24-hour period
  Reversal of normal cycle
  Sleeplessness

Psychomotor behavior
  Hyperactive
  Hypoactive
  Mixed

Language impairment
  Word-finding difficulty/dysnomia/paraphasia
  Dysgraphia
  Altered semantic content
  Severe forms can mimic expressive or receptive aphasia

Altered or labile affect
  Any mood can occur, usually incongruent to context
  Anger or increased irritability common
  Hypoactive delirium often mislabeled as depression
  Lability (rapid shifts) common
  Unrelated to mood preceding delirium

Delirium is considered a syndrome and not a unitary disorder because a wide variety of underlying etiologies can cause it. Identification of these etiologies, often multiple or occurring serially over time, is a key part of clinical management. Despite these varied etiologies and physiology, delirium symptoms are characteristic and thus may represent dysfunction of a final common neural pathway that includes perturbations of the various brain regions responsible for the abnormal cognitions, thinking, sleep, and behaviors (see section "Neuropathogenesis" later in this chapter).

Unlike most other psychiatric disorders, delirium symptoms typically fluctuate in intensity over any 24-hour period. Symptom fluctuation is measurable (Gagnon et al. 2004a, 2004b) and is an important indicator of delirium emphasized in diagnostic classifications such as DSM-IV (American Psychiatric Association 1994, 2000). During this characteristic waxing and waning of symptoms, relative lucid or quiescent periods often occur, which frustrate accurate diagnosis and complicate research severity ratings. In milder cases, such periods involve a significant diminution of delirium symptoms or even a seeming resolution of symptoms, but the latter has not been carefully studied. The underlying reason for this fluctuation in symptom severity is poorly understood—it may relate to shifts between hypoactive and hyperactive periods or fragmentations of the sleep–wake cycle, including daytime rapid eye movement (REM) sleep.

Although not nearly as well studied, the symptom profile of delirium in children appears to be similar to that in adults (Prugh et al. 1980; Turkel et al. 2003, 2004). In the only study of delirium phenomenology in children and adolescents in which a standardized instrument was used, Turkel et al. (2003) retrospectively described 84 consecutively evaluated delirium patients (age 6 months to 19 years) and found scores comparable to those in adults, with the only difference being fewer delusions and hallucinations in younger children. Turkel et al. (2004) also compared delirium symptoms across the life cycle and, despite differences in methodologies, considered them to be largely similar. Prugh et al. (1980) noted the importance of educating nursing staff about the difference between visual hallucinations and imaginary friends. Documentation of all delirium symptoms in preverbal children or noncommunicative adults is difficult. In these patients, more reliance on inference and observation of changed or unusual behaviors—for example, inferring hallucinations or recording sleep–wake cycle changes—is needed.

Delirium symptoms in adults across the age range are comparable, although the co-occurrence of another cognitive mental disorder is particularly likely in the elderly compared with younger adults and is usually related to degenerative or vascular dementia. How the presence of a comorbid dementia alters the phenomenological presentation of delirium in the elderly is not well studied, but existing data suggest that delirium overshadows the dementia symptoms (see section "Differential Diagnosis" later in this chapter). Likewise, diagnosing delirium in mentally retarded patients can be more challenging.

One of the challenges for both clinicians and delirium researchers is the myriad of terms applied to the delirious state. Historically, acute global cognitive disturbances have been labeled according to the setting in which they occurred or the apparent etiology for the confusional state, resulting in the myriad of synonyms (see Table 6–2)

TABLE 6–2.   Terms used to denote delirium

Acute brain failure	Cerebral insufficiency	Organic brain syndrome
Acute brain syndrome	Confusional state	Posttraumatic amnesia
Acute brain syndrome with psychosis	Dysergastic reaction	Reversible cerebral dysfunction
Acute dementia	Encephalopathy	Reversible cognitive dysfunction
Acute organic psychosis	Exogenous psychosis	Reversible dementia
Acute organic reaction	Infective-exhaustive psychosis	Reversible toxic psychosis
Acute organic syndrome	Intensive care unit (ICU) psychosis	Toxic confusion state
Acute reversible psychosis	Metabolic encephalopathy	Toxic encephalopathy
Acute secondary psychosis	Oneiric state	

that exist in practice and the literature. Little evidence supports these as separate entities, and, as such, *delirium* has been adopted as the accepted umbrella term to denote acute disturbances of global cognitive function as defined in both DSM-IV and ICD-10 (World Health Organization 1992) research classification systems. Even though the term *delirium* has been used since classical Greek medical writings, unfortunately, different terms continue to be used by nonpsychiatric physicians (e.g., *ICU psychosis, hepatic encephalopathy, toxic psychosis, posttraumatic amnesia*). These terms inappropriately suggest the existence of independent psychiatric disorders for each etiology rather than recognize delirium as a unitary syndrome. Terms such as *acute brain failure* and *acute organic brain syndrome* highlight the global nature and acute onset of cerebral cortical deficits in patients with delirium, but they lack specificity in regard to other cognitive mental disorders. The term *delirium* subsumes these many other terms, and its consistent use will enhance medical communication, diagnosis, and research.

Little work has been done with the use of daily delirium ratings to better understand the temporal course of this syndrome. In a study of 432 medical inpatients 65 years or older, Rudberg et al. (1997) found that 15% had delirium, and 69% of those had delirium for only a single day. Mean delirium scores on day 1 were significantly higher (i.e., worse) in those whose delirium occurred for multiple days compared with those whose delirium lasted for 1 day (25.4±3.6 vs. 22.6±4.4), suggesting a relation between severity and duration in delirium episodes.

Delirium continues to be understudied compared with other psychiatric disorders, as well as underrecognized and underdiagnosed. It is commonly misdiagnosed as depression by nonpsychiatrists (Nicholas and Lindsey 1995). Misdiagnosis of delirium is more likely when delirium is hypoactive in presentation and when patients are referred from surgical or intensive care settings (S.C. Armstrong et al. 1997). Van Zyl and Davidson (2003) reviewed charts of 31 delirious patients who were referred for psychiatric consultation and received standardized delirium assessments. They found that delirium or a synonym was noted in 55% of the structured discharge summaries and in none of the unstructured summaries, for an overall rate of 16%. It was more likely mentioned when it occurred in women, was more severe, or was the main reason for admission. Johnson et al. (1992) studied consecutive elderly patients admitted to a general hospital and found that delirium was explicitly documented in 5% of the patients and noted as a synonym in 18%, with a variable but poor recognition of individual delirium symptoms. The missed cases were denoted as dementia (25%), a functional psychiatric disorder (25%), or no diagnosis noted (50%).

Nondetection was associated with poorer outcome, including increased mortality, in a study of detection of delirium in emergency department patients (Kakuma et al. 2003). In contrast, explicit recognition of delirium was associated with better outcome in the form of shorter inpatient stays and lower mortality (Rockwood et al. 1994). Detection can be improved by providing formal educational programs, for example, with house staff (Rockwood et al. 1994). Personal attitudes are important among nursing staff, who often play a key role in identifying and reporting symptoms because the symptoms fluctuate, for example, at night (McCarthy 2003). Detection is a challenge in ICU settings, where the sickest patients are at the highest risk for delirium. Ely et al. (2004b) distributed a survey to 912 physicians, nurses, respiratory therapists, and pharmacists attending international critical care meetings and found that 72% thought that ventilated patients experienced delirium, 92% considered delirium a very serious problem, and 78% acknowledged that it was underdiagnosed. Yet only 40% routinely screened for delirium, and only 16% used a specific tool for assessment. Rincon et al. (2001) reported that critical care unit staff underdiagnosed delirium (and other psychiatric disorders) and used psychotropic medications without any clear documentation.

ICU populations have delirium prevalence rates ranging from 40% to 87% (Ely et al. 2001c). ICU delirium is understudied and neglected probably because it is "expected" to happen during severe illness, and medical resources are preferentially dedicated to managing the more immediate "life-threatening" problems.

Related to pressures to reduce acute hospital care costs, elderly patients are discharged, often to nursing homes, before delirium resolves. Kiely et al. (2003) studied 2,158 patients from seven Boston, Massachusetts, area skilled nursing facilities and found that 16% had a full-blown delirium. In general, such facilities are even less equipped with health care professionals to diagnose and manage delirium than are acute care settings.

Delirium can have a profound effect on a patient's morbidity and mortality as well as on his or her caregivers and loved ones. Delirious patients have difficulty comprehending and communicating effectively, consenting to procedures, complying with medical management (e.g., removing intravenous lines, tubes, or catheters), benefiting from many therapies, and maintaining expected levels of self-hygiene and eating. They also are at risk for inadvertent self-harm because of confusion about the environment or in response to hallucinations or paranoid delusions. Delirium-recovered patients were uncomfortable discussing their delirium episodes—even to the extent of denial—because they feared that it meant that they were "senile" or "mad" (Schofield 1997). Breitbart et al. (2002a) prospectively interviewed and rated 101 cancer patients with a resolved delirium episode, their spouses, and their nurses (see Figure 6–1). About half (43%) of the patients recalled their episode, with recall dependent on delirium severity (100% of patients with mild delirium vs. 16% of patients with severe delirium recalled the episode). Mean distress levels were high for patients and nurses but were highest for spouses. However, among patients with delirium who did not recall the episode, the mean distress level was half that of those who did recall. The experience of the delirium was frightening and stressful for all involved, but for somewhat different reasons—for patients, the presence of delusions; for nurses, the presence of perceptual disturbances or overall severe delirium; and for spouses, the low ability to function was predictive of distress level. Spouses perceived the delirium as indicating a high risk for death and loss of the loved one, contributing to bereavement. Medical complications, including decubitus ulcers, feeding problems, and urinary incontinence, are common in patients with delirium (Gustafson et al. 1988). Effects on hospital length of stay, "persistence" of cognitive impairment, increased rate of institutionalization, and reduced ambulation and activities of daily living (ADL) level have been reported.

The Academy of Psychosomatic Medicine Task Force on Mental Disorders in General Medical Practice (Saravay

and Strain 1994) reviewed studies finding that comorbid delirium increased hospital length of stay 100% in general medical patients (R.I. Thomas et al. 1988), 114% in elderly patients (Schor et al. 1992), 67% in stroke patients (Cushman 1988), 300% in critical care patients (Kishi et al. 1995), 27% in cardiac surgery patients, and 200%–250% in hip surgery patients (Berggren et al. 1987). The Academy of Psychosomatic Medicine task force noted that delirium contributed to increased length of stay via medical and behavioral mechanisms, including the following: decreased motivation to participate in treatment and rehabilitation, medication refusal, disruptive behavior, incontinence and urinary tract infection, falls and fractures, and decubiti.

Significantly increased length of stay associated with delirium has been reported in many studies (Cushman 1988; Forman et al. 1995; Francis et al. 1990; Gustafson et al. 1988; Hales et al. 1988; Levkoff et al. 1992; Pompei et al. 1994; Schor et al. 1992; R.I. Thomas et al. 1988) but not all (Cole et al. 1994; George et al. 1997; Jitapunkul et al. 1992; Rockwood 1989). A meta-analysis of eight studies (Cole and Primeau 1993) supported statistically significant differences in length of stay between delirium and control groups. Ely et al. (2004a) found that delirium duration was associated with length of stay in both the medical ICU and the hospital ($P<0.001$) and was the strongest predictor of length of stay even after adjustment for illness severity, age, gender, and days of opiate and narcotic use (see Figure 6–2). McCusker et al. (2003a) studied elderly medical inpatients and found significantly longer length of stay for those with incident, but not prevalent, delirium. Methodological issues often affect interpretation of such studies.

Franco and colleagues (2001) identified the increased costs associated with delirium in a prospective study of 500 elective surgery patients older than 50 years. Delirium occurred in 11.4% of the patients during postoperative days 1–4, and these patients had higher professional, consultation, technical, and routine nursing care costs. Milbrandt and colleagues (2004) compared costs associated with having at least one delirium episode in 183 mechanically ventilated medical ICU patients and nondelirious control subjects after controlling for age, comorbidity of illness, degree of organ dysfunction, nosocomial infection, and hospital mortality. Median ICU costs per patient were $22,346 for delirious and $13,332 for nondelirious patients ($P<0.001$), and total hospital costs were $41,836 and $27,106 ($P=0.002$), respectively; more severe delirium cases resulted in higher costs than did milder ones.

Decreased independent living status and increased institutionalization during follow-up after a delirium epi-

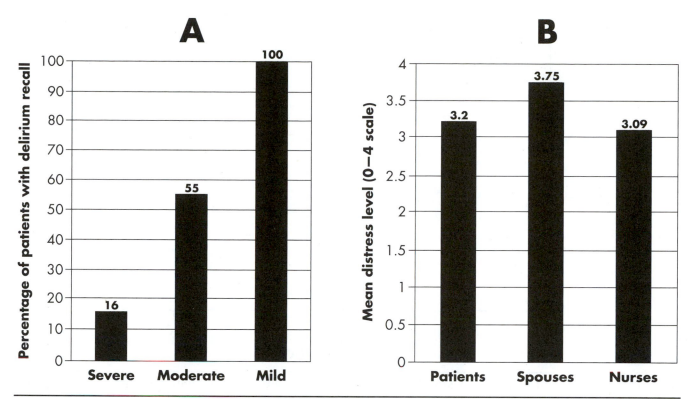

FIGURE 6–1. Relation of delirium severity to patient recall of the episode, and comparison of delirium-related distress levels, in cancer patients with a resolved delirium episode and their families and caregivers.

(A) Percentage of patients who recalled their episode, by delirium severity. **(B)** Mean distress levels of patients, spouses or caregivers, and nurses (rated on a 0–4 rating scale).

Source. Reprinted from Breitbart W, Gibson C, Tremblay A: "The Delirium Experience: Delirium Recall and Delirium-Related Distress in Hospitalized Patients With Cancer, Their Spouses/Caregivers, and Their Nurses." *Psychosomatics* 43:183–194, 2002. Copyright 2002, American Psychiatric Publishing, Inc. Used with permission.

sode were found in many studies, especially in the elderly (Cole and Primeau 1993; George et al. 1997; Inouye et al. 1998). Reduction in ambulation and/or ADL level at follow-up is also commonly reported (Francis and Kapoor 1992; Gustafson et al. 1988; Inouye et al. 1998; Minagawa et al. 1996; Murray et al. 1993). Delirium also has an effect in nursing home settings, where incident cases are associated with poor 6-month outcome, including behavioral decline, initiation of physical restraints, greater risk of hospitalization, and increased mortality (Murphy 1999). Even subsyndromal delirium is reported to increase index admission length of stay and postdischarge dysfunction and mortality after adjustment for age, sex, marital status, previous living arrangement, comorbidity, dementia status, and clinical and physiological severity of illness (Cole et al. 2003b).

In nursing home patients, better cognitive function at baseline was associated with better outcome from delirium (Murphy 1999), supporting the notion that impaired brain reserve is an important predelirium factor that needs to be taken into account in any longitudinal out-

come assessments. Alternatively, longitudinal postdelirium cognitive assessments of younger adults who are not at risk for dementia could help answer the question of persistent cognitive impairment following delirium.

Epidemiology

Delirium can occur at any age, although it is particularly understudied in children and adolescents. Most epidemiological studies have focused on the elderly, who are at higher risk to develop delirium than are younger adults. This is likely because of age-related changes in the brain, including decreased cholinergic functioning, often referred to as *reduced brain reserve*. The frequent occurrence of central nervous system disorders (e.g., stroke, hypertensive and atherosclerotic vessel changes, tumor, dementias) in the elderly further increases their vulnerability to delirium. Elderly medical ICU patients with dementia were 40% more likely to have delirium, even after various indices of medical comorbidity severity were controlled

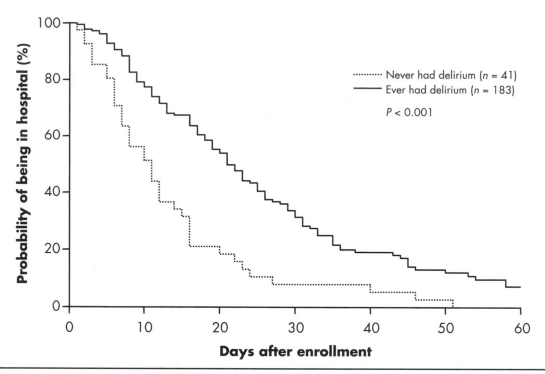

FIGURE 6–2.   **Hospital length of stay in patients with and without prevalent delirium during medical intensive care unit (ICU) stay.**

Source.   Reprinted from Ely EW, Shintani A, Truman B, et al.: "Delirium as a Predictor of Mortality in Mechanically Ventilated Patients in the Intensive Care Unit." *Journal of the American Medical Association* 291:1753–1762, 2004. Used with permission.

for (McNicoll et al. 2003). Frail elderly individuals living in nursing facilities studied for 3 months during and after an acute medical hospitalization had a high incidence of delirium of 55% at 1 month and 25% at 3 months, which persisted until death or hospitalization in 72% (Kelly et al. 2001). Improving our understanding and treatment of delirium is thus a considerable health care challenge in the coming years because the world's population is aging at a dramatic rate.

Most studies of delirium incidence and prevalence report general hospital populations consisting of either referral samples or consecutive admissions to a given service. Little information is available about the rate of delirium in the general population. Specific patient populations, such as elderly patients who require emergent hip surgery, liver transplant candidates, and hospitalized traumatic brain injury patients, may be responsible for disparate rates reported in studies. In addition, not all studies use sensitive and specific diagnostic and measurement techniques, possibly resulting in overestimates or underestimates of the true occurrence of delirium. A review by Fann (2000) of (mostly) prospective studies found that delirium incidence ranged from 3% to 42%, and prevalence ranged from 5% to 44%, in hospitalized patients. Table 6–3 reviews incidence and prevalence studies

of delirium in which DSM diagnostic criteria or rating scales were used. These studies were done in medical, surgical, palliative care, institutional care, intensive care, and community settings, and most focused on geriatric patients.

Up to 60% of nursing home patients older than 65 years may have delirium when assessed cross-sectionally (Sandberg et al. 1998). When admitted to a hospital, 10%–15% of elderly patients have delirium, and another 10%–40% receive diagnoses of delirium during the hospitalization. A clinical "rule of thumb" seems to be that, on average, approximately one-fifth of general hospital patients have delirium sometime during hospitalization. Terminally ill cancer patients have a very high incidence of delirium, with rates from 28% to 42% on admission to a palliative care unit and up to 88% before death (Lawlor et al. 2000a). Also, about 50% of those undergoing stem cell transplantation have a delirium in the postoperative month (Fann et al. 2002).

In a prospective cohort study of older medical ICU patients, McNicoll et al. (2003) found delirium in 31% on admission and an overall prevalence and incidence of delirium of 62% during the ICU stay and of 70% during the entire hospitalization. In addition, 30% had evidence of prior dementia, and these patients were 40% more likely

TABLE 6–3. Incidence and prevalence studies of delirium

Study	N	Sample	Delirium ascertainment	Design	Findings
Erkinjuntti et al. 1986	2,000	Medical inpatients, age ≥55 years	SPMSQ, DSM-III criteria on interview and chart review	Prospective	Prevalence 15%
Cameron et al. 1987	133	Medical inpatients, ages 32–97 years	DSM-III criteria on interview	Prospective	Prevalence 14%, incidence 3%
Gustafson et al. 1988	111	Femoral neck fracture patients, age ≥65 years	OBS Scale, DSM-III criteria on interview	Prospective	Prevalence 33%, incidence 42%
Rockwood 1989	80	Medical inpatients, age ≥65 years	DSM-III criteria on interview	Prospective	Prevalence 16%, incidence 11%
Francis et al. 1990	229	Medical inpatients, age ≥70 years	DSM-III-R criteria on interview and chart review	Prospective	Prevalence 16%, incidence 7%
Johnson et al. 1990	235	Medical inpatients, age >70 years	DSM-III criteria on interview	Prospective	Prevalence 16%, incidence 5%
Folstein et al. 1991	810	Community sample	DSM-III criteria on interview	Cross-sectional	Prevalence 0.4% (1.1%, age ≥55)
Williams-Russo et al. 1992	51	Bilateral knee replacement surgery patients receiving postoperative fentanyl	DSM-III-R criteria on interview and chart review	Prospective	Incidence 41%
Jitapunkul et al. 1992	184	Medical inpatients, age ≥60 years	DSM-III-R criteria on chart review	Prospective	Prevalence 22%
Snyder et al. 1992	42	Acquired immunodeficiency syndrome inpatients	DSM-III-R criteria on interview	Prospective	Prevalence 17%
Schor et al. 1992	325	Medical and surgical inpatients, age ≥65 years	DSI	Prospective	Prevalence 11%, incidence 31%
Leung et al. 1992	569	Male medical inpatients, ages 12–99 years	DSM-III criteria on interview	Prospective	Prevalence 9.5%
Kolbeinsson and Jonsson 1993	331	Medical inpatients, age ≥70 years	MSQ, MMSE, and DSM-III-R criteria on interview	Prospective	Prevalence 14%
Rockwood 1993	168	Geriatric medical inpatients, mean age = 79 years	DRS, DSM-III-R criteria on interview	Prospective	Prevalence 18%, incidence 7%
Marcantonio et al. 1994a	1,341	Noncardiac surgery patients, age ≥50 years	CAM, medical records, nursing intensity index	Prospective	Incidence 9%
Pompei et al. 1994	432	Medical and surgical inpatients, age ≥65 years	Digit Span, Vigilance "A" Test, CAC, CAM, DSM-III-R criteria on interview	Prospective	Prevalence 5%, incidence 10%
Pompei et al. 1994	323	Medical and surgical inpatients, age ≥70 years	CAM	Prospective	Prevalence 15%, incidence 12%
Kishi et al. 1995	238	Critical care medical unit patients	DSM-III-R criteria on clinical evaluation	Prospective	Incidence 16%
Fisher and Flowerdew 1995	80	Elective orthopedic surgery inpatients, age ≥60 years	CAM	Prospective	Incidence 18%

TABLE 6–3. Incidence and prevalence studies of delirium (*continued*)

Study	N	Sample	Delirium ascertainment	Design	Findings
Forman et al. 1995	95	Community hospital inpatients, age ≥65 years	Delirium diagnosis or DSM-III-R criteria on chart review	Retrospective	Incidence 38%
Inouye and Charpentier 1996	196	Medical inpatients, age ≥70 years	CAM	Prospective	Incidence 18%
	312	Medical inpatients, age ≥70 years	CAM	Prospective	Incidence 15%
Minagawa et al. 1996	93	Terminally ill cancer patients admitted to palliative care unit	MMSE and DSM-III-R criteria on interview	Prospective	Prevalence 28%
Glick et al. 1996	195	Patients receiving intra-aortic balloon pump treatment	DSM-III-R criteria on chart review	Retrospective	Prevalence 34%
Rudberg et al. 1997	432	Medical-surgical patients	DSM-III-R and DRS daily ratings	Prospective	Incidence 15%
Sandberg et al. 1998	717	Institutional care patients, age ≥75 years	OBS Scale	Cross-sectional	Prevalence 44%
Gagnon et al. 2000	89	Hospitalized terminal cancer patients	CAM, CRS	Prospective longitudinal	Incidence 33%, prevalence on admission 20%
Lawlor et al. 2000b	104	Hospitalized advanced cancer patients	DSM-IV, MDAS	Prospective	Incidence 45%, prevalence on admission 42%
Caraceni et al. 2000	393	Multicenter palliative care cancer patients	CAM	Prospective	Prevalence 28%
van der Mast et al. 1999	296	Elective cardiac surgery patients, ages 26–83 years	DSM-III-R criteria on interview and chart review	Prospective	Incidence 14%
Fann et al. 2002	90	Hospitalized hematopoietic stem cell transplant patients	DRS, MDAS	Prospective	Incidence 50%, cumulative incidence 73%
Ely et al. 2004a	275	Consecutive mechanically ventilated medical ICU patients	DSM-IV and CAM-ICU	Prospective	Incidence 82%
McNicoll et al. 2003	118	Elderly medical ICU patients	CAM-ICU	Prospective	Incidence on admission 31%, incidence and prevalence combined 62%
Kiely et al. 2003	2,158	Skilled nursing facility elderly patients in Boston area	CAM	Prospective	Prevalence 16%

Note. CAC=Critical Assessment of Confusion; CAM=Confusion Assessment Method; CRS=Confusion Rating Scale; DRS=Delirium Rating Scale; DSI=Delirium Symptom Interview; ICU=intensive care unit; MDAS=Memorial Delirium Assessment Scale; MMSE=Mini-Mental State Examination; MSQ=Mental Status Questionnaire; OBS=Organic Brain Syndrome; SPMSQ=Short Portable Mental Status Questionnaire.

to become delirious, even after comorbidity, baseline functional status, severity of illness, and invasive procedures were controlled for. In a prospective study of 275 consecutive mechanically ventilated medical ICU patients that used daily ratings over 5,353 patient days, 51 (18.5%) were comatose; of the remaining 224 patients, 183 (82%) had a delirium at some point during the hospitalization, with a median duration of 2.1 days (Ely et al. 2004b). Delirious patients had numerically higher admission mean comorbidity and critical illness severity scores compared with those who never became delirious, but mean ages were comparable.

Diagnosis is also an issue for epidemiological studies. Substantial differences in rates can occur—for example, when DSM-III (American Psychiatric Association 1980), DSM-III-R, DSM-IV, and ICD-10 criteria were used, only 25% of the patients with delirium received accurate diagnoses by all four systems (Laurila et al. 2003). Lesser diagnostic emphasis on disorganized thinking in the DSM-IV criteria accounted for that system's greater sensitivity and inclusivity (but lower specificity) in comparison with the other systems, whereas ICD-10 criteria were the least inclusive (Cole et al. 2003a).

Thus, irrespective of the diversity of incidence and prevalence rates reported among studies, delirium is very common, and its rates generally exceed those for any other serious psychiatric disorder in a medical setting.

Risk Factors

Delirium is particularly common during hospitalization when a confluence of both predisposing (vulnerabilities) and precipitating factors is present. Several patient, illness, pharmacological, and environmental factors have been identified as being relevant risk factors for delirium. Although some factors are more relevant in certain settings, age, preexisting cognitive impairment, severe comorbid illness, and medication exposure are particularly strong predictors of delirium risk across a range of populations (Inouye et al. 1999). Terminal illness is a risk factor for delirium (Lawlor et al. 2000a). In stem cell transplant patients, pretransplant risk factors included lower cognition on Trail Making Test B; higher serum levels of urea nitrogen, magnesium, or alkaline phosphatase; and lower physical functioning (Fann et al. 2002).

Stress-vulnerability models for the occurrence of delirium have been long recognized. Henry and Mann (1965) described "delirium readiness." More recent models of causation involve cumulative interactions between predisposing factors and precipitating insults (Inouye and Charpentier 1996; O'Keeffe and Lavan 1996). Baseline

risk is a more potent predictor of delirium likelihood—if baseline vulnerability is low, patients are very resistant to the development of delirium despite exposure to significant precipitating factors, whereas if baseline vulnerability is high, delirium is likely even in response to minor precipitants. Tsutsui et al. (1996), for example, found that in patients older than 80 years, delirium occurred in 52% after emergency surgery and 20% after elective procedures, whereas no case of delirium was noted in patients younger than 50 years undergoing either elective or emergency procedures. In addition to the elderly, children are considered at higher risk for delirium, possibly related to ongoing brain development. For example, maturation of the cholinergic system continues into midadolescence.

Up to two-thirds of the cases of delirium occur superimposed on preexisting cognitive impairment (Wahlund and Bjorlin 1999). Delirium is 2.0–3.5 times more common in patients with dementia compared with nondemented control subjects (Erkinjuntti et al. 1986; Jitapunkul et al. 1992). Delirium risk appears to be greater in Alzheimer's disease of late onset and dementia of vascular origin as compared with other dementias, with this increased risk perhaps reflecting the relatively widespread neuronal disturbance associated with these conditions (Robertsson et al. 1998).

More recently, several studies addressed the influence of genetic factors on delirium vulnerability. To date, these studies have focused on the role of genotype in susceptibility to alcohol withdrawal delirium and suggest positive associations between polymorphisms of both the dopamine transporter gene (Gorwood et al. 2003; Wernicke et al. 2002) and the neuropeptide Y gene (Koehnke et al. 2002) and the risk of delirium tremens.

O'Keeffe and Lavan (1996) stratified patients into four levels of delirium risk based on the presence of three factors (chronic cognitive impairment, severe illness, elevated serum urea) and found that the risk of delirium increased as these factors accumulated. Similarly, Inouye and Charpentier (1996) developed a predictive model that included four predisposing factors (cognitive impairment, severe illness, visual impairment, dehydration) and five precipitating factors (more than three medications added, catheterization, use of restraints, malnutrition, any iatrogenic event). These factors predicted a 17-fold variation in the relative risk of developing delirium. Uremia increases the permeability of the blood-brain barrier, allowing many larger molecules, such as drugs, to enter the brain when they ordinarily would not.

Although the value of reducing risk factors appears self-evident, many may simply be markers of general morbidity; therefore, studies showing preventive effect are important (see section "Prevention Strategies" later in this chapter). Some risk factors are potentially modifiable and thus are targets for prevention. Even just closer observation of patients at high risk for delirium could mean prompter intervention in emerging delirium. For example, thiamine deficiency is an underappreciated cause of and risk factor for delirium in pediatric intensive care and oncology patients (Seear et al. 1992) and nonalcoholic elderly patients (O'Keeffe et al. 1994).

Medication exposure is probably the most readily modifiable risk factor for delirium, implicated as a cause in 20%–40% of cases. Polypharmacy and drug intoxication and withdrawal may be the most common causes of delirium (Hales et al. 1988; Trzepacz et al. 1985). Benzodiazepines, opiates, and drugs with anticholinergic activity have a particular association with delirium (T.M. Brown 2000; Marcantonio et al. 1994b). Many drugs (and their metabolites) can unexpectedly contribute to delirium as a result of unrecognized anticholinergic effects. Ten of the 25 most commonly prescribed drugs for the elderly had sufficient in vitro anticholinergic activity identified by radioreceptor assay to cause memory and attention impairment in nondelirious elderly subjects (Tune et al. 1992). Therefore, drug exposure must be minimized, especially when facing high-risk periods such as the perioperative phase. Although opiates are associated with delirium, Morrison et al. (2003) found in a prospective study of older patients undergoing hip surgery that delirium was nine times more likely in those patients deemed to have undertreated pain.

The temporal relation between exposure to risk factors and development of delirium requires further study. Postoperative delirium (excluding emergence from anesthesia) appears most frequently at day 3. A large multi-center study found age, duration of anesthesia, lower education, second operation, postoperative infection, and respiratory complications to be predictors of postoperative cognitive impairment (Moller et al. 1998).

Low serum albumin is an important risk factor at any age and may signify poor nutrition, chronic disease, or liver or renal insufficiency. Hypoalbuminemia results in a greater bioavailability of many drugs that are transported in the bloodstream by albumin, which is associated with an increased risk of side effects, including delirium (Dickson 1991; Trzepacz and Francis 1990). This increased biological drug activity occurs within the therapeutic range and may not be recognized because increased levels of free drug are not separately reported in most assays. Serum albumin was identified by discriminant analysis, along with Trail Making Test B and EEG dominant posterior rhythm, as sensitively distinguishing delirious from nondelirious liver transplant candidates (Trzepacz et al. 1988b).

Nicotine withdrawal has been implicated as a potential risk factor in the development of delirium, especially in heavy smokers unable to continue their habit during hospital admission. Klein et al. (2002) reported a single case of delirium in such a patient who responded quickly to a transdermal nicotine patch.

Mortality

Delirium appears to be associated with high mortality. Whether this mortality risk is increased during the index admission, at long-term follow-up, or both is not completely clear; this uncertainty is in part related to challenges in research design. It is also not known whether increased mortality is attributable to the underlying etiologies of delirium; to indirect effects on the body related to perturbations of neuronal, endocrine, and immunological function during delirium; or to damaging effects on the brain from neurochemical abnormalities associated with delirium (i.e., similar to glutamate surges after stroke). Additionally, patients with delirium cannot fully cooperate with their medical care or participate in rehabilitative programs during hospitalization. Their behaviors can directly reduce the effectiveness of procedures meant to treat their medical problems (e.g., removing tubes and intravenous lines, climbing out of bed), which adds to morbidity and possibly to further physiological injury and mortality.

Methodological inconsistencies and shortcomings affect the interpretation of studies of mortality risk associated with delirium. Some studies do not compare patients who have delirium with control groups. Many studies include patients with comorbid dementia, and many studies do not control for severity of medical comorbidity (admittedly difficult to measure). In addition, most studies do not address the effects of advanced age as a separate risk factor, and specific delirium rating instruments are rarely used. The effect on reducing mortality risk of treatment for the delirium itself, a potential confound, is also not reported in most studies. Prospective application of DSM criteria by qualified clinicians, attention to whether the sample is incident or prevalent, identification of referral biases, and indication of whether follow-up mortality rates are cumulative to include the original sample are also important issues that vary across study designs. Attention to matching patients to control subjects for numerous factors, including demographics, education and occupation, baseline cognitive functioning, severity of each medical condition, certain laboratory tests, and medications, is a daunting task but probably more accurate than statistical manipulations of data to adjust for confounding factors.

Reported mortality rates during the index hospitalization for a delirium episode range from 4% to 65% (Cameron et al. 1987; Gustafson et al. 1988), depending on the study design and population. One study found significant differences in index mortality among motoric subtypes, with the lowest rate (10%) in hyperactive as compared with hypoactive (38%) and mixed cases (30%) (Olofsson et al. 1996). When delirium present on admission was excluded, index mortality in incident cases was as low as about 1.5% (Inouye et al. 1999). Index mortality for delirious patients did not differ significantly from that for control subjects without delirium in some studies (Forman et al. 1995; George et al. 1997; Gustafson et al. 1988; Inouye et al. 1998, 1999; Kishi et al. 1995), but it did in others (Cameron et al. 1987; Jitapunkul et al. 1992; Pompei et al. 1994; Rabins and Folstein 1982; van Hemert et al. 1994). Many long-term follow-up studies of delirium mortality rates (more than 3 months after discharge) did find worse mortality in delirium groups, including patients with subsyndromal delirium (Cole et al. 2003b). Excess mortality in some reports was attributed to older age (Gustafson et al. 1988; Huang et al. 1998; Kishi et al. 1995; Trzepacz et al. 1985; Weddington 1982), more serious medical problems (Cole and Primeau 1993; Jitapunkul et al. 1992; Magaziner et al. 1989; Trzepacz et al. 1985), and dementia (Cole and Primeau 1993; Gustafson et al. 1988). Some studies did not find cancer as an explanation for higher mortality rates (Rabins and Folstein 1982), whereas studies comparing only cancer inpatients did find significantly poorer survival in patients with delirium as compared with control subjects (Lawlor et al. 2000a; Minagawa et al. 1996). Curyto et al. (2001) found an increased mortality of 75% at 3 years for delirious compared with control (51%) elderly patients despite no differences in prehospital levels of depression, global cognitive performance, physical functioning, or medical comorbidity.

In a prospective study of medically hospitalized elderly, Inouye et al. (1998) found that delirium significantly increased mortality risk, even after controlling for age, gender, dementia, ADL level, and Acute Physiology and Chronic Health Evaluation (APACHE) II scores. Ely et al. (2004a) reported that delirium was independently associated with a greater than 300% increased likelihood of dying at 6 months ($P=0.008$), even after correcting for numerous covariates, including coma and use of psychoactive medications, in a prospective cohort study of medical ICU patients (see Figure 6–3). McCusker et al. (2002) showed that delirium is a significant predictor of 12-month mortality for older inpatients, even after adjusting for age, sex, marital status, living location, comorbidity, acute physiological severity, illness severity, dementia,

and hospital service. Frail elderly living in nursing facilities studied for 3 months during and after an acute medical hospitalization had a high mortality rate of 18% in hospital and 46% at 3 months that was associated with severe and persistent delirium (Kelly et al. 2001).

In a prospective cohort study of prevalent delirium in emergency departments, 30 delirious and 77 nondelirious elderly patients who were discharged to home instead of being admitted to the hospital were assessed at 6-month follow-up intervals until 18 months (Kakuma et al. 2003). After adjustment for age, sex, functional level, cognitive status, comorbidity, and number of medications, delirium was significantly associated with mortality (see Figure 6–4). Those whose delirium was not detected by the emergency department staff had the highest mortality over 6 months compared with those whose delirium was detected, for whom no mortality difference from the nondelirious was found, emphasizing the importance of detection.

Thus, although the mechanism is not understood, the presence of delirium does indeed appear to be an adverse prognostic sign that is associated with an increased risk for mortality, extending well beyond the index hospitalization. To what extent aggressive treatment of both the delirium and its comorbid medical problems would reduce morbidity and mortality is not well studied, but at the very least, such treatment makes good clinical sense.

Reversibility of a Delirium Episode

Delirium traditionally has been distinguished from dementia by its potential for reversal. In most cases, delirium is reversible, except in terminal illness or particular examples of severe brain injury. However, evidence that an index episode of delirium may be associated with enduring cognitive deficits suggests that delirium may be more than a transient state. Longer duration of cognitive impairment linked to coma or delirium following traumatic brain injury is associated with poorer recovery, and more severe or prolonged impairments due to delirium from other causes also may be associated with poorer recovery. This association is supported by evidence for worse cognitive outcome in more severe delirium (Wada and Yamaguchi 1993) and episodes of longer duration (Liptzin and Levkoff 1992), but no neurotoxic mechanism has been identified. Moreover, poorer long-term outcome may be related to preexisting comorbidities, including a previously undiagnosed dementia that progresses after delirium resolution. Terminology is also difficult regarding when chronic delirium becomes a dementia. In addition, that many patients continue to

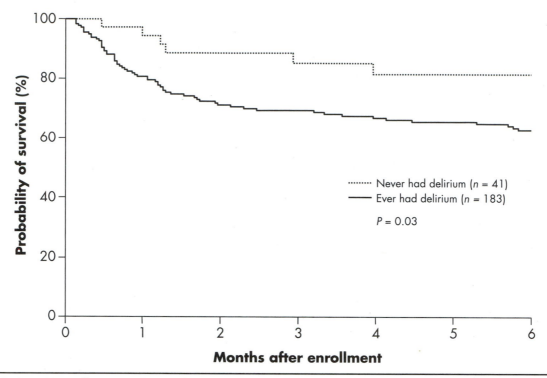

FIGURE 6–3.   **Mortality over 6 months in patients with and without prevalent delirium during medical intensive care unit (ICU) stay.**

Source.   Reprinted from Ely EW, Shintani A, Truman B, et al.: "Delirium as a Predictor of Mortality in Mechanically Ventilated Patients in the Intensive Care Unit." *Journal of the American Medical Association* 291:1753–1762, 2004. Used with permission.

experience delirium symptoms at hospital discharge (Levkoff et al. 1994) raises the question of incomplete treatment during the index hospitalization as the true cause of persisting symptoms.

In a landmark study of delirium, Bedford (1957) indicated that approximately 5% of the patients were still "confused" at 6-month follow-up, but more recent studies suggested that persistent disturbances may be more frequent after an episode of delirium. Levkoff et al. (1994), in a longitudinal study of elderly patients, found that almost one-third still had delirium after 6 months, with most still having some of its features (disorientation, emotional lability, and sleep disturbances). Full resolution of delirium symptoms at hospital discharge of elderly patients may be the exception rather than the rule (Levkoff et al. 1992; Rockwood 1993). Levkoff et al. (1992) found that only 4% of elderly patients with delirium had complete resolution of symptoms at discharge, 21% at 6 weeks, and 18% at 6 months. However, neither of the studies by Levkoff et al. excluded dementia patients. McCusker et al. (2003b) found that 12 months after diagnosis of delirium in elderly medical inpatients, inattention, disorientation, and poor memory were the most persistent individual symptoms both in those with and in those without concomitant dementia.

Alternatively, others interpret "persisting" cognitive deficits as more related to "diminished brain reserve" associated with aging or preexisting dementia that has simply progressed over time (Francis and Kapoor 1992; Koponen et al. 1994). Camus et al. (2000), in a cross-sectional study of consecutive psychogeriatric admissions, found that the only factor significantly linked to incomplete symptom resolution in delirium was the presence of preexisting cognitive impairment. Rahkonen et al. (2000) found that when the index episode of delirium resolved, a new diagnosis of dementia was made in 27% of 51 prospectively studied community-dwelling elderly, and at 2-year follow-up, a total of 55% had a new diagnosis of dementia. Koponen et al.'s (1994) 5-year longitudinal study of delirium in the elderly found persistence and progression of symptoms to be attributed more to the underlying dementia than to the previous delirium episode. Camus et al. (2000) found that preexisting dementia was associated with only partial or no recovery from delirium in hospitalized elderly patients at 3-week follow-up. Kolbeinsson and Jonsson (1993) found that delirium was complicated by dementia at follow-up in 70% of patients. Thus, "persistent" deficits may instead reflect an underlying disorder and not the delirium. Comorbid dementia may go unrecognized at the time of the delirium index episode in

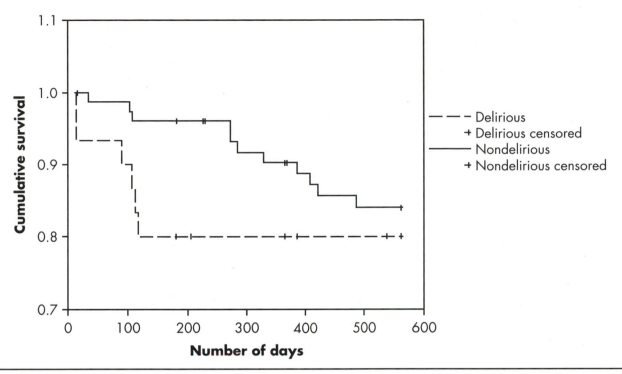

FIGURE 6–4. **Long-term follow-up survival differences in emergency department patients with and without delirium who were discharged to home.**

Source. Reprinted from Kakuma R, du Fort GG, Arsenault L, et al.: "Delirium in Older Emergency Department Patients Discharged Home: Effect on Survival." *Journal of the American Geriatrics Society* 51:443–450, 2003. Copyright 2003. Used with permission.

part because it is methodologically challenging to adequately assess for preexisting dementia retrospectively. Jackson et al. (2003) used a Modified Blessed Dementia Index during surrogate interviews and review of medical records in their study of long-term cognitive outcome of elderly medical ICU patients with delirium.

In contrast, a longitudinal cohort study of 674 community-dwelling elderly patients with hip fractures assessed delirium, proxy prefracture dementia, and 2- and 12-month follow-up for cognition and social and ADL functioning (Gruber-Baldini et al. 2003). They found that 28% had prefracture dementia or impairment on the Mini-Mental State Exam (MMSE), and another 22% had newly detected cognitive impairment while in the hospital. More than 40% of the latter group had persistent cognitive deficits at follow-up, despite no obvious preexisting dementia, accompanied by poorer physical ADLs and social functioning at 12 months in those still cognitively impaired at 2 months. This supports the notion that an index episode of delirium indeed may be associated with persistent cognitive deficits in almost half the patients in elderly hip surgery populations.

A prospective longitudinal cohort study of 90 stem cell transplant patients addressed the relation between delirium and cognitive outcome posttransplant (Fann et al. 2003). The mean age of the patients was 42 years; thus, the dementia confound in elderly studies was avoided. After adjustment for age and gender, delirium and its severity predicted executive cognitive impairment at day 80 despite significant improvements in overall vigor and functioning.

Individual delirium symptoms may predict the duration of an episode. Wada and Yamaguchi (1993), in a study of elderly neuropsychiatry consults, found that a longer duration of delirium (≥1 week) was predicted by the severity of cognitive disturbance, mood lability, and sleep–wake cycle disruption. Treloar and MacDonald (1997) found that the degree of reversibility of an index episode of delirium was predicted by motor activity, speech and thought disturbances, and a fluctuating course. However, their definition of reversibility was more modest than most clinicians would expect.

Biological measures may correlate with reversibility of delirium. Mach et al. (1995) found that higher levels of serum anticholinergic activity were associated with greater likelihood of full resolution of delirium, perhaps implying that the causes of delirium, such as anticholinergic toxicity, were more reversible, although this was not specifically addressed in this study.

The relation between delirium and persistent symptoms at follow-up may be explained by an index episode of delirium being an actual risk factor for, rather than a cause or marker of, other causes of cognitive impairment. Rockwood et al. (1999) reported an 18% annual incidence of dementia in patients with delirium—a risk more than three times higher than in nondelirious patients when the confounding effects of comorbid illness, severity, and age were adjusted for.

Thus, whether delirium itself causes permanent damage remains controversial. Studies to date do not fully account for the role of underlying etiologies, treatment received, preexisting cognitive impairment, or other confounds. Nonetheless, the concept of delirium as an inherently reversible condition is increasingly questioned.

Clinical Features

Phenomenology

The classic descriptive study of 106 "dysergastic reaction" (i.e., delirium) patients by Wolff and Curran (1935) is still consistent with current conceptions of delirium phenomenology. Inconsistent and unclear definitions of symptoms and underuse of standardized symptom assessment tools have hampered subsequent efforts to describe delirium phenomenology or to compare symptom incidences across studies and etiological populations. Nearly all studies are cross-sectional, so we lack an understanding of how various symptoms change over the course of an episode. More recent longitudinal research in which daily delirium ratings were used has reported only total scale scores and not the occurrence of individual symptoms and their pattern over time. Relations between symptoms also have not been studied, except through factor analyses of cross-sectional data in a few reports (Trzepacz and Dew 1995; Trzepacz et al. 1998; van der Mast 1994). Although carried out in different populations, these factor analyses had some striking similarities regarding which symptoms clustered together and also suggested that delirium symptoms overshadow dementia symptoms when they are comorbid.

Despite across-study inconsistencies for symptom frequencies, certain symptoms occur more often than others, consistent with the proposal that delirium has core symptoms irrespective of etiology (Trzepacz 1999b, 2000). Multiple etiologies for delirium may "funnel" into a final common neural pathway (Trzepacz 1999b, 2000), so that the phenomenological expression becomes similar despite a breadth of different physiologies. Candidates for *core symptoms* include attention deficits, memory impairment, disorientation, sleep–wake cycle disturbance,

thought process abnormalities, motor alterations, and language disturbances, whereas *associated* or *noncore symptoms* would include perceptual disturbances (illusions, hallucinations), delusions, and affective changes (Trzepacz 1999b). Analysis of Delirium Rating Scale—Revised–98 (DRS-R-98) blinded ratings supports this separation of so-called core from associated symptoms on the basis of their relative prevalence (Trzepacz et al. 2001a). The occurrence of the less frequent associated symptoms might suggest involvement of particular etiologies and their specific pathophysiologies or individual differences in brain circuitry and vulnerability. Characteristic diagnostic features of delirium, such as altered state of consciousness (e.g., called *clouding* by some) and fluctuation of symptom severity over a 24-hour period, may be epiphenomena and not symptoms per se. These features may be more related to *how* the symptoms are expressed, affecting the observed outward appearance of delirium.

Historically, delirium has been viewed by some neurologists primarily as a disturbance of attention; less importance has been attributed to its other cognitive deficits and behavioral symptoms. Disturbance of attention is a key symptom required for diagnosis of delirium yet is unlikely to explain the breadth of delirium symptoms. Distractibility, inattention, and poor environmental awareness can be evident during interview as well as on formal testing. Impairment in attention was found in 100% of the patients with delirium in a blinded assessment in which the DRS-R-98 was used (Trzepacz et al. 2001a). O'Keeffe and Gosney (1997) found that attention deficits discriminated delirium patients from both patients with dementia and elderly inpatients without dementia when sensitive tests such as the Digit Span Backward and Digit Cancellation tests were used.

Memory impairment occurs often in delirium, affecting both short- and long-term memory, although most reports have not distinguished between types of memory impairment. In subclinical hepatic encephalopathy, attention is intact but nonverbal memory is impaired, suggesting that these cognitive functions may be differentially affected during mild delirium (Tarter et al. 1988). In delirium due to posttraumatic brain injury, procedural and declarative memory are impaired, and procedural memory improves first (Ewert et al. 1985). Patients are often amnestic for some or all of their delirium episodes (Breitbart et al. 2002a). Trzepacz et al. (2001a) found a high correlation between the DRS-R-98 short- and long-term memory items ($r=0.51$, $P=0.01$) in delirious patients, with attention correlating with short-term memory ($r=0.44$, $P=0.03$) but not with long-term memory. This is consistent with normally needing to pay attention before information can enter short-term (working) memory, and then selected data from working memory are stored in long-term memory.

Language disturbances in delirium include dysnomia, paraphasias, impaired comprehension, dysgraphia, and word-finding difficulties. In extreme cases, language resembles a fluent dysphasia. Incoherent speech or speech disturbance is reported commonly. Dysgraphia was once thought to be specific to delirium (Chedru and Geschwind 1972). A more recent comparison with writing samples from patients with other psychiatric disorders reported that dysgraphia was not specific to delirium (Patten and Lamarre 1989). Rather, it appears that the semantic content of language is a more differentiating feature of delirium.

Disorganized thinking was found in 95% of the patients in one study (Rockwood 1993) and was also noted by Cutting (1987) to be different from thought processes in patients with schizophrenia. However, very little work has been done to characterize thought process disorder in patients with delirium, which ranges from tangentiality and circumstantiality to loose associations. When the DRS-R-98 was used, 21% of the patients with delirium exhibited tangentiality or circumstantiality, whereas 58% had loose associations (Trzepacz et al. 2001a).

Disturbances of the sleep–wake cycle are common in patients with delirium. Sleep–wake cycle disturbances may underlie fluctuations in the severity of symptoms during a 24-hour period. Sleep disturbances range from napping and nocturnal disruptions to a more severe disintegration of the normal circadian cycle. The extent to which sleep–wake cycle disturbance confounds the hyperactive–hypoactive subtyping of delirium is not known.

Hallucinations, illusions, and other misperceptions and delusions occur less frequently in delirium than do core symptoms. The type of perceptual disturbance and delusion distinguishes delirium from schizophrenia (Cutting 1987). Clinically, the occurrence of visual (as well as tactile, olfactory, and gustatory) hallucinations heightens the likelihood of delirium, although primary psychiatric disorders occasionally present with visual misperceptions. Visual hallucinations range from patterns or shapes to complex and vivid animations, which may vary according to which part of the brain is affected (Trzepacz 1994). Persecutory delusions that are poorly formed (not systematized) are the most common type in delirium, although other types occur (e.g., somatic or grandiose). Delusions do not seem to be a result of cognitive impairment per se. A retrospective study of 227 patients with delirium found that 26% had delusions, 27% had visual hallucinations, 12% had auditory hallucinations, and 3% had tactile hallucinations (Webster and Holroyd 2000).

Affective lability that changes within minutes is characteristic of delirium. It takes many forms (e.g., anxious, apathetic, angry, dysphoric), changes from one type to another without obvious relation to the context (i.e., incongruent), and is usually not under self-control.

Motor Subtypes

There has been much interest in whether there are subtypes of delirium, derived from various parameters such as underlying physiology, etiology, and symptom profile (Trzepacz 1994), similar to the way heart failure is categorized. It is unclear whether such meaningful subtypes exist. Nonetheless, the most studied possible subtype is based on psychomotor behavior. Although not all patients with delirium exhibit psychomotor change, different presentations of activity have been recognized for centuries. Neurologists have differentiated disorientation with reduced motor activity, referred to as "acute confusion," from the hyperactive disorientation of patients labeled as "delirious" (Mesulam 1985; Mori and Yamadori 1987). In a study of infarctions of the right middle cerebral artery, Mori and Yamadori (1987) suggested that acute confusional states are disturbances of attention resulting from frontostriatal damage, whereas acute agitated deliria are disturbances of emotion and affect resulting from injury to the middle temporal gyrus. However, these distinctions and localizations have not been supported by subsequent studies (Trzepacz 1994).

Lipowski (1990) championed the use of the umbrella term *delirium* and then described three psychomotor subtypes: "hyperactive," "hypoactive," and "mixed." Various definitions of motor subtypes have been subjectively described, are not standardized, and include nonmotor behavioral features such as disturbances of speech, affective changes, and disturbances of thinking and perception (see Table 6–4). With the use of such definitions, motor subtypes are characterized by similar degrees of overall cognitive impairment and EEG slowing (Koponen et al. 1989; Ross et al. 1991) but differ for some nonmotor symptoms. Delusions, hallucinations, mood lability, speech incoherence, and sleep disturbances may be somewhat more frequent in hyperactive patients (Meagher and Trzepacz 2000; Ross et al. 1991). Waxing and waning of symptom severity and sleep–wake cycle abnormalities complicate our understanding of motor subtypes, as does reliance on subjective and retrospective reports of behavior over 24-hour periods. Reports of relative frequencies of motor subtypes vary widely, even when patients with alcohol withdrawal are excluded. In a prospective study of patients with delirium, Meagher (2003) found a remarkably low level of concordance between three different psychomotor schemas. Studies that use objective motor activity level monitoring are needed.

TABLE 6–4. Features of psychomotor subtypes of delirium

	Hyperactive	Hypoactive
Motor symptoms	Increased activity levels Increased speed of actions Loss of control of activity Restlessness and wandering	Decreased activity levels Decreased speed of actions Apathy and listlessness
Nonmotor symptoms	Increased amount, speed, and volume of speech Altered content of verbal output (e.g., singing, shouting, laughing) Aggression, combativeness, uncooperativeness Hallucinations Hyperalertness, increased startle	Decreased amount, speed, and volume of speech Hypoalertness Hypersomnolence Social withdrawal
Electroencephalogram	Diffuse slowing	Diffuse slowing
Cognition	Diffuse deficits	Diffuse deficits
Treatment	Neuroleptic responsive	Neuroleptic responsive
Outcome	? Lower mortality	? Increased mortality and closer to stupor

Note. Mixed subtype requires evidence of both hyperactive and hypoactive delirium.

In many reports, up to half of the patients have a mixed motor subtype during their episode. Detailed longitudinal study of delirium symptoms is necessary before any definitive conclusion can be reached regarding the stability of motor subtypes. Peterson et al. (2003) used the Richmond Agitation and Aggression Scale to longitudinally rate medical ICU delirium patients by nurses three times per shift. They found very few hyperactive (*n*=4) and mostly hypoactive (*n*=138) or mixed (*n*=255) deliria, but the use of sedating medications confounds these results.

Studies to date have not provided convincing evidence that motor subtypes have distinct neurobiological underpinnings. The delirium symptom profile of patients with localized cerebral insults does not reliably link specific motor subtypes to lesions at particular cerebral sites. Neither EEG nor functional neuroimaging findings distinguish motor subtypes (Trzepacz 1994).

Motor subtypes of delirium may be associated with different etiologies, treatment, or outcome. Delirium due to drug-related causes is most commonly hyperactive, whereas delirium due to metabolic disturbances, including hypoxia, is more frequently hypoactive (Meagher and Trzepacz 1998; O'Keeffe and Lavan 1999; Olofsson et al. 1996; Ross et al. 1991). Patients with a hyperactive subtype may have better outcomes after an episode of delirium, with shorter lengths of stay, lower mortality rates, and higher rates of full recovery (Kobayashi et al. 1992; Liptzin and Levkoff 1992; Olofsson et al. 1996). However, these varied outcomes may reflect differences in underlying causes, recognition rates, and/or treatment practices. Underdetection and misdiagnosis are especially common in hypoactive patients. Even when hypoactive subtypes are actively screened for, these patients still may have a poorer outcome (O'Keeffe and Lavan 1999). Meagher et al. (1996) found that the use of psychotropic medication and supportive environmental ward strategies were more closely linked to level of hyperactivity than to the degree of cognitive disturbance. In contrast, Olofsson et al. (1996) reported better outcomes in patients with hyperactive delirium but noted that they received less haloperidol than did nonhyperactive patients. O'Keeffe and Lavan (1999) reported greater use of neuroleptics and shorter hospital stays in hyperactive patients but linked these to less severe illness at the onset of delirium and a lower incidence of hospital-acquired infections and bedsores in those who were hyperactive. Others have found that different motor subtypes were associated with similar outcomes (Camus et al. 2000).

Treatment studies have not been designed specifically to assess response of effectiveness for different motor subtypes. In clinical practice, it is often presumed that psychotropic agents are useful in delirium solely for sedative or antipsychotic purposes and thus more effective for hyperactive patients, but the few available data are mixed (Breitbart et al. 2002b; Platt et al. 1994a; Uchiyama et al. 1996). Overall, the relationships among motor subtype, treatment, and outcome remain unclear and confounded by methodological issues.

Diagnosis and Assessment

Diagnosis

Specific diagnostic criteria for delirium first appeared in DSM-III, around the same time as the first symptom rating scales for delirium. Thus, early clinical reports and research based on the first two editions of DSM (American Psychiatric Association 1952, 1968) or Research Diagnostic Criteria (RDC) were affected by this lack of diagnostic specificity.

DSM-I was first published in 1952 and described acute and chronic brain syndromes (American Psychiatric Association 1952). Most forms of delirium were encompassed within the acute, reversible category and were characterized by impairments of orientation, memory, all intellectual functions, and judgment, as well as lability and shallowness of affect. Other disturbances, such as hallucinations and delusions, were considered secondary to the disturbance of the sensorium. Causes of delirium were specifically noted—for example, "acute brain syndrome associated with cerebrovascular accident." DSM-II (American Psychiatric Association 1968) described two organic brain syndromes, psychotic and nonpsychotic types, each with an acute or a chronic delineation. DSM-II maintained the same five symptoms as DSM-I. DSM-III (American Psychiatric Association 1987) distinguished delirium from dementia and other organic mental disorders, each identified by its own explicit criteria. Some revisions were made in DSM-III-R, especially to the major criterion involving inattention and altered consciousness.

DSM-IV (American Psychiatric Association 1994), and its text revision, DSM-IV-TR (American Psychiatric Association 2000), have five categories of delirium; the criteria are the same for each category except the one for etiology. The categories are 1) delirium due to a general medical condition, 2) substance intoxication delirium, 3) substance withdrawal delirium, 4) delirium due to multiple etiologies, and 5) delirium not otherwise specified. This notation of etiology in DSM-IV is reminiscent of that used in DSM-I.

DSM-III, DSM-III-R, and DSM-IV included efforts to further clarify the major criterion describing altered state of consciousness, considered as either *a disturbance of consciousness* or *inattention*. Liptzin et al. (1993) found disturbed consciousness in 100% of delirious elderly patients irrespective of whether comorbid dementia was present. Impairment of attention distinguishes delirium from dementia. Attention deficits in delirium range from general, nonspecific reduction in alertness to decreased selective focusing or sustaining of attention. The contribution of attention deficits to the altered awareness that occurs in delirium is insufficient by itself to account for other prominent symptoms such as formal thought disorder, language and sleep–wake cycle disturbances, and other cognitive-perceptual deficits.

The temporal course of delirium, with acute onset and fluctuation of symptoms, has been a separate criterion in each of the last three editions of DSM. Temporal features assist in distinguishing delirium from dementia, supported by data derived from the DRS-R-98 (Trzepacz et al. 2002b).

Despite the breadth of the symptoms of delirium, not all have been emphasized in the various editions of DSM. Dysexecutive symptoms (impairment of prefrontal executive cognition) are not mentioned in any DSM edition, despite their clinical importance in delirium (Trzepacz 1994). Psychosis has not received much attention, except in DSM-II, despite the occurrence of delusions in about a fifth of patients with delirium (Ross et al. 1991; Sirois 1988). Characteristic features of delusions (usually paranoid and poorly formed) and hallucinations (often visual) have not been specified in DSM criteria, despite their usefulness to the clinician.

The World Health Organization's research diagnostic criteria for delirium in ICD-10 are similar to the DSM-IV criteria. However, ICD-10 diverges from DSM-IV in that cognitive dysfunction is manifested by both "impairment of immediate recall and recent memory, with intact remote memory" and "disorientation in time, place or person." Additionally, a disturbance in sleep is present and manifested by insomnia, nocturnal worsening of symptoms, or disturbing dreams or nightmares that may continue as hallucinations or illusions when awake, which seems to etiologically link perceptual disturbances to sleep mechanisms. Despite these differences, a study of 80 patients with delirium showed 100% concordance for diagnosis between DSM-III-R and ICD-10 research criteria (Treloar and MacDonald 1997).

Cole et al. (2003a) used DSM-III-R as the gold standard to compare the sensitivity and specificity of DSM-IV, DSM-III, and ICD-10 criteria for delirium in 40 patients with delirium only, 94 with dementia only, and 128 with comorbid delirium and dementia. They found that requiring clouding of consciousness lowered the sensitivity considerably and recommended inattention instead—perhaps because the term *clouding of consciousness* is vague and therefore poorly assessable. Sensitivity and specificity of DSM-IV, DSM-III, and ICD-10 criteria were 100% and 71%, 96% and 91%, and 61% and 91%, respectively. Thus, DSM-IV was found to be the most inclusive.

Cognitive Assessment

Because delirium is primarily a cognitive disorder, bedside assessment of cognition is critical to proper diagnosis. Although all cognitive domains—orientation, attention, short- and long-term memory, visuoconstructional ability, and executive function—are affected in delirium, attention deficits are the most specifically emphasized in DSM. Pattern and timing of deficits assist in differential diagnosis from dementias and amnestic disorders. Use of bedside screening tests (see also Chapter 1, "Psychiatric Assessment and Consultation") such as the well-known MMSE (Folstein et al. 1975) is important clinically to document the presence of a cognitive disorder; however, it is alone insufficient to distinguish delirium from dementia (Trzepacz et al. 1988a). The MMSE is too easy for many people (ceiling effect) and has a limited breadth of items, particularly for prefrontal executive and right-hemisphere functions.

The Cognitive Test for Delirium (CTD; Hart et al. 1996) is a more recent bedside test designed specifically for patients with delirium who are often unable to speak or write in a medical setting (e.g., on a ventilator). Unlike the MMSE, the CTD has many nonverbal (nondominant hemisphere) items and abstraction questions. The CTD correlates highly with the MMSE ($r=0.82$) in patients with delirium and was performable in 42% of the ICU patients in whom the MMSE was not. It has two equivalent forms that correlated highly ($r=0.90$) in patients with dementia, which makes it better suited for repeated measurements. However, it correlates less well with symptom rating scales for delirium that also include noncognitive symptoms—for example, the MCV Nurses Rating Scale for Delirium ($r=-0.02$) (Hart et al. 1996) and the DRS-R-98 ($r=-0.62$) (Trzepacz et al. 2001b). An abbreviated version of the CTD, with just two of its nine items (visual attention span and recognition memory for pictures), retained good reliability and discriminant validity (Hart et al. 1997).

The clock drawing test is a useful screen for cognitive impairment in medically ill patients, but it does not discriminate between delirium and dementia (Manos 1997). A global rating of attentiveness and the Digit Span Backward and Digit Cancellation tests differentiated delirium from dementia among elderly medical inpatients, whereas the Vigilance Test, the MMSE, and the Digit Span Forward test did not (O'Keefe and Gosney 1997). However, patients were excluded from the study if their MMSE score was 10 points or less, which effectively rules out applicability to many patients with delirium.

Delirium Assessment Instruments

Diagnostic criteria are important in diagnosing delirium, and cognitive tests are useful in documenting cognitive impairment. Rating a range of delirium symptoms, however, requires other methods. More than 10 instruments have been proposed to assess symptoms of delirium (Trzepacz 1996b) for screening, diagnosis, or symptom severity rating. Nonvalidated measures, designed for use in a single study, continue to proliferate in the literature. However, relatively few have been used broadly (see later in this section). Three instruments operationalized DSM-III criteria: the Saskatoon Delirium Checklist (Miller et al. 1988), Organic Brain Syndrome Scale (Berggren et al. 1987), and Delirium Assessment Scale (O'Keeffe 1994). In these, DSM-III–derived items are rated along a continuum of mild to moderate to severe. None has been well described or validated. The Delirium Assessment Scale could not distinguish delirium from dementia patients. A more recent severity scale, the Confusional State Evaluation (Robertsson 1999), assessed 22 items, but 12 were determined a priori to be "key symptoms." It was not validated against control groups, and patients with dementia were included in the delirium group.

The Confusion Assessment Method (CAM) is probably the most widely used screening tool for diagnosis of delirium in general hospitals in its 4-item form (Inouye et al. 1990). CAM is based on DSM-III-R criteria and has two forms: 1) a full scale with 11 items rated as present or absent and 2) the more commonly used algorithm that requires the presence of 3 of 4 cardinal symptoms for a diagnosis of delirium. It is intended for use by nonpsychiatric clinicians in hospital settings and is useful for case finding, although nurses' ratings were much less sensitive than those done by physicians (0.13 vs. 1.00) when compared with an independent physician's DSM-III-R diagnosis (Rolfson et al. 1999). One study (Rockwood 1993) suggested that lower specificity and sensitivity are the trade-offs for the test's simplicity, even though in other studies the test performed well compared with physicians' diagnoses in acute hospital settings. It has not been well studied for its ability to distinguish delirium from dementia, depression, or other psychiatric disorders.

Recently, Cole et al. (2003a) assessed the sensitivity and specificity of the full CAM in patients with DSM-III-R–diagnosed delirium, dementia, or comorbid delirium and dementia. With a cutoff of 6 of 11 items present, the authors found 95% sensitivity and 83% specificity in delirium-only patients and 98% sensitivity and 76% specificity in comorbid patients; however, use of fewer items (e.g., a minimum cutoff of 3 symptoms) greatly reduced the specificities to 60% for delirium and 47% for comorbid delirium and dementia. The CAM appears to be useful for screening elderly emergency department patients for delirium (Monette et al. 2001). On the basis of a geriatrician's interview, comparison of ratings from the geriatrician interviewer with those from an observing layperson indicated interrater reliability of 0.91, sensitivity of 0.86, and specificity of 1.00.

A recent extension of the CAM is the CAM-ICU (Ely et al. 2001a, 2001b), aimed at use by nurses for severely medically ill patients in the ICU setting. The CAM-ICU uses specific adjunctive tests and standardized administration to enhance reliability and validity; 95% validity and 0.92–0.96 interrater reliability have been reported, compared with expert psychiatric diagnosis of delirium with DSM-IV criteria, in two different validation studies of 150 patients (Ely et al. 2001a, 2001b).

The delirium assessment tool most commonly used by nurses is the NEECHAM Scale (Neelon et al. 1996). It is scored from 0 to 30, with cutoffs for levels of confusion severity, and was originally validated in elderly acute medical and nursing home settings without a control group. Interrater reliability was 0.96, correlation with the MMSE was 0.81, and correlation with nurses' subjective ratings was 0.46. It has three sections, including a physiological measurement section. Internal consistency was between 0.73 and 0.82 (Cronbach α) in 73 elderly hip surgery patients, in whom factor analysis identified three factors (Johansson et al. 2002). It has been translated into Swedish, Norwegian, and Japanese.

The Delirium Rating Scale (DRS; Trzepacz et al. 1988a) is a 10-item scale assessing a breadth of delirium features and can function both to clarify diagnosis and to assess symptom severity because of its hierarchical nature (Trzepacz 1999a; van der Mast 1994). It is probably the most widely used delirium rating scale and has been translated into Italian, French, Spanish, Korean, Japanese, Mandarin Chinese, Dutch, Swedish, German, Portuguese, and a language of India for international use. It is generally used by those who have some psychiatric training. The DRS has high interrater reliability and validity, even when compared with other psychiatric patient groups, and distinguishes delirium from dementia. Factor analysis finds a two- or three-factor structure (Trzepacz 1999a; Trzepacz and Dew 1995). However, because of some of its items, it does not function as well for frequent repeated measurements and thus has been modified by some researchers to a seven- or eight-item subscale. In one study (Treloar and MacDonald 1997), the DRS and CAM diagnosed delirium in patients with high level of agreement (κ=0.81). More recently, it has been useful in children and adolescents (Turkel et al. 2003).

The DRS-R-98 is a substantially revised version that addresses the shortcomings of the DRS (Trzepacz et al. 2001b). It allows for repeated measurements and includes separate or new items for language, thought processes, motor agitation, motor retardation, and five cognitive domains. The DRS-R-98 has 16 items, with 3 diagnostic items separable from 13 severity items that form a severity subscale that also was validated. Severity for a broad range of symptoms known to occur in delirium is described with standard phenomenological definitions, without a priori assumptions about which occur more frequently. The total scale is used for initial evaluation of delirium to allow discrimination from other disorders. The DRS-R-98 total score distinguished ($P<0.001$) delirium from dementia, schizophrenia, depression, and other medical illnesses during blind ratings, with sensitivities ranging from 91% to 100% and specificities from 85% to 100%, depending on the cutoff score chosen. The DRS-R-98 has high internal consistency (Cronbach α=0.90), correlates well with the DRS (r=0.83) and CTD (r=−0.62), and has high interrater reliability (intraclass correlation coefficient [ICC]=0.99). Translations exist or are in progress for Japanese, Korean, Greek, Portuguese, Danish, Dutch, German, Spanish (Mexico and Spain), French, Lithuanian, Norwegian, Italian, and Chinese versions. Japanese and Spanish (Spain) versions have been validated and published (Fonseca et al., in press; Kishi et al. 2001). A Palm Pilot version has been used for clinical research (Hill et al. 2002).

The Memorial Delirium Assessment Scale (MDAS) is a 10-item severity rating scale for use after a diagnosis of delirium has been made (Breitbart et al. 1997). It was intended for repeated ratings within a 24-hour period, as in treatment studies. The MDAS does not include items for temporal onset or fluctuation of symptoms, which helps to distinguish delirium from dementia. The MDAS correlated highly with the DRS (r=0.88) and MMSE (r=−0.91). The Japanese version of the MDAS was validated in 37 elderly patients with either delirium, dementia, mood disorder, or schizophrenia and found to distinguish among them ($P<0.001$), with mean score of 18 in the delirium group (Matsuoka et al. 2001). It correlated reasonably well with the DRS Japanese version (r=0.74) and Clinician's Global Rating of Delirium (r=0.67) and less well with the MMSE (r=0.54). The Italian version (Grassi et al. 2001) correlated well with the DRS Italian version in a study of 105 consecutive (66 had delirium) cancer patients. With the CAM as the diagnostic standard, the MDAS had high specificity (94%) but low sensitivity (68%), whereas the DRS with a cutoff of 10 had high sensitivity (95%) and low specificity (68%) and with a cutoff of 12 had a sensitivity of 80% and a specificity of

76%. In this same study, the MMSE had a 96% sensitivity but only a 38% specificity. Factor analysis showed a three-factor structure for the DRS and a two-factor structure for the MDAS. Lawlor et al. (2000b) used the MDAS in cancer patients with DSM-IV–diagnosed delirium and found two factors on factor analysis (Cronbach $\alpha = 0.78$ and $r = 0.55$ with the MMSE).

On the basis of issues such as instrument design, purpose, and breadth of use, several of the available instruments are recommended (see Table 6–5). They can be used together or separately, depending on the clinical or research need. For example, a screening tool can be used for case detection, followed by application of DSM criteria, and then a more thorough rating for symptom severity.

Electroencephalography

In the 1940s, Engel and Romano (1944, 1959; Romano and Engel 1944) wrote a series of classic papers that described the relation of delirium, as measured by cognitive impairment, to EEG generalized slowing. In their seminal work, they showed an association between abnormal electrical activity of the brain and symptoms of delirium, the reversibility of both of these conditions, the ubiquity of EEG changes for different underlying disease states, and the improvement in EEG background rhythm that paralleled clinical improvement. In most cases, EEGs are not needed to make a clinical diagnosis of delirium; instead, they are used when seizures are suspected or differential diagnosis is difficult, as in schizophrenic patients with medical illness. Most often, a careful assessment of behaviors, cognition, and history is sufficient to diagnose delirium. Nonetheless, EEG is the only technological method to assist in delirium diagnosis.

EEG characteristics in delirium include slowing or dropout of the dominant posterior rhythm, diffuse theta or delta waves (i.e., slowing), poor organization of the background rhythm, and loss of reactivity of EEG to eye opening and closing (Jacobson and Jerrier 2000). Similarly, quantitative EEG in delirium shows slowing of power bands' mean frequency, especially in posterior regions (see Figure 6–5).

In burn patients, Andreasen et al. (1977) showed that the time course of EEG slowing could precede or lag behind overt clinical symptoms of delirium, although sensitive delirium symptom ratings were not used. EEG dominant posterior rhythm, along with serum albumin and Trail Making Test B, distinguished delirious from nondelirious cirrhosis patients in another study (Trzepacz et al. 1988b). Although generalized slowing is the typical EEG pattern for both hypoactive and hyperactive presentations of delirium and for most etiologies, delirium tremens is most prominently associated with low-voltage fast activity (Kennard et al. 1945) that is superimposed on slow waves. Intoxication with sedative-hypnotics is associated with fast beta waves. Although diffuse slowing is the most common presentation, false-negative results occur when a person's characteristic dominant posterior rhythm does not slow sufficiently to drop from the alpha to the theta range, thereby being read as normal despite the presence of abnormal slowing for that individual. (Generally, a change of more than 1 cycle[s] per second [cps] from an individual's baseline is considered abnormal.) Jacobson and Jerrier (2000) warned that it can be difficult to distinguish delirium from drowsiness and light sleep unless the technologist includes standard alerting procedures during the EEG. Comparison with prior baseline EEGs is often helpful to document that slowing has in fact occurred. Less commonly, but nonetheless important, an EEG may detect focal problems, such as ictal and subictal states or a previously unsuspected tumor that presents with prominent confusion (see Table 6–6). These include toxic ictal psychosis, nonconvulsive status, and complex partial status epilepticus (Drake and Coffey 1983; Trzepacz 1994) or focal lesions (Jacobson and Jerrier 2000). Toxic ictal states include tricyclic antidepressant overdose, in which the seizure threshold is lowered and anticholinergicity contributes to delirium. New-onset complex partial seizures, usually related to ischemic damage (Sundaram and Dostrow 1995), are underrecognized causes of delirium in the elderly, especially when prolonged confusion occurs during status.

Advances in EEG technologies have expanded our knowledge. After spectral analysis of elderly patients with delirium (about 75% of whom also had dementia), Koponen et al. (1989) found significant reductions in alpha percentage, increased theta and delta activity, and slowing of the peak and mean frequencies. All of these findings are consistent with EEG slowing. The study also found a correlation between the severity of cognitive decline and the length of the patient's hospital stay, on the one hand, and the degree of EEG slowing, on the other. Jacobson et al. (1993a) used quantitative EEG to distinguish delirious persons from nondelirious individuals with the relative power of the alpha frequency band and delirious persons from individuals with dementia with the theta activity and relative power of delta. Serial EEGs of patients with delirium showed associations between the relative power of the alpha band and cognitive ability, whereas in patients with dementia, the absolute power of the delta band was associated with cognitive changes (Jacobson et al. 1993b). Quantitative EEG could replace conventional EEG for delirium assessment in the future (Jacobson and Jerrier 2000).

TABLE 6–5. Recommended delirium assessment instruments

Instrument[a]	Type	Rater
NEECHAM (Neelon et al. 1996)	Screen for high-risk patients	Nurses
Confusion Assessment Method (Inouye et al. 1990)	4-item diagnostic screen	Nonpsychiatric clinician
Delirium Rating Scale (Trzepacz et al. 1998)	10-item severity/diagnostic scale	Psychiatrically trained clinician
Memorial Delirium Assessment Scale (Breitbart et al. 1997)	10-item severity scale	Clinician
Delirium Rating Scale—Revised–98 (Trzepacz et al. 2001b)	16-item scale (includes severity subscale)	Psychiatrically trained clinician

[a]See text for descriptions.

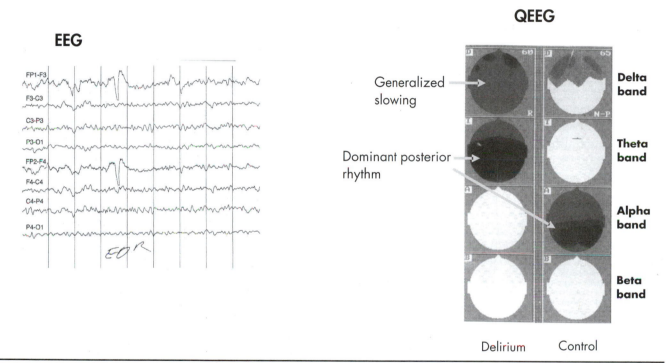

FIGURE 6–5. Typical electroencephalogram (EEG) and quantitative EEG (QEEG) findings in delirium.
Examples of bipolar lead EEG and QEEG in delirium showing diffuse slowing, especially of the dominant posterior rhythm. On QEEG, higher power is shown in darker shading, according to each of the four frequency bands.
Source. Reprinted from Jacobson SA, Jerrier S: "EEG in Delirium." *Seminars in Clinical Neuropsychiatry* 5:86–93, 2000. Used with permission.

Evoked potentials also may be abnormal in delirium. Metabolic causes of delirium precipitate abnormalities in visual, auditory, and somatosensory evoked potentials (Kullmann et al. 1995; Trzepacz 1994), whereas somatosensory evoked potentials are abnormal in patients whose delirium is due to posttraumatic brain injury. In general, normalization of evoked potentials parallels clinical improvement, although evoked potentials are not routinely recorded for clinical purposes.

EEGs and evoked potentials in children with delirium show patterns similar to those in adults, with diffuse slowing on EEG and increased latencies of evoked potentials (J. A. Katz et al. 1988; Prugh et al. 1980; Ruijs et al. 1993, 1994). The degree of slowing on EEGs and evoked potentials performed serially over time in children and adolescents correlates with the severity of delirium and with recovery from delirium (Foley et al. 1981; Montgomery et al. 1991; Onofrj et al. 1991).

TABLE 6–6.   Electroencephalographic patterns in patients with delirium

Electroencephalographic finding	Comment	Causes
Diffuse slowing	Most typical delirium pattern	Many causes, including anticholinergicity, posttraumatic brain injury, hepatic encephalopathy, hypoxia
Low-voltage fast activity	Typical of delirium tremens	Alcohol withdrawal; benzodiazepine intoxication
Spikes/polyspikes, frontocentral	Toxic ictal pattern (nonconvulsive)	Hypnosedative drug withdrawal; tricyclic and phenothiazine intoxication
Left/bilateral slowing or delta bursts; frontal intermittent rhythmic delta	Acute confusional migraine	Usually in adolescents
Epileptiform activity, frontotemporal or generalized	Status with prolonged confusional states	Nonconvulsive status and complex partial status epilepticus

Etiology

Delirium has a wide variety of etiologies, which may occur alone or in combination (see Tables 6–7 and 6–8). These include primary cerebral disorders, systemic disturbances that affect cerebral function, drug and toxin exposure (including intoxication and withdrawal), and a range of factors that can contribute to delirium but have an uncertain role as etiological factors by themselves (psychological and environmental factors). To be considered causal, an etiology should be a recognized possible cause of delirium and be temporally related in onset and course to delirium presentation; also, the delirium should not be better accounted for by other factors. No clear cause is found in approximately 10% of patients, and these cases are categorized as delirium not otherwise specified in DSM-IV-TR.

In those studies in which the possibility of multiple etiologies has been considered, between two and six possible causes are typically identified (Breitbart et al. 1996; Francis et al. 1990; Meagher et al. 1996; O'Keeffe and Lavan 1996; Trzepacz et al. 1985), with a single etiology identified in fewer than 50% of cases (Camus et al. 2000; O'Keeffe and Lavan 1999; Olofsson et al. 1996). Delirium with multiple etiologies is more frequent in the elderly and those with terminal illness. For example, delirium in cancer patients can be due to the direct effect of the primary tumor or the indirect effects of metastases, metabolic problems (organ failure or electrolyte disturbance), chemotherapy, radiation and other treatments, infections, vascular complications, nutritional deficits, and paraneoplastic syndromes. This multifactorial nature has been underemphasized in research—etiological attribution typically is based on clinical impressions that are not standardized (e.g., the most likely cause identified by referring physician) or that are oversimplified by documenting a single etiology for each case. That delirium due to a single etiology is the exception rather than the rule highlights the importance of multidisciplinary approaches to management and the need for continued vigilance to the possibility of further etiological inputs even when a cause has been identified.

Some causes are more frequently encountered in particular populations. Delirium in children and adolescents involves the same categories of etiologies as in adults, although specific causes may differ. Delirium related to illicit drugs is more common in younger populations, whereas delirium due to prescribed drugs and polypharmacy is more common in older populations. Cerebral hypoxia is common at age extremes—chronic obstructive airway disease, myocardial infarction, and stroke are common in older patients, and hypoxia due to foreign-body inhalation, drowning, and asthma are more frequent in younger patients. Poisonings are also more common in children than in adults, whereas young adults have the highest rates of head trauma.

Once delirium is diagnosed, a careful and thorough, but prioritized, search for causes must be conducted. Ameliorations of specific underlying causes are important in resolving delirium; however, this should not preclude treatment of the delirium itself, which can reduce symptoms even before underlying medical causes are rectified (Breitbart et al. 1996).

Neuropathogenesis

Even though delirium has many different etiologies, its constellation of symptoms is largely stereotyped, with some considered core symptoms. Somehow, this diversity of physiological perturbations translates into a common clinical expression that may represent dysfunction of

TABLE 6–7. Selected etiologies of delirium[a]

Drug intoxication
Alcohol
Sedative-hypnotics
Opiates
Psychostimulants
Hallucinogens
Inhalants
Drug withdrawal
Alcohol
Sedative-hypnotics
Metabolic and endocrine disturbance
Volume depletion or volume overload
Acidosis or alkalosis
Hypoxia
Uremia
Anemia
Hepatic failure
Hypoglycemia or hyperglycemia
Hypoalbuminemia
Bilirubinemia
Hypocalcemia or hypercalcemia
Hypokalemia or hyperkalemia
Hyponatremia or hypernatremia
Hypomagnesemia or hypermagnesemia
Hypophosphatemia
Thyroid storm
Hypopituitarism
Other metabolic disorders (e.g., porphyria, carcinoid syndrome)
Traumatic
Traumatic brain injury
Subdural hematoma
Fat emboli
Hypoxic
Pulmonary insufficiency
Pulmonary emboli
Neoplastic disease
Intracranial primary/metastasis/meningeal carcinomatosis
Paraneoplastic syndrome

Intracranial infection
Meningitis
Encephalitis
Abscess
Neurosyphilis
Human immunodeficiency virus
Systemic infection
Bacteremia/sepsis
Fungal
Protozoal
Viral
Cerebrovascular
Stroke, transient ischemic attack
Subarachnoid hemorrhage
Other central nervous system disorders
Cerebral edema
Seizures
Hypertensive encephalopathy
Eclampsia
Autoimmune
Central nervous system vasculitis
Systemic lupus erythematosus
Acute graft rejection
Acute graft vs. host disease
Cardiac
Heart failure
Endocarditis
Other systemic etiologies
Postoperative state
Hyperthermia: heatstroke, neuroleptic malignant syndrome, malignant hyperthermia
Hypothermia
Disseminated intravascular coagulation and other hypercoagulable states
Radiation
Electrocution

[a]See Table 6–8 for drugs causing delirium.

certain neural circuits (as well as neurotransmitters)—that is, a final common neural pathway (Trzepacz 1999b, 2000). The involvement of certain specific regions and pathways is largely based on limited structural and functional neuroimaging data. (For more detailed discussion, refer to Trzepacz 2000 and Trzepacz et al. 2002a.) Dysfunction in both cortical and subcortical regions in delirium has been supported by studies of regional cerebral blood flow, single photon emission computed tomography, positron-emission tomography, EEG, and evoked potentials (Trzepacz 1994; Yokota et al. 2003). Whereas some etiologies of delirium alter neurotransmission via general

metabolism, others may antagonize or interfere with specific receptors and neurotransmitters.

The best-established neurotransmitter alteration accounting for many cases of delirium is reduced cholinergic activity (Trzepacz 1996a, 2000). A wide variety of medications and their metabolites have anticholinergic activity and cause delirium. Some act postsynaptically; others act presynaptically; and still others, such as norfentanyl and normeperidine, have anticholinergic metabolites (Coffman and Dilsaver 1988). Tune and colleagues (1992) measured the anticholinergic activity of many medications in "atropine equivalents." They identified

TABLE 6–8.   Selected drugs causing delirium

Analgesics
  Opiates (especially meperidine, pentazocine)
  Salicylates
Antimicrobials
  Acyclovir, ganciclovir
  Aminoglycosides
  Amphotericin B
  Antimalarials
  Cephalosporins
  Chloramphenicol
  Ethambutol
  Interferon
  Isoniazid
  Metronidazole
  Rifampin
  Sulfonamides
  Vancomycin
Anticholinergic drugs
  Antihistamines, H_1 (e.g., diphenhydramine)
  Antispasmodics
  Atropine and atropine-like drugs (e.g., scopolamine)
  Benztropine
  Biperiden
  Phenothiazines (especially thioridazine)
  Tricyclics (especially amitriptyline)
  Trihexyphenidyl
Anticonvulsants
  Phenobarbital
  Phenytoin
  Valproic acid
Anti-inflammatory drugs
  Corticosteroids
  Nonsteroidal anti-inflammatory drugs
Antineoplastic drugs
  Aminoglutethimide
  Asparaginase
  Dacarbazine (DTIC)
  5-Fluorouracil
  Hexamethylenamine
  Methotrexate (intrathecal)
  Procarbazine
  Tamoxifen
  Vinblastine
  Vincristine

Antiparkinsonian drugs
  Amantadine
  Bromocriptine
  Levodopa
Cardiac drugs
  Beta-blockers
  Captopril
  Clonidine
  Digitalis
  Disopyramide
  Lidocaine
  Methyldopa
  Mexiletine
  Procainamide
  Quinidine
  Tocainide
Sedative-hypnotics
  Barbiturates
  Benzodiazepines
Stimulants
  Amphetamines
  Cocaine
  Ephedrine, epinephrine, phenylephrine
  Theophylline
Miscellaneous drugs
  Antihistamines, H_2 (e.g., cimetidine, ranitidine)
  Baclofen
  Bromides
  Chlorpropamide
  Disulfiram
  Ergotamines
  Lithium
  Metrizamide (intrathecal)
  Podophyllin (by absorption)
  Propylthiouracil
  Quinacrine
  Timolol ophthalmic

medications usually not recognized as being anticholinergic (e.g., digoxin, nifedipine, cimetidine, and codeine). Delirium induced by anticholinergic drugs is associated with generalized EEG slowing and is reversed by treatment with physostigmine or neuroleptics (Itil and Fink 1966; Stern 1983).

Several causes of delirium thought of as having diffuse, nonspecific effects on neuronal function may at least in part be acting through anticholinergic effects. Thiamine deficiency, hypoxia, and hypoglycemia all may reduce acetylcholine by affecting the oxidative metabolism of glucose and the production of acetyl coenzyme A, the rate-limiting step for acetylcholine synthesis (Trzepacz 1994). Parietal cortex levels of choline are reduced in chronic hepatic encephalopathy (Kreis et al. 1991). Serum levels of anticholinergic activity are elevated in patients with postoperative delirium and correlate with severity of cognitive impairment (Tune et al. 1981), improving with resolution of the delirium (Mach et al. 1995). Post–electroconvulsive therapy delirium is also associated with higher serum anticholinergic activity (Mondimore et al. 1983). Alzheimer's and vascular dementias reduce cholinergic activity and are associated with increased risk for delirium. Dementia with Lewy bodies, with its fluctuating symptom severity, confusion, hallucinations (especially visual), delusions, and EEG slowing, mimics delirium and is associated with significant loss of cholinergic nucleus basalis neurons. Its delirium symptoms respond to donepezil (Kaufer et al. 1998). Age-associated changes in cholinergic function also increase delirium propensity. Stroke and traumatic brain injury are associated with decreased cholinergic activity (Yamamoto et al. 1988) and have enhanced vulnerability to antimuscarinic drugs (Dixon et al. 1994). The low cholinergic state seems to correlate temporally with delirium following the acute event. Thus, there is broad support for an anticholinergic mechanism for many seemingly diverse mechanisms of delirium.

However, anticholinergic mechanisms cannot explain all deliria, because cholinergic toxicity from organophosphate insecticides, nerve poisons, and tacrine (Trzepacz et al. 1996) also can cause delirium. Increased dopamine also may play a role in some deliria. Delirium can occur from intoxication with dopaminergic drugs (Ames et al. 1992) and cocaine binges (Wetli et al. 1996). Excessive dopaminergic activity also might play a role in delirium (Trzepacz 2000), including during specific states such as alcohol withdrawal (Sander et al. 1997), opiate intoxication, hypoxia (Broderick and Gibson 1989), and hepatic encephalopathy (Knell et al. 1974). The efficacy of antidopaminergic agents, particularly neuroleptics, in treating delirium, including that arising from anticholinergic causes (Itil and Fink 1966; Platt et al. 1994b), also suggests a neuropathogenetic role for dopamine.

Both increased and decreased gamma-aminobutyric acid (GABA) levels have been implicated in causing delirium. Increased GABAergic activity is one of several putative mechanisms implicated in hepatic encephalopathy (Mousseau and Butterworth 1994). GABA activity is reduced during delirium following withdrawal from ethanol and sedative-hypnotic drugs. Decreased GABA activity is also implicated in the mechanism of antibiotic delirium caused by penicillins, cephalosporins, and quinolones (Akaike et al. 1991; Mathers 1987). Both low and excessive levels of serotonin are also associated with delirium (van der Mast and Fekkes 2000). Serotonin syndrome (see Chapter 37, "Psychopharmacology") is the obvious ex-

ample of the latter, but serotonergic activity may be increased in patients with hepatic encephalopathy (Mousseau and Butterworth 1994; van der Mast and Fekkes 2000) and sepsis (Mizock et al. 1990). Histamine may play a role in delirium through its effects on arousal and hypothalamic regulation of sleep–wake circadian rhythms. Both H_1 and H_2 antagonists can cause delirium, although both also have anticholinergic properties (Picotte-Prillmayer et al. 1995; Tejera et al. 1994). Glutamate release is increased during hypoxia, and glutamatergic receptors may be activated by quinolone antibiotics (P.D. Williams and Helton 1991).

Altered ratios of plasma amino acids during severe illness, surgery, and trauma may affect neurotransmitter synthesis in the brain (Trzepacz and van der Mast 2002; van der Mast and Fekkes 2000). In addition to changes in major neurotransmitter systems, neurotoxic metabolites, such as quinolinic acid from tryptophan metabolism (Basile et al. 1995), and false transmitters, such as octopamine in patients with liver failure, have been implicated in the pathogenesis of delirium. Because glia help to regulate neurotransmitter amounts in the synapse, glial dysfunction also may be involved. Increased blood-brain barrier permeability, as occurs in uremia, is another possible mechanism contributing to delirium. Van der Mast and Fekkes (2000) proposed that surgery induces immune activation and a physical stress response, which is characterized by increased hypothalamic-pituitary-adrenocortical axis activity, low triiodothyronine (T_3) syndrome, and alterations of blood-brain barrier permeability. Cytokines have been implicated as causes of inflammatory or infection-induced delirium, as well as when given as treatment (interferons, interleukins). Cytokines are increased during stress, rapid growth, inflammation, tumor, trauma, and infection (Hopkins and Rothwell 1995; Rothwell and Hopkins 1995; Stefano et al. 1994). The mechanism by which they cause delirium may be as neurotoxins (Lipton and Gendelman 1995), through effects on a variety of neurotransmitters (Rothwell and Hopkins 1995; Stefano et al. 1994), by altering blood-brain barrier permeability, or through effects on glial function.

A final common neural pathway for delirium could have neuroanatomic and neurochemical components. The predominance of evidence supports a low cholinergic–excess dopaminergic state in this final common neural theory (Trzepacz 1999b, 2000). Other neurotransmitter systems are known to be involved for certain etiologies (e.g., hepatic insufficiency or alcohol withdrawal), whereas cholinergic and dopaminergic pathways can be affected by these other neurotransmitters. The role of cholinergic and dopaminergic neurotransmission in delirium has been reviewed in detail elsewhere (Trzepacz 1996a, 2000).

Differential Diagnosis

The presence of delirium is frequently detected late or not at all in clinical practice. Between one-third and two-thirds of cases are missed across a range of care settings and by a variety of specialists, including psychiatrists and neurologists (Johnson et al. 1992). Nonrecognition represents a failure to recognize the symptoms or diagnosis of delirium and is reflected in poorer outcomes (Kakuma et al. 2003; Rockwood et al. 1994). Poor detection rates in part indicate that delirium is an inherently fluctuating disorder involving multiple cognitive and noncognitive disturbances, which confer great clinical variability.

The stereotyped image of delirium (as in delirium tremens) of an agitated psychotic patient does not represent most patients with delirium, who have either mixed or hypoactive symptom profiles (Meagher and Trzepacz 2000). The hypoactive presentation is less appreciated because the quiet, untroublesome patient is often presumed to have intact cognition and is more easily overlooked in the time-pressured technological environment of modern medicine. It is not surprising that nursing staff, who have the greatest amount of patient and family contact, may have better detection rates than do physicians (Gustafson et al. 1991). Detection can be improved by routinely assessing cognitive function, improving awareness of the varied presentations of delirium, and using one of the currently available screening instruments for

delirium (Rockwood et al. 1994), such as the CAM or CAM-ICU.

Delirium has a wide differential diagnosis. It can be mistaken for dementia, depression, psychosis, anxiety, somatoform disorders, and, particularly in children, behavioral disturbance (see Table 6–9). Accurate diagnosis requires close attention to symptom profile and temporal onset and is further supplemented by a variety of tests (e.g., cognitive, laboratory, EEG). Given that delirium can be the presenting feature of serious medical illness, any patient experiencing a sudden deterioration in cognitive function should be examined for possible delirium.

The most difficult differential diagnosis for delirium is dementia—the other cause of generalized cognitive impairment. Indeed, end-stage dementia has been described as a chronic delirious state. Particularly challenging can be diagnosing dementia with Lewy bodies because it mimics delirium with fluctuation of symptom severity, visual hallucinations, attentional impairment, alteration of consciousness, and delusions (Robinson 2002). Despite this substantial overlap, delirium and dementia can be reliably distinguished by a combination of careful history-taking and interviewing for symptom profile onset and clinical investigation. The tendency for abrupt onset and fluctuating course are highly characteristic of delirium. In addition, level of consciousness and attention are markedly disturbed in delirium but remain relatively intact in uncomplicated dementia. Dementia patients often have

TABLE 6–9.   Differential diagnosis of delirium

	Delirium	Dementia	Depression	Schizophrenia
Onset	Acute	Insidious[a]	Variable	Variable
Course	Fluctuating	Often progressive	Diurnal variation	Variable
Reversibility	Usually[b]	Not usually	Usually but can be recurrent	No but has exacerbations
Level of consciousness	Impaired	Clear until late stages	Generally unimpaired	Unimpaired (perplexity in acute stage)
Attention/memory	Inattention, poor memory	Poor memory without marked inattention	Poor attention, memory intact	Poor attention, memory intact
Hallucinations	Usually visual; can be auditory, tactile, gustatory, olfactory	Can be visual or auditory	Usually auditory	Usually auditory
Delusions	Fleeting, fragmented, and usually persecutory	Paranoid, often fixed	Complex and mood congruent	Frequent, complex, systematized, and often paranoid

[a]Except for large strokes.
[b]Can be chronic (paraneoplastic syndrome, central nervous system adverse events of medications, severe brain damage).

nocturnal disturbances of sleep, whereas delirium is characterized by varying degrees of disruption of the sleep–wake cycle, including fragmentation and sleeplessness. Overall, the presentation of delirium does not seem to be greatly altered by the presence of dementia, with delirium symptoms dominating the clinical picture when they co-occur (Trzepacz et al. 1998).

A range of investigative tools can facilitate differentiation of delirium and dementia in clinical practice. The DRS (Trzepacz and Dew 1995), DRS-R-98, and CTD (Hart et al. 1996) have been shown to distinguish delirium from dementia during validation studies. Although abnormalities of the EEG are common to both delirium and dementia, diffuse slowing occurs more frequently in (81% vs. 33%)—and favors a diagnosis of—delirium. EEG slowing occurs later in the course of most degenerative dementias, although slowing occurs sooner with viral and prion dementias. Percentage theta activity on quantitative EEG may aid differentiation of delirium from dementia (Jacobson and Jerrier 2000).

Several studies have addressed the issue of which symptoms may discriminate between patients with delirium and patients with dementia, or patients with both disorders, with varying results (Liptzin et al. 1993; O'Keeffe 1994; Trzepacz and Dew 1995; Trzepacz et al. 1998, 2002b). Overall, their results suggest that when delirium and dementia are comorbid, delirium phenomenology overshadows that of the dementia, but when the two are assessed as individual conditions, several discriminating symptoms are seen. These research findings are consistent with the clinical rule of thumb that "it is delirium until proven otherwise."

Often, the early behavioral changes of delirium are mistaken for adjustment reactions to adverse events, particularly in patients who have experienced major trauma or who have cancer. Hypoactive delirium is frequently mistaken for depression (Nicholas and Lindsey 1995). Some symptoms of major depression occur in delirium (e.g., psychomotor slowing, sleep disturbances, irritability). It has been estimated that 7% of patients with delirium attempt self-harm during an episode. However, in major depression, symptom onset tends to be less acute, and mood disturbances typically dominate the clinical picture, with any cognitive impairment more reflective of poor effort. Dehydration or malnutrition can precipitate delirium in severely depressed patients who are unable to maintain food or fluid intake. The distinction of delirium from depression is particularly important because, in addition to delayed treatment, some antidepressants have anticholinergic activity (paroxetine and tricyclics) that can aggravate delirium. The overactive, disinhibited presentation of some patients with delirium can closely resemble similar disturbances encountered in patients with agitated depression or mania, such as delirious (Bell's) mania and agitated ("lethal") catatonia, which typically include cognitive impairment.

Abnormalities of thought and perception can occur in both delirium and schizophrenia but are more fluctuant and fragmentary in delirium. Delusions in delirium are rarely as fixed or complex as in schizophrenia, and first-rank symptoms are uncommon (Cutting 1987). Unlike schizophrenia, hallucinations in delirium tend to be visual rather than auditory. Consciousness, attention, and memory are generally less impaired in schizophrenia, with the exception of the pseudodelirious picture that can occur as a result of marked perplexity in the acute stage of illness. Careful examination, coupled with EEG and/or an instrument such as the DRS, generally distinguishes delirium from these functional disorders.

Despite the fact that delirium is rarely specifically cited as the reason for a request for psychiatric consultation (Francis et al. 1990; Trzepacz et al. 1985), it is very common among patients referred to psychiatric consultation services because of frequent misdiagnosis by referring clinicians. Overall, approximately 10% of the patients referred to psychiatric consultation have delirium, and about 10% of the general hospital patients with delirium receive a psychiatric consultation (Francis et al. 1990; Sirois 1988), with psychiatrist involvement typically reserved for more difficult cases.

Treatment

Delirium is an example par excellence of a disorder requiring a multifaceted biopsychosocial approach to assessment and treatment. After the diagnosis of delirium is made, the process of identifying and reversing suspected etiologies begins. Rapid treatment is important because of the high morbidity and mortality associated with delirium. Treatments include medication, environmental manipulation, and patient and family psychosocial support (American Psychiatric Association 1999). However, no drug has a U.S. Food and Drug Administration indication for the treatment of delirium, and double-blind, placebo-controlled studies of efficacy and safety of drugs in treating delirium are lacking (American Psychiatric Association 1999).

Psychiatric consultation facilitates identification of predisposing and precipitating factors for delirium. Medication exposure, visual and hearing impairments, sleep deprivation, uncontrolled pain, dehydration, malnutrition, catheterization, and use of restraints are all factors that can be modified, but uncertainty remains as to the precise value of multicomponent interventions that attempt to reduce the incidence and severity of delirium through modification of recognized risk factors (Bogardus et al. 2003; Cole et al. 1998; Inouye et al. 1999) or systematic detection and multidisciplinary care of identified cases (Cole et al. 2002). The effect of such interventions depends on degree of implementation, with evidence that higher adherence leads to lower delirium rates (Inouye et al. 2003). A range of preoperative psychological interventions aimed at patient education and anxiety reduction may have preventive value, but these require more study before they warrant introduction into routine clinical practice.

The principles of management of delirium include ensuring the safety of the patient and his or her immediate surroundings (includes sitters), achieving optimal levels of environmental stimulation, and minimizing the effects of any sensory impediments. The complications of delirium can be minimized by careful attention to the potential for falls and avoidance of prolonged hypostasis. Using orienting techniques (e.g., calendars, night-lights, and reorientation by staff) and familiarizing the patient with the environment (e.g., with photographs of family members) are sometimes comforting, although it is important to remember that environmental manipulations alone do not reverse delirium (American Psychiatric Association 1999; Anderson 1995). It also has been suggested that diurnal cues from natural lighting reduce sensory deprivation and incidence of delirium (Wilson 1972), although sensory deprivation alone is insufficient to cause delirium (Francis 1993). Unfortunately, implementation of these environmental interventions occurs primarily in response to agitation rather than the core disturbances of delirium (Meagher et al. 1996).

Supportive interaction with relatives and caregivers is fundamental to good management of delirium. Relatives can play an integral role in efforts to support and reorient patients with delirium, but ill-informed, critical, or anxious caregivers can add to the burden of a delirious patient. A nontherapeutic triangle can emerge whereby medical staff respond to the distress of relatives by medicating patients, which complicates ongoing cognitive assessment. Clarification of the cause and meaning of symptoms combined with recognition of treatment goals can allow better management of what is a distressing experience for both patient and loved ones (Breitbart et al. 2002a; Meagher 2001).

Prevention Strategies

Nonpharmacological and pharmacological interventions are available to prevent delirium. Preoperative patient ed-

ucation or preparation was helpful in reducing delirium symptom rates (Chatham 1978; Owens and Hutelmyer 1982; M.A. Williams et al. 1985). However, studies of caregiver education and environmental or risk factor interventions have had mixed results, with two not finding any significant effect on delirium rate (Nagley 1986; Wanich et al. 1992). In contrast, Inouye et al. (1999) studied the effect on delirium of preventive measures that minimized six of the risk factors identified in their previous work with hospitalized elderly patients. They used standardized protocols in a prospective study of 852 elderly inpatients to address cognitive impairment, sleep deprivation, immobility, visual impairment, hearing impairment, and dehydration, which resulted in significant reductions in the number (62 vs. 90) and duration (105 vs. 161 days) of delirium episodes relative to control subjects. Effects of adherence on delirium risk were subsequently reported for 422 elderly patients during implementation of this standardized protocol (Inouye et al. 2003). Adherence ranged from 10% for the sleep protocol to 86% for orientation. Higher levels of adherence by staff resulted in lower delirium rates, up to a maximum of an 89% reduction, even after controlling for confounding variables. At 6-month follow-up of 705 survivors from this intervention study of six risk factors, no differences were found between groups for any of the 10 outcome measures, except for less frequent incontinence in the intervention group (Bogardus et al. 2003), suggesting that the intervention's effect was essentially during the index hospitalization without any longer-lasting benefits. When a subset of high-risk patients were compared at baseline, however, the intervention group had significantly better self-rated health and functional status at follow-up.

Milisen et al. (2001) compared delirium rates in two cohorts of elderly hip surgery patients ($N=60$ in each cohort)—before and after implementing an intervention consisting of nurse education, cognitive screening, consultation by a nurse or physician geriatric/delirium specialist, and a scheduled pain protocol. They found no effect on delirium incidence but a shorter duration of delirium (median 1 vs. 4 days) and lower delirium severity in the intervention group. Marcantonio et al. (2001) used a different study design and randomized 62 elderly hip fracture patients to either a perioperative geriatric consultation or usual care. On the basis of daily ratings, they found a lower delirium rate (32% vs. 50%) and fewer cases of severe delirium (12% vs. 29%) in the consultation group. Length of stay was not affected, and the effect of consultation was greatest in those patients without preexisting dementia or poor ADLs.

Some pharmacological prophylaxis trials have been done. Cholinergic agents have engendered the most interest. Citicholine 1.2 mg/day was assessed for delirium prevention in a randomized, placebo-controlled trial of 81 nondemented hip surgery patients, given 1 day before and each of the 4 days after surgery (Diaz et al. 2001). Fewer cases of delirium occurred in the citicholine group (12% vs. 17%), but the difference was not statistically significant. Perioperative piracetam use during anesthesia was reviewed across eight studies, mostly from the 1970s, and was believed to have a positive effect on reducing postoperative delirium symptoms (Gallinat et al. 1999).

Kalisvaart et al. (2003) studied 408 elderly hip surgery patients in a randomized, placebo-controlled comparison of haloperidol and placebo given up to 3 days before and 3 days after surgery. Even though the authors found only a nonsignificant lower numerical difference for delirium incidence (23% vs. 32%) with haloperidol, significant differences were found for shorter delirium duration (4 vs. 12 days), lower DRS scores (13.6 vs. 18.2), and shorter length of stay (12 vs. 24 days) in the active treatment group. This study represents the first double-blind, placebo-controlled trial for delirium prevention with a neuroleptic agent.

Maldonado et al. (2004) reported an interim data analysis showing significantly reduced delirium incidence (5%) when a novel alpha$_2$-adrenergic receptor agonist—dexmedetomidine—was used for postoperative sedation, compared with propofol (54%) or fentanyl/midazolam (46%), in cardiac valve surgery patients. Improved pain control after hepatectomy surgery in elderly patients who used patient-controlled epidural anesthesia with bupivacaine and fentanyl ($n=14$), compared with continuous-epidural mepivacaine ($n=16$), was associated with lower incidences of moderate and severe delirium (36% vs. 75% and 14% vs. 50%, respectively), and antipsychotic drug use also was lower in the former group (Tokita et al. 2001).

Pharmacological Treatment

Current delirium pharmacotherapies have evolved from use in the treatment of mainstream psychiatric disorders; hence, psychiatrists are well acquainted with the practicalities of their use. Medications are implicated as significant contributing factors in more than one-third of cases and can act as either protective or risk factors for delirium, depending on the drug. Pharmacological treatment with a neuroleptic agent (D$_2$ antagonist) is the clinical standard for delirium treatment. A survey of intensivists indicated that delirium was treated in the ICU with haloperidol by 66% of the respondents, lorazepam by 12%, and atypical antipsychotics by fewer than 5%. More than 55% administered haloperidol and lorazepam at daily doses of 10 mg or less, but some used a dosage of more than 50 mg/day of either medication (Ely et al. 2004b).

Haloperidol is the neuroleptic most often chosen for the treatment of delirium. It can be administered orally, intramuscularly, or intravenously (Adams 1984, 1988; Dudley et al. 1979; Gelfand et al. 1992; Moulaert 1989; Sanders and Stern 1993; Tesar et al. 1985), although the intravenous route has not been approved by the U.S. Food and Drug Administration. Intravenously administered haloperidol is twice as potent as that taken orally (Gelfand et al. 1992). Bolus intravenous doses usually range from 0.5 to 20 mg, although larger doses are sometimes given. In severe, refractory cases, continuous intravenous infusions of 15–25 mg/hour (up to 1,000 mg/day) can be given (Fernandez et al. 1988; J.L. Levenson 1995; Riker et al. 1994; Stern 1994).

Based on clinical use, haloperidol traditionally has been considered to be relatively safe in the seriously medically ill and does not cause as much hypotension as droperidol does (Gelfand et al. 1992; Moulaert 1989; Tesar et al. 1985). Haloperidol does not antagonize dopamine-induced increases in renal blood flow (D.H. Armstrong et al. 1986). Even when haloperidol is given intravenously at high doses in delirium, extrapyramidal symptoms (EPS) usually are not a problem, except in more sensitive patients, such as those with HIV or dementia with Lewy bodies (Fernandez et al. 1989; McKeith et al. 1992; Swenson et al. 1989). A case series of five ICU patients receiving 250–500 mg/day of continuous or intermittent intravenous haloperidol had self-limited withdrawal dyskinesia following high-dose haloperidol (Riker et al. 1997). The anticholinergic state of delirium itself may be somewhat protective from EPS (J.L. Levenson, personal communication, January 2004). Intravenous lorazepam is sometimes combined with intravenous haloperidol in critically ill patients to lessen EPS and increase sedation. Cases of prolonged QT$_c$ interval on electrocardiogram and torsades de pointes tachyarrhythmia (multifocal ventricular tachycardia) have been increasingly recognized and attributed to intravenously administered haloperidol (Hatta et al. 2001; Huyse 1988; Kriwisky et al. 1990; Metzger and Friedman 1993; O'Brien et al. 1999; Perrault et al. 2000; Wilt et al. 1993; Zee-Cheng et al. 1985). The American Psychiatric Association (1999) "Practice Guideline for the Treatment of Patients With Delirium" advised that QT$_c$ prolongation greater than 450 msec or to greater than 25% over a previous electrocardiogram may warrant telemetry, cardiac consultation, dose reduction, or discontinuation. They also recommend monitoring use of other drugs that also can prolong the QT$_c$ interval, as well as serum magnesium and potassium, in critically ill patients with delirium whose QT$_c$ is 450 msec or greater.

Empirical treatment studies of neuroleptics in delirium are rare but support their efficacy. Itil and Fink (1966) found that chlorpromazine reversed anticholinergic delirium. With the use of standardized assessment methods and a double-blind, randomized controlled design, Breitbart et al. (1996) found that delirium in patients with AIDS significantly improved with haloperidol or chlorpromazine but not with lorazepam. Platt et al. (1994b) reported that both hypoactive and hyperactive subtypes responded to treatment with haloperidol or chlorpromazine, and they noted improvement within hours of treatment, even before the underlying medical causes were addressed.

Haloperidol use in pediatric patients with delirium is not well documented, despite its use in adult delirium and in many other childhood psychiatric disorders (Teicher and Gold 1990). Clinical experience with haloperidol in pediatric delirium supports its beneficial effects, but no controlled studies have been done. A retrospective report of 30 children (age 8 months to 18 years; mean age=7 years) with burn injuries supported the use of haloperidol for agitation, disorientation, hallucinations, delusions, and insomnia (R.L. Brown et al. 1996). The mean haloperidol dose was 0.47 mg/kg, with a mean maximum dose in 24 hours of 0.46 mg/kg, administered intravenously, orally, and intramuscularly. Haloperidol was not efficacious in 17% of the patients (4 of 5 of these failures were via the oral route). EPS were not observed, and one episode of hypotension occurred with the intravenous route.

Droperidol is sometimes used to treat acute agitation and confusion from a variety of causes, including mania and delirium (Hooper and Minter 1983; Resnick and Burton 1984; H. Thomas et al. 1992), and is superior to placebo (van Leeuwen et al. 1977). After initial use in patients with severe agitated delirium, droperidol can be replaced by haloperidol for continued treatment. Compared with haloperidol, droperidol has a faster onset of action, but it is more sedating, can be used only parenterally in the United States, and is very hypotensive because of potent α-adrenergic antagonism, although continuous intravenous infusion of 1–10 mg/hour causes less hypotension than do intravenous boluses (Moulaert 1989). Having the patient lie supine is helpful. Dosing is similar to that for haloperidol, although droperidol may have less antipsychotic effect and fewer EPS (Frye et al. 1995). Prolonged QT_c intervals can occur with droperidol (Lawrence and Nasraway 1997; Lischke et al. 1994). Oral droperidol (and thioridazine) was recently reported in Europe to significantly prolong the QT_c interval in a dose-related manner (Reilly et al. 2000); therefore, caution is suggested before use in delirium.

Some atypical antipsychotic agents are being used to treat delirium, and the literature to date includes mostly case reports, retrospective case series, and a few small open-label, prospective trials that used standardized measures (Schwartz and Masand 2002; Torres et al. 2001). Poor response to haloperidol was associated with improvement of delirium in several patients after switching to an atypical antipsychotic (Al-Samarrai et al. 2003; Leso and Schwartz 2002; Passik and Cooper 1999). Haloperidol is avoided in posttraumatic brain injury delirium because dopamine blockade is thought by some clinicians to be deleterious for cognitive recovery; two traumatic brain injury patients with delirium given low-dose olanzapine showed remarkable improvement within a short period (Ovchinsky et al. 2002), suggesting a possible role for atypical antipsychotics in this population. Double-blind, placebo-controlled, randomized studies are necessary to truly establish efficacy and safety profiles.

Clozapine would not be a good choice for treatment of delirium because it has significant anticholinergic side effects, causes sinus tachycardia, lowers seizure threshold, and can cause agranulocytosis. Furthermore, clozapine has itself caused delirium in 8%–10% of psychiatric inpatients (Centorrino et al. 2003; Gaertner et al. 1989). Cholinergic agents can reverse clozapine-induced delirium (Schuster et al. 1977).

Risperidone (mean dosage=1.6 mg/day) has been reported to reduce delirium severity in an open-label case series, with the maximum response on the fifth day (Sipahimalani and Masand 1997). In a prospective open trial in patients with delirium who had been taking haloperidol, risperidone was effective in 80% at a mean dose of 1.7 mg/day (range=0.5–3 mg); adverse events included sleepiness in 30% and mild drug-induced parkinsonism in 10% (Horikawa et al. 2003). Another prospective open trial of risperidone (mean dose=1.4 mg/day) in older patients with delirium also showed that it was effective (Mittal et al. 2004). However, risperidone was reported to cause delirium in four patients (Chen and Cardasis 1996; Ravona-Springer et al. 1998). Risperidone has dose-related EPS beginning at a dosage of about 2 mg/day according to double-blind, placebo-controlled studies (I.R. Katz et al. 1999).

An open-label, nonrandomized delirium case series comparing olanzapine (mean dose=8.2 mg) and haloperidol (mean dose=5.1 mg) showed comparable efficacy; however, there were frequent EPS or excessive sedation with haloperidol compared with olanzapine, which did not have these side effects (Masand and Sipahimalani 1998). Breitbart et al. (2002b) described 82 cancer inpatients with delirium, 81% of whom had metastases (20% in the brain), who were given olanzapine (dose range =

2.5–20 mg); delirium resolved in 79% of the patients by day 3, with overall good tolerability. In a prospective study of olanzapine (mean dose=6 mg) by K.-S. Kim et al. (2001), 70% of the patients had a 50% or greater reduction in delirium symptoms, and the drug was well tolerated without EPS. Olanzapine has a favorable EPS profile and does not appear to have a clinically significant effect on the QT_c interval at therapeutic doses in schizophrenic patients (Czekalla et al. 2001).

A small uncontrolled study of older patients with delirium treated with quetiapine (mean dose=93 mg) has provided preliminary evidence that quetiapine is well tolerated and reduces symptoms of delirium (K.Y. Kim et al. 2003). In a retrospective case series, quetiapine (mean dose=211 mg/day, range=25–750 mg/day) also was quite effective in improving delirium scores, with sedation in 30% and discontinuation in two elderly patients because of worsening (Schwartz and Masand 2000). Very little is known about ziprasidone or aripiprazole in delirium.

Very few reports include more than one atypical agent. Hill et al. (2002) measured delirium symptoms daily in 50 patients with delirium treated with either haloperidol, olanzapine, or risperidone. They found a significant main effect of drug and time at 3 days; olanzapine was more effective in reducing delirium severity than was either haloperidol or risperidone.

Unlike haloperidol and droperidol, atypical agents had not been available until recently in the United States in parenteral form, a route often needed in treating agitated, uncooperative patients. Intramuscular olanzapine and ziprasidone have been developed for the treatment of agitation in psychiatric patients, and olanzapine has a rapidly dissolving oral formulation that is placed on the tongue, but none of these has yet been studied in delirium.

Other classes of drugs are indicated in particular situations. Benzodiazepines are generally reserved for delirium due to ethanol or sedative-hypnotic withdrawal; lorazepam or clonazepam (the latter for alprazolam withdrawal) is often used. Some physicians use lorazepam as an adjunctive medication with haloperidol in the most severe cases of delirium or when extra assistance with sleep is needed. Anticholinergic poisoning–induced delirium and/or agitation was controlled and reversed with physostigmine (87% and 96%, respectively), whereas benzodiazepines controlled agitation in only 24% and were ineffective in treating delirium (Burns et al. 2000). Patients who received physostigmine had a lower incidence of complications (7% vs. 46%) and a shorter time to recovery (median=12 vs. 24 hours). Ely et al. (2004a) found a significant aggravating effect of lorazepam on delirium in medical ICU patients, but this effect was not found for propofol, morphine, and fentanyl.

The cholinergic deficiency hypothesis of delirium suggests that treatment with a cholinergic enhancer drug could be therapeutic. Physostigmine reverses anticholinergic delirium (Stern 1983), but its side effects (seizures) and short half-life make it unsuitable for routine clinical treatment of delirium. Tacrine also was shown to reverse central anticholinergic syndrome (Mendelson 1977), although it has not been studied formally. Three case reports found that donepezil improved delirium postoperatively, in dementia with Lewy bodies, and in alcohol dementia (Burke et al. 1999; Wengel et al. 1998, 1999). Physostigmine administered in the emergency department to patients suspected of having muscarinic toxicity resulted in reversal of delirium in 22 of 39, including several patients in whom the cause could not be determined (Schneir et al. 2003); only 1 patient in 39 had an adverse event (brief seizure).

Psychostimulants can worsen delirium and are not recommended when depressed mood is present (J.A. Levenson 1992; Rosenberg et al. 1991). Mianserin, a serotonergic tetracyclic antidepressant, has been used in Japan for delirium in elderly medical and postsurgical patients, administered either orally or as a suppository. Several open-label studies found reductions in the DRS scores similar to those seen with haloperidol (Nakamura et al. 1995, 1997a, 1997b; Uchiyama et al. 1996). A single 8-mg intravenous dose of ondansetron, a serotonin$_3$ receptor antagonist, was reported to reduce agitation in 35 postcardiotomy delirium patients (Bayindir et al. 2000).

Clearly, further delirium treatment research is needed—especially randomized, controlled trials of drug compared with placebo and of drug compared with drug—addressing both efficacy and safety.

References

Adams F: Neuropsychiatric evaluation and treatment of delirium in the critically ill cancer patient. Cancer Bull 36:156–160, 1984

Adams F: Emergency intravenous sedation of the delirious medically ill patient. J Clin Psychiatry 49 (suppl):22–26, 1988

Akaike N, Shirasaki T, Yakushiji T: Quinolone and fenbufen interact with GABA-A receptors in dissociated hippocampal cells of rats. J Neurophysiol 66:497–504, 1991

Al-Samarrai S, Dunn J, Newmark T, et al: Quetiapine for treatment-resistant delirium. Psychosomatics 44:350–351, 2003

American Psychiatric Association: Diagnostic and Statistical Manual: Mental Disorders. Washington, DC, American Psychiatric Association, 1952

American Psychiatric Association: Diagnostic and Statistical Manual of Mental Disorders, 2nd Edition. Washington, DC, American Psychiatric Association, 1968

American Psychiatric Association: Diagnostic and Statistical Manual of Mental Disorders, 3rd Edition. Washington, DC, American Psychiatric Association, 1980

American Psychiatric Association: Diagnostic and Statistical Manual of Mental Disorders, 3rd Edition, Revised. Washington, DC, American Psychiatric Association, 1987

American Psychiatric Association: Diagnostic and Statistical Manual of Mental Disorders, 4th Edition. Washington, DC, American Psychiatric Association, 1994

American Psychiatric Association: Practice guideline for the treatment of patients with delirium. Am J Psychiatry 156 (suppl): 1–20, 1999

American Psychiatric Association: Diagnostic and Statistical Manual of Mental Disorders, 4th Edition, Text Revision. Washington, DC, American Psychiatric Association, 2000

Ames D, Wirshing WC, Szuba MP: Organic mental disorders associated with bupropion in three patients. J Clin Psychiatry 53:53–55, 1992

Anderson SD: Treatment of elderly patients with delirium. Can Med Assoc J 152:323–324, 1995

Andreasen NJC, Hartford CE, Knott JR, et al: EEG changes associated with burn delirium. Dis Nerv Syst 38:27–31, 1977

Armstrong DH, Dasts JF, Reilly TE, et al: Effect of haloperidol on dopamine-induced increase in renal blood flow. Drug Intell Clin Pharm 20:543–546, 1986

Armstrong SC, Cozza KL, Watanabe KS: The misdiagnosis of delirium. Psychosomatics 38:433–439, 1997

Basile AS, Saito K, Li Y, et al: The relationship between plasma and brain quinolinic acid levels and the severity of hepatic encephalopathy in animal models of fulminant hepatic failure. J Neurochem 64:2607–2614, 1995

Bayindir O, Akpinar B, Can E, et al: The use of the 5-HT$_3$-receptor antagonist ondansetron for the treatment of postcardiotomy delirium. J Cardiothorac Vasc Anesth 14:288–292, 2000

Bedford PD: General medical aspects of confusional states in elderly people. BMJ 2:185–188, 1957

Berggren D, Gustafson Y, Eriksson B, et al: Postoperative confusion following anesthesia in elderly patients treated for femoral neck fractures. Anesth Analg 66:497–504, 1987

Bogardus ST, Desai MM, Williams CS, et al: The effects of a targeted multicomponent delirium intervention on postdischarge outcomes for hospitalized older adults. Am J Med 114:383–390, 2003

Breitbart W, Marotta R, Platt MM, et al: A double-blind trial of haloperidol, chlorpromazine, and lorazepam in the treatment of delirium in hospitalized AIDS patients. Am J Psychiatry 153:231–237, 1996

Breitbart W, Rosenfeld B, Roth A, et al: The Memorial Delirium Assessment Scale. J Pain Symptom Manage 13:128–137, 1997

Breitbart W, Gibson C, Tremblay A: The delirium experience: delirium recall and delirium-related distress in hospitalized patients with cancer, their spouses/caregivers, and their nurses. Psychosomatics 43:183–194, 2002a

Breitbart W, Tremblay A, Gibson C: An open trial of olanzapine for the treatment of delirium in hospitalized cancer patients. Psychosomatics 43:175–182, 2002b

Broderick PA, Gibson GE: Dopamine and serotonin in rat striatum during in vivo hypoxic-hypoxia. Metab Brain Dis 4:143–153, 1989

Brown RL, Henke A, Greenhalgh DG, et al: The use of haloperidol in the agitated, critically ill pediatric patient with burns. J Burn Care Rehabil 17:34–38, 1996

Brown TM: Drug-induced delirium. Semin Clin Neuropsychiatry 5:113–125, 2000

Burke WJ, Roccaforte WH, Wengel SP: Treating visual hallucinations with donepezil. Am J Psychiatry 156:1117–1118, 1999

Burns MJ, Linden CH, Graudins A, et al: A comparison of physostigmine and benzodiazepines for the treatment of anticholinergic poisoning. Ann Emerg Med 35:374–381, 2000

Cameron DJ, Thomas RI, Mulvihill M, et al: Delirium: a test of DSM-III criteria on medical inpatients. J Am Geriatr Soc 35:1007–1010, 1987

Camus V, Gonthier R, Dubos G, et al: Etiologic and outcome profiles in hypoactive and hyperactive subtypes of delirium. J Geriatr Psychiatry Neurol 13:38–42, 2000

Caraceni A, Nanni O, Maltoni M, et al: Impact of delirium on the short term prognosis of advanced cancer patients. Cancer 89:1145–1149, 2000

Centorrino F, Albert MJ, Drago-Ferrante G, et al: Delirium during clozapine treatment: incidence and associated risk factors. Pharmacopsychiatry 36:156–160, 2003

Chatham MA: The effect of family involvement on patients' manifestations of postcardiotomy psychosis. Heart Lung 7:995–999, 1978

Chedru F, Geschwind N: Writing disturbances in acute confusional states. Neuropsychologia 10:343–353, 1972

Chen B, Cardasis W: Delirium induced by lithium and risperidone combination. Am J Psychiatry 153:1233–1234, 1996

Coffman JA, Dilsaver SC: Cholinergic mechanisms in delirium. Am J Psychiatry 145:382–383, 1988

Cole MG, Primeau FJ: Prognosis of delirium in elderly hospital patients. Can Med Assoc J 149:41–46, 1993

Cole MG, Primeau FJ, Bailey RF, et al: Systematic intervention for elderly inpatients with delirium: a randomized trial. Can Med Assoc J 151:965–970, 1994

Cole M, Primeau F, Elie L: Delirium: prevention, treatment, and outcome studies. J Geriatr Psychiatry Neurol 28:551–556, 1998

Cole M, McCusker J, Bellavance F, et al: Systematic detection and multidisciplinary care of delirium in older medical inpatients: a randomized trial. Can Med Assoc J 167:753–759, 2002

Cole MG, Dendukuri N, McCusker J, et al: An empirical study of different diagnostic criteria for delirium among elderly medical inpatients. J Neuropsychiatry Clin Neurosci 15:200–207, 2003a

Cole M, McCusker J, Dendukuri N, et al: The prognostic significance of subsyndromal delirium in elderly medical inpatients. J Am Geriatr Soc 51:754–760, 2003b

Cushman LA: Secondary neuropsychiatric implications of stroke: implications for acute care. Arch Phys Med Rehabil 69:877–879, 1988

Curyto KJ, Johnson J, TenHave T, et al: Survival of hospitalized elderly patients with delirium: a prospective study. Am J Geriatr Psychiatry 9:141–147, 2001

Cutting J: The phenomenology of acute organic psychosis: comparison with acute schizophrenia. Br J Psychiatry 151:324–332, 1987

Czekalla J, Beasley CM Jr, Dellva MA, et al: Analysis of the QTc interval during olanzapine treatment of patients with schizophrenia and related psychoses. J Clin Psychiatry 62:191–198, 2001

Dickson LR: Hypoalbuminemia in delirium. Psychosomatics 32:317–323, 1991

Dixon CE, Hamm RJ, Taft WC, et al: Increased anticholinergic sensitivity following closed skull impact and controlled cortical impact traumatic brain injury in the rat. J Neurotrauma 11:275–287, 1994

Drake ME, Coffey CE: Complex partial status epilepticus simulating psychogenic unresponsiveness. Am J Psychiatry 140:800–801, 1983

Dudley DL, Rowlett DB, Loebel PJ: Emergency use of intravenous haloperidol. Gen Hosp Psychiatry 1:240–246, 1979

Ely EW, Inouye SK, Bernard GR, et al: Delirium in mechanically ventilated patients: validity and reliability of the Confusion Assessment Method for the Intensive Care Unit (CAM-ICU). JAMA 286:2703–2710, 2001a

Ely EW, Margolin R, Francis J, et al: Evaluation of delirium in critically ill patients: validation of the Confusion Assessment Method for the Intensive Care Unit (CAM-ICU). Crit Care Med 29:1370–1379, 2001b

Ely EW, Siegel MD, Inouye SK: Delirium in the intensive care unit: an under-recognized syndrome of organ dysfunction. Semin Respiratory and Critical Care Medicine 22:115–126, 2001c

Ely EW, Shintani A, Truman B, et al: Delirium as a predictor of mortality in mechanically ventilated patients in the intensive care unit. JAMA 291:1753–1762, 2004a

Ely EW, Stephens RK, Jackson JC, et al: Current opinions regarding the importance, diagnosis, and management of delirium in the intensive care unit: a survey of 912 healthcare professionals. Crit Care Med 32:106–112, 2004b

Engel GL, Romano J: Delirium, II: reversibility of electroencephalogram with experimental procedures. Arch Neurol Psychiatry 51:378–392, 1944

Engel GL, Romano J: Delirium, a syndrome of cerebral insufficiency. J Chronic Dis 9:260–277, 1959

Erkinjuntti T, Wikstrom J, Parlo J, et al: Dementia among medical inpatients: evaluation of 2000 consecutive admissions. Arch Intern Med 146:1923–1926, 1986

Ewert J, Levin HS, Watson MG, et al: Procedural memory during posttraumatic amnesia in survivors of severe closed head injury: implications for rehabilitation. Arch Neurol 46:911–916, 1985

Fann JR: The epidemiology of delirium: a review of studies and methodological issues. Semin Clin Neuropsychiatry 5:86–92, 2000

Fann JR, Roth-Roemer S, Burington BE, et al: Delirium in patients undergoing hematopoietic stem cell transplantation. Cancer 95:1971–1981, 2002

Fann JR, Roth-Roemer S, Burington BE, et al: Delirium and affective and cognitive outcomes in patients undergoing stem cell transplantation. Annals of Behavioral Medicine S064, 2003

Fernandez F, Holmes VF, Adams F, et al: Treatment of severe, refractory agitation with a haloperidol drip. J Clin Psychiatry 49:239–241, 1988

Fernandez F, Levy JK, Mansell PWA: Management of delirium in terminally ill AIDS patients. Int J Psychiatry Med 19:165–172, 1989

Fisher BW, Flowerdew G: A simple model for predicting postoperative delirium in older patients undergoing elective orthopedic surgery. J Am Geriatr Soc 43:175–178, 1995

Foley CM, Polinsky MS, Gruskin AB, et al: Encephalopathy in infants and children with chronic renal disease. Arch Neurol 38:656–658, 1981

Folstein MF, Folstein SE, McHugh PR: Mini-Mental State: a practical method for grading the cognitive state of patients for the clinician. J Psychiatr Res 12:189–198, 1975

Folstein MF, Bassett SS, Romanoski AJ, et al: The epidemiology of delirium in the community: the Eastern Baltimore Mental Health Survey. Int Psychogeriatr 3:169–176, 1991

Fonseca F, Bulbena A, Navarrete R, et al: Spanish version of the Delirium Rating Scale—Revised-98: reliability and validity. J Psychosom Res (in press)

Forman LJ, Cavalieri TA, Galski T, et al: Occurrence and impact of suspected delirium in hospitalized elderly patients. J Am Osteopath Assoc 95:588–591, 1995

Francis J: Sensory and environmental factors in delirium. Paper presented at Delirium: Current Advancements in Diagnosis, Treatment and Research, Geriatric Research, Education, and Clinical Center (GRECC), Veterans Administration Medical Center, Minneapolis, MN, September 13–14, 1993

Francis J, Kapoor WN: Prognosis after hospital discharge of older medical patients with delirium. J Am Geriatr Soc 40:601–606, 1992

Francis J, Martin D, Kapoor WN: A prospective study of delirium in hospitalized elderly. JAMA 263:1097–1101, 1990

Franco K, Litaker D, Locala J, et al: The cost of delirium in the surgical patient. Psychosomatics 42:68–73, 2001

Frye MA, Coudreaut MF, Hakeman SM, et al: Continuous droperidol infusion for management of agitated delirium in an ICU. Psychosomatics 36:301–305, 1995

Gaertner HJ, Fischer E, Hoss J: Side effects of clozapine. Psychopharmacology 99:S97–S100, 1989

Gagnon P, Allard P, Mâsse B, et al: Delirium in terminal cancer: a prospective study using daily screening, early diagnosis, and continuous monitoring. J Pain Symptom Manage 19:412–426, 2000

Gagnon P, Allard P, Gagnon B, et al: Delirium incidence and associated factors in terminally ill cancer patients. Psychosomatics 45:153, 2004a

Gagnon P, Gandreau JD, Harel F, et al: Delirium incidence and associated factors in hospitalized cancer patients. Psychosomatics 45:154, 2004b

Gallinat J, Möller H-J, Hegert U: Piracetam in der Anästhesie zur Prophylaxe eines postoperativen Delirs. Anasthesiol Intensivmed Notfallmed Schmerzther 34:520–527, 1999

Gelfand SB, Indelicato J, Benjamin J: Using intravenous haloperidol to control delirium (abstract). Hosp Community Psychiatry 43:215, 1992

George J, Bleasdale S, Singleton SJ: Causes and prognosis of delirium in elderly patients admitted to a district general hospital. Age Ageing 26:423–427, 1997

Glick RE, Sanders KM, Stern TA: Failure to record delirium as a complication of intra-aortic balloon pump treatment: a retrospective study. J Geriatr Psychiatry Neurol 9:97–99, 1996

Gorwood P, Limosin F, Batel P, et al: The A9 allele of the dopamine transporter gene is associated with delirium tremens and alcohol-withdrawal seizure. Biol Psychiatry 53:85–92, 2003

Grassi L, Caraceni A, Beltrami E, et al: Assessing delirium in cancer patients: the Italian versions of the Delirium Rating Scale and the Memorial Delirium Assessment Scale. J Pain Symptom Manage 21:59–68, 2001

Gruber-Baldini AL, Zimmerman S, Morrison RS, et al: Cognitive impairment in hip fracture patients: timing of detection and longitudinal follow-up. J Am Geriatr Soc 51:1227–1236, 2003

Gustafson Y, Berggren D, Brahnstrom B, et al: Acute confusional states in elderly patients treated for femoral neck fracture. J Am Geriatr Soc 36:525–530, 1988

Gustafson Y, Brannstrom B, Norberg A, et al: Underdiagnosis and poor documentation of acute confusional states in the elderly hip fracture patient. J Am Geriatr Soc 39:760–765, 1991

Hales RE, Polly S, Orman D: An evaluation of patients who received an organic mental disorder diagnosis on a psychiatric consultation-liaison service. Gen Hosp Psychiatry 11:88–94, 1988

Harrell R, Othmer E: Postcardiotomy confusion and sleep loss. J Clin Psychiatry 48:445–446, 1987

Hart RP, Levenson JL, Sessler CN, et al: Validation of a cognitive test for delirium in medical ICU patients. Psychosomatics 37:533–546, 1996

Hart RP, Best AM, Sessler CN, et al: Abbreviated Cognitive Test for Delirium. J Psychosom Res 43:417–423, 1997

Hatta K, Takahashi T, Nakamura H, et al: The association between intravenous haloperidol and prolonged QT interval. J Clin Psychopharmacol 21:257–261, 2001

Henry WD, Mann AM: Diagnosis and treatment of delirium. Can Med Assoc J 93:1156–1166, 1965

Hill EH, Blumenfeld M, Orlowski B: A modification of the Trzepacz Delirium Rating Scale—Revised-98 for use on the Palm Pilot and a presentation of data of symptom monitoring using haloperidol, olanzapine, and risperidone in the treatment of delirious hospitalized patients. Psychosomatics 43:158, 2002

Hooper JF, Minter G: Droperidol in the management of psychiatric emergencies. J Clin Psychopharmacol 3:262–263, 1983

Hopkins SJ, Rothwell NJ: Cytokines and the nervous system, I: expression and recognition. Trends Neurosci 18:83–88, 1995

Horikawa N, Yamazaki T, Miyamoto K, et al: Treatment for delirium with risperidone: results of a prospective open trial with 10 patients. Gen Hosp Psychiatry 25:289–292, 2003

Huang S-C, Tsai S-J, Chan C-H, et al: Characteristics and outcome of delirium in psychiatric inpatients. Psychiatry Clin Neurosci 52:47–50, 1998

Huyse F: Haloperidol and cardiac arrest. Lancet 2:568–569, 1988

Inouye SK, Charpentier PA: Precipitating factors for delirium in hospitalized elderly patients: predictive model and interrelationships with baseline vulnerability. JAMA 275:852–857, 1996

Inouye SK, van Dyke CH, Alessi CA, et al: Clarifying confusion: the Confusion Assessment Method. Ann Intern Med 113:941–948, 1990

Inouye SK, Rushing JT, Foreman MD, et al: Does delirium contribute to poor hospital outcome? J Gen Intern Med 13:234–242, 1998

Inouye SK, Bogardus ST, Charpentier PA, et al: A multicomponent intervention to prevent delirium in hospitalized older patients. N Engl J Med 340:669–676, 1999

Inouye SK, Bogardus ST Jr, Williams CS, et al: The role of adherence on the effectiveness of non-pharmacologic interventions: evidence from the Delirium Prevention Trial. Arch Intern Med 163:958–964, 2003

Itil T, Fink M: Anticholinergic drug-induced delirium: experimental modification, quantitative EEG, and behavioral correlations. J Nerv Ment Dis 143:492–507, 1966

Jackson JC, Hart RP, Gordon SM, et al: Six-month neuropsychological outcome of medical intensive care unit patients. Crit Care Med 31:1226–1234, 2003

Jacobson SA, Jerrier S: EEG in delirium. Semin Clin Neuropsychiatry 5:86–93, 2000

Jacobson SA, Leuchter AF, Walter DO: Conventional and quantitative EEG diagnosis of delirium among the elderly. J Neurol Neurosurg Psychiatry 56:153–158, 1993a

Jacobson SA, Leuchter AF, Walter DO, et al: Serial quantitative EEG among elderly subjects with delirium. Biol Psychiatry 34:135–140, 1993b

Jitapunkul S, Pillay I, Ebrahim S: Delirium in newly admitted elderly patients: a prospective study. Q J Med 83:307–314, 1992

Johansson IS, Hamrin EK, Larsson G: Psychometric testing of the NEECHAM Confusion Scale among patients with hip fracture. Res Nurs Health 25:203–111, 2002

Johnson JC, Gottlieb GL, Sullivan E, et al: Using DSM-III criteria to diagnose delirium in elderly general medical patients. J Gerontol 45:M113–M119, 1990

Johnson JC, Kerse NM, Gottlieb G, et al: Prospective versus retrospective methods of identifying patients with delirium. J Am Geriatr Soc 40:316–319, 1992

Kakuma R, du Fort GG, Arsenault L, et al: Delirium in older emergency department patients discharged home: effect on survival. J Am Geriatr Soc 51:443–450, 2003

Kalisvaart K: Prophylactic haloperidol cuts delirium. Paper presented at the annual meeting of the American Association of Geriatric Psychiatry, Honolulu, HI, 2003

Katz IR, Jeste DV, Mintzer JE, et al: Comparison of risperidone and placebo for psychosis and behavioral disturbances associated with dementia: a randomized double-blind trial. J Clin Psychiatry 60:107–115, 1999

Katz JA, Mahoney DH, Fernbach DJ: Human leukocyte alpha-interferon induced transient neurotoxicity in children. Invest New Drugs 6:115–120, 1988

Kaufer DI, Catt KE, Lopez OL, et al: Dementia with Lewy bodies: response of delirium-like features to donepezil. Neurology 51:1512–1513, 1998

Kelly KG, Zisselman M, Cutillo-Schmitter T, et al: Severity and course of delirium in medically hospitalized nursing facility residents. Am J Geriatr Psychiatry 9:72–77, 2001

Kennard MA, Bueding E, Wortis WB: Some biochemical and electroencephalographic changes in delirium tremens. Q J Stud Alcohol 6:4–14, 1945

Kiely DK, Bergmann MA, Murphy KM, et al: Delirium among newly admitted postacute facility patients: prevalence, symptoms, and severity. J Gerontol A Biol Sci Med Sci 58:M441–445, 2003

Kim K-S, Pae C-U, Chae J-H, et al: An open pilot trial of olanzapine for delirium in the Korean population. Psychiatry Clin Neurosci 55:515–519, 2001

Kim KY, Bader GM, Kotlyar V, et al: Treatment of delirium in older patients with quetiapine. J Geriatr Psychiatry Neurol 16:29–31, 2003

Kishi Y, Iwasaki Y, Takezawa K, et al: Delirium in critical care unit patients admitted through an emergency room. Gen Hosp Psychiatry 17:371–379, 1995

Kishi Y, Hosaka T, Yoshikawa E, et al: Delirium Rating Scale-Revised-98 (DRS-R-98), Japanese version. Seishin Igaku 43:1365–1371, 2001

Klein M, Payaslian S, Gomez J, et al: Acute confusional syndrome due to acute nicotine withdrawal. Medicina (B Aires) 62:335–336, 2002

Knell AJ, Davidson AR, Williams R, et al: Dopamine and serotonin metabolism in hepatic encephalopathy. BMJ 1:549–551, 1974

Kobayashi K, Takeuchi O, Suzuki M, et al: A retrospective study on delirium type. Jpn J Psychiatry Neurol 46:911–917, 1992

Koehnke MD, Schick S, Lutz U, et al: Severity of alcohol withdrawal symptoms and the T1128C polymorphism of the neuropeptide Y gene. J Neural Transm 109:1423–1429, 2002

Kolbeinsson H, Jonsson A: Delirium and dementia in acute medical admissions of elderly patients in Iceland. Acta Psychiatr Scand 87:123–127, 1993

Koponen H, Partanen J, Paakkonen A, et al: EEG spectral analysis in delirium. J Neurol Neurosurg Psychiatry 52:980–985, 1989

Koponen H, Sirvio J, Lepola U, et al: A long-term follow-up study of cerebrospinal fluid acetylcholinesterase in delirium. Eur Arch Psychiatry Clin Neurosci 243:347–351, 1994

Kreis R, Farrow N, Ross BN: Localized NMR spectroscopy in patients with chronic hepatic encephalopathy: analysis of changes in cerebral glutamine, choline, and inositols. NMR Biomed 4:109–116, 1991

Kriwisky M, Perry GY, Tarchitsky D, et al: Haloperidol-induced torsades de pointes. Chest 98:482–484, 1990

Kullmann F, Hollerbach S, Holstege A, et al: Subclinical hepatic encephalopathy: the diagnostic value of evoked potentials. J Hepatol 22:101–110, 1995

Laurila JV, Pitkala KH, Strandberg TE, et al: The impact of different diagnostic criteria on prevalence rates for delirium. Dement Geriatr Cogn Disord 16:156–162, 2003

Lawlor PG, Gagnon B, Mancini IL, et al: Occurrence, causes and outcome of delirium in patients with advanced cancer. Arch Intern Med 160:786–794, 2000a

Lawlor PG, Nekolaichuk C, Gagnon B, et al: Clinical utility, factor analysis and further validation of the Memorial Delirium Assessment Scale in patients with advanced cancer: assessing delirium in advanced cancer. Cancer 88:2859–2867, 2000b

Lawrence KR, Nasraway SA: Conduction disturbances associated with administration of butyrophenone antipsychotics in the critically ill: a review of the literature. Pharmacotherapy 17:531–537, 1997

Leso L, Schwartz TL: Ziprasidone treatment of delirium. Psychosomatics 43:61–62, 2002

Leung CM, Chan KK, Cheng KK: Psychiatric morbidity in a general medical ward: Hong Kong's experience. Gen Hosp Psychiatry 14:196–200, 1992

Levenson JA: Should psychostimulants be used to treat delirious patients with depressed mood? (letter). J Clin Psychiatry 53:69, 1992

Levenson JL: High-dose intravenous haloperidol for agitated delirium following lung transplantation. Psychosomatics 36:66–68, 1995

Levkoff SE, Evans DA, Liptzin B, et al: Delirium: the occurrence and persistence of symptoms among elderly hospitalized patients. Arch Intern Med 152:334–340, 1992

Levkoff SE, Liptzin B, Evans D, et al: Progression and resolution of delirium in elderly patients hospitalized for acute care. Am J Geriatr Psychiatry 2:230–238, 1994

Lipowski ZJ: Delirium: Acute Confusional States. New York, Oxford University Press, 1990

Lipton SA, Gendelman HE: Dementia associated with the acquired immunodeficiency syndrome. N Engl J Med 332:934–940, 1995

Liptzin B, Levkoff SE: An empirical study of delirium subtypes. Br J Psychiatry 161:843–845, 1992

Liptzin B, Levkoff SE, Gottlieb GL, et al: Delirium. J Neuropsychiatry Clin Neurosci 5:154–160, 1993

Lischke V, Behne M, Doelken P, et al: Droperidol causes a dose-dependent prolongation of the QT interval. Anesth Analg 79:983–986, 1994

Ljubisavljevic V, Kelly B: Risk factors for development of delirium among oncology patients. Gen Hosp Psychiatry 25:345–352, 2003

Mach J, Dysken M, Kuskowski M, et al: Serum anticholinergic activity in hospitalized older persons with delirium: a preliminary study. J Am Geriatr Soc 43:491–495, 1995

Magaziner J, Simonsick EM, Kashner M, et al: Survival experience of aged hip fracture patients. Am J Public Health 79:274–278, 1989

Maldonado JR, van der Starre P, Wysong A, et al: Dexmedetomidine: can it reduce the incidence of ICU delirium in postcardiotomy patients? (abstract). Psychosomatics 45:173, 2004

Manos PJ: The utility of the ten-point clock test as a screen for cognitive impairment in general hospital patients. Gen Hosp Psychiatry 19:439–444, 1997

Marcantonio ER, Goldman L, Mangione CM, et al: A clinical prediction rule for delirium after elective noncardiac surgery. JAMA 271:134–139, 1994a

Marcantonio ER, Juarez G, Goldman L, et al: The relationship of postoperative delirium with psychoactive medications. JAMA 272:1518–1522, 1994b

Marcantonio ER, Flacker JM, Wright J, et al: Reducing delirium after hip fracture: a randomized trial. J Am Geriatr Soc 49:516–522, 2001

Masand PS, Sipahimalani A: Olanzapine in the treatment of delirium. Psychosomatics 39:422–430, 1998

Mathers DA: The GABA-A receptor: new insights from single channel recording. Synapse 1:96–101, 1987

Matsuoka Y, Miyake Y, Arakaki H, et al: Clinical utility and validation of the Japanese version of the Memorial Delirium Assessment Scale in a psychogeriatric inpatient setting. Gen Hosp Psychiatry 23:36–40, 2001

Matsushima E, Nakajima K, Moriya H, et al: A psychophysiological study of the development of delirium in coronary care units. Biol Psychiatry 41:1211–1217, 1997

McCarthy MC: Detecting acute confusion in older adults: comparing clinical reasoning of nurses working in acute, long-term, and community health care environments. Res Nurs Health 26:203–212, 2003

McCusker J, Cole M, Abrahamowicz M, et al: Delirium predicts 12-month mortality. Arch Intern Med 162:457–463, 2002

McCusker J, Cole MG, Dendukuri N, et al: Does delirium increase hospital stay? J Am Geriatr Soc 51:1539–1546, 2003a

McCusker J, Cole MG, Dendukuri N, et al: The course of delirium in older medical inpatients: a prospective study. J Gen Intern Med 18:696–704, 2003b

McKeith I, Fairbairn A, Perry R, et al: Neuroleptic sensitivity in patients with senile dementia of Lewy body type. BMJ 305:673–678, 1992

McNicoll L, Pisani MA, Zhang Y, et al: Delirium in the intensive care unit: occurrence and clinical course in older patients. J Am Geriatr Soc 51:591–598, 2003

Meagher DJ: Delirium: the role of psychiatry. Advances in Psychiatric Treatments 7:433–443, 2001

Meagher DJ: The significance of motoric symptoms and subtypes in delirium. Symposium presented at the 156th annual meeting of the American Psychiatric Association, San Francisco, CA, May 17–22, 2003

Meagher DJ, Trzepacz PT: Delirium phenomenology illuminates pathophysiology, management and course. J Geriatr Psychiatry Neurol 11:150–157, 1998

Meagher DJ, Trzepacz PT: Motoric subtypes of delirium. Semin Clin Neuropsychiatry 5:76–86, 2000

Meagher DJ, O'Hanlon D, O'Mahony E, et al: Use of environmental strategies and psychotropic medication in the management of delirium. Br J Psychiatry 168:512–515, 1996

Mendelson G: Pheniramine aminosalicylate overdosage: reversal of delirium and choreiform movements with tacrine treatment. Arch Neurol 34:313, 1977

Mesulam M-M: Attention, confusional states, and neglect, in Principles of Behavioral Neurology. Edited by Mesulam M-M. Philadelphia, PA, FA Davis, 1985, pp 125–168

Metzger E, Friedman R: Prolongation of the corrected QT and torsades de pointes cardiac arrhythmia associated with intravenous haloperidol in the medically ill. J Clin Psychopharmacol 13:128–132, 1993

Milbrandt EB, Deppen S, Harrison PL, et al: Costs associated with delirium in mechanically ventilated patients. Crit Care Med 32:955–962, 2004

Milisen K, Foreman MD, Abraham IL, et al: A nurse-led interdisciplinary intervention program for delirium in elderly hip fracture patients. J Am Geriatr Soc 49:523–532, 2001

Miller PS, Richardson JS, Jyu CA, et al: Association of low serum anticholinergic levels and cognitive impairment in elderly presurgical patients. Am J Psychiatry 145:342–345, 1988

Minagawa H, Uchitomi Y, Yamawaki S, et al: Psychiatric morbidity in terminally ill cancer patients: a prospective study. Cancer 78:1131–1137, 1996

Mittal D, Jimerson NA, Neely E, et al: Risperidone in the treatment of delirium: results from a prospective open-label trial. J Clin Psychiatry 65:662–667, 2004

Mizock BA, Sabelli HC, Dubin A, et al: Septic encephalopathy: evidence for altered phenylalanine metabolism and comparison with hepatic encephalopathy. Arch Intern Med 150:443–449, 1990

Moller JT, Cluitmans P, Rasmussen LS, et al: Long-term postoperative cognitive dysfunction in the elderly ISPOCD1 study. ISPOCD investigators. International Study of Post-Operative Cognitive Dysfunction. Lancet 351:857–861, 1998 [published erratum appears in Lancet 351:1742, 1998]

Mondimore FM, Damlouji N, Folstein MF, et al: Post-ECT confusional states associated with elevated serum anticholinergic levels. Am J Psychiatry 140:930–931, 1983

Monette J, Galbaud du Fort G, Fung SH, et al: Evaluation of the Confusion Assessment Method (CAM) as a screening tool for delirium in the emergency room. Gen Hosp Psychiatry 23:20–25, 2001

Montgomery EA, Fenton GW, McClelland RJ, et al: Psychobiology of minor head injury. Psychosom Med 21:375–384, 1991

Mori E, Yamadori A: Acute confusional state and acute agitated delirium. Arch Neurol 44:1139–1143, 1987

Morrison RS, Magaziner J, Gilbert M, et al: Relationship between pain and opioid analgesics on the development of delirium following hip fracture. J Gerontol A Biol Sci Med Sci 58:76–81, 2003

Moulaert P: Treatment of acute nonspecific delirium with IV haloperidol in surgical intensive care patients. Acta Anaesthesiol Belg 40:183–186, 1989

Mousseau DD, Butterworth RF: Current theories on the pathogenesis of hepatic encephalopathy. Proc Soc Exp Biol Med 206:329–344, 1994

Murphy KM: The baseline predictors and 6-month outcomes of incident delirium in nursing home residents: a study using the minimum data set. Psychosomatics 40:164–165, 1999

Murray AM, Levkoff SE, Wetle TT, et al: Acute delirium and functional decline in the hospitalized elderly patient. J Gerontol 48:M181–M186, 1993

Nagley SJ: Predicting and preventing confusion in your patients. J Gerontol Nurs 12:27–31, 1986

Nakamura J, Uchimura N, Yamada S, et al: The effect of mianserin hydrochloride on delirium. Hum Psychopharmacol 10:289–297, 1995

Nakamura J, Uchimura N, Yamada S, et al: Does plasma free 3-methoxy-4-hydroxyphenyl(ethylene)glycol increase the delirious state? A comparison of the effects of mianserin and haloperidol on delirium. Int Clin Psychopharmacol 12:147–152, 1997a

Nakamura J, Uchimura N, Yamada S, et al: Mianserin suppositories in the treatment of post-operative delirium. Hum Psychopharmacol 12:595–599, 1997b

Neelon VJ, Champagne MT, Carlson JR, et al: The NEECHAM Scale: construction, validation, and clinical testing. Nurs Res 45:324–330, 1996

Nicholas LM, Lindsey BA: Delirium presenting with symptoms of depression. Psychosomatics 36:471–479, 1995

O'Brien JM, Rockwood RP, Suh KI: Haloperidol-induced torsades de pointes. Ann Pharmacother 33:1046–1050, 1999

O'Keeffe ST: Rating the severity of delirium: the Delirium Assessment Scale. Int J Geriatr Psychiatry 9:551–556, 1994

O'Keeffe ST, Gosney MA: Assessing attentiveness in older hospitalized patients: global assessment vs. test of attention. J Am Geriatr Soc 45:470–473, 1997

O'Keeffe ST, Lavan JN: Predicting delirium in elderly patients: development and validation of a risk-stratification model. Age Ageing 25:317–321, 1996

O'Keeffe ST, Lavan JN: Clinical significance of delirium subtypes in older people. Age Ageing 28:115–119, 1999

O'Keeffe ST, Tormey WP, Glasgow R, et al: Thiamine deficiency in hospitalized elderly patients. Gerontology 40:18–24, 1994

Olofsson SM, Weitzner MA, Valentine AD, et al: A retrospective study of the psychiatric management and outcome of delirium in the cancer patient. Support Care Cancer 4:351–357, 1996

Onofrj M, Curatola L, Malatesta G, et al: Reduction of P3 latency during outcome from post-traumatic amnesia. Acta Neurol Scand 83:273–279, 1991

Ovchinsky N, Pitchumoni S, Skotzko CE: Use of olanzapine for the treatment of delirium following traumatic brain injury. Psychosomatics 43:147–148, 2002

Owens JF, Hutelmyer CM: The effect of postoperative intervention on delirium in cardiac surgical patients. Nurs Res 31:60–62, 1982

Passik SD, Cooper M: Complicated delirium in a cancer patient successfully treated with olanzapine. J Pain Symptom Manage 17:219–223, 1999

Patten SB, Lamarre CJ: Dysgraphia (letter). Can J Psychiatry 34:746, 1989

Perrault LP, Denault AY, Carrier M, et al: Torsades de pointes secondary to intravenous haloperidol after coronary artery bypass graft surgery. Can J Anaesth 47:251–254, 2000

Peterson JF, Truman B, Shintani A, et al: The prevalence of delirium subtypes in medical ICU patients. J Am Geriatr Soc 51:S174, 2003

Picotte-Prillmayer D, DiMaggio JR, Baile WF: H-2 blocker delirium. Psychosomatics 36:74–77, 1995

Platt MM, Breitbart W, Smith M, et al: Efficacy of neuroleptics for hypoactive delirium. J Neuropsychiatry Clin Neurosci 6:66–67, 1994a

Platt MM, Trautman P, Frager G, et al: Pediatric delirium: research update. Paper presented at the annual meeting of the Academy of Psychosomatic Medicine, Phoenix, AZ, November 1994b

Pompei P, Foreman M, Rudberg MA, et al: Delirium in hospitalized older persons: outcomes and predictors. J Am Geriatr Soc 42:809–815, 1994

Prugh DG, Wagonfeld S, Metcalf D, et al: A clinical study of delirium in children and adolescents. Psychosom Med 42:177–195, 1980

Rabins PV, Folstein MF: Delirium and dementia; diagnostic criteria and fatality rates. Br J Psychiatry 140:149–153, 1982

Rahkonen T, Luukkainen-Markkula R, Paanila S, et al: Delirium episode as a sign of undetected dementia among community dwelling elderly subjects: a 2 year follow up study. J Neurol Neurosurg Psychiatry 69:519–521, 2000

Ravona-Springer R, Dohlberg OT, Hirschman S, et al: Delirium in elderly patients treated with risperidone: a report of three cases. J Clin Psychopharmacol 18:171–172, 1998

Reilly JG, Ayis AS, Ferrier IN, et al: QT$_c$-interval abnormalities and psychotropic drug therapy in psychiatric patients. Lancet 355:1048–1052, 2000

Resnick M, Burton BT: Droperidol versus haloperidol in the initial management of acutely agitated patients. J Clin Psychiatry 45:298–299, 1984

Riker RR, Fraser GL, Cox PM: Continuous infusion of haloperidol controls agitation in critically ill patients. Crit Care Med 22:433–440, 1994

Riker RR, Fraser GL, Richen P: Movement disorders associated with withdrawal from high-dose intravenous haloperidol therapy in delirious ICU patients. Chest 111:1778–1781, 1997

Rincon HG, Granados M, Unutzer J, et al: Prevalence, detection and treatment of anxiety, depression and delirium in the adult critical care unit. Psychosomatics 42:391–396, 2001

Robertsson B: Assessment scales in delirium. Dement Geriatr Cogn Disord 10:368–379, 1999

Robertsson B, Blennow K, Gottfries CG, et al: Delirium in dementia. Int J Geriatr Psychiatry 13:49–56, 1998

Robinson MJ: Probable Lewy body dementia presenting as delirium. Psychosomatics 43:84–86, 2002

Rockwood K: Acute confusion in elderly medical patients. J Am Geriatr Soc 37:150–154, 1989

Rockwood K: The occurrence and duration of symptoms in elderly patients with delirium. Journal of Gerontological Medical Science 48:M162–M166, 1993

Rockwood K, Cosway S, Stolee P, et al: Increasing the recognition of delirium in elderly patients. J Am Geriatr Soc 42:252–256, 1994

Rockwood K, Cosway S, Carver D, et al: The risk of dementia and death after delirium. Age Ageing 28:551–556, 1999

Rolfson DB, McElhaney JE, Jhangri GS, et al: Validity of the Confusion Assessment Method in detecting post-operative delirium in the elderly. Int Psychogeriatr 11:431–438, 1999

Romano J, Engel GL: Delirium, I: electroencephalographic data. Archives of Neurology and Psychiatry 51:356–377, 1944

Rosenberg PB, Ahmed I, Hurwitz S: Methylphenidate in depressed medically ill patients. J Clin Psychiatry 52:263–267, 1991

Ross CA, Peyser CE, Shapiro I, et al: Delirium: phenomenologic and etiologic subtypes. Int Psychogeriatr 3:135–147, 1991

Rothwell NJ, Hopkins SJ: Cytokines and the nervous system, II: actions and mechanisms of action. Trends Neurosci 18:130–136, 1995

Rudberg MA, Pompei P, Foreman MD, et al: The natural history of delirium in older hospitalized patients: a syndrome of heterogeneity. Age Ageing 26:169–174, 1997

Ruijs MB, Keyser A, Gabreels FJ, et al: Somatosensory evoked potentials and cognitive sequelae in children with closed head injury. Neuropediatrics 24:307–312, 1993

Ruijs MB, Gabreels FJ, Thijssen HM: The utility of electroencephalography and cerebral CT in children with mild and moderately severe closed head injuries. Neuropediatrics 25:73–77, 1994

Sandberg O, Gustafson Y, Brannstrom B, et al: Prevalence of dementia, delirium and psychiatric symptoms in various care settings for the elderly. Scand J Soc Med 26:56–62, 1998

Sander T, Harms H, Podschus J, et al: Alleleic association of a dopamine transporter gene polymorphism in alcohol dependence with withdrawal seizures or delirium. Biol Psychiatry 41:299–304, 1997

Sanders KM, Stern TA: Management of delirium associated with use of the intra-aortic balloon pump. Am J Crit Care 2:371–377, 1993

Saravay SM, Strain JJ: Academy of Psychosomatic Medicine Task Force on Funding Implications of Consultation/Liaison Psychiatry Outcome Studies: special series introduction: a review of outcome studies. Psychosomatics 35:227–232, 1994

Schneir AB, Offerman SR, Ly BT, et al: Complications of diagnostic physostigmine administration to emergency department patients. Ann Emerg Med 42:14–19, 2003

Schofield I: A small exploratory study of the reaction of older people to an episode of delirium. J Adv Nurs 25:942–952, 1997

Schor JD, Levkoff SE, Lipsitz LA, et al: Risk factors for delirium in hospitalized elderly. JAMA 267:827–831, 1992

Schuster P, Gabriel E, Kufferle B, et al: Reversal by physostigmine of clozapine-induced delirium. Clin Toxicol 10:437–441, 1977

Schwartz TL, Masand PS: Treatment of delirium with quetiapine. Prim Care Companion J Clin Psychiatry 2:10–12, 2000

Schwartz TL, Masand PS: The role of atypical antipsychotics in the treatment of delirium. Psychosomatics 43:171–174, 2002

Seear M, Lockitch G, Jacobson B, et al: Thiamine, riboflavin and pyridoxine deficiency in a population of critically ill children. J Pediatr 121:533–538, 1992

Sipahimalani A, Masand PS: Use of risperidone in delirium: case reports. Ann Clin Psychiatry 9:105–107, 1997

Sirois F: Delirium: 100 cases. Can J Psychiatry 33:375–378, 1988

Snyder S, Reyner A, Schmeidler J, et al: Prevalence of mental disorders in newly admitted medical inpatients with AIDS. Psychosomatics 33:166–170, 1992

Stefano GB, Bilfinger TV, Fricchione GL: The immune-neurolink and the macrophage: post-cardiotomy delirium, HIV-associated dementia and psychiatry. Prog Neurobiol 42:475–488, 1994

Stern TA: Continuous infusion of physostigmine in anticholinergic delirium: a case report. J Clin Psychiatry 44:463–464, 1983

Stern TA: Continuous infusion of haloperidol in agitated critically ill patients. Crit Care Med 22:378–379, 1994

Sundaram M, Dostrow V: Epilepsy in the elderly. Neurologist 1:232–239, 1995

Swenson JR, Erman M, Labelle J, et al: Extrapyramidal reactions: neuropsychiatric mimics in patients with AIDS. Gen Hosp Psychiatry 11:248–253, 1989

Tarter RE, van Thiel DH, Arria AM, et al: Impact of cirrhosis on the neuropsychological test performance of alcoholics. Alcohol Clin Exp Res 12:619–621, 1988

Teicher MH, Gold CA: Neuroleptic drugs: indications and guidelines for their rational use in children and adolescents. J Child Adolesc Psychopharmacol 1:33–56, 1990

Tejera CA, Saravay SM, Goldman E, et al: Diphenhydramine-induced delirium in elderly hospitalized patients with mild dementia. Psychosomatics 35:399–402, 1994

Tesar GE, Murray GB, Cassem NH: Use of high-dose intravenous haloperidol in the treatment of agitated cardiac patients. J Clin Psychopharmacol 5:344–347, 1985

Thomas H, Schwartz E, Petrilli R: Droperidol versus haloperidol for chemical restraint of agitated and combative patients. Ann Emerg Med 21:407–413, 1992

Thomas RI, Cameron DJ, Fahs MC: A prospective study of delirium and prolonged hospital stay. Arch Gen Psychiatry 45:937–946, 1988

Tokita K, Tanaka H, Kawamoto M, et al: Patient-controlled epidural analgesia with bupivacaine and fentanyl. Masui 50:742–746, 2001

Torres R, Mittal D, Kennedy R: Use of quetiapine in delirium: case reports. Psychosomatics 42:347–349, 2001

Treloar AJ, Macdonald AJ: Outcome of delirium, part I: outcome of delirium diagnosed by DSM III-R, ICD-10 and CAMDEX and derivation of the Reversible Cognitive Dysfunction Scale among acute geriatric inpatients. Int J Geriatr Psychiatry 12:609–613, 1997

Trzepacz PT: Neuropathogenesis of delirium: a need to focus our research. Psychosomatics 35:374–391, 1994

Trzepacz PT: Anticholinergic model for delirium. Semin Clin Neuropsychiatry 1:294–303, 1996a

Trzepacz PT: Delirium: advances in diagnosis, assessment, and treatment. Psychiatr Clin North Am 19:429–448, 1996b

Trzepacz PT: The Delirium Rating Scale: its use in consultation/liaison research. Psychosomatics 40:193–204, 1999a

Trzepacz PT: Update on the neuropathogenesis of delirium. Dement Geriatr Cogn Disord 10:330–334, 1999b

Trzepacz PT: Is there a final common neural pathway in delirium? Focus on acetylcholine and dopamine. Semin Clin Neuropsychiatry 5:132–148, 2000

Trzepacz PT, Dew MA: Further analyses of the Delirium Rating Scale. Gen Hosp Psychiatry 17:75–79, 1995

Trzepacz PT, Francis J: Low serum albumin and risk of delirium (letter). Am J Psychiatry 147:675, 1990

Trzepacz PT, van der Mast R: Neuropathophysiology of delirium, in Delirium in Old Age. Edited by Lindesay J, Rockwood K, MacDonald A. Oxford, UK, Oxford University Press, 2002, pp 51–78

Trzepacz PT, Teague GB, Lipowski ZJ: Delirium and other organic mental disorders in a general hospital. Gen Hosp Psychiatry 7:101–106, 1985

Trzepacz PT, Baker RW, Greenhouse J: A symptom rating scale for delirium. Psychiatry Res 23:89–97, 1988a

Trzepacz PT, Brenner R, Coffman G, et al: Delirium in liver transplantation candidates: discriminant analysis of multiple test variables. Biol Psychiatry 24:3–14, 1988b

Trzepacz PT, Ho V, Mallavarapu H: Cholinergic delirium and neurotoxicity associated with tacrine for Alzheimer's dementia. Psychosomatics 37:299–301, 1996

Trzepacz PT, Mulsant BH, Dew MA, et al: Is delirium different when it occurs in dementia? A study using the Delirium Rating Scale. J Neuropsychiatry Clin Neurosci 10:199–204, 1998

Trzepacz PT, Mittal D, Torres R, et al: Delirium phenomenology using the Delirium Rating Scale-Revised-98 (DRS-R-98). J Neuropsychiatry Clin Neurosci 13:154, 2001a

Trzepacz PT, Mittal D, Torres R, et al: Validation of the Delirium Rating Scale–Revised-98: comparison with the Delirium Rating Scale and the Cognitive Test for Delirium. J Neuropsychiatry Clin Neurosci 13:229–242, 2001b [published erratum appears in J Neuropsychiatry Clin Neurosci 13:433, 2001]

Trzepacz PT, Meagher DJ, Wise M: Neuropsychiatric aspects of delirium, in The American Psychiatric Publishing Textbook of Neuropsychiatry and Clinical Neurosciences, 4th Edition. Edited by Yudofsky SC, Hales RE. Washington, DC, American Psychiatric Publishing, 2002a, pp 525–564

Trzepacz PT, Mittal D, Torres R, et al: Delirium vs. dementia symptoms: Delirium Rating Scale-Revised-98 (DRS-R-98) and Cognitive Test for Delirium (CTD) item comparisons. Psychosomatics 43:156–157, 2002b

Tsutsui S, Kitamura M, Higachi H, et al: Development of postoperative delirium in relation to a room change in the general surgical unit. Surg Today 26:292–294, 1996

Tune LE, Dainloth NF, Holland A, et al: Association of postoperative delirium with raised serum levels of anticholinergic drugs. Lancet 2:651–653, 1981

Tune L, Carr S, Hoag E, et al: Anticholinergic effects of drugs commonly prescribed for the elderly: potential means for assessing risk of delirium. Am J Psychiatry 149:1393–1394, 1992

Turkel SB, Braslow K, Tavare CJ, et al: The Delirium Rating Scale in children and adolescents. Psychosomatics 44:126–129, 2003

Turkel SB, Trzepacz PT, Tavare J: Comparison of delirium symptoms across the life cycle (abstract). Psychosomatics 45:162, 2004

Uchiyama M, Tanaka K, Isse K, et al: Efficacy of mianserin on symptoms of delirium in the aged: an open trial study. Prog Neuropsychopharmacol Biol Psychiatry 20:651–656, 1996

van der Mast RC: Detecting and measuring the severity of delirium with the Symptom Rating Scale for Delirium, in Delirium After Cardiac Surgery. Thesis, Erasmus University Rotterdam, Benecke Consultants, Amsterdam, 1994, pp 78–89

van der Mast RC, Fekkes D: Serotonin and amino acids: partners in delirium pathophysiology? Semin Clin Neuropsychiatry 5:125–131, 2000 van der Mast RC, van den Broek WW, Fekkes D, et al: Incidence of and preoperative predictors for delirium after cardiac surgery. J Psychosom Res 46:479–483, 1999

van Hemert AM, van der Mast RC, Hengeveld MW, et al: Excess mortality in general hospital patients with delirium: a 5-year follow-up study of 519 patients seen in psychiatric consultation. J Psychosom Res 38:339–346, 1994

van Leeuwen AMH, Molders J, Sterkmans P, et al: Droperidol in acutely agitated patients: a double-blind placebo-controlled study. J Nerv Ment Dis 164:280–283, 1977

van Zyl LT, Davidson PR: Delirium in hospital: an underreported event at discharge. Can J Psychiatry 48:555–560, 2003

Wada Y, Yamaguchi N: Delirium in the elderly: relationship of clinical symptoms to outcome. Dementia 4:113–116, 1993

Wahlund L, Bjorlin GA: Delirium in clinical practice: experiences from a specialized delirium ward. Dement Geriatr Cogn Disord 10:389–392, 1999

Wanich CK, Sullivan-Marx EM, Gottlieb GL, et al: Functional status outcomes of a nursing intervention in hospitalized elderly. Image J Nurs Sch 24:201–207, 1992

Webster R, Holroyd S: Prevalence of psychotic symptoms in delirium. Psychosomatics 41:519–522, 2000

Weddington WW: The mortality of delirium: an underappreciated problem? Psychosomatics 23:1232–1235, 1982

Wengel SP, Roccaforte WH, Burke WJ: Donepezil improves symptoms of delirium in dementia: implications for future research. J Geriatr Psychiatry Neurol 11:159–161, 1998

Wengel SP, Burke WJ, Roccaforte WH: Donepezil for postoperative delirium associated with Alzheimer's disease. J Am Geriatr Soc 47:379–380, 1999

Wernicke C, Smolka M, Gallinat J, et al: Evidence for the importance of the human dopamine transporter gene for withdrawal symptomatology of alcoholics in a German population. Neurosci Lett 333:45–48, 2002

Wetli CV, Mash D, Karch SB: Cocaine-associated agitated delirium and the neuroleptic malignant syndrome. Am J Emerg Med 14:425–428, 1996

Williams MA, Campbell EB, Raynor WJ, et al: Reducing acute confusional states in elderly patients with hip fractures. Res Nurs Health 8:329–337, 1985

Williams PD, Helton DR: The proconvulsive activity of quinolone antibiotics in an animal model. Toxicol Lett 58:23–28, 1991

Williams-Russo P, Urquhart BL, Sharrock NE, et al: Postoperative delirium: predictors and prognosis in elderly orthopedic patients. J Am Geriatr Soc 40:759–767, 1992

Wilson LM: Intensive care delirium: the effect of outside deprivation in a windowless unit. Arch Intern Med 130:225–226, 1972

Wilt JL, Minnema AM, Johnson RF, et al: Torsades de pointes associated with the use of intravenous haloperidol. Ann Intern Med 119:391–394, 1993

Wolff HG, Curran D: Nature of delirium and allied states: the dysergastic reaction. Archives of Neurology and Psychiatry 33:1175–1215, 1935

World Health Organization: International Statistical Classification of Diseases and Related Health Problems, 10th Revision. Geneva, World Health Organization, 1992

Yamamoto T, Lyeth BG, Dixon CE, et al: Changes in regional brain acetylcholine content in rats following unilateral and bilateral brainstem lesions. J Neurotrauma 5:69–79, 1988

Yokota H, Ogawa S, Kurokawa A, et al: Regional cerebral blood flow in delirium patients. Psychiatry Clin Neurosci 57:337–339, 2003

Zee-Cheng C-S, Mueller CE, Siefert CF, et al: Haloperidol and torsades de pointes (letter). Ann Intern Med 102:418, 1985

7 Dementia

Antonio Lobo, M.D., Ph.D.

Pedro Saz, M.D., Ph.D.

CONCERN IS INCREASING about the frequency and consequences of dementia in Western countries. The high prevalence of dementing conditions in medical settings, often undiagnosed, and the association of dementia with longer hospital stays and greater use of health resources have direct implications for psychosomatic medicine and consultation-liaison psychiatry (Table 7–1). The psychiatric consultant is an invaluable collaborator with other health care professionals in the identification, evaluation, treatment, management, discharge planning, placement, and rehabilitation of the patient with dementia. In this chapter, we focus on the general clinical approach to dementia and its common causes. Some of these and other causes of dementia are also discussed elsewhere in this book: those disorders that are particularly likely to present with other neurological symptoms in Chapter 32, "Neurology and Neurosurgery"; HIV infection in Chapter 28, "HIV/AIDS"; other infections in Chapter 27, "Infectious Diseases"; alcohol and other substance use in Chapter 18, "Substance-Related Disorders"; toxic/metabolic conditions in Chapter 23, "Endocrine and Metabolic Disorders"; rheumatological/inflammatory conditions in Chapter 25, "Rheumatology"; traumatic brain injury in Chapter 35, "Physical Medicine and Rehabilitation"; and paraneoplastic syndromes in Chapter 24, "Oncology."

Concept of Dementia and Clinical Approach

Dementia is a brain condition and a paradigm of the disease model in psychiatry (McHugh and Slavney 1998). Medically ill patients referred to psychiatrists may require special diagnostic criteria (Malt et al. 1996). *Dementia* may be conveniently defined as a syndrome of global deterioration of intellectual function occurring in clear consciousness and caused by a brain condition. The notion of deterioration emphasizes the acquired nature of the impairment in dementia, to distinguish it from mental retardation, and the requirement of clear consciousness underlines the difference from delirium, if dementia is the only diagnosis. The impairment of memory is the most frequent and important sign or symptom, but deterioration in at least two other cognitive domains is required in our operational definition (Table 7–2). It is also required that, precisely because of cognitive decline, personal activities of daily living (ADLs) and social or occupational activities are impaired.

Deterioration in personality and neuropsychiatric symptoms are very frequent in dementia and are most important for psychiatrists, but there is general agreement that only the cognitive psychopathology should be in-

We gratefully acknowledge research grants from the Fondo de Investigación Sanitaria, Ministry of Health, Spain (98/0103, 01/0255); Instituto de Salud Carlos III (Redes Temáticas de Investigación Cooperativa, Project G03/128), Ministry of Health, Spain; and Ministry of Science and Technology, Spain (PM 1999-0084). We also wish to thank Olga Ibáñez for her administrative help.

TABLE 7–1.   Relevance of dementia in psychosomatic medicine and consultation-liaison psychiatry

General relevance

- Worldwide epidemic (Plum 1979; World Health Organization 1985)
- High prevalence: 9.6% in the United States elderly community (Breitner et al. 1999); 74% in nursing homes (Macdonald et al. 2002)
- High incidence: 2.8 per 1,000 person-years (age group=65–69 years), increases to 56.1 per 1,000 person-years in the older than 90-year age group (Kukull et al. 2002)
- Dramatic increase in the projected dementia rates is expected in the next decades (Organization for Economic Cooperation and Development, in press)
- Burden of the disease:
  Patient-related (Teri 1999)
  Caregiver-related (Colvez et al. 2002; Ory et al. 1999)
  Leads to earlier institutionalization (Patterson et al. 1999)
  DAT patients occupy two-thirds of nursing home beds (Macdonald et al. 2002)
  Gross annual cost of community care in the United States (Rice et al. 1993):
      $52,118 for mild to moderate cases; $69,389 for severe cases
      Two-thirds of these amounts go to informal care (e.g., family caregivers)
- Mortality rate at least twice that of individuals without dementia (Dewey and Saz 2001)

Specific relevance to psychosomatic medicine and consultation-liaison psychiatry

- High prevalence in general hospital patients (Erkinjuntti et al. 1986)
- High prevalence in specific medical conditions
- One-third of elderly referrals to consultation-liaison psychiatrists frequently undiagnosed (Huyse et al. 1996; Lobo et al. 1993)
- Most patients have noncognitive, neuropsychiatric symptoms (Ballard et al. 2001a; Lyketsos et al. 2002)
- Most patients with early dementia go undiagnosed in the general population (Larson et al. 1992; Lobo et al. 1997)
- Longer hospital stays, associated with higher costs; greater use of health resources after discharge (Lyketsos et al. 2000; Saravay and Lavin 1994)

Note.   DAT=dementia of the Alzheimer's type.

TABLE 7–2.   The dementia syndrome

A. Global deterioration of intellectual function
    Memory
    At least two other cognitive functions
B. Clear consciousness
C. Impairment of personal activities of daily living and social or occupational activities due to the decline in intellectual function
D. Deterioration in emotional control, motivation, or personality frequent but not necessary for diagnosis
E. Duration of at least 6 months (important exceptions, such as in the general hospital)

---

cluded in the diagnostic criteria. Persistence of the syndrome is important for the diagnosis, and some international committees require that symptoms be present for at least 6 months (World Health Organization 1992). However, exceptions to this norm occur and are important in settings such as the general hospital. Progression of the syndrome is the norm in most cases of dementia but is not included in the concept because some cases of dementia are stable and reversible.

Recent research has identified "a transitional state" between the cognitive changes of normal aging and dementia, known as *mild cognitive impairment* (Petersen et al. 2001a). Mild cognitive impairment refers to documented memory and other cognitive difficulties of mild severity in individuals who are otherwise functioning well that do not meet the clinical criteria for dementia. Several studies have shown that persons without dementia who have cognitive impairment have a higher chance of progressing to dementia and/or have a higher mortality rate. However, mild cognitive impairment is a heterogeneous concept (Wahlund et al. 2003). Not all individuals with mild cognitive impairment progress to dementia; a portion show improvement in cognition (Palmer et al. 2003).

Epidemiology, Risk Factors, and Etiology

Dementia has been etiologically associated with numerous heterogeneous conditions, as listed in Table 7–3. The adjusted prevalence estimate was 9.6% for all dementias in the U.S. population after age 65 and 6.5% for dementia

TABLE 7–3. Disorders that may produce dementia syndromes

Degenerative disorders
  Cortical
    Alzheimer's disease
    Frontotemporal dementia
    Dementia with Lewy bodies
  Subcortical
    Parkinson's disease
    Huntington's disease
    Basal ganglia calcification
      Wilson's disease
      Striatonigral degeneration
      Thalamic dementia
    Progressive supranuclear palsy
    Spinocerebellar degeneration
  Others
    Demyelinating disorders
      Multiple sclerosis
      Others
    Amyotrophic lateral sclerosis
    Hallervorden-Spatz disease
    Lafora myoclonus epilepsy

Vascular dementias
  Multi-infarct dementia
  Multiple large-vessel occlusions
  Strategic infarct dementia
  Lacunar state
  Binswanger's disease
  Chronic ischemia

Hydrocephalic dementias
  Communicating, normal pressure
  Noncommunicating

CNS infection–associated dementias
  HIV-associated dementia
  Creutzfeldt-Jakob disease
  Neurosyphilis
  Chronic meningitis
  Viral encephalitis
  Progressive multifocal leukoencephalopathy
  Fungal meningitis (cryptococcal)

Metabolic disorders
  Anoxia
    Cardiac disease
    Pulmonary failure
    Anemia
    Others
  Chronic renal failure
    Uremic encephalopathy
    Dialysis dementia
  Hepatic failure
    Portosystemic encephalopathy
    Acquired hepatocerebral degeneration
  Endocrinopathies
    Thyroid disturbances
    Cushing's syndrome
    Parathyroid disturbances
    Recurrent hypo- or hyperglycemia
  Porphyria
  Vitamin deficiency states
    Thiamine (B_1)
    Cyanocobalamin (B_{12})
    Folate
    Niacin
  Other chronic metabolic abnormalities
    Hypo- or hypernatremia
    Hematological conditions

Toxic conditions
  Alcohol related
  Drugs
    Polydrug abuse
    Psychotropic agents and anticonvulsants
    Solvents and other inhalants
    Anticholinergic compounds
    Antineoplastic therapies
    Corticosteroids, NSAIDs
    Antihypertensive and cardiac medications
  Metals
    Lead, mercury, arsenic, nickel, others
  Industrial agents and pollutants
    Carbon monoxide
    Organophosphate insecticides
    Organochlorine pesticides
    Perchloroethylene, toluene
    Trichloroethane, trichloroethylene
    Hydrocarbon inhalants
    Others

Neoplastic dementias
  Meningioma
  Glioblastoma
  Metastases
  Paraneoplastic syndromes
    Limbic encephalopathy
    Others
  Others

Traumatic conditions
  Posttraumatic
  Subdural hematoma
  Dementia pugilistica

Chronic inflammatory conditions
  Systemic lupus erythematosus
  Other collagen-vascular disorders

Psychiatric disorders
  Depression
  Others

Note. CNS = central nervous system; NSAIDs = nonsteroidal anti-inflammatory drugs.

of the Alzheimer's type (DAT) (Breitner et al. 1999). Similar rates have been reported in other United States studies (McDowell 2001), as well as in the EURODEM Study completed in 10 different cities across Europe (Lobo et al. 2000). In all these studies, the proportion of elderly patients with dementia increases dramatically with age, approximately doubling every 5 years. DAT is the most common type of dementia, accounting for 55%–75% of cases. Vascular dementia (or mixed DAT and vascular dementia) is the second most common cause, accounting for approximately 15%–30% of cases, and the other dementias listed in Table 7–3 account for the remaining 10%–25% of cases of dementia in the general population.

Reports from institutions such as nursing homes consistently document higher prevalence rates of dementia (74%), particularly of severe dementia (38%) (Macdonald et al. 2002). In general hospitals, recent reports also have confirmed that dementia is common. A large-scale study documented that 9.1% of the patients ages 55 years and older admitted to a teaching hospital medical service had dementia, but the prevalence was 31.2% in patients ages 85 years and older. Vascular dementia (75%) was reported to be the most frequent type (Erkinjuntti et al. 1986). Dementia is frequent in elderly patients with alcoholism (60%–70%) (Kasahara et al. 1996), Parkinson's disease (Aarsland et al. 2001), HIV disease (American Academy of Neurology AIDS Task Force 1991), and traumatic brain injury (TBI) (Kraus and Sorenson 1994). Both dementia with Lewy bodies in elderly patients and frontotemporal dementias (E.K. Perry et al. 1990) in cases of earlier onset may prove to be considerably more common than previously recognized (Campbell et al. 2001). The prevalence of *age-associated memory impairment* ranges from 17% to 34%, but this is probably a more inclusive term than *mild cognitive impairment.* Mild cognitive impairment may account for more than one-third of the patients referred to memory clinics (Wahlund et al. 2003).

Epidemiological studies also have shown that most patients with dementia have noncognitive, neuropsychiatric symptoms at some point in the course of the disease (Ballard et al. 2001a), and their potential for serious adverse consequences must be recognized (Eustace et al. 2002). In a recent population-based study, Lyketsos et al. (2002) found that 75% of the individuals with dementia had at least one neuropsychiatric symptom, and 62% were clinically significant. The most frequent disturbances were apathy (36%), depression (32%), and agitation or aggression (30%). The reported prevalence of depressive syndromes in dementia has ranged widely, from 10% to 54%, across recruitment sites (Devanand et al. 1997; Lobo et al. 1995; Zubenko et al. 2003). Similarly, estimates of the prevalence of psychotic symptoms in DAT vary widely, but this heterogeneity may be due to periods of exacerbation and remission of symptoms (Mohs et al. 2000). No differences in psychotic phenomena have been found between DAT and vascular dementia.

In the first population-based estimate among those with mild cognitive impairment, 43% of the individuals reported neuropsychiatric symptoms during the previous month (29% were rated as clinically significant) (Lyketsos et al. 2002).

Incidence estimates of dementia are provided by ambitious cohort studies that follow transversal studies counting prevalent cases. DAT rates rise from 2.8 per 1,000 person-years (age group, 65–69 years) to 56.1 per 1,000 person-years (age group, older than 90 years) (Kukull et al. 2002). These data are consistent with those in comparable studies in the United States (Brookmeyer et al. 1998; McDowell 2001); studies in Japan (Yoshitake et al. 1995); and cross-national European studies (Fratiglioni et al. 2000). All showed that the risk of developing global dementia, and DAT in particular, increases dramatically with age; the proportion also doubles every 5 years. DAT and vascular dementia are the most frequent incident dementias, accounting for 60%–90% in different studies (Fratiglioni et al. 2000). However, it is difficult to draw firm conclusions about both the prevalence and the incidence of vascular dementia because the rates reported vary substantially, suggesting lack of uniformity in implementing diagnostic criteria (Rocca and Kokmen 1999).

The potential of epidemiological research to test environmental hypotheses related to risk and protective factors that might eventually lead to preventive measures has been illustrated in recent studies. North–South differences in the incidence of dementia in Europe have been found, supporting environmental hypotheses in the etiology of dementia (Fratiglioni et al. 2000). Table 7–4 summarizes the results of recent, sophisticated analytic epidemiological research, including case–control studies in incident cases. Confirmed risk factors for DAT are scarce and limited to age, unalterable genetic factors (the apolipoprotein E4 genotype), and mild cognitive impairment. Mild cognitive impairment has important clinical and preventive implications, because recent studies, tending to confirm previous reports (Petersen et al. 2001a), suggest that when persons with mild cognitive impairment are observed longitudinally, they progress to clinically probable DAT at rates three or more times higher than those in persons without cognitive impairment (H.P. Bennett et al. 2002; Tuokko et al. 2003; Wahlund et al. 2003).

Probable risk factors and protective factors in dementia are also listed in Table 7–4 (Cedazo-Minguez and Cowburn 2001; Dartigues et al. 2002; Esposito et al. 2002; Letenneur et al. 2000; McDowell 2001; Verghese et al. 2003). Recent meta-analytic studies have found evidence to support an association between depression and dementia from both case–control studies and prospective studies (Jorm 2001). Several hypotheses have been put forward to explain the association, but depression has to be seriously considered as a probable risk factor for dementia. The attributable risk of DAT related to cardiovascular risk factors is still debated (Posner et al. 2002),

---

TABLE 7–4.   Risk factors and protective factors in dementias

Risk factors for dementia of the Alzheimer's type	
Age	++
Women	+
Low education	+
First-degree relative	+
Down syndrome	+
Head trauma	+
Apolipoprotein ε4 allele	++
Aluminum level	+/–
Hypertension	+
Depression	+
Mild cognitive impairment	++
Risk factors for vascular dementia	
Age >60 years	+
Men	+
Stroke risk factors	
Hypertension	++
Heart disease/atrial fibrillation	+
Cigarette smoking	++
Diabetes mellitus	++
Excessive alcohol consumption (3 drinks/day)	+
Hyperlipidemia	+
Hyperhomocysteinemia, low serum folate levels	+
Previous mental decline	+/–
Protective factors for dementia of the Alzheimer's type	
Apolipoprotein ε2 allele[a]	++
Low cholesterol level[a]	+/–
Statins[a]	+/–
Antihypertensive drug treatment[a]	+
Moderate alcohol consumption	+/–
Other	
Hormonal replacement therapy (estrogens)	+/–
Aspirin	–
Nonsteroidal anti-inflammatory drugs	+/–
Dietary factors (vitamin E, antioxidants)	+/–
Lifestyle (active life, leisure activities, social support and network)	+/–

Note.   ++=confirmed; +=probable; +/–=controversial; –=negative.
[a]Protective factors also for vascular dementia.

but recent research has suggested that cerebrovascular disease plays an important role in determining the presence of dementia (Vermeer et al. 2003), and specifically DAT (O'Brien et al. 2003; Snowdon et al. 1997). Hypertension may be particularly relevant in this respect because it is very common in the community and may be preventable. Until now, not enough evidence has been found to support some factors hypothesized as increasing the risk for DAT, such as aluminum level, or others thought to be protective, such as low cholesterol level,

moderate alcohol consumption, estrogens, antioxidants in the diet, or lifestyle activities, including leisure and social activities or a supportive social network.

Risk and protective factors for vascular dementia are also listed in Table 7–4. They include hyperhomocysteinemia and low serum folate levels, which are potentially reversible and can be identified early (Kessler et al. 2003; Maxwell et al. 2002).

Genetic knowledge about dementing conditions, most relevant if related to pathophysiology, may be summarized as follows. Huntington's disease is inherited as an autosomal dominant trait with complete penetrance, the mutation responsible being in an elongated and unstable trinucleotide (CAG) repeat on the short arm of chromosome 4 (Haskins and Harrison 2000). In DAT, particularly with early onset, several well-documented cases suggest that the disorder is transmitted in families through an autosomal dominant gene, although such transmission is rare. Possible genetic loci for familial DAT have been documented in chromosomes 21, 19, 14, and 1 (Levy-Lahad et al. 1995; Schellenberg et al. 1992; Whatley and Anderton 1990). Apolipoprotein E is coded on chromosome 19, and evidence is emerging for a late-onset Alzheimer's disease susceptibility gene located on chromosome 12 (Cedazo-Minguez and Cowburn 2001). The gene for beta-amyloid precursor protein is on the long arm of chromosome 21, and a gene carried on chromosome 17 is thought to be related to familial multiple system tauopathy, an early-onset dementia similar to DAT.

Wilson's disease is an autosomal recessively inherited defect in the copper-carrying serum protein ceruloplasmin, resulting in the destructive deposition of copper in the basal nuclei, the defective gene being localized on chromosome 13 (Loudianos and Gitlin 2000). Recent advances in the genetics of other dementias include the identification of *tau* gene mutations on chromosome 17 in some familial cases of frontotemporal dementia (H.J. Rosen et al. 2000) and the identification of genetic loci in other disorders that produce dementia, such as Pick's disease, cerebral autosomal dominant arteriopathy with subcortical infarcts and leukoencephalopathy, some forms of cerebral amyloid angiopathy, alcoholism, major depression, and some forms of Parkinson's disease (Lev and Melamed 2001).

Important changes in the classification of dementia might soon occur following dramatic advances in the genetics of dementia. Tau aggregates and alpha-synucleinopathy aggregates observed in neurodegenerative disorders have generated the concepts of tauopathies and alpha-synucleinopathies, respectively (Goedert 1998). Most cases of frontotemporal dementia tend now to be classified as tauopathies, related to mutations in the *tau* gene (Buee et al. 2000), with a large clinical spectrum including Pick's disease, progressive supranuclear palsy (PSP), corticobasal degeneration, and multisystem atrophy (Lebert et al. 2002). Alpha-synucleinopathies include dementia with Lewy bodies and Parkinson's disease (Ferrer and Puig 2003; Ferrer et al. 2002; Litvan 1999), but the findings of both types of pathological aggregates in several diseases have led to some disagreement in classifications (Iseki et al. 2003; Litvan 1999).

General Clinical Features

The Dementia Syndrome

The clinical picture may differ widely according to the type and severity of dementia, and the characteristics are important in the differential diagnosis. In most cases of degenerative processes—in particular DAT, some types of vascular dementia, and dementias due to endocrinopathies, brain tumors, metabolic disorders, and abuse of medications—the onset of symptoms is gradual, and the signs of the dementia syndrome are subtle and may at first be ignored by both the patient and his or her relatives. In contrast, the onset may be abrupt after severe cerebral infarcts, head trauma, cardiac arrest with cerebral hypoxia, and encephalitis.

The full dementia syndrome progresses through severity levels in degenerative processes and is very characteristic in DAT (Table 7–5). The earliest manifestations, such as impairment of memory, may be very subtle. Individuals with dementia also show impairment in thinking and their capacity for reasoning, but the earliest difficulties can be mistakenly disregarded or explained away as the expression of fatigue, distraction, or discouragement. The deficits may become apparent in the face of more complex problems, or when specifically tested, but patients often attempt to compensate for defects by using strategies to avoid showing failures in intellectual performance. Similarly, language is impoverished if carefully observed, and praxic difficulties for complex tasks may be documented, but special examinations may be necessary. The general loss of efficiency in all aspects of thinking, and disturbances in executive functions necessary to maintain goal-directed behavior, including planning, organizing, and sequencing, may be apparent, and the patient has difficulties in his or her usual occupation and with ADLs, such as using the telephone, managing small amounts of money, cooking, or taking responsibility for medications (Figure 7–1).

The dementia syndrome in degenerative disorders such as DAT relentlessly progresses to severe deteriora-tion (see Table 7–5). Eventually, the patient may retain only the earliest learned information; he or she is totally disoriented, with extreme impoverishment of thought, and communication with the patient is impossible. Apraxia and agnosia are severe. The patient is incontinent of urine and feces and is entirely dependent on caregivers. He or she may be totally disconnected from their environment, with respect to both input and output. The most severe neurological signs, including primitive reflexes, motor system rigidity, and flexion contractures, are then present, and the patient is confined to bed. The patient may experience a final stage of decortication, but death, from pneumonia or some other infection, commonly occurs before this stage.

Changes in personality and behavior are frequent, usually as a result of the disease. The patient may seem to be less concerned than he or she had been about issues of daily life or about the effects of his or her behavior on others. *Catastrophic reactions*, with agitation or extreme emotion, also may be observed, as a reaction to the subjective awareness of the patient's inability to cope with a problem. In the face of poor judgment, the patient is liable to misinterpret situations and may react inappropriately and emotionally.

Neuropsychiatric symptoms are almost universal in the course of dementia, are often quite disturbing for patients and caregivers, and may be quite persistent unless treated (Ballard et al. 2001a). Neuropsychiatric symptoms have been best studied in DAT (Lyketsos et al. 2001), but no important differences have been found in vascular dementia (Leroi et al. 2003). The modern classification of neuropsychiatric symptoms distinguishes delirium, affective syndrome, psychotic syndrome, drive disturbances (sleep and eating), and specific problem behaviors (usually in late stages). Major depressive episodes are frequent in DAT and other types of dementia (Zubenko et al. 2003) and often have serious adverse consequences for patients and their caregivers. The more severe signs and symptoms, including agitated and psychotic behavior, are more characteristic of advanced disease or of patients with frontal lobe involvement. Paranoid ideas are frequent, often representing "logical" conclusions based on misinterpretations, misperceptions, or memory deficits. They may not be persistent, but complex and well-systematized delusions, as well as hallucinations, are also reported (for all modalities).

The course of the syndrome is also variable according to type of dementia and has implications for the differential diagnosis. An incrementally worsening or stepwise course is common in vascular dementia, whereas the deficits may be stable in some types of dementia, such as in dementia related to head trauma (see also Chapter 35,

TABLE 7–5.   Clinical findings in patients with dementia of the Alzheimer's type, by severity level

Mild (MMSE score=18–23; duration of disease=1–3 years)
   Impaired registration and recent memory (early sign); remote recall mildly impaired
   Defective temporal orientation
   Mild impairment of thinking; bewilderment in the face of complexity
   Impoverishment of language; naming problems
   Mild apraxia for complex tasks
   Agnosia not evident unless tested
   Difficulties in planning, sequencing, and executing instrumental activities of daily living
   Frequent personality changes: irritability, less apparent concern about issues of daily life and effects of their behavior on
      others
   Depression in approximately 20% of patients; mild apathy; loss of initiative; lack of energy
   Frequent misinterpretations; psychotic phenomena rare
   Urinary incontinence in fewer than 10%
   Other neurological signs and primitive reflexes rare

Moderate (MMSE score=12–17; duration of disease=2–8 years)
   Recent memory and remote recall more severely impaired
   Severe temporal disorientation, moderate spatial disorientation
   Obvious impairment of thinking; catastrophic reactions if pressured
   Fluent aphasia, anomia, paraphasic errors, empty quality of language, perseveration
   Praxic difficulties to manage dressing, feeding, manipulations
   Agnosia evident: failure to identify objects, including familiar faces
   Difficulties in planning, sequencing, and executing extend to basic activities of daily living
   Evident personality changes: marked irritability, marked lack of concern about issues of daily life and effects of their behavior on
      others
   Dysphoric mood, depression less frequent; apathy; loss of initiative
   Frequent psychotic phenomena (delusions, illusions, hallucinations)
   Restlessness, pacing, wandering occasionally, agitation, sporadic aggressiveness
   Urinary incontinence frequent; fecal incontinence rare
   Gait disorder and frequent primitive reflexes

Severe (MMSE score<12; duration of disease=7–12 years)
   Memory: only earliest learned information retained
   Total disorientation
   Severe impairment of thinking; indifference in the face of failures
   Extreme impoverishment of language; communication impossible
   Complete incapacity to manage dressing, feeding, simple manipulations
   Severe agnosia: does not identify close relatives
   Total dependence for even basic activities of daily living
   Total disconnection from environment
   Affective indifference; severe apathy; loss of initiative
   Double incontinence (urinary and fecal)
   Motor system rigidity and flexion contractures of all limbs; final stage of decortication

Note.   MMSE=Mini-Mental State Examination.

"Physical Medicine and Rehabilitation"). Furthermore, the regression of symptoms is a possibility, once treatment is initiated, in dementias caused by potentially reversible disorders, such as normal-pressure hydrocephalus (NPH); metabolic and toxic conditions; or dementias related to the use of medications, to subdural hematoma, or to brain tumors. These conditions have been called *reversible dementias* and were once considered to be rather frequent (Rabins 1983). In fact, recent studies have found that only 4%–23% of the patients referred to memory clinics had potentially reversible conditions (Freter et al. 1998; Hejl et al. 2002; Norup et al. 2002), and actual reversal of dementia through treatment is rare (Freter et al. 1998; Ovsiew 2003).

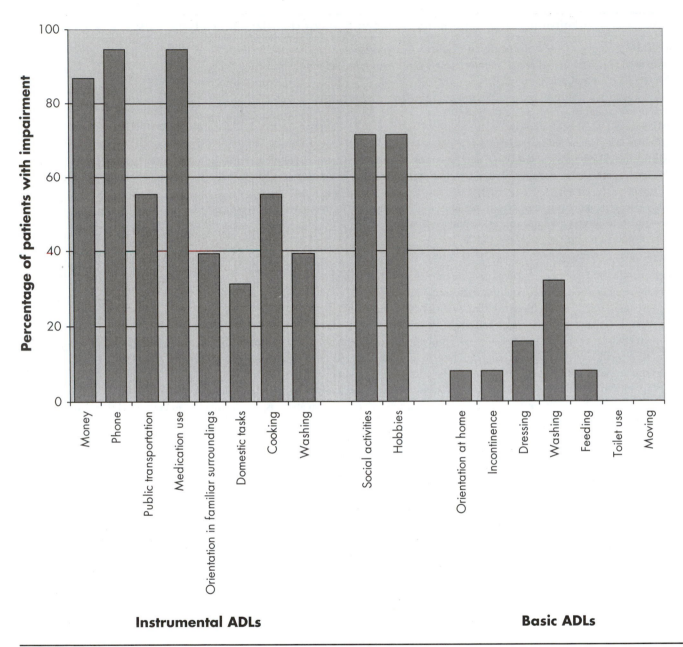

FIGURE 7–1. **Impairment in instrumental[a] and basic[b] activities of daily living (ADLs) in patients with dementia of the Alzheimer's type of mild severity (Mini-Mental State Examination score >18) at time of diagnosis.**

Note. Patients were new referrals to a memory clinic in a psychosomatics/consultation-liaison psychiatry service.

[a]Instrumental items in modified Lawton and Brody Scale.

[b]Basic items in Katz Index.

Source. Adapted from Lobo and Saz (in press).

Clinicopathological Correlations

Some clinical characteristics suggest the involvement of specific brain areas and should help in clinical recognition of entities with different implications, as well as in understanding the underlying pathology of cognitive and noncognitive phenomena (McHugh and Folstein 1979). *Cor-*

tical dementia is the conceptual term for those dementias in which the predominance of dysfunction is in the cortex, even if coexisting pathology exists in subcortical regions (Cummings and Benson 1984). Together with amnesia, not helped by cues to remember, the most characteristic signs are aphasia, apraxia, and agnosia, which are often designated as the *A's* (Table 7–6).

TABLE 7–6.   Clinical characteristics of cortical and subcortical dementia syndromes

	Cortical	Subcortical
Aphasia	Early	No
Agnosia	Late	No
Apraxia	Rather early	Rare
Alexia	Rather late	No
Apathy, inertia	Rare or late	Very marked, early
Loss of initiative	Frequent, late	Marked
Psychomotor retardation	Rare or late	Very marked, early
Amnesia	Recall and recognition not aided by cues to remember	Recognition better preserved, may be aided by cues to remember
Gait	Normal until late	Abnormal, early
Extrapyramidal signs	Rare or late	Very marked, early
Pathological reflexes (grasp, snout, suck, etc.)	Late	Rare
Affective syndromes	Less frequent	Frequent, severe

Subcortical dementia describes the predominant involvement of the white and deep gray matter structures, such as basal ganglia, thalamus, and their frontal lobe projections. McHugh and Folstein (1975) were among the first to emphasize that parts of the brain other than the cortex have a role in cognitive activity and described the distinctive combination of three features in what they called the "subcortical dementia syndrome": a slowly progressive dilapidation of all cognitive powers; prominent psychic apathy and inertia that may worsen to akinetic mutism; and the absence of aphasia, alexia, or agnosia (see Table 7–6). The same authors also emphasized the early appearance in subcortical dementia of prominent noncognitive symptoms, particularly depression and other affective disturbances considered to be a direct consequence of the cerebral pathology. Patients with subcortical dementia commonly present with psychomotor retardation; loss of initiative; and a general loss of vitality, physical energy, and emotional drive (Mandell and Albert 1990). Rabins et al. (1999) have designated some specific features of subcortical dementia as the four *D's*:

Dysmnesia—patients may benefit from cues to remember

Dysexecutive—related to troubles with decision making

Delay—related to slowed thinking and moving

Depletion—patients have reduced complexity of thought

Finally, the term *mixed dementia* describes the involvement of both cortical and subcortical regions. The clinical characteristics include aspects of cortical dementia, such as aphasia and apraxia, and the apathetic state produced by, and characteristic of, lesions in the subcortical areas.

Clinical Types and Pathophysiology of Dementia

Cortical Dementias

Alzheimer's Disease

Most cases of Alzheimer's disease start after age 65, but an earlier onset is not infrequent. Although some authors consider "presenile" and "senile" clinical forms to be different diseases (Jacobs et al. 1994), most consider them the same disorder with varied age at onset. The characteristic general dementia syndrome has been described and includes the cortical signs (see Tables 7–5 and 7–6). The insidious onset and slowly worsening, relentless course are most characteristic and crucial in the diagnostic process. The early clinical phase (see Table 7–5) is now distinguished from a preclinical phase, with mild cognitive impairment being apparent only on testing, preservation of instrumental ADLs, and specific neuroimaging findings. Other characteristic clinical signs and symptoms are also summarized in Table 7–5. They include 1) a "hippocampal type" of memory difficulty, which is not reliably aided by cues on memory testing and has a high number of intrusions and false recognitions (Petersen et al. 1994); 2) language difficulties, including a fluent aphasia with anomia, paraphasic errors, and a tendency of the patient to perseverate (Cummings and Benson 1986); 3) the patient's being able in many cases to retain the ability to recognize objects and to use them appropriately at a time when he or she can no longer name them accurately (Rapcsak et al. 1989); and 4) agnosia for faces, including family faces in late stages of the disease. Gait disorder in the middle stages is also common, as well as frontal signs such as grasping and sucking reflexes, along with a change in muscular tone.

The neuropathology of this condition is its defining characteristic (M.F. Folstein and McHugh 1983); its extent and severity correlate with the type and severity of the cognitive signs and symptoms (Blessed et al. 1968). Cortical atrophy occurs, with widened sulci and ventricular enlargement. The most severe changes occur in the medial temporal lobe, including the hippocampus. Areas of association cortex in the parietotemporal lobes and, to a lesser degree, the frontal lobes are also involved (Pearlson and Powell 1989). Characteristic microscopic findings are neuronal loss; synaptic loss, particularly in the cortex; senile plaques, with a core of amyloid peptide; neurofibrillary tangles, containing abnormally phosphorylated tau proteins; granulovacuolar degeneration of the neurons; and amyloid angiopathy. The location and abundance of microscopic findings determine the postmortem histological diagnosis of Alzheimer's disease (Cummings et al. 1998; Khachaturian 1985).

Several studies have supported the cholinergic deficit hypothesis in DAT, including specific degeneration of cholinergic neurons in the nucleus basalis of Meynert; decreases in acetylcholine and choline acetyltransferase concentrations in the brain; and observations about the role of cholinergic agonists and antagonists. Other hypotheses are suggested by the decrease in norepinephrine activity and, more recently, by reports of decreased levels of many neurotransmitters, including serotonin and the neuroactive peptides somatostatin and corticotropin. Evidence also indicates that the excitatory activity of L-glutamate plays a role in the pathogenesis of DAT (Greenamyre et al. 1988). However, recent research suggests that vascular factors may play an important role in determining the presence and severity of the clinical symptoms of DAT (de la Torre 2002; Mori 2002; O'Brien et al. 2003; Snowdon et al. 1997).

Dementia With Lewy Bodies

Dementia with Lewy bodies is a condition of uncertain nosological status, with cortical signs suggesting DAT alongside the classic, extrapyramidal features of Parkinson's disease (Lishman 1998a; McKeith et al. 1996). However, the typical neuropathological findings of DAT are much less common in this condition. The distinctive feature is the presence of Lewy bodies in the cortex, particularly in limbic areas, whereas in Parkinson's disease they are typically found in subcortical regions (Lishman 1998a). Some authors now include both dementia with Lewy bodies and Parkinson's disease among the alpha-synucleinopathies on the basis of recent pathological findings (Ferrer and Puig 2003; Ferrer et al. 2002; Litvan 1999). Mean age at disease onset varies between 60 and 80 years. Psychotic, hallucinatory syndromes and confusional states are common and may be the presenting symptomatology. Other characteristics include relative preponderance of visuospatial and frontal lobe signs, clear day-to-day fluctuations in symptoms and cognitive performance, and episodes resembling acute confusional states with visual and auditory hallucinations and paranoid delusions. Depressive symptoms also occur frequently. Patients who have dementia with Lewy bodies have frequent falls and/or transient, unexplained episodes of loss of consciousness. They have a characteristic vulnerability to neuroleptics, which frequently exacerbate extrapyramidal dysfunction. Such reactions may be severe and may include acute episodes of rigidity, instability, and falls.

Frontotemporal Dementia

Frontotemporal dementia syndromes, often accompanied by cortical signs, are also the result of neurodegenerative diseases. The most characteristic features that distinguish frontotemporal dementia from DAT are personality changes and neuropsychiatric symptoms, which may be quite marked and precede the cognitive decline by several years (Neary et al. 1998). The psychiatric symptoms in frontotemporal dementia include marked irritability; poor judgment; defective control of impulses, including violent impulses in some cases; disinhibition; and a general disregard for the conventional rules of social conduct. Restlessness and hyperorality also have been reported. Social withdrawal or overt depression may be the first symptom in some patients.

Neuronal loss and gliosis in the frontotemporal areas define this type of neurodegenerative dementia. Pick's disease, characterized by the presence of distinctive intraneuronal Pick bodies and ballooned Pick cells on microscopic examination, may be diagnosed in up to 25% of cases. This disease and the remaining types of frontotemporal dementias tend now to be classified as tauopathies, with a large clinical spectrum including Pick's disease, PSP, corticobasal degeneration, and multisystem atrophy (Lebert et al. 2002). PSP is often classified among subcortical dementias because of the predominance of subcortical signs. Primary progressive aphasia is an atypical dementia typified by insidious and progressive impairment in language, with relative preservation of memory and other cortical functions, once thought to be rare but now recognized as not uncommon (Mesulam 2003).

Subcortical Dementias

Huntington's Disease

Huntington's disease has the three main characteristics of the subcortical dementia syndrome (M.F. Folstein and McHugh 1983), together with the classic choreoathetoid movement disorder and a positive family history. Huntington's disease usually has its onset in the third or fourth decade, although juvenile forms occasionally occur. The psychopathology, both cognitive and noncognitive, may appear before the movement abnormalities (McHugh and Folstein 1975). Both cognitive difficulties and mental apathy may be subtle initially. Once they appear, they tend to steadily progress to the point of very severe cognitive loss and profound self-neglect, resembling an akinetic mute state. Several authors also have reported prominent symptoms that may be difficult to differentiate from primary affective disorder, particularly depression (S.E. Folstein et al. 1979; Lieberman et al. 1979). However, demoralization and depressive reactions are also frequent, and the risk of suicide is increased (Huntington 1872; Reed and Chandler 1958). Suspiciousness and misinterpretations are quite common, but delusions and hallucinations with paranoid and catatonic features also have been described (Dewhurst et al. 1969). Huntington's disease also may include Schneiderian first-rank symptoms, making it difficult to differentiate from schizophrenia (McHugh and Folstein 1975).

The neuropathology in Huntington's disease includes atrophy of the caudate nucleus and loss of gamma-aminobutyric acid (GABA) interneurons (Lishman 1998b). The clinical findings are considered to be caused by imbalance of subcortical cholinergic and dopaminergic systems (T.L. Perry et al. 1973).

Parkinson's Disease

A subcortical, progressive dementia syndrome may occur in approximately one-third of patients with Parkinson's disease (Breteler et al. 1995), but contrary to Huntington's disease, it tends to occur late in the course of the illness, after the motor symptoms have advanced significantly. The classic Parkinson's disease neurological signs in a patient with dementia point to the diagnosis. Apathy is particularly prominent and may advance to an akinetic mute state. Individual parkinsonian patients endure a wide variety of psychopathological symptoms, including frequent emotional reactions to the disease, but a depressive disorder identical to that seen in affective illness and responsive to the usual treatments is found in approximately one-third of patients (Faber and Trimble 1991; Loranger et al. 1972).

Nigral pathology alone is probably not sufficient for the development of dementia in Parkinson's disease and requires the spread of pathology to other subcortical nuclei, the limbic system, and the cerebral cortex. The main degenerative pathology seems to be Lewy body type, principally made of alpha-synuclein (Duyckaerts et al.

2003), and some controversy exists with regard to the frequency and implications of DAT-type pathology found in cases of dementia in Parkinson's disease (Apaydin et al. 2002; Emre 2003). Losses of cholinergic, dopaminergic, and noradrenergic innervation have been suggested to be the underlying neurochemical deficits.

Wilson's Disease

Subcortical dementia with characteristic extrapyramidal signs also may be seen in Wilson's disease (Starosta-Rubinstein et al. 1987). This combination of symptoms, together with onset during adolescence or early adulthood, should suggest the diagnosis. Cognitive deficits are usually mild, and psychosis is infrequent. However, depressive syndromes, irritability, disinhibition, personality changes, and poor impulse control are common, with the severity paralleling the severity of the neurological signs (Dening and Berrios 1989). The psychopathological features result from destructive deposition of copper in the basal nuclei (Starosta-Rubinstein 1995) due to an inherited defect in the copper-carrying serum protein ceruloplasmin (Akil and Brewer 1995).

Normal-Pressure Hydrocephalus

NPH can present as a very characteristic neuropsychiatric syndrome, a triad of clinical symptoms combining motoric and psychopathological features (M.F. Folstein and McHugh 1983; McHugh 1964, 1966): 1) an early gait disturbance, resembling the stiff steps of spastic paraparesis; 2) subcortical dementia with particularly severe apathetic features; and 3) urinary incontinence that may not appear until late in the course. An insidious onset with cognitive difficulties is common. Outbursts of hostile behavior occur sometimes (Sandyk 1984), and eventually the illness may progress to a state resembling akinetic mutism if untreated. The neuropsychiatric deficits are considered to be the result of tissue destruction by stretching as a result of the chronic hydrocephalus (McHugh and Folstein 1979).

Mixed Dementia and Dementia in Disseminated Brain Diseases

Vascular Dementia

Vascular dementia is defined as the dementia resulting from ischemic, ischemic-hypoxic, or hemorrhagic brain lesions due to cerebrovascular or cardiovascular pathology (Roman 2002). Clinical findings in vascular dementia are heterogeneous and depend to a great extent on the speed, total volume, and localization of the lesions. Typically, the onset is in later life, and the dementia syndrome is the result of small brain infarcts, which lead to cognitive deterioration when they have enough cumulative effects on critical areas of the brain. However, cognitive impairment and probably dementia also can be seen in chronic ischemia without frank infarction (Chui et al. 1992). Acute onset usually develops after stroke, either from thrombosis, from an embolism, or rarely from a single massive hemorrhage. Onset and course of dementia are often more gradual in so-called *multi-infarct dementia*, as a consequence of many minor ischemic episodes, which produce an accumulation of lacunae in the cerebral parenchyma.

Cortical dementia occurs when the infarcts affect primarily the cortex, with focal neurological signs being the norm. Subcortical dementia is typically seen in patients with a history of hypertension and foci of ischemic destruction in the deep white matter of the cerebral hemispheres. A variant of vascular dementia is *Binswanger's disease*, or *subcortical arteriosclerotic encephalopathy*, which is associated with pseudobulbar palsy, spasticity, and weakness (D.A. Bennett et al. 1990). In such cases, extensive, diffuse demyelination of white matter can be seen in periventricular regions, and recent neuroimaging techniques have shown that the condition is more frequent than previously suspected. Mixed cortical and subcortical syndromes are also common in vascular dementia, with neuroimaging findings or autopsy findings suggesting the presence of lesions in both cerebral areas. Mild cognitive impairment of the vascular type also has been described, with an outcome worse than in nonvascular mild cognitive impairment (Frisoni et al. 2002).

The course of vascular dementia has classically been described as stepwise and patchy, but advances in brain imaging techniques have shown that patients with vascular dementia may have clinical courses as gradual and smooth as in patients with DAT. Poststroke depression, independent of the disability caused by the disease, is frequent (M.F. Folstein et al. 1977; Robinson 1997). Emotional lability, with transient depressive mood, weeping, or explosive laughter, is also a classic finding in these patients. Personality is usually relatively preserved, but in a proportion of patients, personality changes may be evident, with apathy or disinhibition or the accentuation of previous traits such as egocentricity, paranoid attitude, or irritability.

Most studies have supported the view that the total volume of infarcted brain and the total number of infarctions with additive or multiplicative effects correlate well with the severity of dementia. However, the location of the infarctions also may be important (Liu et al. 1992). In more than two-thirds of vascular dementia patients, the pathological correlate is the lacunar state, characterized by multiple lacunar infarctions in subcortical structures such as the basal ganglia and thalamus. Other pathological findings include watershed infarctions due to reduction in brain perfusion, multiple embolic infarcts, diffuse demyelination of white matter in Binswanger's disease, and a mixture of lesions. The term *vascular cognitive impairment* has been proposed to broaden the current definitions of vascular dementia to recognize the important part cerebrovascular disease plays in several cognitive disorders, including DAT and other degenerative dementias (O'Brien et al. 2003). It is now estimated that the prevalence of mixed cases of vascular dementia and DAT has been underestimated; that pure vascular dementia is rare; and that, in addition to simple coexistence, vascular dementia and DAT may share common pathogenetic mechanisms (Erkinjuntti 2002).

Infection-Associated Dementias

HIV-associated dementia, formerly called *AIDS dementia complex*, is now the most common dementia caused by an infectious disease (see also Chapter 27, "Infectious Diseases," and Chapter 28, "HIV/AIDS"). Cognitive deterioration is frequently observed in infection with HIV-1 and may be severe enough to fulfill criteria for dementia (World Health Organization 1990). Cognitive dysfunction may be the earliest or the only clinical manifestation of AIDS. The heterogeneity of psychopathological manifestations and the occurrence of both cortical and subcortical features suggest disseminated brain pathology in this condition (Van Gorp et al. 1993). Noncognitive psychopathology—in particular depressive syndromes associated with the subcortical cognitive psychopathology (Van Gorp et al. 1993)—is also common in patients infected with HIV-1 (S. Perry and Jacobsen 1986).

Creutzfeldt-Jakob disease is a dementia with an extremely rapid course, caused by a transmissible infectious agent, the *prion* (Prusiner 2001). Cognitive deterioration is progressive, widespread, very severe, and accompanied by pyramidal and extrapyramidal signs, early characteristic myoclonic jerks, muscle rigidity, and ataxia. Death usually occurs in 6–12 months (Will et al. 1996). Pathological findings are widespread in both the cortex and the subcortical structures (Budka et al. 1995). Spongiform change in neurons is characteristic, and neuronal loss and astrocytic proliferation occur.

Neurosyphilis may evolve into different types of dementia if left untreated (Dewhurst 1969). The most severe form is general paresis, which becomes evident 15–20 years after the original infection. The dementia may be easily recognized in the advanced state and is accompanied by characteristic signs, such as pupillary abnormalities, dysarthria, tremor of the tongue, and hypotonia. However, the onset is commonly insidious, and the diagnosis may be suggested when the initial memory difficulties are accompanied by indifference, facial quivering, tremor, and, sometimes, myoclonus. Intellectual deterioration is progressive and severe, with cortical deficits and often signs suggesting frontal lobe involvement, including disinhibited behavior. Psychotic phenomena, such as grandiose or hypochondriacal delusions, are common (Dewhurst 1969).

Chronic meningitis, caused by chronic bacterial, parasitic, or fungal infections, can eventually cause progressive dementia, with fluctuations in arousal and cognitive performance, apathy and lethargy, disorientation, and cranial nerve abnormalities.

Immunosuppressed or debilitated, chronically ill patients are at special risk. *Herpes simplex encephalitis* may cause major neurological and cognitive sequelae. Because herpes encephalitis has a predilection for the temporal lobes, amnestic and aphasic syndromes are common, but dementia also can be seen (Hierons et al. 1978). Other cortical signs reflect damage to other cortical areas (Skoldenberg 1991).

Progressive multifocal leukoencephalopathy (PML) is a rare complication of a common subacute viral disorder, most commonly seen in immunosuppressed patients (von Einsiedel et al. 1993). Clinical signs and symptoms are quite heterogeneous, and the dementia may include both cortical and subcortical signs and symptoms, reflecting widespread lesions in the central nervous system. PML is usually progressive, with motor dysfunction and blindness sometimes developing; death commonly follows in a few months.

Metabolic and Toxic Dementias

Metabolic and toxic dementias (see also Chapter 23, "Endocrine and Metabolic Disorders") form a heterogeneous group of diseases (see Table 7–3) of special interest to the consultant psychiatrist because they are relatively frequent in medical settings and are potentially reversible. Dementia in these conditions has predominantly subcortical features but may have mixed characteristics. Psychomotor slowing may be severe in cases of hypothyroidism. Memory deficits are often accompanied by problems in executive function, with impaired attention and concentration also common. Whether the metabolic and toxic encephalopathies are best conceptualized as reversible dementias or as chronic deliria is unclear, and perhaps the distinction is primarily semantic, particularly in cases of hepatic, renal, and cardiopulmonary failure. Progression of the dementia is usually quite insidious, in relation to the chronicity of the metabolic or toxic condition, and the course tends to be disease-specific.

The neuropathology in these conditions is not well known. Hippocampal neurons are probably most vulnerable to anoxic injury (Zola-Morgan et al. 1986) but are also vulnerable to severe hypercholesterolemia and to repeated or severe episodes of hypoglycemia, such as may occur in type 1 diabetes mellitus (Sachon et al. 1992). Hypothyroidism can produce subcortical damage through a mechanism of relative cerebral hypoxia (Mintzer 1992). Vitamin B_{12} deficiency, as seen in pernicious anemia, has been associated with disseminated degeneration in areas of cortical white matter, the optic tracts, and the cerebellar peduncles (Martin et al. 1992). In pellagra, lack of nicotinic acid and probably other vitamin B deficiencies may lead to neuronal destruction.

Alcoholic dementia, one possible complication of chronic alcoholism, is more frequent after age 50 years and is likely multifactorial in etiology. Thiamine and other vitamin B deficiencies and multiple TBIs have been found in these patients. Pathological findings at autopsy suggest that this condition is probably underdiagnosed. The cognitive deficits are more global here than in pure amnestic syndrome (e.g., Korsakoff's psychosis), and unlike those patients, alcoholic patients with dementia may complain of decreased efficiency of memory and intellectual functioning. Deterioration of visuoperceptual and executive functions is commonly found. Neuropathological changes include cortical atrophy and nerve fiber disintegration with dissolution of myelin sheaths (Kril and Harper 1989). Dementing syndromes are also seen in distinct brain diseases related to chronic alcoholism, such as Marchiafava-Bignami disease, with degeneration of the corpus callosum and anterior commissure, or in acquired hepatocerebral degeneration.

Dementing syndromes also may occur in *chronic intoxication with medications*, which can be either prescribed or abused by patients. The onset is insidious, and the course is progressive; physicians should be alert to the possibility of this reversible dementia. Benzodiazepines, including those with high potency and a short half-life, are known to cause anterograde amnesia and impairment of memory consolidation and subsequent memory retrieval (Scharf et al. 1987). Elderly patients are more vulnerable to developing the dementia syndrome. Syndromes of cognitive deterioration have been reported in cocaine users and also in heavy users of cannabis (Deahl 1991).

Neoplastic-Associated Dementias

Neoplastic disease may affect any part of the brain and produce essentially any kind of neuropsychiatric symptoms, depending on tumor location and extent, as well as rapidity of tumor growth and propensity to cause increased intracranial pressure (see also Chapter 24, "Oncology," and Chapter 32, "Neurology and Neurosurgery"). Dementia is one such syndrome, and certain symptom clusters that occur with regularity may suggest the general location of lesions (M.F. Folstein and McHugh 1983; Hecaen and De Ajuriagueria 1956). Such clusters may be apparent before motor symptoms or a full dementia syndrome is suspected.

Initial symptoms of depression and some cognitive loss, with apathy, negativism, and akinesia, suggest the possibility of frontal lobe tumors such as meningioma or some forms of glioblastoma; a low performance on executive function tests further supports a frontal lobe site. Temporal lobe tumors are prone to produce seizures, and the psychiatric symptomatology may be complex and include features such as sexual disturbances, irritability, aggressiveness, and hallucinations. Tumors in the parietal region often cause characteristic language disorders when the location is in the dominant hemisphere. In the nondominant hemisphere, they tend to produce signs such as unilateral neglect or apraxia. Tumors around the third ventricle, such as craniopharyngiomas and colloid cysts, may obstruct the flow of spinal fluid and cause hydrocephalic, subcortical dementia.

Dementia is one of the *paraneoplastic syndromes* that affect the brain. *Limbic encephalopathy* is a nonmetastatic complication of small cell lung carcinoma (and less commonly some other cancers) and may manifest with dramatic, sudden onset of memory loss (Corsellis et al. 1968). A full dementia syndrome may eventually develop (Bakheit et al. 1990). Mood disturbance, behavior change, and sometimes psychotic symptoms are also common. Pathological findings include neuronal loss, astrocytosis, lymphocytic perivascular infiltration, and glial nodules. The psychiatric symptoms may antedate the diagnosis of malignancy by several years. Early medical intervention might considerably improve the outcome of treatment in some cases (Burton et al. 1988).

Dementia Following Traumatic Brain Injury

A variety of cognitive difficulties are very frequent after TBI (see also Chapter 35, "Physical Medicine and Rehabilitation"). Posttraumatic amnesia is the norm in cases of severe trauma with loss of consciousness. Cognitive deficits become permanent in more than half of the patients if they do not recover memory and orientation within 2 weeks after injury (Levin 1989). Common difficulties include dysmnesia, organic personality disorder, dysphasia, attentional disturbances, and impairments suggestive

of frontal lobe damage (Stuss et al. 1989). Dementia also occurs and may be accompanied by seizures and neurological deficits, as well as secondary psychiatric syndromes, including depression, mania, and psychosis (McAllister 1992). Dementia in boxers (*dementia pugilistica*) commonly starts with signs of ataxia, dysarthria, and Parkinson-like extrapyramidal signs before the global cognitive deficits are appreciated. Dementia due to subdural hematoma is notable because it is potentially reversible. In cases of dementia following TBI, diffuse axonal injury, with anatomic disruption and axonal tearing, has been described (Graham et al. 1987), and contusional foci in cortical areas and intracerebral hemorrhage also have been reported.

Depression

The relation between dementia and depression is complex (Mahendra 1985). *Pseudodementia* is a term used to describe the condition of depressed patients who perform poorly on cognitive tasks because of lack of interest and motivation. However, *dementia syndromes of depression* (DSD) occur during episodes of severe mood disorder (M.F. Folstein and McHugh 1978). DSD are probably associated with potentially reversible neurotransmitter dysfunction. They are more frequent in elderly patients with a history of depression, and the presenting depressive syndrome often includes severe psychomotor retardation and other melancholic symptoms (Emery and Oxman 1992), as well as psychotic features such as delusions. Cortical signs such as language disturbances are uncommon, and in DSD, in contrast to DAT, prompting and organization of material tend to improve memory performance (O'Brien et al. 2001). DSD may be potentially reversible and tends to disappear with successful treatment of depression (Rabins et al. 1984). However, cognitive monitoring and follow-up are recommended because a persistent dementia syndrome may develop in a significant proportion of cases (Alexopoulos et al. 1993; Chen et al. 1999). The concept that cognitive dysfunction in elderly depressed patients should be considered a pseudodementia has been undermined by more recent studies reporting that cognitive dysfunction often persists after treatment of depression, suggesting either that the patient had both diagnoses (depression and dementia) or that "treatable" depression was a secondary manifestation of dementia. Furthermore, depressive symptoms in the elderly and a history of late-onset depression have been associated with the severity of subcortical white matter lesions, suggesting an etiological role for vascular disease (de Groot et al. 2000).

Diagnosis and Differential Diagnosis

Early detection of dementia can play an important role in both the social and the health care dimensions of the disease (Organization for Economic Cooperation and Development, in press). A brief interview can detect dementia with reasonable accuracy (Boustani et al. 2003) and can be taught to nonpsychiatrists. However, a systematic search for dementia should follow general screening principles and should be linked ideally to a system prepared to care for all identified patients (Wilson and Junger 1968). Dementia should be suspected in patients at risk referred to psychiatrists, particularly elderly medical patients with delirium or unexpected behavioral disturbances and patients referred by primary care physicians because of subjective complaints or observations of relatives about memory problems or loss of intellectual efficiency. In both cases, the clinical approach to diagnosis follows a classic sequence: first, to identify characteristic signs and symptoms of cognitive impairment; second, to document whether the signs and symptoms cluster in the defined syndrome and to complete a differential diagnosis by discarding false positive cases; and finally, to search for the etiological type of dementia. A search for associated medical conditions, neuropsychiatric symptoms, and special social needs completes the evaluation process.

Clinical History

A clinical history corroborated through reliable caregivers and a systematic mental status examination lay the foundation of the diagnostic process. Among different medical specialists involved in the field of dementia, psychiatrists have special advantages because of their expertise in assessing psychopathology, as well as the social consequences of the disease included in the diagnostic criteria (see Table 7–2), including DSM-IV-TR criteria (American Psychiatric Association 2000). In taking the history, it is important to search for specific evidence of deterioration in memory and other cognitive functions summarized in the general dementia syndrome (see Table 7–5). Specific, convincing examples should be required as support for the diagnosis of dementia. Furthermore, the consultant must assess the presence, extent, and consequences of the cognitive problems in occupational activities and ADLs (see Figure 7–1). An outside informant is crucial for obtaining data about decline in cognitive function measured against premorbid abilities. The Informant Questionnaire on Cognitive Decline in the Elderly (IQ-CODE) (Jorm and Jacomb 1989)—and in particular the short form (Jorm 1994)—is suggested as a useful, simple questionnaire that has good reliability and validity. The dementia questionnaire for DAT is another useful instrument for the same purpose and is also valid in telephone interviews with informants (Ellis et al. 1998). The onset and pattern of progression of the cognitive difficulties also should be carefully documented. Insidious diseases such as DAT can easily go undetected for years before becoming apparent (Larson et al. 1992). Finally, it is also important to determine whether changes in personality and behavior have accompanied the cognitive difficulties and whether psychopathological signs and symptoms, including apathy and loss of initiative, are present.

Mental Status Examination

A systematic, basic bedside or office mental status examination is a minimum requirement in each case of suspected dementia. The cognitive assessment is relatively easy to complete and should include all relevant domains. Table 1–4 in Chapter 1, "Psychiatric Assessment and Consultation," summarizes the cognitive areas to cover in the assessment and includes specific questions and items that may be used. Figure 7–2 shows the performance on some construction tasks by patients with dementia. It is strongly recommended that the clinician be familiar with a standard assessment method, ideally one supported by efficiency data. Although no standardized instrument is a substitute for sound clinical assessment, some are quite helpful, provided their limitations are kept in mind.

The Mini-Mental State Examination (MMSE) is one such instrument (sensitivity ≥87%; positive predictive value ≥79% in clinical populations) (M.F. Folstein et al. 1975, 2001) and is widely considered to be the standard measure in most clinical and research studies (Gray and Cummings 2002). It fares very well in different cultures, if the standardization has been adequate (Lobo et al. 1999). Data on the efficiency of individual items in the MMSE, remarkable in items such as temporal orientation, may help the consultant in interpreting the results of the test (Table 7–7). The limits of the MMSE relate to both floor and ceiling effects, and population norms have to be considered in adjusting the usual cutoff point (23 of 24) (Crum et al. 1993; Lobo et al. 1999; Tombaugh and McIntyre 1992) to avoid false-positive cases in individuals with limited educational background or, conversely, false-negative cases in highly educated, intelligent patients. The Modified Mini-Mental State (3MS) (Teng and Chui 1987), with minor changes introduced to circumvent these difficulties, works well in clinical practice (McDowell et al. 1997). Executive functions, which are not well covered in the MMSE, may be easily assessed at bedside with the Frontal Assessment Battery (FAB) (Dubois et al.

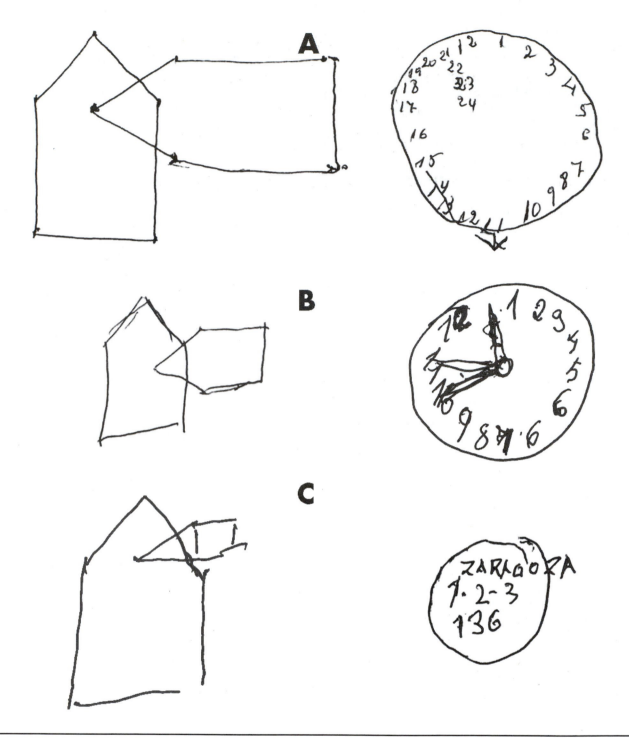

FIGURE 7–2. Performance in construction tasks (commands to draw interlocked pentagons and a clock) by patients with increasing severity levels of dementia.

Impairment in performance appears earlier in clock drawing than in pentagon construction and increases with severity level of dementia. **Clock A** (Mini-Mental State Examination [MMSE] score=18) shows executive deficits in planning and organization; construction deficits to place the numbers; probable perseveration (24 hours); and deficits in judgment to correct errors and to place the hands indicating the time (11:10). **Pentagon A** shows nominal construction deficit. **Clock B** (MMSE score=15) shows subtle construction deficits (mild deviation of numbers, but spacing is correct); executive deficits in planning and judgment to indicate the time; and unsuccessful executive attempts to correct errors (in placing number 6; in placing the hands). **Pentagon B** shows mild construction deficit. **Clock C** (MMSE score=14) shows deficits both in remembering and in understanding the command and probable "stimulus dependence syndrome" (the pen in the patient's hand acts as a stimulus and writes inappropriately inside the circle). **Pentagon C** shows construction and visuomotor coordination deficits.

TABLE 7–7. Validity of individual items of MMSE (administered by lay interviewers)[a]

MMSE items	Cutoff score	Sensitivity (%)	Specificity (%)	PPV (%)[b]	NPV (%)[b]	Misclassifications (%)	AUC
Temporal orientation	3/4	81.3	91.5	93.9	96.3	10.1	0.914
Spatial orientation	4/5	70.8	86.4	45.3	92.5	17.4	0.805
Immediate memory	2/3	14.6	97.7	53.8	86.1	15.2	0.565
Calculation	3/4	78.0	71.4	31.4	95.1	27.6	0.794
Delayed memory	1/2	91.7	49.6	25.4	96.9	43.7	0.774
Nomination	1/2	12.2	98.8	66.7	85.3	15.6	0.555
Articulation	0/1	12.8	94.9	31.6	85.5	17.9	0.540
Verbal commands	2/3	41.7	79.5	27.8	87.8	26.5	0.618
Written commands	0/1	29.0	95.1	45.0	90.8	12.8	0.620
Writing	0/1	60.0	58.6	17.1	91.1	41.2	0.595
Pentagon drawing	0/1	91.9	54.4	24.6	97.6	40.4	0.730

Note. AUC=area under receiver operating characteristics curve; MMSE=Mini-Mental State Examination; NPV=negative predictive value; PPV=positive predictive value.

[a]Gold standard=dementia (diagnosis by psychiatrist, DSM-III-R criteria [American Psychiatric Association 1987], 2-month interval); Lobo et al. (1999).

[b]Predictive values for a prevalence of dementia of 5.5%.

2000). The Mini-Cog, which consists of just the three-item recall from the MMSE and the clock drawing test, may perform as well as other longer measures and thus appeal to primary care physicians as an initial screen (Borson et al. 2000).

Neurological Examination

The neurological examination is also an integral part of, and informs, the diagnosis and differential diagnosis. The examination should be standard but may be focused on the assessment of neurological signs described in the clinical section, including specific gait difficulties, praxias, and pathological reflexes. Other testing should be included if warranted by clinical information.

Differential Diagnosis

Differential diagnosis starts by ruling out false-positive cases of dementia—namely, previous *mental retardation; amnestic syndromes* (such as in Korsakoff's psychosis), without the global deficits required for the diagnosis of dementia; cognitive difficulties due to *general physical frailty,* particularly in elderly patients; and *age-related memory impairment* (or benign senescent forgetfulness), characterized by a minor degree of memory problems observed as a normal part of aging and not significantly interfering with a person's social or occupational behavior. *Pseudodementia syndromes* may be the result of motivational or emotional factors interfering with performance. They include *acute psychotic episodes, conversion disorder, factitious*

disorder, and *malingering,* suggested by reports of relatives, examination, or evidence of primary and/or secondary gains. *Schizophrenia* may present special diagnostic difficulties, both because of the emotional and psychotic features and because of the cognitive deficits (Zakzanis et al. 2003a). The cardinal symptoms of schizophrenia and longitudinal history should help clarify the diagnosis. The central cognitive functions and ADLs that deteriorate in dementia usually are preserved in schizophrenia. *Ganser's syndrome,* or the syndrome of "nearly correct answers," requires special consideration. The complete syndrome, including some disturbance of consciousness and subsequent amnesia, is rare, but "nearly correct answers" are more common. Both the syndrome and its symptoms may occur in association with organic and nonorganic psychiatric disturbances. Association with hysteria or hysterical mechanisms is frequent and must be considered in the differential diagnosis (Lishman 1998c).

Depressive disorders in elderly patients also should be considered because these patients may have memory difficulties, slowed thinking, and lack of spontaneity, which suggest dementia (see discussion of DSD earlier in this chapter in the "Depression" subsection). *Delirium* makes it very difficult to determine whether concurrent dementia is present, and delirium without fluctuating level of consciousness may be very difficult to distinguish from dementia. The diagnosis of delirium is suggested when global cognitive disturbance (including immediate and recent memory) is accompanied by rapid onset, fluctuating level of consciousness, impairment of attention, incoherence of thought, visual illusions or hallucinations or other perceptual disturbances, and disturbances of the sleep–wake cycle, all in the presence of a severe medical condition. Definitive diagnosis often must be postponed until the follow-up after recovery from acute medical illness. A "double" diagnosis of delirium superimposed on dementia is very common in general hospital patients; Lobo and Saz (in press) found that a postdischarge diagnosis of dementia is confirmed in approximately half the cases of uncertain diagnosis.

Mild cognitive impairment merits special consideration because of its high prevalence and the high rate of progression to dementia (Petersen et al. 2001a). The following characteristics are all required for the diagnosis: 1) subjective complaints of memory and/or other cognitive functions, preferably corroborated by an informant; 2) objective impairment of cognitive functions of mild severity compared with age and education norms; and 3) preserved ADLs. Clinical judgment is required for the diagnosis, but neuropsychological assessment is helpful. The screening instruments and rating scales presented in this chapter may be used for this purpose. Scores of 2 or 3 on the Global Deterioration Scale (GDS) (Reisberg et al. 1982) or a score of 0.5 on the Clinical Dementia Rating Scale (CDR) (Hughes et al. 1982) has been considered to correspond to mild cognitive impairment (Petersen et al. 2001b). Neuroimaging findings helpful in the diagnosis are described in the following sections.

Once false-positive cases are ruled out and a dementia syndrome is confirmed, the consultant determines whether the syndrome has characteristics of *cortical, subcortical,* or *mixed* type (see Table 7–6), as described in the previous sections. The onset and progression of the cognitive difficulties, the other psychopathological features, and whether another medical condition is present will give further clues as to the type of dementia. For diagnostic purposes, clinical differences between types of dementia have been emphasized in the clinical section. The search for potentially reversible types of dementia due to medical conditions or toxic effects (see Table 7–3) has long been emphasized and remains an important step in the diagnostic process. Such conditions are more frequent in general hospital patients (Barry and Moskowitz 1988), although the identification of truly reversible causes has become less common than in the past, and true reversibility has been questioned (Weytingh et al. 1995). No standard dementia workup is applicable to every patient. Table 7–8 lists a screening battery of tests that are commonly used to identify conditions associated with dementia, such as infectious, metabolic, and neoplastic diseases and substance-induced dementia. The specific tests used should be determined by various factors, including the patient's age, medical comorbidities, history, and physical

TABLE 7–8. Laboratory tests and other diagnostic procedures in the assessment of dementia

Screening battery[a]
 Complete blood cell count with differential cell type count
 Erythrocyte sedimentation rate
 Blood glucose
 Blood urea nitrogen
 Electrolytes, calcium, magnesium
 Thyrotropin
 Vitamin B_{12} and folate levels
 Urinalysis
 Fluorescent treponemal antibody absorption[b]
 Liver and renal function tests

Neuroimaging
 Computed tomography (CT) head scan
 Magnetic resonance imaging (MRI) head scan[c]
 Single photon emission computed tomography[b,c]

Other tests and procedures[a]
 Blood tests
  Arterial blood gases
  Blood and urine screens for alcohol, drugs, and heavy metals
  Serum HIV test[b,c]
  Homocysteine level
  Antinuclear antibody, C3, C4, anti-double-stranded DNA, anticardiolipin antibody
 Other
  Chest X ray
  Electrocardiogram
  Disease-specific tests (e.g., serum copper and ceruloplasmin for Wilson's disease)
  Lumbar puncture[c] (usually after CT or MRI)

---

[a]Tests may be selected on the basis of patient age.
[b]May require special consent and counseling.
[c]Tests selected on the basis of specific symptoms (history and physical examination) or patient populations.

examination. Neuroimaging is often obtained, and neuropsychological testing may be very useful in some cases (Table 7–9). Lumbar puncture should be considered for patients with early onset or atypical clinical features, as well as for patients with positive syphilis serology or suspected hydrocephalus, central nervous system infection, vasculitis, immunosuppression, or metastatic cancer.

Most cases of dementia are DAT or vascular dementia. The DSM-IV-TR criteria overlap with the ICD-10 criteria (World Health Organization 1992), and the latter also have been adapted for use in general hospital patients (Malt et al. 1996). However, the strict application of the norms in both the American and the World Health Organization classifications in the same sample of patients may lead to important differences in diagnostic estimates (Er-

TABLE 7–9. Neuroimaging findings in dementia syndromes

Syndrome and findings	Neuroimaging modalities
Dementias treatable by surgical procedures	
Normal-pressure hydrocephalus, brain tumors, subdural hematoma	CT, MRI
Dementia of the Alzheimer's type	
Enlarged ventricles	CT, MRI
General atrophy	CT, MRI
Medial temporal lobe or hippocampus atrophy (early markers)	CT, MRI (combined with SPECT)
Temporoparietal (and sometimes frontal) hypoperfusion	SPECT
Temporoparietal (and sometimes frontal) hypometabolism; relative sparing of visual and sensorimotor cortex	PET
Absence of signs of vascular dementia	CT, MRI
Vascular dementia	
Leukoaraiosis in white matter (very frequent)	CT
Areas of infarct (very characteristic, only half the cases)	CT
Hyperintensities in white matter (more sensitive)	MRI
Frontal dementia	
Frontal (and temporal) atrophy	CT, MRI
Frontal (and temporal) hypoperfusion	SPECT
Normal-pressure hydrocephalus	
Very enlarged ventricles	CT, MRI
Huntington's disease	
Atrophy of caudate nucleus	CT, MRI
Alcoholic dementia	
Enlarged ventricles and atrophy	CT, MRI
HIV dementia	
Atrophy	CT, MRI
Demyelination of subcortical white matter	MRI
Hypermetabolism of thalamus and basal ganglia	PET
Depression	
Frontal hypometabolism, asymmetric (reversible)	PET
Mild cognitive impairment	
Hippocampal and entorhinal volume reduction	MRI, CT
Hypoperfusion or hypometabolism	SPECT, PET

Note. Structural imaging: CT=computed tomography; MRI=magnetic resonance imaging. Functional imaging: PET=positron emission tomography; SPECT=single photon emission computed tomography.

kinjuntti et al. 1997). Although stringent diagnostic criteria are fundamental for research purposes, clinicians may need a more flexible application to classify all patients assessed.

Previous diagnostic guidelines tended to emphasize that the diagnosis of DAT was a process of exclusion. It is also accepted that a definitive diagnosis of Alzheimer's disease requires histological evidence in the brain at autopsy (McKhann et al. 1984). Biopsy of brain or extraneural tissues may be recommended only in very special circumstances (Reichman and Cummings 1990). DAT is currently considered to be a very characteristic clinico-

pathological process, amenable to clinical diagnosis (Reisberg et al. 1997). This view is based on the presence of a cortical type of dementia syndrome, an insidious onset with slow deterioration (although plateaus may occur in the progression), and characteristic psychopathological and neurological signs and symptoms (see Table 7–5). The diagnosis is further supported by neuroimaging findings (see Table 7–9); the absence of clinical evidence; or findings from special investigations, which suggest that the mental state may be due to vascular dementia (Table 7–10) or another systemic disease that can induce a dementia syndrome.

TABLE 7–10.   Clinical characteristics suggesting vascular dementia

Mixed type of dementia syndrome
Uneven cognitive deterioration
Relative preservation of insight and judgment
Abrupt onset, stepwise course
Emotional incontinence and lability
History of strokes
History of cardiovascular risk factors
Focal neurological signs and symptoms

Genetic testing for DAT is promising and relies on the fact that two general groups of genes are associated with this disease. Presenilin 1 (PS1) is a fairly accurate predictor of early-onset Alzheimer's disease, but genetic testing for mutations in presenilin has proven to be ineffective as a screening tool because of its low sensitivity (Kurz et al. 2002). The *APOE* genotype is statistically associated with late-onset Alzheimer's disease, but current genetic testing for the *APOE* ε4 allele can at best be used as an adjunct to clinical assessment for symptomatic patients (McConnell et al. 1999).

The clinical characteristics supporting a diagnosis of vascular dementia are summarized in Table 7–10, and Table 7–9 includes the characteristic and differential neuroimaging findings. More stringent diagnostic criteria are also available (Roman et al. 1993) and are widely considered important for research purposes. A diagnosis of a mixed DAT and vascular type of dementia or a double diagnosis is usually made when clinical and imaging characteristics of both coexist. This may happen, for example, when cerebrovascular episodes are superimposed on a clinical picture and history suggesting Alzheimer's disease. Vascular dementia also may precede neurodegenerative changes of DAT, but in such cases, it may not be possible to make the diagnosis of the latter on clinical grounds. The presence of cerebrovascular lesions in patients with DAT has been confirmed by recent evidence, including postmortem findings (Kalaria 2000).

Neuroimaging and Electroencephalography

Neuroimaging has revolutionized the ability of clinicians to diagnose dementia (Burns 1990). It is a useful adjunct to clinical diagnosis and is considered to be mandatory in some stringent diagnostic systems (McKhann et al. 1984; Roman et al. 1993). Computed tomography (CT) and magnetic resonance imaging (MRI) are very useful in ruling out reversible conditions such as NPH, subdural hematoma, and brain tumors. Therefore, these imaging modalities should be routinely considered in patients with history or findings suggesting those conditions, specifically when such patients have cognitive impairment with rapid onset or recent head trauma; focal neurological signs or abnormalities in gait; severe headache, papilledema, or visual field defect; early appearance of incontinence; or history of stroke or seizures without known risk factors.

In DAT, both CT and MRI are helpful diagnostic tools (see Table 7–9). However, the findings are not totally specific, in particular general atrophy, which may be found in elderly patients without dementia. Images of enlarged ventricles are considered to be better discriminators (Giacometti et al. 1994). Early markers of the disease may be the CT—and particularly the MRI—views of the medial temporal lobe and hippocampus (Convit et al. 1997; De Leon et al. 1989). Single photon emission computed tomography (SPECT) is also a promising technique (see Table 7–9), as is positron emission tomography (PET), although not all hospitals have adequate facilities. The utility of both functional techniques has been supported by a recent meta-analytic review (Zakzanis et al. 2003b). However, the costs of tests, and whether the results will make a difference in management of the patient, should be considered before routine recommendation in clinical practice. In vascular dementia, neuroimaging can provide strong support for the diagnosis, especially the MRI finding of hyperintensities in the white matter, and some authors suggest that the diagnosis is excluded in the absence of vascular lesions (Roman 2002). However, some hyperintensities are also found in DAT and other degenerative dementias, as well as in control subjects (Pantoni and Garcia 1995). PET is promising in patients with DSD (Martinot et al. 1990).

A review of the literature suggests that MRI and PET or SPECT are currently the most commonly used neuroimaging modalities in studies focusing on mild cognitive impairment (Wolf et al. 2003). Significant hippocampal and entorhinal cortex volume reductions were consistently found in subjects with mild cognitive impairment as compared with cognitively unimpaired control subjects. However, these measures cannot be regarded as being of high predictive value in an individual case, and neuroimaging measures of change are more informative (Petersen et al. 2001b). In PET and SPECT studies, reduced blood flow and/or glucose metabolism in temporoparietal association areas, posterior cingulate, and hippocampus have been associated with a higher risk of progressive cognitive decline in patients with mild cognitive impairment (Wolf et al. 2003).

The electroencephalogram (EEG) has limited utility in the differential diagnosis of dementia because abnormalities are frequent but relatively nonspecific. Slow wave activity characteristic of delirium does not appear until late in the course of DAT (Reisberg et al. 1997). Characteristic tracings may be seen in patients with Creutzfeldt-Jakob disease (triphasic, periodic burst patterns) and in patients with some metabolic dementias, such as hepatic encephalopathy (triphasic waves) (Brown et al. 1986), although in neither case is the finding pathognomonic.

Neuropsychological Testing

Neuropsychological testing (see also Chapter 2, "Neuropsychological and Psychological Evaluation") is valuable as an adjunct to the clinical examination but is no substitute for sound clinical judgment. Any battery of tests for the evaluation of dementia should assess a wide range of cognitive abilities, with special emphasis on memory (W.G. Rosen 1983). The age, education, and culture of the population must be considered in standardizing the instruments and interpreting the results. Neuropsychological testing may be particularly useful to differentiate dementia from age-related cognitive impairment and to provide both quantitative and qualitative information that helps differentiate types of dementia. Batteries commonly used include measures of memory, intellect, language, and visuospatial function. Some are exhaustive, with the administration taking several hours—a feature that limits their utility. A rather short battery has been standardized by the Consortium to Establish a Registry for Alzheimer's Disease (Welsh et al. 1992) and has been used in different countries.

Dementia Rating Scales

Aside from the MMSE, screening and assessment instruments for dementia include classic scales, such as the Blessed Mental Status Examination (Blessed et al. 1968), and new brief tests for discriminating dementia from nondementia in samples of persons with heterogeneous educational and cultural backgrounds, such as the Mini-Cog (Borson et al. 2000). Instruments for specific purposes have been designed; one such instrument, the Alzheimer's Disease Assessment Scale (ADAS) (W.G. Rosen et al. 1984), is considered to have improved sensitivity for DAT. The use of these instruments does not replace a careful mental status examination. Educational and cultural factors must be taken into account in interpreting the results of cognitive assessment with any of these instruments (Tombaugh and McIntyre 1992). Primary care physicians and nurse practitioners can be trained in their use.

Global staging procedures, such as the GDS (Reisberg et al. 1982) and, in particular, the CDR (Hughes et al. 1982), have come into wide use. Scales for measuring neuropsychiatric symptoms, such as the Neuropsychiatric Inventory (NPI) (Cummings et al. 1994), are also becoming widely used, and some can be recommended for clinical practice. A variety of assessments are also available for documenting functional deficits, such as the classic instruments of Lawton and Brody (1969), the Katz Index (Katz et al. 1970), or the Functional Assessment Staging (FAST) procedure, which can be used in conjunction with the GDS staging system (Reisberg et al. 1993). Some reports suggest that these scales can better assess the temporal variance of DAT than cognitive instruments can (Reisberg et al. 1996).

Clinical Course, Prognosis, and Outcome

The course and prognosis of dementia are generally disease-specific but may be influenced by a variety of factors. Timely surgical treatment, before irreversible brain damage occurs, may have spectacular results in subdural hematoma or brain tumors, depending on type and location. Classical studies suggested the improvement of severe apathy in NPH by surgical shunting, although cognitive improvement was not as evident. However, this remains a controversial issue, and a recent systematic review concluded that no evidence indicates whether placement of a shunt is effective (Esmonde and Cooke 2004). One would expect that dementia associated with medications or metabolic conditions should be reversible, but this is not always the case in practice (Clarfield 1988).

Medical comorbidity may be present in two-thirds of DAT patients and is strongly associated with greater impairment in cognition and in self-care (Doraiswamy et al. 2002). Optimal management of medical illnesses may offer potential to improve cognition in Alzheimer's disease. Dementias associated with infections have disease-specific prognoses. Untreated HIV dementia generally progresses quickly (over months) to severe global dementia, mutism, and death. However, the course may be variable, and with careful antiretroviral treatment, patients may survive for years. The course of dementia in central nervous system syphilis or chronic inflammatory diseases is also variable; cognitive improvement may be seen if early treatment is implemented. Adequate treatment with dopamine agonists and other standard treatments significantly improves the prognosis of dementia in Parkinson's disease. Early treatment with thiamine is vital in alcoholic patients with cognitive dysfunction (Blansjaar and van Dijk 1992).

Important events or changes in a patient's routine may precipitate episodes of behavioral disturbance. Medical illness (most often urinary tract infection or pneumonia) or the use of benzodiazepines or alcohol also may precipitate episodes of delirium. Psychosocial and pharmacological treatments may be beneficial, and the symptoms of degenerative processes may progress slowly for a time or may even recede somewhat. Patients with good premorbid adjustment and greater intelligence and education are in general more able to compensate for intellectual deficits and disability. Support from family and caregivers may determine to an important extent the presence or absence of affective and other psychological symptoms, as well as the course of dementia.

Recent studies suggest that median survival after the onset of DAT is much shorter than has previously been estimated and is strongly associated with age. In the study by Brookmeyer et al. (2002), median survival ranged from 8.3 years for persons who received the diagnosis at age 65 years to 3.4 years for persons who received the diagnosis at age 90 years. No important differences in mean survival have been found between DAT and vascular dementia (Wolfson et al. 2001).

The relative risk of death for DAT is two to three times higher than in persons without DAT, particularly in older women (Dewey and Saz 2001; Dodge et al. 2003). The mean annual rate of progression of cognitive impairment is approximately 2–4 points when degree of impairment is assessed with the MMSE (Ballard et al. 2001b). Although there are some discrepant reports (Mortimer et al. 1992), most researchers have found faster rates of decline in early-onset DAT (Jacobs et al. 1994; Stern et al. 1997). A more recent review (Sarazin et al. 2002) suggested that an increased rate of deterioration was associated with the following factors: low baseline cognitive status, presence of Lewy bodies, language deficits, lower scores on nonverbal neuropsychological tests, extrapyramidal signs, and myoclonus. The relation between *APOE* ε4 and the course of DAT is still debated (Frisoni et al. 1995; Galasko et al. 2000), but the presence of psychotic symptoms at baseline is strongly and independently predictive of a more rapid decline (Levy et al. 1996; Paulsen et al. 2000). However, some reports consider that cognitive decline in such cases might be related to neuroleptic treatment (McShane et al. 1997). Neuropsychiatric symptoms tend to fluctuate in the course of dementia in most patients, but depression, agitation, and aggression may show greater persistence as compared with delusions and hallucinations (Devanand et al. 1997). Dysthymia has been reported to be less persistent in DAT patients (Starkstein et al. 1997).

Functional impairment in DAT is highly correlated with the severity of cognitive impairment (Mohs et al. 2000), but the rate of functional decline may be slower for patients with mild and severe dementia than for patients with moderate dementia (Schmeidler et al. 1998). Instrumental ADLs demand higher cognitive functions than do the basic ADLs, and, as expected, the former are impaired earlier (Green et al. 1993; Lawton and Brody 1969). Functional impairment occurs more quickly in patients with severe neuropsychiatric symptoms (Stern et al. 1997). As expected, nursing home placement has consistently been related not only to severity of dementia but also to severity of both functional impairment and neuropsychiatric symptoms (Smith et al. 2001; Steele et al. 1990; Stern et al. 1997). Strong evidence suggests that caring for patients with dementia has a negative effect on caregivers, often more negative than when caring for a person with physical disabilities (Morris et al. 1988); the ability of caregivers to tolerate neuropsychiatric symptoms reduces the probability of nursing home placement (Smith et al. 2001).

Considerably less evidence is available regarding the course of other degenerative diseases, but clinical experience and some reports suggest that disease progression is similar to that in DAT. Early studies of dementia with Lewy bodies suggested that the mean duration of illness was shorter than in DAT patients, but this finding has been questioned (Ballard et al. 2001b). Duration of dementia with Lewy bodies ranges from 1.8 to 9.5 years (Walker et al. 2000), and early-onset cases might have a more rapid decline. Visual hallucinations tend to be persistent in dementia with Lewy bodies (Ballard et al. 2001b), but psychosis does not appear to predict accelerated decline (Mohs et al. 2000). The increased survival reported in studies might be related to a decrease in the prescription of neuroleptics in patients with dementia with Lewy bodies (McShane et al. 1997), in view of the greater awareness of their negative side effects, which include rapid cognitive decline.

A faster rate of deterioration in executive functions, but not of other cognitive functions, has been reported in patients with frontotemporal dementia when compared with DAT (Galasko et al. 2000). Loss of autonomy appears early in the course of frontotemporal dementia and is frequently accompanied by behavior changes.

In the late stages of subcortical dementias, such as Huntington's disease, apathy may be quite severe and cause profound self-neglect; the patient's condition may resemble the akinetic mute state. Duration of disease varies from 5–10 years in PSP to 10–15 years in Huntington's disease. Survival in Parkinson's disease might be 12–14 years, provided the treatment is adequate, and patients with Wilson's disease may have a normal survival time if their symptoms are adequately treated with penicillamine before irreversible liver and brain damage occur. The course of vascular dementia is typically stepwise but varies significantly depending on the type of vascular problem. Prognosis is poor, and patients usually die as a result of new cardiovascular events or strokes, but considerable individual variation is seen.

Treatment

General Principles

The general principles for treatment of dementia are summarized in Table 7–11. Patients with dementia very often have a broad range of medical problems, neuropsychiatric symptoms, and social needs accompanying their cognitive deterioration. Therefore, they usually need a multimodal plan, which should be adapted to the individual and to the specific stage of the disease. Specific recommendations are discussed in the following sections.

Adequate medical care is crucial in all dementias because both cognitive function and behavior may be adversely influenced by medical problems. Specific and frequent problems that must be addressed include the management of pain, urinary tract infections, and decubitus ulcers. Tube feeding to improve survival in hospitalized patients with advanced dementia is controversial, if not contraindicated, because it lacks demonstrated benefits (Meier et al. 2001). Treatment in nonreversible dementia aims at controlling the underlying condition as much as possible and slowing the progression of symptoms. Increasing evidence indicates that adequate prevention and treatment of vascular problems are also important in both vascular dementia and DAT. The treatment of cognitive loss with new pharmacological agents has become a major focus, but these medications have not supplanted the value of other measures. Identification and treatment of neuropsychiatric symptoms are especially relevant for psychiatrists. General measures include mandatory restrictions on driving. Both patients and families should be informed that dementia increases the risk for accidents, even in the early stages, and patients certainly should not be driving when dementia reaches a moderately severe stage. Psychological and social support and treatment always should be considered for patients. Psychiatrists also should be alert to the potential needs of caregivers. Long-term treatment must be considered in most dementias, and psychiatrists should participate in public health, including public awareness campaigns that stress the importance of early detection and treatment of dementia (Organization for Economic Cooperation and Development, in press).

Pharmacological Treatment

General guidelines for psychotropic medication use in frail elderly patients are applicable (American Psychiatric Association 1997; Ryan et al. 2002; Spar and La Rue 2002). Specific suggestions for dementia patients are summarized in Table 7–12. Systematic evidence to support the effectiveness of particular psychotropic drugs in dementia patients is limited. Therefore, choice of drug class may be based on clinical evidence, and choice of agent is often based on the side-effect profile and on the characteristics of a given patient. Noncognitive, psychopathological, and behavioral manifestations in patients with dementia may be early targets for psychiatric intervention.

Treatment of Psychosis and Agitation

There is some evidence of the effectiveness of antipsychotics to control agitation, aggressiveness, wandering, and psychotic symptoms in patients with dementia (Olin and Schneider 2002; Stoppe et al. 1999). The data suggest that improvement is greater for psychosis than for other symptoms. Antipsychotics are often administered in the evening so that maximum levels occur at sleep time. Most antipsychotics have long half-lives, so once-a-day doses may be sufficient. Oral administration is preferred, except in cases of emergency or when the patient is unable to take the medication by mouth. Initial treatment with low doses of a high-potency agent, such as haloperidol (0.5–2.0 mg/day; maximum dosage = 5 mg/day), may be recommended, and evidence indicates that it is effective in reducing aggressiveness in agitated dementia (Lonergan et al. 2004). However, the atypical antipsychotics cause fewer extrapyramidal effects, and their use in dementia has been supported by studies of risperidone (0.5–2.0 mg/day; maximum dosage = 6 mg/day) (Brodaty et al. 2003), olanzapine (5–10 mg/day) (Motsinger et al. 2003), quetiapine (25–100 mg/day) (Takahashi et al. 2003), and ziprasidone (20–40 mg/day) (Byerly et al. 2001). Another option is clozapine (maximum dose = 100 mg/day), which may be the best choice for Parkinson's disease (Motsinger et al. 2003) or dementia with Lewy bodies (Chacko et al. 1993) but carries risk of agranulocytosis. Thioridazine has been in wide clinical use in some countries for controlling behavior in patients with dementia. However, it has high anticholinergic activity and may cause worrisome QT prolongation. Furthermore, a systematic review suggested that no evidence supports its use in dementia (Kirchner et al. 2004).

There is less empirical support for, but considerable clinical experience with, the use of other medications in cases of agitated behavior, particularly in milder cases or

TABLE 7–11.   General principles for treatment of dementia and bases for consultation-liaison programs

Use a multimodal treatment plan and individualize it for each patient.
Adjust treatment to stage of disease.

Provide adequate care of emergencies.
Evaluate for suicidal potential, self-harm (e.g., falling or wandering), or accidents (e.g., fires).
Treat agitation and potential for violence.

Initiate early treatment of potentially reversible medical or surgical conditions etiologically related to dementia (e.g., hypothyroidism, subdural hematoma).

See patient on regular basis.
Frequent visits when starting therapy; routine follow-up every 4–6 months thereafter (more frequent visits may be required in special circumstances).

Ensure adequate medical care.
Maintain the patient's physical health: nutritious diet, proper exercise.
Identify and treat comorbid medical conditions: cardiopulmonary dysfunction, pain, urinary tract infections, decubitus ulcers, visual and auditory problems, etc.
Care for iatrogenic events, pressure sores, aspiration pneumonia, fecal impaction.
Exert stringent control of unnecessary drugs taken for other medical disorders.

Try to control underlying disease and slow progression in nonreversible dementias.
Prevent and treat vascular problems (in both vascular dementia and dementia of the Alzheimer's type): hypertension, hyperlipidemia, obesity, cardiac disease, diabetes, alcohol dependence, smoking cessation, etc.
Treat cognitive loss: pharmacological, other measures.

Use other general measures.
Use general health measures: recreational and activity therapies, etc.
Restrict driving and use of other dangerous equipment.

Identify neuropsychiatric symptoms; provide vigorous treatment if needed.

Provide psychological support and treatment for patient.
Provide orientation aids (calendars, clocks, television).
Assess activities of daily living and provide assistance as needed.
Use special techniques: stimulation-oriented, reminiscence therapy, cognitive or reality therapy.

Provide social treatment.
Educate family caregivers.
Give advice with arrangements for wills, power of attorney, and general estate matters.
Suggest support groups, community organizations.

Provide support for caregivers and treatment if needed (e.g., for depression).

Arrange long-term treatment and coordinate with care organizations.
Memory clinics
Community resources, geriatric day hospitals
Multidisciplinary rehabilitation in an outpatient setting
Support groups, Alzheimer's Association
Respite care
Long-term facility (including nursing homes, hospice) necessary if caregivers not available
Vigilance regarding neglect or abuse

Incorporate health care strategies.
Public awareness campaigns; campaigns for early detection and treatment of dementia

cases unresponsive to neuroleptics. These medications include trazodone (50–400 mg/day; higher doses have been reported by some clinicians) (Rojas-Fernández et al. 2003), buspirone (15–50 mg/day) (Salzman 2001), carbamazepine (400–1,200 mg/day; maximum blood levels=8–12 ng/mL) (Olin et al. 2001), and gabapentin (400–1,200 mg/day) (Miller 2001). These medications may be particularly useful in cases of dementia with Lewy bodies because the likelihood of severe adverse side effects with the use of neuroleptics is quite high (McKeith et al. 1992).

TABLE 7–12.   Suggested guidelines for psychotropic medication use

Consider that agitation and/or behavioral disturbances may be due to
  A medical condition, pain, other psychiatric condition, or sleep loss, which would resolve with treatment of the primary
    condition.
  Hunger, constipation, stressful atmosphere, change in living conditions, or interpersonal difficulties.

Use strategies to minimize the total amount of medication required.
  Instruction of caregivers to appropriately administer sedatives when warranted.
  Mild symptoms or limited risk often may resolve with support, reassurance, and distraction.

Remember that dementia patients are often physically frail and have decreased renal clearance and slowed hepatic
metabolism.

Be specific in selecting target symptoms.

Use low initial doses, one-quarter to one-third of the usual initial dose; dose increments should be smaller and
between-dose intervals longer. Seek lowest effective dose.

Avoid polypharmacy.

Keep especially alert to
  Medical conditions and drug interactions.
  Frequent and worrying side effects: orthostatic hypotension and central nervous system sedation (may worsen cognition and
    cause falls); susceptibility to extrapyramidal side effects.
  Idiosyncratic drug effects: mental confusion; restlessness; increased sedation; and vulnerability to anticholinergic effects of
    psychotropic medication.

In cases of extrapyramidal effects, reduce the dose or change to another drug rather than use anticholinergic drugs.

Reassess risks and benefits of psychotropic treatment on an ongoing basis.

Anticonvulsants require close monitoring because of potential toxic effects. Several other agents have been proposed for the treatment of agitation in patients with dementia, including benzodiazepines and beta-blockers, but evidence of efficacy is very limited, and potential side effects preclude routine recommendation.

Treatment of Depression

Both well-designed studies (Lyketsos et al. 2003) and reviews of randomized controlled trials (Olin and Schneider 2002) suggest that antidepressants may be effective for treating depressive syndromes in patients with dementia. Improvement of both cognitive function and apathy, especially in frontal lobe dementias, is also a frequent target in the treatment of depression. However, because antidepressants do have side effects, clinicians should prescribe with due caution (Bains et al. 2004). The newer antidepressants, particularly the selective serotonin reuptake inhibitors (SSRIs), are widely considered to be first-line treatment and should be preferred because of their favorable side-effect profile (Giron et al. 2001). SSRIs used in dementia include fluoxetine (initial dosage=5–10 mg/day, increase at several-week intervals to 40–60 mg/day); paroxetine (same dosages, increase every 1–2 weeks because of shorter half-life); sertraline (initial dosage=25 mg/day, increase at 1- to 2-week intervals to 150–200 mg/day); and citalopram (initial dosage=10 mg/day, increase at weekly intervals to a maximum dosage of 40 mg/day). Escitalopram (10–20 mg/day) is promising (Lepola et al. 2003). Aside from well-known gastrointestinal symptoms, some potential SSRI side effects, such as agitation, akathisia and other extrapyramidal symptoms, dizziness, and weight loss, require monitoring in dementia patients. Venlafaxine (initial dosage=18.75–37.50 mg twice a day, increase at weekly intervals to 350–375 mg/day) is also recommended, particularly in apathetic patients because of stimulating effects, but it may elevate blood pressure at higher doses. Trazodone (initial dosage=25–50 mg/day, increase at weekly intervals to 300–400 mg/day) is often recommended when sedation and improved sleep are desired. Trazodone's main risks in elderly patients with dementia are orthostatic hypotension and excessive sedation.

Classic cyclic antidepressants usually are not considered first-line treatment because they have more adverse effects such as orthostatic hypotension, delays in cardiac conduction, anticholinergic effects, impaired cognition, and delirium. However, some clinicians prefer these drugs, particularly in treating severe depressive syndromes. In such cases, because of a more favorable side-effect profile, the recommended drugs are nortriptyline, particularly when sedation is needed (initial dosage=10–25 mg/day, increase at weekly intervals to 100–150 mg/day; blood levels should not exceed 100–150 ng/mL), and desipramine (initial dosage=25–50 mg/day, increase at weekly intervals to 200 mg/day; blood levels should not exceed 150–200 ng/mL). There is also considerable experience with nortriptyline in "organic" depression (Robinson 1998), and clinical experience and some reports support the use of SSRIs and nortriptyline in pathological crying (Robinson et al. 1993). In depressed patients with frontotemporal dementia, both SSRIs (Swartz et al. 1997) and trazodone (Lebert et al. 1999) have shown some benefit.

Evidence is limited on the beneficial effects of other drugs recommended in the treatment of depression or depression-associated symptoms in dementia patients, such as bupropion, which may increase the risk of seizures at high doses, or buspirone for the treatment of agitation and anxiety associated with depression. Monoamine oxidase inhibitors (MAOIs) should be used only if other drugs fail, because postural hypotension is a serious problem in frail elderly, and patients with dementia cannot be trusted to avoid restricted foods. Psychostimulants, such as D-amphetamine and methylphenidate, are sometimes useful in patients with medical illness and depression; potential side effects of restlessness, agitation, sleep disturbances, and appetite suppression are uncommon at low doses. Apathy in depressed dementia patients also has been treated with bromocriptine, whereas potential side effects, such as psychosis, confusion, dyskinesias, and anticholinergic effects, including delirium, have been reported after treatment with amantadine. Clinical experience suggests that electroconvulsive therapy (ECT) may be useful in treating severe depression associated with dementia that does not respond to drugs, but the data are limited. In such cases, ECT should be given twice rather than thrice weekly, and less memory loss has been documented with unilateral than with bilateral placement of electrodes (American Psychiatric Association 1997) (see also Chapter 39, "Electroconvulsive Therapy").

Treatment of Insomnia and Anxiety

Sleep disturbances, which are frequent in patients with dementia, should be primarily managed by careful attention to sleep hygiene. When the disturbances occur in patients with other neuropsychiatric symptoms requiring psychotropic treatment, a drug with sedating properties, given at bedtime, probably should be selected. Otherwise, trazodone (50–100 mg, once at bedtime) is often prescribed. Clinical experience suggests that low-dose antipsychotics (haloperidol 0.5–1.0 mg or the atypical antipsychotics) can be helpful. Chloral hydrate (250–500 mg/day) and zolpidem (5–10 mg at bedtime) are good alternatives for short-term use. Clonazepam (0.5 mg/day, with

increases in dosage up to 2 mg/day) is recommended by some clinicians in patients with frequent awakening or nocturnal wandering. However, all hypnotics have the potential risk of causing nocturnal confusion, daytime sedation, tolerance, rebound insomnia, worsening cognition, disinhibition, and delirium. Triazolam is not recommended because of its association with amnesia. Many patients use diphenhydramine because it is available in a variety of nonprescription preparations and therefore is erroneously believed to be safe. It is not a good choice because of its anticholinergic properties, which may exacerbate confusion and also counteract the effects of cholinesterase inhibitors.

The use of benzodiazepines for anxiety in patients with dementia is controversial because of the side-effect profile described, which also includes ataxia and accidental falls, respiratory depression, and agitation among the most disturbing effects in dementia patients. Low dosages of relatively short-acting drugs, such as lorazepam (0.5–1.0 mg every 4–6 hours) or oxazepam (7.5–15.0 mg four times per day), are preferred when using benzodiazepines and may be beneficial for brief periods. Antidepressants should be considered for long-term treatment, but empirical evidence is very limited regarding their use for anxiety in dementia patients.

Treatment of Cognitive Deficits

Pharmacological treatment of DAT also should aim at restoring cognitive function and associated functional losses. Currently, the main drugs approved act by inhibiting acetylcholinesterase and thus providing cholinergic augmentation. They may improve cognitive and behavioral symptoms, as well as functional ADLs, in patients with mild to moderate DAT. However, the degree of benefit achieved is limited (Doody et al. 2001) or symptomatic (Cochrane reviews, see Table 7–13; Mayeux and Sano 1999)—that is, with little proven effect on the ultimate outcome. Tacrine, which was approved for treating DAT in 1993, has since been replaced by a group of drugs with fewer adverse affects, which include donepezil, rivastigmine, and galantamine (Mayeux and Sano 1999).

To date, there are no head-to-head comparisons of cholinesterase inhibitors, and the main differences between these drugs are in safety profiles and ease of administration (one to two times daily administration) (Grutzendler and Morris 2001). Donepezil is the most widely prescribed, probably because it was the first one to appear (Organization for Economic Cooperation and Development, in press). One cost-effectiveness analysis of cholinesterase inhibitors supported their use (Clegg et al. 2001), but medical guidelines in many countries recommend that cholinergic augmentation therapy be used only in patients with mild to moderate forms of DAT (MMSE score >10 or 12 points or the equivalent score on the Alzheimer's Disease Assessment Scale—cognitive subscale [ADAS-Cog]) (Gillen et al. 2001). However, positive results have been documented in moderate to severe cases of DAT with a new drug, memantine (Reisberg et al. 2003) (see Table 7–13). It blocks the effects of glutamate in stimulating the N-methyl-D-aspartate receptor. A Cochrane review concluded that the evidence to date shows that in moderate to severe DAT, memantine improves measures of cognition and functional decline but does not affect clinically discernible change or improve global measures of dementia (Areosa Sastre and Sherriff 2004). A randomized, placebo-controlled trial of memantine in patients with moderate to severe Alzheimer's disease who were already receiving donepezil found statistically significant but clinically modest benefits (Tariot et al. 2004).

Cholinesterase inhibitors show some promise in the treatment of other dementias, such as dementia with Lewy bodies (McKeith et al. 2000) and Parkinson's disease (Emre 2003). Furthermore, pharmacological studies supporting the use of these and other agents have heuristic value in stimulating research on the pathogenesis of neurodegenerative dementias.

An antioxidant, vitamin E (200–2,000 IU/day), is frequently recommended for DAT patients to prevent further decline (American Psychiatric Association 1997). Recommendations were based on both empirical evidence and clinical experience. Although a recent, systematic review found no evidence to support its use (Tabet et al. 2003), vitamin E appears to be very safe and is still considered by some clinicians for treatment of DAT, particularly in the moderately severe stage, alone or in combination with an anticholinergic agent. Lower dosages should be used in patients with vitamin K deficiency because vitamin E may worsen coagulation deficits.

Positive results with a wide variety of agents to treat DAT have been reported, and systematic reviews support the benefits of nimodipine (90 mg/day), a calcium channel blocker (López-Arrieta and Birks 2004); nicergoline, an ergot derivative (Fioravanti et al. 2004); and selegiline, a monoamine oxidase–B (MAO-B) inhibitor (Birks and Flicker 2004). Selegiline (5–10 mg/day) may delay cognitive deterioration and may be worth considering in patients who are intolerant of, or unresponsive to, cholinesterase inhibitors. It requires no dietary limitations as with other MAOIs, but a major side effect is orthostatic hypotension.

Beneficial effects have been claimed, but not proven, with several agents, including statin therapy for lowering serum cholesterol (Scott and Laake 2004); dehydroepian-

drosterone (Huppert and Van Niekerk 2004); estrogen replacement therapy in postmenopausal women (Hogervorst et al. 2004); and ginkgo biloba, an extract of the leaves of the maidenhair tree (Birks et al. 2003a). No evidence has been found for the use of hydergine, an ergoloid mesylate, in DAT (L. S. Schneider and Olin 1994), but it may be appropriately continued for patients who have experienced benefits (American Psychiatric Association 1997). Preventive treatment with antihypertensive drugs is also controversial, but the results of a large international trial with candesartan in mild hypertension are promising (Forette et al. 1998; Lithell et al. 2003). In view of recent findings related to vascular factors influencing the cognitive symptoms of DAT, the management of these factors has become a focus of attention, discussed later in this section in relation to vascular dementia.

Finally, systematic reviews do not support the use of indomethacin, a nonsteroidal anti-inflammatory drug (Tabet and Feldman 2003); piracetam, a nootropic agent with effects on increasing oxygen and glucose utilization and probable platelet antiaggregation properties (Flicker and Grimley Evans 2004); lecithin, a major dietary source of choline (Higgins and Flicker 2004); D-cycloserine, an antibiotic that enhances glutamate function (Jones et al. 2004); and nicotine (López-Arrieta et al. 2003). Future drugs may strategically aim to retard or prevent amyloid deposition and neuronal degeneration and to stimulate neuroprotection (Cutler and Sramek 2001). The development of an experimental vaccine directed against the formation and accumulation of amyloid plaques has shown promise (Bard et al. 2000).

Drug treatment of mild cognitive impairment is controversial because evidence supporting pharmacological strategies remains limited. Efficacy of nicergoline (Fioravanti and Flicker 2004) and the dopamine receptor agonist piribedil (Nagaraja and Jayashree 2001) has been reported, and results of a meta-analysis support the use of acetyl-L-carnitine (Montgomery et al. 2003). Several long-term clinical trials are still ongoing (antioxidants, nootropics, anticholinesterases). Prevention and disease-modifying strategies raise ethical questions because interventions are focused on nondiseased elderly at risk, which means that long-term safety should be given disproportionate emphasis compared with efficacy. At present, treatment strategies for DAT could be extrapolated to mild cognitive impairment (Jelic and Winblad 2003). We recommend follow-up and monitoring of individuals with mild cognitive impairment, especially when neuroimaging suggests a high probability of conversion to DAT (see section "Neuroimaging and Electroencephalography" earlier in this chapter). Early treatment should be considered as soon as the diagnosis of dementia is clear.

TABLE 7–13. Drug treatments for cognitive and functional losses in dementia of the Alzheimer's type (DAT): Cochrane System Reviews

Drug	Effectiveness[a]	Cognitive[a]	Behavioral[a]	ADL[a]	Indications in DAT	Dosage	Mechanism of action	Side effects
Donepezil[b]	++	++	++	++	Mild or moderate	5–10 mg once daily	AChE inhibitor	Nausea, vomiting, diarrhea
Rivastigmine[c]	++	++	++	++	Mild or moderate	1.5–6 mg twice a day	AChE, BChE inhibitor	Nausea, vomiting, diarrhea
Galantamine[d]	++	++	++	++	Mild or moderate	4–12 mg twice a day	AChE inhibitor	Nausea, vomiting, diarrhea
Memantine[e]	+	++	+	+	Moderate or severe	10–20 mg twice a day	NMDA antagonist	Agitation, urinary incontinence

Note. ADL=activity of daily living; AChE=acetylcholinesterase; BchE=butyrylcholinesterase; NMDA=*N*-methyl-D-aspartate.

[a]++=evidence considerable; +=some evidence, limited number of controlled trials.
[b]Birks et al. 2003b; Feldman et al. 2001.
[c]Birks et al. 2004; Rösler et al. 1999.
[d]Doody et al. 2001; Olin and Schneider 2002.
[e]Areosa Sastre and Sherriff 2004.

Vascular dementia has no standard treatment (Erkinjuntti 2002), but recently, symptomatic cholinergic treatment has shown promise in both Alzheimer's disease with vascular dementia and vascular dementia alone (Erkinjuntti 2002). Systematic reviews give specific support to memantine (Areosa Sastre and Sherriff 2004), nicergoline (Fioravanti and Flicker 2004), and nimodipine (López-Arrieta and Birks 2004) in both vascular dementia and mixed dementia. Evidence is limited on the primary prevention and secondary prevention of vascular dementia (Roman 2002), but treating associated medical conditions and reducing known cardiovascular and cerebrovascular risk factors seem logical steps. Daily aspirin therapy to inhibit platelet aggregation has been recommended but remains controversial (Hebert et al. 2000) and is not supported by the results of a recent systematic review (Rands et al. 2004). The preventive effects of early treatment of even mild hypertension are also promising for vascular dementia (Forette et al. 1998; Lithell et al. 2003), but no convincing evidence has been found so far relating diabetic treatment to the prevention or management of cognitive impairment in type 2 diabetes (Areosa Sastre and Grimley Evans 2004). More studies are needed of the effectiveness and efficacy of prevention and treatment of mild cognitive impairment of vascular origin. In the meantime, good clinical sense recommends symptomatic treatment and control of other treatable risk factors—namely, cardiac disease, hyperlipidemia, obesity, hyperhomocysteinemia, hyperfibrinogenemia, and other conditions that can cause brain hypoperfusion, such as obstructive sleep apnea and orthostatic hypotension (Frisoni et al. 2002). Psychiatrists can play a prominent role in treating and preventing smoking and alcohol dependence. Genetic counseling may be considered in diseases of genetic basis, such as cerebral autosomal dominant arteriopathy with subcortical infarcts and leukoencephalopathy.

Psychological Treatment

Two main goals may be identified in the psychological treatment of dementia: providing support and modifying behavior. Few psychological treatments have been subjected to systematic evaluation, but some research, including single-case studies, along with clinical experience, supports their effectiveness. The supportive techniques are based on the recognition that deterioration of cognitive function and sense of identity has significant psychological meaning for patients with dementia and may be associated with high levels of distress. Patients benefit from specific support and attention to self-esteem issues, as well as assistance in grieving and accepting the extent of their disability. There is some overlap with cognitive-

behavioral techniques because the support is often accompanied by educational measures in which the nature and course of their illness are clearly explained. Psychiatrists also can assist patients and teach other staff to find ways to maximize functioning in preserved areas and to compensate for the defective functions. This includes simple maneuvers, such as taking notes for memory problems or making schedules to help structure activities into a daily routine. In this way, patients with dementia may have a predictable schedule and avoid undue distress, including catastrophic reactions when confronted with unfamiliar activities or environments.

Behavioral treatments are often focused on specific cognitive deficits, and different strategies have been devised. Reality orientation operates through the presentation of orientation-related information (e.g., time-, place-, and person-related), which is thought to provide the person with a greater understanding of his or her surroundings, possibly resulting in an improved sense of control and self-esteem. This technique has been associated with frustration in some patients, but a systematic review found evidence that reality orientation has benefits for both cognition and behavior in dementia (Spector et al. 2004a). Observational studies give some support to other strategies, such as stimulation-oriented treatment, which includes recreational activity, art therapy, dance therapy, and pet therapy. Reminiscence therapy tries to stimulate the patient to talk about the past. Beneficial effects on the patient's mood and/or behavior have been reported with both techniques, but the evidence in systematic reviews is limited (Chung et al. 2004; Spector et al. 2004b). Similarly, evidence is insufficient on the effectiveness of other techniques, such as validation therapy (Neal and Briggs 2004).

Family Support and Social Care

The fate of dementia patients is determined to a large extent by their social framework (Organization for Economic Cooperation and Development, in press). Psychiatrists and other providers should pay attention to the family and social structures, community supports, and the potential need for residential treatment. Strong evidence suggests that informal (i.e., family) caregivers very frequently have psychiatric morbidity and possibly also medical morbidity related to the burden of caring for patients with dementia (Colvez et al. 2002; DeKosky and Orgogozo 2001; Ory et al. 1999; J. Schneider et al. 1999). However, many caregivers feel that caring for an afflicted loved one, even though an unexpected task, is a meaningful, accepted responsibility of which they wish to be an integral part. Empathic interventions may help them understand the complex mixture of feelings associated with caring for a loved one with a dementing illness. Formal psychotherapy may be necessary in some cases. Referral to support groups is often indicated, and associations of families of patients with dementia exist in many countries and often provide critical support. The family also should be educated about the disease and helped with information to facilitate planning for financial decisions and end-of-life care issues, including advance directives. Education for family caregivers of DAT patients has been shown to improve the outcomes for both caregivers and patients (Olin and Schneider 2002). Furthermore, comprehensive support and counseling services for spouse-caregivers decrease the likelihood of placing a spouse in a nursing home (Cohen and Pushkar 1999).

Care Provision

Mental health facilities that specialize in treating dementia are varied. Psychiatrists should participate in supporting access to quality care, but no consensus currently exists about what constitutes quality care and how to assess care provision (Innes 2002). Social service referrals are very helpful to inform the family about available resources. Special care units for patients with dementia may offer models of optimal care, but no empirical evidence indicates that this type of unit achieves better outcomes than do traditional facilities.

The most common facility to care for patients with dementia is the memory clinic (Colvez et al. 2002). Such clinics gain value when attached to a psychosomatic medicine/consultation-liaison service, particularly when liaison is developed with primary care (Lobo and Saz, in press). Community resources include home health services, day care, or nursing homes. Shortage of nursing home beds is reported in most countries, so residential care remains important and in demand (Organization for Economic Cooperation and Development, in press). Geriatric day hospitals provide multidisciplinary rehabilitation in an outpatient setting. A review of studies documented a significant difference in favor of day hospital attendance when compared with no comprehensive elderly care (Forster et al. 2004). However, the general move toward an increased emphasis on community care is also dependent on the availability of informal caregivers. Respite services are considered very important for informal caregivers, although their effectiveness remains inconclusive (Organization for Economic Cooperation and Development, in press).

Long-term care of patients with dementia presents special problems. Delirium, a frequent complication in institutionalized, elderly patients with dementia, is dis-

cussed in Chapter 6, "Delirium." Delirium in patients with dementia is still managed empirically, and no evidence has documented the effectiveness of multidisciplinary team interventions or supported changes in current practice at this time (Britton and Russell 2004). Another complication is wandering, which is very common in long-term dementia patients. They may, at times, put themselves at risk, creating difficult challenges for caregivers and institutional staff. Traditional interventions to prevent wandering include restraint, drugs, and locked doors. Because cognitively impaired patients may respond to environmental stimuli in different ways, new techniques that might reduce wandering include the design of visual and other selective barriers, such as mirrors and grids or stripes of tape. However, a systematic review has found no evidence that these techniques are effective (Price et al. 2004).

The appropriate use of antipsychotic medications and tranquilizers is also an important issue in long-term institutionalized patients. Overuse of medication can lead to worsening of the dementia and to harmful side effects. Available alternatives, such as the search for medical, psychiatric, or environmental factors that may be causing agitation or behavior problems, are discussed in a previous section of this chapter ("Epidemiology, Risk Factors, and Etiology") and should be pursued. However, if a patient's behavior is dangerous, psychotropic medications should be used, and additional measures may be needed if no response occurs. Use of physical restraints should be limited to patients with imminent risk of physical harm to themselves or others and only until more definitive treatment is provided or after other measures have been exhausted (or pose greater risk to the patient). Good clinical practice, and legal regulations in some countries, requires careful consideration and documentation of the indications and available alternatives, monitoring of the response, and reassessment of the need for treatment. Structured educational programs for staff may decrease both the abuse of tranquilizers and the use of physical restraints in the institutionalized elderly.

References

Aarsland D, Andersen K, Larsen JP, et al: Risk of dementia in Parkinson's disease: a community-based, prospective study. Neurology 56:730–736, 2001

Akil M, Brewer GJ: Psychiatric and behavioral abnormalities in Wilson's disease. Adv Neurol 65:171–178, 1995

Alexopoulos GS, Meyers BS, Young RC, et al: The course of geriatric depression with "reversible dementia": a controlled study. Am J Psychiatry 150:1693–1699, 1993

American Academy of Neurology AIDS Task Force: Nomenclature and research case definitions for neurologic manifestations of human immunodeficiency virus-type 1 (HIV-1) infection. Neurology 41:778–785, 1991

American Psychiatric Association: Diagnostic and Statistical Manual of Mental Disorders, 3rd Edition, Revised. Washington, DC, American Psychiatric Association, 1987

American Psychiatric Association: Practice Guideline for the Treatment of Patients With Alzheimer's Disease and Other Dementias of Late Life. Washington, DC, American Psychiatric Association, 1997

American Psychiatric Association: Diagnostic and Statistical Manual of Mental Disorders, 4th Edition, Text Revision. Washington, DC, American Psychiatric Association, 2000

Apaydin H, Ahlskog JE, Parisi JE, et al: Parkinson disease neuropathology: later-developing dementia and loss of the levodopa response. Arch Neurol 59:102–112, 2002

Areosa Sastre A, Grimley Evans J: Effect of the treatment of type II diabetes mellitus on the development of cognitive impairment and dementia (Cochrane Review), in The Cochrane Library, Issue 2. Chichester, UK, Wiley, 2004

Areosa Sastre A, Sherriff F: Memantine for dementia (Cochrane Review), in The Cochrane Library, Issue 2. Chichester, UK, Wiley, 2004

Bains J, Birks JS, Dening TR: Antidepressants for treating depression in dementia (Cochrane Review), in The Cochrane Library, Issue 2. Chichester, UK, Wiley, 2004

Bakheit AMO, Kennedy PGE, Behan PO: Paraneoplastic limbic encephalitis: clinico-pathological correlations. J Neurol Neurosurg Psychiatry 53:1084–1088, 1990

Ballard CG, Margallo-Lana M, Fossey J, et al: A 1-year follow-up study of behavioral and psychological symptoms in dementia among people in care environments. J Clin Psychiatry 62:631–636, 2001a

Ballard CG, O'Brien JT, Morris CM, et al: The progression of cognitive impairment in dementia with Lewy bodies, vascular dementia and AD. Int Psychogeriatr 16:499–503, 2001b

Bard F, Cannon C, Barbour R, et al: Peripherally administered antibodies against amyloid beta-peptide enter the central nervous system and reduce pathology in a mouse model of Alzheimer disease. Nat Med 6:916–919, 2000

Barry PP, Moskowitz MA: The diagnosis of reversible dementia in the elderly: a critical review. Arch Intern Med 148:1914–1918, 1988

Bennett DA, Wilson RS, Gilley DW, et al: Clinical diagnosis in Binswanger's disease. J Neurol Neurosurg Psychiatry 53:961–965, 1990

Bennett HP, Corbett AJ, Gaden S, et al: Subcortical vascular disease and functional decline: a 6-year predictor study. J Am Geriatr Soc 50:1969–1977, 2002

Birks J, Flicker L: Selegiline for Alzheimer's disease (Cochrane Review), in The Cochrane Library, Issue 2. Chichester, UK, Wiley, 2004

Birks J, Grimley Evans J, Van Dongen M: Ginkgo biloba for cognitive impairment and dementia (Cochrane Review), in The Cochrane Library, Issue 1. Chichester, UK, Wiley, 2003a

Birks J, Melzer D, Beppu H: Donepezil for mild and moderate Alzheimer's disease (Cochrane Review), in The Cochrane Library, Issue 1. Chichester, UK, Wiley, 2003b

Birks J, Grimley Evans J, Iakovidou V, et al: Rivastigmine for Alzheimer's disease (Cochrane Review), in The Cochrane Library, Issue 2. Chichester, UK, Wiley, 2004

Blansjaar BA, van Dijk JG: Korsakoff minus Wernicke syndrome. Alcohol 27:435–437, 1992

Blessed G, Tomlinson BE, Roth M: The association between quantitative measures of dementia and of senile change in the cerebral grey matter of elderly subjects. Br J Psychiatry 114:797–811, 1968

Borson S, Scanlan J, Brush M, et al: The mini-cog: a cognitive "vital signs" measure for dementia screening in multilingual elderly. Int J Geriatr Psychiatry 15:1021–1027, 2000

Boustani M, Peterson B, Hanson L, et al: Screening for dementia in primary care: a summary of the evidence for the U.S. Preventive Services Task Force. Ann Intern Med 138:927–937, 2003

Breitner JC, Wyse BW, Anthony JC, et al: APOE-epsilon4 count predicts age when prevalence of AD increases, then declines: the Cache County Study. Neurology 53:321–331, 1999

Breteler MMB, De Groot RRM, Van Romunde LKJ, et al: Risk of dementia in patients with Parkinson's disease, epilepsy and severe head trauma: a register-based follow-up study. Am J Epidemiol 142:1300–1305, 1995

Britton A, Russell R: Multidisciplinary team interventions for delirium in patients with chronic cognitive impairment (Cochrane Review), in The Cochrane Library, Issue 2. Chichester, UK, Wiley, 2004

Brodaty H, Ames D, Snowdon J, et al: A randomized placebo-controlled trial of risperidone for the treatment of aggression, agitation, and psychosis of dementia. J Clin Psychiatry 64:134–143, 2003

Brookmeyer R, Gray S, Kawas C: Projections of Alzheimer's disease in the United States and the public health impact of delaying disease onset. Am J Public Health 88:1337–1342, 1998

Brookmeyer R, Corrada MM, Curriero FC, et al: Survival following a diagnosis of Alzheimer disease. Arch Neurol 59:1764–1767, 2002

Brown P, Cathala F, Castaigne P, et al: Creutzfeldt-Jakob disease: clinical analysis of a consecutive series of 230 neuropathologically verified cases. Ann Neurol 20:597–602, 1986

Budka H, Aguzzi A, Brown P, et al: Neuropathological diagnostic criteria for Creutzfeldt-Jacob disease (CJD) and other human spongiform encephalopathies (prion diseases). Brain Pathol 5:459–466, 1995

Buee L, Bussiere T, Buee-Scherrer V, et al: Tau protein isoforms, phosphorylation and role in neurodegenerative disorders. Brain Res Rev 33:95–130, 2000

Burns A: Cranial computed tomography in dementia of the Alzheimer type. Br J Psychiatry 157:10–15, 1990

Burton GV, Bullard DE, Walther PJ, et al: Paraneoplastic limbic encephalopathy with testicular carcinoma: a reversible neurologic syndrome. Cancer 62:2248–2251, 1988

Byerly MJ, Weber MT, Brooks DL, et al: Antipsychotic medications and the elderly: effects on cognition and implications for use. Drugs Aging 18:45–61, 2001

Campbell S, Stephens S, Ballard C: Dementia with Lewy bodies: clinical features and treatment. Drugs Aging 18:397–407, 2001

Cedazo-Minguez A, Cowburn RF: Apolipoprotein E: a major piece in the Alzheimer's disease puzzle. J Cell Mol Med 5:254–266, 2001

Chacko R, Hurley R, Jankovic J: Clozapine used in diffuse Lewy body disease. J Neuropsychiatry Clin Neurosci 5:206–208, 1993

Chen P, Ganguli M, Mulsant BH, et al: The temporal relationship between depressive symptoms and dementia: a community-based prospective study. Arch Gen Psychiatry 56:261–266, 1999

Chui HC, Victoroff JI, Margolin D, et al: Criteria for the diagnosis of ischemic vascular dementia proposed by the state of California Alzheimer's Disease Diagnostic and Treatment Centers. Neurology 42:473–480, 1992

Chung JCC, Lai CKY, Chung PMB, et al: Snoezelen for dementia (Cochrane Review), in The Cochrane Library, Issue 2. Chichester, UK, Wiley, 2004

Clarfield AM: The reversible dementias: do they reverse? Ann Intern Med 109:476–486, 1988

Clegg A, Bryant J, Nicholson T, et al: Clinical and cost-effectiveness of donepezil, rivastigmine and galantamine for Alzheimer's disease: a rapid and systematic review. Health Technol Assess 5:1–137, 2001

Cohen CA, Pushkar D: Lessons learned from a longitudinal study of dementia care. Am J Geriatr Psychiatry 7:139–146, 1999

Colvez A, Joel ME, Ponton-Sanchez A, et al: Health status and work burden of Alzheimer patients' informal caregivers: comparisons of five different care programs in the European Union. Health Policy 60:219–233, 2002

Convit A, de Leon MJ, Tarshish C, et al: Specific hippocampal volume reductions in individuals at risk for Alzheimer's disease. Neurobiol Aging 18:1–9, 1997

Corsellis JAN, Goldberg GJ, Norton AR: Limbic encephalitis and its associations with carcinoma. Brain 91:481–496, 1968

Crum RM, Anthony JC, Basset SS, et al: Population based norms for the Mini-Mental State Examination by age and educational level. JAMA 269:2386–2391, 1993

Cummings JL, Benson DF: Subcortical dementia: review of an emerging concept. Arch Neurol 41:874–879, 1984

Cummings JL, Benson DF: Dementia of the Alzheimer's type: an inventory of diagnostic clinical features. J Am Geriatr Soc 34:12–19, 1986

Cummings JL, Mega M, Gray KF, et al: The Neuropsychiatric Inventory: comprehensive assessment of psychopathology in dementia. Neurology 44:2308–2314, 1994

Cummings JL, Vinters HV, Cole GM, et al: Alzheimer's disease: etiologies, pathophysiology, cognitive reserve, and treatment opportunities. Neurology 51:S2–S17, 1998

Cutler NR, Sramek JJ: Review of the next generation of Alzheimer's disease therapeutics: challenges for drug development. Prog Neuropsychopharmacol Biol Psychiatry 25:27–57, 2001

Dartigues JF, Letenneur L, Helmer C: Epidemiology of dementia: protective factors, in Alzheimer's Disease and Related Disorders Annual 2002. Edited by Gauthier S, Cummings JL. London, Taylor & Francis Group, 2002, pp 67–76

de Groot JC, de Leeuw FE, Oudkerk M, et al: Cerebral white matter lesions and depressive symptoms in elderly adults. Arch Gen Psychiatry 57:1071–1076, 2000

de la Torre JC: Alzheimer disease as a vascular disorder: nosological evidence. Stroke 33:1152–1162, 2002

De Leon MJ, George AE, Golomb J, et al: Early marker for Alzheimer's disease: the atrophic hippocampus. Lancet 2:672–673, 1989

Deahl M: Cannabis and memory loss. Br J Addict 86:249–252, 1991

DeKosky ST, Orgogozo JM: Alzheimer disease; diagnosis, costs, and dimensions of treatment. Alzheimer Dis Assoc Disord 15 (suppl 1):3–7, 2001

Dening DC, Berrios GE: Wilson's disease: psychiatric symptoms in 195 cases. Arch Gen Psychiatry 46:1126–1134, 1989

Devanand DP, Jacobs DM, Tang MX, et al: The course of psychopathologic features in mild to moderate Alzheimer's disease. Arch Gen Psychiatry 54:257–263, 1997

Dewey ME, Saz P: Dementia, cognitive impairment and mortality in persons aged 65 and over living in the community: a systematic review of literature. Int J Geriatr Psychiatry 16:751–761, 2001

Dewhurst K: The neurosyphilitic psychoses today: a survey of 91 cases. Br J Psychiatry 115:31–38, 1969

Dewhurst K, Oliver J, Trick KL, et al: Neuro-psychiatric aspects of Huntington's disease. Confin Neurol 31:258–268, 1969

Dodge HH, Shen C, Pandav R, et al: Functional transitions and active life expectancy associated with Alzheimer disease. Arch Neurol 60:253–259, 2003

Doody RS, Stevens JC, Beck C, et al: Practice parameter: management of dementia (an evidence-based review). Report of the Quality Standards Subcommittee of the American Academy of Neurology. Neurology 56:1154–1166, 2001 (EBM Reviews–ACP Journal Club abstract)

Doraiswamy PM, Leon J, Cummings JL, et al: Prevalence and impact of medical comorbidity in Alzheimer's disease. J Gerontol A Biol Sci Med Sci 57:M173–M177, 2002

Dubois B, Slachevsky A, Litvan I, et al: The FAB: a Frontal Assessment Battery at bedside. Neurology 55:1621–1626, 2000

Duyckaerts C, Verny M, Hauw JJ: Recent neuropathology of parkinsonian syndromes [in French]. Rev Neurol (Paris) 159 (5 pt 2): 3S11–3S18, 2003

Ellis RJ, Jan K, Kawas C, et al: Diagnostic validity of the dementia questionnaire for Alzheimer disease. Arch Neurol 55:360–365, 1998

Emery VO, Oxman TE: Update on the dementia spectrum of depression. Am J Psychiatry 149:305–317, 1992

Emre M: Dementia associated with Parkinson's disease. Lancet Neurol 2:229–237, 2003

Erkinjuntti T: Diagnosis and management of vascular cognitive impairment and dementia. J Neural Transm Suppl 63:91–109, 2002

Erkinjuntti T, Wikstrom J, Palo J, et al: Dementia among medical inpatients: evaluation of 2000 consecutive admissions. Arch Intern Med 146:1923–1926, 1986

Erkinjuntti T, Ostbye T, Steenhuis R, et al: The effect of different diagnostic criteria on the prevalence of dementia. N Engl J Med 337:1667–1674, 1997

Esmonde T, Cooke S: Shunting for normal pressure hydrocephalus (NPH) (Cochrane Review), in The Cochrane Library, Issue 2. Chichester, UK, Wiley, 2004

Esposito E, Rotilio D, Di Matteo V, et al: A review of specific dietary antioxidants and the effects on biochemical mechanisms related to neurodegenerative processes. Neurobiol Aging 23:719–735, 2002

Eustace A, Coen R, Walsh C, et al: A longitudinal evaluation of behavioural and psychological symptoms of probable Alzheimer's disease. Int J Geriatr Psychiatry 17:968–973, 2002

Faber R, Trimble MR: Electroconvulsive therapy in Parkinson's disease and other movement disorders. Mov Disord 6:293–303, 1991

Feldman H, Gauthier S, Hecker J, et al: A 24-week, randomized, double-blind study of donepezil in moderate to severe Alzheimer's disease. Neurology 57:613–620, 2001 (EBM Reviews–ACP Journal Club abstract)

Ferrer I, Puig B: Novedades neuropatológicas en la enfermedad de Alzheimer y en otras demencias afines. Papel de kinasas en taupatías y alpha-synucleinopathies, in Alzheimer 2003: ¿Qué hay de nuevo? Edited by Martínez Lage JM, Pascual LF. Madrid, Spain, Aula Médica, 2003, pp 21–34

Ferrer I, Barrachina M, Puig B: Glycogen synthase kinase-3 (GSK-3) is associated with neuronal and glial hyper-phosphorylated tau deposits in Alzheimer's disease, Pick's disease, progressive supranuclear palsy and corticobasal degeneration. Acta Neuropathol 104:583–591, 2002

Fioravanti M, Flicker L: Nicergoline for dementia and other age associated forms of cognitive impairment (Cochrane Review), in The Cochrane Library, Issue 2. Chichester, UK, Wiley, 2004

Flicker L, Grimley Evans J: Piracetam for dementia or cognitive impairment (Cochrane Review), in The Cochrane Library, Issue 2. Chichester, UK, Wiley, 2004

Folstein MF, McHugh PR: Dementia syndrome of depression, in Alzheimer's Disease: Senile Dementia and Related Disorders, Aging, Vol 7. Edited by Katzman R, Terry RD, Bick KL. New York, Raven, 1978, pp 87–93

Folstein MF, McHugh PR: The neuropsychiatry of some specific brain disorders, in Handbook of Psychiatry 2, Mental Disorders and Somatic Illness. Edited by Lader MH. London, Cambridge University Press, 1983, pp 107–118

Folstein MF, Folstein SE, McHugh PR: Mini-Mental State: a practical method for grading the cognitive state of patients for the clinician. J Psychiatr Res 12:189–198, 1975

Folstein MF, Maiberger R, McHugh PR: Mood disorder as a specific complication of stroke. J Neurol Neurosurg Psychiatry 40:1018–1020, 1977

Folstein MF, Folstein SE, McHugh PR, et al: MMSE: Mini-Mental State Examination: User's Guide. Odessa, FL, PAR Psychological Assessment Resources, 2001

Folstein SE, Folstein MF, McHugh PR: Psychiatric syndromes in Huntington's disease, in Advances in Neurology, Vol 23. Edited by Chase TN, Wexler NS, Barbeau A. New York, Raven, 1979, pp 281–289

Forette F, Seux M-L, Staessen JA, et al: Prevention of dementia in randomised double-blind placebo-controlled Systolic Hypertension in Europe (Syst-Eur) trial. Lancet 352:1347–1351, 1998

Forster A, Young J, Langhorne P, for the Day Hospital Group: Medical day hospital care for the elderly versus alternative forms of care (Cochrane Review), in The Cochrane Library, Issue 2. Chichester, UK, Wiley, 2004

Fratiglioni L, Launer LJ, Andersen K, et al: Incidence of dementia and major subtypes in Europe: a collaborative study of population-based cohorts. Neurology 54 (suppl 5):10–15, 2000

Freter S, Bergman H, Gold S, et al: Prevalence of potentially reversible dementias and actual reversibility in a memory clinic cohort. Can Med Assoc J 159:657–662, 1998

Frisoni GB, Govoni S, Geroldi C, et al: Gene dose of the epsilon 4 allele of apolipoprotein E and disease progression in sporadic late-onset Alzheimer's disease. Ann Neurol 37:596–604, 1995

Frisoni GB, Galluzzi S, Bresciani L, et al: Mild cognitive impairment with subcortical vascular features: clinical characteristics and outcome. J Neurol 249:1423–1432, 2002

Galasko DR, Gould RL, Abramson IS, et al: Measuring cognitive change in a cohort of patients with Alzheimer's disease. Stat Med 19:1421–1432, 2000

Giacometti AR, Davis PC, Alazraki NP, et al: Anatomic and physiologic imaging of Alzheimer's disease. Clin Geriatr 10:277–298, 1994

Gillen TE, Gregg KM, Yuan H, et al: Clinical trials in Alzheimer's disease: calculating Alzheimer's Disease Assessment Scale—cognitive subsection with the data from the Consortium to Establish a Registry for Alzheimer's Disease. Psychopharmacol Bull 35:83–96, 2001

Giron MS, Forsell Y, Bernsten C, et al: Psychotropic drug use in elderly people with and without dementia. Int J Geriatr Psychiatry 16:900–906, 2001

Goedert M: Neurofibrillary pathology of Alzheimer's disease and other tauopathies. Prog Brain Res 117:287–306, 1998

Graham DI, Adams JH, Gennarelli TA: Pathology of brain damage in head injury, in Head Injury, 2nd Edition. Edited by Cooper PR. Baltimore, MD, Williams & Wilkins, 1987, pp 72–88

Gray KF, Cummings JL: Dementia, in The American Psychiatric Publishing Textbook of Consultation-Liaison Psychiatry: Psychiatry in the Medically Ill, 2nd Edition. Edited by Wise MG, Rundell JR. Washington, DC, American Psychiatric Publishing, 2002, pp 273–306

Green CR, Mohs RC, Schmeidler J, et al: Functional decline in Alzheimer's disease: a longitudinal study. J Am Geriatr Soc 41:654–661, 1993

Greenamyre JT, Maragos WF, Albin RL, et al: Glutamate transmission and toxicity in Alzheimer's disease. Prog Neuropsychopharmacol Biol Psychiatry 12:421–430, 1988

Grutzendler J, Morris JC: Cholinesterase inhibitors for Alzheimer's disease. Drugs 61:41–52, 2001

Haskins BA, Harrison MB: Huntington's disease. Curr Treat Options Neurol 2:243–262, 2000

Hebert R, Lindsay J, Verreault R, et al: Vascular dementia: incidence and risk factors in the Canadian study of health and aging. Stroke 31:1487–1493, 2000

Hecaen H, De Ajuriagueria J: Troubles Mentaux au cours des Tumeurs Intracraniennes [Mental Disturbances in the Course of Intracranial Tumors]. Paris, France, Masson, 1956

Hejl A, Hogh P, Waldemar G: Potentially reversible conditions in 1000 consecutive memory clinic patients. J Neurol Neurosurg Psychiatry 73:390–394, 2002

Hierons R, Janota I, Corsellis JAN: The late effects of necrotising encephalitis of the temporal lobes and limbic areas: a clinico-pathological study of 10 cases. Psychol Med 8:21–42, 1978

Higgins JPT, Flicker L: Lecithin for dementia and cognitive impairment (Cochrane Review), in The Cochrane Library, Issue 2. Chichester, UK, Wiley, 2004

Hogervorst E, Yaffe K, Richards M, et al: Hormone replacement therapy to maintain cognitive function in women with dementia (Cochrane Review), in The Cochrane Library, Issue 2. Chichester, UK, Wiley, 2004

Hughes CP, Berg L, Danziger WL, et al: A new clinical scale for the staging of dementia. Br J Psychiatry 140:566–572, 1982

Huntington G: On chorea. Med Surg Rep 26:317–332, 1872

Huppert FA, Van Niekerk JK: Dehydroepiandrosterone (DHEA) supplementation for cognitive function (Cochrane Review), in The Cochrane Library, Issue 2. Chichester, UK, Wiley, 2004

Huyse FJ, Herzog T, Malt UF, et al: The European Consultation-Liaison Workgroup (ECLW) Collaborative Study, I: general outline. Gen Hosp Psychiatry 18:44–55, 1996

Innes A: The social and political context of formal dementia care provision. Ageing Soc 22:483–499, 2002

Iseki E, Togo T, Suzuki K, et al: Dementia with Lewy bodies from the perspective of tauopathy. Acta Neuropathol (Berl) 105:265–270, 2003

Jacobs D, Sano M, Marder K, et al: Age at onset of Alzheimer's disease: relation to pattern of cognitive dysfunction and rate of decline. Neurology 44:1215–1220, 1994

Jelic V, Winblad B: Treatment of mild cognitive impairment: rationale, present and future strategies. Acta Neurol Scand Suppl 179:83–93, 2003

Jones R, Laake K, Oeksengaard AR: D-Cycloserine for Alzheimer's disease (Cochrane Review), in The Cochrane Library, Issue 2. Chichester, UK, Wiley, 2004

Jorm AF: A short form of the Informant Questionnaire on Cognitive Decline in the Elderly (IQCODE): development and cross-validation. Psychol Med 24:145–153, 1994

Jorm AF: History of depression as a risk factor for dementia: an updated review. Aust N Z J Psychiatry 35:776–781, 2001

Jorm AF, Jacomb PA: The Informant Questionnaire on Cognitive Decline in the Elderly (IQCODE): socio-demographic correlates, reliability, validity and some norms. Psychol Med 19:1015–1022, 1989

Kalaria RN: The role of cerebral ischemia in Alzheimer's disease. Neurobiol Aging 21:321–330, 2000

Kasahara H, Karasawa A, Ariyasu T, et al: Alcohol dementia and alcohol delirium in aged alcoholics. Psychiatry Clin Neurosci 50:115–123, 1996

Katz S, Downs TD, Cash HR, et al: Progress in development of the index of ADL. Gerontologist 10:20–30, 1970

Kessler H, Bleich S, Falkai P, et al: [Homocysteine and dementia]. Fortschr Neurol Psychiatr 71:150–156, 2003

Khachaturian ZS: Diagnosis of Alzheimer's disease. Arch Neurol 42:1097–1105, 1985

Kirchner V, Kelly CA, Harvey RJ: Thioridazine for dementia (Cochrane Review), in The Cochrane Library, Issue 2. Chichester, UK, Wiley, 2004

Kraus JF, Sorenson SB: Epidemiology, in Neuropsychiatry of Traumatic Brain Injury. Edited by Silver JM, Yudofsky SC, Hales RE. Washington, DC, American Psychiatric Press, 1994, pp 3–41

Kril JJ, Harper CG: Neuronal counts from four cortical regions of alcoholic brains. Acta Neuropathol 79:200–204, 1989

Kukull WA, Higdon R, Bowen JD, et al: Dementia and Alzheimer disease incidence: a prospective cohort study. Arch Neurol 59:1737–1746, 2002

Kurz A, Riemenschneider M, Drzezga A, et al: The role of biological markers in the early and differential diagnosis of Alzheimer's disease. J Neural Transm Suppl 62:127–133, 2002

Larson EB, Kukull WA, Katzman RL: Cognitive impairment: dementia and Alzheimer's disease. Annu Rev Public Health 13:431–449, 1992

Lawton MP, Brody E: Assessment of older people: self-maintaining and instrumental activities of daily living. Gerontologist 9:179–186, 1969

Lebert F, Souliez L, Pasquier F, et al: Trazodone in the treatment of behavior in frontotemporal dementia. Hum Psychopharmacol Clin Exp 14:279–281, 1999

Lebert F, Delacourte A, Pasquier F: Treatment of frontotemporal dementia, in Alzheimer's Disease and Related Disorders Annual 2002. Edited by Gauthier S, Cummings JL. London, Taylor & Francis, 2002, pp 171–182

Lepola UM, Loft H, Reines EH: Escitalopram (10–20 mg/day) is effective and well tolerated in a placebo-controlled study in depression in primary care. Int Clin Psychopharmacol 18:211–217, 2003

Leroi I, Voulgari A, Breitner JC, et al: The epidemiology of psychosis in dementia. Am J Geriatr Psychiatry 11:83–91, 2003

Letenneur L, Launer LJ, Andersen K, et al: Education and the risk for Alzheimer´s disease: sex makes a difference. EURODEM pooled analyses. EURODEM Incidence Research Group. Am J Epidemiol 151:1064–1071, 2000

Lev N, Melamed E: Heredity in Parkinson's disease: new findings. Isr Med Assoc J 3:435–438, 2001

Levin HS: Memory deficit after closed-head injury. J Clin Exp Neuropsychol 12:129–153, 1989

Levy ML, Cummings JL, Fairbanks LA, et al: Longitudinal assessment of symptoms of depression, agitation, and psychosis in 181 patients with Alzheimer's disease. Am J Psychiatry 153:1438–1443, 1996

Levy-Lahad E, Wijsman EM, Nemens E, et al: A familial Alzheimer's disease locus on chromosome 1. Science 269:970–973, 1995

Lieberman A, Dziatolowski M, Neophytides A, et al: Dementias of Huntington's and Parkinson's disease, in Advances in Neurology, Vol 23. Edited by Chase TN, Wexler NS, Barbeau A. New York, Raven, 1979, pp 273–289

Lishman WA: Senile dementias, presenile dementias and pseudodementias, in Organic Psychiatry: The Psychological Consequences of Cerebral Disorder, 3rd Edition. London, Blackwell Science, 1998a, pp 450–453

Lishman WA: Senile dementias, presenile dementias and pseudodementias, in Organic Psychiatry: The Psychological Consequences of Cerebral Disorder, 3rd Edition. London, Blackwell Science, 1998b, pp 465–473

Lishman WA: Senile dementias, presenile dementias and pseudodementias, in Organic Psychiatry: The Psychological Consequences of Cerebral Disorder, 3rd Edition. London, Blackwell Science, 1998c, pp 480–483

Lithell H, Hansson L, Skoog I, et al: The Study on Cognition and Prognosis in the Elderly (SCOPE): principal results of a randomized double-blind intervention trial. J Hypertens 21:875–886, 2003

Litvan I: Recent advances in atypical parkinsonian disorders. Curr Opin Neurol 12:441–446, 1999

Liu CK, Miller BL, Cummings JL, et al: A quantitative MRI study of vascular dementia. Neurology 42:138–143, 1992

Lobo A, the European Consultation-Liaison Workgroup for General Hospital Psychiatry and Psychosomatics (ECLW): Delirium and dementia in European general hospitals. Paper presented at the VI Congress of the International Federation of Psychiatric Epidemiology, Lisbon, September 1993

Lobo A, Saz P: Clínica de la memoria y unidad de demencias: un programa de enlace con atención primaria [A memory clinic and dementia unit: a liaison program with primary care]. Cuadernos de Medicina Psicosomática (in press)

Lobo A, Saz P, Marcos G, et al: The prevalence of dementia and depression in the elderly community in a Southern European population: the Zaragoza study. Arch Gen Psychiatry 52:497–506, 1995

Lobo A, Saz P, Marcos G, et al: The Zaragoza Study: Dementia and Depression in the Elderly Community. Barcelona, Spain, Editorial Masson Salvat S.A., 1997

Lobo A, Saz P, Marcos G, et al: Revalidación y normalización del Mini-Examen Cognoscitivo (primera versión en castellano del Mini-Mental State Examination) en la población general geriátrica [Revalidation and standardization of the cognition mini-exam (first Spanish version of the Mini-Mental Status Examination) in the general geriatric population]. Med Clin (Barc) 112:767–774, 1999 [published erratum appears in Med Clin (Barc) 113:197, 1999]

Lobo A, Launer LJ, Fratiglioni L, et al: Prevalence of dementia and major subtypes in Europe: a collaborative study of population-based cohorts. Neurology 54 (suppl 5):4–9, 2000

Lonergan E, Luxenberg J, Colford J: Haloperidol for agitation in dementia (Cochrane Review), in The Cochrane Library, Issue 2. Chichester, UK, Wiley, 2004

López-Arrieta, Birks J: Nimodipine for primary degenerative, mixed and vascular dementia (Cochrane Review), in The Cochrane Library, Issue 2. Chichester, UK, Wiley, 2004

López-Arrieta JM, Rodriguez JL, Sanz F: Efficacy and safety of nicotine on Alzheimer's disease patients (Cochrane Review), in The Cochrane Library, Issue 1. Chichester, UK, Wiley, 2003

Loranger AW, Goodell H, McDowell FH, et al: Intellectual impairment in Parkinson's syndrome. Brain 95:405–412, 1972

Loudianos G, Gitlin JD: Wilson's disease. Semin Liver Dis 2:353–364, 2000

Lyketsos CG, Sheppard JM, Rabins PV: Dementia in elderly persons in a general hospital. Am J Psychiatry 157:704–707, 2000

Lyketsos CG, Breitner JC, Rabins PV: An evidence-based proposal for the classification of neuropsychiatric disturbance in Alzheimer's disease. Int J Geriatr Psychiatry 16:1037–1042, 2001

Lyketsos CG, Lopez O, Jones B, et al: Prevalence of neuropsychiatric symptoms in dementia and mild cognitive impairment: results from the Cardiovascular Health Study. JAMA 288:1475–1483, 2002

Lyketsos CG, DelCampo L, Steinberg M, et al: Treating depression in Alzheimer disease: efficacy and safety of sertraline therapy, and the benefits of depression reduction: the DIADS. Arch Gen Psychiatry 60:737–746, 2003

Macdonald AJ, Carpenter GI, Box O, et al: Dementia and use of psychotropic medication in non-"Elderly Mentally Infirm" nursing homes in South East England. Age Ageing 31:58–64, 2002

Mahendra B: Depression and dementia: the multi-faceted relationship. Psychol Med 15:227–236, 1985

Malt UF, Huyse FJ, Herzog T, et al: The ECLW Collaborative Study, III: training and reliability of ICD-10 psychiatric diagnoses in the general hospital setting—an investigation of 220 consultants from 14 European countries. J Psychosom Res 41:451–463, 1996

Mandell AM, Albert ML: History of subcortical dementia, in Subcortical Dementia. Edited by Cummings JL. New York, Oxford University Press, 1990, pp 17–30

Martin DC, Francis J, Protetch J, et al: Time dependency of cognitive recovery with cobalamin replacement: report of a pilot study. J Am Geriatr Soc 40:168–172, 1992

Martinot JL, Hardy P, Feline A, et al: Left prefrontal glucose hypometabolism in the depressed state: a confirmation. Am J Psychiatry 147:1313–1317, 1990

Maxwell CJ, Hogan DB, Ebly EM: Serum folate levels and subsequent adverse cerebrovascular outcomes in elderly persons. Dement Geriatr Cogn Disord 13:225–234, 2002

Mayeux R, Sano M: Treatment of Alzheimer's disease. N Engl J Med 341:1670–1679, 1999

McAllister TW: Neuropsychiatric sequelae of head injuries. Psychiatr Clin North Am 15:395–413, 1992

McConnell LM, Sanders GD, Owens DK: Evaluation of genetic tests: APOE genotyping for the diagnosis of Alzheimer disease. Genet Test 3:47–53, 1999

McDowell I: Alzheimer's disease: insights from epidemiology. Aging (Milano) 13:143–162, 2001

McDowell I, Kristjansson B, Hill GB, et al: Community screening for dementia: the Mini Mental State Exam (MMSE) and Modified Mini-Mental State Exam (3MS) compared. J Clin Epidemiol 50:377–383, 1997

McHugh PR: Occult hydrocephalus. Q J Med 33:297–308, 1964

McHugh PR: Hydrocephalic dementia. Bull N Y Acad Med 42:907–917, 1966

McHugh PR, Folstein MF: Psychiatric syndromes of Huntington's chorea: a clinical and phenomenologic study, in Psychiatric Aspects of Neurologic Disease. Edited by Benson DF, Blumer D. New York, Grune & Stratton, 1975, pp 267–285

McHugh PR, Folstein MF: Psychopathology of dementia: implications for neuropathology, in Congenital and Acquired Cognitive Disorders. Edited by Katzman R. New York, Raven, 1979, pp 17–30

McHugh PR, Slavney PR: The Perspectives of Psychiatry. Baltimore, MD, Johns Hopkins University Press, 1998

McKeith I, Fairburn A, Perry R, et al: Neuroleptic sensitivity in patients with senile dementia of Lewy body type. BMJ 305:673–678, 1992

McKeith IG, Galasko D, Kosaka K, et al: Consensus guidelines for the clinical and pathologic diagnosis of dementia with Lewy bodies (DLB): report of the Consortium on DLB International Workshop. Neurology 47:1113–1124, 1996

McKeith I, Del Ser T, Spano P, et al: Efficacy of rivastigmine in dementia with Lewy bodies: a randomised, double-blind, placebo-controlled international study. Lancet 356:2031–2036, 2000

McKhann G, Drachman D, Folstein M, et al: Clinical diagnosis of Alzheimer's disease: report of the NINCDS–ADRDA Work Group under the auspices of Department of Health and Human Services Task Force on Alzheimer's Disease. Neurology 34:939–944, 1984

McShane R, Gedling D, Reasing M, et al: A prospective study of psychotic symptoms in dementia sufferers: psychosis in dementia. Int Psychogeriatr 9:57–64, 1997

Meier DE, Ahronheim JC, Morris J, et al: High short-term mortality in hospitalized patients with advanced dementia: lack of benefit of tube feeding. Arch Intern Med 161:594–599, 2001

Mesulam MM: Primary progressive aphasia—a language-based dementia. N Engl J Med 349:1535–1542, 2003

Miller LJ: Gabapentin for treatment of behavioral and psychological symptoms of dementia. Ann Pharmacother 35:427–431, 2001

Mintzer MJ: Hypothyroidism and hyperthyroidism in the elderly. J Fla Med Assoc 79:231–235, 1992

Mohs RC, Schmeidler J, Aryan M: Longitudinal studies of cognitive, functional and behavioral change in patients with Alzheimer's disease. Stat Med 19:1401–1409, 2000

Montgomery SA, Thal LJ, Amrein R: Meta-analysis of double blind randomized controlled clinical trials of acetyl-L-carnitine versus placebo in the treatment of mild cognitive impairment and mild Alzheimer's disease. Int Clin Psychopharmacol 18:61–71, 2003

Mori E: Impact of subcortical ischemic lesions on behavior and cognition. Ann N Y Acad Sci 977:141–148, 2002

Morris RG, Morris LW, Britton PG: Factors affecting the emotional wellbeing of the caregivers of dementia sufferers. Br J Psychiatry 153:147–156, 1988

Mortimer JA, Ebbitt B, Jun SP, et al: Predictors of cognitive and functional progression in patients with probable Alzheimer's disease. Neurology 42:1689–1696, 1992

Motsinger CD, Perron GA, Lacy TJ: Use of atypical antipsychotic drugs in patients with dementia. Am Fam Physician 67:2335–2340, 2003

Nagaraja D, Jayashree S: Randomized study of the dopamine receptor agonist piribedil in the treatment of mild cognitive impairment. Am J Psychiatry 158:1517–1519, 2001

Neal M, Briggs M: Validation therapy for dementia (Cochrane Review), in The Cochrane Library, Issue 2. Chichester, UK, Wiley, 2004

Neary D, Snowden JS, Gustafson L, et al: Frontotemporal lobar degeneration: a consensus on the clinical diagnostic criteria. Neurology 51:1546–1554, 1998

Norup PW, Kufahl JW, Feilberg JB, et al: [The incidence of reversible dementia in 145 patients referred on suspicion of dementia]. Ugeskr Laeger 164:4934–4937, 2002

O'Brien J, Thomas A, Ballard C, et al: Cognitive impairment in depression is not associated with neuropathologic evidence of increased vascular or Alzheimer-type pathology. Biol Psychiatry 49:130–136, 2001

O'Brien JT, Erkinjuntti T, Reisberg B, et al: Vascular cognitive impairment. Lancet Neurol 2:89–98, 2003

Olin J, Schneider L: Galantamine for Alzheimer's disease. Cochrane Database Syst Rev (3):CD001747, 2002 (EBM Reviews–ACP Journal Club abstract)

Olin JT, Fox LS, Pawluczyk S, et al: A pilot randomized trial of carbamazepine for behavioural symptoms in treatment-resistant outpatients with Alzheimer disease. Am J Geriatr Psychiatry 9:400–405, 2001

Organization for Economic Cooperation and Development (OECD): Case Study on Dementia Care. OECD Report. Paris (in press)

Ory MG, Hoffman RR 3rd, Yee JL, et al: Prevalence and impact of caregiving: a detailed comparison between dementia and nondementia caregivers. Gerontologist 39:177–185, 1999

Ovsiew F: Seeking reversibility and treatability in dementia. Semin Clin Neuropsychiatry 8:3–11, 2003

Palmer K, Fratiglioni L, Winblad B: What is mild cognitive impairment? Variations in definitions and evolution of nondemented persons with cognitive impairment. Acta Neurol Scand Suppl 179:14–20, 2003

Pantoni L, Garcia JH: The significance of cerebral white matter abnormalities 100 years after Binswanger's report: a review. Stroke 26:1293–1301, 1995

Patterson CJS, Gauthier S, Bergman H, et al: The recognition, assessment and management of dementing disorders: conclusions from the Canadian Consensus Conference on Dementia. Can Med Assoc J 160 (suppl 12):S1–S15, 1999

Paulsen JS, Salmon DP, Thal LJ: Incidence of and risk factors for hallucinations and delusions in patients with probable AD. Neurology 54:1965–1971, 2000

Pearlson RCA, Powell TPS: The neuroanatomy of Alzheimer's disease. Rev Neurosci 2:101–122, 1989

Perry EK, Kerwin J, Perry RH, et al: Cerebral cholinergic activity is related to the incidence of visual hallucinations in senile dementia of Lewy body type. Dementia 1:2–4, 1990

Perry S, Jacobsen P: Neuropsychiatric manifestations of AIDS-spectrum disorders. Hosp Community Psychiatry 37:135–142, 1986

Perry TL, Hansen S, Kloster M: Huntington's chorea: deficiency of gamma-aminobutyric acid in brain. N Engl J Med 288:337–342, 1973

Petersen RC, Smith GE, Ivnik RJ, et al: Memory function in very early Alzheimer's disease. Neurology 44:867–872, 1994

Petersen RC, Doody R, Kurz A, et al: Current concepts in mild cognitive impairment. Arch Neurol 58:1985–1992, 2001a

Petersen RC, Stevens JC, Ganguli M, et al: Practice parameter: early detection of dementia: mild cognitive impairment (an evidence-based review). Report of the Quality Standards Subcommittee of the American Academy of Neurology. Neurology 56:1133–1142, 2001b

Plum AF: Dementia: an approaching epidemic. Nature 279:372–373, 1979

Posner HB, Tang MX, Luchsinger J, et al: The relationship of hypertension in the elderly to AD, vascular dementia, and cognitive function. Neurology 58:1175–1181, 2002

Price JD, Hermans DG, Grimley Evans J: Subjective barriers to prevent wandering of cognitively impaired people (Cochrane Review), in The Cochrane Library, Issue 2. Chichester, UK, Wiley, 2004

Prusiner SB: Shattuck Lecture: neurodegenerative diseases and prions. N Engl J Med 344:1516–1526, 2001

Rabins PV: Reversible dementia and the misdiagnosis of dementia: a review. Hosp Community Psychiatry 34:830–835, 1983

Rabins PV, Merchan A, Nestadt G: Criteria for diagnosing reversible dementia caused by depression: validation by 2-year follow-up. Br J Psychiatry 144:488–492, 1984

Rabins PV, Lyketsos CG, Steele C: Practical Dementia Care. New York, Oxford University Press, 1999

Rands G, Orrel M, Spector A, et al: Aspirin for vascular dementia (Cochrane Review), in The Cochrane Library, Issue 2. Chichester, UK, Wiley, 2004

Rapcsak SZ, Croswell SC, Rubens AB: Apraxia in Alzheimer's disease. Neurology 39:664–668, 1989

Reed TE, Chandler JH: Huntington's chorea in Michigan, I: demography and genetics. Am J Hum Genet 10:201–225, 1958

Reichman WE, Cummings JL: Diagnosis of rare dementia syndromes: an algorithmic approach. J Geriatr Psychiatry Neurol 3:73–84, 1990

Reisberg B, Ferris SH, de Leon MJ, et al: The Global Deterioration Scale for assessment of primary degenerative dementia. Am J Psychiatry 139:1136–1139, 1982

Reisberg B, Sclan SG, Franssen E, et al: Clinical stages of normal aging and Alzheimer's disease: the GDS staging system. Neurosci Res Commun 13 (suppl 1):551–554, 1993

Reisberg B, Ferris SH, Franssen EH, et al: Mortality and temporal course of probable Alzheimer's disease: a five-year prospective study. Int Psychogeriatr 8:291–311, 1996

Reisberg B, Burns A, Brodaty H, et al: Diagnosis of Alzheimer's disease: report of an International Psychogeriatric Association Special Meeting Work Group Under the Cosponsorship of Alzheimer's Disease International, the European Federation of Neurological Societies, the World Health Organization, and the World Psychiatric Association. Int Psychogeriatr 9 (suppl 1): 11–38, 1997

Reisberg B, Doody R, Stoffler A, et al: Memantine in moderate-to-severe Alzheimer's disease. N Engl J Med 348:1333–1341, 2003

Rice DP, Fox PJ, Max W, et al: The economic burden of Alzheimer's disease care. Health Aff (Millwood) 12:164–176, 1993

Robinson RG: Neuropsychiatric consequences of stroke. Annu Rev Med 48:217–229, 1997

Robinson RG: Treatment of poststroke depression, in The Clinical Neuropsychiatry of Stroke. Edited by Robinson RG. Cambridge, UK, Cambridge University Press, 1998, pp 282–294

Robinson RG, Parikh RM, Lipsey JR, et al: Pathological laughing and crying following stroke: validation of a measurement scale and a double-blind treatment study. Am J Psychiatry 150:286–293, 1993

Rocca WA, Kokmen E: Frequency and distribution of vascular dementia. Alzheimer Dis Assoc Disord 13 (suppl 3):S9–S14, 1999

Rojas-Fernández CH, Eng M, Allie ND: Pharmacologic management by clinical pharmacists of behavioral and psychological symptoms of dementia in nursing home residents: results from a pilot study. Pharmacotherapy 23:217–221, 2003

Roman GC: Vascular dementia revisited: diagnosis, pathogenesis, treatment, and prevention. Med Clin North Am 86:477–499, 2002

Roman GC, Tatemichi TK, Erkinjuntti T, et al: Vascular dementia: diagnostic criteria for research studies. Report on the NINDS-AIREN International Workshop. Neurology 43:250–260, 1993

Rosen HJ, Lengenfelder J, Miller B: Frontotemporal dementia. Neurol Clin 18:979–992, 2000

Rosen WG: Clinical and neuropsychological assessment of Alzheimer disease, in The Dementias. Edited by Melnick VL, Dubler NN. New York, Raven, 1983, pp 51–64

Rosen WG, Mohs RC, Davis KL: A new rating scale for Alzheimer's disease. Am J Psychiatry 141:1356–1364, 1984

Rösler M, Anand R, Cicin-Sain A, et al: Efficacy and safety of rivastigmine in patients with Alzheimer's disease: international randomised controlled trial. BMJ 318:633–640, 1999 (EBM Reviews–ACP Journal Club abstract)

Ryan JM, Kidder SW, Daiello LA, et al: Psychopharmacological interventions in nursing homes: what do we know and where should we go? Psychiatr Serv 53:1407–1413, 2002

Sachon C, Grimaldi A, Digy JP, et al: Cognitive function, insulin-dependent diabetes and hypoglycaemia. J Intern Med 231:471–475, 1992

Salzman C: Treatment of the agitation of late-life psychosis and Alzheimer's disease. Eur Psychiatry 16 (suppl 1):25S–28S, 2001

Sandyk R: Aggressive dementia in normal pressure hydrocephalus. S Afr Med J 65:114, 1984

Saravay SM, Lavin M: Psychiatric comorbidity and length of stay in the general hospital: a critical review of outcome studies. Psychosomatics 35:233–252, 1994

Sarazin M, Horne N, Dubois B: Natural history of Alzheimer's disease and other dementing illnesses, in Alzheimer's Disease and Related Disorders Annual. Edited by Gauthier S, Cummings JL. London, Taylor & Francis, 2002, pp 183–197

Scharf MB, Saskin P, Fletcher K: Benzodiazepine-induced amnesia: clinical laboratory findings. J Clin Psychiatry 5 (monograph):14–17, 1987

Schellenberg GD, Bird TD, Wijsman EM, et al: Genetic linkage evidence for a familial Alzheimer's disease locus on chromosome 14. Science 258:668–671, 1992

Schmeidler J, Mohs RC, Aryan M: Relationship of disease severity to decline on specific cognitive and functional measures in Alzheimer disease. Alzheimer Dis Assoc Disord 12:146–151, 1998

Schneider J, Murray J, Banerjee S, et al: EUROCARE: a cross-national study of co-resident spouse carers for people with Alzheimer's disease, I: factors associated with carer burden. Int J Geriatr Psychiatry 14:651–661, 1999

Schneider LS, Olin JT: Overview of clinical trials of hydergine in dementia. Arch Neurol 51:787–798, 1994 (EBM Reviews–ACP Journal Club abstract)

Scott HD, Laake K: Statins for the prevention of Alzheimer's disease (Cochrane Review), in The Cochrane Library, Issue 2. Chichester, UK, Wiley, 2004

Skoldenberg B: Herpes simplex encephalitis. Scand J Infect Dis Suppl 80:40–46, 1991

Smith GE, O'Brien PC, Ivnik RJ, et al: Prospective analysis of risk factors for nursing home placement of dementia patients. Neurology 57:1467–1473, 2001

Snowdon DA, Greiner LH, Mortimer JA, et al: Brain infarction and the clinical expression of Alzheimer disease: the Nun Study. JAMA 277:813–817, 1997

Spar JE, La Rue A: Concise Guide to Geriatric Psychiatry, 3rd Edition. Washington, DC, American Psychiatric Publishing, 2002

Spector A, Orrell M, Davies S, et al: Reality orientation for dementia (Cochrane Review), in The Cochrane Library, Issue 2. Chichester, UK, Wiley, 2004a

Spector A, Orrell M, Davies S, et al: Reminiscence therapy for dementia (Cochrane Review), in The Cochrane Library, Issue 2. Chichester, UK, Wiley, 2004b

Starkstein SE, Chemerinski E, Sabe L, et al: Prospective longitudinal study of depression and anosognosia in Alzheimer's disease. Br J Psychiatry 171:47–52, 1997

Starosta-Rubinstein S: Treatment of Wilson's disease, in Treatment of Movement Disorders. Edited by Kurlan R. Philadelphia, PA, JB Lippincott, 1995, pp 663–664

Starosta-Rubinstein S, Young AB, Kluin K, et al: Clinical assessment of 31 patients with Wilson's disease. Arch Neurol 44:365–370, 1987

Steele C, Rovner B, Chase GA, et al: Psychiatric symptoms and nursing home placement of patients with Alzheimer's disease. Am J Psychiatry 147:1049–1051, 1990

Stern Y, Tang MX, Albert MS, et al: Predicting time to nursing home care and death in individuals with Alzheimer disease. JAMA 277:806–812, 1997

Stoppe G, Brandt CA, Staedt JH: Behavioral problems associated with dementia: the role of newer antipsychotics. Drugs Aging 14:41–54, 1999

Stuss DT, Stethem LL, Hugenholtz H, et al: Reaction time after head injury: fatigue, divided and focused attention, and consistency of performance. J Neurol Neurosurg Psychiatry 52:742–748, 1989

Swartz JR, Miller BL, Lesser IM, et al: Frontotemporal dementia: treatment response to serotonin selective reuptake inhibitors. J Clin Psychiatry 58:212–216, 1997

Tabet N, Feldman H: Indomethacin for Alzheimer's disease (Cochrane Review), in The Cochrane Library, Issue 2. Chichester, UK, Wiley, 2004

Tabet N, Birks J, Grimley Evans J, et al: Vitamin E for Alzheimer's disease (Cochrane Review), in The Cochrane Library, Issue 2. Chichester, UK, Wiley, 2004

Takahashi H, Yoshida K, Sugita T, et al: Quetiapine treatment of psychotic symptoms and aggressive behavior in patients with dementia with Lewy bodies: a case series. Prog Neuropsychopharmacol Biol Psychiatry 27:549–553, 2003

Tariot PN, Farlow MR, Grossberg GT, et al: Memantine Study Group: memantine treatment in patients with moderate to severe Alzheimer disease already receiving donepezil: a randomized controlled trial. JAMA 291:317–324, 2004

Teng EL, Chui HC: The Modified Mini-Mental State (3MS) Examination. J Clin Psychiatry 48:314–318, 1987

Teri L: Training families to provide care: effects on people with dementia. Int J Geriatr Psychiatr 14:110–116, discussion 116–119, 1999

Tombaugh TN, McIntyre NJ: The Mini-Mental State Examination: a comprehensive review. J Am Geriatr Soc 40:922–935, 1992

Tuokko H, Frerichs R, Graham J, et al: Five-year follow-up of cognitive impairment with no dementia. Arch Neurol 60:577–582, 2003

Van Gorp WG, Hinken C, Satz P, et al: Subtypes of HIV-related neuropsychological functioning: a cluster analysis approach. Neuropsychology 7:62–72, 1993

Verghese J, Lipton RB, Katz MJ, et al: Leisure activities and the risk of dementia in the elderly. N Engl J Med 348:2508–2516, 2003

Vermeer SE, Prins ND, den Heijer T, et al: Silent brain infarcts and the risk of dementia and cognitive decline. N Engl J Med 348:1215–1222, 2003

Von Einsiedel RW, Fife TD, Aksamit AJ, et al: Progressive multifocal leukoencephalopathy in AIDS: a clinicopathologic study and review of the literature. J Neurol 240:391–406, 1993

Wahlund LO, Pihlstrand E, Jonhagen ME: Mild cognitive impairment: experience from a memory clinic. Acta Neurol Scand Suppl 179:21–24, 2003

Walker Z, Allen R, Shergill S, et al: Three years survival in patients with a clinical diagnosis of dementia with Lewy bodies. Int J Geriatr Psychiatry 15:267–273, 2000

Welsh KA, Butters B, Hughes JP, et al: Detection and staging of dementia of Alzheimer's disease: use of the neuropsychological measures developed for the Consortium to Establish a Registry for Alzheimer's Disease. Arch Neurol 49:448–452, 1992

Weytingh MD, Bossuyt PM, van Crevel H: Reversible dementia: more than 10% or less than 1%? A quantitative review. J Neurol 242:466–471, 1995

Whatley SA, Anderton BH: The genetics of Alzheimer's disease. Int J Geriatr Psychiatry 5:145–159, 1990

Will RG, Ironside JW, Zeidler M, et al: A new variant of Creutzfeldt-Jacob disease in the UK. Lancet 347:921–925, 1996

Wilson JMG, Junger G: The Principles and Practice of Screening for Disease (Public Health Papers No 34). Geneva, Switzerland, World Health Organization, 1968

Wolf H, Jelic V, Gertz HJ, et al: A critical discussion of the role of neuroimaging in mild cognitive impairment. Acta Neurol Scand Suppl 179:52–76, 2003

Wolfson C, Wolfson DB, Asgharian M, et al: A reevaluation of the duration of survival after the onset of dementia. N Engl J Med 344:1111–1116, 2001

World Health Organization: Dementia in Later Life: Research and Action: Report of WHO Scientific Group on Senile Dementia (Technical Reports Series). Geneva, World Health Organization, 1985

World Health Organization: Report of the Second Consultation on the Neuropsychiatric Aspects of HIV-1 Infection, Global Programme on AIDS, Geneva, Annex 3 (Ref No WHO/GPA/MNH 90.1). Geneva, World Health Organization, 1990

World Health Organization: The ICD-10 Classification of Mental and Behavioural Disorders: Clinical Descriptions and Diagnostic Guidelines. Geneva, World Health Organization, 1992

Yoshitake T, Kiyohara Y, Kato I, et al: Incidence and risk factors of vascular dementia and Alzheimer's disease in a defined elderly Japanese population: the Hisayama Study. Neurology 45:1161–1168, 1995

Zakzanis KK, Andrikopoulos J, Young DA, et al: Neuropsychological differentiation of late-onset schizophrenia and dementia of the Alzheimer's type. Appl Neuropsychol 10:105–114, 2003a

Zakzanis KK, Graham SJ, Campbell Z: A meta-analysis of structural and functional brain imaging in dementia of the Alzheimer's type: a neuroimaging profile. Neuropsychol Rev 13:1–18, 2003b

Zola-Morgan S, Squire LR, Amaral DG: Human amnesia and the medial temporal region: enduring memory impairment following a bilateral lesion limited to the CA1 field of the hippocampus. J Neurosci 6:2950–2967, 1986

Zubenko GS, Zubenko WN, McPherson S, et al: A collaborative study of the emergence and clinical features of the major depressive syndrome of Alzheimer's disease. Am J Psychiatry 160:857–866, 2003

8 Aggression and Violence

Chiadi U. Onyike, M.D., M.H.S.

Constantine G. Lyketsos, M.D., M.H.S.

AGGRESSION IS UBIQUITOUS in human societies. As an adaptive behavior, it serves the social expression of drives and feelings that are intimately connected with survival needs. It is a complex socialized behavior associated with motivations such as self-preservation (which includes protection of offspring), retaliation, material advantage, and power. Thus, in some circumstances, aggression represents the expression of appetitive drives, and in others, it represents defensive behaviors. From an "everyday" perspective, aggressive behaviors range from assertiveness to coercion (including the use of force) and from hostile attitudes and verbal abuse to threats, belligerence, and violence.

Generally, psychiatry is concerned with forms of aggression that can be attributed to medical or psychological disorders. Even within this narrower context, aggression still encompasses a broad range of behaviors. In this chapter, we cover those aggressive behaviors that are associated with psychiatric, neurological, and general medical conditions. The focus is on fear-inducing and violent behavior: hostility, verbal abuse, and physically aggressive behavior—actions that threaten or inflict harm on an individual or an object. Definitions of aggression, violence, and related terms used in this chapter are presented in Table 8–1. Although most aggression involves intent to harm, the definition used in this chapter does not require such intent because clinically important aggressive behavior can occur in the absence of demonstrable intent—especially in patients with cognitive impairments, delirium, dementia, or mental retardation. Not included here are behaviors that may be characterized as *agitation*, such as nonthreatening verbal outbursts, oppositional and resistive behaviors, intrusiveness, restlessness, pacing, and other aberrant motor behaviors. We do not deal with community violence (e.g., riots, war, terrorism) or criminality.

TABLE 8–1.	Terms used in this chapter
Aggression	Hostile, threatening, and violent behaviors directed at another person or objects, often with no (or trivial) provocation
Violence	Overt physical aggression directed at another person or object
Domestic violence	A continuum of behaviors directed against an intimate partner, ranging from verbal abuse, to threats and intimidation, to sexual assault and violence
Agitation	A state of pathologically intense emotional arousal and motor restlessness
Disinhibition	A behavioral state in which ability of the individual to preemptively evaluate and inhibit behavioral responses is decreased or lost
Impulsivity	A behavioral state characterized by a proneness to act without thought or self-restraint; a habitual tendency toward "hair trigger" actions
Irritability	A state of abnormally low tolerance in which the individual is easily provoked to anger and hostility

Psychiatrists primarily encounter aggression and violence when patients present for treatment in acute states. Aggression occurs as a complication of psychiatric states such as delusional psychoses, dementia, agitated delirium, intoxication, personality disorder (especially conduct, antisocial, borderline, and narcissistic types), and even adjustment disorder. Aggression also may complicate many nonpsychiatric illnesses because it can occur when patients feel disregarded, dissatisfied, frustrated, confused, frightened, thwarted, unable to convey concerns, and angry at perceived unfairness or mistreatment or as a "primary" symptom of the illness. Aggression can manifest in males and females, at any age (except in early infancy), and is seen in all patient care settings—outpatient clinics, inpatient units, rehabilitation programs, residential and custodial care facilities, nursing homes, and emergency departments. Aggressive behavior can result in involuntary confinement (in hospitals and jails), disruption of clinical and custodial care environments, longer hospital stays, and physical injury to patients and their caregivers (family and paid caregivers) and health care professionals. Family, paid caregivers, and health care professionals who are repeatedly exposed to aggression often experience demoralization, which leads to a diminished quality of care for patients.

In this chapter, we focus on aggression and violence in the medically ill, beginning with the epidemiology of aggressive and violent behaviors in diverse clinical settings, including risk factors and the causes and precipitants of aggression; we use the epidemiological causal model of *host*, *agent*, and *environment*. Next, we review the evaluation, formulation, and differential diagnosis of aggression. We conclude with a review of the management of aggressive behavior in the general hospital setting, including the emergency department. The content of this chapter is based on empirical evidence, existing care standards, and clinical experience.

Epidemiology

Violence is common among individuals with psychiatric disorders. In a population-based study from the National Institute of Mental Health Epidemiologic Catchment Area project, 55.5% of the respondents who reported violent behavior in the past year had a psychiatric diagnosis, compared with 19.6% of the nonviolent respondents (Swanson et al. 1990). Only 2.7% of the men and 1.1% of the women without a psychiatric diagnosis reported any violent behavior, compared with 8.9%–21.1% of the men and 3.3%–21.7% of the women with a psychiatric diagnosis; the association was lowest for anxiety disorders and highest for substance use disorders, major affective disorders, and schizophrenia. Having more than one psychiatric diagnosis increased the likelihood of violent behavior in this study; this likelihood increased with each additional diagnosis. However, other data indicate that violence is not the inevitable outcome of mental illness. For example, judging from self-reports by United States community residents, only 4% of the risk for violence can be explained by major mental illness (Swanson 1994).

Most patients with mental illness are not violent, but aggressive and violent subgroups exist. Violent behavior is associated with specific conditions, such as schizophrenia, major depressive disorders, substance abuse, personality disorders (antisocial and borderline), dementia, and traumatic brain injury, as well as with specific states, such as confusion, intoxication (with alcohol or other substances), akathisia, fearfulness, agitation, *paranoid* delusions, and *command* hallucinations (Eronen et al. 1998; Kalunian et al. 1990; Lyketsos 2000; McNiel et al. 2000; Raja et al. 1997; Sheridan et al. 1990; Soyka 2000; Swanson et al. 1997). The mere presence of delusions does not necessarily increase the risk for violent behavior (Appelbaum et al. 2000); however, psychotic illness concurrent with substance use appears to increase synergistically the risk for violent behavior (Scott et al. 1998; Soyka 2000).

Although men are generally more aggressive than women, the gender gap in the frequency and severity of aggressive behavior narrows among individuals with major mental illness and disappears among psychiatric inpatients and patients recently evaluated in an emergency department (Lam et al. 2000; Newhill et al. 1995). Other psychosocial correlates of aggression include younger age, onset of psychiatric illness at a younger age, previous violence, longer duration of hospitalization, and treatment nonadherence and resistance—particularly among patients with psychotic illness (Binder 1999; Ehmann et al. 2001; Swartz et al. 1998; Torrey 1994). Environmental factors such as overcrowding, rigid limits and rules, and staff attitude (Lancee et al. 1995; Ng et al. 2001; Owen et al. 1998; Palmstierna et al. 1991) may predispose psychiatric inpatients to anger and violence. In addition, the patient's background contributes powerfully to the development and expression of violent behavior (Volavka 1999). Social maladjustment and impaired functioning also can accentuate the background risk for aggression and violence, particularly in patients with psychotic illness (Swanson et al. 1998).

All health care professionals, regardless of training and specialty, may encounter aggressive, violent patients. Aggression is observed in all ambulatory, hospital, and custodial (or residential) settings, although the frequency generally varies according to the specific population (i.e., diagnostic mix and acuity levels) and the characteristics of the setting (e.g., crowding, staffing levels). Within settings, the frequency of violence may vary by specific diagnosis, mode of presentation of the patient, illness acuity, and stage of illness. For example, aggression may be more frequent in the immediate postoperative period in surgical settings.

In an analysis of data from consecutive medical emergency calls in a 1-month period, emergency medical service (EMS) personnel were reported to have observed aggression in about 8.5% of encounters (Grange and

Corbett 2002). About half of these episodes were directed at these personnel (rather than at other individuals in the setting), with violence constituting 80% of this directed aggression. Patients were responsible for 90% of the directed aggression (relatives and other bystanders were responsible for the remainder). In adjusted analyses, higher relative odds of aggression were observed in encounters that involved males, police presence, street gangs, suspected psychiatric disorder, and abuse of alcohol or other substances. Clearly, EMS personnel may be victims of violence; because they must stabilize and transport these patients to the emergency department, they are at high risk for injury and psychological stress. In a questionnaire survey of a convenience sample of EMS personnel in California (67% response rate, with members of law enforcement excluded from the analysis), 95% reported having to restrain a patient, and 61% reported ever being assaulted (25% of whom were injured by the assault) (Corbett et al. 1998). Other studies have reported similar or higher prevalence estimates of assault and injury (Mock et al. 1998; Pozzi 1998; Tintinalli and McCoy 1993).

The incidence of violence in the EMS setting (as estimated by reviewing call records) was reported to be about 0.8% of all encounters in a 6-month period (Tintinalli and McCoy 1993), but these data were also limited by the use of a convenience sample and reporting biases. Most commentators agree that exposure to aggression among these workers is frequently compounded by their limited formal training on how to manage aggressive patients and lack of counseling in the aftermath of an assault. Fortunately, the relevant training needs of EMS personnel are beginning to be addressed through journals and other media and the development of a comprehensive training curriculum by the U.S. Department of Transportation (1998).

Aggressive and violent episodes are also common in the emergency department. For many patients, their agitation, aggressiveness, or violent behavior may be the reason that they have been brought to the emergency department, whereas for others who were not agitated or aggressive on arrival, threatening and violent behavior may develop as a result of their acute condition or other factors. Although the data are limited, results from several surveys of large emergency departments (with volumes of 40,000 or more cases annually) indicate that several episodes of staff being threatened by patients occur daily, the use of restraints is frequently indicated, and nearly 50% of these facilities experience at least one episode of staff assault each month—up to 25% of the assaults result in staff injury (Blanchard and Curtis 1999). Although health professionals (particularly nurses) are typ-

ically the victims of patient aggression, sometimes a visitor or another patient is assaulted. In some cases, a family member or other visitor, not the patient, is the perpetrator of an aggressive act. Violence in the emergency department is associated with a wide variety of motivations, predisposing factors, and precipitants. These determinants include the following:

- Patient factors, such as intoxication with substances of abuse, presence of psychiatric disorders (including personality disorders), transport to the hospital involuntarily, negative perceptions of hospital staff, and possession of a weapon at presentation
- Staff factors, such as impoliteness, insensitivity, and inadequate training
- Environmental factors, such as high noise levels, overcrowding, and uncomfortable waiting rooms
- System factors, such as high patient volumes, prolonged waiting and throughput times, inadequate security staff, and absent or inadequate formal training in the management of hostile and aggressive patients

Aggression is also common beyond the emergency department and occurs in a variety of inpatient settings. Of the estimated 20% of hospital staff assaulted by patients, up to 90% of violent incidents directed at hospital staff may occur beyond the emergency department (i.e., on inpatient units) (Whittington et al. 1996). In hospitalized patients, aggressive acts may occur as features or complications of confusion associated with the patients' primary conditions (e.g., thyroid storm, head injuries, hypoxia, encephalitis) or administered treatments (e.g., benzodiazepines or corticosteroids) or may result from co-occurring mental illness. On surgical units, aggression may result from confusion occurring in the immediate postoperative period, undiagnosed alcohol withdrawal, or inadequately controlled postoperative pain. Aggression in the general hospital may also evolve from patients' dissatisfaction with care or frustration from unfulfilled wants and expectations or during patient–staff conflicts.

In a recently reported survey of intensive care units (ICUs) in England and Wales, nurses were subjected to verbal hostility by patients in 87% of the ICUs and by patients' relatives in 74% (Lynch et al. 2003). Nurses were physically assaulted by patients in 77% of the ICUs and by relatives in 17%; rates of hostility and assault directed at physicians were moderately lower. Medical illness severity was associated with aggression committed by patients, whereas emotional distress, alcohol abuse, and sociopathic traits were associated with aggression committed by relatives. A similar pattern of aggressive behaviors may be seen on general medical and surgical wards, although the frequency of aggressive behaviors (particularly those committed by relatives) is likely to be lower.

Substance abuse and sociopathic traits among inpatients may contribute more to aggressive behaviors expressed in hospital wards (as compared with aggression expressed in ICUs). Substance abusers who have a withdrawal syndrome or intense cravings are frequent perpetrators of in-hospital aggression. Even nicotine can be a factor: smokers are no longer allowed to smoke in hospitals, and although nicotine withdrawal and craving are unlikely to directly cause violence, they can inflame conflict between patient and staff and may become the precipitant of aggression in a patient on the verge because of other factors. Because individuals are more likely to show negative affects and personality traits during times of high stress, including serious medical illness, patients with personality styles high in impulsivity, distrust, and aggressiveness (particularly antisocial or borderline personality disorders) may be more likely to commit violent acts during hospitalization.

Aggression and violence have serious consequences for patients and for those who care for them. These include disruption of the care environment, longer duration of hospitalization, higher treatment costs (Greenfield et al. 1989), and stigmatization of the mentally ill and their caregivers. Patients may sustain injuries—for example, from punching walls or glass, handling dangerous objects, falling, fighting with another patient, or resisting restraint. In addition, inpatients who are prone to impulsive aggressive acts tend to be at higher risk for elopement (Bowers et al. 2000) and for impulsive suicidal acts (Volavka 1999).

Although physicians, nurses, and other personnel are all at risk for injury, by far the hospital staff most likely to be injured by violent patients are nurses and clinical assistants (Binder and McNiel 1994; Hillbrand et al. 1996; Whittington et al. 1996). Assaults and injuries cause demoralization, physical and psychological disability, absenteeism (as a result of sick days and disability), and staff turnover or premature retirement among nurses, as well as increased administrative costs and litigation exposure for the care facility. In addition, violence from patients can cause staff to adopt negative attitudes toward their work and their patients, resulting in impaired job performance, poor patient–staff relationships, and patient dissatisfaction with care (Arnetz and Arnetz 2001). Patient violence has a myriad of negative effects on the treatment environment and the overall quality of patient care and can result in a vicious cycle in which a deteriorating environment promotes yet more violence (Arnetz and Arnetz 2001).

Mechanisms of Aggression

Empirical evidence supports the categorization of aggression and violence as either impulsive or premeditated. This evidence includes the association of impulsive aggression (and not the premeditated form) with cognitive deficits, learning disability, lower verbal skills, brain injury, and abnormal patterns of brain glucose use (Brower and Price 2001; Davidson et al. 2000; Volavka 1999). *Impulsive aggression* is relatively unplanned and spontaneous behavior and is sometimes explosive (such as sometimes occurs in patients with frontal lobe injuries), whereas *premeditated aggression* is deliberate behavior that may be predatory (committed for material gain or power) or pathological (a reaction to misperceptions, hallucinations, or delusions). This simple categorization is clinically useful because 1) most aggressive patients will manifest predominantly impulsive or predominantly premeditated behaviors, and 2) clinically relevant aggressive behaviors are generally impulsive or pathological—although some patients with mental disorders have predatory behaviors. It is important to note that impulsive aggression is not necessarily unintentional. Impulsive aggression occurs on a *continuum of intention*, ranging from entirely unintentional reflexive behaviors (e.g., ill-directed shoving and swinging in a patient with postictal confusion) to resistive behaviors (e.g., thrashing, spitting, and biting during placement of lines or tubes in a agitated patient with delirium) to spur-of-the-moment intentional behaviors (e.g., a patient with borderline personality disorder throwing a telephone at the nurse who is scolding her).

From a pathogenetic perspective, aggression is a heterogeneous behavior associated with background genetic, familial, and social determinants, including unfavorable prenatal, perinatal, and rearing experiences (such as childhood experience of neglect or abuse); genetic endowments and predispositions; poor parental role modeling; poor education; and negative cultural and peer influences (Volavka 1999). These factors, and acquired others such as Axis I conditions, brain injury syndromes, and personality disorders, coalesce in the individual to yield a *host* who has a baseline propensity for aggression that interacts with specific provocations (*agents*) and occurs in environments (*circumstances*) to produce aggressive behaviors. Examples of *agents* include threats by others, misperceptions, conflicts, or physical discomfort. *Circumstances* are contexts, such as intense (or distant) interpersonal relationships, losses, or hospitalization for physical illness, that are generally captured in a narrative that shows the patient's maladaptive interactions with his or her environment given his or her dispositional vulnerabilities. This explanatory approach describes the setting and sequence of events leading to an episode of aggressive behavior, while simultaneously placing these events in the context of the specific circumstances and the individual's psychological assets and liabilities.

Integration of the host, agent, and circumstance perspectives allows for enhanced understanding of any patient and his or her observed aggressive behavior. In some cases, an aggressive episode is the latest in a pattern of recurring impulsive, predatory, or pathological acts, which may (or may not) be associated with identifiable triggers, in an individual with cognitive or emotional vulnerabilities. In other cases, the act may be a somewhat understandable complication of the patient's primary condition or a not-so-surprising reaction to distressing circumstances.

Consider the following illustrations:

- Aggression and violence in inpatient settings appear to be relatively frequent in the first 48 hours after admission in acutely psychotic patients and in substance users (Barlow et al. 2000; Sheridan et al. 1990). In contrast, a rapid reduction in the risk of aggression in patients with schizophrenia within a few days after admission also has been reported (Binder and McNiel 1990). Both of these observations can be reconciled by considering that agitation and acute psychosis often lead to more intensive treatment efforts.
- Substance users may become aggressive soon after admission as a result of irritability associated with a withdrawal syndrome. When preemptive treatment for the withdrawal syndrome is initiated, the risk for aggression is minimized.
- Patient–staff conflicts—especially those that involve enforcement of rules, denying of privileges or requests (e.g., discharge, change in medications, off-unit smoking breaks), and involuntary admission or transfer—can precipitate aggressive acts and violence (Sheridan et al. 1990).

Psychosomatic medicine specialists often encounter recurrent impulsive aggression, which occurs as an inexplicable event or a "hair-trigger" response to relatively unimportant stimuli. This form of aggression is usually related to dysfunction of the brain areas involved in the modulation (or suppression) of primitive impulses and drives. It often arises as a consequence of physical illness or injury that directly or indirectly affects these brain areas. It is also true that in the general hospital setting, many episodes of impulsive aggression are not related to physical illness or injury per se but rather arise in an individual in whom impulsivity is a dominant (or prominent)

behavioral *trait*—for example, individuals with antisocial and borderline personality disorders. Since Phineas Gage's injury and its sequelae were described about 150 years ago (Harlow 1848, 1868), studies of patients who express acquired antisocial behavior and impulsive aggression following coarse brain injury have yielded important clues about brain mechanisms that modulate the expression of aggression. These case studies have shown that impulsivity, jocularity, tactless talk, aggressive outbursts, and reckless disregard for others frequently follow injury to frontal-subcortical brain circuits in adults. Acquired antisocial behavior and impulsive aggression also have been noted in war veterans with frontal lobe injury and in individuals who had frontal lobe injuries in childhood and subsequently developed coarse adult personality features, including psychological immaturity, impaired executive cognition, and recurring impulsive aggression (Brower and Price 2001).

Abnormalities in tests of executive cognition have been found repeatedly in studies of impulsively aggressive patients with antisocial personality disorder, frontal lobe injuries, and frontotemporal dementias and in children and adolescents with attention-deficit/hyperactivity disorder (ADHD) or conduct disorder (Brower and Price 2001; Coccaro and Siever 2002; Davidson et al. 2000). These abnormalities include deficits in working memory, abstract thinking, moral reasoning, affective regulation, and behavioral inhibition. Even though many of these patients show normal intelligence and executive cognition when tested, their real-life decisions suggest severe impairments in judgment and foresight (Brower and Price 2001).

The orbitofrontal and ventromedial cortices are involved in the restraint of impulsive behavior and thus play a central role in the regulation of impulsive aggression. The limbic system, particularly the amygdala and the cingulate cortex, is also involved in the regulation of aggression, presumably through a role in the generation of defensive aggressive states. Cases of acquired antisocial behavior and impulsive aggression have been associated with traumatic injuries to the orbitofrontal cortex and also to the ventromedial cortex (see reviews by Brower and Price 2001; Coccaro and Siever 2002; Davidson et al. 2000; Lyketsos 2000; Volavka 1999). It has been postulated that impulsive aggression arises as the result of a low threshold in the amygdala for activation of negative affects (fear, anger, and aggressive responses) or a failure of the orbitofrontal cortex to suppress negative affects in conformity to social rules or cues in the environment (Brower and Price 2001; Davidson et al. 2000). This view is supported by data from neuropsychological, neurophysiological, neurochemical, and functional brain imaging studies of impulsively aggressive patients and violent offenders (Brower and Price 2001; Coccaro and Siever 2002; Davidson et al. 2000; Lyketsos 2000; Volavka 1999).

The neurotransmitter systems involved in the modulation of aggression are primarily those involving serotonin and the catecholamines (norepinephrine and dopamine). Accumulated evidence indicates that impulsive aggression may result from disruption of serotonin neurotransmission, which putatively leads to the loss of inhibitory control of behavior (Berman and Coccaro 1998; Coccaro and Siever 2002; Davidson et al. 2000; Volavka 1999). These data include lower cerebrospinal fluid (CSF) levels of the serotonin metabolite 5-hydroxyindoleacetic acid (5-HIAA) in aggressive psychiatric patients, impulsive violent men (including violent offenders), disruptive and aggressive male children and adolescents, victims of violent suicides, and individuals with type 2 alcoholism (which has been associated with familial alcoholism, antisocial behavior, and impulsive aggression). These findings are further supported by pharmacological challenge studies designed to examine whether low CSF levels of 5-HIAA represented low central serotonin activity. These studies have reported a blunted prolactin response to serotonin agonist challenge (with buspirone or fenfluramine) in aggressive, antisocial, and suicidal individuals, indicating deficient serotonergic neurotransmission in patients with impulsive aggression (Coccaro and Siever 2002; Davidson et al. 2000; Volavka 1999).

Irritable aggression has been linked to catecholamine neurotransmission. High noradrenergic activity and low levels of monoamine oxidase (MAO) and catecholamine-O-methyltransferase (COMT) are associated with hostility and aggression in adults without psychiatric disorders and patients with psychosis (Volavka 1999). Dopaminergic neurotransmission also has been implicated in the expression of aggressive behavior, putatively because lower activity leads to impaired ability to restrain behavior (Berman and Coccaro 1998). However, only a modest role for noradrenergic and dopaminergic neurotransmission has been shown in impulsive aggression because much of the variance in aggression in these studies is accounted for by CSF levels of 5-HIAA (Coccaro and Siever 2002).

Evaluation of Aggression

An episode of belligerence and violence in the general hospital setting typically progresses from a specific clinical state—the *setting*—to a *sequence* of events that culminates in the *outcome*—aggressive behavior (see Figure 8–1). Several factors influence the expression of aggression in

the clinic or hospital: aggression may occur if the patient has specific symptoms, mental states, adverse effects of medicines, dissatisfaction with care, or conflicts with staff. However, aggression can be prevented, its intensity reduced, or its consequences avoided or minimized by prompt intervention (the clinical progression of aggressive behavior in the general hospital is depicted in Figure 8–1). The choice of intervention depends on the specific situation as well as the case formulation and the specific diagnosis the patient has received.

The elucidation of the *setting-sequence-outcome* involves describing the specific aggressive behavior, the sequence of events preceding it, and the symptoms and factors that may be influencing its expression. This approach has been referred to as the *define and decode strategy* (Lyketsos 2000). The effects of the patient's behavior also should be noted by inquiring about injury to the patient or others, damage to property, disruption of the milieu, and so on. Precipitants such as staff–patient conflicts, end of visiting hours, or recent administration of a medication should be carefully sought, and the history also should clarify the setting in which the behavior has occurred and the temporal relation of the aggressive behavior to any co-occurring symptoms. It is also helpful to know whether the patient is febrile, confused, in pain, craving cigarettes, cognitively impaired or disabled, anxious or fearful, hallucinating or delusional, or if he or she has epilepsy (especially a recent seizure). All prescribed medicines (e.g., insulin, benzodiazepines, anticholinergics, neuroleptics) should be noted. The psychiatrist should systematically search for symptoms such as acute confusion, restlessness, akathisia, or agitation, which require urgent intervention.

In addition to collecting a careful history of the aggressive episode, the evaluation requires describing concurrent illnesses; the patient's personal, social, and family history (including current psychosocial functioning); any substance abuse; and the patient's personality and psychiatric status. General medical, neurological, cognitive, and mental status examinations are focused on describing systems that have been implicated in the history but also should include important "inspections," such as the checking of vital signs, airway and cardiovascular status, exclusion of injuries, repeated assessment of alertness, assessment of dangerousness (inquiring about violent or suicidal ideas), and assessment of reality testing.

In the general hospital setting, laboratory data are often essential to accurate differential diagnosis. Blood tests can help to identify infection, anemia, electrolyte disturbances, or biochemical abnormalities that may explain delirium. Likewise, toxicology screens and serum drug concentrations may help to identify acute intoxications and

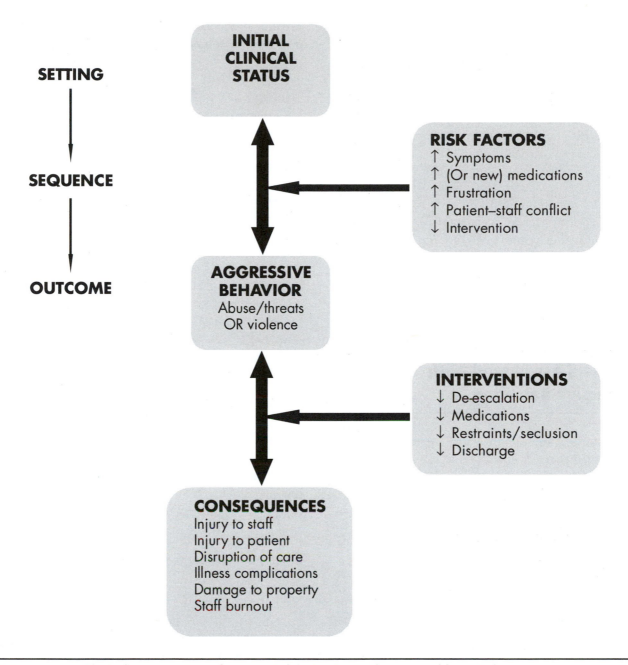

SETTING

SEQUENCE

OUTCOME

INITIAL CLINICAL STATUS

RISK FACTORS
↑ Symptoms
↑ (Or new) medications
↑ Frustration
↑ Patient–staff conflict
↓ Intervention

AGGRESSIVE BEHAVIOR
Abuse/threats
OR violence

INTERVENTIONS
↓ De-escalation
↓ Medications
↓ Restraints/seclusion
↓ Discharge

CONSEQUENCES
Injury to staff
Injury to patient
Disruption of care
Illness complications
Damage to property
Staff burnout

FIGURE 8–1. Clinical progression of aggressive behavior in the general hospital.

chronic substance use. Urinalysis, microbiological cultures (of blood and urine), and chest X ray may be helpful in certain circumstances (e.g., in immunosuppressed patients or patients with dementia). If seizures are a possibility, an electroencephalogram (EEG) should be performed. When obtundation, evidence of recent head trauma, or another reason to suspect an acute intracranial event is present, brain imaging (computed tomography [CT] or magnetic resonance imaging [MRI]) should be obtained. In most circumstances, a brain CT is adequate. A high index of suspicion for intracranial hemorrhage (e.g., subdural hematoma) is appropriate because those

who are violent toward others are at higher risk for being victims of violence themselves.

The integration of the clinical data leads to a case formulation and differential diagnosis, as well as a summary narrative that depicts the *setting-sequence-outcome* of the aggressive episode (and also articulates the contributions of *host*, *agent*, and *circumstance*). The formulation addresses the following questions:

• Does the patient have a mental illness, personality vulnerability, cognitive impairment, delirium, or other condition that predisposes him or her to aggressive behavior?

- Is the aggression linked to specific aspects of illness such as psychomotor agitation, disinhibition, command hallucinations, aphasia, or acute pain?
- Can the aggression be explained by medications causing confusion, akathisia, or intoxication?
- Is the aggression associated with a specific activity or with interpersonal conflicts?
- How is the environment contributing to the behavior?
- Is the environment uncomfortable, noisy, overcrowded, or frightening?

It is also important for psychiatrists to remember that many impulsively aggressive patients have a relatively high risk for suicidal behavior (Volavka 1999). Several psychiatric disorders manifesting aggressive and violent behavior, particularly alcohol dependence and personality disorders, are associated with suicidal behavior. Thus, the evaluation of aggression also must include an assessment of the risk for self-injury and suicide.

Disorders Associated With Aggressive Behavior

Many disorders can manifest with aggression and violence in the general hospital (Table 8–2). Thus, the psychiatrist's task will include a consideration of these disorders in the differential diagnosis of violent behavior in patients.

Psychoses and Chronic Serious Mental Illness

As noted earlier in this chapter, several major mental disorders can produce violent behavior. Irritable patients with mania, depression, schizophrenia, or other major psychoses may commit impulsive violent acts. This risk for impulsive violence is greatest during acute presentations and is particularly high when patients have been brought to treatment against their will. Clinicians should therefore maintain high levels of vigilance when evaluating the irritable psychotic patient, especially when the patient is seen in the emergency department or soon after being involuntarily hospitalized.

Deliberate premeditated violence also can arise from psychotic disorders—usually as a response to delusional beliefs—but generally the content of psychotic patients' delusions is focused on familiar individuals (people in the patients' daily life), public figures, or imaginary persecutors rather than on the health professionals caring for them. It also should be noted that many patients with

TABLE 8–2.   Differential diagnosis of aggressive and violent behavior

Psychoses
 Mania
 Depression
 Schizophrenia
 Delusional disorder

Personality disorders
 Antisocial personality
 Borderline personality
 Paranoid personality
 Narcissistic personality

Other behavior disorders
 Intermittent explosive disorder
 Episodic dyscontrol
 Hypothalamic–limbic rage
 Conduct disorder

Substance use disorders
 Alcohol
 Phencyclidine
 Stimulants
 Cocaine

Epilepsy
 Preictal
 Ictal
 Postictal
 Interictal

Delirium

Executive dysfunction syndromes

Dementia

Developmental disorders
 Mental retardation
 XYY genotype

chronic mental illness have maladaptive coping responses to stress or conflict and thus may react with violence during interpersonal conflicts. Therefore, a crucial aspect of the psychiatrist's role is to educate nonpsychiatric physicians, nurses, and others caring for these patients. When patients with major mental illness are admitted to nonpsychiatric settings, the psychiatrist's role as consultant should include educating the medical team about the illness (its current status and treatment) and the fact that most such patients can communicate their concerns and symptoms, will cooperate with care, and are nonviolent (even when psychotic). Treatment recommendations should include ways of approaching the patient (e.g., approaching the patient from within his or her visual field and calling out a greeting so that he or she is not startled), ensuring that the patient's current psychotropic regimen is prescribed, and pointing out any known habits or preferences that can be accommodated (e.g., arranging for regular smoking breaks, preferred meals, or a favorite television show). The patient's physicians and nurses should be educated about early signs of agitation, such as pacing, restlessness, staring, and refusal of medications, and contingency plans for managing these symptoms or states should be specified—what behavioral approaches, including positive reinforcers, pacifiers, and tranquilization strategies, should be used and how the psychiatrist can be contacted when his or her expertise is urgently needed.

Personality Disorders

Violence associated with personality disorders is usually embedded in the individual's behavioral repertoire. Personality disorders that frequently manifest violent behavior are shown in Table 8–2; of these, antisocial personality is the most likely to be associated with habitual aggression. Antisocial individuals usually are thrill-seeking, have low frustration tolerance, and have high rates of substance abuse, criminal behavior, and violence. They often present to the emergency department with injuries resulting from violence (such as stab and gunshot wounds) and with a variety of medical complications of substance abuse (including severe intoxications, wound infections, head injuries, and hepatitis); they often require admission to the medical or surgical ward for treatment of these conditions. Antisocial patients who are intoxicated can become very dangerous because of their mood instability, lowered frustration tolerance, and behavioral disinhibition. While in the hospital, they may become aggressive when their demands—for pain medication, more food, cigarettes, and so on—are not met. In making these demands, they may verbally threaten, intimidate staff with boasts and gestures, or become violent.

Many antisocial patients are repeatedly hospitalized for treatment of problems arising from their lifestyle, especially the medical complications of addictions and risk-taking behaviors. This often arouses resentment and animosity from physicians and nurses, who may believe that their efforts to care for the patient are unwanted and futile. Health care professionals may be provoked into angry verbal (and, rarely, physical) retaliation. Such patients have earned notoriety from their behavior during earlier hospitalizations, which may put them at risk for punitive interventions such as suboptimal care, inadequate pain treatment, and premature discharge. Staff may understandably prefer to focus care on patients who are seen as cooperative, appreciative, and "innocent victims" of disease. This puts the aggressive antisocial patient at higher risk for missed diagnoses and medical errors. Thus, psy-

chiatrists involved in caring for such patients need to know their reputation on the unit and the feelings of the physicians and nurses caring for them. This information is valuable for formulating a plan of care that ensures adequate evaluation and treatment for the patient and appropriate safeguards for the staff. One of the psychiatrist's responsibilities with such patients is to help physicians, nurses, and other staff appropriately handle their anger and frustration, avoiding both overreaction (e.g., yelling at patients, inappropriate precipitous discharge) and underreaction (e.g., failing to set limits, failing to discharge when indicated). Antisocial patients are not immune to other conditions that may explain aggression, including delirium, substance withdrawal, and psychosis. Therefore, psychiatrists should pursue a systematic psychiatric and general medical assessment whenever antisocial patients are encountered in nonpsychiatric settings.

Borderline personality is characterized by intense emotionality, intense relationships, rejection sensitivity, manipulative behaviors, impulsiveness, recklessness, low self-regard, irritability, aggressiveness, and a tendency to extreme reactions. Most patients with borderline personality disorder are women. Their violent acts usually are impulsive and typically occur during interpersonal conflict. They also have a high potential for self-injury and suicidal acts and thus are often seen in the emergency department. Borderline patients can be very difficult to manage because they may demand specific conditions or individuals before submitting to an interview or examination. They are capable of angrily refusing care or of violent temper tantrums. Thus, a major challenge in their care is maintaining limits on behavior and managing the intense negative countertransference feelings that they may stir up. In caring for them, psychiatrists must maintain an empathic stance and assist the staff in doing so, often despite deliberate provocation.

Individuals with borderline personality seen in the emergency department should be screened for depression, substance abuse, and domestic violence because these conditions are highly comorbid. On medical units, borderline patients can become disruptive when their expectations are not met. Psychiatrists should educate their physicians and nurses about the need to define behavior limits, meet expectations agreed on with the patient, and maintain a consistent approach to the patient's care. This is best accomplished in an interdisciplinary care conference, with the psychiatrist assisting the staff in constructing a written treatment contract to be negotiated with, and signed by, the patient.

Other personality disorders are less frequently associated with violent behavior, although narcissistic individuals may threaten or act (e.g., slap a nurse) in retaliation for perceived slights or to satiate their sense of entitlement, and individuals with paranoid personality may become aggressive in response to perceived mistreatment.

Intermittent Explosive Disorder, Episodic Dyscontrol Syndrome, and Hypothalamic–Limbic Rage Syndrome

Intermittent explosive disorder, episodic dyscontrol syndrome, and hypothalamic–limbic rage syndrome describe disturbances that are characterized by explosive episodes of aggression and violence. *Intermittent explosive disorder*, as defined by DSM-IV (American Psychiatric Association 1994a) and its text revision, DSM-IV-TR (American Psychiatric Association 2000), refers to a disturbance characterized by recurrent episodes of explosive anger not explained by psychosis or some other mental disorder. *Episodic dyscontrol* is a similar construct, denoting recurring episodes of uncontrollable rage. It has been used as a label for males who have a history of conduct disorder, unstable employment, poverty, domestic violence and other sexual assaults, criminal behavior, and substance abuse (typically alcohol) (Cummings and Mega 2003). Neurological signs such as short attention span, poor coordination, and mild gait abnormalities have been found in some cases, and temporal lobe EEG abnormalities have been found in others. Whereas intermittent explosive disorder denotes a relatively narrow clinical spectrum of explosive aggression, episodic dyscontrol refers to episodic, impulsive violence in a broad, ill-defined group of mostly antisocial individuals. Because episodic dyscontrol syndrome overlaps widely with several psychiatric categories (including intermittent explosive disorder, ADHD, conduct disorder, and antisocial personality disorder), it lacks face validity and is of limited clinical usefulness.

Although rare, rage attacks in association with neoplastic and surgical lesions of the hypothalamus and amygdala have been described (Demaree and Harrison 1996; Tonkonogy and Geller 1992). These attacks, which have been repeatedly reproduced in experimental animals with lesion models and neurophysiological methods, have been termed *hypothalamic rage attacks* or *hypothalamic–limbic rage syndrome*. This disorder is characterized by provoked and unprovoked episodes of uncontrollable rage and may represent an acquired form of intermittent explosive disorder. In addition to rage attacks, patients may have symptoms such as hyperphagia, polydipsia, excessive weight gain, or obesity; clinical findings suggesting thyroid, adrenal, or pituitary disease; a history of recently diagnosed pituitary, midbrain, or temporal lobe tumor; or recent brain surgery. Treatment involves correction of the under-

lying condition (including surgical resection of tumors) and behavioral and pharmacological approaches targeted at aggression.

Substance Use Disorders

Alcohol is the psychoactive substance most often associated with violence. Alcohol-related violence may result from a severely intoxicated state that produces gross impairment of self-restraint and judgment and/or a blackout. Pathological intoxication, which occurs in vulnerable individuals following the ingestion of only modest amounts of alcohol, may be associated with disorganized behavior, emotional lability, and violent outbursts. In severe cases, pathological intoxication may be accompanied by a delirium with hyperarousal, hallucinations, delusions, and terror, followed by amnesia for the event after recovery. Alcohol withdrawal also can be accompanied by irritability and low frustration tolerance, which predispose to directed aggression, or by seizures that are followed by aggression during a postictal state. Patients who develop delirium tremens may show poorly coordinated, resistive, or preemptive violence in response to hyperarousal, hallucinations, and terror.

Intoxication with other substances also can result in violence. Cocaine and amphetamine abuse is common and can produce impulsive, disinhibited intoxicated states during which violence may occur. Patients undergoing opioid, sedative, or cocaine withdrawal may experience anxious tension and irritability, during which interpersonal conflict or frustration may result in violent behavior. Although phencyclidine is not commonly abused, phencyclidine intoxication can manifest with severe impulsively directed violence. Even less common is violence that occurs in individuals who have taken Ecstasy, lysergic acid diethylamide (LSD), or other hallucinogens; as an apparent consequence of severe perceptual disturbances; and in patients who abuse anticholinergic agents, in whom delirium may be accompanied by aggressive behavior.

Epilepsy

In evaluating episodes of aggression in patients with epilepsy (see also Chapter 32, "Neurology and Neurosurgery"), psychosomatic medicine psychiatrists must carefully consider whether the aggression is directly related to a seizure, a feature of mental state changes associated with seizures, or a complication of other conditions that increase the risk of aggressive behavior. In addition, psychiatrists must be aware that certain seizures can be misinterpreted as intentional violent behavior. Violent behavior may be observed during complex partial seizures but never during grand mal seizures.

Ictal violence is rare, and most cases are characterized by spontaneous, nondirected, stereotyped aggressive behaviors. Typical characteristics are as follows: 1) the seizure episode occurs suddenly, without provocation, and is of very short duration (usually a few minutes); 2) automatisms and other stereotypic phenomena of the patient's habitual seizures accompany the aggressive act, and the act is associated with these phenomena from one seizure to the next; 3) the patient's consciousness is impaired; 4) the aggressive behavior is poorly directed and involves few skills; and 5) purpose and interpersonal interaction are absent (Marsh and Krauss 2000). In practice, it can be difficult to determine whether a violent behavior should be attributed to a seizure event. This determination requires the integration of findings from interview, clinical history, and video EEG monitoring to make the diagnosis. Abnormal nonseizure EEG phenomena (such as sharp waves) are nonspecific findings and should not be used as evidence that violence is ictal. Widely applicable criteria for attributing a specific violent act to an epileptic seizure have been developed (see Treiman 1986) and are presented in Table 8–3.

Although uncommon, a prodromal state of affective instability preceding a seizure episode by several hours or days may be associated with directed aggression (Marsh and Krauss 2000). The affective symptoms may be specific to the preictal state or an exacerbation of interictal phenomena; these states and their aggressive features usually resolve after the seizure.

Violent behavior in epilepsy is most frequent during postictal confusional states. These states are usually brief but can vary widely in duration because they are influenced by the type and severity of the preceding seizures. Abnormal moods, paranoia, hallucinations, and delirium may occur and result in violence by heightening aggressive propensities or causing misinterpretations of stimuli in the immediate environment. In general, episodes of postictal violence are longer in duration than episodes of ictal violence, are associated with amnesia for the event, and are out of character for the individual. In some males, stereotypic episodes of severe postictal aggression can occur after clusters of seizures (Gerard et al. 1998). Postictal delirium can be detected clinically by assessing the patient's level of consciousness and awareness and performing an EEG—which shows diffuse slowing (and no ictal activity). Typically, the delirium is brief, and a gradual return to normal consciousness follows, but prolonged or repetitive seizures can extend the duration. Violence occurring during postictal delirium is usually relatively undirected; resistive violence is fairly frequent, usually oc-

TABLE 8–3. Criteria for determining whether a violent act resulted from an epileptic seizure

1. Diagnosis of epilepsy established by an expert neurologist[a]
2. Epileptic automatisms documented by clinical history and closed-circuit-television electroencephalogram
3. Aggression during epileptic automatisms documented on closed-circuit-television electroencephalogram
4. The violent behavior is characteristic of the patient's habitual seizures
5. Clinical judgment by the neurologist that the behavior was part of a seizure

[a]A neurologist with special competence in epilepsy.
Source. Adapted from Treiman 1986.

curring when attempts are made to help or restrain a patient after the seizure.

Many episodes of postictal violence are motivated by a postictal psychosis. The psychosis may emerge from postictal confusion or a lucid state and tends to follow a psychosis-free interval of several hours to a few days after a seizure (or cluster of complex partial seizures) (Marsh and Krauss 2000). Postictal psychosis usually manifests as grandiose affective psychoses (mania or depression with mood-congruent psychotic phenomena) or with thought disorder, hallucinations, and paranoid ideational psychoses reminiscent of schizophrenia. Although usually transient (of no longer than several hours' duration), these states may last up to several weeks. Postictal psychosis has a tendency to recur and may become chronic. Violence in the context of postictal psychosis may be motivated by paranoid delusions and hallucinations, in which case it manifests as well-directed violence. In fact, violence is more likely to occur in individuals with postictal psychosis, compared with those with interictal psychosis or postictal confusion (Kanemoto et al. 1999). Most episodes of postictal psychosis resolve spontaneously or following treatment with low doses of a neuroleptic, and improved control of the epilepsy then becomes the focus of treatment. However, some patients require chronic maintenance treatment with neuroleptics (see also Chapter 11, "Mania, Catatonia, and Psychosis," and Chapter 32, "Neurology and Neurosurgery").

Most violent behaviors in patients with epilepsy have no particular association with ictal or postictal states. For example, studies that report higher prevalence rates of epilepsy in prisoners than in nonprisoners rarely identify connections between criminal acts and specific seizure episodes, and prevalence rates for epilepsy are not higher in violent criminals than in nonviolent criminals (Treiman 1986). Thus, the increased risk for violence in prisoners who have epilepsy can be attributed to other factors such as cognitive dysfunction and adverse social circumstances (Treiman 1986). The assessment of violence in patients with epilepsy should therefore also elicit a contextualized description (*setting-sequence-outcome*) of the act and other biological and psychosocial factors that may mediate the expression of aggression. These forms of aggression are well directed and are associated with stressors and triggers. They typically occur around other people and are purposeful, nonstereotyped, and highly coordinated. The aggression is "explained" by the situation at hand, is associated with the buildup of negative emotions concerning some circumstance, and may be of relatively prolonged duration.

Brain injury and cognitive impairment are important risk factors for interictal aggressive behavior. In addition, interictal psychiatric phenomena, such as depression, hallucinations, and delusions, and sociopathic personality traits, such as impulsivity, remorselessness, self-absorption, and superficiality, also predispose patients with epilepsy to aggressive behavior. Furthermore, violence can be learned behavior in patients whose educational and social disadvantages are a correlate or result of their epilepsy.

Delirium

States of heightened arousal often accompany the confusion and fluctuating alertness of delirium and may predispose patients to violent behavior. The presence of hallucinations and delusions also increases the potential for violence in patients with delirium, as it does in patients with epilepsy. The presence of delirium in an aggressive patient should prompt a thorough search for an underlying cause. When ambiguity exists about the presence of delirium, the diagnosis can be established by variable scores on the Mini-Mental State Examination (or other short cognitive battery) in a relatively short period (several hours) or by slowed cerebral activity on the EEG. A more detailed discussion of delirium is presented in Chapter 6, "Delirium."

Executive Dysfunction Syndromes

Executive dysfunction syndromes, more commonly called *frontal lobe syndromes*, are manifestations of brain injury characterized by varying combinations of inattention, impulsivity, disinhibition, emotional dysregulation, absence of insight, impairment of judgment, and diminished initiative (Lyketsos et al. 2004). These frontal-subcortical syndromes result from a range of etiologies, including trauma, infection, neoplasm, stroke, and neurodegenerative disease. Explosive violence is often a feature, particularly in patients in whom impulsivity, disinhibition, or affective dysregulation predominates. In many individuals with habitual impulsive violence, formal neuropsychological testing indicates deficits in executive cognition (see section "Mechanisms of Aggression" earlier in this chapter); these individuals may be viewed as having occult executive dysfunction syndromes. Further discussion of these syndromes is presented in Chapter 35, "Physical Medicine and Rehabilitation."

Dementia

Aggression is common in patients with dementia, with the risk increasing with dementia severity, concurrent medical illness, crowding, noise, poor quality of interpersonal relationships, and sleep disorder (Lyketsos 2000). The presence of motor restlessness, depression, hallucinations, misinterpretations, paranoia, or delusions in patients with dementia also should alert the clinician to the risk for aggressive behavior. Type of dementia appears to have limited influence on the likelihood of aggression, even though patients with vascular dementia and Huntington's disease may be less cognitively impaired than their counterparts with other forms of dementia.

In elders with dementia, aggression generally manifests as relatively simple behaviors such as throwing objects, pushing, shoving, kicking, pinching, biting, and scratching; destruction of property is uncommon (Cohen-Mansfield and Billig 1986). Sometimes male patients engage in sexually aggressive behaviors, such as grabbing the breasts of women or slapping women on the buttocks (Cohen-Mansfield and Billig 1986). It is unusual for elderly persons with dementia to have well-coordinated and goal-directed physical aggression, but such violence does occur and can be serious, especially when committed by younger patients with dementia.

Aggression in patients with dementia often occurs during routine care activities, such as bathing, morning grooming, and toileting. In these situations, the aggression may result from adversarial interactions with caregivers or from unsophisticated caregiving. Thus, it is important for the physician evaluating violence in the patient with dementia to be cognizant of the circumstances of the act and to search carefully for environmental or caregiver factors that may be triggers for aggression. Careful identification of such "external" factors facilitates their removal or modification (see also Chapter 7, "Dementia").

Elder Abuse

Elder mistreatment, in the form of abuse or neglect, also might be a contextual setting for aggression by the mistreated elder. Mistreatment begets aggression, but aggressive elders also are more likely to be mistreated by caregivers, whether at home or in an institutional setting. Psychiatrists must be alert to this possibility and screen for mistreatment if an elder presents with an unusual pattern of agitated behavior—for example, if the elder is only aggressive with a particular caregiver or in a particular setting (e.g., while being bathed or dressed) or if he or she presents with physical signs of mistreatment, such as shin bruises or unexplained persistent skin tears. For a comprehensive discussion of elder mistreatment and how to screen for and manage it, the reader is referred to a recent review published by the National Academies of Sciences (2003).

Domestic Violence

Domestic violence refers to a continuum of behaviors ranging from verbal abuse to threats and intimidation to sexual assault and violence (Golding 2002). The perpetrators do not belong to any particular social class and are often without mental illness, a particular personality type, or a criminal history (Eisenstat and Bancroft 1999). Intimate partners are the usual victims, with more than 90% of the cases involving women being abused by men. Physical intimate partner violence is estimated to occur in 4–6 million relationships in the United States (American Medical Association 1992; Rodriguez et al. 1999). The risk for battery increases (and ongoing battery may worsen) with pregnancy and ill health (Eisenstat and Bancroft 1999; Golding 2002).

Victims of domestic aggression are seen frequently in a variety of ambulatory care settings (Eisenstat and Bancroft 1999): an estimated 25% of women who seek care in the emergency department, 37% of women who are treated for physical injury in the emergency department, 14%–19% of pregnant women (within the past year), 25% of women who are treated for psychiatric symptoms, 25% of those who attempt suicide, and almost 70% of mothers of battered children. Victims of domestic violence experience adverse health outcomes, including risk for serious injury or death, complications of pregnancy and childbirth, sexually transmitted diseases (including human immunodeficiency virus and acquired immunodeficiency syndrome), treatment nonadherence and worse outcomes for existing conditions, somatoform and conversion disorders, eating disorders, substance abuse, anxiety, depression, and suicide (American Medical Association 1992; Coid et al. 2003; Eisenstat and Bancroft 1999). Exposed children sustain emotional injury living in an environment of domestic aggression and may themselves be victims of accidental or intentional violence. Many of these

children will later in life show a wide range of psychopathology and are prone to becoming abusive men and abused women themselves (Eisenstat and Bancroft 1999; Lamberg 2000).

Victims of domestic violence are frequent visitors to clinics and emergency departments, and although some are too afraid to discuss their experiences with a physician, many are willing (Gerbert et al. 1999). Unfortunately, despite this willingness to disclose, most cases remain undetected because few physicians inquire. Several factors account for this lack of inquiry, including inadequate training in the detection and management of domestic violence, physicians' feelings of discomfort and powerlessness, and pressures on physicians to spend less time with patients. Patients' reluctance comes from negative past experiences, fear of retaliation, pessimism, emotional dependency, and low self-confidence.

Vigilant clinicians can recognize patterns suggestive of domestic violence, including repeat visits for vague or minor complaints or chronic pain (especially pelvic), evasive and anxious behavior, inability to recall events, inadequate or baffling explanations for injuries, domineering and obstructionist behavior in a partner, unexplained nonadherence with treatments, and findings of child or elder abuse (Eisenstat and Bancroft 1999). In addition, certain physical findings should raise the possibility of physical abuse: injuries to the head, neck, or mouth; multiple injuries; bruises in various stages of healing; defensive injuries of the forearms; dental trauma; and genital injuries. It is prudent to screen for domestic violence in patients with somatoform, anxiety, and substance abuse disorders and in those with suicidal ideation or attempts.

Routine screening of all women, particularly those seen in emergency departments and in antenatal and gynecology clinics, facilitates early intervention and has been recommended by the American Psychiatric Association (1994b), American Medical Association (1992), and several other professional organizations (American Association of Family Physicians 1994; American College of Emergency Physicians 1995; American College of Obstetrics and Gynecology 1995; Emergency Nurses Association 1998). Women treated for injuries in the emergency department or surgical units and those attending family planning clinics, sexually transmitted disease clinics, and substance abuse programs certainly should be screened for domestic violence. Domestic violence is so common that it is logical to screen all women, regardless of the clinical setting. Mnemonic approaches to screening have been developed and include AVDR (Gerbert et al. 2000):

- **A**sking about abuse
- Providing **V**alidation and emotional support

- **D**ocumenting findings and disclosures
- **R**eferring patients to domestic violence specialists

In Table 8–4, we provide some sample questions that may be used to initiate the screening process. Incorporating screening questions into the routine interview process can minimize physician and patient discomfort.

When ongoing abuse is identified, descriptions of current, recent, and past battery—including dates and circumstances—should be elicited and carefully documented. Legal intervention may rely on this documentation, so all findings should be described in clear and precise language, quoting the specific words spoken by the patient when possible. A complete history and thorough examination should be performed, all injuries should be carefully described (body maps are very useful for this purpose), and photographs should be taken if the patient consents. Strict confidentiality of the disclosure is needed to protect the patient from retaliation; this may require restricted access or sequestration of the disclosure records. On completion of the medical evaluation, a social work evaluation and referral to services such as the National Domestic Violence Hotline (1-800-799-SAFE) and local advocacy organizations should follow (Eisenstat and Bancroft 1999). It is usually best to respect the patient's wishes regarding when to report the violence to legal authorities and when to flee the situation. However, in some states, the physician is required by law to make a report. In the United States, mandatory reporting is the norm whenever evidence of child abuse is found (see also Chapter 3, "Legal Issues").

TABLE 8–4.   Helpful questions for domestic abuse screening by clinicians

1. Do you and your partner argue a lot? Does it ever get physical? Has either one of you hit the other? Has either one of you injured the other?
2. Do you ever feel unsafe at home?
3. Has anyone hit you or tried to injure you in any way?
4. Has anyone ever threatened you or tried to control you?
5. Have you ever felt afraid of your partner?
6. Is there anything particularly stressful going on now? How are things at home?
7. I see patients in my practice who are being hurt or threatened by someone they love. Is this happening to you? Has this ever happened to you?

Source. Question 1 from J.L. Levenson (personal communication, October 2003); Questions 2–5 from Eisenstat and Bancroft 1999; Questions 6–7 from Gerbert et al. 2000.

Developmental Disorders

Violent behavior also occurs in patients with neurodevelopmental syndromes such as mental retardation. Few patients with mental retardation are habitually or impulsively aggressive. However, because many patients with mental retardation also have severe communication or language deficiencies, they may be prone to temper tantrums and violence when frustrated or in discomfort (e.g., from pain). They are also at increased risk for psychiatric symptoms, such as irritability, impulsivity, disinhibition, and low frustration tolerance, and affective and psychotic conditions, which may occasionally contribute to aggressive behavior.

Management of Aggressive Behavior

Education and Relationship Building

Ideally, the management of aggression in the general hospital setting begins well before a particular patient is seen. These early interventions are part of the liaison role of the psychiatrist and consist primarily of education and relationship-building activities. For example, the psychiatrist may give grand rounds and topical seminars or may seize opportunities provided by collaboration in the care of specific patients to conduct bedside teaching with medical colleagues, nurses, nurse's aides, and other health care professionals. The psychiatrist's goal is to convey basic clinical information about psychiatric disturbances and practical strategies for the management of difficult or problem patients, including aggressive and violent ones. The psychiatrist's teaching should include recognition of the early signs suggesting later aggression (e.g., restlessness, staring, pacing) and behavioral interventions, including verbal de-escalation techniques (nonthreatening approaches such as speaking calmly, using gentle eye contact, adopting a problem-solving stance, and knowing when to disengage) and when and how to use "show of force," pharmacological tranquilization, and physical restraint. This teaching serves to broaden the skill set of the medical team members and to increase their confidence in their ability to manage these patients, which can result in fewer aggressive incidents, less likelihood of patient or staff injury during episodes, more effective treatment of the underlying conditions, and more effective collaboration in their care.

Safety of the Environment

The safety of the environment should be ensured before any aggressive patient is evaluated. The psychiatrist should check that actual weapons, such as guns and knives, and potential weapons, such as scissors, belts, and ropes, have been removed. In the emergency department, this is often accomplished by routinely using hand searches and metal detectors and by keeping any discovered items safely locked away. On inpatient units, monitoring and controlling what the patient can keep, conducting periodic room searches, and providing plastic utensils for meals are common interventions. A safe environment also should allow for the examiner's easy escape, as well as observation and easy entry by other health care personnel. The psychiatrist should use what information is available to anticipate what precautions and emergency interventions may be needed before starting the evaluation and should make sure that the medical team is ready to intervene in the event that the patient becomes severely agitated or violent.

Psychiatric Evaluation

Effective management of the aggressive patient requires a comprehensive psychiatric evaluation, ultimately leading to the identification of potentially modifiable factors at which interventions are targeted. In many instances, formulation of the case results in the diagnosis of a psychiatric disorder, and specific treatment is instituted with the expectation that remission of the disorder will lead to resolution of the aggression. For example, when an acute psychosis is believed to be responsible for the aggressive behavior of a patient who has schizophrenia, an antipsychotic is prescribed. However, in many patients with aggression, the psychiatric diagnosis only partially explains the behavior and does not indicate what the appropriate treatment strategy should be. This situation is often observed in patients with personality disorder, brain injury, or dementia but is frequently also true for patients with major mental disorders such as schizophrenia. In most such situations, careful characterization of the patient's background and careful description and decoding of the aggressive behavior will inform the approach to treatment.

Positive Therapeutic Alliance

The first step in the management of the aggressive patient is to develop a positive therapeutic alliance (Beauford et al. 1997). In all cases, and particularly in patients who are chronically aggressive or have recurrent violent episodes, it is crucial to actively seek the patient's collaboration in the treatment process. A positive therapeutic alliance facilitates the patient's compliance with behavioral expectations and with prescribed treatments and makes it easier

to mediate patient–staff conflicts and de-escalate aggressive episodes. Also, a positive alliance facilitates the development of a psychotherapeutic relationship that may enable the psychiatrist to eventually reduce the patient's propensity to violent responses when anticipated precipitants occur in the future (O'Connor 2003).

Behavioral Approaches

Verbal de-escalation techniques (shown in Table 8–5) are often effective for controlling and terminating mild to moderate aggression (threats and belligerence) and are used frequently in the emergency department, psychiatric ICU, and acute psychiatric ward. These techniques can be used in general medical settings by those who have been taught how to use them. Although verbal de-escalation should be conceptualized as a semistructured intervention (see Table 8–5), in practice, it is often deployed as an instinctive, commonsense reaction to the patient's behavior rather than as a systematic intervention. The basic goal of de-escalation is to manage a patient's anger and hostility by conveying empathy and understanding, personalizing the clinician, helping the patient to articulate grievances and frustrations, and actively involving the patient in problem solving and treatment planning (Stevenson 1991). Verbal de-escalation techniques are most use-

---

TABLE 8–5.   Verbal de-escalation techniques

Communication

Nonverbal
- Maintain a safe distance
- Maintain a neutral posture
- Do not stare; eye contact should convey sincerity
- Do not touch the patient
- Stay at the same height as the patient
- Avoid sudden movements

Verbal
- Speak in a calm, clear tone
- Personalize yourself
- Avoid confrontation; offer to solve the problem

Tactics

Debunking
- Acknowledge the patient's grievance
- Acknowledge the patient's frustration
- Shift focus to discussion of how to solve the problem

Aligning goals
- Emphasize common ground
- Focus on the big picture
- Find ways to make small concessions

Monitoring
- Be acutely aware of progress
- Know when to disengage
- Do not insist on having the last word

ful in situations that involve patient–staff conflict but also can be used to manage pathological aggression and to set the stage for pharmacological interventions.

More sophisticated behavioral approaches have been successfully applied to the management of chronic aggression, particularly in patients with dementia and brain injury. These approaches include behavioral analysis, operant conditioning, differential reinforcement strategies, validation, manipulation of ambient light and/or sound, activity programs, and environmental modification (Lyketsos 2000). Evidence for the use of these approaches derives primarily from uncontrolled studies.

Seclusion and Restraint

It is not unusual for de-escalation and other behavioral techniques to fail to calm the patient who is very agitated, particularly in the emergency department and other acute care settings. Also, in some settings, de-escalation techniques may be impractical because the patient is unable to communicate meaningfully (as a result of confusion, cognitive impairment, or communication disorders), is known to be explosive, is too severely agitated to cooperate, or is already engaging in violent behavior. In such cases, the use of physical restraint, which may involve *manual restraint* (wherein the patient is restrained by several health care workers) and *mechanical restraint* (wherein an appliance is used to restrain the patient), may be needed to terminate dangerous behavior. Sometimes, physical restraint is needed to administer tranquilizers or to protect other medical interventions (e.g., to keep the patient from pulling out intravenous lines, chest tubes, urinary catheters, or other vital lines or tubes). For a brief period immediately after the application of physical restraints (or the administration of tranquilizers), it is prudent to observe the patient in isolation (in his or her own room or a designated safe room) to ensure that the violent episode, its consequences, and identifiable triggers have been successfully managed. Because improper use of restraints can result in injury to the patient or to health care workers, such use should be directed and implemented only by experienced personnel. Training courses in the use of manual and physical restraints are widely supported, and many jurisdictions have developed certification programs.

During the past decade, the use of seclusion and physical restraints has come under intense criticism. As a result, governmental and judicial regulation of restraint use has steadily increased (see also Chapter 3, "Legal Issues"). In response to these trends, the Academy of Psychosomatic Medicine issued guidelines (Bronheim et al. 1998, p. S20) that state the following:

Constant observation and restraints should be implemented for the shortest possible time with the least restrictive, though effective, means available; these interventions must not be made solely for the convenience of medical staff. Assessment and treatment of underlying psychiatric conditions that contribute to the patient's need for these measures should be expeditiously undertaken.

These guidelines are consistent with those developed by other medical associations, with regulatory standards, and with the general opinion of the courts. In general, the standards for the clinical use of restraints are as follows: 1) restraints should be used only when necessary to protect the patient or others from harm; 2) restraints should not be used solely to coerce the patient to accept treatments or remain in the treatment setting; and 3) when restraints are being used, the patient should be closely monitored and his or her condition frequently reassessed. The clinical and regulatory issues involved in the use of restraints are complex; thus, it is often necessary for psychiatrists to help other medical colleagues explore the various options for managing an aggressive patient and to address any staff discomfort with the use of restraints, while keeping in mind the clinical and legal risks involved in using or forgoing restraints.

Pharmacological Approaches

Data indicating that neurotransmitter systems modulate aggression have stimulated the development of pharmacological approaches for the clinical management of aggression. This pharmacotherapy for aggression is based more on contemporary intuitions of the neurotransmitter effects of medications and how these effects modulate the expression of aggressive behavior and less on evidence from controlled trials. Medications are particularly indicated for impulsive and pathological forms of aggression. In general, treatment of clinically relevant aggression falls into two broad categories: 1) treatment of *syndromic* aggression separate from the diagnostic context and 2) focused treatment of conditions that manifest *symptomatic* aggression, such as schizophrenia, delusional disorders, major depressive disorders, and delirium. The discussion that follows focuses mainly on the treatment of syndromic aggression; treatments for specific conditions are covered in detail in other chapters of this text.

Pharmacological agents are indicated for both acute and chronic aggression. In the treatment of acute aggression, the goal is typically rapid tranquilization (which refers to the use of medications to achieve a rapid termination of agitated or aggressive behavior). A survey of U.S. psychiatrists who specialize in emergency psychiatry found that benzodiazepines (particularly lorazepam) were the preferred agents for treating acute aggression (Allen et al. 2001) because they are relatively free of adverse effects that are typically associated with neuroleptics, such as the acute dystonias, akathisia, and parkinsonism. However, neuroleptics, especially haloperidol, also were considered first-line agents, particularly for acute aggression associated with psychosis. One controlled trial found the combination of lorazepam and haloperidol to be superior to lorazepam or haloperidol alone for the treatment of acute agitation in patients with psychosis (Battaglia et al. 1997), suggesting that the combination also may be more effective for acute aggression. Newer neuroleptics—the atypical antipsychotics such as risperidone and olanzapine—are also being increasingly used for the management of acute agitation and aggression (Allen et al. 2001). For rapid tranquilization, drugs that can be given parenterally are advantageous. Lorazepam (intramuscular, intravenous) and haloperidol (intramuscular, intravenous) are typically used for this purpose, but other benzodiazepines (e.g., diazepam) and antipsychotics (e.g., fluphenazine, loxapine) are also available. Parenteral formulations of three atypical neuroleptics—ziprasidone, olanzapine, and risperidone—are now available, although the intramuscular formulation of risperidone is a depot injection.

A wider range of pharmacological agents is used for the treatment of chronic aggression (see Table 8–6). Of these agents, neuroleptics are the most widely used. The relative dearth of evidence from placebo-controlled trials and the phenotypic and neurobiological heterogeneity of aggression may explain the diversity of agents used to treat chronic aggression. It is noteworthy that placebo-controlled trials of treatments for agitation and aggression in elderly patients have yielded placebo responses as high as 60% in some studies, underscoring the importance of rigorous methodology in the evaluation of treatments (Lyketsos 2000). However, despite the limited availability of data from controlled trials, considerable empirical support exists for the use of several psychotropic classes in treating aggression.

Neuroleptics are the preferred agents for treating agitation and aggression in the general medical setting, especially when these phenomena arise in a patient with delirium. Neuroleptics are also used to treat aggression in psychotic patients and to tranquilize patients with severe aggression (regardless of cause). Tranquilization may terminate an episode of aggression, but sometimes it does not reduce the frequency or severity of future episodes of impulsive aggression.

In clinical trials of typical neuroleptics for the treatment of impulsive aggression in patients with personality disorders, results have been mixed; however, the atypical agents (which selectively block 5-HT$_2$ receptors—an ac-

tion associated with reduced aggression in animals) may be more effective in treating chronic impulsive aggression (Coccaro and Siever 2002). Consistent with this, studies have found that clozapine (across a wide range of measures) and perhaps risperidone have superior efficacy for treating aggression in patients with schizophrenia (Buckley et al. 1995, 1997; Czobor et al. 1995; Rabinowitz et al. 1996; Ratey et al. 1993). In a randomized comparative study, clozapine was the most efficacious agent (independent of effectiveness in relieving psychosis); olanzapine, risperidone, and haloperidol were equally effective in treating aggression (Citrome et al. 2001). Although these results would seem to recommend clozapine as a first choice for treating aggression in psychotic patients, in practice, the drug is typically reserved for severe or treatment-resistant cases because of its adverse-effect profile.

Neuroleptics are also used to treat aggression in patients with brain diseases. In multicenter trials enrolling patients with dementia, risperidone and olanzapine were found to be superior to haloperidol for the treatment of aggression (Lyketsos 2000). Haloperidol was superior to placebo in those studies.

Data showing that experimental and pharmacological modulation of serotonin neurotransmission can reduce levels of aggression in nonhuman primates and smaller animals (Walsh and Dinan 2001), and other results showing low CSF levels of serotonin metabolites in impulsively aggressive patients, violent offenders, and suicide attempters (discussed earlier, in the section "Mechanisms of Aggression"), constitute compelling reasons to treat impulsive aggression with selective serotonin reuptake inhibitors (SSRIs), lithium, buspirone, and other drugs that may enhance central serotonin levels. In addition, SSRIs, lithium, and buspirone have been effective, in placebo-controlled trials, in reducing impulsive nonviolent aggression in patients with personality disorders, autism, and depressive disorders (Coccaro and Siever 2002).

Anticonvulsants also have received systematic evaluation for treating aggressive behavior. Divalproex sodium has been evaluated in several open studies. A review of available data concluded that aggression is responsive to divalproex sodium (Lindenmayer and Kotsaftis 2000). However, this review found no blinded, placebo-controlled trials, only three open-label studies, and all other data came from anecdotal reports. In blinded, placebo-controlled trials, carbamazepine reduced aggression in nursing home patients with dementia (Tariot et al. 1998) and in patients with personality disorder (Cowdry and Gardner 1988; Gardner and Cowdry 1986). Phenytoin also may be useful for the treatment of aggression because limited data from controlled trials suggest that some cases of impulsive aggression may respond to the medication (Barratt et

TABLE 8–6.   Medications used in the treatment of chronic aggression

Medication	Starting dosage	Usual target dosage
SSRIs		
Sertraline	25 mg/day	150–200 mg/day
Fluoxetine	10 mg/day	60–80 mg/day
Paroxetine	10 mg/day (or bedtime)	20–60 mg/day
Citalopram	10 mg/day	20–40 mg/day
TCAs		
Nortriptyline	10–25 mg at bedtime	Serum level: 50–150 ng/dL
Clomipramine	25 mg at bedtime	Serum level: 150–200 ng/dL
SNRIs		
Venlafaxine XR	37.5 mg/day (or twice daily)	225–300 mg/day
Trazodone	25–50 mg at bedtime	300–500 mg/day
Nefazodone	50 mg at bedtime	500–600 mg/day
Mirtazapine	7.5–15.0 mg at bedtime	15–45 mg/day
Neuroleptics		
Haloperidol	2.5 mg/day (or twice daily)	15–20 mg/day
Fluphenazine	2.5 mg/day (or twice daily)	15–20 mg/day
Loxapine	5–10 mg twice daily	50 mg/day
Thioridazine	50 mg/day	200 mg/day
Risperidone	0.5–1.0 mg/day	4–8 mg/day
Olanzapine	2.5–5.0 mg at bedtime	10–20 mg/day
Clozapine	12.5–25.0 mg/day	150–300 mg/day
Quetiapine	25 mg twice daily	100–250 mg/day
Anticonvulsants		
Divalproex sodium	250 mg twice daily	Serum level: 50–100 ng/dL
Carbamazepine	100 mg twice daily	Serum level: 4–12 ng/dL
Gabapentin	300 mg twice daily	1,800–2,400 mg/day
Phenytoin	100 mg twice daily	300 mg/day
Others		
Lithium	300 mg/day	Serum level: 0.6–1.2 mEq/dL
Buspirone	5.0–7.5 mg twice daily	20–30 mg/day
Propranolol	20–40 mg twice daily	80–160 mg/day
Amantadine	50–100 mg twice daily	200–300 mg/day
Progesterone	10 mg/day	20 mg/day
Leuprolide	2.5–5.0 mg intramuscularly every 2 weeks	10 mg intramuscularly every 2 weeks

Note.   SNRIs=serotonin-norepinephrine reuptake inhibitors; SSRIs=selective serotonin reuptake inhibitors; TCAs=tricyclic antidepressants. Initial and target doses are up to 50% lower when the patient is an elder, is mentally retarded, is taking many medications, has a severe systemic or metabolic illness, or has a dementia.

al. 1997). However, psychiatric experience with phenytoin is very limited. On the contrary, gabapentin is frequently prescribed for impulsive aggression, but no empirical evidence yet supports this practice.

Because overactivity in the noradrenergic system has been implicated in expression of aggression, noradrenergic blockade has emerged as another therapeutic strategy. The typically used agents are propranolol and nadolol, both beta-adrenergic blockers. Clinical trials have found them to be effective in patients with traumatic brain injury, dementia, and psychosis (Allan et al. 1996; Ratey et al. 1992; Shankle et al. 1995; Sorgi et al. 1986). Beta-

blockers may cause hypotension and bradycardia and therefore should be used with caution. In fact, low-dose treatment may be effective for certain patients; one study found that low-dose propranolol (10–80 mg/day) reduced aggression in patients with dementia (Shankle et al. 1995).

Table 8–6 provides a summary of other medications that may be helpful for treating aggression. Progesterone and leuprolide are used for some patients with aggressive sexual behavior (see Chapter 17, "Sexual Disorders"). In routine practice, psychiatrists often use combinations of medications from different classes because the response to single-agent therapy is usually modest.

Conclusion

Aggression is a major clinical and public health problem. In clinical settings, it represents a difficult, disruptive, and dangerous problem for psychiatrists, nonpsychiatric physicians, nurses, and other health care workers. Fortunately, strategies exist to manage this problem. A careful description of the aggressive episode, in the context of a comprehensive psychiatric examination, informs clinical management. Out of the clinical examination comes an appreciation of the fundamental nature of the problem (for instance, whether the aggression is impulsive or premeditated), the factors that have produced and/or sustained it, and the approaches to treatment.

The treatment of aggression requires awareness that psychiatric diagnosis alone is often not enough to inform the treatment—and, therefore, an individualized approach. For most patients, aggression is managed empirically with a combination of approaches—behavioral, environmental, and pharmacological. In the general hospital, the management of aggressive patients involves active collaboration among psychiatrists, nonpsychiatric physicians, nurses, and other health care workers. This collaboration works best when the ground has been prepared beforehand through the teaching efforts of the psychiatrist and will maximize the effectiveness of interventions while minimizing the risk of injury to patients and medical staff.

Finally, it is also important to keep in mind that many aggressive patients, particularly those with impulsive aggression, are also at risk for suicidal behavior and require a careful suicide risk assessment and appropriate interventions. Recent research has yielded much insight into the neurobiology of aggression and violence, but more work is needed to develop predictive methods and more effective preventive and treatment modalities.

References

Allan ER, Alpert M, Sison CE, et al: Adjunctive nadolol in the treatment of acutely aggressive schizophrenic patients. J Clin Psychiatry 57:455–459, 1996

Allen MH, Currier GW, Hughes DH, et al: The Expert Consensus Guideline Series: treatment of behavioral emergencies. Postgrad Med (Spec No):1–88; quiz 89–90, 2001

American Association of Family Physicians: Family violence: an AAFP white paper. The AAFP Commission on Special Issues and Clinical Interests. Am Fam Physician 50:1636–1640, 1644–1646, 1994

American College of Emergency Physicians: Emergency medicine and domestic violence. Ann Emerg Med 25:442–443, 1995

American College of Obstetrics and Gynecology: ACOG technical bulletin: domestic violence (No 209, August 1995; replaces No 124, January 1989). Int J Gynaecol Obstet 51:161–170, 1995

American Medical Association: Violence against women: relevance for medical practitioners. Council on Scientific Affairs, American Medical Association. JAMA 267:3184–3189, 1992

American Psychiatric Association: Diagnostic and Statistical Manual of Mental Disorders, 4th Edition. Washington, DC, American Psychiatric Association, 1994a

American Psychiatric Association: Position statement on women and domestic violence among several approved by APA. Hosp Community Psychiatry 45:185–186, 1994b

American Psychiatric Association: Diagnostic and Statistical Manual of Mental Disorders, 4th Edition, Text Revision. Washington, DC, American Psychiatric Association, 2000

Appelbaum PS, Robbins PC, Monahan J: Violence and delusions: data from the MacArthur Violence Risk Assessment Study. Am J Psychiatry 157:566–572, 2000

Arnetz JE, Arnetz BB: Violence towards health care staff and possible effects on the quality of patient care. Soc Sci Med 52:417–427, 2001

Barlow K, Grenyer B, Ilkiw-Lavalle O: Prevalence and precipitants of aggression in psychiatric inpatient units. Aust N Z J Psychiatry 34:967–974, 2000

Barratt ES, Stanford MS, Felthous AR, et al: The effects of phenytoin on impulsive and premeditated aggression: a controlled study. J Clin Psychopharmacol 17:341–349, 1997

Battaglia J, Moss S, Rush J, et al: Haloperidol, lorazepam, or both for psychotic agitation? A multicenter, prospective, double-blind, emergency department study. Am J Emerg Med 15:335–340, 1997

Beauford JE, McNiel DE, Binder RL: Utility of the initial therapeutic alliance in evaluating psychiatric patients' risk of violence. Am J Psychiatry 154:1272–1276, 1997

Berman ME, Coccaro EF: Neurobiologic correlates of violence: relevance to criminal responsibility. Behav Sci Law 16:303–318, 1998

Binder RL: Are the mentally ill dangerous? J Am Acad Psychiatry Law 27:189–201, 1999

Binder RL, McNiel DE: The relationship of gender to violent behavior in acutely disturbed psychiatric patients. J Clin Psychiatry 51:110–114, 1990

Binder RL, McNiel DE: Staff gender and risk of assault on doctors and nurses. Bull Am Acad Psychiatry Law 22:545–550, 1994

Blanchard JC, Curtis KM: Violence in the emergency department. Emerg Med Clin North Am 17:717–731, 1999

Bowers L, Jarrett M, Clark N, et al: Determinants of absconding by patients on acute psychiatric wards. J Adv Nurs 32:644–649, 2000

Bronheim HE, Fulop G, Kunkel EJ, et al: The Academy of Psychosomatic Medicine practice guidelines for psychiatric consultation in the general medical setting. The Academy of Psychosomatic Medicine. Psychosomatics 39:S8–S30, 1998

Brower MC, Price BH: Neuropsychiatry of frontal lobe dysfunction in violent and criminal behaviour: a critical review. J Neurol Neurosurg Psychiatry 71:720–726, 2001

Buckley P, Bartell J, Donenwirth K, et al: Violence and schizophrenia: clozapine as a specific antiaggressive agent. Bull Am Acad Psychiatry Law 23:607–611, 1995

Buckley PF, Ibrahim ZY, Singer B, et al: Aggression and schizophrenia: efficacy of risperidone. J Am Acad Psychiatry Law 25:173–181, 1997

Citrome L, Volavka J, Czobor P, et al: Effects of clozapine, olanzapine, risperidone, and haloperidol on hostility among patients with schizophrenia. Psychiatr Serv 52:1510–1514, 2001

Coccaro EF, Siever LJ: Pathophysiology and treatment of aggression, in Neuropharmacology: The Fifth Generation of Progress. Edited by Davis KL, Charney D, Coyle JT, et al. Philadelphia, PA, Lippincott, Williams & Wilkins, 2002, pp 1709–1723

Cohen-Mansfield J, Billig N: Agitated behaviors in the elderly, I: a conceptual review. J Am Geriatr Soc 34:711–721, 1986

Coid J, Petruckevitch A, Chung WS, et al: Abusive experiences and psychiatric morbidity in women primary care attenders. Br J Psychiatry 183:332–339, 2003

Corbett SW, Grange JT, Thomas TL: Exposure of prehospital care providers to violence. Prehosp Emerg Care 2:127–131, 1998

Cowdry RW, Gardner DL: Pharmacotherapy of borderline personality disorder: alprazolam, carbamazepine, trifluoperazine, and tranylcypromine. Arch Gen Psychiatry 45:111–119, 1988

Cummings JL, Mega MS: Violence and aggression, in Neuropsychiatry and Behavioral Neuroscience. New York, Oxford University Press, 2003, pp 360–370

Czobor P, Volavka J, Meibach RC: Effect of risperidone on hostility in schizophrenia. J Clin Psychopharmacol 15:243–249, 1995

Davidson RJ, Putnam KM, Larson CL: Dysfunction in the neural circuitry of emotion regulation—a possible prelude to violence. Science 289:591–594, 2000

Demaree HA, Harrison DW: Case study: topographical brain mapping in hostility following mild closed head injury. Int J Neurosci 87:97–101, 1996

Ehmann TS, Smith GN, Yamamoto A, et al: Violence in treatment resistant psychotic inpatients. J Nerv Ment Dis 189:716–721, 2001

Eisenstat SA, Bancroft L: Domestic violence. N Engl J Med 341:886–892, 1999

Emergency Nurses Association: Emergency Nurses Association position statement: forensic evidence collection. J Emerg Nurs 24(5):38A, 1998

Eronen M, Angermeyer MC, Schulze B, et al: The psychiatric epidemiology of violent behaviour. Soc Psychiatry Psychiatr Epidemiol 33 (suppl 1):S13–S23, 1998

Gardner DL, Cowdry RW: Positive effects of carbamazepine on behavioral dyscontrol in borderline personality disorder. Am J Psychiatry 143:519–522, 1986

Gerard ME, Spitz MC, Towbin JA, et al: Subacute postictal aggression. Neurology 50:384–388, 1998

Gerbert B, Bronstone A, Pantilat S, et al: When asked, patients tell: disclosure of sensitive health-risk behaviors. Med Care 37:104–111, 1999

Gerbert B, Moe J, Caspers N, et al: Simplifying physicians' response to domestic violence. West J Med 172:329–331, 2000

Golding AM: Domestic violence. J R Soc Med 95:307–308, 2002

Grange JT, Corbett SW: Violence against emergency medical services personnel. Prehosp Emerg Care 6:186–190, 2002

Greenfield TK, McNiel DE, Binder RL: Violent behavior and length of psychiatric hospitalization. Hosp Community Psychiatry 40:809–814, 1989

Harlow JM: Passage of an iron rod through the head. Boston Med Surg J 39:389–393, 1848

Harlow JM: Recovery from the passage of an iron rod through the head. Publications of the Massachusetts Medical Society 2:327–347, 1868

Hillbrand M, Foster HG, Spitz RT: Characteristics and cost of staff injuries in a forensic hospital. Psychiatr Serv 47:1123–1125, 1996

Kalunian DA, Binder RL, McNiel DR: Violence by geriatric patients who need psychiatric hospitalization. J Clin Psychiatry 51:340–343, 1990

Kanemoto K, Kawasaki J, Mori E: Violence and epilepsy: a close relation between violence and postictal psychosis. Epilepsia 40:107–109, 1999

Lam JN, McNiel DE, Binder RL: The relationship between patients' gender and violence leading to staff injuries. Psychiatr Serv 51:1167–1170, 2000

Lamberg L: Domestic violence: what to ask, what to do. JAMA 284:554–556, 2000

Lancee WJ, Gallop R, McCay E, et al: The relationship between nurses' limit-setting styles and anger in psychiatric inpatients. Psychiatr Serv 46:609–613, 1995

Lindenmayer JP, Kotsaftis A: Use of sodium valproate in violent and aggressive behaviors: a critical review. J Clin Psychiatry 61:123–128, 2000

Lyketsos CG: Aggression, in The American Psychiatric Press Textbook of Geriatric Neuropsychiatry. Edited by Coffey E, Cummings JL. Washington, DC, American Psychiatric Press, 2000, pp 477–488

Lyketsos CG, Rosenblatt A, Rabins P: The forgotten frontal lobe syndrome or "executive dysfunction syndrome." Psychosomatics 45:247–255, 2004

Lynch J, Appelboam R, McQuillan PJ: Survey of abuse and violence by patients and relatives towards intensive care staff. Anaesthesia 58:893–899, 2003

Marsh L, Krauss GL: Aggression and violence in patients with epilepsy. Epilepsy Behav 1:160–168, 2000

McNiel DE, Eisner JP, Binder RL: The relationship between command hallucinations and violence. Psychiatr Serv 51:1288–1292, 2000

Mock EF, Wrenn KD, Wright SW, et al: Prospective field study of violence in emergency medical services calls. Ann Emerg Med 32:33–36, 1998

National Academies of Sciences: Elder Mistreatment: Abuse, Neglect, and Exploitation in an Aging America. Panel to Review Risk and Prevalence of Elder Abuse and Neglect. Washington, DC, National Academies Press, 2003

Newhill CE, Mulvey EP, Lidz CW: Characteristics of violence in the community by female patients seen in a psychiatric emergency service. Psychiatr Serv 46:785–789, 1995

Ng B, Kumar S, Ranclaud M, et al: Ward crowding and incidents of violence on an acute psychiatric inpatient unit. Psychiatr Serv 52:521–525, 2001

O'Connor S: Violent behavior in chronic schizophrenia and inpatient psychiatry. J Am Acad Psychoanal Dyn Psychiatry 31:31–44, 2003

Owen C, Tarantello C, Jones M, et al: Repetitively violent patients in psychiatric units. Psychiatr Serv 49:1458–1461, 1998

Palmstierna T, Huitfeldt B, Wistedt B: The relationship of crowding and aggressive behavior on a psychiatric intensive care unit. Hosp Community Psychiatry 42:1237–1240, 1991

Pozzi C: Exposure of prehospital providers to violence and abuse. J Emerg Nurs 24:320–323, 1998

Rabinowitz J, Avnon M, Rosenberg V: Effect of clozapine on physical and verbal aggression. Schizophr Res 22:249–255, 1996

Raja M, Azzoni A, Lubich L: Aggressive and violent behavior in a population of psychiatric inpatients. Soc Psychiatry Psychiatr Epidemiol 32:428–434, 1997

Ratey JJ, Sorgi P, O'Driscoll GA, et al: Nadolol to treat aggression and psychiatric symptomatology in chronic psychiatric inpatients: a double-blind, placebo-controlled study. J Clin Psychiatry 53:41–46, 1992

Ratey JJ, Leveroni C, Kilmer D, et al: The effects of clozapine on severely aggressive psychiatric inpatients in a state hospital. J Clin Psychiatry 54:219–223, 1993

Rodriguez MA, Bauer HM, McLoughlin E, et al: Screening and intervention for intimate partner abuse: practices and attitudes of primary care physicians. JAMA 282:468–474, 1999

Scott H, Johnson S, Menezes P, et al: Substance misuse and risk of aggression and offending among the severely mentally ill. Br J Psychiatry 172:345–350, 1998

Shankle WR, Nielson KA, Cotman CW: Low-dose propranolol reduces aggression and agitation resembling that associated with orbitofrontal dysfunction in elderly demented patients. Alzheimer Dis Assoc Disord 9:233–237, 1995

Sheridan M, Henrion R, Robinson L, et al: Precipitants of violence in a psychiatric inpatient setting. Hosp Community Psychiatry 41:776–780, 1990

Sorgi PJ, Ratey JJ, Polakoff S: Beta-adrenergic blockers for the control of aggressive behaviors in patients with chronic schizophrenia. Am J Psychiatry 143:775–776, 1986

Soyka M: Substance misuse, psychiatric disorder and violent and disturbed behaviour. Br J Psychiatry 176:345–350, 2000

Stevenson S: Heading off violence with verbal de-escalation. J Psychosoc Nurs Ment Health Serv 29(9):6–10, 1991

Swanson JW: Mental disorder, substance abuse, and community violence: an epidemiologic approach, in Violence in Mental Disorder: Developments in Risk Assessment. Edited by Monahan J, Steadman HJ. Chicago, IL, University of Chicago Press, 1994, pp 101–136

Swanson JW, Holzer CE 3rd, Ganju VK, et al: Violence and psychiatric disorder in the community: evidence from the Epidemiologic Catchment Area surveys. Hosp Community Psychiatry 41:761–770, 1990 [published erratum appears in Hosp Community Psychiatry 42:954–955, 1991]

Swanson J, Estroff S, Swartz M, et al: Violence and severe mental disorder in clinical and community populations: the effects of psychotic symptoms, comorbidity, and lack of treatment. Psychiatry 60:1–22, 1997

Swanson J, Swartz M, Estroff S, et al: Psychiatric impairment, social contact, and violent behavior: evidence from a study of outpatient-committed persons with severe mental disorder. Soc Psychiatry Psychiatr Epidemiol 33 (suppl 1):S86–S94, 1998

Swartz MS, Swanson JW, Hiday VA, et al: Taking the wrong drugs: the role of substance abuse and medication noncompliance in violence among severely mentally ill individuals. Soc Psychiatry Psychiatr Epidemiol 33 (suppl 1):S75–S80, 1998

Tariot PN, Erb R, Podgorski CA, et al: Efficacy and tolerability of carbamazepine for agitation and aggression in dementia. Am J Psychiatry 155:54–61, 1998

Tintinalli JE, McCoy M: Violent patients and the prehospital provider. Ann Emerg Med 22:1276–1279, 1993

Tonkonogy JM, Geller JL: Hypothalamic lesions and intermittent explosive disorder. J Neuropsychiatry Clin Neurosci 4:45–50, 1992

Torrey EF: Violent behavior by individuals with serious mental illness. Hosp Community Psychiatry 45:653–662, 1994

Treiman DM: Epilepsy and violence: medical and legal issues. Epilepsia 27 (suppl 2):S77–S104, 1986

U.S. Department of Transportation: Emergency Medical Technician—Paramedic: National Standard Curriculum, United States Department of Transportation, 1998

Volavka J: The neurobiology of violence: an update. J Neuropsychiatry Clin Neurosci 11:307–314, 1999

Walsh MT, Dinan TG: Selective serotonin reuptake inhibitors and violence: a review of the available evidence. Acta Psychiatr Scand 104:84–91, 2001

Whittington R, Shuttleworth S, Hill L: Violence to staff in a general hospital setting. J Adv Nurs 24:326–333, 1996

9 Depression

Gary M. Rodin, M.D., F.R.C.P.C.

Robert P. Nolan, Ph.D., R.Psych.

Mark R. Katz, M.D., F.R.C.P.C.

MEDICAL AND DEPRESSIVE illnesses are common conditions that frequently coexist in the general population. This association is to be expected both because of coincidence and because the risk of depressive disorders is increased in most medical conditions. This elevated risk is due, in part, to the association of most, or all, serious medical illnesses with a variety of nonspecific risk factors for depression. There also has been much speculation about whether specific biological mechanisms may account for the comorbidity of depression with particular medical conditions.

Depression is frequently undiagnosed and untreated in medical and primary care populations, despite its frequency, negative effect on health, and treatability. Such underdiagnosis may occur for several reasons. One reason is that many of the symptoms of depression are similar to those of medical illness. As a result, it may be problematic to determine whether such symptoms are manifestations of a physical disease or of a comorbid depressive disorder. Furthermore, in the context of a serious medical illness, it can be difficult to differentiate normal, adaptive psychological reactions from dysfunctional psychological states and overt psychiatric illness. For example, distinguishing to what extent passive suicidal ideation in individuals with advanced disease reflects depression and to what extent it reflects the wish to escape from unbearable suffering or from a rational wish to end life may be problematic. False positive diagnoses of depressive disorders also may occur when physical symptoms of medical illness, such as apathy, fatigue, sleep disturbance, and realistic feelings of sadness, are mistakenly attributed to a depressive disorder. Hypoactive delirium associated with apathy and psychomotor retardation also may be mislabeled as depres-

sion. However, it is clearly established that depressive disorders occur with increased frequency in the medically ill, have an adverse effect on quality of life, and increase morbidity and mortality in many medical disorders.

In this chapter, we review the prevalence, clinical features, screening and diagnostic issues, and etiological mechanisms related to depressive disorders in specific medical populations and consider approaches to treatment. In addition, we address some of the potential mechanisms to account for the links between depression and specific medical illnesses affecting the course and outcome.

The Continuum of Depression: From Experience to Disorder

The experience of sadness is a normal, expectable response to the multiple adverse effects of a serious medical illness. These effects include changes in bodily appearance and functioning; pain and physical distress; limitations in the capacity to work and to engage in pleasurable activities; a perceived alteration in the anticipated life trajectory; fears of disability and dependency; alterations in intimate relationships, family life, social relationships, and activities; and neurobiological and hormonal abnormalities.

Initial grief reactions and a subsequent mourning process are common following the onset of a serious or terminal illness (reviewed in detail in Chapter 40, "Palliative Care"). Individuals who have difficulty resolving this process and who have other risk factors are more likely to develop major depressive disorder (MDD). Factors that affect the likelihood of a comorbid depressive disorder include the personal coping style of the individual, the physical effects of the illness and treatment, the support-iveness of the environment, the stigma and personal meaning associated with the medical condition, and the propensity of the individual to respond to stressful life circumstances with depression. Individuals with a personal or family history of depression, and those who are younger and who have low social support, are much more likely to develop clinical depression in the context of a medical illness (Cavanaugh et al. 1983; Craven et al. 1987). Physiological effects of medical illness also may contribute to mood alterations, although the specificity of this relationship has not been well established in most medical conditions. Clinical depression may be the end of a final common pathway resulting from the interaction of multiple risk and protective factors (see Figure 9–1).

We place particular emphasis in this chapter on the syndrome of MDD and on dysthymic disorder, although it is recognized that depressive symptoms occur on a con-tinuum and that distress and impaired functioning may be associated with subthreshold disorders (Kendler and Gardner 1998).

Epidemiology

Depressive disorders are extremely common in the general population. Up to 17% of adults in the United States have had at least one episode of MDD during their lifetime (Blazer et al. 1994; Kessler et al. 2003), and 2%–4% have a current MDD (Burvill 1995). There may be large cross-national differences in the prevalence of depressive disorders on the basis of diagnostic, clinical, and social factors. In a study of more than 25,000 primary care patients in 14 countries, the prevalence of current MDD was found to vary 15-fold across centers (Simon et al. 2002).

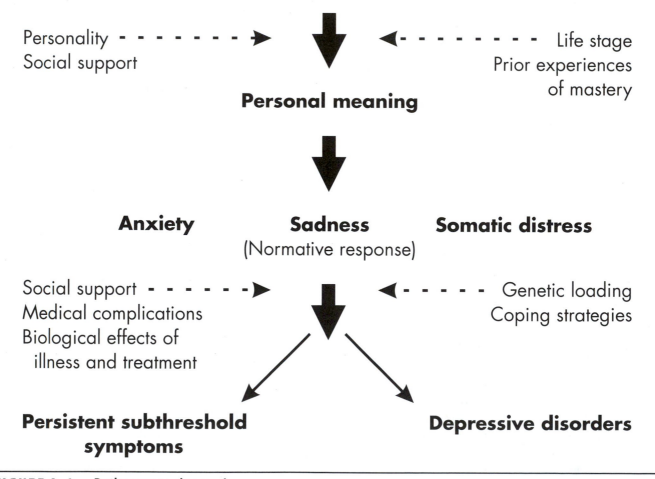

FIGURE 9–1.   Pathways to depression.

Source.   Reprinted from Peveler R, Carson A, Rodin G: "ABC of Psychological Medicine: Depression in Medical Patients." *British Medical Journal* 325:149–152, 2002. Used with permission of the BMJ Publishing Group.

Many medical illnesses have been shown to be associated with an increased risk for MDD. In the Epidemiologic Catchment Area program, the prevalence of affective disorders was 9.4%–12.9% in medically ill patients but only 5.8%–8.4% in a matched control group of healthy individuals (Wells et al. 1988). In another study (Ormel et al. 1993), the decline in functioning secondary to a medical illness was shown to be associated with an increased subsequent risk for the development of major depression. The prevalence of MDD in medical populations varies, to some extent, with the severity of the medical condition. In that regard, the prevalence of MDD has been found to increase progressively from community samples (2%–4%), to primary care settings (5%–10%), to medical inpatient settings (6%–14%) (Burvill 1995). Furthermore, the number of comorbid medical diseases has been shown to be associated with the onset of a depressive episode in both primary care (Barkow et al. 2002) and community samples (Lindeman et al. 2000; Wilhelm et al. 1999). Similar to MDD, minor depressive disorders have been reported in up to 16% of medical outpatients (D.A. Beck and Koenig 1996), a rate several times higher than that in the general population (Burvill 1995). The prevalence of depressive disorders in specific medical conditions is discussed in subsequent sections of this chapter.

Clinical Features and Diagnosis

The four major categories of depressive disorders specified in DSM-IV-TR (American Psychiatric Association 2000) are 1) MDD, 2) dysthymic disorder, 3) adjustment disorder with depressed mood, and 4) mood disorder due to a (specified) general medical condition. The last category refers to mood disorders judged to be the direct physiological consequence of a specific general medical condition. In that regard, medical conditions such as stroke, Parkinson's disease, multiple sclerosis, pancreatic cancer, and diabetes all have been postulated to be a direct cause of depression. However, this category is problematic because the specificity of these relationships is most often difficult or impossible to confirm. A depressed mood in this context has not been shown to be due to the linear effect of any one psychological, biological, or social factor; usually, these interact with one another in the etiology of depression. DSM-IV-TR also delineates the condition of dementia with depressed mood, which is addressed in Chapter 7 ("Dementia") of this text.

The diagnosis of depressive disorders in medical populations is fraught with difficulty for a variety of reasons, including the following:

1. Many symptoms of medical illness (e.g., fatigue, anorexia, weight loss, insomnia, psychomotor retardation, and diminished concentration) resemble those of depression. Following a stroke, a variety of emotional disturbances, such as "emotionalism," pathological crying, apathy, or fatigue, can be mistaken for depression (Bogousslavsky 2003).

2. Thoughts of death and the desire for death may be reported by patients with advanced medical disease in the absence of a depressed mood. A subtle form of suicidality, the desire for hastened death, has been reported by 4% of hospitalized cancer patients (Jones et al. 2003) and by 17% of cancer patients in the last few weeks of life (Breitbart et al. 2000). The desire for hastened death in cancer patients is associated with depressive symptoms but also may be linked to hopelessness and unrelieved pain. Interestingly, with more advanced disease, the desire for hastened death may occur in the absence of self-reported depression (Jones et al. 2003). These findings suggest that loss of the will to live may be a less reliable sign of a depressive disorder in those with advanced medical disease than in nonmedical populations.

3. Physical suffering and disability may diminish the capacity to experience pleasure in many activities, in the absence of comorbid depression. Whereas the loss of interest and pleasure in activities is usually a characteristic symptom of depression, the multiple physical symptoms associated with many serious medical conditions may interfere with pleasure in such activities, independent of a depressed mood. It may not be until pain and other physical symptoms have been adequately treated that the interest, or capacity, to engage in valued activities can resume. A depressed mood or withdrawal from social or physical activities that is disproportionate to physical disability increases the likelihood that depression is present.

4. In medical populations, depressive symptoms may manifest in atypical or masked forms, including the amplification of somatic symptoms and noncompliance with or refusal of medical treatment (Starace et al. 2002). These factors may contribute to both the underdiagnosis and the overdiagnosis of MDD in medical populations.

5. The onset of a serious medical illness may be associated with a profound sense of loss, which may be similar to that observed with bereavement and grief. The boundary between nonpathological grief reactions and clinical depression is frequently difficult to establish, and the 2-week duration of symptoms specified in DSM-IV-TR may be too short to make this distinction. Whether the usual criteria for depression should

apply in this context is unclear, although it has been recommended that when depressive symptoms persist after 2 months, antidepressant treatment should be considered (Whooley and Simon 2000).

Various approaches have been proposed to diminish the effect of confounding medical symptoms in the diagnosis of MDD. DSM-IV-TR suggests an "exclusive" and an "etiological" approach, which specifies that symptoms that are judged by the clinician to be etiologically related to a general medical condition should be excluded from the diagnostic criteria for MDD. An exclusive approach is one in which symptoms are removed from the diagnostic criteria if they are not found to be more frequent in depressed than in nondepressed patients (Bukberg et al. 1984). This approach is intended to avoid attributing symptoms of physical illness to a depressive syndrome. However, the wording in DSM-IV-TR leaves unclear whether this exclusion applies only to the physiological consequences of the medical condition or extends to psychological reactions to the condition (Koenig 1997). In any case, the criteria for determining which symptoms are due to a medical illness and which are due to other factors unrelated to the medical illness are unclear (Rifkin et al. 1985).

Another approach to the diagnosis of MDD in the medically ill is "substitutive" (Endicott 1984). In this approach, symptoms most likely confused with medical illness, such as loss of energy, weight loss, and impaired concentration, are substituted with symptoms that are more likely to be affective in origin, such as irritability, tearfulness, social withdrawal, and feeling punished (Cavanaugh et al. 1983). This substitution eliminates the need to distinguish symptoms of medical illness from those of depression; however, it also excludes some somatic symptoms that are core manifestations of more severe forms of depression. Furthermore, the criteria to determine which symptoms should be substituted are not clearly established, and this approach has not been widely adopted.

Koenig et al. (1997) evaluated the rates of depression in hospitalized elderly medical patients according to six different diagnostic schemes. They found that the prevalence of MDD varied from 10% to 20%, depending on the diagnostic scheme used, and that of minor depression varied from 14% to 25%. However, they concluded that there was no overall single advantage of one diagnostic scheme compared with the others. The exclusive-etiological approach identified the most severe persistent depressions, but an inclusive approach, in which all symptoms are included without making a judgment as to whether they may be related to a comorbid medical disorder, was the most sensitive and reliable approach. In cases that continue to be confusing, a trial of treatment may be indicated to help resolve the uncertainty and to reduce the risk of failing to treat a potentially reversible depressive disorder.

Health Outcomes

It was estimated in the Global Burden of Disease Study (C.J. Murray and Lopez 1997) that MDD was the fourth leading cause of disability in 1990 and that, within two decades, it would be the second leading cause, surpassed only by heart disease. Depressed patients show substantial and long-lasting impairment in multiple domains of functioning (Hays et al. 1995). Depression is also associated with a significant economic burden due, in part, to work-related disability (Druss et al. 2000) and to increased medical costs both in primary care (S.D. Pearson et al. 1999; Simon et al. 1995) and in hospital settings (Druss et al. 1999). After a review of cross-sectional, longitudinal, and treatment studies of patients with and without arthritis, chronic obstructive pulmonary disease, diabetes, or heart disease, Simon (2003) concluded that depression significantly increases the burden of functional impairment in medical illness and that treatment of depression reduces both disability and health service costs.

Medical illness with comorbid MDD is associated with worse medical outcomes and with an increased mortality rate because of several different factors. An increased risk of suicide has been reported in carefully conducted studies of several medical conditions, including cancer (Breitbart and Krivo 1998), multiple sclerosis (Stenager et al. 1996), and Huntington's chorea (Almqvist et al. 1999). In addition to an increased suicide rate (Wulsin 2000), MDD has been associated with increased mortality from other medical disorders (Musselman et al. 1998; Penninx et al. 1998). Mortality in the medically ill has been related to the triad of current MDD, a history of depression, and the severity of the medical illness. The increased mortality rate with MDD persists even when the contribution of factors such as smoking, physical health, and alcohol consumption is controlled (Schulz et al. 2000). Studies of specific medical conditions have found that depression is associated with a more rapid progression of HIV disease (Leserman et al. 1997; Page-Shafer et al. 1996) and with increased mortality in cardiovascular disease (Frasure-Smith et al. 1995; Lesperance et al. 1996; Morris et al. 1993), including poorer 6-month survival rates after myocardial infarction (Frasure-Smith et al. 1993).

Depression may affect health outcomes via several different mechanisms. Biological aspects of depression may increase cardiac mortality through its effects on the autonomic nervous system. Some of these postulated effects are outlined later in this chapter (see subsection "Depression and Coronary Artery Disease"). Noncompliance with medical treatment also may contribute to the increased morbidity and mortality in depressed medical patients. A meta-analysis (DiMatteo et al. 2000) suggested that the odds are three times greater that depressed patients will be noncompliant with medical treatment recommendations compared with nondepressed patients. Depression also has been associated with poor treatment compliance in patients with end-stage renal disease and patients with HIV disease (Starace et al. 2002) and with more impaired metabolic control in patients with type 1 diabetes (Lustman et al. 2000a). Such noncompliance may include not taking treatments that are prescribed, not following diet or lifestyle recommendations, and not attending medical appointments (Wing et al. 2002).

Depression may be associated with a variety of other health risk behaviors such as cigarette smoking, as well as overeating and physical inactivity, both of which may be associated with obesity. These factors may not only increase the risk of depression but also contribute to poorer health outcomes in those who are depressed. Current depressive symptoms are associated with smoking (Breslau et al. 1993), and smokers who are depressed more often tend to fail smoking cessation programs (Anda et al. 1990). Mechanisms that have been postulated to account for the association of depression and smoking include the hypotheses that smoking is used to self-medicate to prevent or to reduce depressive symptoms and that the propensity to smoke and the tendency to become depressed share a common genetic or emotional basis (Dilsaver et al. 1990; Hughes 1985).

The relationships among depression, overeating, inactivity, and obesity are difficult to unravel, partly because many of the studies of obesity are based on selected samples of those who seek treatment (Stunkard et al. 2003). However, current evidence suggests that a childhood history of obesity is associated with depression in adult life (Pine et al. 2001) and that depression is associated with obesity in women but not in men (Istvan et al. 1992). Both binge-eating disorder (Marcus et al. 1995) and night-eating syndrome (Gluck et al. 2001) have been associated with increased rates of MDD, as has physical inactivity (Paluska and Schwenk 2000).

Screening for and Detection of Depression in the Medically Ill

Obstacles to Diagnosis in the Clinic Setting

Depression and other forms of distress are often underdiagnosed and undertreated in medical settings (Newport and Nemeroff 1998; Rodin et al. 1991). This is of concern because missing the diagnosis of MDD, or of a minor depressive disorder, may result in the lost opportunity to improve quality of life, decrease the risk of suicide, shorten hospital stay, and improve treatment compliance in the medically ill (D.A. Beck and Koenig 1996; Hall and Wise 1995; Koenig 1997; Strain 1998).

There are many potential explanations for the poor detection of clinical depression in clinic settings. Most medical visits last less than 15 minutes, and many issues must be addressed in this brief time (Kroenke et al. 1997). Such time constraints and the lack of privacy in the medical setting may limit disclosure or elaboration of symptoms. It is, therefore, not surprising that medical specialists are frequently unaware of which of their patients are emotionally distressed and in need of further evaluation and intervention (Sollner et al. 2001). Some clinicians may fear that they lack sufficient time or skill to manage the emotionality that may be triggered when they inquire about their patients' emotional reaction to the illness experience. Some patients may be reluctant to disclose depressive symptoms because of perceived stigma or perceived lack of interest by their medical caregivers. However, most patients are comfortable discussing psychosocial problems and welcome questions about such issues (Kroenke et al. 1997). Some patients may not recognize depressive symptoms that are present or may attribute such symptoms to the effects of their medical condition. Indeed, both patients and clinicians may have difficulty in differentiating the somatic symptoms of depression from the manifestations of medical disease. In addition, both may normalize or rationalize the depression as an appropriate, understandable reaction to the multiple stresses of medical illness. Unfortunately, the "understandability" of such depressive states may lead to the mistaken belief that treatment is unnecessary or ineffective. Finally, the patient or the clinician may be skeptical about the efficacy and tolerability of antidepressant treatment.

Screening for Depression: General Considerations

An obvious need exists for accurate and rapid methods of screening for depression in medical settings, where assessment might otherwise not be conducted. A screening program allows for standardization in identifying distress and can facilitate psychosocial resource planning and referral of patients for psychosocial and psychiatric treatment. The ideal screening instrument would be easy to administer and score, acceptable to patients, and, most important, accurate (Zabora 1998). The utility of screening for depression also depends on whether it leads to timely and effective intervention. Recent critical reviews of depression screening suggest that such efforts have resulted in increased recognition of depression but not necessarily in better management of depression or in improved outcomes (Schade et al. 1998).

Description of Screening Instruments

The three instruments that have been most widely used to screen for depression in the medically ill are (Bottomley 1998) 1) the Center for Epidemiologic Studies Depression Scale (CES-D) (Radloff 1977), 2) the Hospital Anxiety and Depression Scale (HADS) (Zigmond and Snaith 1983), and 3) the Beck Depression Inventory–II (BDI-II) (A.T. Beck et al. 1996). The Patient Health Questionnaire (PHQ) (Kroenke et al. 2001) is new, and its use is rapidly spreading. A brief discussion of each of these instruments follows.

The CES-D Scale (Radloff 1977) is a 20-item self-report measure of depressive symptoms, in which only 4 of the 20 items are somatic. Originally designed as a measure of depressive distress in nonpsychiatric community samples, it may be the most widely used screening instrument in North America. It also has been extensively used in medically ill samples with evidence of good psychometric properties (Beeber et al. 1998; Devins et al. 1988). A cutoff score of 17 was originally recommended to identify subjects with clinically significant depressive distress (Radloff 1977). However, the sensitivity and specificity of various cutoff scores have been evaluated in a variety of medical populations. Kuptniratsaikul et al. (2002) found that the CES-D was an accurate instrument in screening for depression in spinal cord injury patients. A cutoff score of 21 provided a sensitivity of 80% and a specificity of 70%, with a positive predictive value of 46%. One study in cancer patients found acceptable levels of sensitivity (70%) and specificity (80%) but a low positive predictive value (26%) when a cutoff score of 16 was used (Pasacreta 1997). Another study (Katz et al. 2004) found the CES-D to be accurate in screening for depression in head and neck cancer patients, with a cutoff score of 17 yielding a sensitivity of 100%, a specificity of 85%, and a positive predictive value of 63%. These studies support the value of the CES-D to screen for depression in the medically ill, although the positive predictive value has been relatively low in some studies, and a lack of consensus remains about the optimal cutoff score.

The HADS (Zigmond and Snaith 1983) is a 14-item self-report scale with separate 7-item subscales for anxiety and depression. It was specifically designed for use in the medically ill and has been most widely used in Europe. The Depression subscale places emphasis on anhe-

donia and does not include somatic items; it is brief and highly acceptable to patients (Herrmann 1997) and has been extensively used in the medically ill (Herrmann 1997). The HADS has been shown to have good concurrent and discriminant validity (Bramley et al. 1988; Clark et al. 1998; Flint and Rifat 1996; Snaith and Taylor 1985) and acceptable sensitivity to change (Flint and Rifat 1996). However, it has not been extensively validated as a screening instrument, for which conflicting data exist regarding its accuracy (Herrmann 1997). Some (Berard et al. 1998; Chaturvedi et al. 1996; Kugaya et al. 2000; Razavi et al. 1990) have reported acceptable sensitivity and specificity for the HADS. Katz et al. 2004) found that the HADS was highly accurate in screening for depression in head and neck cancer patients, although their optimal cutoff score was lower than that in other reports in the literature. Others found that the HADS performed very poorly as a screening instrument, with unacceptably low levels of sensitivity, specificity, or positive predictive value (Clarke et al. 1993; Lloyd-Williams et al. 2001; Silverstone 1994). Investigators also disagree about whether the total score (HADS-T) or the depressive subscale (HADS-D) should be used to screen for depression. Although the HADS-D seems more appropriate, according to theory and factor-analytic data (Flint and Rifat 1996; Herrmann 1997), some empirical studies have found that the total score predicts more accurately the presence of MDD or minor depression (Chaturvedi et al. 1996; Razavi et al. 1990).

A lack of consensus exists about the utility of the HADS and about the optimal cutoff scores to screen for MDD and minor depression. Cutoff scores recommended in the literature for the HADS-D have ranged from 7 (Razavi et al. 1990) to 11 (Clarke et al. 1993), with a cutoff score of 8 being the most widely recommended (Berard et al. 1998; Chaturvedi et al. 1996; Silverstone 1994). For the HADS-T, recommended total scores have ranged from 13 (Razavi et al. 1990) to 21 (Clarke et al. 1993), with Chaturvedi et al. (1996) and Kugaya et al. (2000) recommending midrange scores of 16 and 15, respectively.

The BDI-II (A.T. Beck et al. 1996) is the most widely accepted measure of depressive distress. Originally developed for use as a measure of symptom severity in psychiatric patients, this 21-item self-report scale has been used in numerous studies of depression in the medically ill. Concerns have been raised about its validity in patients with medical illness because of the preponderance of somatic items, and about its acceptability to patients because of its forced-choice format and complex response alternatives (Koenig et al. 1992). However, several studies have evaluated the accuracy of the BDI-II as a screening instrument in medically ill samples and found it to be an accurate self-report measure of depressive symptoms (Berard et al. 1998; Clarke et al. 1993; Craven et al. 1988).

A. T. Beck et al. (1996) recommended a BDI-II cutoff score of 10 when screening for mild depression, 16 for mild to moderate depression, 20 for moderate to severe depression, and 30 for severe depression. Studies in the medically ill have recommended cutoff scores ranging from a low of 10 (Nielsen and Williams 1980) to a high of 16 (Berard et al. 1998), with several recommending scores between 13 and 15 (Clarke et al. 1993; Craven et al. 1988; Meakin 1992). Berard et al. (1998) found in a sample of 100 mixed cancer outpatients that an optimal cutoff score of 16 yielded a sensitivity of 86%, specificity of 95%, and positive predictive value of 82%. Katz et al. (2004) found the BDI-II to be an accurate tool in screening for depression in head and neck cancer patients. The optimal cutoff score in this sample was 13, which corresponds to the midlevel cutoff score recommended in the literature. This score yielded a sensitivity of 92%, a specificity of 90%, and a positive predictive value of 69%. As with the CES-D Scale and the HADS, the preponderance of evidence suggests that the BDI-II can be used effectively to screen for depression in the medically ill.

The PHQ-9 is the nine-item depression module of the PHQ, a self-administered version of the PRIME-MD diagnostic instrument for common mental disorders that is specifically designed for primary care settings (Kroenke et al. 2001). The PHQ as a whole has been studied in thousands of primary care and medical specialty outpatients in the United States, Europe, and China. A Spanish language version has been validated as well (Diez-Quevedo et al. 2001). The PHQ-9 scores each of the nine DSM-IV-TR criteria for major depressive episode from 0 (not at all) to 3 (nearly every day). Assessed against an independent structured interview by a mental health professional, in a sample of 6,000 medical outpatients, a PHQ-9 score of 10 or greater had a sensitivity of 88% and a specificity of 88% for major depression. PHQ-9 scores of 5, 10, 15, and 20 represented mild, moderate, moderately severe, and severe depression, respectively. In a large sample of obstetrics-gynecology patients, the PHQ identified 13% as having mood disorders, 80% of which had been unrecognized by their physicians (Spitzer et al. 2000). The PHQ also yields an index of depressive severity, which also highly correlates with mental health professional assessment (Spitzer et al. 1999).

Any of these instruments may be acceptable to screen for depression in the medically ill, although the evidence for the utility of the HADS is less strong than for the BDI-II and the CES-D Scale. The PHQ has better sensitivity and specificity than the HADS (Lowe et al. 2004). The cutoff score used on any of the measures should depend, to some extent, on the purpose of screening and the resources available for follow-up. If the intent is to avoid missing cases of depression, then less stringent cutoff scores should be used, at the risk of capturing more false positive results. If there is concern about limited resources to follow up on the results of the screening, then more stringent cutoff scores should be used, which will result in fewer false positive results.

Single-Item and Very Brief Screening Scales

In addition to the use of depression rating scales in the medical setting, some evidence indicates that single-item screening for depression may have some utility. In a study conducted by Chochinov et al. (1997) with terminally ill patients, single-item screening from the Schedule for Affective Disorders and Schizophrenia (SADS) (Endicott and Spitzer 1978) diagnostic interview correctly identified the eventual diagnostic outcome of MDD, minor depression, or no depression. It should be noted that the single item "Are you depressed?" was not administered on its own but as part of a series of the following questions: "How have you been feeling? Describe your mood.... Have you felt depressed (sad, blue, moody, down, empty, as if you didn't care)? Have you cried or been tearful? (How often? Does it come and go?) . . . (How long does it last?) . . . (How bad is the feeling? Can you stand it?) . . . (What about during the last week?)." This approach is not actually single-item screening, but the publication of these findings nevertheless stimulated interest in single-item or very brief screening measures for depression in the medically ill.

C. Watkins et al. (2001) explored the accuracy of a single question assessing depression from the Yale-Brown Obsessive Compulsive Scale (Goodman et al. 1989) and compared it with clinician-derived diagnoses of depression with the Montgomery-Åsberg Rating Scale for Depression (Montgomery and Åsberg 1979). The specific item used was "Do you often feel sad or depressed?" Stroke patients were asked to simply reply "yes" or "no." They found that this single item had a sensitivity of 86%, a specificity of 78%, and a positive predictive value of 82% in screening for depression. In contrast, Lloyd-Williams et al. (2003) found that asking patients in a palliative care unit the single question "Are you depressed?" with a response choice of "yes" or "no" yielded a sensitivity of only 55% and a specificity of 74% for the diagnosis of MDD. Pomeroy et al. (2001) compared very short screening scales for depression with longer, more widely used scales in elderly medical patients, including the 30-item, 15-item, and 4-item Geriatric Depression Scales (Yesavage et al.

1983) and the 1-item Mental Health Index (Berwick et al. 1991). They found that the 4-item Geriatric Depression Scale and 1-item Mental Health Index were as effective as the longer scales in screening for depression in this population.

Kroenke et al. (2002) recently evaluated the two-item version of the PHQ (PHQ-2), which was itself derived from the nine-item PHQ module for depression (Kroenke et al. 2001). The PHQ-2 includes the first two items of the PHQ-9: "Over the last two weeks, how often have you been bothered by...little interest or pleasure in doing things" and "feeling down, depressed or hopeless?" Using an independent, structured, mental health interview for comparison, Kroenke et al. (2002) found that a PHQ-2 score of 3 or greater had a sensitivity of 83% and a specificity of 92% for MDD in a sample of primary care and obstetrics-gynecology clinic patients.

These studies suggest that very brief structured assessments of depression that focus on the core features of depression and/or anhedonia may be useful in the medically ill and that further study to compare these assessments with the longer, more established scales is warranted. Furthermore, it would appear that the major shortcoming in the detection of depression is not in the nature of the instrument used or in the question posed in the clinical setting but rather in the failure to screen for depression using any method.

Depression in Specific Medical Conditions

Depressive symptoms and depressive disorders have been found to occur at increased rates in virtually all medical conditions in which they have been studied. There have been claims and hypotheses that specific biological mechanisms may cause depression in specific medical populations, including patients with stroke, Parkinson's disease, type 1 diabetes, and some types of cancer. However, such specificity has not been substantiated in any of these conditions, although each has multiple nonspecific risk factors associated with it that may increase the prevalence of depression.

There are a variety of reasons for interest in the association of depressive disorders with specific medical diseases. There has been particular concern about depression in individuals with coronary artery disease (CAD) because of its reported association with increased mortality (see also Chapter 19, "Heart Disease"). In other conditions, such as diabetes mellitus or HIV disease, depression has been of particular interest because of the risk that

it will adversely affect treatment adherence. We do not attempt to review depression in all medical conditions; the reader may refer to the chapters on specific medical conditions in this book for more information. We selectively focus on several representative medical disorders that have been more extensively investigated in relation to depression.

Depression and Coronary Artery Disease

Approximately 27%–35% of patients with CAD present with dysphoric mood, and MDD has been diagnosed in 16%–23% of this population (R.M. Carney et al. 1987; Forrester et al. 1992; Lauzon et al. 2003; Schleifer et al. 1989). Elevated symptoms of depression and MDD are common following the spectrum of CAD events and interventions, including myocardial infarction (MI) (Frasure-Smith et al. 1999), percutaneous transluminal coronary angioplasty (R.M. Carney et al. 1987; Mendes de Leon et al. 1996), coronary artery bypass graft surgery (Connerney et al. 2001), and coronary catheterization (Hance et al. 1996). Depressed mood is also prevalent among patients with congestive heart failure, who represent an older population that is more vulnerable to medical and psychosocial comorbidities (Jiang et al. 2001; Vaccarino et al. 2001).

Depressed mood has been identified as an independent predictor of morbidity and mortality following the onset of CAD (Hemingway and Marmot 1999; Rozanski et al. 1999). A few studies have reported a significantly increased relative risk for coronary events when depressive symptoms that meet DSM-IV-TR criteria for MDD are present (e.g., Lesperance et al. 2002). However, it is also noteworthy that even mild to moderate depression is associated with secondary coronary events (Hemingway and Marmot 1999; Rozanski et al. 1999). The American College of Cardiology regards depression as a secondary risk factor for CAD because of its independent association with CAD but not as a Category I risk factor, which would require evidence that a decrease in symptoms of depression leads to a decrease in morbidity or mortality among patients with CAD (Grundy 1999; T.A. Pearson and Fuster 1996).

The prognostic importance of mild to moderate symptoms of depression raises the possibility that a specific symptom cluster within the MDD profile, rather than the full syndrome, may account for the association between depression and coronary events. For example, vital exhaustion has been observed to predict recurrent coronary events, including MI, following percutaneous transluminal coronary angioplasty (Appels and Mulder 1988; Mendes de Leon et al. 1996). This symptom construct, which overlaps with depression, includes excessive fatigue, low energy, feelings of demoralization, and irritability. It remains to be established whether other depressive symptoms, such as anhedonia, psychomotor retardation, and diminished attention and concentration, are associated with greater disease severity and prolonged disability in CAD patients. Depressive symptoms may increase medical risk because they may adversely affect motivation to initiate and sustain heart-healthy lifestyle changes, such as smoking cessation, modification of diet, and an exercise program.

A subgroup of depressogenic symptoms may trigger a psychophysiological pathway to secondary coronary events by increasing sympathetic tone. CAD patients who are depressed have greater sympathetic and neuroendocrine response to stress, as well as decreased heart rate variability, diminished baroreflex sensitivity, and higher resting heart rate (R.M. Carney et al. 1988; Krantz et al. 2000; Krittayaphong et al. 1997; L.L. Watkins and Grossman 1999). These sympathoexcitatory states lower the threshold for hypertension and progression of the atherosclerotic process (C.B. Eaton et al. 1999) and for clinically significant cardiac events (Dambrink et al. 1994; Huikuri et al. 1999; Lanza et al. 1997; Shusterman et al. 1998; Sroka et al. 1997; Valkama et al. 1995; van den Berg et al. 1997), including sudden cardiac death (Meredith et al. 1991; Wallis et al. 2000).

Two large randomized, controlled trials have assessed the efficacy of antidepressant therapies in reducing morbidity and mortality in a CAD population. The Sertraline Antidepressant Heart Attack Trial (SADHART) assessed the efficacy of sertraline compared with placebo in alleviating depression and reducing recurrent coronary events among 369 patients with CAD whose symptoms met the criteria for MDD (Glassman et al. 2002). Results from SADHART were quite modest, with sertraline failing to significantly enhance left ventricular ejection fraction, ventricular premature complex runs, or other indices of cardiovascular functioning. Fewer severe cardiovascular events were noted in the group that received sertraline rather than placebo, but this reduction did not reach statistical significance. In addition, symptoms of depression were significantly alleviated with sertraline. The Enhancing Recovery in Coronary Heart Disease (ENRICHD) trial was designed to assess the efficacy of interventions for depression and low social support in decreasing morbidity and mortality following MI (Berkman et al. 2003). In this study, 2,841 patients with MI were randomized to receive cognitive-behavioral therapy (CBT) or usual medical care. Antidepressant pharmacotherapy (i.e., selective serotonin reuptake inhibitors [SSRIs]) was prescribed for patients presenting with severe symptoms of depression. The ENRICHD trial failed to significantly lower the prevalence of recurrent MI or mortality over a 4-year interval. However, the intervention group did show a modest but statistically significant improvement in social support and reduced symptoms of depression over the short-term interval of this trial.

Depression and Cancer

Prevalence rates for MDD in cancer have varied widely in the literature, with reported rates ranging from 1.5% to 50% (Raison and Miller 2003). The reasons for such variability include the heterogeneity of cancer and the higher rates of depression associated with some cancer types (e.g., lung, pancreas, brain, and oropharynx tumors) (McDaniel et al. 1995; Zabora et al. 2001). Pancreatic cancer has been considered to have a specific association with depression (Passik and Roth 1999), but one study suggested that this association may have been overestimated and that depressive symptoms in this context are closely linked to pain (Kelsen et al. 1995). Certain chemotherapeutic treatment modalities for cancer, including the cytokines (e.g., interleukin-2, interferon-alfa), corticosteroids (e.g., prednisone, dexamethasone), and *Vinca* alkyloids (e.g., vincristine, vinblastine), are also associated with higher rates of depression (Capuron et al. 2001). It has been suggested that the prevalence rates for depression associated with cancer may be declining as a result of recent improvements in cancer treatments and more frequent provision of psychosocial support for cancer patients (Spiegel and Giese-Davis 2003). However, recent reviews suggest that the overall prevalence rate for MDD and minor depression in cancer patients is still between 10% and 30% (Hotopf et al. 2002). The prevalence rates tend to be higher in cancer patients who have more advanced disease, who are hospitalized, or who have lower performance status (Ciaramella and Poli 2001).

Depression in cancer is associated with many adverse health outcomes. Several recent studies have suggested that depression is an independent predictor of mortality (Herrmann et al. 1998; Loberiza et al. 2002; Stommel et al. 2002; Watson et al. 1999), although others have failed to find such an association (Teno et al. 2000; Tross et al. 1996). Other reported adverse sequelae of depression in cancer patients include decreased compliance with medical treatment, increased length of hospital stays, impaired quality of life, and reduced capacity to cope with pain and other physical symptoms (Massie and Popkin 1998; Pelletier et al. 2002; Pirl and Roth 1999). The emergence of MDD is associated with significantly higher rates of treatment discontinuation in patients with malignant melanoma receiving interferon-alfa (Musselman et al. 2001) and with a heightened desire for hastened death in hospitalized cancer patients (Jones et al. 2003) and terminally ill patients (Chochinov et al. 1995, 1999).

As with other medical illnesses, the diagnosis of depression may be difficult to make in the context of cancer. Fatigue and anorexia are almost universal concomitants of advanced cancer, and the side effects of many chemotherapeutic agents and radiation therapy protocols may be difficult to distinguish from depression-related symptoms. This may be the case with cytokine-induced sickness syndrome, a condition resulting from tissue damage secondary to cytokines such as interferon, which are used in cancer treatments (see Raison and Miller 2003). Despite this symptom overlap, an inclusive approach to diagnosing depression in cancer has been recommended (Chochinov et al. 1997).

Depression and Neurological Disease

The relation between neurological disorders and depression has been of particular interest both because of the frequent comorbidity of these conditions and because of what it might indicate about the neurobiology of depression. High rates of depression have been documented in many neurological illnesses with both cortical and subcortical pathology, including Parkinson's disease, poststroke syndromes, various forms of dementia, epilepsy, Huntington's disease, and multiple sclerosis (see also Chapter 7, "Dementia"). Understanding the interface between depression and disorders of the central nervous system (CNS) provides a potential opportunity to clarify the neuroanatomic pathways involved in depression. Sheline (2003) recently noted that the sites of damage to brain structures, including the frontal cortex, hippocampus, thalamus, amygdala, and basal ganglia, identified in a variety of neurological disorders overlap with some areas implicated in early-onset recurrent MDD. A specific neuroanatomic circuit, the limbic-cortical-striatal-pallidal-thalamic tract, is now thought to be particularly important in the neurobiological mediation of depression. This tract is intimately involved in emotional regulation and has been associated with structural brain abnormalities, particularly volume loss, in computed tomography (CT) and magnetic resonance imaging (MRI) studies of patients with primary unipolar depression. Mechanisms that have been postulated to account for this volume loss in early-onset recurrent depression include chronic stress-induced hypercortisolemic states of glucocorticoid-mediated neurotoxicity, inhibition of neurogenesis, decreased brain-derived growth factor, and loss of neuroplasticity (Sheline 2003).

Parkinson's Disease

Clinically significant depressive symptoms are thought to occur in approximately 50% of the patients with Parkinson's disease (Dooneief et al. 1992), and, indeed, melancholia was described as a feature of the disorder in the original description by James Parkinson in 1817. Most depressed patients with Parkinson's disease do not have MDD but rather dysthymic disorder, minor depression, and nonpsychiatric states of sadness (McDonald et al. 2003). Such depression may be caused by the psychosocial stress of this progressive incurable disorder, its effect on quality of life, and the implications for future functioning. However, other factors, including neurobiological ones, also may play an etiological role. Neurodegeneration of subcortical nuclei and disturbances in the structure and metabolic activity of the circuit connecting basal ganglia to thalamus and frontal cortex have been correlated with clinical symptoms of depression in patients with Parkinson's disease (McDonald et al. 2003). It also has been postulated that degeneration of dopamine-, serotonin-, and norepinephrine-containing neurons in the ventral tegmental area and in the substantia nigra, which project to mesocortical and mesolimbic and striatal areas, may explain some of the depression seen in these patients (McDonald et al. 2003). Finally, treatment of Parkinson's disease with levodopa and other agents may be associated with mood disturbances (Cummings 1992).

The assessment of depression in patients with Parkinson's disease presents many challenging issues. These include differentiating depressive symptoms, such as psychomotor retardation, affective restriction, fatigue, and disturbances in sleep and concentration, from the core features of Parkinson's disease. The akinesia and restricted facial expression that are characteristic of Parkinson's disease also may lead to the overdiagnosis of depression. Also, the dementia that commonly coexists with Parkinson's disease may be associated with apathy and cognitive impairment, which can be mistaken for depression. However, evidence indicates that screening instruments such as the BDI are useful to assess depression in Parkinson's disease, despite the overlap of somatic items with symptoms of Parkinson's disease (Leentjens et al. 2000).

Depressive disorders in patients with Parkinson's disease are one of the most important reversible factors that affect functioning and quality of life. Depressive disorders in Parkinson's disease have been associated with increased impairment of fine motor performance, cognitive function, and perceived quality of life (McDonald et al. 2003). In a randomized, multisite treatment study, depressive symptoms were the single most important determinant of patient quality-of-life ratings, exceeding the effects of both disease severity and medication (Global Parkinson's Disease Survey Steering Committee 2002).

Poststroke Depression

Strokes are the third leading cause of mortality and the most common serious neurological disorder, accounting for 50% of all acute hospitalizations for neurological disease (R.G. Robinson 2003). Pooled data from prevalence studies in the worldwide literature indicate that mean prevalence rates of major depression are 19.3% among hospitalized and 23.3% among ambulatory samples of stroke patients (R.G. Robinson 2003). Depression in these patients affects functional rehabilitation and cognitive functioning in the poststroke period (Herrmann et al. 1998; Kauhanen et al. 1999; Paolucci et al. 1999; Spalletta et al. 2002). Furthermore, poststroke depression may be associated with a heightened risk of mortality 1 year (House et al. 2001) and 10 years (Morris et al. 1993) later, even after medical and other background variables are controlled.

It has been suggested that poststroke depression is associated with lesions in the left anterior and left basal ganglia regions (R.G. Robinson 2003). However, a recent meta-analysis failed to show any association between poststroke depression and left anterior or left hemisphere lesions (Carson et al. 2000). Bogousslavsky (2003) suggested that poststroke depression in the chronic phase tends to be associated with lesions in the subcortical white matter, thalamus, and basal ganglia and brain stem. In a recent review, Whyte and Mulsant (2002) concluded that the available data support the hypothesis that poststroke depression is multifactorial in origin, which is consistent with the biopsychosocial model of illness (Whyte and Mulsant 2002).

Good evidence now shows that tricyclic antidepressants (TCAs), such as nortriptyline, and serotonin reuptake inhibitors, such as citalopram, are effective in treating poststroke depression (Andersen et al. 1994; R.G. Robinson et al. 2000). Preliminary evidence also suggests that cognitive impairment associated with poststroke depression may be improved by treating the depression (Kimura et al. 2000). Finally, two of three randomized, controlled antidepressant trials (Narushima et al. 2002; Rasmussen et al. 2003) suggested that cardiovascular morbidity and mortality may be reduced in stroke patients who receive antidepressant medication, particularly SSRIs.

Dementing Disorders

Depression is one of the most common neuropsychiatric, noncognitive symptoms of Alzheimer's dementia (Lee and Lyketsos 2003). The prevalence of MDD ranges from 20% to 32% in Alzheimer's dementia (Burns et al. 1990; Lyketsos et al. 2002; Migliorelli et al. 1995), with minor depression occurring in an additional 25% (Migliorelli et al. 1995). Symptoms of Alzheimer's dementia, such as emotional lability, may be easily mistaken for depression. Other symptoms, such as apathy, may arise additively from both conditions. Apathy has been found in 27% of Alzheimer's dementia patients and in 56% of Alzheimer's dementia patients with comorbid MDD (Lyketsos et al. 2001). These diagnoses may be even more difficult to distinguish in cognitively impaired patients because of the associated difficulty in communication (Lee and Lyketsos 2003).

The occurrence of late-onset depression and reversible cognitive impairment associated with depression (i.e., pseudodementia) also has been shown to be highly correlated with the eventual diagnosis of Alzheimer's dementia (Alexopoulos et al. 1993). It has been postulated that noradrenergic neuronal loss in the locus coeruleus, and serotonergic cell loss in the dorsal raphe nucleus in Alzheimer's dementia, may contribute to these high rates of reported depression (Forstl et al. 1992). Depression is also thought to be common in other dementing disorders, such as vascular dementia. Subcortical white matter infarcts are thought to be associated with depression in vascular dementia and, to some degree, in Alzheimer's dementia (Alexopoulos et al. 1997).

In Alzheimer's dementia, depression is associated with more adverse outcomes, such as nursing home placement, diminished activities of daily living, more rapid cognitive decline, and increased mortality (Bassuk et al. 1998; Kopetz et al. 2000; Lyketsos et al. 1997). However, the findings regarding the treatment of depression in Alzheimer's dementia have been equivocal. Some studies have found antidepressants to be efficacious in this population, whereas others have reported minimal treatment effects (see Lee and Lyketsos 2003).

Epilepsy

Depression is the most common psychiatric condition found in patients with epilepsy, with prevalence rates linked to the degree of seizure control. MDD has been found in 20%–55% of those with recurrent seizures but in only 3%–9% of those whose seizures are well controlled (Kanner 2003). The relation between depression and epilepsy appears to be bidirectional. Depression may be caused by the seizure disorder, particularly with complex partial seizures (Kanner 2003). It also has been suggested that monoamine depletion, which may occur with depression, may contribute to seizure activity (Jobe et al.

1999). In support of this interrelationship, a history of depression was found to be 17 times more common in patients with complex partial seizures than in control subjects (Forsgren and Nystrom 1990). This increased rate of depression could be partially caused by the effects of certain antiepileptic drugs, such as phenobarbital. Although antidepressants may lower the seizure threshold, this risk is small and more common with TCAs than with SSRIs or venlafaxine (Kanner 2003). Bupropion, maprotiline, and amoxapine are the most likely antidepressants to trigger seizures and should be avoided in this population (Pisani et al. 2002).

Other Neurological Disorders

Depressive disorders may occur in up to 50% of patients with multiple sclerosis, typically during acute exacerbations or as part of a chronic progressive course (Minden and Schiffer 1990). Some evidence indicates that depressed patients with multiple sclerosis are more likely to have white matter demyelinating plaques involving the arcuate fasciculus (Pujol et al. 1997). Interferon-beta-1b, used to treat multiple sclerosis, is associated with depression in up to 40% of patients with multiple sclerosis (Mohr et al. 1996).

Huntington's disease is an autosomal dominant disorder affecting the basal ganglia and is characterized by involuntary movements and cognitive impairment. Huntington's disease has been associated with MDD in up to 32% and with bipolar disorder in 9% of patients (Folstein et al. 1983). These and other neurological disorders are discussed more fully in Chapter 7, "Dementia."

Depression and Type 1 Diabetes

Type 1 diabetes mellitus is a chronic medical condition associated with considerable treatment demands, including multiple daily insulin injections, adherence to a diet that is restrictive, and monitoring of serum glucose levels. Individuals with diabetes must live with this illness and with its risks of multiple medical complications, including blindness, renal failure, amputations, neuropathy, and cardiovascular disease. The burden of this disease and its frequent medical comorbidity might be expected to increase the risk for depression. However, it also has been suggested that the neurochemical changes associated with the metabolic impairment in type 1 diabetes mellitus may contribute to mood disturbances via neurobiological mechanisms (Jacobson et al. 2002).

It is well documented that depressive disorders are at least twice as common in those with type 1 or type 2 diabetes mellitus as in the general population (Anderson et al. 2001; W. W. Eaton 2002; Egede et al. 2002). Further-

more, some studies suggest that depression in individuals with diabetes mellitus is characterized by longer episodes (Peyrot and Rubin 1999), higher recurrence rates, and lower recovery rates (Kovacs et al. 1997). Depression in individuals with diabetes mellitus is an important risk factor because it is associated with poorer adherence to the diabetes mellitus dietary and medication regimen and with poorer quality of life (Ciechanowski et al. 2000; Gary et al. 2000; Hanninen et al. 1999).

Some studies have indicated that MDD is associated with poorer glycemic control (Lustman et al. 1986, 1997, 2000a), whereas others have not confirmed the relationship of hyperglycemia to MDD (N. Robinson et al. 1988) or to depressive symptoms (Jacobson et al. 1990; Peyrot and Rubin 1997, 1999). Both biological and psychological mechanisms have been postulated to account for the potential relationship between depression and metabolic control in diabetes mellitus. The relationship between depression and poor compliance with the diabetes treatment regimen may be reciprocal, with depression leading to lower self-efficacy and to self-neglect. Van Tilburg et al. (2001) found that variations in glycemic control in type 1 diabetes mellitus were associated with clinically meaningful differences in depressive symptoms, which appeared to be at least partly mediated through decreased self-care behavior. It also has been postulated that the metabolic abnormalities associated with diabetes mellitus lead to changes in brain structure and function, which then render individuals more susceptible to develop a depressive disorder (Jacobson et al. 1990).

Whatever the mechanism that accounts for the comorbidity of depression and diabetes, this association clearly has serious health implications. Depression has been associated with an increased risk of diabetes-related medical complications, including sexual dysfunction, retinopathy, nephropathy, heart disease, and stroke (de Groot et al. 2001; Kinder et al. 2002). Because of the reciprocal relationship between depression and metabolic control, attention to both mood disturbances and measures to enhance diabetes management is necessary to prevent or delay the progression of such complications.

Depression Caused by Medications

Depression has been reported as an adverse effect of many different drugs (see Table 9–1). In some cases (e.g., anticonvulsants), depression occurs primarily at high serum levels, whereas other drugs (e.g., interferon) may cause depression frequently at normal doses. Some reports in the literature have been uncritical, either misinterpreting drug-induced symptoms as indicative of de-

---

TABLE 9–1.   Selected drugs reported to cause depression

Angiotensin-converting enzyme inhibitors
Anticonvulsants
Antihypertensives (especially clonidine, methyldopa, thiazides)
Antimicrobials (amphotericin, ethionamide, metronidazole)
Antineoplastic drugs (procarbazine, vincristine, vinblastine, asparaginase)
Beta-blockers
Calcium channel blockers
Corticosteroids
Estrogens
Interferon
Isotretinoin
Metoclopramide
Nonsteroidal anti-inflammatory drugs (especially indomethacin)
Sedative-hypnotics
Statins

---

pression (e.g., weakness, sedation, bradykinesia, fatigue, anorexia, insomnia) or misattributing preexisting depression to the drug. Consequently, controversy surrounds the question of whether some of these drugs do cause depression (e.g., beta-blockers) or how serious a threat is posed (e.g., isotretinoin). Most of these drugs and their psychiatric side effects are discussed in other chapters of this textbook.

Treatment

Both pharmacotherapy and structured forms of psychotherapy have been shown to be effective in the treatment of MDD (Schulberg et al. 1998) and dysthymic disorder or minor depression (Thase 1997; Williams et al. 2000). Some carefully designed studies have shown that the combination of pharmacotherapy and psychotherapy is more effective in the treatment of chronic and more severe forms of depression than either modality alone (Keller 2000; Thase 1997). Psychotherapeutic modalities such as interpersonal therapy (IPT), CBT, and problem-solving interventions also have been shown to be as effective as pharmacotherapy for the treatment of milder depressions (Barrett et al. 2001; Thase 1997). Remission of depressive symptoms in this setting has been associated with improved social and occupational functioning (Ormel et al. 1993; Von Korff et al. 1992). However, despite the evidence for the effectiveness of treatment and for the elevated rates of depression found in medical populations, the rates of treatment for depression are not

higher than those of individuals with depression in the absence of comorbid medical conditions (Koike et al. 2002). In fact, it has been estimated that more than 60% of primary care patients with depression do not receive adequate care for this condition (Kessler et al. 2003).

Most antidepressant treatment studies have been conducted in primary care or psychiatric samples, typically with individuals who do not have a serious medical illness. However, several recent studies have reported that both pharmacological and psychotherapeutic interventions are effective for the treatment of depression associated with medical disorders such as type 1 diabetes mellitus (Lustman et al. 1998), post-MI (Frasure-Smith and Lesperance 2003), chronic obstructive pulmonary disease (Borson et al. 1992), cancer (van Heeringen and Zivkov 1996), and HIV infection and AIDS (Elliot et al. 1998). Evidence to support the effectiveness of psychotherapeutic and psychopharmacological treatment of depression in the medically ill is discussed in the following subsections.

Psychopharmacological Management of Depression in the Medically Ill

SSRIs, heterocyclic antidepressants and TCAs, novel antidepressants, and psychostimulants have been used in the treatment of depression comorbid with medical illness. A recent meta-analysis of the Cochrane database of treatment outcomes provided evidence that SSRIs, TCAs, and other antidepressants improve depressive symptoms in patients with a wide range of physical illnesses significantly more often than does either placebo or no treatment (Gill and Hatcher 2003). All antidepressants are discussed more fully in Chapter 37 ("Psychopharmacology"); we summarize some key points here.

SSRIs

SSRIs are generally regarded as first-line treatment in the management of depression in the medically ill because of their tolerability and relative safety. Randomized, controlled trials have shown various SSRIs to be effective in patients with cardiac disease (Glassman et al. 2002; Strik et al. 2000), stroke (Andersen et al. 1994; Wiart et al. 2000), cancer (Holland et al. 1998; Pezzella et al. 2001), HIV infection (Elliot et al. 1998; Rabkin et al. 1999; Zisook et al. 1998), Alzheimer's disease (Karlsson et al. 2000; Lyketsos et al. 2000), multiple sclerosis (Mohr et al. 2001), and diabetes (Lustman et al. 2000b). Results of open trials indicate that SSRIs may improve depressive symptoms in patients with Parkinson's disease (Hauser and Zesiewicz 1997; Tesei et al. 2000) and in those with renal failure (Levy et al. 1996).

An innovative study reported by Musselman et al. (2001) showed that paroxetine was very effective in preventing depression in melanoma patients receiving high-dose interferon-alfa therapy. Subjects were randomized to paroxetine or placebo at the start of their interferon therapy. MDD subsequently developed in 45% of the placebo group but in only 11% of the paroxetine group. This difference significantly affected health outcomes because 35% of the placebo group, compared with only 5% of the paroxetine group, discontinued interferon-alfa because of severe depressive distress. This study raises important questions about the potential benefit of prophylactic antidepressant treatment in other high-risk medical populations.

With medically ill patients, SSRIs may provide benefits beyond their antidepressant effect. Some evidence suggests that fluoxetine may improve motor function (Dam et al. 1996) and cognitive performance (González-Torrecillas et al. 1995) in stroke patients and may help improve glycemic control in patients with diabetes mellitus (Lustman et al. 2000b). Paroxetine and citalopram may possess analgesic properties in the treatment of diabetic neuropathy (Sindrup et al. 1990, 1992), and fluoxetine and sertraline may be useful as analgesics for chronic pain syndromes (Breitbart 1992; Hynes et al. 1985). Sertraline also was effective in reducing hot flashes in men requiring hormone replacement therapy for advanced prostate cancer (A.J. Roth and Scher 1998). It also has been shown to reduce hot flash frequency and intensity in women with breast cancer who develop chemical menopause associated with tamoxifen use (Loprinzi et al. 2000b; Stearns et al. 2000). Fluoxetine may ameliorate severe refractory or orthostatic hypotension (Grubb et al. 1994).

SSRIs have been regarded generally as safer and less toxic than TCAs. However, significant side effects still may occur with SSRIs in the medically ill (Jansen Steur 1993; Richard et al. 1999). All SSRIs can cause nausea, headache, sexual dysfunction, and tremor. Other frequent side effects include nervousness, insomnia, sedation, diarrhea, constipation, and dry mouth. Rare but potentially serious side effects of SSRIs include the syndrome of inappropriate antidiuretic hormone secretion and platelet dysfunction leading to bleeding (van Walraven et al. 2001). Some reports indicate that SSRIs may worsen motor symptoms in some patients with Parkinson's disease (Richard et al. 1999).

Drug interactions or the presence of hepatic disease may affect SSRI metabolism and excretion and alter antidepressant pharmacokinetics (Beliles and Stoudemire 1998). A reduced initial dose with slow titration of the shorter half-life SSRIs is recommended for patients with hepatic disease because the metabolism of SSRIs is decreased by significant hepatic disease (Beliles and Stoudemire 1998; Joffe et al. 1998). Fluvoxamine should be avoided because of its propensity for drug interactions (Beliles and Stoudemire 1998). Sertraline and citalopram appear to present the lowest risk for drug interactions (Beliles and Stoudemire 1998). Drug interactions are reviewed in detail in Chapter 37 ("Psychopharmacology") and in the specialty and subspecialty chapters.

Novel Antidepressants

Novel antidepressants include venlafaxine, bupropion, mirtazapine, nefazodone, and moclobemide. Venlafaxine, bupropion, and mirtazapine have become increasingly popular as alternatives to SSRIs in the medically ill, although a paucity of empirical evidence exists regarding their use in this population. Evidence shows that moclobemide is efficacious in reducing depressive symptoms in patients with Alzheimer's disease (M. Roth et al. 1996). Results of open trials point to the effectiveness of other novel antidepressants in patients with stroke (venlafaxine) (Dahmen et al. 1999), cancer (mirtazapine) (Theobald et al. 2002), and HIV infection (nefazodone) (Elliot et al. 1999).

Extended-release venlafaxine is a serotonin-norepinephrine reuptake inhibitor that is well tolerated, having side effects similar to those of the SSRIs, but it may be associated with increased blood pressure at higher doses. In depressed patients, this dual-action agent may achieve greater remission rates compared with the SSRIs (Smith et al. 2002; Thase et al. 2001). Extended-release venlafaxine has a wide dose range with few drug interactions and is minimally protein bound. A recent randomized, controlled trial showed efficacy in breast cancer patients with hot flashes (Loprinzi et al. 2000a), and it has been found to be useful for neuropathic pain in cancer and in other populations (Davis and Smith 1999; Dwight et al. 1998).

Mirtazapine increases norepinephrine and serotonin concentrations through blockade of inhibitory receptors. Unlike the SSRIs, mirtazapine does not appear to cause nausea, insomnia, anxiety, or sexual dysfunction (De Boer 1996). Mirtazapine, as a result of its serotonin$_3$ receptor-blocking anti-emetic effects, may be useful in treating medically ill patients who are experiencing nausea. It may rapidly improve insomnia and anorexia, which are commonly seen with depressive disorders in the medically ill. The main side effects of mirtazapine are sedation and weight gain, which may be useful in some cachectic patients (Stimmel et al. 1997). Mirtazapine is also associated with very minimal drug interactions (De Boer 1996).

Bupropion is a norepinephrine and dopamine modulator. It is not sedating, does not cause sexual dysfunction, and has little cardiotoxicity (Golden et al. 1998). It may be particularly useful in treating patients with prominent fatigue. Side effects may include agitation, insomnia, and seizures at higher doses. Because of this latter concern, it is generally recommended that single doses greater than 150 mg and daily doses greater than 300 mg be avoided in patients with brain tumors and a history of seizures (Golden et al. 1998).

TCAs

TCAs have been shown to be efficacious in poststroke depression, cancer, HIV infection, Parkinson's disease, Alzheimer's disease, multiple sclerosis, diabetes, and renal failure (Gill and Hatcher 2003). TCAs have proven to be effective as analgesics in the treatment of chronic pain syndromes, including pain related to cancer (reviewed in Magni et al. 1987). With their analgesic and sedating effects, TCAs may be particularly useful in depressed patients with significant pain and/or insomnia.

TCAs are variably noradrenergic and/or serotonergic. Their side effects are related to their central and peripheral anticholinergic effects, their central antihistaminic properties, and their effects on the cardiac conduction system and the peripheral autonomic nervous system. TCAs should be avoided in patients with cardiac disease because they are associated with hypotension and the potential for arrhythmias (Glassman et al. 1993; Jackson et al. 1987). TCAs should be used with caution in diabetic patients because their anticholinergic, orthostatic hypotensive, and cardiovascular adverse effects can exacerbate complications of diabetes mellitus (C. Carney 1998). Anticholinergic side effects of TCAs may exacerbate cognitive impairment and cause delirium in patients with CNS disorders, especially dementia (Reynolds 1992). TCAs that are more anticholinergic generally are not recommended for the treatment of depression in patients with HIV or AIDS because they promote thrush (Rabkin et al. 1994). TCAs may not be suitable for patients at increased risk for bone fractures, cancer, or skeletal weakness because orthostatic hypotension may cause falls (Shuster et al. 1992). TCAs have been associated with seizures, mainly in overdoses or at high plasma levels (Preskorn and Fast 1992).

Many patients are unable to tolerate tricyclics, and they can be lethal in overdose. For insomnia or pain, lower doses of TCAs may be needed than those required for an antidepressant effect (Potter et al. 1998). If a TCA is desired for medically ill patients, the secondary amines such as nortriptyline or desipramine are preferred because they are better tolerated (Potter et al. 1998). Nortriptyline has reliable serum levels and a defined therapeutic window that may guide clinical management, particularly in patients with liver disease or malabsorption (Potter et al. 1998).

Psychostimulants

Methylphenidate has been shown to alleviate depressive symptoms in a range of medical conditions, including stroke (Grade et al. 1998), HIV disease (Fernandez et al. 1995), and cancer (Grade et al. 1998). Psychostimulants are generally well tolerated and, in relatively low doses, can elevate mood rapidly, increase appetite, diminish fatigue (Homsi et al. 2001; Masand et al. 1991), serve as adjuvant analgesics (Bruera et al. 1987; Forrest et al. 1977), improve attention and concentration, and reduce sedation caused by opiates or other drugs (Homsi et al. 2001). Many would consider psychostimulants to be the antidepressants of choice in the palliative care setting because of their rapid onset of action (Wilson et al. 2000). Side effects are typically mild and dose-related and include agitation, nausea, and insomnia. Rarely, psychotic symptoms or tachycardia and hypertension may occur (Masand et al. 1991). Methylphenidate is typically given in divided doses (2.5–10 mg) in the morning and afternoon.

Electroconvulsive Therapy in the Medically Ill

Electroconvulsive therapy (ECT) is sometimes used in the medically ill as an alternative to antidepressants in the treatment of severe or refractory depression (Beale et al. 1997). ECT has been shown to be an effective treatment of depression in Parkinson's disease and also may improve the symptoms of the Parkinson's disease itself (Poewe and Seppi 2001). It has been shown to improve depression following stroke (Currier et al. 1992; G.B. Murray et al. 1986) and in patients with multiple sclerosis, endocrine disorders, and renal failure (Weiner and Coffey 1993). ECT has been associated with improvements in cognition and mood in patients with dementia (Rao and Lyketsos 2000). ECT is considered safe for epilepsy patients with severe or refractory depression (Lambert and Robertson 1999). ECT should be considered early in the course of psychotic depression and depression associated with severe suicidal ideation or failure to maintain adequate nutritional status (Kaplan and Sadock 1998). ECT and its risks are reviewed in detail in Chapter 39 ("Electroconvulsive Therapy").

Psychotherapeutic Treatment of Depression in the Medically Ill

The relationship with the primary medical caregiver may be the most important psychotherapeutic tool for many patients with a serious medical illness. Patient groups and self-help and other support groups also may protect the patient from depression by diminishing stigma and promoting self-efficacy and a sense of mastery. A referral for specific psychotherapeutic intervention should take into account the severity of the patient's distress, the available support network, the patient's motivation for psychological assistance, and the patient's capacity to learn new coping strategies and to engage in a process that involves introspection and the expression of feelings.

Psychotherapeutic approaches to treatment of depression in medical populations may include the promotion of active coping strategies and the implementation of specific interventions, including CBT, IPT, and supportive-expressive therapy on an individual or a group basis. The need to refer to a mental health professional will depend on the severity of the depression and on the skill, interest, and availability of primary care practitioners. Many psychosocial interventions have been shown to improve psychological well-being and to reduce depressive symptoms in medically ill patients. Some of the studies in which a specific intervention was targeted toward depressive symptoms or toward the diagnosis of MDD or dysthymic disorder are reviewed here.

Barrett et al. (2001) compared the effectiveness of a problem-solving approach to support active coping strategies with that of paroxetine for the treatment of minor depression or dysthymic disorder in a primary care sample. In this randomized, controlled study, both treatment approaches were equally effective for the treatment of dysthymic disorder but were no more effective than watchful waiting for the treatment of minor depression. Teri et al. (1997) found that patients with Alzheimer's disease and depressive symptoms showed significant improvement in depressive symptoms with a behavioral intervention for patient–caregiver dyads focused on either pleasant events or caregiver problem solving.

Some positive results have been found with CBT or IPT for the treatment of depression in the medically ill. Mohr et al. (2000) found that a telephone-administered cognitive-behavioral intervention to assist patients in coping with cancer was associated with a greater reduction in depressive symptoms compared with usual care. Lustman et al. (1998) showed in patients with type 2 diabetes that an intervention that included CBT and diabetes education produced more than a threefold higher remission rate from depression compared with a control condition. This treatment was associated with a significant improvement in glycosylated hemoglobin 6 months after the end of treatment. A randomized trial of CBT plus group therapy when feasible, together with SSRIs, for cardiac patients who had elevated and/or persistent depressive symptoms resulted in an improvement in the treatment group that was greater than in the usual care group. However, this intervention did not result in increased rates of cardiac event–free survival in the treatment group (Berkman et al. 2003). Kelley et al. (1993) found that both cognitive-behavioral and support group brief therapies equally reduced depressive symptoms in depressed HIV-infected individuals. Mohr et al. (2001) found that individuals with multiple sclerosis and MDD had a greater reduction in depressive symptoms when CBT or sertraline was used than did those who received supportive-expressive therapy. In contrast, a randomized trial of CBT for depression following stroke failed to find any significant difference between the treatment group and the control group (Lincoln and Flannaghan 2003). Furthermore, in a recent review of 15 trials of at least fair quality in which the effects of interventions such as CBT, relaxation therapy, and education on depressive symptoms in cancer patients were examined, Newell et al. (2002) identified no significant reduction in depressive symptoms following any of the interventions. However, Markowitz et al. (1998) found that depressed HIV-positive patients had greater improvement in depressive symptoms with IPT or supportive psychotherapy plus imipramine than did subjects who received supportive therapy or CBT alone.

These studies of psychotherapeutic interventions to treat depression indicate some degree of effectiveness in a variety of medical populations, although their effectiveness is often improved when combined with antidepressant medication. Numerous other nonspecific psychotherapeutic and educational interventions also may be effective in reducing depressive symptoms and in protecting individuals from their emergence. However, the range of psychosocial interventions designed to improve adjustment in medical populations is beyond the scope of this chapter.

Conclusion

Clinical depression, particularly MDD and dysthymic disorder, is common in the medically ill and is associated with impaired quality of life, decreased compliance with medical treatment, and increased medical morbidity and mortality. The diagnosis of depressive disorders in medical patients is complicated by the frequent overlap between symptoms of depression and those of medical illness. This overlap may contribute to underdiagnosis, when symptoms of depression are assumed to be features of the medical condition, or to overdiagnosis, when symptoms of a medical illness are attributed to a depressed mood. However, the failure to simply inquire about the symptoms of depression may be the most common reason that the diagnosis of depression is overlooked in a medical population. Screening tests may be useful for drawing the attention of clinicians to these symptoms and identifying patients in medical clinics who are most likely to have depressive disorders.

The increased prevalence of depression in the medically ill is most often the result of multiple nonspecific risk factors, although there has been continued speculation that specific biological mechanisms operate in certain medical conditions.

Psychopharmacological and psychotherapeutic approaches are both effective in the treatment of depressive disorders in the medically ill and can be used together. Medical patients may be more sensitive to the side effects of pharmacological treatments, and careful attention must be paid to the dosage, to the potential for drug interactions, and to impairment in hepatic or renal function, which can affect drug metabolism.

References

Alexopoulos GS, Meyers BS, Young RC, et al: The course of geriatric depression with "reversible dementia": a controlled study. Am J Psychiatry 150:1693–1699, 1993

Alexopoulos GS, Meyers BS, Young RC, et al: "Vascular depression" hypothesis. Arch Gen Psychiatry 54:915–922, 1997

Almqvist EW, Bloch M, Brinkman R, et al: A worldwide assessment of the frequency of suicide, suicide attempts, or psychiatric hospitalization after predictive testing for Huntington disease. Am J Hum Genet 64:1293–1304, 1999

American Psychiatric Association: Diagnostic and Statistical Manual of Mental Disorders, 4th Edition, Text Revision. Washington, DC, American Psychiatric Association, 2000

Anda RF, Williamson DF, Escobedo LG, et al: Depression and the dynamics of smoking: a national perspective. JAMA 264:1541–1545, 1990

Andersen G, Vestergaard K, Lauritzen L: Effective treatment of poststroke depression with the selective serotonin reuptake inhibitor citalopram. Stroke 25:1099–1104, 1994

Anderson RJ, Freedland KE, Clouse RE, et al: The prevalence of comorbid depression in adults with diabetes: a meta-analysis. Diabetes Care 24:1069–1078, 2001

Appels A, Mulder P: Excess fatigue as a precursor of myocardial infarction. Eur Heart J 9:758–764, 1988

Barkow K, Maier W, Ustun TB, et al: Risk factors for new depressive episodes in primary health care: an international prospective 12-month follow-up study. Psychol Med 32:595–607, 2002

Barrett JE, Williams JW Jr, Oxman TE, et al: Treatment of dysthymia and minor depression in primary care: a randomized trial in patients aged 18 to 59 years. J Fam Pract 50:405–412, 2001

Bassuk SS, Berkman LF, Wypij D: Depressive symptomatology and incident cognitive decline in an elderly community sample. Arch Gen Psychiatry 55:1073–1081, 1998

Beale MD, Kellner CH, Parsons PJ: ECT for the treatment of mood disorders in cancer patients. Convuls Ther 13:222–226, 1997

Beck AT, Steer RA, Brown GK: Manual for the Beck Depression Inventory-II. San Antonio, TX, Psychological Corporation, 1996

Beck DA, Koenig HG: Minor depression: a review of the literature. Int J Psychiatry Med 26:177–209, 1996

Beeber LS, Shea J, McCorkle R: The Center for Epidemiologic Studies Depression Scale as a measure of depressive symptoms in newly diagnosed patients. Journal of Psychosocial Oncology 16:1–20, 1998

Beliles K, Stoudemire A: Psychopharmacologic treatment of depression in the medically ill. Psychosomatics 39:S2–S19, 1998

Berard RM, Boermeester F, Viljoen G: Depressive disorders in an out-patient oncology setting: prevalence, assessment, and management. Psychooncology 7:112–120, 1998

Berkman LF, Blumenthal J, Burg M, et al: Effects of treating depression and low perceived social support on clinical events after myocardial infarction: the Enhancing Recovery in Coronary Heart Disease Patients (ENRICHD). JAMA 289:3106–3116, 2003

Berwick DM, Murphy JM, Goldman PA, et al: Performance of a five-item mental health screening test. Med Care 29:169–176, 1991

Blazer DG, Kessler RC, McGonagle KA, et al: The prevalence and distribution of major depression in a national community sample: the National Comorbidity Survey. Am J Psychiatry 151:979–986, 1994

Bogousslavsky J: William Feinberg Lecture 2002: emotions, mood, and behavior after stroke. Stroke 34:1046–1050, 2003

Borson S, McDonald GJ, Gayle T, et al: Improvement in mood, physical symptoms, and function with nortriptyline for depression in patients with chronic obstructive pulmonary disease. Psychosomatics 33:190–201, 1992

Bottomley A: Depression in cancer patients: a literature review. European Journal of Cancer Care 7:181–191, 1998

Bramley PN, Easton AM, Morley S, et al: The differentiation of anxiety and depression by rating scales. Acta Psychiatr Scand 77:133–138, 1988

Breitbart W: Psychotropic adjuvant analgesics for cancer pain. Psychooncology 1:133–145, 1992

Breitbart W, Krivo S: Suicide, in Psycho-Oncology. Edited by Holland JC. New York, Oxford University Press, 1998, pp 541–547

Breitbart W, Rosenfeld B, Pessin H, et al: Depression, hopelessness, and desire for hastened death in terminally ill patients with cancer. JAMA 284:2907–2911, 2000

Breslau N, Kilbey MM, Andreski P: Vulnerability to psychopathology in nicotine-dependent smokers: an epidemiologic study of young adults. Am J Psychiatry 150:941–946, 1993

Bruera E, Chadwick S, Brenneis C, et al: Methylphenidate associated with narcotics for the treatment of cancer pain. Cancer Treat Rep 71:67–70, 1987

Bukberg J, Penman D, Holland JC: Depression in hospitalized cancer patients. Psychosom Med 46:199–212, 1984

Burns A, Jacoby R, Levy R: Behavioral abnormalities and psychiatric symptoms in Alzheimer's disease: preliminary findings. Int Psychogeriatr 2:25–36, 1990

Burvill PW: Recent progress in the epidemiology of major depression. Epidemiol Rev 17:21–31, 1995

Capuron L, Bluthe RM, Dantzer R: Cytokines in clinical psychiatry. Am J Psychiatry 158:1163–1164, 2001

Carney C: Diabetes mellitus and major depressive disorder: an overview of prevalence, complications, and treatment. Depress Anxiety 7:149–157, 1998

Carney RM, Rich MW, Tevelde A, et al: Major depressive disorder in coronary artery disease. Am J Cardiol 60:1273–1275, 1987

Carney RM, Rich MW, Tevelde A, et al: The relationship between heart rate, heart rate variability and depression in patients with coronary artery disease. J Psychosom Res 32:159–164, 1988

Carson AJ, MacHale S, Allen K, et al: Depression after stroke and lesion location: a systematic review. Lancet 356:122–126, 2000

Cavanaugh S, Clark DC, Gibbons RD: Diagnosing depression in the hospitalized medically ill. Psychosomatics 24:809–815, 1983

Chaturvedi SK, Shenoy A, Prasad KM, et al: Concerns, coping and quality of life in head and neck cancer patients. Support Care Cancer 4:186–190, 1996

Chochinov HM, Wilson KG, Enns M, et al: Desire for death in the terminally ill. Am J Psychiatry 152:1185–1191, 1995

Chochinov HM, Wilson KG, Enns M, et al: "Are you depressed?" Screening for depression in the terminally ill. Am J Psychiatry 154:674–676, 1997

Chochinov HM, Tataryn D, Clinch JJ, et al: Will to live in the terminally ill. Lancet 354:816–819, 1999

Ciaramella A, Poli P: Assessment of depression among cancer patients: the role of pain, cancer type and treatment. Psychooncology 10:156–165, 2001

Ciechanowski PS, Katon WJ, Russo JE: Depression and diabetes: impact of depressive symptoms on adherence, function, and costs. Arch Intern Med 160:3278–3285, 2000

Clark DA, Cook A, Snow D: Depressive symptom differences in hospitalized, medically ill, depressed psychiatric inpatients and nonmedical controls. J Abnorm Psychol 107:38–48, 1998

Clarke DM, Smith GC, Herrman HE: A comparative study of screening instruments for mental disorders in general hospital patients. Int J Psychiatry Med 23:323–337, 1993

Connerney I, Shapiro PA, McLaughlin JS, et al: Relation between depression after coronary artery bypass surgery and 12-month outcome: a prospective study. Lancet 358:1766–1771, 2001

Craven JL, Rodin GM, Johnson L, et al: The diagnosis of major depression in renal dialysis patients. Psychosom Med 49:482–492, 1987

Craven JL, Rodin GM, Littlefield C: The Beck Depression Inventory as a screening device for major depression in renal dialysis patients. Int J Psychiatry Med 18:365–374, 1988

Cummings JL: Depression and Parkinson's disease: a review. Am J Psychiatry 149:443–454, 1992

Currier MB, Murray GB, Welch CC: Electroconvulsive therapy for post-stroke depressed geriatric patients. J Neuropsychiatry Clin Neurosci 4:140–144, 1992

Dahmen N, Marx J, Hopf HC, et al: Therapy of early poststroke depression with venlafaxine: safety, tolerability and efficacy as determined in an open, uncontrolled clinical trial. Stroke 30:691–692, 1999

Dam M, Tonin P, De Boni A, et al: Effects of fluoxetine and maprotiline on functional recovery in poststroke hemiplegic patients undergoing rehabilitation therapy. Stroke 27:1211–1214, 1996

Dambrink JH, Tuininga YS, van Gilst WH, et al: Association between reduced heart rate variability and left ventricular dilatation in patients with a first anterior myocardial infarction. CATS Investigators. Captopril and Thrombolysis Study. Br Heart J 72:514–520, 1994

Davis JL, Smith RL: Painful peripheral diabetic neuropathy treated with venlafaxine HCl extended release capsules. Diabetes Care 22:1909–1910, 1999

De Boer TH: Pharmacologic profile of mirtazapine. J Clin Psychiatry 57 (4 suppl):19–25, 1996

de Groot M, Anderson R, Freedland KE, et al: Association of depression and diabetes complications: a meta-analysis. Psychosom Med 63:619–630, 2001

Devins GM, Orme CM, Costello CG, et al: Measuring depressive symptoms in illness populations: psychometric properties of the Center for Epidemiologic Studies Depression (CES-D) Scale. Psychol Health 2:139–156, 1988

Diez-Quevedo C, Rangil T, Sanchez-Planell L, et al: Validation and utility of the Patient Health Questionnaire in diagnosing mental disorders in 1003 general hospital Spanish inpatients. Psychosom Med 63:679–686, 2001

Dilsaver SC, Pariser SF, Churchill CM, et al: Is there a relationship between failing efforts to stop smoking and depression? J Clin Psychopharmacol 10:153–154, 1990

DiMatteo MR, Lepper HS, Croghan TW: Depression is a risk factor for noncompliance with medical treatment: meta-analysis of the effects of anxiety and depression on patient adherence. Arch Intern Med 160:2101–2107, 2000

Dooneief G, Mirabello E, Bell K, et al: An estimate of the incidence of depression in idiopathic Parkinson's disease. Arch Neurol 49:305–307, 1992

Druss BG, Rohrbaugh RM, Rosenheck RA: Depressive symptoms and health costs in older medical patients. Am J Psychiatry 156:477–479, 1999

Druss BG, Rosenheck RA, Sledge WH: Health and disability costs of depressive illness in a major U.S. corporation. Am J Psychiatry 157:1274–1278, 2000

Dwight MM, Arnold LM, O'Brien H, et al: An open clinical trial of venlafaxine treatment of fibromyalgia. Psychosomatics 39:14–17, 1998

Eaton CB, Lapane KL, Garber CE, et al: Effects of a community-based intervention on physical activity: the Pawtucket Heart Health Program. Am J Public Health 89:1741–1744, 1999

Eaton WW: Epidemiologic evidence on the comorbidity of depression and diabetes. J Psychosom Res 53:903–906, 2002

Egede LE, Zheng D, Simpson K: Comorbid depression is associated with increased health care use and expenditures in individuals with diabetes. Diabetes Care 25:464–470, 2002

Elliot AJ, Uldall KK, Bergam K, et al: Randomized, placebo-controlled trial of paroxetine versus imipramine in depressed HIV-positive outpatients. Am J Psychiatry 155:367–372, 1998

Elliot AJ, Russo J, Bergam K, et al: Antidepressant efficacy in HIV-seropositive outpatients with major depressive disorder: an open trial of nefazodone. J Clin Psychiatry 60:226–231, 1999

Endicott J: Measurement of depression in patients with cancer. Cancer 53 (10 suppl):2243–2249, 1984

Endicott J, Spitzer RL: A diagnostic interview: the Schedule for Affective Disorders and Schizophrenia. Arch Gen Psychiatry 35:837–844, 1978

Fernandez F, Levy JK, Samley HR, et al: Effects of methylphenidate in HIV-related depression: a comparative trial with desipramine. Int J Psychiatry Med 25:53–67, 1995

Flint AJ, Rifat SL: Validation of the Hospital Anxiety and Depression Scale as a measure of severity of geriatric depression. Int J Geriatr Psychiatry 11:991–994, 1996

Folstein S, Abbott MH, Chase GA, et al: The association of affective disorder with Huntington's disease in a case series and in families. Psychol Med 13:537–542, 1983

Forrest WH Jr, Brown BW Jr, Brown CR, et al: Dextroamphetamine with morphine for the treatment of postoperative pain. N Engl J Med 296:712–715, 1977

Forrester AW, Lipsey JR, Teitelbaum ML, et al: Depression following myocardial infarction. Int J Psychiatry Med 22:33–46, 1992

Forsgren L, Nystrom L: An incident case-referent study of epileptic seizures in adults. Epilepsy Res 6:66–81, 1990

Forstl H, Burns A, Luthert P, et al: Clinical and neuropathological correlates of depression in Alzheimer's disease. Psychol Med 22:877–884, 1992

Frasure-Smith N, Lesperance F: Depression—a cardiac risk factor in search of a treatment. JAMA 289:3171–3173, 2003

Frasure-Smith N, Lesperance F, Talajic M: Depression following myocardial infarction: impact on 6-month survival. JAMA 270:1819–1825, 1993 [published erratum appears in JAMA 271:1082, 1994]

Frasure-Smith N, Lesperance F, Talajic M: The impact of negative emotions on prognosis following myocardial infarction: is it more than depression? Health Psychol 14:388–398, 1995

Frasure-Smith N, Lesperance F, Juneau M, et al: Gender, depression, and one-year prognosis after myocardial infarction. Psychosom Med 61:26–37, 1999

Gary TL, Crum RM, Cooper-Patrick L, et al: Depressive symptoms and metabolic control in African-Americans with type 2 diabetes. Diabetes Care 23:23–29, 2000

Gill D, Hatcher S: Antidepressants for depression in medical illness (Cochrane Methodology Review), in The Cochrane Library, Issue 4. Chichester, UK, Wiley, 2003

Glassman AH, Roose SP, Bigger JT Jr: The safety of tricyclic antidepressants in cardiac patients: risk-benefit reconsidered. JAMA 269:2673–2675, 1993

Glassman AH, O'Connor CM, Califf RM, et al: Sertraline treatment of major depression in patients with acute MI or unstable angina. JAMA 288:701–709, 2002

Global Parkinson's Disease Survey Steering Committee: Factors impacting on quality of life in Parkinson's disease: results from an international survey. Mov Disord 17:60–67, 2002

Gluck ME, Geliebter A, Satov T: Night eating syndrome is associated with depression, low self-esteem, reduced daytime hunger, and less weight loss in obese outpatients. Obes Res 9:264–267, 2001

Golden RN, Dawkins K, Nicholas L, et al: Trazodone, nefazodone, bupropion, and mirtazapine, in The American Psychiatric Press Textbook of Psychopharmacology, 2nd Edition. Edited by Schatzberg AF, Nemeroff CB. Washington, DC, American Psychiatric Press, 1998, pp 251–269

González-Torrecillas JL, Mendlewicz J, Lobo A: Effects of early treatment of poststroke depression on neuropsychological rehabilitation. Int Psychogeriatr 7:547–560, 1995

Goodman WK, Price LH, Rasmussen SA, et al: The Yale-Brown Obsessive Compulsive Scale, I: development, use, and reliability. Arch Gen Psychiatry 46:1006–1011, 1989

Grade C, Redford B, Chrostowski J, et al: Methylphenidate in early post-stroke recovery: a double blind, placebo-controlled study. Arch Phys Med Rehabil 79:1047–1050, 1998

Grubb BP, Samoil D, Kosinski D, et al: Fluoxetine hydrochloride for the treatment of severe refractory orthostatic hypotension. Am J Med 97:366–368, 1994

Grundy SM: Primary prevention of coronary heart disease: integrating risk assessment with intervention. Circulation 100:988–998, 1999

Hall RC, Wise MG: The clinical and financial burden of mood disorders: cost and outcome. Psychosomatics 36:S11–S18, 1995

Hance M, Carney RM, Freedland KE, et al: Depression in patients with coronary heart disease: a 12-month follow-up. Gen Hosp Psychiatry 18:61–65, 1996

Hanninen JA, Takala JK, Keinanen-Kiukaanniemi SM: Depression in subjects with type 2 diabetes: predictive factors and relation to quality of life. Diabetes Care 22:997–998, 1999

Hauser RA, Zesiewicz TA: Sertraline for the treatment of depression in Parkinson's disease. Mov Disord 12:756–759, 1997

Hays RD, Wells KB, Sherbourne CD, et al: Functioning and well-being outcomes of patients with depression compared with chronic general medical illnesses. Arch Gen Psychiatry 52:11–19, 1995

Hemingway H, Marmot M: Evidence based cardiology: psychosocial factors in the aetiology and prognosis of coronary heart disease: systematic review of prospective cohort studies. BMJ 318:1460–1467, 1999

Herrmann C: International experiences with the Hospital Anxiety and Depression Scale—a review of validation data and clinical results. J Psychosom Res 42:17–41, 1997

Herrmann C, Brand-Driehorst S, Kaminsky B, et al: Diagnostic groups and depressed mood as predictors of 22-month mortality in medical inpatients. Psychosom Med 60:570–577, 1998

Holland JC, Romano SJ, Heiligenstein JH, et al: A controlled trial of fluoxetine and desipramine in depressed women with advanced cancer. Psychooncology 7:291–300, 1998

Homsi J, Nelson KA, Sarhill N, et al: A phase II study of methylphenidate for depression in advanced cancer. Am J Hosp Palliat Care 8:403–407, 2001

Hotopf M, Chidgey J, Addington-Hall J, et al: Depression in advanced disease: a systematic review, part 1. Palliat Med 16:81–97, 2002

House A, Knapp P, Bamford J, et al: Mortality at 12 and 24 months after stroke may be associated with depressive symptoms at 1 month. Stroke 32:696–701, 2001

Hughes JE: Depressive illness and lung cancer. Eur J Surg Oncol 11:15–20, 1985

Huikuri HV, Makikallio T, Airaksinen KE, et al: Measurement of heart rate variability: a clinical tool or a research toy? J Am Coll Cardiol 34:1878–1883, 1999

Hynes MD, Lochner MA, Bemis KG, et al: Fluoxetine, a selective inhibitor of serotonin uptake, potentiates morphine analgesia without altering its discriminative stimulus properties or affinity for opioid receptors. Life Sci 36:2317–2323, 1985

Istvan J, Zavela K, Weidner G: Body weight and psychological distress in NHANES I. Int J Obes Relat Metab Disord 16:999–1003, 1992

Jackson WK, Roose SP, Glassman AH: Cardiovascular toxicity of antidepressant medications. Psychopathology 20 (suppl 1):64–74, 1987

Jacobson AM, Adler AG, Wolfsdorf JI, et al: Psychological characteristics of adults with IDDM: comparison of patients in poor and good glycemic control. Diabetes Care 13:375–381, 1990

Jacobson AM, Samson JA, Weinger K, et al: Diabetes, the brain, and behavior: is there a biological mechanism underlying the association between diabetes and depression? Int Rev Neurobiol 51:455–479, 2002

Jansen Steur ENH: Increase in Parkinson disability after fluoxetine medication. Neurology 43:211–213, 1993

Jiang W, Alexander J, Christopher E, et al: Relationship of depression to increased risk of mortality and rehospitalization in patients with congestive heart failure. Arch Intern Med 161:1849–1856, 2001

Jobe PC, Dailey JW, Wernicke JF: A noradrenergic and serotonergic hypothesis of the linkage between epilepsy and affective disorders. Crit Rev Neurobiol 13:317–356, 1999

Joffe P, Larsen FS, Pedersen V, et al: Single-dose pharmacokinetics of citalopram in patients with moderate renal insufficiency or hepatic cirrhosis compared with healthy subjects. Eur J Clin Pharmacol 54:237–242, 1998

Jones JM, Huggins MA, Rydall AC, et al: Symptomatic distress, hopelessness, and the desire for hastened death in hospitalized cancer patients. J Psychosom Res 55:411–418, 2003

Kanner AM: Depression in epilepsy: prevalence, clinical semiology, pathogenic mechanisms, and treatment. Biol Psychiatry 54:388–398, 2003

Kaplan HI, Sadock BJ: Electroconvulsive therapy, in Kaplan and Sadock's Synopsis of Psychiatry: Behavioral Sciences/Clinical Psychiatry, 8th Edition. Baltimore, MD, Lippincott, Williams & Wilkins, 1998, pp 1115–1122

Karlsson I, Godderis J, Augusto De Mendonca Lima C, et al: A randomized, double-blind comparison of the efficacy and safety of citalopram compared to mianserin in elderly, depressed patients with or without mild to moderate dementia. Int J Geriatr Psychiatry 15:295–305, 2000

Katz MR, Kopek N, Waldron J, et al: Screening for depression in head and neck cancer. Psychooncology 13:269–280, 2004

Kauhanen M, Korpelainen JT, Hiltunen P, et al: Poststroke depression correlates with cognitive impairment and neurological deficits. Stroke 30:1875–1880, 1999

Keller MB: Citalopram therapy for depression: a review of 10 years of European experience and data from U.S. clinical trials. J Clin Psychiatry 61:896–908, 2000

Kelley JA, Murphy DA, Bahr GR, et al: Outcome of cognitive-behavioural and support group brief therapies for depressed, HIV-infected persons. Am J Psychiatry 150:1679–1686, 1993

Kelsen DP, Portenoy RK, Thaler HT, et al: Pain and depression in patients with newly diagnosed pancreas cancer. J Clin Oncol 13:748–755, 1995

Kendler KS, Gardner CO Jr: Boundaries of major depression: an evaluation of DSM-IV criteria. Am J Psychiatry 155:172–177, 1998

Kessler RC, Berglund P, Demler O, et al: The epidemiology of major depressive disorder: results from the National Comorbidity Survey Replication (NCS-R). JAMA 289:3095–3105, 2003

Kimura M, Robinson RG, Kosier JT: Treatment of cognitive impairment after poststroke depression: a double-blind treatment trial. Stroke 31:1482–1486, 2000

Kinder LS, Kamarck TW, Baum A, et al: Depressive symptomatology and coronary heart disease in type I diabetes mellitus: a study of possible mechanisms. Health Psychol 21:542–552, 2002

Koenig HG: Differences in psychosocial and health correlates of major and minor depression in medically ill older adults. J Am Geriatr Soc 45:1487–1495, 1997

Koenig HG, Cohen HJ, Blazer DG, et al: A brief depression scale for use in the medically ill. Int J Psychiatry Med 22:183–195, 1992

Koenig HG, George LK, Peterson BL, et al: Depression in medically ill hospitalized older adults: prevalence, characteristics, and course of symptoms according to six diagnostic schemes. Am J Psychiatry 154:1376–1383, 1997

Koike AK, Unutzer J, Wells KB: Improving the care for depression in patients with comorbid medical illness. Am J Psychiatry 159:1738–1745, 2002

Kopetz S, Steele CD, Brandt J, et al: Characteristics and outcomes of dementia residents in an assisted living facility. Int J Geriatr Psychiatry 15:586–593, 2000

Kovacs M, Obrosky DS, Goldston D, et al: Major depressive disorder in youths with IDDM: a controlled prospective study of course and outcome. Diabetes Care 20:45–51, 1997

Krantz DS, Sheps DS, Carney RM, et al: Effects of mental stress in patients with coronary artery disease: evidence and clinical implications. JAMA 283:1800–1802, 2000

Krittayaphong R, Cascio WE, Light KC, et al: Heart rate variability in patients with coronary artery disease: differences in patients with higher and lower depression scores. Psychosom Med 59:231–235, 1997

Kroenke K, Jackson JL, Chamberlin J: Depressive and anxiety disorders in patients presenting with physical complaints: clinical predictors and outcome. Am J Med 103:339–347, 1997

Kroenke K, Spitzer RL, Williams JB: The PHQ-9: validity of a brief depression severity measure. J Gen Intern Med 16:606–613, 2001

Kroenke K, Spitzer RL, Williams JB: The PHQ-15: validity of a new measure for evaluating the severity of somatic symptoms. Psychosom Med 64:258–266, 2002

Kugaya A, Akechi T, Okuyama T, et al: Prevalence, predictive factors, and screening for psychologic distress in patients with newly diagnosed head and neck cancer. Cancer 88:2817–2823, 2000

Kuptniratsaikul V, Chulakadabba S, Ratanavijitrasil S: An instrument for assessment of depression among spinal cord injury patients: comparison between the CES-D and TDI. J Med Assoc Thai 85:978–983, 2002

Lambert MV, Robertson MM: Depression in epilepsy: etiology, phenomenology, and treatment. Epilepsia 40 (suppl 10):S21–S47, 1999

Lanza GA, Pedrotti P, Rebuzzi AG, et al: Usefulness of the addition of heart rate variability to Holter monitoring in predicting in-hospital cardiac events in patients with unstable angina pectoris. Am J Cardiol 80:263–267, 1997

Lauzon C, Beck CA, Huynh T, et al: Depression and prognosis following hospital admission because of acute myocardial infarction. Can Med Assoc J 168:547–552, 2003

Lee HB, Lyketsos CG: Depression in Alzheimer's disease: heterogeneity and related issues. Biol Psychiatry 54:353–362, 2003

Leentjens AF, Verhey FR, Luijckx GJ, et al: The validity of the Beck Depression Inventory as a screening and diagnostic instrument for depression in patients with Parkinson's disease. Mov Disord 15:1221–1224, 2000

Leserman J, Petitto JM, Perkins DO, et al: Severe stress, depressive symptoms, and changes in lymphocyte subsets in human immunodeficiency virus-infected men: a 2-year follow-up study. Arch Gen Psychiatry 54:279–285, 1997

Lesperance F, Frasure-Smith N, Talajic M: Major depression before and after myocardial infarction: its nature and consequences. Psychosom Med 58:99–110, 1996

Lesperance F, Frasure-Smith N, Talajic M, et al: Five-year risk of cardiac mortality in relation to initial severity and one-year changes in depression symptoms after myocardial infarction. Circulation 105:1049–1053, 2002

Levy NB, Blumenfield M, Beasley CM Jr, et al: Fluoxetine in depressed patients with renal failure and in depressed patients with normal kidney function. Gen Hosp Psychiatry 18:8–13, 1996

Lincoln NB, Flannaghan T: Cognitive behavioral psychotherapy for depression following stroke: a randomized controlled trial. Stroke 34:111–115, 2003

Lindeman S, Hamalainen J, Isometsa E, et al: The 12-month prevalence and risk factors for major depressive episode in Finland: representative sample of 5993 adults. Acta Psychiatr Scand 102:178–184, 2000

Lloyd-Williams M, Friedman T, Rudd N: An analysis of the validity of the Hospital Anxiety and Depression Scale as a screening tool in patients with advanced metastatic cancer. J Pain Symptom Manage 22:990–996, 2001

Lloyd-Williams M, Spiller J, Ward J: Which depression screening tools should be used in palliative care? Palliat Med 17:40–43, 2003

Loberiza FR Jr, Rizzo JD, Bredeson CN, et al: Association of depressive syndrome and early deaths among patients after stem-cell transplantation for malignant diseases. J Clin Oncol 20:2118–2126, 2002

Loprinzi CL, Kugler JW, Sloan JA, et al: Venlafaxine in management of hot flashes in survivors of breast cancer: a randomized controlled trial. Lancet 356:2059–2063, 2000a

Loprinzi CL, Zahasky KM, Sloan JA, et al: Tamoxifen-induced hot flashes. Clin Breast Cancer 1:52–56, 2000b

Lowe B, Spitzer RL, Grafe K, et al: Comparative validity of three screening questionnaires for DSM-IV depressive disorders and physicians' diagnoses. J Affect Disord 78:131–140, 2004

Lustman PJ, Griffith LS, Clouse RE, et al: Psychiatric illness in diabetes mellitus: relationship to symptoms and glucose control. J Nerv Ment Dis 174:736–742, 1986

Lustman PJ, Griffith LS, Freedland KE, et al: The course of major depression in diabetes. Gen Hosp Psychiatry 19:138–143, 1997

Lustman PJ, Griffith LS, Freedland KE, et al: Cognitive behavior therapy for depression in type 2 diabetes mellitus: a randomized, controlled trial. Ann Intern Med 129:613–621, 1998

Lustman PJ, Anderson RJ, Freedland KE, et al: Depression and poor glycemic control: a meta-analytic review of the literature. Diabetes Care 23:934–942, 2000a

Lustman PJ, Freedland KE, Griffith LS, et al: Fluoxetine for depression in diabetes: a randomized double-blind placebo-controlled trial. Diabetes Care 23:618–623, 2000b

Lyketsos CG, Steele C, Baker L, et al: Major and minor depression in Alzheimer's disease: prevalence and impact. J Neuropsychiatry Clin Neurosci 9:556–561, 1997

Lyketsos CG, Sheppard JM, Steele CD, et al: Randomised, placebo-controlled, double-blind clinical trial of sertraline in the treatment of depression complicating Alzheimer's disease: initial results from the Depression in Alzheimer's Disease study. Am J Psychiatry 157:1686–1689, 2000

Lyketsos CG, Sheppard JM, Steinberg M, et al: Neuropsychiatric disturbance in Alzheimer's disease clusters into three groups: the Cache County study. Int J Geriatr Psychiatry 16:1043–1053, 2001

Lyketsos CG, Lopez O, Jones B, et al: Prevalence of neuropsychiatric symptoms in dementia and mild cognitive impairment: results from the cardiovascular health study. JAMA 288: 1475–1483, 2002

Magni G, Conlon P, Arsie D: Tricyclic antidepressants in the treatment of cancer pain: a review. Pharmacopsychiatry 20:160–164, 1987

Marcus MD, Moulton MM, Greeno CG: Binge eating onset in obese patients with binge eating disorders. Addict Behav 20:747–755, 1995

Markowitz JC, Kocsis JH, Fishman B, et al: Treatment of depressive symptoms in human immunodeficiency virus-positive patients. Arch Gen Psychiatry 55:452–457, 1998

Masand P, Pickett P, Murray GB: Psychostimulants for secondary depression in medical illness. Psychosomatics 32:203–208, 1991

Massie MJ, Popkin MK: Depressive disorders, in Psycho-Oncology. Edited by Holland J. New York, Oxford University Press, 1998, pp 518–540

McDaniel JS, Musselman DL, Porter MR, et al: Depression in patients with cancer: diagnosis, biology, and treatment. Arch Gen Psychiatry 52:89–99, 1995

McDonald WM, Richard IH, DeLong MR: Prevalence, etiology, and treatment of depression in Parkinson's disease. Biol Psychiatry 54:363–375, 2003

Meakin CJ: Screening for depression in the medically ill: the future of paper and pencil tests. Br J Psychiatry 160:212–216, 1992

Mendes de Leon CF, Kop WJ, de Swart HB, et al: Psychosocial characteristics and recurrent events after percutaneous transluminal coronary angioplasty. Am J Cardiol 77:252–255, 1996

Meredith IT, Broughton A, Jennings GL, et al: Evidence of a selective increase in cardiac sympathetic activity in patients with sustained ventricular arrhythmias. N Engl J Med 325:618–624, 1991

Migliorelli R, Teson A, Sabe L, et al: Prevalence and correlates of dysthymia and major depression among patients with Alzheimer's disease. Am J Psychiatry 152:37–44, 1995

Minden SL, Schiffer RB: Affective disorders in multiple sclerosis: review and recommendations for clinical research. Arch Neurol 47:98–104, 1990

Mohr DC, Goodkin DE, Likosky W, et al: Therapeutic expectations of patients with multiple sclerosis upon initiating interferon beta-1b: relationship to adherence to treatment. Mult Scler 2:222–226, 1996

Mohr DC, Likosky W, Bertagnolli A, et al: Telephone-administered cognitive-behavioral therapy for the treatment of depressive symptoms in multiple sclerosis. J Consult Clin Psychol 68:356–361, 2000

Mohr DC, Boudewyn AC, Goodkin DE, et al: Comparative outcomes for individual cognitive-behavior therapy, supportive-expressive group psychotherapy, and sertraline for the treatment of depression in multiple sclerosis. J Consult Clin Psychol 69:942–949, 2001

Montgomery S, Åsberg M: A new depression scale designed to be sensitive to change. Br J Psychiatry 134:383–389, 1979

Morris PL, Robinson RG, Samuels J: Depression, introversion and mortality following stroke. Aust N Z J Psychiatry 27:443–449, 1993

Murray CJ, Lopez AD: Alternative projections of mortality and disability by cause 1990–2020: Global Burden of Disease Study. Lancet 349:1498–1504, 1997

Murray GB, Shea V, Conn DK: Electroconvulsive therapy for poststroke depression. J Clin Psychiatry 47:258–260, 1986

Musselman DL, Evans DL, Nemeroff CB: The relationship of depression to cardiovascular disease: epidemiology, biology, and treatment. Arch Gen Psychiatry 55:580–592, 1998

Musselman DL, Lawson DH, Gumnick JF, et al: Paroxetine for the prevention of depression induced by high-dose interferon alfa. N Engl J Med 344:961–966, 2001

Narushima K, Kosier JT, Robinson RG: Preventing poststroke depression: a 12-week double-blind randomized treatment trial and 21-month follow-up. J Nerv Ment Dis 190:296–303, 2002

Newell SA, Sanson-Fisher RW, Savolainen NJ: Systematic review of psychological therapies for cancer patients: overview and recommendations for future research. J Natl Cancer Inst 94:558–584, 2002

Newport DJ, Nemeroff CB: Assessment and treatment of depression in the cancer patient. J Psychosom Res 45:215–237, 1998

Nielsen AC, Williams TA: Depression in ambulatory medical patients: prevalence by self-report questionnaire and recognition by nonpsychiatric physicians. Arch Gen Psychiatry 37:999–1004, 1980

Ormel J, Oldehinkel T, Brilman E, et al: Outcome of depression and anxiety in primary care: a three-wave 3 1/2-year study of psychopathology and disability. Arch Gen Psychiatry 50:759–766, 1993

Page-Shafer K, Delorenze GN, Satariano WA, et al: Comorbidity and survival in HIV-infected men in the San Francisco Men's Health Survey. Ann Epidemiol 6:420–430, 1996

Paluska SA, Schwenk TL: Physical activity and mental health: current concepts. Sports Med 29:167–180, 2000

Paolucci S, Antonucci G, Pratesi L, et al: Poststroke depression and its role in rehabilitation of inpatients. Arch Phys Med Rehabil 80:985–990, 1999

Pasacreta JV: Depressive phenomena, physical symptom distress, and functional status among women with breast cancer. Nurs Res 46:214–221, 1997

Passik SD, Roth AJ: Anxiety symptoms and panic attacks preceding pancreatic cancer diagnosis. Psychooncology 8:268–272, 1999

Pearson SD, Katzelnick DJ, Simon GE, et al: Depression among high utilizers of medical care. J Gen Intern Med 14:461–468, 1999

Pearson TA, Fuster V: Executive Summary. J Am Coll Cardiol 27:957–1047, 1996

Pelletier G, Verhoef MJ, Khatri N, et al: Quality of life in brain tumor patients: the relative contributions of depression, fatigue, emotional distress, and existential issues. J Neuro-oncol 57:41–49, 2002

Penninx BWJH, Guralnik JM, Mendes de Leon CF, et al: Cardiovascular events and mortality in newly and chronically depressed persons >70 years of age. Am J Cardiol 81:988–994, 1998

Peyrot M, Rubin RR: Levels and risks of depression and anxiety symptomatology among diabetic adults. Diabetes Care 20:585–590, 1997

Peyrot M, Rubin RR: Persistence of depressive symptoms in diabetic adults. Diabetes Care 22:448–452, 1999

Pezzella G, Moslinger-Gehmayr R, Contu A: Treatment of depression in patients with breast cancer: a comparison between paroxetine and amitriptyline. Breast Cancer Res Treat 70:1–10, 2001

Pine DS, Goldstein RB, Wolk S, et al: The association between childhood depression and adulthood body mass index. Pediatrics 107:1049–1056, 2001

Pirl WF, Roth AJ: Diagnosis and treatment of depression in cancer patients. Oncology 13:1293–1301, discussion 1301–1302, 1305–1306, 1999

Pisani F, Oteri G, Costa C, et al: Effects of psychotropic drugs on seizure threshold. Drug Saf 25:91–110, 2002

Poewe W, Seppi K: Treatment options for depression and psychosis in Parkinson's disease. J Neurol 248 (suppl 3):12–21, 2001

Pomeroy IM, Clark CR, Philp I: The effectiveness of very short scales for depression screening in elderly medical patients. Int J Geriatr Psychiatry 16:321–326, 2001

Potter WZ, Manji HK, Rudorfer MV: Tricyclics and tetracyclics, in The American Psychiatric Press Textbook of Psychopharmacology, 2nd Edition. Edited by Schatzberg AF, Nemeroff CB. Washington, DC, American Psychiatric Press, 1998, pp 199–218

Preskorn SH, Fast GA: Tricyclic antidepressant-induced seizures and plasma drug concentration. J Clin Psychiatry 53:160–162, 1992

Pujol J, Bello J, Deus J, et al: Lesions in the left arcuate fasciculus region and depressive symptoms in multiple sclerosis. Neurology 49:1105–1110, 1997

Rabkin JG, Rabkin R, Harrison W, et al: Effect of imipramine on mood and enumerative measures of immune status in depressed patients with HIV illness. Am J Psychiatry 151:516–523, 1994

Rabkin JG, Wagner GJ, Rabkin R: Fluoxetine treatment for depression in patients with HIV and AIDS: a randomized, placebo-controlled trial. Am J Psychiatry 156:101–107, 1999

Radloff LS: The CES-D: a self-report depression scale for research in the general population. Applied Psychological Measures 3:385–401, 1977

Raison CL, Miller AH: Depression in cancer: new developments regarding diagnosis and treatment. Biol Psychiatry 54:283–294, 2003

Rao V, Lyketsos CG: The benefits and risks of ECT for patients with primary dementia who also suffer from depression. Int J Geriatr Psychiatry 15:729–735, 2000

Rasmussen A, Lunde M, Poulsen DL, et al: A double-blind, placebo-controlled study of sertraline in the prevention of depression in stroke patients. Psychosomatics 44:216–221, 2003

Razavi D, Delvaux N, Farvacques C, et al: Screening for adjustment disorders and major depressive disorders in cancer inpatients. Br J Psychiatry 156:79–83, 1990

Reynolds CF III: Treatment of depression in special populations. J Clin Psychiatry 53 (suppl):45–53, 1992

Richard IH, Maughn A, Kurlan R: Do serotonin reuptake inhibitor antidepressants worsen Parkinson's disease? A retrospective case series. Mov Disord 14:155–157, 1999

Rifkin A, Reardon G, Siris S, et al: Trimipramine in physical illness with depression. J Clin Psychiatry 46:4–8, 1985

Robinson N, Fuller JH, Edmeades SP: Depression and diabetes. Diabet Med 5:268–274, 1988

Robinson RG: Poststroke depression: prevalence, diagnosis, treatment, and disease progression. Biol Psychiatry 54:376–387, 2003

Robinson RG, Schultz SK, Castillo C, et al: Nortriptyline versus fluoxetine in the treatment of depression and in short-term recovery after stroke: a placebo-controlled, double-blind study. Am J Psychiatry 157:351–359, 2000

Rodin G, Craven J, Littlefield C: Depression in the Medically Ill: An Integrated Approach. New York, Brunner/Mazel, 1991

Roth AJ, Scher HI: Sertraline relieves hot flashes secondary to medical castration as treatment of advanced prostate cancer. Psychooncology 7:129–132, 1998

Roth M, Mountjoy CQ, Amrein R: Moclobemide in elderly patients with cognitive decline and depression: an international double-blind, placebo-controlled trial. Br J Psychiatry 168:149–157, 1996

Rozanski A, Blumenthal JA, Kaplan J: Impact of psychological factors on the pathogenesis of cardiovascular disease and implications for therapy. Circulation 99:2192–2217, 1999

Schade CP, Jones ER Jr, Wittlin BJ: A ten-year review of the validity and clinical utility of depression screening. Psychiatr Serv 49:55–61, 1998

Schleifer SJ, Macari-Hinson MM, Coyle DA, et al: The nature and course of depression following myocardial infarction. Arch Intern Med 149:1785–1789, 1989

Schulberg HC, Katon W, Simon GE, et al: Treating major depression in primary care practice: an update of the Agency for Health Care Policy and Research Practice Guidelines. Arch Gen Psychiatry 55:1121–1127, 1998

Schulz R, Beach S, Ives D, et al: Association between depression and mortality in older adults: the Cardiovascular Health Study. Arch Intern Med 160:1761–1768, 2000

Sheline YI: Neuroimaging studies of mood disorder effects on the brain. Biol Psychiatry 54:338–352, 2003

Shuster JL, Stern TA, Greenberg DB: Pros and cons of fluoxetine for the depressed cancer patient. Oncology 6:45–50, 1992

Shusterman V, Aysin B, Gottipaty V, et al: Autonomic nervous system activity and the spontaneous initiation of ventricular tachycardia. J Am Coll Cardiol 32:1891–1899, 1998

Silverstone PH: Poor efficacy of the Hospital Anxiety and Depression Scale in the diagnosis of major depressive disorder in both medical and psychiatric patients. J Psychosom Res 38: 441–450, 1994

Simon GE: Social and economic burden of mood disorders. Biol Psychiatry 54:208–215, 2003

Simon G, Ormel J, VonKorff M, et al: Health care costs associated with depressive and anxiety disorders in primary care. Am J Psychiatry 152:352–357, 1995

Simon GE, Goldberg DP, Von Korff M, et al: Understanding cross-national differences in depression prevalence. Psychol Med 32:585–594, 2002

Sindrup SH, Gram LF, Brosen K, et al: The selective serotonin reuptake inhibitor paroxetine is effective in the treatment of diabetic neuropathy symptoms. Pain 42:135–144, 1990

Sindrup SH, Bjerre U, Dejgaard A, et al: The selective serotonin reuptake inhibitor citalopram relieves the symptoms of diabetic neuropathy. Clin Pharmacol Ther 52:547–552, 1992

Smith D, Dempster C, Glanville J, et al: Efficacy and tolerability of venlafaxine compared with selective serotonin reuptake inhibitors and other antidepressants: a meta-analysis. Br J Psychiatry 180:396–404, 2002

Snaith RP, Taylor CM: Rating scales for depression and anxiety: a current perspective. Br J Clin Pharmacol 19 (suppl):17S–20S, 1985

Sollner W, DeVries A, Steixner E, et al: How successful are oncologists in identifying patient distress, perceived social support, and need for psychosocial counselling? Br J Cancer 84:179–185, 2001

Spalletta G, Guida G, De Angelis D, et al: Predictors of cognitive level and depression severity are different in patients with left and right hemispheric stroke within the first year of illness. J Neurol 249:1541–1551, 2002

Spiegel D, Giese-Davis J: Depression and cancer: mechanisms and disease progression. Biol Psychiatry 54:269–282, 2003

Spitzer RL, Kroenke K, Williams JB: Validation and utility of a self-report version of PRIME-MD: the PHQ primary care study. JAMA 282:1737–1744, 1999

Spitzer RL, Williams JB, Kroenke K, et al: Validity and utility of the PRIME-MD Patient Health Questionnaire in assessment of 3000 obstetric-gynecologic patients. Am J Obstet Gynecol 183:759–769, 2000

Sroka K, Peimann CJ, Seevers H: Heart rate variability in myocardial ischemia during daily life. J Electrocardiol 30:45–56, 1997

Starace F, Ammassari A, Trotta MP, et al: Depression is a risk factor for suboptimal adherence to highly active antiretroviral therapy. J Acquir Immune Defic Syndr 31 (suppl 3): S136–S139, 2002

Stearns V, Isaacs C, Rowland J, et al: A pilot trial assessing the efficacy of paroxetine hydrochloride (Paxil) in controlling hot flashes in breast cancer survivors. Ann Oncol 11:17–22, 2000

Stenager EN, Koch-Henriksen N, Stenager E: Risk factors for suicide in multiple sclerosis. Psychother Psychosom 65:86–90, 1996

Stimmel GL, Dopheide JA, Stahl SM: Mirtazapine: an antidepressant with noradrenergic and specific serotonergic effects. Pharmacotherapy 17:10–21, 1997

Stommel M, Given BA, Given CW: Depression and functional status as predictors of death among cancer patients. Cancer 94:2719–2727, 2002

Strain JJ: Adjustment disorders, in Psycho-Oncology. Edited by Holland J. New York, Oxford University Press, 1998, pp 509–517

Strik JJ, Honig A, Lousberg R, et al: Efficacy and safety of fluoxetine in the treatment of patients with major depression after first myocardial infarction: findings from a double-blind, placebo-controlled trial. Psychosom Med 62:783–789, 2000

Stunkard AJ, Faith MS, Allison KC: Depression and obesity. Biol Psychiatry 54:330–337, 2003

Teno JM, Harrell FE Jr, Knaus W, et al: Prediction of survival for older hospitalized patients: the HELP survival model. J Am Geriatr Soc 48 (suppl 5):16–24, 2000

Teri L, Logsdon R, Yesavage J: Measuring behavior, mood, and psychiatric symptoms in Alzheimer disease. Alzheimer Dis Assoc Disord 11 (suppl 6):50–59, 1997

Tesei S, Antonini A, Canesi M, et al: Tolerability of paroxetine in Parkinson's disease: a prospective study. Mov Disord 15: 986–989, 2000

Thase ME: Psychotherapy of refractory depressions. Depress Anxiety 5:190–201, 1997

Thase ME, Entsuah AR, Rudolph RL: Remission rates during treatment with venlafaxine or selective serotonin reuptake inhibitors. Br J Psychiatry 178:234–241, 2001

Theobald DE, Kirsh KL, Holtsclaw E, et al: An open-label, crossover trial of mirtazapine (15 and 30 mg) in cancer patients with pain and other distressing symptoms. J Pain Symptom Manage 23:442–447, 2002

Tross S, Herndon J 2nd, Korzun A, et al: Psychological symptoms and disease-free and overall survival in women with stage II breast cancer. J Natl Cancer Inst 88:661–667, 1996

Vaccarino V, Kasl SV, Abramson J, et al: Depressive symptoms and risk of functional decline and death in patients with heart failure. J Am Coll Cardiol 38:199–205, 2001

Valkama JO, Huikuri HV, Koistinen MJ, et al: Relation between heart rate variability and spontaneous and induced ventricular arrhythmias in patients with coronary artery disease. J Am Coll Cardiol 25:437–443, 1995

van den Berg MP, Haaksma J, Brouwer J, et al: Heart rate variability in patients with atrial fibrillation is related to vagal tone. Circulation 96:1209–1216, 1997

van Heeringen K, Zivkov M: Pharmacological treatment of depression in cancer patients: a placebo-controlled study of mianserin. Br J Psychiatry 169:440–443, 1996

Van Tilburg MA, McCaskill CC, Lane JD, et al: Depressed mood is a factor in glycemic control in type 1 diabetes. Psychosom Med 63:551–555, 2001

van Walraven C, Mamdani MM, Wells PS, et al: Inhibition of serotonin reuptake by antidepressants and upper gastrointestinal bleeding in elderly patients: a retrospective cohort study. BMJ 323:1–6, 2001

Von Korff M, Ormel J, Katon W, et al: Disability and depression among high utilizers of health care: a longitudinal analysis. Arch Gen Psychiatry 49:91–100, 1992

Wallis EJ, Ramsay LE, Ul H, et al: Coronary and cardiovascular risk estimation for primary prevention: validation of a new Sheffield table in the 1995 Scottish Health Survey population. BMJ 320:671–676, 2000 [published erratum appears in BMJ 320:1034, 2000]

Watkins C, Daniels L, Jack C, et al: Accuracy of a single question in screening for depression in a cohort of patients after stroke: comparative study. BMJ 323:1159, 2001

Watkins LL, Grossman P: Association of depressive symptoms with reduced baroreflex cardiac control in coronary artery disease. Am Heart J 137:453–457, 1999

Watson M, Haviland JS, Greer S, et al: Influence of psychological response on survival in breast cancer: a population-based cohort study. Lancet 354:1331–1336, 1999

Weiner RD, Coffey CE: Electroconvulsive therapy in the medical and neurologic patients, in Psychiatric Care of the Medical Patient. Edited by Stoudemire A, Fogel BS. New York, Oxford University Press, 1993, pp 207–224

Wells KB, Golding JM, Burnam MA: Psychiatric disorder in a sample of the general population with and without chronic medical conditions. Am J Psychiatry 145:976–981, 1988

Whooley MA, Simon GE: Primary care: managing depression in medical outpatients. N Engl J Med 343:1942–1950, 2000

Whyte EM, Mulsant BH: Post stroke depression: epidemiology, pathophysiology, and biological treatment. Biol Psychiatry 52:253–264, 2002

Wiart L, Petit H, Joseph PA, et al: Fluoxetine in early poststroke depression: a double-blind placebo-controlled study. Stroke 31:1829–1832, 2000

Wilhelm K, Parker G, Dewhurst-Savellis J, et al: Psychological predictors of single and recurrent major depressive episodes. J Affect Disord 54:139–147, 1999

Williams JW Jr, Barrett J, Oxman T, et al: Treatment of dysthymia and minor depression in primary care: a randomized controlled trial in older adults. JAMA 284:1519–1526, 2000

Wilson KG, Chochinov HM, de Fay BJ, et al: Diagnosis and management of depression in palliative care, in Handbook of Psychiatry in Palliative Medicine. Edited by Chochinov HM, Breitbart W. New York, Oxford University Press, 2000, pp 25–49

Wing RR, Phelan S, Tate D: The role of adherence in mediating the relationship between depression and health outcomes. J Psychosom Res 53:877–881, 2002

Wulsin LR: Does depression kill? Arch Intern Med 160:1731–1732, 2000

Yesavage JA, Brink TL, Rose TL, et al: Development and validation of a geriatric depression screening scale: a preliminary report. J Psychiatr Res 17:37–49, 1983

Zabora J: Screening procedures for psychosocial distress, in Psycho-Oncology. Edited by Holland J. New York, Oxford University Press, 1998, pp 507–517

Zabora J, BrintzenhofeSzoc K, Curbow B, et al: The prevalence of psychological distress by cancer site. Psychooncology 10:19–28, 2001

Zigmond AS, Snaith RP: The Hospital Anxiety and Depression Scale. Acta Psychiatr Scand 67:361–370, 1983

Zisook S, Peterkin J, Goggin KJ, et al: Treatment of major depression in HIV-seropositive men. J Clin Psychiatry 59:217–224, 1998

10 Suicidality

John Michael Bostwick, M.D.

James L. Levenson, M.D.

ONE OF THE most common questions posed to any psychiatrist, including psychosomatic medicine specialists, is whether a patient is suicidal. Suicidal ideation, frequent and ubiquitous in medical settings, challenges the psychiatrist to discern what drives the patient's suicidal statement. Compared with suicidal ideation, completed suicide is rare in psychiatric patients and rarer still in medically ill patients.

Completed suicides are statistically rare events. Many risk factors are recognized, but none has a high positive predictive value (Mann 1987). As a low-base-rate phenomenon, screening for suicide risk has a high rate of false-positive results. Demographic risk factors alone will identify many more subjects potentially at risk than imminently in danger of dying (Goldberg 1987).

Despite hundreds of studies over decades that made dozens of epidemiological correlations between suicide and particular descriptors, no effective screening paradigm has been identified. This situation is no different with suicidality in medical illness. Many medical illnesses have been associated with increased suicide attempts—for example, in one study, lung disease (odds ratio [OR] = 1.8) and peptic ulcer (OR = 2.1) (Goodwin et al. 2003). A Canadian study showed elevated ORs for completed suicide in cancer (1.73), prostate disease (1.70), and chronic pulmonary disease (1.86) (Quan et al. 2002). In a Swedish study, visual impairment (OR = 7.00), neurological disorders (OR = 3.8), and malignancy (OR = 3.4) were independently associated with suicide (Waern et al. 2002). Nevertheless, these increased rates are still too low to use the medical diagnosis to predict suicide. Moreover, no epidemiological risk factor represents an individual's suicide intent—the essential, highly personal variable in suicide prediction (Davidson 1993). Fortunately, the field of suicidology has shifted from trying to predict individual suicides to a more realistic goal of estimating probabilities of risk for particular subpopulations (Hughes and Kleespies 2001). Such data can then be used to inform the psychiatrist's assessment of an individual patient's suicide threat while also considering the personal meaning of the patient's communication.

A focus on probabilities of risk and general categories of psychiatric symptoms rather than individual diagnoses lends itself well to understanding suicidality in the medically ill. Medical illness by itself is rarely a sole determinant of suicide potential. Comorbid factors drive what is best understood as a multidetermined act (Hughes and Kleespies 2001). Shneidman (1989), the father of American suicidology, conceptualized a cubic model of suicidal states, incorporating *perturbation* (the state of being stirred up or upset), *pain* (psychological pain resulting from frustrated psychological needs), and *press* (genetic and developmental susceptibility to particular events). Moscicki (1995) envisioned two distinct but interactive groups of risk factors, with recent events—"proximal risk factors"—unfolding on a substrate of underlying "distal" conditions. According to both models, the assessment of a medically ill person—as with any suicidal person—demands attention to what past characterological, temperamental, or experiential features push someone toward suicide.

In Mann's (1998) diathesis–stress model of suicidal behavior, *stresses* resemble Moscicki's proximal factors, and *diatheses* resemble her distal ones (Figure 10–1). Noting that two groups of patients, each with the same severity of depressive illness, attempt suicide at different rates, Mann proposed suicide diathesis components, including genetic predisposition, early life experience, chronic illness, chronic substance abuse, and certain dietary factors. Extreme stress alone, which Mann defined as acute psychiatric illness, intoxication, medical illness, or family and

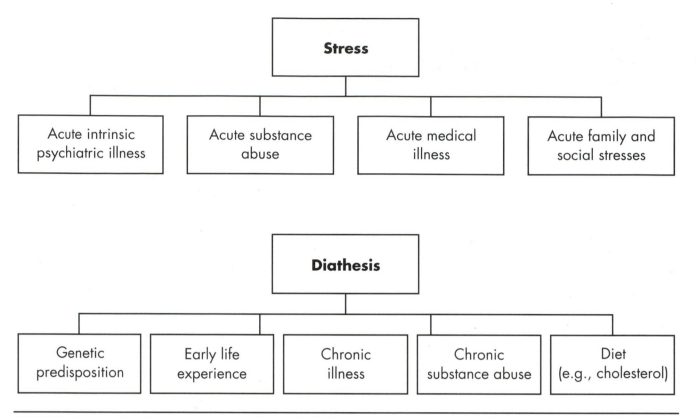

FIGURE 10–1.   **Diathesis–stress model of suicidal behavior: components of stress and diathesis.**

Source.   Adapted from Mann JJ: "The Neurobiology of Suicide." *Nature Medicine* 4:25–30, 1998. Copyright 1998. Used with permission.

social stresses, is not typically enough to invoke suicidal behavior. A suicidal individual already has the predisposition, or diathesis, on which the stress is superimposed, resulting in the suicide attempt (Mann 1998).

Mann's subcategories adapt readily to the medically ill. Acute intrinsic psychiatric illness is represented by dementia, depression, delirium, and anxiety in the context of a general medical illness. Acute substance abuse appears in the form of intoxication or withdrawal syndromes. Acute medical illness includes not only the disease itself but also the effects of treatments. Acute family and social stresses could include fears of becoming a burden, financial consequences such as expense of treatment and lost income, and disruption in the family members' lives. These state phenomena occur against the background of trait characteristics, which Mann labels as *diathesis*. Diatheses include genetic predisposition to illness, coping styles and personality characteristics (e.g., pain tolerance), and the long-term effects of chronic physical illness or substance abuse.

The Mann model, though comprehensive, does not inform the psychiatrist whether a patient is at immediate risk for suicide. Litman (1989) noted that the 95% prevalence of psychiatric illness among individuals who commit suicide is derived from psychological autopsies and retrospective studies, the scientific equivalent of Monday-morning quarterbacking. At any moment, very few of those who are "at risk" will die by suicide. Identifying the medical patient at high risk is just a first step in evaluation. The search for possible biological markers for suicide has focused on the midbrain dorsal and median raphe nuclei, with their serotonergic inputs to the ventral prefrontal cortex. Responsible for dampening aggressive or impulsive behavior, the ventral prefrontal cortex exerts its inhibitory effects on suicidal behavior less effectively when serotonergic hypofunction occurs (Kamali et al. 2001). A history of child abuse, a familial depression history, substance abuse, head injury, genetic variants, and low cholesterol levels are all associated with both lower serotonergic activity and greater suicide risk (Mann 1998). No practical test based on these psychobiological research advances currently exists. If a test were available, it would likely provide only one more risk factor in a complex biopsychosocial formulation.

Kishi and Kathol (2002) identified four "pragmatic reasons" for suicidality: 1) psychosis, 2) depression, 3) poor impulse control, and 4) philosophical reasons. White and colleagues (1995) subdivided the suicidal medically ill into three general categories: 1) patients admitted to a medical–surgical bed after a suicide attempt, 2) patients with delirium and resultant agitation and impulsivity, and 3) patients with chronic medical illness causing frustration or hopelessness.

In this chapter, we integrate these two approaches first by reviewing the general epidemiology of suicide and suicide attempts and then by discussing psychodynamic factors. The next section concerns the management of the medical and surgical consequences of a suicide attempt and the care of high-risk patients on medical inpatient units. Suicide in the medically ill is reviewed next, exemplified by a focus on cancer, end-stage renal disease, and AIDS. Finally, we address physician-assisted suicide.

Epidemiology

Suicide assessment begins with demographic clues to the patient's relative risk of suicide. Both descriptive and dynamic risk factors are important. In this section, we review descriptive risk factors—comparatively static characteristics of the individual. As the subsequent sections make clear, however, changes in psychiatric status coupled with recent life events are crucial in understanding suicidality in the medically ill.

Completed Suicide

Reported suicide was the eleventh leading cause of death in the United States in 2001, equal to 1.3% of all deaths (McIntosh 2003). The known suicide rate is nearly identical to what it was in 1900 (Monk 1987), but the epidemiology of suicide has been shifting over the last decade. Between 1990 and 2001, suicide rates have decreased in every age category, with the overall annual rate in the United States declining from 12.4 to 10.8 per 100,000. In 2001, annual suicide rates per 100,000 individuals increased throughout life—from 0.7 in 5- to 14-year-olds and 9.9 in 15- to 24-year-olds to 17.5 in those ages 85 years and older. In 15- to 24-year-olds, suicide ranks behind only accidents and homicide as a leading cause of death (McIntosh 2003). The suicide rate among men is three times higher than among women. Nonwhite Americans killed themselves in 2001 at less than half the rate of white Americans.

Over the course of the life cycle, men and women show different patterns of suicide. For men, suicide rates gradually rise during adolescence, increase sharply in early adulthood, and then decrease before starting an upward trajectory in midlife, increasing into the 75- to 84-year age bracket and beyond (Shneidman 1989). Suicide rates for women peak in midlife and then decrease, in contrast to the bimodal peaks for men. Men's suicide methods tend to be more violent and lethal; men are more likely to die by hanging, drowning, and shooting. Women are less likely to die in suicide attempts because they are more likely to choose the less lethal methods of wrist cutting and overdose (Kaplan and Klein 1989; A. Morgan 1989). Traditionally, epidemiological studies have shown that suicide attempters are more likely to be younger, female, and married and to use pills, whereas completers are more likely to be older, male, and single and to use violent means (Fawcett and Shaughnessy 1988). However, anyone at any age may contemplate or execute suicide.

History of a suicide attempt is an important predictor of future suicide risk (Pokorny 1983). One of every 100 suicide attempt survivors will die by suicide within 1 year of the index attempt, a suicide risk approximately 100 times that for the general population (Hawton 1992). Twenty-five percent of chronically self-destructive or suicidal patients will eventually kill themselves (Litman 1989). Of those who complete suicide, 25%–50% have tried before (Patterson et al. 1983). A Danish study of patients admitted to a psychiatric unit after a suicide attempt reported that 12% successfully completed suicide within the next 5 years, 75% within 6 months of their last admission (Nielsen et al. 1990). Bostwick and Pankratz (2000) found that depressed patients who had suicidal ideation or who had just made a suicide attempt had a lifetime prevalence of suicide of 8.6%. Palmer et al. (in press) found that three-fourths of suicides in schizophrenic patients occur within 10 years of the first admission or first diagnosis.

It has been repeatedly shown in general population American and European retrospective psychological autopsy studies over the last half-century that psychiatric illness—particularly depression and alcoholism—is associated with the vast majority of completed suicides (Barraclough et al. 1974; Dorpat and Ripley 1960; Robins et al. 1959; Roy 1989). Most patients had not been identified before death as being psychiatrically ill and had not received treatment.

Many suicides are committed by patients with active alcohol use disorders. In one study, 43% of the suicide attempters were using alcohol at the time of the attempts (Hall et al. 1999). In another study, nearly 20% of the subjects completing suicide were legally intoxicated at their deaths (Buzan and Weissberg 1992). Although alcohol abusers may kill themselves at any age, especially when acute intoxication clouds their judgment and disinhibits them, those with chronic alcoholism tend to commit suicide after their relationships, work performance, and health are all in decay. Murphy and Weitzel (1990) estimated that 3.4% of alcoholic patients kill themselves, a rate that is nearly three times the lifetime risk in the general population (Murphy and Weitzel 1990). Most of the higher suicide rates among men may be accounted for by the higher rates of alcoholism among men (Klerman 1987).

Alcoholic patients often commit suicide in response to crises in their personal lives. One-third of alcoholic patients who kill themselves have lost a close relationship within the previous 6 weeks, and another one-third anticipate such a loss (Murphy 1992). Alcoholic patients frequently have numerous other suicide risk factors, many resulting from their substance abuse, including comorbid major depression, estrangement from family and social supports, unemployment, and serious medical illness. People who abuse other psychoactive substances also have high suicide rates. For example, opiate-dependent patients kill themselves at 20 times the expected rate (Miles 1977), although inadvertent overdoses may constitute part of this number.

Attempted Suicide

An estimated 735,000 suicide attempts occurred in the United States in 2001, 25 times more than completed suicides. Although there are important differences, attempted suicides are not a discrete category from completed ones, particularly in the medically ill. Suicide attempts occur across spectra of lethality of intent and lethality of effect, which may or may not coincide. Some patients deliberately plan death but naively choose a nonlethal method (e.g., benzodiazepine overdose), whereas others only intend gestures but unwittingly select a fatal method (e.g., acetaminophen overdose). At the more severe end of the spectrum, suicide attempters resemble completers. In a New Zealand study, Beautrais (2001) compared individuals who died by suicide with those who made very serious attempts. She found that they shared the same predictors, including current psychiatric disorder, history of suicide attempts, previous psychiatric care and contact, social disadvantage, and exposure to recent stressful life events.

Nonetheless, some characteristics distinguish surviving attempters from those who die. In the study by Hall et al. (1999) of serious suicide attempters, the patients, by and large, did not have long-standing mental illness or carefully considered plans. They did not have command hallucinations and were not particularly ruminative about their suicidal intent. Whereas 80% had symptoms of an anxiety or a depressive disorder, few had chronic symptoms. Patients who overdose are more likely to survive because they have time after the act to reconsider (or be found) and undergo medical treatment, infrequent options after a jump or a gunshot wound. As with completed

suicides, demographics change over the life cycle. The ratio of attempts to death in the young is 100–200:1, but by old age, it narrows precipitously to 4:1.

Hackett and Stern (1991) reported that 1%–2% of all patients evaluated in the Massachusetts General Hospital emergency department had overdosed, and 47% of these required admission—one-half to medical–surgical wards and one-half to psychiatric units. Of the patients, 85% had overdosed on benzodiazepines, alcohol, nonnarcotic analgesics, antidepressants, barbiturates, or antihistamines/anticholinergics.

Medical illness is a common factor in suicide attempters admitted to general psychiatry units. In a 1-year sample of admissions to a Danish psychiatry unit, 52% of the individuals had a somatic disease, and 21% took daily analgesic medications for pain. The somatic group was older, and most had neurological or musculoskeletal conditions in conjunction with depression that was more severe than in the nonsomatic group (Stenager et al. 1994). In the study by Hall et al. (1999) of 100 serious suicide attempters, 41% had a chronic, deteriorating medical illness, and 9% had recently received a diagnosis of a life-threatening illness.

Psychodynamic Factors

Litman (1989) described a *presuicidal syndrome*, a change in cognitive set, that characterizes lethal attempts and completed suicides. The presuicidal patient in crisis has constricted choices and perception, a tunnel vision of life as hopeless, physical tension, and emotional perturbation. The tension and distress may be relieved by a fantasy of death. The hopelessness is combined with help rejection and distrust. Often the patient has a long-term disposition toward impulsive action, an all-or-nothing approach to problems, and the characterological attitude "my way or no way."

Klerman (1987) framed the presuicidal crisis in terms of a medical model—as the result of an underlying condition, the patient has lost the capacity for rational thought. The hopelessness and helplessness of severe depression may have reached irrational proportions. Hallucinations may be commanding self-harm. Clouded sensorium, impaired judgment, and the disinhibition and misperceptions of delirium, intoxication, or substance withdrawal all may be causing the patient to act in self-destructive or dangerous ways that he or she would be unlikely to resort to when his or her mind was clear.

Gardner and Cowdry (1985) divided suicidal behavior into four categories, each with its own affective state, motivation, and outcome:

1. *True suicidal acts* are characterized by intense melancholia and despair, a wish for release from emotional pain, and the highest risk of completed suicide, given the likelihood of careful planning and a high-risk to low-rescue ratio.
2. *Retributive rage* is characterized by impulsiveness, vengefulness, and a nihilistic, constricted capacity to see other immediate options.
3. *Parasuicidal gesturing*, often repetitive and tinged with strong dependency needs, appears to be a form of communication, designed to extract a response from a significant other.
4. *Self-mutilation* serves the purpose of relieving dysphoria, a form of "indirect self-destructive behaviors" (N. Farberow 2000).

Only the first category includes the *intent* to die, but any of the four can be lethal.

An early study of personality factors and suicide among medically ill patients identified a "dependent-dissatisfied" behavior pattern among the patients who committed suicide (L. Farberow et al. 1966). Many subsequent investigators have added to the picture of the types of personality structure or cognitive styles that lend themselves to suicidal ideation or behavior. Berger (1995) observed that rational-seeming suicides were unusual in his study of the medically ill and instead were correlated with maladaptive emotional reactions. Describing the role of hopelessness in the thinking of terminally ill cancer patients who wished for hastened death, Breitbart et al. (2000) found the hopelessness to represent a pessimistic cognitive style rather a patient's assessment of a poor prognosis. That is, patients wished to speed death not because they were mortally ill but because they were chronically pessimistic. A similar finding came from Goodwin and Olfson's study (2002) of suicidal ideation in nearly 2,600 patients with physical illness diagnoses. Perception of poor health was a significant predictor of suicidal ideation, even after controlling for psychiatric disorders, physical conditions, and other factors.

The tendency of patient and medical provider alike to attribute the hopelessness to the disease—the proximal factor—has resulted in a failure to recognize the mental disorder or personality type—the distal condition—that is actually speaking. "There has been a tendency to regard the suicide of a victim of severe medical illness, such as cancer, as a rational alternative to the distress caused by the disease," concluded Suominen and colleagues (2002) after analyzing a year's worth of suicides in Finland. "On the other hand, most suicide victims with physical illness have suffered from concurrent mental disorder....Mental disorders may thus have a mediating role between medical disorder and suicide" (p. 412).

Suicide is often a response to a loss, real or imagined. To help assess the meaning of suicidal ideation or behavior, psychiatrists must inquire about recent or anticipated losses and coping strategies that the patient has used with past losses (Davidson 1993). Fantasies of revenge, punishment, reconciliation with a rejecting object, relief from the pain of loss, or reunion with a dead loved one may be evident (Furst and Ostow 1979).

A patient's degree of autonomy and extent of dependency on external sources of emotional support can shed light on the level of psychic resilience (Buie and Maltsberger 1989). A recent loss of a loved one or a parental loss during childhood increases suicide risk. Holidays and anniversaries of important days in the life and death of the deceased person, when the loved one's absence is experienced more intensely, also increase the risk for suicide. In medical settings, what may be lost is a part of one's self. It may be tangible—an organ, a limb, sexual potency—or intangible—a sense of youthfulness, health, or invincibility. Glickman (1980) believed that a suicidal patient cannot be judged safe until he or she has either regained the lost object, accepted its loss, or replaced it with a new object.

Psychiatrists must monitor themselves for reactions and countertransference feelings toward suicidal patients. In medical settings, consulting psychiatrists help other health care professionals identify and overcome their countertransference reactions as well. These include the classic reactions of "countertransference hate" (Maltsberger and Buie 1974), in which aversion to the suicidal patient (conscious or unconscious) leads to acting angrily toward the patient or withdrawing to an aloof passivity, both of which increase the risk for suicide. Overidentification with seriously medically ill patients may lead to other countertransference reactions. For example, in response to a hopeless patient, the psychiatrist may become overly pessimistic or too reassuring.

Management in Medical Inpatient Settings

For a patient who survives a recent suicide attempt, the emergency department usually is the first stop for assessment and triage. If the patient is medically cleared, ideally a psychiatrist, but sometimes another mental health professional, evaluates the patient and decides whether psychiatric inpatient or outpatient management is the appropriate disposition. It is important for psychiatrists to form their own judgment about whether patients are truly medically stable enough for transfer out of the medical setting because countertransference to suicidal states frequently causes nonpsychiatric physicians to minimize the role of medical contributions and prematurely "clear" patients. For a patient with self-induced injuries severe enough to require additional medical or surgical care, admission follows, and a psychiatrist is consulted. Patients who are admitted to medical–surgical beds after suicide attempts represent a particularly dangerous subset of suicidal patients. Considering data from all of New Zealand's public hospitals, Conner et al. (2003) showed that individuals hospitalized with self-induced injuries have a relative risk of 105.4 for suicide within the next year and a relative risk of 175.7 for additional self-injury hospitalizations, compared with the New Zealand general population.

Divergent conditions such as delirium, psychosis, personality disorder, and intoxication and withdrawal syndromes have in common the impulsivity that must be anticipated and managed in medical settings. Withdrawal—particularly from alcohol or sedative-hypnotics—epitomizes impulsivity syndromes that can be deadly and must be recognized and aggressively managed with detoxification protocols. In the absence of a suitably equipped psychiatric unit, the psychiatrist will need to arrange medical admission.

In addition to trying to make the environment safe, egress must be controlled. In the general medical hospital, patients should be prevented access to open stairwells, roofs, and balconies, and all windows should be secured (Berger 1995). In a classic study of the dangers of hospitalizing impulsive patients in an unsecured environment, Reich and Kelly (1976) described 17 medical inpatients who attempted suicide while on the medical and surgical wards at Peter Bent Brigham Hospital between 1967 and 1973 and survived. They judged 15 of the 17 patients to have mental disorders, but the cardinal characteristics of depression and hopelessness were not present in this sample. "All…were impulsive acts, none of the patients gave warnings, left notes, expressed suicidal thoughts or appeared to be seriously depressed" (Reich and Kelly 1976, p. 300). The investigators considered most of these 17 attempts to be reactions motivated by anger at perceived loss of emotional support, usually from staff. They attributed this underlying impaired impulse control to personality disorders in 8 of the patients, to psychosis in 7, and to delirium in 3.

When a suicidal or an impulsive patient is too medically ill to be cared for on a locked general psychiatry unit, a medical–psychiatry unit—if a hospital has one—is the ideal disposition for such a patient. In the absence of such a specialty unit, medical intensive care units are more likely to provide one-to-one nursing care, although critical care physicians may argue that such observation in the absence of need for critical care is an inappropriate use of their service.

> Ms. C, a 22-year-old woman addicted to crack cocaine, developed severe cardiomyopathy after the birth of her third child. Four months later, no longer able to climb the two flights of stairs to her apartment without becoming short of breath, she was admitted to the hospital with congestive heart failure. A toxicology screen was positive for alcohol and cocaine.
>
> After she arrived on the medical floor, Ms. C curled up in a fetal position and refused to speak to her nurse until she was found lighting a cigarette while receiving oxygen. When the nurse attempted to stop her, Ms. C began cursing and shrieked that if she were not allowed to smoke, she would overdose on digitalis she had hidden in the room.
>
> Ms. C refused to submit to a room search. The psychiatric consultant recommended that security be called so that Ms. C could not leave before he could perform an emergency evaluation. Ms. C had to be placed in leather restraints when she assaulted the officers. After speaking with the psychiatrist, Ms. C agreed to take medication (5 mg of haloperidol and 1 mg of lorazepam). She then consented to a search of her belongings. A bottle of 50 digitalis tablets was found in her suitcase. Because of her threats and impulsivity, the psychiatrist recommended constant observation with sitters.

As Ms. C's case shows, the first task in the medical setting is ensuring the patient's safety (Gutheil and Appelbaum 2000). A safe environment must be created and maintained until the patient is stable enough for psychiatric transfer.

Patients who are most intent on suicide, as well as those who are most impulsive and unpredictable, may attempt suicide in the hospital. The patient's room must be secured—that is, anything that patients could potentially use to injure themselves must be removed. Luggage and possessions should be searched with a suspicious eye and a morbid imagination. Staff must ferret out sharp objects, lighters, belts, caches of pills—anything that could inflict damage in either an impulsive or a carefully planned way. Objects that are being brought into the room must be regarded as potential hazards (e.g., the phlebotomist's needles, the pop-tops from soft drink cans, the custodian's disinfectants). The rooms of the general medical hospital lack many of the safeguards that are routine on inpatient psychiatric units, such as locked unit entrances and collapsible shower heads, curtain rods, and light fixtures. Normally, in the former, scissors and a variety of paraphernalia that can be "creatively" used for self-harm are easily accessible. The culture on medical inpatient units also differs from that on psychiatric units. On medical units, staff do not usually consider elopement a risk; they assume that patients are fundamentally compliant and that they will press their call buttons when they need help (Kelly et al. 1999).

Early reports focused on jumping as a means of suicide in medically hospitalized patients (N. Farberow and Litman 1970; Glickman 1980; Pollack 1957), a usually lethal method regardless of whether the patient actually intends to die. In the most recent study, White and colleagues (1995) identified impulsivity and agitation in many of the 12 patients who jumped from an Australian general hospital during a 12-year period. Five had been noted to be delirious on the day of the jump, 7 were dyspneic, and 10 were in pain. Ten of the 12 had two of these factors, and 1 had all three factors.

Modern hospitals are deliberately built without open stairwells and without windows that open or break easily; however, many older buildings remain in service, indicating the persistent need for corrective precautions. The inpatient suicide rate in a New York hospital dropped fivefold during the first 11 years after the hospital secured the windows and implemented educational programs encouraging staff members to pay closer attention to disruption in the doctor–patient relationship (Pisetsky and Brown 1979; Sanders 1988).

Shah and Ganesvaran (1997) found that one-third of 103 suicides committed by psychiatric inpatients at their hospital involved patients away on pass, and another one-third involved patients away from the hospital without permission. Methods readily available near the hospital include jumping in front of vehicles, leaping from buildings or bridges, and drowning in nearby bodies of water (H. Morgan and Priest 1991). Although these authors studied psychiatric inpatients, the same dangers exist with patients on medical units. Passes are rarely given from contemporary medical units, but elopements are all too common, with resultant ready access to potentially lethal means of suicide.

Constant observation by a one-to-one sitter is indicated for patients judged at high risk for impulsive self-harm. This may require compromising patients' privacy. Patients permitted to use the bathroom unobserved have been known to hang or cut themselves behind the closed door. A moment of privacy granted to the patient out of misplaced civility, or a few minutes of inattention or absence by the sitter, may be all the time a suicidal person needs to execute a suicide plan. All staff guarding suicidal patients should know how to summon security personnel as reinforcements when they perceive that they have lost control of the patient or the situation. In an era of cost cutting, the consultant may feel pressure to limit the use of constant observation. Economizing on sitters could mean the life of a suicidal patient. On the other hand, staff anxiety may lead to overuse, initiating one-to-one sitters for every patient who has expressed any suicidal thoughts. In addition to wasting resources, overuse of sitters may desensitize them to the constant awareness needed for their role. The decision to use constant observation should be made on clinical grounds. Prudent risk management supports avoiding under- and overuse of one-to-one sitters.

After the environment is secured, the medical psychiatrist should search for reversible contributors to the impulsive state, including delirium (see Chapter 6, "Delirium"), medical illness or medications that may be contributing to mood (see Chapter 9, "Depression"), anxiety (see Chapter 12, "Anxiety Disorders"), and psychotic disorders (see Chapter 11, "Mania, Catatonia, and Psychosis").

Agitation and active suicide attempts in the hospital often require chemical restraints and, rarely, physical restraints. Neuroleptics should be used in patients with delirium or psychosis, and neuroleptics and/or benzodiazepines should be given to other agitated, anxious patients. Physical restraints may be required if other measures prove inadequate. In some cases, emergent electroconvulsive therapy may be necessary (see Chapter 39, "Electroconvulsive Therapy").

Suicide in the Medically Ill

Physical disease is present in a high proportion of people who commit suicide. A recent review cited several large studies that reported that medical illness was present in 30%–40% of the patients who committed suicide (Hughes and Kleespies 2001). However, most of these suicides do not occur during medical hospitalization. About 2% of Finnish suicides occurred in medical or surgical inpatients (Suominen et al. 2002). In Montreal, Quebec, about 3% of the suicides were in general hospital inpatients, of which one-third (1%) were medical–surgical patients (Proulx et al. 1997). During a 10-year period in a 3,000-bed Chinese medical hospital, there were 75 self-destructive acts, only 15 of which proved fatal (Hung et al. 2000).

Sanders (1988) reviewed six studies of inpatients at a general hospital who committed suicide. Most had one or more chronic or terminal illnesses or sequelae that were painful, debilitating, or both, including dyspnea, ostomies, or disfiguring surgery. Harris and Barraclough (1994) compiled a list of 63 medical disorders noted in the medical literature as potentially having elevated suicide risk. In their meta-analysis, they concluded that the only disorders that actually elevated suicide risk were HIV and

AIDS, Huntington's disease, cancer (particularly head and neck), multiple sclerosis, peptic ulcer disease, end-stage renal disease, spinal cord injuries, and systemic lupus erythematosus. More recent studies confirm or add to a seemingly arbitrary list of medical conditions associated with risk for suicide. In a Canadian study, cancer, prostate disease, and chronic pulmonary disease were associated with suicide ORs of 1.70–1.86 among adults older than 55 years with versus without the diseases (Quan et al. 2002). In the previously cited Chinese study of patients who committed suicide in a general hospital, 40% had cancer, 13% had neurological disease, 13% had cardiovascular disease, and 7% had liver failure (Hung et al. 2000). In the Montreal study, associated diagnoses included cardiovascular disease, abdominal pain, cerebrovascular disease, Parkinson's disease, and rheumatoid arthritis (Proulx et al. 1997). Of 12 patients who jumped from an Australian hospital between 1980 and 1991, 4 had delirium, 4 had terminal cancer, 2 had advanced lung disease, and 1 had irreversible cardiac failure (White et al. 1995). However, these studies were small and did not capture suicides in the medically ill attempted or completed outside the hospital, so they cannot be used to construct a list of "most suicidal" medical disorders.

A recent study drawing on the U.S. National Comorbidity Survey identified a dozen general medical diagnostic categories with statistically significantly elevated ORs for suicide attempts, most ranging from 1.1 to 3.2, except for AIDS (133.9) and hernia (10.4) (Goodwin et al. 2003). Clinically, however, use of a diagnosis alone in estimating suicide risk is not helpful. Even though the OR in each of the 12 categories achieved statistical significance, substituting a rate only slightly higher than the very low base rate offers little to guide clinical decision making, particularly if this is the only indicator being used to predict suicide.

What does appear useful is that suicides in the medically ill—as in the general population—appear to be related to frequently unrecognized comorbid psychiatric illnesses, including depression, substance-related disorders, delirium, dementia, and personality disorder (Davidson 1993; Kellner et al. 1985). In their study of the role of physical disease in 416 Swedish suicides, Stensman and Sundqvist-Stensman (1988) concluded that somatic disease was one important factor in the complexity of the suicidal act, but psychiatric conditions such as depression and alcohol abuse were more significant. Rather than focus on particular medical diagnoses, it will be more fruitful for the medical psychiatrist to determine whether a suicide-prone psychiatric condition is present in a medically ill patient, whether the patient is at a particularly emotionally difficult time in his or her illness course, and whether secondary effects of the medical illness—pain, physical disfigurement, cognitive dysfunction, and disinhibition—are present that add to the risk.

It must be emphasized that no matter how horrific the medical condition, significant suicide risk is not the rule. According to Brown et al. (1986), most terminally ill patients do not develop severe depression, and suicidality is closely associated with the presence of a depressive disorder. In the study of terminally ill cancer patients by Breitbart et al. (2000), only 17% had a high desire for hastened death, for which depression and hopelessness were the strongest predictors. An important empirical finding in a Canadian study was that the will to live in the terminally ill fluctuates, mostly predicted by depression, anxiety, shortness of breath, and sense of well-being (Chochinov et al. 1999).

Three diagnoses—cancer, end-stage renal disease, and AIDS—are discussed here to illustrate these points further. These comparatively common conditions underscore principles that can be extrapolated to the breadth of diagnoses and situations encountered in medical settings.

Cancer

Three large studies have found an increased suicide rate among patients with cancer. Luohivuori and Hakama (1979) studied 63 suicides among 28,857 Finnish cancer patients and found relative risks (compared with the general population) of 1.3 for women and 1.9 for men, with the highest excess mortality associated with gastrointestinal tumors. Fox et al. (1982) studied 192 suicides between 1940 and 1973 among 144,530 patients in the Connecticut Tumor Registry and calculated no increased suicide risk for women but a 2.3 relative risk for men. In the largest study of the relation between cancer and suicide, Allebeck and colleagues (1985) gathered statistics on 963 suicides between 1962 and 1979 among 424,127 Swedes with a diagnosis of cancer and found an overall 1.9 relative risk for men and a 1.6 relative risk for women. Gastrointestinal tumors (excluding colorectal cancers) in men (relative risk=3.1) and lung tumors in either sex (relative risk=3.1 for men and 3.5 for women) were associated with the highest rate of death due to suicide.

Cancer patients who die by suicide are psychiatrically similar to noncancer patients, particularly when the cancer is in remission. In a case–control study of 60 suicides in individuals with cancer and 60 age- and sex-matched comparison suicides in individuals without a cancer history, Henriksson et al. (1995) found that most of the patients with cancer who committed suicide—as well as the control subjects without cancer—had a diagnosable psychiatric disorder. Terminally ill cancer patients had lower rates of depression and alcohol dependence than did patients in remission (72% vs. 96%), but nearly three-quarters still met criteria for a depressive disorder. As a group, cancer patients had fewer psychotic disorders than did control subjects. Allebeck et al. (1985) observed that the longer the time from diagnosis of cancer, the lower the relative risk for suicide in a Swedish cohort. In the first year after diagnosis, the relative risk was 16.0 for men and 15.4 for women. From 1 to 2 years, the ratio decreased to 6.5 for men and 7.0 for women. By 3–6 years, the ratio was 2.1 for men and 3.2 for women. By 10 years after diagnosis, the rate, at 0.4, was actually less than one-half that in the general population. A study of Japanese cancer patients found the highest risk of suicide soon after patients had been discharged from the hospital, with an elevated relative risk the first 5 years after diagnosis compared with the general population and disappearing thereafter (Tanaka et al. 1999).

The fear of pain, disfigurement, and loss of function that cancer evokes in the patients' imagination can precipitate suicide, especially early in the patients' courses. In a large cohort of Italians with cancer, suicide accounted for only 0.2% of the deaths, but the relative risk during the first 6 months after diagnosis was 27.7 (Crocetti et al. 1998). The high relative risk of suicide just after diagnosis comes at a time of overwhelming fear and cognitive overload. In individual patients, important contributing factors (Filiberti et al. 2001) can include overly pessimistic prognosis, exaggerated impressions of anticipated suffering, a physician unintentionally undermining hope, fear of loss of control, or nihilism about treatment. Patients may fear or experience inadequate pain control, lost dignity, compromised privacy, or guilt at having habits that caused the disease. Surgical treatments may be disfiguring, chemotherapy debilitating, and side effects defeminizing or emasculating. As cancer patients live longer with their disease, most become less frightened and less susceptible to suicide.

End-Stage Renal Disease

More formidable than the suicide risk among cancer patients was the purported increase in relative risk of suicide among patients with end-stage renal disease. Abrams and colleagues (1971) reported very high rates of suicide and suicidal behavior among 3,478 renal dialysis patients studied at 127 dialysis centers. In their sample, 20 deaths were the result of suicide; 17 suicide attempts were unsuccessful; 22 patients withdrew from the program, knowing that doing so would hasten their deaths; and 117 deaths were attributed to noncompliance with treatment. The authors' calculated suicide rate of 400 times that in the general population has been widely quoted but is misleading. In arriving at a 5% figure for suicidal behavior in dialysis patients, they used an extremely broad definition of suicide that encompassed death caused by a wide range of causes, from willful acts of self-destruction to noncompliance.

Most of the cases that Abrams and colleagues called suicide would never come to the attention of psychiatry today. Although their report has been widely cited, no other subsequent study (there have been nearly 20) has defined suicide so broadly (Bostwick and Pankratz 2000). In extreme cases, noncompliance is better understood as a function of personality-disordered behavior; in less dramatic examples, it can be an understandable human response to a burdensome treatment. Deciding to forgo dialysis is not equivalent to suicide (see also Chapter 22, "Renal Disease"). A recent United States study concluded that "most patients who decide to stop dialysis do not seem to be influenced by major depression or ordinary suicidal ideation" (Cohen et al. 2002, p. 889). Treatment withdrawal, negotiated among the patient, significant others, and the treatment team, has become routine as quality of life during dialysis fades.

In 1,766 Minnesota dialysis patients followed up for 17 years, for example, only 3 killed themselves by frank suicide, representing only 2% of the 155 cases in which dialysis was discontinued (Neu and Kjellstrand 1986). The suicide rate in this sample of dialysis patients was only about 15 times that in the general population, which is a considerable rate but much lower than Abrams and colleagues' figure. Haenel et al. (1980) also found less dramatic suicide rates among European patients undergoing chronic dialysis between 1965 and 1978. In Switzerland, dialysis patients killed themselves at about 10 times the rate in the general population. When patients who refused therapy and died as a result were included in the suicide group, the rate was 25 times higher. They also found no statistically significant difference between suicide rates among patients with functioning cadaveric renal transplants and patients undergoing maintenance dialysis, suggesting that transplantation may not in and of itself be associated with decreased suicide risk. Overall, among dialysis patients pooled from all countries belonging to the European Dialysis and Transplant Association, the suicide rate was 108 per 100,000 per year (Haenel et al. 1980). Whether compared with the general population suicide rate of 4–5 per 100,000 in Mediterranean countries or 20–25 per 100,000 in central European or Scandinavian countries, the figure of 108 per 100,000 represents a higher suicide rate, although not orders of magnitude greater than that in the general population.

AIDS

AIDS patients also have a higher relative risk of suicide, even though the risk appears to have decreased since the disease emerged. The existing data are primarily based on men who had sex with men in the United States in the 1980s. Extrapolation to the present is problematic because of many changes, including the demographics and geographic distribution of AIDS, advances in treatment, availability of mental health services, public education, and reduction in stigma and social hysteria. The perspective of suicide has changed as AIDS has evolved from a terminal illness to a chronic one. Another caveat in interpreting studies of suicidality in persons with HIV is that results will be confounded because the study populations (e.g., men who have sex with men, injection drug abusers, and poor minority heterosexual women) all differ in their sociodemographics and psychiatric epidemiology.

Marzuk et al. (1988) found a suicide rate in persons with AIDS 36 times that in an age-matched sample of men without AIDS and 66 times that in the general population in New York City in 1985. Marzuk and colleagues (1997) reexamined this question based on all suicides in New York City in 1991–1993 and concluded that positive HIV serostatus was associated, at most, with a modest elevation in suicide risk. In California, in 1986, the rate was 21 times higher than that in the general population (Kizer et al. 1988). In the largest study to date, Cote et al. (1991) charted a continuous decrease in suicide rates over 3 years among AIDS patients in 45 states and the District of Columbia. From 1987 to 1989, a total of 165 suicides among AIDS patients were reported to the National Center for Health Statistics. Of these, 164 were committed by men. The relative suicide risk calculated for AIDS patients was 10.5 in 1987, 7.4 in 1988, and 6.0 in 1989. The authors attributed the decrease to advances in medical care, diminishing social stigma, and improved psychiatric services, while noting probable underreporting of deaths due to both AIDS and suicide (Cote et al. 1991). In a review of 100 publications with information about suicide and HIV, Palmer et al. (in press) concluded that there has been a distinctive downward trend in HIV-related suicidality in the United States since the beginning of the epidemic.

Frierson and Lippman (1988) suggested that suicide risk also may be increased among HIV-positive but asymptomatic people who fear the eventual illness, HIV-negative people who are worried about contracting the disease, and people who enter suicide pacts with dying loved ones. Rundell and colleagues (1992) compared 15 HIV-infected active-duty members of the air force who attempted suicide with 15 who did not and identified several risk factors equivalent to risk factors for suicide in general, including social isolation, perceived lack of social support, adjustment disorder, personality disorder, alcohol abuse, interpersonal or occupational problems, and history of depression.

Recent studies reflect both the changing demographics of HIV and AIDS and the stable classic risk factors for suicidality. Roy (2003) found that almost half of a cohort of HIV-positive substance-dependent patients had attempted suicide. Those who had attempted suicide were younger; were more likely to be female; and were more likely to have more childhood trauma, more depression, more family history of suicidal behavior, and higher neuroticism. A survey in HIV-infected Americans living in rural areas found that 38% had thoughts of suicide during the past week, associated with greater depression and more stigma-related stress and less coping self-efficacy (Heckman et al. 2002).

Finally, two recent studies, one in Italy (Grassi et al. 2001) and one in Brazil (Malbergier and de Andrade 2001), found that although psychiatric morbidity and suicidal ideation or attempts are common in HIV-positive intravenous drug abusers, they are equally common in those who are HIV-negative. A Swiss study of men having sex with men found a high rate of suicide attempts in both HIV-negative and HIV-positive individuals, with moderately more suicidal ideation in those who were HIV-positive (Cochand and Bovet 1998). Dannenberg et al. (1996) compared 4,147 HIV-positive United States military service applicants and 12,437 HIV-negative applicants disqualified from military service because of other medical conditions (matched on age, race, sex, and screening date and location) with the matched general population; the relative risk for suicide was similar for each group: 2.08 in the HIV-positive and 1.67 in the HIV-negative applicants. These studies reinforce the point that psychopathology is implicated more potently than any specific medical diagnosis in suicidality.

Prevention and Treatment

The first priority in preventing suicide in the medically ill is the early detection and treatment of the comorbid psychiatric disorders covered throughout this book. Patient and family education about the medical disease course and its treatment can help prevent excessive fear and pessimism. Direct questions and frank discussion about suicidal thoughts, ideally part of every primary physician's care for any patient with a serious disease, can reduce suicidal pressures. One important role for psychiatrists is to restrain other physicians from automatically prescribing antidepressants for every medically ill patient who expresses a wish to die. Overdiagnosis of depression can lead to inappropriate pharmacotherapy, pathologization of normal feelings, or neglect of relevant personality traits potentially amenable to psychotherapeutic intervention. Soliciting patients' wishes and preferences regarding pain management and end-of-life care early on may reduce the fear of having no control of their dying that lures some patients toward suicide.

Palliative care for the terminally ill is essential in offering relief to those for whom life has become (or is feared) unbearable (see Chapter 40, "Palliative Care"). Psychiatrists can help elicit fears, guilt, impulses, and history that patients may be reluctant to share with their primary physicians. In addition to treating psychiatric symptoms, psychiatrists can monitor for illicit drug use, medication side effects, and emergent neuropsychiatric complications of the underlying medical illness. Psychotherapy can facilitate the exploration and expression of grief and restore a sense of meaning in life (Chochinov 2002; Frierson and Lippman 1988; see also Chapter 38, "Psychotherapy," and Chapter 40, "Palliative Care"). Psychotherapy also may be psychoeducational, reinforcing patients' and family members' accurate knowledge about the disease. Attention to patients' spiritual needs is very important as well; spiritual well-being offers some protection against end-of-life despair (McClain et al. 2003). Finally, for both patients and family, support groups and other community resources may be critical in making the difference between feeling life is worth living and giving up.

Physician-Assisted Suicide

In an editorial in *Medicine*, McHugh (1994) argued that assisted suicides and "naturalistic" ones occurred in different groups of people. Conceptually, physician-assisted suicide follows a rational request from a competent, hopelessly ill patient whose decision is not driven by psychiatric illness. It is legal in very few jurisdictions, where there are practice guidelines and legal safeguards.

In a pair of unanimous 1997 decisions, the U.S. Supreme Court ruled that there is no constitutional right to physician-assisted suicide and that states can prohibit physician conduct in which the primary purpose is to hasten death (Burt 1997). Only one state, Oregon, has legalized physician-assisted suicide; its Death With Dignity Act was passed in 1994 and enacted in 1997. Terminally ill Oregonians can ask their primary care physicians to prescribe lethal doses of medication, but the patients must be able to administer the killing doses themselves.

The safeguards built into the Oregon process closely resemble criteria in place in the Netherlands since 1973,

outside the law for nearly three decades, until the Dutch Parliament passed the Termination of Life on Request and Assistance With Suicide Act in 2001 (Cohen-Almagor 2002). To meet the guidelines of the act, the patient must experience his or her situation as intolerable and voluntarily and repeatedly ask the physician for assistance with suicide. The request must be informed, uncoerced, and consistent with the patient's values, and all treatment options must have been exhausted or refused. Finally, the initial physician must seek a second opinion to confirm the diagnosis and prognosis and report the death to the designated municipal authorities (Cohen-Almagor 2002; de Wachter 1989; Singer and Siegler 1990). Quill and colleagues (1992) suggested an addition to these more legalistic safeguards—that physician-assisted suicide should be carried out only in the context of a meaningful doctor-patient relationship.

The Oregon law is both more conservative and more specific than its Dutch counterpart. It requires supplicants to have the capacity to make their own health care decisions. They must have an illness expected to lead to death within 6 months and must make their requests to the physician in the form of one written and two oral statements separated by 15 days from each other. The primary physician and the consultant giving a second opinion not only must agree on capacity, diagnosis, and terminal prognosis but also have the option of referring the patient for a mental health evaluation if either suspects that depression or another psychiatric disorder is affecting the patient's judgment. The primary physician is required to inform the patient of all feasible options, such as comfort care, hospice care, and pain management; only then can the patient be given a lethal prescription (Chin et al. 1999). The law specifically forbids active euthanasia, which is distinguished from physician-assisted suicide by the physician actively performing the killing act. Physician-assisted suicide is thus denied to patients who lack motor capacity (e.g., patients with amyotrophic lateral sclerosis) (Rowland 1998). Such individuals may still wish for physician-assisted suicide; Ganzini et al. (2002) reported that one-third of amyotrophic lateral sclerosis patients discussed wanting assisted suicide in the last month of life, particularly those with greater distress at being a burden and those with more insomnia, pain, and other discomfort.

Although he postulated that a request for suicide could be rational, Muskin (1998) advocated a psychodynamic approach to a dialogue between the patient and the physician, a dialogue he believed any such request demands. He saw the query as "an opportunity for patient and physician to more fully understand and know one another" (p. 327) and asserted that "every request to die should be subjected to careful scrutiny of its multiple potential meanings" (p. 323). For example, is the patient asking the physician to provide a reason to live? Does the patient harbor revenge fantasies? Is the patient driven by inadequately treated pain or depression, by guilt or hopelessness, or by feelings of already being dead?

In contrast to Muskin's fundamentally intrapsychic approach, Hackett and Stern (1991) outlined diverse interpersonal factors to be considered in evaluating a patient requesting physician-assisted suicide, potentially life-threatening analgesics, or withdrawal of life support. The attending physician and consulting psychiatrist each must take sufficient time to understand the wishes of the patient. What has the patient pictured his or her clinical course to be? What are his or her values? What notions exist about the end of life? Is the patient clinically depressed? Where does the family stand? Does the family understand the patient's request, and how do they affect it? At what point does the patient specify that the potential for meaning in his or her life has been exhausted? Does the patient fear that he or she will become a financial burden, a caregiving burden, or both? Has any of this been discussed with the family? If the patient considers life devoid of value and meaning for himself or herself, does it have meaning for significant others? Does that affect the patient's thinking? Has the patient made any effort to achieve family consensus so that death can actually be a meaningful shared family experience?

The psychiatrist's role in physician-assisted suicide is to be available for consultation. In that psychiatrists are almost never primary care providers for terminally ill patients other than dementia patients, who—by definition—lack capacity and are thus not eligible for physician-assisted suicide, Oregon psychiatrists have not been writing lethal prescriptions (Linda Ganzini, personal communication, 2003). Moreover, mental health evaluation is not among the mandatory safeguards in the Oregon law. Despite numerous investigators who have opined that primary care physicians are usually ill-equipped to tease out factors confounding a truly informed decision to take an active role in the timing of one's death (Billings and Block 1996; Conwell and Caine 1991; Hendin and Klerman 1993), only 20% of potential Oregon physician-assisted suicide patients have a mental health evaluation (Ganzini et al. 2000).

Block and Billings (1995) outlined five key clinical questions for psychiatrists to explore in clarifying decision-making capacity in terminally ill patients requesting euthanasia or assisted suicide:

1. Does the patient have physical pain that is undertreated or uncontrolled?

2. Does the patient have psychological distress driven by inadequately managed psychiatric symptoms?
3. Does the patient have social disruption resulting from interpersonal relationships strained by fears of burdening others, losing independence, or exacting revenge?
4. Does the patient have spiritual despair in the face of taking the measure of a life nearing its end while coming to terms with personal beliefs about the presence or absence of God?
5. Does the patient have iatrogenic anxiety about the dying process itself and the physician's availability as death encroaches?

Regardless of the status of the law, Block and Billings argued that requests to hasten death will come, and they explicitly acknowledged in a case example—as others have done in notorious publications ("A Piece of My Mind: It's Over, Debbie" 1988; Quill 1991)—that some physicians participate in extralegal physician-assisted suicide. They enjoin the psychiatrist to perform several functions for a nonpsychiatric colleague wrestling with such a request, including "offering a second opinion on the patient's psychological status, providing a sophisticated evaluation of the patient's decision-making capacity, validating that nothing treatable is being missed, and helping create a setting in which the primary physician and team can formulate a thoughtful decision about how to respond" (Block and Billings 1995, pp. 454–455).

Making time and space for a comprehensive mental health evaluation for the presence of a treatable psychiatric disorder can result in a patient deciding to live longer and withdraw the physician-assisted suicide request (Hendin and Klerman 1993), particularly if "the demoralizing triad" of depression, anxiety, and preoccupation with death is confronted and dispelled. The Oregon experience has shown that intervening in any or all of Block and Billings's five realms can forestall a physician-assisted suicide request actually being carried to completion. Only 1 in 6 requests resulted in the physician issuing a prescription, and only 1 in 10 of those initially requesting physician-assisted suicide ultimately used the medication to hasten death (Ganzini et al. 2001).

Although the U.S. Supreme Court in its 1997 decision specifically denied that physician-assisted suicide was a constitutional right, it endorsed making palliative care more available and acknowledged the legal acceptability of providing pain relief, even if it hastened death (Burt 1997; Quill et al. 1997). Terminal sedation (in which a patient is given narcotics, even to the point of unconsciousness) accompanied by withdrawal or withholding life-prolonging therapies such as ventilatory support (see

Chapter 20, "Lung Disease"), antibiotics, food, and water has become normative end-of-life management (see Chapter 40, "Palliative Care").

The distinctions among, and propriety of, physician-assisted suicide, active euthanasia, and passive euthanasia remain controversial and beyond the scope of this chapter, but some clarifications should be noted. At present, all 50 states in the United States continue to outlaw active euthanasia, and since the 1997 Supreme Court ruling, no state is required to permit physician-assisted suicide within its borders. Some have worried that making physician-assisted suicide legal would undermine the availability of appropriate care, partly driven by financial exigencies such as strained health care resources. In the Netherlands, the availability of euthanasia appears to have stunted the evolution of palliative care (Cohen-Almagor 2002), but in Oregon, the reverse appears to have happened. The availability of physician-assisted suicide has coincided there with a dramatic increase in the use of hospice. In 1994, when voters approved physician-assisted suicide, 22% of Oregonians died in hospice care. By 1999, that figure had risen to 35% without any appreciable increase in the geographic distribution or number of hospice beds in the state (Ganzini et al. 2001). The fear that physician-assisted suicide would become a ubiquitous and convenient way of prematurely disposing of Oregon's dying patients also appears not to have been borne out: in 1999, fewer than 1 in 1,000 Oregon deaths resulted from physician-assisted suicide (Ganzini et al. 2001). Another concern among the public is whether allowing patients to decide to die through refusal of fluids and nutrition will cause undue suffering. The evidence clearly shows that this is not the case (Ganzini et al. 2003).

Psychiatrists will continue to be consulted frequently when patients request withdrawal of treatment or assisted suicide. Evaluation of the patient's capacity for decision making follows the same principles as for other medical decisions (see Chapter 3, "Legal Issues," and Chapter 4, "Ethical Issues"), but psychiatrists should strive to distinguish those who wish to die despite remediable contributors to their despair from those who primarily find the burdens of treatment outweighing the offered benefits. As with any "competency consultation," the psychiatrist should always broaden the scope of examination to a full understanding of the patient and his or her predicament.

Conclusion

Compared with suicidal ideation, completed suicide is rare in psychiatric patients and rarer still in the medically ill. Although there are identifiable demographic factors associated with increased risk for suicide, by themselves these factors will identify many more persons potentially at risk than imminently in danger of dying. Many medical illnesses have been associated with increased suicide attempts, but medical illness by itself is rarely the sole determinant of suicide potential. The assessment of a suicidal medically ill person—as with any suicidal person—demands attention to the role played by characterological, temperamental, or experiential features in the individual's immediate push toward suicide. Management begins with a search for reversible contributors to impulsivity, such as delirium, psychosis, and intoxication. A priority in preventing suicide in the medically ill is the early detection and treatment of comorbid psychiatric disorders.

One of the most frequent reasons for psychiatric consultation in medical hospitals is for evaluation for transfer of care of patients who have made suicide attempts. Because countertransference issues not infrequently lead nonpsychiatric physicians to prematurely "clear" patients, it is critical for psychiatrists to form their own judgments about whether patients are truly medically stable enough for transfer out of the medical setting. If a suicidal patient must remain on a medical floor, the psychiatric consultant should keep in mind that rooms in the general medical hospital may lack safeguards routinely found on inpatient psychiatric units. Constant observation by a one-on-one sitter is indicated for patients judged to be at high risk.

Suicide is not synonymous with refusal of lifesaving treatment or with requests to hasten death in terminal illness. Psychiatrists are frequently consulted when patients request withdrawal of treatment or assisted suicide; in these situations, the clinician should evaluate the patient's capacity for decision making, the adequacy of pain management, and the role that treatable psychiatric illness may be playing in the request. Psychological distress, social disruption of interpersonal relationships, and spiritual despair must also be explored and addressed. Responding to these issues with concern and comfort may transform a desire for hastened death into a graceful and timely exit from life.

References

Abrams H, Moore G, Westervelt F: Suicidal behavior in chronic dialysis patients. Am J Psychiatry 127:1199–1204, 1971

Allebeck P, Bolund C, Ringback F: Increased suicide rate in cancer patients. J Clin Epidemiol 42:611–616, 1985

A piece of my mind: it's over, Debbie (case report). JAMA 259:272, 1988

Barraclough B, Bunch J, Nelson B, et al: A hundred cases of suicide: clinical aspects. Br J Psychiatry 125:355–373, 1974

Beautrais A: Suicides and serious suicide attempts: two populations or one? Psychol Med 31:837–845, 2001

Berger D: Suicide risk in the general hospital. Psychiatry Clin Neurosci 49:585–589, 1995

Billings JA, Block SD: Slow euthanasia. J Palliat Care 12:21–30, 1996

Block S, Billings J: Patient requests for euthanasia and assisted suicide in terminal illness: the role of the psychiatrist. Psychosomatics 36:445–457, 1995

Bostwick J, Pankratz V: Affective disorders and suicide risk: a re-examination. Am J Psychiatry 157:1925–1932, 2000

Breitbart W, Rosenfeld B, Pessin H, et al: Depression, hopelessness, and desire for hastened death in terminally ill patients with cancer. JAMA 284:2907–2911, 2000

Brown J, Henteleff P, Barakat S, et al: Is it normal for terminally ill patients to desire death? Am J Psychiatry 143:208–211, 1986

Buie D, Maltsberger J: The psychological vulnerability to suicide, in Suicide: Understanding and Responding. Edited by Jacobs D, Brown H. Madison, CT, International Universities Press, 1989, pp 59–71

Burt R: The Supreme Court speaks—not assisted suicide but a constitutional right to palliative care. N Engl J Med 337:1234–1236, 1997

Buzan R, Weissberg M: Suicide: risk factors and therapeutic considerations in the emergency department. J Emerg Med 10:335–343, 1992

Chin A, Hedberg K, Higginson G, et al: Legalized physician-assisted suicide in Oregon—the first year's experience. N Engl J Med 340:577–583, 1999

Chochinov H: Dignity-conserving care—a new model for palliative care: helping the patient feel valued. JAMA 287:2253–2260, 2002

Chochinov H, Tataryn D, Clinch J, et al: Will to live in the terminally ill. Lancet 354:816–819, 1999

Cochand P, Bovet P: HIV infection and suicide risk: an epidemiological inquiry among male homosexuals in Switzerland. Soc Psychiatry Psychiatr Epidemiol 33:230–234, 1998

Cohen L, Dobscha S, Hails K, et al: Depression and suicidal ideation in patients who discontinue the life-support treatment of dialysis. Psychosom Med 64:889–896, 2002

Cohen-Almagor R: Dutch perspectives on palliative care in the Netherlands. Issues Law Med 18:111–126, 2002

Conner K, Langley J, Tomaszewski K, et al: Injury hospitalization and risks for subsequent self-injury and suicide: a national study from New Zealand. Am J Public Health 93:1128–1131, 2003

Conwell Y, Caine E: Rational suicide and the right to die. N Engl J Med 324:1100–1103, 1991

Cote T, Biggar R, Dannenberg A: Risk of suicide among persons with AIDS: a national assessment. JAMA 268:2066–2068, 1991

Crocetti E, Arniani S, Acciai S, et al: High suicide mortality soon after diagnosis among cancer patients in central Italy. Br J Cancer 77:1194–1196, 1998

Dannenberg A, McNeail J, Brundage J, et al: Suicide and HIV infection: mortality follow-up of 4147 HIV-seropositive military service applicants. JAMA 276:1743–1746, 1996

Davidson L: Suicide and aggression in the medical setting, in Psychiatric Care of the Medical Patient. Edited by Stoudemire A, Fogel B. New York, Oxford University Press, 1993, pp 71–86

de Wachter M: Active euthanasia in the Netherlands. JAMA 262:3316–3319, 1989

Dorpat T, Ripley H: A study of suicide in the Seattle area. Compr Psychiatry 1:349–359, 1960

Farberow L, McKelligott J, Cohen S, et al: Suicide among patients with cardiorespiratory illnesses. JAMA 195:422–428, 1966

Farberow N: Indirect self-destructive behavior, in Comprehensive Textbook of Suicidology. Edited by Maris R, Berman A, Silverman M. New York, Guilford, 2000, pp 427–455

Farberow N, Litman R: Suicide prevention in hospitals, in The Psychology of Suicide. Edited by Shneidman E, Farberow N, Litman R. New York, Science House, 1970, pp 423–458

Fawcett J, Shaughnessy R: The suicidal patient, in Psychiatry: Diagnosis and Therapy. Edited by Flaherty J, Channon R, Davis J. Norwalk, CT, Appleton & Lange, 1988, pp 49–56

Filiberti A, Ripamonti C, Totis A, et al: Characteristics of terminal cancer patients who committed suicide during a home palliative care program. J Pain Symptom Manage 22:544–553, 2001

Fox BH, Stanek EJ 3rd, Boyd SC, et al: Suicide rates among cancer patients in Connecticut. J Chronic Dis 35:89–100, 1982

Frierson R, Lippman S: Suicide and AIDS. Psychosomatics 29:226–231, 1988

Furst S, Ostow M: The psychodynamics of suicide, in Suicide: Theory and Clinical Aspects. Edited by Hankoff L, Einsidler B. Littleton, MA, PSG Publishing, 1979, pp 165–178

Ganzini L, Nelson H, Schmidt T, et al: Physicians' experiences with the Oregon Death with Dignity Act. N Engl J Med 342:557–563, 2000

Ganzini L, Nelson H, Lee M, et al: Oregon physicians' attitudes about and experiences with end-of-life care since passage of the Oregon Death with Dignity Act. JAMA 285:2363–2369, 2001

Ganzini L, Silveira M, Johnston W: Predictors and correlates of interest in assisted suicide in the final month of life among ALS patients in Oregon and Washington. J Pain Symptom Manage 24:312–317, 2002

Ganzini L, Goy E, Miller L, et al: Nurses' experiences with hospice patients who refuse food and fluids to hasten death. N Engl J Med 349:359–365, 2003

Gardner DL, Cowdry RW: Suicidal and parasuicidal behavior in borderline personality disorder. Psychiatr Clin North Am 8:389–403, 1985

Glickman L: The suicidal patient, in Psychiatric Consultation in the General Hospital. New York, Marcel Dekker, 1980, pp 181–202

Goldberg R: The assessment of suicide risk in the general hospital. Gen Hosp Psychiatry 9:446–452, 1987

Goodwin R, Olfson M: Self-perception of poor health and suicidal ideation in medical patients. Psychol Med 32:1293–1299, 2002

Goodwin R, Marusic A, Hoven C: Suicide attempts in the United States: the role of physical illness. Soc Sci Med 56:1783–1788, 2003

Grassi L, Mondardini D, Pavanati M, et al: Suicide probability and psychological morbidity secondary to HIV infection: a control study of HIV-seropositive, hepatitis C virus (HCV)-seropositive and HIV/HCV-seronegative injecting drug users. J Affect Disord 64:195–202, 2001

Gutheil T, Appelbaum P: Legal issues in emergency psychiatry, in Clinical Handbook of Psychiatry and the Law. Philadelphia, PA, Lippincott Williams & Wilkins, 2000, pp 39–82

Hackett T, Stern T: Suicide and other disruptive states, in The Massachusetts General Hospital Handbook of General Hospital Psychiatry. Edited by Cassem N. St. Louis, MO, Mosby-Year Book, 1991, pp 281–307

Haenel T, Brunner F, Battegay R: Renal dialysis and suicide: occurrence in Switzerland and Europe. Compr Psychiatry 21:140–145, 1980

Hall R, Platt D, Hall R: Suicide risk assessment: a review of risk factors for suicide in 100 patients who made severe suicide attempts. Psychosomatics 40:18–27, 1999

Harris E, Barraclough B: Suicide as an outcome for medical disorders. Medicine 73:281–296, 1994

Hawton K: Suicide and attempted suicide, in Handbook of Affective Disorders. Edited by Paykel E. New York, Guilford, 1992, pp 635–650

Heckman T, Miller J, Kochman A, et al: Thoughts of suicide among HIV-infected rural persons enrolled in a telephone-delivered mental health intervention. Ann Behav Med 24:141–148, 2002

Hendin H, Klerman G: Physician-assisted suicide: the dangers of legalization. Am J Psychiatry 150:143–145, 1993

Henriksson M, Isometsa E, Hietanen P, et al: Mental disorders in cancer suicides. J Affect Disord 36:11–20, 1995

Hughes D, Kleespies P: Suicide in the medically ill. Suicide Life Threat Behav 31 (suppl):48–59, 2001

Hung C, Liu C, Liao M, et al: Self-destructive acts occurring during medical general hospitalization. Gen Hosp Psychiatry 22:115–121, 2000

Kamali M, Oquendo M, Mann J: Understanding the neurobiology of suicidal behavior. Depress Anxiety 14:164–176, 2001

Kaplan A, Klein R: Women and suicide, in Suicide: Understanding and Responding. Edited by Jacobs D, Brown H. Madison, CT, International Universities Press, 1989, pp 257–282

Kellner C, Best C, Roberts J, et al: Self-destructive behavior in hospitalized medical and surgical patients. Psychiatr Clin North Am 8:279–289, 1985

Kelly M, Mufson M, Rogers M: Medical settings and suicide, in The Harvard School Guide to Suicide Assessment and Intervention. Edited by Jacobs D. San Francisco, CA, Jossey-Bass, 1999, pp 491–519

Kishi Y, Kathol RG: Assessment of patients who attempt suicide. Prim Care Companion J Clin Psychiatry 4:132–136, 2002

Kizer K, Green M, Perkins C, et al: AIDS and suicide in California (letter). JAMA 260:1881, 1988

Klerman G: Clinical epidemiology of suicide. J Clin Psychiatry 48:33–38, 1987

Litman R: Suicides: what do they have in mind? in Suicide: Understanding and Responding. Edited by Jacobs D, Brown H. Madison, CT, International Universities Press, 1989, pp 143–154

Luohivuori K, Hakama M: Risk of suicide among cancer patients. Am J Epidemiol 109:59–65, 1979

Malbergier A, de Andrade A: Depressive disorders and suicide attempts in injecting drug use with and without HIV infection. AIDS Care 13:141–150, 2001

Maltsberger J, Buie D: Countertransference hate in the treatment of suicidal patients. Arch Gen Psychiatry 30:625–633, 1974

Mann J: Psychobiological predictors of suicide. J Clin Psychiatry 48:39–43, 1987

Mann J: The neurobiology of suicide. Nat Med 4:25–30, 1998

Marzuk PM, Tierney H, Tardiff K, et al: Increased risk of suicide in persons with AIDS. JAMA 259:1333–1337, 1988

Marzuk PM, Tardiff K, Leon A, et al: HIV seroprevalence among suicide victims in New York City, 1991–1993. Am J Psychiatry 154:1720–1725, 1997

McClain C, Rosenfeld B, Breitbart W: Effect of spiritual well-being on cnd-of-life despair in terminally ill cancer patients. Lancet 361:1603–1607, 2003

McHugh P: Suicide and medical afflictions. Medicine 73:297–298, 1994

McIntosh J: U.S.A. Suicide: Suicide Data, p 2001. Washington, DC, American Association of Suicidology, 2003

Miles C: Conditions predisposing to suicide: a review. J Nerv Ment Dis 164:231–246, 1977

Monk M: Epidemiology of suicide. Epidemiol Rev 9:51–69, 1987

Morgan A: Special issues of assessment and treatment of suicide risk in the elderly, in Suicide: Understanding and Responding. Edited by Jacobs D, Brown H. Madison, CT, International Universities Press, 1989, pp 239–255

Morgan H, Priest P: Suicide and other unexpected deaths among psychiatric inpatients. Br J Psychiatry 158:368–374, 1991

Moscicki E: Epidemiology of suicide. Int Psychogeriatr 7:137–148, 1995

Murphy G: Recognizing the alcoholic risk for suicide. Lifesavers: Newsletter of the American Suicide Foundation 4:3, 1992

Murphy G, Weitzel R: The lifetime risk of suicide in alcoholism. Arch Gen Psychiatry 47:383–392, 1990

Muskin P: The request to die: role for a psychodynamic perspective on physician-assisted suicide. JAMA 279:323–328, 1998

Neu S, Kjellstrand C: Stopping long-term dialysis: an empirical study of withdrawal of life-supporting treatment. N Engl J Med 314:14–20, 1986

Nielsen B, Wang A, Brille-Brahe U: Attempted suicide in Denmark, IV: a five-year follow-up. Acta Psychiatr Scand 81:250–254, 1990

Palmer B, Pankratz V, Bostwick J: The risk of suicide in schizophrenia: a meta-analysis. Arch Gen Psychiatry (in press)

Patterson W, Dohn H, Bird J, et al: Evaluation of suicidal patients: the SAD PERSONS scale. Psychosomatics 24:348–349, 1983

Pisetsky J, Brown W: The general hospital patient, in Suicide: Theory and Clinical Aspects. Edited by Hankoff L, Einsidler B. Littleton, MA, PSG Publishing, 1979, pp 279–290

Pokorny A: Prediction of suicide in psychiatric patients: report of a prospective study. Arch Gen Psychiatry 40:249–257, 1983

Pollack S: Suicide in a general hospital, in The Psychology of Suicide. Edited by Shneidman E, Farberow N. New York, McGraw-Hill, 1957, pp 152–176

Proulx F, Lesage A, Grunberg F: One hundred in-patient suicides. Br J Psychiatry 171:247–250, 1997

Quan H, Arboleda-Florez J, Fick G, et al: Association between physical illness and suicide among the elderly. Soc Psychiatry Psychiatr Epidemiol 37:190–197, 2002

Quill T: Death and dignity—a case of individualized decision making. N Engl J Med 324:691–694, 1991

Quill T, Cassel C, Meier D: Care of the hopelessly ill: proposed clinical criteria for physician-assisted suicide. N Engl J Med 327:1380–1384, 1992

Quill T, Lo B, Brock D: Palliative options of last resort: a comparison of voluntarily stopping eating and drinking, terminal sedation, physician-assisted suicide, and voluntary active euthanasia. JAMA 278:2099–2104, 1997

Reich P, Kelly M: Suicide attempts by hospitalized medical and surgical patients. N Engl J Med 294:298–301, 1976

Robins E, Murphy G, Wilkinson R, et al: Some clinical considerations in the prevention of suicide based on a study of 134 successful suicides. Am J Public Health 49:888–899, 1959

Rowland L: Assisted suicide and alternatives in amyotrophic lateral sclerosis. N Engl J Med 339:987–989, 1998

Roy A: Emergency psychiatry: suicide, in Comprehensive Textbook of Psychiatry/V. Edited by Kaplan H, Sadock B. Baltimore, MD, Williams & Wilkins, 1989, pp 1414–1427

Roy A: Characteristics of HIV patients who attempt suicide. Acta Psychiatr Scand 107:41–44, 2003

Rundell J, Kyle K, Brown G, et al: Risk factors for suicide attempts in a human immunodeficiency virus screening program. Psychosomatics 33:24–27, 1992

Sanders R: Suicidal behavior in critical care medicine: conceptual issues and management strategies, in Problems in Critical Care Medicine. Edited by Wise M. Philadelphia, PA, JB Lippincott, 1988, pp 116–133

Shah A, Ganesvaran T: Inpatient suicides in an Australian mental hospital. Aust N Z J Psychiatry 31:291–298, 1997

Shneidman E: Overview: a multidimensional approach to suicide, in Suicide: Understanding and Responding. Edited by Jacobs D, Brown H. Madison, CT, International Universities Press, 1989, pp 1–30

Singer P, Siegler M: Euthanasia—a critique. N Engl J Med 322:1881–1883, 1990

Stenager EN, Stenager E, Jensen K: Attempted suicide, depression, and physical diseases: a 1-year follow-up study. Psychother Psychosom 61:65–73, 1994

Stensman R, Sundqvist-Stensman U: Physical disease and disability among 416 suicide cases in Sweden. Scand J Soc Med 16:149–153, 1988

Suominen K, Isometsa E, Heila H, et al: General hospital suicides—a psychological autopsy study in Finland. Gen Hosp Psychiatry 24:412–416, 2002

Tanaka H, Tsukuma H, Masaoka T, et al: Suicide risk among cancer patients: experience at one medical center in Japan, 1978–1994. Jpn J Cancer Res 90:812–817, 1999

Waern M, Rubenowitz E, Runeson B, et al: Burden of illness and suicide in elderly people: case-control study. BMJ 324:1355–1358, 2002

White R, Gribble R, Corr M, et al: Jumping from a general hospital. Gen Hosp Psychiatry 17:208–215, 1995

11 Mania, Catatonia, and Psychosis

Prakash S. Masand, M.D.

Eric J. Christopher, M.D.

Greg L. Clary, M.D.

Rajnish Mago, M.D.

James L. Levenson, M.D.

Ashwin A. Patkar, M.D.

IN THIS CHAPTER, we review the impact of mania, catatonia, and psychosis on medical care and treatment in patients with serious medical illness. The etiology and differential diagnosis of secondary mania, catatonia, and psychosis are also reviewed. Mania, catatonia, and psychosis attributed to a medical condition or substance use are termed secondary disorders. Although the terms *primary* and *secondary* are not formally used in DSM-IV and DSM-IV-TR (American Psychiatric Association 1994, 2000), many clinicians prefer to use them to distinguish between syndromes that result from psychiatric disorders such as schizophrenia and affective disorders and those that are due to general medical conditions, psychoactive substances, or medications.

Mania in the Medically Ill

Bipolar illness is common in the general population, with a lifetime prevalence rate between 1% and 3% (Kessler et al. 1997; Regier et al. 1990). It is often underrecognized; it also is often misdiagnosed as major depression, anxiety disorder, or schizophrenia, and in medical inpatients it may be mistaken for delirium. While evaluating patients for secondary causes of mania, clinicians should always consider the possibility that the patient may have a primary bipolar disorder. In general, the treatment of primary mania in the medically ill should follow established guidelines, except when the medical condition (e.g., impaired hepatic metabolism) requires modifications in the medications used (see Chapter 37, "Psychopharmacology").

Diagnosis

A classification system of six subtypes of bipolar disorder published in 1978 included type IV, defined as manic symptoms with etiology related to general medical illness or the use or abuse of prescription or illicit drugs (Krauthammer and Klerman 1978). In DSM-III, this condition was referred to as "organic mania" (American Psychiatric Association 1980). In current DSM-IV-TR terminology, secondary mania, or manic symptoms attributed to an organic etiology, is referred to as mood disorder secondary to a general medical condition (American Psychiatric Association 2000). The diagnosis of secondary mania requires a prominent and persistent elevated, expansive, or irritable mood and evidence from the history, physical examination, or laboratory findings that the disturbance is the direct physiological consequence of a general medical condition.

An overlap of the clinical presentation of secondary mania with delirium can complicate diagnosis and treatment. Both can present with abrupt onset, inattention, agitation, disordered sleep, and psychosis. Delirium differs from secondary mania in its waxing and waning course, clouding of consciousness, and visual hallucinations and illusions, whereas secondary mania is suggested by manic affect, hypersexuality, and pressured speech.

The course of secondary mania has not been well defined, nor are its prevalence and incidence known. With primary bipolar illness, the course is usually chronic and recurrent, but in secondary mania, the episode may begin within hours or days of the organic or toxic insult. The differentiation between primary mania and secondary mania is often based primarily on a temporal correlation between an organic factor and the manic behavior. In determining whether such a correlation is substantive, it is important to obtain a careful history of psychiatric symptoms before what is believed to be the initiating event, looking for previously unrecognized cyclical episodes of affective illness. Age at presentation can be a significant factor in determining the difference between secondary mania and primary bipolar disorder (see subsection "Mania in the Elderly" later in chapter). Bipolar illness most commonly has onset during the first three decades of life (Goodwin and Jamison 1990). Initial bipolar episodes rarely occur after age 50 years, although there is a growing literature describing late-life bipolar illness (Krishnan 2002).

In contrast to patients with primary mania, patients with secondary mania may have some cognitive dysfunction (American Psychiatric Association 1994). The likelihood that mania is secondary is greater when there is no prior personal or family history of bipolar disorder, when cognitive dysfunction or focal neurological signs are present, or when affective symptoms fail to respond to treatment. The distinction between primary and secondary mania may not be possible in some patients who have a preexisting vulnerability to bipolar disorder and in whom the medical illness or drug appears to have precipitated mania. The presence of a family history of affective disorder suggests but does not prove that a patient's mania is primary (Jorge et al. 1993). For example, approximately 30% of brain-injured patients with mania have at least one relative with unipolar depression (Shukla et al. 1987; Snowdon 1991; Starkstein et al. 1987). A personal or family history of affective illness could indicate either that the mania is primary or that the patient was more vulnerable to developing secondary mania after brain injury. Postpartum mania is another example in which the primary–secondary distinction is often ambiguous, because precipitous hormonal change and preexisting bipolar vulnerability may both play a role (see Chapter 33, "Obstetrics and Gynecology")

Etiology

The etiology of secondary mania is heterogeneous, and it is likely that several different distinct mechanisms contribute to its pathophysiology. Secondary mania unrelated to primary bipolar illness has been attributed to various conditions, including drug use, central nervous system (CNS) trauma, neoplasms, vascular and degenerative diseases, epilepsy, infections, and metabolic conditions (Table 11–1) (Clayton 1981; Krauthammer and Klerman 1978; Stasiek and Zetin 1985). In cases of secondary mania caused by medications such as psychostimulants or dopamine agonists, behavioral changes are typically totally reversible. However, symptoms may persist in patients with mania secondary to CNS injury (from either traumatic injury or stroke), neoplasm, infection, or underlying neurodegenerative diseases such as Huntington's disease or multiple sclerosis (Evans et al. 1995; Rundell and Wise 1989).

Mania in the Elderly

It is particularly appropriate to consider secondary mania in elderly patients with new-onset mania; they have been reported to be twice as likely to have a neurological disorder as patients with prior episodes of mania (Shulman and Post 1980; Shulman et al. 1987, 1992).

The relationships between bipolar disorder, old age, and dementia are not well defined (Shulman and Post 1980; Shulman et al. 1987, 1992). Bipolar patients above age 65 are not necessarily only those who have had bipolar disorder since they were much younger. A bimodal distribution of bipolar disorder for women has been noted, with the greatest peak before age 30 and a second peak in the late 40s (Goodwin and Jamison 1990). In men there is an increased incidence of mania in old age, with a peak in the eighth or ninth decade (Sibisi 1990; Spicer et al. 1973). There is increasing evidence of subtle vascular disease in elderly patients with mania (McDonald et al. 1991). It has been reported that a high prevalence of deep subcortical ischemic changes occurs in patients with late-life bipolar disorder. There is some evidence for genetic loading in elderly patients with bipolar disorder, but the number of affectively ill relatives is greater in the group with early-onset illness than in those with late-onset bipolar illness (Krishnan 2002).

Neurological impairment appears to create a diathesis for the development of late-onset mania. In a retrospective review of 50 patients age 65 or older admitted for an episode of mania (Shulman et al. 1992), the rate of con-

TABLE 11–1. Selected causes of secondary mania

Neurological conditions

Cryptococcal meningoencephalitis
Human immunodeficiency virus (HIV) encephalopathy
Huntington's disease
Kleine-Levin syndrome
Klinefelter's syndrome
Multiple sclerosis
Neurosyphilis
Psychomotor seizures
Strokes (temporal, right hemispheric)
Traumatic brain injury
Tumors (gliomas, meningiomas, thalamic metastases)
Viral encephalitis (acute or postinfection)
Wilson's disease

Other systemic conditions

Cushing's syndrome
Hyperthyroidism
Niacin deficiency
Postoperative delirium
Puerperal psychosis
Uremia
Vitamin B_{12} deficiency

Selected medications

Amantadine
Amphetamines
Anabolic steroids
Antidepressants
Benzodiazepines (triazolam, alprazolam)
Bromocriptine
Cimetidine and other H_2 antagonists
Cocaine
Corticosteroids; corticosteroid withdrawal
Cyclobenzaprine
Cyproheptadine
Dextromethorphan
Dronabinol
Hypericum (St. John's wort)
Isoniazid
Levodopa
Methylphenidate and other stimulants
Monoamine oxidase inhibitors (MAOIs)
Procarbazine
Sympathomimetic amines (e.g., ephedrine)
Yohimbine
Zidovudine

current neurological disorders was significantly higher than in a group of depressed patients (36% vs. 8%). Fourteen of the 50 patients (28%) presented with a first episode of mania after age 65. Patients with new-onset mania were twice as likely to have had a comorbid neurological disorder than were elderly patients with multiple episodes

of mania (71% vs. 28%). Neuroimaging studies of a very small number of patients suggest that the right frontal lobe or limbic connecting areas might be involved in the development of secondary mania and that the underlying mechanism may be related to interruption of the frontotemporal pathways (Gafoor and O'Keane 2003). Mania in the elderly is also associated with an increased mortality rate. During a mean follow-up period of 5.6 years, the mortality rate was significantly higher among elderly manic patients than among elderly patients without mania (50% vs. 20%) (Shulman et al. 1992).

Neurological Causes of Secondary Mania

Many neurological disorders—including stroke, movement disorders, some demyelinating diseases, epilepsy, and head trauma—can manifest manic symptoms (Evans et al. 1995; Rundell and Wise 1989). Neurological disorders appear to be particularly important as risk factors for new onset of mania in the elderly (Krauthammer and Klerman 1978; Stasiek and Zetin 1985). In a retrospective review of the charts of 92 consecutively admitted manic patients older than 65 years, almost a quarter of the patients manifested cerebral disease (Parkinson's disease, cerebrovascular disease, or epilepsy) (Stone 1989). Patients with comorbid neurological diseases had significantly later age at onset and were less likely to have a family history of affective illness. Neurological mania is more likely to manifest as a single episode than as multiple recurrent episodes of mania or as bipolar disorder (Starkstein et al. 1987, 1991).

Some patients who develop secondary mania after brain injury have been reported to have focal brain lesions in the right hemisphere, usually involving the structures of the limbic system (R.G. Robinson et al. 1988; Starkstein et al. 1987). It is postulated that lesions affecting the right hemisphere and limbic structures may produce euphoria, hypersexuality, insomnia, hyperactivity, and irritability (Starkstein et al. 1991). Despite these observations, specific lesion locations have not been clearly established in secondary neurological mania. In part, this is because secondary mania associated with stroke is believed to be quite rare (R.G. Robinson et al. 1988; Wiart 1997). In one study, only two cases of mania were observed among more than 700 consecutive stroke patients (R.G. Robinson et al. 1988). Although patients with primary bipolar disorder have more focal lesions on magnetic resonance imaging (MRI) studies compared with control subjects, no specific lesion locations have been identified (Swayze et al. 1990).

Huntington's disease. Psychiatric symptoms in Huntington's disease are variable, but depression, irritability, and anxiety are common (Glosser 2001). (See Chapter 7, "Dementia," and Chapter 32, "Neurology and Neurosurgery.") Some patients may display irritability, elevated mood, overactivity, decreased need for sleep, and increased risk of suicide, consistent with a diagnosis of secondary mania (Rosenblatt and Leroi 2000). According to one estimate, 4.8% of patients with Huntington's disease have mania (Mendez 2000). In another study, episodes of hypomania and mania were observed in up to 10% of patients with Huntington's disease (Folstein and Folstein 1983).

Multiple sclerosis.   Multiple sclerosis is the most common demyelinating autoimmune disease (see Chapter 32, "Neurology and Neurosurgery"). It is believed that strategically located multiple sclerosis lesions could be the cause of psychosis in multiple sclerosis, with a mean duration of neurological symptoms before onset of psychosis of 8.5 years (Feinstein et al. 1992). Patients with multiple sclerosis may have euphoria, pathological laughing and weeping, and other frontal lobe disinhibition symptoms (Minden 2000). It has been reported that the incidence of bipolar disorder is greater in patients with multiple sclerosis than among the general population (Schiffer et al. 1986), but it is not clear to what extent this represents primary or secondary bipolar disorder. Diffuse, multifocal white matter lesions might "unmask" primary bipolar disorder or cause secondary mania (Kellner et al. 1984). However, most cases of secondary mania in multiple sclerosis patients may have been due to corticosteroid treatment rather than multiple sclerosis (E.S. Brown et al. 1999).

Depression occurs in multiple sclerosis far more often than mania and affects up to 40%–60% of patients (Patten and Metz 1997). In addition to CNS lesions, causes of depression in multiple sclerosis patients include the psychological experience of an unpredictable debilitating disease and treatment with corticosteroids or interferons (Mohr et al. 1999). The rate of suicide in patients with multiple sclerosis has been reported to be 7.5 times that in the age-matched general population (Sadovnick et al. 1991). It is not known if mania is a risk factor for suicide in multiple sclerosis, but extrapolations from observations of patients with primary mania indicate that caution is warranted. Regardless of the cause, the symptoms of mood disorders in people with multiple sclerosis generally benefit from standard treatments (Minden 2000).

Traumatic brain injury.   Mood disorders have been estimated to occur in 6%–7.7% of all patients with traumatic brain injury (TBI) (Rao and Lykestsos 2002), and secondary mania has been estimated to occur in 3%–10% (Jorge et al. 1993) (see also Chapter 35, "Physical Medicine and Rehabilitation"). Estimates of the frequency of aggressive behaviors during the acute period after TBI have ranged from 11% to 96% (Tateno et al. 2003). Despite the frequency of TBI, the literature regarding TBI-associated bipolar disorder is limited to case reports and small series. In the largest case series of TBI patients with manic symptoms, 66 TBI patients were observed for 1 year after their initial injury (Jorge et al. 1993). Approximately 9% (6 of 66) met the DSM-III-R criteria for bipolar disorder (American Psychiatric Association 1987). Symptoms included expansive mood, irritability, increased motor or verbal activity, evidence of thought disorder, increased sexual interest, aggressive behavior, decreased need for sleep, and grandiose delusions. The duration of each manic episode was relatively brief (lasting only 2 months on average). Neuroimaging revealed a greater prevalence of anterior temporal lobe lesions.

The study by Jorge et al. (1993) found no apparent association between secondary mania of TBI origin and family history of mood disorder, personal history of psychiatric illness, severity of brain injury, degree of physical or cognitive impairment, social support, social level of functioning, or posttraumatic epilepsy. However, in one study of 20 patients with a history of TBI who were referred for schizoaffective or manic symptoms, 30% had at least one relative with a history of depression (Shukla and Cook 1987). The interval between injury and onset of symptoms ranged from less than 1 year to 12 years, although in 14 of 20 cases it was less than 2 years.

HIV infection.   HIV infection is an important risk factor for the development of secondary mania, which is believed to result from brain infection with HIV (see also Chapter 28, "HIV/AIDS"). Secondary mania associated with HIV infection may be differentiated from primary mania in HIV-infected patients by its late onset in the course of the infection and its association with cognitive decline and AIDS dementia. Although mania has been reported to occur in 4%–8% of HIV-infected individuals, the prevalence of mania that is directly attributable to an HIV-related focus is not known (Kilbourne et al. 2001; Lyketsos et al. 1993a). Advanced disease is an ever-increasing risk factor for the evolution of HIV-related mania. Patients with later onset of manic symptoms (presumed to be secondary mania) were less likely than those with early-onset mania to have had a personal or family history of affective disorder but were more likely to have a concurrent diagnosis of dementia (Lyketsos et al. 1993a).

The mood of patients with secondary mania due to HIV infection is most often described as a combination of elevated, irritable, and labile (Ellen et al. 1999; Lyketsos et al. 1993a, 1993b, 1997). Imaging studies of one group of HIV-infected patients with secondary mania revealed neurological abnormalities in 53%. The most common finding was bilateral white matter foci, usually in the periventricular areas (Ellen et al. 1999).

Endocrine Abnormalities

A variety of endocrine disorders, including Cushing's disease and thyroid abnormalities, are associated with secondary mania (Brownlie et al. 2000) (see also Chapter 23, "Endocrine and Metabolic Disorders"). Mania has been reported in patients with hyperthyroidism (Corn and Checkley 1983; Villani and Weitzel 1979). Hypothyroidism does not cause mania per se, but it is well known to induce rapid cycling in patients with primary bipolar disorder. Treatment with corticosteroids is probably the most common cause of secondary mania (Rundell and Wise 1989). Depression is more common than mania as a steroid side effect, but mixed states also occur. Steroid-induced mood disorder can be severe; in one study, 51% of patients exhibiting either hypomania or depression developed psychotic symptoms (K. Wada et al. 2001).

Substance-Induced Mania

Many other classes of illicit substances and prescription medications have induced well-documented cases of secondary mania (see Table 11–1 for full list). As mentioned above, corticosteroids and dopaminergic agonists (e.g., levodopa, bromocriptine, and amantadine) are frequent causes of secondary mania. Over-the-counter sympathomimetic agents and cocaine have precipitated severe cases of manic behavior. Because they inhibit monoamine oxidase, isoniazid and procarbazine have caused mania even in patients without histories of any mood disorder. Cimetidine and other histamine H_2 receptor antagonists have also been reported to cause secondary mania.

Other compounds that have been reported to lead to the development of mania include cyclobenzaprine; yohimbine; baclofen; phencyclidine; and several of the benzodiazepines, including alprazolam and triazolam (Goodman and Charney 1987; Weilberg et al. 1987).

Evaluation

All patients with suspected secondary mania should have a complete evaluation, including a careful history and physical examination and appropriate laboratory and imaging studies. Depending on the likelihood of particular etiologies, testing may include metabolic and endocrine tests (especially cortisol and thyroid-stimulating hormone), complete blood cell count, HIV test, fluorescent treponemal antibody test, urine toxicology screen, computed tomography (CT) or MRI brain scan, lumbar puncture, and other investigations.

Treatment of Primary and Secondary Mania in the Medically Ill

There are essentially no data from controlled trials of drug treatments for secondary manic syndromes, so clinical practice has been guided by case reports and clinical experience (Evans et al. 1995; Halman et al. 1993; Shulman et al. 1987). The first step, whenever possible, is to treat the underlying disorder or eliminate the offending agent. When this is not possible (e.g., with steroid-induced mania in a patient with lupus), symptomatic treatment is indicated. Medications that are recommended are essentially the same as those used in primary bipolar disorder, with only occasional caveats.

As with primary mania, lithium, divalproex sodium, and carbamazepine are the mainstays of treatment and can be used prophylactically to prevent drug-induced mania (e.g., due to steroids). Lithium is difficult to use safely in patients with unstable fluid/electrolyte status or hyperthyroidism. Lithium is effective not only for manic symptoms but also for depression induced by corticosteroids (K. Wada et al. 2001), but it may be contraindicated by the underlying medical disorder (e.g., renal disease in systemic lupus erythematosus; see Chapter 25, "Rheumatology"). Some of the more recently developed anticonvulsants may also prove helpful in patients who do not respond to or cannot tolerate first-line drugs.

Both the older typical and newer antipsychotic drugs appear to have antimanic effects and may provide mood stability in secondary mania regardless of whether the patient also has psychosis. For patients with acute secondary mania, particularly when it is expected to be temporary, antipsychotics may be more helpful than lithium or anticonvulsants because of faster onset of benefit. In neurological secondary mania, atypical antipsychotics are generally preferable because of their lower risk of extrapyramidal side effects (Gupta et al. 1999; Masand and Gupta 2000). Buspirone may also be helpful in treating disruptive behaviors in patients with Huntington's disease or other neurological disorders (Bhandary and Masand 1997). Treatment of HIV mania is addressed in Chapter 28, "HIV/AIDS."

Catatonia in the Medically Ill

Although it is a relatively rare condition, catatonia may be acute or chronic and can be caused by psychiatric disorders, medical illnesses, or drugs. Catatonia occurs as a subtype of schizophrenia but more often as part of severe affective illness. We focus here primarily on secondary catatonia caused by medical illness or drugs and on the medical complications encountered in chronic catatonia of any cause.

Secondary Catatonia

Diagnosis

The core features of catatonia are stupor, motoric immobility, mutism, negativism, excitement, catalepsy, and posturing. The core features are the same regardless of whether the condition occurs in the context of a mood, psychotic, or medical state. The latter is recognized in DSM-IV-TR as the category of catatonia secondary to a general medical condition. A full history and those aspects of the physical examination requiring cooperation are usually not obtainable from a catatonic patient, so information must be sought from family members and other sources.

Other disease states can mimic catatonia and should be considered in the differential diagnosis. These conditions include stiff-person syndrome, akinetic Parkinson's disease, malignant hyperthermia, locked-in syndrome, elective mutism, and hyperkinetic and hypokinetic states (Fink and Taylor 2003). Stiff-person syndrome is an uncommon autoimmune disorder with progressive muscle stiffness, rigidity, and spasm, slowly progressive over the course of years (Helfgott 2003). Akinetic Parkinson's disease also can produce a state similar to catatonia, but it usually occurs after the diagnosis of Parkinson's disease has been well established. Malignant hyperthermia often includes some of the characteristics of catatonia, but it occurs in the context of anesthesia. Elective mutism shares only that one feature of catatonia and is usually associated with conversion or underlying personality disorders (Fink and Taylor 2003). Hyperkinetic (e.g., Gilles de la Tourette's syndrome, cerebral palsy) and hypokinetic (e.g., Huntington's disease, Wilson's disease) movement disorders can have some features of catatonia as well.

Etiology

Catatonia has been associated with a number of medical conditions, including metabolic, neurological, and substance disorders (Table 11–2). In a review of the literature from 1966 to 1993, 261 cases of catatonia were identified (Carroll et al. 1994). In 76% of these cases, there was no relevant psychiatric disorder associated with the catatonic state. CNS injury or dysfunction—resulting from stroke, trauma, CNS tumor, seizures, infection, or anoxia—is the most common cause of secondary catatonia. Strokes involving the anterior cerebral circulation have the propensity to cause akinetic and apathetic states (Kumral et al. 2002). Bilateral infarction of the cingulate gyri of the medial frontal lobes can lead to a lack of spontaneous motor movement and mutism (Reichman 1995). CNS tumors such as astrocytomas may initially present with catatonia (Muqit et al. 2001). Catatonia may also be caused by epilepsy or by endocrine or metabolic disorders, including hypothyroidism, adrenal insufficiency, and vitamin B_{12} deficiency (Catalano et al. 1998).

TABLE 11–2.   Selected causes of secondary catatonia

Neurological causes

Angiomas
Basilar artery thrombosis
Bilateral infarction of the anterior cingulate gyrus
Bilateral infarction of the temporal lobes
Cerebral anoxia
Closed head injury
Encephalitis or other central nervous system infection (e.g., neurosyphilis)
Gliomas
HIV encephalopathy
Normal-pressure hydrocephalus
Seizure disorders
Surgery near the hypothalamus

Other medical causes

Addison's disease
Bacterial sepsis
Cushing's disease
Encephalitis (acute or postinfectious)
HIV encephalopathy
Hyperthyroidism
Malaria
Neurosyphilis
Postoperative states
Postpartum psychosis
Systemic lupus erythematosus
Typhoid fever
Uremia
Viral hepatitis
Vitamin deficiencies

Medications and toxic substances

Corticosteroids
Cyclobenzaprine
Disulfiram
3,4-Methylenedioxymethamphetamine (MDMA; Ecstasy)
Phencyclidine (PCP)
Sedative-hypnotic withdrawal
Tetraethyl lead poisoning

A number of drugs and toxins may cause catatonia (see Table 11–2). Persons under the influence of hallucinogens, such as phencyclidine (PCP) or 3,4-methylenedioxymethamphetamine (MDMA; Ecstasy) (Masi et al. 2002), may present in an excited catatonic state. Carbon monoxide toxicity can cause catatonia due to damage to the putamen, caudate nucleus, or globus pallidus.

Neuroleptics may cause a parkinsonian catatonic state. Serotonergic agents can cause serotonin syndrome, and antidopaminergic agents can cause neuroleptic malignant syndrome. Both serotonin syndrome and neuroleptic malignant syndrome may cause catatonia in addition to their other symptoms. Neuroleptic malignant syndrome can be particularly difficult to distinguish from severe agitated primary catatonia, often called lethal catatonia (Mann et al. 1986). If a patient with catatonia of any etiology is treated with a neuroleptic, it can be difficult, if not impossible, to discriminate the original catatonia from neuroleptic-induced catatonia and neuroleptic malignant syndrome.

Complications

The care of patients in a chronic or relapsing catatonic state can be challenging from both a medical and a psychiatric standpoint. Although catatonia can encompass varying states of psychomotor abnormalities from excitement to rigid stupor, patients are often bedridden and undernourished, which contributes to their frequent long-term medical complications. The inability of catatonic patients to report their symptoms requires clinicians to be vigilant regarding such complications. In a chart review (1985–1991) of patients with catatonia, Carroll (1996) described complications, including deep venous thrombosis, nonfatal pulmonary embolism, urinary tract infection, urosepsis, cachexia, hypernatremia, rhabdomyolysis, acute tubular necrosis, aspiration pneumonia, and flexion contractures.

Cardiovascular complications.   One problem for catatonic patients is cardiovascular deconditioning, especially orthostatic intolerance, which occurs after only a few weeks of bed rest. In addition to vascular changes, cardiopulmonary efficiency is also reduced. The use of psychotropic medications that have central and peripheral cardiovascular effects may further aggravate cardiovascular dysfunction in patients with catatonia (Gupta et al. 2001).

A significant source of morbidity and mortality in patients with catatonia is deep venous thrombosis and subsequent pulmonary embolism (Barbuto 1983; McCall et al. 1995; Morioka et al. 1997; Regestein et al. 1977; Sukov 1972). Prolonged immobilization and dehydration are

risk factors that promote venous thrombosis. Carroll (1996) observed that about 6% of catatonic patients developed venous thrombosis. Prevention of thrombosis and subsequent pulmonary embolism has been studied extensively in acute medical conditions associated with immobility, as well as after various surgical procedures (Turpie et al. 2002). Maintenance of hydration, physical therapy, support hose, and prophylactic anticoagulation have all been suggested for prevention. Although subcutaneous heparin and low-molecular-weight heparin are well supported by studies in patients following orthopedic surgery, a time when the risk of venous thromboembolism is high, the increased risk is much lower in chronically immobilized patients (Heit et al. 2002). Whether heparin would reduce morbidity and mortality in catatonia is unknown and is worthy of study.

Pulmonary system complications.   The most frequent pulmonary complication seen in chronic catatonia is aspiration (Levenson and Pandurangi 2004), which is also the most common cause of death in patients with dysphagia caused by neurological disorders and the most common cause of death in patients nourished by tube feeding (Marik 2001). Aspiration can result in pneumonitis or pneumonia. Aspiration pneumonitis is the regurgitation of gastric contents into the pulmonary tree with an accompanying inflammatory response. Aspiration pneumonia is an infection by aspirated bacteria, usually from oropharyngeal secretions. Aspiration pneumonitis can be considered a chemical pneumonitis caused by gastric acid. Although antacids, histamine H_2 blockers, and proton-pump inhibitors can decrease stomach acidity, their use prevents the sterility of gastric contents and can make aspiration of gastric contents more likely and more severe (Marik 2001). Conventional neuroleptics may also increase the risk of aspiration, perhaps via the effects of dystonia on swallowing (H. Wada et al. 2001). Daily oral hygiene can lessen the risk of aspiration pneumonia (Shay 2002). Unfortunately, this is not a priority in the care of the chronically ill and is usually overlooked in patients with catatonia. Anticholinergic psychiatric medications that reduce salivation may also promote pathogenic oral flora. Prophylactic antibiotics are not recommended (Levenson and Pandurangi 2004).

Gastrointestinal system complications.   Maintaining nutrition is a challenge in persistently catatonic patients. When required, enteral feeding can be provided either by nasally or surgically placed tubes. Nasogastric or nasoenteric tubes are preferred in patients who will need invasive feeding for 30 days or less (Koretz et al. 2001). Placement of these tubes is not benign. Patients with altered mental status are especially at risk because of the inability to co-operate with the procedure and the presence of a decreased gag reflex. Cases of malpositioning, pulmonary intubation, and death have all been reported with the use of enteral feeding tubes (Raff et al. 1987). Also, contrary to common belief, nasoenteric feeding tubes do not prevent aspiration (Finucane et al. 1999). For chronically catatonic patients requiring ongoing artificial feeding, surgical gastrostomy and jejunostomy are options. However, pathogenic colonization occurs in patients fed by either nasogastric or percutaneous enterogastric tubes (Leibovitz et al. 2003). In patients with acute or periodic catatonia, tube feeding with nutritional supplements is appropriate. However, the chronic catatonic patient presents an ethical dilemma (similar to that encountered in other chronic debilitating diseases such as dementia, amyotrophic lateral sclerosis, or Parkinson's disease) that requires careful weighing of the benefits of enteral feedings versus their complications and effects on general health and quality of life (Finucane et al. 1999; Levenson and Pandurangi 2004; Li 2002). These factors should all be considered before the initiation of tube feedings in any severely chronically ill patient.

Dermatological complications. Pressure ulcers (also called decubitus ulcers) are common in patients with chronic catatonia, and their complications include sepsis, osteomyelitis, and increased mortality risk (Thomas 2001). Frequent turning is necessary but is not always sufficient to prevent pressure ulcers. Although malnutrition is associated with risk of development of pressure ulcers, nutritional supplementation has not been proven to prevent their occurrence (Thomas 2001). The use of pressure-relieving beds helps, but no one device has proven to be superior (S.J. Brown 2001). Maintaining clean, dry skin prevents maceration and breakdown of the skin. Compared with diapering, the use of Foley catheters may actually increase the risk of pressure ulcers (Thomas 2001). Fecal contamination is a major risk in the development of pressure ulcers.

Musculoskeletal system complications. Skeletal muscle deconditioning occurs in patients with chronic catatonia as in other immobilized patients. Catatonic patients with muscle rigidity are particularly vulnerable to the development of flexion contractures in response to loss of muscle use and shortening of the ligaments. The best treatment is prevention through physical therapy; once contractures develop, treatment benefits are limited (Fox et al. 2000). Finally, prolonged immobility is a risk for the development of rhabdomyolysis. Although rhabdomyolysis is a recognized complication of lethal catatonia and neuro-

leptic malignant syndrome, its frequency in chronic catatonia is unknown (Levenson and Pandurangi 2004).

Treatment of Secondary Catatonia

If a medical or neurological condition is determined to be the cause of catatonia, treatment should be directed at the underlying condition. When this is not possible or when catatonia persists or interferes with treatment, benzodiazepines and electroconvulsive therapy (ECT) are the mainstays of treatment (Bush et al. 1996). Benzodiazepines may provide almost immediate benefit for the motor and speech signs of catatonia. Bush and associates (1996) prospectively used lorazepam in 21 patients with catatonia and found symptom remission in 16 patients. After a 5-day trial of lorazepam, patients who were still not responding were administered ECT, with remission occurring in 4 of the remaining 5 patients. ECT is the most effective treatment for catatonia (American Psychiatric Association 2001) and can be used safely in almost all medically ill individuals (Christopher 2003) (see Chapter 39, "Electroconvulsive Therapy").

Psychosis in the Medically Ill

In addition to their occurrence in major psychiatric disorders such as schizophrenia and mood disorders, psychotic symptoms frequently occur as a part of several medical illnesses. Psychotic symptoms may also be induced by psychoactive substances or by medications that are used to treat medical disorders. Psychotic symptoms in medically ill patients can complicate the diagnosis and management of the medical condition in several ways but can usually be ameliorated with appropriate interventions.

Primary Psychosis

Because schizophrenia and related disorders occur in 1%–2% of the general population, the possibility of a primary psychotic disorder should be considered in a medically ill patient who manifests psychotic symptoms before attributing them to the medical illness. In general, the usual medications for treatment of primary psychosis can be used in the medically ill, but selection of a particular drug and determination of the dosage depend on the underlying medical illness.

There are a number of potential complications of primary psychotic disorders in the medically ill. Schizophrenia itself carries an increased risk for several medical comorbidities, such as obesity and diabetes (Dixon et al. 2000; Ryan et al. 2003), relative to the risk of these conditions in the general population (Gupta et al. 1997; Jeste et al. 1996). Most antipsychotics add to these risks, causing weight gain (Allison et al. 1999; Masand 1999, 2000c), elevated glucose levels, and hyperlipidemia (Wirshing et al. 2003). Patients with schizophrenia often have poor health habits, such as inadequate nutrition, physical inactivity, and high rates of smoking and substance abuse (Dixon 2003; Patkar et al. 2002). Poverty, institutionalization, self-neglect, and social isolation may all adversely affect health in chronic psychosis. Patients with chronic schizophrenia often have problems with access to health care and with adherence to complex treatment regimens. Among the homeless, those with schizophrenia have fewer medical visits and documented medical complaints than those with depression and are less likely to have careful physical examinations and screenings for medical disorders (Folsom et al. 2002). Somatic delusions and hallucinations, psychotic denial, and thought disorder may lead to physical symptoms being misperceived or ignored by patients and clinicians, leading to delay in medical treatment (Reeves and Torres 2003). Psychosis may negatively affect the patient's relationship with health care providers, interfering with communication and eliciting a variety of negative countertransference reactions. Finally, poor integration between the mental health care and general health care systems disrupts continuity of care for these patients.

Secondary Psychosis

Diagnosis

When psychotic symptoms are observed in a patient who has a concurrent medical illness, the following possibilities should be considered:

1. Preexistence, exacerbation, or new onset of a "primary" psychotic disorder (e.g., schizophrenia, bipolar disorder)
2. Delirium or dementia
3. Psychotic disorder due to a general medical condition (American Psychiatric Association 2000)
4. Psychoactive substance use or withdrawal (including medications)

In a medically ill patient, an attempt should be made to distinguish between a primary and a secondary psychotic disorder on the basis of the patient's history and clinical features (Table 11–3). Distinguishing the two is often challenging because of the similarities in the clinical features and difficulties in establishing a cause-and-effect relationship between a putative etiological medical condition or medication and psychotic symptoms. Certain his-

torical information makes a secondary psychosis more likely; this includes first onset of psychotic symptoms at an older age, absence of a past or family history of primary psychotic disorders, a concomitant medical condition known to cause psychotic symptoms, active substance use or withdrawal, and atypical clinical features. Visual hallucinations are more frequent in secondary psychoses, as are olfactory, gustatory, and tactile hallucinations. Cognitive deficits and focal abnormalities on the neurological examination also point toward secondary psychosis. The temporal pattern of the symptoms should be carefully delineated and may be the most important factor in making the diagnosis. Onset of psychotic symptoms much earlier than the putative cause usually suggests primary psychosis, but the possibility that the psychosis was the first symptom of an evolving medical condition should be considered. If the onset and resolution of the psychotic symptoms parallel the course of the putative causative factor, a diagnosis of secondary psychosis is more likely. Rapid and complete resolution of psychotic symptoms on elimination of the suspected factor may confirm the causative relationship. The diagnosis often becomes more obvious with the evolution of the syndrome. Specific tests (see subsection "Evaluation" below) may also provide useful information to distinguish between primary and secondary psychoses.

Etiology

Selected medical conditions that may cause psychotic symptoms are listed in Table 11–4. Although many medications can cause psychotic symptoms at toxic doses, Table 11–5 lists selected medications that have caused psychotic symptoms at therapeutic doses.

Delirium and dementia are perhaps the most common causes of psychotic symptoms in the medically ill. Delusions occur in approximately 20% of patients with delirium and 45% of those with dementia (Rabins et al. 1982). Psychosis is also discussed in Chapter 6, "Delirium," and Chapter 7, "Dementia."

Psychotic symptoms due to brain disease or injury occur most often with subcortical or temporal lobe lesions. Psychosis related to seizure disorders is more common during the interictal phase, after a long history of seizures, and when there is evidence of temporal lobe lesions or left-sided foci (Cummings 1985). Psychotic symptoms can occur ictally, postictally, or interictally. Brief psychotic symptoms can occur in nonconvulsive status epilepticus, most commonly with partial complex status (Sachdev 1998). In such cases, automatisms (e.g., lip smacking, picking at clothes), mutism, altered consciousness, or amnesia may be present. Postictal psychosis follows an increase in the frequency of seizures, usually with

TABLE 11–3.   Clinical features differentiating primary from secondary psychotic disorders

	Primary psychosis (e.g., schizophrenia, mood disorder)	Secondary psychosis (due to a general medical condition or substance related)
Gross cognitive function	Relatively normal	Abnormal
Level of consciousness	Normal	Often abnormal or fluctuating
Focal neurological signs	Absent	May be present
Hallucinations	Auditory most common	Visual most common
	Tactile/olfactory/gustatory uncommon	Tactile/olfactory/gustatory may be present
Delusions	Often complex	Usually simple
Thought disorder	May be prominent in schizophrenia (thought process often includes loose associations and idiosyncratic language)	Not prominent (thought process may be concrete or perseverative)
Incontinence	Usually absent	May be present
Vital signs	Usually normal	Often abnormal

TABLE 11–4.   Selected medical disorders that may cause psychosis

Brain diseases
Central nervous system vasculitis
Encephalitis or other central nervous system infection (e.g., neurosyphilis)
HIV encephalopathy
Huntington's disease
Paraneoplastic encephalitis
Psychomotor seizures (ictal, postictal, or interictal)
Stroke
Tumor
Wilson's disease

Endocrine disorders
Cushing's syndrome
Hypothyroidism or hyperthyroidism

Metabolic disorders
Acute intermittent porphyria
Hepatic encephalopathy
Hypoglycemia
Hyponatremia
Uremia
Vitamin deficiency (e.g., Korsakoff's psychosis with thiamine deficiency, B_{12} deficiency)

a nonpsychotic period of 1–7 days between the last seizure and the psychosis. Finally, interictal psychosis can occur even in the absence of frequent seizures, but it usually occurs in patients with poorly controlled seizures. It is typically self-limiting but can last for a few weeks. Unlike postictal psychosis, interictal psychosis is sometimes ameliorated by the occurrence of one or more seizures (Sachdev 1998). Chronic interictal psychosis differs from schizophrenia by the presence of better preservation of affect, mood swings, mystical experiences, and visual hallucinations (Slater et al. 1963; see also Chapter 32, "Neurology and Neurosurgery").

Substance-induced psychotic disorder (see Chapter 18, "Substance-Related Disorders") is commonly caused by intoxication with cocaine, amphetamines, or phencyclidine and may persist after the elimination of the drug or its metabolites (Hill et al. 2001; Serper et al. 1995). A negative drug screen does not exclude the possibility that psychotic symptoms were caused by drugs that are not routinely tested for (e.g., hallucinogens) or that may have been eliminated from the body or are otherwise undetectable. Although transient paranoia may be observed in association with cannabis use, cannabis-induced psychotic disorder is rare. Substances most likely to cause psychotic symptoms during withdrawal are sedative-hypnotics and alcohol.

Evaluation

A careful workup of secondary psychosis includes chart review, history, physical examination, and laboratory and radiological investigations (Patkar and Kunkel 1997). Some tests that are performed are considered routine, and others are obtained only if there are more specific reasons to justify them. Usually included in the former category are complete blood cell count, metabolic panel, serum calcium, liver function tests, thyroid-stimulating hormone level, syphilis test, urinalysis, and urine toxicology screen. Common optional tests include chest radiograph, serum drug levels (e.g., theophylline), arterial blood gases, vitamin B_{12} and folate levels, HIV, CT or MRI scan, and lumbar puncture. Additional investigations may be necessary depending on the clinical features and course of symptoms (e.g., if porphyria is suspected).

TABLE 11–5. Selected medications that may cause psychotic symptoms

Type of medication	Examples
Psychotropic	Antidepressants
	Anticholinergics (e.g., benztropine, diphenhydramine)
	Disulfiram
Cardiovascular	Antiarrhythmics (lidocaine, mexiletine, procainamide, quinidine, tocainide)
	Beta-blockers
	Digitalis
Antihistaminic	Cimetidine, ranitidine, diphenhydramine
Antineoplastic	Asparaginase, cytarabine, fluorouracil, ifosfamide, methotrexate, vincristine
Anti-infective	Antimalarials
	Antituberculars (cycloserine, isoniazid)
	Antivirals (acyclovir, interferon, vidarabine, zidovudine)
	Ciprofloxacin
Anticonvulsant	Carbamazepine, ethosuximide, lamotrigine, phenytoin, valproate
Anti-inflammatory	Corticosteroids, indomethacin
Dopaminergic	Amantadine, bromocriptine, levodopa, pramipexole, ropinirole
Opioid	Meperidine, pentazocine
Sympathomimetic	Ephedrine, pseudoephedrine
Other	Baclofen, cyclosporine, metrizamide, methysergide

Complications

Perhaps the most important complication associated with secondary psychosis in the medically ill is when the diagnosis is missed and the patient is treated as if he or she had schizophrenia or another primary psychotic disorder. As noted earlier, psychosis of any cause can adversely affect the doctor–patient relationship and the patient's ability to cooperate with medical evaluation and treatment.

Treatment

The overall goals are to maintain the safety of the patient and others, to identify and treat the underlying medical condition, and to treat the psychotic symptoms. Close collaboration between the psychiatrist and the medical staff involved in the care of the patient is required. Constant observation, restraints, or both may be necessary to prevent self-injury or disruptive behavior (see Chapter 8, "Aggression and Violence"). To ensure safety of the patient and staff, involuntary treatment may be necessary (see Chapter 3, "Legal Issues"). Psychological support includes reassurance and education of the patient and the family about the symptoms and their causes, if known. Vital signs, nutritional status, and fluid-electrolyte balance should be closely monitored.

Treatment of Patients With Primary Psychosis

Psychotic patients who are unstable should not undergo repeated interviews by groups of trainees or by other personnel (Adler and Griffith 1991). Simple, straightforward

information is indicated rather than detailed technical descriptions of medical interventions. Whenever feasible, efforts should be made to psychiatrically stabilize any acutely psychotic patient before any medical or surgical procedures are performed. Close collaboration between psychiatric and medical staff is needed to coordinate the patient's medical care and determine whether inpatients are best treated on a medical unit with psychiatric consultation or on a psychiatric unit with medical consultation. Treatment of psychosis during pregnancy and the postpartum period is discussed in Chapter 33, "Obstetrics and Gynecology."

Antipsychotic agents. The elderly and the medically ill are particularly sensitive to the adverse effects of antipsychotics (Masand 2000a, 2000b), but they also tend to respond to lower doses. The time-honored principle of "start low and go slow" is particularly important in the medically ill. However, the dosage should be individualized, and increasing the dosage should be considered if the patient's response is inadequate. The use of antipsychotics in the medically ill is covered in detail in Chapter 37, "Psychopharmacology," but we review some highlights here.

In general, antipsychotics are selected on the basis of potential side effects, some of which may be desired. Of the typical antipsychotics, haloperidol is preferred in medically ill patients because of extensive experience with its use and because it has minimal sedative and anticholinergic properties, has little or no effect on respiration, and can be administered parenterally. Although there are few data from controlled studies, clinical experience suggests that atypical antipsychotics may be safe and effective in the medically ill and have the advantages of fewer extrapyramidal side effects compared with older agents (Caley and Cooper 2002; Duggan et al. 2003; Marder et al. 2003; Masand 1998; Nasrallah and Tandon 2002). Therefore, atypicals are preferred, especially if there is a history of extrapyramidal side effects, tardive dyskinesia, or a coexisting movement disorder (e.g., Parkinson's disease). For agitated patients, atypical agents with sedative properties, such as quetiapine, may be appropriate. On the other hand, when sedation is not necessary, an agent such as risperidone, aripiprazole, or ziprasidone should be considered.

The patient's medical status may require a particular method of drug administration. It may be preferable to give the antipsychotic as a liquid (e.g., haloperidol, risperidone, ziprasidone) or as an orally disintegrating tablet (e.g., olanzapine, risperidone) to patients who have difficulty swallowing pills (Kelleher et al. 2002). For treatment of patients who are not allowed oral medication, at present only haloperidol, olanzapine, and ziprasidone are available for intramuscular injection. If many doses are required, intramuscular administration is not practicable, and intravenous haloperidol should be considered.

Antipsychotics can be used in cardiac patients even after an acute myocardial infarction. Haloperidol has generally been used safely but has been implicated as causing torsades de pointes when used intravenously in patients with cardiomyopathy (M.J. Robinson and Levenson 2000).

Although cholestatic hepatitis has been reported with atypical antipsychotics and with some low-potency typical antipsychotics, liver disease does not appear to increase the risk of hepatotoxicity of antipsychotic agents. Mild elevations in liver enzymes do not contraindicate the use of antipsychotics, because these changes may be transient and do not always lead to more severe hepatotoxicity (Stoudemire et al. 1991). All antipsychotics are metabolized in the liver to a large extent, and therefore they should be used more cautiously in patients with hepatic failure. Reduction in quetiapine dosage has been recommended for the elderly and for patients with hepatic impairment (Nemeroff et al. 2002). Mild to moderate hepatic impairment does not significantly alter the pharmacokinetics of ziprasidone (Everson et al. 2000), and the pharmacokinetics of risperidone were not significantly altered even in patients with cirrhosis (Snoek et al. 1995).

In renal failure, clearance of risperidone is decreased. Therefore, risperidone should be started at lower doses than usual and the dose increases should be gradual in pa-

tients with renal failure (Snoek et al. 1995). Although the manufacturers do not specifically recommend dose adjustments for other atypical antipsychotics in renal failure, it is prudent to be similarly cautious when treating renal patients because of their comorbidities. Mild to moderate impairment in renal function and hemodialysis do not seem to have a significant effect on the pharmacokinetics of ziprasidone (Aweeka et al. 2000). Dehydration increases the risk of neuroleptic malignant syndrome, so fluid intake should be carefully monitored when medically ill patients are given antipsychotics.

The presence of any type of brain injury increases the likelihood of seizures, and therefore the use of antipsychotics that lower seizure threshold to a greater extent (e.g., clozapine) should be avoided (Stoudemire et al. 1991).

Benzodiazepines.   Benzodiazepines are sometimes used for agitation in medically ill patients with psychosis. Lorazepam and oxazepam are desirable because of their lack of active metabolites, their shorter half-lives, and their minimal hepatic metabolism. In general, however, benzodiazepines should be avoided (except in alcohol or sedative withdrawal), particularly in patients with brain injuries, because these agents may paradoxically aggravate agitation. If a benzodiazepine is used for control of severe agitation, intramuscular lorazepam (1 mg, repeated after 1 hour if needed) is preferred because of its reliable absorption. It can also be given intravenously (0.5–1.0 mg administered over 2 minutes).

Other medications.   Anticonvulsants are not specifically indicated for the treatment of psychotic symptoms (except for those attributed to seizure disorder) but may be used for the treatment of bipolar disorder, a potential cause of psychotic symptoms.

Treatment of Secondary Psychosis in the Medically Ill

In addition to the measures discussed in the previous subsections, there are some additional considerations in patients with secondary psychosis. All nonessential medications should be discontinued or reduced in dosage if they are possible contributors. Antipsychotics should be used when psychotic symptoms interfere with treatment, present risk of harm to the patient or others, or cause personal distress (American Psychiatric Association 1999). In using antipsychotics, the patient's condition should be assessed repeatedly. If there is a rapid and complete resolution of symptoms, the possibility that an "organic" cause has been reversed should be considered and the antipsychotic tapered.

Second-generation antipsychotics are being increasingly used in the treatment of delirium (Schwartz and Masand 2002). There are open-label data to support the use in delirium for olanzapine (Breitbart et al. 2002; Sipahimalani and Masand 1998; Skrobik et al. 2004), low-dose risperidone (Horikawa et al. 2003; Sipahimalani et al. 1997), and quetiapine (Pae et al. 2004; Sasaki et al. 2003). Haloperidol, however, remains the first choice if repeated parenteral administration is needed or cost is a significant factor (Masand et al. 2002).

In dementia with psychotic symptoms, low-potency typical antipsychotics or adjunctive anticholinergics should be avoided. Second-generation antipsychotics are being increasingly used for psychosis or agitation in patients with dementia. At present, double-blind studies support the use of risperidone (Katz et al. 1999) and olanzapine (De Deyn et al. 2004; Schatz 2003 [review of four studies]).

Benzodiazepines are used in alcohol or sedative-hypnotic withdrawal and in seizure disorders. Anticonvulsants are indicated for the treatment of psychosis associated with seizure disorders, but antipsychotics and/or benzodiazepines may be necessary in addition. At this time, there is no evidence to suggest that more recently developed anticonvulsants—including gabapentin, topiramate, and levetiracetam—provide specific benefits for the treatment of psychosis.

Conclusion

The diagnosis and treatment of psychiatric symptoms in medically ill patients can be challenging, not only because of the wider differential diagnosis that must be considered but also because of the complex interactions of psychiatric symptoms, medical illnesses, and medications. However, with careful attention to obtaining accurate and complete clinical data, consideration of the effects of medical and psychiatric illnesses on each other, and comprehensive treatment planning, tremendous benefit can accrue to these often very sick and suffering patients.

References

Adler LE, Griffith JM: Concurrent medical illness in the schizophrenic patient: epidemiology, diagnosis, and management. Schizophr Res 4:91–107, 1991

Allison DB, Mentore JL, Heo M, et al: Antipsychotic-induced weight gain: a comprehensive research synthesis. Am J Psychiatry 156:1686–1696, 1999

American Psychiatric Association: Diagnostic and Statistical Manual of Mental Disorders, 3rd Edition. Washington, DC, American Psychiatric Association, 1980

American Psychiatric Association: Diagnostic and Statistical Manual of Mental Disorders, 3rd Edition, Revised. Washington, DC, American Psychiatric Association, 1987

American Psychiatric Association: Diagnostic and Statistical Manual of Mental Disorders, 4th Edition. Washington, DC, American Psychiatric Association, 1994

American Psychiatric Association: Practice guidelines for the treatment of patients with delirium. Am J Psychiatry 156 (5 suppl):1–20, 1999

American Psychiatric Association: Diagnostic and Statistical Manual of Mental Disorders, 4th Edition, Text Revision. Washington, DC, American Psychiatric Association, 2000

American Psychiatric Association: The Practice of Electroconvulsive Therapy: Recommendations for Treatment, Training, and Privileging: A Task Force Report of the American Psychiatric Association, 2nd Edition. Washington, DC, American Psychiatric Association, 2001

Aweeka F, Jayeskara D, Horton M, et al: The pharmacokinetics of ziprasidone in subjects with normal and impaired renal function. Br J Clin Pharmacol 49 (suppl 1):27S–33S, 2000

Barbuto J: Preventing sudden death during a catatonic episode. Hosp Community Psychiatry 34:72–73, 1983

Bhandary A, Masand PS: Buspirone in the management of disruptive behaviors due to Huntington's disease and other neurological disorders. Psychosomatics 38:389–391, 1997

Breitbart W, Tremblay A, Gibson C: An open trial of olanzapine for the treatment of delirium in hospitalized cancer patients. Psychosomatics 43:175–182, 2002

Brown ES, Khan DA, Nejtek VA: The psychiatric side effects of corticosteroids. Ann Allergy Asthma Immunol 83:495–503, 1999

Brown SJ: Bed surfaces and pressure sore prevention: an abridged report. Orthop Nurs 20:38–40, 2001

Brownlie BEW, Rae AM, Walshe JW, et al: Psychoses associated with thyrotoxicosis—"thyrotoxic psychosis." A report of 18 cases, with statistical analysis of incidence. Eur J Endocrinol 142:438–444, 2000

Bush G, Fink M, Petrides G, et al: Catatonia. II. Treatment with lorazepam and electroconvulsive therapy. Acta Psychiatr Scand 93:137–143, 1996

Caley CF, Cooper CK: Ziprasidone: the fifth atypical antipsychotic. Ann Pharmacother 36:839–851, 2002

Carroll BT: Complications of catatonia (letter). J Clin Psychiatry 57:95, 1996

Carroll BT, Anfinson TJ, Kennedy JC, et al: Catatonic disorder due to general medical conditions. J Neuropsychiatr 6:122–133, 1994

Catalano G, Catalano MC, Rosenberg EI, et al: Catatonia, another neuropsychiatric presentation of vitamin B deficiency? Psychosomatics 39:456–460, 1998

Christopher EJ: Electroconvulsive therapy in the medically ill. Curr Psychiatry Rep 5:225–230, 2003

Clayton PJ: The epidemiology of bipolar affective disorder. Compr Psychiatry 22:31–43, 1981

Corn TH, Checkley SA: A case of recurrent mania with recurrent hyperthyroidism. Br J Psychiatry 143:74–76, 1983

Cummings JL: Organic delusions: phenomenology, anatomical correlations, and review. Br J Psychiatry 146:184–197, 1985

De Deyn PP, Carrasco MM, Deberdt W, et al: Olanzapine versus placebo in the treatment of psychosis with or without associated behavioral disturbances in patients with Alzheimer's disease. Int J Geriatr Psychiatry 19:115–126, 2004

Dixon L: Health, medical comorbidities and diabetes in schizophrenia. Drug Benefit Trends 4 (suppl):6–11, 2003

Dixon L, Weiden P, Delahanty J, et al: Prevalence and correlates of diabetes in national schizophrenia samples. Schizophr Bull 26:903–912, 2000

Duggan L, Fenton M, Dardennes RM, et al: Olanzapine for schizophrenia. Cochrane Database Syst Rev (1):CD001359, 2003

Ellen SR, Judd FK, Mijch AM, et al: Secondary mania in patients with HIV infection. Aust N Z J Psychiatry 33:353–360, 1999

Evans DL, Byerly MJ, Greer RA: Secondary mania: diagnosis and treatment. J Clin Psychiatry 56:31–37, 1995

Everson G, Lasseter KC, Anderson KE, et al: The pharmacokinetics of ziprasidone in subjects with normal and impaired hepatic function. Br J Clin Pharmacol 49 (suppl 1): 21S–26S, 2000

Feinstein A, du Boulay G, Ron MA: Psychotic illness in multiple sclerosis: a clinical and magnetic resonance imaging study. Br J Psychiatry 161:680–685, 1992

Fink M, Taylor MA: Catatonia: A Clinician's Guide to Diagnosis and Treatment. New York, Cambridge University Press, 2003

Finucane TE, Christmas C, Travis K: Tube feeding in patients with advanced dementia: a review of the evidence. JAMA 282:1365–1370, 1999

Folsom DP, McCahill M, Bartels SJ, et al: Medical comorbidity and receipt of medical care by older homeless people with schizophrenia or depression. Psychiatr Serv 53:1456–1460, 2002

Folstein SE, Folstein MF: Psychiatric features of Huntington's disease: recent approaches and findings. Psychiatr Dev 1:193–205, 1983

Fox P, Richardson J, McInnes B, et al: Effectiveness of a bed positioning program for treating older adults with knee contractures who are institutionalized. Phys Ther 80:363–372, 2000

Gafoor R, O'Keane VO: Three case reports of secondary mania: evidence supporting a right frontotemporal locus. Eur Psychiatry 18:32–33, 2003

Glosser G: Neurobehavioral aspects of movement disorders. Neurol Clin 19:535–551, 2001

Goodman WK, Charney DS: A case of alprazolam, but not lorazepam, inducing manic symptoms. J Clin Psychiatry 48:117–118, 1987

Goodwin FK, Jamison KR: Manic-Depressive Illness. New York, Oxford University Press, 1990

Gupta S, Masand PS, Kaplan D, et al: The relationship between schizophrenia and irritable bowel syndrome (IBS). Schizophr Res 23:265–268, 1997

Gupta S, Mosnik D, Black DW, et al: Tardive dyskinesia: review of treatments past, present, and future. Ann Clin Psychiatry 11:257–266, 1999

Gupta S, Masand PS, Kothari AJ: Cardiovascular side effects of novel antipsychotics. CNS Spectr 6:912–918, 2001

Halman MM, Worth JL, Sanders KM, et al: Anticonvulsant use in the treatment of manic syndromes with HIV-1 infection. J Neuropsychiatry Clin Neurosci 5:430–434, 1993

Heit JA, O'Fallon WM, Petterson TM, et al: Relative impact of risk factors for deep vein thrombosis and pulmonary embolism: a population-based study. Arch Intern Med 162:1245–1248, 2002

Helfgott SM: Stiff-man syndrome, in UpToDate. Edited by Rose BD. Wellesley, MA, UpToDate, 2003

Hill KP, Patkar AA, Weinstein SP: Folie a famille associated with amphetamine use. Jefferson Journal of Psychiatry 16:26–31, 2001

Horikawa N, Yamazaki T, Miyamoto K, et al: Treatment for delirium with risperidone: results of a prospective open trial with 10 patients. Gen Hosp Psychiatry 25:289–292, 2003

Jeste DV, Gladsjo JA, Lindamer LA, et al: Medical comorbidity in schizophrenia. Schizophr Bull 22:413–430, 1996

Jorge RE, Robinson RG, Starkstein SE, et al: Secondary mania following traumatic brain injury. Am J Psychiatry 150:916–921, 1993

Katz IR, Jeste DV, Mintzer JE, et al: Comparison of risperidone and placebo for psychosis and behavioral disturbances associated with dementia: a randomized, double-blind trial. Risperidone Study Group. J Clin Psychiatry 60:107–115, 1999

Kelleher JP, Centorrino F, Albert MJ, et al: Advances in atypical antipsychotics for the treatment of schizophrenia: new formulations and new agents. CNS Drugs 16:249–261, 2002

Kellner CH, Davenport Y, Post RM, et al: Rapidly cycling bipolar disorder and multiple sclerosis. Am J Psychiatry 141:112–113, 1984

Kessler RC, Rubinow DR, Holmes C, et al: The epidemiology of DSM-III-R bipolar I disorder in a general population survey. Psychol Med 27:1079–1089, 1997

Kilbourne AM, Justice AC, Rabeneck L, et al: General medical and psychiatric comorbidity among HIV-infected veterans in the post-HAART era. J Clin Epidemiol 54 (suppl):S22–S28, 2001

Koretz RL, Lipman TO, Klein S: American Gastroenterological Association technical review on parenteral nutrition. Gastroenterology 121:970–1001, 2001

Krauthammer C, Klerman GL: Secondary mania: manic syndromes associated with antecedent physical illness or drugs. Arch Gen Psychiatry 35:1333–1339, 1978

Krishnan KR: Biological risk factors in late life depression. Biol Psychiatry 52:185–192, 2002

Kumral E, Bayulkem G, Evyapan D, et al: Spectrum of anterior cerebral artery territory infarction: clinical and MRI findings. Eur J Neurol 9:615–624, 2002

Leibovitz A, Plotnikov G, Habot B, et al: Pathogenic colonization of oral flora in frail elderly patients fed by nasogastric tube or percutaneous enterogastric tube. J Gerontol A Biol Sci Med Sci 58:52–55, 2003

Levenson JL, Pandurangi AK: Prognosis and complications, in Catatonia: From Psychopathology to Neurobiology. Edited by Caroff SN, Mann SC, Francis A, et al. Washington, DC, American Psychiatric Publishing, 2004, pp 161–172

Li I: Feeding tubes in patients with severe dementia. Am Fam Physician 65:1605–1610, 2002

Lyketsos CG, Hanson AL, Fishman M, et al: Manic syndrome early and late in the course of HIV. Am J Psychiatry 150:326–327, 1993a

Lyketsos CG, Hanson AL, Fishman M, et al: Mood disorders in HIV infection: prevalence and risk factors in a non-epicenter of the AIDS epidemic. Am J Psychiatry 150:326–327, 1993b

Lyketsos CG, Schwartz J, Fishman M: AIDS mania. J Neuropsychiatry Clin Neurosci 9:277–279, 1997

Mann SC, Caroff SN, Bleier HR: Lethal catatonia. Am J Psychiatry 143:1374–1380, 1986

Marder SR, McQuade RD, Stock E, et al: Aripiprazole in the treatment of schizophrenia: safety and tolerability in short-term, placebo-controlled trials. Schizophr Res 61:123–136, 2003

Marik PE: Aspiration pneumonitis and aspiration pneumonia. N Engl J Med 344:665–671, 2001

Masand PS: Atypical agents in nonschizophrenic disorders. J Clin Psychiatry 59:322–328, 1998

Masand PS: Weight gain with psychotropics: size does matter. J Clin Psychiatry 60:3–4, 1999

Masand PS: Atypical antipsychotics for elderly patients with neurodegenerative disorders and medical conditions. Psychiatr Ann 30:202–208, 2000a

Masand PS: Side effects of antipsychotics in the elderly. J Clin Psychiatry 61:43–49, 2000b

Masand PS: Weight gain associated with psychotropics. Expert Opin Pharmacother 1:377–389, 2000c

Masand PS, Gupta S: Long term adverse effects of novel antipsychotics. Journal of Psychiatric Practice 6:299–309, 2000

Masand PS, Schwartz TL, Wang X, et al: Prescribing conventional antipsychotics in the era of novel antipsychotics: informed consent issues. Am J Ther 9(6):484–487, 2002

Masi G, Mucci M, Floriani C: Acute catatonia after a single dose of ecstasy (letter). J Am Acad Child Adolesc Psychiatry 41:892, 2002

McCall WV, Mann SC, Shelp FE, et al: Fatal pulmonary embolism in the catatonic syndrome: two case reports and a literature review. J Clin Psychiatry 56:21–25, 1995

McDonald WM, Krishnan KR, Doraiswamy PM, et al: Occurrence of subcortical hyperintensities in elderly subjects with mania. Psychiatry Res 40:211–220, 1991

Mendez MF: Mania in neurologic disorders. Curr Psychiatry Rep 2:440–445, 2000

Minden SL: Mood disorders in multiple sclerosis: diagnosis and treatment. J Neurovirol 6 (suppl 2):S160–S167, 2000

Mohr DC, Likosky W, Dwyer P, et al: Course of depression during the initiation of interferon beta-1a treatment for multiple sclerosis. Arch Neurol 56:1263–1265, 1999

Morioka H, Nagatomo I, Yamada K, et al: Deep venous thrombosis of the leg due to psychiatric stupor. Psychiatry Clin Neurosci 51:323–326, 1997

Muqit MMK, Rakshi JS, Shakir RA, et al: Catatonia or abulia? A difficult differential diagnosis. Mov Disord 16:360–362, 2001

Nasrallah HA, Tandon R: Efficacy, safety, and tolerability of quetiapine in patients with schizophrenia. J Clin Psychiatry 63 (suppl 13):12–20, 2002

Nemeroff CB, Kinkead B, Goldstein J: Quetiapine: preclinical studies, pharmacokinetics, drug interactions, and dosing. J Clin Psychiatry 63 (suppl 13):5–11, 2002

Pae CU, Lee SJ, Lee CU, et al: A pilot trial of quetiapine for the treatment of patients with delirium. Hum Psychopharmacol 19:125–127, 2004

Patkar AA, Kunkel EJS: Treating delirium among elderly patients. Psychiatr Serv 48:46–48, 1997

Patkar AA, Gopalakrishnan R, Lundy A, et al: Relationship between tobacco smoking and positive and negative symptoms in schizophrenia. J Nerv Ment Dis 190:604–610, 2002

Patten SB, Metz LM: Depression in multiple sclerosis. Psychother Psychosom 66:286–292, 1997

Rabins PV, Mase NL, Lucas MJ: The impact of dementia on the family. JAMA 248:333–335, 1982

Raff MH, Cho S, Dale R: A technique for positioning nasoenteral feeding tubes. JPEN J Parenter Enteral Nutr 11:210–213, 1987

Rao V, Lyketsos CG: Psychiatric aspects of traumatic brain injury. Psychiatr Clin North Am 25:43–69, 2002

Reeves RR, Torres RA: Exacerbation of psychosis by misinterpretation of physical symptoms. South Med J 96:702–704, 2003

Regestein QR, Alpert JS, Reich P: Sudden catatonic stupor with disastrous outcome. JAMA 238:618–620, 1977

Regier DA, Farmer ME, Rae DS, et al: Comorbidity of mental disorders with alcohol and other drug abuse. Results from the Epidemiologic Catchment Area (ECA) study. JAMA 264:2511–2518, 1990

Reichman WE: Neuropsychiatric aspects of cerebrovascular diseases and tumors, in Comprehensive Textbook of Psychiatry/VI, 6th Edition. Edited by Kaplan HI, Sadock BJ. Baltimore, MD, Williams & Wilkins, 1995, pp 189–190

Robinson MJ, Levenson JL: The use of psychotropics in the medically ill. Curr Psychiatry Rep 2:247–255, 2000

Robinson RG, Boston JD, Starkstein SE, et al: Comparison of mania and depression after brain injury: causal factors. Am J Psychiatry 145:172–178, 1988

Rosenblatt A, Leroi I: Neuropsychiatry of Huntington's disease and other basal ganglia disorders. Psychosomatics 41:24–30, 2000

Rundell JR, Wise MG: Causes of organic mood disorder. J Neuropsychiatry 1:398–400, 1989

Ryan MC, Collins P, Thakore JH: Impaired fasting glucose tolerance in first-episode, drug-naive patients with schizophrenia. Am J Psychiatry 160:284–289, 2003

Sachdev P: Schizophrenia-like psychosis and epilepsy: the status of the association. Am J Psychiatry 155:325–336, 1998

Sadovnick AD, Eisen K, Ebers GC, et al: Cause of death in patients attending multiple sclerosis clinics. Neurology 41:1193–1196, 1991

Sasaki Y, Matsuyama T, Inoue S, et al: A prospective, open-label, flexible-dose study of quetiapine in the treatment of delirium. J Clin Psychiatry 64:1316–1321, 2003

Schatz RA: Olanzapine for psychotic and behavioral disturbances in Alzheimer disease. Ann Pharmacother 37:1321–1324, 2003

Schiffer RB, Wineman NM, Weitkamp LR: Association between bipolar affective disorder and multiple sclerosis. Am J Psychiatry 143:94–95, 1986

Schwartz TL, Masand PS: The role of atypical antipsychotics in the treatment of delirium. Psychosomatics 43:171–174, 2002

Serper MR, Alert M, Richardson N, et al: Clinical effects of recent cocaine use on patients with acute schizophrenia. Am J Psychiatry 152:1464–1469, 1995

Shay K: Infectious complications of dental and periodontal diseases in the elderly population. Clin Infect Dis 34:1215–1223, 2002

Shukla S, Cook BL, Muherjee S, et al: Mania following head trauma. Am J Psychiatry 144:93–96, 1987

Shulman K, Post F: Bipolar affective disorder in old age. Br J Psychiatry 136:26–32, 1980

Shulman KI, Mackenzie S, Hardy B: The clinical use of lithium carbonate in old age: a review. Prog Neuropsychopharmacol Biol Psychiatry 11:159–164, 1987

Shulman KI, Tohen M, Satlin A, et al: Mania compared with unipolar depression in old age. Am J Psychiatry 149:341–345, 1992

Sibisi CD: Sex differences in the age of onset of bipolar affective illness. Br J Psychiatry 156:842–845, 1990

Sipahimalani A, Masand PS: Olanzapine in the treatment of delirium. Psychosomatics 39:422–430, 1998

Sipahimalani A, Sime R, Masand PS: Treatment of delirium with risperidone. International Journal of Geriatric Psychopharmacology 1:24–26, 1997

Skrobik YK, Bergeron N, Dumont M, et al: Olanzapine vs haloperidol: treating delirium in a critical care setting. Intensive Care Med 30:444–449, 2004

Slater E, Beard AW, Glithero E: The schizophrenialike psychoses of epilepsy. Br J Psychiatry 109:95–150, 1963

Snoek E, Van Peer A, Sack M: Influence of age, renal and liver impairment on the pharmacokinetics of risperidone in man. Psychopharmacology (Berl) 122:223–229, 1995

Snowdon J: A retrospective case-note study of bipolar disorder in old age. Br J Psychiatry 158:485–490, 1991

Spicer CC, Hare EH, Slater E: Neurotic and psychotic forms of depressive illness: evidence from age-incidence in a national sample. Br J Psychiatry 123:535–541, 1973

Starkstein SE, Robinson RG, Price TR: Comparison of cortical and subcortical lesions in the production of poststroke mood disorders. Brain 110:1045–1059, 1987

Starkstein SE, Federoff P, Robinson RG: Manic-depressive and pure manic states after brain lesions. Biol Psychiatry 29:149–158, 1991

Stasiek C, Zetin M: Organic manic disorders. Psychosomatics 26:394–402, 1985

Stone K: Mania in the elderly. Br J Psychiatry 155:220–224, 1989

Stoudemire A, Moran MG, Fogel BS: Psychotropic drug use in the medically ill. Part II. Psychosomatics 32:34–46, 1991

Sukov RJ: Thrombophlebitis as a complication of severe catatonia. JAMA 220:587–578, 1972

Swayze VW, Andreasen NC, Alliger RJ, et al: Structural brain abnormalities in bipolar affective disorder. Arch Gen Psychiatry 47:1054–1059, 1990

Tateno A, Jorge RE, Robinson RG: Clinical correlates of aggressive behavior after traumatic brain injury. J Neuropsychiatry Clin Neurosci 15:155–160, 2003

Thomas DR: Prevention and treatment of pressure ulcers: what works? what doesn't? Cleve Clin J Med 68:704–721, 2001

Turpie AG, Chin BS, Lip GY: Venous thromboembolism: pathophysiology, clinical features, and prevention. BMJ 325:887–890, 2002

Villani S, Weitzel WD: Secondary mania (letter). Arch Gen Psychiatry 36:1031, 1979

Wada H, Nakajoh K, Satoh-Nakagawa T, et al: Risk factors of aspiration pneumonia in Alzheimer's disease patients. Gerontology 47:271–276, 2001

Wada K, Yamada N, Sato T, et al: Corticosteroid-induced psychotic and mood disorders. Psychosomatics 42:461–466, 2001

Weilberg JB, Sachs G, Falk WE: Triazolam-induced brief episodes of secondary mania in a depressed patient. J Clin Psychiatry 48:492–493, 1987

Wiart L: Post-cerebrovascular stroke depression. Encephale 3:51–54, 1997

Wirshing DA, Pierre JM, Erhart SM, et al: Understanding the new and evolving profile of adverse drug effects in schizophrenia. Psychiatr Clin North Am 26:165–190, 2003

12 Anxiety Disorders

Steven A. Epstein, M.D.

Daniel Hicks, M.D.

ANXIETY IS AN extremely common problem in primary care and specialty medical settings. Because the lifetime prevalence rate of any anxiety disorder in the general population is approximately 25% (Kessler et al. 1994), many medically ill patients will have concurrent anxiety unrelated to the experience of medical illness. The profound physical and psychological stressors of medical illness often precipitate anxiety, particularly in individuals with preexisting vulnerability. Therefore, when evaluating a medically ill patient, the psychosomatic medicine psychiatrist should always determine if anxiety symptoms are present. Although the presence of anxiety may reflect a mood disorder or other psychiatric disorder, formal assessment for the presence of an anxiety disorder should be considered in all patients. Unfortunately, medical professionals often neglect to screen for these highly treatable disorders. Even when they recognize anxiety, some practitioners minimize its significance by considering it to be a "normal" response to the uncertainty and adversity associated with having a disease.

Once the psychiatrist has determined that a patient has anxiety, the more complex task of determining etiology must be undertaken. Although it is advisable to use a biopsychosocial approach to formulation, there are surprisingly few data regarding medical and pharmacological causes of anxiety. Nonetheless, the psychiatrist must carefully assess their potential etiological roles. Finally, it is important to consider medical comorbidity when designing pharmacological and psychotherapeutic treatment plans. In this chapter, we discuss each of these topics. For detailed reviews of anxiety among individuals with specific medical comorbidities, the reader is referred to the corresponding chapters in this text.

General Features and Diagnostic Considerations

The symptom of anxiety may reflect the presence of an anxiety disorder but may also be a symptom of another psychiatric disorder such as depression. In the medical setting, it is also important to remember that anxiety may be a symptom of delirium, dementia, or a somatoform disorder such as hypochondriasis. Anxiety may also be due to a medical disorder (e.g., hyperthyroidism) or a medication side effect. Furthermore, some symptoms and signs of medical disorders (e.g., tachycardia, dyspnea, and diaphoresis) may be mistaken for anxiety.

An interview using DSM-IV-TR criteria (American Psychiatric Association 2000) is the gold standard for diagnosis of an anxiety disorder. In primary care settings, it is often useful to ask brief screening questions to determine whether a full diagnostic assessment is necessary. The Primary Care Evaluation of Mental Disorders (PRIME-MD) Patient Health Questionnaire is a valuable screening instrument. This self-administered survey includes screening questions for panic disorder, general health worries, and posttraumatic stress disorder (Spitzer et al. 1999). Other scales specifically designed to assess anxiety include the Hamilton Rating Scale for Anxiety (Hamilton 1959), State-Trait Anxiety Inventory (Spielberger et al. 1970), Beck Anxiety Inventory (Beck et al. 1988), Panic Disorder Severity Scale (Houck et al. 2002), Clinician-Administered PTSD Scale (Weathers et al. 2001), and Yale-Brown Obsessive Compulsive Scale (Goodman et al. 1989).

Many patients with anxiety do not present to mental health providers. Of all anxiety disorder visits in the National Ambulatory Medical Care Survey in 1998, 48% were to primary care physicians (Harman et al. 2002). Among a sample of 3,000 adult primary care patients, 11% were diagnosed with an anxiety disorder (Spitzer et al. 1999). Individuals with chronic medical conditions such as arthritis, heart disease, diabetes, and hypertension are more likely to have anxiety disorders (Wells et al. 1988, 1989). Unfortunately, many individuals treated in primary care settings do not receive appropriate care for anxiety (Roy-Byrne et al. 1999; Young et al. 2001). Some physicians lack the skill or time to treat anxiety. In addition, some primary care patients are reluctant to consider either psychosocial or pharmacological treatment for their conditions (Hazlett-Stevens et al. 2002).

Anxiety disorders have clearly been shown to impair functioning and well-being among individuals with chronic medical conditions (Sherbourne et al. 1996). Anxiety may be a risk factor for the development of medical illness and may physiologically exacerbate some conditions (e.g., angina, arrhythmias, movement disorders, labile hypertension, and irritable bowel syndrome). There is some evidence that phobic anxiety is a risk factor for fatal coronary artery disease (Kawachi et al. 1994), but some studies have shown no relationship between anxiety and mortality (e.g., Herrmann et al. 2000; Lane et al. 2001). Anxiety may also lead to increased risk of developing hypertension in the future (Jonas et al. 1997). Although depression is more clearly a predictor of poor adherence to medical treatment (DiMatteo et al. 2000), in some individuals excessive anxiety about one's health might reduce adherence (e.g., due to fear of visiting a physician). Anxiety may lead some individuals to refuse diagnostic procedures or surgery and even to sign out of the hospital against medical advice.

Specific Anxiety Disorders

Panic Disorder

Primary care patients with panic attacks (see Table 12–1 for diagnostic criteria) are high utilizers of medical care (Roy-Byrne et al. 1999). In particular, many patients who present with chest pain are found to have panic disorder. For example, in one recent study panic disorder was found in approximately 25% of 441 patients presenting to an emergency room with chest pain (Fleet et al. 1996). Researchers estimate that at least one-third of individuals with chest pain and normal coronary arteries have panic disorder (e.g., Beitman et al. 1989; Cormier et al. 1988; Fleet et al. 1998; Maddock et al. 1998). These rates contrast with lifetime prevalence rates of 3.5% found in the

---

TABLE 12–1.   DSM-IV-TR criteria for panic attack

Physical symptoms
Palpitations, pounding heart, or accelerated heart rate
Sweating
Trembling or shaking
Sensations of shortness of breath or smothering
Feeling of choking
Chest pain or discomfort
Nausea or abdominal distress
Feeling dizzy, unsteady, lightheaded, or faint
Paresthesias (numbness or tingling sensations)
Chills or hot flushes

Cognitive symptoms
Derealization (feelings of unreality) or depersonalization (being detached from oneself)
Fear of losing control or going crazy
Fear of dying

Source.   American Psychiatric Association 2000.

National Comorbidity Survey (Kessler et al. 1994). A recent meta-analysis identified five variables that correlate with higher rates of panic disorder among individuals seeking treatment for chest pain in emergency rooms or cardiology clinics: 1) absence of coronary artery disease; 2) atypical quality of chest pain; 3) female sex; 4) younger age; and 5) a high level of self-reported anxiety (Huffman and Pollack 2003).

Patients with benign palpitations have high rates of panic disorder (Barsky et al. 1994; Ehlers et al. 2000). One explanation for such high rates is that individuals with panic disorder may have heightened cardiac sensitivity to symptoms such as chest pain and palpitations (Barsky 2001; Mayou 1998). Panic symptoms may also be linked to physiological changes in peripheral organ systems. For example, low vagal tone and decreased heart rate variability may be biological traits that predispose an individual to the development of panic disorder (Friedman and Thayer 1998). Panic attacks may be difficult to distinguish symptomatically from paroxysmal atrial tachycardia; both occur frequently in young, otherwise healthy women, and they are frequently comorbid. Before palpitations are attributed to anxiety, it is important for patients to undergo cardiac evaluation (e.g., ambulatory electrocardiographic monitoring) to rule out arrhythmias (Lessmeier et al. 1997; Zimetbaum and Josephson 1998).

Panic disorder also leads patients to present to other medical specialists. For example, patients who present for evaluation of dizziness have elevated rates of this disorder (Simon et al. 1998; M.B. Stein et al. 1994). Panic disorder is also common among individuals with irritable bowel syndrome who present for treatment (Walker et al. 1995).

In patients with irritable bowel syndrome, anxiety may be due to locus coeruleus activation by afferent signals from the bowel. Thus, with irritable bowel syndrome and other medical disorders such as asthma, anxiety symptoms may be due to central nervous system responses to afferent information from the viscera (Zaubler and Katon 1998).

Recent work has shown that collaborative care interventions can improve outcomes for primary care patients with panic disorder. In one model, collaborative care consisted of patient education, treatment with paroxetine, two visits with an on-site consulting psychiatrist, and follow-up telephone calls. Patients who received this intervention, compared with those receiving usual primary care, had significantly fewer days with anxiety (Katon et al. 2002; Roy-Byrne et al. 2001).

For an excellent review of panic disorder in the general medical setting, see the article by Zaubler and Katon (1998). (For further discussion of panic disorder in cardiac patients, see Chapter 19, "Heart Disease.")

Posttraumatic Stress Disorder

The National Comorbidity Survey estimated the lifetime prevalence of DSM-III-R (American Psychiatric Association 1987) posttraumatic stress disorder (PTSD) in the general population to be 7.8% (Kessler et al. 1995). Prevalence in medical settings appears to be higher. For example, in one primary care sample the current prevalence of PTSD was approximately 12% (M.B. Stein et al. 2000). Trauma victims and individuals with PTSD are frequent users of health care. Factors contributing to increased medical symptom reporting and health care utilization include increased levels of somatization, comorbidity with depression, the association of hyperarousal with cardiovascular complaints, and heightened perception of autonomic changes (Golding 1994; Wolfe et al. 1994).

It is not surprising that PTSD symptoms are common among individuals who experience acute physical traumas. For example, burn victims have been reported to have PTSD at rates ranging from 20% to 45% (Difede et al. 2002; Perry et al. 1992; Roca et al. 1992; Yu and Dimsdale 1999). In one study, 30%–40% of survivors of a motor vehicle crash or an assault reported PTSD symptoms for months after the trauma. Higher symptom levels were associated with female gender, stimulant intoxication, and greater prior trauma (Zatzick et al. 2002). PTSD has also been reported among individuals with automatic implantable cardioverter defibrillators (Hamner et al. 1999). Intensive care unit experiences can result in PTSD symptoms. In one study, recall of "delusional memories" (paranoia, hallucinations, or nightmares presumably due to delirium) from an intensive care unit

hospitalization was shown to be associated with the development of PTSD symptoms (C. Jones et al. 2001). PTSD symptoms may occur after many other medical conditions or treatments, including myocardial infarction and the diagnosis of HIV infection. For a comprehensive review, see the article by Tedstone and Tarrier (2003).

Acute stress disorder may also occur after life-threatening illnesses or injuries. In one study, 19% of 83 hospitalized adult burn patients developed acute stress disorder within 2 weeks of injury. The presence of acute stress disorder strongly predicted the presence of PTSD at least 6 months later (Difede et al. 2002). Similarly, the degree of fright experienced at the time of myocardial infarction was associated with PTSD symptoms 3 months later (Bennett et al. 2001).

Life-threatening illness such as cancer is a stressor that can precipitate PTSD (Kangas et al. 2002; M.Y. Smith et al. 1999). However, this trauma is different from more usual PTSD stressors such as rape in two principal ways: 1) the threat arises from one's own body; and 2) once the patient has been treated, the ongoing stressor is often not the memory of past events, but the fear of recurrence (B.L. Green et al. 1997). Some researchers have speculated that the trauma associated with the diagnosis and treatment of serious medical illness might be sufficient to cause PTSD even in the absence of a catastrophic event. The rate of current PTSD in cancer survivors is approximately 3%–5%, but many more patients experience some symptoms of PTSD (Alter et al. 1996; Andrykowski and Cordova 1998; B.L. Green et al. 1998). The likelihood of developing PTSD symptoms after cancer treatment has been shown to be increased among individuals with past trauma, prior psychiatric diagnoses, lower levels of social support, and recent life stressors (B.L. Green et al. 2000; Jacobsen et al. 2002). As is the case with other medical illnesses, severity of cancer is not a strong predictor of the development of PTSD.

Other Anxiety Disorders

There are relatively few studies regarding the characteristics and significance of other anxiety disorders in medical settings. Although the 12-month prevalence rate of generalized anxiety disorder (GAD) in community samples is approximately 3% (Kessler et al. 1994), an international study found the 1-month prevalence rate in primary care to be 7.9%. In that study, GAD was usually comorbid with other psychiatric conditions (Maier et al. 2000). GAD may also lead to excess health care utilization (G.N. Jones et al. 2001). GAD symptoms such as fatigue, muscle tension, and insomnia often lead the patient to present initially to a primary care physician. As is the case with depression, it is important for physicians to consider GAD in the differential diagnosis for such patients. A simple screening question can be extremely useful in helping the physician to determine if GAD may be present, for example, "In the past 4 weeks how often have you been bothered by feeling nervous, anxious, on edge, or worrying a lot about different things?" (Spitzer et al. 1999).

Although specific phobias are quite common, they rarely come to the attention of medical professionals. Exceptions include blood-injection-injury phobias and claustrophobia. Blood-injection-injury phobias may lead to fainting during medical procedures or to avoidance of injections and blood tests. In the Baltimore Epidemiologic Catchment Area study, approximately 3% of the sample was found to have one of these phobias. Of that sample of 60 individuals, 23% reported fear of blood; 47%, fear of injections; and 78%, fear of dentists. Although this condition may have serious implications for an affected individual, little is known about its public health significance (Bienvenu and Eaton 1998). Syncope or presyncope in individuals with health care phobias may be due to an underlying predisposition toward neurally mediated syncope (Accurso et al. 2001). Claustrophobia comes to medical attention most commonly when individuals need a magnetic resonance imaging (MRI) procedure. The procedure commonly causes anxiety that is severe enough to require sedation (e.g., with a short-acting benzodiazepine such as midazolam or lorazepam; McIsaac et al. 1998; Murphy and Brunberg 1997). Behavioral techniques such as relaxation exercises may also be helpful.

Compulsive skin picking or scratching may be a manifestation of obsessive-compulsive disorder (OCD). In one study of 31 individuals with self-injurious skin picking, 52% were found to have OCD (Wilhelm et al. 1999). However, in another study of 34 patients with psychogenic excoriation, OCD was not a common disorder (Arnold et al. 1998). (For further discussion, see Chapter 29, "Dermatology.")

Causes of Anxiety in the Medically Ill

In evaluating an anxious patient who is also medically ill, it is essential for the psychiatrist to consider the full range of potential causes of anxiety. In addition to the possibility of a preexisting primary anxiety disorder, three categories of causes of anxiety should be considered for every patient. First, is the patient having a psychological reaction to the experience of medical illness? Second, is the patient's anxiety directly due to the biological effects of a substance? Third, is the patient's anxiety directly due to

the biological effects of a medical illness? As is the case for many medically ill patients, the etiology of anxiety is often multifactorial and may vary with the course of illness.

Anxiety as a Psychological Reaction to the Experience of Illness

The importance of one's health added to the often unavoidable uncertainty associated with medical illness leads many medically ill patients to feel anxious. Particularly for individuals with a predisposition to anxiety, the psychosocial stress of illness may be sufficient to induce an anxiety disorder. Just as when evaluating a depressed patient, psychiatrists should never make assumptions regarding the cause of anxiety in an individual patient. For example, it is easy to assume that the patient who is awaiting cardiac surgery is afraid of dying, when in fact the patient might actually be more concerned about potential disability. When approaching the anxious patient, the psychiatrist should consider all potential psychological causes of anxiety. The following discussion reviews the major causes among medically ill populations. For seminal reviews of this topic, the reader is referred to the work of Strain and Grossman (1975) and Kahana and Bibring (1964) (see also Chapter 5, "Psychological Responses to Illness").

Uncertainty Regarding Medical Diagnosis

Some individuals worry excessively that they might have a serious illness. Routine evaluations may cause anxiety, especially in those with a personal or family history of illness. For example, an individual with a family history of breast cancer might become quite anxious in the period preceding routine mammography. In one study, 8% of first-degree relatives of women with breast cancer were so anxious that they performed daily breast self-examinations (Epstein et al. 1997). Anxiety may also occur during the period between initial evaluation and receipt of the definitive result—for example, after the physician tells the patient, "It's probably nothing, but let's perform a brain MRI just to be sure." Prolonged uncertainty regarding diagnosis is even more anxiety-provoking, such as when the patient is told, "Your PSA [prostate-specific antigen] is slightly elevated, but at this point we should simply wait and reevaluate your level in a few months." Although physicians are acutely aware that there is significant uncertainty inherent in medical diagnoses, patients are generally not reassured by this fact.

Uncertainty Regarding Medical Prognosis

For most medical illnesses and medical procedures, prognosis is uncertain. Many patients will experience ongoing fears of recurrence, especially when they have illnesses that frequently do recur (e.g., arrhythmias, cancer, and multiple sclerosis). Similarly, many fear that their treatments will fail, even if they are initially successful. Examples include fear of rejection of a transplanted organ and development of graft-versus-host disease. Physicians often realize that the potential for a poor prognosis—for example, in cases of relatively advanced cancer—often leads to anxiety. However, it is important to keep in mind that patients who have favorable prognoses often experience anxiety. For example, a 95% cure rate is reassuring to many patients, but some will have difficulty coping with the prospect of a 5% recurrence rate. Complicating the problem is the fact that prognoses may be inaccurate when they are derived from aggregate data, which may have been based on treatments that are now outmoded. For patients who learn about their prognoses through personal medical searches, physicians may be able to provide reassurance by reminding the anxious patients of this information: "You are not a statistic; those data were published before the newest treatments became available."

Anxiety About One's Body

Many individuals experience anxiety regarding the future effects of illness on their bodies (see Strain and Grossman 1975). Patients may fear that they will lose body parts (e.g., due to amputation). Ongoing fears of amputation are particularly problematic for some patient populations (e.g., those with diabetes mellitus and peripheral vascular disease). Others may fear that they will lose functional capacities or that they will become overly dependent on others. For example, individuals with diabetes mellitus may fear eventual blindness, patients with chronic obstructive pulmonary disease may fear "being hooked to a breathing machine," and men with prostate cancer may fear impotence. Others are afraid of the experience of pain. For example, individuals with metastatic cancer are often afraid that they will have unremitting, severe pain. Knowledge of these fears can help the physician to provide appropriate reassurances (e.g., that pain will be aggressively treated).

Fear of Death

All individuals, regardless of their physical health, fear death at some time in their lives. The experience of physical illness often heightens that fear, because everyone either has faced life-threatening illness or has known someone who has died from a physical illness. Physicians must be comfortable assessing fears of death in both patients and their families. This assessment must include an exploration of specific reasons for fear of death (e.g., a patient may fear death from childbirth because that occurred many years earlier to a close relative). Exploration of the reasons for an irrationally high estimate of risk of death may lead to straightforward reassurance. Assessment of death anxiety should also include the opportunity for individuals to discuss existential thoughts about dying (e.g., reflections about the meaning of one's life [Adelbratt and Strang 2000]). When interviewing the patient with a fear of dying, the physician should assess for particular dying-related fears (e.g., a patient may actually be at peace with dying but may be afraid that her family will not be able to survive without her). In that case, involvement of the family may lead to reassurance and a more peaceful dying process (see also Chapter 40, "Palliative Care").

Anxiety About the Impact of Illness on Identity and Livelihood

Even if illness alone is not sufficient to cause anxiety, patients may be concerned about the potential impact of illness on their ability to work, to perform essential household functions, or to maintain income. Uncertainties regarding medical reimbursements may make insured individuals justifiably concerned. The uninsured are often so anxious about how they would pay for medical procedures that they avoid medical visits altogether. Patients may be anxious that the costs of medical treatment might cause financial burdens for their families, and they may decline treatment for this reason. In these situations, meetings with family members and health care financial counselors may help to assuage unjustifiable fears that treatments will cause more harm than good.

Anxiety Regarding Strangers and Being Alone in the Hospital

Individuals with medical illnesses become anxious even when their own personal physician performs a medical procedure. Thus, it is not unusual for an acutely ill patient to become intensely anxious when asked to trust his or her life to the new physician he or she has just met in the emergency room or the intensive care unit. Patients who are so anxious that they refuse a medical procedure may be labeled as noncompliant when, in fact, fear is the underlying explanation. As noted by Muskin (1995), acceptance of the involvement of unfamiliar clinicians may be particularly difficult for individuals with preexisting problems with trust (e.g., those with paranoia or borderline personality disorder). Similarly, it is often difficult for some patients to tolerate being alone in the hospital. Because many individuals regress while hospitalized, it is not surprising that patients with dependency needs might become unduly anxious when left alone in an unfamiliar environment.

Anxiety Regarding Negative Reactions From Physicians

Many individuals with medical illness worry about their physician's opinion of them. Excessive concern may lead to reluctance to seek health care. Persons who feel guilty for not following their physician's recommendations might cancel appointments for fear of being scolded (e.g. for failure to lose weight, stop smoking, or check blood sugar levels more reliably). Similarly, some individuals' anxiety might lead them to deny or fail to disclose important information (e.g., regarding sexual risk factors or level of alcohol intake). Anxiety may be particularly prominent among patients who have caused or aggravated their own illness. It is important for the physician to be vigilant for clues that a patient might have excessive anxiety. Awareness of negative countertransference is essential; it is appropriate to provide consistent, firm reminders of the need for proper medical care, but harsh criticism is unwarranted and may contribute to poor adherence.

Substance-Induced Anxiety

In evaluating the anxious medical patient, it is important to consider whether medications or medication withdrawal might be contributory. Because they can be obtained without prescriptions, caffeine and over-the-counter sympathomimetics are common causes of anxiety in the general population. Caffeine is widely used and commonly causes anxiety. It may be present in significant quantities in coffee, tea, caffeinated soda, caffeinated water (e.g., Java-Water), and coffee ice cream, as well as in over-the-counter preparations for alertness (e.g., NoDoz), weight loss, and headache (e.g., Excedrin). Even at low doses, caffeine may induce anxiety in susceptible individuals (Bruce et al. 1992). In individuals with anxiety disorders, reduction of caffeine intake often reduces anxiety symptoms (G. A. Smith 1988). Over-the-counter sympathomimetics used as decongestants (e.g., pseudoephedrine) frequently cause anxiety, and tachyphylaxis develops rapidly. Some individuals may use large quantities in the form of nasal spray. Similarly, the widely used herbal preparation ephedra may also cause anxiety.

The most important medication classes that are associated with anxiety are summarized in Table 12–2, which includes examples of specific medications in each class. Where appropriate, notes have been added for further clarification. General references in this area are the book by Brown and Stoudemire (1998), *The Medical Letter on Drugs and Therapeutics* ("Drugs That May Cause Psychiatric Symptoms" 2002), and the *Physicians' Desk Reference* (2003).

Anxiety Secondary to General Medical Conditions

Many medical problems have been reported to cause anxiety, but their significance is in some cases uncertain due to reporting bias and lack of controlled studies (Caine and Lyness 2000; Popkin and Tucker 1992). Nonetheless, it is important for the psychosomatic medicine physician to consider medical causes of anxiety when evaluating an anxious patient. It is particularly important to evaluate medical causes when the history is not typical for a primary anxiety disorder (e.g., lack of personal or family history, lack of psychosocial stressors) and when the onset of anxiety is at a later age (Pollack et al. 1998). In addition, it is important to evaluate medical causes when the anxiety is accompanied by disproportionate physical symptoms (e.g., marked dyspnea, tachycardia, or tremor) or atypical physical symptoms (e.g., syncope, confusion, or focal neurological symptoms).

It is important for the clinician to keep in mind the distinction between anxiety that is physiologically secondary to a general medical condition and anxiety that is comorbid with, or a psychological reaction to, a general medical condition. (For example, hyperthyroidism appears to biologically cause anxiety, whereas diabetes mellitus usually does not.) The DSM-IV-TR diagnosis of anxiety due to a general medical condition refers to the former, not the latter. This difference has not been clearly articulated in some reviews in this area, and it can also be confusing for patients. One source of confusion results from the assumption of causality when there is an epidemiological association between anxiety and a specific medical condition. For example, in one young adult cohort, the odds ratio of any anxiety disorder among individuals with migraine was 2.7 (Merikangas et al. 1990), but the onset of anxiety disorders generally precedes that of migraine (Merikangas and Stevens 1997).

Components of the medical evaluation of the anxious patient should be determined by the patient's specific medical symptoms. For example, it may be necessary to obtain electroencephalograms and a neurological consultation for a patient with seizure-like episodes. The general evaluation of all anxious patients should include the following elements (Colon and Popkin 2002; Pollack et al. 1998):

1. History and physical examination, including neurological examination
2. Evaluation of the potential role of medications and substances (see Table 12–2)
3. Screening diagnostic studies (e.g., routine blood chemistries, complete blood cell count, calcium concentration, thyroid hormone levels, electrocardiogram)

TABLE 12–2.   Substances that may cause anxiety

Class	Examples	Notes
Androgens	Nandrolone Methyltestosterone	Most problems occur when abused
Angiotensin-converting enzyme inhibitors	Captopril Lisinopril	Often stimulating
Anticholinergics	Atropine Benztropine Dicyclomine Hyoscyamine	
Antidepressants	Serotonin reuptake inhibitors Bupropion Tricyclic agents	
Antiemetics	Prochlorperazine Promethazine	Anxiety may actually be akathisia
Antimigraine agents	Sumatriptan Naratriptan	
Antimycobacterial agents	Isoniazid	
Antineoplastic agents	Vinblastine Ifosfamide	
Antipsychotics	Thiothixene Haloperidol	Anxiety may actually be akathisia
Antiviral agents	Acyclovir Didanosine Foscarnet Ganciclovir Efavirenz	
Beta-adrenergic agonists	Albuterol Metaproterenol	
Cannabinoids	Dronabinol	
Class I antiarrhythmics	Lidocaine Procainamide Quinidine	
Corticosteroids	Prednisone Methylprednisolone	
Dopaminergic agents	Carbidopa-levodopa Amantadine Pergolide	
Estrogens	Conjugated estrogens Ethinyl estradiol Levonorgestrel implant	May cause panic attacks and depression
Gonadotropin-releasing hormone active agents	Leuprolide	
Histamine H_2 receptor antagonists	Cimetidine Famotidine Nizatidine	
Interferons	Interferon-alfa Interferon-beta	
Methylxanthines	Caffeine Theophylline	

TABLE 12–2. Substances that may cause anxiety *(continued)*

Class	Examples	Notes
Sympathomimetics	Ephedrine Epinephrine Phenylephrine nasal Pseudoephedrine	
Nonsteroidal anti-inflammatory drugs	Indomethacin Naproxen Salicylates	
Opiates	Meperidine	Owing to drug withdrawal, meperidine may directly cause anxiety with progression to delirium (Kaiko et al. 1983)
Opioid antagonists	Naltrexone	Observe for opiate withdrawal
Progestins	Medroxyprogesterone acetate Norethindrone	
Prokinetic agents	Metoclopramide	Anxiety may be due to akathisia
Psychostimulants	Methylphenidate Dextroamphetamine	
Sedative-hypnotics	Benzodiazepines Barbiturates Alcohol	Anxiety due to drug withdrawal

In the following subsections, we discuss common medical conditions that are associated with anxiety for which data are strongly supportive of a causal relationship.

Thyroid Disease

Anxiety symptoms commonly occur among individuals with thyroid disease (Jadresic 1990). Trzepacz et al. (1988) found that 7 of 13 patients with untreated Graves' disease met research diagnostic criteria for GAD and major depression. In another study, 15 of 32 hyperthyroid patients reported increased anxiety symptoms compared with baseline levels (Kathol and Delahunt 1986) (see also Chapter 23, "Endocrine and Metabolic Disorders").

Hyperthyroidism may be difficult to distinguish from a primary anxiety disorder. Signs that may be suggestive of thyrotoxicosis include persistent tachycardia, palms that are warm and dry (not cold and clammy), and fatigue accompanied by the desire to be active (Colon and Popkin 2002). However, data differentiating the two are not definitive in this regard (see Iacovides et al. 2000), and much of the research in this area is not current. Some individuals with hyperthyroidism may also have cognitive impairment. Improvement in anxiety usually parallels successful treatment of the hyperthyroidism (Kathol et al. 1986). Therefore, specific antianxiety treatment may not be necessary. Nonetheless, antianxiety treatment should be considered during normalization of thyroid hormone levels, particularly for individuals with moderate to severe symptoms. Beta-blockers, which are used routinely for acute treatment of hyperthyroidism, will relieve peripheral manifestations of anxiety.

Because thyroid dysfunction is so common among individuals with anxiety, a screening thyroid-stimulating hormone (TSH) assay should be considered for patients with new-onset anxiety disorders and treatment-resistant anxiety, particularly when the anxiety is generalized and accompanied by prominent physical symptoms. If the TSH level is abnormal, further evaluation of the thyroid axis is recommended (e.g., free thyroxine index or free thyroxine measurement).

There are a number of putative mechanisms for the association between abnormalities of the thyroid axis and mood or anxiety symptoms. A blunted TSH response to thyrotropin-releasing hormone stimulation occurs in up to one-third of depressed patients, many of whom may have concomitant anxiety symptoms (Joffe 2000). The adrenergic overreactivity that accompanies hyperthyroidism provides a ready explanation for its association with anxiety. Finally, thyroid hormones interact with brain neurotransmitters (e.g., the serotonergic and noradrenergic systems; Altshuler et al. 2001). Nonetheless, the association between the thyroid axis and anxiety is not well understood.

Anxiety has been reported to be a symptom of hypothyroidism (Hall and Hall 1999), but data are minimal. Its association may be better explained by the association between depression and hypothyroidism, in which anxiety is conceptualized as a symptom of depression as opposed to a direct biological result of a hypothyroid state.

Pulmonary Disease

Patients with pulmonary disease often experience symptoms of anxiety. Rates of panic disorder among individuals with asthma and chronic obstructive pulmonary disease are higher than among the general population (e.g., Bussing et al. 1996; Yellowlees et al. 1987). The psychological stress and uncertainty of living with asthma certainly make important contributions to this association. In addition, it is essential to consider physiological factors intrinsic to asthma (Yellowlees and Kalucy 1990). For example, both hypercapnia and hyperventilation may lead to symptoms of a panic attack; in one model, hypercapnia may lead to increased locus coeruleus activity, which could cause panic and hyperventilation (Carr 1998; Zaubler and Katon 1998). Furthermore, carbon dioxide inhalation has been shown to precipitate panic attacks among individuals with panic disorder. Asthma may also be associated with panic attacks through a process of classical conditioning. In this paradigm, because a severe asthma attack is so terrifying, a future sensation of mild dyspnea might precipitate a full-blown panic episode (Carr et al. 1992). In addition, anxiety may worsen asthma, thereby contributing to a vicious circle in which pulmonary and anxiety symptoms exacerbate each other (Carr 1998). Several asthma medications may cause anxiety (see Table 12–2). Pulmonary emboli may also lead to symptoms of anxiety (Tapson 2000); this diagnosis is more easily missed when the emboli are small (see also Chapter 20, "Lung Disease").

Parkinson's Disease

Anxiety is often seen in individuals with Parkinson's disease (Walsh and Bennett 2001). Most studies of the prevalence of anxiety disorders among patients with Parkinson's disease involve small samples, but they indicate that these disorders are much more common among Parkinson's disease patients than in the general population (Richard et al. 1996). Anxiety often appears after the manifestations of symptoms of Parkinson's disease. For example, some individuals may develop social anxiety disorder symptoms because they are embarrassed about manifestations of the Parkinson's disease (e.g., tremor) (American Psychiatric Association 2000). Anxiety may also be due to the uncertainty associated with Parkinson's disease, with respect to both day-to-day functioning and long-term prognosis. Some authors have found that anxiety may be worse during "off" periods compared with "on" periods, but findings are not definitive (Richard et al. 1996; Siemens et al. 1993; Vazquez et al. 1993).

Depression and anxiety symptoms often coexist among individuals with Parkinson's disease (Henderson et al. 1992; Vazquez et al. 1993). In one study of 42 patients with Parkinson's disease, of the 12 patients with an anxiety disorder (5 of whom had panic disorder and 5 of whom had GAD), 11 had a depressive disorder. In the same study, of the 18 patients with a depressive disorder, 12 also had an anxiety disorder (Menza et al. 1993).

The neurobiology of anxiety in Parkinson's disease has not been clearly delineated, but there is limited evidence supporting the roles of neurotransmitter abnormalities, particularly in central noradrenergic systems (Richard et al. 1996). The dopaminergic neural circuits implicated in Parkinson's disease have intimate connections with systems involved with anxiety (e.g., serotonin). Anxiety may also be due to medications used to treat Parkinson's disease, such as levodopa and pergolide (see Table 12–2; Vazquez et al. 1993). Anxiety may also occur with declining dopamine levels (Factor et al. 1995).

Poststroke Anxiety

Poststroke anxiety may occur as a symptom of the more widely described syndrome of poststroke depression (Robinson and Starkstein 2002; Wise and Rundell 1999). Less commonly, anxiety may appear alone. When they appear after a stroke, anxiety symptoms have been shown to persist in many individuals. For example, in one study, 31% of patients had GAD at 3 months, and 19% had it at 3 years (Astrom 1996). Anxiety has been associated with right-hemisphere lesions, whereas depression and mixed depression and anxiety are more commonly associated with left-hemisphere lesions (Astrom 1996; Castillo et al. 1993).

Seizures

Anxiety symptoms may be caused by seizures. For example, complex partial seizures may be accompanied by symptoms of panic disorder, including fear, depersonalization, derealization, dizziness, and paresthesias (Tucker 2002; Wise and Rundell 1999). One group used ambulatory electroencephalographic monitoring with sphenoidal electrodes to study patients with atypical panic attacks (i.e., panic attacks with concomitant neurological symptoms such as change in level of consciousness, aphasia, and focal paresthesias). Focal paroxysmal electroencephalographic changes were found in 5 of 11 patients who had panic attacks during monitoring (Weilburg et al. 1995). Animal models provide some support for the hypothesis that limbic kindling might lead to interictal anxiety (Depaulis et al. 1997).

For further discussion of neurophysiological and neuroanatomic aspects of anxiety disorders, the reader is referred to Chapter 32, "Neurology and Neurosurgery," and D.J. Stein and Hugo (2002).

Other Conditions

In addition to the disorders discussed above, anxiety has reportedly been caused by many other medical conditions. For example, anxiety may be associated with hypocalcemia and hypomagnesemia. Relatively rare conditions for which there are only limited data supporting a causal relationship include carcinoid syndrome, hyperparathyroidism, and pheochromocytoma (Colon and Popkin 2002). In the absence of other findings suggestive of one of these rare disorders, it is not advisable to screen for them (e.g., serotonin metabolites to rule out carcinoid, parathyroid hormone levels to rule out hyperparathyroidism, or catecholamine metabolites to rule out pheochromocytoma).

Treatment of Anxiety in the Medically Ill

Psychotherapy

An overemphasis on psychopharmacology in the care of medically ill patients may result in overlooking the value of psychotherapy. The first step in the treatment of anxiety is to spend time listening to and talking with the patient. Just as in psychotherapy with any patient, empathic listening is a powerful tool to relieve distress. With medically ill patients, the goal is to help patients understand and discuss their emotional reactions to their illness so that they can then manage these feelings by using their own coping mechanisms (S. Green 1994). Psychotherapeutic approaches include supportive, psychodynamic, and cognitive-behavioral therapies.

Supportive Therapy

Supportive therapy involves listening and providing reassurance, sympathy, education about the medical process and the underlying illness, advice, and suggestions (Generalized anxiety disorder 2003). The process includes listening for fears and misperceptions about illness or its treatment and giving patients appropriate information so that they can be as prepared as possible (House and Stark 2002). Effective communication, using language the patient and family can understand, can lead to a great decrease in anxiety. It is also helpful to give patients as much choice in their treatment decisions as possible so that they

feel they have some control over the course of their treatment.

Reassurance is an important skill that all physicians use in treating patients. In some highly anxious patients, however, simple reassurance can actually cause increased anxiety and lead to a cycle of maladaptive behavior. For example, if a patient who has been told that a procedure is simple or painless subsequently experiences pain or untoward results, the resulting anxiety can lead to more reassurance-seeking behavior, mistrust, and decreased cooperation. Many anxious patients tend to interpret bodily symptoms as evidence of serious disease, and as a result, they may seek multiple consultations for reassurance. Understanding the patient's beliefs, concerns, and perceptions can be helpful in challenging misperceptions, educating the patient about his or her illness, and devising a realistic plan to monitor symptoms. Having a realistic plan to help patients differentiate minor symptoms from those that may need medical attention will reduce anxiety and decrease the excessive need for reassurance (Stark and House 2000). It is also important that the physician not assume that a patient's anxiety is due to fear of dying. When reassurance is directed at the wrong fear, it may accentuate anxiety and lead patients to believe that their physician does not understand them.

The consultant can also serve as a liaison between the patient and the health care team. For example, the psychiatrist might help the primary physician understand the importance of clarifying the risks and benefits of treatment and of informing the anxious patient when there are delays in scheduling. It also may be helpful for the treatment team to consult directly with the psychiatrist about how to care for the anxious patient. Facilitating communication among the patient and the treatment team can help avoid misperceptions or mistrust that will only serve to heighten anxiety.

Another important aspect of supportive therapy is the involvement of the patient's support system of family, friends, and religious community. Working with the support network is important to ensure that their anxiety and misperceptions do not add to the stress of the patient. Helping a patient to expand his or her social network can be an important component of a supportive program. In addition, hospital staff such as nurses, chaplains, social workers, volunteers, and other allied professionals can help provide support and encouragement to the medically ill patient (Colon and Popkin 2002).

Patients confronting life-threatening or terminal illnesses such as cancer may experience death anxiety (Yalom 1980). Relief of physical pain, dyspnea, and other physical symptoms is critical for the alleviation of anxiety

(Payne and Massie 2000). Some patients have strong religious or spiritual beliefs that may help reduce their distress, and pastoral counseling is often beneficial (Alvarado et al. 1995). Open discussions with patients about death help to reduce anxiety and distress (Spiegel et al. 1981), and psychological interventions alone can help patients manage their death anxiety (Payne and Massie 2000). Maintaining hope is an important aspect of minimizing anxiety, although goals can change from full recovery to having more time to accomplish specific short-term goals. Helping patients find meaning and value in their lives, despite their illness and suffering, helps to relieve emotional distress (Frankl 1987). For example, anxiety can be reduced when patients see that they are still important to their families or that they still have unfinished business to address. The hospice movement has been instrumental in helping provide relief for many patients (Byock 1997). Despite recent improvements in physician education, caregivers need more training to be able to overcome their own death anxiety so that they can provide comfort to end-of-life patients (Adelbratt and Strang 2000) (see Chapter 40, "Palliative Care").

Supportive group interventions are very effective in reducing anxiety and distress in medically ill patients (Fawzy et al. 1995). HIV, cancer, cardiac, and other support groups have proliferated in recent years. They can be quite helpful in providing emotional support and education in stress management, coping skills, and other behavioral techniques (Payne and Massie 2000). Participants have been shown to have decreased stress levels and improved functioning (Spiegel et al. 1989).

Cognitive-Behavioral Therapy

Cognitive-behavioral therapy has been proven to be as effective as medication in treating many anxiety disorders, including GAD and panic disorder (Generalized anxiety disorder 2003). Cognitive techniques are used to uncover and correct misinterpretations and irrational thoughts that lead to increased anxiety and distress. Behavioral techniques, such as systematic desensitization, can also be used to help overcome irrational fears that can interfere with effective treatment, such as blood or needle phobias and claustrophobia during MRI (Goldberg and Posner 2000). Since cognitive-behavioral therapy techniques usually take several sessions to be effective, medications may be needed initially to help reduce anxiety. A brief course of cognitive-behavioral therapy can have long-lasting effects, but occasional "booster" sessions may be needed.

A variety of therapies that involve teaching self-awareness and self-regulation of body functions have been found effective in reducing anxiety and physical symptoms in medically ill patients. These include muscle relaxation techniques (such as Jacobson's progressive muscle relaxation), autogenic training (such as biofeedback, which uses technology to control internal processes), and relaxation techniques (such as meditation, breathing exercises, and self-hypnosis). Muscular conditions such as tension headaches and musculoskeletal disorders may respond better to muscle relaxation; migraine headaches and hypertension, to autogenic training; and anxieties and phobias, to more cognitive techniques; however, further research is needed (Lehrer et al. 1994). When used by a skilled practitioner with a patient who is open to this approach, all of these techniques may be helpful in reducing symptoms of various conditions exacerbated by anxiety and stress. Guided imagery with relaxation and hypnosis has also been an effective technique to reduce anxiety (Payne and Massie 2000). Relaxation techniques have been used to decrease the use of medications in hypertensive patients, to decrease pain in patients with chronic pain, and to expedite recovery and decrease complications in postsurgical patients (Benson 1988). Meditation has been shown to reduce panic attacks (Kabat-Zinn et al. 1992), and biofeedback and relaxation have been used to help wean patients from the ventilator (Acosta 1988) as well as to reduce dyspnea and anxiety in patients with chronic obstructive pulmonary disease (Renfroe 1988; Smoller et al. 1999).

Psychodynamic Therapy

For patients who are not too ill and who have sufficient emotional resilience, brief dynamic psychotherapy can be useful in uncovering the conscious and unconscious meaning of the illness to the patient. Understanding patients' developmental history, interpersonal dynamics, and defense mechanisms can help the psychiatrist to assist them in finding healthier ways to cope with medical illness (Viederman 2000). What coping strategies have helped in the past? When did the individual feel most fulfilled in his or her life? How can those memories and skills be used now, even in the presence of significant medical illness? Psychotherapy can uncover areas leading to increased distress, such as real or imagined guilt, unhealthy coping strategies like avoidance and denial, and recognition of past conflicted relationships that may be repeated in the current doctor–patient relationship. An understanding of the patient's underlying dynamics can help identify and resolve conflicts with the treatment team that may be interfering with recovery. Psychotherapy started in the hospital may then be continued on an outpatient basis, to help patients cope with their illness and achieve optimal functioning (Colon and Popkin 2002). An understanding of psychodynamic principles can also help psychiatrists in working with the primary treatment team that is caring for the anxious patient.

Countertransference reactions can cause a number of problems for providers of anxious patients. For example, physicians may overidentify with their patients, leading to frustration because of lack of progress or poor prognosis. As a result, they may then overcompensate by offering excessive reassurance, or they may minimize or overlook symptoms in an unconscious attempt to reduce their own anxiety. Caregivers may also become withdrawn and distant, providing care mechanically with little empathy or awareness of the emotional needs of the patient. Psychiatrists can play a role in helping the health care team to be cognizant of these defenses so they do not interfere with the provision of optimal patient care (S. Green 1994). (See Chapter 38, "Psychosocial Treatments," for further discussion of psychotherapy for the medically ill.)

Pharmacotherapy

Psychotherapeutic techniques are often not sufficient to manage anxiety in the medically ill. An increasingly broad range of psychopharmacological agents can be used safely with this population. (For further details, see Chapter 37, "Psychopharmacology," and specific discussions in Chapter 19, "Heart Disease," through Chapter 35, "Physical Medicine and Rehabilitation.")

Benzodiazepines

For acute anxiety symptoms, the most immediately effective and frequently used agents are the benzodiazepines (Table 12–3). Diazepam and chlordiazepoxide were among the first of these to be used. They also have established efficacy for other conditions—diazepam as an anticonvulsant and muscle relaxant and chlordiazepoxide for alcohol detoxification. Diazepam can be given orally or intravenously but should not be given intramuscularly. However, newer benzodiazepines have better safety profiles and shorter half-lives, so they tend to be used more frequently.

TABLE 12–3. Selected benzodiazepines used for anxiety in the medically ill

Medication	Route	Dosage	Elimination half-life	Comments
Alprazolam	Oral	0.25–1.0 mg tid	9–20 hours	Rapid onset. Interdose withdrawal a problem, but new extended-release form is available.
Chlordiazepoxide	Oral, intramuscular	5–25 mg qid	28–100 hours (including metabolites)	Useful for alcohol withdrawal.
Clonazepam	Oral	0.25–1 mg bid-tid	19–60 hours	Also used for absence seizures, periodic leg movements, and neuropathic pain.
Diazepam	Oral, intravenous	2–10 mg qid	30–200 hours (including metabolites)	Also used as an anticonvulsant and muscle relaxant.
Lorazepam	Oral, intramuscular, intravenous	0.5–2.0 mg up to qid	8–24 hours	Intravenous availability is an advantage. Metabolized by conjugation. Also approved for chemotherapy-related nausea and vomiting.
Midazolam	Intramuscular, intravenous	Intramuscular: 5 mg single dose Intravenous: 0.02–0.10 mg/kg per hour	1–20 hours (including metabolites)	Used for preoperative sedation and intravenous induction.
Oxazepam	Oral	10–30 mg qid	3–25 hours	Metabolized by conjugation. May also be useful for alcohol withdrawal.

Source. Adapted from *Physician's Desk Reference* 2003; Bezchlibnyk-Butler and Jeffries 2002.

Alprazolam works rapidly and is eliminated quickly, but as a result there may be rebound anxiety and withdrawal symptoms. Because lorazepam can be given orally, intravenously, or intramuscularly and does not have an active metabolite, it is often a preferred medication in hospitalized patients. Lorazepam can be given in an intravenous bolus or drip, but as doses increase to provide sedation and treat delirium tremens, respiratory status must be watched closely. Like lorazepam, oxazepam and the hypnotic temazepam are metabolized through conjugation and so are less problematic in patients with liver disease than the other benzodiazepines, which are oxidatively metabolized (Stoudemire 1996). Midazolam, a benzodiazepine with a very short half-life that can only be given intravenously or intramuscularly, is used for short-term procedures such as bone marrow biopsies, endoscopies, and MRI scans in claustrophobic patients (Goldberg and Posner 2000).

For patients who need long-term benzodiazepines, it is often helpful to change to a medication with a longer half-life, such as clonazepam (Katon 1994).

Hypnotics are commonly used in medically ill patients who are kept awake by their anxiety. Triazolam has been used less frequently in recent years because it can cause retrograde amnesia. Temazepam is occasionally still used for persons who tend to awaken when taking the shorter-acting hypnotics. Newer agents such as zolpidem and zaleplon are nonbenzodiazepines that act on the benzodiazepine receptor. They are preferred for short-term use because they have very short half-lives and as a result cause less daytime sedation, impaired coordination, and cognitive disturbance. Generally all of the hypnotics are best used for short intervals to decrease the chance of side effects, to maintain effectiveness (i.e., prevent tolerance), and to prevent dependence.

All benzodiazepines can cause excessive sedation. They may also cause motor and cognitive disturbances, especially in older persons and individuals with impaired brain functioning (e.g., due to dementia, head injury, or mental retardation; Salzman et al. 1993). Therefore, they should be used with caution, if at all, in these patients. Anxiety in delirious patients is usually better treated with antipsychotics than with benzodiazepines (Breitbart et al. 1996). Benzodiazepines can cause respiratory suppression, so they should be used cautiously in persons with pulmonary disease who retain carbon dioxide, or in patients with sleep apnea. Because of potential teratogenicity, benzodiazepines should be avoided in the first trimester of pregnancy. They should also be avoided at the very end of pregnancy, because there are reports of sedation and withdrawal symptoms in the fetus (McGee and Pies 2002). All benzodiazepines can lead to tolerance and de-

pendence, so they should be avoided or used judiciously (i.e., for detoxification) in persons with a substance abuse history. However, compared with barbiturates and earlier sedative-hypnotics such as meprobamate, they are much safer in overdose and have fewer side effects. In persons who are conscientious and do not have a history of chemical dependence, benzodiazepines can often be safely used for years without causing problems or tolerance. As an individual ages, use should be reevaluated. Similarly, long-term benzodiazepine use may need to be reduced or discontinued among patients who develop specific medical conditions (e.g., end-stage liver disease, dementia, chronic obstructive pulmonary disease, and cerebellar dysfunction).

Antidepressants

The pharmacological treatment of choice for GAD, panic disorder, posttraumatic stress disorder, obsessive-compulsive disorder, and social anxiety disorder is one of the selective serotonin reuptake inhibitors (SSRIs): fluoxetine, sertraline, paroxetine, citalopram, escitalopram, and fluvoxamine. Venlafaxine, which inhibits both serotonin and norepinephrine reuptake, has been approved for GAD and social anxiety disorder and will probably also be shown to be effective for other anxiety disorders (Gorman 2002). These medications have few side effects and therefore are generally quite safe for the medically ill; they do not result in cardiac conduction problems, orthostatic hypotension, or physical dependence. Because antidepressants may take 2–6 weeks to relieve anxiety, the patient may need initial treatment with benzodiazepines. Once the patient has been stabilized on the antidepressant medication, the benzodiazepines can usually be gradually withdrawn without recurrence of anxiety. The antidepressant should be used for at least 3–6 months before stopping it, and it should be tapered to avoid discontinuation symptoms. Antidepressants can be used safely on a long-term basis if anxiety returns.

One of the main drawbacks of the SSRIs and venlafaxine is a relatively high incidence of sexual dysfunction in both men and women. This side effect may be particularly problematic for persons with medical problems already associated with sexual dysfunction, such as diabetes or vascular disease (see Chapter 17, "Sexual Disorders"). In addition, psychiatrists must be concerned about the potential for drug interactions, for example, with fluoxetine and paroxetine (cytochrome P450 2D6 inhibitors) and fluvoxamine (a cytochrome P450 3A4 inhibitor; see Chapter 37, "Psychopharmacology"). Serotonin reuptake inhibitors may cause initial gastrointestinal distress and nausea, so they are generally given with food. It is important to reassure the patient with gastrointestinal disease that these side effects are almost always transient. SSRIs are also associated with the syndrome of inappropriate secretion of antidiuretic hormone, especially in older patients. In a small percentage of patients, venlafaxine produces a unique side effect of sustained blood pressure elevation, which is dose-related. Blood pressure should be monitored when this drug is being initiated and with each dosage increase. If diastolic blood pressure increases occur, the dosage should be reduced or the drug stopped. Although SSRIs may help some individuals with migraine headaches, they can also exacerbate headaches. It has been reported that SSRIs can exacerbate parkinsonism in individuals with Parkinson's disease; however, this appears to be an uncommon side effect (Dell'Agnello et al. 2001). Because all SSRIs are equally efficacious in studies, medication choice is often based on side-effect profile. For example, the more sedating SSRIs (e.g., fluvoxamine and paroxetine) may be advantageous for the highly anxious patient with insomnia, whereas fluoxetine may be more stimulating. For medically ill patients taking multiple medications, agents with the fewest drug interactions are preferred: sertraline, citalopram, escitalopram, and venlafaxine.

Mirtazapine—an alpha-adrenoceptor antagonist and an antagonist at serotonin 5-HT$_{2A}$, 5-HT$_{2C}$, and 5-HT$_3$ receptors—may be helpful in reducing anxiety. Its use in medically ill patients has increased recently for two reasons: 1) it has few drug interactions, and 2) the side effects of sedation and increased appetite are helpful in patients who have insomnia and anorexia with weight loss. Nefazodone is another unique antidepressant with some anxiolytic properties, but it can be problematic for medically ill patients because of its inhibition of the cytochrome P450 3A4 enzyme, the need for gradual dose adjustment, and its recent black-box warning of rare liver toxicity. Neither of these medications causes sexual dysfunction.

Tricyclic antidepressants and monoamine oxidase inhibitors are well established as effective treatments for anxiety disorders as well as for depression. Tricyclics can be efficacious for the treatment of anxiety in the medically ill (e.g., in patients with chronic pain or diarrhea-predominant irritable bowel syndrome). The main reasons these medications are currently not used frequently as first-line treatment are their numerous side effects and their toxicity in overdose. Tricyclics often cause dry mouth, weight gain, constipation, sedation, orthostatic hypotension, urinary retention, and falls, especially in elderly patients. In addition, because of their quinidine-like effects, they can cause heart block and arrhythmias. Because there is a relatively small margin of safety between efficacy and toxicity, overdose can be dangerous and even fatal. Persons with liver and kidney disease may develop toxicity due to

impaired metabolism and excretion (Stoudemire and Moran 1993). Monoamine oxidase inhibitors can cause dizziness, orthostatic hypotension, and weight gain. These side effects, as well as the potential for serious hypertensive crises, limit their usefulness in medically ill patients.

Antipsychotics

Antipsychotic medications are not approved for the treatment of anxiety, although there are limited data clearly supporting their efficacy (El-Khayat and Baldwin 1998). Nonetheless, psychiatrists often find them to be efficacious and safe to use in selected medical populations. Because antipsychotics do not cause confusion or respiratory compromise, they may be preferable to benzodiazepines for the more severe anxiety associated with agitation or delirium or in patients with respiratory compromise. For example, antipsychotics may be helpful in assisting the anxious patient who is being weaned from a ventilator (Cassem and Murray 1997). Of the older, or typical, antipsychotics, the agent used most often in medically ill patients is haloperidol, which can be given orally, intramuscularly, or intravenously. In acutely agitated patients who may be violent or psychotic, 5–10 mg of haloperidol is often given orally or intramuscularly, usually in conjunction with a benzodiazepine such as lorazepam, and sometimes with benztropine to prevent a dystonic reaction. In medically ill patients who are delirious, haloperidol rarely causes extrapyramidal side effects or dystonia. For mild agitation, 0.5–2.0 mg might be given, but much higher doses can be used. If a high-potency typical antipsychotic such as haloperidol is used in treating anxiety, it is important to monitor for akathisia because it can be mistaken for worsening anxiety. Newer atypical antipsychotics such as olanzapine, risperidone, quetiapine, ziprasidone, and aripiprazole are also used selectively in the management of anxiety, especially in lower doses. Ziprasidone is the only one available in intramuscular formulation at this time. Compared with the older agents, they have relatively favorable side-effect profiles. There are no data regarding their use for anxiety in general and specifically in medically ill populations, but they can be a safe alternative for those who might not do well with benzodiazepines, such as delirious patients or those with respiratory compromise.

Buspirone

Buspirone is a partial serotonin agonist approved for treatment of GAD. It may be useful in treating medically ill patients with anxiety because there are few drug interactions; it does not cause sedation, respiratory depression, or cognitive problems; and its metabolism is not greatly affected by liver disease (Stoudemire and Moran 1993). The main drawbacks with buspirone are that it may take 2–4 weeks to become effective, and its benefits seem modest. Because of its short half-life, buspirone needs to be given 2–3 times a day. Some patients complain of dizziness and excessive sedation when first beginning the medication, but it is usually well tolerated.

Beta-Blockers

Beta-adrenergic blockers produce anxiolytic effects by blocking autonomic hyperarousal (elevated pulse, elevated blood pressure, sweating, tremors) associated with anxiety responses. They work best for specific anxiety-producing situations, such as performance anxiety and public speaking, and are less efficacious for panic disorder and social phobias. All beta-blockers are contraindicated in persons with asthma or chronic obstructive lung disease, and they can worsen peripheral vascular disease (Barnes 2000). Patients with insulin-dependent diabetes should not be prescribed nonselective beta-blockers; because those medications block the sympathetic nervous system response to hypoglycemia, the patient may be unaware of symptoms and may be less likely to respond appropriately (Kaplan 2001). Central nervous system side effects such as nightmares, hallucinations, and sleep disturbance are infrequent. They may be more likely to occur with lipophilic drugs such as propranolol and pindolol, which cross the blood-brain barrier, and less likely to occur with atenolol, nadolol, and timolol (McAinsh and Cruickshank 1990). The reported association between beta-blockers and depression has not been supported by data from clinical trials (Ko et al. 2002).

Antihistamines

Sedating histamine H_1 receptor blockers are sometimes used to treat anxiety and insomnia. Hydroxyzine has been shown to be as effective and safe as benzodiazepines in treating anxiety (Llorca et al. 2002) in a general study population. Diphenhydramine, which is often used to treat insomnia, is available in over-the-counter preparations. Because these medications are not addicting, many physicians consider them to be benign. However, they can cause dizziness, excessive sedation, incoordination, and confusion, especially when used with alcohol or other central nervous system depressants. Elderly patients and those with brain disease or injury are more sensitive to these medications and may become delirious even with low doses. Despite these risks, these medications are still an option when benzodiazepines must be avoided due to concerns about dependence or respiratory depression (Stoudemire 1996).

Anticonvulsants

Anticonvulsants are primarily prescribed by psychiatrists for patients with bipolar disorder who cannot tolerate or do not respond to lithium, but they can also be helpful for some individuals with anxiety. Patients with recurrent panic attacks and temporal lobe electroencephalographic abnormalities may respond to anticonvulsants (McNamara and Fogel 1990). Gabapentin works on the gamma-aminobutyric acid system and can be effective for relief of neuropathic pain. It has also been shown to have efficacy for panic disorder (Pande et al. 2000) and social anxiety disorder (Pande et al. 1999). Because gabapentin is not metabolized through the liver, it has few drug interactions and can be used safely in persons with liver disease. Side effects include sedation, headache, and dizziness. Divalproex sodium and carbamazepine have been found to be helpful in calming agitated, anxious patients, especially those with brain injury, mental retardation, or dementia. The newer anticonvulsants lamotrigine, topiramate, and tiagabine show some promise in treatment of mood disorders and may also prove to be beneficial for the treatment of anxiety.

Conclusion

The experience of medical illness often leads to clinically significant anxiety symptoms. Despite the fact that many individuals with medical illnesses have anxiety disorders, these disorders are often underrecognized and undertreated. Both psychotherapy and pharmacotherapy can significantly ameliorate anxiety symptoms, even among patients with severe medical problems. Thus, careful assessment and treatment of anxiety disorders are important components of the psychiatric care of the medically ill.

References

Accurso V, Winnicki M, Shamsuzzaman AS, et al: Predisposition to vasovagal syncope in subjects with blood/injury phobia. Circulation 104:903–907, 2001

Acosta F: Biofeedback and progressive relaxation in weaning the anxious patient from the ventilator: a brief report. Heart Lung 17:299–301, 1988

Adelbratt S, Strang P: Death anxiety in brain tumour patients and their spouses. Palliat Med 14:499–507, 2000

Alter CL, Pelcovitz D, Axelrod A, et al: Identification of PTSD in cancer survivors. Psychosomatics 37:137–143, 1996

Altshuler LL, Bauer M, Frye MA, et al: Does thyroid supplementation accelerate tricyclic antidepressant response? A review and meta-analysis of the literature. Am J Psychiatry 158:1627–1622, 2001

Alvarado DA, Templer DI, Bressler C, et al: The relationship of religious variables to death depression and death anxiety. J Clin Psychol 51:202–207, 1995

American Psychiatric Association: Diagnostic and Statistical Manual of Mental Disorders, 3rd Edition, Revised. Washington, DC, American Psychiatric Association, 1987

American Psychiatric Association: Diagnostic and Statistical Manual of Mental Disorders, 4th Edition, Text Revision. Washington, DC, American Psychiatric Association, 2000

Andrykowski MA, Cordova MJ: Factors associated with PTSD symptoms following treatment for breast cancer: test of the Andersen model. J Trauma Stress 11:189–203, 1998

Arnold LM, McElroy SL, Mutasim DF, et al: Characteristics of 34 adults with psychogenic excoriation. J Clin Psychiatry 59:509–514, 1998

Astrom M: Generalized anxiety disorder in stroke patients: a 3-year longitudinal study. Stroke 27:270–275, 1996

Barnes PJ: Airway pharmacology, in Textbook of Respiratory Medicine, 3rd Edition. Edited by Murray JF, Nadel JA. Philadelphia, PA, WB Saunders, 2000, pp 267–296,

Barsky AJ: Palpitations, arrhythmias, and awareness of cardiac activity. Ann Intern Med 134:832–837, 2001

Barsky AJ, Cleary PD, Coeytaux RR, et al: Psychiatric disorders in medical outpatients complaining of palpitations. J Gen Intern Med 9:306–313, 1994

Beck AT, Brown G, Epstein N, et al: An inventory for measuring clinical anxiety: psychometric properties. J Consult Clin Psychiatry 56:893–897, 1988

Beitman BD, Mukerji V, Lamberti JW, et al: Panic disorder in patients with chest pain and angiographically normal coronary arteries. Am J Cardiol 63:1399–1403, 1989

Bennett P, Conway M, Clatworthy J, et al: Predicting posttraumatic symptoms in cardiac patients. Heart Lung 30:458–465, 2001

Benson H: The relaxation response: a bridge between medicine and religion. Harv Ment Health Lett 4 (March):4–6, 1988

Bezchlibnyk-Butler KZ, Jeffries JJ: Benzodiazepines, in Clinical Handbook of Psychotropic Drugs, 12th Edition. Seattle, WA, Hogrefe & Huber, 2002, pp 109–120

Bienvenu OJ, Eaton WW: The epidemiology of blood-injection-injury phobia. Psychol Med 28:1129–1136, 1998

Breitbart W, Marotta R, Platt M, et al: A double-blind trial of haloperidol, chlorpromazine, and lorazepam in the treatment of delirium in hospitalized AIDS patients. Am J Psychiatry 153:231–237, 1996

Brown TM, Stoudemire A: Psychiatric Side Effects of Prescription and Over-the-Counter Medications: Recognition and Management. Washington, DC, American Psychiatric Press, 1998

Bruce M, Scott N, Shine P, et al: Anxiogenic effects of caffeine in patients with anxiety disorders. Arch Gen Psychiatry 49:867–869, 1992

Bussing R, Burket RC, Kelleher ET: Prevalence of anxiety disorders in a clinic-based sample of pediatric asthma patients. Psychosomatics 37:108–115, 1996

Byock I: Dying Well: The Prospect for Growth at the End of Life. New York, Riverhead Books, 1997

Caine ED, Lyness JM: Delirium, dementia and amnestic and other cognitive disorders, in Kaplan and Sadock's Comprehensive Textbook of Psychiatry, 7th Edition. Edited by Sadock BJ, Sadock VA. Philadelphia, PA, Lippincott Williams & Wilkins, 2000, pp 854–923

Carr RE: Panic disorder and asthma: causes, effects and research implications. J Psychosom Res 44:43–52, 1998

Carr RE, Lehrer PM, Hochron SM: Panic symptoms in asthma and panic disorder: a preliminary test of the dyspnea-fear theory. Behav Res Ther 30:251–261, 1992

Cassem NH, Murray GB: Delirious patients, in Massachusetts General Hospital Handbook of General Hospital Psychiatry, 4th Edition. Edited by Cassem NH, Stern TA, Rosenbaum JF, et al. St. Louis, MO, CV Mosby, 1997, pp 101–122

Castillo CS, Starkstein SE, Fedoroff JP, et al: Generalized anxiety disorder after stroke. J Nerv Ment Dis 181:100–106, 1993

Colon EA, Popkin MK: Anxiety and panic, in The American Psychiatric Publishing Textbook of Consultation-Liaison Psychiatry, 2nd Edition. Edited by Wise MG, Rundell JR. Washington, DC, American Psychiatric Publishing, 2002, pp 393–415

Cormier LE, Katon W, Russo J, et al: Chest pain with negative cardiac diagnostic studies. Relationship to psychiatric illness. J Nerv Ment Dis 176:351–358, 1988

Dell'Agnello G, Ceravolo R, Nuti A, et al: SSRIs do not worsen Parkinson's disease: evidence from an open-label, prospective study. Clin Neuropharmacol 24:221–227, 2001

Depaulis A, Helfer V, Deransart C, et al: Anxiogenic-like consequences in animal models of complex partial seizures. Neurosci Biobehav Rev 21:767–774, 1997

Difede J, Ptacek JT, Roberts J, et al: Acute stress disorder after burn injury: a predictor of posttraumatic stress disorder? Psychosom Med 64:826–834, 2002

DiMatteo MR, Lepper HS, Croghan TW: Depression is a risk factor for noncompliance with medical treatment: meta-analysis of the effects of anxiety and depression on patient adherence. Arch Intern Med 160:2101–2107, 2000

Drugs that may cause psychiatric symptoms. Med Lett Drugs Ther 44:59–62, 2002

Ehlers A, Mayou RA, Sprigings DC, et al: Psychological and perceptual factors associated with arrhythmias and benign palpitations. Psychosom Med 62:693–702, 2000

El-Khayat R, Baldwin DS: Antipsychotic drugs for nonpsychotic patients: assessment of the benefit/risk ratio in generalized anxiety disorder. J Psychopharmacol 12:323–329, 1998

Epstein SA, Lin TH, Audrain J, et al: Excessive breast self-examination among first-degree relatives of newly diagnosed breast cancer patients. High-Risk Breast Cancer Consortium. Psychosomatics 38:253–261, 1997

Factor SA, Molho ES, Podskalny GD, et al: Parkinson's disease: drug-induced psychiatric states, in Behavioral Neurology of Movement Disorders (Advances in Neurology, Vol 65). Edited by Weiner WJ, Lang AE. New York, Raven Press, 1995, pp 115–138

Fawzy FI, Fawzy NW, Arndt LA, et al: Critical review of psychosocial interventions in cancer care. Arch Gen Psychiatry 52:100–113, 1995

Fleet RP, Dupuis G, Marchand A, et al: Panic disorder in emergency department chest pain patients: prevalence, comorbidity, suicidal ideation, and physician recognition. Am J Med 101:371–380, 1996

Fleet RP, Dupuis G, Marchand A, et al: Panic disorder in coronary artery disease patients with noncardiac chest pain. J Psychosom Res 44:81–90, 1998

Frankl V: Man's Search for Meaning. London, Hoddard-Stoughton, 1987

Friedman BH, Thayer JF: Autonomic balance revisited: panic anxiety and heart rate variability. J Psychosom Res 44:133–151, 1998

Generalized anxiety disorder: toxic worry. Harv Ment Health Lett 19(7):1–5, 2003

Goldberg R, Posner D: Anxiety in the medically ill, in Psychiatric Care of the Medical Patient, 2nd Edition. Edited by Stoudemire A, Fogel BS, Greenberg DB, New York, Oxford University Press, 2000, pp 165–180

Golding JM: Sexual assault history and physical health in randomly selected Los Angeles women. Health Psychol 13:130–138, 1994

Goodman WK, Price LH, Rasmussen SA, et al: The Yale-Brown Obsessive-Compulsive Scale. I. Development, use and reliability. Arch Gen Psychiatry 46:1006–1011, 1989

Gorman J: Treatment of generalized anxiety disorder. J Clin Psychiatry 63 (suppl 8):17–23, 2002

Green BL, Epstein SA, Krupnick JL, et al: Trauma and medical illness: assessing trauma-related disorders in medical settings, in Assessing Psychological Trauma and PTSD. Edited by Wilson JP, Keane TM. New York, Guilford, 1997, pp 160–191

Green BL, Rowland JH, Krupnick JL, et al: Prevalence of posttraumatic stress disorder in women with breast cancer. Psychosomatics 39:102–111, 1998

Green BL, Krupnick JL, Rowland JH, et al: Trauma history as a predictor of psychologic symptoms in women with breast cancer. J Clin Oncol 18:1084–1093, 2000

Green S: Supportive psychologic care of the medically ill: a synthesis of the biopsychosocial approach in medical care, in Human Behavior: An Introduction for Medical Students, 2nd Edition. Edited by Stoudemire A. Philadelphia, PA, JB Lippincott, 1994, pp 323–337

Hall RC, Hall RC: Anxiety and endocrine disease. Semin Clin Neuropsychiatry 4:72–83, 1999

Hamilton M: The assessment of anxiety states by rating. Br J Med Psychol 32:50–55, 1959

Hamner M, Hunt N, Gee J, et al: PTSD and automatic implantable cardioverter defibrillators. Psychosomatics 40:82–85, 1999

Harman JS, Rollman BL, Hanusa BH, et al: Physician office visits of adults for anxiety disorders in the United States, 1985–1998. J Gen Intern Med 17:165–172, 2002

Hazlett-Stevens H, Craske MG, Roy-Byrne PP, et al: Predictors of willingness to consider medication and psychosocial treatment for panic disorder in primary care patients. Gen Hosp Psychiatry 24:316–321, 2002

Henderson R, Kurlan R, Kersun JM, et al: Preliminary examination of the comorbidity of anxiety and depression in Parkinson's disease. J Neuropsychiatry Clin Neurosci 4:257–264, 1992

Herrmann C, Brand-Driehorst S, Buss U, et al: Effects of anxiety and depression on 5-year mortality in 5,057 patients referred for exercise testing. J Psychosom Res 48:455–462, 2000

Houck P, Spiegel DA, Shear MK, et al: Reliability of the self-report version of the panic disorder severity scale. Depress Anxiety 15:183–185, 2002

House A, Stark D: Anxiety in medical patients. BMJ 325:207–209, 2002

Huffman JC, Pollack MH: Predicting panic disorder among patients with chest pain: an analysis of the literature. Psychosomatics 44:222–236, 2003

Iacovides A, Fountoulakis K, Grammaticos P, et al: Difference in symptom profile between generalized anxiety disorder and anxiety secondary to hyperthyroidism. Int J Psychiatry Med 30:71–81, 2000

Jacobsen PB, Sadler IJ, Booth-Jones M, et al: Predictors of posttraumatic stress disorder symptomatology following bone marrow transplantation for cancer. J Consult Clin Psychol 70:235–240, 2002

Jadresic DP: Psychiatric aspects of hyperthyroidism. J Psychosom Res 34:603–615, 1990

Joffe RT: Thyroid hormones, in Kaplan & Sadock's Comprehensive Textbook of Psychiatry, 7th Edition. Edited by Sadock BJ, Sadock VA. Philadelphia, PA, Lippincott Williams & Wilkins, 2000, pp 2478–2481

Jonas BS, Franks P, Ingram DD: Are symptoms of anxiety and depression risk factors for hypertension? Longitudinal evidence from the National Health and Nutrition Examination Survey I Epidemiologic Follow-up Study. Arch Fam Med 6:43–49, 1997

Jones C, Griffiths RD, Humphris G, et al: Memory, delusions, and the development of acute posttraumatic stress disorder-related symptoms after intensive care. Crit Care Med 29:573–580, 2001

Jones GN, Ames SC, Jeffries SK, et al: Utilization of medical services and quality of life among low-income patients with generalized anxiety disorder attending primary care clinics. Int J Psychiatry Med 31:183–198, 2001

Kabat-Zinn J, Massion A, Kristeller J, et al: Effectiveness of a meditation-based stress reduction program in the treatment of anxiety disorders. Am J Psychiatry 149:936–943, 1992

Kahana RJ, Bibring GL: Personality types in medical management, in Psychiatry and Medical Practice in a General Hospital. Edited by Zinberg N. New York, International Universities Press, 1964, pp 108–123

Kaiko RF, Foley KM, Grabinski PY, et al: Central nervous system excitatory effects of meperidine in cancer patients. Ann Neurol 13:180–185, 1983

Kangas M, Henry JL, Bryant RA: Posttraumatic stress disorder following cancer. A conceptual and empirical review. Clin Psychol Rev 22:499–524, 2002

Kaplan N: Systemic hypertension: therapy, in Heart Disease: A Textbook of Cardiovascular Medicine, 6th Edition. Edited by Braunwald E, Zipes DP, Libby P. Philadelphia, PA, WB Saunders, 2001, pp 27–28

Kathol RG, Delahunt JW: The relationship of anxiety and depression to symptoms of hyperthyroidism using operational criteria. Gen Hosp Psychiatry 8:23–28, 1986

Kathol RG, Turner R, Delahunt J: Depression and anxiety associated with hyperthyroidism: response to antithyroid therapy. Psychosomatics 27:501–505, 1986

Katon W: Treatment of panic disorder, in Panic Disorder in the Medical Setting (NIH Publ No 94-3482). Washington, DC, U.S. Government Printing Office, 1994, pp 83–106

Katon WJ, Roy-Byrne P, Russo J, et al: Cost-effectiveness and cost offset of a collaborative care intervention for primary care patients with panic disorder. Arch Gen Psychiatry 59:1098–1104, 2002

Kawachi I, Colditz GA, Ascherio A, et al: Prospective study of phobic anxiety and risk of coronary heart disease in men. Circulation 89:1992–1997, 1994

Kessler RC, McGonagle KA, Zhao S, et al: Lifetime and 12-month prevalence of DSM-III-R psychiatric disorders in the United States: results from the National Comorbidity Survey. Arch Gen Psychiatry 51:8–19, 1994

Kessler RC, Sonnega A, Bromet E, et al: Posttraumatic stress disorder in the National Comorbidity Survey. Arch Gen Psychiatry 52:1048–1060, 1995

Ko DT, Hebert PR, Coffey CS, et al: Beta-blocker therapy and symptoms of depression, fatigue, and sexual dysfunction. JAMA 288:351–357, 2002

Lane D, Carroll D, Ring C, et al: Mortality and quality of life 12 months after myocardial infarction: effects of depression and anxiety. Psychosom Med 63:221–230, 2001

Lehrer PM, Carr R, Sargunaraj D, et al: Stress management techniques: are they all equivalent, or do they have specific effects? Biofeedback Self Regul 19:353–401, 1994

Lessmeier TJ, Gamperling D, Johnson-Liddon V, et al: Unrecognized paroxysmal supraventricular tachycardia. Potential for misdiagnosis as panic disorder. Arch Intern Med 157:537–543, 1997

Llorca PM, Spadone C, Sol O, et al: Efficacy and safety of hydroxyzine in the treatment of generalized anxiety disorder: a 3-month double-blind study. J Clin Psychiatry 63:1020–1027, 2002

Maddock RJ, Carter CS, Tavano-Hall L, et al: Hypocapnia associated with cardiac stress scintigraphy in chest pain patients with panic disorder. Psychosom Med 60:5205, 1998

Maier W, Gansicke M, Freyberger HJ, et al: Generalized anxiety disorder (ICD-10) in primary care from a cross-cultural perspective: a valid diagnostic entity? Acta Psychiatr Scand 101:29–36, 2000

Mayou R: Chest pain, palpitations and panic. J Psychosom Res 44:53–70, 1998

McAinsh J, Cruickshank JM: Beta-blockers and central nervous system side effects. Pharmacol Ther 46:163–197, 1990

McGee M, Pies R: Benzodiazepines in primary practice: risks and benefits. Resid Staff Physician 48:42–49, 2002

McIsaac HK, Thordarson DS, Shafran R, et al: Claustrophobia and the magnetic resonance imaging procedure. J Behav Med 21:255–268, 1998

McNamara ME, Fogel BS: Anticonvulsant-responsive panic attacks with temporal lobe EEG abnormalities. J Neuropsychiatry Clin Neurosci 2:193–196, 1990

Menza MA, Robertson-Hoffman DE, Bonapace AS: Parkinson's disease and anxiety: comorbidity with depression. Biol Psychiatry 34:465–470, 1993

Merikangas KR, Stevens DE: Comorbidity of migraine and psychiatric disorders. Neurol Clin 15:115–123, 1997

Merikangas KR, Angst J, Isler H: Migraine and psychopathology: results of the Zurich cohort study of young adults. Arch Gen Psychiatry 47:849–853, 1990

Murphy KJ, Brunberg JA: Adult claustrophobia, anxiety, and sedation in MRI. Magn Reson Imaging 15:51–54, 1997

Muskin PR: The medical hospital, in Psychodynamic Concepts in General Psychiatry. Edited by Schwartz HJ. Washington, DC, American Psychiatric Press, 1995, pp 69–88

Pande AC, Davidson JR, Jefferson JW, et al: Treatment of social phobia with gabapentin: a placebo-controlled study. J Clin Psychopharmacol 19:341–348, 1999

Pande AC, Pollack MH, Crockatt J, et al: Placebo-controlled study of gabapentin treatment of panic disorder. J Clin Psychopharmacol 20:467–471, 2000

Payne D, Massie MJ: Anxiety in palliative care, in Handbook of Psychiatry in Palliative Medicine. Edited by Chochinov HM, Breitbart W. New York, Oxford University Press, 2000, pp 63–74

Perry S, Difede J, Musngi G, et al: Predictors of posttraumatic stress disorder after burn injury. Am J Psychiatry 149:931–935, 1992

Physicians' Desk Reference. Montvale, NJ, Thomson, 2003

Pollack MH, Smoller JW, Lee DK: Approach to the anxious patient, in MGH Guide to Psychiatry in Primary Care. Edited by Stern TA, Herman JB, Slavin PL. New York, McGraw-Hill, 1998, pp 23–37

Popkin MK, Tucker GJ: "Secondary" and drug-induced mood, anxiety, psychotic, catatonic, and personality disorders: a review of the literature. J Neuropsychiatry Clin Neurosci 4:369–385, 1992

Renfroe K: Effect of progressive relaxation on dyspnea and state anxiety in patients with chronic obstructive pulmonary disease. Heart Lung 17:408–413, 1988

Richard IH, Schiffer RB, Kurlan R: Anxiety and Parkinson's disease. J Neuropsychiatry Clin Neurosci 8:383–392, 1996

Robinson RG, Starkstein SE: Neuropsychiatric aspects of cerebrovascular disorders, in The American Psychiatric Publishing Textbook of Neuropsychiatry and Clinical Neurosciences, 4th Edition. Edited by Yudofsky SC, Hales RE. Washington, DC, American Psychiatric Publishing, 2002, pp 723–752

Roca RP, Spence RJ, Munster AM: Posttraumatic adaptation and distress among adult burn survivors. Am J Psychiatry 149:1234–1238, 1992

Roy-Byrne PP, Stein MB, Russo J, et al: Panic disorder in the primary care setting: comorbidity, disability, service utilization, and treatment. J Clin Psychiatry 60:492–499, 1999

Roy-Byrne PP, Katon W, Cowley DS, et al: A randomized effectiveness trial of collaborative care for patients with panic disorder in primary care. Arch Gen Psychiatry 58:869–876, 2001

Salzman C, Miyawaki E, le Bars P, et al: Neurobiologic basis of anxiety and its treatment. Harv Rev Psychiatry 1:197–205, 1993

Sherbourne CD, Wells KB, Meredith LS, et al: Comorbid anxiety disorder and the functioning and well-being of chronically ill patients of general medical providers. Arch Gen Psychiatry 53:889–895, 1996

Siemens ER, Shekhar A, Quaid K, et al: Anxiety and motor performance in Parkinson's disease. Mov Disord 8:501–506, 1993

Simon NM, Pollack MH, Tuby KS, et al: Dizziness and panic disorder: a review of the association between vestibular dysfunction and anxiety. Ann Clin Psychiatry 10:75–78, 1998

Smith GA: Caffeine reduction as an adjunct to anxiety management. Br J Clin Psychol 27(Pt 3):265–266, 1988

Smith MY, Redd WH, Peyser C, et al: Post-traumatic stress disorder in cancer: a review. Psychooncology 8:521–537, 1999

Smoller JW, Simon NM, Pollack MH, et al: Anxiety in patients with pulmonary disease: comorbidity and treatment. Semin Clin Neuropsychiatry 4:84–97, 1999

Spiegel D, Bloom J, Yalom I: Group support for patients with metastatic cancer. Arch Gen Psychiatry 38:527–533, 1981

Spiegel D, Bloom J, Kraemer HC: The beneficial effect of psychosocial treatment on survival of metastatic breast cancer patients. Lancet 2:888–891, 1989

Spielberger CD, Gorsuch RL, Luchene RE: Manual for the State-Trait Anxiety Inventory. Palo Alto, CA, Consulting Psychologist Press, 1970

Spitzer RL, Kroenke K, Williams JB: Validation and utility of a self-report version of PRIME-MD: the PHQ primary care study. Primary Care Evaluation of Mental Disorders. Patient Health Questionnaire. JAMA 282:1737–1744, 1999

Stark D, House A: Anxiety in cancer patients. Br J Cancer 83:1261–1267, 2000

Stein DJ, Hugo FJ: Neuropsychiatric aspects of anxiety disorders, in The American Psychiatric Publishing Textbook of Neuropsychiatry and Clinical Neurosciences, 4th Edition. Edited by Yudofsky SC, Hales RE. Washington, DC, American Psychiatric Publishing, 2002, pp 1049–1068

Stein MB, Asmundson GJ, Ireland D, et al: Panic disorder in patients attending a clinic for vestibular disorders. Am J Psychiatry 151:1697–1700, 1994

Stein MB, McQuaid JR, Pedrelli P, et al: Posttraumatic stress disorder in the primary care medical setting. Gen Hosp Psychiatry 22:261–269, 2000

Stoudemire A: Epidemiology and psychopharmacology of anxiety in medical patients. J Clin Psychiatry 57 (suppl 7):64–72, 1996

Stoudemire A, Moran M: Psychopharmacologic treatment of anxiety in the medically ill elderly patient. J Clin Psychiatry 54:27–36, 1993

Strain JJ, Grossman S: Psychological Care of the Medically Ill. New York, Appleton-Century-Crofts, 1975

Tapson VF: Pulmonary embolism, in Cecil Textbook of Medicine, 21st Edition. Edited by Goldman L, Bennett JC. Philadelphia, PA, WB Saunders, 2000, pp 441–449

Tedstone JE, Tarrier N: Posttraumatic stress disorder following medical illness and treatment. Clin Psychol Rev 23:409–448, 2003

Trzepacz PT, McCue M, Klein I, et al: A psychiatric and neuropsychological study of patients with untreated Graves' disease. Gen Hosp Psychiatry 10:49–55, 1988

Tucker GJ: Neuropsychiatric aspects of seizure disorders, in The American Psychiatric Publishing Textbook of Neuropsychiatry and Clinical Neurosciences, 4th Edition. Edited by Yudofsky SC, Hales RE. Washington, DC, American Psychiatric Publishing, 2002, pp 673–695

Vazquez A, Jimenez-Jimenez FJ, Garcia-Ruiz P, et al: "Panic attacks" in Parkinson's disease. A long-term complication of levodopa therapy. Acta Neurol Scand 87:14–18, 1993

Viederman M: The supportive relationship, the psychodynamic narrative, and the dying patient, in Handbook of Psychiatry in Palliative Medicine. Edited by Chochinov HM, Breitbart W. New York, Oxford University Press, 2000, pp 215–222

Walker EA, Gelfand AN, Gelfand MD, et al: Psychiatric diagnoses, sexual and physical victimization, and disability in patients with irritable bowel syndrome or inflammatory bowel disease. Psychol Med 25:1259–1267, 1995

Walsh K, Bennett G: Parkinson's disease and anxiety. Postgrad Med J 77:89–93, 2001

Weathers FW, Keane TM, Davidson JR: Clinician-administered PTSD scale: a review of the first ten years of research. Depress Anxiety 13:132–156, 2001

Weilburg JB, Schacter S, Worth J, et al: EEG abnormalities in patients with atypical panic attacks. J Clin Psychiatry 56:358–362, 1995

Wells KB, Golding JM, Burnam MA: Psychiatric disorder in a sample of the general population with and without chronic medical conditions. Am J Psychiatry 145:976–981, 1988

Wells KB, Golding JM, Burnam MA: Affective, substance use, and anxiety disorders in persons with arthritis, diabetes, heart disease, high blood pressure, or chronic lung conditions. Gen Hosp Psychiatry 11:320–327, 1989

Wilhelm S, Keuthen NJ, Deckersbach T, et al: Self-injurious skin picking: clinical characteristics and comorbidity. J Clin Psychiatry 60:454–459, 1999

Wise MG, Rundell JR: Anxiety and neurological disorders. Semin Clin Neuropsychiatry 4:98–102, 1999

Wolfe J, Schnurr PP, Brown PJ, et al: Posttraumatic stress disorder and war-zone exposure as correlates of perceived health in female Vietnam War veterans. J Consult Clin Psychol 62:1235–1240, 1994

Yalom I: Death and Dying. New York, Basic Books, 1980

Yellowlees PM, Kalucy RS: Psychobiological aspects of asthma and the consequent research implications. Chest 97:628–634, 1990

Yellowlees PM, Alpers JH, Bowden JJ, et al: Psychiatric morbidity in patients with chronic airflow obstruction. Med J Aust 146:305–307, 1987

Young AS, Klap R, Sherbourne CD, et al: The quality of care for depressive and anxiety disorders in the United States. Arch Gen Psychiatry 58:55–61, 2001

Yu B-H, Dimsdale JE: Posttraumatic stress disorder in patients with burn injuries. J Burn Care Rehabil 20:426–433, 1999

Zatzick DF, Kang SM, Muller HG, et al: Predicting posttraumatic distress in hospitalized trauma survivors with acute injuries. Am J Psychiatry 159:941–946, 2002

Zaubler TS, Katon W: Panic disorder in the general medical setting. J Psychosom Res 44:25–42, 1998

Zimetbaum P, Josephson ME: Evaluation of patients with palpitations. N Engl J Med 338:1369–1373, 1998

13 Somatization and Somatoform Disorders

Susan E. Abbey, M.D., F.R.C.P.C.

SOMATIZATION IS A poorly understood "blind spot" of medicine (Quill 1985). Somatoform disorders remain neglected by psychiatrists despite their associated significant functional impairments and economic burden (Bass et al. 2001). Important conceptual and clinical questions exist about the validity and utility of the concepts, particularly in clinical settings, and new paradigms might lead to more effective management (Epstein et al. 1999; Mayou et al. 2003; Sharpe and Carson 2001).

Somatization and somatoform disorders challenge consulting psychiatrists, who often wade into emotionally charged clinical situations in which diagnosis is difficult, both the referring physician and the patient are frustrated and angry, and the involvement of a psychiatrist may be stigmatizing. The complex set of emotions that patients with somatoform disorders engender has resulted in the application of disparaging names both to these patients (e.g., "crocks") (Lipsitt 1970) and to the discipline (e.g., "psychoceramic medicine"). The evidence base for diagnosing and treating these patients remains suboptimal, but there is a strong clinical literature that can help psychiatrists to work effectively with these patients, produce substantial improvements in the patients' and their families' well-being, and decrease direct and indirect costs of their illness. The medical training of psychosomatic medicine psychiatrists facilitates management of difficult cases, such as patients who somatize or have a somatoform disorder and have a concurrent general medical condition with overlapping symptoms.

This chapter begins with a discussion of the process of somatization, followed by a review of the DSM-IV-TR (American Psychiatric Association 2000) somatoform disorders. The chapter focuses on adults. Somatization and somatoform disorders in children are discussed in Chapter 34, "Pediatrics," and in several reviews (Garralda 1999; Silber and Pao 2003). Conversion disorder is also discussed in Chapter 32, "Neurology and Neurosurgery."

Somatization as a Process

Somatization can be conceptualized in a variety of different ways, but fundamentally it appears to be a way of responding to stress. It is a ubiquitous human phenomenon that at times becomes problematic and warrants clinical attention. Somatization is extremely common in medical settings and among the patients referred to psychosomatic medicine psychiatrists. Not all somatizing patients have a somatoform disorder. Many have another Axis I disorder or transiently somatize in the context of significant life stress.

Definitions and Clinically Useful Theoretical Concepts

The area of somatization is complicated by a lack of uniformity in the use of terminology. Theoretical concepts that are clinically useful in management are described below.

Somatization

Historically, *somatization* was defined by Steckel as a deep-seated neurosis that produced bodily symptoms (Lipowski 1988). In the past 20 years, the term *somatization* has been used to describe the tendency of certain patients to experience and communicate psychological and interpersonal problems in the form of somatic distress and medically unexplained symptoms for which they seek medical help (Katon et al. 1984; Kleinman 1986; Lipowski 1988). Although it has become a widely used term, Sharpe (2002) cautions that its use should be restricted to cases in which the somatic symptoms are an expression of an identifiable emotional disorder. In essence, somatization is a culturally sanctioned idiom of psychosocial distress (Katon et al. 1984; Kleinman 1986). Kirmayer and Young (1998) note that, depending on circumstances, somatization "can be seen as an index of disease or disorder, an indication of psychopathology, a symbolic condensation of intrapsychic conflict, a culturally coded expression of distress, a medium for expressing social discontent, and a mechanism through which patients attempt to reposition themselves within their local worlds" (p. 420).

Three components of somatization described by Lipowski (1988) can offer targets for intervention: experiential, cognitive, and behavioral (Table 13–1).

Medically Unexplained Symptoms

Somatization is frequently implicated in *medically unexplained symptoms*, defined as symptoms that are not attributable to or are out of proportion to identifiable physical disease (Sharpe 2002). Medically unexplained symptoms are discussed in other chapters in this volume, including noncardiac chest pain (see Chapter 19, "Heart Disease"), hyperventilation syndrome (see Chapter 20, "Lung Disease"), irritable bowel and functional upper gastrointestinal tract disorders (see Chapter 21, "Gastrointestinal Disorders"), chronic fatigue syndrome and fibromyalgia (see Chapter 26, "Chronic Fatigue and Fibromyalgia Syndromes"), idiopathic pruritus (see Chapter 29, "Dermatology"), chronic pelvic pain and vulvodynia (see Chapter 33, "Obstetrics and Gynecology"), and pain syndromes (see Chapter 36, "Pain").

TABLE 13–1. Clinical implications of the components of somatization

Component	Potential intervention
Experiential	Techniques to decrease somatic sensations (e.g., biofeedback, pharmacotherapy for concomitant psychiatric disorder)
Cognitive	Reattribution of sensation from sinister to benign cause Distraction techniques
Behavioral	Operant techniques to reduce medication consumption Contract to "save" symptoms for regular visit with primary care physician rather than visiting emergency room

Somatosensory Amplification

Symptoms are the result of bodily sensations and their subsequent cortical interpretation. *Somatosensory amplification* refers to the tendency to experience somatic sensations as intense, noxious, or disturbing (Barsky et al. 1988b). It is composed of three elements: 1) hypervigilance to bodily sensations, 2) predisposition to select out and concentrate on weak or infrequent bodily sensations, and 3) reaction to sensations with cognitions and affect that intensify them and make them more alarming (Barsky et al. 1988b). It has both trait and state components.

Illness Versus Disease

The distinction between illness and disease (Eisenberg 1977) is useful for psychosomatic medicine psychiatrists. *Illness* is the response of the individual and his or her family to symptoms; this contrasts with *disease*, which is defined by physicians and is associated with pathophysiological processes and documentable lesions. Mismatches between illness and disease are common and are at the root of many management problems. Hypertensive patients may not perceive themselves as ill and therefore might not comply with treatment regimens. Patients with somatoform disorders view themselves as very ill despite not having a disease. In somatizing patients with some disease component, their subjective illness experience is assessed to be disproportionate to the degree of disease.

Illness Behavior and Abnormal Illness Behavior

Illness behavior refers to "the manner in which individuals monitor their bodies, define and interpret their symptoms, take remedial action, and utilize sources of help as well as the more formal health care system. It also is concerned with how people monitor and respond to symptoms and symptom change over the course of an illness and how this affects behavior, remedial actions taken, and response to treatment" (Mechanic 1986, p. 1). Illness behavior may be regarded as a syndrome, as a symptom, as a dimension, or as an explanation of behavior (Mayou 1989). Illness behavior is affected by a wide variety of social, psychiatric, and cultural factors and can be used "to achieve a variety of social and personal objectives having little to do with biological systems of the pathogenesis of disease" (Mechanic 1986, p. 3).

Abnormal illness behavior is identified by a physician when there is an "inappropriate or maladaptive mode of perceiving, evaluating or acting in relation to one's own health status, which persists despite the fact that a doctor (or other appropriate social agent) has offered an accurate and reasonably lucid explanation of the nature of the illness and the appropriate course of management to be followed, based on a thorough examination of all parameters of functioning, and taking into account the individual's age, educational and sociocultural background" (Pilowsky 1987, p. 89). It may be somatically or psychologically focused and may be either illness affirming or illness denying. The construct has been criticized as dangerous in that it places physicians in the position of defining what is normal and what is "abnormal." It has been counterargued that a corresponding medical behavior of "abnormal treatment behavior" may be described.

Somatization as a Clinical Problem

Somatization becomes clinically significant when it is associated with significant occupational and social dysfunction or with excessive health care use. The relation between acute and persistent forms of somatization is unclear; they may form a continuum or may be discrete conditions. A longitudinal study of primary care "somatizers" (defined as patients with emotional disorder presenting with recent-onset physical symptoms) found that 16 of 44 patients went on to develop chronic somatoform disorders over a 2-year follow-up period (Craig et al. 1993). Somatization and somatoform disorders pose a significant economic burden (Bass et al. 2001). In addition to the higher-than-average inpatient, ambulatory, and physician service costs of care of such patients, there are social costs, including decreased occupational productivity. Many patients with somatization also have severe distress, particularly depression and anxiety. In addition, somatizing patients are at increased risk of iatrogenic disease and injury. For example, in pseudoseizures, the most frequent cause of morbidity and death is the misdiagnosis of epilepsy and resulting aggressive treatment with anticonvulsants (Kanner 2003).

Relation Among Psychiatric Disorders, Somatization, and Medically Unexplained Symptoms

Strong interrelations exist among somatization, psychiatric disorders, and health care utilization. Four models (Figure 13–1) have been advanced to explain these relations (Simon 1991). Different models may apply to different patients.

Somatization as a Masked Presentation of Psychiatric Illness

Physical symptoms are an integral part of most psychiatric disorders. Somatizing patients focus on these symptoms to the exclusion of psychological symptoms. They may then attribute the psychological symptoms to the distress resulting from the physical symptoms (e.g., "Yes, doctor, I am sad, but you would be too if you couldn't sleep or eat and had no energy!"). This masking of the psychiatric syndrome is important, because major depressive disorder and anxiety disorders are significantly underrecognized in patients presenting with somatic complaints (Kirmayer et al. 1993). Somatization does not appear to be a defense against acknowledging the presence of a psychiatric disorder (Hotopf et al. 2001).

Depression and somatization. Physical symptoms are common in major depressive disorder (Simon et al. 1999; see also Chapter 9, "Depression"). The mechanism by which they are produced is unclear and may be related to 1) psychophysiological concomitants of depression, 2) somatosensory amplification, and 3) a depressive attributional style in which symptoms are perceived as indicating poor health. Primary care patients with depression have higher health care utilization and report more somatic symptoms than do patients without depression (Kroenke 2003). It is estimated that 50% or more of the patients presenting in primary care with major depressive disorder do so with predominantly somatic complaints rather than with cognitive or affective symptoms of depression (Simon and Gureje 1999). These somatic presentations of depression have been referred to as *masked depression* or *depressive equivalents*. Somatic symptoms in depression are related to concomitant anxiety, the tendency to amplify somatic distress, and difficulty identifying and communicating emotional distress (Sayar et al. 2003). Comorbidity among depression, somatization, and somatoform disorders is high (G.R. Smith 1992). Consequently, it has been argued that medically unexplained symptoms are a manifestation of an affective-spectrum disorder (Hudson et al. 2003).

Anxiety and somatization. Anxiety disorders are also accompanied by prominent physical symptoms and are frequently mistaken for or associated with somatization in patients presenting in primary care and medical subspecialty settings (Sullivan et al. 1993; see also Chapter 12, "Anxiety Disorders"). Somatization and hypochondriacal fears and beliefs are common among patients with panic disorder, particularly those who also have agoraphobia and focus more on seeking an explanation for, than on treatment of, their symptoms (Starcevic et al. 1992). In addition, posttraumatic stress disorder often presents with somatic complaints (Andreski et al. 1998; Moreau and Zisook 2002).

Other Axis I diagnoses. Substance abuse is associated with somatization (Mehrabian 2001) and is reported in

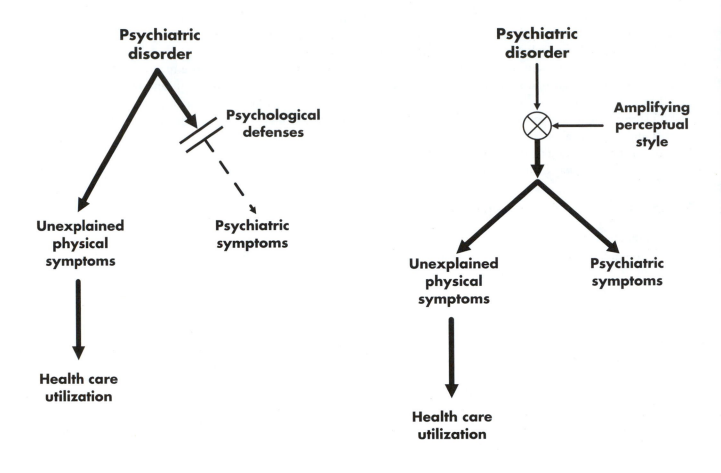

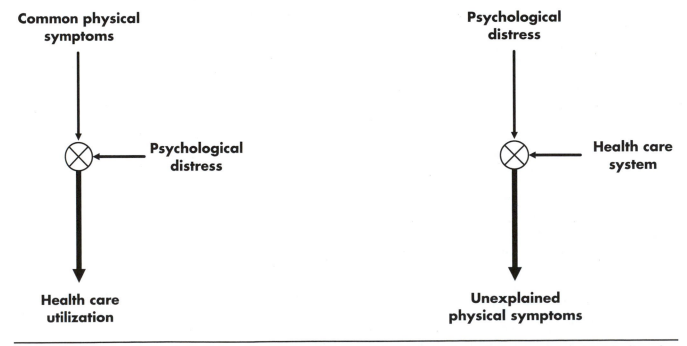

FIGURE 13–1.   Four models of the relation between psychiatric symptomatology and psychiatric disorder.
Source.   Reprinted from Simon GE: "Somatization and Psychiatric Disorder," in *Current Concepts of Somatization: Research and Clinical Perspectives.* Edited by Kirmayer LJ, Robbins JM. Washington, DC, American Psychiatric Press, 1991, pp. 37–62. Used with permission.

subsets of patients with substance abuse. Finally, somatization is also prevalent in patients with schizophrenia and is associated with emotional distress, medication side effects, and expressed emotion within families. A recent study found that more than a quarter of patients with schizophrenia had five or more unexplained medical symptoms, both at admission and 12 months later (Ritsner 2003). Psychotic somatic symptoms (somatic delusions, hallucinations, and misperceptions) are common in schizophrenia and in somatic delusional disorders such as delusions of parasitosis (see Chapter 29, "Dermatology").

Somatization as an Amplifying Personal Perceptual Style

An amplifying personal perceptual style may be a stable personality trait or a consequence of abnormal neuropsychological information processing (Barsky et al. 1988a). Some somatizing patients show a lowered threshold for reporting physical symptoms (Barsky et al. 1988b; Pennebaker and Watson 1991).

Somatization as a Tendency to Seek Care for Common Symptoms

This model posits that emotional distress prompts people to seek care for common symptoms for which they would not seek care in the absence of emotional distress. It is supported by research in patients with a variety of medically unexplained symptoms in whom medical help seeking is associated with higher levels of emotional distress rather than physical symptoms (Drossman 1999; McBeth and Silman 2001).

Somatization as a Response to the Incentives of the Health Care System

The health care system tends to reinforce illness behavior and symptom reporting and may produce "iatrogenic somatization" (Simon 1991).

Etiological Factors in Somatization and Somatoform Disorders

Pathophysiological Mechanisms

Understanding and acknowledging the physiological as well as the psychological mechanisms associated with somatization helps both patient and physician to avoid dualistic "mind versus body" thinking—which often devolves into stigmatized notions of "imaginary" versus "real" symptoms—and to develop a therapeutic alliance (Sharpe and Bass 1992). Some of the proposed patho-

physiological mechanisms of somatization are summarized in Table 13–2.

Genetic Factors

Somatization and somatization disorder appear to have a genetic component (Guze 1993; Kendler et al. 1995). Adoption studies of Swedish men suggested that the psychiatric processes associated with somatization in men and women may be qualitatively different (Cloninger et al. 1986). More studies addressing this question are needed.

Developmental Factors

The cognitive appraisals patients make of somatic symptoms often have some of their roots in early family experiences. Physical symptoms are a major form of interpersonal communication in some families (Stuart and Noyes 1999). Childhood exposure to parental chronic illness or abnormal illness behavior appears to increase the risk of somatization in later life (Bass and Murphy 1995; Craig et al. 1993). Negative parenting styles are associated with somatization in irritable bowel syndrome patients (Lackner et al. 2004). Anxious attachment behavior arising from early life experiences may also be the basis for persistent care-seeking behavior that frustrates both health care professionals and family members (Noyes et al. 2003; Stuart and Noyes 1999).

TABLE 13–2. Pathophysiological mechanisms of somatization

Physiological mechanisms
Autonomic arousal
Muscle tension
Hyperventilation
Vascular changes
Cerebral information processing
Physiological effects of inactivity
Sleep disturbance

Psychological mechanisms
Perceptual factors
Beliefs
Mood
Personality factors

Interpersonal mechanisms
Reinforcing actions of relatives and friends
Health care system
Disability system

Source. Adapted from Mayou 1993; Sharpe and Bass 1992.

Cognitive Theories

Cognitive distortions and preferential memory bias for disorder-congruent information have been demonstrated in patients with somatoform disorders (Brown et al. 1999; Pauli and Alpers 2002).

Personality Characteristics

A variety of psychological traits or personality factors have been linked with somatization, although it is unclear whether they primarily influence symptom production and help-seeking behavior or are a consequence of living with chronic symptoms. Introspectiveness (i.e., the tendency to think about oneself) is associated with increased symptom reporting, greater physical and psychological distress, and more medical help seeking (Mechanic 1986). Negative affectivity, a construct based on negative mood, poor self-concept, and pessimism, is also associated with increased symptom reporting and with greater worry about perceived symptoms (Pennebaker and Watson 1991).

Psychodynamic Factors

Bodily symptoms have been interpreted as metaphors through which a patient expresses emotional distress or psychic conflict (McDougall 1989). Self psychologists argue that bodily preoccupation develops in response to a fragmented sense of self and can be best understood as an attempt to restore a sense of integration (Rodin 1984). *Alexithymia* refers to impairment in the ability to verbalize affect and elaborate fantasies that results from deficits in the cognitive processing and regulation of emotions (Taylor 2000). It has been implicated as a mechanism of some forms of somatization. Although repressed anger or aggression was thought by classical psychodynamic theorists to be important, Kellner et al. (1985) found no evidence that anger or hostility plays a specific etiological role in somatization and hypochondriasis.

Sexual and Physical Abuse

Sexual and physical abuse, in both childhood and adulthood, has been linked with somatization, medically unexplained symptoms, and somatoform disorders in numerous studies since the late 1980s. The development of insight into the relation of the abuse to subsequent somatization is helpful for some patients and may decrease subsequent health care use (Walling et al. 1994). The mechanisms by which physical and sexual trauma is associated with somatization are poorly understood. Sexual abuse negatively affects "embodiment" (i.e., the experience of the self in and through the body) (Young 1992). Abuse also causes a tendency to dissociate, and dissocia-

tion is associated with a tendency to report increased physical symptoms (Salmon et al. 2003). Higher hypnotic susceptibility, a marker of the capacity to self-evoke dissociative experiences, has been found to partially mediate the relationship between abuse and conversion symptoms in patients with conversion disorder (Roelofs et al. 2002).

Sociocultural Factors

Somatization was originally thought to be more common among non-Western cultures, but recent work suggests that somatization is ubiquitous, although prevalence and specific features vary across cultures (Kirmayer and Young 1998). The World Health Organization Cross-National Study of Mental Disorders in Primary Care found that all sites (14 countries) reported high rates of somatization (Gureje et al. 1997) and correlation of somatic symptoms and emotional distress (Simon et al. 1996). The stigmatization of psychiatric distress may be a powerful factor promoting somatization. "Organic" or physical illnesses are seen as more real and less blameworthy than psychiatric disorders, which are seen as being under voluntary control and are often associated with connotations of malingering and weak moral fiber (Kirmayer and Robbins 1991). Somatization may be the only form of communication permissible for the socially powerless.

Gender

The relation between gender and somatization is complex and poorly understood. Although it has traditionally been believed that women somatize more than men, the literature is problematic (Barsky et al. 2001). A recent international study of somatization in primary care found few sex differences (Piccinelli and Simon 1997). A longitudinal study of primary care attendees found that somatizers were more likely to be men (Kirmayer and Robbins 1996), whereas data from the Epidemiologic Catchment Area study found that women report more unexplained symptoms overall (Liu et al. 1997).

Iatrogenesis

The health care insurance and disability systems may foster somatization by providing reinforcement (Ford 1983; Simon 1991). Insurance policies with better coverage and fewer barriers for nonpsychiatric medical care than mental health care also provide incentives to somatize (Ford 1992). Well-intentioned but uninformed actions by physicians may also contribute, through unnecessary diagnostic testing and treatments (and their adverse effects) and reinforcement of the sick role (Page and Wessely 2003).

Assessment and Diagnosis of Somatization

Assessment for somatization or somatoform disorders is often difficult and requires special interviewing skills (Creed and Guthrie 1993; Sharpe et al. 1992).

Building an Alliance With the Patient

Early in the interview, the patient's ambivalence about seeing a psychiatrist must be addressed, as well as what the patient has been told about the consultation process. The specific approach to the examination will vary according to the patient. For very resistant patients, the initial interview is often dominated by gaining sufficient cooperation to allow a more detailed assessment to take place at a later time. The initial phase of the assessment should focus on the history of physical symptoms. Allowing the patient to report a detailed history of his or her physical symptoms provides reassurance that the symptoms are being taken seriously, which aids immeasurably in later phases of the assessment and treatment process. The psychiatrist's use of empathic comments such as "You have had a terrible time" or "The symptoms sound very difficult" help to build an alliance and may lead the patient to volunteer information (Creed and Guthrie 1993). The question "How has this illness or symptom affected your life?" may go a long way toward answering the question "How has your life affected this illness?" Making interpretive or linking statements that bring together the patient's physical and emotional states may encourage the patient to be more forthcoming with regard to emotional distress and may further the sense of engagement (Creed and Guthrie 1993). However, caution must be exercised because premature or maladroit interpretations can be detrimental to the developing trust between patient and physician. For especially skeptical patients, the psychiatrist can emphasize his or her expertise in helping people develop the skills they need to cope with symptoms, regardless of the "cause."

Collaborating With the Referral Source

Collaboration with the referral source is essential for a clear understanding of the reason for referral and of what the patient has been told about it. Psychiatrists can provide guidance about how to explain the psychiatric referral to the patient to make it more acceptable.

Reviewing the Medical Records

Medical records should be reviewed before the consultation to help the psychiatrist devise an approach to the patient. Familiarity with the history fosters an alliance. The type, number, and frequency of the patient's symptoms, as well as comments about the patient's prior attitude toward symptoms and behavior, should be documented (Creed and Guthrie 1993). The importance of a thorough chart review cannot be overestimated, because the psychosomatic medicine psychiatrist may be the first person to thoroughly review the typically thick chart and thus may be in a better position than any other member of the medical team to reach a diagnosis of either a general medical condition or a psychiatric disorder.

Gathering Collateral Information From Family and Friends

Collateral information can be invaluable to the accurate assessment of current and past functional capacity and current and past psychosocial stressors.

Performing a Psychiatric and Mental Status Examination

In addition to routine psychiatric observations, the examination of the patient with somatic symptoms should include observations about abnormal illness behavior, symptom amplification, and the quality of the patient's description of his or her symptoms. It is essential to evaluate the individual's ideas about the meaning, cause, implications, and significance of his or her symptoms and the individual's emotional response to his or her situation (Barsky 1998; Creed and Guthrie 1993; Sharpe et al. 1992). If it is performed after taking a history of the physical complaints (but not before), a mental status examination is usually acceptable to the patient.

Performing a Physical Examination

A physical examination of the patient is a prerequisite for accurate diagnosis and treatment for several reasons. In some cases, elements of the physical examination should be performed by the psychiatrist (see Chapter 1, "Psychiatric Assessment and Consultation"), who may be in the best position to diagnose a general medical condition because "something about the patient (personality, behavior, affect, odd cognition) has effectively distracted the primary physician and other consultants from the diagnosis" (Cassem and Barsky 1991, p. 132). A case example follows.

> Ms. P, a 42-year-old woman who had had a renal transplant 2 months earlier, was referred for psychiatric evaluation of "suspected conversion disorder in a patient with history of obsessive-compulsive disorder" after she developed "constant rocking movement that she can voluntarily stop." The psychiatrist found on examination that the patient had an obvious resting rhythmic truncal tremor. The psychiatrist's examination revealed

subtle choreiform movements in the patient's tongue and fingers. Noting that metoclopramide had been started at the time of the transplant, the psychiatrist diagnosed a movement disorder, which resolved after drug discontinuation.

The physician who is managing a persistently somatizing patient must also tolerate the patient's perpetual concern about symptoms with some degree of equanimity. A medical education that repeatedly emphasizes the danger of "missed diagnoses" and the current medicolegal climate mean that the physician must be confident that a thorough medical evaluation has been completed.

The physical examination may also help to establish a positive diagnosis of somatization disorder. For example, awareness of physical signs associated with stress (e.g., tender anterior chest wall, tender abdomen, spurious breathing, short breath-holding time) leads to a more confident diagnosis rather than a diagnosis of exclusion, the latter of which always has an implication of doubt associated with it (Sharpe and Bass 1992). A variety of physical signs may be useful, but some are controversial in making a diagnosis of a somatoform disorder (see Fishbain et al. 2003). A somatoform disorder should be diagnosed (as the sole diagnosis) only if the examination also confirms normal functioning of the system being tested (Newman 1993).

Clinical Management of Somatization

The key to clinical management is to adopt caring rather than curing as a goal. Management is a much more realistic goal than cure in this population (Bass and Benjamin 1993; Creed and Guthrie 1993; Epstein et al. 1999; Sharpe et al. 1992; G.C. Smith et al. 2000). Management must be tailored to the individual's somatic symptoms, thoughts and beliefs, behavior, and emotional state (Epstein et al. 1999). Three potential management approaches to the patient with somatization disorder have been described:

1. A *reattribution approach* emphasizes helping the patient to link his or her physical symptoms with psychological or stressful factors in his or her life. This is accomplished via a three-step process that links psychosocial stressors (e.g., marital strife) through physiological mechanisms (e.g., increased muscle tension) to physical symptoms (e.g., headache) (Goldberg et al. 1989).
2. A *psychotherapeutic approach* concentrates on developing a close and trusting relationship with the patient (Guthrie et al. 1991).
3. A *directive approach* treats the patient as though he or she has a physical problem, and interventions are framed in a medical model (Benjamin 1989).

The three management approaches vary in their suitability for different patients. The reattribution approach is particularly useful in primary care settings, in medical-surgical inpatient settings with patients who have a fair degree of insight, and in psychiatric settings with patients who have less lengthy histories of somatization. The reattribution technique can be easily taught to primary care practitioners (Goldberg et al. 1989). The psychotherapeutic approach is most suitable for patients with persistent somatization who are willing to explore the effect of psychosocial factors on their symptoms. The directive approach is most useful for hostile patients who deny the importance of psychological or social factors in their symptomatology.

Principles of Management

The fundamental principles of management are similar for patients with somatization and with somatoform disorders.

Providing a positive explanation of symptoms. In order to engage in treatment, patients require a sense that their primary physician is taking them seriously, appreciates the magnitude of their distress, and has a rationale for the proposed management plan. Most somatizing patients hold explanatory models of their symptoms that are in conflict with their physician's model (Salmon et al. 1999). The clinical challenge is therefore to provide explanations that empower patients with tangible mechanisms, exculpation, and encouragement of self-management rather than explanations that reject or collude with the patient's model (Salmon et al. 1999). Reassurance is helpful to many patients (Page and Wessely 2003), but it must be carefully dosed and targeted. Facile or excessive reassurance may exacerbate disease fears or cause patients to redouble efforts to prove they are sick and may undermine the doctor–patient relationship (Warwick 1992). It is important to emphasize to patients that the psychiatrist is not dismissing their symptoms as being "all in their head" but rather sees the symptoms as being "real" and "in their body" and wants to explore all opportunities for symptom control. The use of metaphors and analogies is often helpful. The metaphor of a radio has been reported to be particularly useful (N.H. Cassem, personal communication, July 1985). The radio channel playing is the symptom that is of concern, and given that it cannot be changed by medical or surgical interventions, the patient must gain greater control over the volume control knob (i.e., factors that exacerbate or relieve symptoms) or the sensitivity of the antenna (i.e., factors that amplify symptoms). Physiological mechanisms underlying symptoms may be usefully explained (see Table 13–2) (Sharpe and Bass 1992). Understanding the personal meaning of the symptoms to the patient and tailoring one's explanations and reassurance in light of this meaning may improve the doctor–patient relationship (Epstein et al. 1999; Priel et al. 1991).

Ensuring regular follow-up. Regular follow-up is the key to effective management; it results in decreased health care utilization overall and is less stressful for both patients and physicians than symptom-driven visits. The best choice for most patients is management by their primary care practitioner in consultation with a psychiatrist. However, the psychiatrist may provide primary follow-up if significant comorbid Axis I or Axis II pathology is present or if the primary care physician cannot manage the symptoms.

Treating mood or anxiety disorders. Mood or anxiety disorders have significant morbidity in their own right and interfere with participation in rehabilitation and psychotherapy. Their physiological concomitants may fuel the somatization process or heighten somatic amplification.

Minimizing polypharmacy. Polypharmacy may produce iatrogenic complications. Unnecessary medications should be tapered and withdrawn using a staged approach over time with small, realistically achievable steps.

Providing specific therapy when indicated. A variety of specific therapies have been recommended for the somatoform disorders and are discussed below under "Management of Somatoform Disorders." For example, physiotherapy or massage may be helpful in diminishing musculoskeletal pain for patients with somatoform disorders.

Changing social dynamics that reinforce symptoms. Many patients' lives come to revolve around their symptoms and their use of the health care system. Regularly scheduled follow-up means that the patient no longer has to present a symptom as a "ticket of admission" to the physician's office. Important members of the patient's social support system may be persuaded to consistently reward non-illness-related behaviors. Social skills building, life skills training, assertiveness training, and physical reactivation programs may be indicated. Group therapy may be useful because it provides social support, increases interpersonal skills, and provides a nonthreatening environment in which to learn to experience and express emotions and desires more directly.

Resolving difficulties in the doctor–patient relationship. Somatizing patients often have difficult relationships with their caregivers because of attention seeking, demands, and anger. These difficulties have multiple determinants, including problematic early attachment (Stuart and Noyes 1999), differences in expectations and beliefs about the meaning and management of symptoms, and prior frustrating experiences with the health care system (Page and Wessely 2003). Consequently, addressing shortcomings in doctor–patient interactions can be helpful (Page and Wessely 2003).

Recognizing and controlling negative reactions or countertransference. Somatizing patients can evoke powerful emotional responses in physicians, which may result in less than optimal clinical care (Hahn et al. 1994; Sharpe et al. 1994). The range of emotions experienced by physicians may include guilt for failing to help the patient, fear that the patient will make a complaint, and anger at the patient's entitlement. The physician may be dismissive of the patient or, alternatively, may collude with the patient in excessive investigations to exclude physical disease in "a suspension of professional judgment" (Bass and Murphy 1990). Excessive investigation might result from a conscious attempt to avoid a "painful, embarrassing and time-consuming confrontation" (Bass and Murphy 1990) or may represent an unconscious solution to the conflicts and emotions that the patient evokes in the physician. The treating physician should seek to identify something about the patient that is either likable or interesting that will help to sustain his or her involvement—in the most difficult patients, it may simply be a sense of amazement at the degree of somatization. A physician caring for these patients must also set clear limits as to his or her availability. If all else fails, the physician should transfer the care of the patient to a colleague, either temporarily or permanently.

Somatoform Disorders

The DSM-IV-TR somatoform disorders are somatization disorder, undifferentiated somatoform disorder, conversion disorder, pain disorder, hypochondriasis, body dysmorphic disorder, and somatoform disorder not otherwise specified (American Psychiatric Association 2000). The feature they have in common is the presence of unexplained physical symptoms that are not intentionally produced. In DSM-IV-TR it is emphasized that these disorders are grouped together because of the need to exclude medical and substance-induced etiologies (American Psychiatric Association 2000).

Somatoform disorders are more common in ambulatory than in inpatient settings. They have been diagnosed in 3%–4% of psychiatric consultations in general hospitals in Australia (G.C. Smith et al. 2000) and the Netherlands (Thomassen et al. 2003). In the latter study the somatoform diagnoses were conversion disorder, 40%; hypochondriasis, 24%; somatoform pain disorder, 20%; and somatization disorder, 17%. Studies of the general population have reported more variable rates. A recent study of German adolescents and young adults found a lifetime rate for somatoform disorders of 3%; a further 11% of subjects had subsyndromal conditions (Lieb et al. 2000).

There are a number of difficulties in the clinical application of the somatoform diagnoses as defined in the DSM. First, excluding a medical cause for symptoms is problematic, particularly for those with comorbid medical diseases. The focus on exclusion promotes dualistic thinking, but failure to demonstrate a medical cause for symptoms does not necessarily mean the patient has a psychiatric disorder (Kirmayer and Young 1998). Second, the question of intentionality or consciousness in symptom production is a vexing one. Distinguishing somatoform disorders from the factitious disorders and malingering is discussed in Chapter 14 ("Deception Syndromes: Factitious Disorders and Malingering"), but these disorders can overlap. Third, dimensional rather than categorical approaches may be more helpful in describing hypochondriacal preoccupation, medically unexplained symptoms, and help seeking. Fourth, the clinical descriptions of specific disorders are largely derived from tertiary care or psychiatric hospital samples and emphasize chronicity.

Finally, the separate existence of a discrete category of somatoform disorders reinforces the mind–body dualism of Western medicine and implies a separation of affective, anxiety, dissociative, and somatic symptoms (Kirmayer and Young 1998). In fact, somatic symptoms and somatization cut across DSM-IV-TR diagnostic categories. Some recent critics have suggested extensive reformulation, reclassification, and even abolition of the somatoform disorders (Mayou et al. 2003; Phillips et al. 2003).

Somatization Disorder

Definition

Somatization disorder is based on the earlier diagnosis of Briquet's syndrome, which required 25 of 59 physical symptoms, an illness onset before age 30 years, and a pattern of recurrent physical complaints, and was shown to have validity, reliability, and internal consistency (Feighner et al. 1972). The long-term stability of the diagnosis

was documented by the finding that 80%–90% of patients continued to meet diagnostic criteria at 6- to 8-year follow-up (Guze et al. 1986). DSM-III criteria for somatization disorder were a modification of Feighner's criteria, with a total symptom count of 14 symptoms in women and 12 symptoms in men from a total list of 36 physical symptoms (American Psychiatric Association 1980). In DSM-III-R the criteria were further modified by simplifying the requirement to 13 of 35 physical symptoms and specifically excluding symptoms occurring only during a panic attack (American Psychiatric Association 1987). The diagnostic criteria were again simplified in DSM-IV, and they have been found to be concordant with prior criteria (Yutzy et al. 1995).

Epidemiology

The lifetime prevalence of somatization disorder has varied widely across studies, ranging from 0.2% to 2.0% among women and less than 0.2% in men (American Psychiatric Association 2000), reflecting variations in research methodology and study samples. Because patients with somatization disorder actively seek medical help, their prevalence in medical settings is higher than in the general population. Somatization disorder has been diagnosed in 1%–5% of primary care patients (Simon and Gureje 1999). Changes in practice patterns have likely led to fewer somatization disorder patients being admitted to hospitals. Patients with somatization disorder accounted for 0.7% of Dutch psychiatric consultations (Thomassen et al. 2003) and 0.2% of Australian consultations to medical and surgical inpatients (G.C. Smith et al. 2000). Recent work has emphasized the instability of recall of somatic symptoms, with implications for underdiagnosing somatization disorder (Simon and Gureje 1999). By definition, the syndrome must begin before age 30, but most often symptoms begin in the teens, often with menarche, or less commonly in the early 20s. The risk for depression, alcohol abuse, and antisocial personality disorder is increased in the first-degree relatives of individuals with somatization disorder (Golding et al. 1992).

Specific Culture and Gender Factors

There is cultural variability in the presentation of somatization disorder. Symptoms used in DSM-IV-TR are those that have been found to be most diagnostic in the United States (American Psychiatric Association 2000). The disorder is uncommon in American men (Golding et al. 1991), although in an American sample women and men with somatization disorder had similar clinical characteristics, including comorbid psychopathology (Golding et al. 1991). Women with somatization disorder are more likely to have a history of sexual abuse than are women with primary mood disorders (Morrison 1989).

> Ms. L is a 28-year-old woman referred for psychiatric assessment based on 25 primary care visits, 18 emergency room visits, and 2 hospitalizations in the past 12 months for a variety of symptoms, including unexplained headaches, pelvic pain, dysmenorrhea, back pain, nausea, dysphagia, and irregular menses. She has been "sickly" since childhood; is unemployed as a result of her multiple medical problems; and is socially isolated, having had difficulties in interpersonal relationships for many years.

Clinical Features

The classic patient with somatization disorder is a woman who subjectively is "sickly" and who began to experience medically unexplained symptoms in early adolescence. Her condition has shown a waxing and waning course over the years, with a medical history that documents repeated, unexplained physical complaints. Patients with somatization disorder are often difficult historians who provide dramatic and colorful but vague descriptions of their medical history (Cassem and Barsky 1991) and may present as odd or anxious (Rost et al. 1992). There is often more to be learned in a review of their medical records.

Associated Features

Patients with somatization disorder have high rates of psychiatric comorbidity. As many as 75% of patients with somatization disorder have comorbid Axis I diagnoses (Katon et al. 1991), of which the most common are major depressive disorder, dysthymia, panic disorder, simple phobia, and substance abuse. Because patients with somatization disorder have a low threshold for endorsing symptoms, in some cases comorbid diagnoses may reflect an amplifying response tendency rather than significant symptomatology. However, many patients do have bona fide comorbid Axis I disorders with significant negative impact on functioning. Personality disorders appear to be especially common in patients with somatization disorder. The most common comorbid Axis II diagnoses in psychiatric settings are Cluster B diagnoses, whereas in primary care settings Cluster C and paranoid personality diagnoses are more frequent (Rost et al. 1992). The association between personality disorder and somatization disorder may result from a common biological substrate or social-environmental factors such as childhood abuse (G.R. Smith 1991). Patients with somatization disorder often have multiple social problems and chaotic lifestyles characterized by poor interpersonal relationships, disruptive or difficult behavior, and substance abuse (Cassem and Barsky 1991) and show significant occupational and social impairment.

Clinical Course and Prognosis

Somatization disorder is "a chronic but fluctuating disorder that rarely remits completely. A year seldom passes without the individual's seeking some medical attention prompted by unexplained somatic complaints" (American Psychiatric Association 2000, p. 488). Patients may experience iatrogenic disease or injury secondary to unnecessary diagnostic investigations, polypharmacy, and polysurgery. They are particularly at risk for abuse and dependence on drugs prescribed for symptom control (e.g., analgesics, sedative-hypnotics).

Differential Diagnosis

Occult medical diseases affecting multiple organ systems and manifesting with vague or nonspecific symptoms (e.g., systemic lupus erythematosus, sarcoidosis, lymphoma) should be excluded. Patients with these diagnoses, in contrast to somatization disorder, look chronically ill and usually have abnormal physical examinations or laboratory tests. *Panic disorder* may be mistakenly diagnosed as somatization disorder, given a history of many physicians and extensive diagnostic investigations, although symptom patterns differ, with panic disorder patients describing acute symptoms occurring simultaneously, in contrast to the chronic, protean, and fluctuating symptoms of somatization disorder. Chronic physical symptoms may be a part of a *depressive disorder* but occur in the context of the mood disturbance without the long duration and dramatic symptom fluctuations seen in somatization disorder. Some patients with *schizophrenia* or *delusional disorder* develop multiple somatic delusions, distinguished from somatization disorder by their bizarre content. By definition, somatization disorder includes symptoms compatible with other *somatoform disorders*, and diagnostic overlap is common. Somatization disorder differs from *factitious disorder* and *malingering* by the lack of intentional symptom production.

Undifferentiated Somatoform Disorder

Definition

Undifferentiated somatoform disorder is a residual category for individuals who do not meet the full criteria for somatization disorder or another somatoform disorder. The diagnosis requires one or more physical complaints persisting for more than 6 months that cannot be accounted for by a general medical condition, direct effects of a substance, or another psychiatric disorder.

Epidemiology

No studies of undifferentiated somatoform disorder per se have been conducted, but investigators have studied variously defined subsyndromal somatization syndromes. Using a cutoff score of four DSM-III somatization symptoms for men and six symptoms for women, a group of patients were identified whose characteristics, including increased medical utilization, resembled those of patients meeting the full criteria for somatization disorder (Escobar et al. 1987, 1989). Studies of distressed high utilizers of medical care documented significant increased health care utilization by patients endorsing functional somatic symptoms falling below the DSM-III-R cutoff score of 13 symptoms (Katon et al. 1991). It is estimated that 4%–11% of the population have multiple medically unexplained symptoms that are consistent with a subsyndromal form of somatization disorder (Escobar et al. 1987, 1989).

Alternative diagnoses have been proposed as being more clinically useful than undifferentiated somatoform disorder. "Multisomatoform disorder" is characterized by three or more medically unexplained, currently bothersome physical symptoms in addition to a greater than 2-year history of somatization (Kroenke et al. 1997). "Specific somatoform disorder" requires at least one unexplained physical impairment and a substantial impairment in more than one life domain (Rief and Hiller 1998, 1999) and identifies a more impaired group than does the DSM-IV-TR diagnosis of undifferentiated somatoform disorder (Grabe et al. 2003).

Clinical Course, Prognosis, and Differential Diagnosis

It is likely that the course of this heterogeneous disorder is variable, although there has been little systematic study (American Psychiatric Association 2000). The differential diagnosis is similar to that of somatization disorder.

Conversion Disorder

Definition

Conversion symptoms have been described since antiquity (Mace 1992). DSM-IV-TR diagnostic criteria for conversion disorder include neurological (voluntary motor or sensory) symptoms or deficits that are associated with psychological factors (American Psychiatric Association 2000). Conversion presentations can be quite dramatic and can include paralysis, pseudoseizures, amnesia, ataxia, or blindness (see Chapter 32, "Neurology and Neurosurgery").

Controversies surrounding the diagnosis of conversion disorder include whether 1) it is a symptom rather than a disorder, because it has not been validated on the basis of longitudinal or family studies (Martin 1992); 2) it

is better classified with the dissociative disorders as in ICD-10 (Phillips et al. 2003; Toone 1990); and 3) the determination that the symptom is unconsciously produced can be a valid and reliable judgment. Critics have also questioned what constitutes "relevant psychological conflict," how malingering is excluded, and the extent to which organic disorders can and should be excluded (Halligan et al. 2000).

Epidemiology

The reported prevalence of conversion disorder has varied and is likely influenced by several factors. Toone's 1990 review noted rates of 0.3% in the general population, 1%–3% in medical outpatients, and 1%–4.5% in hospitalized neurological and medical patients. Settings such as combat, in which substantial secondary gain may be involved, have increased rates of conversion. Studies of associations with social class and urban versus rural distribution have yielded equivocal findings (Murphy 1990).

Onset is typically in adolescence or early adulthood, but cases have been described in children as well as in older adults. An often-quoted early study cautioned that many patients given a conversion disorder diagnosis subsequently received a diagnosis of a neurological or medical condition that explained the symptom (Slater and Glithero 1965). Recent studies have found lower (5%–12%) rates of explanatory neurological diagnoses (Crimlisk et al. 1998; Moene et al. 2000). These more recent findings may be partially explained by increasing caution on the part of clinicians in making a diagnosis of conversion disorder and by modern neuroimaging and electrophysiological tests. The relationship between childhood traumatization, particularly physical and sexual abuse, and the subsequent development of conversion disorder was first described by Freud and is supported by recent empirical research (e.g., Roelofs et al. 2002), although this association has not been found in all samples (Binzer and Eisemann 1998). Clinically, this association appears especially frequently among patients with pseudoseizures, with trauma reported by 84%, which included sexual abuse by 67%, physical abuse by 67%, and other traumas by 73% in one study (Bowman and Markand 1996).

Specific Culture and Gender Factors

Much higher prevalence rates have been described in developing countries (Murphy 1990) and in isolated rural American settings (Ford 1983). Women outnumber men with the disorder in a ratio varying from 2:1 to 10:1 (Murphy 1990). Men are more likely to present with conversion symptoms related to military service and industrial accidents (Ford 1983).

Mr. T is a 36-year-old male payroll officer presenting with frequent seizures despite a 10-year history of excellent anticonvulsant control after originally developing seizures following a severe head injury sustained in a motor vehicle accident. There is a strong family history of epilepsy and a history of childhood febrile seizures. Anticonvulsant levels remained therapeutic, and there were no changes in his neurological examination. Detailed history taking revealed markedly increased workplace stress with little chance of changing jobs and a precarious marital relationship. His wife noted that the first seizure occurred on the morning after he had been reprimanded at work.

Clinical Features

Conversion symptoms typically begin abruptly and dramatically. Common conversion symptoms include motor symptoms (e.g., paralysis, disturbances in coordination or balance, localized weakness, akinesia, dyskinesia, aphonia, urinary retention, and dysphagia), sensory symptoms (e.g., blindness, double vision, anesthesia, paresthesia, deafness), and seizures or convulsions that may have voluntary motor or sensory components. Unilateral symptoms may be more likely to occur on the left side of the body, as may be true for other somatoform disorders, although the neurophysiological basis for this finding is unclear (Toone 1990) and not all data support it (Roelofs et al. 2000). Some patients with conversion symptoms also have or had the same symptoms from a neurological disease (e.g., conversion pseudoseizures in a patient with epilepsy, as in the case illustration above; Iriarte et al. 2003). In many patients with conversion disorder there is a discrepancy between the presumably frightening symptoms and the patient's bland, even cheerful emotional response ("la belle indifférence"), but this is not a pathognomonic sign and if present does not have prognostic value (Toone 1990).

Psychological factors are associated with symptom onset or exacerbation. Psychodynamic views of conversion focus on the etiological role of *primary gain*, which refers to "the effectiveness of the conversion symptom in providing a satisfactory symbolic expression for the repressed wishes" (Engel 1970, p. 660). For example, a conflict about aggression might be symbolically expressed through a paralyzed arm. *Secondary gain* refers to the potential tangible benefits accruing from the sick role, which may include alterations in the behavior of significant others that are deemed positive by the patient (e.g., increased attentiveness) and permission to withdraw from disliked responsibilities. Secondary gain is believed to occur, but not to be consciously sought, in patients with conversion disorder. This contrasts with malingering, in which symptoms are produced intentionally and are mo-

tivated by external incentives, or factitious disorders, in which symptoms are produced intentionally from the unconscious motivation of assuming the sick role. Caution must be exercised in making judgments about secondary gain because it is intrinsic to the sick role and may be found in patients with any medical or psychiatric illness.

Associated Features

There has been little systematic study of comorbid Axis I diagnoses. The literature on associated personality features suggests that "hysterical personality may be seen, but only in a minority of conversion cases; other forms of personality disorder of immature, dependent type are more usual" (Toone 1990, p. 229). Protracted conversion reactions may be associated with secondary physical changes (e.g., disuse atrophy).

Clinical Course and Prognosis

The course of conversion disorder is difficult to predict. Individual episodes of conversion are usually of short duration with sudden onset and resolution, although recurrence of symptoms over time is common (American Psychiatric Association 2000; Murphy 1990). In some cases, conversion symptoms may last years. Factors reported to predispose to conversion disorder are antecedent physical disorders in the individual or a close contact, which provides a model for the symptoms occurring; and severe social stressors, including bereavement, rape, incest, warfare, and other forms of psychosocial trauma (Toone 1990). The prognosis depends on a number of factors, including acuity of onset, presence of major stressors, duration of symptoms before treatment, symptom pattern, personality, and sociocultural context within which the illness developed. Most patients show a rapid response to treatment, but some do not. Patients with pseudoseizures, tremor, and amnesia are particularly likely to have a poor outcome (Toone 1990).

Differential Diagnosis

The differential diagnosis of conversion disorder includes *neurological conditions* that present with evanescent signs and symptoms (e.g., multiple sclerosis, complex partial seizures, myasthenia gravis). *Pain disorder* is diagnosed if pain is the only conversion symptom. Conversion symptoms may occur in *other psychiatric disorders* (e.g., pseudoseizures as a manifestation of panic disorder or posttraumatic stress disorder; Bowman and Coons 2000) or during *bereavement*. Psychogenic amnesia, fugue, or stupor may represent conversion or *dissociative disorders*, although this appears to be an arbitrary semantic distinction. As with other somatoform disorders, symptoms are generated unconsciously, whereas they are intentional in *factitious disorder* and *malingering*, although in practice the distinction may be blurry.

Pain Disorder

Pain disorder in DSM-IV-TR is the latest incarnation of somatoform pain disorder (DSM-III-R) and psychogenic pain disorder (DSM-III) (see Chapter 36, "Pain").

Hypochondriasis

Definition

Hypochondriasis is characterized by persistent fears of having a disease or the belief that one has a serious disease based on the misinterpretation of one or more bodily symptoms that persist despite medical reassurance (American Psychiatric Association 2000). The validity of the construct in medical outpatients has been documented (Barsky et al. 1986b; Noyes et al. 1993). Secondary hypochondriasis (i.e., hypochondriasis developing in the context of another Axis I psychiatric disorder, a major life stress, or a medical disorder) has been described (Barsky et al. 1992), although it is not recognized in DSM-IV-TR.

Epidemiology

No large-scale epidemiological studies of hypochondriasis have been conducted. Prevalence rates for primary and secondary forms of hypochondriasis of 3%–13% have been reported for study samples from medical and psychiatric settings (Kellner 1986) and 4%–6% of general medical outpatients (Barsky 2001). The prevalence in the general population is 1%–5% (American Psychiatric Association 2000). The disorder can begin at any age, but onset is most commonly in early adulthood (American Psychiatric Association 2000).

Specific Culture and Gender Factors

The reported data on ethnic and cultural differences are equivocal (Barsky et al. 1986a; Kellner 1986), and these factors may be most important when an individual's concerns are reinforced by a traditional or alternative healer who disagrees with the medical reassurance provided (American Psychiatric Association 2000). Gender has received little attention.

> Mr. J, a 44-year-old sales manager, was referred for assessment of anxiety by an infectious disease doctor who felt that the patient did not have chronic fatigue syndrome. Mr. J was reluctant to speak with a psychiatrist but was grateful to have someone listen in detail to his various medical concerns. On the second assessment in-

terview, he confided that he was convinced that he had multiple sclerosis or amyotrophic lateral sclerosis and that he repeatedly measured the muscle mass in his legs, tested for changes in strength, and watched for "muscle twitches." His preoccupation with his health had negatively affected his work, because he spent much of the day searching the Internet for information, and he reported feeling distant from his wife and children as he "prepared to go downhill and die."

Clinical Features

The core feature of hypochondriasis is fear of disease or a conviction that one has a disease despite normal physical examination results and investigations and physician reassurance. Bodily preoccupation (i.e., increased observation of and vigilance toward bodily sensations) is common. The preoccupation may be with a particular bodily function or experience (e.g., heartbeat); a trivial abnormal physical state that is taken as evidence of disease (e.g., cough); a vague physical sensation; or a particular organ (e.g., heart) or diagnosis (e.g., cancer). Patients with hypochondriasis believe that good health is a relatively symptom-free state, and compared with control patients, they are more likely to consider symptoms to be indicative of disease (Barsky et al. 1993). The concern about the feared illness "often becomes a central feature of the individual's self-image, a topic of social discourse, and a response to life stresses" (American Psychiatric Association 2000, p. 504).

Associated Features

Patients with hypochondriasis have a high rate of psychiatric comorbidity, with the most common comorbid diagnoses being generalized anxiety disorder, dysthymia, major depressive disorder, somatization disorder, and panic disorder (Barsky et al. 1992). Personality disorders as assessed by questionnaire were three times more likely to be diagnosed in hypochondriacal patients compared with a control group (Barsky et al. 1992). High medical utilization is common, and the potential exists for iatrogenic damage from repeated investigations. Involvement with complementary health care practices is common. Interpersonal relationships typically deteriorate because of the preoccupation with disease. Occupational functioning is often compromised, with increased time taken off from work and decreased performance when the individual is at work because of the preoccupation with disease.

Clinical Course and Prognosis

The clinical course and prognosis of hypochondriasis are poorly understood. There appear to be multiple pathways to the diagnosis. Primary hypochondriasis appears to be a chronic condition, and therefore some have argued that it might be better classified as a personality style or trait (Barsky and Klerman 1983; Fallon and Feinstein 2001; Mayou et al. 2003; Tyrer et al. 1990). In DSM-IV-TR the course is described as "usually chronic, with waxing and waning symptoms, but complete recovery sometimes occurs" (American Psychiatric Association 2000, p. 506). Positive prognostic features include an acute onset, brief duration, mild symptoms, absence of secondary gain, presence of a comorbid general medical condition, and absence of psychiatric comorbidity (American Psychiatric Association 2000). Secondary hypochondriasis may develop in the context of either current or past serious illness in the patient or family, bereavement, and psychosocial stressors or during the course of another Axis I disorder, principally a mood or anxiety disorder characterized by prominent somatic symptoms. Some forms of secondary hypochondriasis remit with resolution or treatment of the underlying condition (e.g., major life stressors, mood or anxiety disorders). A prospective study found that hypochondriacal patients had a considerable decline in symptoms and improvement in role functioning over 4–5 years, but two-thirds still met diagnostic criteria (Barsky et al. 1998).

Differential Diagnosis

The differential diagnosis of hypochondriasis includes *general medical conditions*, particularly the early stages of a variety of rheumatological, immunological, endocrine, and neurological diseases in which the patient may notice symptoms that may not be associated with signs detectable on physical examination or with abnormal laboratory investigation. Of course, hypochondriasis may coexist with medical pathology (Barsky et al. 1986a). Transient hypochondriacal preoccupations related to medical illness do not constitute hypochondriasis (American Psychiatric Association 2000). Hypochondriacal concerns may accompany *other psychiatric diagnoses* characterized by prominent somatic symptoms (e.g., *major depressive disorder, dysthymia, panic disorder, generalized anxiety disorder, obsessive-compulsive disorder*). *Psychotic disorders* are characterized by the fixed quality of the patient's delusional belief, in contrast to the hypochondriacal patient, who is convinced of the veracity of his or her concerns but is able to consider the possibility that the feared disease is not present. In clinical practice sorting out delusional from nondelusional hypochondriasis is sometimes difficult.

Body Dysmorphic Disorder

Definition

The hallmark of body dysmorphic disorder (BDD) is the preoccupation with an imagined defect in appearance (if a slight physical anomaly is present, the individual's concern with it is judged to be markedly excessive) that is accompanied by significant distress or impairment in social or occupational functioning (American Psychiatric Association 2000). Although BDD is classified in DSM-IV-TR as a somatoform disorder, it is increasingly seen as an obsessive-compulsive spectrum disorder (Phillips 1998, 2001; Phillips and Hollander 1996; Phillips et al. 2003). There have been several recent reviews of the topic (A. Allen and Hollander 2000; Cororve and Gleaves 2001; Phillips 2001; Sarwer et al. 2003).

Epidemiology

The prevalence of BDD is greater than many clinicians recognize (Phillips 1998). BDD has been reported to occur in about 5% of patients seeking cosmetic surgery in the United Kingdom (Veale et al. 2003), 5% of female Turkish college students (Cansever et al. 2003), and 9% of Turkish patients presenting for acne treatment (Uzun et al. 2003). Otto et al. (2001) estimated a point prevalence of 0.7% in a community sample of women ages 36–44 years in Boston, Massachusetts. Structured interviewing is more likely to identify cases (Zimmerman and Mattia 1998), supporting the claim that it is an underrecognized disorder. Onset is typically in adolescence (Phillips 1998), although the disorder may begin in childhood (Albertini and Phillips 1999). Many years may pass before diagnosis because of the individual's reluctance to reveal symptoms (American Psychiatric Association 2000).

Specific Culture and Gender Factors

Cultural variation in BDD has received relatively little attention, although it is clear that concerns about physical appearance vary across cultures and likely color the presentation in different cultures. A comparative study of American and German college students concluded that body image concerns and preoccupation were significantly greater in American than in German students, although the prevalence of probable BDD was not (Bohne et al. 2002). The sex distribution of BDD varies across case series (Phillips 1998). Men and women describe differential preoccupations in line with cultural norms: women are more likely to be preoccupied with their hips and weight, and men with body build, genitals, and thinning hair (Phillips and Diaz 1997).

> Ms. Y is a 32-year-old woman who was referred to a psychiatrist for "support" by a plastic surgeon whom she had consulted regarding revisions of a rhinoplasty ("still not right") and breast augmentation ("I don't look balanced"). The breast augmentation had been complicated by infection, and there was an objective imbalance

and excessive scarring, but her nose appeared aesthetically pleasing. She believed that plastic surgery would make her more attractive, thus "allowing" her to leave her married abusive boyfriend and find a new partner. Collateral information from her mother revealed longstanding bodily preoccupation dating from early adolescence, difficulties in relationships with men, and poor occupational functioning and underemployment.

Clinical Features

Most patients with BDD have concerns about more than one body part (Phillips 1998). The intensity of the preoccupation with the bodily "defect" has been described as "torturing" and "tormenting," dominating the patients' lives and severely limiting social and occupational functioning. Many patients engage in compulsive "checking" behaviors, such as observing themselves in the mirror or measuring the body part of concern. Medical intervention, including surgery, is sought by many patients—75% in one study, with 66% receiving treatment (Phillips et al. 2001b). Delusional BDD—classified as delusional disorder, somatic type—may reflect a difference in insight rather than a distinct syndrome (Phillips et al. 1994).

Associated Features

BDD has substantial comorbidity. Major depressive disorder is the most common comorbid disorder, with a current comorbidity rate of about 60% and a lifetime rate of more than 80% (Phillips and Diaz 1997). Other disorders with lifetime rates of more than 30% include social phobia, substance use disorders, and obsessive-compulsive disorder. Some case series have lower rates of comorbidity (Veale et al. 1996a). Social phobia usually begins before the onset of BDD, whereas depression and substance use disorders typically develop after the onset of BDD (Gunstad and Phillips 2003). Personality disorder is common (Phillips 2001), with the most common diagnosis being avoidant personality disorder (Veale et al. 1996a). Psychosocial dysfunction is often profound, with social withdrawal and occupational functioning below capacity (Phillips 1998) as well as suicidal behavior (Phillips et al. 1993). BDD can profoundly reduce quality of life; in a study using the SF-36 questionnaire, BDD subjects' scores in all mental health domains were worse than norms for patients with depression, diabetes, or a recent myocardial infarction (Phillips 2000).

Clinical Course and Prognosis

No long-term prospective studies of clinical course have been conducted, but case series suggest that BDD is usually chronic, with few symptom-free intervals. The intensity of the symptoms may vary over time (American Psychiatric Association 2000). Patients with BDD often seek and obtain inappropriate medical and surgical treatment (Phillips et al. 2001b). Cosmetic surgeons have begun to recognize the importance of identifying BDD, because it occurs in 7%–15% of those seeking surgery, and operating on BDD patients may worsen the BDD, placing the surgeon at risk of litigation and physical harm (Sarwer et al. 2003).

Differential Diagnosis

A diagnosis of BDD is not made when another *Axis I disorder* (e.g., *mood disorder, schizophrenia, anorexia nervosa*) better accounts for the behavior. Distinguishing between BDD and *delusional disorder, somatic type*, can be difficult (Phillips 2001; Phillips et al. 1993), as can sorting out "*normal body dissatisfaction*" (Murphy 1990), because concerns about appearance are common and are reinforced by unrealistic media ideals.

Management of Somatoform Disorders

Management of the somatoform disorders shares many features with the management of somatization described earlier in this chapter. Limit setting and caring rather than curing have been the traditional foci, although newer pharmacological and psychotherapeutic approaches offer the potential for substantial improvement in some patients. Because many patients with somatoform disorders refuse mental health treatment, the psychiatrist's role is often that of a consultant developing a management plan that integrates multiple treatment modalities and different health care disciplines. In this section, issues specific to the management of somatoform disorders are summarized. Several recent reviews have discussed psychosocial treatments for unexplained physical symptoms (L.A. Allen et al. 2002; Looper and Kirmayer 2002). Cost-effective integrated programs have shown decreased health care utilization (Hiller et al. 2003). Treatment interventions can be tailored to the relevant underlying mechanisms in specific patients, as illustrated in Figure 13–2 (Looper and Kirmayer 2002).

Approach to the Patient

In addition to the general approach to the somatizing patient discussed earlier in this chapter, specific management strategies have been described for patients with conversion disorder, including 1) explaining to the patient that his or her conversion symptoms are not caused

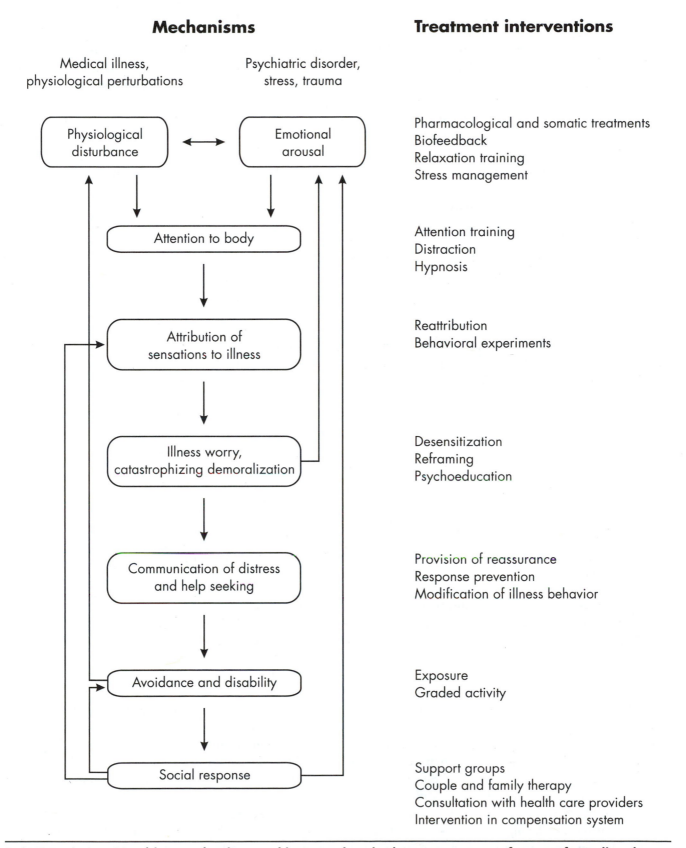

FIGURE 13–2.   Matching mechanisms and interventions in the management of somatoform disorders.

Source.   Reprinted from Looper KJ, Kirmayer LJ: "Behavioral Medicine Approaches to Somatoform Disorders." *Journal of Consulting and Clinical Psychology* 70:810–827, 2002, p. 812. Copyright 2002, the American Psychological Association. Used with permission.

by a serious disease, 2) refraining from confronting the patient, and 3) providing some form of "face-saving" mechanism for symptom resolution such as physical therapy or the suggestion that the patient will improve over a specified period. Eisendrath (1989) observed that "when dealing with behavior with prominent unconscious motivation such as conversion reactions...the therapist provides no benefit by revealing understanding of the psychological processes too early in the treatment" (p. 386). Although many clinicians feel uncomfortable about the risks inherent in "legitimizing" the illness, this approach seems justified based on considerable anecdotal experience of good outcome with treatment and prolonged disability without it. The consulting psychiatrist often must help the referring physician and other health care professionals manage their emotional responses to these patients, whom they may view as deceiving them. The choice of words in talking to patients is very important: terms such as *stress-related seizures* or *functional seizures* are much more acceptable, while remaining truthful, than *pseudoseizures* or *psychogenic seizures*, which may be seen as offensive or pejorative (Stone et al. 2003).

There has been little study of the treatment preferences of patients. Walker et al. (1999) studied 23 volunteers with a diagnosis of hypochondriasis and found that cognitive-behavioral therapy (CBT) was rated as more acceptable than medications and was perceived as more likely to be effective in the short and long term. CBT was the first choice of 74% of participants, in contrast to medication in 4% and equal preference in 22%. Of note, 48% reported they would accept only CBT.

Pharmacotherapy

Pharmacotherapy for somatoform disorders is in its infancy and is limited to studies of small heterogeneous samples, chart reviews, and open-label trials. There is great interest in the potential role of antidepressants in ameliorating somatic symptoms associated with depression, as well as functional somatic symptoms in nondepressed patients (Stahl 2003). Norepinephrine and serotonin have important functions in mediating physical symptoms, and therefore their modulation with antidepressants may bring about changes in somatic experiences (Stahl 2003). An open-label trial of fluoxetine found moderate improvement in 61% of 29 patients with a variety of somatoform disorders (Noyes et al. 1998). In a European placebo-controlled trial, opipramol (a histamine H_1, serotonin 5-HT_2, and dopamine D_2 blocker) demonstrated efficacy in a diverse group of somatoform patients with high rates of depressive and anxiety comorbidity (Volz et al. 2000).

Pharmacotherapy has limited effectiveness in somatization disorder except for treatment of comorbid mood and anxiety disorders. Drugs that have been studied for hypochondriasis include high-dose fluoxetine, which was reported to improve the condition in 10 of 16 patients meeting DSM-III-R criteria who did not have marked depressive features (Fallon et al. 1993), and paroxetine in an open-label study (Oosterbaan et al. 2001) in which 8 of 9 patients (from a sample of 11) who finished the study demonstrated clinical improvement (and 5 of these subjects showed scores consistent with the normal population). Secondary hypochondriasis in patients with depression has been treated with amitriptyline (Kellner et al. 1986). A number of studies of BDD have reported success with selective serotonin reuptake inhibitors (SSRIs) in about two-thirds of patients treated (Phillips 1998; Phillips et al. 2001a). It has also been reported that augmentation strategies and changing antidepressants may be helpful in nonresponders (Phillips et al. 2001a). High relapse rates were reported with discontinuation of pharmacotherapy (Phillips et al. 2001a). Clomipramine (a potent serotonin reuptake inhibitor) was more effective than desipramine (a norepinephrine reuptake inhibitor) in treating BDD in a 16-week double-blind crossover trial (Hollander et al. 1999). The SSRIs appear to be effective even among patients with a delusional variant of BDD (Hollander et al. 1999; Phillips et al. 2001a). The time to response is longer than with major depression for at least one-third of patients.

Physical Reactivation and Physical Therapy

Physical reactivation via a gradually escalating program of exercise (e.g., walking, swimming) often improves the quality of life in patients with a variety of somatoform disorders. It may be difficult to engage patients in exercise, but once they become more active, they often find it pleasurable and report feelings of accomplishment, reduced stress, and greater confidence in their body. Physical reactivation should start at a level just below what the patient can do on his or her worst day, and the patient should then strive for consistency with activity at least 5 days a week. Physical therapy is invaluable for patients who have conversion disorder and may be the only treatment required to restore physical function in some cases (Delargy et al. 1986; Dvonch et al. 1991). In a recent report of 34 consecutive referrals for inpatient rehabilitation treatment of conversion disorder patients with motor paralysis, 9 had complete recovery, 10 had partial recovery, and 15 remained unchanged (Heruti et al. 2002).

Relaxation Therapies, Meditation, and Hypnotherapy

Various forms of relaxation therapies, biofeedback, meditation, and hypnotherapy have been used with somatoform disorder patients. Relaxation therapies modulate somatic sensations and may be used as part of a more comprehensive group treatment program for hypochondriasis (Barsky et al. 1988a). These therapies may be used either as a primary form of treatment based on a psychophysiological model or as an adjuvant to other forms of treatment. Hypnosis has been used diagnostically and therapeutically in patients with conversion disorder (see review by Van Dyck and Hoogduin 1989), and it showed sustained benefits for 6 months in a randomized, controlled trial (Moene et al. 2003). Hypnotherapy may be combined with intravenous sedation (Toone 1990) and eclectic behavioral treatment programs (Moene et al. 2003). Although abreaction or catharsis under hypnosis or sedation has had dramatic anecdotal effects in some individuals in whom the conversion was precipitated by extreme trauma, such interventions are not helpful for most patients (Toone 1990).

Behavioral Treatment

Learning theory models have been proposed for the treatment of several somatoform disorders. Hypochondriasis has been treated with exposure and response prevention individually tailored to the patient's specific problem behaviors (Visser and Bouman 1992, 2001; Warwick and Marks 1988). Prevention of reassurance seeking was a key component of treatment because it is conceptualized as an anxiety-reducing ritual that is reinforced by the reassurance received (Warwick 1992). This program, which required a median of seven treatment sessions and 11 therapist hours, was associated with improvement that was maintained in half of the patients at follow-up (mean duration, 5 years; range, 1–8 years). Exposure therapy may decrease hypochondriacal fears and beliefs in agoraphobic patients (Fava et al. 1988). Exposure plus response prevention for hypochondriasis was found to be as effective as cognitive therapy, and both treatments demonstrated results that were superior to a waiting-list control group (Visser and Bouman 2001). Behavioral stress management is helpful in treating hypochondriasis (Clark et al. 1998). In some patients BDD has been successfully treated with behavioral techniques such as desensitization, live and fantasy exposure, and assertiveness training (Marks and Mishan 1988), although behavioral and cognitive-behavioral approaches remain poorly studied in BDD (Phillips 2001).

Suggestion and Reassurance

The use of suggestion or reassurance requires clinical acumen in framing the intervention and ensuring that one does not give an explanation that is heard as "It's all in your head." Explanations should empower patients, reframe the symptoms, and emphasize the possibility of improvement over time, particularly with active involvement from the patient. For example, the psychiatrist may tell the patient, "The sudden weakness in your legs really laid you up. The good news is that you don't have multiple sclerosis, a stroke, a tumor, or anything else like that. This sort of weakness typically disappears as mysteriously as it initially appears, but our experience is that you can speed up your recovery through physical therapy."

Cognitive Therapy

Cognitive therapy has been used in both individual and group formats for functional somatic symptoms and several somatoform disorders (see critical review of controlled trials by Kroenke and Swindle 2000). It may be the preferred form of treatment for patients with hypochondriasis (Walker et al. 1999). The use of cognitive therapy is predicated on cognitive models such as the one shown in Figure 13–3 for hypochondriasis. A cognitive model directs attention to factors that maintain preoccupation with worries about health, including attentional factors, avoidant behaviors, beliefs, and misinterpretation of symptoms, signs, and medical communications (Salkovskis 1989). Cognitive therapy has been helpful in decreasing health care visits and physical complaints in patients with multiple unexplained physical symptoms (Sumathipala et al. 2000). In an 8-week randomized, controlled study of a group cognitive-behavioral treatment, primary care patients with somatization disorder showed improvements in somatization, bodily preoccupation, and medication use at 6-month (Lidbeck 1997) and 18-month follow-up visits (Lidbeck 2003). A controlled treatment study using both individual and group CBT demonstrated cost-effectiveness and decreased health care utilization in a mixed group of patients with somatoform disorder (Hiller et al. 2003).

Cognitive therapy programs for hypochondriasis have been described in considerable detail (Salkovskis 1989) and are based on a model of hypochondriasis as a disorder of perception and cognition in which somatic sensations are perceived as abnormally intense and are attributed to serious medical disease. Barsky and colleagues (1988a) described a 6-week group program for patients with hypochondriasis. A recent randomized usual-care control trial of a 6-session individual CBT intervention demonstrated significant, persistent reductions at 12-month follow-up of

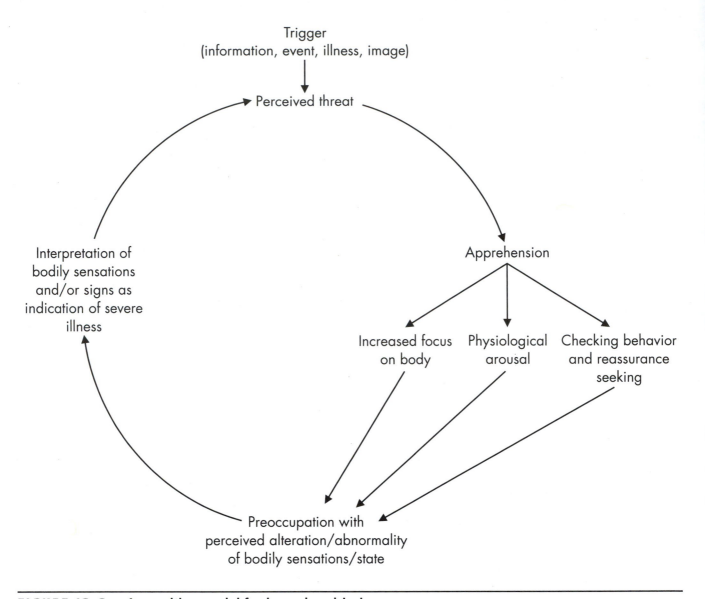

FIGURE 13–3.   A cognitive model for hypochondriasis.

Source.   Reprinted from Salkovskis PM: "Somatic Problems," in *Cognitive Behaviour Therapy for Psychiatric Problems.* Edited by Hawton K, Salkovskis PM, Kirk J, et al. New York, Oxford University Press, 1989, pp. 235–276. Copyright 1989, Oxford University Press (www.oup.com). Used with permission.

hypochondriacal symptoms, beliefs, and attitudes and health-related anxiety, as well as less impairment in social role functioning and activities of daily living, but no improvement in hypochondriacal somatic symptoms (Barsky and Ahern 2004). In a randomized, controlled trial, Clark et al. (1998) demonstrated that cognitive therapy (up to 16 weekly 1-hour sessions and up to 3 booster sessions over the next 3 months) is an effective specific treatment for hypochondriasis. Cognitive therapy was as effective as exposure plus response prevention in treating hypochondriasis (Visser and Bouman 2001). Cognitive therapy may also be helpful in treating BDD (Phillips 2001; Veale et al. 1996b).

Dynamic Psychotherapy

Psychotherapy has a role in the management of some somatoform disorders. In general, psychoeducational and supportive techniques predominate, although insight-oriented therapy may be indicated in some patients. Explanatory therapy for hypochondriasis has been described (Kellner 1986) and showed an impact superior to the waiting-list control condition (Fava et al. 2000). Explanatory therapy has been described as "providing accurate information, teaching the principles of selective perception (attention to one part of the body makes the patient more aware of sensations in that part of the body than in other parts), reassurance, clarification and repetition" (Fava et al. 2000). Unlike CBT, explanatory therapy is simpler, uses fewer therapeutic components, does not introduce specific behavioral techniques, and is not based on a specific theoretical framework (Fava et al. 2000). Insight-oriented psychotherapy for somatizing patients has been advocated (McDougall 1989; Rodin 1984), but there is no empirical evidence supporting it, and it will appeal to only a minority of patients.

Group Psychotherapy

Group therapy may be particularly useful in the management of somatoform disorders. When social and affiliative needs are gratified via the group, patients' need to somatize to establish or maintain relationships may be reduced (Ford 1984). Confrontation by fellow group members about secondary gain is usually better tolerated than that by an individual therapist or primary physician. Anger at physicians and family and dependence needs may be better tolerated in the group setting, which tends to diffuse intense affects. Group therapy also may be useful in increasing interpersonal skills and in enhancing more direct forms of communication regarding thoughts, feelings, and desires (Ford 1984). Helplessness has been identified as a central psychotherapeutic issue that can be effectively addressed in group therapy for patients with somatoform disorder (Levine et al. 1993). Various forms of group therapy have been reported for patients with somatoform disorder (see review by Levine et al. 1993). Short-term group therapy appears to be effective in primary care patients with somatization disorder (Kashner et al. 1995).

Marital and Family Therapy

Most families will benefit from information and psychoeducational approaches. More intensive forms of therapy are required when patients have significant marital or family pathology and when somatic symptoms are an important form of social communication within the family. It is important to identify the family's attitude and response because they may have a conscious or unconscious interest in maintaining a symptom in a patient.

References

Albertini RS, Phillips KA: Thirty-three cases of body dysmorphic disorder in children and adolescents. J Am Acad Child Adolesc Psychiatry 38:453–459, 1999

Allen A, Hollander E: Body dysmorphic disorder. Psychiatr Clin North Am 23:617–628, 2000

Allen LA, Escobar JI, Lehrer PM, et al: Psychosocial treatments for multiple unexplained physical symptoms: a review of the literature. Psychosom Med 64:939–950, 2002

American Psychiatric Association: Diagnostic and Statistical Manual of Mental Disorders, 3rd Edition. Washington, DC, American Psychiatric Association, 1980

American Psychiatric Association: Diagnostic and Statistical Manual of Mental Disorders, 3rd Edition, Revised. Washington, DC, American Psychiatric Association, 1987

American Psychiatric Association: Diagnostic and Statistical Manual of Mental Disorders, 4th Edition, Text Revision. Washington, DC, American Psychiatric Association, 2000

Andreski P, Chilcoat H, Breslau N: Post-traumatic stress disorder and somatization symptoms: a prospective study. Psychiatry Res 79:131–138, 1998

Barsky AJ: A comprehensive approach to the chronically somatizing patient. J Psychosom Res 45:301–306, 1998

Barksy AJ: The patient with hypochondriasis. N Engl J Med 345:1395–1399, 2001

Barsky AJ, Ahern DK: Cognitive behavior therapy for hypochondriasis: a randomized controlled trial. JAMA 291:1464–1470, 2004

Barsky AJ, Klerman GL: Overview: hypochondriasis, bodily complaints, and somatic styles. Am J Psychiatry 140:273–283, 1983

Barsky AJ, Wyshak G, Klerman GL: Hypochondriasis: an evaluation of the DSM-III criteria in medical outpatients. Arch Gen Psychiatry 43:493–500, 1986a

Barsky AJ, Wyshak G, Klerman GL: Medical and psychiatric determinants of outpatient medical utilization. Med Care 24:548–560, 1986b

Barsky AJ, Geringer E, Wood CA: A cognitive-educational treatment for hypochondriasis. Gen Hosp Psychiatry 10:322–327, 1988a

Barsky AJ, Goodson JD, Lane RS, et al: The amplification of somatic symptoms. Psychosom Med 50:510–519, 1988b

Barsky AJ, Wyshak G, Klerman GL: Psychiatric co-morbidity in DSM-III-R hypochondriasis. Arch Gen Psychiatry 49:101–108, 1992

Barsky AJ, Coeytaux RR, Sarnie MK, et al: Hypochondriacal patients' beliefs about good health. Am J Psychiatry 150:1085–1089, 1993

Barsky AJ, Fama JM, Bailey ED, et al: A prospective 4- to 5-year study of DSM-III-R hypochondriasis. Arch Gen Psychiatry 55:737–744, 1998

Barsky AJ, Peekna HM, Borus JF: Somatic symptom reporting in women and men. J Gen Intern Med 16:266–275, 2001

Bass C, Benjamin S: The management of chronic somatisation. Br J Psychiatry 162:472–480, 1993

Bass C, Murphy M: The chronic somatizer and the Government White Paper. J R Soc Med 83:203–205, 1990

Bass C, Murphy M: Somatoform and personality disorders; syndromal comorbidity and overlapping developmental pathways. J Psychosom Res 39:403–427, 1995

Bass C, Peveler R, House A: Somatoform disorders: severe psychiatric illnesses neglected by psychiatrists. Br J Psychiatry 179:11–14, 2001

Benjamin S: Psychological treatment of chronic pain: a selective review. J Psychosom Res 33:121–131, 1989

Binzer M, Eisemann M: Childhood experiences and personality traits in patients with motor conversion symptoms. Acta Psychiatr Scand 98:288–295, 1998

Bohne A, Keuthen NJ, Wilhelm S, et al: Prevalence of symptoms of body dysmorphic disorder and its correlates: a cross-cultural comparison. Psychosomatics 43:486–490, 2002

Bowman ES, Coons PM: The differential diagnosis of epilepsy, pseudoseizures, dissociative identity disorder, and dissociative disorder not otherwise specified. Bull Menninger Clin 64:164–180, 2000

Bowman ES, Markand ON: Psychodynamic and psychiatric diagnoses of pseudoseizure subjects. Am J Psychiatry 153:57–63, 1996

Brown HD, Kosslyn SM, Delamater B, et al: Perceptual and memory biases for health-related information in hypochondriacal individuals. J Psychosom Res 47:67–78, 1999

Cansever A, Uzun O, Donmex E, et al: The prevalence and clinical features of body dysmorphic disorder in college students: a study in a Turkish sample. Compr Psychiatry 44:60–64, 2003

Cassem NH, Barsky AJ: Functional somatic symptoms and somatoform disorders, in Massachusetts General Hospital Handbook of General Hospital Psychiatry, 3rd Edition. Edited by Cassem NH. St. Louis, MO, Mosby Year Book, 1991, pp 131–157

Clark DM, Salkovskis PM, Hackmann A, et al: Two psychological treatments for hypochondriasis: a randomised controlled trial. Br J Psychiatry 173:218–225, 1998

Cloninger CR, Martin RL, Guze SB, et al: A prospective follow-up and family study of somatization in men and women. Am J Psychiatry 143:873–878, 1986

Cororve MB, Gleaves DH: Body dysmorphic disorder: a review of conceptualizations, assessment, and treatment strategies. Clin Psychol Rev 21:949–970, 2001

Craig TK, Boardman AP, Mills K, et al: The South London somatisation study, I: longitudinal course and the influence of early life experiences. Br J Psychiatry 163:579–588, 1993

Creed F, Guthrie E: Techniques for interviewing the somatising patient. Br J Psychiatry 162:467–471, 1993

Crimlisk HL, Bhatia K, Cope H, et al: Slater revisited: 6-year follow-up study of patients with medically unexplained motor symptoms. BMJ 316:582–586, 1998

Delargy MA, Peatfield RC, Burt AA: Successful rehabilitation in conversion paralysis. BMJ 292:1730–1731, 1986

Drossman DA: Do psychosocial factors define symptom severity and patient status in irritable bowel syndrome? Am J Med 107(5A):41S–50S, 1999

Dvonch VM, Bunch WH, Siegler AH: Conversion reactions in pediatric athletes. J Pediatr Orthop 11:770–772, 1991

Eisenberg L: Disease and illness: distinctions between professional and popular ideas of sickness. Cult Med Psychiatry 1:9–23, 1977

Eisendrath SJ: Factitious physical disorders: treatment without confrontation. Psychosomatics 30:383–387, 1989

Engel GL: Conversion symptoms, in Signs and Symptoms: Applied Pathologic Physiology and Clinical Interpretation, 5th Edition. Edited by MacBryde CM. Philadelphia, PA, JB Lippincott, 1970, pp 650–668

Epstein RM, Quill TE, McWhinney IR: Somatization reconsidered: incorporating the patient's experience of illness. Arch Intern Med 159:215–222, 1999

Escobar JI, Burnam MA, Karno M, et al: Somatization in the community. Arch Gen Psychiatry 44:713–718, 1987

Escobar JI, Manu P, Matthews D, et al: Medically unexplained physical symptoms, somatization disorder and abridged somatization: studies with the Diagnostic Interview Schedule. Psychiatr Dev 3:235–245, 1989

Fallon BA, Feinstein S: Hypochondriasis, in Somatoform and Factitious Disorders (Review of Psychiatry Series, Vol 20, No 3; Oldham JM and Riba MB, series editors). Edited by Phillips KA. Washington, DC, American Psychiatric Press, 2001, pp 27–66

Fallon BA, Liebowitz MR, Salman E, et al: Fluoxetine for hypochondriacal patients without major depressive disorder. J Clin Psychopharmacol 13:438–441, 1993

Fava GA, Kellner R, Zielezny M, et al: Hypochondriacal fears and beliefs in agoraphobia. J Affect Disord 14:239–244, 1988

Fava GA, Silvana G, Rafanelli C, et al: Explanatory therapy in hypochondriasis. J Clin Psychiatry 61:317–322, 2000

Feighner JP, Robins E, Guze SB, et al: Diagnostic criteria for use in psychiatric research. Arch Gen Psychiatry 26:57–63, 1972

Fishbain DA, Cole B, Cutler RB, et al: A structured evidence-based review on the meaning of nonorganic physical signs: Waddell signs. Pain Med 4:141–181, 2003

Ford CV: The Somatizing Disorders: Illness as a Way of Life. New York, Elsevier, 1983

Ford CV: Somatizing disorders, in Helping Patients and Their Families Cope With Medical Problems. Edited by Roback HB. Washington, DC, Jossey-Bass, 1984, pp 39–59

Ford CV: Illness as a lifestyle: the role of somatization in medical practice. Spine 17:S338–S343, 1992

Garralda ME: Assessment and management of somatisation in childhood and adolescence: a practical perspective. J Child Psychol Psychiatry 40:1159–1167, 1999

Goldberg D, Gask L, O'Dowd T: The treatment of somatization: teaching techniques of reattribution. J Psychosom Res 33:689–695, 1989

Golding JM, Smith GR Jr, Kashner TM: Does somatization disorder occur in men? Clinical characteristics of women and men with multiple unexplained somatic symptoms. Arch Gen Psychiatry 48:231–235, 1991

Golding JM, Rost K, Kashner TM, et al: Family psychiatric history of patients with somatization disorder. Psychiatr Med 10:33–47, 1992

Grabe HJ, Meyer C, Hapke U, et al: Specific somatoform disorder in the general population. Psychosomatics 44:304–311, 2003

Gunstad J, Phillips KA: Axis I comorbidity in body dysmorphic disorder. Compr Psychiatry 44:270–276, 2003

Gureje O, Simon GE, Ustun TB, et al: Somatization in cross-cultural perspective: a World Health Organization study in primary care. Am J Psychiatry 154:989–995, 1997

Guthrie EA, Creed F, Dawson D, et al: A controlled trial of psychological treatment for the irritable bowel syndrome. Gastroenterology 100:450–457, 1991

Guze SB: Genetics of Briquet's syndrome and somatization disorder. A review of family, adoption, and twin studies. Ann Clin Psychiatry 5:225–230, 1993

Guze SB, Cloninger CR, Martin RL, et al: A follow-up and family study of Briquet's syndrome. Br J Psychiatry 149:17–23, 1986

Hahn SR, Thompson KS, Wills TA, et al: The difficult doctor-patient relationship: somatization, personality and psychopathology. J Clin Epidemiol 47:647–657, 1994

Halligan PW, Bass C, Wade DT: New approaches to conversion hysteria. BMJ 320:1488–1489, 2000

Heruti RJ, Reznik J, Adunski A, et al: Conversion motor paralysis disorder: analysis of 34 consecutive referrals. Spinal Cord 40:335–340, 2002

Hiller W, Fichter MM, Rief W: A controlled treatment study of somatoform disorders including analysis of healthcare utilization and cost-effectiveness. J Psychosom Res 54:369–380, 2003

Hollander E, Allen A, Kwon J, et al: Clomipramine vs desipramine crossover trial in body dysmorphic disorder. Arch Gen Psychiatry 56:1033–1039, 1999

Hotopf M, Wadsworth M, Wessely S: Is "somatisation" a defense against the acknowledgement of psychiatric disorder? J Psychosom Res 50:119–124, 2001

Hudson JL, Mangweth B, Pope HG, et al: Family study of affective spectrum disorder. Arch Gen Psychiatry 60:170–177, 2003

Iriarte J, Parra J, Urrestarazu E, et al: Controversies in the diagnosis and management of psychogenic pseudoseizures. Epilepsy Behav 4:354–359, 2003

Kanner AM: More controversies on the treatment of psychogenic pseudoseizures: an addendum. Epilepsy Behav 4:360–364, 2003

Kashner TM, Rost K, Cohen B, et al: Enhancing the health of somatization disorder patients: effectiveness of short-term group therapy. Psychosomatics 36:462–470, 1995

Katon W, Ries RK, Kleinman A: The prevalence of somatization in primary care. Compr Psychiatry 25:208–215, 1984

Katon W, Lin E, Von Korff M, et al: Somatization: a spectrum of severity. Am J Psychiatry 148:34–40, 1991

Kellner R: Somatization and Hypochondriasis. New York, Praeger, 1986

Kellner R, Slocumb J, Wiggins RG, et al: Hostility, somatic symptoms and hypochondriacal fears and beliefs. J Nerv Ment Dis 173:554–560, 1985

Kellner R, Fava GA, Lisansky J, et al: Hypochondriacal fears and beliefs in DSM-III melancholia: changes with amitriptyline. J Affect Disord 10:21–26, 1986

Kendler KS, Walters EE, Truett KR, et al: A twin-family study of self-report symptoms of panic-phobia and somatization. Behav Genet 25:499–515, 1995

Kirmayer LJ, Robbins JM (eds): Current Concepts of Somatization: Research and Clinical Perspectives. Washington, DC, American Psychiatric Press, 1991

Kirmayer LJ, Robbins JM: Patients who somatize in primary care: a longitudinal study of cognitive and social characteristics. Psychol Med 26:937–951, 1996

Kirmayer LJ, Young A: Culture and somatization: clinical, epidemiological and ethnographic perspectives. Psychosom Med 60:420–430, 1998

Kirmayer LJ, Robbins JM, Dworkind M, et al: Somatization and the recognition of depression and anxiety in primary care. Am J Psychiatry 150:734–741, 1993

Kleinman A: Social Origins of Distress and Disease: Depression, Neurasthenia, and Pain in Modern China. New Haven, CT, Yale University Press, 1986

Kroenke K: Patients presenting with somatic complaints: epidemiology, psychiatric comorbidity and management. Int J Methods Psychiatr Res 12:34–43, 2003

Kroenke K, Swindle R: Cognitive-behavioral therapy for somatization and symptom syndromes: a critical review of controlled clinical trials. Psychother Psychosom 69:205–215, 2000

Kroenke K, Spitzer RL, deGruy FV, et al: Multisomatoform disorder: an alternative to undifferentiated somatoform disorder for the somatizing patient in primary care. Arch Gen Psychiatry 54:352–358, 1997

Lackner JM, Gudleski GD, Blanchard EB: Beyond abuse: the association among parenting style, abdominal pain, and somatization in IBS patients. Behav Res Ther 42:41–56, 2004

Levine JB, Irving KK, Brooks JD, et al: Group therapy and the somatoform patient: an integration. Psychotherapy 30:625–634, 1993

Lidbeck J: Group therapy for somatization disorders in general practice: effectiveness of a short cognitive-behavioural treatment model. Acta Psychiatr Scand 96:14–24, 1997

Lidbeck J: Group therapy for somatization disorders in primary care: maintenance of treatment goals of short cognitive-behavioural treatment one-and-a-half-year follow-up. Acta Psychiatr Scand 107:449–456, 2003

Lieb R, Pfister H, Mastaler M, et al: Somatoform syndromes and disorders in a representative population sample of adolescents and young adults: prevalence, comorbidity and impairments. Acta Psychiatr Scand 101:194–208, 2000

Lipowski ZJ: Somatization: the concept and its clinical application. Am J Psychiatry 145:1358–1368, 1988

Lipsitt DR: Medical and psychological characteristics of "crocks." Psychiatr Med 1:15–25, 1970

Liu G, Clark MR, Eaton WW: Structural factor analyses for medically unexplained somatic symptoms of somatization disorder in the Epidemiologic Catchment Area study. Psychol Med 27:617–626, 1997

Looper KJ, Kirmayer LJ: Behavioral medicine approaches to somatoform disorders. J Consult Clin Psychol 70:810–827, 2002

Mace CJ: Hysterical conversion, I: a history. Br J Psychiatry 161:369–377, 1992

Marks I, Mishan J: Dysmorphophobic avoidance with disturbed bodily perception: a pilot study of exposure therapy. Br J Psychiatry 152:674–678, 1988

Martin RL: Diagnostic issues for conversion disorder. Hosp Community Psychiatry 43:771–773, 1992

Mayou R: Illness behavior and psychiatry. Gen Hosp Psychiatry 11:307–312, 1989

Mayou R: Somatization. Psychother Psychosom 59:69–83, 1993

Mayou R, Levenson J, Sharpe M: Somatoform disorders in DSM-V. Psychosomatics 44:449–451, 2003

McBeth J, Silman AJ: The role of psychiatric disorders in fibromyalgia. Curr Rheumatol Rep 3:157–164, 2001

McDougall J: Theaters of the Body: A Psychoanalytic Approach to Psychosomatic Illness. New York, WW Norton, 1989

Mechanic D: The concept of illness behaviour: culture, situation and personal predisposition. Psychol Med 16:1–7, 1986

Mehrabian A: General relations among drug use, alcohol use, and major indexes of psychopathology. J Psychol 135:71–86, 2001

Moene FC, Landberg EH, Hoogduin KAL: Organic syndromes diagnosed as conversion disorder: identification and frequency in a study of 85 patients. J Psychosom Res 46:7–12, 2000

Moene FC, Spinhoven P, Hoogduin KA, et al: A randomized controlled clinical trial of a hypnosis-based treatment for patients with conversion disorder, motor type. Int J Clin Exp Hypn 51:29–50, 2003

Moreau C, Zisook S: Rationale for a posttraumatic stress spectrum disorder. Psychiatr Clin North Am 25:775–790, 2002

Morrison J: Childhood sexual histories of women with somatization disorder. Am J Psychiatry 146:239–241, 1989

Murphy MR: Classification of the somatoform disorders, in Somatization: Physical Symptoms and Psychological Illness. Edited by Bass C. Boston, MA, Blackwell Scientific, 1990, pp 10–39

Newman NJ: Neuro-ophthalmology and psychiatry. Gen Hosp Psychiatry 15:102–114, 1993

Noyes R Jr, Kathol RG, Fisher MM, et al: The validity of DSM-III-R hypochondriasis. Arch Gen Psychiatry 50:961–970, 1993

Noyes R Jr, Happel RL, Muller BA, et al: Fluvoxamine for somatoform disorders: an open trial. Gen Hosp Psychiatry 20:339–344, 1998

Noyes R Jr, Stuart SP, Langbehn DR, et al: Test of an interpersonal model of hypochondriasis. Psychosom Med 65:292–300, 2003

Oosterbaan DB, VanBalkom AJLM, VanBoeijen CA, et al: An open study of paroxetine in hypochondriasis. Prog Neuropsychopharmacol Biol Psychiatry 25:1023–1033, 2001

Otto MW, Wilhelm S, Cohen LS, et al: Prevalence of body dysmorphic disorder in a community sample of women. Am J Psychiatry 158:2061–2063, 2001

Page LA, Wessely S: Medically unexplained symptoms: exacerbating factors in the doctor-patient encounter. J R Soc Med 96:223–227, 2003

Pauli P, Alpers GW: Memory bias in patients with hypochondriasis and somatoform pain disorder. J Psychosom Res 52:45–53, 2002

Pennebaker JW, Watson D: The psychology of somatic symptoms, in Current Concepts of Somatization: Research and Clinical Perspectives. Edited by Kirmayer LJ, Robbins JM. Washington, DC, American Psychiatric Press, 1991, pp 21–36

Phillips KA: Body dysmorphic disorder: clinical aspects and treatment strategies. Bull Menninger Clin 62 (4 suppl A): A33–A48, 1998

Phillips KA: Quality of life for patients with body dysmorphic disorder. J Nerv Ment Dis 188:170–175, 2000

Phillips KA: Body dysmorphic disorder, in Somatoform and Factitious Disorders (Review of Psychiatry Series, Vol 20, No 3; Oldham JM and Riba MB, series editors). Edited by Phillips KA. Washington, DC, American Psychiatric Press, 2001, pp 67–94

Phillips KA, Diaz SF: Gender differences in body dysmorphic disorder. J Nerv Ment Dis 185:570–577, 1997

Phillips KA, Hollander E: Body dysmorphic disorder, in DSM-IV Sourcebook, Vol 2. Edited by Widiger RA, Frances AJ, Pincus R, et al. Washington, DC, American Psychiatric Association, 1996, pp 949–960

Phillips KA, McElroy SL, Keck PE, et al: Body dysmorphic disorder: 30 cases of imagined ugliness. Am J Psychiatry 150: 302–308, 1993

Phillips KA, McElroy SL, Keck PE, et al: A comparison of delusional and nondelusional body dysmorphic disorder in 100 cases. Psychopharmacol Bull 30:179–186, 1994

Phillips KA, Albertini RS, Siniscalchi JM: Effectiveness of pharmacotherapy for body dysmorphic disorder: a chart-review study. J Clin Psychiatry 62:721–727, 2001a

Phillips KA, Grant J, Siniscalchi J, et al: Surgical and nonpsychiatric medical treatment of patients with body dysmorphic disorder. Psychosomatics 42:504–510, 2001b

Phillips KA, Price LH, Greenberg BD, et al: Should the DSM diagnostic groupings be changed? in Advancing DSM: Dilemmas in Psychiatric Diagnosis. Edited by Phillips KA, First MB, Pinucs HA. Washington, DC, American Psychiatric Association, 2003, pp 57–84

Piccinelli M, Simon G: Gender and cross-cultural differences in somatic symptoms associated with emotional distress. An international study in primary care. Psychol Med 27:433–444, 1997

Pilowsky I: Abnormal illness behavior. Psychiatr Med 5:85–91, 1987

Priel B, Rabinowitz B, Pels RJ: A semiotic perspective on chronic pain: implications for the interaction between patient and physician. Br J Med Psychol 64:65–71, 1991

Quill TE: Somatization disorder: one of medicine's blind spots. JAMA 254:3075–3079, 1985

Rief W, Hiller W: Somatization—future perspectives on a common phenomenon. J Psychosom Res 44:529–536, 1998

Rief W, Hiller W: Toward empirically based criteria for classification of somatoform disorders. J Psychosom Res 46:507–518, 1999

Ritsner M: The attribution of somatization in schizophrenia patients: a naturalistic follow-up study. J Clin Psychiatry 64:1370–1378, 2003

Rodin G: Somatization and the self: psychotherapeutic issues. Am J Psychother 38:257–263, 1984

Roelofs K, Naring GW, Moene FC, et al: The question of symptom lateralization in conversion disorder. J Psychosom Res 49:21–25, 2000

Roelofs K, Keijsers GP, Hoogduin KA, et al: Childhood abuse in patients with conversion disorder. Am J Psychiatry 159:1908–1913, 2002

Rost KM, Akins RN, Brown FW, et al: The comorbidity of DSM-III-R personality disorders in somatization disorder. Gen Hosp Psychiatry 14:322–326, 1992

Salkovskis PM: Somatic problems, in Cognitive Behaviour Therapy for Psychiatric Problems. Edited by Hawton K, Salkovskis PM, Kirk J, et al. New York, Oxford University Press, 1989, pp 235–276

Salmon P, Peters S, Stanley I: Patients' perceptions of medical explanations for somatisation disorders: qualitative analysis. BMJ 318:372–376, 1999

Salmon P, Skaife K, Rhodes J: Abuse, dissociation, and somatization in irritable bowel syndrome: towards an explanatory model. J Behav Med 26:1–18, 2003

Sarwer DB, Crerand CE, Didie ER: Body dysmorphic disorder in cosmetic surgery patients. Facial Plast Surg 19:7–17, 2003

Sayar K, Kirmayer LJ, Taillefer SS: Predictors of somatic symptoms in depressive disorder. Gen Hosp Psychiatry 25:108–114, 2003

Sharpe M: Medically unexplained symptoms and syndromes. Clin Med 2:501–504, 2002

Sharpe M, Bass C: Pathophysiological mechanisms in somatization. Int Rev Psychiatry 4:81–97, 1992

Sharpe M, Carson A: "Unexplained" somatic symptoms, functional syndromes, and somatization: do we need a paradigm shift? Ann Intern Med 134:926–930, 2001

Sharpe M, Peveler R, Mayou R: The psychological treatment of patients with functional somatic symptoms: a practical guide. J Psychosom Res 36:515–529, 1992

Sharpe M, Mayou R, Seagroatt V, et al: Why do doctors find some patients difficult to help? Q J Med 87:187–193, 1994

Silber TJ, Pao M: Somatization disorders in children and adolescents. Pediatr Rev 24:255–264, 2003

Simon GE: Somatization and psychiatric disorders, in Current Concepts of Somatization: Research and Clinical Perspectives. Edited by Kirmayer LJ, Robbins JM. Washington, DC, American Psychiatric Press, 1991, pp 37–62

Simon GE, Gureje O: Stability of somatization disorder and somatization symptoms among primary care patients. Arch Gen Psychiatry 56:90–95, 1999

Simon G, Gater R, Kisely S, et al: Somatic symptoms of distress: an international primary care study. Psychosom Med 58:481–488, 1996

Simon GE, VonKorff M, Piccinelli M, et al: An international study of the relation between somatic symptoms and depression. N Engl J Med 341:1329–1335, 1999

Slater E, Glithero E: A follow-up of patients diagnosed as suffering from "hysteria." J Psychosom Res 9:9–13, 1965

Smith GR: Somatization Disorder in Medical Settings. Washington, DC, American Psychiatric Press, 1991

Smith GR: The epidemiology and treatment of depression when it coexists with somatoform disorders, somatization, or pain. Gen Hosp Psychiatry 14:265–272, 1992

Smith GC, Clarke DM, Handrinos D, et al: Consultation-liaison psychiatrists' management of somatoform disorders. Psychosomatics 41:481–489, 2000

Stahl SM: Antidepressants and somatic symptoms: therapeutic actions are expanding beyond affective spectrum disorders to functional somatic syndrome. J Clin Psychiatry 64:745–746, 2003

Starcevic V, Kellner R, Uhlenhuth EH, et al: Panic disorder and hypochondriacal fears and beliefs. J Affect Disord 24:73–85, 1992

Stone J, Campbell K, Sharma N, et al: What should we call pseudoseizures? The patient's perspective. Seizure 12:568–572, 2003

Stuart S, Noyes R: Attachment and interpersonal communication in somatization. Psychosomatics 40:34–43, 1999

Sullivan M, Clark MR, Katon WJ, et al: Psychiatric and otologic diagnoses in patients complaining of dizziness. Arch Intern Med 153:1479–1484, 1993

Sumathipala A, Hewege R, Hanwella R, et al: Randomized controlled trial of cognitive behaviour therapy for repeated consultations for medically unexplained complaints: a feasibility study in Sri Lanka. Psychol Med 30:747–757, 2000

Taylor GJ: Recent developments in alexithymia theory and research. Can J Psychiatry 45:134–142, 2000

Thomassen R, van Hemert AM, Huyse FJ, et al: Somatoform disorders in consultation-liaison psychiatry: a comparison with other mental disorders. Gen Hosp Psychiatry 25:8–13, 2003

Toone BK: Disorders of hysterical conversion, in Somatization: Physical Symptoms and Psychological Illness. Edited by Bass C. Boston, MA, Blackwell Scientific, 1990, pp 207–234

Tyrer P, Fowler-Dixon R, Ferguson B, et al: A plea for the diagnosis of hypochondriacal personality disorder. J Psychosom Res 34:637–642, 1990

Uzun O, Basoglu C, Akar A, et al: Body dysmorphic disorder in patients with acne. Compr Psychiatry 44:415–419, 2003

Van Dyck R, Hoogduin K: Hypnosis and conversion disorders. Am J Psychother 43:480–493, 1989

Veale D, Boocock A, Gournay K, et al: Body dysmorphic disorder. A survey of fifty cases. Br J Psychiatry 169:196–201, 1996a

Veale D, Gournay K, Dryden W, et al: Body dysmorphic disorder: a cognitive-behavioural model and pilot randomized controlled trial. Behav Res Ther 34:717–729, 1996b

Veale D, De Haro L, Lambrou C: Cosmetic rhinoplasty in body dysmorphic disorder. Br J Plast Surg 56:546–551, 2003

Visser S, Bouman TK: Cognitive-behavioural approaches in the treatment of hypochondriasis: six single case cross-over studies. Behav Res Ther 30:301–306, 1992

Visser S, Bouman TK: The treatment of hypochondriasis: exposure plus response prevention vs cognitive therapy. Behav Res Ther 39:423–442, 2001

Volz HP, Moller HJ, Reimann I, et al: Opipramol for the treatment of somatoform disorders results from a placebo-controlled trial. Eur Neuropsychopharmacol 10:211–217, 2000

Walker J, Vincent N, Furer P, et al: Treatment preference in hypochondriasis. J Behav Ther Exp Psychiatry 30:251–258, 1999

Walling MK, O'Hara MW, Reiter RC, et al: Abuse history and chronic pain in women, II: a multivariate analysis of abuse and psychological morbidity. Obstet Gynecol 84:200–206, 1994

Warwick H: Provision of appropriate and effective reassurance. Int Rev Psychiatry 4:76–80, 1992

Warwick HMC, Marks IM: Behavioural treatment of illness phobia and hypochondriasis: a pilot study of 17 cases. Br J Psychiatry 152:239–241, 1988

Young L: Sexual abuse and the problem of embodiment. Child Abuse Negl 16:89–100, 1992

Yutzy SH, Cloninger CR, Guze SB, et al: DSM-IV field trial: testing a new proposal for somatization disorder. Am J Psychiatry 152:97–101, 1995

Zimmerman M, Mattia JI: Body dysmorphic disorder in psychiatric outpatients: recognition, prevalence, comorbidity, demographic, and clinical correlates. Compr Psychiatry 39:265–270, 1998

14

Deception Syndromes: Factitious Disorders and Malingering

Charles V. Ford, M.D.

Disease has been simulated in every age, and by all classes of society. The monarch, the mendicant, the unhappy slave, the proud warrior, the lofty statesman, even the minister of religion as well as the condemned malefactor and boy "creeping like snail unwillingly to school," have sought to disguise their purposes, or obtain their desires, by feigning mental or bodily infirmities (Gavin 1838, p. i)

The above introductory paragraph to Hector Gavin's 1838 book *On the Feigned and Factitious Diseases of Solders and Seamen*, in which he described clinical features of factitious disorders and malingering, indicates the pervasiveness of simulated disease. Also noteworthy is that in the second century A.D., the Roman physician Galen devoted a chapter to simulated disease in one of his medical texts (Adams 1846).

In the current diagnostic classification, that of DSM-IV-TR (American Psychiatric Association 2000), simulated diseases such as somatization disorder are placed within the category of *somatoform disorders*. These disorders are considered to be of unconscious etiology. *Factitious disorders*, considered to be of conscious production but of unconscious motivation, are included among Axis I diagnoses in a separate category. *Malingering*, considered to be of both conscious production and motivation, is assigned a V code. Imprecise criteria (e.g., conscious vs. unconscious motivation) are bound to result in imprecise diagnoses, and in fact illness behavior is frequently motivated by a variety of conscious and unconscious objectives. Furthermore, a person may feign illness to achieve different goals at different times (Eisendrath 1996). Thus, an originally unconsciously motivated symptom may evolve into a consciously driven symptom so that the patient may achieve secondary gains.

Illness behavior includes a wide continuum of symptoms and motivations. At one extreme are behaviors that might be considered normal in view of their commonality, such as using a complaint of a physical symptom (e.g., a headache) to avoid some undesired social obligation. This chapter focuses on the other extreme of consciously motivated illness behavior: factitious disorders and malingering. As noted above, the primary difference between these two forms of illness behavior is the perceived role of conscious versus unconscious motivation. Such a distinction is useful for textbook descriptions, but unfortunately in actual clinical situations the determination of motivation becomes a highly subjective process. A complicating factor is the unreliability of information provided by persons who are, by definition, deceptive.

There are two primary forms of factitious behavior. The first is self-induced or simulated disease, known at times by the eponym Munchausen syndrome, and the second is factitious disease behavior induced in others, also more commonly known as Munchausen syndrome by proxy. Although these two forms of factitious illness overlap at certain points, they are discussed separately here to provide clarity on various important clinical and legal issues. Malingering, not a medical diagnosis per se, is discussed separately from the factitious disorders.

Interest in factitious disorders has increased markedly since the publication of Asher's sentinel paper in 1951. By 2003 there had been approximately 1,500 publications in the medical literature focusing on factitious disorders. There have been descriptions of a number of other syndromes related to factitious disorder, such as factitious allegations of sexual abuse (Feldman et al. 1994; Feldman-Schorrig 1996; Gibbon 1998), the use of Internet chat rooms and support groups to create a fictional identity (Feldman 2000), the "angel of death" syndrome (Yorker 1996) (in which a nurse creates emergency situations in his or her patients), and even production of disease in one's pets (Munro and Thrusfield 2001).

Hardie and Reed (1998) described the overlaps in characteristics of persons who demonstrate pseudologia fantastica (Table 14–1), create factitious disorders, and engage in impostorship. They proposed the term *deception syndrome* to describe these syndromes—a concept that would provide more unity than does the current tendency to create increasing numbers of new syndromes and eponyms.

Factitious Disorders

Persons who have factitious disorders intentionally feign, exaggerate, aggravate, or self-induce symptoms or disease. They are conscious of their behaviors, although the underlying motivation may be unconscious. By convention, this diagnosis is also characterized by the surreptitious nature of the behavior. Patients who acknowledge that they have produced their own self-harm (e.g., self-mutilators) are not included in this diagnostic group. Inherent in factitious disorders is a paradox: the patient presents to a physician or other health care provider with the request for medical care but simultaneously conceals the known cause of the problem.

Risk factors for factitious disorder vary according to the subtype of the clinical syndrome. The most common subtype is common factitious disorder (or nonperegrinating factitious disorder), in which the person does not use aliases or travel from hospital to hospital. In this syndrome, female gender, unmarried status, age in the 30s, prior work or experience in the health care professions (e.g., nursing), and Cluster B personality disorders with borderline features are frequently found. For full-blown Munchausen syndrome, in which the patient uses aliases and travels from hospital to hospital (and often from state to state), risk factors include male gender, single marital status, age often in the 40s, and a personality disorder of the Cluster B type with at least some antisocial features. In their review of 93 cases of factitious disorder diagnosed at the Mayo Clinic, Krahn and colleagues (2003) found that 72% were women, of whom 65.7% had some association with health-related occupations. The mean age for women was 30.7 years, and the mean age for men was 40.0 years.

TABLE 14–1.   Pseudologia fantastica

A form of pathological lying characterized by
  Matrix of fact and fiction
  An enduring repetitive quality
  Presentation of the storyteller in a grandiose manner and/or
    as a victim
The syndrome is often associated with
  Cognitive dysfunction
  Learning disabilities
  Factitious disorders
  Childhood traumatic experiences

Epidemiological features of factitious disorder are largely determined by inference rather than any specific research data. One mechanism for estimating frequency is the use of the findings of Gault and colleagues (1988), who analyzed material submitted by patients as kidney stones. Of these stones, 3.5% were obviously nonphysiological and artifactitious. Even when false stones that might have been presented innocently were eliminated, 2.6% remained as representing probable attempts to deceive physicians. This number of 2.6% obviously represents an extremely high estimate, and most investigators believe that factitious disorder is a relatively uncommon but not extremely rare disorder. For example, Sutherland and Rodin (1990) noted that 10 of 1,288 psychiatric consultations at a large teaching hospital in Toronto, Ontario, included a diagnosis of factitious disorder. A similar percentage of 0.6% was reported for a German university hospital psychiatric consultation service (Kapfhammer et al. 1998). These differing methods of determining incidence reflect a very large range. If the number of diagnoses established by psychiatric consultation is used as an estimate, then—with the assumption that no more than 1 in 10 medical inpatients is seen in psychiatric consultation—the incidence would be less than 1 in 10,000 admissions to medical–surgical services. However, many patients with factitious disorder may successfully evade detection and thereby go through the system undiagnosed.

Clinical Features: Phenomenology, Course, and Prognosis

Self-induced factitious disorders fit into two major syndromes. Unfortunately, the terminology in the general medical literature is inconsistent, and the terms *Munchausen syndrome* and *factitious disorder* are often used interchangeably (Fink and Jensen 1989). In this chapter, *Munchausen syndrome* refers specifically to the subtype of factitious disorders originally described by Richard Asher in 1951.

Classic Munchausen syndrome consists of three essential components: the simulation or self-induction of disease, pseudologia fantastica, and travel from hospital to hospital, often using aliases to disguise identity. These patients frequently present in the emergency room with dramatic symptoms such as hemoptysis, acute chest pain suggesting a myocardial infarction, or coma from self-induced hypoglycemia. Munchausen patients may make a career out of illness and hospitalizations; as many as 423 separate hospitalizations for an individual patient have been reported (von Maurer et al. 1973).

The types of symptoms and different diseases that have been simulated defy the imagination (Table 14–2). Essentially every subspecialty journal has published case reports of self-induced illness related to that particular subspecialty. Among the most common presentations have been chest pain, endocrine disorders such as hyperthyroidism, coagulopathies, infections, and neurological symptoms. The Munchausen patient often presents during evening or weekend hours, presumably in order to be evaluated by less senior or experienced clinicians. The patient is frequently admitted to an inpatient service, where he or she may become the "star patient" in view of the dramatic nature of the symptoms or the rarity of the presumed diagnosis. In addition, the patient may call attention to himself or herself by providing false information such as claiming to be a former professional football player, a recipient of the Medal of Honor, or perhaps the president of a foreign university. Despite such reputed prominence, these patients and their physicians rarely receive telephone calls from concerned family members or friends. The Munchausen patient is usually willing to undergo multiple diagnostic studies. When inconsistencies in history, medical findings, or laboratory examinations create suspicions, caregivers often become more confrontational. At this point the patient generally responds with irritation, new complaints, disruptive behavior, or threats to file a lawsuit. He or she may request discharge against medical advice or may simply disappear. Embarrassed and angry clinicians on the treatment team may console themselves by preparing a case presentation for grand rounds or perhaps for publication.

Munchausen syndrome is the most dramatic form of factitious behavior, and the eponym certainly has great popularity, but much more frequently seen is what has been termed *common factitious disorder*. In this syndrome, the patient does not use aliases and tends to repetitively seek treatment with the same physician or within the same health system. She may carry a diagnosis—which, on careful reflection, was made with imprecise criteria—such as bleeding coagulopathy or a collagen disease. These patients, usually young women, are often well known to care providers because of their frequent hospital admissions. They may even come to the hospital bringing stuffed animals or special sheets (e.g., Mickey Mouse) for their hospital beds. In retrospect, when the true diagnosis is discovered, it can be determined that their history, both medical and personal, was inaccurate. They are not, however, as inclined to pseudologia fantastica as are patients with full-blown Munchausen syndrome.

TABLE 14–2. Examples of factitious diseases

Symptom/disease	Method of production	Diagnostic clue
Infections	Injections of saliva or feces	Polymicrobial cultures
Hypoglycemic coma	Self-injection of insulin	Low C-peptide
	Oral hypoglycemic agents	Glyburide in urine
Fever of unexplained etiology[a]	Manipulation of thermometer	Dissociation of fever/pulse
Neurological disease	Anisocoria secondary to anticholinergic eyedrops	Variable reactivity of pupils
Diarrhea	Laxative abuse	Laxative in stool
Pheochromocytoma	Epinephrine in urine	Low blood chromogranin A
Electrolyte imbalance	Diuretics	High urinary potassium
Vomiting	Ipecac	Increased urinary potassium with low chloride
Coagulopathies	Warfarin	Serum assay
Anemia	Self-bloodletting	No bleeding site or iron malabsorption
Pancytopenia	Methotrexate	Serum assay
Proteinuria	Egg white in urine	Large daily variations of urine protein
Purpura	Quinidine	Serum or urinary assay
Hyperthyroidism	Exogenous thyroid	Low serum thyroglobulin
Hematuria	Finger prick blood to urine	

[a]Now uncommon because of the use of instantaneous electronic thermometers.
Source. Adapted from Wallach 1994.

Symptoms and signs for patients with common factitious disorder tend to be less dramatic, and their complaints are often more chronic or subjective. Some common symptoms include joint pain, recurrent abscesses, failure to heal from surgical operations, hypoglycemic episodes, simulated renal colic, and blood dyscrasias. Factitious disorder as a cause for these patients' symptoms may not be suspected for months or even years. When the diagnosis is finally established, there may be disbelief among the medical care providers. "Splitting" behavior, in which the patient plays one group of providers against another group, is frequently seen.

Factitious Disorder With Psychological Symptoms

The large majority of published cases of factitious disorder describe physical symptoms alone. When factitious psychological symptoms are recognized, they are generally in association with either authentic or fabricated physical complaints. The reason for this may be that subspecialists in psychosomatic medicine are more likely to encounter patients with factitious psychological symptoms who are hospitalized on medical–surgical wards, or in the emergency room, than to see such patients on psychiatric units. Patients with factitious psychological symptoms fabricate a wide range of symptoms. The most commonly reported include depression and suicidal thinking tied to claims of bereavement (Phillips et al. 1983; Snowden et al. 1978). The patient reports that his or her emotional distress is due to the death of someone close such as a parent or child. Distress appears genuine, is often accompanied by tears, and characteristically elicits sympathy from medical personnel. Later, staff members may discover that the mourned person is very much alive, that the circumstances of the death were less dramatic than the patient reported, or that the death was many years in the past. Case reports of the factitious psychological symptoms also describe feigned multiple personality disorder, substance dependence, dissociative and conversion reactions, memory loss, and posttraumatic stress disorder. Multiple feigned psychological symptoms may be present in the same patient (Parker 1993). Some authors urge caution in diagnosing factitious disorder with predominantly psychological symptoms, especially factitious psychosis, because some patients with these symptoms eventually manifest clear-cut severe mental illness (Nicholson and Roberts 1994; Rogers et al. 1989).

Ganser's syndrome is closely related to factitious disorder, with predominantly psychological symptoms. This syndrome is characterized by the provision of approximate answers (*Vorbeireden*) to questions (e.g., the examiner asks, "What is the color of snow," and the patient answers, "Green"). Complaints of amnesia, disorientation, and perceptual disturbance are generally present as well. This syndrome was originally described by the nineteenth-century German psychiatrist Sigbert Ganser (1965) as a form of malingering seen in prisoners, but it has also been described in other settings, including general hospital units (Dalfen and Anthony 2000; Weiner and Braiman 1955). Ganser's syndrome was described in one patient who also had clear-cut factitious physical and psychological symptoms (Parker 1993). The etiology of this syndrome remains in question, and malingering, dissociation, and organic brain disease (Sigal et al. 1992) have been proposed as contributing factors.

When the patient presents with both physical and psychological factitious symptoms and neither predominates, the appropriate diagnosis is factitious disorder with combined physical and psychological symptoms. The aforementioned case reported by Parker (1993) included pseudodementia (Ganser's syndrome), feigned bereavement, factitious rape, pseudoseizures, and simulated renal failure.

The prognosis of patients with factitious symptoms is unclear. Some patients may, at some point in their life, abandon their behavior. Death, probably as a result of the patient's miscalculations of the risk of the behavior, has also been reported (Nichols et al. 1990).

Diagnosis and Assessment

The diagnosis of factitious disorder may be suggested by inconsistent laboratory results, physical findings that do not conform with reported symptoms, failure to respond as predicted to effective treatment for the disorder in question, or, most frequently, the accidental discovery of medical paraphernalia on the patient's person or in the room. For example, a syringe may be found taped onto the inside portion of a toilet lid or a nurse may come into a patient's room unannounced and find the patient digging in a surgical wound with a foreign body. Ultimately, the diagnosis of factitious disorder is made via detective work by health care providers based on a high index of suspicion. A review of past medical records from other institutions may be essential to establish the diagnosis (Krahn et al. 2003). On the surface the patient may appear normal, and a psychiatric interview per se cannot establish the diagnosis unless there is a "confession." The patient, even when confronted with irrefutable evidence of factitious behavior, typically denies that the illness was self-induced.

The differential diagnoses of factitious disorder include unusual, rare, or as-yet undescribed and unknown diseases, somatoform disorders, and overt malingering.

Etiology

The reasons why a person might engage in factitious illness behavior are to a large extent speculative. Even when seen in long-term treatment, these patients are resistant to articulating their motivations. Proposed underlying motivations are outlined in Table 14–3.

The large majority of patients with factitious disorder have an underlying severe personality disorder, usually of the Cluster B type. Factitious behavior can be seen as a form of acting out, similar to other acting-out behaviors seen in Cluster B personality disorders. Axis I comorbidity, including major depression and schizophrenia, has been described but is not common. However, it must be kept in mind that psychiatric symptoms may also be simulated.

Few patients have been extensively studied with regard to developmental history because very few will agree to see a psychotherapist and even fewer open up honestly. In the very select few who have, a childhood history of parental illness, death, or abandonment or issues of personal illness or institutionalization are common (Ford 1973). As a result of these childhood issues, factitious behavior may be viewed, at least in some circumstances, as a learned coping mechanism.

The possible role of cerebral dysfunction for at least some patients has been proposed. Pankratz and Lezak (1987) reported that approximately one-third of the Munchausen patients in their series had deficits in conceptual organization. Abnormal findings on brain imaging have also been reported (Babe et al. 1992; Fenelon et al. 1991). Brain dysfunction has also been reported in approximately 20%–25% of persons with pseudologia fantastica and/or Munchausen syndrome (Ford 1996b; King and Ford 1988).

Management and Treatment

In the past it was suggested that blacklists should be created, disseminated, and maintained at various hospitals to identify Munchausen patients when they present for care (Mohammed et al. 1985). A variant of this concept for an individual hospital is to mark the old chart in some conspicuous manner to identify the patient when he or she presents to an emergency room. Such blacklists have found disfavor in the United States largely because of legal and ethical concerns and would be considered a violation of regulations under the Health Insurance Portability and Accountability Act of 1996 (P.L. 104-191).

A major question in management is how to deal with a patient once a definitive diagnosis of factitious disorder has been established. No matter how understandable the

TABLE 14–3. Proposed motivations for factitious disorder

Need to be the center of attention
Longing to be cared for
Maladaptive reaction to loss or separation
Anger at physicians or displaced onto physicians
Pleasure derived from deceiving others ("duping delight")

anger at these deceptive patients might be, the temptation to "let them have it" must be resisted. To act out in an angry way only plays into the patient's pathology by drawing the physician into a dramatized scene. A direct, accusative confrontation is likely to result in anger from the patient and in his or her subsequent departure from the hospital, often against medical advice, or with threats to bring a lawsuit for defamation. It has been suggested that the confrontation be more indirect, in a manner that allows face-saving for the patient or an opportunity for therapy. For example, a patient may be told, "When some patients are very upset, they often do something to themselves to create illness as a way of seeking help. We believe that something such as this must be going on, and we would like to help you focus on the true nature of your problem, which is emotional distress." Unfortunately, such an approach, although logical and humane, does not usually result in the patient's acknowledgment of factitious illness behavior and acceptance of psychological treatment. Another approach is to provide the patient with a paradoxical confrontation. In this technique, the patient is told that there is some question as to whether or not the illness is factitious in nature but that definitive treatment for the physical symptoms has been administered and if the patient fails to respond within a set time period then that would indicate that the problem is factitious in nature. This technique has the obvious clinical and ethical drawbacks of dishonestly treating a dishonest patient, which may be self-defeating.

When present, comorbid psychiatric disorders such as depression (if not believed to be also factitious) should be appropriately treated; in at least one case in the literature, remission of factitious behavior with antidepressant medication was reported (Earle and Folks 1986). Psychotherapy with the patient who engages in factitious behavior is, at best, extremely difficult. Treatment for these patients should be conceptualized essentially as being for a severe underlying personality disorder manifested by acting-out defenses. Stone (1977) proposed vigorous persistent confrontation of the behavior, but most clinicians who have had experience with these patients find that such confrontation results in abandonment of treatment or increase in acting-out behaviors. Instead of direct confrontation, the patient may be provided with indirect confrontation or interpretation in ongoing supportive psychotherapy (Eisendrath 2001). This technique is based on the premise that if the patient can maintain a relationship with a physician that is not contingent on development of new physical symptoms, factitious behavior may be reduced. Such a treatment approach must be viewed as primarily symptomatic with no expectation of changes in the basic personality structure that predisposes a person to factitious illness behavior. Experience with this type of treatment indicates that there may be remissions that last a few months but that they are often followed by the patient leaving treatment without warning and reengaging in factitious illness behavior elsewhere.

In the medical care of patients with any somatizing disorder (including factitious illness and malingering), the physician should proceed with invasive diagnostic and treatment procedures based only on objective evidence. Furthermore, physicians must be cautious when prescribing any potentially dangerous or habituating medication (Ford 1992).

Legal and ethical issues frequently arise in the assessment and treatment of patients with factitious disorder. In the past, the paternalistic model of medicine suggested that the physician was permitted to do essentially anything that would help establish the diagnosis. For example, patients' rooms were searched for medical paraphernalia, drugs, and so forth. In one situation, when a bottle of insulin was found during such a search, it was spiked with a radioactive compound and the diagnosis proved by later finding radioactivity in the patient (Berkowitz et al. 1971). More recently, particularly in the United States, medical practice has emphasized patients' rights and informed consent. This creates a dilemma. On one hand, a failure to do all that is necessary to establish the diagnosis might be regarded as abdication of medical responsibility and ultimately harmful to the patient. On the other hand, even patients suspected of factitious behavior have rights to personal privacy, including privacy in one's belongings, confidentiality, and informed consent. One approach is to tell the patient that factitious illness behavior is suspected and request permission to rule this out. This has the risk of alienating a patient who does not have factitious illness. It may result in the patient with factitious disorder refusing permission, leaving the hospital, and perpetuating the same behavior at another medical facility.

Physicians may believe that the patient's outrageous behavior of factitious disease production would leave them free from the risk of malpractice suits. This is untrue, and there have been numerous reports of lawsuits initiated by these patients (Eisendrath 1996; Ford 1996a; Janofsky 1994; Lipsitt 1986). The reasons for lawsuits may include overt greed, rage at a physician who was previously idealized (borderline behavior), or perhaps the opportunity to change one's highly dramatized role as a patient in a hospital to an equally dramatized role as a plaintiff in a courtroom. In one case in which I was an expert witness, it became obvious during the malpractice trial that the patient had produced her postsurgical wound infections. The patient and her attorney then took a new tack, claiming malpractice on the part of the surgeon for failure to recognize that the patient had a factitious disorder!

Because patients with factitious disorder do create legal and ethical problems, it is prudent for the psychiatric consultant to suggest that the management plan require careful multidisciplinary collaboration and appropriate consultation with hospital administrators, hospital and personal attorneys, and the hospital ethics committee. It cannot be overemphasized that any decision to deviate from usual medical practice with such patients should not be made by a solitary individual. Such decisions should be carried out and their rationale noted with the patient's best interests at heart and should be documented in the chart. When factitious disorder is suspected, chart documentation in a factual, nonspeculative manner is highly recommended.

In view of these patients' self-destructive nature, many physicians, including psychiatrists, may question whether involuntary psychiatric hospitalization is indicated. Thresholds for involuntary commitment vary from state to state and from country to country. In the United States, because factitious disorder represents chronic behavior, which is not immediately suicidal, these patients usually do not meet the criteria for involuntary psychiatric hospitalization. In one case in Oregon, outpatient commitment resulted in lower medical costs and less iatrogenic morbidity for a patient with factitious disorder (McFarland et al. 1983).

Factitious Disorders by Proxy (Factitious Disorder Not Otherwise Specified)

In DSM-IV-TR the diagnostic code *factitious disorder not otherwise specified* includes a variety of factitious diseases and symptoms described or induced by another person. This particular syndrome is far better known by the eponym Munchausen syndrome by proxy, and most case reports describe parents (particularly mothers) who have induced disease in their children. There are, however, some reports of adults inducing disease in other adults, particularly when in a caretaker setting, for example, a nurse caring for a bedridden patient (Meadow 1998; Yorker 1996).

Munchausen syndrome by proxy is an invidious behavior that, when it involves children, should be considered a form of child abuse. The syndrome was initially described by Meadow (1977), who coined the term; subsequent to his initial report there have been numerous reports from around the world, including non-Western cultures (Bappal et al. 2001).

The incidence of Munchausen syndrome by proxy is sufficiently high that children's hospitals see several cases per year. Denny et al. (2001) found the incidence in New Zealand to be 2.0/100,000 in children under age 16 years. McClure et al. (1996) computed the annual incidence in the United Kingdom to be at least 2.8/100,000 for children younger than 1 year and 0.5/100,000 for those between 1 and 16. Meadow (1999) reviewed cases of sudden infant death and was of the opinion that many of these deaths fit the phenomenological pattern of Munchausen syndrome by proxy. It is possible that many cases of Munchausen syndrome by proxy are misdiagnosed as spontaneous illness.

Clinical Features: Phenomenology, Course, and Prognosis

The typical presentation of Munchausen syndrome by proxy is that of a child admitted to a hospital with symptoms such as seizures, bleeding, diarrhea, or respiratory or apneic difficulties. The mother, who often has a history of some medical training, characteristically assists the nurses and readily consents to any invasive diagnostic procedures proposed for the child. Discovery of the mother's role in the production of the child's symptoms may occur accidentally, such as by finding her smothering the child with a pillow or introducing a toxic substance into the child's mouth or intravenous tubing. Suspicions also may arise if symptoms or episodes of the illness occur only when the mother is alone with the child, if another child in the family has had unexplained illnesses, or if the child's medical problems do not have a predictable response to appropriate treatment.

Sheridan (2003) reviewed and summarized published data from 451 cases of Munchausen syndrome by proxy. Her findings indicate no gender bias of the child victims, who were usually age 4 years or younger. In the majority of situations the perpetrator actively produced symptoms by smothering or poisoning the child, although in some instances there was exaggeration or lying about symptoms. The most frequently noted symptoms of the child victims were, in order, apnea, anorexia, feeding problems, diarrhea, seizures, and cyanosis. The mortality rate for identified children victims was 6.0%, but 25% of known siblings were known to be dead! This implies a much higher mortality rate (than 6.0%) when the diagnosis is unrecognized. Other reports have also emphasized the high mortality rate associated with Munchausen syndrome by proxy (Bools et al. 1993; Rosenberg 1987).

Diagnosis and Assessment

As noted in the previous subsection, the diagnosis may become apparent by fortuitous findings such as the discovery of secret paraphernalia or drugs or the accidental observation of the mother smothering the child. However, when Munchausen syndrome by proxy is suspected but not confirmed, several procedures to confirm the diagnosis have been proposed. These include 1) a review of medical records of other siblings, looking for a pattern of chronic illness or unexplained death; 2) separation of the child from the parent to determine whether or not there is a change in the child's course of illness (e.g., many children suddenly recover when separated from the parent for several days or weeks); and 3) the controversial technique of video surveillance using a hidden camera. Ethical and legal questions may arise as to whether video surveillance involves an invasion of privacy. Such a procedure should be undertaken only after appropriate consultation with hospital legal staff, administration, and child protective services. Rules for privacy may be somewhat different to protect a helpless child rather than for an adult. In this situation it is the child who is the patient, not the parents. Hall and colleagues (2000) reported that a diagnosis of Munchausen syndrome by proxy was made in 23 of 41 patients monitored by covert video surveillance. In another 4 patients, surveillance was instrumental in establishing the innocence of the parents. It must be kept in mind that such techniques actually place the child at risk, and there should be continuous monitoring of the video screen and preestablished plans for intervention as soon as any danger to the child is detected (Southall et al. 1997).

Ayoub et al. (2002) state that perpetrators of factitious disorder by proxy should be diagnosed with factitious disorder not otherwise specified, DSM-IV-TR code 300.19. However, providing a DSM-IV-TR diagnosis to any person who perpetuates factitious behavior is controversial, because an official diagnosis might imply mitigation for misbehavior—criminal behavior in the case of Munchausen syndrome by proxy. Ford and Zaner (1987) questioned whether persons perpetuating factitious behavior should be entitled to the status and rights of patienthood.

The differential diagnosis of Munchausen syndrome by proxy, of course, always includes the possibility of underlying genuine physical disease and the fact that at times an older child may produce illness in himself or herself (Libow 2000) (Table 14–4). There also may be "blended cases" in which the child or adolescent self-produces symptoms but with the active help of the parent, who may coach the behavior (Libow 2002). At present most pediatricians and child protection caseworkers are well aware of Munchausen syndrome by proxy, and there is a risk of becoming overly zealous in making the diagnosis. Rand and Feldman (1999) reported 4 cases of misdiagnosed Munchausen syndrome by proxy and identified another 11 cases in their review of more than 200 articles and books.

Etiology

In Munchausen syndrome by proxy, the identified patient is the victim of misbehavior by another. Adults who perpetrate this disorder may superficially seem quite normal, and frequently evaluation of them does not result in a psychiatric diagnosis. Others may meet criteria for a somatoform disorder or a personality disorder or have previously produced factitious disease in themselves (Bools et al. 1994). Most explanations for perpetrating this behavior revolve around the idea that the perpetrator is motivated by the need to become the center of attention by playing the role of concerned parent in the high drama of life and death in a hospital.

Characteristics of perpetrators as computed by Sheridan (2003) include motherhood (76.5%); some features of personal Munchausen syndrome (29.3%); a psychiatric diagnosis (22.8%), usually depression or personality disorder; and a personal history of abuse (21.0%).

Family dynamics and the individual psychodynamics of the perpetrator are believed to be important, but there has not been any large-scale systematic study (Mercer and Perdue 1993). Griffith (1988) studied some families with Munchausen syndrome by proxy and proposed several commonly observed features: 1) enmeshment of parent–child relationships; 2) multigenerational themes of dominance and submission in parent–child relationships; 3) intense family-group loyalty with little protective concern for the needs of the developing child; 4) multigenerational pattern of abnormal illness behavior on the maternal side of the family; and 5) a gender reversal of typical sex roles for power and caretaking within the parental couple such that the wife is more dominant and aggressive and the husband is more caretaking and supportive. In their view of family dynamics, Mercer and Perdue (1993) suggest that the mother may be both victim and perpetrator, and her behavior is an attempt to gain power and control in a powerless existence.

TABLE 14–4. Differential diagnosis of Munchausen syndrome by proxy

Pediatric somatization syndromes

Somatoform disorder by proxy (parent's anxiety projected/ displaced onto child)

Infanticide/murder

Psychosis in parent

Child abuse (garden variety)

Factitious behavior initiated by child

Malingering by child (e.g., school rejection)

Unrecognized physical disease

Management and Treatment

Ethical and Legal Issues

The primary and immediate goal in treatment of Munchausen syndrome by proxy is cessation of the behavior that perpetrates symptoms. Separation between the perpetrator and the victim is usually necessary to accomplish cessation of the behavior. In the most common form of factitious disorder by proxy (parent-perpetrated), it is necessary to place the child into some type of foster care. Such placement requires a legal hearing and involvement of the agencies that have responsibility for protecting child welfare. It is amazing to see how a chronically sick child blooms when separated from the perpetrating parent. Permanent separation of parent and child is a major legal and ethical issue; courts are understandably reluctant to act in such a manner without very serious consideration. The key question is whether the parent has been sufficiently rehabilitated to reduce risk to the child, but the nature of the support system (other parent, other family members, availability of caseworkers) is also crucial.

Therapy for the Perpetrator

The perpetrator, who is usually the mother, should receive psychological treatment. The effectiveness of such intervention is dependent on the perpetrator's open and honest acknowledgment of his or her behavior. Unfortunately, this does not usually occur.

Treatment of the Victim

It is recognized that victims of factitious disorder by proxy experience a high incidence of varied psychiatric disorders (Bools et al. 1993; Bryk and Siegel 1997). To date there are no systematic studies of treatment. The specifics of treatment are dependent on the nature of the problem. One role of psychotherapy is to help the victim deal with feelings about an abusive parent.

Hospital Epidemics of Factitious Disorder by Proxy

The term *angel of death syndrome* was first used in newspaper reports (later proven to be inaccurate) in which a Las Vegas, Nevada, nurse was accused of tampering with patients' life-support equipment. The motivation was allegedly to help friends win a betting pool dealing with times of patients' deaths (Kalisch et al. 1980).

Although the case against the Las Vegas nurse was disproved, there have been multiple subsequent reports in which health care providers have been accused of causing epidemics of acute cardiac/pulmonary arrests and unusual patterns of deaths (Yorker 1996). Tragically, many of these epidemics have been shown to be caused by the very persons entrusted with the patients' care. In her detailed review of multiple hospital epidemics, Yorker (1996) concludes that the perpetrators are usually nurses or nurse's aides and that the victims were physically compromised: critically ill, elderly, or very young.

The epidemics tended to cluster on evening and night shifts and also involved a large number of—often successful—resuscitations. Yorker proposed that one motive of the perpetrators is the excitement and exhilaration derived from participating in codes.

This kind of behavior constitutes serial murder, and prosecution has resulted in a number of convictions. Epidemiologal techniques have been used to identify probable perpetrators, but such evidence is circumstantial and cannot be used alone to establish guilt (Sacks et al. 1988).

Malingering

By definition, individuals with malingering are motivated by specific, recognizable external incentives to produce, exaggerate, or simulate physical or psychological illness (American Psychiatric Association 2000; Gorman 1982). Such incentives may be deferment for military service, avoidance of hazardous work assignments, escape from incarceration (e.g., being judged not guilty by reason of insanity), or procurement of controlled substances. Perhaps the most common incentive is financial gain, such as the receipt of disability payments or the hope of damages to be awarded in a lawsuit. It must be kept in mind that malingering is less a diagnosis than a socially unacceptable behavior with legal ramifications (Szasz 1956). Malingering often must be considered in a differential diagnosis, but much caution must be exercised in making such a "diagnosis."

Malingering is most common in settings where there are external and tangible gains accrued by illness. Among these settings are prisons, military service, courtroom settings that involve personal or industrial injury, and the offices of physicians who perform disability evaluations. Flicken (1956) estimated that approximately 5% of persons who are conscripted for military service attempt to avoid it by feigning or manufacturing symptoms. Kay and Morris-Jones (1998) found clear-cut surveillance videotape evidence that at least 20% of the litigants registered in a pain clinic were overtly malingering their symptoms. Financial incentives *do* make a difference in symptoms and disability. In their meta-analysis of 2,353 subjects, Binder and Rohling (1996) found more abnormality and disability in patients with mild closed head injury who had financial incentives than in those who did not have such an incentive. Similarly, Paniak and colleagues (2002) found that when financial compensation was at issue, patients with mild traumatic brain injury had significantly increased symptoms. In contrast, Mayou (1995) conducted a prospective study in the United Kingdom on the outcome of persons involved in motor vehicle accidents and found that malingering to gain compensation was remarkably uncommon. He suggested that the high rates found in some tertiary care centers represent atypical and selected samples. The legal climate regarding lawsuits varies widely from country to country.

Clinical Features: Phenomenology, Course, and Prognosis

Malingering symptoms fall into four major categories: production or simulation of an illness, exacerbation of a previous illness, exaggeration of symptoms, and falsification of laboratory samples or laboratory reports. Embellishment of previous or concurrent illness is probably the form of malingering most frequently encountered by psychosomatic subspecialists. Symptoms are usually subjective and difficult to quantify and include feigned dizziness, weakness, seizures or spells, and features of posttraumatic stress disorder (Sparr and Pankratz 1983). Patients may intensify their complaints when they are asked directly about their symptoms or when they think they are being observed. When distracted, they become physically more relaxed and at times may be seen to engage in physical activities incompatible with their symptom reports.

The malingered symptom generally disappears when the person either obtains the desired goal or is confronted with irrefutable evidence of malingering. However, it has been noted that some malingered symptoms persist even after these occurrences. It may be that the person maintains symptoms as a face-saving mechanism, or perhaps the symptom has in some way been incorporated as a habit into the individual's lifestyle.

Diagnosis and Assessment

As noted above, identification of malingering is more an issue of socially unacceptable behavior, an accusation of a person's external motives, than a psychiatric diagnosis. The clinician should consider malingering when symptom complaints and objective data are incongruent. However, the presence of secondary gains, concurrent litigation, and seeking disability are *not* evidence of malingering per se. Thus, there must be not only verification of an external motivation but also objective evidence to demonstrate the probability of malingering. For example, a patient who cannot walk independently when seen in the consultation suite might later be seen walking normally on a sidewalk outside the hospital. Insurance companies at times engage private investigators who use video surveillance to obtain objective evidence of malingering. For example, a man who claimed an inability to raise his arms above his shoulder was videotaped climbing a ladder onto his roof and installing a television antenna.

Psychological testing is often helpful in identifying malingering patients. The Minnesota Multiphasic Personality Inventory–2 is a useful test for patients who distort their presentations (Lees-Haley and Fox 1990; McCaffrey and Bellamy-Campbell 1989; Wetzler and Marlowe 1990). This test and others have diagnostic value in assessing those who exaggerate physical and psychological symptoms (Cliffe 1992; Rawling 1992). Screening instruments with face validity such as the Beck Depression Inventory and the Hopkins Symptom Checklist–90 are easily distorted by patients who embellish their symptoms (Lees-Haley 1989a, 1989b), and these instruments have very limited value in the determination of malingering. Forced-choice psychological tests may be valuable in detecting malingering. If a person makes more errors than would be expected by chance, a statistical probability can be determined as to whether the person actually knew the correct answers.

No single evaluation technique will unequivocally identify malingerers. This is particularly true when the examiner makes a subjective assessment of a feature such as sincerity of effort (Lechner et al. 1998; Main and Waddell 1998). Rather, patients must be evaluated from a complete physical and psychosocial perspective that includes various other possibilities, such as "pseudomalingering" (Ford 1983). Pseudomalingering arises when the patient uses an external incentive as a rationalization for malingered symptoms, thereby shielding himself or herself from awareness of unconscious determinants (Ford 1983; Schneck 1962). For example, a genuinely psychotic person may believe he or she is feigning psychosis to escape punishment for a crime. By believing that one is feigning the psychosis, the person is defensively shielded from conscious awareness of actual mental illness and thus incorrectly believes that he or she is in control of his or her thought processes. Another form of pseudomalingering may exist when a person consciously exaggerates a symptom because he or she truly believes that there is an underlying problem. An underlying problem may exist, but the examiner who picks up on the malingering may mistakenly attribute the entire problem to malingering.

The differential diagnosis of malingering includes somatoform disorders as well as factitious disorders. These clinical syndromes have indistinct boundaries, and a person may meet criteria for different disorders at different times (Ford 1992; Jonas and Pope 1985; Nadelson 1985). Furthermore, conversion disorder and malingering are on a continuum (Cameron 1947), representing opposite poles of purely unconscious and purely conscious motivation. At any one moment it is difficult for the diagnostician to know the patient's location on this continuum. Relevant factors that may play a role in assessment include evidence of past somatization as well as coexistence of anxiety, mood, substance, or personality disorders. Patients with unconsciously determined somatoform disorders (e.g., conversion) are usually consistent in their symptom presentation irrespective of their audience or whether they believe they are being observed.

Etiology

By definition, the etiology of malingering is to obtain external gain as a result of the symptoms. However, malingering does tend to be more common in persons who may have hysteroid features. Because of personality characteristics (e.g., histrionic or sociopathic) or cognitive style, some persons may be more inclined toward simulated illness.

Management and Treatment

Malingering is more a management problem than a therapeutic issue. With this in mind, the primary physician and psychosomatic subspecialist must be circumspect in their approach to the patient. Every note must be written with the thought in mind that it may become a courtroom exhibit. Malingering is often listed among diagnostic possibilities but is rarely proved conclusively in medical settings.

The person who is suspected of malingering, as a rule, should not be confronted with a direct accusation. Instead, subtle communication can indicate that the physician is "on to the game" (Kramer et al. 1979). One technique is to mention, almost in passing, that diagnostic tests indicate no "serious" basis for the symptoms. The malingerer may feel freer to discard the symptom if the physician suggests that patients with similar problems usually recover after a certain procedure is performed or a particular length of time has passed. Such suggestions are often followed by perceptible improvement, if not recovery. This technique provides face-saving mechanisms for the patient to discard the symptom. Still, some patients, particularly those seeking drugs, will leave treatment and seek medical care elsewhere. Others, in an effort to prove the existence of their disease, may vastly intensify their symptoms. In doing so, they may create such caricatures of illness that their efforts to malinger become obvious to all.

Conclusion

Requests for psychiatric consultation on patients with suspected factitious disorder or malingering are relatively infrequent. However, when the psychosomatic medicine subspecialist does become involved with one of these cases, a disproportionate amount of time is typically required. Issues of diagnosis, legal and ethical considerations, and the need to provide liaison services for members of the medical staff may make one of these patients the primary focus of one's clinical activities for several days. Nevertheless, they are fascinating patients who demonstrate the extreme end of the continuum of abnormal illness behavior. They are rarely forgotten.

References

Adams F: The Seven Books of Paulus Aegineta, Vol 2. London, England, Sydenham Society, 1846

American Psychiatric Association: Diagnostic and Statistical Manual of Mental Disorders, 4th Edition, Text Revision. Washington, DC, American Psychiatric Association, 2000

Asher R: Munchausen's syndrome. Lancet 1:339–341, 1951

Ayoub CC, Alexander R, Beck D, et al: Position paper: definitional issues in Munchausen by proxy. Child Maltreat 7:105–111, 2002

Babe KS Jr, Peterson AM, Loosen PT, et al: The pathogenesis of Munchausen syndrome: a review and case report. Gen Hosp Psychiatry 14:273–276, 1992

Bappal B, George M, Nair R, et al: Factitious hypoglycemia: a tale from the Arab world. Pediatrics 107:180–181, 2001

Berkowitz S, Parrish JE, Field JB: Factitious hypoglycemia: why not diagnose before laparotomy. Am J Med 51:669–674, 1971

Binder LM, Rohling ML: Money matters: a meta-analytic review of the effects of financial incentives on recovery after closed-head injury. Am J Psychiatry 153:7–10, 1996

Bools CN, Neale BA, Meadow SR: Follow up of victims of fabricated illness (Munchausen syndrome by proxy). Arch Dis Child 69:625–630, 1993

Bools C, Neale B, Meadow R: Munchausen syndrome by proxy: a study of psychopathology. Child Abuse Negl 18:773–788, 1994

Bryk M, Siegel PT: My mother caused my illness: the story of a survivor of Munchausen by proxy syndrome. Pediatrics 100:1–7, 1997

Cameron NA: The Psychology of Behavior Disorders. Boston, MA, Houghton Mifflin, 1947

Cliffe MJ: Symptom-validity testing of feigned sensory or memory deficits: a further elaboration for subjects who understand the rationale. Br J Clin Psychol 31:207–209, 1992

Dalfen AK, Anthony F: Head injury, dissociation and the Ganser syndrome. Brain Inj 14:1101–1105, 2000

Denny SJ, Grant CC, Pinnock R: Epidemiology of Munchausen syndrome by proxy in New Zealand. J Paediatr Child Health 37:340–343, 2001

Earle JR Jr, Folks DG: Factitious disorder and coexisting depression: a report of a successful psychiatric consultation and case management. Gen Hosp Psychiatry 8:448–450, 1986

Eisendrath SJ: When Munchausen becomes malingering: factitious disorders that penetrate the legal system. Bull Am Acad Psychiatry Law 24:471–481, 1996

Eisendrath SJ: Factitious disorders and malingering, in Treatments of Psychiatric Disorders, 3rd Edition, Vol 2. Edited by Gabbard GO. Washington, DC, American Psychiatric Press, 2001, pp 1825–1842

Feldman MD: Munchausen by Internet: detecting factitious illness and crisis on the Internet. South Med J 93:669–672, 2000

Feldman MD, Ford CV, Stone T: Deceiving others/deceiving oneself: four cases of factitious rape. South Med J 87:736–738, 1994

Feldman-Schorrig S: Factitious sexual harassment. Bull Am Acad Psychiatry Law 24:387–482, 1996

Fenelon G, Mahieux F, Roullet E, et al: Munchausen's syndrome and abnormalities on magnetic resonance imaging of the brain. BMJ 302:996–997, 1991

Fink P, Jensen J: Clinical characteristics of the Munchausen syndrome: a review and 3 new case histories. Psychother Psychosom 52:164–171, 1989

Flicken DJ: Malingering: a symptom. J Nerv Ment Dis 123:23–31, 1956

Ford CV: The Munchausen syndrome: a report of four new cases and a review of psychodynamic considerations. Psychiatr Med 4:31–45, 1973

Ford CV: The Somatizing Disorders: Illness as a Way of Life. New York, Elsevier, 1983

Ford CV: Illness as a lifestyle: the role of somatization in medical practice. Spine 17:S338–S343, 1992

Ford CV: Ethical and legal issues in factitious disorders: an overview, in The Spectrum of Factitious Disorders. Edited by Feldman MD, Eisendrath SJ. Washington, DC, American Psychiatric Press, 1996a, pp 51–66

Ford CV: Lies! Lies!! Lies!!! The Psychology of Deceit. Washington, DC, American Psychiatric Press, 1996b

Ford CV, Zaner RM: Response to the article "Ethical and management considerations in factitious illness: one and the same" by John Z Sadler. Gen Hosp Psychiatry 9:37–39, 1987

Ganser SJM: A peculiar hysterical state. Br J Criminol 5:120–126, 1965

Gault MH, Campbell NR, Aksu AE: Spurious stones. Nephron 48:274–279, 1988

Gavin H: On the Feigned and Factitious Diseases of Soldiers and Seamen. Edinburgh, Scotland, University Press, 1838

Gibbon KL: Munchausen's syndrome presenting as an acute sexual assault. Med Sci Law 38:202–205, 1998

Gorman WF: Defining malingering. J Forensic Sci 27:401–407, 1982

Griffith JL: The family systems of Munchausen syndrome by proxy. Fam Process 27:423–437, 1988

Hall DE, Eubanks L, Meyyazhagan LS, et al: Evaluation of covert video surveillance in the diagnosis of Munchausen syndrome by proxy: lessons from 41 cases. Pediatrics 105:1305–1312, 2000

Hardie TJ, Reed A: Pseudologia fantastica, factitious disorder and impostership: a deception syndrome. Med Sci Law 38:198–201, 1998

Health Insurance Portability and Accountability Act of 1996, Pub. L. No. 104-191

Janofsky JS: The Munchausen syndrome in civil forensic psychiatry. Bull Am Acad Psychiatry Law 22:489–497, 1994

Jonas JM, Pope HG: The dissimulating disorders: a single diagnostic entity? Compr Psychiatry 26:58–62, 1985

Kalisch PA, Kalisch BJ, Livesay E: The "Angel of Death": the anatomy of 1980s major news story about nursing. Nurs Forum 19:212–241, 1980

Kapfhammer HP, Rothenhauster HB, Dietrich E, et al: Artifactual disorders—between deception and self mutilation: experiences in consultation psychiatry at a university clinic (in German with English abstract). Nervenarzt 69:401–409, 1998

Kay NR, Morris-Jones H: Pain clinic management of medicolegal litigants. Injury 29:305–308, 1998

King BH, Ford CV: Pseudologia fantastica. Acta Psychiatr Scand 77:1–6, 1988

Krahn LE, Li H, O'Connor MK: Patients who strive to be ill: factitious disorder with physical symptoms. Am J Psychiatry 160:1163–1168, 2003

Kramer KK, La Piana FG, Appleton B: Ocular malingering and hysteria: diagnosis and management. Surv Ophthalmol 24:89–96, 1979

Lechner DE, Bradbury SF, Bradley LA: Detecting sincerity of effort: a summary of methods and approaches. Phys Ther 78:867–888, 1998

Lees-Haley PR: Malingering emotional distress on the SCL-90-R: toxic exposure and cancerphobia. Psychol Rep 65:1203–1208, 1989a

Lees-Haley PR: Malingering traumatic mental disorder on the Beck Depression Inventory: cancerphobia and toxic exposure. Psychol Rep 65:623–626, 1989b

Lees-Haley PR, Fox DD: MMPI subtle-obvious scales and malingering: clinical vs simulated scores. Psychol Rep 66:907–911, 1990

Libow JA: Child and adolescent illness falsification. Pediatrics 105:336–342, 2000

Libow JA: Beyond collision: active illness falsification. Child Abuse Negl 26:525–536, 2002

Lipsitt DR: The factitious patient who sues (letter). Am J Psychiatry 143:1482, 1986

Main CJ, Waddell G: Behavioral responses to examination: a reappraisal of the interpretation of "non-organic" signs. Spine 23:2367–2371, 1998

Mayou R: Medico-legal aspects of road traffic accidents. J Psychosom Res 39:789–798, 1995

McCaffrey RJ, Bellamy-Campbell R: Psychometric detection of fabricated symptoms of combat-related post-traumatic stress disorder: a systematic replication. J Clin Psychol 45:76–79, 1989

McClure RF, Davis PM, Meadow SR, et al: Epidemiology of Munchausen syndrome by proxy, non-accidental poisoning and non-accidental suffocation. Arch Dis Child 75:57–61, 1996

McFarland BH, Resnick M, Bloom JD: Ensuring continuity of care for a Munchausen patient through a public guardian. Hosp Community Psychiatry 34:65–67, 1983

Meadow R: Munchausen syndrome by proxy: the hinterland of child abuse. Lancet 2:343–345, 1977

Meadow R: Munchausen syndrome by proxy perpetrated by men. Arch Dis Child 78:210–216, 1998

Meadow R: Unnatural sudden infant death. Arch Dis Child 80:7–14, 1999

Mercer SO, Perdue JD: Munchausen syndrome by proxy: social work's role. Soc Work 38:74–81, 1993

Mohammed R, Goy JA, Walpole BG, et al: Munchausen's syndrome: a study of the casualty "black books" of Melbourne. Med J Aust 143:561–563, 1985

Munro HM, Thrusfield MV: "Battered pets" Munchausen syndrome by proxy (factitious illness by proxy). J Small Anim Pract 42:385–389, 2001

Nadelson T: False patients/real patients: a spectrum of disease presentation. Psychother Psychosom 44:175–184, 1985

Nichols GR II, Davis GJ, Corey TS: In the shadow of the Baron: sudden death due to Munchausen syndrome. Am J Emerg Med 8:216–219, 1990

Nicholson SD, Roberts GA: Patients who (need to) tell stories. Br J Hosp Med 51:546–549, 1994

Paniak C, Reynolds S, Toller-Lobe G, et al: A longitudinal study of the relationship between financial compensation and symptoms after treated mild traumatic brain injury. J Clin Exp Neuropsychol 24:187–193, 2002

Pankratz L, Lezak MD: Cerebral dysfunction in the Munchausen syndrome. Hillside J Clin Psychiatry 9:195–206, 1987

Parker PE: A case report of Munchausen syndrome with mixed psychological features. Psychosomatics 34:360–364, 1993

Phillips MR, Ward NG, Ries RK: Factitious mourning: painless patienthood. Am J Psychiatry 140:420–425, 1983

Rand DC, Feldman MD: Misdiagnosis of Munchausen syndrome by proxy, a literature review and four new cases. Harv Rev Psychiatry 7:94–101 1999

Rawling PJ: The Simulation Index: a reliability study. Brain Inj 6:381–383, 1992

Rogers R, Bagby RM, Rector N: Diagnostic legitimacy of factitious disorder with psychological symptoms. Am J Psychiatry 146:1312–1314, 1989

Rosenberg DA: Web of deceit: a literature review of Munchausen syndrome by proxy. Child Abuse Negl 11:547–563, 1987

Sacks JJ, Herndon JL, Lieg SH, et al: A cluster of unexplained deaths in a nursing home in Florida. Am J Public Health 78:806–808, 1988

Schneck JM: Pseudo-malingering. Dis Nerv Syst 23:396–398, 1962

Sheridan MS: The deceit continues: an updated literature review of Munchausen syndrome by proxy. Child Abuse Negl 27:431–451, 2003

Sigal M, Altmark D, Alfici S, et al: Ganser syndrome: a review of 15 cases. Compr Psychiatry 33:134–138, 1992

Snowden J, Solomons R, Druce H: Feigned bereavement: twelve cases. Br J Psychiatry 133:15–19, 1978

Southall DP, Plunkett MC, Banks MW, et al: Covert video recordings of life-threatening child abuse: lessons for child protection. Pediatrics 199:735–760, 1997

Sparr L, Pankratz LD: Factitious posttraumatic stress disorder. Am J Psychiatry 140:1016–1019, 1983

Stone MH: Factitious illness: psychological findings and treatment recommendations. Bull Menninger Clin 41:239–254, 1977

Sutherland AJ, Rodin GM: Factitious disorders in a general hospital setting: clinical features and a review of the literature. Psychosomatics 31:392–399, 1990

Szasz TS: Malingering: diagnosis or social condemnation? Analysis of the meaning of diagnosis in the light of some interrelations of social structure, value judgment, and the physician's role. AMA Arch Neurol Psychiatry 76:432–443, 1956

von Maurer K, Wasson KR, DeFord JW, et al: Munchausen's syndrome: a thirty year history of peregrination par excellence. South Med J 66:629–632, 1973

Wallach J: Laboratory diagnosis of factitious disorders. Arch Intern Med 154:1690–1696, 1994

Weiner H, Braiman A: The Ganser syndrome. Am J Psychiatry 111:767–773, 1955

Wetzler S, Marlowe D: "Faking bad" on the MMPI, MMPI-2, and Millon-II. Psychol Rep 67:1117–1118, 1990

Yorker BC: Hospital epidemics of factitious disorder by proxy, in The Spectrum of Factitious Disorders. Edited by Feldman MD, Eisendrath SJ. Washington, DC, American Psychiatric Press, 1996, pp 157–174

15 Eating Disorders

Michael J. Devlin, M.D.

Joel P. Jahraus, M.D.

Ilyse J. Dobrow, B.A.

ALTHOUGH FULL-SYNDROME eating disorders are relatively rarely diagnosed in medical settings, eating disorder symptoms—such as uncontrolled eating, excessive dieting, and marked body image distress—occur quite commonly. Two important trends may account, at least in part, for the upsurge in these symptoms: 1) the well-documented increase in the prevalence of overweight and obesity in the United Stated (Mokdad et al. 2001, 2003); and 2) the marked decrease in percentage of body fat of the culturally defined "ideal woman," as exemplified by Miss America pageant winners (Rubinstein and Caballero 2000). Caught between the reality of an obesity-promoting environment and an increasingly unattainable body image ideal, it is perhaps unsurprising that growing numbers of individuals, particularly women, engage in the desperate attempts to lose weight and the dysregulated eating that characterize the eating disorders.

The mortality and morbidity rates in eating disorders are considerable. Anorexia nervosa is among the most lethal of psychiatric disorders, with mortality rates of approximately 5% per decade of illness in the longest follow-up studies (Nielsen 2001). Although the lethality of bulimia nervosa is much less than that of anorexia nervosa, the purging behaviors characteristic of this disorder can lead to significant medical and dental morbidity. Binge eating, to the degree that it contributes to the onset or maintenance of obesity, may contribute to obesity-related morbidity and death (Calle et al. 1999; Kopelman 2000). But perhaps the greater costs of eating disorders are the time and energy spent on the pursuit of thinness, often to the exclusion of interpersonal, vocational, and recreational sources of satisfaction; the shame and secrecy that often accompany these illnesses; and the ultimate loss of function when the symptoms remain untreated.

Among the most puzzling of psychiatric illnesses for practitioners who regard eating as a healthy and satisfying part of life, eating disorders are also among the most difficult to treat. Yet, as summarized in this chapter, progress is being made in the conceptualization, characterization, and treatment of eating disorders.

Definitions and Clinical Features

The diagnosis and treatment of disordered eating in the medical setting are among the most poorly studied and most important areas for ongoing clinical research. To fully appreciate the spectrum of eating disorders presenting in primary care and general medical settings, it is useful to apply both a categorical and a dimensional approach. The major eating disorder syndromes, including the DSM-IV-TR diagnostic categories for eating disorders (American Psychiatric Association 2000a), are discussed in the subsections that follow. Paradoxically, the most common eating disorder, eating disorder not otherwise specified (NOS), is also the most poorly defined and studied, and the dimensional approach to assessment may be of particular use in patients with this diagnosis.

Anorexia Nervosa and Bulimia Nervosa

Anorexia Nervosa

Anorexia nervosa is first and foremost a syndrome of voluntary starvation. However, the term *voluntary* must be interpreted with caution. Although it is true that patients with anorexia nervosa in some sense choose to restrict their eating, this choice is greatly influenced by genetic vulnerabilities, cultural forces, and life events. Patients in the late stages of anorexia nervosa will often clearly describe that any sense of free will they once may have had regarding their condition has, to a great degree, vanished.

The phenomenon of unexplained starvation, or "nervous consumption," in an otherwise healthy individual was reported as long ago as the late seventeenth century (Morton 1689). Although the practice of extreme food restriction for reasons generally unrelated to body image occurred before the nineteenth century (Brumberg 1988), it was not until the 1870s that the modern syndrome of anorexia nervosa was recognized nearly simultaneously by Lasègue (1873) and Gull (1874), the latter of whom coined the term *anorexia nervosa*. This modern concept was further refined in the 1960s by psychiatrist Hilde Bruch (1973) and others, who recognized low self-esteem and body image distortion as core features of the disorder.

In keeping with earlier conceptions, the current definition of anorexia nervosa is centered on the behavioral feature of starvation. To be diagnosed with anorexia nervosa, patients must manifest weight loss, or the absence of expected weight gain, leading to a state of significant undernourishment, as reflected by a weight markedly (i.e., at least 15%) lower than expected for gender and height. However, to meet modern (DSM-IV-TR) criteria for anorexia nervosa, an individual must manifest the more recently identified psychological features. The diagnosis requires an overconcern with weight and shape, which may or may not take the form of an actual misperception of body fatness but must reflect an overinvestment in thinness as a central feature of one's self-worth. In addition, amenorrhea is a requirement for postmenarchal women.

Although patients with anorexia nervosa often view their illness as that which makes them unique or special, there is a surprising uniformity in the way these patients present, and there are a number of associated features that occur quite predictably. In addition to severely restricting their intake of food, many individuals with anorexia nervosa are also compulsive exercisers. Some anorexic patients engage in strict dieting without any binge eating or purging (restricting type), whereas others periodically engage in purging (e.g., vomiting, laxative abuse) or uncontrolled binge eating (binge-eating/purging type). Patients with anorexia nervosa are often rigid and perfectionistic, not only in their adherence to restrictive eating and compulsive exercise practices but also in other areas of life. Interestingly, the narrowing of interests, increasing focus on food, and peculiar food-related rituals (toying with food, consumption of unusual food combinations, possessiveness toward food) were also observed in the Minnesota semistarvation study subjects. These subjects were male World War II conscientious objectors who volunteered to participate in a study of the physiological and psychological effects of starvation, eventually losing 25% of their body weight (Franklin et al. 1948). The fact that these men, who had no prior histories of eating disorders, exhibited behaviors so reminiscent of those seen in anorexia nervosa suggests the degree to which these features of the illness are driven by the physiological effects of starvation.

Bulimia Nervosa

The other major eating disorder currently defined in DSM-IV-TR is bulimia nervosa, popularly known as the binge-purge syndrome. This syndrome, first described as a variant of anorexia nervosa (Russell 1979) and later applied to individuals of normal weight, comprises regular uncontrolled consumption of objectively large amounts of food (binge eating), regular use of unhealthy compensatory methods intended to undo the effects of eating, and preoccupation with weight and/or shape as a central component of self-worth. Eating binges typically consist of more than 2,000 kcal and, contrary to popular belief, are not primarily composed of carbohydrate (Walsh et al. 1989). Compensatory behaviors include purging methods (i.e., elimination of food and fluids from the body by the use of vomiting, laxatives, diuretics, or enemas) and nonpurging methods (such as fasting or excessive exercise) for preventing weight gain. Patients with diabetes mellitus who have bulimia nervosa may attempt to purge by reducing or omitting their insulin dosage to promote glycosuria, thereby eliminating calories from the body. Although most individuals who present for treatment for bulimia nervosa are of normal weight, the diagnosis can also be made in overweight or obese individuals. Under the current diagnostic system, individuals who simultaneously meet criteria for anorexia nervosa and bulimia nervosa are diagnosed as having anorexia nervosa, binge-eating/purging type. In fact, the progression from anorexia nervosa to bulimia nervosa is quite common, occurring in about one-half of patients with restricting anorexia nervosa (Bulik et al. 1997). Normal-weight patients with bulimia nervosa progress to anorexia nervosa much less frequently.

Psychiatric Comorbidity of Anorexia Nervosa and Bulimia Nervosa

Individuals with anorexia nervosa and bulimia nervosa often manifest comorbid symptoms of depression and anxiety. Many studies suggest that, at least in clinical samples, a majority or significant minority of individuals with eating disorders also have a lifetime diagnosis of affective or anxiety disorder (Mitchell et al. 1991). Among affective disorders, major depressive disorder occurs most frequently. Among anxiety disorders, obsessive-compulsive disorder (OCD) has been of particular interest because eating- and exercise-related practices, particularly in individuals with anorexia nervosa, may include the repetitive, ritualized behaviors characteristic of OCD. Although in some cases anxiety or depressive symptoms may be secondary to disordered eating, it is likely that shared etiological factors largely account for the observed comorbidity (Bulik 2002). In any case, a diagnosis of depression or anxiety disorder, particularly in an individual at risk for an eating disorder (i.e., adolescent and young adult women) should raise the clinician's level of suspicion that an eating disorder may also be present. In addition, the comorbid diagnosis must of course be taken into account in devising the treatment plan. In general, treatment can proceed simultaneously with the emphasis, for individuals with anorexia nervosa, on weight restoration as a precondition for successful treatment of comorbid conditions.

The relationship between eating disorders and substance use disorders is of great theoretical as well as practical interest, because the idea of "food addiction" suggests the possibility of common underlying pathophysiological mechanisms (Del Parigi et al. 2003). It is certainly the case that eating and substance abuse disorders co-occur at a rate significantly higher than that explainable by chance (Holderness et al. 1994). However, in contrast to the data on the overlap between eating, affective, and anxiety disorders, the available data on familial transmission of eating and substance abuse disorders fail to support the existence of common genetic risk factors (Wilson 2002). Nonetheless, the experience of patients with eating disorders, and even the terminology patients use (e.g., "compulsive" exercise, "going on a binge") can often mimic the argot of substance abuse. Of course, the one major difference is that, to the degree that food is considered the abused substance, abstinence is not a therapeutic option. For patients with comorbid eating and substance use disorders, it is recommended that the substance abuse problem be prioritized. For patients in whom substance abuse is not severe, treatment for the two disorders may proceed simultaneously (Wilson 2002). Substance use disorders may significantly affect the outcome of eating disorders. In a recent large-scale study, severity of alcohol use disorder was a significant predictor of death in anorexia nervosa, with a significant minority of patients apparently developing alcoholism subsequent to the onset of their eating disorder. This finding suggests that patients with eating disorders should be carefully assessed over time for the emergence or worsening of a substance use disorder (Keel et al. 2003).

Eating Disorders and Obesity

Although obesity is not, in and of itself, an eating disorder (Devlin et al. 2000), obese individuals may have eating disorders such as binge-eating disorder (BED) and night-eating syndrome (Stunkard and Allison 2003). BED (uncontrolled binge eating in the absence of regular compensatory behavior) has been a particular focus of research since it was identified in Appendix B of DSM-IV (American Psychiatric Association 1994) as a criteria set requiring further study. Although the status of BED is uncertain (Devlin et al. 2003), the phenomenon of binge eating among the obese has been clearly identified, and its associated features have been studied (Dingemans et al. 2002). In particular, binge eating in the obese has been found to be associated with higher rates of major medical disorders, greater health dissatisfaction, and a higher lifetime prevalence of depression, panic, phobias, and alcohol dependence (Bulik et al. 2002).

Night-eating syndrome—characterized by morning anorexia, evening hyperphagia, and insomnia—has been much less thoroughly studied, but preliminary studies suggest that it has distinct behavioral/psychological (Gluck et al. 2001) and physiological (Birketvedt et al. 1999) features. Nocturnal sleep-related eating disorders among the obese represent a similar phenomenon but are often characterized by partial or complete amnesia for the nighttime eating episode and by associated sleep disorders (Schenk and Mahowald 1994). Although the best methods for sequencing or combining treatments for obesity and eating disorders have not yet been fully worked out, approaches for simultaneously treating eating disorders and obesity have been described (Devlin 2001).

Atypical Eating Disorders

A final category of eating disorders in DSM-IV-TR is eating disorder NOS, defined as a clinically significant eating disorder that does not meet diagnostic criteria for any defined eating disorder diagnosis. Examples are 1) regular occurrence of subjective binge episodes (i.e., uncontrolled consumption of amounts of food not deemed large) followed by purging, 2) strict dieting and weight loss without amenorrhea, or 3) continuous uncontrolled snacking throughout the day with no discrete binge episodes. In addition, patients with behaviors typical of eating disorders, such as food avoidance or vomiting, but who deny body image concern—attributing their symptoms instead to somatic symptoms like bloating, nausea, intolerable fullness, or extreme discomfort after eating—may be diagnosed as having eating disorder NOS once medical etiologies have been ruled out. Community-based studies have typically found that these atypical eating disorders are more common than anorexia nervosa and bulimia nervosa. Nonetheless, they have received relatively little attention in the literature and are poorly understood at this point. Although much of the literature is based on samples seen in eating disorder clinics that are geared toward treating patients with full-blown anorexia nervosa and bulimia nervosa, individuals seen in the medical setting who are not specifically presenting for treatment of an eating disorder may be particularly likely to manifest eating disorder NOS.

Given this state of affairs, it is perhaps useful to consider a transdiagnostic or dimensional approach to the eating disorders (Fairburn et al. 2003). One dimension of the patient's condition is *nutritional*, with the spectrum ranging from undernourished to severely obese. A second dimension is *behavioral*, with behaviors of interest including binge eating, nighttime eating, uncontrolled eating of some other variety, extreme dieting, purging, and so forth. A third dimension is *psychological*. This dimension includes body image distress—perhaps the most unifying feature of individuals with eating disorders, be they emaciated, of normal weight, or obese—and psychiatric comorbidity. In addition to assessing the psychological dimension, it is important to assess the patient's *motivation for change*. In contrast to anorexia nervosa, which is often embraced by patients as a lifestyle choice that they are ambivalent about relinquishing, patients with bulimia nervosa are generally more motivated to break the binge–purge cycle, although they may be less enthusiastic about confronting the dieting and body obsession that underlie the behavior. Obese patients with eating disorders may be highly motivated to lose weight but may have unrealistic expectations of thinness that continually undermine their weight-control attempts. A consideration of the various dimensions of a given patient's eating disorder syndrome and the particular history of the patient (e.g., chronicity, rapidity of change, and functional impairment) may assist the practitioner in the difficult task of applying findings from clinical studies of typical eating disorders to the atypical eating disorders more commonly observed in the medical setting.

Eating Disorders in Children

Eating disorders in children and adolescents represent a particular concern because, if not diagnosed and treated, they may have life-long psychological and medical consequences (see also Chapter 34, "Pediatrics"). Disordered eating patterns occurring before puberty include food avoidance emotional disorder, selective eating, pervasive

refusal syndrome, functional dysphagia, and full-syndrome anorexia nervosa (Lask and Bryant-Waugh 1997; Rosen 2003). *Food avoidance emotional disorder* is similar to but less severe than anorexia nervosa and carries a better prognosis. *Selective eating* is diagnosed in children who eat only a small number of foods but whose growth and development are generally normal. *Pervasive refusal syndrome* is a severe disorder in which refusal to eat is accompanied by refusal to function in other spheres (e.g., walking, talking, self-care) and is probably not best viewed as an eating disorder. Children with *functional dysphagia* avoid food due to a fear of swallowing, choking, or vomiting for which no organic etiology can be identified. Bulimia nervosa is thought to occur quite rarely before puberty. Problems of food refusal, selective eating, phobias, failure to thrive, pica, and rumination in children are discussed in detail in Chapter 34, "Pediatrics." However, it is notable that symptoms such as eating conflicts, struggles with food, and unpleasant meals in early childhood have been found to be associated with the later development of eating disorders (Kotler et al. 2001) and therefore should be followed closely.

As reviewed in a recent position paper from the Society for Adolescent Medicine (Rome et al. 2003), dieting among school-age girls is increasingly common, and prevention and screening for eating disorders may avert the progression from pathological dieting to clinically significant eating disorders. Thus, the identification of a significant eating disorder symptom, even in the absence of a formal diagnosis, should trigger some form of intervention to address the problem rather than a "wait-and-see" approach, which may allow the problem to become more entrenched. Pathological dieting is in some cases difficult to differentiate from normative dieting, but extreme distress about weight or shape, rapid weight loss, frequent weight or size checking, rigid adherence to dietary or exercise regimens, and use of unhealthy dietary practices are all worrisome signs. From a prevention standpoint, eating disorder NOS should probably be the most commonly diagnosed eating disorder in this group.

Feeding Disorders of Infancy or Early Childhood

Quite distinct from the eating disorders described in the preceding subsections are the feeding disorders seen in infants and children, including pica, rumination disorder, and feeding disorder of infancy or early childhood. *Pica* refers to the consumption of nonnutritive substances such as hair, dirt, pebbles, or clay, sometimes but not always occurring in individuals with mental retardation, but meriting a separate diagnosis only if it is sufficiently severe to warrant independent clinical attention. Pica may be associated with poisoning (e.g., from lead paint) or mechanical obstruction. *Rumination* refers to the regurgitation, rechewing, and reswallowing of ingested food. Although most commonly seen in infants, rumination may also be seen in older children with mental retardation. Interestingly, a small proportion of adolescent and adult patients with anorexia nervosa and bulimia nervosa report rumination.

Finally, feeding disorder of infancy or early childhood is usually diagnosed in the first year of life but sometimes in children up to 3 years of age, for whom food intake is inadequate to support normal growth and development. As recently reviewed by Rudolph and Link (2002), the early recognition of feeding problems and diagnostic workup to exclude gastrointestinal, metabolic, sensory, or other general medical etiologies can lead to more appropriate management of affected children and their families.

Epidemiology

A number of researchers have attempted to establish incidence and prevalence rates for anorexia nervosa, bulimia nervosa, and (to a lesser extent) BED, and findings have been well summarized in recent reviews (Fairburn and Harrison 2003; Nielsen 2001). Anorexia nervosa is thought to have a prevalence of approximately 0.7% among teenage girls and to be approximately one-tenth as common in males as in females. Incidence estimates in Western countries are roughly 10 females and 1 male per 100,000 population per year, with the risk of new onset greatest in white adolescents. It has been suggested, although it has not yet been conclusively proved, that anorexia nervosa has become a more common illness in recent years. Alternative explanations for an apparent increase include greater recognition among patients and clinicians and increased help seeking.

Bulimia nervosa is a more prevalent illness than anorexia nervosa, with a prevalence of 1%–2% in teenage and young adult women. Incidence is roughly 15 females and 0.5 male per 100,000 population per year. Like anorexia nervosa, bulimia nervosa is much less common in men than in women and most often affects Western Caucasian adolescents and young adults. Evidence of an increase in cases of bulimia nervosa over the past few decades is considerably stronger than evidence of an increase in anorexia nervosa. Some research has suggested that certain segments of the population, such as elite athletes (Smolak et al. 2000) and dancers (Dotti et al. 2002), are at particular risk for developing symptoms of bulimia nervosa or anorexia nervosa.

There have been few studies of the epidemiology of BED. The limited data that have been collected suggest that BED has a lifetime prevalence similar to that of bulimia nervosa. Roughly 5%–10% of those seeking treatment for obesity have BED. Unlike anorexia nervosa and bulimia nervosa, approximately a quarter of those with BED are male, and most patients with BED present with the illness in their 40s.

In establishing epidemiological data for eating disorders, it is important to consider not only individuals who meet diagnostic criteria for anorexia nervosa, bulimia nervosa, and BED but also the large numbers of individuals who are diagnosed with eating disorder NOS or who do not fulfill all DSM-IV-TR criteria for an eating disorder but nonetheless have serious eating pathology. In terms of eating disorder NOS, Fairburn and Harrison (2003) cited three community-based case series studies that all found eating disorder NOS to be a more common diagnosis than anorexia nervosa or bulimia nervosa. In addition, studies of subsyndromal anorexia nervosa, bulimia nervosa, and BED indicate that these subthreshold diagnoses are strikingly similar to their diagnostic counterparts in terms of distress and functional impairment. Therefore, to make a truly accurate assessment of the degree of eating pathology in the general population, epidemiologists must consider both eating disorder NOS and subthreshold eating disorders in addition to anorexia nervosa, bulimia nervosa, and BED.

Course and Outcome

Studies of the long-term course of anorexia nervosa suggest that there is no one typical outcome. Rather, the illness tends to require long-term treatment, with some patients achieving full recovery, others experiencing a longer course of partially remitted or unremitted illness, and some dying as a direct or indirect result of the illness (Pike 1998). Mortality rates are as high as 5% per decade of illness in the longest follow-up studies (Nielsen 2001); of surviving patients, fewer than half recover fully, one-third recover partially, and one-fifth remain chronically ill (Steinhausen 2002). The outcome of patients treated as adolescents appears to be more favorable (Strober et al. 1997), underscoring the importance of early intervention or, ideally, prevention. Bulimia nervosa generally has a more favorable course than anorexia nervosa. However, long-term follow-up studies suggest that 10 years after presentation, nearly one-third of patients continue to binge and purge regularly (Keel et al. 1999). The outcome of eating disorder NOS is less well defined. However, it is clear that these atypical eating disorders often represent partial recovery from full-syndrome eating disorders or evolve into fully developed anorexia nervosa and bulimia nervosa (Fairburn and Harrison 2003); careful diagnosis and aggressive treatment are therefore warranted. Several studies have identified specific historical and medical factors that predict good versus poor outcome in eating disorders (Table 15–1).

Assessment and Diagnosis

Assessment

The assessment of patients with symptoms suggestive of eating disorders presents several challenges. The clinical presentation may be confusing in that it may be difficult to determine whether behaviors such as food restriction or vomiting are driven by psychological or somatic distress, and the medical history is often vague and nonspecific. Moreover, as summarized above under "Psychiatric Comorbidity of Anorexia Nervosa and Bulimia Nervosa," comorbid psychiatric conditions frequently occur and may further complicate the presentation. It is often difficult to ascertain whether the comorbid psychiatric illness

is causally related to the eating disorder or is more indirectly involved in the manifestation of the eating disorder. As an illustration of the latter, an individual with comorbid social phobia may experience a flare-up of eating disorder symptoms in social situations.

Probably the single most important component of the workup for eating disorders is a thorough history, covering the nutritional, behavioral, psychological, and motivational features discussed above under "Atypical Eating Disorders." The history should include past and recent patterns of eating, abnormal weight control behavior, associated beliefs and attitudes, timing of emergence of issues with eating and weight, lifetime weight course, and attitudes toward body image. Although obesity and extreme emaciation are readily apparent, the behaviors associated with these bodily states are not. Normal-weight patients with eating disorders may appear entirely healthy, and patients with anorexia nervosa may attempt to persuade the clinician that they are "naturally thin." Patients with eating disorders may hide their symptoms for several reasons. Behaviors such as binge eating and purging are often experienced by patients as shameful or disgusting. Patients with anorexia nervosa often feel that they must

TABLE 15–1. Prognostic factors in eating disorders

Factors predicting negative outcome	Factors predicting favorable outcome
Anorexia nervosa	
History of premorbid development or clinical abnormalities	Early age at onset
Binge eating and/or purging	Hospitalization for an affective disorder before baseline assessment
Long duration of illness	Short interval between symptom onset and beginning of treatment
Weight ≤60% ideal body weight or body mass index <13 kg/m^2	Conflict-free child-parent relationships
High serum uric acid level	Histrionic personality traits
High serum creatinine level	
Low serum albumin level	
Obsessive-compulsive personality traits	
Comorbid affective disorder	
Comorbid substance abuse	
Severity of alcohol use disorder during follow-up	
Bulimia nervosa	
Poor pretreatment global functioning	Younger age
Premorbid parental obesity	Shorter duration of symptoms
History of substance abuse	Less severe symptoms
History of obesity	Absence of concurrent disruptive pathology
Comorbid major depression	Strong motivation for treatment
High self-directedness	
Comorbid personality disorders (particularly borderline)	
Posttreatment food restriction	

Source. Adapted from Bulik et al. 1998; Hebebrand et al. 1997; D.B. Herzog et al. 2000; W. Herzog et al. 1997; Keel et al. 2003; Richards et al. 2000; Steinhausen 2002.

hide their restrictive dieting and compulsive exercise to avoid being prevented from continuing them. Obese patients with eating disorders may be particularly likely to minimize contact with health care providers because they fear being blamed or because they blame themselves for their obesity. Bearing this in mind, clinicians should employ a nonjudgmental assessment style that recognizes the patient's ambivalence and engages the patient in a medically informed discussion of the nature of the illness and the options for treatment. A useful approach to the assessment of eating disorder symptoms in a primary care setting was described by Kreipe and Yussman (2003).

Of particular importance to psychosomatic medicine specialists is the medical evaluation of patients with eating disorders. When the patient displays behaviors and attitudes characteristic of eating disorders (e.g., a classic binge–purge pattern, an unhealthy and excessive dieting regimen, or a lack of concern about weight loss or abnormal eating behaviors), the workup to establish a diagnosis of an eating disorder need not be exhaustive in ruling out primary organic disorders. No laboratory testing is required to make the diagnosis of an eating disorder unless the historical or physical evidence suggests the possibility of an organic etiology. However, for patients with an atypical presentation or those in whom an eating disorder is essentially a diagnosis of exclusion, the workup should be more extensive and the level of suspicion for an underlying organic etiology should remain high. In patients known to have an eating disorder, physical examination and laboratory testing are key in evaluating any medical complications (see below) or comorbid medical illnesses and in guiding treatment.

When the medical provider is seeing the patient for the first time, he or she must, in collaboration with the mental health provider, determine the level of care that is needed and the urgency of intervention. As outlined in the American Psychiatric Association (2000b) "Practice Guideline for the Treatment of Patients With Eating Disorders," the physical assessment of the patient should include 1) a complete physical examination, with attention to evidence of dehydration, acrocyanosis, lanugo, salivary gland enlargement, and scarring on the dorsum of the hands (Russell's sign); 2) vital signs with orthostatic determination of blood pressure and pulse; 3) assessment of physical and sexual growth and development, including height and weight (for pediatric patients a review of the patient's growth chart may be helpful); and 4) dental examination.

Laboratory evaluation should be individualized for the particular patient. In accordance with the American Psychiatric Association (2000b) "Practice Guideline for the Treatment of Patients With Eating Disorders," the routine workup should include serum electrolytes, blood urea nitrogen and creatinine, liver enzymes, serum albumin, thyroid function tests, complete blood cell count, and urinalysis. Severely malnourished patients should receive additional blood chemistry assessments—including calcium, magnesium, and phosphate levels—and an electrocardiogram. Patients who are chronically underweight should be assessed for osteopenia and osteoporosis using dual-energy X-ray absorptiometry, and serum estradiol (or testosterone in males) may be assessed. Other tests that are not performed routinely but may be indicated in particular clinical situations include serum amylase, luteinizing hormone (LH) and follicle-stimulating hormone (FSH) levels; computed tomography or magnetic resonance imaging (MRI) of the brain; and screening stool for blood. Although elevated serum amylase concentration is a frequent concomitant of vomiting, this test is not sufficiently sensitive or specific to serve as a useful screening tool for unreported vomiting (Walsh et al. 1990).

Large-scale screening for eating disorders may be a priority in some settings, particularly those in which the prevalence is known to be relatively high, such as high school or university health services. Although a variety of self-report and interview-based assessment tools are frequently used in research settings, one well-established instrument that can be recommended for its brevity and ease of use is the Eating Attitudes Test (EAT-26), originally developed to assess attitudes and behaviors characteristic of anorexia nervosa and also useful in detecting bulimia nervosa (Garner et al. 1982). Another more recently developed screening tool is the SCOFF, a five-item scale that, in initial studies, has good sensitivity and specificity for detecting anorexia nervosa and bulimia nervosa (Morgan et al. 1999). The SCOFF questions are 1) Do you make yourself **S**ick because you feel uncomfortably full?; 2) Do you worry you have lost **C**ontrol over how much you eat?; 3) Have you recently lost more than **O**ne stone (14 lb) in a 3-month period?; 4) Do you believe yourself to be **F**at when others believe you are too thin?; and 5) Would you say **F**ood dominates your life?

Differential Diagnosis

Hyperphagia, hypophagia, and altered eating patterns occur as features of a variety of medical and psychiatric illnesses and do not, in and of themselves, constitute formal eating disorders according to the standard of DSM-IV-TR. Table 15–2 lists some medical and psychiatric illnesses to consider in the differential diagnosis of an eating disorder. Two conditions of particular interest are Prader-Willi syndrome and Kleine-Levin syndrome.

TABLE 15–2.   Medical and psychiatric differential diagnosis of eating disorders

System	Diagnosis
Endocrine	Diabetes mellitus, hyperthyroidism, Addison's disease, Sheehan's syndrome (postpartum pituitary necrosis), panhypopituitarism
Gastrointestinal	Malabsorption, pancreatitis, cystic fibrosis, inflammatory bowel disease, peptic ulcer disease, superior mesenteric artery syndrome, Zenker's diverticulum, dysmotility disorders
Neurologic	Psychomotor or limbic seizures, degenerative neurological conditions (Pick's disease, Alzheimer's disease, Huntington's disease, Parkinson's disease), hypothalamic or diencephalic tumor
Other medical	Malignancies (especially lymphoma and gastrointestinal cancers), collagen vascular disorders, chronic infections (especially tuberculosis, human immunodeficiency virus, fungal disease), parasitic infections, chronic renal failure, drug-induced appetite/weight change (e.g., corticosteroids, novel antipsychotics)
Psychiatric	Body dysmorphic disorder, melancholic major depression, atypical depression, obsessive-compulsive disorder, substance use disorder, dementia, factitious disorder, somatization disorder, psychotic disorder

Prader-Willi syndrome (PWS) is a multisystem disorder characterized by neonatal hypotonia, later obesity, hyperphagia, hypogonadotropic hypogonadism, and mental retardation. It has recently been reported that, in contrast to most obese individuals, those with PWS have markedly elevated levels of ghrelin, an enteric hormone that stimulates growth hormone secretion and food intake (Haqq et al. 2003). PWS occurs sporadically, as a result of either microdeletion of chromosome 15p (70%) or maternal disomy of chromosome 15 (30%). Care of individuals with PWS can be challenging, primarily due to hyperphagia, food seeking and obesity, and conduct disorder, particularly manifested as tantrums or oppositional behavior (Couper 1999).

Kleine-Levin syndrome is a rare self-limited disorder of unknown origin that usually affects adolescent males and is characterized by episodic hypersomnia, increased appetite, and behavioral and psychiatric disturbances. Individuals typically function normally between episodes (Papacostas and Hadjivasilis 2000).

The presence of body image disturbance or intentional weight manipulation is usually quite useful in differentiating true eating disorders from other eating-related disorders. In the absence of these features, the diagnosis of an eating disorder should be regarded as provisional, and medical disorders such as those listed in Table 15–2 should be thoroughly considered in the differential diagnosis.

Etiology and Risk Factors

As research on the etiology of eating disorders has progressed, it has become clear that the onset of an eating disorder results from a confluence of factors: sociocultural, biological, and genetic. Most of what is currently known about the etiology of eating disorders focuses on anorexia nervosa and bulimia nervosa. Risk factors for BED may overlap with—but are not the same as—those for anorexia

nervosa and bulimia nervosa and are considered briefly below under "Etiology of Binge-Eating Disorder."

Culture

Although eating disorders were once thought to affect mainly upper-class, Western women from majority cultures, they are increasingly prevalent among individuals from lower socioeconomic sectors and minority ethnic groups, both in the United States and in other countries (Gard and Freeman 1996; Striegel-Moore 1997). The one factor that seems to unite all the cultures in which eating disorders are prevalent is a relative abundance of food. In such cultures, thinness becomes an ideal, presented by the media as a quality for which everyone, particularly women, should strive.

Clearly, however, not everyone who lives in a culture of abundance develops an eating disorder. As Polivy and Herman (2002) explain, the "idealization of thinness" in cultures of abundance may trigger for some an intense focus on their body shape and weight. This intense focus, in turn, may precipitate the development of eating disorder pathology. Thus, a culture of abundance (and the thin ideal that comes with that culture) may be a necessary, but not sufficient, precursor to the development of eating disorders.

Some have suggested that the process of cultural change may be associated with increased vulnerability to eating disorders, especially as developing cultures embrace the modern Western body ideal of thinness. Such change may occur across time within a given society or on an individual level (Miller and Pumariega 2001).

Family and Individual Environment

Along with cultural pressures toward thinness, familial and peer pressures to uphold the thin ideal have been cited as potential contributors to eating disorder pathology (Branch and Eurman 1980; Levine et al. 1994; Shisslak et al. 1998; Stice 1998; Wertheim et al. 1997). Furthermore, it has been argued that certain types of familial environments—namely, those in which parents are overly critical, hostile, and coercive and are overly enmeshed in their children's lives (e.g., Haworth-Hoeppner 2000; Minuchin et al. 1978)—may more readily breed eating disorder behaviors. However, none of these assertions concerning the role of peers and family in the development of eating disorders have been proved conclusively, and therefore further study is necessary (Stice 2002). A predisposition to eating disorders has also been noted among individuals who participate in certain activities that promote thinness, such as ballet dancing, modeling, and some sports that emphasize weight and body shape (Kann et al. 2000). Although a history of sexual abuse or trauma appears to be a risk factor for developing eating problems (Everill and Waller 1995; Kendler et al. 2000; Kent and Waller 2000), there is currently not enough consistent evidence to support such a history as a specific risk factor for eating disorders (Stice 2002).

Genetics

Although the research discussed above under "Culture" implicates culture as an important risk factor for the development of eating disorders, it is clear that individual vulnerabilities play a substantial role. Specifically, such traits as perfectionism, impulsivity, negative affect, and low self-esteem have all been cited as potential risk factors (Fairburn et al. 1999; Polivy and Herman 2002; Stice 2002) and may account for the fact that only a minority of young women in a high-risk cultural environment actually develop clinical eating disorders. In addition, a vulnerability to obesity appears to increase risk for bulimia nervosa and BED (Fairburn et al. 1997, 1998), possibly by promoting dieting. Many such trait vulnerabilities may be largely genetically determined, and the genetics of eating disorders is a rapidly developing area of interest (Collier 2002).

Results of some genetic studies have suggested that anorexia nervosa, bulimia nervosa, and atypical eating disorders aggregate in families, and it appears that at least some of the risk factors are common to both anorexia nervosa and bulimia nervosa. In other words, relatives of persons with an eating disorder are significantly more likely than members of the general population to develop either the same or an alternative eating disorder. Twin studies have also suggested that genetic factors contribute substantially to the development of eating disorders (Bulik et

al. 2000). In light of the evidence supporting the importance of genetic risk factors for eating disorders, the challenge of identifying biological abnormalities that reflect the expression of the particular genes associated with eating disorders has become an important part of the research agenda. A reported association between a polymorphism in the promoter region of the serotonin$_{2A}$ receptor gene and risk for anorexia nervosa has not been consistently confirmed, and the current status of this research is uncertain (Collier 2002). In addition, a report (Branson et al. 2003) of an association between BED and a mutation in the melanocortin$_4$ receptor gene, a candidate gene for appetite and weight regulation, represents a potentially important clue to the means by which genetic risk contributes to binge eating. A recent study, however, failed to replicate this finding (Helebrand et al. 2004). Finally, a polymorphism in the gene for agouti-related peptide, a melanocortin receptor inverse agonist, has also been reported to be associated with anorexia nervosa (Adan et al. 2003). Clearly, the clarification of the particular genetic risks for eating disorders awaits further study and replication.

Neurotransmitters, Neuropeptides, and Neuroanatomy

A great deal of research has focused on abnormalities in the functioning of neurotransmitters, particularly serotonin, in the development and maintenance of eating pathology (Kaye and Strober 1999). A confluence of evidence suggests that serotonergic activity is increased in women who have recovered from anorexia nervosa and bulimia nervosa but is decreased in underweight individuals with anorexia nervosa and actively symptomatic women with bulimia nervosa. These findings are consistent with the idea that at baseline these patients are characterized by perfectionism and behavioral overcontrol, but that when symptomatic, they may be more impulsive and undercontrolled (Kaye 2002).

More recently, researchers have been interested in the role of appetite- and weight-regulating peptides, including those that stimulate appetite (such as neuropeptide Y, peptide YY, and galanin) and those that reduce appetite (such as leptin and corticotropin-releasing hormone). Most, but not all, of the reported abnormalities normalize after recovery, suggesting that they may reflect the operation of physiological mechanisms triggered by malnutrition or weight loss. However, increased cerebrospinal fluid concentrations of peptide YY in women who have recovered from bulimia nervosa and reduced cerebrospinal fluid concentrations of galanin in women with anorexia nervosa who have had long-term weight restoration may represent trait abnormalities rather than transient states resulting from eating disorder symptoms. The role of these peptides in the etiology of eating disorders requires further study (Kaye 2002).

One relatively new avenue of research into the biological underpinnings of eating disorders is brain imaging, recently reviewed by Chowdhury and Lask (2001). Computed tomographic and MRI studies have consistently detected ventricular enlargement and diffuse atrophy in underweight patients with anorexia nervosa. Most reported abnormalities appear to reverse with weight restoration, suggesting that they represent secondary effects of malnutrition, although one study reported gray matter volume reduction that persisted even after weight regain (Lambe et al. 1997). Although it is unlikely to be etiological, this persistent abnormality may reflect the effect of long-term malnutrition on the brain and may be related to the high rate of relapse in recovered anorexia nervosa patients.

Functional imaging studies have not yet provided a consistent picture of the relationship between abnormal functioning in particular brain regions and eating disorder symptoms, but provocative findings are beginning to emerge. For example, one recent study of early-onset anorexia nervosa in children and adolescents used single photon emission computed tomography to assess regional cerebral blood flow. The researchers found that most patients in the study had abnormally low cerebral blood flow, predominantly affecting the temporal lobe. The authors concluded that these abnormalities may affect limbic-system function and may be associated with eating disorder psychopathology in these patients (Chowdhury et al. 2003).

Etiology of Binge-Eating Disorder

It should be noted that risk factors for BED may differ in degree and kind from those for anorexia nervosa and bulimia nervosa. A case–control community study found that risk factors for the development of BED were less numerous and weaker than those for anorexia nervosa and bulimia nervosa. Specific risk factors for BED include parental depression, vulnerability to obesity, and repeated exposure to negative comments about shape, weight, and eating (Fairburn et al. 1998). Genetic and environmental factors appear to interact in determining whether an individual progresses toward bulimia nervosa or BED. Genetic risk factors for binge eating and bulimia nervosa may be similar, whereas nonshared environment may be important in influencing the risk for bulimia nervosa once binge eating is initiated (Wade et al. 2000).

Medical Complications

The pathological processes associated with eating disorders are multisystemic in nature and result from the altered eating and compensatory behaviors that characterize these disorders. Medical morbidity in eating disorders results from severe restriction with extensive weight loss; self-induced vomiting; use of laxatives, diuretics, or appetite suppressants; or binge eating with excessive weight gain. These symptoms and the resultant pathological processes may occur singly, as in patients with restricting anorexia nervosa or normal-weight bulimia nervosa, or may co-occur, as in patients with anorexia nervosa purging subtype or eating disorder NOS. It is important to note that individuals with normal or above-normal body weight who lose an excessive amount of weight may manifest similar changes in medical status as those who start at normal or low body weight and lose even more. Eating-disorder symptoms and their effects on medical status are summarized in Table 15–3. Medical morbidity related to obesity has been extensively reviewed elsewhere (Pi-Sunyer 2002) and is beyond the scope of this chapter.

System-Focused Review of Medical Complications

Metabolic/Endocrine

The primary pathophysiological response to starvation is reduced energy expenditure as a physiological adaptation (Dulloo and Jacquet 1998) (see also Chapter 23, "Endocrine and Metabolic Disorders"). This reduction in energy expenditure has been clearly demonstrated in anorexia nervosa. Underlying the reduced metabolic rate is a change in thyroid hormone synthesis characterized by normal thyroid-stimulating hormone level, low or normal thyroxine (T_4) concentration, low or normal levels of triiodothyronine (T_3), and elevated concentration of reverse T_3—a pattern known as the euthyroid sick syndrome. The concept of bulimia nervosa and BED as states of intermittent starvation is controversial, and the data on energy expenditure in these conditions are inconsistent (de Zwaan et al. 2002). The typical endocrine features of starvation (increased cortisol and growth hormone levels; decreased estrogen, LH, and FSH levels in women; decreased testosterone level in men) are also seen in anorexia nervosa and resolve with weight restoration (Devlin and Walsh 1988).

Starvation is also associated with a reduction in noradrenergic activity in the central and peripheral nervous systems of patients with eating disorders. This reduction can

TABLE 15–3. Eating disorder symptoms and medical effects

Symptom	Medical effect
Restrictive eating	Cognitive dysfunction, fatigue, cold intolerance, constipation, dizziness, hypoglycemia, acrocyanosis, orthostatic pulse and blood pressure, edema, amenorrhea
Vomiting	Dehydration, metabolic alkalosis, hypokalemia, arrhythmias, esophagitis/gastritis, esophageal tears, dental caries, parotid/submandibular gland hypertrophy, gastroesophageal reflux disease, pharyngitis
Binge eating/overeating (with increasing weight)	Obesity, dyslipidemia, hypertension, type 2 diabetes, coronary artery disease, stroke, gallbladder disease, osteoarthritis, sleep apnea, respiratory disorders
Laxative abuse	Cathartic colon, dehydration, hypokalemia, metabolic acidosis or mild metabolic alkalosis
Diuretic abuse	Dehydration, electrolyte imbalance (hypokalemia and hypomagnesemia)
Appetite-suppressant abuse	Hypertension, tremor, arrhythmias
Ipecac abuse	Generalized myopathy, cardiomyopathy
Compulsive exercise	Bradycardia, overuse syndrome, stress fractures
Water loading	Hyponatremia, headache, nausea, dizziness, seizure

lead to hypotension, bradycardia, hypothermia, and depression (Pirke 1996). It is not uncommon for body temperature to drop to 95°F (35°C) or even lower with continued weight loss, and marked bradycardia is common in underweight patients and in those who exercise extensively. Altered autonomic control of heart rate and blood pressure appears to return to normal with refeeding and resolution of eating disorder–related symptoms (Rechlin et al. 1998).

Other metabolic concomitants of starvation include low serum albumin and high serum uric acid levels, both poor prognostic indicators in anorexia nervosa (W. Herzog et al. 1997). Hypoglycemia is often seen in underweight patients with anorexia nervosa (Bhanji and Mattingly 1988) and sometimes in normal-weight patients with bulimia nervosa (Devlin et al. 1990); symptomatic hypoglycemia is uncommon, but there are case reports of coma and death attributed to severe hypoglycemia in anorexia nervosa. Finally, the potential for zinc deficiency in patients with anorexia nervosa due to insufficient dietary intake has led to a small number of zinc supplementation trials, the results of which have been mixed (Roerig et al. 2002).

Renal Failure, Loss of Fluids, and Electrolyte Imbalance

Eating disorder–related behaviors such as vomiting, laxative or diuretic use, fluid restriction, or water loading may result in substantial fluctuations in fluid status and lead to life-threatening states such as severe dehydration with hypotension, acid–base disturbances, and electrolyte imbalances. Fluid loss, particularly from vomiting, often leads to metabolic alkalosis. Patients who abuse laxatives often develop metabolic acidosis. The most common electrolyte imbalance is hypokalemia, which, if chronic and persistent, can lead to nephropathy and chronic renal failure requiring dialysis, as well as intestinal ileus and skeletal muscle myopathy. Cardiac arrhythmias secondary to hypokalemia can be life-threatening; patients with arrhythmias must be given supplemental potassium as soon as possible to correct the imbalance. An electrocardiogram should be obtained and the patient should be placed on cardiac monitoring with intravenous potassium replacement if there are significant electrocardiographic abnormalities. Otherwise, oral potassium replacement is usually safe and effective if retention of the medication after ingestion can be assured. Hypomagnesemia may also be present and may interfere with potassium normalization. Hypocalcemia is uncommon, but when present it may be associated with prolongation of the QTc interval (see "Cardiovascular" below).

Serum phosphate levels also must be monitored because they are frequently low in patients with eating disorders, particularly those with low body weight. Although total body phosphate can be depleted through malnutrition, refeeding can also cause a drop to dangerous levels, and oral phosphate replacement is typically needed. During the first week of refeeding in inpatients, electrolyte levels should be obtained at baseline and then monitored at least every other day for the remainder of the week. Thereafter, they can be monitored less frequently if they remain stable (P.S. Mehler and Andersen 1999). Hyponatremia can result from purging behaviors or from water loading. Significant hyponatremia is associated with increased seizure risk and therefore requires prompt detection, treatment, and close monitoring. Free water intake may need to be restricted until the sodium imbalance is corrected. Patients with normal kidney function will typically correct their fluid imbalance via spontaneous diuresis.

Fluid losses caused by vomiting or abuse of diuretics, laxatives, or caffeine stimulate the renin-angiotensin system. Particularly in laxative abusers, this stimulation results in an increase in aldosterone concentration and subsequent fluid retention that may persist for weeks, leading to significant weight gain and even frank edema that is difficult for patients to tolerate. Maintenance of proper fluid status over time will correct the fluid retention, and diuresis will eventually ensue. Erratic release of vasopressin from the posterior pituitary may result in symptoms of diabetes insipidus, including excessive urination and hypernatremia (Gold et al. 1983). Blood urea nitrogen is an unreliable indicator of hydration because it may be both reduced by inadequate protein intake and elevated by dehydration or increased protein catabolism. Renal insufficiency may occur in cases of extreme starvation.

Central Nervous System

Both structural and functional changes in the brain are seen in adults and adolescents with anorexia nervosa. Studies have shown evidence of ventricular and cortical sulcal enlargement as well as functional impairment in attention and concentration, visual associative learning, visuospatial abilities, problem solving, and attentional-perceptual motor functions. Other impairments include psychomotor slowing, poor planning, and lack of insight. Some reversal of these changes have been demonstrated with weight restoration; however, it is unknown if they are completely reversible (Chowdhury and Lask 2001; Kerem and Katzman 2003; Kingston et al. 1996; Lambe et al. 1997).

Cardiovascular

Individuals with very low body weight lose significant cardiac muscle over time. This loss limits their cardiac output and may lead to congestive heart failure. Undernourished individuals may also develop clinically silent pericardial effusions (Silvetti et al. 1998), as well as conduction abnormalities with arrhythmias or a prolonged QTc interval. The latter has been shown to be a marker for risk of sudden death and therefore requires close monitoring (Cooke and Chambers 1995). Prolongation of the QTc interval is often associated with hypokalemia, hypocalcemia, or hypomagnesemia but may also be caused or exacerbated by medication (Al-Khatib et al. 2003; Halmi 2002). It typically normalizes within days after nutritional

restoration begins (Swenne and Larsson 1999). The most common abnormality is sinus bradycardia secondary to vagal hyperactivity. Mitral valve prolapse has also been noted, although its clinical significance is not fully known. This occurs more commonly in patients with anorexia nervosa and is perhaps secondary to physical remodeling of the heart with starvation (Cooke and Chambers 1995). The cardiovascular system is particularly vulnerable to substances used by patients with eating disorders for weight loss, including ipecac, diuretics, and appetite suppressants. The effects of these substances are noted in Table 15–3. Long-term use of ipecac is particularly dangerous, because it can be associated with the development of cardiomyopathy. In one study, chest pain was found to be a relatively common symptom in patients with eating disorders. Typical and atypical angina were surprisingly common and were thought to reflect underlying coronary artery disease. Increasing age, smoking history, and a family history of chest pain were correlated with the presence of angina (Birmingham et al. 1999).

Gastrointestinal

Gastrointestinal complications of eating disorders vary according to the specific eating disorder symptoms the patient manifests. Restrictive eating with marked weight loss leads to a slowing of gastrointestinal motility, resulting in gastroparesis and constipation. Impaired gastrointestinal motility may also result from ongoing abuse of laxatives, often in escalating amounts due to the development of tolerance. This condition, known as *cathartic colon*, can be associated with hemorrhoids and rectal prolapse from chronic straining. Even in the absence of weight loss, patients with bulimia nervosa have delayed gastric emptying (Devlin et al. 1997), which may explain in part the prolonged sensation of uncomfortable fullness commonly reported by these patients. As recently summarized by Roerig et al. (2002), prokinetic agents such as cisapride (now no longer available due to cardiac conduction effects) have been shown to reduce gastrointestinal complaints but do not enhance weight gain in patients with anorexia nervosa. Elevation of hepatic transaminases is common in underweight patients with anorexia nervosa and may transiently increase during early refeeding.

Vomiting may cause complications related to acid reflux such as enlargement of salivary glands, dental caries, esophagitis, and gastritis. Gastrointestinal dysmotility, when present, is often related to hypokalemia. Forced vomiting may result in hematemesis, which may be secondary to a pharyngeal scratch from induction of vomiting but may also be secondary to gastritis, esophagitis, or (less frequently) gastric or esophageal tears. Binge eating in bulimia or anorexia can cause acute gastric dilatation, as can rapid refeeding in anorexia nervosa. This requires decompression with a nasogastric tube and fluid and electrolyte replacement.

Genitourinary

In women with anorexia nervosa, amenorrhea is due to hypothalamic amenorrhea syndrome, in which pulsatile secretion of gonadotropin-releasing hormone (GnRH) is diminished. This reduced secretion in turn causes lower levels of LH and FSH along with low blood levels of estradiol, estrone, progesterone, and testosterone, leading to a physiological return to the prepubertal state. Although weight loss is a common precipitant of amenorrhea, a minority of patients develop amenorrhea before the onset of weight loss, indicating that other factors such as caloric restriction, excessive exercise, or psychogenic stress may also be important contributors (Morgan 1999). Menstrual cycling typically resumes with weight restoration at approximately 90% of standard body weight, but there may be a delay of up to 6 months after initial weight restoration (P.S. Mehler and Andersen 1999). Except in cases in which ovulation is induced, pregnancy is rare in women with active anorexia nervosa. However, in a study of 140 women with this eating disorder, at 10-year follow-up 50 had conceived, of whom 20% appeared to have done so while actively anorectic (Brinch et al. 1988).

About half of women with bulimia nervosa become amenorrheic or oligomenorrheic despite having no apparent change in percentage body fat. As in anorexia nervosa, this condition is commonly associated with impaired follicular maturation due to reduced LH concentrations and pulse frequency. Women with abnormal menstrual cycles in bulimia nervosa appear to be underweight in relationship to their own lifetime high body weight but not to average or expected body weight for their age and height (Devlin et al. 1989; Morgan 1999). Despite the profound effects of eating disorders on reproductive function, outcome studies suggest that with full recovery, fertility may not be compromised (Crow et al. 2002; Mitchell-Gieleghem et al. 2002).

Musculoskeletal

Severe protein-energy malnutrition gives rise to a metabolic myopathy with significant loss of muscle mass and function. Cases of rhabdomyolysis have been reported in anorexia nervosa. However, muscle is very responsive to refeeding. One study found that muscle performance improved long before the nutritional compromise was entirely corrected, with some improvement noted as early as the eighth day of refeeding (Rigaud et al. 1997).

Osteopenia and osteoporosis are relatively unique among complications of starvation in that they appear not to be readily reversible with weight recovery. These conditions are chronic rather than acute effects of starvation, because clinically significant bone loss does not usually begin until 12 months after onset of illness. In their study of adolescent women with anorexia nervosa, Castro et al. (2000) noted the following factors related to development of osteopenia: more than 12 months since onset of the disorder, more than 6 months of amenorrhea, body mass index less than 15 kg/m^2, calcium intake less than 600 mg/day, and less than 3 hours/week of physical activity. It is estimated that osteopenia or osteoporosis occurs in more than half of adolescent and young adult females who struggle with anorexia nervosa. These conditions can result in painful fractures, disfiguring kyphosis, and loss of height. The pathophysiology of bone loss in anorexia nervosa is complex (Golden 2003; P.S. Mehler 2003; Rosenblum and Forman 2002). Estrogen deficiency has long been thought to mediate bone loss in anorexia nervosa via an increase in osteoclast function, which promotes bone resorption. However, there are other factors integral to this process as well. Insulin-like growth factor-1 (IGF-1), a nutritionally dependent bone trophic hormone that stimulates osteoblasts to increase bone formation, is decreased in anorexic females, possibly due to decreased dehydroepiandrosterone (DHEA) in adolescent and young women with anorexia nervosa. Osteopenia and osteoporosis occur in men with anorexia nervosa as well, perhaps due to a relative lack of testosterone, which is a major substrate for estrogen production (Andersen et al. 2000).

The treatment of low bone density in anorexia nervosa requires, first and foremost, refeeding. Weight restoration is found to be effective in increasing bone mass, although not to pre-illness levels. Moderate exercise has been shown to be protective, but strenuous activity is detrimental. The uncertain status of pharmacological treatment for osteoporosis in these individuals has recently been well reviewed (Golden 2003; P.S. Mehler 2003). Hormonal treatment has generally not been found to yield improvement in bone mass in anorexia nervosa, although patients with extremely low weight may derive some benefit (Klibanski et al. 1995), and the combination of IGF-1 and oral contraceptives may be useful in some cases (Grinspoon et al. 2002). The use of estrogen in adolescents should be undertaken with caution because of the potential for fusion of the epiphyses with resultant compromise in final adult height. If estrogen is given, low doses (30–35 µg) should be used. Depot medroxyprogesterone acetate (Depo-Provera) may cause further bone loss and should be avoided. The benefit of supplemental calcium is not clear; however, the current standard practice in the treatment of anorexia nervosa is to give daily calcium (1,500 mg/day) with meals and vitamin D (400 IU/day). The efficacy of oral bisphosphonates in anorexia nervosa is not proven. Raloxifene, a selective estrogen receptor modulator, suppresses bone turnover. Although it is effective for the prevention and treatment of osteoporosis, it has not been studied specifically for use in anorexia nervosa. Likewise, there is no evidence supporting the use of calcitonin in anorexia nervosa.

Integument

The cutaneous signs of eating disorders result from malnutrition and self-induced vomiting. Findings related to malnutrition include dry, scaly skin; lanugo hair; carotenodermia; brittle nails; and hair loss. Those related to self-induced vomiting include calluses on the dorsum of the hands from constant abrasion against the front teeth with induction of vomiting (Russell's sign), and purpura and petechiae from recurrent Valsalva maneuvers to induce vomiting. Purpura and petechiae can also be seen as a result of thrombocytopenia secondary to malnutrition (Sharp and Freeman 1993).

Other

Bone marrow suppression with leukopenia, anemia, and thrombocytopenia is common in states of starvation, but these reach clinically significant levels only in the most severe cases. Pulmonary complications of eating disorders are rare but include pneumomediastinum and aspiration pneumonitis from forced vomiting. Dyspnea in long-standing malnourished states is often secondary to respiratory muscle weakness, which does not always show prompt recovery with refeeding and improved nutrition (Birmingham and Tan 2003).

Eating Disorders and Pregnancy

Eating disorders affect women during the period of reproductive functioning. In one study, a full 17% of female patients seen at an infertility clinic had eating disorders (Stewart et al. 1990). However, pregnant women with eating disorders rarely disclose their eating disorder to their obstetrician. Poor maternal or fetal weight gain should serve as red flags to the clinician regarding the possibility of a hidden eating disorder (Morgan 1999). The diagnosis of an eating disorder has clinical significance, and the timely identification of an eating disorder may enable the clinician to more effectively manage the patient and optimize outcome.

Although the majority of women with eating disorders have normal pregnancies resulting in healthy babies, and eating disorder symptoms may improve during pregnancy, rates of caesarean section and of postpartum depression are elevated in women with eating disorders (Franko et al. 2001). Low prepregnancy weight and low weight gain during pregnancy are associated with low infant birth weight and a higher incidence of congenital malformations. Other maternal complications include an increase in bulimic symptoms during pregnancy as well as restrictive eating. Both low and high maternal weight gain may occur, miscarriage is more common, and hypertension is reported more often among bulimic women. Considerations for hospital admission include degree of weight loss, hypokalemia and other electrolyte abnormalities, and electrocardiographic changes, as well as fetal growth and physiological profile. Birth complications for both anorexia nervosa and bulimia nervosa include stillbirth, low birth weight, low Apgar scores, and cleft lip and palate (Mitchell-Gieleghem et al. 2002).

Breast-feeding problems in women with eating disorders have been noted. These include complaints of insufficient lactation or of allergies or negative reactions to breast milk in the infant, resulting in early transition to bottle feeding. For women whose eating disorder treatment includes medication, the risks and benefits of breast-feeding should be carefully reviewed. Child-rearing practices may also be affected by the presence of an unresolved eating disorder in the mother. In a small proportion of cases, inadequate feeding of children has been reported with a secondary effect on the child's growth (Fairburn and Harrison 2003; Mitchell-Gieleghem et al. 2002).

Eating Disorders and Diabetes Mellitus

Some evidence suggests that there is an increase in disordered eating in chronic medical conditions for which dietary restraint is part of the treatment plan (see also Chapter 23, "Endocrine and Metabolic Disorders"). This is particularly true of type 1 diabetes mellitus. The presence of a comorbid eating disorder is associated with markedly worse outcome. A recent study of mortality of individuals with type 1 diabetes and anorexia nervosa reported crude mortality rates of 2.5% for type 1 diabetes, 6.5% for anorexia nervosa, and 34.8% for concurrent cases (Nielsen et al. 2002). Individuals with anorexia nervosa and bulimia nervosa may withhold their daily insulin to prevent uptake of glucose and, in effect, purge. However, they may also manifest other symptoms such as restricting, laxative use, vomiting, use of appetite suppressants, and compulsive exercise. Blood glucose level is typically elevated, and there is an increased risk of ketoacidosis and other complications (Rodin 2002). In one study (Rydall et al. 1997), disordered eating behavior was found to be associated with a threefold increase in diabetic retinopathy at follow-up. In fact, eating disorders were more predictive of retinopathy than was the duration of diabetes. Another study demonstrated that mean glycosylated hemoglobin was higher in subjects with diabetes mellitus who had an eating disorder (9.4%) compared with those without an eating disorder (8.6%) (Affenito and Adams 2001). The multidisciplinary team treatment of these individuals should include close endocrinological supervision. There is an ongoing need for frequent insulin changes with progression of the meal plan and activity level, or with symptom fluctuation.

Treatment

Given the contributions of cultural, familial, environmental, and genetic factors to the development of eating disorders, it is not difficult to appreciate why a biopsychosocial approach to understanding eating disorders and a multidisciplinary approach to treatment are seen as the foundation of current practice. This approach includes, at a minimum, team members to provide psychotherapy and medication management, medical monitoring and treatment, dietary management, and social service needs. The intensity of treatment and of the setting in which treatment is delivered may vary from self-help or support groups for the least symptomatic patients to weekly outpatient treatment, intensive outpatient treatment, day hospital treatment, or inpatient treatment for the most severely compromised (Kaplan et al. 2001). Patients with anorexia nervosa who are significantly underweight often require inpatient treatment, at least in the initial phase of weight restoration. Those with bulimia nervosa and BED can most often be treated as outpatients, although medical or psychiatric instability or failure of outpatient treatment options may indicate hospitalization. The American Psychiatric Association (2000b) "Practice Guideline for the Treatment of Patients With Eating Disorders" provides a useful set of standards for determining the appropriate initial level of care.

Nutritional Approaches

Nutritional rehabilitation is a fundamental and often extremely challenging component of treatment. Body weight may range from extremely low in patients with anorexia nervosa to high or markedly unstable in patients with bulimia nervosa and BED. Dietary history at intake may reveal various abnormalities, including avoidance of particular foods, overconsumption of low-calorie foods such as artificial sweeteners, uncontrolled binge eating, or food rituals. The latter are common and include preferences for unusually seasoned foods or combinations of foods, prolonged mealtimes, and eating alone. Strikingly, even in patients who eat very little themselves, food obsessions and a tendency to work around food are common (Rock and Curran-Celentano 1996).

Weight restoration is of primary importance for the individual with low body weight, whereas weight stabilization may be needed in individuals with normal or above-normal body weight. For obese patients, weight loss may be a goal, but this is usually best deferred until treatment for the eating disorder is well under way. An inpatient program should be considered for the most seriously nutritionally compromised patients, including those whose weight is less than 75% of ideal body weight or for those, especially children and adolescents, whose weight loss may not be as severe but who are losing weight at a rapid rate. The initial plan calls for establishment of a healthy weight target and a plan to restore weight safely and effectively while addressing body image and related concerns. A target weight for discharge from inpatient treatment is typically set at a range greater than or equal to approximately 90% of average for age and height. It is important that patients understand that this is a *minimum acceptable* rather than a recommended weight range.

Body composition is characterized by an extremely low percentage of body fat in emaciated patients with anorexia nervosa that increases rapidly with refeeding. Measurement of skinfold thickness provides a reliable estimate of body fat in these patients (Probst et al. 2001). Studies of body composition during the process of refeeding in patients with anorexia nervosa reveal that most of the nonfluid weight regained is represented by fat, accounting for 32%–77% of total weight gained (Rock and Curran-Celentano 1996), whereas muscle mass appears to lag behind (Polito et al. 1998). The initial distribution of weight regain is often disproportionately centripetal (Grinspoon et al. 2001), with redistribution occurring in the months following achievement of target weight.

Patients with anorexia nervosa may be unwilling or unable to accept food, at least initially. According to the American Psychiatric Association (2000b) "Practice Guideline for the Treatment of Patients With Eating Disorders," intake levels should usually start at 30–40 kcal/kg/day (approximately 1,000–1,600 kcal/day) and should be advanced progressively to yield a rate of weight gain of 2–3 lb/week for inpatients and 0.5–1 lb/week for outpatients. Patients may require levels of energy intake as high as 70–100 kcal/kg/day or more to accomplish this rate of weight gain, and nutritional supplements are often used in patients with high caloric requirements for weight regain. Although the oral feeding route is preferred, nasogastric feeding is utilized in the initial stage of treatment in some treatment centers. In particular, recent reports support progressive nocturnal nasogastric supplemental feeding for individuals with low body weight as a means of minimizing somatic and psychological distress during initial weight regain and of speeding weight restoration (Robb et al. 2002; Zuercher et al. 2003). As weight gain progresses, regular meal portion sizes are gradually increased until nasogastric supplements are no longer required. Parenteral nutrition may be utilized in extreme circumstances; however, parenteral feedings are usually not given because of the associated risks of infection and increased risk of refeeding syndrome (described below in this subsection). Although weight regain is rarely steady, a particularly erratic weight-gain pattern or inability to gain weight despite increasing caloric intake may reflect covert disposal of food, exercise, purging, or water loading to make weight, and more stringent monitoring may be in order.

Physical activity during weight restoration should be adapted to the food intake and energy expenditure of the patient, taking into account the patient's history of excessive exercise. Adherence to the refeeding protocol is often linked with greater freedom to participate in activities and other rewards. Increases in physical activity must be balanced with medical stability, weight restoration, and control of eating disorder symptoms, including excessive activity. Strict limitations are needed for individuals who struggle with compulsive exercise, and more intensive monitoring may be needed for those found to be exercising covertly. In most programs, activity is progressively advanced to include regimens of stretching, strengthening, and aerobic activity when appropriate (Rosenblum and Foreman 2002).

Careful medical monitoring is essential throughout the refeeding period and typically includes monitoring of vital signs, food and fluid intake and output, and routine electrolytes plus magnesium, calcium, and phosphate. In addition, patients should be observed for edema and rapid weight regain. If present, these may suggest fluid overload or congestive heart failure. Gastrointestinal symptoms of constipation and bloating should also be monitored. Cardiac monitoring may be indicated for severely malnourished individuals (below 70% of ideal body weight), especially children and adolescents and those individuals with severe electrolyte disturbances, arrhythmias, or prolonged QTc interval (Al-Khatib et al. 2003).

One of the most serious complications of weight restoration is the refeeding syndrome, characterized by marked fluid and electrolyte abnormalities, including low serum phosphate levels. The combination of depletion of total body phosphate stores during catabolic starvation and increased cellular influx of phosphate during anabolic refeeding leads to severe extracellular hypophosphatemia. This well-recognized complication of refeeding, particularly in individuals with very low body weight, can lead to cardiac arrhythmias, delirium, and even sudden death (Solomon and Kirby 1990). This syndrome has most often been noted in refeeding with total parenteral nutrition but can be seen with oral and nasogastric refeeding regimens as well (Fisher et al. 2000).

Cholesterol levels in anorexia nervosa are usually normal or high despite low cholesterol intake. These levels do not result from the de novo synthesis of cholesterol. Rather, abnormal thyroid hormone status, low serum estrogen levels, hypercortisolism, and impaired clearance of cholesterol explain or contribute to hypercholesterolemia in this setting. Weight restoration is typically accompanied by reduction in cholesterol level and apolipoprotein B (Feillet et al. 2000), and no effort should be made to further reduce dietary fat or cholesterol (Rock and Curran-Celentano 1996). Other laboratory abnormalities that characterize starvation and early recovery such as low white blood cell count or elevated liver transaminases typically normalize with weight recovery.

As refeeding progresses, specific laboratory markers can be used to assess improvement or deterioration in nutritional status and in effect measure the transition from protein catabolism to anabolism. A number of different parameters have been used, including serum albumin, prealbumin, retinol-binding protein, transferrin, and C-reactive protein. Serum prealbumin has a short half-life and responds rapidly to low energy intake even in the presence of adequate protein intake, making it an excellent marker of nutritional response to refeeding in severely malnourished individuals. Serum prealbumin levels of 20–40 mg/dL are considered normal, levels in the range of 10–15 mg/dL indicate mild malnutrition, levels of 5–10 mg/dL indicate moderate malnutrition, and levels of less than 5 mg/dL suggest severe depletion (Mears 1996). More recently Caregaro et al. (2001) studied the use of IGF-1 as a biochemical marker of malnutrition and a sensitive index of nutritional repletion in patients with eating disorders.

For patients with binge eating and/or purging, nutritional rehabilitation is geared toward the establishment of a regular eating pattern, moderation of dietary restraint, and elimination of unhealthy dieting practices. Inpatients with bulimia nervosa may require constant observation after meals to keep them from vomiting and to help them learn to tolerate the sensation of fullness following a meal.

For obese patients with bulimia nervosa, weight loss may be medically indicated after resolution of the eating disorder. It is an important principle of treatment that cessation of binge eating/purging and simultaneous weight loss are incompatible goals (Rock and Curran-Celentano 1996). In contrast, for obese patients with BED, some have proposed treatments that concurrently target both obesity and binge eating (Devlin 2001).

Psychopharmacological Approaches

A number of studies have evaluated the efficacy of medications in the treatment of eating disorders, and findings are thoroughly summarized in recent reviews of medication for eating disorders (Bacaltchuk et al. 2000; Wilson and Fairburn 2002). An important related area, the psychopharmacological management of obesity associated with mental disorders, is beyond the scope of this chapter but has recently been reviewed (Malhotra and McElroy 2002).

The most widely studied class of drugs for eating disorders is antidepressants, including tricyclics, monoamine oxidase inhibitors (MAOIs), and selective serotonin reuptake inhibitors (SSRIs). For patients with bulimia nervosa, antidepressants are significantly more effective than placebo in reducing binge-eating and purging behaviors. Furthermore, it appears that all antidepressants work equally effectively; however, SSRIs yield fewer side effects than MAOIs and tricyclics, and fluoxetine is the only medication approved by the U.S. Food and Drug Administration for the treatment of bulimia nervosa. However, longer-term studies of antidepressant treatment with bulimia nervosa suggest that these medications alone are not sufficient to facilitate long-term remission (Romano et al. 2002; Walsh et al. 1991). Research on pharmacotherapy for BED has suggested that antidepressants may reduce binge frequency, at least in the short term; however, this finding has not been as clearly demonstrated for BED as for bulimia nervosa. For patients with anorexia nervosa, antidepressant treatment has, for the most part, not proved effective (Attia et al. 1998).

Although they are less well studied than antidepressants, other classes of drugs have been reported to be useful in the treatment of BED and bulimia nervosa. Anticonvulsants (carbamazepine, phenytoin, valproate) and other psychotropic medications (lithium, naltrexone, methylphenidate) have been reported to be effective in reducing binge eating in bulimia nervosa or BED, but their routine use has not been clearly established. Most recently, topiramate has been found to curb binge-eating episodes in patients with BED (McElroy et al. 2003) and bulimia nervosa and also to cause weight loss in obese pa-

tients, a potentially useful side effect that has not been observed with other medications used for these disorders (Malhotra and McElroy 2002). In addition to topiramate, appetite suppressant medications have been thought to be a potentially useful treatment for BED. One study (Stunkard et al. 1996) demonstrated that D-fenfluramine, a drug that is now off the market, was effective in reducing binge eating in patients with BED. In a recently completed trial, sibutramine (Meridia) was found to be significantly more effective than placebo in reducing binge frequency in obese patients with BED. In addition, individuals taking sibutramine lost a clinically significant amount of weight (Appolinario et al. 2003).

In general, patients with anorexia nervosa have not responded favorably to pharmacotherapy (Wilson and Fairburn 2002). However, recent evidence suggests that the antipsychotic medication olanzapine may be a useful tool in the treatment of anorexia nervosa, both for its ability to target the delusions, anxiety, and obsessions that often characterize those with anorexia nervosa and its documented side effect of weight gain (C. Mehler et al. 2001; Powers et al. 2002). Double-blind, randomized trials of olanzapine are necessary before firm conclusions about its efficacy can be drawn. In addition, some studies have found that fluoxetine is a useful tool for relapse prevention in weight-restored patients with prior anorexia nervosa (Kaye et al. 1991, 2001). Again, more research is necessary to validate the use of fluoxetine for this population. Finally, a recent pilot study using recombinant human growth hormone (rhGH) in adolescent patients with anorexia nervosa reported more rapid medical stabilization and numerical but not statistically significant improvements in weight gain and length of hospitalization in the rhGH group (Hill et al. 2000).

Psychotherapeutic Approaches

Mental health professionals employ a wide variety of therapeutic techniques in their efforts to treat the symptoms of anorexia nervosa, bulimia nervosa, and BED. However, only a few of these psychotherapies, such as cognitive-behavioral therapy (CBT) and interpersonal therapy, have been systematically studied in randomized, controlled trials. In addition, certain other types of therapy have been studied for the treatment of only one eating disorder diagnosis, such as manualized family therapy and inpatient treatment for those with anorexia nervosa and behavioral weight loss for patients with BED.

CBT, the most widely studied method of psychotherapy for eating disorders, targets the two broad areas of eating disorder symptoms: 1) cognitive and attitudinal disturbances, such as low self-esteem and overemphasis on and distortion of weight and shape; and 2) behavioral aspects of eating and weight regulation, such as purging and food intake restriction. The goals of CBT are to challenge rigid rules about eating and weight that patients with eating disorders have imposed on themselves and to help these patients develop healthier behaviors and cognitions. CBT for bulimia nervosa was first put into manualized format in the early 1990s (Fairburn et al. 1993b) and has subsequently been modified for patients with anorexia nervosa and BED (Garner et al. 1997; Marcus 1997). CBT has been administered in an individual format, in a group setting, and via a self-help manual.

Most studies of CBT have examined patients with bulimia nervosa. In general, it has been shown that CBT is more effective than minimal treatment, supportive psychotherapy, and purely behavioral interventions in reducing both the behavioral and cognitive disturbances of patients with bulimia nervosa. Studies assessing the effectiveness of CBT alone, medication alone, and their combination in the treatment of bulimia nervosa have shown that CBT alone is more effective than medication alone and leads to more successful long-term maintenance of change. Furthermore, the combination of CBT and antidepressant medication is significantly superior to medication alone (Wilson and Fairburn 2002). Medication may confer modest additional benefits to CBT and may be most useful for targeting comorbid symptoms of depression and anxiety (Walsh et al. 1997). Studies of CBT in patients with BED have shown that CBT is significantly more effective than no treatment (American Psychiatric Association 2000b), but it appears to be no more effective than other types of treatment, such as behavioral weight-loss programs (Agras et al. 1994) or interpersonal therapy (Wilfley et al. 2002). Studies of CBT for anorexia nervosa have been too small in scope and methodologically unsound to yield firm conclusions about the use of CBT in this population.

Interpersonal therapy was originally developed as a treatment for depression (Klerman et al. 1984) and was subsequently adapted for use with bulimia nervosa and BED (Fairburn 1997; Wilfley et al. 1993). Interpersonal therapy focuses on a person's interpersonal relationships rather than on the specific behavioral or attitudinal disturbances of the eating disorder. Studies comparing CBT and interpersonal therapy for bulimia nervosa have shown that although CBT appears to exert its effects more quickly, the two treatments both lead to significant long-term symptom change (Agras et al. 2000; Fairburn et al. 1993a). In patients with BED, CBT and interpersonal therapy appear to be equally effective (Wilfley et al. 2002).

A few additional nonpharmacological forms of treatment for eating disorders deserve mention. One form of

treatment for BED is behavioral weight loss, with the goal of improving the patient's diet and exercise regimen and restricting his or her caloric intake. In general, it appears that behavioral weight loss is effective in the short term in reducing episodes of binge eating and yielding clinically significant weight loss (Agras et al. 1994; Marcus et al. 1995; Nauta et al. 2000). However, few studies have examined the long-term effects of behavioral programs, a key issue in obesity treatment. Some patients who have BED associated with obesity may also pursue weight-loss surgery, the most common procedure being the Roux-en-Y gastric bypass (see Chapter 30, "Surgery"). For these patients, the long-term prognostic significance of an eating disorder is uncertain and merits further study.

There have been few systematic studies of treatment for anorexia nervosa. Patients with anorexia nervosa can be treated either on an inpatient or an outpatient basis. Often treatment is sequenced, starting out with inpatient therapy or partial hospitalization followed by outpatient therapy aimed at relapse prevention. Inpatient therapy usually involves some combination of individual therapy, family therapy, nutritional counseling, and occupational/recreational therapy, typically with behavioral incentives in place for encouraging weight gain. Outpatient therapies used for anorexia nervosa have been eclectic, ranging from nutritional counseling to supportive psychotherapy to CBT. Recently, researchers have begun to empirically evaluate some forms of anorexia nervosa outpatient treatment. For example, a group from the Maudsley Hospital in London developed a manualized outpatient family therapy for adolescents with anorexia nervosa that seeks to empower parents to refeed their child at home (Lock et al. 2001). Results from a number of studies suggest that the Maudsley method is extremely effective for long-term weight restoration in adolescents with an early onset of anorexia nervosa and a short duration of illness (Eisler et al. 1997, 2000; Russell et al. 1987).

Involuntary Treatment

A critical issue concerning treatment for eating disorders, particularly anorexia nervosa, is the question of involuntary hospitalization for critically ill patients. Patients with anorexia nervosa often experience their illness as an important component of their identity, and they are therefore quite reluctant to undertake treatment. Many patients are hospitalized against their will by loved ones or health care providers with serious concerns about their medical stability. Some countries (e.g., the United Kingdom) have established clear guidelines outlining the conditions under which compulsory treatment for anorexia nervosa is indicated. However, the United States has no such guidelines, and American clinicians treating patients with anorexia nervosa must therefore consult more general standards for involuntary treatment.

The question of whether involuntary treatment for anorexia nervosa is ethical is a controversial one. Supporters of involuntary treatment claim that extremely low-weight patients with anorexia nervosa are incapable of making treatment decisions for themselves, due to both the cognitive effects of semistarvation and their distorted thinking surrounding food and body image. Detractors of involuntary treatment cite a host of concerns. Some believe that conceptualizing anorexia nervosa as an illness meriting compulsory treatment overemphasizes its medical aspects and ignores the many pertinent emotional and social factors that may contribute to the illness. Others argue that prospective patients are generally neither psychotic nor grossly impaired in cognitive function and therefore do not lack capacity to make treatment decisions. An additional concern is that patients who are forced into treatment will not be willing to continue treatment once their dire medical situation is resolved and that clinicians who take action to commit their patients against their wishes will destroy the therapeutic relationship (Russell 2001).

Three studies, only one of which took place in the United States, compared the outcomes of patients who had been hospitalized involuntarily with those of voluntary patients (Griffiths et al. 1997; Ramsay et al. 1999; Watson et al. 2000). In the short term, voluntary and involuntary patients made equally strong progress in terms of weight gain, although in some cases involuntary patients required a longer hospital stay to achieve their target weights. No systematic follow-up was done on the patients in these three samples, so the question of long-term effects of involuntary treatment remains open. However, based on the examination of a national mortality register roughly 5 years after hospitalization, one group reported higher mortality rates in involuntary patients. Further study of both the ethical basis and the practical utility of involuntary treatment is needed.

Conclusion

Disordered eating is an important component of the clinical presentation of a variety of patients with weights ranging from emaciated to severely obese. In some cases, disordered eating is of sufficient severity to warrant an eating disorder diagnosis in its own right, whereas in other cases, eating disorder symptoms may complicate the clinical picture of patients with other medical or psychiatric illness. Although the most common eating disorder diagnosis is eating disorder NOS, it is also the most inadequately studied. However, a knowledge of the assessment, differential diagnosis, medical complications, and treatment of the classic eating disorders will aid the psychiatric practitioner in developing a treatment approach for patients with a wide range of eating disorder symptoms and in contributing to the multidisciplinary treatment of severely ill patients who are medically compromised by their eating disorder.

References

Adan RA, Hillebrand JJ, De Rijke C, et al: Melanocortin system and eating disorders. Ann N Y Acad Sci 994:267–274, 2003

Affenito SG, Adams CH: Are eating disorders more prevalent in females with type 1 diabetes mellitus when the impact of insulin omission is considered? Nutr Rev 59:179–182, 2001

Agras WS, Telch CF, Arnow B, et al: Weight loss, cognitive-behavioral, and desipramine treatments in binge eating disorder. An additive design. Behav Ther 25:209–224, 1994

Agras WS, Walsh BT, Fairburn CG, et al: A multicenter comparison of cognitive-behavioral therapy and interpersonal psychotherapy for bulimia nervosa. Arch Gen Psychiatry 57:459–466, 2000

Al-Khatib SM, LaPointe NM, Kramer JM, et al: What clinicians should know about the QT interval. JAMA 289:2120–2127, 2003

American Psychiatric Association: Diagnostic and Statistical Manual of Mental Disorders, 4th Edition. Washington, DC, American Psychiatric Association, 1994

American Psychiatric Association: Diagnostic and Statistical Manual of Mental Disorders, 4th Edition, Text Revision. Washington, DC, American Psychiatric Association, 2000a

American Psychiatric Association: Practice guideline for the treatment of patients with eating disorders (revision). Am J Psychiatry 157 (suppl 1):1–39, 2000b

Andersen AE, Watson T, Schlechte J: Osteoporosis and osteopenia in men with eating disorders (letter). Lancet 355:1967–1968, 2000

Appolinario JC, Bacaltchuk J, Sichieri R, et al: A randomized, double-blind, placebo-controlled study of sibutramine in the treatment of binge-eating disorder. Arch Gen Psychiatry 60:1109–1116, 2003

Attia E, Haiman C, Walsh BT, et al: Does fluoxetine augment the inpatient treatment of anorexia nervosa? Am J Psychiatry 155:548–551, 1998

Bacaltchuk J, Hay P, Mari JJ: Antidepressants vs. placebo for the treatment of bulimia nervosa: a systematic review. Aust N Z J Psychiatry 34:310–317, 2000

Bhanji S, Mattingly D: Medical Aspects of Anorexia Nervosa. Boston, MA, Wright, 1988

Birketvedt G, Florholmen J, Sundsfjord J, et al: Behavioral and neuroendocrine characteristics of the night-eating syndrome. JAMA 282:657–663, 1999

Birmingham CL, Tan AO: Respiratory muscle weakness and anorexia nervosa. Int J Eat Disord 33:230–233, 2003

Birmingham CL, Stigant C, Goldner EM: Chest pain in anorexia nervosa. Int J Eat Disord 25:219–222, 1999

Branch CHH, Eurman LJ: Social attitudes toward patients with anorexia nervosa. Am J Psychiatry 137:631–632, 1980

Branson R, Potoczna N, Kral JG, et al: Binge eating as a major phenotype of melanocortin 4 receptor gene mutations. N Engl J Med 348:1096–1103, 2003

Brinch M, Isager T, Tolstrup K: Anorexia nervosa and motherhood: reproduction pattern and mothering behavior of 50 women. Acta Psychiatr Scand 77:98–104, 1988

Bruch H: Eating Disorders. Obesity, Anorexia Nervosa, and the Person Within. New York, Basic Books, 1973

Brumberg JJ: Fasting Girls: The Emergence of Anorexia Nervosa as a Modern Disease. Cambridge, MA, Harvard University Press, 1988

Bulik CM: Anxiety, depression, and eating disorders, in Eating Disorders and Obesity: A Comprehensive Handbook, 2nd Edition. Edited by Fairburn CG, Brownell KD. New York, Guilford, 2002, pp 193–198

Bulik CM, Sullivan PF, Fear J, et al: Predictors of the development of bulimia nervosa in women with anorexia nervosa. J Nerv Ment Dis 185:704–707, 1997

Bulik CM, Sullivan PF, Joyce PR, et al: Predictors of 1-year treatment outcome in bulimia nervosa. Compr Psychiatry 39:206–214, 1998

Bulik CM, Sullivan PF, Wade TD, et al: Twin studies of eating disorders: a review. Int J Eat Disord 27:1–20, 2000

Bulik CM, Sullivan PF, Kendler KS: Medical and psychiatric morbidity in obese women with and without binge eating. Int J Eat Disord 32:72–78, 2002

Calle EE, Thun MJ, Petrelli JM, et al: Body-mass index and mortality in a prospective cohort of U.S. adults. N Engl J Med 341:1097–1105, 1999

Caregaro L, Favaro A, Santonastaso P, et al: Insulin-like growth factor 1 (IGF-1), a nutritional marker in patients with eating disorders. Clin Nutr 20:251–257, 2001

Castro J, Lazaro L, Pons F, et al: Predictors of bone mineral density reduction in adolescents with anorexia nervosa. J Am Acad Child Adolesc Psychiatry 39:1365–1370, 2000

Chowdhury U, Lask B: Clinical implications of brain imaging in eating disorders. Psychiatr Clin North Am 24:227–234, 2001

Chowdhury U, Gordon I, Lask B, et al: Early onset anorexia nervosa: is there evidence of limbic system imbalance? Int J Eat Disord 33:388–395, 2003

Collier DA: Molecular genetics of eating disorders, in Eating Disorders and Obesity: A Comprehensive Handbook, 2nd Edition. Edited by Fairburn CG, Brownell KD. New York, Guilford, 2002, pp 243–246

Cooke RA, Chambers JB: Anorexia and the heart. Br J Hosp Med 54:313–317, 1995

Couper R: Prader-Willi syndrome. J Paediatr Child Health 35: 331–334, 1999

Crow SJ, Thuras P, Keel PK, et al: Long-term menstrual and reproductive function in patients with bulimia nervosa. Am J Psychiatry 159:1048–1050, 2002

Del Parigi A, Chen K, Salbe AD, et al: Are we addicted to food? Obes Res 11:493–495, 2003

Devlin MJ: Binge eating disorder and obesity—a combined treatment approach. Psychiatr Clin North Am 24:325–335, 2001

Devlin MJ, Walsh BT: The neuroendocrinology of anorexia nervosa, in Neuroendocrinology of Mood (Current Topics in Neuroendocrinology, Vol 8). Edited by Ganten D, Pfaff D. New York, Springer-Verlag, 1988, pp 291–307

Devlin MJ, Walsh BT, Katz JL, et al: Hypothalamic-pituitary-gonadal function in anorexia nervosa and bulimia. Psychiatry Res 28:11–24, 1989

Devlin MJ, Walsh BT, Kral JB, et al: Metabolic abnormalities in bulimia nervosa. Arch Gen Psychiatry 47:144–148, 1990

Devlin MJ, Walsh BT, Kissileff HR, et al: Postprandial cholecystokinin release and gastric emptying in patients with bulimia nervosa. Am J Clin Nutr 65:114–120, 1997

Devlin MJ, Yanovski SZ, Wilson GT: Obesity: what mental health professionals need to know. Am J Psychiatry 157: 854–866, 2000

Devlin MJ, Goldfein JA, Dobrow I: What is this thing called BED? Current status of binge eating disorder nosology. Int J Eat Disord 34 (suppl):S2–S18, 2003

de Zwaan M, Aslam Z, Mitchell JE: Research on energy expenditure in individuals with eating disorders: a review. Int J Eat Disord 31:361–369, 2002

Dingemans AE, Bruna MJ, van Furth EF: Binge eating disorder: a review. Int J Obes 26:299–307, 2002

Dotti A, Fioravanti M, Balotta M, et al: Eating behavior of ballet dancers. Eat Weight Disord 7:60–67, 2002

Dulloo AG, Jacquet J: Adaptive reduction in basal metabolic rate in response to food deprivation in humans: a role for feedback signals from fat stores. Am J Clin Nutr 68:599–606, 1998

Eisler I, Dare C, Russell GF, et al: Family and individual therapy in anorexia nervosa: a 5-year follow-up. Arch Gen Psychiatry 54:1025–1030, 1997

Eisler I, Dare C, Hodes M, et al: Family therapy for adolescent anorexia nervosa: the results of a controlled comparison of two family interventions. J Child Psychol Psychiatry 41: 727–736, 2000

Everill JT, Waller G: Reported sexual abuse and eating psychopathology: a review of the evidence for a causal link. Int J Eat Disord 18:1–11, 1995

Fairburn CG: Interpersonal psychotherapy for bulimia nervosa, in Handbook of Treatment for Eating Disorders, 2nd Edition. Edited by Garner DM, Garfinkel PE. New York, Guilford, 1997, pp 278–294

Fairburn CG, Harrison PJ: Eating disorders. Lancet 361:407–416, 2003

Fairburn CG, Jones R, Peveler RC, et al: Psychotherapy and bulimia nervosa: the longer-term effects of interpersonal psychotherapy, behavior therapy, and cognitive behavior therapy. Arch Gen Psychiatry 50:419–428, 1993a

Fairburn CG, Marcus MD, Wilson GT: Cognitive-behavioral therapy for binge eating and bulimia nervosa: a comprehensive treatment manual, in Binge Eating: Nature, Assessment, and Treatment. Edited by Fairburn CG, Wilson GT. New York, Guilford, 1993b, pp 361–404

Fairburn CG, Welch SL, Doll HA, et al: Risk factors for bulimia nervosa: a community-based case-control study. Arch Gen Psychiatry 54:509–517, 1997

Fairburn CG, Doll HA, Welch SL, et al: Risk factors for binge eating disorder: a community-based, case-control study. Arch Gen Psychiatry 55:425–432, 1998

Fairburn CG, Cooper Z, Doll HA, et al: Risk factors for anorexia nervosa: three integrated case-control comparisons. Arch Gen Psychiatry 56:468–476, 1999

Fairburn CG, Cooper Z, Shafran R: Cognitive behaviour therapy for eating disorders: a "transdiagnostic" theory and treatment. Behav Res Ther 41:509–528, 2003

Feillet F, Feillet-Coudray C, Bard JM, et al: Plasma cholesterol and endogenous cholesterol synthesis during refeeding in anorexia nervosa. Clin Chim Acta 294:45–56, 2000

Fisher M, Simpser E, Schneider M: Hypophosphatemia secondary to oral refeeding in anorexia nervosa. Int J Eat Disord 28:181–187, 2000

Franklin JC, Schiele BC, Brozek J, et al: Observations of human behavior in experimental semistarvation and rehabilitation. J Clin Psychol 4:28–45, 1948

Franko DL, Blais MA, Becker AE, et al: Pregnancy complications and neonatal outcomes in women with eating disorders. Am J Psychiatry 158:1461–1466, 2001

Gard MCE, Freeman CP: The dismantling of a myth: a review of eating disorders and socioeconomic status. Int J Eat Disord 20:1–12, 1996

Garner DM, Olmsted MP, Bohr Y, et al: The Eating Attitudes Test: psychometric features and clinical correlates. Psychol Med 12:871–878, 1982

Garner DM, Vitousek KM, Pike KM: Cognitive-behavioral therapy for anorexia nervosa, in Handbook of Treatment for Eating Disorders, 2nd Edition. Edited by Garner DM, Garfinkel PE. New York, Guilford, 1997, pp 94–144

Gluck ME, Geliebter A, Satov T: Night eating syndrome is associated with depression, low self-esteem, reduced daytime hunger, and less weight loss in obese outpatients. Obes Res 9:264–267, 2001

Gold PW, Kaye W, Robertson GL, et al: Abnormalities in plasma and cerebrospinal-fluid arginine vasopressin in patients with anorexia nervosa. N Engl J Med 308:1117–1123, 1983

Golden N: Osteopenia and osteoporosis in anorexia nervosa. Adolesc Med 14:97–108, 2003

Griffiths RA, Beumont PJV, Russell J et al: The use of guardianship legislation for anorexia nervosa: a report of 15 cases. Aust N Z J Psychiatry 31:525–531, 1997

Grinspoon S, Thomas L, Miller K, et al: Changes in regional fat redistribution and the effects of estrogen during spontaneous weight gain in women with anorexia nervosa. Am J Clin Nutr 73:865–869, 2001

Grinspoon S, Thomas L, Miller K, et al: Effects of recombinant human IGF-1 and oral contraceptive administration on bone density in anorexia nervosa. J Clin Endocrinol Metab 87:2883–2891, 2002

Gull WW: Anorexia nervosa (apepsia hysterica, anorexia hysterica). Transactions of the Clinical Society of London 7:22–28, 1874

Halmi KA: Physiology of anorexia nervosa and bulimia nervosa, in Eating Disorders and Obesity: A Comprehensive Handbook, 2nd Edition. Edited by Fairburn CG, Brownell KD. New York, Guilford, 2002, pp 267–271

Haqq AM, Farooqi S, O'Rahilly S, et al: Serum ghrelin levels are inversely correlated with body mass index, age, and insulin concentrations in normal children and are markedly increased in Prader-Willi syndrome. J Clin Endocrinol Metab 88:174–178, 2003

Haworth-Hoeppner S: The critical shapes of body image: the role of culture and family in the production of eating disorders. J Marriage Fam 62:212–227, 2000

Hebebrand J, Himmelmann GW, Herzog W, et al: Prediction of low body weight at long-term follow-up in acute anorexia nervosa by low body weight at referral. Am J Psychiatry 154:566–569, 1997

Hebebrand J, Geller F, Dempfle A, et al: Binge-eating episodes are not characteristic of carriers of melanocortin-4 receptor gene mutations. Mol Psychiatry 9:796–800, 2004

Herzog DB, Greenwood DN, Dorer DJ, et al: Mortality in eating disorders: a descriptive study. Int J Eat Disord 28:20–26, 2000

Herzog W, Deter HC, Fiehn W, et al: Medical findings and predictors of long-term physical outcome in anorexia nervosa: a prospective, 12-year follow-up study. Psychol Med 27:269–279, 1997

Hill K, Bucuvalas J, McClain C, et al: Pilot study of growth hormone administration during the refeeding of malnourished anorexia nervosa patients. J Child Adolesc Psychopharmacol 10:3–8, 2000

Holderness CC, Brooks-Gunn J, Warren MP: Co-morbidity of eating disorders and substance abuse: review of the literature. Int J Eat Disord 16:1–34, 1994

Kann L, Kinchen SA, Williams BI, et al: Youth risk behavior surveillance—United States, 1999. MMWR CDC Surveill Summ 49(5):1–96, 2000

Kaplan AS, Olmsted MP, Carter JC, et al: Matching patient variables to treatment intensity—the continuum of care. Psychiatr Clin North Am 24:281–292, 2001

Kaye WH: Central nervous system neurotransmitter activity in anorexia nervosa and bulimia nervosa, in Eating Disorders and Obesity: A Comprehensive Handbook, 2nd Edition. Edited by Fairburn CG, Brownell KD. New York, Guilford, 2002, pp 272–277

Kaye W, Strober M: Neurobiology of eating disorders, in Neurobiology of Mental Illness. Edited by Charney DS, Nestler EJ, Bunney BS. New York, Oxford University Press, 1999, pp 891–906

Kaye WH, Weltzin TE, Hsu LK, et al: An open trial of fluoxetine in patients with anorexia nervosa. J Clin Psychiatry 52:464–471, 1991

Kaye WH, Nagata T, Weltzin TE, et al: Double-blind placebo-controlled administration of fluoxetine in restricting- and restricting-purging-type anorexia nervosa. Biol Psychiatry 49:644–652, 2001

Keel PK, Mitchell JE, Miller KB, et al: Long-term outcome of bulimia nervosa. Arch Gen Psychiatry 56:63–69, 1999

Keel PK, Dorer DJ, Eddy KT, et al: Predictors of mortality in eating disorders. Arch Gen Psychiatry 60:179–183, 2003

Kendler KS, Bulik CM, Silberg J, et al: Childhood sexual abuse and adult psychiatric and substance use disorders in women: an epidemiological and cotwin control analysis. Arch Gen Psychiatry 57:953–959, 2000

Kent A, Waller G: Childhood emotional abuse and eating psychopathology. Clin Psychol Rev 20:887–903, 2000

Kerem NC, Katzman DK: Brain structure and function in adolescents with anorexia nervosa. Adolesc Med 14:109–118, 2003

Kingston K, Szmukler G, Andrewes D, et al: Neuropsychological and structural brain changes in anorexia nervosa before and after refeeding. Psychol Med 26:15–28, 1996

Klerman GL, Weissman MM, Rounsaville BJ, et al: Interpersonal psychotherapy of depression. New York, Basic Books, 1984

Klibanski A, Biller BMK, Schoenfeld DA, et al: The effect of estrogen on trabecular bone loss in young women with anorexia nervosa. J Clin Endocrinol Metab 80:898–904, 1995

Kopelman P: Obesity as a medical problem. Nature 404:635–643, 2000

Kotler LA, Cohen P, Davies M et al: Longitudinal relationships between childhood, adolescent, and adult eating disorders. J Am Acad Child Adolesc Psychiatry 40:1434–1440, 2001

Kreipe RE, Yussman SE: The role of the primary care practitioner in the treatment of eating disorders. Adolesc Med 14:133–147, 2003

Lambe EK, Katzman DK, Mikulis DJ, et al: Cerebral grey matter volume deficits after weight recovery from anorexia nervosa. Arch Gen Psychiatry 54:537–542, 1997

Lasègue C: De l'anorexie hystérique. Archives Générales de Médecine 1:384–403, 1873

Lask B, Bryant-Waugh R: Prepubertal eating disorders, in Handbook of Treatment for Eating Disorders, 2nd Edition. Edited by Garner DM, Garfinkel PE. New York, Guilford, 1997, pp 476–483

Levine MP, Smolak L, Moodey AF, et al: Normative developmental challenges and dieting and eating disturbances in middle school girls. Int J Eat Disord 15:11–20, 1994

Lock J, le Grange D, Agras WS, et al: Treatment Manual for Anorexia Nervosa: A Family Based Approach. New York, Guilford, 2001

Malhotra S, McElroy SL: Medical management of obesity associated with mental disorders. J Clin Psychiatry 63 (suppl 4): 24–32, 2002

Marcus MD: Adapting treatment for patients with binge-eating disorder, in Handbook of Treatment for Eating Disorders, 2nd Edition. Edited by Garner DM, Garfinkel PE. New York, Guilford, 1997, pp 484–493

Marcus MD, Wing RR, Fairburn CG: Cognitive behavioral treatment of binge eating vs. behavioral weight control on the treatment of binge eating disorder (abstract). Ann Behav Med 17:S090, 1995

McElroy SL, Arnold LM, Shapira NA, et al: Topiramate in the treatment of binge eating disorder associated with obesity: a randomized, placebo-controlled trial. Am J Psychiatry 160:255–261, 2003

Mears E: Outcomes of continuous process improvement of a nutritional care program incorporating serum prealbumin measurements. Nutrition 12:479–484, 1996

Mehler C, Wewetzer C, Schulze U, et al: Olanzapine in children and adolescents with chronic anorexia nervosa. A study of five cases. Eur Child Adolesc Psychiatry 10:151–157, 2001

Mehler PS: Osteoporosis in anorexia nervosa: prevention and treatment. Int J Eat Disord 33:113–126, 2003

Mehler PS, Andersen AE: Eating Disorders—A Guide to Medical Care and Complications. Baltimore, MD, Johns Hopkins University Press, 1999

Miller MN, Pumariega AJ: Culture and eating disorders: a historical and cross-cultural review. Psychiatry 64:93–110, 2001

Minuchin S, Rosman BL, Baker L: Psychosomatic families: anorexia nervosa in context. Cambridge, MA, Harvard University Press, 1978

Mitchell JE, Specker S, De Zwaan J: Comorbidity and medical complications of bulimia nervosa. J Clin Psychiatry 52:13–20, 1991

Mitchell-Gieleghem A, Mittelstaedt ME, Bulik CM: Eating disorders and childbearing: concealment and consequences. Birth 29:182–191, 2002

Mokdad AH, Bowman BA, Ford ES, et al: The continuing epidemics of obesity and diabetes in the United States. JAMA 286:1195–1200, 2001

Mokdad AH, Ford ES, Bowman BA, et al: Prevalence of obesity, diabetes, and obesity-related health risk factors, 2001. JAMA 289:76–79, 2003

Morgan JF: Eating disorders and reproduction. Aust N Z J Obstet Gynaecol 39:167–73, 1999

Morgan JF, Reid F, Lacey JH: The SCOFF questionnaire: assessment of a new screening tool for eating disorders. BMJ 319:1467–1468, 1999

Morton R: Phthisiologia, seu exercitationes de phthisi. London, S. Smith, 1689

Nauta H, Hospers H, Kok G, et al: A comparison between a cognitive and a behavioral treatment for obese binge eaters and obese non-binge eaters. Behav Ther 31:441–462, 2000

Nielsen S: Epidemiology and mortality of eating disorders. Psychiatr Clin North Am 24:201–214, 2001

Nielsen S, Emborg C, Molbak AG: Mortality in concurrent type 1 diabetes and anorexia nervosa. Diabetes Care 25:309–312, 2002

Papacostas SS, Hadjivasilis V: The Kleine-Levin syndrome. Report of a case and review of the literature. Eur Psychiatry 15:231–235, 2000

Pike KM: Long-term course of anorexia nervosa: response, relapse, remission, and recovery. Clin Psychol Rev 18:447–475, 1998

Pirke KM: Central and peripheral noradrenalin regulation in eating disorders. Psychiatry Res 62:43–49, 1996

Pi-Sunyer FX: Medical complications of obesity in adults, in Eating Disorders and Obesity: A Comprehensive Handbook, 2nd Edition. Edited by Fairburn CG, Brownell KD. New York, Guilford, 2002, pp 467–472

Polito A, Cuzzolaro M, Raguzzini A, et al: Body composition changes in anorexia nervosa. Eur J Clin Nutr 52:655–662, 1998

Polivy J, Herman CP: Causes of eating disorders. Annu Rev Psychol 53:187–213, 2002

Powers PS, Santana CA, Bannon YS: Olanzapine in the treatment of anorexia nervosa: an open label trial. Int J Eat Disord 32:146–154, 2002

Probst M, Goris M, Vandereycken W, et al: Body composition of anorexia nervosa patients assessed by underwater weighing and skinfold-thickness measurements before and after weight gain. Am J Clin Nutr 73:190–197, 2001

Ramsay R, Ward A, Treasure J, et al: Compulsory treatment in anorexia nervosa: short-term benefits and long-term mortality. Br J Psychiatry 175:147–153, 1999

Rechlin T, Weis M, Ott C, et al: Alterations of autonomic cardiac control in anorexia nervosa. Biol Psychiatry 43:358–363, 1998

Richards PS, Baldwin BM, Frost HA, et al: What works for treating eating disorders? A synthesis of 28 outcome reviews. Eating Disorders: The Journal of Treatment and Prevention 8:189–206, 2000

Rigaud D, Moukaddem M, Cohen B, et al: Refeeding improves muscle performance without normalization of muscle mass and oxygen consumption in anorexia nervosa patients. Am J Clin Nutr 65:1845–1851, 1997

Robb AS, Silber TJ, Orrell-Valente JK, et al: Supplemental nocturnal nasogastric refeeding for better short-term outcome in hospitalized adolescent girls with anorexia nervosa. Am J Psychiatry 159:1347–1353, 2002

Rock CL, Curran-Celentano JC: Nutritional management of eating disorders. Psychiatr Clin North Am 19:701–713, 1996

Rodin GM: Eating disorders in diabetes mellitus, in Eating Disorders and Obesity: A Comprehensive Handbook, 2nd Edition. Edited by Fairburn CG, Brownell KD. New York, Guilford, 2002, pp 286–290

Roerig JL, Mitchell JE, Myers TC, et al: Pharmacotherapy and medical complications of eating disorders in children and adolescents. Child Adolesc Psychiatr Clin N Am 11:365–385, 2002

Romano SJ, Halmi KA, Sarkar NP, et al: A placebo-controlled study of fluoxetine in continued treatment of bulimia nervosa after successful acute fluoxetine treatment. Am J Psychiatry 159:96–102, 2002

Rome ES, Ammerman S, Rosen DS, et al: Children and adolescents with eating disorders: the state of the art. Pediatrics 111:e98–e108, 2003

Rosen DS: Eating disorders in children and young adolescents: etiology, classification, clinical features, and treatment. Adolesc Med 14:49–59, 2003

Rosenblum J, Forman S: Evidence-based treatment of eating disorders. Curr Opin Pediatr 14:379–383, 2002

Rubinstein S, Caballero B: Is Miss America an undernourished role model? (letter) JAMA 283:1569, 2000

Rudolph CD, Link DT: Feeding disorders in infants and children. Pediatr Clin North Am 49:97–112, 2002

Russell GFM: Bulimia nervosa: an ominous variant of anorexia nervosa. Psychol Med 9:429–448, 1979

Russell GFM: Involuntary treatment in anorexia nervosa. Psychiatr Clin North Am 24:337–349, 2001

Russell GFM, Szmukler GI, Dare C, et al: An evaluation of family therapy in anorexia nervosa and bulimia nervosa. Arch Gen Psychiatry 44:1047–1056, 1987

Rydall AC, Rodin GM, Olmsted MP, et al: Disordered eating behavior and microvascular complications in young women with insulin-dependent diabetes mellitus. N Engl J Med 336:1849–1854, 1997

Schenk CH, Mahowald MW: Review of nocturnal sleep-related eating disorders. Int J Eat Disord 15:343–356, 1994

Sharp CW, Freeman PL: The medical complications of anorexia nervosa. Br J Psychiatry 162:452–462, 1993

Shisslak CM, Crago M, McKnight KM, et al: Potential risk factors associated with weight control behaviors in elementary and middle school girls. J Psychosom Res 44:301–313, 1998

Silvetti MS, Magnani M, Santilli A, et al: The heart of anorexic adolescents [in Italian]. G Ital Cardiol 28:131–139, 1998

Smolak L, Murnen SK, Ruble AE: Female athletes and eating problems: a meta-analysis. Int J Eat Disord 27:371–380, 2000

Solomon SM, Kirby DF: The refeeding syndrome: a review. JPEN J Parenter Enteral Nutr 14:90–97, 1990

Steinhausen HC: The outcome of anorexia nervosa in the 20th century. Am J Psychiatry 159:1284–1293, 2002

Stewart DE, Robinson E, Goldbloom DS, et al: Infertility and eating disorders. Am J Obstet Gynecol 163:1196–1199, 1990

Stice E: Modeling of eating pathology and social reinforcement of the thin-ideal predict onset of bulimic symptoms. Behav Res Ther 36:931–944, 1998

Stice E: Risk and maintenance factors for eating pathology: a meta-analytic review. Psychol Bull 128:825–848, 2002

Striegel-Moore R: Risk factors for eating disorders. Ann N Y Acad Sci 817:98–109, 1997

Strober M, Freeman R, Morrell W: The long-term course of severe anorexia nervosa in adolescents: survival analysis of recovery, relapse, and outcome predictors over 10–15 years in a prospective study. Int J Eat Disord 22:339–360, 1997

Stunkard AJ, Allison KC: Two forms of disordered eating in obesity: binge eating and night eating. Int J Obes Relat Metab Disord 27:1–12, 2003

Stunkard A, Berkowitz R, Tanrikut C, et al: d-Fenfluramine treatment of binge eating disorder. Am J Psychiatry 153:1455–1459, 1996

Swenne I, Larsson PT: Heart risk associated with weight loss in anorexia nervosa and eating disorders: risk factors for QTc interval prolongation and dispersion. Acta Paediatr 88: 304–309, 1999

Wade TD, Bulik CM, Sullivan FP, et al: The relation between risk factors for binge eating and bulimia nervosa: a population-based female twin study. Health Psychol 19:115–123, 2000

Walsh BT, Kissileff HR, Cassidy SM, et al: Eating behavior of women with bulimia. Arch Gen Psychiatry 46:54–58, 1989

Walsh BT, Wong LM, Pesce MA, et al: Hyperamylasemia in bulimia nervosa. J Clin Psychiatry 51:373–377, 1990

Walsh BT, Hadigan CM, Devlin MJ, et al: Long-term outcome of antidepressant treatment for bulimia nervosa. Am J Psychiatry 148:1206–1212, 1991

Walsh BT, Wilson GT, Loeb KL, et al: Medication and psychotherapy in the treatment of bulimia nervosa. Am J Psychiatry 154:523–531, 1997

Watson TL, Bowers WA, Andersen AE: Involuntary treatment of eating disorders. Am J Psychiatry 157:1806–1810, 2000

Wertheim EH, Paxton SJ, Schutz HK, et al: Why do adolescent girls watch their weight? An interview study examining sociocultural pressures to be thin. J Psychosom Res 42:345–355, 1997

Wilfley DE, Agras WS, Telch CF, et al: Group cognitive-behavioral therapy and group interpersonal psychotherapy for the nonpurging bulimic: a controlled comparison. J Consult Clin Psychol 61:296–305, 1993

Wilfley DE, Welch RR, Stein RI, et al: A randomized comparison of group cognitive-behavioral therapy and group interpersonal psychotherapy for the treatment of overweight individuals with binge eating disorder. Arch Gen Psychiatry 59:713–721, 2002

Wilson GT: Eating disorders and addictive disorders, in Eating Disorders and Obesity: A Comprehensive Handbook, 2nd Edition. Edited by Fairburn CG, Brownell KD. New York, Guilford, 2002, pp 199–203

Wilson GT, Fairburn CG: Treatments for eating disorders, in A Guide to Treatments That Work. Edited by Nathan PE, Gorman JM. New York, Oxford University Press, 2002, pp 559–592

Zuercher JN, Cumella EJ, Woods BK, et al: Efficacy of voluntary nasogastric tube feeding in female inpatients with anorexia nervosa. JPEN J Parenter Enteral Nutr 27:268–276, 2003

16 Sleep Disorders

Lois E. Krahn, M.D.

Jarrett W. Richardson, M.D.

OBTAINING SUFFICIENT QUANTITY and quality of sleep is important for good health. Chronic partial sleep deprivation, also known as insufficient sleep, is common in our society. The consequences include depressed mood, interpersonal irritability, decreased daytime vigilance, and cognitive impairment (Pilcher and Huffcutt 1996). However, determining the appropriate amount of required sleep is difficult for several reasons. Sleep duration gradually decreases from a starting length of 16 hours per 24-hour day as human beings make the transition from infancy to adulthood. Interindividual differences in the optimal amount of sleep range from 6 to 12 hours with a mean of 7.5 hours for adults. When a primary sleep disorder, such as obstructive sleep apnea, is present, the continuity and depth of sleep may be compromised independently of sleep duration. These complexities preclude a simplistic identification of a precise target of sleep duration for any individual. Nonetheless, there is consensus that chronically inadequate sleep is detrimental.

Physiological Mechanisms of Normal Sleep

Sleep can be subdivided into two major components: rapid eye movement sleep (REM), which is characterized by high levels of cortical activation in the presence of muscle atonia to prevent corresponding movements, and non–rapid eye movement sleep (NREM), which consists of four stages. Table 16–1 summarizes the characteristics and percentage of time spent in each sleep stage by healthy, middle-aged adults.

Normal sleep progresses from wakefulness to stage I NREM sleep. From this stage of twilight sleep, a patient can be easily awakened by environmental stimuli. Stage II NREM sleep is deeper, and moderate environmental stimuli, such as a crack of thunder, no longer cause arousal but rather result in a distinctive electrophysiological event, the K complex. Sleep spindles and K complexes are used to identify stage II sleep. When the electroencephalographic (EEG) tracing slows until at least 20% of the activity consists of higher-voltage slow waves, the sleep is rated stage III or IV. These two deeper sleep stages are also known collectively as *delta wave sleep*, *deep sleep*, and *slow wave sleep*. A person awakes from this sleep only when environmental stimuli are marked, such as the prolonged loud noise of an alarm.

As the normal sleep cycle progresses, the EEG activity gradually returns to the most common stage, stage II sleep. Stage II sleep evolves into the first REM sleep episode of the night. REM sleep consists of high-frequency EEG activity, episodic bursts of vertical eye movements, muscle atonia, and penile tumescence. The first REM episode is often brief and typically occurs 70–100 minutes after the person falls asleep. There is marked interindividual variability in arousal threshold in REM sleep (Carskadon and Dement 1994). The sleep cycle repeats four or five times during the night, subsequent REM episodes being of longer duration. In general, slow wave sleep is more common early in the night, and REM periods become longer toward morning. Because the last REM episode occurs at the very end of the major sleep period, people recall their dreams, and men experience morning erections.

The data in Table 16–1 are useful as normative data because sleep study reports typically describe the percentage of the night spent in each complete stage, and thus subjects with normal sleep patterns can be compared with subjects who are patients. In healthy elderly subjects, the

TABLE 16–1. Sleep stages in healthy adults

Stage	Percentage	Polysomnographic characteristics	Physiological changes
Stage I	2–5	Slow eye movements	Easy to arouse
Stage II	45–55	Spindles, K complexes	More difficult to arouse
Stage III/IV	13–23	Slow EEG frequency	Difficult to arouse
REM	20–25	Rapid eye movements	Variable arousal threshold
		Muscle atonia	Penile engorgement
		Increased EEG frequency	

Note. EEG=electroencephalographic; REM=rapid eye movement.

relative percentage of time spent in slow wave sleep decreases, and sleep is generally more fragmented. Patients with disrupted sleep often spend most of the night in stages I and II and have little slow wave or REM sleep. The exact roles of slow wave sleep and REM sleep in a refreshing night's sleep are not well understood, but significant reductions in either state can lead to undesirable results, including daytime sleepiness, depressed mood, and cognitive impairment. In animal studies, prolonged absolute sleep deprivation has resulted in death attributed to sepsis because of suspected underlying compromise of immune function (Bergmann et al. 1996).

Evaluating Sleep

Office Evaluation

A detailed diagnostic interview and physical examination remain the foundation of the sleep evaluation. Table 16–2 lists the many issues that must be evaluated in an assessment for a possible sleep disorder. The decision to refer for a specialty evaluation and diagnostic testing is based on the findings at the history and physical examination conducted by the primary care provider or referring physician. Sleep studies are not absolutely necessary for some

disorders (e.g., restless legs syndrome) and can be avoided if the classic symptoms of the disease are identified in the absence of any other factors. Clinicians need to obtain both thorough medical and thorough psychiatric histories because many illnesses and disorders can alter sleep. As people age, sleep complaints become more common, not because of primary sleep disorders but because of comorbid conditions (Vitiello et al. 2002). Tables 16–3 and 16–4 list disorders that may lead to sleep problems. Treatment should therefore be concentrated on stabilizing the underlying disease.

Because many patients minimize excessive daytime sleepiness or slowly adapt to it, they may lose insight into the degree of their excessive daytime sleepiness. History from other sources, such as family members, may be necessary. Daytime symptoms related to excessive sleepiness can be evaluated with the brief and convenient Epworth Sleepiness Scale (Table 16–5) (Johns 1991). Unfortunately, no similar scale or questionnaire has been used widely in clinical practice to screen for nocturnal sleep symptoms and disorders.

A detailed interview with a bed partner is of great value, if feasible, especially in regard to snoring and respiratory pauses. The more observant the bed partner, the more likely it is the clinician will be able to obtain a useful history of what actually happens while the patient sleeps.

TABLE 16–2. Selected causes of excessive daytime sleepiness

Primarily neurologic

Restless legs syndrome	Periodic limb movement disorder
Idiopathic narcolepsy or hypersomnia	Narcolepsy caused by lesion near the third ventricle
Delirium	Central sleep apnea
Kleine-Levin syndrome	Prader-Willi syndrome

Primarily medical

Obstructive sleep apnea	Gastroesophageal reflux

Primarily psychiatric

Medication-induced disorder (alcohol, hypnotic, sedative, etc.)	Stimulant withdrawal
Mood disorder	Altered sleep–wake schedule

TABLE 16–3. Selected causes of insomnia

Primarily medical

Obstructive sleep apnea	Angina
Chronic obstructive pulmonary disease	Hypoglycemia
Asthma	Congestive heart failure (orthopnea, paroxysmal nocturnal dyspnea)
Gastroesophageal reflux	Hyperthyroidism
Acute pain	Chronic pain

Primarily neurologic

Central sleep apnea	Restless legs syndrome
Dementia	Fatal familial insomnia

Primarily psychiatric

Medication-induced (xanthines, psychostimulants, etc.)	Withdrawal-related (alcohol, benzodiazepines, etc.)
Psychophysiological insomnia	Sleep state misperception
Anxiety disorders	Mood disorders (depression, mania)
Altered sleep–wake schedule	

Primarily environmental

Community noise (traffic, alarms, neighbors, gunshots, etc.)	Altered temperature (too hot, too cold)

TABLE 16–4. Essential issues in a sleep diagnostic interview of patients and bed partners

Presenting complaint?	Previous sleep evaluations?
Sleep schedule—Parenting issues?	Work schedule—Rotating shifts?
Nap schedule—Frequent or prolonged?	Exercise schedule—Late in the evening?
Sleep environment—Bed partner? Bright light? Noisy? Too hot/cold? Pets?	Insomnia—Early? Middle? Late?
Nocturnal movements?	Sleep walking? Somnambulism? Enuresis?
Excessive daytime somnolence?	Motor vehicle accident?
Cataplexy? Sleep paralysis? Hallucinogenic experiences?	Alcohol, street drug, or caffeine use, abuse, or dependence?
Observed apnea?	Sleep position?
Gastrointestinal reflux—Diagnosed? Partially treated?	Pain—Chronic? Acute? Medications wear off?
Erectile problems?	Snoring?
Depression, mania, or panic attacks?	Vivid dreams, nightmares?
Prescription drug use, abuse, or dependence?	Herbal preparations?
Family sleep history	Childhood sleep history

Sometimes, even if the patient sleeps alone, a family member can provide useful information if the partner moved out of a shared bedroom because of intolerable snoring or unusual behaviors. Although this interview results in limited specific information about current symptoms, it can clearly raise suspicion that a pathological condition is present.

During the physical examination, the examiner should note the patient's level of alertness (in the waiting room and during the appointment), body mass index, neck circumference, nasopharyngeal abnormalities, thyroid size, pulmonary findings, findings at cardiac auscultation, and cognition. Valuable laboratory tests include measurement of thyroid-stimulating hormone, ferritin, cobalamin, and folate and a complete blood cell count. The findings of

TABLE 16–5. Epworth Sleepiness Scale

Each item is rated 0–3 by the patient

_____ Sitting and reading

_____ Sitting inactive in a public place

_____ Passenger in a car (>60 minutes)

_____ Lying down to rest in the afternoon

_____ Sitting and talking

_____ Sitting after lunch (without alcohol)

_____ Sitting in traffic

Source. Adapted from Johns 1991.

these studies are helpful in identifying medical disorders that can enter into the differential diagnosis of several sleep disorders.

Because of the cost and inconvenience of sleep studies, a clear need exists for cost-effective screening tools for determining which patients are good candidates for more definitive diagnostic testing. In children, careful visualization of tonsillar size has been found highly sensitive and specific as a screening test for obstructive sleep apnea (A. Li et al. 2002). In adults, other factors, the most significant of which is body mass index, confound clinical prediction models that rely solely on the findings of the nasopharyngeal examination. In one large-scale study with a community-based sample, investigators found that in adults, male sex, older age, higher body mass index, greater neck circumference, snoring, and repeated respiratory pauses were all independent correlates of moderate to severe breathing-related sleep disorder (Young et al. 2002b).

Diagnostic Procedures

Techniques for measuring sleep and body functions during sleep have evolved since the initial description of REM sleep in 1953. Currently, most sleep studies are conducted in facilities using sophisticated computerized equipment that is steadily replacing the older paper-and-ink polygraph units. These recording devices typically monitor and store the multiple physiological measurements considered essential for a polysomnographic study (Table 16–6). Trained technologists attend the patient during the study, making adjustments and assisting as needed. Sleep disorders centers designed for the evaluation and treatment of the full spectrum of sleep disorders are free-standing or located in a hospital. Although there is considerable interest in portable systems with which sleep studies can be performed in the patient's home, these systems are not widely available owing to quality and reimbursement issues.

In some tertiary care hospitals, portable polysomnographic equipment can be deployed to the medical–surgical floor or intensive care unit. In selected cases of a primary sleep disorder coexisting with another process, such as severe chronic obstructive pulmonary disease, identifying and treating the sleep disorder may be necessary before a patient can be stabilized and discharged (Olson 2001). Less research has been conducted on how to screen or test for primary sleep disorders in the patient's home or other settings, such as nursing homes. Sleep diaries can be used but often are inaccurate owing to the patient's poor recall of sleep parameters, lack of adherence to daily documentation, or distorted recall (Mercer et al. 2002).

Use of devices such as wrist actigraphs has been studied in the hospital setting, but these devices are used mostly in ambulatory practices (Krahn et al. 1997). Precise determination of sleep–wake status is impossible with actigraphs because the equipment counts limb movements and does not record EEG activity. In addition, specific sleep stages cannot be identified. One distinct advantage of actigraphy, however, is that the compact device can be worn 24 hours per day for 1–4 weeks. This longitudinal monitoring also allows identification of irregular sleep–wake patterns while the patient is living in the community.

Other portable monitoring devices, which do not enable the full complement of measures obtained with polysomnography, have been marketed, but all have limitations. Several models monitor only respiratory function without EEG data. Similarly, overnight pulse oximetry measures only oxygen saturation and heart rate. With this equipment, the clinician does not know heart rhythm, body position, or whether the patient is asleep or awake or in NREM versus REM sleep (Netzer et al. 2001). False-negative results can be obtained from patients with obstructive sleep apnea so severe that that they cannot fall asleep. Oxygen saturation looks deceptively normal while patients are lying awake in bed at night. Only after patients fall asleep do they begin to experience significant oxygen desaturation. The setting of the oximeter unit can greatly influence the appearance of the compressed overnight printout and contribute to false-positive and false-negative impressions regarding sleep-related breathing conditions (Davila et al. 2002). The results should specify the time settings. Setting up the equipment to acquire data with briefer time periods—for example, 3 seconds rather than 12 seconds—is preferable in screening for breathing-related sleep disorder.

TABLE 16–6.   Components of polysomnography

Essentials

Electroencephalography (typically three channels)
Electromyography (surface)—chin and lower extremity
Electro-oculography (two channels)
Electrocardiography
Respiratory effort measurement
Airflow monitoring (nasal pressure or temperature)
Pulse oximetry

Options

Videotaping (conventional or digital) with infrared lighting
Transcutaneous carbon dioxide monitoring
Esophageal pressure monitoring
Esophageal pH monitoring
Additional electromyography (upper extremities, intercostal muscles)
Additional electroencephalography (seizure detection)

Portable equipment that does monitor EEG activity is prone to malfunction owing to displacement during sleep if sleep technologists are not available to rectify a faulty signal or respond to the patient's needs. Given the importance of an accurate diagnosis for determining long-term prognosis and sometimes expensive treatments, the cost of a high-quality, reliable, and monitored sleep study, such as polysomnography, in a sleep laboratory is worthwhile for appropriately chosen patients (Reuven et al. 2001). Polysomnography yields the highest diagnostic accuracy and reduces uncertainty in the evaluation of patients with sleep disorders. Continuous videotaping is helpful for assessing possible parasomnias or unusual nocturnal movements. Sleep technologists can record body position and describe snoring intensity.

The multiple sleep latency test is used to identify disorders of excessive daytime sleepiness, including narcolepsy (Krahn et al. 2001). Patients must first undergo an overnight sleep study for exclusion of other sleep disorders caused by disrupted nocturnal sleep. If the patient has had, at minimum, 6 hours of sleep to preclude sleep deprivation, then a valid multiple sleep latency test can be conducted the next day. Patients are asked to take four or five scheduled naps wearing a simplified set of leads including only EEG, electromyographic, and electrooculographic leads. The test is used to measure initial sleep latency and initial REM latency, if present, for each nap. Patients are asked to stay awake between naps, to refrain from stimulants such as caffeine and prescribed medications, and to undergo drug screening for occult sedative use. The maintenance of wakefulness test is a similar procedure with slight modifications. Instead of being asked to fall asleep, patients are asked to stay awake during four specified daytime sessions (Mitler et al. 1982). The data can be used to document that a patient with a treated sleep disorder such as obstructive sleep apnea or narcolepsy can sustain wakefulness sufficiently to drive or operate equipment requiring sustained vigilance. The result of this test is sometimes used as a marker of successful treatment outcome.

Sleep Disorders

Several disorders that are closely tied to sleep or the 24-hour sleep–wake schedule are generally classified as sleep disorders. Many other disease states, such as tumor growth and chemotherapy tolerability, vary according to a 24-hour schedule, but circadian rhythmicity is not the most prominent feature (Mormont and Levi 2003).

Narcolepsy and Other Disorders of Excessive Daytime Sleepiness

Narcolepsy is a prime example of a disorder with dysfunction of a specific sleep state, in this case REM sleep. Isolated fragments of REM sleep intrude into wakefulness, and the result is the characteristic symptoms that invariably cause excessive daytime sleepiness. Narcolepsy in humans was first described in 1880 by the French neurologist Gelineau (Gelineau 1880). Since that time, this sleep disorder has been observed in several dog breeds as well as in horses and sheep. These naturally occurring animal models have greatly facilitated investigations into the pathophysiological mechanisms of narcolepsy.

Prevalence

Narcolepsy is a more common disorder than many recognize. As a result, the need to identify and treat it offers a valuable opportunity to prevent medical, occupational, and social complications. When patients present with sleepiness, many other conditions, including insufficient sleep and breathing-related sleep disorder, are suspected before narcolepsy is considered. The average delay between onset of symptoms and diagnosis is 10 years.

In a U.S. community sample, narcolepsy was observed to have prevalence of 0.06% (Silber et al. 2001). All cases of narcolepsy met the diagnostic criteria on the basis of excessive daytime sleepiness and laboratory findings. In 64% of these cases the patient had cataplexy. Incidence data from the same study confirmed the long-standing impression that narcolepsy is slightly more common in men (1.72 per 100,000) than women (1.05 per 100,000). The disease most commonly starts in the second decade of life and is a chronic condition.

Narcolepsy is no longer believed to be a familial disease, although a small number of affected families have been identified (Overeem et al. 2001). When narcolepsy is familial, the mode of inheritance is not a simple recessive or dominant one. The debate centers on whether narcolepsy is the result of an autoimmune or neurodegenerative process. The association between 85% of cases of narcolepsy with cataplexy and a specific HLA allele (DQB1*0602) is the basis of postulation about an autoimmune mechanism; despite several investigations, no confirmatory evidence had been found as of early 2004 (Black et al. 2001). The possibility of the presence of an extremely selective degenerative process stems from the autopsy finding of gliosis in the hypothalamus of narcolepsy patients (Thannickal et al. 2000).

Clinical Features

Narcolepsy is characterized by chronic excessive daytime sleepiness with episodic sleep attacks. Approximately 65%–75% of patients with narcolepsy have cataplexy, which is a condition in which an emotional trigger, most commonly laughter, provokes abrupt muscle atonia without loss of consciousness. Other associated symptoms of narcolepsy include sleep paralysis (isolated loss of muscle tone associated with REM in normal sleep) and hypnagogic and hypnopompic hallucinations (vivid dreaming occurring at the time of sleep onset and awakening that can be difficult to distinguish from reality). When related to the dissociated components of REM sleep, such as muscle atonia (cataplexy and sleep paralysis) and vivid dreams (hypnagogic and hypnopompic hallucinations), these phenomena can intrude into wakefulness. Disturbed nocturnal sleep has been added as a fifth part of this constellation of symptoms.

Pathophysiological Mechanism

In 2000, patients with narcolepsy were reported to have undetectable levels of a newly identified neuropeptide, hypocretin (also known as orexin), in cerebrospinal fluid. Hypocretin is synthesized by a small number of neurons in the anterior hypothalamus that project widely throughout the central nervous system (CNS). After studies of other sleep and neurological disorders, the absence of this neuropeptide appears to be highly specific (99%) for narcolepsy (Mignot et al. 2002). Hypocretin influences sleep, appetite, and temperature. As of early 2004, the relevance of hypocretin as a neuromodulator in diseases other than narcolepsy was unknown. The genes for the ligands and receptors for hypocretin have been knocked out in mice with the development of excessive sleepiness, cataplexy, and obesity (Smart and Jerman 2002).

Investigation

The most important part of an evaluation for narcolepsy is a careful interview conducted as a screen for long-standing excessive daytime sleepiness and spells triggered by emotions. The definitive bedside test for cataplexy is demonstrating the transient absence of deep tendon reflexes during the episode (Krahn et al. 2000). This procedure also aids in differentiating cataplexy from pseudocataplexy (Krahn et al. 2001b). However, cataplexy is difficult to provoke, and the episode is often too short-lived to allow a physical examination.

In most cases diagnostic testing in a sleep disorders center is necessary to supplement the clinical interview. The diagnosis must be as certain as possible before a life-long course of treatment is begun. An overnight sleep study is important for ruling out other causes of excessive daytime sleepiness. This study is ideally preceded by wrist actigraphy to confirm adequate sleep in the weeks before testing and to eliminate sleep deprivation as the cause. If polysomnography reveals that the patient has obstructive sleep apnea or another primary sleep disorder, these conditions must be stabilized before reliable daytime testing can be conducted. The multiple sleep latency test quantifies the time to fall asleep during daytime naps and confirms the presence of inappropriate daytime REM sleep. Testing for hypocretin in the cerebrospinal fluid is not yet part of clinical practice.

Complications

Narcolepsy is associated with a reduction in quality of life beyond that of epilepsy (Broughton and Broughton 1994). Without treatment, patients are at risk of motor vehicle accidents and occupational injuries related to sleepiness. Patients with narcolepsy have a higher-than-expected rate of obstructive sleep apnea, REM sleep behavior disorder, and periodic limb movements (Krahn et al. 2001a). New data indicate that patients with narcolepsy have higher rates of obesity, which may be linked to the hypocretin deficiency. Current pharmacological treatments for sleepiness do not appear to have a significant mitigating effect on weight gain (Schuld et al. 2002).

Treatment

Treatment options for narcolepsy include methylphenidate or amphetamines, which target excessive daytime sleepiness (Mitler and Hayduk 2002). More-extended-release preparations of methylphenidate and amphetamines have the advantage of continuous drug delivery, which reduces the daytime variability in alertness that may occur with the immediate-release forms, which are taken twice or three times a day. Modafinil is a unique wake-promoting medication that was approved by the U.S. Food and Drug Administration (FDA) in 1999. Modafinil is not considered a psychostimulant and lacks sympathomimetic activity, and the mechanism of action is not well understood (U.S. Modafinil in Narcolepsy Multicenter Study Group, 1998). The newest treatment option is sodium oxybate (also known as gamma-hydroxybutyrate), which was approved by the FDA in 2002. This novel hypnotic is approved specifically for the treatment of cataplexy. An endogenous substance, sodium oxybate increases the amount of slow wave sleep and improves the continuity of sleep (Lammers et al. 1993). Improving the quality of nocturnal sleep appears to reduce the severity of all of the classic narcolepsy symptoms. Because of the expense and inconvenience of consuming a liquid medication at sleep onset and 4 hours later, this medication is reserved for patients whose condition is more refractory to treatment. Taken as prescribed, sodium oxybate is well tolerated in general. Risks arise from combining it with other sedative agents and taking it in excessive amounts. Tricyclic antidepressants and, to a lesser degree, selective serotonin reuptake inhibitors (SSRIs) historically have been used to treat cataplexy. These agents increase the level of norepinephrine in the brain and thus suppress REM sleep–related symptoms. Patient education should emphasize the importance of a consistent sleep–wake schedule, the need for adequate sleep, the value of brief daytime naps, and refraining from driving a car when sleepy.

Idiopathic Hypersomnia

Idiopathic hypersomnia is a disorder of unknown etiology characterized by excessive daytime sleepiness without other specific symptoms. Patients typically have a prolonged duration of nocturnal sleep as well as unrefreshing daytime naps. The prevalence of idiopathic hypersomnia is unknown, but the condition appears to develop at equal rates in both male and female patients. As in narcolepsy, symptoms first appear in adolescence or young adulthood. This condition increases the risk of motor vehicle accidents and occupational or educational problems due to sleepiness. Depression may be another consequence (Bassetti and Aldrich 1997).

The clinical interview should concentrate on the duration of excessive daytime sleepiness, the sleep–wake schedule, and the presence of mood disorders. The presence of a mood disorder complicates the evaluation because both depression and antidepressant medications can alter sleep architecture. The evaluation for idiopathic hypersomnia consists of wrist actigraphy, polysomnography, multiple sleep latency testing, and drug screening. Special attention is paid to respiratory arousals, which can indicate the presence of upper airway resistance syndrome or subclinical sleep-related breathing disorder as the cause of persisting excessive daytime sleepiness. The diagnosis of idiopathic hypersomnia is established on the basis of the finding of quantifiable excessive daytime sleepiness on the multiple sleep latency test. Unlike patients with narcolepsy, those with idiopathic hypersomnia have no sleep-onset REM episodes and have normal levels of hypocretin in the cerebrospinal fluid.

The treatment approach to idiopathic hypersomnia, which includes patient education and medications, is similar to that used for narcolepsy. Daytime naps are not encouraged because they are not refreshing, as they are for patients with narcolepsy. Once sleep tests are completed,

use of an antidepressant is appropriate and does not cause problems if the results at evaluation suggest the presence of a coexisting mood disorder.

Kleine-Levin syndrome, also known as recurrent hypersomnia, is an important part of the differential diagnosis of idiopathic hypersomnia. Patients with recurrent hypersomnia are generally male adolescents who engage in binge eating and have periodic hypersomnia that lasts several weeks (Minvielle 2000).

Parasomnias

Parasomnias are disorders in which patients have inappropriate intermittent motor behaviors during sleep. REM sleep behavior disorder is arguably of most interest because of the relationship with other neurological conditions. Patients with REM sleep behavior disorder appear to "act out their dreams" by yelling or gesturing during REM sleep. They lack the muscle atonia normally found in REM sleep and move in response to dream imagery. REM sleep behavior disorder appears more common than originally suspected, although the prevalence has not been established. Risk factors for this sleep disorder are male sex (90% of patients described in the literature) and advanced age (most patients have been 50 years or older) (Olson et al. 2000). SSRIs and venlafaxine have been suggested as possible triggers. Patients and their bed partners can be seriously injured by hitting, kicking, rolling, and other more complex behaviors. REM sleep behavior disorder is associated with several neurological disorders, including Parkinson's disease (15%–33% of patients), multiple system atrophy (69%–90%), and dementia with Lewy bodies (prevalence of REM sleep behavior disorder unknown) (Comella et al. 1998; Plazzi et al. 1997). These neurodegenerative disorders share the pathological finding of cerebral intracellular inclusion bodies containing alpha-synuclein.

Polysomnography with extra electromyographic leads and synchronized videotaping can be useful for documenting increased electromyographic tone during REM sleep. Some patients have an inappropriate degree of muscle tone without reports of disruptive or inappropriate behaviors. These patients are not yet considered to have REM sleep behavior disorder, but the disease may evolve. Polysomnography also helps identify complicating disorders, such as obstructive sleep apnea, which is of particular importance if benzodiazepines are used later. Nocturnal seizures should be excluded from the diagnosis. Treatment includes modifying the bedroom to reduce injury to the patient and bed partner. Bed partners often choose to sleep apart. Clonazepam has become the medication of choice because it reduces the muscle movement that occurs during REM sleep, reducing the risk of injury (Schenck and Mahowald 1990).

NREM parasomnias, unlike REM sleep behavior disorder, are markedly more common in children and adolescents than in adults. Patients act unusually, walk, or eat when not fully alert. Polysomnography is not always needed because the behaviors are often intermittent and therefore difficult to observe with a single night of monitoring. Sleep deprivation, shifting bedtimes, and consumption of alcohol can precipitate episodes in susceptible individuals. In one study sleep deprivation was used as a trigger of sleepwalking. The intriguing results indicated that this test may be a means of confirming the diagnosis or increasing the likelihood that an episode will occur during polysomnography (Joncas et al. 2002).

Treatment of NREM parasomnias includes modifying the sleeping environment to promote safety, a consistent sleep schedule, and, if warranted, medications such as hypnotics to prevent arousal (Mahowald and Schenck 1996). The relationship between parasomnias and posttraumatic stress disorder is unclear and merits further study.

Nocturnal panic disorder is increasingly regarded as a rare disorder. However, panic disorder with attacks occurring both during the day and at night is not rare. Treatment of this condition ideally includes a combination of medications and behavioral measures. When panic or anxiety exists exclusively at night, most typically in NREM sleep, a broad differential diagnosis should be used to screen for breathing-related sleep disorder, nightmares, and medical disorders (e.g., arrhythmia, angina, and gastroesophageal reflux) triggering the anxiety. Confirmed treatment of nocturnal panic disorder relies on medications because behavioral measures are less feasible when an attack develops while the patient sleeps. Hypnosis at bedtime has been tried (Hauri et al. 1989).

Whenever a patient presents with unusual behavior at night, the differential diagnosis must include epilepsy. In particular, seizures arising from a locus in the frontal lobe can result in stereotypical but bizarre events during slow wave sleep (Dyken et al. 2001).

Sleep-Related Breathing Disorder and Snoring

Sleep-related breathing disorder comprises obstructive sleep apnea, central sleep apnea, and obesity hypoventilation syndrome. Obstructive sleep apnea is the most notable of these conditions because of its high prevalence and association with numerous medical conditions if untreated (Walker 2001). Obstructive apnea is defined as cessation of airflow that lasts at least 10 seconds owing to impedance of respiratory effort as the result of airway obstruction. Hypopnea is defined as reduction in airflow resulting in at least a 4% decrease in oxygen saturation. Table 16–7 outlines the diagnostic criteria for obstructive sleep apnea. Apnea and hypopnea both are considered clinically significant markers of disease and as a result are reported together as the apnea–hypopnea index. Since these criteria were published, sleep specialists have recognized that hypopnea with an oxygen desaturation greater than or equal to 4% must be quantified in addition to pure apnea.

Prevalence

Patients with obstructive sleep apnea are the largest subgroup of patients referred to sleep disorders centers. This disorder, which affects at least 2% of women and 4% of men ages 30–60 years (Young et al. 1993), is strongly associated with obesity. Obstructive sleep apnea is more common without marked obesity in several racial groups, including Asians, in whom craniofacial anatomic features can produce a narrower nasopharyngeal airway (K. Li et al. 2000). Advanced age, male sex, and postmenopausal state are all associated with a higher prevalence of this condition (Young et al. 2002a). In subpopulations of patients with hypertension, heart disease, and adult-onset diabetes mellitus, as many as 30%–40% of patients can have obstructive sleep apnea (Partinen 1995).

TABLE 16–7. American Academy of Sleep Medicine diagnostic criteria for obstructive sleep apnea

Essential signs and symptoms
1. Excessive daytime sleepiness
2. Obstructed breathing during sleep

Essential polysomnographic findings
1. More than five episodes of apnea (>10 seconds) per hour of sleep with evidence of respiratory muscle effort and one of the following:
   a. Apnea causing frequent arousals
   b. Apnea causing oxygen desaturation ≥4%
   c. Bradytachycardia

Source. Adapted from American Academy of Sleep Medicine 1997.

Clinical Features

Most patients with obstructive sleep apnea snore. Family members may observe disruptive snoring intermixed with quiet periods and reduced respiration. Although essentially all patients with obstructive sleep apnea snore, the reverse is not the case. Snoring is an extremely common phenomenon in the community, affecting 25% of men and 15% of women. For this reason, screening for obstructive sleep apnea must rely on more than simply a history of snoring. Patients may have restless sleep at times, to the point they are believed to have a parasomnia such as REM sleep behavior disorder. Excessive sweating and morning headaches can be present. Patients may report choking or being awakened by their snoring. An increased rate of nocturia has been described, possibly because the patient is more aware of bladder fullness when awakened by the breathing disorder (Pressman et al. 1996). Obstructive apnea can lead to respiratory arousals and oxygen desaturation, which can cause transient elevations in blood pressure initially at night (Dart et al. 2003). Hypertension is common, especially in patients with severe obstructive sleep apnea. Initially, blood pressure increases follow each obstructive event, but if apneic or hypopneic episodes are frequent, blood pressure can remain elevated throughout the night and day. Pulmonary hypertension also has been an associated finding, particularly with severe obstructive sleep apnea.

The hemodynamic alterations of obstructive sleep apnea include systemic hypertension, increased right and left ventricular afterload, and increased cardiac output. Earlier reports attributed the association between obstructive sleep apnea and cardiovascular disease to the common risk factors such as age, sex, and obesity. However, newer epidemiological data confirm an independent association between obstructive sleep apnea and these cardiovascular diseases. Possible mechanisms include a combination of intermittent hypoxia and hypercapnia, repeated arousals, sustained increase in sympathetic tone, increased platelet aggregation, reduced baroreflex sensitivity, and elevated plasma fibrinogen and homocysteine levels (Bananian et al. 2002).

Pathophysiological Mechanism

Patients with obstructive sleep apnea experience intermittent compromise of the upper airway. The most common site of obstruction is the pharynx, a hollow tube that collapses during swallowing and speech. The pharyngeal musculature serves to keep the upper airway open and opposes the subatmospheric pressure in the pharynx itself. The genioglossus muscles also pull forward to keep the upper airway clear of obstruction. This balance is further influenced by anatomic structures (adipose tissue, tongue size, mandibular length, soft palate, and tonsils) and neuromuscular mechanisms (activity of the pharyngeal muscles affected by sleep state, muscle relaxant, and hypnotic medications) (Rama et al. 2002). The obstructed upper airway leads to cessation or reduction of airflow that results in the finding of an arousal on the EEG tracing. Some patients have marked respiratory arousals without actual apnea or partial apnea (hypopnea). Snoring or increased effort to ventilate due to narrowing but not full

collapse of the airway is called *upper airway resistance syndrome*, a potentially distressing but subclinical form of obstructive sleep apnea that occurs more often in women than in men (Guilleminault et al. 2001).

Diagnostic Testing

Results of polysomnography conducted in a sleep disorders center are the standard of reference for the diagnosis of breathing-related sleep disorder (Bresnitz et al. 1994). Other screening techniques, such as overnight pulse oximetry and use of portable devices, have not been demonstrated to be cost-effective, reliable, or sufficiently sensitive. Many centers use "split-night" sleep studies, often in response to reimbursement issues. Under these circumstances, patients are observed for at least 2 hours while they are sleeping, ideally experiencing both NREM and REM sleep in both the supine and nonsupine positions. Once a diagnosis of breathing-related sleep disorder is established, the technologist introduces treatments such as nasal continuous positive airway pressure (CPAP). Nasal CPAP is applied through a nasal mask connected to a blower that can be adjusted so that pressurized air is delivered to the upper airway. Having positive pressure keep open the airway is particularly important during expiration, when the airway most commonly collapses in patients with obstructive sleep apnea. The nasal CPAP pressure setting can be carefully titrated in response to airway narrowing during the rest of the sleep study. In the morning, the patient can be asked about comfort and acceptance of this therapy. A split-night study is an opportunity for clinician and patient to compare the untreated versus the newly treated state. The procedure is controversial because of the limited time available for both the diagnostic study and the treatment trial. In most cases, a split-night study eliminates the need for a second night in the laboratory (Strollo et al. 1996).

Complications

The complications of obstructive sleep apnea lead to significant morbidity and mortality. Risk factors for obstructive sleep apnea (see section "Evaluating Sleep" earlier in this chapter) are male sex, older age, high body mass index, greater neck circumference, snoring, and observed pauses in breathing at night (Young et al. 2002b). Untreated obstructive sleep apnea has been associated with systemic hypertension, right-sided heart failure, and cerebrovascular accidents (Dyken et al. 1996). The excessive daytime sleepiness that can result from untreated obstructive sleep apnea can put patients at risk of motor vehicle accidents, cognitive problems, and interpersonal difficulties. An association once was found between obstructive sleep apnea and gastroesophageal reflux; however, more recent work indicated that one condition does not appear to cause the other. Nevertheless, treatment with antireflux medication reduces arousals but not apneic episodes, and intervention for obstructive sleep apnea with nasal CPAP does reduce reflux (Ing et al. 2000).

Treatment

Since the early 1980s, the treatment of obstructive sleep apnea has been revolutionized by the use of nasal CPAP. This treatment involves delivering pressurized air (typically 3–18 cm of water pressure) to sites of upper airway collapse (generally the oropharynx and less commonly the nasopharynx) and forcing the airway open. Apnea and snoring are eliminated, allowing the patient to sleep continuously without being aroused to breathe. Nasal CPAP is generally introduced when the patient is sleeping in the sleep laboratory, where staff can adjust the pressure appropriately and assist with mask fit. Newer technology entails the use of self-titrating devices that modify the pressure setting breath by breath without requiring technologist involvement (Berry et al. 2002). The extent to which these more sophisticated machines may replace nasal CPAP titrations conducted in a sleep laboratory is not clear.

Patients with severe obstructive sleep apnea often report marked improvement, within days, in their mood and energy. This improvement is positive reinforcement that leads to good compliance with nasal CPAP treatment (Sullivan and Grunstein 1994). Patients with mild to moderate obstructive sleep apnea have more adherence problems, the compliance rate being estimated at 10%–50%. Even patients who use this device nightly typically use it for only several hours (Clark et al. 1996).

Patients with obstructive sleep apnea who consume alcohol close to bedtime pose a challenge, because alcohol has been observed to decrease the neuromuscular tone of the upper airway. These patients often need higher nasal CPAP settings to prevent apnea. In addition, if the sleep study is done when the patient has not been consuming alcohol often, the selected pressure settings are insufficient on nights when the patient has ingested alcohol (Berry et al. 1991). Certain medications, especially long-acting benzodiazepines, can exert a similar effect and can depress the reticular activating system to reduce the arousal threshold and prevent arousals that effectively interrupt prolonged episodes of apnea (Dolly and Block 1982).

Another treatment of obstructive sleep apnea is bilevel positive airway pressure. This therapy represents a modification of CPAP whereby the positive pressure fluctuates depending on whether the airflow is inspiratory or expiratory. Bilevel pressure therapy is considerably more ex-

pensive than conventional CPAP and is reserved for patients who cannot tolerate CPAP because of discomfort or emergence of central apnea at necessary pressure settings. Supplemental oxygen alone is inadequate for obstructive sleep apnea because the oxygen cannot pass the obstruction to reach the lungs. Patients with both breathing-related sleep disorder and intrinsic lung disease who have persistent hypoxia despite CPAP can benefit from supplemental oxygen delivered through the nasal CPAP mask.

For patients who have apnea only in the supine position, effective treatment may include having them use a device such as a T-shirt with an attached cloth tube of tennis balls (George et al. 1988). This soft lump keeps patients from lying on their backs. Inflatable devices resembling backpacks can serve the same purpose. Few data are available regarding long-term adherence with these practical interventions. Some patients who refuse CPAP and have severe apnea during REM sleep have been offered a REM-suppressant medication such as a monoamine oxidase inhibitor. No published data are available regarding this practice. Abrupt discontinuation of the pharmacological agent should be avoided because of REM rebound, which can increase the risk of apnea.

Weight loss through diet and exercise is an important component of the treatment plan for any overweight patient with breathing-related sleep disorder (Flemons 2002). Motivated patients can succeed. Weight loss should be primary treatment only of patients with mild to moderate disease, particularly if they are not interested in other modalities. Gastric bypass surgery can be especially important for management of medically complicated obesity (see Chapter 30, "Surgery"). In general, a 10-pound weight loss can reduce the required CPAP pressure; however, many patients eventually seem to gain rather than lose weight with the result that CPAP pressure needs to be increased.

Patients with abnormalities of the soft tissue or skeletal structures surrounding the upper airway may consider surgery. Surgical procedures include laser-assisted uvulopalatopharyngoplasty, tonsillectomy, mandibular advancement, and tracheostomy (Littner et al. 2001; Lojander et al. 1996). Patients must be carefully selected. They must have upper airway obstructions that are resectable, for example, large tonsils, and have no other comorbid conditions, such as an elevated body mass index that compromises upper airway patency at multiple points.

There have been promising results with oral appliances that pull the tongue or mandible forward (Clark et al. 1996). Hypnotic agents may be used to treat patients with obstructive sleep apnea, particularly if adherence to nasal CPAP is suboptimal because of discomfort causing insomnia. Medications such as zolpidem and zaleplon have been well tolerated. Benzodiazepines should be used cautiously in the care of patients with obstructive sleep apnea. These agents may prevent a patient from arousing during an episode of apnea and taking a compensatory breath. Some clinicians fear that if patients using benzodiazepines remove the nasal CPAP mask, they may experience longer apnea because they are not aroused when hypoxia develops. Furthermore, nightly use of benzodiazepines may decrease the amount of slow wave sleep and lead to physical dependence.

Central Sleep Apnea and Obesity Hypoventilation

Central sleep apnea and obesity hypoventilation are two additional breathing-related sleep disorders of interest. Central sleep apnea is more likely to be asymptomatic than is obstructive sleep apnea, given that it is less likely to be associated with sleep disruption. Because the patient's airway is not narrowed and vibrating, snoring is not a warning sign. Patients often present with insomnia rather than excessive daytime sleepiness. Patients with central sleep apnea are often older and have associated cardiac or cerebrovascular disease. Central sleep apnea can be differentiated from obstructive sleep apnea by the absence of snoring, this differentiation being confirmed by the presence of polysomnographic features of the apnea (Quaranta et al. 1997). Treatment can include a hypnotic agent to decrease arousals or supplemental oxygen to reduce hypoxia (Guilleminault and Robinson 1998). When central apnea and obstructive sleep apnea coexist, treatment may include CPAP or bilevel positive airway pressure therapy.

In some patients with marked obesity, obstructive sleep apnea with repetitive desaturation is occasionally absent, but patients still have a sleep-related breathing condition. Particularly during REM sleep, when muscle atonia affects all muscles but the diaphragm, patients may be unable to properly ventilate because of the difficulty in expanding their lungs owing to their body mass. In obesity hypoventilation, polysomnography shows persisting oxygen desaturation without the fluctuating cessation of airflow and oxygen desaturation that occur in obstructive sleep apnea. Arterial blood gas panels typically reveal hypercapnia (Kessler et al. 2002). Obese patients commonly have both obesity hypoventilation and obstructive sleep apnea, in which case CPAP is indicated. Other treatment options include weight loss, avoiding any factor that may aggravate hypoventilation (e.g., discontinuing sedatives), CPAP with supplemental oxygen, and bilevel positive airway pressure therapy.

Restless Legs Syndrome and Periodic Limb Movements

Patients with restless legs syndrome describe subjective discomfort of the lower extremities that worsens at night. Patients can have an irresistible need to move their legs in bed or during prolonged periods of sedentary activity, such as airplane flights. This condition was first described by Ekblom in 1945. As a result of these distressing symptoms, patients can experience insomnia or have unrefreshing sleep.

Prevalence

Restless legs syndrome is often unrecognized but is far from rare. For years, all data about this condition were collected in clinical settings and the prevalence in community samples was essentially unknown. A community-based survey showed a prevalence of restless legs syndrome of 3% in respondents ages 18–29 years, 10% in those ages 30–79 years, and 19% in those age 80 years and older. The overall prevalence was 10% with equal rates for male and female respondents. In the study, risk factors for restless legs syndrome were identified as greater age and high body mass index as well as nicotine dependence, diabetes mellitus, and lack of exercise (Phillips et al. 2000). Another survey of community-dwelling adults in five European countries had slightly different findings. The prevalence of restless legs syndrome according to the criteria of the International Classification of Sleep Disorders (Table 16–8) was 5.5% and associated with older age, female sex, musculoskeletal disease, hypertension, use of an SSRI, and engaging in physical activities close to bedtime (Ohayon and Roth 2002).

Restless legs syndrome sometimes occurs in association with anemia and iron deficiency. The condition can develop during the third trimester of pregnancy, likely because of the presence of functional anemia (Allen and Earley 2001a). Case reports have shown that patients with restless legs syndrome who donate blood may have an exacerbation of the condition, which warrants more medication. Patients with restless legs syndrome should care-

---

TABLE 16–8. Clinical characteristics of restless legs syndrome

Desire to move the limbs because of subjective discomfort

Motor restlessness

Symptoms worse or exclusively associated with sedentary activities

Symptoms at least partially relieved by activity

Symptoms worse in the evening or night

fully consider the condition a risk of donating blood (Silber and Richardson 2003).

Restless legs syndrome is known to be secondary to diabetes, peripheral neuropathy, and uremia; 20%–30% of patients with renal failure experience restless legs syndrome (Winkelmann et al. 1996). Familial occurrence of restless legs syndrome has been described. In several large families, an autosomal dominant mode of inheritance has been observed. In a large French Canadian kindred, restless legs syndrome was mapped to chromosome 12q (Desautels et al. 2001). In familial restless legs syndrome, the disorder can have a childhood onset.

Clinical Features

Periodic limb movement disorder is a condition that frequently overlaps with restless legs syndrome. Approximately 80% of patients with restless legs syndrome have intermittent muscle twitches called periodic limb movements (Montplaisir et al. 1997). These movements are involuntary leg jerks that occur at night. They can cause insomnia and, as a result, excessive daytime sleepiness. Almost all patients with restless legs syndrome have periodic limb movements, but many patients with periodic limb movements have no symptoms (Chaudhuri et al. 2001). The periodic limb movements can affect a variety of muscles in the legs or arms. Periodic limb movements in the absence of subjective symptoms of restlessness are of uncertain clinical significance (Nicolas et al. 1999).

Periodic limb movements must be differentiated from nocturnal leg cramps, which are extremely painful sustained muscle contractions, particularly involving the gastrocnemius and soleus muscles. Predisposing factors include pregnancy, diabetes mellitus, electrolyte disturbances, and prior vigorous exercise. Nocturnal leg cramps are not periodic and usually occur, at most, several times a night. The differential diagnosis of restless legs syndrome and periodic limb movement disorder includes neuropathic pain, arthritis, restless insomnia, and drug-induced akathisia.

Complications

Patients with restless legs syndrome experience irritability, depressed mood, or cognitive disturbance due to disturbed sleep; headache, especially on awakening; depressed mood; social isolation; and reduced libido (Ulfberg et al. 2001).

Pathophysiological Mechanism

Restless legs syndrome is believed to be a condition associated with decreased dopamine levels. Treatment with dopamine antagonists aggravates the symptoms, and this syndrome occurs with increased frequency in Parkinson's disease. Positron emission tomographic studies of restless legs syndrome have shown decreased dopaminergic functioning in the caudate and putamen regions of the brain (Ruottinen et al. 2000). Treatment with dopaminergic agonists, even low doses, leads to marked improvement. Restless legs syndrome has been strongly associated with anemia. Deficient iron stores appear to play a role in the pathophysiological mechanism because iron is hypothesized to be a cofactor for tyrosine hydroxylase, the enzyme for the rate-limiting step in the synthesis of dopamine (Earley et al. 2000).

Diagnostic Testing

A rating scale for restless legs syndrome has facilitated diagnosis (Allen and Earley, 2001b). Attempts to develop a self-administered screening survey for restless legs syndrome in dialysis populations have been less successful because of low specificity and a high false-positive rate (Cirignotta et al. 2002).

An overnight sleep study is not essential, because the diagnosis of restless legs syndrome can be based on the patient's history. Polysomnography is valuable when a patient may have a coexisting sleep disorder, such as obstructive sleep apnea, or if the patient does not respond to treatment of restless legs syndrome diagnosed on the basis of history alone. Useful laboratory tests include complete blood count to assess for anemia and ferritin, especially when levels are less than 50 μg/L.

Treatment

Treatment of restless legs syndrome is primarily with dopaminergic medications. Direct dopamine receptor agonists, such as pramipexole, have become first-line agents (Comella 2002). These drugs have replaced low-dose, controlled-release carbidopa and levodopa because of a lower incidence of side effects and improved efficacy. There have been encouraging reports about the benefits of gabapentin (Garcia-Borreguero et al. 2002). Long-acting benzodiazepines, such as clonazepam, and opioids, including codeine and methadone, also have been used. Medications that can lead to physical dependence require careful monitoring for tolerance. As a result, these drugs are not preferred treatment choices. Most clinicians use drug treatment of restless legs syndrome. Nonpharmacological options include physical therapy.

Insomnia

As outlined in Table 16–4, insomnia can be caused by a variety of medical, neurological, psychiatric, and environmental conditions. If possible, any factors that cause or exacerbate insomnia, such as gastric regurgitation, should be corrected (Konermann et al. 2002; Ohayon and Roth 2003). However, many patients have no specific triggers of insomnia, and insomnia is not a symptom of an underlying disorder.

Patients with the classic type of, or psychophysiological (conditioned), insomnia learn to associate sleeplessness with certain circumstances, such as their own bedrooms. These patients become progressively more tense as bedtime approaches. The prevalence of this condition is unknown. Polysomnography is not generally useful in establishing the diagnosis. Sometimes a patient's best sleep in years occurs in the unfamiliar setting of the sleep disorders center (Chesson et al. 2000).

Treatment

Treatment of insomnia includes improvement in sleep hygiene with the techniques listed in Table 16–9; behavioral techniques, such as relaxation strategies including tapes, self-hypnosis, and music; and occasional doses of hypnotic medication (Toney and Ereshefsky 2000).

More medications are now available that were specifically developed as hypnotics. The newer nonbenzodiazepine hypnotics zolpidem and zaleplon have a short half-life that reduces the morning hangover effect. Patients have been shown to have alertness adequate for driving and other activities that require sustained vigilance (Richardson et al. 2001). Physical dependence has not been reported with the short-term use approved by the FDA. Benzodiazepines, although less expensive than nonbenzodiazepine hypnotics, can cause dependence and alter cognition the morning after use. Several antidepressants with prominent sedative side effects, such as mirtazapine and trazodone, are valuable therapeutic options, especially if the patient has a coexisting mood or anxiety disorder. Mirtazapine has prominent antihistaminergic side effects at doses of 15 mg or less; however, undesirable weight gain can occur (Artigas et al. 2002). Because of cardiac and anticholinergic side effects, tricyclic antidepressants should seldom be used expressly for insomnia. Antihistamines such as diphenhydramine are generally a poor choice because they quickly lose effectiveness and can exacerbate confusion in the medically ill. Hypnotic medications have an important role in the management of short-term or intermittent insomnia, but most sleep specialists prefer a meaningful trial of nonpharmacological interventions in the care of patients with the chronic form of primary insomnia. The intent is to alter the thoughts and behaviors that lead to the development of poor-quality nocturnal sleep.

TABLE 16–9.   Sleep hygiene

Circadian issues

Avoid daytime naps

Limit time in bed to 8 hours

Get daily exercise, preferably finishing at least 4 hours before bedtime

Keep regular sleep–wake cycle 7 days per week

Avoid bright light in the evening or at night

Seek bright light in the morning

Reducing sleep disruption

Avoid large quantities of fluids in the evening

Minimize caffeine; a hot drink without caffeine may be beneficial

Avoid alcoholic drinks

Keep the bedroom quiet, dark, and at a comfortable temperature

Develop a relaxing bedtime ritual

Avoid worrying in bed by using tools such as list writing during the day

Manage stress optimally during the day

Do not use the bed and bedroom except for sleep and for sexual activity

Get assistance with pets and children

Avoid large meals soon before bedtime

Pursue medical intervention for problems such as gastroesophageal reflux, pain, and nausea

More specific behavioral studies have produced basic information about sleep habits that can be helpful to patients who have disturbed sleep. These sleep hygiene factors have been found to have particular efficacy in the care of patients with chronic insomnia. Establishing a regular waking time 7 days a week optimizes biological rhythms. This regimen is particularly helpful for patients who need to keep morning commitments but tend to naturally be "night owls" or have problems falling asleep at the needed bedtime. However, the clock tends to drift rapidly back to the old schedule as soon as there is variability in arising time (Brown et al. 2002). Discipline and consistency are important.

When regular exercise is an option, exercising in the late afternoon several hours before bedtime may improve sleep. One postulated mechanism is that a decrease in body temperature is associated with sleep, and body temperature decreases approximately 4 hours after exercise (Montgomery and Dennis 2002). Avoiding "clock watching" can help reduce the arousal effects of becoming annoyed when tracking the slow passage of time throughout the night. Most people recall only periods of wakefulness at night, so clock watching can reinforce the perception that no sleep has occurred. Patients should avoid alcohol, nonprescribed sedatives, and stimulants, including nicotine and caffeine at any time during the day. Patients, particularly patients prone to gastroesophageal reflux, should not sleep on a full stomach. Introducing relaxing routines around bedtime can be helpful to many patients with sleep complaints. Treating gastroesophageal reflux with antacids and histamine$_2$-blocking medication before sleep can be beneficial.

More specific behavioral evaluation may lead to suggestions that a patient learn relaxation techniques or develop stress management strategies (Morin et al. 1999). Psychotherapy can be helpful for sleep-related anxiety. One of the techniques recommended to those who find that they spend inordinate amounts of time worrying when awake at night is called "worry time" or "thinking time." This technique entails the recommendation that patients take 15–30 minutes in the late afternoon or early evening (not near sleep onset) during which there is time to devote attention to worries. Patients are expected to use this time to list their concerns and then identify which they may be able to have some control over and which they do not. When patients awaken at night and begin to worry about a "new" problem, this worry is added to the list, to be included in the next day's session. Eventually the energy and time spent worrying at night diminish, and wakefulness is not perpetuated by anxious thought content (Hauri and Esther 1990).

Stimulus control techniques have been used to help patients with psychophysiological, or conditioned, insomnia (Bootzin and Perlis 1992). These patients find they are sleepy near bedtime, but as soon as they enter the sleeping environment, they become aroused and unable to sleep. This conditioned association between sleeplessness and the bedroom may need to be interrupted by instructing patients to avoid "trying to sleep." Patients who find they are hyperaroused while lying in bed should not try to sleep. They are advised instead to get up and go to a different setting and engage in a different activity (e.g., reading a book, watch relaxing television, or listening to music) until they become sleepy again and return to bed. They should repeat this process as often and as long as needed to extinguish the arousal state conditioned to the bedroom. Some patients find that rather than getting out of bed or leaving the bedroom, they can achieve the same results by watching a monotonous videotape in the bedroom with the VCR set to turn off automatically (Pallesen et al. 2003).

For patients with severe persistent insomnia, a sleep restriction management method may be helpful. In this modality, patients are instructed to allow no more hours in bed than they estimated they slept the previous night. Initially this period may be considerably less than 7.5 hours. When they are able to sleep for essentially all the time in bed for several nights, patients are advised to increase their time in bed by half-hour increments until they achieve optimal sleep time and sleep efficiency. Although pharmacological and behavioral treatments are effective for insomnia management over the initial weeks of treatment, results of a randomized, controlled trial of these treatments in the care of elderly patients suggested that behavioral treatment was associated with more sustained improvement than was pharmacological therapy (Morin et al. 1999). Other findings suggested that, if possible, behavioral techniques ought to be tried without concomitant hypnotic medications because patients taking hypnotics appeared not to have as good an outcome as those who did not take the drugs (Hauri 1997). The availability of medication may reduce patients' motivation and confidence in behavioral techniques.

Sleep State Misperception

Sleep state misperception is a rare type of primary insomnia. Patients with this disorder report subjective sleep disturbance that is not consistent with objective data. For the criteria for this diagnosis to be met, polysomnography must demonstrate normal duration and quality of sleep (American Academy of Sleep Medicine 1997). As the understanding of sleep increases, specific sleep disorders may eventually be diagnosed in some of these patients. Treatment involves discussing with the patient the discrepancy between subjective and objective data. Behavioral techniques and hypnotic medications have been used successfully in this group of patients.

Medications and Sleep

Any substance that crosses the blood-brain barrier will very likely have an effect on CNS receptors that affect sleep and wakefulness. Essentially all drugs that have been studied have been found to have such effects, and many that have not been studied are known by clinicians to influence sleep and wakefulness. Growing understanding of the physiological mechanisms of normal and abnormal sleep indicates that in addition to the classically understood brainstem sleep influences, the hypothalamus is a key center for sleep regulation. Sleep mechanisms were thought to be predominantly due to the interactions of acetylcholine, dopamine, serotonin, and norepinephrine primarily within the brainstem. More recent research findings indicated that the hypothalamic neurotransmitters adenosine, dopamine, gamma-aminobutyric acid (GABA), histamine, and hypocretin also play an important role in the physiological mechanisms of sleep. The latest observations suggest that connections between the thalamus (cortical activation, sleep spindle formation, and

EEG synchronization), hypothalamus (sleep–wake switch), suprachiasmatic nucleus (circadian clock), and the brain stem (ascending cortical activation and REM sleep–wake switch) organize circadian, ultradian, and intrinsic sleep function (Mignot et al. 2002).

Some CNS substances primarily affect the circadian pacemaker system, which is controlled by the suprachiasmatic nucleus (arginine-vasopressin, GABA, melatonin, gastrin-releasing peptide, neuropeptide Y, peptide histidine isoleucine, vasoactive intestinal peptide, glutamate, pancreatic polypeptide, and corticosteroids). Other substances affect intrinsic sleep parameters, such as sleep latency, awakenings, percentage of various stages of sleep, nocturnal wakefulness, and evidence of sleep interruptions manifested primarily at a sleep EEG study. Many drugs have known effects on primary sleep disorders such as restless legs syndrome, obstructive sleep apnea, and insomnia from many causes. The known effects of drugs on sleep are summarized in Table 16–10 (Armitage 2000; Dietrich 1997; Gursky and Krahn 2000; Nicholson 1994; Nicholson et al. 1994; Novak and Shapiro 1997; Obermeyer and Benca 1996; Parrino and Terzano 1996; Pascoe 1994; Placidi et al. 2000; Winokur et al. 2001).

Few drugs have unadulterated beneficial effects on sleep, and effects on healthy study subjects and on patients may not coincide. Rather than assume that these various factors are too complex to be useful in the psychiatric care of a medically ill patient, the consultation psychiatrist can learn the few basic groups of drugs with empirically demonstrated significant effects on sleep (see Table 16–11 for summary of hypnotic effects). Combining this information with knowledge of the physiological mechanisms of sleep will allow the clinician to logically infer the effects of most other drugs on sleep.

The following are general rules about drugs that can help in application of sleep knowledge to patient care.

1. Most CNS drugs decrease slow wave and REM sleep, at least acutely. It is reasonable to learn the relatively short list of drugs known to increase REM sleep and assume that others will suppress or disrupt normal REM sleep function. The medications that increase REM sleep are reserpine, yohimbine (and other alpha-antagonists), and physostigmine (and other cholinomimetic drugs, perhaps including cholinesterase inhibitors such as donepezil) (Slatkin et al. 2001).

2. Many drugs cause daytime sedation. It is reasonable to learn the short list of drugs that cause increased daytime alertness and perhaps anxiety as well (psychostimulants, modafinil, and caffeine) and to presume that most others will either be neutral or negative toward daytime alertness.

3. Stopping drugs suddenly commonly produces adverse effects. The entity suppressed will likely rebound. Thus stopping drugs that suppress REM sleep (most CNS agents) will often lead to REM sleep rebound, which can be associated with insomnia, nightmares, and even hallucinations.

4. Stopping drugs that stimulate the CNS (and have depleted or displaced stimulating neurotransmitters) can lead to temporary depression. This effect is surprisingly uncommon even in patients who have taken high doses of stimulants for a long time. Depression and decreased alertness are common but usually are transient.

5. Many drugs continue their activity on sleep and wakefulness far beyond the intended therapeutic time. Many medications used to promote sleep are associated with some "hangover" experience the next day. The few exceptions are drugs with an ultrashort half-life, such as zaleplon (definitely demonstrated) and perhaps triazolam and zolpidem (less clearly demonstrated) (see Table 16–11).

6. Alternative therapies and herbal preparations may be helpful. Although effort similar to FDA efficacy and safety guidelines is increasingly being put into examining alternative therapies and herbal preparations, little definitive information is available. Many of these agents are pharmacologically active in the CNS, and many have interactions with prescribed medications.

Herbal Agents

Aside from the likelihood that herbal preparations may be contaminated with unknown substances (e.g., anti-inflammatory agents, steroids, diuretics, antihistamines, tranquilizers, hormones, and heavy metals), more information is becoming available about potential adverse effects of herbal preparations taken as sleep aids, as daytime stimulants, and for other purposes. A review of complementary therapies from an Eastern perspective describes in detail an extensive list of Chinese herbal treatments and their potential toxicities (Cheng 2000). A number of authors have reviewed the safety of complementary therapies as they apply to the practice of emergency medicine (Nelson and Perrone 2000) and oncology (Markman 2002). Melatonin, 5-hydroxytryptamine, catnip, chamomile, gotu kola, hops, L-tryptophan, lavender, passionflower, skullcap, and valerian are agents that have been used to manage sleep disorders (Cauffield and Forbes 1999). The toxicities of herbal substances most commonly used for sedative or stimulant purposes among consultation-liaison populations are shown in Table 16–12 (Crone and Wise 1998).

TABLE 16–10.   Effects of medications on sleep

Substance	TST	A	SL	II	SWS	REM	REML	Insomnia	Vigilance	Sedation	Nightmares, parasomnias
Acetylcholinesterase inhibitors							+	+/–			
Alcohol											
Alcohol, acute	+	–	–		+	–	+	+/–			+
Alcohol, W/D	–	+	+		–	+	–	+	+		+
Analgesics											
Opioids, acute	+/–	+	–	–	–	–		+/–		+	+
Opioids, W/D	–	+	+			–		+/–			
Antibiotics											
Quinolones								+			
Anticholinergics		–		+	–	–	+			+/–	+/–
Anticonvulsants											
Felbamate								+			
Gabapentin					++						
Lamotrigine		–			–	+					
Phenytoin			–		–	–					
Tiagabine					+						
Valproate										+	
Vigabatrin		+			+						
Antidepressants											
Bupropion	–							+	–		
MAOI, acute	–	–			+	–	+				
Mirtazapine		–	–		+	+	+			–	+
Nefazodone	–	–				+/–	+/–	–			
SRI	+/–	+/–	+/–			–	+	+/–		+/–	
Trazodone		–	–		+	+	+			+	
Tricyclics	+	–	+/–	+		–	–				
Tricyclics, W/D	–	+	+			+	+	+			
Venlafaxine		+			–	–	+				
Antihistamines											
Histamine₁ agonists		++								+	
Histamine₁ antagonists		–									

TABLE 16–10. Effects of medications on sleep (*continued*)

Substance	TST	A	SL	II	SWS	REM	REML	Insomnia	Vigilance	Sedation	Nightmares, parasomnias
Antihypertensives											
ACE inhibitors											+
Alpha$_2$ agonists	+		+	+	+	−	+			+	+
Alpha$_1$ antagonists										+	
Beta-blocker, lipophilic		+				−			−		+
Calcium channel agonist								+			
5-HT$_2$ agonist				−	+	−					
Methyldopa				−	−						
Reserpine		−				+	−				+
Antineoplastic											
Aminoglutethimide							+			+	+
Flutamide								+		+	+
Procarbazine								+		+	+
Interferon					+			+			
Antiparkinsonism											
L-Dopa, acute					+			−			
L-Dopa, chronic	−	+	−		−	−	+	+			+
Amantadine								+			
Pramipexole										+[a]	
Selegiline	+	−						−			
Antipsychotic											
Acute	+	−	−		+	−	+			+	
W/D	−	+	+			+					
Anxiolytics											
Buspirone								+			
Barbiturates and benzodiazepines, acute	+	−	−	−	−	+					
Barbiturates and benzodiazepines, W/D	−	+	+		+			+			
Barbiturates and benzodiazepines, caffeine	−	+	+					+			

TABLE 16–10. Effects of medications on sleep (continued)

Substance	TST	A	SL	II	SWS	REM	REML	Insomnia	Vigilance	Sedation	Nightmares, parasomnias
Other drugs											
Corticosteroids		+						+		+	+
Lithium	+	−		+	+	−	+			+	
Nicotine, acute	−	−	+			−					
Nicotine, W/D		+								+	
Stimulants	−	+	+			−	+	+	+		
Tetrahydrocannabinol		+			−						
Yohimbine						+		+			

Note. A=number of arousals; ACE=angiotensin converting enzyme; 5-HT_2=serotonin$_2$ receptor; MAOI= monoamine oxidase inhibitor; REM=percentage of rapid eye movement (REM) sleep; REML=initial REM latency; SL=sleep latency; SRI=serotonin reuptake inhibitor; SWS=percentage of slow wave sleep; TST=total sleep time; II=percentage of stage II sleep; W/D=withdrawal; +=drug is known to produce an increase in the sleep parameter or phenomenon; −=drug is known to produce a decrease in the sleep parameter or phenomenon; +/−=drug is known to produce variable effects on the sleep parameter or phenomenon; no symbol=there are no reliable data on the effect of this drug on sleep parameters.

aAt high doses.

TABLE 16–11. Hypnotic drug effects on sleep, including effects of active metabolites

Drug	Half-life (h)	SL	REML	TST	WASO	SWS	REMS	Rebound?	Tolerance?	Carryover
Chloral hydrate	4–12	−	−	+	−	?	−	?	Yes	Yes
Flurazepam	40+	−	+	+	−	−	−	Yes	Yes	Yes
Quazepam	25–41	−	+/−	+	−	?		No	Yes	No
Temazepam	10+	−	+	+	−	−	−	Yes	Yes	No
Trazodone (25–50 mg)	4–7	−	+	+	−	?	?	?	?	Yes
Triazolam	1–5	−	+/−	+	−	?	?	Yes	Yes	No
Zolpidem	1–2	−	−	+	−	+/−	+/−	Yes	Yes	Yes
Zaleplon	1	−	?	+	?	?	?	No	?	No

Note. REML=initial rapid eye movement (REM) latency; REMS=REM sleep; +=increased; SL=sleep latency; SWS=slow wave sleep; TST=total sleep time; WASO=wakefulness after sleep onset; −=decreased; +/−=variable effects.

TABLE 16–12. Herbal medications with sleep–wake toxicity

	Toxicity
Herbal medications used as sedatives	
Broom (*Cytisus scoparius*)	Vomiting, uterine contractions, and bradycardia
Kava kava (*Piper methysticum*)	Dermatitis, hallucinations, and shortness of breath
Passionflower (*Passiflora caerulea*)	Seizures, hypotension, and hallucinations
Valerian (*Valeriana officinalis*)	Dystonic reactions and hepatotoxicity
Miscellaneous herbal preparations with excessive stimulation and insomnia as side or toxic effects	
Echinacea (*Echinacea angustifolia* or *E. purpurea*)	Central nervous system stimulation, dermatitis, and anaphylaxis
Ginseng (*Panax ginseng*)	Hypertension, mastalgia, agitation, anxiety, depression, and insomnia
Golden seal (*Hydrastis canadensis*)	Nausea and vomiting, central nervous system stimulation, paralysis and paresthesia, and respiratory failure
Ma huang (*Ephedra sinica*)	Mania and psychosis, hypertension, and tachycardia
Yohimbine bark (*Pausinystalia yohimbine* or *Corynanthe yohimbe*)	Hallucinations and anxiety, hypertension and tachycardia, and nausea and vomiting

Melatonin

Because melatonin is readily available and patients commonly self-administer it, a brief review of this agent is pertinent. Melatonin is sold over the counter in airports, health food stores, and other venues and is widely used to manage jet lag and insomnia in general. This agent is also being used as an antioxidant. The safety and efficacy of health-food-store melatonin have been studied formally in only a limited way. In one analysis of three commercially prepared over-the-counter melatonin preparations, investigators found several contaminants in each preparation. The substances found included structural analogues of contaminants found in preparations of L-tryptophan that had been associated with eosinophilia-myalgia syndrome (Williamson et al. 1997). Other evidence suggests that even with pharmacologically pure preparations, the varying bioavailability of oral doses of melatonin results in as much as a 20-fold difference in plasma levels of the agent (Di et al. 1997).

A careful review of the literature on jet lag indicates that melatonin is remarkably effective in preventing jet lag, and occasional short-term use appears to be safe. However, the pharmacological and toxicological mechanisms of melatonin need systematic study, and routine pharmacological quality control of melatonin products must be established. There is evidence that a low dose (0.5 mg) of melatonin improves initial sleep quality in selected elderly persons with insomnia. However, large, randomized, controlled trials are yet to be conducted (Olde Rikkert and Rigaud 2001). The literature contains reports of many adverse effects that have yet to be systematically defined so that an appropriate risk–benefit discussion can take place. The reports include autoimmune hepatitis, optic neuropathy, fragmented sleep, psychosis, nystagmus, seizures, headache, skin eruption, and confusion from overdose (Morera et al. 2001).

The mechanisms of action of melatonin are not clearly defined, although there is evidence of an active feedback process between the pineal gland and the suprachiasmatic nucleus. The known interaction in the dopaminergic system has led to investigation of melatonin as an agent in the treatment of parkinsonism, neurodegenerative disorders, tardive dyskinesia (Zisapel 2001), and postoperative delirium (Hanania and Kitain 2002).

In summary, the long-term use of over-the-counter melatonin has not been demonstrated to be safe or effective, and studies of pure preparations of this hormone in carefully controlled research settings have not yet established appropriate indications or risk–benefit assessments. Preferential use of other medications and methods of improving sleep for medically ill patients is recommended.

Conclusion

Sleep takes up one-third of a typical day. Obtaining adequate quantity and quality of sleep is optimal for good health and the prevention of complications. We have addressed the major sleep disorders by discussing their clinical features, diagnostic testing, and treatment. Sleep medicine is a vibrant medical specialty with many developments promoting understanding of the mechanisms of sleep disorders and their treatment. Intervention can prevent undesirable medical, psychiatric, and social consequences. The chief goal at present is to help educate the medical community and the general public about these conditions so that patients can benefit from these discoveries by having dysfunctional sleep recognized and carefully assessed. Once the diagnosis of a specific sleep disorder is made, numerous treatment options are available.

References

Allen R, Earley C: Restless legs syndrome: a review of clinical and pathophysiologic features. J Clin Neurophysiol 18:128–147, 2001a

Allen R, Earley C: Validation of the Johns Hopkins Restless Legs Severity Scale (JHRLSS). Sleep Med 3:239–242, 2001b

American Academy of Sleep Medicine: International Classification of Sleep Disorders, Revised. Rochester, MN, American Academy of Sleep Medicine, 1997

Armitage R: The effects of antidepressants on sleep in patients with depression. Can J Psychiatry 45:803–809, 2000

Artigas F, Nutt D, Shelton R: Mechanism of action of antidepressants. Psychopharmacol Bull 36 (suppl 2):123–132, 2002

Bananian S, Lehrman S, Maguire G: Cardiovascular consequences of sleep-related breathing disorders. Heart Dis 4:296–305, 2002

Bassetti C, Aldrich M: Idiopathic hypersomnia: a series of 42 patients. Brain 120:1423–1435, 1997

Bergmann B, Gilliland M, Feng P, et al: Are physiological effects of sleep deprivation in the rat mediated by bacterial invasion? Sleep 19:554–562, 1996

Berry R, Deas M, Light R: Effect of ethanol on the efficacy of nasal continuous positive airway pressure as a treatment for obstructive sleep apnea. Chest 99:339–341, 1991

Berry R, Parish J, Hartse K: The use of auto-titrating continuous positive airway pressure for the treatment of adult obstructive sleep apnea: an American Academy of Sleep Medicine review. Sleep 25:148–173, 2002

Black J, Krahn L, Silber M: A pilot study of serologic markers of autoimmunity in patients with narcolepsy (abstract). Sleep 24 (suppl):A318–A319, 2001

Bootzin R, Perlis M: Nonpharmacologic treatments of insomnia. J Clin Psychiatry 53 (suppl):37–41, 1992

Bresnitz E, Goldberg R, Kosinski R: Epidemiology of obstructive sleep apnea. Epidemiol Rev 16:210–227, 1994

Broughton W, Broughton R: Psychosocial impact of narcolepsy. Sleep 17 (8 suppl):s45–s49, 1994

Brown FC, Buboltz WC Jr, Soper B: Relationship of sleep hygiene awareness, sleep hygiene practices, and sleep quality in university students. Behav Med 28:33–38, 2002

Carskadon M, Dement W: Normal human sleep: an overview, in Principles and Practice of Sleep Medicine, 2nd Edition. Edited by Kryger M, Roth T, Dement W. Philadelphia, PA, WB Saunders, 1994, pp 16–25

Cauffield J, Forbes H: Dietary supplements used in the treatment of depression, anxiety, and sleep disorders. Lippincotts Prim Care Pract 3:290–304, 1999

Chaudhuri K, Appiah-Kubi L, Trenkwalder C: Restless legs syndrome. J Neurol Neurosurg Psychiatry 71:143–146, 2001

Cheng JT: Review: drug therapy in Chinese traditional medicine. J Clin Pharmacol 40:445–450, 2000

Chesson A Jr, Hartse K, Anderson W, et al: Practice parameters for the evaluation of chronic insomnia: an American Academy of Sleep Medicine report—Standards of Practice Committee of the American Academy of Sleep Medicine. Sleep 23:237–241, 2000

Cirignotta F, Mondini S, Santoro A, et al: Reliability of a questionnaire screening restless legs syndrome in patients on chronic dialysis. Am J Kidney Dis 40:302–306, 2002

Clark G, Blumenfeld I, Yoffe N, et al: A crossover study comparing the efficiency of continuous positive airway pressure with anterior mandibular positioning devices on patients with obstructive sleep apnea. Chest 109:1477–1483, 1996

Comella C: Restless legs syndrome: treatment with dopaminergic agents. Neurology 58 (suppl 1):S87–S92, 2002

Comella CL, Nardine TM, Diedrich NJ, et al: Sleep-related violence, injuries and REM behavior disorder in Parkinson's disease. Neurology 51:526–529, 1998

Crone C, Wise T: Use of herbal medicines among consultation-liaison populations: a review of current information regarding risks, interactions, and efficacy. Psychosomatics 39:3–13, 1998

Dart R, Gregoire J, Gutterman D, et al: The association of hypertension and secondary cardiovascular disease with sleep-disordered breathing. Chest 123:244–260, 2003

Davila D, Richards K, Marshall B, et al: Oximeter performance: the influence of acquisition parameters. Chest 122:1654–1660, 2002

Desautels A, Turecki G, Montplaisir J, et al: Identification of a major susceptibility locus for restless legs syndrome on chromosome 12q. Am J Hum Genet 69:1266–1270, 2001

Di W, Kadva A, Johnston A, et al: Variable bioavailability of oral melatonin (letter). N Engl J Med 336:1028–1029, 1997

Dietrich B: Polysomnography in drug development. J Clin Pharmacol 37 (1 suppl):70S–78S, 1997

Dolly F, Block A: Effect of flurazepam on sleep-disordered breathing and nocturnal oxygen desaturation in asymptomatic subjects. Am J Med 73:239–243, 1982

Dyken M, Somers V, Yamada T, et al: Investigating the relationship between stroke and obstructive sleep apnea. Stroke 27:401–407, 1996

Dyken M, Yamada T, Lin-Dyken D: Polysomnographic assessment of spells in sleep: nocturnal seizures versus parasomnias. Semin Neurol 21:377–390, 2001

Earley C, Allen R, Beard J, et al: Insight into the pathophysiology of restless legs syndrome. J Neurosci Res 62:623–628, 2000

Ekblom K: Restless legs. Acta Med Scand Suppl 158:1–123, 1945

Flemons W: Obstructive sleep apnea. N Engl J Med 347:498–504, 2002

Garcia-Borreguero D, Larrosa O, de la Llave Y, et al: Treatment of restless legs syndrome with gabapentin: a double-blind, cross-over study. Neurology 59:1573–1579, 2002

Gelineau J: De la narcolepsie. Lancette Francaise 53:626–628, 1880

George C, Millar T, Kryger M: Sleep apnea and body position during sleep. Sleep 11:90–99, 1988

Guilleminault C, Robinson A: Central sleep apnea. Otolaryngol Clin North Am 31:1049–1065, 1998

Guilleminault C, Do Kim Y, Chowdhuri S, et al: Sleep and daytime sleepiness in upper airway resistance syndrome compared to obstructive sleep apnoea syndrome. Eur Respir J 17:838–847, 2001

Gursky J, Krahn L: The effects of antidepressants on sleep: a review. Harv Rev Psychiatry 8:298–306, 2000

Hanania M, Kitain E: Melatonin for treatment and prevention of postoperative delirium. Anesth Analg 94:338–339, 2002

Hauri P: Can we mix behavioral therapy with hypnotics when treating insomniacs? Sleep 20:1111–1118, 1997

Hauri P, Esther M: Insomnia. Mayo Clinic Proc 65:869–882, 1990

Hauri P, Friedman M, Ravaris C: Sleep in patients with spontaneous panic attacks. Sleep 12:323–337, 1989

Ing A, Ngu M, Breslin A: Obstructive sleep apnea and gastroesophageal reflux. Am J Med 108 (suppl 4a):120S–125S, 2000

Johns M: A new method for measuring daytime sleepiness: the Epworth Sleepiness Scale. Sleep 14:540–545, 1991

Joncas S, Zadra A, Paquet J, et al: The value of sleep deprivation as a diagnostic tool in adult sleepwalkers. Neurology 58:936–940, 2002

Kessler R, Chaouat A, Schinkewitch P, et al: The obesity-hypoventilation syndrome revisited: a prospective study of 34 consecutive cases. Chest 120:369–376, 2002

Konermann M, Radu H, Teschler H, et al: Interaction of sleep disturbances and gastroesophageal reflux in chronic laryngitis. Am J Otolaryngol 23:20–26, 2002

Krahn L, Lin S, Wisbey J, et al: Assessing sleep in psychiatric inpatients: nurse and patient reports versus wrist actigraphy. Ann Clin Psychiatry 19:203–210, 1997

Krahn L, Boeve B, Olson E, et al: A standardized test for cataplexy. Sleep Med 1:125–130, 2000

Krahn L, Black J, Silber M: Narcolepsy: new understanding of irresistible sleep. Mayo Clinic Proc 76:185–194, 2001a

Krahn L, Hansen M, Shepard J: Pseudocataplexy. Psychosomatics 42:356–358, 2001b

Lammers G, Arends J, Declerck A, et al: Gammahydroxybutyrate and narcolepsy: a double blind placebo-controlled study. Sleep 16:216–220, 1993

Li A, Wong E, Kew J, et al: Use of tonsil size in the evaluation of obstructive sleep apnoea. Arch Dis Child 87:156–159, 2002

Li K, Kushida C, Powell N, et al: Obstructive sleep apnea syndrome: a comparison between Far-East Asian and white men. Laryngoscope 110:1689–1693, 2000

Littner M, Kushida C, Hartse K, et al: Practice parameters for the use of laser-assisted uvulopalatoplasty: an update for 2000. Sleep 24:603–619, 2001

Lojander P, Maasilta P, Partinen M, et al: Nasal-CPAP and conservative management for treatment of obstructive sleep apnea syndrome: a randomized study. Chest 110:114–119, 1996

Mahowald M, Schenck C: NREM sleep parasomnias. Neurol Clin 14:675–696, 1996

Markman M: Safety issues in using complementary and alternative medicine. J Clin Oncol 20 (18 suppl):39S–41S, 2002

Mercer J, Bootzin R, Lack L: Insomniacs' perception of wake instead of sleep. Sleep 25:564–571, 2002

Mignot E, Lammers G, Ripley B, et al: The role of cerebrospinal fluid hypocretin measurement in the diagnosis of narcolepsy and other hypersomnias. Arch Neurol 59:1553–1562, 2002

Minvielle S: Klein-Levin syndrome: a neurological disease with psychiatric symptoms. Encephale 26:71–74, 2000

Mitler M, Hayduk R: Benefits and risks of pharmacotherapy for narcolepsy. Drug Saf 25:790–809, 2002

Mitler M, Gujavarty K, Sampson M, et al: Multiple daytime nap approaches to evaluating the sleepy patient. Sleep 5 (suppl 2):S119–S127, 1982

Montgomery P, Dennis J: Physical exercise for sleep problems in adults aged 60+. Cochrane Database Syst Rev (3): CD003404, 2002

Montplaisir J, Boucher S, Poirier G, et al: Clinical, polysomnographic and genetic characteristics of restless legs syndrome: a study of 133 patients with new standard criteria. Mov Disord 12:61–65, 1997

Morera A, Henry M, de La Varga M: Safety in melatonin use [in Spanish]. Actas Esp Psiquiatr 29:334–347, 2001

Morin C, Hauri P, Espie C, et al: Nonpharmacologic treatment of chronic insomnia: an American Academy of Sleep Medicine review. Sleep 22:1134–1156, 1999

Mormont M, Levi F: Cancer chronotherapy: principles, applications, and perspectives. Cancer 97:155–169, 2003

Nelson L, Perrone J: Herbal and alternative medicine. Emerg Med Clin North Am 18:709–722, 2000

Netzer N, Eliasson A, Netzer C, et al: Overnight pulse oximetry for sleep-disordered breathing in adults: a review. Chest 120:625–633, 2001

Nicholson A: Hypnotics clinical pharmacology and therapeutics, in Principles and Practice of Sleep Medicine, 2nd Edition. Edited by Kryger M, Roth T, Dement W. Philadelphia, PA, WB Saunders, 1994, pp 355–363

Nicholson A, Bradley C, Pascoe P: Medications: effects on sleep and wakefulness, in Principles and Practice of Sleep Medicine, 2nd Edition. Edited by Kryger M, Roth T, Dement W. Philadelphia, PA, WB Saunders, 1994, pp 364–373

Nicolas A, Michaud M, Lavigne G, et al: The influence of sex, age and sleep/wake state on characteristics of periodic leg movements in restless legs syndrome patients. J Clin Neurophysiol 110:1168–1174, 1999

Novak M, Shapiro C: Drug-induced sleep disturbances: focus on nonpsychotropic medications. Drug Saf 16:133–149, 1997

Obermeyer W, Benca R: Effects of drugs on sleep. Neurol Clin 14:827–840, 1996

Ohayon M, Roth T: Prevalence of restless legs syndrome and periodic movement disorder in the general population. J Psychosom Res 53:547–554, 2002

Ohayon M, Roth T: Place of chronic insomnia in the course of depressive and anxiety disorders. J Psychiatr Res 37:9–15, 2003

Olde Rikkert MG, Rigaud AS: Melatonin in elderly patients with insomnia: a systematic review. Z Gerontol Geriatr 34:491–497, 2001

Olson E: Obstructive sleep apnea consultation in hospitalized patients: review of a center's experience. Sleep 24 (abstract suppl):A310, 2001

Olson E, Boeve B, Silber M: Rapid eye movement sleep behavior disorder: demographic, clinical and laboratory findings in 93 cases. Brain 123:331–339, 2000

Overeem S, Mignot E, Gert van Dijk J, et al: Narcolepsy: clinical features, new pathophysiologic insights, and future perspectives. J Clin Neurophysiol 18:78–105, 2001

Pallesen S, Nordhus I, Kvale G, et al: Behavioral treatment of insomnia in older adults: an open clinical trial comparing two interventions. Behav Res Ther 41:31–48, 2003

Parrino L, Terzano M: Polysomnographic effects of hypnotic drugs: a review. Psychopharmacology 126:1–16, 1996

Partinen M: Epidemiology of obstructive sleep apnea syndrome. Curr Opin Pulm Med 1:482–487, 1995

Pascoe P: Drugs and the sleep-wakefulness continuum. Pharmacol Ther 61:227–236, 1994

Phillips B, Young T, Finn L, et al: Epidemiology of restless legs syndrome in adults. Arch Intern Med 160:2137–2141, 2000

Pilcher J, Huffcutt A: Effects of sleep deprivation on performance: a meta-analysis. Sleep 19:318–326, 1996

Placidi F, Scalise A, Marciani M, et al: Effect of antiepileptic drugs on sleep. Clin Neurophysiol 111 (suppl 2):S115–S119, 2000

Plazzi G, Corsini R, Provini F, et al: REM behavior disorder in multiple system atrophy. Neurology 48:1094–1097, 1997

Pressman M, Figueroa W, Kendrick-Mohamed J, et al: Nocturia: a rarely recognized symptom of sleep apnea and other occult sleep disorders. Arch Intern Med 156:545–550, 1996

Quaranta A, D'Alonzo G, Krachman S: Cheyne-Stokes respiration during sleep in congestive heart failure. Chest 111:467–473, 1997

Rama A, Tekwani S, Kushida C: Sites of obstruction in obstructive sleep apnea. Chest 122:1139–1147, 2002

Reuven H, Schweitzer E, Tarasiuk A: A cost-effectiveness analysis of alternative at-home or in-laboratory technologies for the diagnosis of obstructive sleep apnea syndrome. Med Decis Making 21:451–458, 2001

Richardson G, Roth T, Hajak G, et al: Consensus for the pharmacological management of insomnia in the new millennium. Int J Clin Pract 55:42–52, 2001

Ruottinen H, Partinen M, Hublin C, et al: An FDOPA positron emission tomography study in patients with periodic limb movement disorder and restless legs syndrome. Neurology 54:502–504, 2000

Schenck C, Mahowald M: Polysomnographic, neurologic, psychiatric, and clinical outcome report on 70 consecutive cases with the REM behavior disorder (RBD): sustained clonazepam efficacy in 89.5% of 57 treated patients. Cleve Clin J Med 57:S10–S24, 1990

Schuld A, Blum W, Pollmacher T: Low CSF hypocretin (orexin) and altered energy metabolism in human narcolepsy. Ann Neurol 51:660–661, 2002

Silber M, Richardson J: Multiple blood donations associated with iron deficiency in patients with restless legs syndrome. Mayo Clin Proc 78:52–56, 2003

Silber M, Krahn L, Olson E, et al: Epidemiology of narcolepsy in Olmsted County, Minnesota: a population-based study. Sleep 24 (abstract suppl):A98, 2001

Slatkin N, Rhiner M, Bolton T: Donepezil in the treatment of opioid-induced sedation: report of six cases. J Pain Symptom Manage 21:425–438, 2001

Smart D, Jerman J: The physiology and pharmacology of the orexins. Pharmacol Ther 94:51–61, 2002

Strollo PJ, Sanders M, Costantino J, et al: Split-night studies for the diagnosis and treatment of sleep-disordered breathing. Sleep 19 (10 suppl):S255–S259, 1996

Sullivan C, Grunstein R: Continuous positive airway pressure in sleep-disordered breathing, in Principles and Practice of Sleep Medicine, 2nd Edition. Edited by Kryger M, Roth T, Dement W. Philadelphia, PA, WB Saunders, 1994, pp 694–705

Thannickal T, Moore R, Nienhuis R, et al: Reduced number of hypocretin neurons in human narcolepsy. Neuron 27:469–474, 2000

Toney G, Ereshefsky L: Sleep disorders: assisting patients to a good night's sleep. J Am Pharm Assoc (Wash) 40 (5 suppl 1):S46–S47, 2000

Ulfberg J, Nystrom B, Carter N, et al: Prevalence of restless legs syndrome among men aged 18 to 64 years: an association with somatic disease and neuropsychiatric symptoms. Move Disord 16:1159–1163, 2001

US Modafinil in Narcolepsy Multicenter Study Group: Randomized trial of modafinil for the treatment of pathological somnolence in narcolepsy. Ann Neurol 43:88–97, 1998

Vitiello M, Moe K, Prinz P: Sleep complaints cosegregate with illness in older adults: clinical research informed by and informing epidemiological studies of sleep. J Psychosom Res 53:555–559, 2002

Walker R: Long-term health consequences of mild to moderate obstructive sleep apnea. Arch Otolaryngol Head Neck Surg 127:1397–1400, 2001

Williamson B, Tomlinson A, Naylor S, et al: Contaminants in commercial preparations of melatonin (letter). Mayo Clin Proc 72:1094–1095, 1997

Winkelmann J, Chertow G, Lazarus J: Restless legs syndrome in end-stage renal disease. Am J Kidney Dis 28:372–378, 1996

Winokur A, Gary K, Rodner S, et al: Depression, sleep physiology, and antidepressant drugs. Depress Anxiety 14:19–28, 2001

Young T, Palta M, Dempsey J, et al: The occurrence of sleep-disordered breathing among middle-aged adults. N Engl J Med 328:1230–1235, 1993

Young T, Peppard P, Gottlieb D: Epidemiology of obstructive sleep apnea: a population health perspective. Am J Respir Crit Care Med 165:1217–1239, 2002

Young T, Shahar E, Nieto F, et al: Predictors of sleep-disordered breathing in community dwelling adults: the Sleep Heart Health Study. Arch Intern Med 162:893–900, 2002

Zisapel N: Melatonin-dopamine interactions: from basic neurochemistry to a clinical setting. Cell Mol Neurobiol 21:605–616, 2001

17 Sexual Disorders

George R. Brown, M.D.

Richard C. Haaser, M.D.

SEXUALITY IS AN important component of quality of life, but it is often overlooked or relegated to a minor role by those caring for the medically ill. When physicians do focus on sexuality, they usually do so from the perspective of sexual dysfunction rather than sexual health. All phases of the human sexual response are subject to influence by a variety of medical and psychiatric conditions. Whether sexual dysfunction occurs as a direct consequence of medical or surgical illness (e.g., erectile dysfunction from spinal cord injury or diabetic neuropathy), a reflection of psychological struggle arising from illness (e.g., negative body image in psoriasis), a comorbid psychiatric illness (Rosen et al. 1999), or a combination of two or more factors, the psychiatrist has the unique opportunity to address these complex interactions (Nankervis 1989). However, it is not a simple matter to determine the relative contributions of somatic disorders and psychological processes in diagnosing sexual problems in the medically ill.

Fagan et al. (1990) suggested the following seven factors that may indicate a psychological source of sexual dysfunction in patients with discrete medical illnesses:

1. History of sexual trauma or abnormal sexual development
2. Restrictive religious or moral sexual attitudes
3. Preexisting sexual dysfunction
4. Situational or partner-specific dysfunction
5. Evidence of morning or masturbatory full tumescence
6. Evidence of masturbatory arousal and orgasm in women
7. Sexual dysfunction following the onset of another psychiatric disorder

Patients' wishes for privacy or their feelings of embarrassment may collude with their physicians' avoidance of sexual issues and a businesslike tendency to focus on the purely medical aspects of the illness. Consequently, sexual dysfunction can easily escape evaluation and treatment. Patients' physicians might avoid discussing sexual health because of time limitations, discomfort with the topic, or fear of having little to offer even if a problem is identified. Therefore it is important for psychiatrists to routinely address the issue as part of assessment.

We discuss specific medical, surgical, and pharmacological deterrents to healthy sexual functioning. DSM-IV (American Psychiatric Association 1994), and its text revision, DSM-IV-TR (American Psychiatric Association 2000), list specific categories for sexual dysfunction due to a general medical condition. These diagnoses are to be used when patients exhibit clinically significant sexual dysfunctions judged to be etiologically related to a general medical or surgical condition. If psychological factors play a role in initiating, maintaining, or aggravating the sexual dysfunction, the specific sexual dysfunction is diagnosed, and the subtype "due to combined factors" is added to the formal diagnosis. Substance-induced sexual dysfunction is another specific category often seen in hospitalized patients. All too often physicians approach sexual dysfunction in their patients with the question, "Is it physical or psychogenic?" Although this question is a natural one, the reality is that in many, if not the majority, of medically ill patients with sexual problems, biological, psychological, and social factors all contribute. This diagnosis covers not only sexual dysfunction due to the use of intox-

---

Disclaimer. The views expressed in this chapter are those of the authors and do not necessarily reflect those of the United States Government or the Department of Veterans Affairs.

icants, alcohol, and illicit drugs but also the commonly undetected iatrogenic effects of prescribed medications. In addition to the sexual consequences of common medical and surgical disease entities, we discuss primary sexual and gender identity disorders that may be encountered in medical settings and the treatments that are available for patients with these disorders. Many references are cited and provided with the caveat that sexual functioning often involves a personal, highly subjective set of parameters. The many biological, psychological, social, and spiritual complicating factors with which it is fraught make sexual functioning difficult to assess in studies of groups of patients with possibly little more in common than a specific disease, illness, or surgical procedure.

Sexual Expression in Hospitalized Patients

Although sexual expression in hospitalized patients has received little attention in the medical literature, the focus has been on the "problem" of "inappropriate" sexual behaviors by patients in hospitals and nursing homes (Ehrenfeld et al. 1999). These behaviors might not be dysfunctional but merely uncomfortable for staff members. Patients who are hospitalized for extended periods might well have intact sexual function and sexual expression, whether it is through masturbation or with an intimate partner. This activity poses problems for the staff, because hospital settings rarely offer the necessary privacy. The need for privacy might not be appropriate for very ill patients who need close monitoring, but when the hospitalization becomes protracted and the acuity level lower, treatment plans could readily incorporate protected private time. What may appear to be a request to deal with "inappropriate sexuality" may in fact represent an impasse between a patient in need of privacy and a staff member unwilling to accept the reality that sexual needs may transcend the circumstances of hospitalization. The psychiatrist may then act as a mediator in recognizing the "real" issue and brokering a deal between the patient and the treatment team that is mutually beneficial.

Inappropriate expressions of sexual behaviors are indeed common. These activities include attempted involvement by patients with staff (e.g., spinal cord injury patients who are adapting poorly and patients with boundary issues or personality disorders admitted for treatment of medical conditions) and sexual expression by delirious or demented patients, frontal lobe injury patients, and patients who are intoxicated or disinhibited from other causes.

Sexual Functioning in Medical Illness

Heart Disease

Most studies of patients with heart disease that have addressed sexual functioning have focused on men; however, evidence suggests that the general findings might not be substantially different in women (Skinner 1979). Although study designs and specific findings vary, general conclusions have been supported consistently. Sexual activity decreases and the perception of sexual dysfunction increases after myocardial infarction (Nankervis 1989; Skinner 1979). In a study of 276 Israeli men having a first acute myocardial infarction, 12% of subjects had not resumed sexual activity within 3–6 months. Of the men who did resume sexual activity, 35% reported reduced frequency and 35% reported reduced satisfaction (Drory et al. 1998). Resuming post–myocardial infarction sexual activity with one's prior partner and in the usual setting does not increase morbidity (Silber 1987). Results of previous studies have suggested that most impediments to a satisfying sexual life after myocardial infarction are psychological rather than physiological (Drory et al. 1998; Skinner 1979). Drory et al. (1998) found that the frequency and satisfaction of sexual activity after myocardial infarction were explained by the frequency and satisfaction with sexual activity before myocardial infarction. Depression, age, and education contributed in a smaller but significant way (Drory et al. 1998). Physical limitations can be important, too. Patients with low ejection fraction in advanced heart disease experience marked reductions in libido and in ability to perform sexually (Jaarsma 1996).

The percentage of heart disease patients wanting to discuss resumption of sexual functioning far exceeds the percentage of patients who believe that they have been informed adequately (Bedell et al. 2002a). Male patients are more likely to have their sexual concerns addressed (Bedell et al. 2002a). In one study only 24% of patients ever specifically discussed sildenafil with their cardiologists before the drug was prescribed (Bedell et al. 2002b). Guidelines for stratifying cardiac risk in resuming sexual activity should facilitate the discussion of sexual function between cardiologists and other physicians and their heart disease patients (DeBusk et al. 2000). These guidelines should reassure most patients who fall into the low-risk category (controlled hypertension; mild, stable angina; successful coronary revascularization; history of uncomplicated myocardial infarction; mild valvular disease; no symptoms; and fewer than three cardiovascular risk factors) that they can safely resume sexual activity or receive treatment of sexual dysfunction (DeBusk et al. 2000).

Erectile dysfunction (ED) is highly prevalent among patients with coronary artery disease and has most of the same risk factors (Feldman et al. 2000; Jensen et al. 1999; Johannes et al. 2000; Martin-Morales et al. 2001; McVary et al. 2001). The link between hypertension, smoking, diabetes, obesity, dyslipidemia, and ED is sufficiently strong to prompt some investigators to consider ED a marker of covert coronary artery disease (Jensen et al. 1999; Kirby et al. 2001; O'Kane and Jackson 2001). In a prospective study of middle-aged men, increasing exercise reduced the risk of ED, but weight reduction, cessation of smoking, and reduction of alcohol use did not (Derby et al. 2000). The study did not address the outcome that would have occurred had lifestyles been modified in the young adult years.

The advent of effective treatments of ED (Padma-Nathan and Giuliano 2001) shifted the discussion beyond the question of when cardiac patients can safely resume sexual activity to the question of how and when to treat sexual dysfunction in such patients. Sildenafil has been shown to be safe and effective in patients with stable angina or congestive heart failure providing that they do not take oral, topical, or sublingual nitrates (Arruda-Olson et al. 2002; Bocchi et al. 2002; Jackson 2000). In a prospective, placebo-controlled trial with patients in New York Heart Association classes II and III congestive heart failure, sildenafil not only was safe and effective but also provided relief of depressive symptoms and improvement in perceived quality of life (Webster et al. 2004). Sildenafil does not change the onset, extent, or severity of ischemia, as measured by exercise electrocardiography and echocardiography, in men with coronary artery disease and ED (Arruda-Olson et al. 2002). DeBusk (2002) found, however, that most serious sex-related coronary events are not caused by ischemia produced by arterial obstruction but rather are caused by the rupture of vulnerable coronary arteries. The risk of a coronary event is the consequence of the increased cardiac workload inherent in sexual activity, resumption of which is facilitated by sildenafil but is not caused by sildenafil directly (Marwick 2002). Careful assessment of the patient's functional capacity for work therefore is needed before sildenafil is prescribed.

Sexual dysfunction in cardiac patients has prompted some physicians and patients to avoid otherwise-indicated drugs, such as the beta-blockers. Newer research findings suggest this concern is exaggerated (Ko et al. 2002; Lama 2002). In a prospective, randomized, placebo-controlled study, metoprolol did not worsen ED as was expected (Franzen et al. 2001).

An increasing number of patients are living after receiving heart transplants. As survival after heart transplantation continues to improve, attention to subsequent quality of life has increased. Mulligan et al. (1991) reported that libido that was generally strong before surgery re-mained strong afterward, and a majority of the 71 male respondents perceived that their partner's libido increased postoperatively. Sixty percent of the respondents reported posttransplantation anorgasmia. Pretransplantation erectile disability and anorgasmia appeared to increase 3 and 12 months after transplantation. Twenty-seven percent of patients in a sample in Italy reported unsatisfactory sexuality after transplantation (Balestroni et al. 2002). Patients commonly experience sexual concerns after transplantation but rarely pursue their questions (Tabler and Frierson 1990), which are usually similar to those of patients who have undergone cardiac surgery. A unique concern among heart transplant recipients is the absence of acceleration in heart rate during sexual excitement or orgasm owing to denervation of the new heart.

Malignancy

The high prevalence of sexual dysfunction among cancer patients calls for the routine assessment and treatment of sexual problems in oncology centers (Bokhour et al. 2001; Gallo-Silver 2000; McKee and Schover 2001; Monturo et al. 2001; Rice 2000). Particularly in men, a concept of sexual function that goes beyond the traditional focus on ED and intercourse frequency is being recognized (Bokhour et al. 2001; Fox et al. 1999). Educational materials and discussions regarding sexual function and sexual adverse effects allow for improved informed consent before cancer treatments (Gallo-Silver 2000; McKee and Schover 2001). Advanced-practice nurses making home visits can improve communication between men with prostate cancer, their partners, and the treatment team about sexual dysfunction and its treatment after cancer treatments (Monturo et al. 2001).

Breast, cervical, ovarian, endometrial, and vulvar cancers threaten female sexual function through a variety of mechanisms, including altered body image, radiation sequelae, loss of libido, and loss of lubrication (Schover et al. 1987). More effort is being expended to address these factors, but it cannot alter premorbid sexual adjustment and function, which also contribute greatly to sexual function and satisfaction after oncology treatments (Schover 1991).

The sexual effects of breast cancer surgery have been explored in detail. In a study of 18 women undergoing lumpectomy or mastectomy, loss was the predominating theme (Wilmoth 2001). Loss of body part, loss of the perception of youth, loss of sexual sensations, and loss of womanhood were specifically noted. Wilmoth (2001) found that women who actively sought information about the sexual side effects of cancer surgery and who had strong intimate relationships achieved the most successful adjustment. Breast-conserving treatment (lumpectomy) correlates with better sexual satisfaction and body image (Amichetti and Caffo 2001; Greendale et al. 2001). A strong correlation between the quality of cosmesis and sexual functioning has been found for breast-conserving treatment of breast cancer (Al-Ghazal et al. 1999).

It has been expected that breast reconstruction after mastectomy would lead to improved body image and, consequently, improved sexual function, but this connection is not clear. Body image and perceived sexual attractiveness did not improve in women who underwent mastectomy and breast reconstruction compared with women who underwent mastectomy alone (Rowland et al. 2000; Yurek et al. 2000). On the other hand, Al-Ghazal et al. (2000) documented improved body image, self-esteem, sexual feeling of attractiveness, and sexual satisfaction when breast reconstruction was performed immediately after mastectomy rather than being delayed. Regardless of body image and perceived attractiveness, women had equivalent sexual functioning after breast-conserving treatment, modified radical mastectomy, and modified radical mastectomy with breast reconstruction (Rowland et al. 2000; Yurek et al. 2000). The studies cited were not randomized, so the respective groups may not be entirely comparable. As is likely true in all studies of sexuality, whatever the findings for a given study group, breast-conserving treatment will have more or less sexual importance for particular individuals that is difficult, if not impossible, to capture in group studies.

Chemotherapy for breast cancer affects sexual functioning. Premature menopause is often induced by chemotherapy, and hormone replacement therapy is contraindicated (Greendale et al. 2001). The result is vaginal dryness, decreased libido, dyspareunia, and difficulty in achieving orgasm (Young-McCaughan 1996). The negative sexual impact of chemotherapy for breast cancer can be ameliorated through assessment of menopausal symptoms, education and counseling, and specific pharmacological and behavioral interventions (Ganz et al. 2000; Rogers and Kristjanson 2001).

Marked deterioration in sexual functioning after gynecological surgery has not been typical. Prospective multicenter studies have not shown significant changes in frequency of sexual contact or satisfaction after treatment of early gynecological cancers (Kylstra et al. 1999; Leenhouts et al. 2002). Another study, in which findings for 20 women undergoing radical hysterectomy for stage 1B cervical cancer, 18 women undergoing hysterectomy for a benign gynecological condition, and 20 gynecologically healthy women were compared, showed no significant difference in sexuality (Grumann et al. 2001). Even so,

psychosexual counseling after gynecological cancer surgery may provide benefits (Maughan and Clarke 2001).

Sexual functioning after treatment of prostate cancer remains the best-studied issue for men. Many men believe their choice is between death if they are untreated and sexual dysfunction if they are treated (Bertero 2001). The impact of prostate cancer treatments on ED has been well described. Most men (85%) have ED after prostatectomy or radiotherapy (Schover et al. 2002), but the effects go much farther. Twelve to 24 months after treatment, Bokhour et al. (2001) recorded decreases in quality of sexual intimacy, in quality of everyday interactions with women, in extent of sexual imagining and fantasy, and in perception of masculinity. Results of a large survey study revealed that distress from the loss of desire and anorgasmia equaled the distress from ED (Schover et al. 2002). Better sexual outcomes were correlated with younger age, no history of neoadjuvant chemotherapy, no current antiandrogen treatments, nerve-sparing surgical and brachytherapy treatments, better pretreatment in regard to mental and physical health, and a history of normal erections before treatment.

Antiandrogen treatments of prostate cancer severely hinder sexual function. Sexual activity was lost in 92% of men prescribed flutamide and 88% of men prescribed cyproterone over 2 years (Schroder et al. 2000). Cryosurgery appears to be somewhat more sparing of sexual functioning. Observed over 36 months, 5 of 38 men regained erectile function and 13 of 38 men were sexually active with the help of aids after cryosurgery (Robinson et al. 2002). Treatments that better preserve sexual functioning are being explored. Bilateral nerve-sparing prostatectomy (Ofman and Auchincloss 1992; Schover et al. 2002) and three-dimensional conformal radiotherapy (Wilder et al. 2000) reduce the prevalence of ED. Two-thirds of men treated with this form of radiotherapy maintained erectile function after 3 years of observation (Wilder et al. 2000). Sildenafil improved erections in 74% of men left with ED following ^{125}I seed implantation radiotherapy (Raina et al. 2003).

Testicular cancer is another commonly encountered cancer in men. In a demographically distinct group of young men with testicular cancer, 30% of the men indicated that sexual performance difficulties were bothersome 1 year after diagnosis (Rieker et al. 1989). However, their concerns about performance were less prominent than their concerns about retrograde ejaculation and infertility. Electroejaculation has been successful in the treatment of infertility in this context (Ohl et al. 1991). Intramuscular injection of androgens appears to enable good sexual and psychosocial adjustment in men who have undergone bilateral orchiectomy for testicular cancer (Fossa et al. 1999). In a study of men who underwent orchiectomy followed by radiotherapy for seminoma, 20% of the subjects indicated reductions of interest in sex, sexual activity, and pleasure in sex but not to a degree significantly different from that of age-matched healthy controls (Incrocci et al. 2002). In both prostate and testicular cancer, psychiatrists may be called on to assist the patient in choosing between treatments that are effective but are harmful to sexual function and treatments that spare sexual functioning at the expense of cancer-fighting efficacy (Singer et al. 1991).

Tumors of nongenital sites, such as bladder, colon, and rectum, and lymphoma also can be associated with sexual dysfunction, either as a direct consequence of treatments (e.g., retroperitoneal lymph node dissection) or as a result of the negative effects on a patient's self-esteem and body image. For example, ostomy patients might have a particularly difficult struggle with regaining comfortable sexual expression (Ofman and Auchincloss 1992) (see Chapter 30, "Surgery"). ED, ejaculatory difficulties, and dyspareunia all are reported to occur in ostomy patients (Sprunk and Alteneder 2000). New surgical techniques are being explored for preserving sexual functioning in bladder cancer patients (Colombo et al. 2004; Horenblas et al. 2001).

The chemotherapies used to treat cancers distant from the genitourinary system, such as lung cancer, can negatively affect sexual function (Schwartz and Plawecki 2002). All cancer patients should be asked specifically about sexual issues and sexual history, and questions should be addressed to the patient's partner when possible. Health care professionals should not make any assumptions about sexual orientation and should convey a sense of openness to the range of human sexual expression. Negative attitudes in society, among professionals, and within the health care culture, can contribute to the sexual dysfunction of cancer patients by promoting neglect of this aspect of a quality life (Rice 2000). A positive stance should be taken, and an informed capacity for basic counseling and further referral when indicated is necessary (Auchincloss 1989).

Diabetes Mellitus

Many physicians are aware of the nearly threefold increase in ED among diabetic patients (Dey and Shepherd 2002). However, sexual dysfunction in diabetic patients is considerably more pleomorphic than commonly recognized. Fairburn et al. (1982a, 1982b) noted a variety of sexual problems in addition to ED, including a range of ejaculatory disturbances, loss of sexual interest, persistent morning erections in one-half of subjects, and spontaneous erections in one-third. ED in men with type 1 diabetes

correlates with increasing age, duration of diabetes, chronic diabetic complications, and reduced levels of androgens (Alexopoulou et al. 2001). ED in diabetic men also correlates with smoking, obesity, and high levels of glycosylated hemoglobin (Dey and Shepherd 2002).

Psychological factors (e.g., premorbid sexual difficulties and marital discord) may contribute significantly to the presence of ED. Forsberg et al. (1989) conducted a study in which the subjects were 37 diabetic men with ED. The investigators concluded that psychosocial factors were the sole cause of ED in only two patients. Nevertheless, despite identification of neuropathic, hormonal, and vascular contributions in the other 35 men, nearly two-thirds of them had psychosocial factors of importance. One-half of these factors were judged to be of great importance in the diagnosis and treatment of sexual dysfunction.

Lustman and Clouse (1990) further examined the unfortunate but common assumption that diabetic ED is wholly "organic." They used a standardized interview to study 37 diabetic men who had established peripheral neuropathy, peripheral vascular disease, or both. All eight men with neuropathy who met criteria for either current major depression or generalized anxiety disorder had ED. Among the 20 men with neuropathy but neither of the psychiatric diagnoses, only six had ED. Although the study was retrospective and causality was not established, the results suggested that the association between neuropathy and ED often may be dependent on the psychiatric status of the patient.

A meta-analysis of the literature showed that depression was significantly associated with a variety of diabetic complications, including sexual dysfunction (De Groot et al. 2001). Thase et al. (1988) showed that depression alone can produce abnormal findings in nocturnal penile tumescence studies. These observations strengthened the call for caution in assigning undue emphasis to diabetic "organicity" solely on the basis of time-honored evaluations such as nocturnal penile tumescence studies. In a placebo-controlled study in which the subjects were 268 men with diabetes and ED, Rendell et al. (1999) found that 56% of the men reported improved erections using sildenafil and that 10% reported improved erections using placebo. This response rate was 20%–40% lower than that found in a study of sildenafil response in a urology clinical practice (Marks 1999). Taken together with the correlation between psychiatric diagnosis and ED, the need for a comprehensive psychosocial evaluation during assessment and treatment of sexual dysfunction in diabetic patients is emphasized (Sarica et al. 1994).

Sildenafil has been proved beneficial in treating ED in diabetic men (Hatzichristou 2002). Intracavernosal alprostadil injection also is effective treatment. In an open-label, flexible dose-escalating study in which the subjects were diabetic men with ED, 99% of the men reported satisfactory erectile response with intracavernosal alprostadil injection (Heaton et al. 2001). The treatment was well tolerated, albeit with a 24% rate of penile pain. In a survey of 400 diabetes treatment centers in Italy, intracavernosal alprostadil injection was the primary treatment of 85% of diabetic men with ED (Fedele et al. 2001).

The sexual functioning of diabetic women has come under increasing study. In one study, Forsberg et al. (1989) concluded that diabetic women do not have a greater incidence of sexual dysfunction than women in the general population. Webster (1994), however, found that problems with libido, arousal, and orgasm were common to both men and women with diabetes. Erol et al. (2002) found lack of libido in 77% of young women with type 2 diabetes. These investigators also found the patients reported diminished clitoral sensation (62.5%), vaginal discomfort (41.6%), and vaginal dryness (37.5%). In another study, 27% of women with type 1 diabetes reported diminished sexual function; only 15% of control subjects reported this problem (Enzlin et al. 2002). Sexual dysfunction was correlated with the degree of diabetic complications and reduced vaginal lubrication. Quality of marriage and number of endorsed depression symptoms correlated with the presence of sexual dysfunction in both diabetic subjects and healthy control subjects.

Renal Failure

Sexual dysfunction is common in both women and men with renal failure. ED, menstrual abnormalities, and reduced libido and fertility in men and women are highly prevalent (Palmer 1999). The widespread impact of renal failure on multiple organ systems produces a variety of physiological disturbances implicated in sexual dysfunction.

Endocrinological changes in uremic men include decreased testosterone level, increased estradiol level, and excess parathyroid hormone, and all these disorders are linked to sexual dysfunction (Campese and Liu 1990). In men, the impact of renal failure appears to be expressed primarily at the testicular end of the hypothalamic-pituitary-gonadal axis. In women, the impact appears to be more marked in the central nervous system (Palmer 1999). Autonomic dysfunction (Vita et al. 1999), elevated cholesterol level (Cerqueira et al. 2002), and vascular insufficiency (Campese and Liu 1990) all contribute to ED arising from renal failure. More than one-half of uremic women report decreased sexual interest and anorgasmia (Finkelstein and Steele 1978). Medications commonly used in chronic renal failure (e.g., antihypertensives) may further aggravate sexual dysfunction. The anemia of renal failure can drain patients of the desire and energy for sexual activity. Erythropoietin treatment of anemia in men with end-stage renal disease has been shown to improve both gonadotropic hormone levels and sexual function (Wu S et al. 2001).

Entry into long-term dialysis does not appear to alleviate sexual dysfunction. The prevalence of sexual dysfunction is high among renal failure patients undergoing hemodialysis (Naya et al. 2002) and peritoneal dialysis (Juergense et al. 2001). Rates of 62.9% and 75% among men and women, respectively, have been reported for hemodialysis and rates of 69.8% and 66.7% among men and women, respectively, for peritoneal dialysis (Diemont et al. 2000). The prevalence of ED appears to gradually worsen with dialysis treatment (Dillard et al. 1989; Malavaud et al. 2000). Some research findings suggest the possibility of ethnic differences. Older white hemodialysis patients reported greater sexual dysfunction than did matched black counterparts (Kutner et al. 2000).

The prevalence of sexual dysfunction declines after renal transplantation. Rates of 48.3% in men and 44.4% in women have been reported (Diemont et al. 2000). As is the case before transplantation, penile arterial and venous insufficiency plays a substantial role in the pathogenesis of ED in male transplantation patients (Abdel-Hamid et al. 2002). The effect of renal transplantation on sexual functioning remains mixed. In one study (Schover et al. 1990) in which the subjects were 54 men and 36 women who had undergone successful transplantation during the previous 5 years, sexual desire increased significantly for both men and women. Many men also reported substantial improvement in the ability to achieve an erection and experience orgasm. Women enjoyed less definitive improvement in their capacity for orgasm. Although the frequency of sexual activity in women after transplantation doubled to once per week, this rate did not achieve statistical significance. Overall sexual satisfaction levels remained constant before and after transplantation. Approximately 25% of the sample retained sexual dysfunction after transplantation. Tsujimura et al. (2002a) found that 35.5% of posttransplantation patients reported improvement in overall sexual functioning, but 28.1% described overall worsening. Notably, 15 of 20 patients with no intercourse history before transplantation initiated intercourse after transplantation. All 15 patients were younger than 40 years, suggesting a need for earlier transplantation intervention.

Development of end-stage renal disease before adulthood is reached creates obstacles to the achievement of intimate relationships. Schover et al. (1990) found that

37% of people in whom end-stage renal disease developed before adulthood did not marry, compared with only 7% of people in whom end-stage renal disease developed after the person reached adulthood. Although 75% of young patients with renal disease expressed a broad interest in information on sexuality, only one-third of them had received it. This finding points to a particular—and often unmet—need for sexual education and counseling of younger patients with end-stage renal disease to facilitate their development of committed relationships.

As in other illnesses, sildenafil has been used in the treatment of ED in patients with renal disease. The drug has been reported to be safe, reliable, and effective in patients undergoing hemodialysis or peritoneal dialysis (Turk et al. 2001). However, one study showed a benefit among only 13% of peritoneal dialysis patients treated with sildenafil (Juergense et al. 2001), but only one-half of the subjects offered participation chose to take sildenafil. Sildenafil treatment proved to be safe and effective in a group of renal transplantation patients (Prieto Castro et al. 2001). Sildenafil has not been shown to alter immunosuppressant drug levels despite clearance through the same metabolic pathways (Christ et al. 2001; Prieto Castro et al. 2001). Christ et al. (2001) did recommend the lowest possible starting dose of sildenafil and a downward adjustment of preexisting antihypertensive medications because of instances of low blood pressure during concomitant use of sildenafil and tacrolimus.

HIV/AIDS

Patients with early stages of HIV infection, defined as >400 CD4 cells/mm^3 of blood and usually no physical symptoms, may express sexual concerns that have become both quality-of-life and relationship issues for themselves and their partners. New onset of hypoactive sexual desire disorder—operationally defined for this population as at least a one-third decrease in baseline levels of sexual fantasies or desire for sexual activity of any type persistently present for at least 1 month and beginning at least 1 month after notification of HIV seroconversion (among other specific criteria) (Brown et al. 1992)—is one of the most common psychiatric diagnoses in both men and women with early-stage HIV disease. For example, 21.7% of 442 men (Brown et al. 1992) and 31%–41% of 25 women (Brown and Rundell 1990, 1993) were found to have disorders of sexual desire in a U.S. Air Force population. Impaired sexual desire also has been reported in men with HIV disease in Australia (32% of men) (Dunbar et al. 1991) and the Netherlands (23% of men) (Van Buuren et al. 1991). Additionally, the prevalence of depression, with its impact on sexual desire, is higher in men who have sex with men, independent of HIV status (Mills et al. 2004). Rosser et al. (1997) reviewed the sexual issues of gay men living with HIV.

Among women with early HIV disease who are not chemically dependent, marital problems and hypoactive sexual desire disorder may be the only psychiatric problems with substantially increased clinical frequency (Brown and Rundell 1993). Later stages of the illness are associated with increased rates of depression and anxiety disorders, both of which complicate sexual functioning (Morrison et al. 2002). When hypoactive sexual desire disorder is present in HIV-infected women, the women usually describe it in a typical manner 4–18 months after learning of their HIV seropositivity: gradual onset over a 2- to 6-month period, usually in the presence of a willing partner and in the absence of comorbid medical or psychiatric conditions (Brown et al. 1995). The sexual desire problems usually are not a component of mood or anxiety disorders, although such disorders should be ruled out. Most patients in whom hypoactive sexual desire disorder develops a year or more after notification of seropositivity are puzzled by the symptoms and frequently convey that these symptoms threaten previously established levels of intimacy in important relationships. This phenomenon, possibly due to direct infection of the brain by HIV, has been found in women from middle-class backgrounds free of poverty and drug abuse as well as in the inner city populations of intravenous drug users, who often face the challenges of poverty and instability in all areas of life (Goggin et al. 1998).

Patients with late-stage HIV disease (AIDS) may be physically debilitated by the opportunistic infections, wasting, and fatigue that often bring them into the hospital (Tindall et al. 1994). Depression is a frequent concomitant of later HIV disease and contributes not only to sexual dysfunction but also to heightened susceptibility to infectious diseases and diminished longevity in both men (Leserman et al. 1999) and women (Morrison et al. 2002). Testosterone supplementation in HIV-infected men with both mood symptoms and decreased libido has proved effective in controlled studies (Rabkin et al. 1999, 2000).

Sexual health is often overlooked in both the psychiatric and medical care of HIV-infected patients. Patients with positive results of serological tests for HIV may be reluctant to discuss their sexual dysfunction, especially when the topic is not broached by their physicians. Communication is further hampered when the primary physician suggests that complete abstinence from interpersonal sexuality is the only acceptable "safe" alternative. Such absolutism serves only to jeopardize informed, collaborative decision making about sexual and reproductive behavior (Minkoff and Moreno 1990). With the success of prenatal and postnatal antiretroviral treatments that has been replicated in numerous trials, perinatal transmission in the United States has been reduced to less than 7%, making the decision by HIV-positive women to have children substantially safer than in the early years of the epidemic. Negative or moralistic attitudes on the part of the consultant can also lead to dangerous sexual "acting out." HIV/AIDS in developed countries has become a chronic illness managed over possibly decades of infection, covering many years of the reproductive life span. For those who have access to these life-prolonging treatments, there is evidence that this availability may increase the likelihood that uninfected patients engage in risky sexual behaviors (Strathdee et al. 2000; Vanable et al. 2000). Psychiatrists can make a useful contribution by opening a dialogue on sexual issues and communicating the view that sexual health may incorporate responsible, "safer sex" approaches that can limit HIV transmission. Patients should be informed that an undetectable viral load, for example, does not eliminate transmission risk, as is often perceived to be the case (Martin et al. 2001). Additional didactic information may include the potential benefits of masturbation and mutual masturbation with a partner. Major depression and dementia (Atkinson et al. 1988) may also complicate all stages of HIV infection, especially later stages. Sexual desire disorders and, less commonly, secondary ED may accompany these independently treatable conditions.

Psychiatrists caring for HIV/AIDS patients must be aware of the clear connection between increased high-transmission risk behaviors (e.g., unprotected intercourse with seronegative partners) and substance use (Vittinghoff et al. 2001). Use of volatile nitrites ("poppers") at the point of orgasm to intensify the experience has been linked to higher-risk behaviors (Ostrow et al. 1991), as have alcohol and illicit drug use (Crosby et al. 1991; Ostrow and McKirnan 1997). Methamphetamine use by gay and bisexual male patients is strongly linked to higher probabilities of medical illness and unsafe sexual activity (Shoptaw et al. 2002). In the 1990s there appeared to be a decrease in the use of high-risk sexual behaviors, possibly linked to declines in illicit drug use. However, more recent surveys of men having sex with men revealed a continuing strong association between drug and alcohol intoxication and unprotected anal intercourse in a new generation of men who have not known a world without HIV (Stueve et al. 2002). There is evidence to support the concept that at least some men who have sex with men, especially those who are not gay-identified, use substances to deal with internalized homophobia or with anxiety over the risk of contracting HIV infection (Dolezal et al. 2000).

Sexual Functioning in Neurological Disorders

Disorders involving the nervous system can have profound effects on sexuality, involving all phases of the sexual response cycle. Sipski (2001) reviewed sexual functioning in women with neurological disorders, including spinal cord injuries, multiple sclerosis (MS), and dementia, and cerebrovascular accidents (CVAs).

Spinal Cord Injury

The central, peripheral, and autonomic nervous systems are all essential to sexual functioning. Injury to one or more components can disrupt an individual's patterns of function. When spinal cord injury occurs at the cervical or thoracic level, ascending sensory and descending upper motor neuron tracts are compromised. The capability of psychogenic erection or clitoral engorgement is compromised. However, the genital spinal cord reflex allows genital arousal and orgasm to occur in response to mechanical stimulation (Higgins 1978). The patient, however, cannot feel genital sensations, and the reflexive erections usually are unpredictable and often insufficient to sustain intercourse. If the injury occurs at the lumbar or sacral level, the genital spinal cord reflex is lost, and reflexogenic erections do not occur. However, if the injury has spared the autonomic nervous system, the capability of psychogenic genital arousal is preserved. The loss of sensation varies according to the lesion (Kaufman 1990; Stewart 1991).

The erectile disabilities and anorgasmia of spinal cord injury patients are compounded by the potential for bowel and bladder incontinence, the frequent necessity for urinary catheters, and the loss of accustomed mobility and normal sensation. Stewart (1991) properly emphasized the value of discussing sexual possibilities with spinal cord injury patients to affirm the reality of some retained sexual behavior and feelings after the injury, a reality the patient often doubts. This overture also presents the opportunity for patients to share sadness over what has been lost in both the sexual and nonsexual spheres of life (Stewart 1991). A physical therapist with experience in the sexual problems of spinal cord injury can provide invaluable practical assistance.

Spinal cord injuries occur most often in active people younger than 40 years who are usually otherwise healthy. Premorbid sexual and reproductive functioning in most cases is normal. Although women with spinal cord injuries commonly report sexual dysfunction in all phases of the sexual response cycle (including desire-phase disorders, diminished lubrication and swelling, and anorgasmia), most of the literature focuses on ED in paraplegic and quadriplegic men.

Sildenafil may improve the quality of erections after spinal cord injury without the need for a complicated autoinjection regimen. Derry et al. (1998) studied a group of 27 patients who maintained at least a partial reflexogenic erectile response to penile vibratory stimulation after sustaining T6–L5 lesions. After 28 days, 75% of the patients taking sildenafil and 7% taking placebo reported that treatment had improved their erections. In a study of 170 outpatient men with spinal cord injuries, sildenafil improved erections as evidenced by the reports of 88% of the men and 85% of their partners, regardless of the baseline characteristics of the spinal cord injury (Ramos et al. 2001). Similarly, a double-blind, placebo-controlled, crossover study of sildenafil in men with ED secondary to spinal cord injury showed 78% of the men reported improved erections (Giuliano et al. 1999). Derry et al. (2002) performed a comprehensive review of the use of sildenafil in men with spinal cord injury. Women with spinal cord injury also appear to gain benefit with sildenafil. In a double-blind, placebo-controlled, crossover study of 19 women with spinal cord injury, Sipski et al. (2000) found significant increases in the women's subjective report of arousal, particularly when the active drug was paired with a program of visual and manual sexual stimulation. Spinal cord injury patients should generally use a trial of oral therapy with sildenafil or other nitric oxide synthetase inhibitors before resorting to pharmacological erection programs or autoinjections.

Because the etiology of ED in men with spinal cord injuries usually is neurogenic, these men may be candidates for intracavernosal pharmacotherapy. These treatments are best accomplished in the form of home autoinjections for paraplegic men with adequate motivation and dexterity or as a partner-assisted erection program for quadriplegic men (Gerstenberg et al. 1992).

If oral treatment is not effective or appropriate for a patient with spinal cord injury, pharmacological erection programs (Padma-Nathan and Kanellos 1992; Padma-Nathan et al. 1987) may prove a viable option for safely restoring adequate erectile function for intercourse. Originally, fixed combinations of phentolamine mesylate and papaverine hydrochloride were administered by injection with a 0.5-inch (1.27 cm), 28-gauge needle into the lateral base of the penis at the level of the corpus cavernosum. A firm erection for an hour after treatment was the targeted outcome. Corporal scarring (3%) and extended priapism (variable rates) were the major side effects. Advances in this therapy entail a more physiological combination of prostaglandin E_1 and phentolamine mesylate or a triple mixture of papaverine, phentolamine, and alprostadil (prostaglandin E_1) (Chao and Clowers 1994). Test doses are increased until the optimal dose is achieved (erection of sufficient rigidity for intercourse for about 1 hour). The pharmacologically induced erection is often enhanced in both duration and rigidity by sexual stimulation, which then allows a decrease in medication dose. Although priapism remains a risk, the incidence of corporal scarring has been greatly reduced with the substitution of prostaglandin E_1. The average frequency of autoinjection or partner-assisted injection has been reported to be seven times per month, and the partner and patient satisfaction rating is more than 90% (Padma-Nathan and Kanellos 1992).

Other treatments available to patients with spinal cord injuries and ED include a variety of penile prostheses, topical applications of nitroglycerin (Meyhoff et al. 1992), and use of a negative-pressure, or vacuum erection, device (Witherington 1988). Vacuum devices produce negative pressure by using suction and causing mechanical entrapment of blood in the penis. Care must be exercised in the application of such devices owing to the lack of protective sensitivity in the genitals.

Inappropriate sexual behavior on the part of young, male spinal cord injury patients is not uncommon. Impulsive, excitement-seeking individuals are overrepresented in this clinical population (e.g., they have been injured in motorcycle accidents, falling from heights while intoxicated, and in high-speed car crashes). Some of these men do not readily adapt to the literal and figurative impotence associated with spinal cord injury and act out sexually toward the staff they depend on for their care. This behavior jeopardizes the quality of care these patients receive, because the staff may begin avoiding them (consciously or unconsciously) to avoid these uncomfortable interactions. The psychiatrist can gently but firmly discuss this issue with the patient, pointing out that such behavior drives away caregivers and thus deprives the patient of the good care he deserves. The psychiatrist can deliver this message while making it clear that the behavior is unacceptable but without scolding or shaming the patient.

Multiple Sclerosis

MS generally affects individuals between the ages of 20 and 40 years, a time when base rates of sexual dysfunction are otherwise relatively low. Because MS has a variable course and is associated with primary and secondary psychiatric disorders, psychiatrists are often involved in the care of MS patients. Sexual dysfunction is rarely the initial symptom of MS but regularly appears during the course of illness. Deleterious effects on sexuality have been found in 60%–91% of men and 52%–77% of women (Hulter and Lundberg, 1995; Zorzon et al. 2001). Even in cases of "mild" MS with minimal chronic neurological manifestations of the disease, the frequency of sexual dysfunction in both men and women may be high (43% of men, 52% of women) compared with the frequency among the general population (Minderhoud et al. 1984). In a case–control study of 108 MS patients, Zorzon et al. (1999) found anorgasmia or hyporgasmia (37% women), reduced vaginal lubrication (35.7%), diminished libido (39.5% men, 31.4% women), ED (63.2%), and ejaculatory and orgasmic dysfunction (50% men). ED is the most common sexual problem among men with MS; at least 90% of cases are diagnosed as neurogenic and less than 10% as "mainly psychogenic" (Kirkeby et al. 1988). In contrast, disorders in the orgasm phase (48%) and desire phase (58%) are most common in women. A minority of both men and women report that pelvic sensory defects (21% men, 29% women) and fatigue (26% men, 29% women) contribute to sexual dysfunction.

Longitudinal studies of both male and female patients with MS indicated that the number of patients with at least one type of sexual dysfunction increases with time in both sexes (Stenager et al. 1996). On the other hand, in light of the high baseline rates of sexual dysfunction early in the disease process, Zorzon et al. (2001), in a 2-year prospective study of the longitudinal course of MS, found no progression of the greater than 70% baseline prevalence of sexual dysfunction, even as the extent and severity of neurological symptoms advanced. After removal of psychological factors by multivariate analysis, bladder dysfunction was the physical symptom with an independent relationship to sexual dysfunction. Among psychological factors, depression is most closely linked to sexual dysfunction in MS (Janardhan and Bakshi 2002).

The impact of sexual dysfunction cannot be overestimated: sexual problems were predictive of self-reported low quality of life even among MS patients whose neurological disabilities were otherwise mild (Nortvedt et al. 2001). In patients with MS, changes in sexual functioning are not highly correlated with overall ability to ambulate but are correlated with neurological symptoms that can be traced to the sacral segments and to the presence of vertigo and ataxia (Hulter and Lundberg 1995).

Few patients with MS report that the importance of sexual activity decreases after diagnosis, and only 5% endorse the view that chronic illness constitutes a "good reason" for reduced sexual interest and activity (Minderhoud et al. 1984). It has been reported that rare patients with MS paradoxically develop transient hypersexuality (Gondim and Thomas 2001) and, in one case, paraphilia (Frohman et al. 2002). As in most of the other conditions discussed in this chapter, sexual dysfunction in one sexual partner can jeopardize intimacy in spousal or other supportive relationships. Dupont (1996) has thoroughly reviewed sexual functioning in patients with MS.

Dementia

The emergence of disruptive sexual behavior in patients with dementing diseases causes significant distress for family members and hospital staff. Psychiatrists are asked to evaluate patients with compulsive public masturbation, frequent genital exposures, fondling of other patients and staff, and dangerous sexual behaviors (e.g., vaginal or rectal insertions of sharp objects or chair legs). In a study of 133 consecutive admissions to a dementia unit, caretakers in 15% of cases reported inappropriate sexual behaviors without correlation to age, age at dementia onset, gender, educational level, Mini-Mental State Examination score, or type of dementia (Tsai et al. 1999). Patients with Klüver-Bucy syndrome, resulting from bilateral lesions of the temporal lobes, frequently act in inappropriate, hypersexual ways. Normal inhibitory controls appear to be impaired, and primitive sexual displays result. Problems related to hypersexuality may be the cause of hospital admission in patients with Huntington's chorea. A longitudinal study of patients with Huntington's chorea revealed abnormal sexual behavior in 63% of patients, including exhibitionism, sexual aggression, voyeurism, and hypersexuality (Dewhurst and Oliver 1970). Sexual "acting out" by patients with Alzheimer's disease or multi-infarct dementia may frequently reflect disordered frontotemporal inhibitory mechanisms and cause a release phenomenon (Cooper 1987). Behavior is rarely predatory or dangerous but may involve inadvertent self-harm (e.g., during episodes of compulsive or aggressive masturbation). For example, we evaluated a patient with Alzheimer's disease who was hospitalized after public masturbation in a shopping mall. During the admission, the patient was found publicly masturbating while inserting the leg of his desk chair rectally.

Antiandrogen treatment may be effective in some men with dementia and sexual disorders. This treatment may decrease dangerous sexual behaviors. In one study, 300 mg of medroxyprogesterone acetate (MPA) administered intramuscularly each week suppressed dangerous and troublesome sexual behaviors within 14 days in four elderly demented patients, ages 75–84 years (Cooper 1987). After 1 year, MPA was discontinued and three of four patients' behavior remained under control for a 1-year, drug-free follow-up period even though serum testosterone levels had returned to baseline normal levels within 4 weeks of discontinuation. Gonadotropin-releasing hormone analogues, such as triptorelin, goserelin, and others, may be considered in treatment when these behaviors are severe. If this type of treatment is used, caregivers need to be aware that an initial increase in testosterone level after the initial injections is followed by a rapid decline. In this early treatment phase, it is possible for the offending behaviors to temporarily worsen. Because of the ethical and legal issues associated with using pharmacological agents for behavioral "control" of patients with dementia, physicians are advised to seek informed consent from guardians, next of kin, or the courts.

Other Neurological Conditions

There is a growing literature on sexual problems in other neurological conditions. For example, more than 50% of patients who have sustained traumatic brain injury have a decrease in sexual arousal after injury (Crowe and Ponsford 1999). After correction for the level of postinjury depression, reduced cognitive capacity for forming sexual imagery was found to correlate with reduced sexual arousal. The sleep fragmentation in obstructive sleep apnea has been demonstrated to cause diminished levels of luteinizing hormone and testosterone, thereby reducing libido in men with this disorder (Luboshitzky et al. 2002). Awareness of the central role of temporal lobe structures in sexual functioning is growing. In a study of 60 epileptic patients, temporal lobe seizure was related to the development of sexual dysfunction (Souza et al. 2000). Mendez et al. (2000) reported two cases of increasing sexual behavior and late-life-onset homosexual pedophilia developing in the context of brain disease. Positron emission tomographic scanning highlighted right temporal lobe hypometabolism in both men. Krueger and Kaplan (2000) reviewed disorders of sexual impulse control in various neuropsychiatric conditions.

Parkinson's disease commonly causes sexual dysfunction. In their study of 115 patients with Parkinson's disease, Sakakibara and colleagues (2001) found decreased libido in 84% and 83% and decreased sexual intercourse in 55% and 88% of women and men, respectively. These investigators also reported reductions in orgasm (87%), erections (79%), and ejaculation (79%) in the men. Sildenafil had good efficacy in a randomized, placebo-controlled, crossover trial involving 12 men with Parkinson's disease and 12 men with multiple-system atrophy (Hussain et al. 2001). The authors cautioned that exacerbation of hypotension was a problem in using sildenafil to treat men with multiple system atrophy. Sildenafil also was found efficacious in an open-label trial in which the subjects were men with Parkinson's disease and depression (Raffaele et al. 2002). There was both improvement in erections (85% of patients) and alleviation of depressive symptoms (75%).

Cerebrovascular Accident (Stroke)

Unlike those with MS or spinal cord injuries, most patients who experience a CVA are older than 50 years. Because American society tends to "asexualize" elderly and medically ill people, it is not surprising that studies of sexuality in elderly CVA patients have been few, despite the fact that CVA is one of the most common causes of long-term disability. Approximately one-third of patients die of the acute consequences of CVA; one-third are seriously disabled; and one-third largely recover. Sexual functioning after a CVA is generally characterized by reduced desire and decreased frequency of activity in both men and women. There is no general agreement, however, on the causes of decline in sexual functioning, and the relative contributions of the lesion and psychosocial factors are unclear.

In two large studies, all phases of sexual response were impaired after CVA (Table 17–1). In an early study of CVA patients whose average age was approximately 68 years, Monga et al. (1986) found poststroke decreases in desire (54%), erection (56%), lubrication (34%), and orgasm (51% men, 32% women) compared with baseline measurements. Korpelainen et al. (1999) replicated these findings in a sample in Finland, finding that both CVA patients and their spouses were highly likely to experience major disruptions in sexual interest (57%–65%), regularity of intercourse (55%, including cessation altogether in 33%), erectile capacity (75%), vaginal lubrication (46%), and overall sexual satisfaction compared with prestroke baseline values. In a study of Italian patients 1 year after stroke, Giaquinto et al. (2003) found that both patients and their partners were quite forthcoming with information about the significant decline in sexual activity and the reasons for it when directly queried. These investigators also found that the average decline in "frequency of performance" compared with baseline was 83% irrespective of age. More than one-half of men reported severe ED, although 3% reported an increase in sexual activity after stroke. All of these men had a right-sided temporal lesion. This increase was true hypersexuality, not to be confused with the occasional increase in libido noted in some patients when the location of the lesion appears to be irrelevant. For example, Korpelainen et al. (1999) found that 19 of 192 patients experienced an increase in libido in the months after CVA compared with their baseline values. These investigators found that none of the patients were pathologically hypersexual. The investigators speculated that the enhancement in sexual interest was within the normal range and was most likely linked to the improved relationship experienced by these patients and their spouses during rehabilitation.

TABLE 17–1. Changes in sexual functioning after stroke

Phase	Before CVA (%)	After CVA (%)
Normal desire, male	75	21
Normal desire, female	60	34
Normal erection	94	38
Normal lubrication	63	29
Normal orgasm, male	73	22
Normal orgasm, female	43	11
Anorgasmia, female	34	77
Premature ejaculation	13	43

Note. CVA=cerebrovascular accident.
Source. Adapted from Monga T, Lawson J, Inglis J: "Sexual Dysfunction in Stroke Patients." *Archives of Physical Medicine and Rehabilitation* 67:19–22, 1986. Copyright 1986, WB Saunders. Used with permission.

In women, right-hemisphere lesions appear to cause less sexual dysfunction than left-hemisphere CVA. The reverse may be true for men. In one study, 75% of men with unilateral right-hemisphere CVA had sexual dysfunction compared with 29% of those with left-hemisphere CVA (Coslett and Heilman 1986). It has been hypothesized that limbic activation of the dominant hemisphere for sexual function is required for intact sexual functioning in men. Other investigators have not found that changes in sexual functioning in general are based on the location of the lesion (Korpelainen et al. 1999).

In addition to experiencing loss of independence or control over some body movements, CVA patients often experience the loss of their sexual life (Hawton 1984). Monga et al. (1986) found that 95% of men and 76% of women in their late 60s were satisfied with their sexual lives before CVA, whereas only 26% of men and 37% of women remained satisfied after CVA. The most common self-reported cause of both decreased satisfaction and increased dysfunction is fear of having another CVA initiated by blood pressure elevations associated with sexual activity. Other reported causes include diminished self-esteem, anxiety about sexual performance, fear of partner rejection, and pharmacotherapy toxic to sexual functioning (e.g., antianxiety, hypotensive, antidepressant, and hypnotic medications). In a review of poststroke urogenital and sexual problems, Marinkovic and Badlani (2001) found that an additional concern is urinary incontinence, which is considered the best single indicator of future disability, having 60% sensitivity and 78% specificity (Taub et al. 1994). Unlike patients with MS and spinal cord injury, much of whose sexual dysfunction has a clear neurogenic etiology, those surviving one or more CVAs appear more likely to have substantial psychological concerns

that may account for or contribute to their post-CVA sexual problems. Giaquinto et al. (2003) identified that the main issues regarding sexual dysfunction 1 year poststroke were based far more on psychosocial and marital issues than on the location or size of the lesion. These issues included fear of recurrence on the part of the patient or partner, belief that sex is limited to those who are healthy, and the partner's being "turned off" by the idea of having intercourse with a "sick person."

Emotional incontinence is a frequent sequela of CVA and MS and has been linked to both subacute and chronic sexual dysfunction. The presence of emotional incontinence 3 months after stroke was predictive of decreased sexual interest, frequency of intercourse, and erectile capacity at 2 years (Choi-Kwon and Kim 2002).

Although no guarantees can be offered, patients can be informed that the changes in heart rate, blood pressure, and oxygen uptake during most forms of conventional sexual activity with an established partner are similar to those experienced during light to moderate short-term exercise (Bohlen et al. 1984). Orgasm lasting only seconds is associated with the greatest increases in these physiological parameters, which then quickly return to baseline values during the resolution phase of the sexual response cycle. To further decrease stroke risk for men, it has been suggested that couples engage in longer foreplay and minimize or eliminate use of the man-on-top coital position. Self-stimulation and partner stimulation to orgasm using noncoital techniques may further limit the risk of adverse circulatory events.

Psychiatrists should be aware that sexual morbidity after CVA may be largely unrelated to the CVA itself. Diabetes, coronary artery disease, peripheral vascular disease, and hypertension are all very common in CVA patients. Premorbid relationship problems, including loss of interest in sex or in the partner, may be important contributors, the CVA presenting a convenient and socially acceptable reason to exempt oneself from a previously unsatisfactory sexual relationship. In these situations, it is often the spouse who seeks assistance for the identified patient's sexual dysfunction. In addition, loss of sexual desire is a common symptom of major depressive syndromes, for which patients have a heightened risk after stroke.

Medications and Sexual Functioning

Many medications are associated with sexual dysfunction in all phases of the human sexual response cycle. DSM-IV included a new diagnostic category that can be used to differentiate these disorders of substance-induced sexual dysfunctions from nonprescribed substance use. Hospitalized patients are frequently taking several of the medications listed in Table 17–2 that may contribute to sexual dysfunction, but patients may be hesitant to discuss these problems.

Fluoxetine and paroxetine, typical of the selective serotonin reuptake inhibitor (SSRI) drugs, can delay or prevent normal orgasm. This fact has led to use of these drugs in treating premature ejaculation (Waldinger et al. 1997). Sildenafil citrate (Viagra) has revolutionized the treatment of ED in men with physiological compromise, whether vascular or neurologically induced (Eid 2000). The extraordinary prevalence of ED—39% of 40-year-olds, 67% of 70-year-olds (Feldman et al. 1994)—has resulted in the resounding success of this medication in the licit and illicit marketplaces. Sildenafil has become the medication most frequently marketed by illegal Internet "pharmacies."

Sildenafil has a proven record of efficacy compared with placebo in a variety of contexts producing ED. ED arising from diabetes, cardiovascular disease, spinal cord injury, and MS is amenable to sildenafil treatment, and sildenafil shows promise for ED resulting from prostate cancer and its treatments, end-stage renal disease, Parkinson's disease, spina bifida, and multiple organ transplantation (Sadovsky et al. 2001). Sildenafil is effective for aging men, 65.7% having a good response (Tsujimura et al. 2002b). Pooled safety data from 18 studies involving more than 3,700 men showed a remarkable safety profile (Gregoire 1998). Patients with renal and hepatic disease can be treated with this generally safe agent. Typical side effects are minor and include headaches, flushing, nasal congestion, transient changes in color vision, and dyspepsia. However, in one study only 2% of men discontinued treatment because of side effects (Gregoire 1998).

The success of sildenafil has substantially changed practice patterns. Some authors have argued that the medical evaluation of ED no longer requires such historically standard procedures as duplex ultrasonography, nocturnal penile tumescence studies, and penile pharmacotesting (Aversa and Fabbri 2001). Oral therapy with sildenafil or apomorphine (administered in Europe) is the recommended first-line treatment of ED because it is effective and lacks invasiveness (Aversa and Fabbri 2001). Notably, 75% of men with successfully established regimens of intracavernosal alprostadil injection for ED respond well to sildenafil, and when they are given the choice of sildenafil or intracavernosal alprostadil injection, 64% prefer sildenafil (Hatzichristou et al. 2000). Topical alprostadil cream is efficacious and provides an alternative for men who cannot take phosphodiesterase inhibitors and who will not tolerate the invasiveness of intracavernosal injection (Becher 2004).

Drug treatment without consideration of psychological and relationship factors will have much less chance of sustained success than a more comprehensive approach that takes into account both physical and psychological contributions to the problem. For example, 50%–60% of men discontinue successful pharmacological treatment of ED (Althof 2002). Wise (1999) reported the destabilization of a relationship, previously characterized by long-term sexual abstinence, after the introduction of sildenafil. It should be noted that sildenafil is ineffective in the absence of physical sexual stimuli, a fact not always shared with patients.

Because of its success in men, sildenafil has been used to treat women with sexual arousal disorder, and results of the initial open-label research were promising (J. R. Berman et al. 2001; Kaplan et al. 1999). In general, randomized, controlled trials of sildenafil in the treatment of women with sexual arousal disorder have not shown benefit (Basson et al. 2002; Caruso et al. 2001; Laan et al. 2002). A clinical trial of sildenafil in women with spinal cord injuries did demonstrate benefit (Sipski et al. 2000) (see earlier section, "Spinal Cord Injury").

The negative efficacy of sildenafil in arousal disorders in women highlights the need for a global, biopsychosocial approach. For example, women with a childhood history of sexual abuse, a developmental insult highly correlated with later adult sexual dysfunction, did not benefit from sildenafil (L. A. Berman et al. 2001). Because of the recent heavy emphasis on oral medication, Bancroft (2002) admonished physicians not to "medicalize" female sexual dysfunction. He noted that female sexual functioning is, in general, more broadly affected by social and psychological factors than is the sexual functioning of men and that many behaviors labeled as sexual dysfunction in women are actually healthy adaptations to difficult circumstances, such as stress, depression, fatigue, or the "continuing presence of negative or threatening patterns of behavior in the partner" (Bancroft 2002, p. 454).

The future of sexual pharmacology appears bright. A variety of oral erectogenic agents are in late-phase development, including the centrally active dopamine agonist sublingual apomorphine and the peripheral nonselective alpha-blocker oral phentolamine (Rosen 2000). The recently available phosphodiesterase inhibitor vardenafil has proven its efficacy and tolerability in randomized, placebo-controlled studies and offers the advantage of rapid onset of action (Kendirci et al. 2004). In an open-label, short-term, multicenter trial of 147 men taking sildenafil for ED, 90.5% opted to remain with tadalafil after a 9-week crossover phase (Stroberg et al. 2003). In a multicenter, randomized, double-blind crossover study of 215 men, 66% preferred initiation with tadalafil to sildenafil (Govier et al. 2003).

TABLE 17–2.   Medications and substances associated with sexual dysfunction

Medication	Reported adverse effect
Alcohol	Chronic abuse: decreased libido, ED, abnormal ejaculation, dyspareunia
α_1-Adrenergic antagonists	ED, decreased libido, abnormal ejaculation
Amiloride	ED, decreased libido
Aminocaproic acid	Dry ejaculation
Amiodarone	Decreased libido
Amphetamines	Chronic abuse: ED, abnormal ejaculation, anorgasmia (women)
Amyl nitrite	Decreased libido, ED
Anabolic steroids	ED, decreased libido, testicular atrophy
Angiotensin-converting enzyme inhibitors (captopril, trandolapril)	ED, decreased libido, abnormal ejaculation
Anticholinergic agents	ED
Anticholinergic ganglion blockers	ED, decreased libido
Antidepressants	
Mirtazapine	Decreased libido, ED
Nefazodone	Spontaneous ejaculation
Selective serotonin reuptake inhibitors	Anorgasmia, ED, decreased libido, abnormal ejaculation
Trazodone	Priapism, clitoral priapism, decreased libido, abnormal ejaculation, anorgasmia
Tricyclic	Decreased libido, ED, abnormal ejaculation, abnormal orgasm
Venlafaxine	Decreased libido, ED, abnormal ejaculation, delayed orgasm
Antihyperlipidemic (fibrate) agents	Decreased libido, ED
Antipsychotics	
Conventional	Abnormal ejaculation, ED, priapism, decreased libido
Second generation	Abnormal ejaculation, ED, decreased libido, priapism
Atorvastatin calcium	Decreased libido, ED, abnormal ejaculation
Baclofen	ED, no ejaculation
Barbiturates	Decreased libido, ED
Benzodiazepines	Decreased libido, anorgasmia, abnormal ejaculation
Beta-blockers	ED, decreased libido, abnormal ejaculation
Bromocriptine	Painful clitoral tumescence, ED
Buspirone	Priapism
Busulfan	ED
Calcium-channel blockers	ED
Cannabis	Increased libido
Carbamazepine	ED
Carbidopa-levodopa	Priapism, increased libido
Cetirizine hydrochloride	Decreased libido
Chlorambucil	ED
Clonidine	ED, abnormal ejaculation, decreased libido
Cocaine	Priapism
Cyclophosphamide	ED
Cyproterone acetate	Decreased libido
Cytosine arabinoside	ED, decreased libido, dyspareunia
Danazol	Increased or decreased libido
Delavirdine mesylate	Decreased libido, ED
Diethylpropion	ED, delayed ejaculation, anorgasmia (women)
Digoxin	Decreased libido, ED
Disopyramide	ED
Disulfiram	ED
Donepezil	Increased libido

TABLE 17–2.   **Medications and substances associated with sexual dysfunction** *(continued)*

Medication	Reported adverse effect
Estrogens	Increased or decreased libido
Ethosuximide	Increased libido
Ethoxzolamide	Decreased libido
Etretinate (and acitretin)	ED, decreased libido
Fat emulsion	Priapism
Finasteride	Decreased libido, ED, ejaculatory failure
Glutethimide	Decreased libido
Gonadotropin releasing factor analogues	ED, decreased libido, loss of sexual fantasy
Guanabenz	ED
Guanadrel	Decreased libido, abnormal ejaculation, delayed orgasm (women)
Guanfacine	ED
Histamine$_2$ blockers	ED
HIV protease inhibitors	ED, decreased libido, priapism
Hydralazine	ED, priapism
Indapamide	Decreased libido, ED
Interferon-α	Decreased libido, ED
Ketoconazole	ED, decreased libido
Levodopa	Increased libido
Lithium	Decreased libido, ED
LSD	Increased or decreased libido, ED, abnormal ejaculation
Mazindol	ED, spontaneous ejaculation, painful testes
MDA	Increased or decreased libido, ED, abnormal ejaculation
Melphalan	ED
Methaqualone	ED, abnormal ejaculation, decreased libido (women)
Methotrexate	ED
Methyldopa	Decreased libido, ED, abnormal ejaculation, delayed or no orgasm (women)
Metoclopramide	ED, decreased libido
Metyrosine	ED, no ejaculation
Mexiletine	ED, decreased libido
Midodrine	ED
Monoamine oxidase inhibitors	ED, abnormal ejaculation
Naltrexone	Delayed ejaculation, ED
Naratriptan hydrochloride	Decreased libido, inflammation of breast, vagina and fallopian tubes
Nilutamide	Decreased libido, testicular atrophy
Nonsteroidal anti-inflammatory drugs	ED, decreased libido, abnormal ejaculation
Omeprazole	Painful nocturnal erections
Opioids	Decreased libido, ED, abnormal ejaculation
Papaverine	Priapism, especially with neurological disorders
Pergolide	Hypersexuality, priapism, spontaneous ejaculation
Phencyclidine	Increased or decreased libido, ED, abnormal ejaculation
Phenmetrazine	ED, delayed ejaculation
Phenoxybenzamine	Dry ejaculation
Phentolamine	ED
Phenytoin	Decreased libido, ED, priapism
Pramipexole dihydrochloride	Decreased libido, ED
Primidone	Decreased libido, ED
Probucol	ED
Procarbazine	Decreased libido, ED, dyspareunia

TABLE 17–2. Medications and substances associated with sexual dysfunction *(continued)*

Medication	Reported adverse effect
Progestins	ED
Propofol	Sexual disinhibition
Riluzole	Increased or decreased libido, ED
Selegiline	Transient anorgasmia, decreased penile sensation
Sildenafil citrate	Abnormal ejaculation, genital edema, anorgasmia
Spironolactone	Decreased libido, ED
Steroids	Increased or decreased libido
Sulfasalazine	ED
Sulfonamide carbonic anhydrase inhibitors	ED, decreased libido
Tamoxifen	Priapism
Testosterone	Priapism
Thiabendazole	ED
Thiazide diuretics (and chlorthalidone)	ED
Tiagabine	Increased or decreased libido, ED
Tolcapone	Increased or decreased libido, ED
Trimethaphan	ED
Trovafloxacin mesylate	Decreased libido, ED
Valsartan	ED
Vinblastine	Decreased libido, ED, dyspareunia
Zolpidem tartrate	Decreased libido, ED, anorgasmia

Note. ED=erectile dysfunction; MDA=methylenedioxyamphetamine.

Psychotropic Medication–Induced Sexual Dysfunction

SSRIs are often associated with one or more types of sexual dysfunction, including decreased libido, diminished genital sensation, ED, decreased lubrication, and delayed or inhibited orgasms (Rosen et al. 1999). A review of five randomized, controlled trials showed SSRIs to be associated with a high incidence of sexual dysfunction, between 30% and 60% (Gregorian et al. 2002). Bupropion (immediate and sustained release), mirtazapine, and nefazodone are associated with significantly less risk of inducing sexual dysfunction and might therefore prove superior first choices for depressed medically ill patients who express a desire to remain or attain "normal" sexual functioning (Coleman et al. 1999; Croft et al. 1999).

A variety of strategies are available for dealing with medication-induced sexual dysfunction in patients who are doing well with their antidepressants and are reluctant to relinquish them (Clayton 2002; Rosen et al. 1999). Observation to determine whether the sexual problem is a primary depressive symptom or a medication side effect is the first step. Watchful waiting in the latter case generally demonstrates the tenacity of this side effect, which is un-

like the other, typically acute, side effects of SSRI treatment (Rothschild 2000). As a second step, the psychiatrist should consider lowering the dose, if possible, or changing the timing of the dose to be as distant as possible from anticipated sexual activity. The etiology of sexual dysfunction appears to be based on levels of drug in the periphery and is therefore related to dose and half-life. For patients in stable remission from depression and who are taking short-half-life SSRIs such as paroxetine, fluvoxamine, and sertraline, a drug holiday might be considered (Rothschild 1995). Central nervous system levels of short-half-life SSRIs remain high well after the peripheral levels have dropped to the point at which sexual function can occur normally. Several "antidote" approaches to dealing with SSRI-induced sexual dysfunction have been reported. The drugs include amantadine (Balon 1996; Shrivastava et al. 1995), cyproheptadine, yohimbine, and bupropion. Although results of an open-label study indicated reduced SSRI-induced sexual dysfunction with the addition of bupropion (Kennedy et al. 2002), results from two placebo-controlled trials were contradictory (Clayton et al. 2004; Masand et al. 2001). Findings from open-label studies and case reports suggested that sildenafil might have a beneficial role to play in reversing antidepressant-induced sexual dysfunction in men and women (Nurnberg et al. 1999; Salerian et al. 2000; Shen et al. 1999). Results of a randomized, controlled trial demonstrated in men the efficacy of sildenafil in reversing sexual dysfunction from serotonin reuptake–inhibiting antidepressants (Nurnberg et al. 2003).

Priapism, long associated with trazodone use in men but also reported to occur with use of other antidepressants and antipsychotics, must be considered carefully in hospitalized patients who may have other reasons for sluggish blood flow through cavernosal erectile tissues. These factors include leukemia, sickle cell disease, and other hypercoagulable states in both men and women (clitoral priapism). Concurrent treatments with alpha-blockers such as prazosin may make this potentially dangerous side effect even more likely.

The sexual side effects of antipsychotic medications have been underestimated and understudied (Compton and Miller 2001) but most often are related to hyperprolactinemia or autonomic dysfunction (Smith et al. 2002). Side effects have been reported with the new second-generation antipsychotic medications (Wirshing et al. 2003).

Primary Sexual and Gender Disorders That May Be Present in Medical–Surgical Patients

Gender Identity Disorders

Genital self-mutilation was first reported in the medical literature more than 100 years ago (Stroch 1901) and is a rare but highly disturbing reason that surgeons request consultation. Dramatic examples of autocastration and autopenectomy (Fisch 1987; McGuire et al. 1998; Mellon et al. 1989), autoamputation of the labia majora (Wise et al. 1989), and self-inflicted vulvar and vaginal lacerations (Standage et al. 1974) have appeared since the mid 1960s. The patients often have gender dysphoric symptoms with or without psychosis. Clinical considerations in the differential diagnosis of gender dysphoria include the conditions listed in Table 17–3 (Brown 2001). Schizophrenia, with or without gender identity disorder, is a major consideration in patients who have self-inflicted genital wounds (Agoub 2000), although most patients who desperately engage in this behavior are not acutely psychotic at the time. We are aware of several cases of incarcerated persons with gender identity disorder who removed their testicles, penises, or both as a result of not receiving hormonal and surgical treatment of the primary condition. These prisoners were not psychotic at the time and had indicated in advance that they would "self-treat" in this

TABLE 17–3. Differential diagnosis of gender dysphoria

Primary and secondary transsexualism (DSM-IV-TR gender identity disorder)

Transvestic fetishism with depression or regression

Homophobic homosexuality (sexual disorder not otherwise specified)

Schizophrenia with gender identity disorder

Borderline personality disorder

Body dysmorphic disorder

Gender identity disorder not otherwise specified

Ambiguous or androgynous gender role adaptation

Pseudohermaphroditism

Malingering or factitious disorder

Career female impersonator in crisis

Transgenderist (nonoperative transsexual) in crisis (DSM-IV-TR gender identity disorder NOS)

manner by eliminating the "offending" organs. Catalano et al. (2002) reviewed published case reports of repetitive genital self-mutilation and found differences between those who engaged in this activity repeatedly and those who did so once or twice as a form of self-treatment. Among the differences was that the patients who engaged in repeated activity had a propensity to depressive disorders and "unusual" masturbatory practices.

In hospitals where surgical procedures are performed as part of a comprehensive gender confirmation program, consultation may be requested in the preoperative and perioperative periods. Standards of care for all mental health professionals involved in the evaluation and treatment of patients with gender identity disorder have been established and should be reviewed before consultation (Brown 2001; Meyer et al. 2001). These standards are not full practice guidelines but are minimum requirements of care for both the evaluation and treatment of patients with gender identity disorder. Table 17–4 lists the common somatic treatments of patients with gender identity disorders. When a consultation is requested, patients may be at various stages of physical transition and are likely to be receiving one or more treatments, including cross-sex hormonal treatments that may interact with other medications ordered while the patient is in the hospital (Brown 2001; Lothstein and Brown 1992). Futterweit (1998) discussed the complications of cross-sex hormonal treatments, which are often medically necessary and critical to the mental and physical well-being of these patients. Psychosis in the period immediately after castration, penectomy, and neovaginal construction is rare but is a concern. Rejection by family members or loved ones contributes to depressive symptoms in some patients with gender iden-

TABLE 17–4. Medical and surgical treatments of gender identity disorders[a]

Adult natal men with gender identity disorder

Estrogen treatment (lifelong; reduced dose after orchiectomy)

Electrolysis (25–300 hours of manual treatment or four to six sessions of laser treatment)

Laryngeal cartilage shaving

Vocal cord shortening or other voice alteration operations

Liposuction

Rhinoplasty

Jaw reconfiguration

Other facial cosmetic procedures

Penectomy

Neovaginal construction

Augmentation mammoplasty

Adult natal women with gender identity disorder

Testosterone treatment (lifelong; reduced dose after oophorectomy)

Facial cosmetic procedures

Hysterectomy

Oophorectomy

Bilateral mastectomy

Chest wall contouring

Neophallus construction (multiple stages)

Testicular implants

Genitoplasty (maximization of hypertrophied clitoral prominence)

[a]Not all patients need all treatments.

tity disorders both before and after irreversible genital surgery. At times, antidepressant treatment has limited effectiveness, whereas cross-gender hormonal treatment, alone or in combination with antidepressants, can result in dramatic positive responses, including resolution of chronic suicidality.

Patients admitted to surgical or urological services for major genital surgery ideally should already be receiving care from a mental health professional familiar with the case. Because patients often undergo these procedures at a considerable distance from their homes, local psychiatric consultation may be requested. Psychiatrists who are not familiar with these patients should examine their potential negative countertransference reactions in advance (Lothstein 1977). For example, Lothstein (1978) reported that countertransference anxiety in a male anesthesiologist nearly resulted in the death of a male transsexual patient during penectomy and orchiectomy. Brown (1988) and Lothstein (1982) discussed ethical dilemmas surrounding the appropriateness of providing or withholding irreversible genital surgical procedures for gender-dysphoric patients. Although most psychiatrists are not well-versed in the evaluation and treatment of patients

with gender identity disorder, they can still assist the treatment team by providing referral sources and support group contacts for patients with this chronic and severe condition, such as the Harry Benjamin International Gender Dysphoria Association (Meyer et al. 2001).

Other Sexual Disorders

The paraphilias do not often come to clinical attention in medical settings. "Accidental" injuries in the course of practicing paraphilic activities are cause for admission to medical and surgical units. Comorbidity with other sexual disorders, mood disorders, substance use disorders, and attention-deficit disorders are common (Kafka 2001; Kafka and Prentky 1998). We discuss some of these disorders.

Potentially harmful genital manipulation may be present as an active form of autoerotic behavior (a type of fetishistic interest) or as masochistic instrumentation (i.e., a form of factitious disorder). Catalano et al. (2002) reported the case of a man who repeatedly injected air into his scrotum as part of a paraphilic masturbatory ritual. Wise (1982) reported seven cases of urethral manipulation, including those of a woman with borderline personality disorder who repeatedly inserted razor blades into her urethra and a 14-year-old boy who lodged a pencil in his bladder after urethral masturbation. Complete urinary tract obstruction due to the self-infusion of an expandable foam sealant through the urethra is another example of an unusual situation meriting psychiatric consultation (Kim et al. 2002).

In contrast to active forms of urethral manipulation, Wise (1982) described individuals who frequently presented with recurrent inability to void or persistent pain with urination, readily accepted repeated cystoscopy and catheterization, and may have visited several emergency departments for these interventions. Patients who exhibit this type of behavior often have a less obvious psychopathological condition (e.g., obsessional behavior, sadomasochistic fantasies, or monosymptomatic hypochondriasis) than do "active instrumenters" (those with borderline personality disorder, schizophrenia, or multiple paraphilias). Psychiatric consultation usually is requested after medical and urological evaluations uncover no apparent physical causes of the complaints or when foreign objects are discovered in the bladder. Active inserters may initially deny self-instrumentation, but tactful and nonjudgmental questioning may yield a more complete clinical picture. Psychotherapy may be the treatment of choice and involves a dynamic understanding of "libidinal, structural, and ego psychological constructs" (Wise 1982, p. 225). Although these behaviors appear to have fetishistic and sadomasochistic elements, analogies to factitious disorder (Munchausen syndrome) are clear, and engaging such patients in treatment may be very difficult (Ford and Feldman 2002).

The paraphilia classified hypoxyphilia in DSM-IV, coded sexual masochism in DSM-IV-TR, and labeled in the literature as *asphyxiophilia, autoerotic asphyxia,* and *eroticized repetitive hangings* involves the deliberate induction of cerebral anoxia during masturbation to heighten orgasmic intensity (Hucker and Stermac 1992). Practitioners of this potentially lethal sexual behavior rarely seek treatment, but near-fatal self-strangulation may be mistaken for a suicide attempt when encountered in the hospital setting (Johnstone and Huws 1997). However, evidence of suicidal intent was present in only 2 of 157 fatal cases of hypoxyphilia (Hazelwood et al. 1983). Although this behavior is practiced more by men than women, identical "accidental autoerotic death" scenes involving women have been reported (Behrendt et al. 2002).

The literature provides few examples of specific treatment interventions for hypoxyphilia and no results of long-term outcome studies (Hucker 1990). Treatment strategies for other paraphilias used to manage hypoxyphilia include behavior therapy with covert sensitization (Haydn-Smith et al. 1987) and antiandrogenic hormonal treatment (Hucker and Stermac 1992). Lithium carbonate also has been reported to be useful (Cesnick and Coleman 1989). Uva reviewed the literature on this disorder (Uva 1995).

New onset of paraphilic behavior after the age of 30 (assuming the history is accurate and reliable) is extremely uncommon and when present often is associated with structural lesions of the brain. For example, Frohman and colleagues (2002) described a man with known MS who suddenly experienced a paraphilia involving an insatiable urge to touch women's breasts. New lesions in the right sides of the hypothalamus, mesencephalon, red nucleus, substantia nigra, and internal capsule were found. Developmental disorders such as Asperger's syndrome also may be associated with the onset of paraphilias (Milton et al. 2002).

Finally, patients with other paraphilias may seek emergency medical treatment for a variety of inadvertent injuries, including trauma from zoophilic contacts with animals (Kirov et al. 2002) and burns due to sadomasochistic activities involving fire, branding, or application of hot waxes (Tanabe et al. 2002). Transvestic fetishists (i.e., cross-dressers) (Brown 2001) who engage in high-risk public behaviors may be assaulted or even killed by homophobic men who engage in violence directed toward transgender, gay, or bisexual persons.

Pharmacological Treatments of Paraphilic Disorders

Patients who have severe paraphilias necessitating medical or surgical treatment are likely to need pharmacological intervention in addition to psychotherapeutic treatment (Kafka 2001). Antiandrogenic medications are used as an adjunctive treatment of some malignant diseases to limit tumor growth (e.g., prostate cancer) and as primary treatment of moderate to severe sexual disorders and paraphilias (Bradford and Greenberg 1996). "Pure" antiandrogens, including flutamide and nilutamide, block the action of androgen only at the target organs, and the result is greatly elevated gonadotropin and circulating testosterone levels. These drugs are not adequate for monotherapy for paraphilias. Other antiandrogens, including cyproterone acetate (CPA; not available in the United States) and MPA, have progestogenic and antigonadotropic properties, which result in both inhibition of androgen biosynthesis and inhibition of androgen action in the periphery (Bradford 2001; Reilly 2000). In addition, CPA and MPA appear to block central androgen receptor sites that may be important in the generation of deviant sexual fantasies (Cooper 1986, 1987). Results of placebo-controlled trials support the use of antiandrogens for the treatment of moderate to severe paraphilias (Cooper 1981; Kafka 2001), and clinical use of antiandrogens in properly selected and informed patients with paraphilias can yield dramatic results (Neumann and Kalmas 1991; Thibaut et al. 1996). Long-term treatment with MPA is associated with weight gain, increases in systolic blood pressure, gallstone formation, and infertility and possibly with changes in glucose tolerance.

Leuprolide is a synthetic gonadotropin-releasing hormone analogue (luteinizing hormone–releasing hormone agonist) approved by the U.S. Food and Drug Administration in 1985 for the treatment of prostatic cancer. Leuprolide initially stimulates release of luteinizing hormone, follicle-stimulating hormone, and, therefore, testosterone, but further release of luteinizing hormone and follicle-stimulating hormone is blocked after 3–5 days (Allolio et al. 1985). Serum levels of testosterone then decrease to the castrate level. The most common side effect is hot flashes and an initial worsening of sexual symptoms because of the transient increase in testosterone. A depot preparation allows for once-monthly subcutaneous injections in most patients (Krueger and Kaplan 2001). Triptorelin and goserelin are long-acting gonadotropin-releasing hormone analogues that have shown substantial promise in centrally blocking the production of testosterone. Goserelin has been widely used in prostate cancer treatment (Brogden et al. 1995). Both agents are being used increasingly in the treatment of patients with severe sexual disorders that respond to marked lowering of circulating testosterone levels (see Dickey 1992; Rosler and Witztum 1998). The initial month of treatment is associated with increased levels of testosterone before a rapid depletion of testicular stores occurs. Long-term use of these potent agents is associated with bone demineralization due to the effects of loss of testosterone (Krueger and Kaplan 2001), although it appears that this side effect can be mitigated with bone-saving treatments (Dickey 2002).

In addition to antiandrogens and gonadotropin-releasing hormone agents, orally administered estrogens (e.g., ethinyl estradiol, 0.10 mg/day) have been used as monotherapy for some sexual disorders. Success rates have not been as good as with CPA and MPA, but more important is that the side-effect profile of estrogen is distinctly unfavorable compared with the profiles of CPA and MPA. Specifically, estrogen treatment results in feminization (breast growth, decreased upper-body muscle mass, increased hip fat, and changes in body hair), nausea, vomiting, and the risk of breast cancer in men. These side effects may be desired by some patients with either gender identity disorder or transvestic fetishism, because many of these patients seek feminization as a primary treatment end point (Brown 2001; Meyer et al. 2001). Use of hormonal agents is not without some controversy despite their efficacy in many cases. Cordier et al. (1996) reviewed some of these issues.

Because they have nonspecific effects and significant risks, neuroleptic medications are no longer recommended. Results of small, uncontrolled trials of fluoxetine for a variety of paraphilic and nonparaphilic "sexual addictions" have suggested that this medication may have promise in decreasing the compulsivity associated with these disorders (Kafka 2001). However, many patients who have responded have also met criteria for a mood disorder (Kafka and Prentky 1992). Additional studies are necessary before any definitive statements can be made about the efficacy of SSRIs in the management of sexual disorders, alone or in combination with hormonal treatments (Fedoroff 1995; Levitsky and Owens 1999). The consensus, however, appears to be that these treatments are far more benign than hormonal manipulations and should be considered an initial attempt at treatment in doses similar to those used for obsessive-compulsive disorder. Psychiatrists considering this modality should review published treatment algorithms before initiating treatment (Bradford 2001; Krueger and Kaplan 2000; Reilly et al. 2000).

Conclusion

All phases of the human sexual response are subject to influence by a variety of medical diseases and medications. The question, "Is the sexual dysfunction physical or psychogenic?" is commonly raised, but in every case, consideration should be given to the possible contributions of biological, psychological, and social factors. As this chapter illustrates, it is not a simple matter to determine the relative contributions of somatic disorders and psychological processes in diagnosing sexual problems in the medically ill.

This chapter has reviewed sexual issues in heart disease, cancer, diabetes, renal failure, HIV, and a variety of neurological disorders, but sexuality is affected by most chronic medical illnesses. Nevertheless, because of both patient and physician avoidance, sexual dysfunction can easily escape evaluation and treatment. A disconnect remains between physician application of new knowledge and the patients who need it, because of embarrassment and stigma. Yet, effective psychological and pharmacological treatments are available. Recent advances, such as the use of oral medications for erectile dysfunction, SSRIs for premature ejaculation, bupropion for arousal problems or to treat sexual side effects of other medications, and other drugs that hold promise for the near future, should help close the gap between knowledge and practice.

References

Abdel-Hamid I, Eraky I, Fouda M, et al: Role of penile vascular insufficiency in erectile dysfunction in renal transplant recipients. Int J Impot Res 14:32–37, 2002

Agoub M: Male genital self-mutilation in patients with schizophrenia. Can J Psychiatry 45:670, 2000

Alexopoulou O, Jamart J, Maiter D, et al: Erectile dysfunction and lower androgenicity in type I diabetic patients. Diabetes Metab 27:329–336, 2001

Al-Ghazal S, Fallowfield L, Blamey R: Does cosmetic outcome from treatment of primary breast cancer influence psychosocial morbidity? Eur J Surg Oncol 25:571–573, 1999

Al-Ghazal S, Sully L, Fallowfield L, et al: The psychological impact of immediate rather than delayed breast reconstruction. Eur J Surg Oncol 26:17–19, 2000

Allolio B, Keffel D, Deuss U, et al: Treatment of sex behavior disorders with LH-RH superagonists. Deutsch Med Wochenschr 110:110–117, 1985

Althof SE: When an erection alone is not enough: biopsychosocial obstacles to lovemaking. Int J Impot Res 14 (suppl 1): S99–S104, 2002

American Psychiatric Association: Diagnostic and Statistical Manual of Mental Disorders, 4th Edition. Washington, DC, American Psychiatric Association, 1994

American Psychiatric Association: Diagnostic and Statistical Manual of Mental Disorders, 4th Edition, Text Revision. Washington, DC, American Psychiatric Association, 2000

Amichetti M, Caffo O: Quality of life in patients with early stage breast carcinoma treated with conservation surgery and radiotherapy: an Italian monoinstitutional study. Tumori 87:78–84, 2001

Arruda-Olson A, Mahoney D, Nehra A, et al: Cardiovascular effects of sildenafil during exercise in men with known or probable coronary artery disease. JAMA 287:719–725, 2002

Atkinson J, Grant I, Kennedy C, et al: Prevalence of psychiatric disorders among men infected with human immunodeficiency virus. Arch Gen Psychiatry 45:859–864, 1988

Auchincloss S: Sexual dysfunction in cancer patients: issues in evaluation and treatment, in Handbook of Psychooncology: Psychological Care of the Patient With Cancer. Edited by Holland JC, Rowland JH. New York, Oxford University Press, 1989, pp 383–413

Aversa A, Fabbri A: New oral agents for erectile dysfunction: what is changing in our practice? Asian J Androl 3:175–179, 2001

Balestroni G, Bosimini E, Centofanti P, et al: Lifestyle and adherence to the recommended treatments after cardiac transplantation. Ital Heart J 3 (6 suppl):652–658, 2002

Balon R: Intermittent amantadine for fluoxetine-induced anorgasmia. J Sex Marital Ther 22:290–292, 1996

Bancroft J: The medicalization of female sexual dysfunction: the need for caution. Arch Sex Behav 31:451–455, 2002

Basson R, McInnes R, Smith MD, et al: Efficacy and safety of sildenafil citrate in women with sexual dysfunction associated with female sexual arousal disorder. J Womens Health Gend Based Med 11:367–377, 2002

Becher E: Topical alprostadil cream for the treatment of erectile dysfunction. Expert Opin Pharmacother 5:623–632, 2004

Bedell S, Duperval M, Goldberg R: Cardiologists' discussions about sexuality with patients with chronic coronary artery disease. Am Heart J 144:239–242, 2002a

Bedell S, Graboys T, Duperval M, et al: Sildenafil in the cardiologist's office: patients' attitudes and physicians' practices toward discussions about sexual functioning. Cardiology 97:79–82, 2002b

Behrendt N, Buhl N, Seidl S: The lethal paraphiliac syndrome: accidental autoerotic deaths in four women and a review of the literature. Int J Legal Med 116:148–152, 2002

Berman JR, Berman LA, Lin H, et al: Effect of sildenafil on subjective and physiologic parameters of the female sexual response in women with sexual arousal disorder. J Sex Marital Ther 27:411–420, 2001

Berman LA, Berman JR, Bruck D, et al: Pharmacotherapy or psychotherapy? effective treatment for FSD related to unresolved childhood sexual abuse. J Sex Marital Ther 27:421–425, 2001

Bertero C: Altered sexual patterns after treatment for prostate cancer. Cancer Pract 9:245–251, 2001

Bocchi E, Guilherme G, Mocelin A, et al: Sildenafil effects on exercise, neurohormonal activation, and erectile dysfunction in congestive heart failure. Circulation 106:1097–1103, 2002

Bohlen J, Held J, Sanderson M, et al: Heart rate, rate pressure-product and oxygen uptake during four sexual activities. Arch Intern Med 144:1745–1748, 1984

Bokhour B, Clark J, Inui T, et al: Sexuality after treatment for early prostate cancer: exploring the meanings of "erectile dysfunction." J Gen Intern Med 16:649–655, 2001

Bradford J: The neurobiology, neuropharmacology, and pharmacological treatment of the paraphilias and compulsive sexual behavior. Can J Psychiatry 46:26–34, 2001

Bradford J, Greenberg D: Pharmacological treatment of deviant sexual behavior. Ann Rev Sex Res 7:283–303, 1996

Brogden R, Faulds D: Goserelin: a review of its pharmacodynamic and pharmacokinetic properties and therapeutic efficacy in prostate cancer. Drugs Aging 6:324–343, 1995

Brown G: Bioethical issues in the management of gender dysphoria. Jefferson J Psychiatry 6:33–44, 1988

Brown G: Transvestism and gender identity disorders, in Treatments of Psychiatric Disorders, 3rd Edition. Edited by Gabbard GO. Washington, DC, American Psychiatric Publishing, 2001, pp 2007–2067

Brown G, Ceniceros S: Human sexuality in health and disease, in Behavior and Medicine, 3rd Edition. Edited by Wedding D. Seattle, WA, Hogrefe & Huber, 2001, pp 171–183

Brown G, Rundell J: Prospective study of psychiatric morbidity in HIV-seropositive women without AIDS. Gen Hosp Psychiatry 12:30–35, 1990

Brown G, Rundell J: A prospective study of psychiatric aspects of early HIV disease in women. Gen Hosp Psychiatry 15:139–147, 1993

Brown G, Rundell J, McManis S, et al: Prevalence of psychiatric disorders in early stages of HIV infection. Psychosom Med 54:588–601, 1992

Brown G, Kendall S, Ledsky R: Sexual dysfunction in HIV-seropositive women without AIDS. J Psychol Human Sex 7:73–97, 1995

Campese VM, Liu CM: Sexual dysfunction in uremia: endocrine and neurological alterations. Contrib Nephrol 77:1–14, 1990

Caruso S, Intelisano G, Lupo L, et al: Premenopausal women affected by sexual arousal disorder treated with sildenafil: a double-blind, cross-over, placebo-controlled study. BJOG 108:623–628, 2001

Catalano G, Catalano M, Carroll K: Repetitive male genital self-mutilation: a case report and discussion of possible risk factors. J Sex Marital Ther 28:27–37, 2002

Cerqueira J, Moraes M, Glina S: Erectile dysfunction prevalence and associated variables in patients with chronic renal failure. Int J Impot Res 14:65–71, 2002

Cesnick J, Coleman E: Use of lithium carbonate in the treatment of autoerotic asphyxia. Am J Psychother 43:277–286, 1989

Chao R, Clowers DE: Experience with intracavernosal trimixture for the management of neurogenic erectile dysfunction. Arch Phys Med Rehabil 75:276–278, 1994

Choi-Kwon S, Kim J: Poststroke emotional incontinence and decreased sexual activity. Cerebrovasc Dis 13:31–37, 2002

Christ B, Brockmeier D, Hauck E, et al: Interactions of sildenafil and tacrolimus in men with erectile dysfunction after kidney transplantation. Urology 58:589–593, 2001

Clayton A: Female sexual dysfunction related to depression and antidepressant medications. Curr Womens Health Rep 2:182–187, 2002

Clayton AH, Warnock JK, Kornstein SG, et al: A placebo-controlled trial of bupropion SR as an antidote for selective serotonin reuptake inhibitor-induced sexual dysfunction. J Clin Psychiatry 65:62–67, 2004

Coleman C, Cunningham L, Foster V, et al: Sexual dysfunction associated with the treatment of depression: a placebo-controlled comparison of buproprion sustained release and sertraline treatment. Ann Clin Psychiatry 11:205–215, 1999

Colombo R, Bertini R, Salonia A, et al: Overall clinical outcomes after nerve and seminal sparing radical cystectomy for the treatment of organ confined bladder cancer. J Urol 171:1819–1822; discussion 1822, 2004

Compton M, Miller A: Sexual side effects associated with conventional and atypical antipsychotics. Psychopharmacol Bull 35:89–108, 2001

Cooper A: A placebo-controlled trial of the antiandrogen cyproterone acetate in deviant hypersexuality. Compr Psychiatry 22:458–465, 1981

Cooper A: Progestogens in the treatment of male sex offenders: a review. Can J Psychiatry 31:73–79, 1986

Cooper A: Medroxyprogesterone acetate (MPA) treatment of sexual acting out in men suffering from dementia. J Clin Psychiatry 48:368–370, 1987

Cordier B, Thibaut F, Kuhn J, et al: Hormonal treatments for disorders of sexual conduct. Bull Acad Natl Med 180:599–605, 1996

Coslett H, Heilman K: Male sexual function: impairment after right hemisphere stroke. Arch Neurol 43:1036–1039, 1986

Croft H, Settle E, Houser T, et al: A placebo-controlled comparison of the antidepressant efficacy and effects on sexual functioning of sustained-release bupropion and sertraline. J Clin Ther 21:643–658, 1999

Crosby M, Paul J, Midanik L, et al: A new method of measuring the association between alcohol use, drug use, and high-risk sex, in Proceedings of the 7th International Conference on AIDS, Florence, Italy, June 16–21, 1991, MD 4044, p 401

Crowe S, Ponsford J: The role of imagery in sexual arousal disturbances in the male traumatically brain injured individual. Brain Inj 13:347–354, 1999

DeBusk R: Sildenafil and physical exertion in men with coronary artery disease. JAMA 287:2359, 2002

DeBusk R, Drory Y, Goldstein I, et al: Management of sexual dysfunction in patients with cardiovascular disease: recommendations of the Princeton consensus panel. Am J Cardiol 86:175–181, 2000

De Groot M, Anderson R, Freedland K, et al: Association of depression and diabetes complications: a meta-analysis. Psychosom Med 63:619–630, 2001

Derby C, Mohr B, Goldstein I, et al: Modifiable risk factors and erectile dysfunction: can lifestyle changes modify risk? Urology 56:302–306, 2000

Derry F, Dinsmore W, Frazer M, et al: Efficacy and safety of oral sildenafil (Viagra) in men with erectile dysfunction caused by spinal cord injury. Neurology 51:1629–1633, 1998

Derry F, Hultling C, Seftel A, et al: Efficacy and safety of sildenafil citrate (Viagra) in men with erectile dysfunction and spinal cord injury: a review. Urology 60 (2 suppl 2):49–57, 2002

Dewhurst K, Oliver J: Huntington's disease of young people. Eur Neurol 3:278–279, 1970

Dey J, Shepherd M: Evaluation and treatment of erectile dysfunction in men with diabetes mellitus. Mayo Clin Proc 77:276–282, 2002

Dickey R: The management of a case of treatment resistant paraphilia with a long-acting LHRH agonist. Can J Psychiatry 37:567–569, 1992

Dickey R: Case report: the management of bone demineralization associated with long-term treatment of multiple paraphilias with long-acting LHRH agonists. J Sex Marital Ther 28:207–210, 2002

Diemont W, Vruggink P, Meuleman E, et al: Sexual dysfunction after renal replacement therapy. Am J Kidney Dis 35:845–851, 2000

Dillard F, Miller B, Sommer B, et al: Erectile dysfunction posttransplant. Transplant Proc 21:3961–3962, 1989

Dolezal C, Carballo-Dieguez A, Nieves-Rosa L, et al: Substance use and sexual risk behavior: understanding their association among four ethnic groups of Latino men who have sex with men. J Subst Abuse 11:323–336, 2000

Drory Y, Kravetz S, Florian V, et al: Sexual activity after first acute myocardial infarction in middle-aged men: demographic, psycholgical and medical predictors. Cardiology 90:207–211, 1998

Dunbar N, Perdices M, Grunseit A, et al: The relationship between HIV symptomatology and affect, in Proceedings of the 7th International Conference on AIDS, Florence, Italy, June 16–21, 1991, MD 4044, MB 2126, p 213

Dupont S: Sexual function and ways of coping in patients with multiple sclerosis and their partners. Sex Marital Ther 11:359–372, 1996

Ehrenfeld M, Bronner G, Tabak N, et al: Sexuality among institutionalized elderly patients with dementia. Nurs Ethics 6:144–149, 1999

Eid J: Sildenafil citrate: current clinical experience. Int J Impot Res 12 (suppl 4):S62–S66, 2000

Enzlin P, Mathieu C, Van den Bruel A, et al: Sexual dysfunction in women with type I diabetes: a controlled study. Diabetes Care 25:672–677, 2002

Erol B, Tefekli A, Ozbey I, et al: Sexual dysfunction in type II diabetic females: a comparative study. J Sex Marital Ther 28 (suppl 1):55–62, 2002

Fagan PJ, Wise T, Schmidt C: Sexual problems in spinal cord disease, in Current Therapy in Neurologic Disease, 3rd Edition. Edited by Johnson RT. Philadelphia, PA, BC Decker, 1990, pp 168–172

Fairburn C, Wu F, McCulloch D, et al: The clinical features of diabetic impotence: a preliminary study. Br J Psychiatry 140:447–452, 1982a

Fairburn CG, McCulloch DK, Wu FC, et al: The effects of diabetes on male sexual function. Clin Endocrinol Metab 11:749–757, 1982b

Fedele D, Coscelli C, Cucinotta D, et al: Management of erectile dysfunction in diabetic subjects: results from a survey of 400 diabetes centers in Italy. Diabetes Nutr Metab 14:277–282, 2001

Fedoroff J: Antiandrogens vs. serotonergic medications in the treatment of sex offenders: a preliminary compliance study. Can J Hum Sex 4:111–122, 1995

Feldman H, Goldstein I, Hatzichristou D, et al: Impotence and its medical and psychosocial correlates: results of the Massachusetts Male Aging Study. J Urol 151:54–61, 1994

Feldman H, Johannes C, Derby C, et al: Erectile dysfunction and coronary risk factors: prospective results from the Massachusetts male aging study. Prev Med 30:328–338, 2000

Finkelstein F, Steele T: Sexual dysfunction and chronic renal failure: a psychosocial study. Dial Transplant 7:877–878, 1978

Fisch R: Genital self-mutilation in males: psychodynamic anatomy of a psychosis. Am J Psychother 41:453–458, 1987

Ford C, Feldman M: Factitious disorders and malingering, in Textbook of Consultation-Liaison Psychiatry, 2nd Edition. Edited by Wise M, Rundell J. Washington, DC, American Psychiatric Publishing, 2002, pp 519–531

Forsberg L, Hojerback T, Olsson A, et al: Etiologic aspects of impotence diabetes. Scand J Urol Nephrol 23:173–175, 1989

Fossa S, Opjordsmoen S, Haug E: Androgen replacement and quality of life in patients treated for bilateral testicular cancer. Eur J Cancer 35:1220–1225, 1999

Fox S, Collins M, Haney L, et al: Male genitourinary cancer sexuality questionnaire. Urol Nurs 19:101–107, 1999

Franzen D, Metha A, Seifert N, et al: Effects of beta-blockers on sexual performance in men with coronary heart disease: a prospective, randomized and double blinded study. Int J Impot Res 13:348–351, 2001

Frohman E, Frohman T, Moreault A: Acquired sexual paraphilia in patients with multiple sclerosis. Arch Neurol 59:1006–1010, 2002

Futterweit W: Endocrine therapy of transsexualism and potential complications of long-term treatment. Arch Sex Behav 27:209–226, 1998

Gallo-Silver L: The sexual rehabilitation of persons with cancer. Cancer Pract 8:10–15, 2000

Ganz P, Greendale G, Petersen L, et al: Managing menopausal symptoms in breast cancer survivors: results of a randomized controlled trial. J Natl Cancer Inst 92:1054–1064, 2000

Gerstenberg T, Metz P, Ottesen B, et al: Intracavernous self-injection with vasoactive intestinal polypeptide and phentolamine in the management of erectile failure. J Urol 147:1277–1279, 1992

Giaquinto S, Buzzelli S, Di Francesco L, et al: Evaluation of sexual changes after stroke. J Clin Psychiatry 64:302–307, 2003

Giuliano F, Hultling C, El Masry W, et al: Randomized trial of sildenafil for the treatment of erectile dysfunction in spinal cord injury. Ann Neurol 46:15–21, 1999

Goggin K, Engelson E, Rabkin J, et al: The relationship of mood, endocrine, and sexual disorders in human immuno-deficiency virus positive (HIV+) women: an exploratory study. Psychosom Med 60:11–16, 1998

Gondim F, Thomas F: Episodic hyperlibidinism in multiple sclerosis. Mult Scler 7:67–70, 2001

Govier F, Potempa AJ, Kaufman J, et al: A multicenter, randomized, double-blind, crossover study of patient preference for tadalafil 20 mg or sildenafil citrate 50 mg during initiation of treatment for erectile dysfunction. Clin Ther 25:2709–2723, 2003

Greendale G, Petersen L, Zibecchi L, et al: Factors related to sexual function in postmenopausal women with a history of breast cancer. Menopause 8:111–119, 2001

Gregoire A: Viagra: on release. Evidence on the effectiveness of sildenafil is good. BMJ 317:759–760, 1998

Gregorian R, Golden K, Bahce A, et al: Antidepressant-induced sexual dysfunction. Ann Pharmacother 36:1577–1589, 2002

Grumann M, Robertson R, Hacker N, et al: Sexual functioning in patients following radical hysterectomy for stage IB cancer of the cervix. Int J Gynecol Cancer 11:372–380, 2001

Hatzichristou D: Sildenafil citrate: lessons learned from 3 years of clinical experience. Int J Impot Res 14 (suppl 1):S43–S52, 2002

Hatzichristou DG, Apostolidis A, Tzortzis V, et al: Sildenafil versus intracavernous injection therapy: efficacy and preference in patients on intracavernous injection for more than 1 year. J Urol 164:1197–1200, 2000

Hawton K: Sexual adjustment of men who have strokes. J Psychosom Res 28:243–249, 1984

Haydn-Smith P, Marks I, Buchaya A, et al: Behavioral treatment of life-threatening masochistic asphyxiation: a case study. Br J Psychiatry 150:518–519, 1987

Hazelwood R, Dietz P, Burgess A: Autoerotic Fatalities. Lexington, MA, Lexington Books, 1983

Heaton J, Lording D, Liu S, et al: Intracavernosal alprostadil is effective for the treatment of erectile dysfunction in diabetic men. Int J Impot Res 13:317–321, 2001

Higgins G: Sexual response in spinal cord injured adults: a review. Arch Sex Behav 8:173–196, 1978

Horenblas S, Meinhardt W, Ijzerman W, et al: Sexuality preserving cystectomy and neobladder: initial results. J Urol 166:837–840, 2001

Hucker S: Sexual asphyxia, in Principles and Practice of Forensic Psychiatry. Edited by Bluglass R. London, Churchill-Livingstone, 1990, pp 717–721

Hucker S, Stermac L: The evaluation and treatment of sexual violence, necrophilia, and asphyxiophilia. Clin Forensic Psychiatry 15:703–719, 1992

Hulter B, Lundberg P: Sexual function in women with advanced multiple sclerosis. J Neurol Neurosurg Psychiatry 59:83–86, 1995

Hussain I, Brady C, Swinn M, et al: Treatment of erectile dysfunction with sildenafil citrate (Viagra) in parkinsonism due to Parkinson's disease or multiple system atrophy with observations on orthostatic hypotension. J Neurol Neurosurg Psychiatry 71:371–374, 2001

Incrocci L, Hop W, Wijnmaalen A, et al: Treatment outcome, body image, and sexual functioning after orchiectomy and radiotherapy for stage I-II testicular seminoma. Int J Radiat Oncol Biol Phys 53:1165–1173, 2002

Jaarsma T, Dracup K, Walden J, et al: Sexual function in patients with advanced heart failure. Heart Lung 25:262–270, 1996

Jackson G: Sexual intercourse and stable angina pectoris. Am J Cardiol 86:35F-37F, 2000

Janardhan V, Bakshi R: Quality of life in patients with multiple sclerosis: the impact of fatigue and depression. J Neurol Sci 205:51–58, 2002

Jensen J, Lendorf A, Stimpel H, et al: The prevalence and etiology of impotence in 101 male hypertensive outpatients. Am J Hypertens 12:271–275, 1999

Johannes C, Araujo A, Feldman H, et al: Incidence of erectile dysfunction in men 40 to 69 years old: longitudinal results from the Massachusetts male aging study. J Urol 163:460–463, 2000

Johnstone J, Huws R: Autoerotic asphyxia: a case report. J Sex Marital Ther 23:326–332, 1997

Juergense P, Botev R, Wuerth D, et al: Erectile dysfunction in chronic peritoneal dialysis patients: incidence and treatment with sildenafil. Perit Dial Int 21:355–359, 2001

Kafka M: Paraphilias and paraphilia-related disorders, in Treatments of Psychiatric Disorders, 3rd Edition. Edited by Gabbard GO. Washington, DC, American Psychiatric Press, 2001, pp 1951–2005

Kafka M, Prentky R: Fluoxetine treatment of nonparaphiliac sexual addictions and paraphilias in men. J Clin Psychiatry 53:351–358, 1992

Kafka M, Prentky R: Attention-deficit/hyperactivity disorder in males with paraphilias and paraphilia-related disorders: a comorbidity study. J Clin Psychiatry 59:388–396, 1998

Kaplan SA, Reis RB, Kohn IJ, et al: Safety and efficacy of sildenafil in postmenopausal women with sexual dysfunction. Urology 53:481–486, 1999

Kaufman DM: Neurologic aspects of sexual function, in Clinical Neurology for Psychiatrists, 3rd Edition. Edited by Kaufman DM. Philadelphia, PA, WB Saunders, 1990, pp 321–336

Kendirci M, Bivalacqua TJ, Hellstrom WJ: Vardenafil: a novel type 5 phosphodiesterase inhibitor for the treatment of erectile dysfunction. Expert Opin Pharmacother 5:923–932, 2004

Kennedy SH, McCann SM, Masellis M, et al: Combining bupropion SR with venlafaxine, paroxetine, or fluoxetine: a preliminary report on pharmacokinetic, therapeutic, and sexual dysfunction effects. J Clin Psychiatry 63:181–186, 2002

Kim E, Moty A, Wilson D, et al: Treatment of a complete lower urinary tract obstruction secondary to an expandable foam sealant. Urology 60:164, 2002

Kirby M, Jackson G, Betteridge J, et al: Is erectile dysfunction a marker for cardiovascular disease? Int J Clin Pract 55:614–618, 2001

Kirkeby H, Poulsen E, Petersen T, et al: Erectile dysfunction in multiple sclerosis. Neurology 38:1366–1371, 1988

Kirov G, Losanoff J, Kjossev K: Zoophilia: a rare cause of traumatic injury to the rectum. Injury 33:367–368, 2002

Ko D, Hebert P, Coffey C, et al: Beta-blocker therapy and symptoms of depression, fatigue, and sexual dysfunction. JAMA 288:351–357, 2002

Korpelainen J, Nieminen P, Myllyla V: Sexual functioning among stroke patients and their spouses. Stroke 30:715–719, 1999

Krueger R, Kaplan M: Disorders of sexual impulse control in neuropsychiatric conditions. Semin Clin Neuropsychiatry 5:266–274, 2000

Krueger R, Kaplan M: Depot-leuprolide acetate for treatment of paraphilias: a report of twelve cases. Arch Sex Behav 30:409–422, 2001

Kutner N, Brogan D, Fielding B, et al: Black/white differences in symptoms and health satisfaction reported by older hemodialysis patients. Ethn Dis 10:328–333, 2000

Kylstra W, Leenhouts G, Everaerd W, et al: Sexual outcomes following treatment for early stage gynecological cancer: a prospective multicenter study. Int J Gynecol Cancer 9:387–395, 1999

Laan E, van Lunsen RH, Everaerd W, et al: The enhancement of vaginal vasocongestion by sildenafil in healthy premenopausal women. J Womens Health Gend Based Med 11:357–365, 2002

Lama P: Systemic adverse effects of beta-adrenergic blockers: an evidence-based assessment. Am J Ophthalmol 134:749–760, 2002

Leenhouts G, Kylstra W, Everaerd W, et al: Sexual outcomes following treatment for early stage gynecological cancer: a prospective and cross-sectional multi-center study. J Psychosom Obstet Gynecol 23:123–132, 2002

Leserman J, Jackson E, Petitto J, et al: Progression to AIDS: the effects of stress, depressive symptoms, and social support. Psychosom Med 61:397–406, 1999

Levitsky A, Owens N: Pharmacologic treatment of hypersexuality and paraphilias in nursing home residents. J Am Geriatr Soc 47:231–234, 1999

Lothstein L: Countertransference reactions to gender dysphoric patients: implications for psychotherapy. Psychother Theory Res Pract 24:21–31, 1977

Lothstein L: The psychological management and treatment of hospitalized transsexuals. J Nerv Ment Dis 166:255–262, 1978

Lothstein L: Sex reassignment surgery: historical, bioethical, and theoretical issues. Am J Psychiatry 139:417–426, 1982

Lothstein L, Brown GR: Sex reassignment surgery: current concepts. Integr Psychiatry 8:21–30, 1992

Luboshitzky R, Aviv A, Hefetz A, et al: Decreased pituitary-gonadal secretion in men with obstructive sleep apnea. J Clin Endocrinol Metab 87:3394–3398, 2002

Lustman P, Clouse R: Relationship of psychiatric illness to impotence in men with diabetes. Diabetes Care 13:893–895, 1990

Malavaud B, Rostaing L, Rischmann P, et al: High prevalence of erectile dysfunction after renal transplantation. Transplantation 69:2121–2124, 2000

Marinkovic S, Badlani G: Voiding and sexual dysfunction after cerebrovascular accidents. J Urol 165:359–370, 2001

Marks L, Duda C, Dorey F, et al: Treatment of erectile dysfunction with sildenafil. Urology 53:19–24,1999

Martin D, Riopelle D, Steckart M, et al: Support group participation, HIV viral load and sexual risk behavior. Am J Health Behav 25:513–527, 2001

Martin-Morales A, Sanchez-Cruz J, de Tejada I, et al: Prevalence and independent risk factors for erectile dysfunction in Spain: results of the Epidemiologia de la Disfuncion Erectil Masculina Study. J Urol 166:569–574, 2001

Marwick T: Safe sex for men with coronary artery disease. JAMA 287:766–767, 2002

Masand PS, Ashton AK, Gupta S, et al: Sustained-release bupropion for selective serotonin reuptake inhibitor-induced sexual dysfunction: a randomized, double-blind, placebo-controlled, parallel-group study. Am J Psychiatry 158:805–807, 2001

Maughan K, Clarke C: The effect of a clinical nurse specialist in gynaecological oncology on quality of life and sexuality. J Clin Nurs 10:221–229, 2001

McGuire B, Ahmed E, Nazeer S: Genital self-mutilation: a literature review and case report. Sex Marital Ther 13:201–205, 1998

McKee A, Schover L: Sexuality rehabilitation. Cancer 92 (4 suppl): 1008–1012, 2001

McVary K, Carrier S, Wessells H, et al: Smoking and erectile dysfunction: evidence based analysis. J Urol 166:1624–1632, 2001

Mellon C, Barlow C, Cook J, et al: Autocastration and autopenectomy in a patient with transsexualism and schizophrenia. J Sex Res 26:125–130, 1989

Mendez M, Chow T, Ringman J, et al: Pedophilia and temporal lobe disturbances. J Neuropsychiatry Clin Neurosci 12:71–76, 2000

Meyer W, Bockting W, Cohen-Kettenis P, et al: The HBIGDA Standards of Care for Gender Identity Disorders, Version 6. Minneapolis, MN, Harry Benjamin International Gender Dysphoria Association, 2001. Available at: www.hbigda. org. Accessed May 15, 2004.

Meyhoff H, Rosenkilde P, Bodker A: Non-invasive management of impotence with transcutaneous nitroglycerin. Br J Urol 69:88–90, 1992

Mills TC, Paul J, Stall R, et al: Distress and depression in men who have sex with men: the Urban Men's Health Study. Am J Psychiatry 161:278–285, 2004 (erratum in Am J Psychiatry 161:776, 2004)

Milton J, Duggan C, Latham A, et al: Case history of comorbid Asperger's syndrome and paraphilic behaviour. Med Sci Law 42:237–244, 2002

Minderhoud J, Leemhuis J, Kremer J, et al: Sexual disturbances arising from multiple sclerosis. Acta Neurol Scand 70:299–306, 1984

Minkoff H, Moreno J: Drug prophylaxis for human immunodeficiency virus-infected pregnant women: ethical considerations. Am J Obstet Gynecol 163:1111–1114, 1990

Monga T, Lawson J, Inglis J: Sexual dysfunction in stroke patients. Arch Phys Med Rehabil 67:19–22, 1986

Monturo C, Rogers P, Coleman M, et al: Beyond sexual assessment: lessons learned from couples post radical prostatectomy. J Am Acad Nurse Pract 13:511–516, 2001

Morrison M, Petitto J, Ten Have T, et al: Depressive and anxiety disorders in women with HIV infection. Am J Psychiatry 159:789–796, 2002

Mulligan T, Sheehan H, Hanrahan J: Sexual function after heart transplantation. J Heart Lung Transplant 10:125–128, 1991

Nankervis A: Sexual function in chronic disease. Med J Aust 151:548–549, 1989

Naya Y, Soh J, Ochiai A, et al: Significant decrease of the International Index of Erectile Function in male renal failure patients treated with hemodialysis. Int J Impot Res 14:172–177, 2002

Neumann F, Kalmas J: Cyproterone acetate in the treatment of sexual disorders: pharmacology base and clinical experience. Exp Clin Endocrinol 98:71–80, 1991

Nortvedt M, Riise T, Myhr K, et al: Reduced quality of life among multiple sclerosis patients with sexual disturbance and bladder dysfunction. Mult Scler 7:231–235, 2001

Nurnberg H, Hensley P, Lauriello J, et al: Sildenafil for women patients with antidepressant-induced sexual dysfunction. Psychiatr Serv 50:1076–1078, 1999

Nurnberg H, Hensley P, Gelenberg A, et al: Treatment of antidepressant-associated sexual dysfunction with sildenafil: a randomized controlled trial. JAMA 289:56–64, 2003

Ofman U, Auchincloss S: Sexual dysfunction in cancer patients. Curr Opin Oncol 4:605–613, 1992

Ohl D, Denil J, Bennett C, et al: Electroejaculation following retroperitoneal lymphadenectomy. J Urol 145:980–983, 1991

O'Kane P, Jackson G: Erectile dysfunction: is there silent obstructive coronary artery disease? Int J Clin Pract 55:219–220, 2001

Ostrow D, McKirnan D: Prevention of substance-related high-risk sexual behavior among gay men: critical review of the literature and proposed harm reduction approach. J Gay Lesbian Med Assoc 1:97–110, 1997

Ostrow D, Beltran E, Chaniel J, et al: Predictors of volatile nitrite use among the Chicago MACS cohort of homosexual men, in Proceedings of the 7th International Conference on AIDS, Florence, Italy, June 16–21, 1991, MD 4043, p 400

Padma-Nathan H, Giuliano F: Oral drug therapy for erectile dysfunction. Urol Clin North Am 28:321–334, 2001

Padma-Nathan H, Kanellos A: The management of erectile dysfunction following spinal cord injury. Semin Urol 10:133–137, 1992

Padma-Nathan H, Payton T, Goldstein I: Intracavernosal pharmacotherapy: the pharmacologic erection program (PEP). World J Urol 5:160–166, 1987

Palmer B: Sexual dysfunction in uremia. J Am Soc Nephrol 10:1381–1388, 1999

Prieto Castro R, Anglada Curado F, Regueiro Lopez JC, et al: Treatment with sildenafil citrate in renal transplant patients with erectile dysfunction. BJU Int 88:241–243, 2001

Rabkin J, Wagner G, Rabkin R: Testosterone therapy for human immunodeficiency virus-positive men with and without hypogonadism. J Clin Psychopharmacol 19:19–27, 1999

Rabkin J, Wagner G, Rabkin R: A double-blind, placebo-controlled trial of testosterone therapy for HIV-positive men with hypogonadal symptoms. Arch Gen Psychiatry 57:141–147, 2000

Raffaele R, Vecchio I, Giammusso B, et al: Efficacy and safety of fixed-dose oral sildenafil in the treatment of sexual dysfunction in depressed patients with idiopathic Parkinson's disease. Eur Urol 41:382–386, 2002

Raina R, Agarwal A, Goyal KK, et al: Long-term potency after iodine-125 radiotherapy for prostate cancer and role of sildenafil citrate. Urology 62:1103–1108, 2003

Ramos A, Vidal J, Jauregui M, et al: Efficacy, safety and predictive factors of therapeutic success with sildenafil for erectile dysfunction in patients with different spinal cord injuries. Spinal Cord 39:637–643, 2001

Reilly D, Delva N, Hudson R: Protocols for the use of cyproterone, medroxyprogesterone, and leuprolide in the treatment of paraphilia. Can J Psychiatry 45:559–563, 2000

Rendell M, Rajfer J, Wicker P, et al: Sildenafil for treatment of erectile dysfunction in men with diabetes: a randomized controlled trial. Sildenafil Diabetes Study Group. JAMA 281:421–426, 1999

Rice A: Sexuality in cancer and palliative care 2: exploring the issues. Int J Palliat Nurs 6:448–453, 2000

Rieker R, Fitzgerald E, Kalish L, et al: Psychosocial factors, curative therapies, and behavioral outcomes: a comparison of testis cancer survivors and a control group of healthy men. Cancer 64:2399–2407, 1989

Robinson J, Donnelly B, Saliken J, et al: Quality of life and sexuality of men with prostate cancer 3 years after cryosurgery. Urology 60 (2 suppl 1):12–18, 2002

Rogers M, Kristjanson L: The impact on sexual functioning of chemotherapy-induced menopause in women with breast cancer. Cancer Nurs 25:57–65, 2001

Rosen RC: Sexual pharmacology in the 21st century. J Gend Specif Med 3:45–52, 2000

Rosen R, Lane R, Menza M: Effects of SSRIs on sexual function: a critical review. J Clin Psychopharmacol 19:67–85, 1999

Rosler A, Witztum E: Treatment of men with paraphilia with a long-acting analogue of gonadotropin-releasing hormone. N Engl J Med 338:416–422, 1998

Rosser B, Metz M, Bockting W, et al: Sexual difficulties, concerns, and satisfaction in homosexual men: an empirical study with implications for HIV prevention. J Sex Marital Ther 23:61–73, 1997.

Rothschild A: Selective serotonin reuptake inhibitor-induced sexual dysfunction: efficacy of a drug holiday. Am J Psychiatry 152:1514–1516, 1995

Rothschild A: Sexual side effects of antidepressants. J Clin Psychiatry 61 (suppl 11):28–36, 2000

Rowland J, Desmond K, Meyerowitz B, et al: Role of breast reconstructive surgery in physical and emotional outcomes among breast cancer survivors. J Natl Cancer Inst 92:1422–1429, 2000

Sadovsky R, Miller T, Moskowitz M, et al: Three-year update of sildenafil citrate (Viagra) efficacy and safety. Int J Clin Pract 55:115–128, 2001

Sakakibara R, Shinotoh H, Uchiyama T, et al: Questionnaire-based assessment of pelvic organ dysfunction in Parkinson's disease. Auton Neurosci 92:76–85, 2001

Salerian AJ, Deibler WE, Vittone BJ, et al: Sildenafil for psychotropic-induced sexual dysfunction in 31 women and 61 men. J Sex Marital Ther 26:133–140, 2000

Sarica K, Arikan N, Serel A, et al: Multidisciplinary evaluation of diabetic impotence. Eur Urol 26:314–318, 1994

Schover L: The impact of breast cancer on sexuality, body image, and intimate relationships. CA Cancer J Clin 41:112–120, 1991

Schover L, Evans R, von Eschenbach A: Sexual rehabilitation in a cancer center: diagnosis and outcome in 384 cases. Arch Sex Behav 16:445–461, 1987

Schover L, Novick A, Steinmuller D, et al: Sexuality, fertility and renal transplantation: a survey of survivors. J Sex Marital Ther 16:3–13, 1990

Schover L, Fouladi R, Warneke C, et al: Defining sexual outcomes after treatment for localized prostate carcinoma. Cancer 95:1773–1785, 2002

Schroder F, Collette L, de Reijke T, et al: Prostate cancer treated by anti-androgens: is sexual function preserved? Br J Cancer 82:283–290, 2000

Schwartz S, Plawecki H: Consequences of chemotherapy on the sexuality of patients with lung cancer. Clin J Oncol Nurs 6:212–216, 2002

Shen W, Urosevich Z, Clayton D: Sildenafil in the treatment of female sexual dysfunction induced by selective serotonin reuptake inhibitors. J Reprod Med 44:535–542, 1999

Shoptaw S, Reback C, Freese T: Patient characteristics, HIV serostatus, and risk behaviors among gay and bisexual males seeking treatment for methamphetamine abuse and dependence in Los Angeles. J Addict Dis 21:91–105, 2002

Shrivastava R, Shrivastava S, Overweg N, et al: Amantadine in the treatment of sexual dysfunction associated with selective serotonin reuptake inhibitors. J Clin Psychopharmacol 15:83–84, 1995

Silber E (ed): The treatment of ischemic heart disease, in Heart Disease, 2nd Edition. New York, Macmillan, 1987, pp 1663–1665

Singer P, Tasch E, Stocking C, et al: Sex or survival: trade-offs between quality and quantity of life. J Clin Oncol 9:328–334, 1991

Sipski M: Sexual function in women with neurologic disorders. Phys Med Rehabil Clin N Am 12:79–90, 2001

Sipski M, Rosen R, Alexander C, et al: Sildenafil effects on sexual and cardiovascular responses in women with spinal cord injury. Urology 55:812–815, 2000

Skinner J: Sexual relations and the cardiac patient, in Heart Disease and Rehabilitation. Edited by Pollock ML, Schmidt DH. Boston, MA, Houghton Mifflin, 1979, pp 587–599

Smith S, O'Keane V, Murray R: Sexual dysfunction in patients taking conventional antipsychotic medication. Br J Psychiatry 181:49–55, 2002

Souza E, Keiralla D, Silveira D, et al: Sexual dysfunction in epilepsy: identifying the psychological variables. Arq Neuropsiquiatr 58:214–220, 2000

Sprunk E, Alteneder R: The impact of an ostomy on sexuality. Clin J Oncol Nurs 4:85–88, 2000

Standage K, Moore J, Cale M: Self-mutilation of the genitalia by a female schizophrenic. Can Psychiatr Assoc J 19:17–20, 1974

Stenager E, Stenager EN, Jensen K: Sexual function in multiple sclerosis: a 5-year follow-up study. Ital J Neurol Sci 17:67–69, 1996

Stewart TD: The spinal cord-injured patient, in Handbook of General Hospital Psychiatry. Edited by Cassem NH. St Louis, MO, Mosby–Year Book, 1991, pp 484–486

Strathdee S, Martindale S, Cornelisse P, et al: HIV infection and risk behaviours among young gay and bisexual men in Vancouver. CMAJ 162:21–25, 2000

Stroberg P, Murphy A, Costigan T: Switching patients with erectile dysfunction from sildenafil citrate to tadalafil: results of a European multicenter, open-label study of patient preference. Clin Ther 25:2724–2737, 2003

Stroch D: Self-castration. JAMA 36:270, 1901

Stueve A, O'Donnell L, Duran R, et al: Being high and taking sexual risks: findings from a multisite survey of urban young men who have sex with men. AIDS Educ Prev 14:482–495, 2002

Tabler J, Frierson R: Sexual concerns after heart transplantation. J Heart Lung Transplant 9:397–403, 1990

Tanabe H, Yoshida N, Sayama S, et al: A case of burn due to sadomasochism. J Dermatol 29:463–464, 2002

Taub N, Wolfe C, Richardson E, et al: Predicting the disability of first-time stroke sufferers at 1 year: 12-month follow-up of a population-based cohort in Southeast England. Stroke 25:352–357, 1994

Thase M, Reynolds C, Jennings J, et al: Nocturnal penile tumescence is diminished in depressed men. Biol Psychiatry 24:33–46, 1988

Thibaut F, Cordier B, Kuhn J: Gonadotropin hormone releasing hormone agonist in cases of severe paraphilia: a lifetime treatment? Psychoneuroendocrinology 21:411–419, 1996

Tindall B, Forde S, Goldstein D, et al: Sexual dysfunction in advanced HIV disease. AIDS Care 6:105–107, 1994

Tsai S, Hwang J, Yang C, et al: Inappropriate sexual behaviors in dementia: a preliminary report. Alzheimer Dis Assoc Disord 13:60–62, 1999

Tsujimura A, Matsumiya K, Tsuboniwa N, et al: Effect of renal transplantation on sexual function. Arch Androl 48:467–474, 2002a

Tsujimura A, Yamanaka M, Takahashi T, et al: The clinical studies of sildenafil for the ageing male. Int J Androl 25:28–33, 2002b

Turk S, Karalezli G, Tonbul H, et al: Erectile dysfunction and the effects of sildenafil treatment in patients on hemodialysis and continuous ambulatory peritoneal dialysis. Nephrol Dial Transplant 16:1818–1822, 2001

Uva J: Review: autoerotic asphyxiation in the United States. J Forensic Sci 40:534–581, 1995

Vanable P, Ostrow D, McKirnan K, et al: Impact of combination therapies on HIV risk perceptions and sexual risk among HIV-positive and HIV-negative gay and bisexual men. Health Psychol 19:134–135, 2000

Van Buuren H, Lunter C, Groenhuijzen H: Prevalence of psychiatric complications among HIV-infected people in the Netherlands, in Proceedings of the 1st International Conference on Biopsychosocial Aspects of HIV Infection, Amsterdam, The Netherlands, September 22–25, 1991, p 24

Vita G, Bellinghieri G, Trusso, et al: Uremic autonomic neuropathy studied by spectral analysis of heart rate. Kidney Int 56:232–237, 1999

Vittinghoff E, Hessol N, Bacchetti P, et al: Cofactors for HIV disease progression in a cohort of homosexual and bisexual men. J Acquir Immune Defic Syndr 27:308–314, 2001

Waldinger M, Hengeveld M, Zwinderman A: Ejaculation-retarding properties of paroxetine in patients with primary premature ejaculation. Br J Urol 79:592–595, 1997

Webster L: Management of sexual problems in diabetic patients. Br J Hosp Med 51:465–468, 1994

Webster LJ, Michelakis ED, Davis T, et al: Use of sildenafil for safe improvement of erectile function and quality of life in men with New York Heart Association classes II and III congestive heart failure: a prospective, placebo-controlled, double-blind crossover trial. Arch Intern Med 164:514–520, 2004

Wilder RB, Chou RH, Ryu JK, et al: Potency preservation after three-dimensional conformal radiotherapy for prostate cancer: preliminary results. Am J Clin Oncol 23:330–333, 2000

Wilmoth M: The aftermath of breast cancer: an altered sexual self. Cancer Nurs 24:278–286, 2001

Wirshing D, Pierre J, Erhart S, et al: Understanding the new and evolving profile of adverse drug effects in schizophrenia. Psychiatr Clin North Am 26:165–190, 2003

Wise T: Urethral manipulation: an unusual paraphilia. J Sex Marital Ther 8:222–227, 1982

Wise T: Psychosocial side effects of sildenafil therapy for erectile dysfunction. J Sex Marital Ther 25:145–150, 1999

Wise T, Dietrich A, Segall E: Female genital self-mutilation: case reports and literature review. J Sex Marital Ther 15:269–274, 1989

Witherington R: Suction device therapy in the management of erectile impotence. Urol Clin North Am 15:123–128, 1988

Wu SC, Lin SL, Jeng FR: Influence of erythropoietin treatment on gonadotropic hormone levels and sexual function in male uremic patients. Scand J Urol Nephrol 35:136–140, 2001

Young-McCaughan S: Sexual functioning in women with breast cancer after treatment with adjuvant therapy. Cancer Nurs 19:308–319, 1996

Yurek D, Farrar W, Andersen B: Breast cancer surgery: comparing surgical groups and determining individual differences in postoperative sexuality and body change stress. J Consult Clin Psychol 68:697–709, 2000

Zorzon M, Zivadinov R, Bosco A, et al: Sexual dysfunction in multiple sclerosis: a case-control study, I: frequency and comparison of groups. Mult Scler 5:418–427, 1999

Zorzon M, Zivadinov R, Bragadin L, et al: Sexual dysfunction in multiple sclerosis: a 2-year follow-up study. J Neurol Sci 187:1–5, 2001

18

Substance-Related Disorders

John E. Franklin Jr., M.D., M.Sc.

James L. Levenson, M.D.

Elinore F. McCance-Katz, M.D., Ph.D.

THE ABILITY TO recognize and treat substance use disorders (SUDs) is a core competence in psychosomatic medicine. SUDs are common in both inpatient and outpatient medical settings. Alcohol and tobacco use alone contribute to a host of medical illnesses. Illegal drug use taxes the health care system. Drug and alcohol dependence disorders are best characterized as chronic medical illnesses (McLellan et al. 2000). Hepatitis C is an example of a potential long-term complication of even brief drug use, injection drug users being at increased risk. Emergency departments have seen a steady increase in overdoses of drugs, including "club drugs" not prevalent until recently. The long-term effects of perinatal drug abuse are becoming known (Baer et al. 2003; Buka et al. 2003; Thapar et al. 2003). Devastating complications result from the internal concealment of illicit drugs (e.g., body packing) (Traub et al. 2003). Core competence in addiction medicine includes the ability to make accurate diagnoses, initiate treatment, and plan and coordinate services. Some hospitals have specialized addiction consultation services (Fleming et al. 1995; Fuller and Jordan 1994; McDuff et al. 1997), but there is a shortage of board-certified addiction psychiatry specialists. All psychiatrists working in general medical settings are on the front lines of substance abuse and must be sufficiently knowledgeable.

The span of issues for psychiatrists in medical settings includes drug overdose, withdrawal regimens, diagnosis, engaging patients in the therapeutic process, interface with pain management, assessing transplantation candidates, care of trauma and burn patients (who have a high frequency of drug dependency), substance abuse among pregnant women, drug abuse in geriatric or adolescent patients, and referral to substance abuse specialists. American Psychiatric Association practice guidelines (1995a, 1995b) are valuable resources for the treatment of alcohol, cocaine, and opioid use disorders, and the U.S. Veterans Health Administration has published more recent guidelines (Management of Substance Use Disorders Working Group 2001). Ideally, the psychiatrist is part of an integrated, multidisciplinary approach to thorough medical evaluation and education, nutritional assessment, housing and family assessment, and complex legal issues.

In this chapter, we provide an update on addiction medicine and highlight issues that arise on general medical units, including intoxication and withdrawal and their complications; psychological and psychiatric factors; treatment resistance; recovery environment; and relapse potential.

DSM-IV-TR Substance-Related Disorders

In DSM-IV-TR (American Psychiatric Association 2000), the broad diagnostic category "substance-related disorders" includes disorders caused by substances taken by individuals to alter mood or behavior, disorders caused by unintentional use of a substance, and medication side effects. Substance-related disorders are divided into *substance use disorders*, which include abuse and dependence, and *substance-induced disorders*, which include intoxication, withdrawal, delirium, dementia, sexual dysfunction, and amnestic, psychotic, mood, anxiety, and sleep disorders.

Substance abuse is a diagnosis of exclusion, to be used only when a patient does not meet, and has never met, criteria for substance dependence. This distinction can be confusing, because the term *substance abuse* is often used in a nondiagnostic sense to refer to a broad spectrum of substance use patterns.

Definitions

Abuse is the harmful use of a substance. *Misuse* is the use of a prescription drug for other than accepted medical practice. *Addiction* is characterized by impaired control over drug use, compulsive use, continued use despite harm, and craving. *Physical dependence* is a state of adaptation that manifests as a specific withdrawal syndrome. *Psychological dependence* is the feeling of need for a specific substance, either for its positive effects or to avoid negative effects associated with abstinence from it.

Withdrawal is a substance-specific constellation of symptoms that may occur after cessation or a decrease in use of alcohol or drugs by individuals who are physiologically dependent. Withdrawal syndromes are characterized by symptoms opposite to those characteristic of use of the substance. Withdrawal syndromes vary in severity and are not necessarily proportional to the amount of substance use. Some withdrawal syndromes are associated with significant morbidity and, possibly, mortality if not recognized and treated aggressively (e.g., alcohol and benzodiazepines), whereas others are associated with considerable discomfort but are not life-threatening (e.g., opioids). Withdrawal can sometimes precipitate delirium, psychosis, mood disturbances, anxiety, and disordered sleep. It has been postulated that after acute withdrawal from alcohol, opiates, and stimulants, many milder physiological and psychological disruptions can persist for weeks to months (e.g., disordered sleep and mood disturbance). The concept of a protracted substance-specific withdrawal syndrome has been proposed, but its existence and management remain controversial (Begleiter and Porjesz 1979; Geller 1994; Satel et al. 1993).

Tolerance is the need for increasing amounts of a substance to obtain the desired effect (e.g., intoxication) or lesser effect of a substance with continued use of the same amount over time. For example, a series of alcoholic patients in an emergency department had an average blood alcohol concentration of 467 mg/dL—a level known to cause coma or death in an alcohol-naive individual, yet 88% of these patients were oriented to time, person, and place (Minion et al. 1989).

General Principles

General principles of management for patients with SUDs in medical settings are summarized in Table 18–1. In general hospitals, there are a number of barriers to detection and treatment of SUDs. The psychiatrist may enter a clinical situation in which considerable misunderstanding and animosity have developed between the patient and the medical care team. Nurses and physicians may overestimate or underestimate the impact of a patient's substance use or may be overly frustrated by rebuffs of attempts to engage an unmotivated patient. Health care professionals may become nihilistic or angry at patients who are repetitively hospitalized with complications of substance use (e.g., alcoholic pancreatitis). Intense negative emotional responses toward patients with SUDs can interfere with proper care (e.g., giving lower rather than higher than usual doses of narcotics for postoperative pain to a heroin addict). Patients may acknowledge their substance use but either not realize or deny its relation to their medical and psychosocial problems. The social network of those with SUDs may be either chaotic or unsupportive or composed mainly of other substance abusers. Patients with SUDs typically do not request psychiatric assistance and often are not told that a psychiatric consultation has been requested. In general, earlier consultations are more desirable, especially if treatment linkage is necessary. While acutely medically ill, patients are often more open to treatment recommendations. Because some patients are reluctant to fully disclose substance abuse or dependence owing to possible legal problems (e.g., issues relating to motor vehicle collisions) or fear of job loss, information gathering can be difficult.

In medical settings, a high index of suspicion for drug and alcohol use disorders is warranted because of their

---

TABLE 18–1.   General principles of management for patients with substance use disorders in medical settings

Have a high index of suspicion for drug abuse
Use early urine toxicological screens.

Carefully assess for detoxification
Determine the need for inpatient versus outpatient care.
Tailor detoxification for medically ill patients (this approach often needed in this patient population).
Carry out alcohol and sedative detoxification first in case of polysubstance dependence.
Order challenge tests or use conservative estimates if the initial detoxification dose is not clear.

prevalence in the medically ill and their adverse physiological and behavioral effects on disease outcome. Urine toxicological screening should be performed early in the diagnostic evaluation. Tailored detoxification is often needed by medically ill patients; for example, although alcohol detoxification does not routinely necessitate hospitalization, it may for a patient with unstable angina. In polysubstance dependence, alcohol and sedative detoxification is the priority because of the higher risk of morbidity and mortality than with other substances. As a rule, challenge tests or conservative estimates should be used if there is doubt about the initial detoxification dose.

Acute Assessment

The elements of a basic substance use history are listed in Table 18–2. Important additional aspects of assessment include identifying significant negative countertransference, triage, and establishing patient eligibility for follow-up care (this function is an administrative one, but a consultant must not make unrealistic recommendations). It is often difficult and sometimes impossible during the initial consultation to differentiate the effects of substance intoxication, withdrawal, or chronic use from other psychiatric disorders. A carefully obtained history provides clues that can aid diagnostic differentiation between substance-induced disorders and major mental disorders with comorbid substance abuse or dependence, including the historical sequence of substance use and symptoms of a mental disorder. Elements in the history also indicate whether the psychiatric symptoms have occurred during periods of prolonged sobriety. The family history is important given increasing evidence of the heritability of SUDs. Evaluation of the patient's family is essential as a source of collateral information, for learning the extent of the substance use and its consequences, and because a family system that accommodates the patient's substance use also may reinforce it. Including the family in treatment increases the chances that the patient will remain abstinent.

Treatment

Proper implementation of treatment always involves patients and their other medical providers. The steps include 1) educating the patient, 2) motivating the patient to accept the recommended treatment plan, 3) encouraging others to work collaboratively with the patient, 4) suggesting pharmacological treatments, when needed, 5) integrating substance abuse treatment into the overall medical and psychiatric treatment plans, and 6) facilitating transfers to appropriate treatment facilities when appropriate.

TABLE 18–2. Elements of the substance use history

Chief complaint

History of present illness

Current medical signs and symptoms

Substance abuse review of symptoms for all psychoactive substances

Dates of first use, regular use, heaviest use, longest period of sobriety, pattern, amount, frequency, time of last use, route of administration, circumstances of use, reactions to use

Medical history, medications, HIV status, hepatitis B and C status

History of past substance abuse treatment, response to treatment

Family history, including substance abuse history

Psychiatric history

Legal history

Object-relations history

Personal history

Source. Adapted from Frances RJ, Franklin JE Jr: *Concise Guide to Treatment of Alcoholism and Addictions.* Washington, DC, American Psychiatric Press, 1989, p. 62. Used with permission.

Detoxification alone does not constitute treatment of addiction. Some patients with mild substance abuse may resolve drug- or alcohol-related problems without additional treatment (Sobell et al. 1996) or with brief intervention by the consultant or another physician (Barnes and Samet 1997). Brief interventions by primary care physicians have shown promise for heavy drinkers in early addiction patterns (Aalto et al. 2000; Beich et al. 2003; Fleming et al. 2002). Substance dependence, however, is best viewed as a chronic medical illness (McLellan et al. 2000), and many substance-dependent patients benefit from referral to specialized treatments that may be required long-term. Failure to refer can reinforce denial of substance-related problems and enable continued addiction. Treatment of SUDs integrated with regular medical care may reduce inpatient hospitalization rates (Laine et al. 2001).

It is difficult to arrange proper aftercare during a short hospitalization or when financial resources are limited. Insurance coverage varies considerably. In the United States, Medicare and many state Medicaid programs do not cover treatment of SUDs. Many private insurance plans require preauthorization and use a very limited panel of providers. Patients with little or no coverage usually must wait until public treatment slots are available. While waiting, patients often continue use or have relapses. This problem is especially prevalent among patients who have a poor support system and problems with housing, employment, and income (Humphreys et al. 1996).

Recovery is a process in which patients must develop responsibility for their own addiction. Therefore, the role of the psychiatrist and other health care providers is to empathically confront the patient about substance-related problems and to provide support, information, and access to resources, but not to assume total responsibility for patient follow-up. Education and a motivational approach, rather than continuous confrontation, usually work best. The psychiatric consultant is typically not directly involved in a patient's aftercare, so a brief intervention model is needed. An early treatment goal is to have patients accept that their substance use is causing them problems and that some form of treatment is needed.

The most common referrals are to a specialized substance abuse treatment program or to a 12-step group such as Alcoholics Anonymous (AA). Most drug and alcohol treatment programs in the United States emphasize a combination of psychoeducation, participation in a 12-step program, and individual, group, and family counseling. Although resource availability is often a determining factor in follow-up treatment recommendations, guidelines such as those developed by the American Society of Addiction Medicine (Mee-Lee et al. 1994) can be used in referring patients to different levels of care. Because most treatment programs require that patients themselves call for services, the role of the consultant is to inform patients and encourage them to contact programs directly.

AA is a worldwide self-help group of recovering alcoholic individuals that was started in 1936 by Bill Wilson and Robert Smith (Dr. Bob). The only requirement for membership is a desire to stop drinking. Meetings provide members with acceptance, understanding, forgiveness, confrontation, and a means for positive identification. AA uses a 12-step program—12 tenets of recovery that members work through on their way to overcoming addiction. The steps include admitting powerlessness over alcohol, conducting a personal assessment, making amends, and eventually helping others. Members may contact one another outside meetings for sobriety support, and newer members team up with more experienced AA members, sponsors who guide them through the process. Although AA is not affiliated with any religion (25% of AA members identify themselves as atheists), the organization encourages spiritual reevaluation. Members frequently remain active in AA for many years, and AA involvement is generally associated with favorable outcome (Connors et al. 2001; Humphreys et al. 1996; McKellar et al. 2003; Owen et al. 2003; Vaillant 1995) comparable with that of other standard treatment approaches (Ouimette et al. 1997). A prospective study of employed alcoholic patients found that treatment plus AA participation was more effective than AA involvement alone in helping such

individuals attain and continue abstinence (Walsh et al. 1991). In some hospitals, AA members visit inpatients, and many general hospitals host AA meetings.

Other organizations have been modeled on AA. Narcotics Anonymous (NA), founded in 1947, and Cocaine Anonymous (CA), founded in 1982, are two examples. Contacts for AA, NA, and CA can usually be found in local telephone directories or on the organizations' respective Web sites. Patients should be told that some self-help groups address special issues for participants and that it may be necessary for them to attend several different meetings in their area before they find a group that suits them or they make a decision that self-help is not beneficial.

Patients with a substance-related disorder and another psychiatric disorder have better outcomes when both disorders are treated simultaneously and all stakeholders (patients, clinicians, families, and community leaders) are invested (Mueser et al. 1997; Nunes and Quitlin 1997; Torrey et al. 2002). Nevertheless, integrated long-term treatment programs for such patients can be difficult to find. Many psychiatric inpatient units, psychiatric halfway houses, outpatient clinics, and other mental health facilities in the community are unable or unwilling to treat psychiatric patients who also have SUDs. In many substance abuse treatment facilities, there is little if any contact with psychiatrists, and treatment is provided by counselors who have minimal psychiatric training. Integrated programs combine rehabilitation, psychiatric evaluation, and the appropriate use of other treatment modalities, such as psychotherapy and pharmacotherapy. AA, NA, and CA officially support the use of psychotropic medications when necessary. Dual-diagnosis or "double-trouble" groups also use a 12-step approach.

Recommendations for patients after a suicide attempt and a recent history of alcohol or drug use or abuse range from discharge with outpatient mental health and substance abuse follow-up to inpatient psychiatric involuntary commitment (i.e., if there is a strong suicidal risk). When ambivalence exists about the correct disposition, a brief inpatient psychiatric stay for further evaluation usually is prudent.

Patients with concomitant chronic medical illnesses that limit participation in formal substance treatment programs pose special problems. Patients, families, and medical staff may focus so much on the medical illness that substance use is neglected as an issue. Patients may encounter difficulties with transportation or difficulty sustaining the concentration necessary to take full advantage of formal rehabilitation programs. For example, a clinical trial of alcoholism treatment after liver transplantation failed in part because of the patients' infirmity and need for intensive medical management (Weinrieb et al. 2001). Medically ill patients often feel estranged from the "world of the well." Devising aftercare programs tailored to such patients' needs is often difficult. Patients are sometimes seen individually and attend meetings of AA or professional groups as tolerated.

Additional difficulties occur when patients have spinal cord injuries, blindness, deafness, or other physical disabilities. For example, some caregivers involved in the treatment of paraplegic patients experience excessive sympathy that causes them to ignore significant substance abuse problems. However, it is possible to successfully integrate paraplegic patients into standard treatment programs. Deaf patients often need specialized services, such as sign language interpreters, to utilize standard rehabilitation services. Some communities have AA groups for deaf or blind people. Patients with significant cognitive limitations, including mental retardation, traumatic brain injury, and dementia, pose a difficult problem because they are not able to benefit from standard psychosocial treatment approaches, all of which rely on capacity to communicate and learn.

Patients in recovery from addiction and who are abstinent often face the dilemma of whether to take mood-altering substances (e.g., narcotics for pain or anxiolytics for sedation) in the course of the planned treatment. Recovery teaches people to avoid all mood-altering substances because use of these substances can lead to relapse or a substitute addiction. If the hospitalization is elective, such as for ambulatory surgery, the issue can be discussed with drug treatment staff members or AA sponsors. It may be possible to use pain management techniques that avoid the use of narcotics (see Chapter 36, "Pain"). When the issue is discussed in advance and adequate support is provided, most patients do not have relapses. The clinician should encourage AA members and sponsors to visit the patient and should halt treatment with mood-altering medication as soon as medically indicated. Continued or increased need for narcotic medications in the face of improving medical response to the treatment or the development of a pattern of continuing complications resulting in ongoing narcotic requests should lead to an evaluation for recurrence of a SUD.

Treatment Outcome

Long-term studies have consistently shown that treatment of substance dependence is beneficial and cost-efficient from a public health or societal perspective (McLellan et al. 1996). Predicting which individual patients are more apt to benefit from which type of treatment has been a greater problem. Patients who are more compliant with and receive more treatment generally do better, as do patients who receive additional treatment directed at specific ancillary problems, such as housing, employment, and comorbid psychiatric illness (McLellan et al. 1997). In Project Match, a large randomized trial of alcohol treatment modalities and predictive pretreatment variables, investigators did not find a robust association between specific treatments and specific indicators (Project Match Research Group 1998). In a similar study, the COMBINE study, investigators are evaluating the efficacy of naltrexone and acamprosate alone or together in combination with different intensities of behavioral therapy (COMBINE Study Research Group 2003). Other potential predictors, such as severity of addiction, social status, number of previous treatment attempts, coping style, family history, and patient self-selection of treatment type, have not been shown to have consistent associations with treatment outcome.

Relapse prevention is essential in treating substance dependence. The goals of relapse prevention are to address ambivalence, reduce drug or alcohol availability, minimize high-risk situations, develop coping strategies, recognize conditioned cues to craving and decision patterns that lead to use, establish alternatives to drug or alcohol use, and avoid the attitude that all is lost if drug use occurs in the context of treatment (Carroll et al. 1991).

Alcohol-Related Disorders

Workers in the addiction field have attempted to more clearly define alcohol use problems, and accuracy is especially important for making a diagnosis in a medical setting. Several hospitalizations for alcohol-related illness can occur before a direct connection is made between a patient's alcohol use and medical problems. Alcoholic patients tend to experience many alcohol-related problems before seeking professional help or attending AA meetings (Bucholz and Homan 1992). Stigma associated with the term *alcoholism* frequently inhibits physicians and patients from exploring the connections between abuse and biopsychosocial consequences. Psychiatrists participating in a hospital survey positively identified alcohol abuse two-thirds of the time, whereas physicians treating gynecology patients diagnosed the disorder only 10% of the time (Moore et al. 1989). In primary care settings similar underdiagnosis is common; however, in studies that rely on chart review or screening instruments, investigators may underestimate what physicians really suspect to be the case (Rumpf et al. 2001; Rydon et al. 1992).

The official psychiatric nomenclature for alcohol abuse and dependence evolved from the view of alcoholism as a personality disorder (American Psychiatric Association 1952), through recognition of episodic, habitual abuse (American Psychiatric Association 1968), to the more recent definitions in DSM-III (American Psychiatric Association 1980), DSM-III-R (American Psychiatric Association 1987), DSM-IV (American Psychiatric Association 1994), and DSM-IV-TR (American Psychiatric Association 2000). The newer definitions emphasize the complex of psychosocial consequences as well as physiological tolerance and withdrawal as hallmarks of the disease process. The diagnosis of alcohol dependence has been shown over 5 years to be predictive of a chronic, significant course of illness (Schuckit et al. 2001). The National Council on Alcoholism and Drug Dependence and the American Society of Addiction Medicine define alcoholism as a disease process (Morse and Flavin 1992) and disease as an involuntary disability. This definition states that alcoholism is a primary, chronic disease with genetic, psychosocial, and environmental factors influencing its development and manifestations. The disease is often progressive and fatal. It is characterized by impaired control over drinking, preoccupation with alcohol, use of alcohol despite adverse consequences, and distortions in thinking, most notably denial. Each of these symptoms may be continuous or periodic (Morse and Flavin 1992).

Epidemiological Characteristics

The Epidemiologic Catchment Area study showed that the lifetime prevalence of alcohol abuse or dependence in the general population was 13.6% (Robins et al. 1984). Follow-up data from the same Epidemiologic Catchment Area population revealed a 1-year prevalence for alcohol disorders of 7.4%. Only 22% of these people ever used any mental health or addiction services, and of those, approximately one-half were seen by specialty mental health or addiction professionals. The other half were examined by general medical professionals (Regier et al. 1993). In other words, people who seek consultation for alcohol problems are as likely to see general physicians as they are to see mental health or drug abuse specialists. The revised 1-year prevalence estimates for the 18–54 age group, based on both the Epidemiologic Catchment Area and the National Comorbidity Survey and focusing more on clinical significance, are 6.5% for alcohol use disorders and 2.4% for drug abuse disorders (Narrow et al. 2002). Binge drinking is on the rise among adults and is associated with impaired driving (Naimi et al. 2003).

Alcohol-related problems usually begin between the ages of 16 and 30 years. Data suggest that sales to underage drinkers and adult heavy drinkers account for 50% of alcoholic beverages sold (Foster et al. 2003). Regier et al.

(1990) reported that 53% of persons with an alcohol or drug abuse disorder also have a comorbid psychiatric disorder. Women are more likely than men to present for treatment in mental health or medical settings (Weisner and Schmidt 1992). Men are more likely than women to receive treatment in jails and drug treatment programs. Alcoholism among elderly individuals is increasing and is often difficult to diagnose because the symptoms are often less dramatic than they are among younger persons.

A conservative estimate is that 25% of general hospital inpatients and 20% of medical outpatients have alcohol-related disorders (Cleary et al. 1988; Moore et al. 1989). Diagnosis of these disorders in patients in general hospitals is challenging. For example, a patient may present with cirrhosis and severe gastritis after several years of "moderate" alcohol intake, but no psychosocial sequelae are reported. Detailed, repeated, or collateral history is necessary before the diagnosis of alcohol dependence becomes clear.

Patients with alcoholism usually resist and avoid doctors because of denial, embarrassment, stigma, problems with authority figures, or poor self-care. The medical condition occasionally is the only apparent indication of alcohol abuse. Results of a seminal study by Vaillant (1995) highlighted the fact that medical complications sometimes are the main reason for abstinence, as when alcohol use precipitates gastrointestinal bleeding, a traumatic injury, a sickle-cell crisis, or a seizure.

Medical and Other Complications

Common alcohol-related medical conditions include gastritis and peptic ulcer, pneumonia, alcoholic hepatitis and cirrhosis, trauma (e.g., traumatic brain injury, subdural hematoma, fractures), pancreatitis, cardiomyopathy, hemorrhagic stroke, labile hypertension, anemia, peripheral neuropathy, fetal alcohol syndrome, amnestic syndrome (Korsakoff's psychosis), and alcoholic dementia (Lieber 1995; Rehm and Bondy 1998; Reynolds et al. 2003).

Liver disease is the ninth leading cause of death, and alcoholism is a major cause of liver disease. It has been estimated that 75% of patients with chronic pancreatitis are alcohol dependent (Van Thiel et al. 1981). Alcohol use also contributes to increased rates of oral cavity, laryngeal, esophageal, liver, and breast cancers (Cole and Rodu 2001; Singletary and Gapstur 2001). Heavy alcohol use adversely effects the natural course of chronic hepatitis C (Bhattacharya and Shuhart 2003). Women experience increased mortality risk at a lower level of alcohol intake than men. Although in some epidemiological studies limited alcohol consumption, compared with abstinence, has been associated with lower risk of myocardial infarction, ischemic cerebrovascular disease, and dementia (Mukamal et al. 2003a, 2003b, 2003c), such correlations require replication and may not be simply causal. More important, these results are based on samples from the general population, not the medically ill, and may be misused by alcohol-dependent patients to rationalize continued use of alcohol. The goal for patients with substance abuse and medical conditions should be abstinence, and patients benefit most from integrated primary care and addiction treatment (Weisner et al. 2001).

The total spending for health care services to manage alcohol problems and the medical consequences of alcohol consumption was estimated at $22.5 billion for 1995, with a total economic cost of $166.5 billion (National Institute on Drug Abuse and National Institute on Alcohol Abuse and Alcoholism 2001). There is an association between alcohol use and violent crime, including assault, rape, child molestation, and murder. In one study involving 2,095 trauma victims, Meyers et al. (1990) found that 41% of the patients were drinking before sustaining the injuries. In a more recent study, Schermer et al. (2003a) found that 45% of trauma surgery patients had positive screening results for problem alcohol use. Alcohol problems are underrecognized and undertreated on trauma services and burn units (Bernstein et al. 1992; Schermer et al. 2003b) (see Chapter 30, "Surgery"). Orthopedic injuries in alcohol and drug users are more severe and require longer hospitalizations than in nonusers (Levy et al. 1996).

Alcoholism, which is strongly associated with suicide, increases the suicide rate 60–120 times compared with the rate in the nonalcoholic population, particularly in synergy with other predisposing factors such as unemployment, impulsivity, and aggression (Caces and Harford 1998; Mann et al. 1999). The lifetime risk of suicide among alcoholic patients is estimated to be 2.0%–3.4% (Murphy and Wetzel 1990). Alcoholic patients who attempt suicide may have more severe alcohol problems and greater comorbidity than those who do not attempt suicide (Murphy et al. 1992).

Predisposition and Risk Factors

Alcoholism probably results from a complex interaction among biological vulnerability, family, environment, and culture. Studies involving men and women showed that genetic variables significantly influence incidence, although the mechanism of genetic transmission is unknown (Johnson et al. 1998; Merikangas et al. 1998b). Hypothesized heritable factors include abnormalities in the serotonergic (Lappalainen et al. 1998; Mantere et al. 2002), dopaminergic (Edenberg et al. 1998), and opioid

systems (Camí and Farré 2003; Wand et al. 1998). Functional neuroimaging points to particular areas of the brain associated with craving, intoxication, and withdrawal (Tapert et al. 2003). Inherited variations in alcohol-metabolizing enzymes, such as those common in Asian populations, confer reduced risk of alcoholism (Schuckit 1999). Genotypic variation in neurotransmitter alleles may effect vulnerability to alcohol dependence and its phenotypes (Enoch et al. 2003; Nurnberger et al. 2001). The P300 component of the event-related potential continues to be investigated as a marker of alcoholism (Justus et al. 2001; Suresh et al. 2003).

In a prospective study, Vaillant (1995) found no personality style to be predictive of alcoholism; however, alcoholism occurs more commonly when other psychiatric disorders are present. Neurobehavioral disinhibition in childhood and conduct disorder in adolescence may be risk factors (Tarter et al. 2003), and increased tolerance of alcohol during the teen years may be a marker for future dependence (Schuckit and Smith 2001). There is a rich literature on the relationship between alcohol use and depression (Hasin et al. 2002) and on the shared genetic vulnerability between alcohol dependence and other psychiatric disorders (de Graaf et al. 2002; Fu et al. 2002; Hasin and Grant 2002; Hasin et al. 2002). Alcoholic patients are at increased risk of bipolar disorder, panic disorder, and social phobia but not of non-substance-induced major depressive disorder (Schuckit et al. 1997). In a study involving general hospital patients with borderline personality disorder, 67% of the patients had an SUD (Dulit et al. 1990). Antisocial personality disorder also is associated with alcohol use disorders and with poorer treatment outcome (Kranzler et al. 1996). Debate continues over the explanations for these associations (Jacobsen et al. 2001; Kopelman 1995; Merikangas et al. 1998a). Alcohol use is common in patients with schizophrenia, in whom such use may transiently decrease social anxiety, dysphoria, insomnia, and other nonpsychotic but unpleasant experiences. Alcohol use may also contribute to poor outcome in this population (Cantor-Graae et al. 2001; Drake et al. 1989; Noordsy et al. 1991).

Specific Disorders

Intoxication

The effects of alcohol intoxication range from mild inebriation to respiratory depression, coma, and, rarely, death. Gamma-aminobutyric acid (GABA), *N*-methyl-D-aspartate (NMDA), and second-messenger systems all mediate physiological effects (Nestler and Self 1997). Alcohol activates GABA-mediated chloride ion channels, inhibits NMDA-activated ion channels, and potentiates serotonin 5-HT$_3$ receptor–activated ion channels. GABA subunits may change structurally as tolerance and dependence develop. Alcohol may combine with endogenous and exogenous chemicals such as dopamine and cocaine to produce toxic metabolites (McCance-Katz et al. 1995, 1998).

The body metabolizes alcohol at the rate of approximately 100 mg/kg/hour. Approximately 1.5 hours are required to metabolize 1 ounce (30 mL) of whiskey. Among individuals who have not developed tolerance, a blood alcohol concentration of 0.03 mg% can lead to euphoria, 0.05 mg% can cause mild coordination problems, and 0.1 mg% usually causes ataxia. Anesthesia, coma, and death are associated with a blood alcohol concentration greater than 0.4 mg% (Adams et al. 1997). In patients who engage in chronic heavy drinking and have developed tolerance, high blood levels are reached with fewer of these effects. The first-pass metabolism of alcohol is lower in women because they have lower amounts of gastric alcohol dehydrogenase than do men. This phenomenon may explain the increased bioavailability of alcohol, higher rates of cirrhosis, and lower thresholds for intoxication among women (Frezza et al. 1990).

Uncomplicated Withdrawal

In individuals who have developed tolerance, alcohol withdrawal symptoms develop when a relative decrease in blood alcohol level occurs; therefore, symptoms can occur while drinking continues. A coarse, high-frequency generalized tremor may appear that increases during motor activity or stress (e.g., when the hand or the tongue is extended). The tremor typically peaks 24–48 hours after the last drink and subsides after 5–7 days of abstinence. Patients also often have signs of autonomic hyperactivity, including hypertension, tachycardia, sweating, malaise, nausea, vomiting, anxiety, and disturbed sleep.

Histories can be difficult to obtain during medical emergencies. A patient who is not believed to have alcohol dependence often suddenly develops withdrawal symptoms 1–3 days after surgery. It is often difficult to differentiate withdrawal from other causes of postoperative delirium (see Chapter 30, "Surgery"). Changes in vital signs may have many other explanations in acute medical illness, and concurrent medications (e.g., sedative-hypnotics, beta-blockers, and anticonvulsants) may partially obscure or suppress signs of withdrawal, seriously delaying recognition and full appropriate treatment of withdrawal. The diagnosis is particularly at risk of being missed in patients who are critically ill. The Clinical Institute Withdrawal Assessment for Alcohol—Revised

(CIWA-Ar) is a valuable clinical scale for quantifying withdrawal and following symptoms over time (Sullivan et al. 1991). The CIWA-Ar must be carefully interpreted in the medically ill, because symptoms of other systemic disease may overlap with symptoms of withdrawal (Lambert 2003; Lapid and Bostwick 2002).

Withdrawal Seizures

Withdrawal seizures typically occur 7–38 hours after last alcohol use, peak frequency occurring at approximately 24 hours after last use (Adams et al. 1997). However, a significant fraction (16%) of first seizures in drinkers fall outside the conventionally defined withdrawal period, coming while the person is still drinking or as long as a week after the last drink (Ng et al. 1988). Although the relation of seizures to alcohol use is dose dependent and appears to be causal, the timing of seizures is seemingly random (Ng et al. 1988). Among patients with chronic alcoholism, 10% experience multiple seizures (Espir and Rose 1987). Hypomagnesemia, hypokalemia, respiratory alkalosis, and hypoglycemia all potentially contribute to alcohol withdrawal seizures. As many as one-third of patients who experience withdrawal seizures develop alcohol withdrawal delirium.

Withdrawal Delirium (Delirium Tremens)

Delirium tremens (DT) is characterized by confusion, disorientation, fluctuating or clouded consciousness, and perceptual disturbances. Typical signs and symptoms include delusions, hallucinations, agitation, insomnia, mild fever, and marked autonomic arousal. Patients frequently report vivid visual hallucinations of insects or small animals or other perceptual distortions. These hallucinations are typically (but not invariably) associated with feelings of terror and agitation. Symptoms of DT usually appear 2–3 days after cessation of heavy drinking, peak intensity occurring on the fourth to fifth day. Patients often have a repetitive pattern of DT each time they withdraw from alcohol (Turner et al. 1989). Withdrawal symptoms, which can wax and wane, usually subside after 3 days of adequate treatment, but even well-managed DT can continue to wax and wane for several weeks (Hersh et al. 1997). Untreated DT can last as long as 4–5 weeks. Compared with other alcoholic patients, those with a history of DT or withdrawal seizures report a greater maximum number of drinks per day, more lifetime withdrawal episodes, more sedative-hypnotic abuse, and a greater number of medical problems (Schuckit et al. 1995). DT occurs more frequently and is particularly dangerous in patients who have infections, subdural hematomas, trauma, liver disease, or metabolic disorders. In earlier literature, mortality rates of 15%–20% among patients with DT were cited, but deaths have become uncommon with adequate treatment (Foy et al. 1997). One study showed that of 334 alcohol-dependent patients presenting with alcohol withdrawal, 6.9% developed DT despite benzodiazepine treatment (Palmstierna 2001). All of the patients with DT had the following five risk factors: 1) current infectious disease, 2) heart rate greater than 120 beats/minute on admission, 3) withdrawal symptoms despite an alcohol concentration greater than 1 g/L body fluid by Breathalyzer test, 4) history of seizures, and 5) history of delirious withdrawal episodes. In a case–control study, Fiellin et al. (2002) identified elevated blood pressure, previous DT or withdrawal seizure, and medical comorbidity as contributing to the risk of DT. In the hospital, physical restraints and 24-hour sitters are sometimes needed to protect the patient and to ensure that intravenous lines are maintained.

Alcohol-Induced Psychotic Disorder

Alcoholic hallucinosis, designated *alcohol-induced psychotic disorder* in DSM-IV-TR, is defined as vivid auditory hallucinations that last at least 1 week and occur soon after the cessation or reduction of heavy alcohol ingestion. The hallucinosis presents with a relatively clear sensorium and few autonomic signs or symptoms. As many as 10%–20% of cases may become chronic (Soyka 1996). The hallucinations sometimes include familiar noises or clear voices. The patient usually responds to these hallucinations with fear, anxiety, and agitation (Victor 1992). Diagnosis is based on a history of recent heavy alcohol use and the absence of schizophrenia or mania. Auditory hallucinations and delusions in alcoholic hallucinosis can closely resemble those in schizophrenia and can make differential diagnosis difficult in the absence of adequate historical findings (Soyka 1990).

Alcohol-Induced Amnestic Disorder

Persisting alcohol-induced amnestic disorder (Wernicke-Korsakoff syndrome) often begins with an abrupt onset of truncal ataxia, ophthalmoplegia, and delirium (Wernicke's encephalopathy), but it can occur in the absence of the classic symptom constellation (Brew 1986). The etiology of the disorder is thiamine deficiency due to poor nutritional, medical, or other factors. Thiamine deficiency can cause death or, more commonly, persisting, severe, anterograde amnesia (Korsakoff's psychosis) in which memory is not transferred from immediate to long-term memory storage. Approximately 80% of patients with Wernicke's encephalopathy who are treated and survive develop this persisting amnesia (Reuler et al. 1985). Postmortem examinations show lesions in the brainstem, diencephalon, and frontal lobes (Kopelman 1995) (see also Chapter 7, "Dementia"; Chapter 23, "Endocrine and Metabolic Disorders"; and Chapter 32, "Neurology and Neurosurgery").

Neurological Disease

Alcohol-induced dementia is another example of a neuropsychiatric disorder found in patients with chronic alcoholism (see Chapter 7, "Dementia"). Because alcoholic patients have complicated medical histories and are often poor historians, the diagnosis is often presumptive. Other disorders affecting the nervous system associated with chronic alcoholism include polyneuropathy, hepatic encephalopathy, acute or chronic subdural hematoma, and cerebellar degeneration with truncal ataxia. Rare conditions such as central pontine myelinolysis, Marchiafava-Bignami disease, and nutritional amblyopia also occur.

Liver Disease

Alcohol has direct toxic effects on the liver (Lieber 1988). Alcohol dehydrogenase, a liver enzyme, metabolizes alcohol to toxic acetaldehyde. Aldehyde dehydrogenase catalyzes the transformation of acetaldehyde. Acetic acid, lactic acid, uric acid, and fat are by-products of this process. The first stage of alcoholic liver injury is mild alcoholic hepatitis, which is reversible with abstinence but with continued drinking progresses to cirrhosis. Severe alcoholic hepatitis has a mortality approaching 50% (Haber et al. 2003). Cirrhosis is irreversible and results in hepatic encephalopathy (see Chapter 6, "Delirium"), liver failure, portal hypertension, ascites, and gastrointestinal bleeding. The only definitive way to diagnose alcohol-induced cirrhosis is by liver biopsy. Hepatitis C can accelerate liver damage caused by alcohol consumption, and vice versa.

Cirrhosis decreases the activity and levels of hepatic enzymes, including the cytochrome P450 system. Decreased albumin concentration, common in alcoholic patients with liver disease, increases the bioavailability of most psychotropic drugs. In patients with impaired liver function, the doses of hepatically metabolized medications may have to be reduced. Blood levels of the drugs should be monitored when possible (see Chapter 37, "Psychopharmacology").

Liver Transplantation

Despite early reluctance to perform liver transplantation on alcoholic patients, approximately 30% of the 3,000 orthotopic liver transplantations in the United States each year are performed on patients with alcoholism. There is reliable evidence that properly screened alcoholic patients rarely return to drinking and that they have rates of survival and a quality of life comparable with those of nonalcoholic patients (DiMartini et al. 1998, 2002; Lucey et al. 1997). The psychiatric evaluation should include consideration of history of drinking, insight into illness, family insight and support, willingness to consider treatment, social stability, and long-term sobriety predictors such as substitute activities, a sense of hope, and comorbidity with drug use or antisocial personality (DiMartini et al. 2002; Franklin and Paine 2003; Roggla et al. 1996; Tringali et al. 1996). Transplantation and substance abuse are discussed in detail in Chapter 31 ("Organ Transplantation").

Interaction Between Alcohol and Medications

The interaction between alcohol and medications can have a wide range of effects (i.e., from lethal overdoses to undermedication) (Table 18–3). Alcohol is partly metabolized through the hepatic microsomal enzyme system that metabolizes other drugs. In the acute phase, alcohol can slow metabolism and increase blood levels of medications, such as oral anticoagulants, diazepam, and phenytoin, which compete for cytochrome P450 enzymes. In the chronic phase, because of cytochrome P450 enzyme induction, alcohol can lead to increased metabolism and decreased blood levels of these medications. Chronic alcohol intake with associated cytochrome P450 enzyme induction can also promote acetaminophen toxicity as a result of the accumulation of toxic metabolites

Conversely, some medications can influence the metabolism of alcohol. For example, chlorpromazine, chloral hydrate, and cimetidine increase blood alcohol levels by inhibiting alcohol dehydrogenase. Alcohol enhances diazepam absorption, which decreases its safety margin and increases the possibility of overdose. In addition, alcohol increases the potency of other central nervous system (CNS) depressants and has unpredictable effects when used with CNS stimulants. Mild disulfiram-like reactions can occur with oral hypoglycemics (e.g., tolbutamide and chlorpropamide), griseofulvin, metronidazole, and quinacrine. Long-term use of salicylates or nonsteroidal anti-inflammatory drugs and alcohol can lead to gastrointestinal bleeding. Because some alcoholic beverages contain tyramine, monoamine oxidase inhibitors are best avoided in the treatment of active or recovering alcoholic patients.

Physical Examination and Laboratory Testing

Spider nevi, palmar erythema, cigarette burns between the index and middle fingers, poor dental care, jaundice, enlarged liver, abdominal pain, peripheral neuropathy, and muscle weakness are clinical signs of alcoholism. When alcoholic patients present as severely intoxicated, semicomatose, or comatose, complications of alcoholism must be considered, including head injury (e.g., subdural hematoma), stroke, metabolic derangements (e.g., hypoglycemia), hepatic encephalopathy, postictal state, aspiration, and cardiac arrhythmia as well as the possibility of polydrug intoxication.

TABLE 18–3.   Medication interactions with alcohol

Medication	Effects
Disulfiram (Antabuse)	Flushing, diaphoresis, vomiting, pounding headache, anxiety, confusion
Anticoagulants (oral)	Increased anticoagulation effect with acute alcohol intoxication, decreased effect after chronic alcohol use
Griseofulvin	Minor disulfiram-alcohol-like reaction
Metronidazole	Minor disulfiram-alcohol-like reaction
Oral hypoglycemics	Minor disulfiram-alcohol-like reaction
Tranquilizers, narcotics, antihistamines	Increased central nervous system (CNS) depression
Diazepam	Increased absorption of diazepam, synergistic CNS depression
Phenytoin	Increased anticonvulsant effect with acute intoxication; with chronic alcohol use, alcohol intoxication or withdrawal may lower seizure threshold
Salicylates, nonsteroidal anti-inflammatory drugs	Gastrointestinal bleeding
Chlorpromazine	Increased levels of alcohol
Cimetidine	Increased levels of alcohol
Monoamine oxidase inhibitors	Hypertensive crisis possibly due to adverse reaction to tyramine in some alcoholic beverages

Source.   Adapted from Mack AH, Franklin JE Jr, Frances RJ: "Substance Use Disorders," in *The American Psychiatric Publishing Textbook of Clinical Psychiatry*, 4th Edition. Edited by Hales RE, Yudofsky SC. Washington, DC, American Psychiatric Publishing, 2003, p. 362. Used with permission.

For years investigators have searched for reliable laboratory markers of recent heavy alcohol use (see Table 18–4). Serum gamma-glutamyltransferase (SGGT) levels are increased in more than 50% of patients who have an alcohol problem and in 80% of alcoholic patients with liver dysfunction (Trell et al. 1984). Aspartate aminotransferase (AST) levels are increased in 46% of patients with alcoholism. Decreased white blood cell count and increased mean corpuscular volume and uric acid, triglyceride, alanine aminotransferase (ALT), and blood urea nitrogen (BUN) levels are also common in alcoholism. However, in patients with advanced cirrhosis, liver enzyme levels are sometimes normal, but prothrombin time is increased, and BUN level may be low. One-third of patients with alcoholism have increased blood glucose levels, but it is not uncommon for alcoholic patients with inadequate calorie intake to have hypoglycemia and hypoalbuminemia.

Both the total amount of carbohydrate-deficient transferrin and the ratio of carbohydrate-deficient transferrin to total serum transferrin can help identify heavy alcohol use over time. Stowell et al. (1997) found the test to be approximately 80% sensitive and 90% specific in the detection of chronic consumption of more than 60 g of alcohol daily in a population of male drinkers. Although results may be influenced by tobacco use, age, cirrhosis, sex, and other factors (Stowell et al. 1997; Whitfield et al. 1998), the test may be useful for monitoring for relapse in men and women, particularly when combined with measurement of SGGT concentration (Allen et al. 1999, 2001; Anton et al. 1998). However, no single test or combination of laboratory measures has been found sufficiently sensitive and specific for identification of occult alcohol dependence.

Screening Tests

Two widely used brief screening tests for the detection of alcoholism are the self-administered Michigan Alcoholism Screening Test (MAST) and the clinician-administered CAGE questionnaire (Table 18–5). The MAST is a 25-question form that is 90% sensitive; the CAGE is a four-item test. The CAGE has been studied in a variety of populations. In a study of pretraumatic and posttraumatic brain injury, sensitivity and specificity both were more than 90% (Ashman et al. 2004). The four-question Rapid Alcohol Problems Screen, the five-question TWEAK test, and the 10-question Alcohol Use Disorders Identification Test have been found more useful than the CAGE in women and ethnically diverse populations (Bradley et al. 1998; Cherpitel 2002; Steinbauer et al. 1998). The Alcohol Use Disorders Identification Test is more sensitive than the CAGE for identification of nondependent hazardous drinking (McCusker et al. 2002). The Patient Health Questionnaire, a brief self-administered screen for psychiatric disorders designed for primary care, also helps identify alcohol use disorders (Spitzer et al. 1999). A single positive response is reasonably effective in identifying problem drinking (Hodgson et al. 2003). The addiction severity index is a treatment planning assessment tool that examines seven areas of patient functioning, including drug and alcohol abuse (McLellan et al. 1980). A review of the various screening instruments is available online through the Center for Substance Abuse Treatment, Treatment Improvement Protocol series (Center for Substance Abuse Treatment 2004).

Acute Management and Treatment

Intoxication

Intoxicated behavior is managed by decreasing external stimuli, interrupting alcohol ingestion, and protecting

---

TABLE 18–4.   Laboratory findings associated with alcohol abuse

Increased mean corpuscular volume
Increased AST, ALT, and lactate dehydrogenase levels
Increased SGGT level (particularly sensitive)
Increased serum carbohydrate-deficient transferrin level
Decreased albumin, vitamin B_{12}, and folic acid levels
Increased uric acid and amylase levels, evidence of bone
   marrow suppression
Prolonged prothrombin time (cirrhosis)

Note.   ALT=alanine aminotransferase; AST=aspartate aminotransferase; SGGT=serum gamma-glutamyltransferase.
Source.   Adapted from Mack AH, Franklin JE Jr, Frances RJ: *Concise Guide to Treatment of Alcoholism and Addictions*, 2nd Edition. Washington, DC, American Psychiatric Publishing, 2001, p. 97. Used with permission.

TABLE 18–5.   CAGE questionnaire for the diagnosis of alcoholism

Have you ever…

C   Thought you should CUT back on your drinking?
A   Felt ANNOYED by people criticizing your drinking?
G   Felt GUILTY or bad about your drinking?
E   Had a morning EYE-OPENER to relieve hangover or nerves?

Note.   Two or three positive responses=high index of suspicion; four positive responses=pathognomonic.
Source.   Reprinted from Ewing JA: "Detecting Alcoholism: The CAGE Questionnaire." *Journal of the American Medical Association* 252:1905–1907, 1984. Copyright 1984, American Medical Association. Used with permission.

individuals from harming themselves and others until the toxic effects of alcohol disappear. Psychiatrists most often encounter acutely intoxicated patients in the emergency department. No antidote is available in the United States, but elsewhere metadoxine has been found safe and effective in accelerating elimination of alcohol and reducing signs of intoxication (Addolorato et al. 2003). In cases of potentially fatal overdoses, hemodialysis is sometimes attempted.

Withdrawal

The choice of inpatient versus outpatient treatment of withdrawal usually depends on the severity of symptoms, the stage of withdrawal, the presence of medical and psychiatric comorbidity, the presence of polysubstance abuse, patient cooperation, ability to follow instructions, social support systems, patient history, and, increasingly, insurance reimbursement policies. Consultation requests often involve patients whose withdrawal symptoms have been only partially eliminated during detoxification or patients who are not yet beyond danger of serious medical complications.

Not all alcohol-dependent patients need medication for detoxification. Benzer (1990) found that only 10.6% of hospitalized alcohol-dependent patients had withdrawal symptoms severe enough to necessitate medication. Full detoxification, a modified detoxification schedule, or as-needed medication is used depending on the severity of dependence, medical condition, detoxification history, vital signs, and mental status. For routine cases, as-needed (symptom-triggered) oxazepam was found as safe and effective as a fixed-schedule protocol (Daeppen et al. 2002). In alcoholic patients with histories of withdrawal seizures, DT, or otherwise complicated withdrawals or with other serious medical conditions (e.g., coronary artery disease), full medical detoxification should proceed; one should not rely on as-needed medications alone. Safe detoxification occurs when autonomic signs and symptoms are adequately controlled. Sedation is a clinically useful indicator of adequate treatment in early withdrawal.

Benzodiazepines are recommended for the treatment and prevention of withdrawal symptoms (Mayo-Smith 1997). Benzodiazepines are safe, easy to administer, have anticonvulsant properties, and are efficacious. Chlordiazepoxide is commonly used because of its long-acting metabolites. Benzodiazepines such as lorazepam (the only one that can reliably be given orally, intramuscularly, or intravenously) and oxazepam should be used in the treatment of patients with severe liver disease and of elderly patients, because these drugs are metabolized via conjugation rather than oxidation. Otherwise, no clear differ-

ences in efficacy have been found among benzodiazepines. Diazepam is less frequently used in detoxification because of its reported euphorigenic properties in some patients. The benzodiazepines with longer half-lives, such as chlordiazepoxide and clonazepam, may require less frequent administration. Anticonvulsants are being used increasingly in the treatment of alcohol withdrawal and have been shown in a number of studies to be as efficacious as benzodiazepines (Malcolm et al. 2001). A few consultants prefer to use phenobarbital because of its very long half-life, which offers some degree of protection in patients who leave a facility before completing detoxification. Despite the evidence that administration of ethanol is a poor choice for treating alcohol withdrawal in the hospital, the practice continues, primarily among surgeons (Rosenbaum and McCarty 2002). A survey showed that 91% of hospitals still had alcohol in their formularies and that most ethanol was dispensed for alcohol withdrawal (Blondell et al. 2003). Use of alcohol for alcohol detoxification is not considered standard-of-care treatment.

Ideal candidates for outpatient detoxification have good social supports, are highly motivated, and need to be able to make daily clinic visits during the withdrawal period. Furthermore, they have CIWA-Ar scores of 10 or less (Table 18–6), have no history of withdrawal seizures or DT, and do not have medical illnesses that may complicate the withdrawal process (e.g., history of gastrointestinal bleeding or cirrhosis). Optimal inpatient withdrawal follows a symptom-triggered medication protocol with a standardized withdrawal rating scale, such as the CIWA-Ar (Table 18–6). Ward staff must be trained in using such scales, but withdrawal generally is faster and requires less medication with use of the scales (Saitz et al. 1994). Patients initially found to need withdrawal medication on the basis of CIWA-Ar results should be considered for a medication-tapering schedule for safe detoxification.

Nutritional deficiencies of thiamine, vitamin B_{12}, and folic acid should be corrected with oral thiamine (100 mg/day), folic acid (1 mg/day orally), daily multivitamins, and adequate nutrition. It is uncertain how long vitamin supplementation should be continued, but because vitamins are inexpensive and harmless, some clinicians recommend continuing them indefinitely. Thiamine 100–200 mg should be given intramuscularly or intravenously to patients with very poor nutrition or who are unable to tolerate oral intake. Intravenous thiamine should be given before glucose infusion, because glucose depletes thiamine stores, which can precipitate acute Wernicke's encephalopathy. Magnesium, potassium, and phosphate all may have to be repleted.

TABLE 18–6. Pharmacological management of alcohol withdrawal

Symptom-triggered medication regimens

Administer one of the following medications every 2–4 hours when the CIWA-Ar score is ≥10:

Consider the patient's history, recent alcohol intake, and weight in determining dosage

Chlordiazepoxide (50–100 mg orally)

Oxazepam (30–60 mg orally)

Lorazepam (1–2 mg orally)

Repeat the CIWA-Ar 2–4 hours after every dose to assess the need for further medication

Structured medication regimens

Chlordiazepoxide 50 mg orally every 6 hours for four doses, then 50 mg every 12 hours for two doses, then 25 mg orally every 12 hours for 2 doses, then one dose of 25 mg and discontinue

Lorazepam 2 mg orally every 6 hours for four doses, then 1 mg every 6 hours for eight doses

For severe withdrawal (CIWA-Ar >20), lorazepam up to 2–4 mg every 6 hours may be necessary with taper based on symptoms over several days

---

Note. CIWA-Ar=Clinical Institute Withdrawal Assessment for Alcohol—Revised.

Individuals with a history of epilepsy may need additional anticonvulsant medication. For uncomplicated withdrawal seizures, the addition of anticonvulsants to benzodiazepines is not always necessary (D'Onofrio et al. 1999); however, for those who experience a seizure or who have a history of alcohol withdrawal seizures, the addition of carbamazepine or valproate, tapered over 1–2 weeks, can be helpful. Diazepam, 10 mg intravenously, usually aborts status epilepticus; however, the addition of phenytoin is occasionally necessary. Lorazepam has been found to be effective in the emergency setting (Alldredge et al. 2001).

Alcohol-Induced Psychotic Disorder

When patients experience alcoholic hallucinosis during detoxification, a potent antipsychotic such as haloperidol, 2–5 mg orally twice a day, is typically needed to control agitation and hallucinations, but newer atypical antipsychotics may be efficacious. Although there is a theoretical concern that antipsychotics lower the seizure threshold, this problem is unlikely as long as the patient also is receiving a benzodiazepine. The clinician should reassess the use of antipsychotic medication soon after cessation of symptoms. Continued administration of antipsychotics is seldom needed unless the patient has a chronic alcoholic psychosis (Korsakoff's psychosis).

Delirium Tremens

The best treatment of DT is prevention through careful assessment and aggressive treatment of significant signs and symptoms of withdrawal. Once it is evident, DT may follow a course of its own. The first principle of management is protection of patients from themselves and others. Sedation and reduced stimulation are needed, and physical restraints may be necessary. Large doses of benzodiazepines usually are required but occasionally are ineffective. A switch to phenobarbital has proved effective in some cases. Propofol has been reported effective in cases of DT refractory to high doses of benzodiazepines (McCowan and Marik 2000). Patients in danger of severe damage due to muscular agitation may need to be pharmacologically paralyzed for their protection and receive mechanical ventilation.

Long-Term Medication Management

Although disulfiram (Antabuse) has not been shown to be generally effective in controlled trials in which adherence has not been monitored (Fuller et al. 1986), this agent may be a useful adjunct for some patients with alcoholism. However, disulfiram therapy should be used only in patients who have made a commitment to long-term treatment, so administration of the drug is rarely initiated in the treatment of general hospital inpatients. Contraindications to disulfiram treatment include severe liver disease, pregnancy, heart disease, and psychosis. Disulfiram also is associated with important drug–drug interactions (e.g., increased levels of phenytoin and isoniazid).

Naltrexone has been shown to reduce the risk of relapse to heavy drinking in alcohol-dependent patients (Garbutt et al. 1999; Volpicelli et al. 1992). The usual dosage is 50 mg orally once a day. In patients with polysubstance dependence, the dose may have to be increased (Oslin et al. 1999). Side effects include headache, nausea, and mild dysphoria. These effects can be minimized if administration is initiated at a dose of 25 mg. Because it is an opioid antagonist, naltrexone cannot be used in the treatment of patients receiving opioid analgesics. Medication compliance significantly affects efficacy. Kranzler et al. (1998) performed preliminary investigations of an injectable, sustained-release form of naltrexone. Large, double-blind, placebo-controlled trials of oral naltrexone have produced mixed results in different populations (Guardia et al. 2002; Krystal et al. 2001; Morris et al. 2001).

Treatment Outcome

Approximately 33% of patients with alcoholism stop drinking without formal treatment intervention, 33% improve with treatment, and 33% never achieve sobriety. Patients who are simply handed lists of community-based substance abuse programs rarely follow through with treatment. Motivational interviewing techniques are important skills that help guide patients to recognize their addiction, resolve ambivalence about changing behaviors, and instill patient ownership of the change process (Miller et al. 2003).

Sedative-, Hypnotic-, and Anxiolytic-Related Disorders

Abuse and Dependence

Sedative-hypnotic and alcohol intoxications are similar in symptoms and complications. Because sedative-hypnotic use is so frequent in hospitalized patients, the detection of sedative abuse can be difficult. Abuse rarely starts as a result of treatment of acute anxiety or insomnia in a hospitalized patient. The risk of sedative abuse in chronically medically ill outpatients is far greater. There are three major classes of benzodiazepine abusers: polysubstance abusers, pure sedative abusers, and therapeutic users who have lost control. Individuals prone to polysubstance abuse tend to use sedatives for their calming effects (i.e., to come down after use of a stimulant such as cocaine) and for their ability to decrease dysphoric affects, including anxiety, or to potentiate euphoric effects of other drug classes (e.g., benzodiazepines in combination with methadone to boost euphoria).

Pure sedative abusers usually have significant underlying psychopathological conditions (Martinez-Cano et al. 1999), and relapse is common. In a long-term follow-up study involving subjects with primary sedative-hypnotic dependence, 46% of the subjects continued to abuse drugs after in-hospital rehabilitation treatment (Allgulander et al. 1987). Anyone can develop physiological dependence with low-dose use over several years or high-dose use over weeks to months (Dietch 1983). Patients with a history of other SUDs are at increased risk of benzodiazepine abuse (Ross and Darke 2000). In addition, children of alcoholic individuals may respond differently to benzodiazepines than others and may be more prone to benzodiazepine abuse (Ciraulo et al. 1996).

In general, drugs with short half-lives are more likely to cause abuse, withdrawal, dependence, and addiction than are similar drugs with long half-lives, such as alprazolam versus clonazepam and butalbital versus phenobarbital. However, despite their short half-lives, the nonbenzodiazepine hypnotics zolpidem and zopiclone are reported to cause much less abuse and dependence than benzodiazepines, although they both pose risk in patients with prior substance abuse (Hajak et al. 2003). Rarely prescribed older sedatives such as carisoprodol (Soma), chloral hydrate (Noctec), ethchlorvynol (Placidyl), glutethimide (Doriden), meprobamate (Miltown), methaqualone (Quaalude), and methyprylon (Noludar) have high abuse liability and are associated with severe withdrawal syndromes.

Complications

Most cases of gross benzodiazepine intoxication are self-limiting and are best treated supportively. In severe cases and in overdose, the benzodiazepine antagonist flumazenil can reverse coma (Basile et al. 1991), but use of this agent may be associated with seizures, especially if the patient is benzodiazepine dependent. Elderly patients taking even low-dose sedative-hypnotics are at increased risk of confusion, loss of balance, and falls (Frels et al. 2002). Cognitive deficits are not uncommon with benzodiazepine abuse. These deficits may improve or persist for months after detoxification (Tonne et al. 1995). In one study involving more than 4,000 elderly patients, more than 9% of the patients had been treated with benzodiazepines in the preceding year, and benzodiazepine use was associated with impaired functional status independent of age and other medical conditions (Ried et al. 1998).

The high-potency benzodiazepine flunitrazepam (Rohypnol) has been used illegally to incapacitate women for the purpose of sexual assault and can induce anterograde amnesia. Covert flunitrazepam intoxication should be suspected in sexual assault victims who are amnestic for the assault (Anglin et al. 1997).

Withdrawal

The length of time between last use of a drug and onset of withdrawal is a function of the elimination half-life of the drug. For example, withdrawal symptoms occur 7–10 days after abrupt cessation of diazepam but 1–2 days after cessation of alprazolam. Withdrawal symptoms are similar to those produced by alcohol. Seizures may herald withdrawal and are a potential complication of high-dose, unexpected, or poorly managed benzodiazepine withdrawal. Severe withdrawal can produce psychosis and may result in death.

Treatment of sedative-hypnotic withdrawal is similar to that of withdrawal from alcohol. Because of the high prevalence of polysubstance abuse, a detailed substance use history should be obtained to determine the likelihood of polysubstance withdrawal (Busto et al. 1996). A cross-tolerant sedative is given to prevent benzodiazepine withdrawal symptoms, and the daily dose is gradually decreased; long-acting benzodiazepines are recommended. Alprazolam is particularly difficult to taper after long-term use or high-dose abuse, and it is usually best to convert treatment to a longer-acting benzodiazepine such as clonazepam, which can be easily withdrawn. For some high-dose abusers, particularly those with serious medical comorbidity, inpatient detoxification may be necessary. Addition of an anticonvulsant (e.g., carbamazepine or valproate) can add an additional margin of safety over the course of a difficult withdrawal process.

The most important factor in minimizing complications during benzodiazepine withdrawal is to decrease the dose by approximately 10% per day; the terminal 10% should be tapered slowly to zero over a 3- to 4-day period. In general, detoxification is accomplished within a 10- to 14-day period, but certain individuals need longer detoxification. Tapering may take weeks or months when patients have been taking benzodiazepines for many years or when the drug is resistant to tapering (e.g., alprazolam).

Certain personality traits, such as dependency and passivity, are associated with higher daily doses, more severe withdrawal symptoms, and treatment failure (Schweizer et al. 1998). Detoxification with shorter-acting benzodiazepines, such as oxazepam or lorazepam, often is used in the treatment of elderly patients and patients with liver or pulmonary disease. Anticonvulsants and propranolol are reportedly useful adjuncts in treating prolonged withdrawal symptoms when long-term benzodiazepine therapy is discontinued (Schweizer et al. 1991).

Prevention and Acute Management

Preventing habituation to sedative-hypnotic drugs is the best prevention of abuse and dependence. Limited prescriptions, single-source policies (i.e., obtaining prescriptions from one provider), and appropriate follow-up all are helpful. General guidelines for anxiolytic treatment are reviewed in Chapter 12 ("Anxiety Disorders") and hypnotic use in Chapter 16 ("Sleep Disorders"). Sedative-hypnotics should usually be avoided in the treatment of patients with alcoholism and those with a history of substance abuse.

Opioid-Related Disorders

Opioid abuse manifests in various ways in patients in medical settings. Psychiatrists are frequently consulted regarding opioid therapy for patients who are prescribed methadone, are thought or known to be dependent on prescription or illicit narcotics, engage in drug-seeking behavior, exhibit personality problems that interfere with medical care, or have overdosed. Suspicion is heightened by exaggerated pain complaints, by visits to multiple providers for multiple pain complaints requiring a narcotic prescription (e.g., migraine, back pain, dental pain, fibromyalgia, and endometriosis), and by claims to be "allergic" to every analgesic except for particular opioids (e.g., hydrocodone or oxycodone).

Opioid-dependent patients often provoke angry reactions from staff, which can result in discharging a patient prematurely or underprescribing pain medications. Chronic pain patients who develop tolerance to opioids and experience opiate withdrawal on cessation of use are often mislabeled addicts (see Chapter 36, "Pain"). Tolerance and withdrawal alone are not sufficient for the diagnosis of either substance abuse or dependence. For example, cancer patients with painful bone metastatic lesions may need high doses of narcotics and are unlikely to become psychologically dependent or engage in addictive behaviors.

Deaths related to heroin overdose are common and recently have been on the rise, resulting from variations in purity and the presence of contaminants (Office of Applied Studies 2003). Although most heroin is taken intravenously, snorting has become more popular among users who fear contracting HIV infection or hepatitis C. Polysubstance abuse is extremely common among people addicted to opiates. The combination of heroin and cocaine ("speedballing") is one of the most frequent combinations, and concomitant alcohol use is common. Heroin abuse exists among working middle- and upper-class individuals as well as the poor. Rates of misuse of, and death from, use of controlled-release oxycodone and similar prescription drugs doubled between 1992 and 2000 (Office of Applied Studies 2004). Synthetic opioids such as fentanyl are abused by individuals who have easy access, such as nurses, physicians, and especially anesthesiologists.

Epidemiological Characteristics

Estimates of opioid abuse derive from overdose reports, surveys, the prevalence of medical complications, reports of arrests, and data on admissions into treatment programs. In the United States most of the approximately 1 million individuals with chronic opioid dependence are not in treatment. Difficult-to-reach addicts are an intense focus for HIV and tuberculosis education programs and intervention.

Pathophysiological Mechanism

There are three major subtypes of opioid receptors: mu, sigma, and kappa. Opioids that bind at the mu receptor produce analgesia, altered mood (often euphoria), sedation, respiratory depression, reduced gastrointestinal motility, inhibition of certain spinal polysynaptic reflexes, cough suppression, suppression of corticotropin-releasing factor and adrenocorticotropic hormone, miosis, pruritis, and nausea and vomiting. Certain individuals may be prone to addiction because of a hypothesized hypoactivity of the endogenous opioid system. In one study of 3,372 male twin pairs, genetic factors were calculated to account for 38% of the variance in heroin abuse (Tsuang et al. 1998).

Comorbidity

Among people addicted to opiates, the prevalence of other psychiatric disorders is high (Frei and Rehm 2002; Rounsaville et al. 1982). However, it is often difficult to separate the symptoms of chronic intoxication and withdrawal from those of preexisting Axis I and II pathological conditions. During initial rehabilitation, symptoms of depression are not as likely to remit as they are in alcoholic patients. Rounsaville and Kleber (1985) found that opiate-dependent people who sought treatment in community programs were more often depressed than an untreated community sample and had poorer social functioning, increased nonspecific anxiety symptoms, and more drug-related legal problems. These factors probably facilitate crises that lead patients to treatment.

Contaminated needles and impure drugs can cause endocarditis, septicemia, pulmonary emboli, pulmonary hypertension, skin infections, hepatitis C and B, and HIV infection. Of persons injecting drugs for at least 5 years, 60%–80% are infected with hepatitis C (Centers for Disease Control and Prevention 2002). Intravenous drug use and sexual contact with those who use are major routes of transmission of HIV in the United States and elsewhere (see Chapter 28, "HIV/AIDS"). Chronic constipation is common in chronic opioid users and can cause recurrent abdominal pain simulating intestinal obstruction (Rogers and Cerda 1989).

Intoxication and Withdrawal

Physical signs of intoxication include pupillary constriction (so-called pinpoint pupils), decreased gastrointestinal motility, marked sedation, slurred speech, and impairment in attention and memory. Daily use of opioids for days to weeks, depending on the dosage and potency of the drug, can produce intensely uncomfortable but non-life-threatening withdrawal syndromes after cessation.

The onset of opioid withdrawal depends on the half-life of the opioid and the chronicity of use; symptoms begin approximately 8–10 hours after the last dose of short-acting opioids such as morphine and heroin. Opioid withdrawal presents as a flulike syndrome. The symptoms include anxiety, dysphoria, yawning, sweating, rhinorrhea, lacrimation, pupillary dilatation, piloerection (the origin of the term "cold turkey"), mild hypertension, tachycardia, disruption of sleep, hot and cold flashes, deep muscle and joint pain, nausea, vomiting, diarrhea, abdominal pain, weight loss, and fever. Subacute, protracted withdrawal symptoms can last for several weeks.

Urine toxicological screening should be performed whenever opioid abuse is suspected. In many hospital toxicological screens, synthetic opioids are not detected as part of the initial screen, so specific testing may be needed if this problem is suspected. Quinolone antibiotics can produce false positive opiate results (Baden et al. 2001).

An opioid overdose should be considered in any patient who presents in a coma, especially when respiratory depression, pupillary constriction, or needle marks are present. Naloxone (0.4 mg) should be given immediately, even without certainty that the coma is due to opioids, because this drug is harmless (except for the risk that excessive naloxone can precipitate severe withdrawal in opioid-dependent individuals). In cases in which it does appear that an opioid overdose is the cause of coma, administration of naloxone is repeated because the drug has a short duration of action. In overdose of long-acting opioids such as methadone, treatment in an intensive care unit and a naloxone intravenous drip may be instituted.

In pregnant women, methadone doses of more than 20 mg/day are associated with moderate to severe withdrawal in newborns (Ostrea and Welch 1991). However, in the care of pregnant women already receiving methadone treatment, opioid withdrawal is not recommended (Center for Substance Abuse Treatment 1993). In the United States the standard of care for the treatment of pregnant women found to be heroin addicted is methadone therapy. The outcome of infant withdrawal improves when mothers are supervised in methadone maintenance programs (Harris-Allen 1991) compared with when mothers are opiate addicted but are not in methadone maintenance programs.

Acute Management and Treatment

Two methods of treatment are available for actively using opioid-dependent individuals in a general hospital—detoxification and agonist maintenance. Detoxification is often needed for general hospital patients who are abusing street drugs such as heroin or prescription drugs such as oxycodone, meperidine, and codeine. Agonist maintenance is rarely initiated in the general hospital unless it is part of pain management; more often, the consulting psychiatrist is asked to advise on the continuation or modification of ongoing outpatient maintenance. When opioid dependence is questionable, the consultant can perform a naloxone challenge test by administering naloxone 0.4 mg intravenously. Abrupt onset or worsening of withdrawal symptoms strongly supports a diagnosis of opioid dependence.

Agonist Maintenance

Dole and Nyswander in 1965 first postulated that methadone would diminish drug-seeking behavior, increase personal productivity, and decrease illicit activities because wide fluctuations in opioid blood levels would cease. In "hard-core addicts" (i.e., opioid-addicted patients who have been using drugs two or more times per day for more than a year or who are continuously involved in drug street life), methadone therapy continues to contribute to improved health, decreased crime, increased employment, and decreased risk of HIV infection (Office of National Drug Control Policy 2001).

Methadone is relatively long acting with a half-life of 24–36 hours. The long half-life prevents extreme fluctuation in opioid blood levels. Methadone, at doses of approximately 80 mg daily, also blunts the euphoric response to heroin. Unlike heroin, which has a half-life of 8–12 hours, methadone is taken once daily, usually orally, but it can be given intramuscularly (in divided doses) or intravenously (one-third of oral maintenance dose). Once-daily administration provides a structure for rehabilitation and is superior to drug-free treatment of hard-core addicts (Sees et al. 2000). With ongoing participation in psychosocial therapies in addition to methadone maintenance, the goal of treatment is that the addicted person no longer engages in illegal activities to support a costly habit and is able to successfully obtain and keep gainful employment and attend to family and social responsibilities. Common side effects of methadone are sedation, mild euphoria, constipation, and reduced sweating.

A frequent mistake made by medical staff is to base an initial methadone dose solely on how a patient looks, how a patient says he or she feels, and vital signs. The Clinical Opiate Withdrawal Scale is a useful, standardized, clinician-administered rating scale that combines signs and symptoms for assessment of severity of withdrawal (Wesson and Ling 2003). Hospitalized patients receiving methadone maintenance should continue to receive methadone on the basis of their preadmission dose, which should be verified with the methadone clinic, unless methadone is medically contraindicated. An average maintenance dosage is 80 mg/day, but occasionally higher maintenance doses are given.

Several medications, including rifampin, phenobarbital, phenytoin, and carbamazepine (Gourevitch and Friedland 2000), efavirenz (McCance-Katz et al. 2002), and lopinavir/ritonavir (McCance-Katz et al. 2003), increase methadone metabolism, placing patients at risk of opiate withdrawal. Methadone also increases plasma desipramine concentration (Kosten et al. 1990). Methadone should not be combined with monoamine oxidase inhibitors. Methadone maintenance is possible in patients with liver disease until late stages of the disease. The dose should be reduced by at least one-half in patients with impaired hepatic function.

Buprenorphine, a long-acting mu opioid receptor partial agonist, was approved by the U.S. Food and Drug Administration in 2003 as a Schedule III narcotic for the treatment of opioid dependence. At lower doses buprenorphine functions as an opioid agonist, but at higher doses it has antagonist properties. This drug has shown promise in clinical trials for use in outpatient maintenance therapy for opioid dependence, with sublingual administration daily to three times a week, at an average dosage of 9 mg/day (Ling et al. 1998). However, the average clinical dosage is 16 mg/day and ranges from 8 to 32 mg/day. Clinical trials support the feasibility and effectiveness of having trained primary care physicians in private offices prescribe buprenorphine or buprenorphine/naloxone administered sublingually for the treatment of opioid dependence (Fudala et al. 2003). Prescribing physicians must apply for and receive a waiver from the Center for Substance Abuse Treatment. A physician can obtain the waiver by meeting one of the qualifications listed in the enabling legislation or by participating in an 8-hour training program. Buprenorphine/naloxone in a 4:1 ratio is the formulation to be used for maintenance therapy (e.g., 8/2 mg is 8 mg of buprenorphine and 2 mg of naloxone). The addition of naloxone prevents diversion of the drug to injected use by those who are opioid dependent. Because of the partial agonist properties of buprenorphine, opioid-dependent patients must show objective signs of opiate withdrawal before dosing. This requirement usually means that at least 6 hours have elapsed since the previous dose of opioid was self-administered. Induction is conducted over several hours on day 1, with patients receiving up to 4/1 mg initially and observation. The initial dose is followed by another 4/1 mg if opioid withdrawal symptoms persist after 2 hours for a total dose on day 1 not to exceed 8/2 mg. This dose can be increased to 16/4 mg if needed on day 2. Most patients need 16/4 mg daily (R.E. Johnson et al. 2003). The hope is that this approach will increase access to treatment not only for heroin addicts but also for persons addicted to prescription opioids, because the office setting is less stigmatizing and more anonymous than that of methadone clinics. The utility of buprenorphine for short-term detoxification in medical or psychiatric settings is receiving study in the National Drug Abuse Treatment Clinical Trials Network (see http://www.nida.nih.gov/CTN/brochures/pat_info_ctn_001.html). Buprenorphine is new, and many details of how to best use it require further investigation (Gowing et al. 2000).

Methadone Detoxification

Methadone detoxification is a viable option for patients who have good pretreatment functioning, have long-term success with a low dose of methadone, are less connected to "street culture," or are addicted to opioids other than heroin. Slow outpatient detoxification (i.e., decreasing by 10% per week until the daily dose is 10–20 mg and then decreasing by 3% per week) reduces relapse rates. Clonidine or buprenorphine can be substituted toward the end of methadone detoxification, when the methadone dose is 20 mg or less

Detoxification From Heroin and Other Opiates

For opioid-dependent patients hospitalized on a general medical unit who are not already taking methadone, 30–40 mg/day in divided doses over the first 24 hours is a reasonable methadone detoxification dosage. Agonist detoxification from heroin, morphine, meperidine, and weaker opioids (e.g., codeine and oxycodone) is generally accomplished by giving sufficient methadone to reduce withdrawal symptoms and then decreasing the dose by 20% each day over a 5- to 7-day period. Patients may need other medications for symptoms of opiate withdrawal, including diarrhea, muscle and stomach cramps, and insomnia (e.g., dicyclomine, ibuprofen, attapulgite [Kaopectate], and lorazepam).

Detoxification With Clonidine

Clonidine blocks the autonomic manifestations of opioid withdrawal. Results of several studies have confirmed the usefulness of clonidine for inpatient detoxification from opioids (Charney et al. 1981). A clinical trial in hospitalized heroin-dependent patients with HIV infection showed clonidine to be as effective as methadone or buprenorphine. Results have been less impressive in outpatient trials (Kleber et al. 1985, McCann et al. 1997). In clinical trials in which the subjects were outpatients, clonidine was inferior to buprenorphine (Fingerhood et al. 2001;

Gowing et al. 2000; O'Connor et al. 1997). Although it suppresses autonomic signs of withdrawal, clonidine is less effective in relieving subjective discomfort (Jasinski et al. 1985). Clonidine may be administered orally, transdermally (via the Catapres TTS-1, -2, or -3 patch), or in combination. The advantage of the patch is once-a-week application, which is usually adequate. The patch is more difficult to use in the care of elderly patients because it can cause orthostasis. In addition, the patch can have adverse interactions with other drugs and may not be effective in cases of severe dependence. Sedation and hypotension are common side effects and limit the dose of clonidine. Although clonidine is widely used, U.S. Food and Drug Administration has not approved if for the management opioid detoxification. As with agonist detoxification, patients detoxified with clonidine may need adjunctive medications for reduction of auxiliary withdrawal symptoms.

Detoxification With Clonidine and Naltrexone

A combination of clonidine and low-dose naltrexone can be used for opiate detoxification. Detoxification with this combination is more effective than detoxification with clonidine alone (O'Connor et al. 1997). The combination may shorten the withdrawal period to 3 or 4 days, clonidine diminishing the naltrexone-associated withdrawal. Higher doses of clonidine often are necessary for successful use of this combination in outpatients (Stine and Kosten 1992).

Opiate Addiction and Pain

The general principles of evaluation and treatment of pain in opioid-dependent individuals are similar to those for other patients with pain and are reviewed in Chapter 36 ("Pain"). However, treatment complexities can arise when opioid-addicted patients develop acute or chronic pain syndromes. The consultant must ensure that adequate pain medications are prescribed and that as-needed medication schedules are avoided. Opioid-dependent patients need higher doses of narcotics for acute pain control as a result of tolerance. When given only standard doses, addicted patients legitimately state they need more narcotic, but the staff may misinterpret this request as drug seeking. On the other hand, some opioid-dependent patients are inappropriately demanding and truly drug seeking. Explicit expectations and behavioral limits must be established early and ideally by means of a written contract with the patient. When they are used for analgesia, such as for postoperative pain, opioids should be tapered at the same percentage rate in both non-opioid-dependent and opioid-dependent patients.

Cocaine-Related Disorders

DSM-IV-TR describes both *cocaine use disorders* (cocaine dependence and cocaine abuse) and *cocaine-induced disorders* (cocaine intoxication, cocaine withdrawal, cocaine intoxication delirium, cocaine-induced sexual dysfunction, cocaine-induced psychotic, mood, anxiety, and sleep disorders).

Epidemiological Characteristics

An estimated 193,034 U.S. emergency department visits solely for cocaine use were documented in the 2001 Drug Abuse Warning Network (Office of Applied Studies 2003), and cocaine is the most frequently reported drug in emergency department visits. Frequent reasons for psychiatric consultation in the medical setting are cocaine overdose, positive results of a urine toxicological screen, cocaine-induced depression, cocaine-induced cardiac problems, and cocaine-induced psychosis. According to the 1998 National Household Survey on Drug Abuse, 1.8 million individuals in the United States had used cocaine during a 1-month period (Office of Applied Studies 1999). Use of crack cocaine is especially high in poor urban areas (Rees Davis et al. 2003), but its use is widespread among other populations, such as rural migrant workers. Many cocaine users are polysubstance abusers (Community Epidemiology Working Group 2001).

Pharmacological Characteristics

Cocaine hydrochloride is a white crystalline powder derived from the coca plant. It is usually diluted to 20% purity by mixing with other local anesthetics, such as lidocaine or procaine, or various sugars. Freebase cocaine is prepared from the hydrochloride salt by alkalinization and extraction with organic solvents. Crack or rock cocaine is a prepackaged freebase form of cocaine that is ready for smoking. "Freebasing" is smoking freebase cocaine; intense euphoria begins within seconds. Because freebased cocaine is absorbed directly from the lungs, it goes immediately to the brain, bypassing the liver. Euphoric effects depend on blood levels and on the slope to peak concentration. Most cocaine is hydrolyzed in the body to benzoylecgonine, which is detectable in the urine up to 36 hours after use. High doses are detectable for up to 3 weeks. Rapid tolerance develops to the euphoric effects of cocaine. Cocaine and alcohol may combine to make a toxic metabolite called *cocaethylene*, which is potentially quite cardiotoxic (McCance-Katz et al. 1995, 1998).

Pathophysiological Mechanism

Cocaine blocks reuptake of neuronal dopamine, serotonin, and norepinephrine. With repeated cocaine use, tolerance develops rapidly as a result of decreased reuptake inhibition and release of catecholamines and altered receptor sensitivity. Hypotheses to explain the severe craving associated with cocaine dependence have included cortical kindling (Halikas et al. 1991), altered opioid receptor binding (Zubieta et al. 1996), altered dopaminergic or serotonergic function (Satel et al. 1995), and hedonistic deregulation (Koob et al. 1997). Neuropsychological deficits and cortical tissue loss (measured by magnetic resonance imaging) are reported (Franklin et al. 2002; Gottschalk et al. 2001). Functional neuroimaging is focusing on dysfunction of dopaminergic systems in the orbitofrontal and memory circuits (Goldstein and Volkow 2002, Volkow et al. 2002), and genetic risk factors may also be important in determining cocaine abuse (Kendler et al. 2003a, 2003b).

Intoxication

Intoxication is characterized by euphoria, hyperalertness, grandiosity, and impaired judgment. Individuals are more gregarious or withdrawn; may have increased anxiety, restlessness, and vigilance; and exhibit stereotypical behavior. Maladaptive behavior includes fighting, psychomotor agitation, and impaired social or occupational functioning.

Cocaine binges can last for a few hours to several days. Tolerance to the euphoric effects develops during the course of a binge. Physical signs of use include tachycardia, pupillary dilation, increased blood pressure, perspiration, chills, nausea and vomiting, and visual and tactile hallucinations. Paranoia occurs with high doses and chronic or binge use of cocaine and is usually of brief duration. In one study, experienced cocaine users given intravenous cocaine became uniformly paranoid (Sherer et al. 1988). These symptoms usually remit, but heavy, prolonged use or a preexisting psychopathological disorder may result in persistent psychosis. Bizarre obsessive and ritualistic behaviors, such as skin picking, are reported.

Withdrawal or Abstinence

Medically uncomplicated withdrawal occurs with cessation of or decreases in cocaine use after regular, high doses.

Medical and Other Complications

Cocaine use is associated with acute and chronic medical ailments (e.g., chronic intranasal use leads to septal necrosis). Anesthetic properties of cocaine can lead to oral numbness and dental neglect. Cocaine binges can cause malnutrition, severe weight loss, and dehydration. Intravenous cocaine use, because of contaminants, can result in endocarditis, septicemia, HIV infection, local vasculitis, hepatitis B and C, emphysema, pulmonary emboli, and granuloma. Freebasing of cocaine is associated with decreased pulmonary gas exchange, and pulmonary dysfunction can persist (Itkomen et al. 1984).

In New York City, one of every five individuals who committed suicide during a 1-year period used cocaine immediately before his or her death (Marzuk et al. 1992). Congenital deficiency of pseudocholinesterase slows metabolism of cocaine, and the slowed metabolism can result in toxic levels, sudden delirium, and hyperthermia. Cocaine can cause acute agitation, diaphoresis, tachycardia, metabolic and respiratory acidosis, cardiac dysrhythmia, grand mal seizures, and, ultimately, respiratory arrest. Cardiac complications include acute chest pain, myocardial infarction, congestive heart failure, arrhythmias, endocarditis, aortic dissection, and cardiomyopathy. Approximately 25% of cases of myocardial infarction in adults younger than 45 years are attributable to cocaine (Qureshi et al. 2001). Cardiac disease has been found commonly (38%), even in young asymptomatic chronic cocaine users (Roldan et al. 2001). Cocaine is associated with increased risk of hemorrhagic and ischemic stroke (Pettiti et al. 1998) as well as acute rhabdomyolysis (Ruttenber et al. 1999). Neuropsychological deficits may persist after 1 year of abstinence (Toomey et al. 2003). Death from cocaine toxicity is not linearly correlated with dose, and deaths have occurred among recreational, low-dose users. Pregnant women who use cocaine are at increased risk of abruptio placentae. A "crack baby" syndrome including both physical and psychological abnormalities was widely described in offspring of mothers who used cocaine during pregnancy (Eyler et al. 1998a, 1998b). However, authors of a systematic literature review concluded that "there is no convincing evidence that prenatal cocaine exposure is associated with developmental toxic effects that are different in severity, scope, or kind from the sequelae of multiple other risk factors…, including prenatal exposure to tobacco, marijuana, or alcohol, and the quality of the child's environment" (Frank et al. 2001, p. 1614).

Acute Management and Referral

Agitation and anxiety associated with cocaine intoxication are treated with benzodiazepines. Beta-blockers are contraindicated for this purpose because they cause unopposed alpha-adrenergic stimulation. Dihydropyridine-class calcium channel antagonists have been proposed for the treatment of cocaine-induced stroke (Johnson et al. 2001). Patients with cocaine-associated chest pain who do not have acute cardiac complications after 9–12 hours may require only a brief observation period in the hospital (Weber et al. 2003). Haloperidol is usually effective in the treatment of cocaine-associated psychosis. Withdrawal depression generally does not necessitate use of antidepressant medication. McCance (1997) noted that although more than 30 medications have undergone clinical trials, no medication has shown consistent efficacy in the treatment of cocaine dependence or in the reduction of craving for the drug. Medications investigated include tricyclic antidepressants, selective serotonin reuptake inhibitors, anticonvulsants, dopamine agonists and antagonists, and miscellaneous agents such as bupropion, naltrexone, methylphenidate, and tyrosine. Baclofen, a GABAergic agent, has shown promise as a treatment for cocaine dependence and is undergoing clinical trials (Shoptaw et al. 2003). When a comorbid psychiatric disorder, such as major depression, bipolar disorder, or schizophrenia, is present, optimal concurrent treatment of that disorder is essential to rehabilitation of cocaine users.

Treatment Outcome

Treatment outcome is affected by severity of psychosocial problems, family support, intensity of withdrawal, and degree of antisocial features in addition to initial motivation for treatment. In a randomized multicenter trial Crits-Christoph et al. (1999) compared four manual-guided psychotherapeutic treatments of cocaine dependence. Individual drug counseling combined with group drug counseling proved more effective in reducing cocaine use than cognitive psychotherapy, supportive-expressive psychotherapy, or group drug counseling alone. Positive and community reinforcement therapy with vouchers is also promising (Higgins et al. 2003). Not surprisingly, relapse rates after treatment are lowest among patients with the fewest psychosocial problems (Simpson et al. 1999). People who abuse cocaine must avoid alcohol and other mood-altering drugs, which disinhibit behavior and lead to relapse. This concept is difficult for cocaine-dependent individuals to accept, because they merely want to quit cocaine use. Treatment of clearly defined attention-deficit/hyperactivity disorder (Levin et al. 1998) should proceed in concert with treatment of cocaine dependence, but methylphenidate has not been proved to have any effect on cocaine use itself (Schubiner et al. 2002), and stimulants carry their own risk of abuse.

Amphetamine-Related Disorders

Amphetamines (speed) have stimulant and reinforcing properties similar to those of cocaine. Amphetamines cause catecholamine release, especially of dopamine. The signs and symptoms of amphetamine intoxication include tachycardia, increased blood pressure, pupillary dilatation, agitation, elation, loquacity, and hypervigilance. In contrast to cocaine, amphetamines rarely cause myocardial infarction (Costa et al. 2001). Amphetamine psychosis can resemble acute paranoid schizophrenia. Visual hallucinations are common. Binge episodes ("runs"), which are similar to those experienced with cocaine use, often alternate with symptoms of a severe crash. Polysubstance use is common.

CNS stimulants, such as dextroamphetamine and methylphenidate, are prescribed for the treatment of narcolepsy, attention-deficit/hyperactivity disorder, and fatigue in multiple sclerosis, but the doses used infrequently cause adverse effects such as insomnia, irritability, confusion, and hostility. Amphetamine abuse can start in an attempt to lose weight or to enhance energy.

Epidemiological Characteristics and Complications

Abuse of methamphetamine ("ice") is a particular problem in the midwestern, western, and southwestern United States but has been spreading into other parts of the country (Community Epidemiology Working Group 2001)—2.1% of the population has tried methamphetamine at least once. Among the so-called club drugs, methamphetamine abuse accounted for the largest share of reported emergency visits 15,000 in the United States in 2001 (Ball and Kissin 2002, 2003). Methamphetamine can be readily manufactured ("cooked") in small kitchen or bathroom "labs," and the process can result in explosions, fires, and exposure of household residents to toxic chemicals. The effects include increases in blood pressure, body temperature, activity, alertness, and risky sexual behaviors (Frosch et al. 1996). Toxicity can include stroke, seizures, arrhythmias, coma, and death. Methamphetamine has a relatively long half-life, and chronic methamphetamine users can exhibit prolonged psychosis. Evidence suggests the presence of long-term neurotoxicity in methamphetamine abusers after they become abstinent (Ernst et al. 2000). Withdrawal can produce a "crash" similar to cocaine withdrawal and accompanied by depression and anergia. Intravenous amphetamine abuse can present with the same complications as those of intravenous use of other illicit substances.

Acute Management

Treatment of individuals who abuse amphetamines is similar to that of cocaine users. However, the effects of amphetamine may last longer. The consultant may be asked to assist with management of psychosis, aggressive behavior, or withdrawal depression and suicidality. Acidification of urine speeds elimination. Antipsychotic medications should be used to treat paranoid or delusional symptoms, which can continue for days to weeks after the drug is no longer present in the urine. Rehabilitation requires a comprehensive treatment approach, as described for other substances earlier (see section "General Principles" earlier in this chapter).

Phencyclidine-Related Disorders

Phencyclidine (PCP) is an anesthetic agent that first appeared as a street drug in the 1960s; PCP abuse peaked between 1978 and 1980. In 2002, 3.2% of the population 12 years or older had used PCP at least once and 1.1% of high school seniors had used PCP within the past year (Johnston et al. 2004). Current street samples sold as PCP vary greatly in purity. Smoking marijuana cigarettes laced with PCP is the most common form of administration. PCP is a noncompetitive NMDA/glutamate receptor antagonist and has effects on serotonergic and dopaminergic systems as well (Jentsch and Roth 1999; Nabeshima et al. 1996).

Medical and Other Complications

The psychoactive effects of PCP generally begin within 5 minutes and plateau 30 minutes after use. Volatile emotionality is the predominant behavioral presentation. PCP clinical effects are unpredictable, and people who repeatedly seek these experiences may have an underlying psychiatric disorder. Affects range from intense euphoria to anxiety, and behavior can include stereotypical repetitive activities and bizarre aggression. Distorted perceptions, numbness, and confusion are also common. Associated physical signs include hypertension, muscle rigidity, ataxia, and nystagmus (particularly vertical nystagmus). At higher doses, dilated pupils, hypersalivation, hyperthermia, involuntary movements, and coma can occur (Davis 1982; Deutsch et al. 1998).

Acute Management

Acute reactions generally require pharmacological intervention. Intravenous diazepam is the drug of first choice; antipsychotics are occasionally necessary. Because supportive treatment may also be needed, management in a medical setting is preferred. After ingestion of PCP, the urine test result may be positive for 7 days; false-negative results can occur. PCP elimination is initially enhanced by ammonium chloride and subsequently by ascorbic acid or cranberry juice (Aronow et al. 1980).

Club Drugs and Hallucinogens

The term *club drugs* comes from the association of several drugs with use in dance clubs or all night dance parties ("raves"). Popular club drugs are methamphetamine (see earlier section, "Amphetamine-Related Disorders"), lysergic acid diethylamide (LSD; "acid"), 3,4-methylenedioxymethamphetamine (MDMA; "Ecstasy" or "X"), gamma-hydroxybutyrate (GHB; "liquid X"), ketamine ("special K"), Rohypnol ("roofies"), and dextromethorphan ("DMX") (Bialer 2002). Emergency department visits due to MDMA and GHB use increased dramatically starting in the late 1990s. In the United States in 2002, emergency department visits for MDMA-related disorders numbered 4,026 and for GHB-related disorders numbered 3,330 (Ball and Kissin 2002). Hallucinogenic drugs include LSD, mescaline, psilocybin, and synthetic derivatives such as 3,4-methylenedioxyamphetamine (MDA). The popularity of hallucinogens began to wane in the mid-1970s, but a modest resurgence in use occurred in the early 1990s, particularly among youth.

MDMA ("Ecstasy")

MDMA, called "Ecstasy," was promoted in the 1960s and 1970s as a "mood drug" without the distracting perceptual changes of other hallucinogens (Grinspoon and Bakalar 1986). MDMA is usually taken orally but can be taken intranasally (snorted). The purity of the drug in tablets or pills can vary dramatically, and it is often "cut" with numerous stimulants. Desired effects include feelings of empathy, connectedness, extroversion, euphoria, and self-confidence. MDMA is thought to cause increased release of serotonin as well as serotonin reuptake inhibition. Serotonin neurotoxicity and parkinsonian syndromes have occurred in association with MDMA use, and neuropsychological deficits may persist; however, the actual relationship to drug use is hotly debated (Daumann et al. 2003; Halpern and Pope 1999; Reneman et al. 2001; Ricaurte et al. 2002; Rickert et al. 1999; Simon and Mattick 2002). MDMA use has been associated with derealization, depersonalization, and racing thoughts. Serious medical complications have included hyperthermia, seizures, cardiac arrhythmias, myocardial infarction, hyponatremia, fulminant liver failure (necessitating transplantation in several cases), and death (Burgess et al. 2000; Caballero et al. 2002; Kunitz et al. 2003; Qasim et al. 2001; Schifano et al. 2003; Shannon 2000; Vollenweider et al. 2002).

GHB

GHB is a CNS depressant that is increasingly being used for recreational purposes. As recently as 1990, GHB was sold in health food stores as an antianxiety agent. On the street GHB is usually sold as a liquid. GHB users describe pleasurable effects similar to those of alcohol, and the adverse CNS effects of GHB are also similar to those of alcohol. After recognition of the toxicity of GHB, the U.S. government restricted access to this agent; however, this prohibition was followed by the appearance of 1,4-butanediol and gamma-butyrolactone, industrial solvents that are precursors of GHB. These substances began to be marketed as dietary supplements and have been taken recreationally, to enhance bodybuilding, and to treat depression or insomnia (Zvosec et al. 2001). Serious cases of toxicity with GHB and these two precursor solvents have included vomiting, incontinence, agitation, fluctuating consciousness, respiratory depression, and death (Zvosec et al. 2001). Regular daily GHB use can produce tolerance, physiological dependence, and addiction. The signs and symptoms of GHB withdrawal are similar to those of alcohol and benzodiazepine withdrawal (Dyer et al. 2001; Rosenberg et al. 2003). Treatment of GHB withdrawal and delirium is approached similarly to that of alcohol withdrawal with supportive care and high-dose sedatives (McDaniel et al. 2001).

Ketamine

Ketamine hydrochloride was originally used as a human and animal anesthetic but recently has become part of the rave scene. Much of the ketamine sold on the street is diverted from veterinarians' offices. Ketamine is odorless and flavorless, so it can be added to beverages without detection. The drug also is a potent NMDA antagonist (Haas and Harper 1992). Ketamine produces dissociative feelings and sedation, immobility, amnesia, increase in body temperature, and analgesia (Dillon et al. 2003; Freese et al. 2002). Ketamine can be taken orally, smoked, snorted, or injected but generally is snorted or swallowed. Most of the effects of ketamine are dose-related. When taken at higher doses, ketamine can cause vomiting, amnesia, slurred speech, incoordination, agitation, delirium, and out-of-body experiences. Ketamine flashbacks, similar to flashbacks with hallucinogens, are common. Treatment is supportive.

LSD and Other Hallucinogens

LSD is derived from ergot, a fungus, and is a potent mood-altering drug. Studies in the United States have shown a 5.9% annual prevalence of use by 12th graders

(Johnston et al. 2004), and 13% of women ages 14–26 years (Rickert et al. 2003) report ever having used LSD. LSD is sold on the street in capsules, tablets, and occasionally in liquid form.

LSD induces intense changes in perception of time, space, and body image. Physical signs of intoxication include tachycardia, dilatation of pupils, and sweating. An individual's response to LSD, mescaline, and related drugs varies greatly with the user's expectations and the circumstances of use. Individuals having "bad trips" can present with severe anxiety or paranoia. The chance of a bad trip is increased by emotional distress before use, reluctant use, or an aversive setting. Flashbacks, usually visual, occasionally occur after cessation of hallucinogenic drug use.

Management

Hallucinogen-intoxicated patients should be placed in a quiet setting with minimal stimuli. Spoken to in a soft, calm voice, the individual is then "talked down" from frightening experiences. Diazepam sometimes is needed as an adjunct. Antipsychotics are rarely necessary. In studies involving small numbers of patients, clonidine, naltrexone, and sertraline have been used successfully to treat flashbacks (Lerner et al. 1998, 2000), but risperidone reportedly worsens symptoms (Morehead 1997).

Cannabis-Related Disorders

The main psychoactive constituent in marijuana is delta-9-tetrahydrocannabinol (Δ^9-THC), one of 60 cannabinoids. Marijuana sold on the street contains 5%–17% Δ^9-THC (Drug Enforcement Administration 2001). Hashish is a resin from the cannabis plant that contains a higher percentage of Δ^9-THC than does marijuana. Δ^9-THC binds to cannabinoid receptors, located primarily in hippocampal and striatal regions. An endogenous ligand for these receptors, anandamide, has been identified (Ameri 1999). Results of several studies suggested that there is a genetic vulnerability to cannabis use and dependence (Kendler et al. 2002; Merikangas et al. 1998b; Tsuang et al. 1998). Medical use of marijuana is still a hotly debated scientific and political issue (Watson et al. 2000).

Laboratory Findings

Cannabinoids can be detected in the urine of chronic abusers 21 days or more after cessation of chronic, heavy use, because of slow release from fat stores. In most occasional users, urine drug screen results remain positive for 1–5 days (Schwartz and Hawks 1985).

Intoxication

Peak intoxication after smoking cannabis generally occurs in 10–30 minutes. Intoxication usually lasts 2–4 hours, depending on the dose; however, behavioral and psychomotor impairment may continue several hours longer. Δ^9-THC and its metabolites, which are highly liquid soluble, tend to accumulate in fat cells. This phenomenon extends the half-life to approximately 50 hours. Personality, past experience with the drug, and setting can alter the experience dramatically, although higher doses of Δ^9-THC increase the chances of a toxic reaction. Users experience slowed sense of time, increased appetite and thirst, and a keener sense in all modes of perception. They also experience euphoria, heightened introspection, absorbing sensual experiences, feelings of relaxation and floating, and increased self-confidence. Psychosis, derealization, and aggression occur rarely. Conjunctivitis, a strong odor of cannabis, dilated pupils, tachycardia, dry mouth, and coughing are physical signs of recent use.

Withdrawal

In chronic high-dose users, reported withdrawal symptoms from cannabis include anxiety, irritability, insomnia, anorexia, and myalgia, but no stereotypic syndrome has been described (Haney et al. 1999).

Long-Term Use

Controversy surrounds the existence of an "amotivational syndrome" associated with chronic cannabis use. This syndrome is characterized by passivity, decreased drive, diminished goal-directed activity, fatigue, and apathy. Research into this amotivational syndrome is plagued by methodological problems, including selection bias and lack of control subjects. Long-term marijuana users may have residual cognitive deficits (Pope et al. 2001; Solowij et al. 2002) and other comorbid psychiatric symptoms (Troisi et al. 1998). There is little evidence that cannabis causes chronic psychosis in individuals who do not have symptoms (Gruber and Pope 1994).

Δ^9-THC is used in some medical settings to control severe nausea and vomiting, mainly in association with AIDS, cancer chemotherapy, and bone marrow transplantation. Δ^9-THC is no longer an approved treatment of glaucoma, because more effective treatments are available. Other medical use remains highly controversial (Joy et al. 1999). A report by the Institute of Medicine comprehensively evaluated the scientific evidence for benefits and risks of using marijuana as a medicine (Watson et al. 2000).

Acute Management

Marijuana intoxication does not usually require professional attention. Anxiolytic agents are occasionally needed, and neuroleptics are used in rare cases of protracted paranoia. Patients with cardiovascular disease may not tolerate the increased heart rate and blood pressure that are caused by marijuana.

Long-Term Management

Treatment of people who abuse marijuana follows the general principles established for other substances, but special attention is paid to developmental issues in adolescent abusers. Adolescent drug programs typically focus on promoting age-appropriate behavior and communication skills.

Nicotine-Related Disorders

Tobacco addiction is the most preventable health problem in the United States. In 1993, approximately 60 million Americans smoked tobacco, and 400,000 deaths and $50 billion in direct medical-care expenditures were attributable to tobacco (Medical-Care Expenditures Attributable to Cigarette Smoking 1994). In the United States, approximately 30% of men and 26% of women smoke cigarettes. The percentage of young adults smoking cigarettes significantly increased between 1994 (35%) and 1998 (42%) (Office of Applied Studies 1999). Since 1965, the prevalence of cigarette smoking among adults in the United States has declined almost half. Cigarette smoking prevalence declined in the late 1970s, leveled off in the 1980s, and increased in the 1990s (Giovino 2002). Similar trends have occurred in other Western countries, but the prevalence of smoking has been increasing in Asia.

Nicotine is a psychoactive substance with euphoric and positive reinforcement properties, similar to those of cocaine and opiates (Benowitz 1988; Henningfield 1984). The individual develops tolerance to nicotine and experiences significant withdrawal symptoms, including craving for tobacco, irritability, anxiety, difficulty concentrating, restlessness, decreased heart rate, increased eating with a weight gain of 5–10 pounds (2.3–4.5 kg), and sleep disturbance. Subjects with higher nicotine tolerance have more withdrawal discomfort. Because most general hospitals are smoke-free, nicotine withdrawal should be considered in the differential diagnosis of any anxious or dysphoric inpatient.

Predisposition or Risk Factors and Comorbidity

Cigarette smokers generally begin smoking as teenagers, because of peer tobacco use, parental tobacco use, and symptoms of anxiety, depression, or conduct disorder. A strong association exists between smoking and other drug abuse, especially alcohol abuse. However, alcoholic patients stop smoking at the same rate as do nonalcoholic patients.

Genetic factors play a major role in the initiation of smoking and the transition to nicotine dependence (Sullivan and Kendler 1999). There is a well-established relationship between nicotine dependence and major depressive disorder. For example, Kendler et al. (1993) found a strong association between average lifetime daily cigarette smoking and lifetime prevalence of depression. Nicotine withdrawal is typically more severe in persons with histories of major depression or anxiety disorders. Patients with histories of major depressive disorder are prone to recurrence of depression after smoking cessation (Covey et al. 1997) and should therefore be more closely monitored.

Effects

The adverse health effects of both active and passive smoking, as well as intrauterine exposure, are well-known and documented extensively in the literature. Tobacco use can produce a calming, euphoric effect in chronic users. This effect is more pronounced after a period of tobacco deprivation. Symptoms of acute nicotine poisoning include nausea, salivation, abdominal pain, vomiting and diarrhea, headaches, dizziness, and sweating. Inability to concentrate, confusion, and tachycardia also can occur (Hughes and Hatsukami 1986).

Tobacco smoke also contains polycyclic hydrocarbons that alter hepatic metabolism of many drugs (Carrillo et al. 1996; Hughes 1993). Patients who resume smoking after prolonged stays in smoke-free hospitals may experience clinically significant alterations in therapeutic blood levels of prescribed medications (Zevin and Benowitz 1999).

Management

The success rate with every attempt to stop smoking is 5%, and 50% of individuals eventually stop. Behavioral, cognitive, educational, self-help, and pharmacological approaches are all used to treat nicotine dependence (American Psychiatric Association 1996). Cognitive-behavioral treatments may be particularly suitable for patients with histories of depression (Hall et al. 1998). However, 95% of individuals who stop smoking receive no formal intervention; research is needed to clarify how and why these individuals discontinue use. Fear of weight gain frequently delays smoking cessation. Cognitive-behavioral strategies, pharmacological strategies, or exercise regimens are sometimes used to treat weight gain associated with cessation.

Nicotine replacement therapy should be considered for medically ill hospitalized patients with heavy nicotine addiction, because 50% experience marked withdrawal. Most general hospitals have antismoking rules, but it is unfortunate that few have adequate smoking cessation programs. Nicotine replacement is available in a number of forms, including gum, transdermal patch, intranasal spray, and inhaler.

Bupropion improves abstinence rates independently of its antidepressant effect (Hayford et al. 1999). Jorenby et al. (1999) found that combining bupropion with the transdermal patch further improves abstinence rates while reducing weight gain. The efficacy of bupropion is modest, and probably not unique, although not all antidepressants provide benefit in smoking cessation. Earlier smaller controlled trials showed beneficial effects of nortriptyline, doxepin, and cognitive behavioral therapy. The results of large controlled trials of fluoxetine and sertraline were never published. In a multiple-arm clinical trial Hall et al. (2002) found nortriptyline, bupropion, and psychological intervention each produced better abstinence rates than simple medical management, but all three had limited efficacy in producing sustained abstinence.

Inhalant-Related Disorders

Inhalants are a diverse group of chemicals and include gasoline, airplane glue, aerosols (e.g., spray paint), lighter fluid, fingernail polish remover, typewriter correction fluid, a variety of solvents, amyl and butyl nitrites, and nitrous oxide. Inhalant use has been increasing among both male and female adolescents (Neumark et al. 1998). A high rate of abuse has also been found among Native Americans (Reed and May 1984). Nitrous oxide abuse occurs among medical and dental personnel. Inhalants are inexpensive and easily obtained. Fumes of glues and paint products are usually inhaled from bags or rags.

Intoxication

Typical signs and symptoms of inhalant intoxication include grandiosity, a sense of invulnerability and immense strength, euphoria, slurred speech, and ataxia. Visual distortions and faulty space perception are also common. Inhalant intoxication is associated with aggressive, disruptive, and antisocial behavior. Among adolescents, inhalant abuse is associated with arrests, poor school performance, increased family disruption, and other drug abuse (Santos de Barona and Simpson 1984).

Intoxication can last from a few minutes to as long as 2 hours. Impaired judgment, poor insight, violence, and psychosis are common sequelae (Cohen 1984). Paint stains around the face are a clear indication of inhalant abuse. Central respiratory depression, cardiac arrhythmia, and accidents can cause death, and long-term damage to bone marrow, kidneys, liver, muscles, and the nervous system has been reported (Brouette and Anton 2001; Espeland 1995). The lifetime course of an inhalant abuser is not clear. Reports suggest that inhalants are primarily abused by youths. Inhalant abusers are likely to move on to other substances in later life.

References

Aalto M, Saksanen R, Laine P, et al: Brief intervention for female heavy drinkers in routine general practice: a 3-year randomized, controlled study. Alcohol Clin Exp Res 24:1680–1686, 2000

Adams RD, Victor M, Ropper AH: Principles of Neurology, 6th Edition. New York, McGraw-Hill, 1997

Addolorato G, Ancona C, Capristo E, et al: Metadoxine in the treatment of acute and chronic alcoholism: a review. Int J Immunopathol Pharmacol 16:207–214, 2003

Alldredge BK, Gelb AM, Isaacs SM, et al: A comparison of lorazepam, diazepam, and placebo for the treatment of out-of-hospital status epilepticus. N Engl J Med 345:631–637, 2001

Allen JP, Sillamaukee P, Anton R: Contribution of carbohydrate deficient transferrin to gamma glutamyl transpeptidase in evaluating progress of patients in treatment for alcoholism. Alcohol Clin Exp Res 23:115–120, 1999

Allen JP, Litten RZ, Fertig JB, et al: Carbohydrate-deficient transferrin: an aid to early recognition of alcohol relapse. Am J Addict 10 (suppl):24–28, 2001

Allgulander C, Ljungberg L, Fisher LD: Long-term prognosis in addiction on sedative and hypnotic drugs analyzed with the Cox regression model. Acta Psychiatr Scand 75:521–531, 1987

Ameri A: The effects of cannabinoids on the brain. Prog Neurobiol 58:315–348, 1999

American Psychiatric Association: Diagnostic and Statistical Manual: Mental Disorders. Washington, DC, American Psychiatric Association, 1952

American Psychiatric Association: Diagnostic and Statistical Manual of Mental Disorders, 2nd Edition. Washington, DC, American Psychiatric Association, 1968

American Psychiatric Association: Diagnostic and Statistical Manual of Mental Disorders, 3rd Edition. Washington, DC, American Psychiatric Association, 1980

American Psychiatric Association: Diagnostic and Statistical Manual of Mental Disorders, 3rd Edition, Revised. Washington, DC, American Psychiatric Association, 1987

American Psychiatric Association: Diagnostic and Statistical Manual of Mental Disorders, 4th Edition. Washington, DC, American Psychiatric Association, 1994

American Psychiatric Association: Practice guideline for psychiatric evaluation of adults. Am J Psychiatry 152:63–80, 1995a

American Psychiatric Association: Practice guideline for the treatment of patients with substance use disorders: alcohol, cocaine, opioids. Am J Psychiatry 152:1–59, 1995b

American Psychiatric Association: Practice guideline for the treatment of patients with nicotine dependence. Am J Psychiatry 153:1–31, 1996

American Psychiatric Association: Diagnostic and Statistical Manual of Mental Disorders, 4th Edition, Text Revision. Washington, DC, American Psychiatric Association, 2000

Anglin D, Spears KL, Hutson HR: Flunitrazepam and its involvement in date or acquaintance rape. Acad Emerg Med 4:323–326, 1997

Anton RF, Stout RL, Roberts JS, et al: The effect of drinking intensity and frequency on serum carbohydrate-deficient transferrin and gamma-glutamyl transferase levels in outpatient alcoholics. Alcohol Clin Exp Res 22:1456–1462, 1998

Aronow R, Miceli JN, Done AK: A therapeutic approach to the acutely overdosed PCP patient. J Psychedelic Drugs 12:259–267, 1980

Ashman TA, Schwartz ME, Cantor JB, et al: Screening for substance abuse in individuals with traumatic brain injury. Brain Inj 18:191–202, 2004

Baden LR, Horowitz G, Jacoby H, et al: Quinolones and false-positive urine screening for opiates by immunoassay technology. JAMA 286:3115–3119, 2001

Baer JS, Sampson PD, Barr HM, et al: A 21-year longitudinal analysis of the effects of prenatal alcohol exposure on young adult drinking. Arch Gen Psychiatry 60:377–385, 2003

Ball J, Kissin W: The DAWN Report: Major Drugs of Abuse in ED Visits, 2001 update. Rockville, MD, Substance Abuse and Mental Health Services Administration, 2002

Ball J, Kissin W: The DAWN Report: Trends in Drug-Related Emergency Department Visits, 1994–2001 at a glance. Rockville, MD, Substance Abuse and Mental Health Services Administration, 2003

Barnes HN, Samet JH: Brief interventions with substance-abusing patients. Med Clin North Am 81:867–879, 1997

Basile AS, Hughes RD, Harrison PM, et al: Elevated brain concentrations of 1,4-benzodiazepines in fulminant hepatic failure. N Engl J Med 325:473–478, 1991

Begleiter H, Porjesz B: Persistence of a subacute withdrawal syndrome following chronic ethanol intake. Drug Alcohol Depend 4:353–357, 1979

Beich A, Thorsen T, Rollnick S: Screening in brief intervention trials targeting excessive drinkers in general practice: systematic review and meta-analysis. BMJ 327:536–542, 2003

Benowitz NL: Drug therapy: pharmacologic aspects of cigarette smoking and nicotine addiction. N Engl J Med 319:1318–1330, 1988

Benzer D: Quantification of the alcohol withdrawal syndrome in 487 alcoholic patients. J Subst Abuse Treat 7:117–123, 1990

Bernstein L, Jacobsberg L, Ashman T, et al: Detection of alcoholism among burn patients. Hosp Community Psychiatry 43:255–256, 1992

Bhattacharya R, Shuhart MC: Hepatitis C and alcohol: interactions, outcomes, and implications. J Clin Gastroenterol 36:242–252, 2003

Bialer PA: Designer drugs in the general hospital. Psychiatr Clin North Am. 25:231–243, 2002

Blondell RD, Dodds HN, Blondell MN, et al: Ethanol in formularies of US teaching hospitals. JAMA 289:552, 2003

Bradley KA, Boyd-Wickizer J, Powell SH, et al: Alcohol screening questionnaires in women: a critical review. JAMA 280:166–171, 1998

Brew BJ: Diagnosis of Wernicke's encephalopathy. Aust N Z J Med 16:676–678, 1986

Brouette T, Anton R: Clinical review of inhalants. Am J Addict 10:79–94, 2001

Bucholz KK, Homan SM: When do alcoholics first discuss drinking problems? J Stud Alcohol 53:582–589, 1992

Buka SL, Shenassa ED, Niaura R: Elevated risk of tobacco dependence among offspring of mothers who smoked during pregnancy: a 30-year prospective study. Am J Psychiatry 160:1978–1984, 2003

Burgess C, O'Donohoe A, Gill M: Agony and ecstasy: a review of MDMA effects and toxicity. Eur Psychiatry 15:287–294, 2000

Busto UE, Romach MK, Sellers EM: Multiple drug use and psychiatric comorbidity in patients admitted to the hospital with severe benzodiazepine dependence. J Clin Psychopharmacol 16:51–57, 1996

Caballero F, Lopez-Navidad A, Cortorruelo J et al: Ecstasy-induced brain death and acute hepatocellular failure: multiorgan donor and liver transplantation. Transplantation 74:532–537, 2002

Caces F, Harford T: Time series analysis of alcohol consumption and suicide mortality in the United States, 1934–1987. J Stud Alcohol 59:455–461, 1998

Camí J, Farré M: Drug addiction. N Engl J Med 349:975–986, 2003

Cantor-Graae E, Nordstrom LG, McNeil TF: Substance abuse in schizophrenia: a review of the literature and a study of correlates in Sweden. Schizophr Res 48:69–82, 2001

Carrillo JA, Dahl ML, Svensson JO, et al: Disposition of fluvoxamine in humans is determined by the polymorphic CYP2D6 and also by the CYP1A2 activity. Clin Pharmacol Ther 60:183–190, 1996

Carroll KM, Rounsaville BJ, Keller DS: Relapse prevention strategies for the treatment of cocaine abuse. Am J Drug Alcohol Abuse 17:249–265, 1991

Center for Substance Abuse Treatment: Treatment Improvement Protocol for Pregnant, Substance-Using Women. Rockville, MD, Center for Substance Abuse Treatment, 1993

Center for Substance Abuse Treatment: Treatment Improvement Protocols. Available at: http://www.treatment.org/Externals/tips.html. Accessed February 15, 2004.

Centers for Disease Control and Prevention: Viral hepatitis and injection drug users (IDU/HIV Prevention fact sheet). September 2002. Available at: http://www.cdc.gov/idu/hepatitis/viral_hep_drug_use.pdf. Accessed February 15, 2004.

Charney DS, Sternberg DE, Kleber HD, et al: The clinical use of clonidine in abrupt withdrawal from opiates. Arch Gen Psychiatry 38:1273–1277, 1981

Cherpitel CJ: Screening for alcohol problems in the U.S. general population: comparison of the CAGE, RAPS4, and RAPS4-QF by gender, ethnicity, and service utilization: rapid alcohol problems screen. Alcohol Clin Exp Res 26:1686–1691, 2002

Ciraulo DA, Sarid-Segal O, Knapp C, et al: Liability to alprazolam abuse in daughters of alcoholics. Am J Psychiatry 153:956–958, 1996

Cleary PD, Miller M, Bush BT, et al: Prevalence and recognition of alcohol abuse in a primary care population. Am J Med 85:466–471, 1988

Cohen S: The hallucinogens and inhalants. Psychiatr Clin North Am 4:681–688, 1984

Cole P, Rodu B: Analytic epidemiology: cancer causes, in Cancer: Principles and Practice of Oncology, 6th Edition. Edited by Devita VT, Hellman S, Rosenberg SA. Philadelphia, PA, Lippincott Williams & Wilkins, 2001, pp 241–252

COMBINE Study Research Group: Testing combined pharmacotherapies and behavioral interventions in alcohol dependence: rationale and methods. Alcohol Clin Exp Res. 27:1107–1122, 2003

Community Epidemiology Working Group: Epidemiologic trends in drug abuse (NIH Publ No. 01-4916A). Bethesda, MD, National Institute on Drug Abuse, 2001

Connors GJ, Tonigan JS, Miller WR; MATCH Research Group: A longitudinal model of intake symptomatology, AA participation and outcome: retrospective study of the Project MATCH outpatient and aftercare samples. J Stud Alcohol 62:817–825, 2001

Costa GM, Pizzi C, Bresciani B, et al: Acute myocardial infarction caused by amphetamines: a case report and review of the literature. Ital Heart J 2:478–480, 2001

Covey LS, Glassman AH, Stetner F: Major depressive disorder following smoking cessation. Am J Psychiatry 154:263–265, 1997

Crits-Christoph P, Siqueland L, Blaine J, et al: Psychosocial treatments for cocaine dependence: National Institute on Drug Abuse Collaborative Cocaine Treatment Study. Arch Gen Psychiatry 56:493–502, 1999

Daeppen JB, Gache P, Landry U, et al: Symptom-triggered vs fixed-schedule doses of benzodiazepine for alcohol withdrawal: a randomized treatment trial. Arch Intern Med. 162:1117–1121, 2002

Daumann J, Fimm B, Willmes K, et al: Cerebral activation in abstinent ecstasy (MDMA) users during a working memory task: a functional magnetic resonance imaging (fMRI) study. Brain Res Cogn Brain Res 16:479–487, 2003

Davis BL: The PCP epidemic: a critical review. Int J Addict 17:1137–1155, 1982

de Graaf R, Bijl RV, Smit F, et al: Risk factors for 12-month comorbidity of mood, anxiety, and substance use disorders: findings from the Netherlands mental health survey and incidence study. Am J Psychiatry 159:620–629, 2002

Deutsch SI, Mastropaolo J, Rosse RB: Neurodevelopmental consequences of early exposure to phencyclidine and related drugs. Clin Neuropharmacol 21:320–332, 1998

Dietch J: The nature and extent of benzodiazepine abuse: an overview of recent literature. Hosp Community Psychiatry 34:1139–1145, 1983

Dillon P, Copeland J, Jansen K: Patterns of use and harms associated with non-medical ketamine use. Drug Alcohol Depend 69:23–28, 2003

DiMartini A, Jain A, Irish W, et al: Outcome of liver transplantation in critically ill patients with alcoholic cirrhosis: survival according to medical variables and sobriety. Transplantation 66:298–302, 1998

DiMartini A, Weinrieb R, Fireman M: Liver transplantation in patients with alcohol and other substance use disorders. Psychiatr Clin North Am 25:195–209, 2002

Dole VP, Nyswander ME: A medical treatment of heroin addiction. JAMA 193:646–650, 1965

D'Onofrio G, Rathlev N, Ulrich A, et al: Lorazepam for the prevention of recurrent seizures related to alcohol. N Engl J Med 340:915–919, 1999

Drake RE, Osher FC, Wallach MA: Alcohol use and abuse in schizophrenia: a prospective community study. J Nerv Ment Dis 177:408–414, 1989

Drug Enforcement Administration: Cannabis, in Drugs of Abuse. Available at: http://www.usdoj.gov/dea/concern/abuse/chap6/marijuan.htm. Accessed January 5, 2001.

Dulit RA, Fyer MR, Haas GL, et al: Substance use in borderline personality disorder. Am J Psychiatry 147:1002–1007, 1990

Dyer JE, Roth B, Hyma BA: Gamma-hydroxybutrate withdrawal syndrome. Ann Emerg Med 37:147–153, 2001

Edenberg HJ, Foroud T, Koller DL, et al: A family based analysis of the association of the dopamine D2 receptor (DRD2) with alcoholism. Alcohol Clin Exp Res 22:505–512, 1998

Enoch MA, Schuckit MA, Johnson BA, et al: Genetics of alcoholism using intermediate phenotypes. Alcohol Clin Exp Res 27:169–176, 2003

Ernst T, Chang L, Leonido-Yee M, et al: Evidence for long-term neurotoxicity associated with methamphetamine abuse: a 1H-MRS study. Neurology. 54:1344–1349, 2000

Espeland K: Identifying the manifestations of inhalant abuse. Nurse Pract 20:49–50, 53, 1995

Espir ML, Rose FC: Alcohol, seizures and epilepsy. J R Soc Med 9:542–543, 1987

Eyler FD, Behnke M, Conlon M, et al: Birth outcome from a prospective, matched study of prenatal crack/cocaine use, I: interactive and dose effects on health and growth. Pediatrics 101:229–237, 1998a

Eyler FD, Behnke M, Conlon M, et al: Birth outcome from a prospective, matched study of prenatal crack/cocaine use, II: interactive and dose effects on neurobehavioral assessment. Pediatrics 101:237–241, 1998b

Fiellin DA, O'Connor PG, Holmboe ES, et al: Risk for delirium tremens in patients with alcohol withdrawal syndrome. Subst Abus 23:83–94, 2002

Fingerhood MI, Thompson MR, Jasinski DR: A comparison of clonidine and buprenorphine in the outpatient treatment of opiate withdrawal. Subst Abus 22:193–199, 2001

Fleming MF, Wilk A, Kruger J, et al: Hospital-based alcohol and drug specialty consultation service: does it work? South Med J 88:275–282, 1995

Fleming MF, Mundt MP, French MT, et al: Brief physician advice for problem drinkers: long-term efficacy and benefit-cost analysis. Alcohol Clin Exp Res 26:36–43, 2002

Foster SE, Vaughan RD, Foster WH, et al: Alcohol consumption and expenditures for underage drinking and adult excessive drinking. JAMA 289:989–995, 2003

Foy A, Kay J, Taylor A: The course of alcohol withdrawal in a general hospital. QJM 90:253–261, 1997

Frank DA, Augustyn M, Knight WG, et al: Growth, development, and behavior in early childhood following prenatal cocaine exposure: a systematic review. JAMA 285:1613–1625, 2001

Franklin JE, Paine RM: Psychiatric issues in organ transplantation, in Handbook of Organ Transplantation, 3rd Edition. Edited by Stuart F, Abecassis MM, Kaufman DB. Georgetown, TX, Landes Bioscience, 2003, pp 378–398

Franklin TR, Acton PD, Maldjian JA, et al: Decreased gray matter concentration in the insular, orbitofrontal, cingulate, and temporal cortices of cocaine patients. Biol Psychiatry 51:134–142, 2002

Freese TE, Miotto K, Reback CJ: The effects and consequences of selected club drugs. J Subst Abuse Treat 23:151–156, 2002

Frei A, Rehm J: [The prevalence of psychiatric co-morbidity among opioid addicts]. Psychiatr Prax 29:258–262, 2002

Frels C, Williams P, Narayanan S, et al: Iatrogenic causes of falls in hospitalised elderly patients: a case-control study. Postgrad Med J 78:487–489, 2002

Frezza M, Di Padova G, Pozzato G, et al: High blood alcohol levels in women: the role of decreased gastric alcohol dehydrogenase activity and first-pass metabolism. N Engl J Med 322:95–99, 1990

Frosch D, Shoptaw S, Huber A, et al: Sexual HIV risk among gay and bisexual male methamphetamine abusers. J Subst Abuse Treat 13:483–486, 1996

Fu Q, Heath AC, Bucholz KK, et al: Shared genetic risk of major depression, alcohol dependence, and marijuana dependence: contribution of antisocial personality disorder in men. Arch Gen Psychiatry 59:1125–1132, 2002

Fudala PJ, Bridge TP, Herbert S, et al: Office-based treatment of opiate addiction with a sublingual-tablet formulation of buprenorphine and naloxone. N Engl J Med 349:949–958, 2003

Fuller MG, Jordan ML: The substance abuse consultation team: addressing the problem of hospitalized substance abusers. Gen Hosp Psychiatry 16:73–77, 1994

Fuller RK, Branchey L, Brightwell DR, et al: Disulfiram treatment of alcoholism. JAMA 256:1449–1455, 1986

Garbutt JC, West SL, Carey TS, et al: Pharmacological treatment of alcohol dependence: a review of the evidence. JAMA 281:1318–1325, 1999

Geller A: Management of protracted withdrawal, in Principles of Addiction Medicine. Edited by Miller NS. Chevy Chase, MD, American Society of Addiction Medicine, 1994, pp 1–6

Giovino GA: Epidemiology of tobacco use in the United States. Oncogene 21:7326–7340, 2002

Goldstein RZ, Volkow ND: Drug addiction and its underlying neurobiological basis: neuroimaging evidence for the involvement of the frontal cortex. Am J Psychiatry 159:1642–1652, 2002

Gottschalk C, Beauvais J, Hart R, et al: Cognitive function and cerebral perfusion during cocaine abstinence. Am J Psychiatry 158:540–545, 2001

Gourevitch MN, Friedland GH: Interactions between methadone and medications used to treat HIV infection: a review. Mt Sinai J Med 67(5–6):429–436, 2000

Gowing L, Ali R, White J: Buprenorphine for the management of opioid withdrawal. Cochrane Database Syst Rev (2): CD002025, 2000

Grinspoon L, Bakalar JB: Psychedelics and arylcyclohexylamines, in Psychiatry Update: The American Psychiatric Association Annual Review, Vol 5. Edited by Frances AJ, Hales RE. Washington, DC, American Psychiatric Press, 1986, pp 212–225

Gruber AJ, Pope HG Jr: Cannabis psychotic disorder: does it exist? Am J Addict 3:72–83, 1994

Guardia J, Caso C, Arias F, et al: A double-blind, placebo-controlled study of naltrexone in the treatment of alcohol-dependence disorder: results from a multicenter clinical trial. Alcohol Clin Exp Res 26:1381–1387, 2002

Haas DA, Harper DG: Ketamine: a review of its pharmacologic properties and use in ambulatory anesthesia. Anesth Prog 39:61–68,1992

Haber PS, Warner R, Seth D, et al: Pathogenesis and management of alcoholic hepatitis. J Gastroenterol Hepatol 18:1332–1344, 2003

Hajak G, Muller WE, Wittchen HU, et al: Abuse and dependence potential for the non-benzodiazepine hypnotics zolpidem and zopiclone: a review of case reports and epidemiological data. Addiction 98:1371–1378, 2003

Halikas JA, Crosby RD, Carlson GA, et al: Cocaine reduction in unmotivated crack users using carbamazepine versus placebo in a short term, double-blind crossover design. Clin Pharmacol Ther 50:81–95, 1991

Hall SM, Reus VI, Munoz RF, et al: Nortriptyline and cognitive-behavioral therapy in the treatment of cigarette smoking. Arch Gen Psychiatry 55:683–690, 1998

Hall SM, Humfleet GL, Reus VI, et al: Psychological intervention and antidepressant treatment in smoking cessation. Arch Gen Psychiatry. 59:930–936, 2002

Halpern JH, Pope HJ: Do hallucinogens cause residual neuropsychological toxicity? Drug Alcohol Depend 53:247–256, 1999

Haney M, Ward AS, Comer SD, et al: Abstinence symptoms following smoked marijuana in humans. Psychopharmacology (Berl) 141:395–404, 1999

Harris-Allen M: Detoxification considerations in the medical management of substance abuse in pregnancy. Bull N Y Acad Med 67:270–276, 1991

Hasin DS, Grant BF: Major depression in 6050 former drinkers: association with past alcohol dependence. Arch Gen Psychiatry 59:794–800, 2002

Hasin D, Liu X, Nunes E, et al: Effects of major depression on remission and relapse of substance dependence. Arch Gen Psychiatry 59:375–380, 2002

Hayford KE, Patten CA, Rummans TA, et al: Efficacy of bupropion for smoking cessation in smokers with a former history of major depression or alcoholism. Br J Psychiatry 174:173–178, 1999

Henningfield JE: Pharmacologic basis and treatment of cigarette smoking. J Clin Psychiatry 45:24–34, 1984

Hersh D, Kranzler HR, Meyer RE: Persistent delirium following cessation of heavy alcohol consumption: diagnostic and treatment implications. Am J Psychiatry 154:846–851, 1997

Higgins ST, Sigmon SC, Wong CJ, et al: Community reinforcement therapy for cocaine-dependent outpatients. Arch Gen Psychiatry 60:1043–1052, 2003

Hodgson RJ, John B, Abbasi T, et al: Fast screening for alcohol misuse. Addict Behav 28:1453–1463, 2003

Hughes JR: Tobacco abstinence and psychiatric treatment. J Clin Psychiatry 54:110–114, 1993

Hughes JR, Hatsukami D: Signs and symptoms of tobacco withdrawal. Arch Gen Psychiatry 43:289–294, 1986

Humphreys K, Moos RH, Finney JW: Life domains, Alcoholics Anonymous, and role incumbency in the 3-year course of problem drinking. J Nerv Ment Dis 184:475–481, 1996

Itkomen J, Schnoll S, Glassroth J: Pulmonary dysfunction in freebase cocaine users. Arch Intern Med 144:2195–2197, 1984

Jacobsen LK, Southwick SM, Kosten TR: Substance use disorders in patients with posttraumatic stress disorder: a review of the literature. Am J Psychiatry 158:1184–1190, 2001

Jasinski DR, Johnson RE, Kocher TR: Clonidine in morphine withdrawal. Arch Gen Psychiatry 42:1063–1066, 1985

Jentsch JD, Roth RH: The neuropsychopharmacology of phencyclidine: from NMDA receptor hypofunction to the dopamine hypothesis of schizophrenia. Neuropsychopharmacology 20:201–225, 1999

Johnson BA, Devous MD, Ruiz P, et al: Treatment advances for cocaine-induced ischemic stroke: focus on dihydropyridine-class calcium channel antagonists. Am J Psychiatry 158:1191–1198, 2001

Johnson FW, Gruenewald PJ, Treno AJ, et al: Drinking over the life course within gender and ethnic groups: a hyperparametric analysis. J Stud Alcohol 59:568–580, 1998

Johnson RE, Strain EC, Amass L. Buprenorphine: how to use it right. Drug Alcohol Depend 70 (2 suppl):S59–S77, 2003

Johnston LD, O'Malley PM, Bachman JG, et al: Monitoring the Future national results on adolescent drug abuse: overview of key findings, 2003 (NIH Publ No. 04-5506). Bethesda, MD, National Institute on Drug Abuse, 2004

Jorenby DE, Leischow SJ, Nides MA, et al: A controlled trial of sustained-release bupropion, a nicotine patch, or both for smoking cessation. N Engl J Med 340:685–691, 1999

Joy JE, Watson SJ, Benson J (eds): Marijuana and Medicine: Assessing the Science Base. Washington, DC, National Academy Press, 1999

Justus AN, Finn PR, Steinmetz JE: P300, disinhibited personality, and early-onset alcohol problems. Alcohol Clin Exp Res 25:1457–1466, 2001

Kendler KS, Neale MC, MacLean CJ, et al: Smoking and major depression: a causal analysis. Arch Gen Psychiatry 50:36–43, 1993

Kendler KS, Neale MC, Thornton LM, et al: Cannabis use in the last year in a US national sample of twin and sibling pairs. Psychol Med. 32:551–554, 2002

Kendler KS, Jacobson KC, Prescott CA, et al: Specificity of genetic and environmental risk factors for use and abuse/dependence of cannabis, cocaine, hallucinogens, sedatives, stimulants, and opiates in male twins. Am J Psychiatry 160:687–695, 2003a

Kendler KS, Prescott CA, Myers J, et al: The structure of genetic and environmental risk factors for common psychiatric and substance use disorders in men and women. Arch Gen Psychiatry 60:929–937, 2003b

Kleber HD, Riordan CE, Rounsaville B, et al: Clonidine in outpatient detoxification from methadone maintenance. Arch Gen Psychiatry 42:391–394, 1985

Koob GF, Le Moal M: Drug abuse: hedonic homeostatic dysregulation. Science 278:52–58, 1997

Kopelman MD: The Korsakoff syndrome. Br J Psychiatry 166:154–173, 1995

Kosten TR, Gawin FH, Morgan C: Evidence for altered desipramine disposition in methadone-maintained patients treated for cocaine abuse. Am J Drug Alcohol Abuse 16:329–336, 1990

Kranzler HR, Del Boca FK, Rounsaville BJ: Comorbid psychiatric diagnosis predicts three-year outcomes in alcoholics: a posttreatment natural history study. J Stud Alcohol 57:619–626, 1996

Kranzler HR, Modesto-Lowe V, Nuwayser ES: Sustained-release naltrexone for alcoholism treatment: a preliminary study. Alcohol Clin Exp Res 22:1074–1079, 1998

Krystal JH, Cramer JA, Krol WF, et al: Naltrexone in the treatment of alcohol dependence. N Engl J Med 345:1734–1739, 2001

Kunitz O, Ince A, Kuhlen R, et al: [Hyperpyrexia and rhabdomyolysis after ecstasy (MDMA) intoxication]. Anaesthesist 52:511–515, 2003

Laine C, Hauck WW, Gourevitch MN, et al: Regular outpatient medical and drug abuse care and subsequent hospitalization of persons who use illicit drugs. JAMA 285:2355–2361, 2001

Lambert MT: Alcohol withdrawal in severe hypothyroidism. Psychosomatics 44:79–81, 2003

Lapid MI, Bostwick JM: CIWA-ar false positives: is this scale appropriate for use in the medically ill? (letter). Psychosomatics 43:2, 2002

Lappalainen J, Long JC, Eggert M, et al: Linkage of antisocial alcoholism to the serotonin 5-HT1B receptor gene in 2 populations. Arch Gen Psychiatry 55:989–994, 1998

Lerner AG, Finkel B, Oyffe I, et al: Clonidine treatment for hallucinogen persisting perception disorder (letter). Am J Psychiatry 155:1460, 1998

Lerner A, Gelkopf M, Oyffe I, et al: LSD-induced hallucinogen persisting perception disorder treatment with clonidine: an open pilot study. Int Clin Psychopharmacol 15:35–37, 2000

Levin FR, Evans SM, McDowell DM, et al: Methylphenidate treatment for cocaine abusers with adult attention-deficit/hyperactivity disorder: a pilot study. J Clin Psychiatry 59:300–305, 1998

Levy RS, Hebert CK, Munn BG, et al: Drug and alcohol use in orthopedic trauma patients: a prospective study. J Orthop Trauma 10:21–27, 1996

Lieber C: Biochemical and molecular basis of alcohol-induced injury to liver and other tissues. N Engl J Med 319:1639–1647, 1988

Lieber CS: Seminars in medicine of the Beth Israel Hospital, Boston: medical disorders of alcoholism. N Engl J Med 333:1058–1065, 1995

Ling W, Charuvastra C, Collins JF, et al: Buprenorphine maintenance treatment of opiate dependence: a multicenter, randomized clinical trial. Addiction 93:475–486, 1998

Lucey MR, Carr K, Beresford TP, et al: Alcohol use after liver transplantation in alcoholics: a clinical cohort follow-up study. Hepatology 25:1223–1227, 1997

Malcolm R, Myrick H, Brady KT, Ballenger JC: Update on anticonvulsants for the treatment of alcohol withdrawal. Am J Addict 10 (suppl):16–23, 2001

Management of Substance Use Disorders Working Group: VHA/DoD clinical practice guideline for the management of substance use disorders. Washington, DC, Veterans Health Administration, Department of Defense, 2001

Mann JJ, Waternaux C, Haas GL, et al: Toward a clinical model of suicidal behavior in psychiatric patients. Am J Psychiatry 156:181–189, 1999

Mantere T, Tupala E, Hall H, et al: Serotonin transporter distribution and density in the cerebral cortex of alcoholic and nonalcoholic comparison subjects: a whole-hemisphere autoradiography study. Am J Psychiatry 159:599–606, 2002

Martinez-Cano H, de Iceta Ibanez de Gauna M, Vela-Bueno A, et al: DSM-III-R co-morbidity in benzodiazepine dependence. Addiction 94:97–107, 1999

Marzuk PM, Tardiff K, Leon AC: Prevalence of cocaine use among residents of New York City who committed suicide during a one-year period. Am J Psychiatry 3:371–375, 1992

Mayo-Smith MF: Pharmacological management of alcohol withdrawal: a meta-analysis and evidence-based practice guideline—American Society of Addiction Medicine Working Group on Pharmacological Management of Alcohol Withdrawal. JAMA 278:144–151, 1997

McCance EF: Overview of potential treatment medications for cocaine dependence, in Medications Development for the Treatment of Cocaine Dependence: Issues in Clinical Efficacy Trials. Edited by Tai B, Chiang N, Bridge P. Rockville, MD, National Institute on Drug Abuse, 1997, pp 36–72

McCance-Katz EF, Price LH, Kosten TR, et al: Cocaethylene: pharmacology, physiology, and behavioral effects in humans. J Pharm Exp Ther 274:215–223, 1995

McCance-Katz EF, Kosten TR, Jatlow P: Concurrent use of cocaine and alcohol is more potent and potentially more toxic than use of either drug alone: a multiple dose study. Biol Psychiatry 44:250–259, 1998

McCance-Katz EF, Gourevitch MN, Arnsten J, et al: Modified directly observed therapy (MDOT) for injection drug users with HIV disease. Am J Addict 11:271–278, 2002

McCance-Katz EF, Rainey P, Friedland G, et al: The protease inhibitor lopinavir/ritonavir may produce opiate withdrawal in methadone-maintained patients. Clin Infect Dis 37:476–482, 2003

McCann MJ, Miotto K, Rawson RA, et al: Outpatient nonopioid detoxification for opioid withdrawal: who is likely to benefit? Am J Addict 6:218–223, 1997

McCowan C, Marik P: Refractory delirium tremens treated with propofol: a case series. Crit Care Med 28:1781–1784, 2000

McCusker MT, Basquille J, Khwaja M, et al: Hazardous and harmful drinking: a comparison of the AUDIT and CAGE screening questionnaires. QJM 95:591–595, 2002

McDaniel CH, Miotto KA: Gamma hydroxybutyrate (GHB) and gamma butyrolactone (GBL) withdrawal: five case studies. J Psychoactive Drugs 33:143–149, 2001

McDuff DR, Solounias BL, Beuger M, et al: A substance abuse consultation service: enhancing the care of hospitalized substance abusers and providing training in addiction psychiatry. Am J Addict 6:256–265, 1997

McKellar J, Stewart E, Humphreys K: Alcoholics anonymous involvement and positive alcohol-related outcomes: cause, consequence, or just a correlate? a prospective 2-year study of 2,319 alcohol-dependent men. J Consult Clin Psychol 71:302–308, 2003

McLellan AT, Luborsky L, Woody GE, et al: An improved diagnostic evaluation instrument for substance abuse patients: Addiction Severity Index. J Nerv Ment Dis 168: 26–33, 1980

McLellan AT, Woody GE, Metzger D, et al: Evaluating the effectiveness of addiction treatments: reasonable expectations, appropriate comparisons. Milbank Q 74:51–85, 1996

McLellan AT, Grissom GR, Zanis D, et al: Problem-service "matching" in addiction treatment: a prospective study in 4 programs. Arch Gen Psychiatry 54:730–735, 1997

McLellan AT, Lewis DC, O'Brien CP, et al: Drug dependence, a chronic medical illness: implications for treatment, insurance, and outcomes evaluation. JAMA 284:1689–1695, 2000

Medical-care expenditures attributable to cigarette smoking—United States, 1993. MMWR Morb Mortal Wkly Rep 43: 469–472, 1994

Mee-Lee D, Shulman G, Gartner L: ASAM Patient Placement Criteria for the Treatment of Psychoactive Substance-Related Disorders, 2nd Edition. Chevy Chase, MD, American Society of Addiction Medicine, 1994

Merikangas KR, Mehta RL, Molnar BE, et al: Comorbidity of substance use disorders with mood and anxiety disorders: results of the International Consortium in Psychiatric Epidemiology. Addict Behav 23:893–907, 1998a

Merikangas KR, Stolar M, Stevens DE, et al: Familial transmission of substance use disorders. Arch Gen Psychiatry 55:973–979, 1998b

Meyers HB, Zepeda SG, Murdock MA: Alcohol and trauma: an endemic syndrome. West J Med 153:149–153, 1990

Miller WR, Yahne CE, Tonigan JS: Motivational interviewing in drug abuse services: a randomized trial. J Consult Clin Psychol 71:754–763, 2003

Minion GE, Slovid CM, Boutiette L: Severe alcohol intoxication: a study of 204 consecutive patients. J Toxicol Clin Toxicol 27:375–384, 1989

Moore RD, Bone LR, Geller G, et al: Prevalence, detection and treatment of alcoholism in hospitalized patients. JAMA 261:403–407, 1989

Morehead DB: Exacerbation of hallucinogen-persisting perception disorder with risperidone (letter). J Clin Psychopharmacol 17:327–328, 1997

Morris PL, Hopwood M, Whelan G, et al: Naltrexone for alcohol dependence: a randomized controlled trial. Addiction 96:1565–1573, 2001

Morse R, Flavin D: The definition of alcoholism. JAMA 268: 1012–1014, 1992

Mueser KT, Drake RE, Miles KM: The course and treatment of substance use disorders in persons with severe mental illness, in Treatment of Drug-Dependent Individuals With Comorbid Mental Disorders. Edited by Onken LS, Blaine JD, Genser S, et al. Rockville, MD, NIH, 1997, pp 86–109

Mukamal KJ, Conigrave KM, Mittleman MA, et al: Roles of drinking pattern and type of alcohol consumed in coronary heart disease in men. N Engl J Med 348:109–118, 2003a

Mukamal KJ, Kronmal RA, Mittleman MA, et al: Alcohol consumption and carotid atherosclerosis in older adults: the Cardiovascular Health Study. Arterioscler Thromb Vasc Biol 23:2252–2259, 2003b

Mukamal KJ, Kuller LH, Fitzpatrick AL, et al: Prospective study of alcohol consumption and risk of dementia in older adults. JAMA 289:1405–1413, 2003c

Murphy GE, Wetzel R: The lifetime risk of suicide in alcoholism. Arch Gen Psychiatry 47:383–392, 1990

Murphy GE, Wetzel RD, Robine E, et al: Multiple risk factors predict suicide in alcoholism. Arch Gen Psychiatry 49:459–463, 1992

Nabeshima T, Kitaichi K, Noda Y: Functional changes in neuronal systems induced by phencyclidine administration. Ann N Y Acad Sci 801:29–38, 1996

Naimi TS, Brewer RD, Mokdad A, et al: Binge drinking among US adults. JAMA 289:70–75, 2003

Narrow WE, Rae DS, Robins LN, et al: Revised prevalence estimates of mental disorders in the United States: using a clinical significance criterion to reconcile 2 surveys' estimates. Arch Gen Psychiatry 59:115–123, 2002

National Institute on Drug Abuse and National Institute on Alcohol Abuse and Alcoholism: The economic costs of alcohol and drug abuse in the United States—1992. Available at: http://www.nida.nih.gov/EconomicCosts/Table7_6. html. Accessed January 5, 2001.

Nestler EJ, Self DW: Neurobiologic aspects of ethanol and other chemical dependencies, in The American Psychiatric Press Textbook of Neuropsychiatry, 3rd Edition. Edited by Yudofsky SC, Hales RE. Washington, DC, American Psychiatric Press, 1997, pp 773–798

Neumark YD, Delva J, Anthony JC: The epidemiology of adolescent inhalant drug involvement. Arch Pediatr Adolesc Med 152:781–786, 1998

Ng SK, Hauser WA, Brust JC, et al: Alcohol consumption and withdrawal in new-onset seizures. N Engl J Med. 319:666–673, 1988

Noordsy DL, Drake RE, Teague GB, et al: Subjective experiences related to alcohol use among schizophrenics. J Nerv Ment Dis 179:410–414, 1991

Nunes EV, Quitlin FM: Treatment of depression in drug dependent patients: effects on mood and drug use, in Treatment of Drug-Dependent Individuals With Comorbid Mental Disorders. Edited by Onken LS, Blaine JD, Genser S, et al. Rockville, MD, National Institutes of Health, 1997, pp 61–85

Nurnberger JI, Foroud T, Flury L, et al: Evidence for a locus on chromosome 1 that influences vulnerability to alcoholism and affective disorder. Am J Psychiatry 158:718–724, 2001

O'Connor PG, Carroll KM, Shi JM, et al: Three methods of opioid detoxification in a primary care setting: a randomized trial. Ann Intern Med 127:526–530, 1997

Office of Applied Studies: Summary Findings From the 1998 National Household Survey on Drug Abuse. Rockville, MD, Substance Abuse and Mental Health Services Administration, 1999

Office of Applied Studies: Emergency department trends from the Drug Abuse Warning Network: final estimates 1995–2002 (DAWN series D-24; DHHS Publ No. SMA 03-3780). Rockville, MD, Substance Abuse and Mental Health Services Administration, 2003

Office of Applied Studies: Treatment Admissions in Urban and Rural Areas Involving Abuse of Narcotic Painkillers: The DASIS Report. Rockville, MD, Substance Abuse and Mental Health Services Administration, 2004

Office of National Drug Control Policy: Consultation document on opioid agonist treatment. Available at: http://www.whitehousedrugpolicy.gov/scimed/methadone/contents.html. Accessed January 5, 2001.

Oslin DW, Pettinati HM, Volpicelli JR, et al: The effects of naltrexone on alcohol and cocaine use in dually addicted patients. J Subst Abuse Treat 16:163–167, 1999

Ostrea EM Jr, Welch RA: Detection of prenatal drug exposure in the pregnant woman and her newborn infant. Clin Perinatol 18:629–645, 1991

Ouimette PC, Finney JW, Moos RH: Twelve-step and cognitive-behavioral treatment for substance abuse: a comparison of treatment effectiveness. J Consult Clin Psychol 65:230–240, 1997

Owen PL, Slaymaker V, Tonigan JS, et al: Participation in alcoholics anonymous: intended and unintended change mechanisms. Alcohol Clin Exp Res 27:524–532, 2003

Palmstierna T: A model for predicting alcohol withdrawal delirium. Psychiatr Serv 52:820–823, 2001

Petitti DB, Sidney S, Quesenberry C, et al: Stroke and cocaine or amphetamine use. Epidemiology. 9:596–600, 1998

Pope HG, Gruber AJ, Hudson SM, et al: Neuropsychological performance in long term cannabis users. Arch Gen Psychiatry 58:909–915, 2001

Project MATCH Research Group: Matching alcoholism treatments to client heterogeneity: treatment main effects and matching effects on drinking during treatment. J Stud Alcohol 59:631–639, 1998

Qasim A, Townend J, Davies M: Ecstasy induced acute myocardial infarction. Heart 85:E10, 2001

Qureshi AI, Suri MF, Guterman LR, et al: Cocaine use and the likelihood of nonfatal myocardial infarction and stroke: data from the Third National Health and Nutrition Examination Survey. Circulation 103:502–506, 2001

Reed BT, May PA: Inhalant abuse and juvenile delinquency: a control study in Albuquerque, New Mexico. Int J Addict 19:789–803, 1984

Rees Davis W, Johnson BD, Randolph D, et al: An enumeration method of determining the prevalence of users and operatives of cocaine and heroin in Central Harlem. Drug Alcohol Depend 72:45–58, 2003

Regier DA, Farmer ME, Rae DS, et al: Comorbidity of mental disorders with alcohol and other drug abuse: results from the Epidemiologic Catchment Area (ECA) study. JAMA 264:2511–2518, 1990

Regier DA, Narrow WE, Rae DS, et al: The de facto US Mental and Addictive Disorders Service System: Epidemiologic Catchment Area prospective 1-year prevalence rates of disorders and services. Arch Gen Psychiatry 50:85–94, 1993

Rehm J, Bondy S: Alcohol and all-cause mortality: an overview. Novartis Found Symp 216:223–232, 1998

Reneman L, Lavalaye J, Schmand B, et al: Cortical serotonin transporter density and verbal memory in individuals who stopped using 3,4-methylenedioxymethamphetamine (MDMA or "ecstasy"). Arch Gen Psychiatry 58:901–906, 2001

Reuler JB, Girard DE, Cooney TG: Wernicke's encephalopathy. N Engl J Med 312:1035–1039, 1985

Reynolds K, Lewis LB, Nolen JDL, et al: Alcohol consumption and risk of stroke: a meta-analysis. JAMA 289:579–588, 2003

Ricaurte GA, Yuan J, Hatzidimitriou G, et al: Severe dopaminergic neurotoxicity in primates after a common recreational dose regimen of MDMA ("ecstasy"). Science 297:2260–2263, 2002

Rickert VI, Wiemann CM, Berenson AB: Prevalence, patterns, and correlates of voluntary flunitrazepam use. Pediatrics 103:E6, 1999

Rickert VI, Siqueira LM, Dale T, et al: Prevalence and risk factors for LSD use among young women. J Pediatr Adolesc Gynecol 16:67–75, 2003

Ried LD, Johnson RE, Gettman DA: Benzodiazepine exposure and functional status in older people. J Am Geriatr Soc 46:71–76, 1998

Robins LN, Helzer JE, Weissman MM, et al: Lifetime prevalence of specific psychiatric disorders in three sites. Arch Gen Psychiatry 41:949–958, 1984

Rogers M, Cerda JJ: The narcotic bowel syndrome. J Clin Gastroenterol 11:132–135, 1989

Roggla H, Roggla G, Muhlbacher F: Psychiatric prognostic factors in patients with alcohol-related end-stage liver disease before liver transplantation. Wien Klin Wochenschr 108:272–275, 1996

Roldan CA, Aliabadi D, Crawford MH: Prevalence of heart disease in asymptomatic chronic cocaine users. Cardiology 95:25–30, 2001

Rosenbaum M, McCarty T: Alcohol prescription by surgeons in the prevention and treatment of delirium tremens: historic and current practice. Gen Hosp Psychiatry 24:257–259, 2002

Rosenberg MH, Deerfield LJ, Baruch EM: Two cases of severe gamma-hydroxybutyrate withdrawal delirium on a psychiatric unit: recommendations for management. Am J Drug Alcohol Abuse 29:487–496, 2003

Ross J, Darke S: The nature of benzodiazepine dependence among heroin users in Sydney, Australia. Addiction 95:1785–1793, 2000

Rounsaville BJ, Kleber HD: Untreated opiate addicts: how do they differ from those seeking treatment? Arch Gen Psychiatry 42:1072–1077, 1985

Rounsaville BJ, Weissman MM, Kleber H, et al: The heterogenicity of psychiatric diagnoses in treated opiate addicts. Arch Gen Psychiatry 39:161–166, 1982

Rumpf HJ, Bohlmann J, Hill A, et al: Physicians' low detection rates of alcohol dependence or abuse: a matter of methodological shortcomings? Gen Hosp Psychiatry 23:133–137, 2001

Ruttenber AJ, McAnally HB, Wetli CV: Cocaine-associated rhabdomyolysis and excited delirium: different stages of the same syndrome. Am J Forensic Med Pathol 20:120–127, 1999

Rydon P, Redman S, Sanson-Fisher RW, et al: Detection of alcohol-related problems in general practice. J Stud Alcohol 53:197–202, 1992

Saitz R, Mayo-Smith MF, Roberts MS, et al: Individualized treatment for alcohol withdrawal: a randomized double-blind controlled trial. JAMA 272:519–523, 1994

Santos de Barona M, Simpson DD: Inhalant users in drug abuse prevention programs. Am J Drug Alcohol Abuse 10:503–518, 1984

Satel SL, Kosten TR, Schuckit MA, et al: Should protracted withdrawal from drugs be included in DSM-IV? Am J Psychiatry 150:695–704, 1993

Satel SL, Krystal JH, Delgado PL, et al: Tryptophan depletion and attenuation of cue-induced craving for cocaine. Am J Psychiatry 152:778–783, 1995

Schermer CR, Bloomfield LA, Lu SW, et al: Trauma patient willingness to participate in alcohol screening and intervention. J Trauma 54:701–706, 2003a

Schermer CR, Gentilello LM, Hoyt DB, et al: National survey of trauma surgeons' use of alcohol screening and brief intervention. J Trauma 55:849–856, 2003b

Schifano F, Oyefeso A, Webb L, et al: Review of deaths related to taking ecstasy, England and Wales, 1997–2000. BMJ 326:80–81, 2003

Schubiner H, Saules KK, Arfken C, et al: Double-blind placebo-controlled trial of methylphenidate in the treatment of adult ADHD patients with comorbid cocaine dependence. Exp Clin Psychopharmacol 10:286–294, 2002

Schuckit MA: New findings in the genetics of alcoholism. JAMA 281:1875–1876, 1999

Schuckit MA, Smith TL: The clinical course of alcohol dependence associated with a low level of response to alcohol. Addiction 96:903–910, 2001

Schuckit MA, Tipp JE, Reich T, et al: The histories of withdrawal convulsions and delirium tremens in 1648 alcohol dependent subjects. Addiction 90:1335–1347, 1995

Schuckit MA, Tipp JE, Bucholz KK, et al: The lifetime rates of three major mood disorders and four major anxiety disorders in alcoholics and controls. Addiction 92:1289–1304, 1997

Schuckit MA, Smith TL, Danko GP, et al: Five-year clinical course associated with DSM-IV alcohol abuse or dependence in a large group of men and women. Am J Psychiatry 158:1084–1090, 2001

Schwartz RH, Hawks RL: Laboratory detection of marijuana use. JAMA 254:788–792, 1985

Schweizer E, Rickels K, Case WG, et al: Carbamazepine treatment in patients discontinuing long-term benzodiazepine therapy: effects on withdrawal severity and outcome. Arch Gen Psychiatry 48:448–452, 1991

Schweizer E, Rickels K, De Martinis N, et al: The effect of personality on withdrawal severity and taper outcome in benzodiazepine dependent patients. Psychol Med 28:713–720, 1998

Sees KL, Delucchi KL, Masson C, et al: Methadone maintenance vs 180-day psychosocially enriched detoxification for treatment of opioid dependence: a randomized controlled trial. JAMA 283:1303–1310, 2000

Shannon M: Methylenedioxymethamphetamine (MDMA, "ecstasy"). Pediatr Emerg Care 16:377–380, 2000

Sherer MA, Kumor KM, Cone EJ, et al: Suspiciousness induced by four-hour intravenous infusions of cocaine: preliminary findings. Arch Gen Psychiatry 45:673–677, 1988

Shoptaw S, Yang X, Rotheram-Fuller EJ, et al: Randomized placebo-controlled trial of baclofen for cocaine dependence: preliminary effects for individuals with chronic patterns of cocaine use. J Clin Psychiatry 64:1440–1448, 2003

Simon NG, Mattick RP: The impact of regular ecstasy use on memory function. Addiction 97:1523–1529, 2002

Simpson DD, Joe GW, Fletcher BW, et al: A national evaluation of treatment outcomes for cocaine dependence. Arch Gen Psychiatry 56:507–514, 1999

Singletary KW, Gapstur SM: Alcohol and breast cancer: review of epidemiologic and experimental evidence and potential mechanisms. JAMA 286:2143–2151, 2001

Sobell LC, Cunningham JA, Sobell MB: Recovery from alcohol problems with and without treatment: prevalence in two population surveys. Am J Public Health 86:966–972, 1996

Solowij N, Stephens RS, Roffman RA, et al: Cognitive functioning of long-term heavy cannabis users seeking treatment. JAMA. 287:1123–1131, 2002

Soyka M: Psychopathological characteristics in alcohol hallucinosis and paranoid schizophrenia. Acta Psychiatr Scand 81:255–259, 1990

Soyka M: [Alcohol-induced hallucinosis: clinical aspects, pathophysiology and therapy.] Nervenarzt 67:891–895, 1996

Spitzer RL, Kroenke K, Williams JB: Validation and utility of a self-report version of PRIME-MD: the PHQ primary care study—Primary Care Evaluation of Mental Disorders, Patient Health Questionnaire. JAMA 282:1737–1744, 1999

Steinbauer JR, Cantor SB, Holzer CE 3rd, et al: Ethnic and sex bias in primary care screening tests for alcohol use disorders. Ann Intern Med 129:353–362, 1998

Stine SM, Kosten TR: Use of drug combinations in treatment of opioid withdrawal. J Clin Psychopharmacol 3:203–209, 1992

Stowell LI, Fawcett JP, Brooke M, et al: Comparison of two commercial test kits for quantification of serum carbohydrate-deficient transferrin. Alcohol Alcohol 32:507–516, 1997

Sullivan JT, Swift RM, Lewis DC: Benzodiazepine requirements during alcohol withdrawal syndrome: clinical implications of using a standardized withdrawal scale. J Clin Psychopharmacol 11:291–295, 1991

Sullivan PF, Kendler KS: The genetic epidemiology of smoking. Nicotine Tob Res 1 (suppl 2):S51–S57, 1999

Suresh S, Porjesz B, Chorlian DB, et al: Auditory P3 in female alcoholics. Alcohol Clin Exp Res 27:1064–1074, 2003

Tapert SF, Cheung EH, Brown GG, et al: Neural response to alcohol stimuli in adolescents with alcohol use disorder. Arch Gen Psychiatry 60:727–735, 2003

Tarter RE, Kirisci L, Mezzich A, et al: Neurobehavioral disinhibition in childhood predicts early age at onset of substance use disorder. Am J Psychiatry 160:1078–1085, 2003

Thapar A, Fowler T, Rice F, et al: Maternal smoking during pregnancy and attention deficit hyperactivity disorder symptoms in offspring. Am J Psychiatry 160:1985–1989, 2003

Tonne U, Hiltunen AJ, Vikander B, et al: Neuropsychological changes during steady-state drug use, withdrawal and abstinence in primary benzodiazepine-dependent patients. Acta Psychiatr Scand 91:299–304, 1995

Toomey R, Lyons MJ, Eisen SA, et al: A twin study of the neuropsychological consequences of stimulant abuse. Arch Gen Psychiatry 60:303–310, 2003

Torrey WC, Drake RE, Cohen M, et al: The challenge of implementing and sustaining integrated dual disorders treatment programs. Community Ment Health J 38:507–521, 2002

Traub SJ, Hoffman RS, Nelson LS: Body packing—the internal concealment of illicit drugs. N Engl J Med 349:2519–2526, 2003

Trell E, Kristenson H, Fex G: Alcohol-related problems in middle-aged men with elevated serum gamma-glutamyltransferase: a preventive medical investigation. J Stud Alcohol 45:302–309, 1984

Tringali RA, Trzepacz PT, DiMartini A, et al: Assessment and follow-up of alcohol-dependent liver transplantation patients: a clinical cohort. Gen Hosp Psychiatry 18:70S–77S, 1996

Troisi A, Pasini A, Saracco M, et al: Psychiatric symptoms in male cannabis users not using other illicit drugs. Addiction 93:487–492, 1998

Tsuang MT, Lyons MJ, Meyer JM, et al: Co-occurrence of abuse of different drugs in men: the role of drug-specific and shared vulnerabilities. Arch Gen Psychiatry 55:967–972, 1998

Turner RG, Lichstein PR, Peden JG, et al: Alcohol withdrawal syndromes: a review of pathophysiology, clinical presentations and treatment. J Gen Intern Med 4:432–444, 1989

Vaillant GE: The Natural History of Alcoholism Revisited. Cambridge, MA, Harvard University Press, 1995

Van Thiel DH, Lipsitz HD, Porter LE, et al: Gastrointestinal and hepatic manifestations of chronic alcoholism. Gastroenterology 81:594–615, 1981

Victor M: The effects of alcohol on the nervous system, in Medical Diagnosis and Treatment of Alcoholism. Edited by Mendelson JH, Mello NK. New York, McGraw-Hill, 1992, pp 201–262

Volkow ND, Fowler JS, Wang GJ, et al: Role of dopamine, the frontal cortex and memory circuits in drug addiction: insight from imaging studies. Neurobiol Learn Mem 78:610–624, 2002

Vollenweider FX, Liechti ME, Gamma A, et al: Acute psychological and neurophysiological effects of MDMA in humans. J Psychoactive Drugs 34:171–184, 2002

Volpicelli JR, Alterman AI, Hayashida M, et al: Naltrexone in the treatment of alcohol dependence. Arch Gen Psychiatry 49:876–880, 1992

Walsh DC, Ringson RW, Merrigan DM, et al: A randomized trial of treatment options for alcohol abusing workers. N Engl J Med 325:775–782, 1991

Wand GS, Mangold D, El Deiry S, et al: Family history of alcoholism and hypothalamic opioidergic activity. Arch Gen Psychiatry 55:1114–1119, 1998

Watson SJ, Benson JA Jr, Joy JE: Marijuana and medicine: assessing the science base: a summary of the 1999 Institute of Medicine report. Arch Gen Psychiatry. 57:547–552, 2000

Weber JE, Shofer FS, Larkin GL, et al: Validation of a brief observation period for patients with cocaine-associated chest pain. N Engl J Med 348:510–517, 2003

Weinrieb RM, Van Horn DHA, McLellan AT, et al: Alcoholism treatment after liver transplantation: lessons learned from a clinical trial that failed. Psychosomatics 42:110–116, 2001

Weisner C, Schmidt L: General disparities in treatment for alcohol problems. JAMA 268:1872–1876, 1992

Weisner C, Mertens J, Parthasarathy S, et al: Integrating primary medical care with addiction treatment: a randomized controlled trial. JAMA 286:1715–1723, 2001

Wesson DR, Ling W: The clinical opiate withdrawal scale (COWS). J Psychoactive Drugs 35:253–259, 2003

Whitfield JB, Fletcher LM, Murphy TL, et al: Smoking, obesity, and hypertension alter the dose-response curve and test sensitivity of carbohydrate-deficient transferrin as a marker of alcohol intake. Clin Chem 44:2480–2489, 1998

Zevin S, Benowitz NL: Drug interactions with tobacco smoking: an update. Clin Pharmacokinet 36:425–438, 1999

Zubieta JK, Gorelick DA, Stauffer R, et al: Increased mu opioid receptor binding detected by PET in cocaine-dependent men is associated with cocaine craving. Nat Med 2:1225–1229, 1996

Zvosec DL, Smith SW, McCutcheon JR, et al: Adverse events, including death, associated with the use of 1,4-butanediol. N Engl J Med. 344:87–94, 2001

PART III

Specialties and Subspecialties

19 Heart Disease

Peter A. Shapiro, M.D.

CARDIOVASCULAR DISEASE IS the cause of death for one-third of American adults, and it is the leading cause of death in the developed world. Although some patients experience sudden fatal illness, many have a disease with chronic course that has a marked impact on their life. The relationships between psychiatry and cardiovascular disease are complex, including both the effects of psychosocial factors on the heart and vascular system and the effects of cardiovascular system changes on mental states. Many psychological states and traits have been identified as contributing to risk for the development or exacerbation of heart disease, including anxiety, anger, type A behavior pattern, depression, stress, and, recently, sleep disorders. Behavioral disorders such as overeating, smoking, and alcohol abuse also add to the risk of heart disease. Conversely, the experience of heart disease seems to contribute to risk for numerous psychiatric problems, especially depression, anxiety, and cognitive disorders. Not only are the psychological effects of dealing with cardiac illness complicated and profound, but the medications and other treatments for heart diseases also often have psychiatric effects. Because heart disease is so common, psychiatrists must expect to deal with the effects of cardiovascular comorbidity in the care of their patients, evaluating the role of medical factors in their mental health and recognizing the potential impact of psychiatric interventions on the cardiovascular system.

Coronary Artery Disease

Aggressive attention to primary prevention measures has reduced the incidence of coronary artery disease (CAD) in the United States over the past 20 years. Traditional CAD risk factors include hypertension, smoking, hypercholesterolemia, diabetes, male sex, and family history. National campaigns to raise awareness about modifiable coronary risk factors and promote treatment have re-sulted in reduction in the prevalence of some of these factors. Nevertheless, the incidence of acute myocardial infarction (MI) is about 500,000 cases per year in the United States (Rosamond et al. 1998). One-third of patients die within the first hour after the onset of symptoms, before receiving any treatment. Aggressive use of thrombolysis and revascularization procedures, beta-adrenergic blockers, angiotensin-converting enzyme (ACE) inhibitors, statins, and antiplatelet agents has reduced mortality in those who survive long enough to receive acute care. Estimated 28-day survival after acute MI for patients who survive to hospital admission is about 91% (Rosamond et al. 1998).

Congestive Heart Failure

The point prevalence of congestive heart failure (CHF) in the United States is over 2%—a figure essentially unchanged over the past 2 decades. In individuals older than 65 years, the incidence of heart failure approaches 1% per year. By and large, heart failure is characterized by an inexorable if gradual downhill course. The 5-year mortality of congestive heart failure is 50%, generally within 1 year after the onset of symptoms. The primary modes of death in heart failure are pump failure and cardiac arrhythmias (Jessup and Brozena 2003). Treatment with beta-adrenergic blockers, ACE inhibitors, angiotensin$_2$ receptor blockers, spironolactone, and implantable cardiac defibrillators reduces the risk of death, whereas inotropic agents have largely failed to do so, although they improve functional status in severely ill patients (Cohn 1996; Jessup and Brozena 2003). New treatments in heart failure include the use of biventricular pacing and long-term ventricular assist devices, which hold the promise of improving survival and quality of life (Jessup and Brozena 2003; Lazeau et al. 2001; Rose et al. 2001).

Psychiatric Disorders in Heart Disease

The development of cardiac disease in a previously well individual is associated with a variety of psychological reactions. Perhaps most fundamentally, it is difficult to maintain denial about one's mortality after a cardiac event. Viewing oneself as having heart disease has effects at every level of psychological development: increasing concerns about dependency, autonomy, control, and ability to provide for others; provoking loss of self-esteem and concern about loss of love; and inciting fears about vitality, sexuality, and mortality. The maintenance of denial has been associated with mental well-being (Levenson et al. 1989; Levine et al. 1987) and may be manifest as minimizing the severity of the event ("I just had a small attack") or attributing symptoms to a noncardiac source ("gas pains"), but excessive denial can be detrimental to health because of the failure to accept the need to maintain a treatment regimen or a delay in seeking treatment (Cassem 1985). In contrast, inadequate denial or exaggeration of the illness can lead to invalidism or mental disorder in the cardiac patient.

Attention to one's heartbeat, conscious experience of twinges of chest pain or palpitations, and other preoccupations with minor physical symptoms may result in hypochondriacal avoidance of activity and increased visits to the doctor and emergency room. Research with hypochondriacal, somatizing, and panic patients, who make up a large portion of patients presenting to emergency rooms with noncardiac chest pain, has demonstrated the high level of somatic awareness common in such patients (Barsky 1992; Barsky et al. 1994a, 1996).

Depression

Depression in Coronary Artery Disease

Depression appears to be the most common psychiatric disorder in CAD patients (Glassman and Shapiro 1998). Numerous surveys of patients with established coronary disease, acute MI, and unstable angina indicate a point prevalence of depression consistently in the range of 15%–20% (Shapiro et al. 1997). In a study of 200 patients interviewed after diagnostic coronary angiography confirmed a diagnosis of CAD, 16% met the criteria for major depressive disorder, and 17% met the criteria for minor depression. Most patients with major depression and about half of those with minor depression were found to have major depression at 1-year follow-up (Hance et al. 1996). Studies in post-MI patients in Europe, Canada, and the United States also converge on a point prevalence

of depression of about 15% (Frasure-Smith et al. 1993; Ladwig et al. 1991; Schleifer et al. 1989). This figure is remarkable in light of national surveys indicating a lifetime prevalence of depression of approximately 16% in the general population (Kessler et al. 2003). Three studies of patients following coronary artery bypass graft surgery also demonstrate a point prevalence of depression in the range of 20%–30% (Blumenthal et al. 2003; Connerney et al. 2001; Shapiro et al. 1998). Elevated symptom scores on depression rating scales such as the Beck Depression Inventory (BDI) are even more common and may predict subsequent major depression (Frasure-Smith et al. 1995a, 1995b).

Many studies indicate the failure to diagnose and treat depression in CAD patients (Frasure-Smith 1993; Luutonen et al. 2002). In a Finnish study (Luutonen et al. 2002) of 85 consecutive post-MI patients with 18-month follow-up, the prevalence of BDI scores of 10 or greater was 21% in hospital, 30% at 6 months, and 33.9% at 18 months. Only 6 patients received mental health treatment; 2 received benzodiazepines; none received adequate antidepressant therapy (Luutonen et al. 2002). In the Montreal Heart Institute sample, none of 35 patients identified with major depression by research interviews in the post-MI hospital stay received antidepressants (Frasure-Smith et al. 1993). In another study of patients with newly diagnosed CAD, one-sixth of the sample met the criteria for major depression; at 1-year follow-up, only one-sixth of those who were depressed had received treatment (Hance et al. 1996). The availability of good social support reduces the likelihood of persistent depression after an acute coronary event (Frasure-Smith et al. 1995b, 2000).

Depression in Congestive Heart Failure

Fewer studies have examined the prevalence of depression in patients with CHF, but as in patients with coronary disease, a point prevalence of depression approaching 20% is suggested by available data (Faris et al. 2002; Freedland et al. 1998; Jiang et al. 2001). A recent study of 347 hospitalized CHF patients demonstrated a 14% point prevalence for major depression, and 35% of patients had a BDI score over 10, commonly regarded as a threshold of significant depressive symptoms (Jiang et al. 2001). Other studies have estimated a prevalence of significant depressive symptoms in 20%–30% of CHF patients. In the REMATCH trial, a study comparing left ventricular assist device (LVAD) implantation with medical therapy for patients with chronic, end-stage congestive heart failure, the mean baseline BDI score was over 16, and more than two-thirds of patients had a score over 10 (Rose et al. 2001).

Anxiety

Anxiety in Coronary Artery Disease

The prevalence of anxiety disorders in CAD has not been as well studied as that of depression, but anxiety symptoms are clearly elevated in patients with acute coronary disease and in 5%–10% of patients with chronic heart disease (Sullivan et al. 2000). Many patients with coronary disease have a family history of death of the parent of the same sex as a result of the same illness. This history is often associated with the conscious fantasy that the patient's death at the age at which the parent died is inevitable, leading to considerable vigilance, avoidance, and other anxiety behaviors.

Anxiety in Congestive Heart Failure

There is a marked absence of studies on the frequency of anxiety disorders in CHF patients (MacMahon and Lip 2002). In a survey of ambulatory outpatients with dilated cardiomyopathy, anxiety symptoms rated by the Hospital Anxiety and Depression Scale were significantly increased in comparison to population norms, suggesting a substantial prevalence of anxiety disorders, but no diagnostic information was obtained (Steptoe et al. 2000).

Panic and Mitral Valve Prolapse

An association of mitral valve prolapse with panic was proposed in the past on the basis of symptoms associated with prolapse (fluttering or palpitation experiences) in patients with panic disorder and echocardiographic findings of prolapse (Carney et al. 1990; Gorman et al. 1988). Depending on the echocardiographic criteria employed, 5%–20% or more of patients with panic disorder have mitral valve prolapse (Dager et al. 1986; Liberthson et al. 1986; Margraf et al. 1988). Individuals with mitral valve prolapse may be asymptomatic or may experience occasional palpitations or "fluttering" sensations in the precordium, and it has been proposed that these sensations give rise to catastrophic cognitions that stimulate panic attacks in predisposed individuals (Barlow 1988). The nature of the link between panic and mitral valve prolapse has been questioned, however, because panic does not occur at higher-than-expected rates in patients with echocardiographic mitral valve prolapse and because mitral valve prolapse occurs in many other psychiatric disorder populations. Confusion has been created by varying criteria for mitral valve prolapse, small sample sizes, and poorly controlled studies. A possible link, in at least some cases, comes from recent genetic studies in panic disorder that have identified a syndrome of joint hyperlaxity, bladder and renal abnormalities, mitral valve prolapse, and panic that is linked to chromosome 13 (Hamilton et al. 2003; Martin-Santos et al. 1998).

Anxiety and Automatic Implantable Cardioverter-Defibrillators

Malignant ventricular arrhythmias account for a substantial fraction of fatal events in patients with ischemic heart disease and CHF. The use of automatic implantable cardioverter-defibrillators (AICDs) reduces mortality (DiMarco 2003), but the experience of defibrillation is unpleasant, likened to being "kicked in the chest." Implantable defibrillator discharges are associated with iatrogenic anxiety, particularly in patients who experience repetitive, frequent, or early discharges after device implantation (Heller et al. 1998). Early experience indicated a 50% incidence of psychiatric disorders after AICD implant (adjustment disorders, major depression, and panic disorder) (Morris et al. 1991), but the incidence of psychopathology has apparently diminished over time (Crow et al. 1998). In the Antiarrhythmics Versus Implantable Defibrillators (AVID) trial, patients who reported shocks during the follow-up period had reduced mental well-being and physical functioning and more anxiety than patients who did not receive shocks (Schron et al. 2002). In the Canadian Implantable Defibrillator Study (CIDS), adverse effects on quality of life were observed in patients who had received four or more shocks. Patients who did not receive shocks reported quality of life equal or superior to that of arrhythmia patients being treated with drug therapy who did not complain of side effects of the drug therapy (Irvine et al. 2002). Although full-fledged posttraumatic stress disorder appears to occur in fewer than 5% of AICD patients, symptoms of the disorder such as avoidance, hypervigilance, and reexperiencing are common, especially if patients experience multiple sequential shocks while conscious, which they endure with a sense of helplessness. A variety of other reactions to implanted defibrillators have been described, including feelings of invulnerability, dependency, and withdrawal (Fricchione et al. 1989). Nevertheless, most patients with implanted defibrillators report satisfaction with their experience with the device.

A recent trial of defibrillator-delivered pacing and shock therapy for atrial fibrillation found improvement in quality of life at a 6-month follow-up to implantation. In patients in whom the device fired during the follow-up period, there was no decrement in quality of life compared with that of patients who did not experience defibrillator discharges (D.M. Newman et al. 2003).

Anxiety and Supraventricular Tachycardia

Patients with supraventricular tachycardias often experience anxiety, especially with paroxysmal arrhythmias (e.g., paroxysmal supraventricular tachycardia—see the section "Diagnostic Issues" later in this chapter).

Delirium and Neurocognitive Dysfunction

In the cardiac surgery intensive care unit (ICU), delirium, like beauty, is very much in the eye of the beholder. After coronary bypass graft surgery and open-heart procedures, it is evident that many patients have altered mental status with impaired level of consciousness for some days. Whether these patients are identified as experiencing delirium appears to depend on the sensitivity of the observer and on the degree to which the patient's obtundation or agitation interferes with the clinical management of the postoperative state. Pioneering studies in the 1960s of the psychiatric aspects of heart disease included observations of the psychiatric complications of mitral commissurotomy and mitral and aortic valve replacement (Kornfeld et al. 1965). These studies documented a high prevalence of delirium in early open-heart surgery patients, which led to changes in ICU design and attention to preservation of sleep–wake cycles and appropriate use of narcotic analgesia in open-heart surgery. Studies demonstrating the importance of emboli from valvular structures or intracardiac thrombus, and from the cardiopulmonary bypass circuit, for subsequent cognitive impairment led to alterations of surgical technique and bypass circuit filters (S. Newman 1989; S. Newman et al. 1988; Willner and Rodewald 1991).

Frequency of adverse cerebral effects after coronary-artery bypass graft (CABG) was estimated at 6% at hospital discharge in a multicenter study of 2,104 patients, with about half of these events being focal neurological events; other problems included persistent cognitive impairment, diminished level of consciousness, and seizures (Roach 1996). Risk factors included advanced age, history of alcohol abuse, systolic hypertension, pulmonary disease, and aortic arch atherosclerosis. A longitudinal study of 261 patients found that 53% of post-CABG patients demonstrated neurocognitive impairment 1 week after surgery; the prevalence of impairment fell to 24% at 6 months (M. F. Newman et al. 2001) Predictors of delirium after open-heart surgery include older age, cerebrovascular disease, prolonged sedation, and narcotic use. Off-pump coronary bypass surgery has been studied as a means of reducing delirium and neuropsychological impairment after surgery (Diegeler et al. 2000). Avoidance of the heart-lung bypass machine reduces the production of inflammatory cytokines and reduces emboli to the brain; these factors appear to correlate with modestly improved neuropsychological outcome (Lee et al. 2003; Van Dijk et al. 2002).

Psychiatric Side Effects of Cardiac Drugs

A few cardiac medications have psychiatric side effects. These include digoxin, ACE inhibitors, amiodarone, lidocaine, and beta-blockers. Beta-blockers are frequently blamed for depression, fatigue, and sexual dysfunction; however, a recent analysis demonstrated that fatigue, but not depression, is likely to be exacerbated by beta-blockers (Ko et al. 2002). An exhaustive review is available (Brown and Stoudemire 1998) (see Table 19–1).

TABLE 19–1. Selected psychiatric side effects of cardiac drugs

Drug/Class	Effects
Digoxin	Visual hallucinations (classically, yellow rings around objects); delirium; depression
Beta-blockers	Fatigue, sexual dysfunction more common than depression per se; possibly less effect with atenolol
Alpha-blockers	Depression
Lidocaine	Agitation, delirium
Carvedilol	Fatigue, insomnia
Methyldopa	Depression, confusion, insomnia
Reserpine	Depression
Clonidine	Depression
ACE inhibitors	Mood elevation or depression (rare)
Pressors (dobutamine, milrinone, dopamine)	Rarely cause psychiatric effects
Angiotensin II receptor blockers	Rarely cause psychiatric effects
Amiodarone	Mood disorders secondary to thyroid effects
Diuretics	Hypokalemia, hyponatremia can result in anorexia, weakness, apathy

Note. ACE=angiotensin-converting enzyme.

Cardiac Neurosis

Development of cardiac neurosis can occur after a patient experiences symptoms attributed to heart disease, whether or not actual heart disease exists. In some patients, apparent clinging to symptoms of disease, and the resulting disability, serve as an unconscious, face-saving means to escape otherwise intolerable life stress related to work, troubled intimate relationships, or other demands. Remaining in the sick role provides respite from negative affects related to one's previous psychosocial role. Such patients may have a previous history of hard work; denial of dependent needs; and relatively poor capacity for introspection, psychological insight, and verbalization of affects (alexithymia). In other patients preexisting hypochondriasis, somatization, or panic is directed toward awareness of cardiac symptoms after an initial episode of symptoms. Less commonly, a patient with depression or a chronic psychosis becomes fixated and delusional about cardiac disease. Factitious illness and malingering must also be considered in the differential diagnosis for patients who appear to cling to cardiac disability.

Sexual Dysfunction

Sexual dysfunction after the onset of heart disease occurs as a consequence of both physical and psychological factors. Physical factors include medications, comorbid medical conditions such as peripheral vascular disease and diabetes mellitus, and low cardiac output. Psychological factors include depression, anxiety, and fear of inducing a heart attack. Coital angina makes up 5% of angina attacks, but it is rare in patients who do not have angina during strenuous physical exertion. The metabolic demand of coitus is about 2–4 metabolic equivalents in men age 33 years, about equal to the demand of walking 2–3 miles/hour. The metabolic demand may be less in older men (DeBusk 2003) (see Chapter 17, "Sexual Disorders").

Effects of Psychological Factors on the Heart and Heart Disease Risk

Depression and Risk of Coronary Heart Disease

Community prospective studies of several different populations demonstrate that a history of depressive disorder or elevated symptoms of depression as evaluated by questionnaire ratings is associated with increased risk for the subsequent development of ischemic heart disease and for coronary disease death. In studies of American, Danish, and Swedish populations, the estimated magnitude of the risk of incident disease associated with depression is 1.5- to 2.0-fold (Anda et al. 1993; Barefoot and Schroll 1996; Barefoot et al. 1996). In patients with preexisting CAD, the risk of death for patients with depression is three- to fourfold higher than that for nondepressed coronary patients (Carney et al. 2003; Frasure-Smith et al. 1993, 1995a; Ladwig et al. 1991).

Following CABG surgery, depression predicts recurrent cardiac events at 12 months (Connerney et al. 2001), and a recent study with 817 patients showed that moderate to severe depression symptoms on the day before surgery or even mild depression persisting from baseline to 6-month follow-up after surgery was a predictor of mortality over mean follow-up of 5.2 years, with hazard ratios of more than 2.0 (Blumenthal et al. 2003).

Depression clearly adversely affects patients' perceptions of their heart disease status and quality of life. A recent study (Ruo et al. 2003) examined 1,024 patients with stable CAD to evaluate the contributions of depressive symptoms and objective measures of cardiac function to their health status. The patients who had depressive symptoms (20%) were more likely to report coronary disease symptom burden, physical limitations, diminished quality of life, and fair to poor health. In multivariate analyses, depression symptoms had significant independent association with these health status outcomes. In contrast to exercise capacity, left ventricular ejection fraction and myocardial ischemia (measured by stress echocardiography) were not related to worse health status. These findings suggest that efforts to improve subjective health status in coronary disease patients should address depression symptoms.

Mechanisms Linking Depression and Coronary Artery Disease

Candidate psychophysiological mechanisms linking depression to adverse coronary disease outcomes include platelet dysfunction, autonomic dysfunction, and abnormalities of inflammation (Carney et al. 2002). Persons with depression have increased platelet reactivity to orthostatic challenge (Musselman et al. 1996) and heightened circulating levels of beta-thromboglobulin and platelet factor 4, two markers of platelet activation (Laghrissi-Thode et al. 1997; Pollock et al. 2000). This implies that depressed patients have increased likelihood of thrombus formation in response to thrombogenic stimuli. Serotonin is stored in platelets, and serotonin release is a crucial intermediate step in platelet aggregation and thrombus formation. Serotonin storage in platelets is dependent on a serotonin transporter protein on the platelet cell membrane. Serotonin reuptake inhibitors may reduce the capacity of platelets to store serotonin, and thereby reduce their capacity to initiate thrombus formation. A large case–control study of first MI patients demonstrated that use of serotonergic antidepressants with high affinity for the serotonin transporter protein reduced the risk of MI in comparison to the risk for those using other antidepressant agents (Sauer et al. 2003).

Several measures of cardiac autonomic control, derived from time series or power spectral analyses of heart rate variability, are also deranged in depression. These measures indicate elevated sympathetic activation, suppression of vagal tone, and increased propensity to cardiac arrhythmias (Carney et al. 2001; Stein et al. 2000). Similar changes in heart rate variability have been described as common in CAD patients and predict mortality after MI (Bigger et al. 1992, 1993).

Inflammation has only recently been widely recognized as another process involved in the development of atherosclerosis and acute coronary events (Libby et al. 2002). Inflammatory cytokines are elevated in coronary disease patients, and the extent of elevation of specific markers such as interleukin-6 (IL-6), tumor necrosis factor–α, and C reactive protein (CRP), predicts coronary and cerebrovascular disease events and progression of heart failure (Cesari et al. 2003). Depression has been shown to be associated with increases in circulating levels of IL-6 and CRP (Miller et al. 2002).

Depression may also exert a negative effect on cardiovascular outcomes through its negative effects on adherence to treatment recommendations. Demonstrated effects of depression in coronary disease patients include lower rates of smoking cessation, exercise, dietary modification, and adherence to medication regimen (Glassman 1993; Ziegelstein et al. 2000). However, the magnitude of the adherence effects does not appear sufficiently large to account for the differential effect of depression on survival and morbidity in cardiac patients.

The ENRICHD and SADHART Trials

If depression exerts a negative effect on cardiac outcomes in coronary disease, a natural and important question is whether treatment of depression improves coronary disease outcomes. Two recent trials have investigated this subject—in particular, in patients with depression after MI. In the SADHART trial (Glassman et al. 2002), 369 patients with major depression after hospitalization for unstable angina or acute MI were randomized in a double-blind study to receive treatment with sertraline, 50–200 mg/day, or placebo. The primary goal of the trial was to assess the safety of sertraline treatment, but a secondary goal was to obtain an estimate of the effect on cardiac outcomes. Although the trial was not powered to ade-

quately test an effect on morbidity or mortality (i.e., only seven deaths occurred during the follow-up period), sertraline was superior in absolute numerical terms to placebo in the rate of recurrent MI, mortality, heart failure, and angina, suggesting that a larger study of treatment effects on mortality would be worthwhile.

Concurrent with the SADHART trial, the ENRICHD (Enhancing Recovery in Coronary Heart Disease) trial was directed primarily at addressing the effects of treatment on mortality in post-MI patients (Writing Committee for the ENRICHD Investigators 2003). In ENRICHD, patients with low social support or depression after MI were enrolled in usual care or a cognitive-behavioral therapy (CBT) intervention group. Patients in the intervention group received 6–10 sessions of treatment over 6 months following acute MI. Mortality was assessed at 30-month follow-up. A confounding element of the trial was the use of antidepressants, usually sertraline, in both arms of the trial in patients with more severe depressive symptoms. The CBT intervention was not effective in reducing mortality, and subgroup analyses did not demonstrate an effect of the intervention even in the depression subgroup. Although the use of sertraline was not randomized, it was notable that all-cause mortality in the sertraline-treated patients was only 7.4%, compared with 15.3% and 10.6% in patients who did not receive drug therapy and patients treated with tricyclic antidepressants, respectively. However, sertraline did not reduce the risk of recurrent nonfatal MI.

Suggestive convergent evidence of a possible benefit of selective serotonin reuptake inhibitor (SSRI) treatment of depression on cardiovascular disease outcomes in cardiovascular disease patients comes from a study of prophylaxis of depression after stroke (Rasmussen et al. 2003). In this study, 137 patients with acute ischemic stroke who were not depressed at screening assessment within 4 weeks of the index stroke were randomized to placebo or sertraline treatment for 12 months. The study demonstrated a strong prophylactic effect of sertraline on the incidence of depression, and cardiovascular adverse events during the 12-month follow-up were reduced by two-thirds in the sertraline group, compared with the patients receiving placebo.

Depression Effects on CHF Outcome

Depression also appears to carry increased mortality risk in patients with CHF. In one cohort, major depression more than doubled the risk of 3-month and 1-year mortality (Jiang et al. 2001), although the effect did not quite achieve the level of statistical significance after adjustment for other medical variables associated with mortality risk. Depression did continue in multivariate analyses to predict hospital readmissions at 1-year follow-up. "Mild depression," defined as a BDI score of 10 or greater in the absence of a major depressive disorder, did not confer an increased risk of mortality or readmission. A retrospective assessment in an English center, with 5-year follow-up of 396 patients with congestive heart failure caused by nonischemic dilated cardiomyopathy, found that 21% of the patients were clinically depressed; of these, 60% were receiving antidepressants. Mortality at 5 years was 36% in depressed versus 16% in nondepressed patients, yielding a significant hazard ratio of 3.0 (Faris et al. 2002).

A multicenter study of 460 outpatients with CHF showed that, compared with nondepressed patients, patients with significant depression symptoms had both worse health status at baseline and more deterioration in health status over short-term follow-up. Depression predicted worsening of heart failure symptoms, physical and social functioning, and quality of life. Depression symptoms were the strongest predictor of decline in health status (Rumsfeld et al. 2003).

Anxiety and CAD Risk

There is little evidence in nonclinical samples that anxiety symptoms increase the risk of coronary disease or heart-disease-related mortality, with the exception of sudden cardiac death. Two prospective epidemiological studies do demonstrate an association of anxiety with sudden cardiac death. In a study involving 33,999 male, middle-aged health professionals with 2-year follow-up, there were 168 new cases of coronary heart disease, including 40 fatal and 128 nonfatal events. Nonfatal events were not associated with anxiety, but the risk of fatal CHD increased with the level of phobic anxiety, and high phobic anxiety carried a threefold increased relative risk of fatality compared with the risk in subjects with low anxiety; the excess risk was limited to cases of sudden cardiac death, with a sixfold increased risk associated with high anxiety (Kawachi et al. 1994a). The second study assessed 2,280 men free of chronic disease at baseline, with 32-year follow-up. Subjects completed an anxiety symptom rating scale at baseline. During the follow-up, there were 26 sudden cardiac deaths and 105 nonsudden CHD deaths. In multivariate analysis, after adjustment for potential confounding variables, men with anxiety scores above the ninety-eighth percentile had a 4.46-fold increased risk of sudden cardiac death, and a 1.94-fold increased risk of fatal coronary heart disease, but no excess risk for angina or nonfatal MI. These hazard ratios are strongly suggestive of an association of anxiety and sudden cardiac death (Kawachi et al. 1994b).

In a clinical study of hospitalized acute MI patients, scores above the median on the anxiety subscale of the Brief Symptom Inventory were associated with a more than twofold increased risk of death during the hospitalization (Moser and Dracup 1996). In the long run after MI, anxiety does confer mortality risk independently of depression in some studies (Frasure-Smith et al. 1995b; Strik et al. 2003), but some reviewers have expressed concern that inadequate adjustment for confounding medical disease severity accounts for these positive findings (Lane et al. 2003).

Panic disorder was associated with increased cardiovascular morbidity (MI and stroke) in a community sample using a subset of the Epidemiologic Catchment Area Study data, but the study had significant methodological limitations, including retrospective self-report of cardiovascular outcomes without external validation (Weissman et al. 1990). In an anxiety disorders clinic sample, panic disorder was associated with an excess of cardiovascular deaths in men, but not in women, and the total number of deaths was too small to provide reliable estimates (Coryell 1988; Coryell et al. 1986).

Anger, Type A Behavior, and Hostility

Type A behavior pattern—characterized by anger, impatience, aggravation, and irritability—was linked to incident coronary disease in men in the 1970s. The Western Collaborative Group Study of more than 3,000 middle-aged men demonstrated that type A behavior was associated with a more than twofold increased risk of incident MI and of fatal coronary events (Rosenman et al. 1975). One of the few large-scale clinical trials in psychosomatic cardiology, the Recurrent Coronary Prevention Project, examined the effect of group counseling to reduce type A behavior pattern on mortality and recurrent infarction. Patients were survivors of an acute MI and were randomized to usual care or added type A behavior modification groups. Follow-up in 4.5 years demonstrated a significant reduction in recurrent infarction in those assigned to type A counseling (Friedman et al. 1986). Subsequent studies of type A behavior pattern and CAD have been inconclusive or negative, perhaps because of the difficulty in measuring type A behavior or changes in cardiovascular therapeutics, especially the widespread use of beta-adrenergic blockers in patients with coronary disease (Booth-Kewley and Friedman 1987).

Anger and hostility, considered as "toxic components" within the type A concept, have also been studied as risk factors for coronary disease but with mixed results in longitudinal observations (Barefoot et al. 1994, 1995). Low hostility is protective against incident coronary disease

(Shekelle et al. 1983), but high anger and high hostility are less clearly linked to increased cardiovascular risk. In the Normative Aging Study analysis, anger predicted the incidence of a combined endpoint of coronary death, nonfatal MI, and angina, but it did not predict coronary death or nonfatal MI to a statistically significant degree (Kawachi et al. 1996).

Acute Mental Stress

George Engel, who championed the biopsychosocial model in medicine, provided vivid examples from the news media of acute mental stress preceding acute coronary events (Engel 1976), and epidemiological studies of disasters have helped to confirm the relationship of acute stress to risk for sudden cardiac death (Leor et al. 1996). In animal experimental models of sudden cardiac death, acute mental stress has been one of the most studied psychosomatic factors. Animals conditioned to anticipate unpleasant restraint experience increased ventricular ectopy and ventricular tachycardia-fibrillation when exposed to the threat of restraint. Interestingly, this effect depends on the presence of myocardial ischemia and can be disrupted by the use of intracerebral β-adrenergic blockade (DeSilva 1983, 1993; Lown 1990; Lown et al. 1980; Skinner 1985; Skinner et al. 1975, 1981). The Northridge, California, earthquake in 1994 caused a surge in sudden cardiac deaths over the subsequent 2 days in individuals who were not physically endangered by the earthquake but resided in the immediate area (Leor et al. 1996). A preliminary, similar finding has been reported in the aftermath of the destruction of the World Trade Center in New York in 2001 (Qureshi et al. 2003). Acute stress in the laboratory, provoked by standardized tasks such as mirror-drawing, the Stroop color word test, mental arithmetic, video games, and public speaking, results in elevation in heart rate and blood pressure and alteration in indices of cardiac autonomic regulation, with diminished parasympathetic and elevated sympathetic activation, in both healthy volunteers and patients with CAD (Blumenthal et al. 1995; Manuck and Krantz 1986; Rozanski et al. 1988, 1999; Sheps et al. 2002). In addition, coronary vasospasm appears to be a mechanism of mental stress-induced ischemia in at least some cases (Yeung et al. 1991). One-third to one-half of patients with CAD experience ischemia during mental stress testing, and ischemia occurs at lower levels of rate-pressure product elevation during mental stress than during exercise stress. Most patients with mental stress-induced ischemia also have exercise-induced ischemia. Wall motion abnormality appears to be a more sensitive indicator of ischemia than ST segment depression, for unknown reasons (Strike and Steptoe 2003). Mental stress–induced ischemia is usually silent (Blumenthal et al. 1995; Rozanski et al. 1988, 1999). The technique of ecological momentary assessment has been used to demonstrate that emotional arousal, and especially anger during daily events, is associated with similar alterations in hemodynamic and autonomic state, and it has been estimated that acute emotional stress is a trigger for up to 20%–30% of acute coronary events (Muller et al. 1994). In patients with coronary disease, mental stress–induced ischemia, indicated by wall motion abnormalities on radionuclide ventriculography or echocardiography, is associated with increased risk of death, even after adjusting for other prognostic variables (Jiang et al. 1996; Sheps et al. 2002).

Sleep Apnea

Sleep apnea is associated with hypertension and CHF (Bradley and Floras 2003a, 2003b). Two studies of chronic heart failure patients found the prevalence of obstructive sleep apnea to range from 11% to 37%, and the presence of sleep apnea increases the risk of developing heart failure. Obstructive apnea results in hypoxia, elevated intrathoracic pressure, and sympathetic nervous system activation, with increases in heart rate and blood pressure. These physiological derangements may contribute to the development of heart failure, ischemic events, and arrhythmias (Shamsuzzaman et al. 2003). A recent randomized trial showed that continuous positive airway pressure for 1 month leads to improvement in the number of apneas, systolic blood pressure, heart rate, left ventricular end-systolic dimension, and left ventricular ejection fraction (Kaneko et al. 2003). Central sleep apnea does not severely exacerbate negative intrathoracic pressure, but it does produce periodic sympathetic arousals and increased afterload and myocardial work (Bradley and Floras 2003b) (see also Chapter 16, "Sleep Disorders").

Stress Management and Health Education Interventions in CAD Patients

A large meta-analysis of a variety of health-education and stress-reduction interventions in patients with CAD concluded that these interventions reduce the incidence of recurrent MI (29% reduction) and death (34% reduction) at 2- to 10-year follow-up. The mechanism of the effect is unclear; these analyses do not consistently demonstrate a reduction in mental symptoms (i.e., anxiety and depression ratings are not reduced) (Dusseldorp et al. 1999).

Psychoeducational programs may include varying components of health education, stress management, and supervised exercise training; and many individual reports fail to give specific details of the interventions. Successful effects on proximal targets such as systolic blood pressure, cholesterol, body weight, smoking behavior, physical exercise, and emotional distress or some combination of these mediate the beneficial effects for mortality. For recurrent MI, protective effects of psychoeducational intervention were associated with beneficial effects on systolic blood pressure, smoking behavior, physical exercise, and emotional distress. Patients who participate in psychoeducational programs are three times more likely to be successful in quitting smoking (Dusseldorp et al. 1999). Longer intervention programs with more hours of intervention and more tailoring of program content to individual needs appear to have greater long-term effect on cardiac outcomes (Linden 2000; Linden et al. 1996).

Diagnostic Issues

Most psychiatric diagnoses are reached in a straightforward fashion in patients with heart disease, but confusion may arise because of the overlap of symptoms of heart disease with symptoms of psychiatric disorder and because treatments for heart disease may cause psychiatric side effects. The most frequent problem in psychiatric diagnosis is the attribution of symptoms of depression to the underlying cardiac disease or to a "normal" reaction to the illness, with the resultant underdiagnosis of depression. Generally in practice, however, an inclusive approach is appropriate, counting symptoms such as fatigue and poor sleep toward a diagnosis of depression even if the symptoms might also be attributable to the patient's cardiac condition (Cohen-Cole and Kauffman 1993) (see also Chapter 9, "Depression"). In an analysis of the 222 acute MI patients included in the landmark Montreal Heart Institute depression-mortality study, the investigators considered the specificity of various symptoms from the depression criteria set for a diagnosis of depression. Sleep disturbance and appetite disturbance did not help to distinguish between patients who met criteria for depressive episode and those who did not (i.e., these symptoms were common in both depressed and nondepressed patients), but fatigue and especially sadness and loss of pleasure occurred almost exclusively in patients who met criteria for a major depressive episode (Lesperance et al. 1996). This suggests that patients reporting somatic symptoms of depression should be evaluated for the presence of the cardinal mood and interest symptoms, and they should be considered depressed if these symptoms are also present.

Patients with advanced heart failure often develop appetite loss and cachexia, but in the absence of loss of self-esteem, interest in ordinarily interesting events, or depressed mood, these patients should not be diagnosed with a depressive disorder.

Paroxysmal supraventricular tachycardia (PSVT) occurs in young and middle-aged adults and may manifest with symptoms of shortness of breath, chest discomfort, and apprehension. Because these features may overlap with those of generalized anxiety symptoms and panic attacks, there is a significant risk of misdiagnosis. In a retrospective study of 107 patients with PSVT, DSM-IV criteria for panic disorder were met in 59 patients (67%) (American Psychiatric Association 1994); PSVT had been unrecognized after initial medical evaluation in 55% and remained unrecognized for a median of 3.3 years. Prior to the eventual identification of PSVT, nonpsychiatric physicians attributed symptoms to panic, anxiety, or stress in 32 (54%) of the 59 patients (Lessmeier et al. 1997). Of course, some patients may have both PSVT and an anxiety disorder, with symptomatic attacks including elements of each.

Atypical Chest Pain and Palpitations

Typical anginal chest pain in CAD occurs with exertion or after eating; is not exacerbated by palpation of the chest or inspiration; is described as dull, pressurelike, or burning rather than sharp or stabbing; and is experienced across the precordium rather than in a pinpoint area of the left side of the chest. Many patients present for evaluation of atypical chest pain. While atypical features do not rule out a diagnosis of CAD, 40%–70% of patients with no history of documented CAD and few CAD risk factors have panic disorder, somatoform disorders, or depression (Alexander et al. 1994; Fleet et al. 2000). In the absence of CAD, characteristics of chest pain patients predicting panic disorder include female sex, atypical chest pain quality, younger age, lower education and income, and high self-reported anxiety (Dammen et al. 1999; Huffman and Pollack 2003). A study of 199 outpatient cardiology clinic chest pain patients found that a three-item questionnaire (Table 19–2), with a cutoff score of 5 points, correctly identified 74% of patients with panic disorder with a sensitivity of 55% and a specificity of 86%. Panic disorder is twice as likely in chest pain patients without CAD as in patients with CAD (Dammen et al. 1999; Fleet et al. 2000).

Psychiatric disorders are also common in patients complaining of palpitations. In one study using structured diagnostic interviews and self-report questionnaires for patients undergoing ambulatory electrocardiogram (ECG)

TABLE 19–2. Screening questions for panic disorder in patients with atypical chest pain

When nervous or frightened, patient thinks he or she will pass out.	(never = 1, always = 5)
In past 7 days, patient has been bothered by pain in the heart or chest.	(not at all = 0, extremely = 4)
Pain is experienced as tiring or exhausting.	(no = 0, severe = 3)

Note. A cutoff score of 5 correctly identifies 74% of patients with panic disorder in the outpatient setting.
Source. Dammen et al. 1999.

monitoring, the lifetime prevalence of any disorder was 45%, and 25% of the patients had a current disorder. The lifetime prevalence of panic disorder and major depression was 27% and 21%, respectively. Current prevalence of panic disorder was 19% (Barsky et al. 1994b). These rates are probably somewhat higher than in the general population, because they derive from a tertiary care clinic setting.

Special Issues

Heart Transplantation

Heart transplantation has been the treatment of last resort for patients with severe heart failure, and occasionally for patients with intractable recurrent myocardial ischemia or ventricular arrhythmias, for the past 2 decades (see also Chapter 31, "Organ Transplantation"). Because of donor scarcity, the number of heart transplants performed annually in the United States has reached a plateau of approximately 3,000/year. Patients eligible for heart transplantation typically have an expected survival of less than 2 years unless they receive a transplant. With transplantation, expected 5-year survival is now better than 75%. Complications can occur, and the care regimen for heart transplant patients is complicated, especially in the first few months after surgery, so transplant programs generally screen patients and exclude from candidacy those with absolute contraindications or excessive relative contraindications.

These facts provide the context for the "normal" psychological experience of patients entering the process. Patients generally fear that they are close to death, or will experience a sudden catastrophic deterioration in the future, and believe that a transplant is their best hope for survival. Although they may be anxious about the dangers of transplantation, they are even more often anxious about being excluded from candidacy. Consequently, the evaluation period is a time of heightened concern, and pa-

tients meeting with a psychiatrist as part of the evaluation process wonder whether they will "pass" this examination. Patients awaiting transplantation often experience depression symptoms, because they perceive themselves as helpless to fundamentally affect their own chances of survival. During the waiting period, depression is often enhanced by a sense of guilt over wishes for the death of a suitable donor. Patients sometimes describe a kind of psychological ambulance chasing, hearing a siren and wondering whether this might signal the availability of a donor. Before, at the time of evaluation, and up to the time of receiving a transplant, patients may also display variable levels of denial of the seriousness of their illness and ambivalence about undergoing transplant surgery. This minimization or denial of illness can fluctuate and coexist with other emotional responses, including fear, depression, and anxiety. Patients who come to heart transplantation after an acute catastrophic cardiac event, without a prior chronic heart failure syndrome, are especially prone to experience a combination of denial, shock, anger, and fear all at the same time, as they must rapidly assimilate an altered view of their health status, appreciate the associated risks, and appraise the possible risks and benefits of transplantation, before having much opportunity to mourn the loss of their previous health and associated social role. If they are sedated or in a state of altered consciousness because of cardiogenic shock, medication, or metabolic disarray, their capacity to psychologically adjust is further reduced, with more adaptation forced on them after the fact.

Following heart transplant surgery, patients receive multiple immunosuppressive antirejection medications, along with vitamins; minerals; antibacterial, antifungal, and antiviral medications; and treatments as needed for hypertension, arrhythmias, fluid retention, or other conditions. Most patients are hospitalized for 10–20 days after surgery, undergoing surveillance for allograft rejection as the immunosuppressive medication doses are adjusted. (These medications are discussed in Chapter 31, "Organ Transplantation.") High doses of intravenous and then oral corticosteroids are the rule in the initial weeks after transplant surgery, and predictably they induce increased appetite, fluid retention, and mood lability. Most patients experience an initial euphoria at awakening from surgery, knowing that they have now been delivered from end-stage heart failure, but the emotional reaction depends in part on the patient's previous expectations in comparison with the state of subjective well-being in the early days after surgery. Positive feelings tend to subside as complications occur and as the patient settles into the work of rehabilitation and adjustment to the new medication regimen. One or more episodes of rejection are not uncommon in the early period after surgery; if transient corticosteroid dose increases are employed to treat rejection episodes, a medication-exacerbated emotional roller coaster may ensue.

Psychiatric complications after heart transplantation are fairly common. In addition to postoperative delirium, steroid-induced mood disorders and depression not attributable to steroids occur in perhaps 20%–40% of patients in the first year after surgery. Many cases occur in the setting of medical complications, but role transitions are often difficult for the recovering patient, and stressors such as increased demand for autonomous function or the need to provide for others in the family, difficulty negotiating return to work, or financial concerns that were previously ignored often stimulate increased emotional distress (Shapiro 1990; Shapiro and Kornfeld 1989). Some heart transplant patients experience transplantation-related posttraumatic stress disorder following particularly frightening or troubling episodes during their care, appear psychologically fixated on these events and subjectively distressed, and are impaired in their daily functioning long after the transplant (Dew et al. 2001).

Left Ventricular Assist Devices

The shortage of available donors of hearts for transplantation and the large number of patients dying of congestive heart failure provided impetus even early in the era of heart transplantation for the development of artificial heart technology (Goldstein and Oz 2000). In addition to attempting to devise a total artificial heart, researchers have developed and tested a variety of ventricular assist pumps over the past decade. To date, experience with total artificial hearts has been characterized by limited success—limited patient survival compromised by stroke, infection, and poor quality of life. Ventricular assist devices, however, have been more successful and are in widespread use as rescue devices—that is, bridges to heart transplantation or in some cases bridges to recovery after acute myocardial injury (Goldstein and Oz 2000). Early experience with use of left ventricular assist devices (LVADs) designed to be used for periods of weeks to months as a bridge to transplantation indicated that significant neuropsychiatric issues were delirium, stroke, cognitive impairment, pain, and depressed mood. Depression seemed especially linked to frustration with ongoing limitations in function as a result of tethering to the device, and cerebrovascular and cognitive problems were associated with a history of even minor or transient cerebrovascular disease symptoms before LVAD surgery (Shapiro et al. 1996). For most patients, quality of life with LVADs was superior to that while they were in severe heart failure (Dew et al. 1998,

1999a, 1999b). Ongoing improvements in device design have reduced the mechanical problems of attachment to an external device to a considerable degree and are likely to continue to do so (Goldstein and Oz 2000).

The success of LVAD use as a bridge to transplantation led to study of permanent ("destination") LVAD treatment for patients with end-stage heart failure who could not receive a heart transplant (Rose et al. 1999). The REMATCH trial, a randomized clinical trial providing either optimized medical therapy or LVAD therapy for patients with severe chronic heart failure, demonstrated a substantial survival benefit associated with LVADs, along with improved quality of life outcomes (Rose et al. 2001). Interestingly, somatic dimensions of quality of life were substantially better in LVAD recipients, but mental-emotional components did not differ from those of medically treated heart failure patients (Shapiro et al. 2002). Postoperative delirium was the most important psychiatric problem seen in the LVAD patients in this study (Lazar et al. 2004). The success of LVAD treatment in extending survival without worsening quality of life in the REMATCH trial led to approval by the U.S. Food and Drug Administration of destination LVAD therapy for nonexperimental use in the United States in 2002. Although issues of cost, patient selection, and criteria for approval of cardiac surgical centers by regulatory agencies continue to limit availability, it is likely that destination ventricular assist device therapy will become more widespread in the next several years. Continuous device modifications make it difficult to extrapolate the neuropsychiatric and quality-of-life implications from past data.

Hypertension

The relationship of psychological factors to the development of hypertension has been a subject of controversy, with mixed findings in large-scale observational studies.

In a cross-sectional correlation of psychological variables with mild hypertension measured in clinic visits or by ambulatory monitoring in 283 middle-aged men, there were no significant differences between normotensive and hypertensive men in any of the psychological variables assessed, including type A behavior, state and trait anger, anger expression, anxiety, psychological distress, locus of control, or attributional style (Friedman et al. 2001). In one study that noted an increased prevalence of panic disorder in patients with hypertension compared with normotensive comparison primary care patients, the onset of panic occurred after the diagnosis of hypertension in most cases. Thus the study does not support the idea that panic gives rise to hypertension (Davies et al. 1999).

A 15-year prospective study of psychosocial risk factors for hypertension based on a follow-up of over 3,000 young white and black adults from four metropolitan areas of the United States used multivariate analysis, including age, sex, gender, body mass index, race, and baseline blood pressure, and found that two components of type A behavior—namely, "time urgency–impatience" and "hostility"—were each associated with almost double the rate of incident hypertension at 15-year follow-up. In contrast, anxiety symptoms, depression symptoms, and "achievement-striving-competitiveness" (another type A component) did not predict hypertension (Yan et al. 2003). In another large longitudinal study, however, results differed.

A population-based cohort of 3310 normotensive persons without chronic diseases from the NHANES I Epidemiologic Follow-up Study was followed for four waves, up to 22 years. Using Cox proportional hazards regression analysis, controlling for baseline blood pressure (BP), age, sex, race, education, smoking, alcohol use, body mass index (BMI), and change in BMI over time, and using combined symptoms of depression and anxiety ("negative affect") as the primary independent variable, increased negative affect was associated with increased risk for hypertension. The risk for treated hypertension was increased in both men and women and was most pronounced (over threefold) in black women (Jonas and Lando 2000).

In addition to these individual large-scale studies, a recent review (Rutledge and Hogan 2002) examined 15 prospective studies of psychological traits affecting the development of hypertension. These studies included samples of 78 to 4,650 subjects, and most cohorts were primarily male- and white-dominated. The length of follow-up varied from 2.5 to 21 years. Psychological variables included anger, anxiety, depression, defensiveness, neuroticism, and "psychopathology." Small but significant effects were observed for anger, anxiety, depression, and other variables, with an overall magnitude of effect suggesting an 8% increase in prospective hypertension risk associated with a high level of one or more of the psychological variables. A smaller number of studies separately reported the effect of psychological factors on hypertension in African Americans and in women. In African Americans the same psychological predictors appeared to be associated with hypertension. In women, the results were equivocal.

The main psychiatric consequence of hypertension seems to be long-term neurocognitive impairment and increased risk of dementia (Frishman 2002). Treatment that successfully controls blood pressure reduces the risk (Forette et al. 2002; Guo et al. 1999; Launer et al. 1995). The data demonstrate that dihydropyridine calcium chan-

nel blockers reduce the risk of dementia of probable Alzheimer's disease, as well as vascular or mixed dementia, and improve or maintain cognitive function in patients with impaired cognition.

Congenital Heart Disease

The prevalence of psychiatric disorders in adult survivors of congenital heart disease is unknown. The existence of this clinical population depends largely on advances in pediatric cardiac surgery over the past 3 decades, and adult survivors have not been systematically studied from a psychiatric standpoint. Clinical experience suggests that although many patients appear to have excellent psychological adjustment, anxiety is common.

Some studies have examined children and adolescents. One evaluated 243 children, age 5 years, who had been treated for congenital heart defects. Full-Scale IQ, Verbal IQ, and Performance IQ were all in the normal range. Lower socioeconomic status and velocardiofacial syndrome predicted lower Full-Scale IQ. Single ventricle diagnosis, longer ICU stay, and duration of hypothermic circulatory arrest showed trends toward association with lower Full-Scale IQ (Forbess et al. 2002). For cyanotic conditions, but not for acyanotic lesions, delayed repair appears to exacerbate intellectual impairment (Newburger et al. 1984). Other common psychological problems for children and young adults with congenital heart disease include concerns about exclusion from participation in peer-group activities such as sports and gym class, problems with appearance (short stature, cyanosis, drug side effects on appearance), concerns about attractiveness, capacity to develop intimate relationships, exclusion from work, and fears about mortality (Kendall et al. 2001).

Treatment Issues

Psychotherapy

Psychological reactions to the experience of heart disease include feelings of anxiety and sadness and concerns about survival, well-being, and effects on social roles, relationships, and the impact on loved ones. Denial is nearly universal as an initial reaction to illness, and it can be helpful in staving off depressed and anxious mood or hurtful because of nonadherence to the treatment program. Conversely, preoccupation with disease can lead to abnormal illness behavior, unnecessary disability, and impaired quality of life. Few systematic studies of psychotherapy have been reported that specifically targeted psychological symptoms or psychiatric disorders in heart patients. As was described previously, a larger number of studies have described stress management or health education effects on cardiac outcomes in cardiac rehabilitation settings; meta-analyses of these studies do show beneficial effects on cardiac outcomes and suggest that reducing emotional distress may be correlated with better cardiac disease outcomes (Dusseldorp et al. 1999; Linden et al. 1996).

The ENRICHD trial tested the effects of a CBT intervention versus usual care in patients who had a recent MI and either low social support and/or major depression or minor depression with a history of prior major depression in a randomized trial. Patients in the intervention arm participated in either individual or group therapy sessions; treatment was manualized; and therapist adherence to treatment methods was assessed during the trial. Most patients received 6–10 therapy sessions. The trial demonstrated a modest benefit of the CBT intervention on measures of social support and depression. However, the improvement on these measures seen in the usual-care group was higher than expected, so that the effect of treatment, although statistically significant, was of small magnitude (Writing Committee for the ENRICHD Investigators 2003).

As described previously, the Recurrent Coronary Prevention Project tested the effect of group type A behavior modification on the extent of type A behavior in a cohort of post-MI patients on recurrent coronary events (Friedman et al. 1986). In retrospect, although the term was not used at the time, this was clearly a cognitive-behavioral psychotherapy intervention. The intervention had a strong beneficial effect on type A behavior as rated using a videotaped structured interview for the assessment of type A behavior.

Interpersonal psychotherapy (IPT) of depression focuses on present-day interpersonal problems linked to depressed mood, such as interpersonal disputes, grief after object loss, interpersonal deficits, and social role transitions. One such role transition may occur with the change in social role imposed by development of a chronic or acute medical illness (Klerman et al. 1984). Therefore IPT would seem to be readily applicable to the treatment of patients who experience depression after the onset or exacerbation of heart disease. Although a case has been reported (Stuart and Cole 1996), controlled trials of IPT in heart disease patients have not appeared.

Psychopharmacological Treatment

Common adverse cardiac effects of psychiatric drugs are shown in Table 19–3 (see also Chapter 37, "Psychopharmacology").

Antidepressants

Antidepressants must be used in therapeutically effective doses in cardiac patients with depression, and it is counterproductive to use inadequate doses out of fear of side effects or prolongation of metabolism. Unless the patient has severe right heart failure resulting in hepatic congestion, ascites, and jaundice, it is unlikely that metabolism of oral psychotropic medication (except for lithium) will be substantially impaired because of heart disease.

Tricyclic antidepressants (TCAs) cause orthostatic hypotension, cardiac conduction delay (bundle branch block or complete AV nodal block), and, in overdose, ventricular arrhythmias (ventricular premature depolarization, ventricular tachycardia, and ventricular fibrillation). QRS interval prolongation results from interference with phase 1 depolarization (slow Na^+ channel activity) of the action potential across the membrane of the specialized conduction tissue of the ventricle. Prolongation of the QT interval is predominantly caused by prolongation of the

TABLE 19–3. Selected cardiac side effects of psychotropic drugs	
Drug	**Cardiac effects**
Lithium	Sinus node dysfunction and arrest
SSRIs	Slowing of heart rate; occasional sinus bradycardia or sinus arrest
TCAs	Orthostatic hypotension; atrioventricular conduction disturbance; type IA antiarrhythmic effect; proarrhythmia in overdose and in setting of ischemia
MAOIs	Orthostatic hypotension
Phenothiazines	Orthostatic hypotension, QT interval prolongation; rare instances of torsade de pointes
Second-generation antipsychotics	Variable; QT interval prolongation
Carbamazepine	Type IA antiarrhythmic effects; AV block
Cholinesterase inhibitors	Decreased heart rate

Note. AV=atrioventricular; MAOI=monoamine oxidase inhibitor; SSRI=selective serotonin reuptake inhibitor; TCA=tricyclic antidepressant.

QRS interval, and ventricular tachycardia or fibrillation can occur if marked prolongation of the QT interval (over 500 msec) results in the R-on-T phenomenon. Nortriptyline and desipramine tend to cause less orthostatic hypotension than tertiary-amine tricyclic drugs and are better tolerated by patients with cardiac disease (Roose and Glassman 1989; Roose et al. 1986, 1987, 1989). Cardiac pacemakers can obviate the risk of heart block associated with TCAs. More commonly problematic, however, is orthostatic hypotension, which can result in syncope and falls.

TCAs have quinidine-like effects on cardiac conduction and are classified as type 1A antiarrhythmic agents. Drugs of this class have been shown to increase rather than decrease mortality in post-MI patients with premature ventricular contractions (CAST Investigators 1989; CAST II Investigators 1992; Morganroth and Goin 1991), an effect believed to be mediated by episodic myocardial ischemia (Lynch et al. 1987). Consequently, TCAs should generally not be used as first-line agents for treatment of depression in ischemic heart disease patients. This is not to say that they should never be used, however, because their efficacy may offset the risk for selected patients. Consideration should be given to the totality of the clinical situation, including the severity of depression, past treatment responses, concomitant medications, and ECG (Glassman et al. 1993).

SSRIs have little to no cardiac effect in healthy subjects. The most commonly observed effect is slowing of heart rate, generally by a clinically insignificant 1–2 beats/minute. Occasional cases of sinus bradycardia or sinus arrest, with lightheadedness or syncope, have been reported (Roose et al. 1994, 1998a, 1998b). The combination of beta-adrenergic blockade and serotonin reuptake inhibitors may result in additive effects on slowing of heart rate with increased risk of symptoms. In addition, some SSRIs (fluoxetine, paroxetine, fluvoxamine) inhibit metabolism through the cytochrome P450 2D6 pathway responsible for metabolism of many beta-blockers. Therefore, the blood level and effect of beta-adrenergic blockers may be increased.

In patients with preexisting heart disease, the effects of SSRIs on cardiac function have been evaluated in several studies (Sheline et al. 1997). Some studies using fluoxetine and paroxetine in mixed groups of stable patients with ischemic and nonischemic heart disease demonstrate that ejection fraction may actually improve to a small extent in patients with preexisting ventricular dysfunction. The effects on heart rate are similar to those seen in patients who are free of cardiac disease, and no blood pressure, cardiac conduction, or arrhythmia effects have been noted (Roose et al. 1994, 1998a, 1998b). The SADHART

study, as described previously, was a double-blind, placebo-controlled, randomized trial examining the effect of sertraline in patients with major depression immediately after an acute coronary syndrome. Sertraline had no effect on heart rate, blood pressure, arrhythmias, ejection fraction, or cardiac conduction, and adverse events were rare. All patients in SADHART began medication within 30 days of the index acute coronary event (Glassman et al. 2002). Sertraline was effective for treatment of depression in those patients with a prior history of depression, but it did not differ from placebo in response rate for those patients with no prior history of depression.

The cardiovascular effects of other antidepressants have been less fully studied, especially in patients with cardiac disease. Bupropion appears to have few cardiovascular effects in small studies but may cause hypertension in some patients (Roose et al. 1991). The serotonin-norepinephrine reuptake inhibitor venlafaxine behaves as an SSRI at low doses and displays a noradrenergic effect at higher doses. The main cardiovascular effect of this dual action is a tendency to increase blood pressure in a dose-dependent fashion at a dosage of 150 mg/day or higher. There may be a diminution of this hypertensive effect of venlafaxine with its extended-release formulation. The effect on patients with preexisting heart disease or hypertension has not been evaluated. Clinical experience with mirtazapine in patients with hypertension has also demonstrated instances of worsening hypertension, but the frequency of this adverse effect is unknown. Monoamine oxidase inhibitors (MAOIs) cause hypotension and orthostatic hypotension; dietary indiscretions resulting in high circulating levels of tyramine cause hypertensive crises. Consequently, there has been little interest in use of MAOIs in patients with heart disease. Sympathomimetic agents increase blood pressure in patients on MAOIs, though hypertensive crises are actually infrequent. Caution with the use of intravenous pressors (epinephrine, isoproterenol, norepinephrine, dopamine, dobutamine) is required (Krishnan 1995).

Antipsychotics

Antipsychotics are used in cardiac disease patients in cases of comorbid schizophrenia or other psychotic disorders and in the management of delirium in acute cardiac care settings, such as after cardiac surgery or in ICU management of pulmonary edema, arrhythmias, or acute MI. Although first-generation antipsychotic medications are losing primacy as agents of choice for management of chronic psychosis because of their extrapyramidal side effects, they continue to play a role in management of acute psychotic symptoms in delirium. In part this is because of the availability of parenteral formulations for haloperidol, few cardiovascular effects, and extensive experience with use of intravenous haloperidol in the critically ill (see Chapter 6, "Delirium").

For chronically psychotic patients with heart disease, the choice of antipsychotic is based on side-effect profile. The principal cardiovascular effects of antipsychotic agents are orthostatic hypotension and QT interval prolongation. Orthostatic hypotension secondary to antipsychotic drugs is related to their α-adrenergic receptor blocking effect, seen especially with the low-potency antipsychotic agents such as chlorpromazine and often accompanied by sedative effects. There are few data about the frequency or clinical significance of orthostatic effects of antipsychotic drugs in patients with heart disease. More attention has been paid to the less common but much more dramatic and dangerous side effect of cardiac arrest secondary to ventricular tachyarrhythmias in patients on antipsychotic drugs. The characteristic tachyarrhythmia is *torsade de pointes*, a polymorphic tachycardia with the appearance of "twisting of the points" of the QRS complex. Risk factors for torsade include QT interval prolongation of more than 500 msec, family history of sudden death, female sex, hypokalemia, hypomagnesemia, and low ejection fraction. QT prolongation as a result of antipsychotic agents, unlike that caused by TCAs, appears to be an effect of impaired repolarization of the ventricular conduction tissue at the end of systole, specifically an effect on the so-called potassium rectifier channel. The QT interval normally is less than 450 msec. Because the normal QT interval is dependent on heart rate, evaluation customarily adjusts for heart rate to yield a corrected QT interval (QTc). Thioridazine is the agent most commonly associated with torsade and sudden cardiac death, and sertindole was withdrawn in the United States because of its QT prolongation effects and the rate of sudden cardiac deaths observed overseas. Intravenous haloperidol is frequently employed in delirious open-heart surgery patients, and although it does have the potential to prolong the QT interval, its use in dosages up to 1,000 mg/24 hours has been reported without complications (Tesar et al. 1985). Clearly, electrocardiographic monitoring is important in ICU settings, and patients with a QTc interval greater than 450 msec should be closely monitored. A QTc interval over 500 msec is generally considered a contraindication to use of haloperidol and other QT-prolonging agents.

Not all antipsychotic drugs have been associated with sudden cardiac death or QT prolongation, and the correlation of QT interval prolongation with risk of sudden death is not exact. For example, ziprasidone prolongs the QT interval but has not been associated with sudden death. Olanzapine, risperidone, and quetiapine have not been associated with QT prolongation or sudden death. In considering the use of drugs that may prolong the QT interval, factors to be reviewed in the history include familial long QT syndrome; family or personal history of sudden cardiac death, syncope, or unexplained seizure; arrhythmias; personal history of hypertension; medications that prolong the QT interval; medications that may interfere with metabolism of other QT-prolonging agents; valvular heart disease; and bradycardia. Laboratory values of particular importance are magnesium and potassium levels. Class IA and III antiarrhythmic drugs, dolasetron, droperidol, tacrolimus, levomethadyl acetate, other antipsychotic agents, many antibiotics ("floxacins"), and antifungal agents may increase the risk of torsade de pointes (Al-Khatib 2003; Glassman and Bigger 2001; Moss 2003).

Anxiolytics

Benzodiazepines have no specific cardiac effects. Reduction of anxiety tends to reduce sympathetic nervous system activation and, therefore, to slow heart rate, reduce myocardial work, and reduce myocardial irritability. Before the introduction of beta-blockers to acute coronary care, benzodiazepines were widely used for prophylaxis of infarct extension and arrhythmias in acute coronary syndrome patients, but this practice has largely been abandoned. Lorazepam can be given by intramuscular (or intravenous) injection; for most other benzodiazepines this route should be avoided because of poor absorption. Buspirone has no cardiovascular effects.

Stimulants

Stimulants are often useful for treating of depressed, medically ill patients, particularly those with pronounced apathy, fatigue, or psychomotor slowing. At dosages of 5–30 mg/day, dextroamphetamine and methylphenidate are well tolerated by heart disease patients, including patients with cardiac arrhythmias and angina (Masand and Tesar 1996), and have no effects on heart rate and blood pressure. Clinical response generally occurs within days rather than weeks.

Lithium

Lithium occasionally causes sinus node dysfunction and even sinus arrest (Mitchell and Mackenzie 1982). There are no studies of the use of lithium in patients with heart disease. Generally, even in patients with heart disease with reduced cardiac output, lithium can be safely used by adjusting the dosage downward. Because renal function is sometimes impaired in advanced heart failure, lithium dosing requires further reduction. Caution is necessary for patients taking diuretics, especially thiazides, and those on salt-restricted diets. In patients with acute congestive heart failure exacerbations and acute coronary syndromes, rapid electrolyte and fluid balance shifts can occur; lithium is best avoided during such episodes because of the difficulty managing fluctuations in lithium level as cardiac therapy is adjusted.

Other Mood Stabilizers

Valproic acid and lamotrigine have no cardiovascular effects. Carbamazepine resembles TCAs in having a quinidine-like type IA antiarrhythmic effect and may cause atrioventricular conduction disturbances.

Cholinesterase Inhibitors and NMDA Receptor Antagonists

The elderly are prone to co-occurrence of dementia and heart disease, and relatively new treatments for dementia, including cholinesterase inhibitors (donepezil, rivastigmine, galantamine) and NMDA inhibitors (memantine), are likely to be used increasingly in patients with concurrent heart disease. The procholinergic effect of cholinesterase inhibitors may cause vagotonic effects, including bradycardia or heart block. For memantine, hypertension is the only cardiac effect described by the manufacturer on the basis of premarketing controlled trials.

Electroconvulsive Therapy

Electroconvulsive therapy (ECT) leads to an initial sympathetic discharge, with tachycardia and hypertension, followed by a parasympathetic reflex response, with instances of bradycardia and arrhythmia. Asystole can occur rarely but can be prevented by premedication with atropine. Excessive sympathetic response may evoke myocardial ischemia; for the elderly or those with known coronary disease, monitoring the ECG is essential, and

treatment with intravenous beta-blockers is sometimes required. Cardiac effects of ECT are discussed in Chapter 39, "Electroconvulsive Therapy". ECT has been used safely in patients with ischemic heart disease, heart failure, and heart transplants. Acute MI or recent malignant tachyarrhythmias are relatively strong contraindications.

Cardiac–Psychiatric Drug Interactions

A few drug interactions between psychotropic and cardiovascular drugs are worth noting (see Table 19–4). Many psychotropic drugs lower blood pressure; their interaction with antihypertensive medications, vasodilators, and diuretics may potentiate hypotension. TCAs and antipsychotic drugs that prolong the QT interval may interact with antiarrhythmic agents such as quinidine, procainamide, moricizine, and amiodarone and result in further QT prolongation or atrioventricular block.

Drug Interactions: Cytochrome P450 Issues

Cytochrome P450 2D6 is responsible for the metabolism of many beta-blockers, carvedilol, and antiarrhythmic agents; this metabolic pathway is inhibited by haloperidol, fluoxetine, and paroxetine, with resulting elevation of blood levels of 2D6 substrates. Conversely, amiodarone is a 2D6 inhibitor and can elevate blood levels of amitriptyline, nortriptyline, clomipramine, codeine, desipramine, fluoxetine, and risperidone. Cytochrome P450 3A4 is responsible for metabolism of alprazolam, midazolam, triazolam, zolpidem, buspirone, carbamazepine, and haloperidol and of calcium channel blockers, cyclosporine, many statin agents, and tacrolimus. The 3A4 system is inhibited by amiodarone, diltiazem, verapamil, grapefruit juice, and nefazodone, and to a lesser degree by fluoxetine and sertraline. The combination of nefazodone

TABLE 19–4. Selected psychotropic drug interactions with cardiovascular drugs

Psychotropic agent	Cardiovascular agent	Effect
SSRIs	Beta-blockers	Additive bradycardic effects
SSRIs	Warfarin	Increased bleeding risk, despite little effect on INR
MAOIs	Epinephrine, dopamine	Hypertension
Lithium	Thiazide diuretics	Increased lithium level
TCAs	Guanethidine	Reduced antihypertensive efficacy of guanethidine
TCAs	Type IA antiarrhythmic agents, amiodarone	Prolong QT interval, increase AV block
Lithium	ACE inhibitors	Increase lithium level
Phenothiazines	Beta-blockers	Hypotension

Note. ACE=angiotensin-converting enzyme; AV=atrioventricular; INR=international normalized ratio; MAOI=monoamine oxidase inhibitor; SSRI=selective serotonin reuptake inhibitor; TCA=tricyclic antidepressant.

and haloperidol might increase the risk of ventricular arrhythmias, because increased haloperidol levels may result in greater QT prolongation. Carbamazepine and St. John's wort are inducers of 3A4 activity. An evolving reference listing for P450 interactions is available on the World Wide Web (Flockhart 2003), and these interactions are also reviewed in Chapter 37, "Psychopharmacology".

References

Alexander PJ, Prabhu SG, Krishnamoorthy ES, et al: Mental disorders in patients with noncardiac chest pain. Acta Psychiatr Scand 89:291–293, 1994

Al-Khatib SM, LaPointe NMA, Kramer JM, et al: What clinicians should know about the QT interval. JAMA 289:2120–2127, 2003

American Psychiatric Association: Diagnostic and Statistical Manual of Mental Disorders, 4th Edition. Washington, DC, American Psychiatric Association, 1994

Anda R, Williamson D, Jones D, et al: Depressed affect, hopelessness, and the risk of ischemic heart disease in a cohort of U.S. adults. Epidemiology 4:285–294, 1993

Barefoot J, Schroll M: Symptoms of depression, acute myocardial infarction, and total mortality in a community sample. Circulation 93:1976–1980, 1996

Barefoot JC, Patterson JC, Haney TL, et al: Hostility in asymptomatic men with angiographically confirmed coronary artery disease. Am J Cardiol 74:439–442, 1994

Barefoot JC, Larsen S, Von der Lieth L, et al: Hostility, incidence of acute myocardial infarction, and mortality in a sample of older Danish men and women. Am J Epidemiol 142:477–484, 1995

Barefoot JC, Helms MJ, Mark DB, et al: Depression and long term mortality risk in patients with coronary artery disease. Am J Cardiol 78:613–617, 1996

Barlow DH: Anxiety and Its Disorders. New York, Guilford, 1988

Barsky AJ: Palpitations, cardiac awareness, and panic disorder. Am J Med 92 (suppl. 1A):31S–34S, 1992

Barsky AJ, Cleary PD, Sarnie MK, et al: Panic disorder, palpitations, and the awareness of cardiac activity. J Nerv Ment Dis 182:63–71, 1994a

Barsky AJ, Cleary PD, Coeytaux RR, et al: Psychiatric disorders in medical outpatients complaining of palpitations. J Gen Intern Med 9:306–313, 1994b

Barsky AJ, Delamater BA, Clancy SA, et al: Somatized psychiatric disorder presenting as palpitations. Arch Intern Med 156:1102–1108, 1996

Bigger JT, Fleiss JL, Steinman RC, et al: Frequency domain measures of heart period variability and mortality after myocardial infarction. Circulation 85:164–171, 1992

Bigger JT, Fleiss JL, Rolnitzky LM, et al: Frequency domain measures of heart period variability to assess risk late after myocardial infarction. J Am Coll Cardiol 21:729–736, 1993

Blumenthal JA, Jiang W, Waugh RA, et al: Mental stress-induced ischemia in the laboratory and ambulatory ischemia during daily life. Association and hemodynamic features. Circulation 92:2102–2108, 1995

Blumenthal JA, Lett HS, Babyak MA, et al: Depression as a risk factor for mortality after coronary artery bypass surgery. Lancet 362:604–609, 2003

Booth-Kewley S, Friedman HS: Psychological predictors of heart disease: a quantitative review. Psychol Bull 101:343–362, 1987

Bradley TD, Floras JS: Sleep apnea and heart failure, I: obstructive sleep apnea. Circulation 107:1671–1678, 2003a

Bradley TD, Floras JS: Sleep apnea and heart failure, II: central sleep apnea. Circulation 107:1822–1826, 2003b

Brown TM, Stoudemire A: Cardiovascular agents, in Psychiatric Side Effects of Prescription and Over the Counter Drugs. Washington, DC, American Psychiatric Press, 1998, pp 209–238

Carney RM, Freedland KE, Ludbrook PA, et al: Major depression, panic disorder, and mitral valve prolapse in patients who complain of chest pain. Am J Med 89:757–760, 1990

Carney RM, Blumenthal JA, Stein PK, et al: Depression, heart rate variability, and acute myocardial infarction. Circulation 104:2024–2028, 2001

Carney RM, Freedland KE, Miller GE, et al: Depression as a risk factor for cardiac mortality and morbidity. A review of potential mechanisms. J Psychosom Res 53:897–902, 2002

Carney RM, Blumenthal JA, Catellier D, et al: Depression as a risk factor for mortality after acute myocardial infarction. Am J Cardiol 92:1277–1281, 2003

Cassem NH. The person confronting death, in The New Harvard Guide to Psychiatry. Edited by Nicholi AM Jr. Cambridge, MA, Harvard University Press, 1985, pp 728–758

CAST Investigators: Preliminary report: effect of encainide and flecainide on mortality in a randomized trial of arrhythmia suppression after myocardial infarction. N Engl J Med 321:406–412, 1989

CAST II Investigators: Effect of the antiarrhythmic agent moricizine on survival after myocardial infarction. New Engl J Med 327:227–233, 1992

Cazeau S, Leclercq C, Lavergne T, et al: Effects of multisite biventricular pacing in patients with heart failure and intraventricular conduction delay. N Engl J Med 344:873–880, 2001

Cesari M, Penninx BWJH, Newman AB, et al: Inflammatory markers and onset of cardiovascular events: results from the health ABC study. Circulation 108:2317–2322, 2003

Cohen-Cole SA, Kauffman KG: Major depression in physical illness: diagnosis, prevalence, and antidepressant treatment. A ten year review: 1982–1992. Depression 1:181–204, 1993

Cohn JN: The management of chronic heart failure. N Engl J Med 335:490–498, 1996

Connerney I, Shapiro PA, McLaughlin JS, et al: Relation between depression after coronary artery bypass surgery and 12-month outcome: a prospective study. Lancet 358:1766–1771, 2001

Coryell W: Panic disorder and mortality. Psychiatr Clin North Am 2:433–440, 1988

Coryell W, Noyes R, House JD: Mortality among outpatients with anxiety disorders. Am J Psychiatry 143:508–510, 1986

Crow SJ, Collins J, Justic M, et al: Psychopathology following cardioverter defibrillator implantation. Psychosomatics 39: 305–310, 1998

Dager SR, Comess KA, Dunner DL: Differentiation of anxious patients by two-dimensional echocardiographic evaluation of the mitral valve. Am J Psychiatry 143:533–535, 1986

Dammen T, Ekeberg O, Arnesen H, et al: The detection of panic disorder in chest pain patients. Gen Hosp Psychiatry 21:323–332, 1999

Davies SJ, Ghahramani P, Jackson PR, et al: Association of panic disorder and panic attacks with hypertension. Am J Med 107:310–316, 1999

DeBusk RF: Sexual activity in patients with angina. JAMA 290: 3129–3132, 2003

DeSilva RA: Central nervous system risk factors for sudden cardiac death. J S C Med Assoc 561–572, 1983

DeSilva RA: Cardiac arrhythmias and sudden cardiac death, in Medical-Psychiatric Practice. Edited by Stoudemire A, Fogel BS. Washington, DC, American Psychiatric Press, 1993, pp 199–236

Dew MA, Kormos RL, Nastala C, et al: Psychiatric and psychosocial issues and intervention among ventricular assist device patients, in Quality of Life and Psychosomatics in Mechanical Circulation and Heart Transplantation. Edited by Albert W, Bittner A, Hetzer R. New York, Springer, 1998, pp 17–27

Dew MA, Kormos RL, Winowich S, et al: Human factors in ventricular assist device recipients and their family caregivers. Paper presented at the American Society for Artificial Internal Organs, San Diego CA, June 1999a

Dew MA, Kormos RL, Winowich S, et al: Quality of life outcomes in left ventricular assist system inpatients and outpatients. ASAIO J 45:218–225, 1999b

Dew M, Kormos R, DiMartini A, et al: Prevalence and risk of depression and anxiety-related disorders during the first three years after heart transplantation. Psychosomatics 42: 300–313, 2001

Diegeler A, Hirsch R, Schneider F, et al: Neuromonitoring and neurocognitive outcome in off-pump versus conventional coronary bypass operation. Ann Thoracic Surg 69:1162–1166, 2000

DiMarco JP: Implantable cardioverter-defibrillators. N Engl J Med 349:1836–1847, 2003

Dusseldorp E, Van Elderen T, Maes S, et al: A meta-analysis of psychoeducational programs for coronary heart disease patients. Health Psychol 18:506–519, 1999

Engel GL: Psychologic factors in instantaneous cardiac death. N Engl J Med 294:664–665, 1976

Faris R, Purcell H, Henein MY, et al: Clinical depression is common and significantly associated with reduced survival in patients with non-ischaemic heart failure. Eur J Heart Fail 4:541–551, 2002

Fleet R, Lavoie K, Beitman PD: Is panic disorder associated with coronary artery disease? J Psychosom Res 48:347–356, 2000

Flockhart DA: Drug interactions. Indianapolis, IN, Indiana University School of Medicine, Division of Clinical Pharmacology, 2003. Available at: http://www.drug-interactions.com. Accessed December 2003

Forbess JM, Visconti KJ, Hancock-Friesen C, et al: Neurodevelopmental outcome after congenital heart disease surgery: results from an institutional registry. Circulation 106 (12 suppl 1):I95–I102, 2002

Forette F, Seux ML, Staessen JA, et al: Systolic Hypertension in Europe Investigators. The prevention of dementia with antihypertensive treatment: new evidence from the Systolic Hypertension in Europe (Syst-Eur) study. Arch Intern Med 162:2046–2052, 2002

Frasure-Smith N, Lesperance F, Talajic M: Depression following myocardial infarction. Impact on 6-month survival. JAMA 270:1819–1825, 1993

Frasure-Smith N, Lesperance F, Talajic M: Depression and 18-month prognosis following myocardial infarction. Circulation 91:999–1005, 1995a

Frasure-Smith N, Lesperance F, Talajic M: The impact of negative emotions on prognosis following myocardial infarction: is it more than depression? Health Psychol 14:388–398, 1995b

Frasure-Smith N, Lesperance F, Gravel G, et al: Social support, depression, and mortality during the first year after myocardial infarction. Circulation 101:1919–1924, 2000

Freedland KE, Carney RM, Davila-Roman VG, et al: Major depression and survival in congestive heart failure. Psychosom Med 60:118, 1998

Fricchione GL, Olson LC, Vlay SC: Psychiatric syndromes in patients with the automatic internal cardioverter defibrillator: Anxiety, psychological dependence, abuse, and withdrawal. Am Heart J 117:1411–1414, 1989

Friedman M, Thoresen CE, Gill JJ, et al: Alteration of type A behavior and its effect on cardiac recurrences in post myocardial infarction patients: summary results of the recurrent coronary prevention project. Am Heart J 112:653–665, 1986

Friedman R, Schwartz JE, Schnall PL, et al: Psychological variables in hypertension: relationship to casual or ambulatory blood pressure in men. Psychosom Med 63:19–31, 2001

Frishman WH: Are antihypertensive agents protective against dementia? A review of clinical and preclinical data. Heart Dis 4:380–386, 2002

Glassman AH: Cigarette smoking: implications for psychiatric illness. Am J Psychiatry 150:546–553, 1993

Glassman AH, Bigger JT Jr: Antipsychotic drugs: prolonged QTc interval, Torsade de Pointes and sudden death. Am J Psychiatry 158:1774–1782, 2001

Glassman AH, Shapiro PA: Depression and the course of coronary artery disease. Am J Psychiatry 155:4–11, 1998

Glassman AH, Roose SP, Bigger JT Jr: The safety of tricyclic antidepressants in cardiac patients. Risk-benefit reconsidered. JAMA 269:2673–2675, 1993

Glassman AH, O'Connor CM, Califf RM, et al: Sertraline treatment of major depression in patients with acute MI or unstable angina. JAMA 288:701–709, 2002

Goldstein DJ, Oz MC: Cardiac Assist Devices. Armonk, NY, Futura, 2000

Gorman JM, Goetz RR, Fyer M, et al: The mitral valve prolapse-panic disorder connection. Psychosom Med 50:114–122, 1988

Guo Z, Fratiglioni L, Zhu L, et al: Occurrence and progression of dementia in a community population aged 75 years and older: relationship of antihypertensive medication use. Arch Neurol 56:991–996, 1999

Hamilton SP, Fyer AJ, Durner M, et al: Further genetic evidence for a panic disorder syndrome mapping to chromosome 13q. Proc Natl Acad Sci USA 100:2550–2555, 2003

Hance M, Carney RM, Freedland KE, et al: Depression in patients with coronary heart disease. Gen Hosp Psychiatry 18:61–65, 1996

Heller SS, Ormont MA, Lidagoster LC, et al: Psychosocial outcome after ICD implantation: a current perspective. Pacing Clin Electrophysiol 21:1207–1215, 1998

Huffman JC, Pollack MH: Predicting panic disorder among patients with chest pain: an analysis of the literature. Psychosomatics 44:222–236, 2003

Irvine J, Dorian P, Baker B, et al: Quality of life in the Canadian Implantable Defibrillator Study (CIDS). Am Heart J 144:282–289, 2002

Jessup M, Brozena S: Heart failure. N Engl J Med 348:2007–2018, 2003

Jiang W, Babyak M, Krantz DS, et al: Mental stress-induced myocardial ischemia and cardiac events. JAMA 275:1651–1656, 1996

Jiang W, Alexander J, Christopher E, et al: Relationship of depression to increased risk of mortality and rehospitalization in patients with congestive heart failure. Arch Intern Med 161:1849–1856, 2001

Jonas BS, Lando JF: Negative affect as a prospective risk factor for hypertension. Psychosom Med 62:188–196, 2000

Kaneko Y, Floras JS, Usui K, et al: Cardiovascular effects of continuous positive airway pressure in patients with heart failure and obstructive sleep apnea. N Engl J Med 348:1233–1241, 2003

Kawachi I, Colditz GA, Ascherio A, et al: Prospective study of phobic anxiety and risk of coronary heart disease in men. Circulation 89:1992–1997, 1994a

Kawachi I, Sparrow D, Vokonas PS, et al: Symptoms of anxiety and risk of coronary heart disease. The normative aging study. Circulation 90:2225–2229, 1994b

Kawachi I, Sparrow D, Spiro A III, et al: A prospective study of anger and coronary heart disease: the normative aging study. Circulation 94:2090–2095, 1996

Kendall L, Lewin RJ, Parsons JM, et al: Factors associated with self-perceived state of health in adolescents with congenital cardiac disease attending paediatric cardiologic clinics. Cardiology in the Young 11:431–438, 2001

Kessler RC, Berglund P, Demler O, et al: The epidemiology of major depressive disorder: results from the national comorbidity survey replication (NCS-R). JAMA 289:3095–3105, 2003

Klerman GL, Weissman MM, Rounsaville BJ, et al: Interpersonal psychotherapy of depression. New York, Basic Books, 1984

Ko DT, Hebert PR, Coffey CS, et al: Beta-blocker therapy and symptoms of depression, fatigue, and sexual dysfunction. JAMA 288:351–357, 2002

Kornfeld DS, Zimberg S, Malm JR: Psychiatric complications of open heart surgery. N Engl J Med 273:287–292, 1965

Krishnan KRR: Monoamine oxidase inhibitors, in American Psychiatric Press Textbook of Psychopharmacology. Edited by Schatzberg AF, Nemeroff CB. Washington, DC, American Psychiatric Press, 1995, pp 183–193

Ladwig KH, Kieser M, Konig J, et al: Affective disorders and survival after acute myocardial infarction. Results from the post-infarction late potential study. Eur Heart J 12:959–964, 1991

Laghrissi-Thode F, Wagner WR, Pollack BG, et al: Elevated platelet factor 4 and beta-thromboglobulin plasma levels in depressed patients with ischemic heart disease. Biol Psychiatry 42:290–295, 1997

Lane D, Carroll D, Lip GY: Anxiety, depression, and prognosis after myocardial infarction. Is there a causal association? J Am Coll Cardiol 42:1808–1810, 2003

Launer LJ, Masaki K, Petrovitch H, et al: The association between midlife blood pressure levels and late-life cognitive function. The Honolulu-Asia Aging Study. JAMA 274:1846–1851, 1995

Lazar RM, Shapiro PA, Jaski BE, et al: Neurological events during long-term mechanical circulatory support for heart failure: the REMATCH experience. Circulation 109:2423–2427, 2004

Lee JD, Lee SJ, Tsushima WT, et al: Benefits of off-pump bypass on neurologic and clinical morbidity: a prospective randomized trial. Ann Thorac Surg 76:18–25, 2003

Leor WJ, Poole WK, Kloner RA: Sudden cardiac death triggered by an earthquake. N Engl J Med 334:413–419, 1996

Lesperance F, Frasure-Smith N, Talajic M: Major depression before and after myocardial infarction: its nature and consequences. Psychosom Med 58:99–110, 1996

Lessmeier TJ, Gamperling D, Johnson-Liddon V, et al: Unrecognized paroxysmal supraventricular tachycardia. Potential for misdiagnosis as panic disorder. Arch Intern Med 157:537–543, 1997

Levenson JL, Mishra A, Bauernfeind RA: Denial and medical outcome in unstable angina. Psychosom Med 51:27–35, 1989

Levine J, Warrenberg S, Kerns R: The role of denial in recovery from coronary heart disease. Psychosom Med 49:109–117, 1987

Libby P, Ridker PM, Maseri A: Inflammation and atherosclerosis. Circulation 105:1135–1143, 2002

Liberthson R, Sheehan DV, King ME, et al: The prevalence of mitral valve prolapse in patients with panic disorders. Am J Psychiatry 143:511–515, 1986

Linden W: Psychological treatments in cardiac rehabilitation: review of rationales and outcomes. J Psychosom Res 48:443–454, 2000

Linden W, Stossel C, Maurice J: Psychosocial interventions for patients with coronary artery disease. Arch Intern Med 156:745–752, 1996

Lown B: Role of higher nervous activity in sudden cardiac death. Jpn Circ J 54:581–602, 1990

Lown B, De Silva RA, Reich P, et al: Psychophysiologic factors in sudden cardiac death. Am J Psychiatry 137:1325–1335, 1980

Luutonen S, Holm H, Salminen JK, et al: Inadequate treatment of depression after myocardial infarction. Acta Psychiatr Scand 106:434–439, 2002

Lynch JJ, Dicarlo LA, Montgomery DG, et al: Effects of flecainide acetate on ventricular tachyarrhythmia and fibrillation in dogs with recent myocardial infarction. Pharmacology 35:181–193, 1987

MacMahon KMA, Lip GYH: Psychological factors in heart failure: a review of the literature. Arch Intern Med 162:509–516, 2002

Manuck SB, Krantz DS: Psychophysiologic reactivity in coronary heart disease and essential hypertension, in Handbook of Stress, Reactivity, and Cardiovascular Disease. Edited by Matthews KA, Weiss SM, Detre T, et al. New York, Wiley, 1986

Margraf J, Ehlers A, Roth WT: Mitral valve prolapse and panic disorder: a review of their relationship. Psychosom Med 50:93–113, 1988

Martin-Santos R, Bulbena A, Porta M, et al: Association between joint hypermobility syndrome and panic disorder. Am J Psychiatry 155:1578–1583, 1998

Masand PS, Tesar GE: Use of stimulants in the medically ill. Psychiatr Clin North Am 19:515–548, 1996

Miller GE, Stetler CA, Carney RM, et al: Clinical depression and inflammatory risk markers for coronary heart disease. Am J Cardiology 90:1279–1283, 2002

Mitchell JE, Mackenzie TB: Cardiac effects of lithium therapy in man: a review. J Clin Psychiatry 43:47–51, 1982

Morganroth J, Goin JE: Quinidine-related mortality in the short-to-medium-term treatment of ventricular arrhythmias. Circulation 84:1977–1983, 1991

Morris PL, Badger J, Chmielewski C, et al: Psychiatric morbidity following implantation of the automatic implantable cardioverter defibrillator. Psychosomatics 32:58–64, 1991

Moser DK, Dracup K: Is anxiety early after myocardial infarction associated with subsequent ischemic and arrhythmic events? Psychosom Med 58:395–401, 1996

Moss AJ: Long QT syndrome. JAMA 289:2041–2044, 2003

Muller JE, Abela GS, Nesto RW, et al: Triggers, acute risk factors and vulnerable plaques: the lexicon of a new frontier. J Am Coll Cardiol 23:809–813, 1994

Musselman DL, Tomer A, Manatunga AK, et al: Exaggerated platelet reactivity in major depression. Am J Psychiatry 153:1313–1317, 1996

Newburger JW, Silbert AR, Buckley LP, et al: Cognitive function and age at repair of transposition of the great arteries in children. N Engl J Med 310:1495–1499, 1984

Newman DM, Dorian P, Paquette M, et al: Effect of an implantable cardioverter defibrillator with atrial detection and shock therapies on patient-perceived, health-related quality of life. Am Heart J 145:841–846, 2003

Newman MF, Kirchner JL, Phillips-Bute B, et al: Longitudinal assessment of neurocognitive function after coronary-artery bypass surgery. N Engl J Med 344:395–402, 2001

Newman S: Incidence and nature of neuropsychological morbidity following cardiac surgery. Perfusion 4:93–100, 1989

Newman S, Pugsley W, Klinger L, et al: Neuropsychological consequences of circulatory arrest with hypothermia. J Clin Exp Neuropsychol 11:529–538, 1988

Pollock BG, Laghrissi-Thode F, Wagner WR: Evaluation of platelet activation in depressed patients with ischemic heart disease after paroxetine or nortriptyline treatment. J Clin Psychopharmacol 20:137–140, 2000

Qureshi EA, Merla V, Steinberg J, et al: Terrorism and the heart: implications for arrhythmogenesis and coronary artery disease. Card Electrophysiol Rev 7:80–84, 2003

Rasmussen A, Lunde M, Poulsen DL, et al: A double-blind, placebo-controlled study of sertraline in the prevention of depression in stroke patients. Psychosomatics 44:216–221, 2003

Roach GW, Kanchuger M, Mangano CM, et al: Adverse cerebral outcomes after coronary bypass surgery. N Engl J Med 335:1857–1863, 1996

Roose SP, Glassman AH: Cardiovascular effects of tricyclic antidepressants in depressed patients with and without heart disease. J Clin Psychiatry 50:S1–S18, 1989

Roose SP, Glassman AH, Giardina EGV, et al: Nortriptyline in depressed patients with left ventricular impairment. JAMA 256:3253–3257, 1986

Roose SP, Glassman AH, Giardina EGV, et al: Tricyclic antidepressants in depressed patients with cardiac conduction disease. Arch Gen Psychiatry 44:273–275, 1987

Roose SP, Glassman AH, Dalack GW: Depression, heart disease, and tricyclic antidepressants. J Clin Psychiatry 50:12–16, 1989

Roose SP, Dalack GW, Glassman AH, et al: Cardiovascular effects of bupropion in depressed patients with heart disease. Am J Psychiatry 148:512–516, 1991

Roose SP, Glassman AH, Attia E, et al: Comparative efficacy of selective serotonin reuptake inhibitors and tricyclics in the treatment of melancholia. Am J Psychiatry 151:1735–1739, 1994

Roose SP, Glassman AH, Attia E, et al: Cardiovascular effects of fluoxetine in depressed patients with heart disease. Am J Psychiatry 155:660–665, 1998a

Roose SP, Laghrissi-Thode F, Kennedy JS, et al: Comparison of paroxetine and nortriptyline in depressed patients with ischemic heart disease. JAMA 279:287–291, 1998b

Rosamond WD, Chambless LE, Folsom, AR et al: Trends in the incidence of myocardial infarction and in mortality due to coronary heart disease, 1987 to 1994. N Engl J Med 339: 861–867, 1998

Rose EA, Moskowitz AJ, Packer M, et al: The REMATCH trial: rationale, design, and end points. Ann Thorac Surg 67:723–730, 1999

Rose EA, Gelijns AC, Moskowitz AJ, et al: Long-term mechanical circulatory support for end stage heart failure: the REMATCH trial. N Engl J Med 345:1435–1443, 2001

Rosenman RH, Brand RJ, Jenkins CD, et al: Coronary heart disease in the Western Collaborative Group Study. Final follow-up experience of 8½ years. JAMA 233:872–877, 1975

Rozanski A, Bairey CN, Krantz DS, et al: Mental stress and the induction of silent myocardial ischemia in patients with coronary artery disease. N Engl J Med 318:1005–1012, 1988

Rozanski A, Blumenthal JA, Kaplan J: Impact of psychological factors on the pathogenesis of cardiovascular disease and implications for therapy. Circulation 99:2192–2217, 1999

Rumsfeld JS, Havranek E, Masoudi FA, et al: Depressive symptoms are the strongest predictors of short-term declines in health status in patients with heart failure. J Am Coll Cardiol 42:1811–1817, 2003

Ruo B, Rumsfeld JS, Hlatky MA, et al: Depressive symptoms and health-related quality of life. The Heart and Soul Study. JAMA 290:215–221, 2003

Rutledge T, Hogan BE: A quantitative review of prospective evidence linking psychological factors with hypertension development. Psychosom Med 64:758–766, 2002

Sauer WH, Berlin JA, Kimmel SE: Effect of antidepressants and their relative affinity for the serotonin transporter on the risk of myocardial infarction. Circulation 108:32–36, 2003

Schleifer SJ, Macari-Hinson MM, Coyle DA, et al: The nature and course of depression following myocardial infarction. Arch Intern Med 149:1785–1789, 1989

Schron EB, Exner DV, Yao Q, et al: Quality of life in the antiarrhythmics versus implantable defibrillators trial: impact of therapy and influence of adverse symptoms and defibrillator shocks. Circulation 105:589–594, 2002

Shamsuzzaman ASM, Gersh BJ, Somers VK: Obstructive sleep apnea: implications for cardiac and vascular disease. JAMA 290:1906–1914, 2003

Shapiro PA: Life after heart transplantation. Prog Cardiovasc Dis 32:405–418, 1990

Shapiro PA, Kornfeld DS: Psychiatric outcome of heart transplantation. Gen Hosp Psychiatry 11:352–357, 1989

Shapiro PA, Levin HR, Oz MC: Left ventricular assist devices: psychosocial burden and implications for heart transplant programs. Gen Hosp Psychiatry 18:30S–35S, 1996

Shapiro PA, Lidagoster L, Glassman AH: Depression and heart disease. Psychiatr Ann 27:347–352, 1997

Shapiro PA, DePena M, Lidagoster L, et al: Depression after coronary artery bypass graft surgery (abstract). Psychosom Med 60:108, 1998

Shapiro PA, Park SJ, Gupta L, et al: Quality of life outcomes in heart failure patients treated with optimal medical management vs. long-term mechanical assist device therapy: results from the REMATCH trial. Circulation 106 (suppl II):606–607, 2002

Shekelle RB, Gale M, Ostfeld AM, et al: Hostility, risk of coronary heart disease, and mortality. Psychosom Med 45:109–114, 1983

Sheline YI, Freedland KE, Carney RM: How safe are serotonin reuptake inhibitors for depression in patients with coronary heart disease? Am J Med 102:54–59, 1997

Sheps DS, McMahon RP, Becker L, et al: Mental stress-induced ischemia and all-cause mortality in patients with coronary artery disease: results from the Psychophysiological Investigations of Myocardial Ischemia study. Circulation 105: 1780–1784, 2002

Skinner JE: Regulation of cardiac vulnerability by the cerebral defense system. J Am Coll Cardiol 5:88B–94B, 1985

Skinner JE, Reed JC: Blockade of a frontocortical-brainstem pathway prevents ventricular fibrillation of the ischemic heart in pigs. Am J Physiol 240:H156–H163, 1981

Skinner JE, Lie JT, Entman ML: Modification of ventricular fibrillation latency following coronary artery occlusion in the conscious pig. Circulation 51:656–667, 1975

Stein PK, Carney RM, Freedland KE, et al: Severe depression is associated with markedly reduced heart rate variability in patients with stable coronary heart disease. J Psychosom Res 48:493–500, 2000

Steptoe A, Mohabir A, Mahon NG, et al: Health related quality of life and psychological well-being in patients with dilated cardiomyopathy. Heart 83:645–650, 2000

Strik JJ, Denollet J, Lousberg R, et al: Comparing symptoms of depression and anxiety as predictors of cardiac events and increased health care consumption after myocardial infarction. J Am Coll Cardiol 42:1801–1807, 2003

Strike PC, Steptoe A: Systematic review of mental stress induced myocardial ischemia. Eur Heart J 24:690–703, 2003

Stuart S, Cole V: Treatment of depression following myocardial infarction with interpersonal psychotherapy. Ann Clin Psychiatry 8:203–206, 1996

Sullivan M, LaCroix AX, Spertus JS, et al.: Effects of anxiety and depression on symptoms and function in patients with coronary heart disease: A five-year prospective study. Psychosomatics 41:187, 2000

Tesar GE, Murray GB, Cassem NH: Use of high dose intravenous haloperidol in the treatment of agitated cardiac patients. J Clin Psychopharmacol 5:344–347, 1985

Van Dijk D, Jansen EWL, Hijman R, et al: Cognitive outcome after off-pump and on-pump coronary artery bypass graft surgery: a randomized trial. JAMA 287:1405–1412, 2002

Weissman MM, Markowitz JS, Ouellette R, et al: Panic disorder and cardiovascular/cerebrovascular problems: results from a community survey. Am J Psychiatry 147:1504–1508, 1990

Willner A, Rodewald G: The Impact of Cardiac Surgery on the Quality of Life: Neurological and Psychological Aspects. New York, Plenum, 1991

Writing Committee for the ENRICHD Investigators: Effects of treating depression and low perceived social support on clinical events after myocardial infarction: the enhancing recovery in coronary heart disease patients (ENRICHD) randomized trial. JAMA 289:3106–3116, 2003

Yan LL, Liu K, Matthews KA, et al: Psychosocial factors and risk of hypertension: the coronary artery risk development in young adults (CARDIA) study. JAMA 290:2138–2148, 2003

Yeung AC, Vekshstein VI, Krantz DS, et al: The effect of atherosclerosis on the vasomotor response of coronary arteries to mental stress. N Engl J Med 325:1551–1556, 1991

Ziegelstein RC, Fauerbach JA, Stevens SS, et al: Patients with depression are less likely to follow recommendations to reduce cardiac risk during recovery from a myocardial infarction. Arch Intern Med 160:1818–1823, 2000

20 Lung Disease

Kathy Coffman, M.D.
James L. Levenson, M.D.

IN THIS CHAPTER, we review psychiatric aspects of the major pulmonary disorders, as well as lung transplantation and the use of psychiatric drugs in pulmonary patients. Diseases affecting the lungs occur across the life span. Asthma and cystic fibrosis usually have an early onset; sarcoidosis may begin in early to midlife; and emphysema, chronic bronchitis, and pulmonary fibrosis are usually diagnosed in midlife to senescence. Tuberculosis, hyperventilation syndrome, and vocal cord dysfunction may affect people of any age. For end-stage patients who are not candidates for lung transplantation, terminal weaning may be considered. Despite the large number of people with lung disease, many conditions have not been well studied from the psychosomatic standpoint.

Common Pulmonary Disorders

Asthma

Asthma is now the most common chronic disease in the United States, affecting 5%–7% of the population, or roughly 17 million people (American Lung Association 2000; Barnes and Woolcock 1998). This chapter focuses on asthma in adults (see Chapter 34, "Pediatrics," for discussion of asthma in children). Mortality has risen steadily since the early 1980s. Age-adjusted mortality of asthma varies among ethnic groups: Puerto Ricans, 40.9 per million; non-Hispanic blacks, 38.1 per million; Cuban Americans, 15.8 per million; non-Hispanic whites, 14.7 per million; and Mexican Americans, 9.2 per million (National Center for Health Statistics 2000).

Comorbidity With Psychiatric Disorders

Asthma symptoms overlapping with those of other disorders can complicate diagnosis. Asthma may be misdiagnosed as an anxiety disorder, and some anxiety disorders (panic, social anxiety) may be mislabeled as asthma. In one study, 31% of patients who had been given an asthma diagnosis had a negative methacholine inhalation challenge test, indicating no airway hyperresponsiveness. Social anxiety symptoms were a strong predictor of mislabeling the patient as asthmatic. Among patients without bronchial reactivity, social phobia was 10 times more common than in patients who actually had asthma (Schmaling et al. 1999). Therefore, clinicians should ask whether symptoms only occur in certain circumstances such as social settings. Methacholine inhalation challenge was useful in identifying three cases of factitious asthma (Downing et al. 1982).

Of course, patients may frequently have both asthma and anxiety. Anxiety is increased by sudden and unexpected attacks of asthma, anticipation of attacks in response to certain triggers, and side effects of medications for treatment of asthma. Anxiety can affect the patient's response to an attack, as well as use of medications and quality of life (ten Thoren and Petermann 2000).

Some have reported a high comorbidity between asthma and panic disorder and other anxiety disorders. Those with asthma and panic disorder have more perceived breathlessness after an inhalation challenge test than those without panic disorder. Perceived discomfort, rather than actual bronchoconstriction, predicts use of bronchodilators (Schmaling et al. 1999). Several recent studies have indicated that anxiety and depression are more common in asthma patients than in the general population, particularly in women and those with less education (Centanni et al. 2000). A study of 230 outpatients with asthma revealed that almost half had a positive screen for depressive symptoms (Mancuso et al. 2000). Most recently, Goodwin and colleagues (2003) systematically screened a general adult population sample of more than 13,000 Germans for asthma and DSM-IV mental disorders. They found that current asthma and lifetime history of severe asthma were each associated with significantly elevated odds ratios of anxiety disorders, including panic, social phobia, generalized anxiety, and specific phobias.

Psychological Factors in Asthma

Psychosomatic theories about asthma were proposed by French and Alexander in 1939–1941, based on the hypothesis that a central conflict revolved around unconscious dependency issues with the mother and fear of separation. However, these theories have little empirical support (Greenberg et al. 1996).

Few prospective studies of the relationship of psychosocial variables to pulmonary function in patients with asthma have been reported. One small study showed that 50% of subjects had significant associations between pulmonary function and a variety of psychosocial factors (Schmaling et al. 2002).

Asthma is a primary respiratory disease with varying immunological and autonomic pathophysiological changes. No particular personality type is more susceptible to development of asthma. Asthma was once regarded as a classic psychosomatic disorder, and it is still widely believed that psychological factors (particularly anxiety) play an important role in the precipitation and aggravation of asthma. However, respiratory distress itself may be misinterpreted as anxiety and can also cause anxiety symptoms (panic attacks, generalized and anticipatory anxiety, phobic avoidance). In addition, most of the drugs used to treat asthma can cause anxiety. *Brittle* asthma patients, like brittle diabetic patients, are more likely to have current or past psychiatric disorders, particularly anxiety disorders, than other asthma patients are; but which comes first has not been established (Garden and Ayres 1993). Anxiety and depression are associated with more respiratory symptom complaints in asthma patients but with no differences in objective measures of respiratory function (Janson et al. 1994; Rietveld et al. 1999).

Similar to panic disorder, those with asthma have a tendency to hold catastrophic beliefs. In a study of 50 subjects and their partners, there was a significant association between catastrophic cognitions and more asthma symptoms such as irritability, panic and fear, and rapid breathing even when severity of asthma was considered (Giardino et al. 2002).

Asthma attacks have long been thought to be provoked by psychological distress. There was a 27% increase in severity of asthma symptoms in patients surveyed in New York City 5–9 weeks after the September 11, 2001, terrorist attacks (Centers for Disease Control and Prevention 2002), and PTSD was a significant predictor of asthma symptom severity (Fagan et al. 2003).

Psychological factors and psychosocial problems in hospitalized asthma patients were a more powerful predictor of which patients required intubation than any other examined variable (e.g., smoking, infection, prior hospitalization) (LeSon and Gershwin 1996). Several psychological factors in asthma patients may be associated with asthma deaths. A case–control study involving 533 cases showed an increased risk of death associated with health behaviors such as poor adherence with follow-up visits and poor inhaler technique. Three independent psychosocial factors appeared to increase the odds of death: psychosis, financial problems, and learning difficulties. Two factors associated with reduced risk were sexual problems and prescription of antidepressant drugs. Surprisingly, factors such as bereavement, domestic abuse, family problems, and social isolation did not correlate with risk of asthma death (Sturdy et al. 2002).

By what mechanisms might psychological factors affect asthma? From a physiological perspective, the vagus nerve is thought to mediate airway reactivity to emotion (Isenberg et al. 1992). The upper airways innervated by cholinergic neurons may be affected more by suggestion and emotion than smaller airways (Lehrer et al. 1986). Recent research has shown that various emotions and types of stress can increase respiratory resistance in asthma (Ritz et al. 2000).

Psychological factors may also influence asthma through behavioral mechanisms. Noncompliance with medications is common among asthma patients and may increase likelihood of hospitalization. Psychological morbidity is associated with high levels of denial and delays in seeking medical care, which may be life-threatening in severe asthma (D.A. Campbell et al. 1995; Miles et al. 1997), as well as less medication adherence and consequently poorer control of asthma (Cluley and Cochrane 2001). Not surprisingly, then, psychopathology in persons with severe asthma is associated with increased health care utilization, including hospitalizations and outpatient and emergency room (ER) visits, independent of asthma severity (ten Brinke et al. 2001). One study of 85 asthma patients showed higher prevalence of self-reported noncompliance with treatment among those who were ever hospitalized than those that had never been hospitalized. Emotional distress associated with disease and treatment was related to noncompliance (Put et al. 2000).

Interventions With Asthma Patients

Adjuvant forms of treatment for asthma may involve psychological interventions such as biofeedback, education programs, hypnosis, stress management, symptom perception, and yoga (Lehrer et al. 2002). Patient education programs can reduce anxiety and improve self-management. Problem checklists and patient diaries of asthma attacks can be useful in determining signs of an attack, triggers of attacks, helpful steps for the patient or others to take during an attack, and the impact of the illness on social and academic development and family life (Weiss 1994).

Whether behavioral interventions can affect asthma morbidity was investigated in a randomized, controlled study of 16 young, non-steroid-dependent asthma patients who participated in biofeedback-assisted relaxation. This small study found that the intervention produced improvement in FEV1/FVC (ratio of forced expiratory volume after 1 second to forced vital capacity) at posttest and decreased severity of asthma and bronchodilator usage with changes in white blood cell populations over time, suggesting decreased inflammation (Kern-Buell et al. 2000).

Cystic Fibrosis

In the United States, cystic fibrosis (CF) affects over 18,000 children under the age of 18 (1 in 2,500 births). CF is the most common hereditary disease in white children, and it is also seen in other races. The disease typically results in chronic progressive lung disease and pancreatic insufficiency. Survival improved from a median age of 12 years in 1966 to 40 years by 2001 (Jaffe and Bush 2001), so adults living with CF are a relatively recent and growing population. (See Chapter 34, "Pediatrics," for information on CF in children.)

The regimen of therapy necessary to maintain health in patients with cystic fibrosis is extremely time-consuming and may involve the whole family, especially in early childhood. Treatment includes a nebulizer with bronchodilators followed by physiotherapy three times a day, frequent antibiotic treatment via portacath, pancreatic enzyme replacement, inhalers, and, in cases of severe malnutrition, gastrostomy tubes with a kangaroo pump (Llewellyn 1998).

Psychological Factors in Cystic Fibrosis

Several authors have described growing up with CF from a child's perspective. Different issues arise during various stages of psychological development. In adolescence, for example, teens may come to grips with the illness, put it into a new perspective because of their growing cognitive abilities, and hopefully assume responsibility for their health care. Knowing the key issues involved can enhance effectiveness of therapeutic interventions (Christian and D'Auria 1997; Hains et al. 1997; Llewellyn 1998).

One recent study looked at the impact of recent pulmonary exacerbations on quality of life in patients ages 5–45 with mild-to-moderate CF. Among the 162 patients who participated, recent exacerbations had an impact on health-related quality of life that was not accounted for by lung function, nutritional status, or demographic factors (Britto et al. 2002).

There are few studies of psychological functioning in adults with CF. One recent study included 34 adults with CF who completed the Minnesota Multiphasic Personality Inventory–2, Beck Depression Inventory (BDI), and State-Trait Anxiety Inventory; the patients did not display significant levels of depression, anxiety, or any other psychopathology. Males reported higher depression and anxiety scores than females. Lower anxiety correlated with better pulmonary function (D.L. Anderson et al. 2001).

Coping responses and reasons for nonadherence to medical regimens in 60 adult CF patients were systematically explored. Four ways of coping with CF were described: optimistic acceptance, hopefulness, distraction, and avoidance. Not surprisingly, the adherent patients scored higher on the optimistic acceptance and hopefulness scales, whereas the nonadherent patients used avoidant strategies significantly more often. Those patients who relied heavily on distraction fell in the middle regarding adherence (Abbott et al. 2001).

A comparison of pre–lung transplant quality of life in 58 patients with CF versus 52 patients with other types of end-stage lung disease revealed some interesting differences. The CF patients had lower levels of anxiety, were more likely to be working, and used more functional coping methods. This suggests that adults with CF had developed better adaptation to their illness than had those with other chronic lung disease (Burker et al. 2000).

However, other investigators found psychiatric problems, mainly related to anxiety, in 50%–60% of CF patients (Hains et al. 1997). Increases in depressive symptoms have been seen in older teenagers and young adults (Benner 1993). Noncompliance with the medical regimen has been estimated to be at least 35% (Czajkowski and Koocher 1987).

Chronic Obstructive Pulmonary Disease

Almost 16 million Americans have chronic obstructive pulmonary disease (COPD): 14 million with chronic bronchitis and 2 million with emphysema. COPD ranks fourth as a cause of death in the United States after heart disease, cancer, and stroke. Whereas many other types of lung disease affect minority groups disproportionately, COPD shows a higher age-adjusted death rate for whites (21.9 per 100,000) than blacks (17.7 per 100,000). Cigarette smokers are 10 times as likely to die of COPD as nonsmokers.

COPD results in progressive and usually irreversible declines in arterial oxygen, with carbon dioxide increasing late in the course of the disease. Hypoxia causes confusion, disorientation, altered consciousness, muscle twitching, tremor, and seizures. Mild hypoxia can be accompanied by irritability, mental slowing, and impairment of memory with poor reasoning and perseveration. Prolonged hypoxia can result in permanent memory deficits or dementia, that is, hypoxic encephalopathy (Lishman 1987). Chronic or severe hypoxia can lead to extrapyramidal symptoms, pseudobulbar palsy, or visual agnosia. If hypoxia is accompanied by hypercapnia and respiratory acidosis, as in chronic bronchitis or status asthmaticus, patients may be lethargic and have auditory and visual hallucinations (Lishman 1987).

Comorbidity With Psychiatric Disorders

Nicotine dependence is the most commonly associated psychiatric condition in COPD patients. More than 80% of COPD cases are associated with tobacco smoking (Tashkin et al. 2001). Alcohol abuse aggravates COPD, in part because of a higher rate of severe community-acquired pneumonia, particularly aspiration pneumonia (Ewig and Torres 1999).

Sexual dysfunction is also common in COPD. In a study of Spanish male COPD patients on long-term oxygen, 67% of the patients and 94% of their wives said they had sexual problems, including lack of desire and impotence (Ibanez et al. 2001). There are intriguing reports of decreased dyspnea and improvement in spirometry after sildenafil for treatment of erectile dysfunction (Charan 2001).

Major depression is also very common in patients with COPD, although this finding is in part a result of its increased prevalence in smokers (Aydin and Ulasahin 2001; Withers et al. 1999; Yohannes et al. 2000). In one recent study, clinical depression was found in 42% of the patients, of whom 30% were mildly depressed; 68%, moderately depressed; and 2%, severely depressed (Yohannes et al. 2000). Only about one-fifth of COPD patients with major depression are treated with antidepressants. Depression not only may adversely impact rehabilitation but also may contribute to difficulty ceasing tobacco use, and the depression may recur when tobacco is discontinued (Borson et al. 1998).

Anxiety is also common in COPD (Aydin and Ulasahin 2001; Withers et al. 1999; Yohannes et al. 2000). The prevalence of panic disorder in COPD patients remains controversial, because some groups claim a higher rate among COPD patients, and others dispute this finding. Many studies mention panic attacks without stating whether the patients met DSM or ICD criteria for panic disorder.

In one study, 37% of COPD patients reported having had a panic attack. These patients also reported significantly more agoraphobic cognitions and more concern with bodily sensations than those who did not have panic (Porzelius et al. 1992). Another study found that COPD patients had symptoms similar to those of agoraphobic patients, though not as intense (Klonoff and Kleinhenz 1993).

Cognitive dysfunction is also very common in COPD, because of hypoxemia, and is improved by supplemental oxygen. Two decades ago, it was demonstrated that 42% of COPD patients with neuropsychological deficits showed modest improvement after 6 months of oxygen therapy. Those receiving continuous oxygen treatment (COT) had better neuropsychological performance and survival at 12 months than did those receiving nocturnal oxygen treatment only (Heaton et al. 1983). Rates of neuropsychological impairment rose from 27% in those with mild hypoxemia to 61% in those with severe hypoxemia (Grant et al. 1987). Higher scores on the Benton Visual Motor Retention Test and Digit Symbol subtest of the Wechsler Adult Intelligence Scale (associated with better oxygenation) predicted significantly better survival (Fix et al. 1985). More recent studies have shown slower reaction times, (Della Sala et al. 1992) and decreased visual attention related to the nadir of nocturnal saturation of oxygen (Vos et al. 1995). About 30% of COPD patients showed immediate memory impairment (Fioravanti et al. 1995). Of the COPD patients tested at discharge after a first episode of acute respiratory failure requiring mechanical ventilation, 47% showed Mini-Mental Status Examination (MMSE) scores below 24, compared with 3% of stable COPD control subjects receiving continuous oxygen treatment. Retesting 6 months later showed that 17% of the hospitalized patients still scored below 24 on the MMSE versus 5% of the comparison group (Ambrosino et al. 2002). Anterior cerebral hypoperfusion has been demonstrated on SPECT in hypoxemic COPD patients, with below-normal scoring on verbal attainment, attention, and deductive reasoning, which could presage frontal-type cognitive decline with worsening hypoxemia (Antonelli Incalzi et al. 2003).

Psychological Factors in COPD

As with other medical illnesses, measurement of physical symptoms in COPD may be confounded by psychological symptoms, and vice versa. Psychological distress in COPD amplifies dyspnea, usually without causing changes in objective pulmonary functions. One study of COPD patients showed that patients with more severe physical symptoms had more negative mood symptoms. In particular, fatigue was found to account for 28% of the variance on the Negative Mood Scale. Surprisingly, dyspnea, congestion, and peripheral-sensory disturbances did not factor into the equation for negative mood in this study (Small and Graydon 1992).

Results have not been consistent in correlating quality of life and various measures of pulmonary function. A recent study found that quality of life was related to perceived self-efficacy with functional activities in COPD rather than strictly to pulmonary function (Kohler et al. 2002). Those with higher levels of positive social support had better quality of life with less depression and anxiety. Lower quality of life was seen when catastrophic withdrawal coping strategies were employed by the patients (McCathie et al. 2002).

Depression and anxiety in COPD patients have led to lower exercise tolerance (Withers et al. 1999), noncompliance with treatment (Bosley et al. 1996), and increased disability (Aydin and Ulusahin 2001). Psychological factors may predict whether a patient with obstructive pulmonary disease is at higher risk of relapse after emergency treatment. In one study, those with anxiety or depression had a higher rate of relapse within 1 month (53%) compared with those in the group without anxiety or depression (19%) (Dahlen and Janson 2002).

On the basis of clinical experience, Dudley et al. (1985) observed that when patients and physicians face COPD, they may feel helpless. The patient may be viewed by others as weak and lacking motivation. The physician may feel impotent when a patient cannot be cured. The patient and family may be angry and frustrated that this illness cannot be fixed. The patients may feel guilty if smoking resulted in the disease, and he or she may feel like a burden to spouse and family. The patient may avoid emotional expression because it exacerbates his or her sense of dyspnea. Denial, suppression of affect, repression, and isolation are frequently used as coping strategies in COPD patients (Dudley et al. 1985). Consequently, the patient's spouse or family may feel that the patient is emotionally distant and unavailable. This may perpetuate a cycle of confrontation and avoidance, leading to unresolved anger and despair as neither the needs of the patient nor those of the family are met. Patients may fear loss of control or loss of independence. Other losses may include loss of job, social status, role in the family, and changes in appearance because of steroids. Chronic steroid use may also exacerbate depression, emotional lability, or irritability, which in turn further strains interpersonal relationships.

Dependence on supplemental oxygen can be socially stigmatizing and make the patient feel unattractive. The oxygen tank may or is feared to be a liability in the patient's occupation. Some cannot accept the need for oxygen because of denial about the illness. Others become psychologically dependent on oxygen, exceeding the amount prescribed, posing a risk of carbon dioxide retention, which leads to lethargy.

The Veterans Administration Normative Aging Study found that optimism in older men with COPD predicted higher levels of pulmonary function and a slower rate of pulmonary function decline (independent of smoking status). Significantly higher forced expiratory volume in 1 second (FEV_1) and forced vital capacity (both $P<0.01$) were found in those with more optimism, measured 8 years earlier (Kubzansky et al. 2002).

Interventions With COPD Patients

Psychotherapeutic, psychopharmacological, and rehabilitation intervention trials in COPD have been recently reviewed in detail elsewhere (Brenes 2003). The first priority in the rehabilitation of patients with COPD is smoking cessation. Other interventions include pharmacotherapy, physical therapy, psychosocial interventions, nutritional therapy, and, for those who are hypoxemic, long-term oxygen therapy surgery. A small fraction of patients may benefit from bilateral lung volume reduction surgery (Wurtemberger and Hutter 2001).

COPD is a chronic debilitating disease that limits lifestyle and progressively compromises quality of life. The goals of treatment are to relieve symptoms, improve physical functioning via rehabilitation, and improve patients' coping skills (Small and Graydon 1992). Patients may interpret dyspnea as a signal to avoid all activity and thus become homebound and isolated. Exercise may allow patients to build endurance, improve their range of activities, and learn to pace themselves. Some patients avoid exercise groups so as to avoid confronting their illness or seeing others who may be sicker, foreshadowing their own eventual decline. These patients may do better with individual physical therapy. Through participating in a structured exercise program, the patient may gain control and learn that mild dyspnea is not necessarily life-threatening. A treatment plan with realistic and attainable goals and rewards can counteract helplessness (Dudley et al. 1985).

A meta-analysis of 23 randomized, controlled trials of pulmonary rehabilitation for COPD concluded that pulmonary rehabilitation significantly decreased dyspnea and fatigue, although the improvement in exercise capacity was modest (Lacasse et al. 2002).

Pulmonary rehabilitation may decrease dyspnea and anxiety symptoms significantly and increase global quality of life (Buchi et al. 2000). An uncontrolled study of the impact of inpatient pulmonary rehabilitation found 29.2% of patients with significant anxiety on admission and 15% with significant depression. Scores for both anxiety and depression were significantly lower after pulmonary rehabilitation and at 6-month follow-up. Those with high initial anxiety scores made significantly greater improvement in exercise capacity than those with low initial scores (Withers et al. 1999). Pulmonary rehabilitation can increase patients' sense of control over COPD, a key issue in this progressive chronic illness (Lacasse et al. 2002).

Predictors of nonadherence with an outpatient pulmonary rehabilitation program were investigated by Young et al. (1999). Noncompleters were more likely to be currently smoking, divorced, living alone in rented accommodations, and less likely to use inhaled corticosteroids. In this study, noncompleters were not more anxious, depressed, or prone to hyperventilation or worse quality of life, and were not more physiologically impaired (Young et al. 1999).

Rose et al. (2002) reviewed 25 published studies of psychological treatments for reduction of anxiety in patients with COPD. Only 6 were randomized, and methodological limitations across all studies led the authors to conclude that there is an insufficient evidence base to recommend a specific psychological treatment for anxiety in COPD. However, some clinicians have found relaxation techniques useful in motivated patients, and there seems to be no reason to believe that psychological interventions for anxiety would be harmful in COPD (Rose et al. 2002). Pharmacological treatment of anxiety is discussed later in this chapter.

Sarcoidosis

Although sarcoidosis was first reported by Jonathan Hutchinson in 1872 (Scadding 1967), its etiology is still undetermined. Sarcoidosis is characterized by noncaseating granulomatous involvement of lymph nodes, lymphatic channels in the lung and other tissues. Sarcoidosis affects black patients more than whites in the United States (40 per 100,000 vs. 5 per 100,000). In Europe, Swedes and Danes have high prevalence rates (American Lung Association 2000). Onset of the illness is usually between ages 20 and 40. Diagnosis may be delayed by failure to recognize the slowly progressive symptoms until characteristic findings are recognized on a chest X ray. The disease often follows a relapsing and remitting course, with recovery in 80% of patients, but about 5% die from sarcoidosis. Patients may be asymptomatic, but often they have a dry cough, shortness of breath, fatigue, and weight loss. Lesions can affect the skin, bones, joints, skeletal muscles, and heart. Fatal complications include progressive respiratory impairment, infection, cardiac disease, and renal failure.

Central Nervous System Sarcoidosis

Sarcoidosis affects the central nervous system (CNS) in as many as 5% of patients. Neurosarcoidosis may cause brain lesions, involve cranial nerves (especially VII), and cause peripheral neuropathies (and rarely choreoathetosis). In as many as 30% of cases, the cerebrospinal fluid may be normal, and the diagnosis is made on clinical grounds (Stoudemire et al. 1983). Arachnoiditis may cause increased intracranial pressure and hydrocephalus, and meningitis can cause headache. Hypothalamic involvement can cause obesity, hyperthermia, memory dysfunction, personality changes, and somnolence. Pituitary involvement may result in diabetes insipidus, or conversely syndrome of inappropriate antidiuretic hormone secretion (SIADH) with hyponatremia, hypercalcemia, hyperprolactinemia, menstrual cycle changes, or hypogonadism (see Bullman et al. 2000; Delaney 1977; Mino et al. 2000; Sharma 1975).

CNS disease may cause disturbance of orientation, sensorium, memory, and cognitive functions (Mathews 1965; Silverstein et al. 1965). Various psychiatric symptoms, such as apathy, dementia, hallucinosis, irritability, and neglect, have been noted (Hook 1954). CNS sarcoidosis can mimic depressive stupor, Wernicke-Korsakoff psychosis, classic paranoid psychosis, and schizophreniform disorder (Hook 1954; Sabaawi et al. 1992; Suchenwirth and Dold 1969; Zerman 1952). Psychotic symptoms rapidly remit with steroids. Patients with CNS sarcoidosis may also present with seizures (Thompson and Checkley 1981).

Psychological Factors in Sarcoidosis

Sarcoidosis has been rarely investigated from the psychological standpoint. One small study found that increased life stress predicted subsequent impairment of lung function. The only psychological variable that consistently correlated with lung function was the mean score for day-to-day hassles, suggesting the potential benefit of relaxation exercises and stress management (Klonoff and Kleinhenz 1993). Some patients ultimately diagnosed with sarcoidosis have been mistakenly labeled as having somatization disorder, which can happen with any occult multisystem disease (DeGruy et al. 1987).

Hoitsma et al. (2003) studied pain in 821 Dutch patients with sarcoidosis without other medical comorbidity. They found that 72% of patients had pain, including arthralgia (53.8%), muscle pain (40.2%), headache (28%), and chest pain (26.9%), suggesting that psychological and pharmacological pain management may also be beneficial. Wirnsberger et al. (1998) found that sarcoidosis has considerable impact on quality of life, especially via fatigue, although fatigue was not related to any measured psychological variable.

Pulmonary Fibrosis

The etiology of idiopathic pulmonary fibrosis (IPF) is unknown, but the prevalence is roughly 3–5 per 100,000. Pulmonary fibrosis also may be caused by inhalation of a variety of agents (especially via occupational exposure), radiation, and rheumatological disorders, especially systemic sclerosis. Patients with IPF develop gradual progressive loss of lung function and declining exercise tolerance.

Psychological factors have received surprisingly little attention in IPF. Dyspnea is the most important factor in determining quality of life in IPF. Dyspnea correlated with quality-of-life variables, as did some pulmonary parameters (Martinez et al. 2000). DeVries et al. (2001) studied patients with IPF, comparing them with control subjects, and found that the subjective sense of breathlessness appeared related to depressive symptoms and quality of life.

Tuberculosis

The incidence of tuberculosis (TB) had been declining for more than 70 years but began to rise again over the last decade in the United States, Western Europe, Asia, and Africa. Causes for this trend include the rise of AIDS and increasing homelessness, as well as the failure to fund public health systems to provide treatment. The World Health Organization estimates there are 2.9 million deaths per year and nearly 8 million new cases per year in the world. About one-third of the world's population is infected with *Mycobacterium tuberculosis* and at risk for the disease. Roughly one-fifth of all adult deaths in developing nations are caused by tuberculosis (Bloom et al. 1996). See Chapter 27, "Infectious Diseases," for a discussion of CNS tuberculosis.

Psychiatrists may be asked to make capacity determinations in patients who are nonadherent with TB treatment and need to be confined for treatment of TB (O'Dowd et al. 1998). One survey of TB detainees showed that 81% had drug or alcohol abuse, 46% were homeless, and 28% had mental illness (Oscherwitz et al. 1997). The prevalence of mental illness in the homeless ranges from 25%–33% in Ireland and Spain to 80%–95% in the United States, Australia, Canada, Norway, and Germany (Martens 2001). Screening of the homeless in Spain showed that 75% were infected with TB, 14% had radiographic evidence of inactive pulmonary TB, and 1% had active pulmonary TB (Solsona et al. 2001). In San Francisco,

homeless patients showed an incidence of TB of 270 per 100,000 associated with older age, less education, HIV infection, and nonwhite ethnicity (Moss et al. 2000). Positive purified protein derivative (PPD) tests were found in 17% of the severely mentally ill in New York City, but none had active TB (McQuistion et al. 1997). In New Orleans, PPD screening of homeless men with psychotic disorders showed a relative risk of 4.48 compared with the general population. It is very difficult to effectively treat TB in homeless, infected individuals with severe chronic mental illness, particularly in the absence of adequate mental health treatment and social and residential resources (Sakai et al. 1998).

Alcoholic patients are more susceptible to TB (Sternbach 1990), and drug dependence is also a risk factor (Reichman et al. 1979). Thus, access to adequate substance abuse treatment may be essential to achieving recovery from TB and preventing relapse. Measures to control TB in homeless, mentally ill, alcoholic, or drug-addicted persons include screening in clinics, hotels, and shelters; directly observed therapy; and incentive programs (Malotte et al. 1999).

Psychiatrists must also be attuned to the possibility of iatrogenic neuropsychiatric symptoms during treatment with isoniazid, such as mania and psychosis (Alao and Yolles 1998), probably related to its being a weak inhibitor of monoamine oxidase. Predisposing factors identified include alcoholism, diabetes, hepatic insufficiency, old age, slow acetylation, and family and personal history of mental illness (Djibo and Lawan 2001). Pyridoxine deficiency may also play a role in the etiology of isoniazid-related psychosis. Acute overdosage with isoniazid, causing convulsions (controlled by giving pyridoxine), has been reported (Ebadi et al. 1982). Pellagra encephalopathy has also been seen, especially with poor nutrition, because isoniazid inhibits conversion of tryptophan to niacin. Clinicians should suspect pellagra if TB patients taking isoniazid show gastrointestinal, mental, or neurological symptoms (Ishii and Nishihara 1985).

Hyperventilation

A syndrome of hyperventilation was first recognized in 1871 by DaCosta. Hyperventilation is a common presenting complaint in ERs leading to psychiatric consultation (Nguyen et al. 1992). These patients experience an increase in the rate and depth of breathing briefly for a few minutes and may have dizziness or syncope from the respiratory alkalosis and cerebral vasoconstriction that result. Accompanying symptoms of carpopedal spasm, myoclonic jerks, or paresthesias may frighten the patient or relatives and result in an ER visit.

Hyperventilation syndrome (HVS) has been defined by three criteria: the patient hyperventilates and has a low pCO_2, somatic diseases causing hyperventilation have been ruled out, and the patient has somatic complaints because of hypocapnia (Folgering 1999). HVS occurs across the life span, from children to the elderly (Hodgens et al. 1988; Teramoto et al. 1997). The incidence of HVS may be as high as 6%–11% of the general population (Lachman et al. 1992). In one Japanese study, HVS attacks recurred in half of patients and continued to recur over 3 years in 10% (Hirokawa et al. 1995). Differential diagnosis for hyperventilation includes medical and psychiatric disorders. Evaluation in the ER, to avoid mislabeling patients as having HVS, may include a chest X ray, blood chemistries, a complete blood count, and thyroid functions (Saisch et al. 1996).

Medical illnesses that can cause hyperventilation and be confused with HVS include angina, arrhythmia, asthma (Demeter and Cordasco 1986), carbon monoxide poisoning (Skorodin et al. 1986), diabetic ketoacidosis (Treasure et al. 1987), pulmonary emboli (Hoegholm et al. 1987), epilepsy, hypoglycemia, ingestion of salicylates (Rognum et al. 1987), Meniere disease, tetany (Hehrmann 1996), and vasovagal syncope. In HVS patients, unilateral neurological symptoms, often left-sided, may mimic a cerebral vascular accident; and loss of consciousness and pseudoseizures caused by hyperventilation may be misdiagnosed as epilepsy (North et al. 1990; Perkin and Joseph 1986). However, there have also been reports of neurological causes of hyperventilation, including thalamic infarct (Scialdone 1990), Cheyne-Stokes breathing (Liippo et al. 1992), and traumatic vestibular hyperreactivity after whiplash injury (Fisher et al. 1995).

Hyperventilation syndrome may be present in many patients with cardiac chest pain (Castro et al. 2000; Freeman and Nixon 1985; Hegel et al. 1989). Hyperventilation syndrome and medical disorders are not mutually exclusive; they frequently occur together both because some disorders promote hyperventilation physically *and* psychologically (i.e., asthma, angina, pulmonary embolism), and because the metabolic consequences of hyperventilation may precipitate pathological events (i.e., arrhythmia, seizures, muscle spasm). Medications reported to cause central hyperventilation include carbamazepine, salicylates, and topiramate. Central hyperventilation resolves promptly within a day or two after discontinuation of these drugs (Lasky and Brody 2000; Mizukami et al. 1990).

Psychiatric disorders to consider in HVS include conversion disorder, histrionic personality disorder, panic disorder, phobic disorders, hypochondriasis, and substance abuse. Hyperventilation syndrome has also occurred as part of mass psychogenic illness (Araki and Honma

1986). Estimates of the overlap between HVS and panic disorder are between 35% and 50%, and in one study 83% of the patients had panic disorder with agoraphobia, and 82% had generalized anxiety disorder (Cowley and Roy-Byrne 1987; deRuiter et al. 1989; Hoes et al. 1987). The relationship between HVS and panic disorder is controversial. Bass has argued that the concept of a discrete hyperventilation syndrome is no longer tenable and that there is no evidence to support the view that panic attacks and hyperventilation are synonymous (Bass 1997). Patients with HVS may benefit from exploration of stressful life events, relationships, and self-esteem (Hanna et al. 1986; Robinson et al. 1988; Roncevic et al. 1994).

Various treatments for HVS have been employed over the years. Some methods are anecdotal, such as use of antidepressants (Saarijarvi and Lehtinen 1987), intravenous sedatives (Hirokawa et al. 1995), group therapy (Fensterheim and Wiegand 1991), and resolution of grief through individual psychotherapy (Paulley 1990). Methods with some evidence of effectiveness include beta-blockers (Van De Ven et al. 1995), breathing retraining (DeGuire et al. 1992, 1996; Pinney et al. 1987), and hypnosis (Conway et al. 1988).

Although having patients with acute hyperventilation rebreathe into a brown paper bag is a traditional technique used in the ER, there may be some hazards associated with its use. Death resulted in three cases where this treatment was mistakenly applied to patients with hypoxia or myocardial ischemia. A study of the effects of paper bag rebreathing in normally breathing volunteers showed that a few subjects reached CO_2 levels as high as 50, (though many never reached 40), and the mean maximal drop in O_2 was 26 mmHg (Callaham 1989). A small study showed that CO_2 restoration during a paper bag rebreathing paradigm for HVS is subject to the effects of expectation and suggestion (Van den Hout et al. 1988). A large nonrandomized outcome study showed that half of the HVS patients recovered without treatment, while the others recovered with either paper bag rebreathing or intravenous sedatives (Hirokawa et al. 1995).

Vocal Cord Dysfunction

Vocal cord dysfunction (VCD) is a respiratory syndrome often confused with asthma, although they often occur together (Neman et al. 1995). It is not unusual for VCD to be misdiagnosed as steroid-resistant asthma (Thomas et al. 1999). VCD may also co-occur with HVS. The syndromal picture of VCD was first described 200 years ago by Osler (Brugman 2003), yet it is still not well understood. VCD has been called by many different names—for example, episodic laryngeal dyskinesia, paradoxical vocal cord motion, hysterical croup, adductor spastic dysphonia, factitious asthma, and functional upper airway obstruction. The disorder may present in childhood, adolescence, or adulthood. Patients may appear in severe respiratory distress yet have relatively normal blood gas levels, or respiratory alkalosis from hyperventilation, only rarely presenting with hypoxemia. In contrast to asthma, in VCD wheezing will be loudest over the larynx and more pronounced in the inspiratory phase, but the chest is otherwise clear. Also unlike asthma, VCD attacks typically have rapid onset and equally rapid resolution. VCD may lead to frequent ER visits and hospitalizations, high doses of (ineffective) asthma medications, and unnecessary intubation (Bahrainwala and Simon 2001). The differential diagnosis of VCD includes asthma, HVS, neurological disorders (e.g., spasmodic dysphonia and laryngeal nerve injury), and angioedema (Brugman 2003).

For many years, VCD was considered a conversion disorder, but VCD should be considered as a symptom. In most patients, VCD appears not to be a primary psychiatric disorder but rather a conditioned response or functional disorder, which may result in secondary anxiety, which then further aggravates the condition. The onset of VCD is typically preceded by allergy, asthma, reflux, irritant exposure (Perkner et al. 1998), or a dyspneic episode in athletes (Newsham et al. 2002). The psychiatric literature reflects referral bias but nevertheless captures part of the VCD spectrum. Case reports and retrospective case series noted strong dependency needs and fears of separation in patients with VCD and its acute precipitation following psychosocial stress. One study of tertiary care VCD patients found that the majority had a history of childhood sexual abuse (Freedman et al. 1991), but this has not been substantiated (Brugman 2003). There is only one prospective controlled blinded study using standardized measurements, comparing adolescent patients with VCD to matched asthma patients without VCD (Gavin et al. 1998). Anxiety disorders and depression were much more common in VCD patients. Psychiatrists are most likely to see those patients with VCD who develop panic attacks and phobic symptoms. Wamboldt et al. (in press) note the considerable overlap among VCD, HVS, and panic disorder, and they postulate that VCD is linked to Klein's "faulty suffocation alarm" (Klein 1993). Other referred cases of VCD may represent conversion disorder, posttraumatic stress disorder, somatization disorder, factitious illness, or another psychiatric disorder.

There is no empirically proven treatment for VCD. Most patients with uncomplicated VCD respond well to speech therapy alone (Brugman 2003). Those with associated psychopathology should receive treatment appropriate to their psychiatric diagnosis, for example, psycho-

therapy or antipanic pharmacotherapy. Biofeedback has recently been reported as helpful (Earles et al. 2003).

Lung Cancer

Lung cancer is the most common cause of cancer death in the United States and the world. Smoking tobacco is the primary cause of most lung cancers (Strauss 1998).

A review of quality of life in lung cancer patients from 1970 to 1995 noted that over 80% of lung cancer patients died within a year of diagnosis, because many were diagnosed late (Montazeri et al. 1998). More than 50 instruments have been used to measure quality of life in patients with lung cancer. Psychological distress and lower quality of life have been correlated with even moderate weight loss (Ovesen et al. 1993). Symptoms of psychological distress are common in lung cancer. One study showed that newly diagnosed lung cancer patients had frequent insomnia (52%), loss of libido (48%), loss of interest or ability to work (33%), concerns about their families (29%), and poor concentration (19%) (Ginsburg et al. 1995). Another study found that predictors of psychological distress in ambulatory lung cancer patients included being female, living alone, having no children as confidants, relying on nursing staff as confidants, and having a helpless or hopeless coping style (Akechi et al. 1998).

A study of newly diagnosed patients with unresectable non–small cell cancer of the lung described the most common psychiatric diagnoses as nicotine dependence (67%), adjustment disorders (14%), alcohol dependence (13%), and major depression (5%). Depression did not increase over the course of the illness. Pain management was key in relieving depression (Akechi et al. 2001). Uchitomi et al. (2003) also studied non–small cell lung cancer patients (n = 212) and found that the prevalence of depression in the year after curative resection did not significantly decrease, suggesting that ongoing psychosocial support is needed even after curative resection of non–small cell cancer of the lung. Type of lung cancer may influence the rate of depression. In one study, the rate of depression was nearly three times higher in those with small-cell cancer (25%) than in those with non–small cell cancer (9%). The most important risk factor for depression was functional impairment (Hopwood and Stephens 2000).

Fatigue is more common at diagnosis with lung cancer than most other cancers: 50% of those with inoperable non–small cell cancer reported severe fatigue. Key factors contributing to fatigue include disease burden, dyspnea, pain, and psychological distress (Stone et al. 2000). Adaptive behaviors can reduce fatigue even with low hemoglobin levels. Lung or colon cancer subjects who used nonadaptive routines—namely, disorganization, inertia, and overexertion—reported more fatigue (Olson et al. 2002).

Tanaka et al. (2002) found that dyspnea, very common in advanced lung cancer, was significantly correlated with cough, pain, and psychological distress. Given the high rate of dyspnea in lung cancer patients, one might expect that many patients would cease tobacco use. However, this is not the case, despite evidence that continued smoking after lung cancer diagnosis decreases treatment efficacy, increases complications, increases risk of recurrence and occurrence of another primary tumor, and decreases survival time. Schnoll et al. (2002) noted that in 74 cancer patients decreased readiness to quit smoking was associated with emotional distress, fatalistic beliefs, greater nicotine dependence, less self-efficacy, and having relatives at home who also smoke.

Do psychological factors alter the course of lung cancer? One study of lung cancer patients found that self-report of depressive coping was an independent predictor of decreased survival time at 8- and 10-year follow-up (Faller and Bulzebruck 2002; Faller et al. 1997). Psychological factors may also influence response to treatment in other ways. For example, one small study concluded that anxiety or depression predicted increased nausea scores after chemotherapy (Takatsuki et al. 1998).

Little has been written on coping in lung cancer. One study noted four common coping strategies among 50 patients with stages III and IV adenocarcinoma of the lung: seeking social support, problem solving, self-control, and positive reappraisal. There was no correlation between coping, mood, or perceived stress and the side effects of chemotherapy (Chernecky 1999).

Lung Transplantation

Indications and Contraindications

The first lung transplant was performed in 1963, but it was 20 years before the first successful operation in 1983 (Ochoa and Richardson 1999) (see also Chapter 31, "Organ Transplantation"). The most common indication is COPD (including alpha-I-antitrypsin deficiency), which accounts for about 45% of lung transplants (Hosenpud et al. 1998). Transplants are also performed for those with CF, IPF, Eisenmenger syndrome, primary pulmonary hypertension, and a number of other pulmonary diseases (Etienne et al. 1997). Patients are generally listed when their quality of life has declined and transplant would confer a survival benefit, given the waiting time of up to 2 years once the patient is listed for transplant (Maurer et al. 1998).

Exclusion criteria vary from one transplant center to another. Absolute contraindications typically include serious cardiac, renal, or hepatic insufficiency; cancer; chronic infections (e.g., cytomegalovirus, hepatitis B virus, or hepatitis C virus); or weight less than 70% or greater than 130% of ideal body weight. Psychiatric factors that are considered to be absolute contraindications to lung transplantation include active alcoholism, drug abuse or cigarette use, severe psychiatric illness, and noncompliance with treatment (Aris et al. 1997; Paradowski 1997; Snell et al. 1993).

Generally, lungs are allocated differently than hearts and livers. Presently in the United States, only waiting time, not severity of disease, is considered, but a prioritization scheme is currently being developed (Hauptman and O'Connor 1997). There are four main approaches to lung transplantation, including single-lung transplantation (the type most commonly performed), bilateral sequential transplantation, heart-lung transplantation, and single-lobe donation from living donors (Arcasoy and Kotloff 1999). Living donor donation has been controversial because of the uncertainty regarding risks to the donor. An analysis of one series of 120 donors reported four serious complications requiring return to surgery but no deaths. Loss of one lobe only decreased the lung volume by 15%, because the remaining lung expands to compensate, which does not impact long-term function in the donor (Barr et al. 1998).

Medical and Surgical Outcome

Patient survival in the United States at 1 year and 3 years after lung transplant is currently 77% and 58%, respectively. Median survival is 3.7 years. For comparison, the corresponding survival figures after heart transplant are 85% and 77% (United Network for Organ Sharing 2003). For patients with CF and IPF, there appears to be increased survival relative to the natural history of the underlying illness. However, for patients with COPD, no survival advantage has been demonstrated, although transplant does appear to improve quality of life and functional ability. Exercise capacity improves, with about 80% of recipients reporting no limitations in activity within 1 year of transplant. Only 4% of lung recipients require total care at 1 year posttransplant. Quality of life remains stable for the first few years if the course is uncomplicated, but those who develop bronchiolitis obliterans show a sharp decline in quality of life. Despite improvements in exercise tolerance and quality of life, 40% or fewer of lung transplant recipients return to work. This finding may be a result of employer bias, a fear of losing health insurance or disability benefits, or a change in priorities after a life-threatening illness (Paris et al. 1998).

Early complications after lung transplantation include primary graft failure, stenosis of the anastomosis, and a higher rate of infectious complications than in other solid organ transplantation, including bacterial pneumonia, cytomegalovirus pneumonitis, and complications of infection by *Aspergillus* and other pathogens (Christie et al. 1998; Kramer et al. 1993).

The incidence of acute rejection is greatest in the first 100 days after transplantation and declines over the first year (Bando et al. 1995). Chronic rejection is more common in lung transplant recipients, resulting in bronchiolitis obliterans (fibrotic obliteration of small airways) (Estenne and Hertz 2002).

Psychological Factors and Quality of Life

Until recently, there were few studies in this area because of the small numbers of lung transplants being performed and the dearth of long-term survivors to study. All available studies are limited by small size. Cohen et al. (1998) described 32 recipients reporting better quality of life posttransplant. No pretransplant psychological variables were found to be associated with the length of survival posttransplant. Pretransplant trait anxiety did predict posttransplant quality of life. Those with higher levels of pretransplant trait anxiety had poorer mental health as well as more state anxiety, subjective sleep disturbances, and cardiac and pulmonary symptoms posttransplant (Cohen et al. 1998).

Stilley et al. (1999) studied 36 lung recipients and 14 heart–lung recipients, noting no differences in psychological data between the two transplant types. Recipients showed lower hostility than a normative sample. On the Hopkins Symptom Checklist–90 (SCL-90), recipients had about double the rates of depression and anxiety compared with the control group, with lung recipients having higher rates than heart–lung recipients. Lower global quality of life was more often seen in those recipients with low caregiver support, lower educational level, and higher level of health-related concerns when other variables were controlled (Stilley et al. 1999).

Limbos et al. observed that although many lung transplant recipients continued to have impaired psychological functioning posttransplant, most reported significant improvement in general health, self-esteem, social functioning, quality of life, anxiety, and depression. They noted no significant differences in sexual functioning between pretransplant and posttransplant subjects (Limbos et al. 2000).

A group in the Netherlands followed 28 lung transplant recipients for at least 55 months. Until about 43 months after transplant, there were significant improvements in anxiety, depression, quality of life, and activities of daily living, but after that time there was a decline in all of these measures (Vermeulen et al. 2003).

Psychological Interventions

Napolitano et al. (2002) tested the efficacy of inexpensive telephone-based supportive and cognitive behavioral therapy for lung transplant candidates. The telephone-intervention group reported significantly higher general well-being, general quality of life, disease-specific quality of life, and levels of social support.

Teichman et al. (2000) studied adherence to treatment regimens after lung transplant and found that the level of family support was significantly correlated with self-reported compliance. Patients became less compliant the further from the time of transplant, suggesting that periodic reeducation after transplantation may improve adherence.

Terminal Weaning

Patients with end-stage pulmonary disease caused by amyotrophic lateral sclerosis, COPD, CF, IPF, lung cancer, or other diseases may request terminal weaning to avoid futile interventions. The term *terminal weaning* has been viewed by some as an oxymoron for several reasons. *Terminal* implies that the withdrawal of ventilator support will inevitably end in death, yet *weaning* carries the implication of achieving independence from the ventilator. Another problem with the term is that patients do not always die shortly after discontinuation of ventilatory support. In one study, 8% of patients survived and were discharged (M.L. Campbell 1994). In the Karen Quinlan case, the U.S. Supreme Court supported her parents' right to have her ventilator withdrawn. Physician experts for both sides testified that she would die shortly afterward, but she lived 10 years after extubation. The phrase "discontinuation of ventilator support" or "withdrawal of mechanical ventilation" may be used when talking with the patient, family, and staff caring for the patient (Apelgren 2000; Daly et al. 1993).

Ethicists and legal experts concur that competent patients have the right to refuse treatment, regardless of whether it is "life saving," and that there is no moral difference between not initiating treatment and withdrawing treatment in response to the patient's request. However, physicians and nurses find withdrawing treatment, especially a ventilator, more difficult because this is viewed as a more active intervention, which may cause a greater sense of culpability. The patient must be aware that death is the most likely outcome when ventilator support is discontinued (although not every patient dies) and make the decision after due deliberation. The patient may view mechanical ventilation as an intolerable intrusion that diminishes the quality of life and renders death the preferred option (Daly et al. 1993).

The patient's goals should guide the process of withdrawing ventilator support (J. Anderson and O'Brien 1995). If the patient shows ambivalence about terminal weaning, or it is unclear whether the patient has sufficient mental capacity to make a well-thought-out decision, consultation from a psychiatrist should be obtained. The first step in evaluation is to explore why the patient has requested discontinuation of ventilator support. Some patients may be depressed and will agree to a trial of antidepressants prior to finalizing the decision for terminal weaning. Some have concluded (often correctly) that they can never be weaned successfully and prefer death to spending whatever is left of their lives on a ventilator in the hospital. Some are delirious, and their request is inconsistent and confused. Some are worried about burdening their families with hospital bills. Others may be struggling with whether giving up on the ventilator violates their religion's prohibition of suicide. Those health care workers caring for the patient should have an opportunity to discuss the decision as a team. In difficult cases, in addition to the psychiatrist, involvement of the hospital's ethics committee, chaplain, social worker, and legal counsel may be helpful. A brief delay after the decision has been made to withdraw ventilator support may reassure staff and family that the patient made a decision that was not based on temporary frustration or discomfort.

Patients should be told that the weaning process may be stopped at any time if they wish and that they may decide who will be present during the weaning process. Family members should be asked if they want to be present if the patient is incompetent or unresponsive. Withdrawal of the ventilator may follow the withdrawal of pressors, antibiotics, and enteral feeding (Brody et al. 1997). In a comatose patient whose family does not wish to be present, the physician may opt for extubation. In a conscious patient, a gradual decrease in FIO_2, with decreased positive end-expiratory pressure (PEEP) and decrease in respiratory rate over several hours has been advocated (Grenvik 1983).

No matter which method is used, adjunctive medication may alleviate distress. Opiates have been used for pain relief and to decrease gasping, coughing, or the sensation of shortness of breath; to provide sedation; and to decrease anxiety in the patient. Documentation of the physician's intent in administering opiates is important to show that the medication is being used as a comfort measure and not to hasten death. One protocol suggests giving a bolus of 5–10 mg morphine intravenously followed by a drip of 2.5–5.0 mg per hour of morphine. Benzodiazepines may decrease anxiety and prevent myoclonus or twitching that may be unsettling to the family (Faber-Langendoen 1994). Phenobarbital may control twitching not relieved by benzodiazepines. Low-dose haloperidol may be used intravenously for anxiety not relieved by benzodiazepines or if the patient is delirious.

The family should be educated prior to the procedure that although the patient may have reflexive gasping or twitching, the medications used will prevent the patient from having awareness of these bodily events, and they may induce euphoria. Although patients in a persistent vegetative state may grimace when extubated, without higher cortical function there is no awareness of discomfort.

Use of paralytic agents is discouraged because they may prevent the patient from signaling if there is any distress. In patients who retain carbon dioxide, decreasing tidal volume or respiratory rate on intermittent mechanical ventilation may allow the CO_2 to gradually rise, resulting in drowsiness, at which point mechanical ventilation may be stopped. The process should take place over just a few hours, preventing a prolonged bedside vigil that is exhausting for the family. The comfort of the family should be considered, for example, by providing ample seating and tissues, dimming the lights if desired, and turning off patient monitors if the family finds constantly beeping alarms disruptive or the electrocardiogram (ECG) readout upsetting. Staff members should remain at the bedside in a supportive, unobtrusive way, to attend to the patient and provide comfort to the family. Expressions of concern about how the withdrawal of ventilator support is affecting family members are appropriate. Physicians should take cues from the family and may step out to allow privacy or for religious ceremonies to be performed without interference (Benner 1993; Daly et al. 1993).

Psychopharmacology in Pulmonary Disease

Anxiety

Anxiety in pulmonary patients may be caused by symptoms of lung disease such as breathlessness, bronchospasm, excessive secretions, or hypoxia, so the first step in treatment of anxiety is optimization of management of the patient's respiratory illness. Many drugs used to treat pulmonary disease may themselves cause anxiety (Table 20–1). Theophylline, a methylxanthine, can cause anxiety, nausea, tremor, and restlessness, especially at higher doses. Beta-adrenergic bronchodilators used in treatment of asthma or other obstructive lung disease can cause marked anxiety, tachycardia, and tremor, particularly in patients who overuse their inhalers. Nonprescription asthma preparations contain nonselective sympathomimetics, which are even more likely to cause anxiety. At high doses, they may cause psychosis and seizures.

TABLE 20–1. Psychiatric side effects of common pulmonary drugs

Anticholinergics	Auditory and visual hallucinations, anxiety, confusion, delirium, depersonalization, amnesia, paranoia
Antileukotrienes	Anxiety
Beta-agonists (selective)	Anxiety in susceptible patients
Beta-agonists (nonselective)	Anxiety, psychosis
Corticosteroids (inhaled)	None
Corticosteroids (systemic)	Depression, mania
Cromolyn	Irritability
Cycloserine	Agoraphobia, anxiety, depression, psychosis
Isoniazid	Amnesia, anxiety, depression, hallucinations, mania, psychosis
Theophylline	Anxiety, delirium, insomnia, mutism, restlessness, tremor

Source. Adapted from *The Medical Letter* 1998, 2002.

In anxious pulmonary patients with hypercapnia, buspirone is preferred for treatment of anxiety, but it may have a slow onset of action (Craven and Sutherland 1991). Buspirone may improve exercise tolerance and dyspnea, can be used safely in patients with sleep apnea (Mendelson et al. 1991), and can be combined with theophylline and terbutaline (Kiev and Domantay 1988).

In COPD patients who do not retain carbon dioxide, prudent doses of benzodiazepines may decrease breathlessness. In elderly or debilitated patients, shorter-acting benzodiazepines with no active metabolites, such as alprazolam, lorazepam, and oxazepam, are preferred. Zolpidem does not alter respiratory drive in COPD patients, but rebound insomnia or withdrawal similar to triazolam may result. Diazepam has no effect on breathlessness and may decrease exercise tolerance. Although some have advocated promethazine to decrease breathlessness and increase exercise tolerance in COPD, this drug is a phenothiazine and has the same spectrum of adverse effects as chlorpromazine. Selective serotonin reuptake inhibitors (SRRIs) may also be helpful in treating panic symptoms and do not have pulmonary side effects. If panic does not respond to these measures, then neuroleptics may be effective in low doses. Beta-blockers should not be used for anxiety in asthma patients, because of resulting bronchoconstriction.

Depression

When choosing an antidepressant, the side-effect profile and cytochrome P450 interactions with pulmonary drugs should be considered. Generally, SSRIs other than fluvoxamine are effective and have few drug interactions that are problematic in pulmonary patients, and SSRIs may decrease dyspnea and even increase arterial oxygen concentration in some patients (Ciraulo and Shader 1990; Smoller et al. 1998).

Many pulmonary patients are elderly with comorbid conditions and may be on other medications that can pro-

long the QT interval, so reviewing the ECG is prudent when considering treatment with a tricyclic antidepressant. In elderly patients or in patients with COPD or sleep apnea, nortriptyline or desipramine is preferred over the more sedating tertiary amines, which may cause delirium or hypotension. Protriptyline may be helpful in sleep apnea by increasing respiratory drive, but the half-life is very long (54–92 hours), three to four times longer than that of nortriptyline, and there is no evidence that protriptyline is more effective than other tricyclics for sleep apnea (DeVane 1998). Doxepin may be a mild bronchodilator because of its anticholinergic qualities (Cooper 1988).

Psychosis

Pulmonary patients may have primary psychotic disorders, such as bipolar disorder or schizophrenia, or may become psychotic because of medications such as beta-agonists, cycloserine, isoniazid, or corticosteroids. The incidence of steroid psychosis is dose-related, seen in less than 1% of patients taking 40 mg or less of prednisone per day versus 28% taking 80 mg daily (Boston Collaborative Drug Surveillance Program 1972).

Typical neuroleptics such as haloperidol at high doses may cause laryngospasm, akathisia, and paradoxical intercostal muscle movements that, in turn, may cause restlessness and interfere with breathing. Tardive dyskinesia sometimes affects the diaphragm and other muscles used in breathing, and in severe cases, this effect can result in respiratory insufficiency. For chronic treatment, newer drugs with lower incidence of extrapyramidal side effects may be preferred.

Drug Interactions Between Psychotropic and Pulmonary Drugs

The psychiatrist should consider potential interactions when prescribing psychotropic medications to patients with pulmonary disease (Table 20–2). Theophylline levels

TABLE 20–2. Drug interactions

Pulmonary drug	Psychotropic drug	Adverse effect
Isoniazid	TCAs	MAOI effect of isoniazid
Rifampin	Donepezil	Decreased donepezil effect
Rifampin	Diazepam	Induced diazepam metabolism
Rifampin	Valproate	Decreased valproate level
Rifampin	TCAs, MAOIs	Induced TCA, MAOI metabolism
Sympathomimetic drugs[a]	TCAs, MAOIs	Hypertensive crisis
Theophylline	Alprazolam	Decreased benzodiazepine effect
Theophylline	Carbamazepine	Decreased carbamazepine level
Theophylline	Clozapine	Increased theophylline level
Theophylline	Fluvoxamine	Increased theophylline level
Theophylline	Lithium	Reduced lithium level 20%–30%

Note. MAOI=monoamine oxidase inhibitor; TCA=tricyclic antidepressant.
[a]Epinephrine, ephedrine, pseudoephedrine.
Source. Adapted from Cozza KL, Armstrong SC, Oesterheld JR: *Drug Interaction Principles Pocket Guide.* Washington, DC, American Psychiatric Publishing, 2003.

may be reduced from 50%–80% by tobacco smoking. Nicotine gum does not have this effect. Alcohol can reduce clearance of theophylline as much as 30% for up to 24 hours. Most pulmonary medications do not affect lithium levels, except theophylline, which can lower lithium levels by 20%–30%. Patients with chronic pulmonary disease may develop right-sided heart failure, and they may receive diuretics that raise or lower lithium levels depending on choice of diuretic. Theophylline preparations administered concurrently with electroconvulsive therapy can prolong seizure duration, especially if the theophylline level is above the accepted therapeutic range, even if the level is below that typically associated with seizures (Peters et al. 1984).

Rifampin is a cytochrome P450 3A4 substrate and so may compete with many psychotropic drugs, including the antidepressants amitriptyline, imipramine, fluoxetine, sertraline, bupropion, venlafaxine, and trazodone. Rifampin may compete through the same site with anticonvulsants (e.g., carbamazepine, tiagabine, and valproate) and with benzodiazepines, zolpidem, and haloperidol. Montelukast sodium may have similar interactions to those of rifampin, because of metabolism via 3A4 and 2C9.

References

Abbott J, Dodd M, Gee L, Webb K: Ways of coping with cystic fibrosis: implications for treatment adherence. Disabil Rehabil 23:315–24, 2001

Akechi T, Kugaya A, Okamura H, et al: Predictive factors for psychological distress in ambulatory lung cancer patients. Support Care Cancer 6:281–286, 1998

Akechi T, Okamura H, Nishiwaki Y, et al: Psychiatric disorders and associated and predictive factors in patients with unresectable nonsmall cell lung carcinoma: a longitudinal study. Cancer 92:2609–2622, 2001

Alao AO, Yolles JC: Isoniazid-induced psychosis. Ann Pharmacother 32:889–891, 1998

Ambrosino N, Bruletti G, Scala V, et al: Cognitive and perceived health status in patients with chronic obstructive pulmonary disease surviving acute or chronic respiratory failure: a controlled study. Intensive Care Med 28:170–177, 2002

American Lung Association: Minority Lung Disease Data 2000. Available at: www.lungusa.org. Accessed January 2000.

Anderson J, O'Brien M: Challenges for the future: the nurse's role in weaning patients from mechanical ventilation. Intensive Crit Care Nurs 11:2–5, 1995

Anderson DL, Flume PA, Hardy KK: Psychological functioning of adults with cystic fibrosis. Chest 119:1079–1084, 2001

Antonelli Incalzi R, Marra C, Giordano A, et al: Cognitive impairment in chronic obstructive pulmonary disease—a neuropsychological and SPECT study. J Neurol 250:325–332, 2003

Apelgren KN: "Terminal" wean is the wrong term. Crit Care Med 28:3576–3577, 2000

Araki S, Honma T: Mass psychogenic systemic illness in school children in relation to the Tokyo photochemical smog. Arch Environ Health 41:159–162, 1986

Arcasoy SM, Kotloff RM: Lung transplantation. N Engl J Med 340:1081–1091, 1999

Aris RM, Gilligan PH, Neuring IP, et al: The effect of panresistant bacteria in cystic fibrosis patients on lung transplant outcome. Am J Respir Crit Care Med 155:1699–1704, 1997

Aydin IO, Ulusahin A: Depression, anxiety comorbidity, and disability in tuberculosis and chronic obstructive pulmonary disease patients: applicability of GHQ-12. Gen Hosp Psychiatry 23:77–83, 2001

Bahrainwala AH, Simon MR: Wheezing and vocal cord dysfunction mimicking asthma. Curr Opin Pulm Med 7:8–13, 2001

Bando K, Paradis IL, Similo S, et al: Obliterative bronchiolitis after lung and heart-lung transplantation: an analysis of risk factors and management. J Thorac Cardiovasc Surg 110:4–14, 1995

Barnes PJ, Woolcock AJ: Difficult asthma. Eur Respir J 12:1209–1218, 1998

Barr ML, Schenkel FA, Cohen RG, et al: Recipient and donor outcomes in living related and unrelated lobar transplantation. Transplant Proc 30:2261–2263, 1998

Bass C: Hyperventilation syndrome: a chimera? J Psychosom Res 423:421–426, 1997

Benner KL: Terminal weaning: a loved one's vigil. Am J Nurs 93:22–25, 1993

Bloom BB, Humphries DE, Kuang PP, et al: Structure and expression of the promoter for the R4/ALK5 hu type I transforming growth factor-beta receptor: regulation by TGF-beta. Biochim Biophys Acta 1312:243–248, 1996

Borson S, Claypoole K, McDonald GJ: Depression and chronic obstructive pulmonary disease: treatment trials. Semin Clin Neuropsychiatry 3:115–130, 1998

Bosley CM, Corden ZM, Rees PJ, et al: Psychological factors associated with use of home nebulized therapy for COPD. Eur Respir J 9:2346–2350, 1996

Boston Collaborative Drug Surveillance Program: Acute adverse reaction to prednisone in relation to dosage. Clin Pharmacol Ther 13:694–697, 1972

Brenes GA: Anxiety and chronic obstructive pulmonary disease: prevalence, impact, and treatment. Psychosom Med 65:963–970, 2003

Britto MT, Kotagal UR, Hornung RW, et al: Impact of recent pulmonary exacerbations on quality of life patients with cystic fibrosis. Chest 1211:64–72, 2002

Brody H, Campbell ML, Faber-Langendoen, et al: Withdrawing intensive life-sustaining treatment—recommendations for compassionate clinical management. N Engl J Med 336:652–657, 1997

Brugman SM: The many faces of vocal cord dysfunction: what 36 years of literature tell us. Am J Respir Crit Care Med 167:A588, 2003

Buchi S, Brandli O, Klingler K, et al: Inpatient rehabilitation in inpatients with chronic obstructive lung disease: effect on physical capacity for work, psychological wellbeing and quality of life. Schweiz Med Wochenschr Suppl 130:135–432, 2000

Bullman C, Faust M, Hoffmann A, et al: Five cases with central diabetes insipidus and hypogonadism as first presentation of neurosarcoidosis. Eur J Endocrinol 142:365–372, 2000

Burker EJ, Carels RA, Thompson LF, et al: Quality of life in patients awaiting lung transplant: cystic fibrosis versus other end-stage lung diseases. Pediatr Pulmonol 30:453–460, 2000

Callaham M: Hypoxic hazards of traditional paper bag rebreathing in hyperventilating patients. Ann Emerg Med 18:622–628, 1989

Campbell DA, Yellowlees PM, McLennan G, et al: Psychiatric and medical features of near fatal asthma. Thorax 50:254–259, 1995

Campbell ML: Terminal weaning: it's not simply "pulling the plug." Nursing 24:34–39, 1994

Castro PF, Larrain G, Perez O, et al: Chronic hyperventilation syndrome associated with syncope and coronary vasospasm. Am J Med 109:78–80, 2000

Centanni S, DiMarco F, Castagna F, et al: Psychological issues in the treatment of asthmatic patients. Respir Med 94:742–749, 2000

Centers for Disease Control and Prevention: Self-reported increase in asthma severity after the September 11 attacks on the World Trade Center—Manhattaan, New York, 2001. MMWR Morb Mortal Wkly Rep 51:781–784, 2002

Charan NB: Does sildenafil also improve breathing? Chest 120:305–306, 2001

Chernecky C: Temporal differences in coping, mood, and stress with chemotherapy. Cancer Nurs 22:266–276, 1999

Christian BJ, D'Auria JP: The child's eye: memories of growing up with cystic fibrosis. J Pediatr Nurs 12:3–12, 1997

Christie JD, Bavaria JE, Palevsky HI, et al: Primary graft failure following lung transplantation. Chest 114:51–60, 1998

Ciraulo DA, Shader RI: Fluoxetine drug-drug interactions II. J Clin Psychopharmacol 10:213–217, 1990

Cluley S, Cochrane GM: Psychological disorder in asthma is associated with poor control and poor adherence to inhaled steroids. Respir Med 95:37–39, 2001

Cohen L, Littlefield C, Kelly P, et al: Predictors of quality of life and adjustment after lung transplantation. Chest 113:633–644, 1998

Conway AV, Freeman LJ, Nixon PG: Hypnotic examination of trigger factors in the hyperventilation syndrome. Am J Clin Hypn 30:286–304, 1988

Cooper GL: The safety of fluoxetine—an update. Br J Psychiatry Suppl 3:77–86, 1988

Cowley DS, Roy-Byrne PP: Hyperventilation and panic disorder. Am J Med 83:929–937, 1987

Cozza KL, Armstrong SC, Oesterheld JR: Drug Interaction Principles Pocket Guide. Washington, DC, American Psychiatric Publishing, 2003

Craven J, Sutherland A: Buspirone for anxiety disorders in patients with severe lung disease (letter). Lancet 338:249, 1991

Czajkowski DR, Koocher GP: Medical compliance and coping with cystic fibrosis. J Child Psychol Psychiatry 28:311–319, 1987

Dahlen I, Janson C: Anxiety and depression are related to the outcome of emergency treatment in patients with obstructive pulmonary disease. Chest 122:1633–1637, 2002

Daly BJ, Newlon B, Montenegro HD, et al: Withdrawal of mechanical ventilation: ethical principles and guidelines for terminal weaning. Am J Crit Care 2:217–223, 1993

Degruy F, Crider J, Hashimi DK, et al: Somatization disorder in a university hospital. J Fam Pract 25:579–584, 1987

DeGuire S, Gevirtz R, Kawahara Y, et al: Hyperventilation syndrome and the assessment of treatment for functional cardiac symptoms. Am J Cardiol 70:673–677, 1992

DeGuire S, Gevirtz R, Hawkinson D, et al: Breathing retraining: a 3-year follow-up study of treatment for hyperventilation syndrome and associated functional cardiac symptoms. Biofeedback Self Regul 21:191–198, 1996

Delaney P: Neurologic manifestations in sarcoidosis: review of the literature, with a report of 23 cases. Ann Intern Med 87: 336–345, 1977

Della Sala S, Donner CF, Sacco C, et al: Does chronic lung failure lead to cognitive failure? Schweiz Arch Neurol Psychiatr 143:343–354, 1992

Demeter SL, Cordasco EM: Hyperventilation syndrome and asthma. Am J Med 81:989–994, 1986

deRuiter C, Garssen B, Rijken H, et al: The hyperventilation syndrome in panic disorder, agoraphobia and generalized anxiety disorder. Behav Res Ther 27:447–452, 1989

DeVane CL: Principles of pharmacokinetics and pharmacodynamics, in Textbook of Psychopharmacology, 2nd Edition. Edited by Schatzberg AF, Nemeroff CB. American Psychiatric Press, Washington, DC, London, pp 155–169, 1998

DeVries J, Kessels BL, Drent M: Quality of life of idiopathic pulmonary fibrosis patients. Eur Respir J 17:954–961, 2001

Djibo A, Lawan A: Behavioral disorders after treatment with isoniazid. Bull Soc Pathol Exot 94(2):112–114, 2001

Downing ET, Braman SS, Fox MJ, et al: Factitious asthma. Physiological approach to diagnosis. JAMA 248:2878–2881, 1982

Dudley DL, Sitzman J, Rugg M: Psychiatric aspects of patients with chronic obstructive pulmonary disease. Adv Psychosom Med 14:64–77, 1985

Earles J, Kerr B, Kellar M: Psychophysiologic treatment of vocal cord dysfunction. Ann Allergy Asthma Immunol 90:669–671, 2003

Ebadi M, Gessert CF, Al-Sayegh A: Drug-pyridoxal phosphate interactions. Q Rev Drug Metab Drug Interact 4:289–331, 1982

Estenne M, Hertz MI: Bronchiolitis obliterans after human lung transplantation. Am J Respir Crit Care Med 166:440–444, 2002

Etienne B, Bertocchi M, Gamondes JP, et al: Successful double-lung transplantation for bronchioalveolar carcinoma. Chest 112:1423–1424, 1997

Ewig S, Torres A: Severe community-acquired pneumonia. Clin Chest Med 20:575–587, 1999

Faber-Langendoen K: The clinical management of dying patients receiving mechanical ventilation: a survey of physician practice. Chest 106:880–888, 1994

Fagan J, Galea S, Ahern J, et al: Relationship of self-reported asthma severity and urgent health care utilization to psychological sequelae of the September 11, 2001 terrorist attacks on the World Trade Center among New York City area residents. Psychosom Med 65:993–996, 2003

Faller H, Bulzebruck H: Coping and survival in lung cancer: a 10-year follow-up. Am J Psychiatry 159:2105–2107, 2002

Faller H, Bulzebruck H, Schilling S, et al: Do psychological factors modify survival of cancer patients? II: results of an empirical study with bronchial carcinoma patients. Psychother Psychosom Med Psychol 47:206–218, 1997

Fensterheim H, Wiegand B: Group treatment of the hyperventilation syndrome. Int J Group Psychother 41:399–403, 1991

Fioravanti M, Nacca D, Amati S, et al: Chronic obstructive pulmonary disease and associated patterns of memory decline. Dementia 6:39–48, 1995

Fischer AJ, Huygen PL, Folgering HT, et al: Vestibular hyperreactivity and hyperventilation after whiplash injury. J Neurol Sci 132:35–43, 1995

Fix AJ, Daughton D, Kass I, et al: Cognitive functioning and survival among patients with chronic obstructive pulmonary disease. Int J Neurosci 27:13–17, 1985

Folgering H: The pathophysiology of hyperventilation syndrome. Monaldi Arch Chest Dis 54:356–372, 1999

Freedman MR, Rosenberg SJ, Schmaling KB: Childhood sexual abuse in patients with paradoxical vocal cord dysfunction. J Nerv Ment Dis 179:295–298, 1991

Freeman LJ, Nixon PG: Are coronary artery spasm and progressive damage to the heart associated with the hyperventilation syndrome? Br Med J (Clin Res Ed) 291:851–852, 1985

Garden GM, Ayres JG: Psychiatric and social aspects of brittle asthma. Thorax 48:501–505, 1993

Gavin LA, Wamboldt M, Brugman S, et al: Psychological and family characteristics of adolescents with vocal cord dysfunction. J Asthma 35:409–417, 1998

Giardino ND, Schmaling KB, Afari N: Relationship satisfaction moderates the association between catastrophic cognitions and asthma symptoms. J Asthma 39:749–756, 2002

Ginsburg ML, Quirt C, Ginsburg AD, et al: Psychiatric illness and psychosocial concerns of patients with newly diagnosed lung cancer. CMAJ 152:1961–1963, 1995

Goodwin RD, Jacobi F, Thefeld W: Mental disorders and asthma in the community. Arch Gen Psychiatry 60:1125–1130, 2003

Grant I, Prigatoano GP, Heaton RK, et al: Progressive neuropsychological impairment and hypoxemia. Relationship in chronic obstructive pulmonary disease. Arch Gen Psychiatry 44:999–1006, 1987

Greenberg, DB, Halperin P, Kradin RL, et al: Internal medicine and medical subspecialties, in Textbook of Consultation-Liaison Psychiatry. Washington, DC, American Psychiatric Press, 1996, pp 565–566

Grenvik A: "Terminal weaning": discontinuance of life-support therapy in the terminally ill patient. Crit Care Med 11:394–395, 1983

Hains AA, Davies WH, Behrens D, et al: Cognitive behavioral interventions for adolescents with cystic fibrosis. J Pediatr Psychol 22:669–687, 1997

Hanna DE, Hodgens JB, Daniel WA: Hyperventilation syndrome. Pediatr Ann 15:708–712, 1986

Hauptman PJ, O'Connor KJ: Procurement and allocation of solid organs for transplantation. N Engl J Med 336:422–431, 1997

Heaton RK, Grant I, McSweeney AJ, et al: Psychologic effects of continuous and nocturnal oxygen therapy in hypoxemic chronic obstructive pulmonary disease. Arch Intern Med 143:1941–1947, 1983

Hegel MT, Abel GG, Etscheidt M, et al: Behavioral treatment of angina-like chest pain in patients with hyperventilation syndrome. J Behav Ther Exp Psychiatry 20:31–39, 1989

Hehrmann R: Hypocalcemic crisis. Hypoparathyroidism—non-parathyroid origin—the most frequent form: hyperventilation syndrome [in German]. Fortschr Med 114:223–226, 1996

Hirokawa Y, Kondo T, Ohta Y, et al: Clinical characteristics and outcome of 508 patients with hyperventilation syndrome. Nihon Kyobu Shikkan Gakkai Zasshi 33:940–946, 1995

Hodgens JB, Fanurik D, Hanna DE: Adolescent hyperventilation syndrome. Ala J Med Sci 25:423–436, 1988

Hoegholm A, Clementsen P, Mortensen SA: Syncope due to right atrial thromboembolism: diagnostic importance of two-dimensional echocardiography. Acta Cardiol 42:469–473, 1987

Hoes MJ, Colla P, Van Doorn P et al: Hyperventilation and panic attacks. J Clin Psychiatry 48:435–437, 1987

Hoitsma E, DeVries J, van Santen-Hoeufft M, et al: Impact of pain in a Dutch sarcoidosis patient population. Sarcoidosis Vasc Diffuse Lung Dis 20:33–39, 2003

Hook O: Sarcoidosis with involvement of the nervous system. Report of nine cases. Arch Neurol Psychiatry 71:554–575, 1954

Hopwood P, Stephens RJ: Depression in patients with lung cancer: prevalence and risk factors derived from quality-of-life data. J Clin Oncol 18:893–903, 2000

Hosenpud JD, Bennett LE, Keck BM, et al: The registry of the international society for heart and lung transplantation: fifteenth official report—1998. J Heart Lung Transplant 17:656–668, 1998

Ibanez M, Aguilar JJ, Maderal MA, et al: Sexuality in chronic respiratory failure: coincidences and divergences between patients and primary caregiver. Respir Med 95:975–979, 2001

Isenberg SA, Lehrer PM, Hochron S: The effects of suggestion and emotional arousal on pulmonary function in asthma: a review and a hypothesis regarding vagal mediation. Psychosom Med 54:192–216, 1992

Ishii N, Nishihara Y: Pellagra encephalopathy among tuberculous patients: its relation to isoniazid therapy. J Neurol Neurosurg Psychiatry 48:628–634, 1985

Jaffe A, Bush A: Cystic fibrosis: a review of the decade. Monaldi Arch Chest Dis 56:240–247, 2001

Janson C, Bjornsson E, Hetta J, et al: Anxiety and depression in relation to respiratory symptoms and asthma. Am J Respir Crit Care Med 149 (4 pt 1):930–934, 1994

Kern-Buell CL, McGrady AV, Conran PB, et al: Asthma severity, psychophysiological indicators of arousal, and immune function in asthma patients undergoing biofeedback-assisted relaxation. Appl Psychophysiol Biofeedback 25:79–91, 2000

Kiev A, Domantay AG: A study of buspirone coprescribed with bronchodilators in 82 anxious ambulatory patients. J Asthma 25:281–284, 1988

Klein DF: False suffocation alarms, spontaneous panics, and related conditions. An integrative hypothesis. Arch Gen Psychiatry 50:306–317, 1993

Klonoff EA, Kleinhenz ME: Psychological factors in sarcoidosis: the relationship between life stress and pulmonary function. Sarcoidosis Vasc Diffuse Lung Dis 10:118–124, 1993

Kohler CL, Fish L, Greene PG: The relationship of perceived self-efficacy to quality of life in chronic obstructive pulmonary disease. Health Psychol 21:610–614, 2002

Kramer MR, Marshall SE, Starnes VA, et al: Infectious complications in heart-lung transplantation: analysis in 200 episodes. Arch Intern Med 153:2010–2016, 1993

Kubzansky LD, Wright RJ, Cohen S, et al: Breathing easy: a prospective study of optimism and pulmonary function in the normative aging study. Ann Behav Med 24:345–353, 2002

Lacasse Y, Brosseau L, Milne S, et al: Pulmonary rehabilitation for chronic obstructive pulmonary disease. Cochrane Database Syst Rev 3:CD003793, 2002

Lachman A, Gielis O, Thys P, et al: Hyperventilation syndrome: current advances. Rev Mal Respir 9:277–285, 1992

Lasky JA, Brody AR: Interstitial fibrosis and growth factors. Environ Health Perspect 108 (suppl 4):751–762, 2000

Lehrer PM, Hochron SM, McCann B, et al: Relaxation decreases large-airway but not small-airway asthma. J Psychosom Res 30:13–25, 1986

Lehrer P, Feldman J, Giardino N, et al: Psychological aspects of asthma. J Consult Clin Psychol 70:691–711, 2002

LeSon S, Gershwin ME: Risk factors for asthmatic patients requiring intubation. J Asthma 33:27–35, 1996

Liippo K, Puolijoki H, Tala E: Periodic breathing imitating hyperventilation syndrome. Chest 102:638–639, 1992

Limbos MM, Joyce DP, Chan CK, et al: Psychological functioning and quality of life in lung transplant candidates and recipients. Chest 118:408–416, 2000

Lishman WA: Endocrine diseases and metabolic disorders, in Organic Psychiatry. London, Blackwell, 1987, pp 466–467, 651

Llewellyn K: CF and me. Interview by Anna Sidey. Paediatr Nurs 10:21–22, 1998

Malotte CK, Hollingshead JR, Rhodes F: Monetary versus nonmonetary incentives for TB skin test reading among drug users. Am J Prev Med 16:182–188, 1999

Malotte CK, Hollingshead JR, Larro M: Incentives vs outreach workers for latent tuberculosis treatment in drug users. Am J Prev Med 20:103–107, 2001

Mancuso CA, Peterson MG, Charlson ME: Effects of depressive symptoms on health-related quality of life in asthma patients. J Gen Intern Med 15:301–310, 2000

Martens WH: A review of physical and mental health in homeless persons. Public Health Rev 29:13–33, 2001

Martinez TY, Pereira CA, Dos Santos ML, et al: Evaluation of the short-form 36-item questionnaire to measure health-related quality of life in patients with idiopathic pulmonary fibrosis. Chest 117:1627–1632, 2000

Mathews WB: Sarcoidosis of the nervous system. J Neurol Neurosurg Psychiatry 28:23–29, 1965

Maurer JR, Frost AE, Estenne M et al: International guidelines for the selection of lung transplant candidates. J Heart Lung Transplant 17:703–709, 1998

McCathie HC, Spence SH, Tate RL: Adjustment to chronic obstructive pulmonary disease: the importance of psychological factors. Eur Respir J 19:47–53, 2002

McQuistion HL, Colson P, Yankowitz R, et al: Tuberculosis infection among people with severe mental illness. Psychiatr Serv 48:833–835, 1997

Mendelson WB, Maczaj M, and Holt J: Buspirone administration to sleep apnea patients. J Clin Psychopharmacol 11:71–72, 1991

Miles JF, Garden GM, Tunnicliffe WS, et al: Psychological morbidity and coping skills in patients with brittle and non-brittle asthma: a case-control study. Clin Exp Allergy 27:1151–1159, 1997

Mino M, Narita N, Ikeda H: A case of a pituitary mass in association with sarcoidosis. No To Shinkei 52:253–257, 2000

Mizukami K, Naito Y, Yoshida M, et al: Mental disorders induced by carbamazepine. Jpn J Psychiatry Neurol 44:59–63, 1990

Montazeri A, Gillis CR, McEwen J: Quality of life in patients with lung cancer: a review of literature from 1970 to 1995. Chest 113:467–481, 1998

Moss AR, Hahn JA, Tulsky JP, et al: Tuberculosis in the homeless. A prospective study. Am J Respir Crit Care Med 162 (2 pt1): 460–464, 2000

Napolitano MA, Babyak MA, Palmer S, et al: Effects of a telephone-based psychosocial intervention for patients awaiting lung transplantation. Chest 122:1176–1184, 2002

National Center for Health Statistics: Vital And Health Statistics: Current Estimates from the National Health Interview Survey. U.S. Department of Health and Human Services, 1990–1993. National Vital Statistics Reports 48:26, 2000

Newman KB, Mason UG 3rd, Schmaling KB: Clinical features of vocal cord dysfunction. Am J Respir Crit Care Med 152 (4 pt 1):1382–1386, 1995

Newsham KR, Klaben BK, Miller VJ, et al: Paradoxical vocal-cord dysfunction: management in athletes. J Athl Train 37:325–328, 2002

Nguyen VQ, Byrd RP, Fields CL, et al: DaCosta's syndrome: chronic symptomatic hyperventilation. J Ky Med Assoc 90:221–334, 1992

North KN, Ouvier RA, Nugent M: Pseudoseizures caused by hyperventilation resembling absence epilepsy. J Child Neurol 5:288–294, 1990

Ochoa LL, Richardson GW: The current status of lung transplantation: a nursing perspective. AACN Clin Issues 10:229–239, 1999

O'Dowd MA, Jaramillo J, Dubler N, et al: A noncompliant patient with fluctuating capacity. Gen Hosp Psychiatry 20:317–324, 1998

Olson K, Tom B, Hewitt J, et al: Evolving routines: preventing fatigue associated with lung and colorectal cancer. Qual Health Res 12:655–670, 2002

Oscherwitz T, Tulsky JP, Roger S, et al: Detention of persistently nonadherent patients with tuberculosis. JAMA 278:843–846, 1997

Ovesen L, Hannibal J, Mortensen EL: The interrelationship of weight loss, dietary intake, and quality of life in ambulatory patients with cancer of the lung, breast, and ovary. Nutr Cancer 19:159–167, 1993

Paradowski LJ: Saprophytic fungal infections and lung transplantation revisited. J Heart Lung Transplant 16:524–531, 1997

Paris WP, Diercks M, Bright J, et al: Return to work after lung transplantation. J Heart Lung Transplant 17:430–436, 1998

Paulley JW: Hyperventilation. Recenti Prog Med 81:594–600, 1990

Perkin GD, Joseph R: Neurological manifestations of the hyperventilation syndrome. J R Soc Med 79:448–450, 1986

Perkner JJ, Fennelly KP, Balkissoon R, et al: Irritant-associated vocal cord dysfunction. J Occup Environ Med 40:136–143, 1998

Peters SG, Wochos DN, Peterson GC: Status epilepticus as a complication of concurrent electroconvulsive and theophylline therapy. Mayo Clin Proc 59:568–570, 1984

Pinney S, Freeman LJ, Nixon PG: Role of the nurse counselor in managing patients with the hyperventilation syndrome. J R Soc Med 80:216–218, 1987

Porzelius J, Vest M, Nochomovitz M: Respiratory function, cognitions, and panic in chronic obstructive pulmonary patients. Behav Res Ther 30:75–77, 1992

Put C, Van den Bergh O, Demedts M, et al: A study of the relationship among self-reported noncompliance, symptomatology, and psychological variables in patients with asthma. J Asthma 37:503–510, 2000

Reichman LB, Felton CP, Edsall JR: Drug dependence, a possible new risk factor for tuberculosis disease. Arch Intern Med 139:337–339, 1979

Rietveld S, van Beest I, Everaerd W: Stress-induced breathlessness in asthma. Psychol Med 29:1359–1366, 1999

Ritz T, Steptoe A, DeWilde S, et al: Emotions and stress increased respiratory resistance in asthma. Psychosom Med 62:402–412, 2000

Robinson DP, Greene JW, Walker LS: Functional somatic complaints in adolescents: relationship to negative life events, self-concept, and family characteristics. J Pediatr 112:588–593, 1988

Rognum TO, Olaisen B, Teige B: Hyperventilation syndrome. Could acute salicylic acid poisoning be the cause? [in Norwegian]. Tidsskr Nor Laegeforen 107:1043, 1050, 1987

Roncevic N, Stojadiic A, Simic I, et al: The hyperventilation syndrome in children. Med Pregl 47(5–6):213–215, 1994

Rose C, Wallace L, Dickson R, Ayres J, Lehman R, Searle Y, Burge PS: The most effective psychologically-based treatments to reduce anxiety and panic in patients with chronic obstructive pulmonary disease (COPD): a systematic review. Patient Educ Couns 47:311–318, 2002

Saarijarvi S, Lehtinen P: The hyperventilation syndrome treated with antidepressive agents. Duodecim 103:417–420, 1987

Sabaawi M, Gutierrez-Nunez J, Fragala MR: Neurosarcoidosis presenting as schizophreniform disorder. Int J Psychiatry Med 22:269–274, 1992

Saisch SG, Wessely S, Gardner WN: Patients with acute hyperventilation presenting to an inner-city emergency department. Chest 110:952–957, 1996

Sakai J, Kim M, Shore J, Hepfer M: The risk of purified protein derivative positivity in homeless men with psychotic symptoms. South Med J 91:345–348, 1998

Scadding JG: Sarcoidosis. London, Eyre and Spottiswood, 1967

Schmaling KB, Niloofar A, Barnhart S, et al: Medical and psychiatric predictors of airway reactivity. Respir Care 44:1452–1457, 1999

Schmaling KB, McKnight PE, Afari N: A prospective study of the relationship of mood and stress to pulmonary function among patients with asthma. J Asthma 39:501–510, 2002

Schnoll RA, Malstrom M, James C, et al: Correlates of tobacco use among smokers and recent quitters diagnosed with cancer. Patient Educ Couns 46:137–145, 2002

Scialdone AM: Thalamic hemorrhage imitating hyperventilation. Ann Emerg Med 19:817–819, 1990

Sharma, OP: Sarcoidosis: A Clinical Approach. Springfield, IL, Charles C Thomas, 1975

Silverstein A, Feuer M, Siltzback L: Neurologic sarcoidosis. Arch Neurol 12:1–11, 1965

Skorodin MS, King F, Sharp JT: Carbon monoxide poisoning presenting as hyperventilation syndrome. Ann Intern Med 105:631–632, 1986

Small SP, Graydon JE: Perceived uncertainty, physical symptoms, and negative mood in hospitalized patients with chronic obstructive pulmonary disease. Heart Lung 21:568–574, 1992

Smoller JW, Pollack MH, Systrom D, et al: Sertraline effects on dyspnea in patients with obstructive airways disease. Psychosomatics 39:24–29, 1998

Snell G, deHoyos A, Krajden M, et al: *Pseudomonas capacia* in lung transplantation recipients with cystic fibrosis. Chest 103:466–471, 1993

Solsona J, Cayla JA, Nadal J, et al: Screening for tuberculosis upon admission to shelters and free-meal services. Eur J Epidemiol 17:123–128, 2001

Sternbach GL: Infections in alcoholic patients. Emerg Med Clin North Am 8:793–803, 1990

Stilley C, Dew MA, Stukas AA, et al: Psychological symptom levels and their correlates in lung and heart-lung transplant recipients. Psychosomatics 40:503–509, 1999

Stone P, Richards M, A'Hern R, et al: A study to investigate the prevalence, severity and correlates of fatigue among patients with cancer in comparison with a control group of volunteers without cancer. Ann Oncol 11:561–567, 2000

Stoudemire A, Linfors E, Houpt JL, et al: Central nervous system sarcoidosis. Gen Hosp Psychiatry 5:129–132, 1983

Strauss GM: Bronchogenic carcinoma, in Textbook of Pulmonary Disease, 6th Edition. Edited by Baum GL, Grapo JD, Celli BR. Philadelphia, PA, Lippincott-Raven, 1998, p 1329

Sturdy PM, Victor CR, Anderson HR, et al: Mortality and severe morbidity working group of the national asthma task force. Psychological, social and health behavior risk factors for deaths certified as asthma: a national case-control study. Thorax 57:1034–1039, 2002

Suchenwirth R, Dold V: Functional psychoses in sarcoidosis. Verh Dtsch Ges Inn Med 75:757–759, 1969

Takatsuki K, Kado T, Satouchi M, et al: Psychiatric studies of chemotherapy and chemotherapy-induced nausea and vomiting of patients with lung or thymic cancer. Gan To Kagaku Ryoho 25:403–408, 1998

Tanaka K, Akechi T, Okuyama T, et al: Factors correlated with dyspnea in advanced lung cancer patients: organic causes and what else? J Pain Symptom Manage 23:490–500, 2002

Tashkin D, Kanner R, Bailey W, et al: Smoking cessation in patients with chronic obstructive pulmonary disease: a double-blind, placebo-controlled, randomised trial. Lancet 357:1571–1575, 2001

Teichman BJ, Burker EJ, Weiner M, et al: Factors associated with adherence to treatment regimens after lung transplantation. Prog Transplant 10:113–121, 2000

ten Brinke A, Ouwerkerk ME, Zwinderman AH, et al: Psychopathology in patients with severe asthma is associated with increased health utilization. Am J Respir Crit Care Med 163:1093–1096, 2001

ten Thoren C, Petermann F: Reviewing asthma and anxiety. Respir Med 94:409–415, 2000

Teramoto S, Sugai M, Saito E, et al: Hyperventilation in a very old woman. Nippon Ronen Igakkai Zasshi 43:226–229, 1997

Thomas PS, Geddes DM, Barnes PJ: Pseudo-steroid resistant asthma. Thorax 54:352–356, 1999

Thompson C, Checkley S: Short term memory deficit in a patient with cerebral sarcoidosis. Br J Psychiatry 139:160–161, 1981

Treasure RA, Fowler PB, Millington HT, et al: Misdiagnosis of diabetic ketoacidosis as hyperventilation syndrome. BMJ (Clin Res Ed) 294:630, 1987

Uchitomi Y, Mikami I, Nagai K, et al: Depression and psychological distress in patients during the year after curative resection of non-small cell lung cancer. J Clin Oncol 21:69–77, 2003

Van den Hout MA, Boek C, van der Molen GM, et al: Rebreathing to cope with hyperventilation: experimental tests of the paper bag method. J Behav Med 11:303–310, 1988

Van De Ven LL, Mouthan BJ, Hoes MJ: Treatment of the hyperventilation syndrome with bisoprodol: a placebo-controlled clinical trial. J Psychosom Res 39:1007–1013, 1995

Vermeulen KM, Ouwens JP, van der Bij W, et al: Long-term quality of life in patients surviving at least 55 months after lung transplantation. Gen Hosp Psychiatry 25:95–102, 2003

Vos PJ, Folgering HT, van Herwaarden CL: Visual attention in patients with chronic obstructive pulmonary disease. Biol Psychol 41:295–305, 1995

Weiss ST: The origins of childhood asthma. Monaldi Arch Chest Dis 49:154–158, 1994

Wirnsberger RM, deVries J, Breterler MH, et al: Evaluation of quality of life in sarcoidosis patients. Respir Med 92:750–756, 1998

Withers NJ, Rudkin ST, White RJ: Anxiety and depression in severe chronic obstructive pulmonary disease: the effects of pulmonary rehabilitation. J Cardiopulm Rehabil 19:362–365, 1999

Wurtemberger G, Hutter BO: The significance of health related quality of life for the evaluation of interventional measures in patients with COPD. Pneumologie 55:91–99, 2001

Yohannes AM, Baldwin RC, Connolly MJ: Depression and anxiety in elderly outpatients with chronic obstructive pulmonary disease: prevalence, and validation of the BASDEC screening questionnaire. Int J Geriatr Psychiatry 15:1090–1096, 2000

Young P, Dewse M, Fergusson W, Kolbe J: Respiratory rehabilitation in chronic obstructive pulmonary disease: predictors of nonadherence. Eur Respir J 13:855–859, 1999

Zerman W: Die Meningoencephalitis. Nervenarzt 23:43–52, 1952

21 Gastrointestinal Disorders

Francis Creed, M.D., F.R.C.P.C., F.R.C.Psych., F.Med.Sci.

Kevin W. Olden, M.D.

THE CLOSE RELATIONSHIP between the gut and the psyche means that there are many examples of biopsychosocial relationships in the patient population seen by gastroenterologists. The consulting psychiatrist can expect to see a large number of patients with functional gastroenterological disorders, such as functional dyspepsia and irritable bowel syndrome. Functional disorders like these compose approximately half of all patients seen by gastroenterologists (Thompson et al. 2000). Life stressors and mood disorders are thought to play a large part in the symptoms, presentation, and course of the disorders. Psychiatrists in medical settings can also expect to see patients with organic diseases, such as liver disease and inflammatory bowel disease, where the relationship with stress is less clear but where psychiatric disorders can influence management and outcome. Some patients are seen routinely by psychiatrists prior to liver transplant (see Chapter 31, "Organ Transplantation") or before commencing interferon treatment for chronic hepatitis C.

Functional Gastrointestinal Disorders

The broad categorization of disorders into *functional* and *organic* (or *structural*) has some advantages and many disadvantages. The distinction has helped to facilitate research into the psychological factors that are important in the etiology, presentation, and outcome of the so-called functional disorders. This research has been multidisciplinary, with gastroenterologists, physiologists, psychiatrists, and psychologists working to understand underlying mechanisms. This has led to a useful adaptation of the biopsychosocial model in gastroenterology (Drossman 1998; Drossman et al. 1999).

The most prominent disadvantage of the functional and organic terminology is the reinforcement of dualistic thinking—the separation of mind and body. Thus, peptic ulcer was previously regarded as a psychosomatic condition until the importance of *Helicobacter pylori* was discovered and then interest in the psychological aspects of peptic ulcers waned (Levenstein 2000). Another problem is that some gastroenterologists falsely equate *functional* with *psychiatric*, which leads them to ignore psychiatric disorders in patients with organic disease.

For convenience, the term *functional gastrointestinal disorder* will be used in this chapter. However, a multifactorial view of illness should be maintained. Therefore, readers should bear in mind the frequent comorbidity of psychiatric disorders with all gastrointestinal (GI) disorders.

In clinical practice, the identification and treatment of psychiatric disorders in patients with GI disorders can be very rewarding. Many patients with functional GI disorders may experience considerable improvement in their symptoms when a concurrent psychiatric disorder is successfully identified and treated. In structural (organic) disorders, the GI symptoms may not change as dramatically when coexisting depression or anxiety is treated, but patients may experience substantial improvement in their health-related quality of life—that is, they can cope with their symptoms, treatment, and lifestyle changes much more successfully.

Epidemiology of Psychiatric Disorders and Their Relationship With Gastrointestinal Diseases

Our understanding of the relationship between psychiatric and GI disorders has developed considerably over the last 2 decades, as more refined clinical studies have used better diagnostic systems. The development of the *Diagnostic and Statistical Manual of Mental Disorders* (DSM; American Psychiatric Association 1980, 1994, 2000) has been mirrored by a similar symptom-based classification of the functional GI disorders, the so-called Rome criteria. (Drossman et al. 2000a). Such a classification has caused much discussion among gastroenterologists, who are used to making diagnoses on the basis of observable structural abnormalities. This has implications for clinical practice because some gastroenterologists may give the impression to patients that complaints based on structural abnormalities of the gut are "real," whereas complaints without any abnormalities seen on endoscopy or imaging studies may be dismissed as they turn out to be "only" functional. When this occurs, the psychiatrist must first deal with patients feeling angry or devalued before a full clinical appraisal of symptoms is commenced (Creed and Guthrie 1993; Guthrie and Creed 1996).

Recent epidemiological research in gastroenterology has included population-based samples. This is important because it may challenge ideas developed in the clinical setting. For example, *H. pylori* and nonsteroidal anti-inflammatory drug (NSAID) usage have been considered to be the underlying agents responsible for most cases of peptic ulcer. Certainly, eradication of *H. pylori* or NSAID discontinuation usually leads to ulcer healing, but population-based studies have shown that many people carry *H. pylori* without any evidence of peptic ulcer. Host factors are also important in the etiology of peptic ulcer (Levenstein 1999). We need to understand the nature of these host factors if patients with refractory ulcers, as well as ulcers with no obvious cause, are to be helped. Population-based studies have clarified the relationship between GI and psychiatric disorders; in particular, it is recognized that psychological variables are important determinants of treatment seeking.

The prevalence of psychiatric disorders in patients attending gastroenterology clinics has been studied repeatedly with reasonably consistent results. Approximately half of patients with functional disorders and 15%–30% of patients with structural gut disorders have mood, anxiety, or related disorders. The proportions are particularly high in certain groups, such as people with chronic hepatitis C virus (HCV) infection.

Peptic Ulcer

It has been estimated that approximately 10% of individuals in Western countries will develop a peptic ulcer sometime during their lifetime (Rosenstock and Jorgensen 1995). The two major risk factors associated with the development of both gastric and duodenal ulcers are the use of NSAIDs and the presence of infection with *H. pylori* (Kurata et al. 1997). Interestingly, since the late 1960s the overall incidence of peptic ulcer disease has begun to decline. This trend is believed to be a result of declining rates of infection with *H. pylori* (Parsonnet 1995). Although gastric ulcers and ulcers of the duodenum were seen as two different disorders in the past, more recently they are being conceptualized as part of the same disease spectrum attributed almost exclusively to NSAID use and/or infection with *H. pylori*. However, despite the revolution in our understanding of peptic ulcer, significant psychosocial dimensions remain to be considered with this disorder.

Prevalence of Psychiatric Disorders

The number of sound studies concerning the prevalence of psychiatric disorders in peptic ulcer disease is relatively limited (see Table 21–1). A comprehensive review of the relevant literature in 1995 concluded that there was insufficient evidence to be certain that the prevalence of anxiety and mood disorders was greater in clinical populations of people with duodenal ulcers compared with the general population (Lewin and Lewis 1995). This lack of evidence reflects the methodological problems of most studies, which have used small, clinic-based samples in cross-sectional design. One of the most comprehensive studies included patients with peptic ulcer and inflammatory bowel diseases of recent onset (Craig 1989); 16% of patients had definite psychiatric disorders, and a further 32% had borderline ("subthreshold") psychiatric disorders. These data illustrate an important point for psychosomatic medicine: subthreshold disorders may impair health-related quality of life and lead to a worse prognosis, so psychiatric or psychological treatments should not be confined to people who meet the DSM criteria for a psychiatric disorder. Many other studies have found somewhat higher prevalence figures for psychiatric disorders in peptic ulcer patients; this probably reflects the selection of people with chronic or relapsing disease seen in specialty clinics (Lewin and Lewis 1995; Tennant et al. 1986). There have been relatively few studies in recent years on this topic because the research literature has been focused heavily on *H. pylori* as well as NSAID use as the major causes of peptic ulcer disease.

One large-scale population-based study found a specific association between self-reported peptic ulcer disease and generalized anxiety disorder (but not with any other psychiatric disorder) (Goodwin and Stein 2002). Another has shown a specific association with neuroticism (Goodwin and Stein 2003), which held even after adjustment for cigarette smoking. Such studies concur with the

TABLE 21–1. Prevalence of psychiatric disorder in peptic ulcer disease

Study	Psychiatric disorder measure	Peptic ulcer disease, no.	Control subjects, no.	Statistical significance
Langeluddecke et al. 1987	STAI, ZDS	63	50 (medically ill patients)	No significant difference from MI patients
Langeluddecke et al. 1987	STAI, ZDS	83	59 (dyspepsia patients)	Less anxious than dyspepsia patients
Tennant et al. 1986	STAI, ZDS	87	Population normative data	Higher anxiety and depression scores than norms
Craig 1989	PSE	—[a]	—[b]	Prevalence of psychiatric disorder was less than in patients with functional GI disorder and more than in healthy control subjects
Magni et al. 1982	KSSRT	25 (duodenal ulcer) 36 (acute gastroduodenitis)	61 (matched control subjects)	Both groups more anxious than control subjects. Only acute gastroduodenitis group had higher depression and somatization scores

Note. GI=gastrointestinal; KSSRT=Kellner-Sheffield Symptom Rating Test; MI=myocardial infarction; PSE=Present State Examination; STAI=State-Trait Anxiety Inventory; ZDS=Zung Depression Scale.
[a]16% had psychiatric disorders.
[b]34% of patients with functional GI disorder and 8% of control subjects had psychiatric disorders.

research and clinical observations that anxiety or depression appears to be associated with persistence of peptic ulcer (Levenstein et al. 1996).

The relationship between stress and peptic ulcer disease has been a topic of interest for many years. Early studies focused on personality profile as a predisposing factor for development of peptic ulcer, but there is no convincing evidence of a causal link between a particular personality type and duodenal ulcer (Lewin and Lewis 1995). In a classic study, Weiner et al. (1957) successfully predicted which men in a large cohort of U.S. Army draftees would have duodenal ulcers by combining psychological criteria with the biological criterion of high baseline pepsinogen secretion. Subsequent studies have found convincing evidence that the onset, perpetuation, and recurrence of peptic ulcers are associated with stressful life events. This has been demonstrated after earthquakes, where stress and the presence of *H. pylori* interacted (Matsushima et al. 1999). Other studies have demonstrated that with more chronic stressors that involve goal frustration—that is, in which the individual is repeatedly prevented from reaching a much sought-after goal—peptic ulcer disease was more persistent (Craig 1989; Ellard et al. 1990). The latter may reflect a personality type, associated with continuing at a task or toward a goal even when the odds are against success.

Some studies have focused on a group of patients who show the personality traits of social withdrawal, suspi-ciousness, hostility, and dependency (Jess et al. 1989; Levenstein et al. 1992). Their ulcers appear to develop when stress leads to increased cigarette and alcohol consumption (Levenstein 2000). In clinical practice, it is worth assessing these personality attributes in persons who have recurrent or persistent ulcers, in whom discussion about possible preventive measures is important (Levenstein et al. 1996).

More recent studies have examined possible host factors that might interact with NSAID use and *H. pylori* to provide a more complete explanation of the relationship between *H. pylori* and ulcer development (Levenstein 2000). In addition to *H. pylori*, NSAIDs, smoking, and psychological stress (indirectly measured by anxiolytic use) appear to be independent risk factors for ulcer development (Anda et al. 1992; Levenstein et al. 1997; Rosenstock et al. 2003). Psychosomatic medicine specialists should be prepared to discuss these finding with patients as part of a strategy to prevent recurrent ulcers. Some patients understand the association between *H. pylori* and peptic ulcer as a one-to-one relationship, excluding the possibility that outcome might be influenced by their own behavior.

Health-Related Quality of Life

Health-related quality of life is impaired in people with gastric or duodenal ulcers, which are exacerbated by anxiety or depression (Dimenas et al. 1995). Depression also adversely affects the outcome of standard treatment for peptic ulcer (Xuan et al. 1999).

Inflammatory Bowel Disease

Idiopathic inflammatory bowel disease (IBD) represents a spectrum of illnesses from ulcerative colitis and Crohn's disease to the less common but emerging disorders of microscopic colitis, collagenous colitis, and lymphocytic colitis. The latter three disorders tend to produce more subtle inflammation of the bowel, which usually can only be visualized on histological examination of colonic mucosa. Ulcerative colitis is a systemic disorder that can produce inflammation in the skin (pyoderma gangrenosum and erythema nodosum), eyes (conjunctivitis and uveitis), and joints (arthritis). In the bowel, ulcerative colitis involves only the colon. In the colon, its inflammatory effect tends to involve only the mucosa and is not transmural (i.e., not extending through all layers of the bowel). Crohn's disease, however, can involve any portion of the gut from the oropharynx to the perirectal area, and it tends to be transmural. Crohn's disease can frequently produce fistulae, fissures, and strictures of the bowel. It is difficult to judge the prevalence of IBD because many subtle cases go undiagnosed. Likewise, many episodes of diarrhea diagnosed as infectious colitis often actually represent minor flare-ups of IBD. Taking into account these limitations, the incidence of Crohn's disease in the United States is 3.6–8.8 per 100,000 (Mendeloff and Calkins 1995), and the incidence of ulcerative colitis is 3–15 cases per 100,000. The incidence of Crohn's disease has increased sixfold in the past 50 years (Nunes and Ahlquist 1983), whereas the incidence of ulcerative colitis has remained reasonably stable.

Prevalence of Psychiatric Disorders

Patients with IBD show a higher prevalence of psychological disorder than the general population, but a lower prevalence of psychological disorder than patients with functional bowel disorder (Walker et al. 1995). The rate, mostly in the range of 21% to 35%, is similar to that found in other chronic physical illnesses (Creed et al. 2002). Mood disorder appears to be more common in older patients and in those with a previous history of psychiatric disorder (Acosta-Ramirez et al. 2001).

Stress, Psychiatric Disorder, and Gastrointestinal Function

The relationship between psychiatric disorder and IBD is unclear (Table 21–2). Some investigators have suggested that certain patients with IBD may be particularly vulnerable to developing psychiatric disorder because of experiences which are independent of the disease process (e.g., childhood victimization and abuse) (Walker et al. 1996). One study showed that relapses occur at times of stress (Duffy et al. 1991), but most other studies have failed to find an association with stress (North et al. 1991). Many authors report psychiatric disorder only in close relationship with increased disease activity, suggesting that the former is a consequence of an IBD flare (North et al. 1991); however, one study suggests that relapse is predicted by depression (Mittermaier et al. 2004).

Evidence from a population-based sample indicates an excess of anxiety and depression both immediately before and shortly after onset—findings that support both the etiological and psychological reaction theories relating psychological state to inflammatory bowel disease (Kurina et al. 2001). A recent cross-sectional study suggests that high levels of psychological distress are associated with recently diagnosed active disease, recent stressful life events, and, in those with many stressors, low social support (Sewitch et al. 2001).

Some patients with IBD may avidly attribute their symptoms to stress. This can be maladaptive if patients conclude the disease is somehow their (or someone else's) fault or if patients use it to rationalize avoidance of chronic drug therapy. It should be pointed out that general stress reduction measures may be helpful, but they are not an alternative to close adherence to the prescribed medications (Maunder and Esplen 2001; Maunder et al. 1997).

Health-Related Quality of Life

There is clear evidence that anxiety and depression impair health-related quality of life in IBD (Guthrie et al. 2002; Nordin et al. 2002; Turnbull and Vallis 1995; Walker et al. 1996). This pattern is demonstrated in Figure 21–1, which shows the effect of anxiety and depressive disorders, including subthreshold disorders, on the four *physical* components of health-related quality of life. It can be seen that even after adjustment for severity of IBD, patients with possible anxiety or depressive disorders have significantly worse physical function, role limitation (physical), health perception, and pain than patients with very few or no psychiatric symptoms. Although some studies have reported a worse health-related quality of life in patients with Crohn's disease as compared with those with ulcerative colitis, this difference disappears after adjustment for gender and severity of IBD (Andrews et al. 1987; de Boer et al. 1998; Guthrie et al. 2002; Walker et al. 1995).

When IBD relapses, both physical and emotional symptoms are prominent. In remission, the former may

TABLE 21–2. Prevalence of psychiatric disorder in patients with inflammatory bowel disease

| Study | Psychiatric disorder measure | Ulcerative colitis and Crohn's disease patients | | Comment |
		Total no.	% with psychiatric disorder	
Helzer et al. 1982	Standardized psychiatric interview/Feighner criteria	50	26	Prevalence similar to that in other medically ill patients (30%)
Andrews et al. 1987	DSM-III	162	33	No difference between Crohn's disease and ulcerative colitis groups
Tarter et al. 1987	DIS/DSM-III	53	26 (anxiety) 15 (panic) 10 (depression)	Greater prevalence than in control subjects
Magni et al. 1991		50	22 (lifetime) 62 (current)	More than in control subjects
Walker et al. 1996	DIS	40	35	No difference between IBD groups
De Boer et al. 1998	CES-D	224	32	No difference between IBD groups
Guthrie et al. 2002	HADS	112	26	No difference between IBD groups
Rose et al. 2002	CES-D	66	21	No control group

Note. CES-D = Center for Epidemiologic Studies Depression Scale; DIS = Diagnostic Interview Schedule; HADS = Hospital Anxiety and Depression Scale; IBD = inflammatory bowel disease.

remit, but impairment due to emotional distress may remain and require attention (Casellas et al. 2001). Failure to attend to this distress may leave the patient anxious and depressed and possibly at a higher risk of relapse (Andrews et al. 1987; Kurina et al. 2001). There is preliminary evidence that health-related quality of life improves if psychiatric morbidity is treated (Walker et al. 1996), and this should be the main aim of psychiatric treatment in people with concurrent psychiatric disorders and IBD.

The presence of psychiatric disorder in patients with IBD is also associated with many GI symptoms that are typical of irritable bowel syndrome—abdominal pain that is relieved by defecation; bloating; and altered bowel habits. People with IBD who also have these comorbid irritable bowel syndrome symptoms have the greatest impairment of health-related quality of life of all patients with IBD (Simren et al. 2002). Clinicians should therefore ask about irritable bowel syndrome–type symptoms even in patients with IBD and anticipate that these symptoms may improve with psychiatric treatment.

Relationship Between Health Care Utilization and Psychological and Disease-Related Variables

Although the severity of IBD is the main predictor of health service use, especially hospitalization, a number of psychological and social variables are also important independent predictors. These include depression (de Boer et al. 1998; Guthrie et al. 2002), emotional and social functioning, and patients' concerns (Drossman et al. 1989,

1991). Because many patients with IBD are young and striving to lead a normal life, any intervention that reduces the time spent visiting doctors is beneficial—another reason for energetically treating any concurrent psychiatric disorder.

Functional Gastrointestinal Disorders: Irritable Bowel Syndrome and Functional Dyspepsia

Functional GI disorders represent a spectrum of disorders of function, which encompasses the functional esophageal disorders, such as noncardiac chest pain and functional dysphagia; functional dyspepsia (previously called nonulcer dyspepsia); irritable bowel syndrome; as well as functional constipation, functional diarrhea, and functional abdominal pain. The sine qua non of a functional GI disorder is the lack of structural or biochemical abnormalities that could explain the patient's symptoms, which requires that the diagnosis of functional GI disorders be symptom based.

In an attempt to improve the nomenclature, international working teams have been formed to address the issue of diagnostic criteria for the functional GI disorders. Based in Rome, these so-called Rome committees function in a manner similar to the DSM committees of the American Psychiatric Association. Diagnostic criteria for the various functional GI disorders have been created (Thompson et al. 2000).

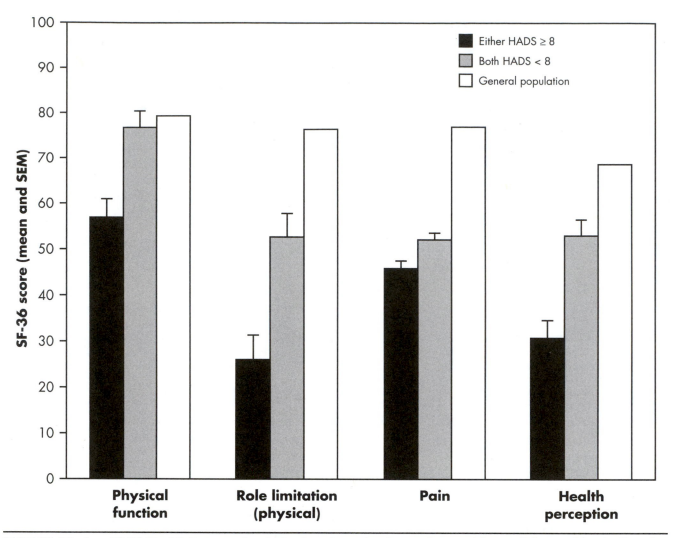

FIGURE 21–1. SF-36 Health Survey physical subscale scores for patients with possible psychiatric disorder (HADS ≥ 8) versus patients without psychiatric disorder (HADS < 8).

Note. Mean subscale scores for the general population are included for reference. HADS=Hospital Anxiety and Depression Scale.
Source. Guthrie et al. 2002.

The most common functional GI disorder is irritable bowel syndrome (IBS), which comes in three general clinical forms: with constipation, with diarrhea, and with an alternating pattern of diarrhea and constipation. The diagnostic criteria for IBS are outlined in Table 21–3. The creation of standardized diagnostic criteria for the functional bowel disorders has led to significant improvements in research and clinical practice. Many patients with vague, unexplainable GI complaints were previously diagnosed as having IBS, when many of them in fact had other functional GI disorders. The various functional GI disorders have different natural histories, psychosocial correlates, and prognoses. Advances in nomenclature have greatly improved our ability to understand and study these disorders, which have significant psychosocial dimensions (Budavari and Olden 2003).

Prevalence of Psychiatric Disorders

The prevalence of anxiety and mood disorders, particularly panic disorder, in patients attending gastroenterology clinics with functional bowel disorders (50%–60%) is approximately twice that of IBD (Drossman et al. 2000a, 2002). There appears to be little difference across diagnostic groups such as patients with IBS, functional dyspepsia, functional abdominal pain, and noncardiac chest pain (Biggs 2004; Dimenas et al. 1995). Anxiety is more prominent in first-time attenders, but depression seems more prominent in those who have chronic symptoms and who have been attending the clinic over a long period without remission (Guthrie et al. 1992). Panic disorder is frequent in some specialist settings (Lydiard et al. 1993). High levels of psychological distress are found in people who have numerous bodily symptoms outside of the GI

TABLE 21–3.   Rome II criteria for irritable bowel syndrome

At least 12 weeks or more, which need not be consecutive, in the preceding 12 months of abdominal discomfort or pain that has two out of the following three features:
- Relieved with defecation
- Onset associated with a change in frequency of stool
- Onset associated with a change in form (appearance) of stool

Symptoms that cumulatively support the diagnosis of irritable bowel syndrome:
- Abnormal stool frequency (for research purposes, "abnormal" may be defined as more than three bowel movements per day and less than three bowel movements per week)
- Abnormal stool form (lumpy/hard or loose/watery stool)
- Abnormal stool passage (straining, urgency, or feeling of incomplete evacuation)
- Passage of mucus
- Bloating or feeling of abdominal distension

tract (so-called extraintestinal symptoms), including fibromyalgia (Sperber et al. 2000; Whitehead et al. 2002).

The onset of anxiety or mood disorder precedes or coincides with the onset of the bowel disorder in approximately two-thirds of IBS patients (Craig 1989; Ford et al. 1987). This suggests a close link between the psychiatric disorder and gut symptoms. The presence of (untreated) psychiatric disorder predicts a poor outcome, and conversely, reduction of psychiatric symptoms is associated with reduction of bowel symptoms (Creed 1999).

Stress, Psychiatric Disorder, and Gastrointestinal Function

A number of studies have shown that stress precedes the onset of functional bowel disorders, whether there is concurrent psychiatric disorder or not (Creed et al. 1988; Drossman 1998). The most common stresses relate to difficult personal relationships—marital separations, divorce, and other relationship breakups. Many patients tend to deny the importance of such events and claim that any psychological or social difficulties are the result of the bowel disorder rather than stress. Careful history taking with sufficient attention paid to time course of events will usually demonstrate the correct sequence.

Social stress is also the single most important predictor of outcome in patients with IBS who attend a gastroenterology clinic (Bennett et al. 1998). Failure to address the stressor(s) may therefore lead to persistent symptoms. Some patients are reluctant to discuss social stress, protesting that it is unrelated to the bowel disorder (Creed and Guthrie 1993). For most patients, however, a clear

explanation of the purpose of doing so leads to a fruitful discussion. For example, a series of patients with dyspepsia were asked to list their main complaints, and about two-thirds spontaneously mentioned "anxiety" before "dyspepsia"; therefore, an open question may enable the psychiatrist to rapidly elicit a person's concerns (Haug et al. 1995).

Health-Related Quality of Life

Anxiety and mood disorders play a large part in the impairment of health-related quality of life observed in IBS (Creed et al. 2001; Walker et al. 1995; Whitehead et al. 1996). As in other medical conditions, the effects of physical and psychological symptoms are approximately additive in terms of their effect on quality of life (Creed et al. 2001, 2002; Wells et al. 1989). In dyspepsia, psychological distress is a better predictor of health-related quality of life than severity of the dyspepsia (Quartero et al. 1999), and the considerable impairment of health-related quality of life attributed to IBS may be the result of concurrent psychiatric disorders (Creed et al. 2001; Drossman et al. 2000b, 2000c; Talley et al. 1995a). In other words, there is a good prospect of improvement of health-related quality of life when the anxiety or mood disorder is satisfactorily treated, as has been demonstrated with both antidepressants and psychotherapy (Creed et al. 2003; Drossman et al. 2003; Guthrie et al. 1991; Hamilton et al. 2000). In severe functional GI disorders, a proportion of people are unemployed because of ill health; the disorder is closely associated with psychiatric status and may respond to appropriate psychological treatment (Creed et al. 2001, 2003).

Relationship Between Health Care Utilization and Psychological and Disease-Related Variables

Many people with functional dyspepsia or IBS do not consult a doctor (Drossman et al. 1988). Those who do so have more severe abdominal pain than nonconsulters, but they also have more anxiety and depression and, in particular, more worries about their health—especially fears of cancer (Creed 1999; Gomborone et al. 1995; Kettell et al. 1992; Koloski et al. 2003; Lydiard and Jones 1989). Adequately addressing these worries in the gastroenterology clinic may lead to fewer subsequent visits (van Dulmen et al. 1995). Psychiatrists should routinely ask about such fears and be prepared to deal with them directly, because they often persist even after diagnostic investigations have been normal. Some gastroenterologists seem puzzled when a patient has not been reassured adequately by the normal investigations; often insufficient time and effort has been spent explaining the significance of negative results to patients and, when appropriate, to their partner or family members.

There are two reports of greatly increased health anxiety immediately prior to upper endoscopy (Lucock et al. 1997; Quadri and Vakil 2003). There is some reduction of health anxiety after endoscopy, which lasts for a year in the majority of patients. In one-third of people, after upper endoscopy, however, worries about serious illness have returned to their preendoscopy level 1 year later (Lucock et al. 1997). The sources of health anxiety in such people are not fully understood, but lack of social support and early life experience, including illness in the family, abuse, or neglect, both may play a part (Biggs et al. 2003; Whitehead et al. 1982). It is crucial for the psychiatrist to fully explore concerns about serious illness with the patient; such concerns are often related to illness in family members or remarks made to the individual by a physician that play on the patient's mind.

Sexual Abuse and Functional Gastrointestinal Disorders

There is an established literature that demonstrates an association between IBS and a history of childhood sexual abuse (Delvaux et al. 1997; Drossman et al. 1990, 1995; Leserman et al. 1996, 1998; Walker et al. 1995). However, these findings have not been replicated consistently in studies of consecutive clinic attenders, rather than selected clinic series (Biggs 2004; Talley et al. 1995a), or in population-based studies (Talley et al. 1998). It appears that a history of sexual abuse might be a predictor of chronicity and severity of a disorder (Longstreth et al. 1993) and may not be specific to IBS (Katon et al. 2001). A history of sexual abuse does appear to be more prevalent in people with chronic IBS than in those with IBD and is associated with adverse effects on adult sexual functioning and other aspects of health-related quality of life (Guthrie et al. 1987; Walker et al. 1995).

Reported childhood sexual abuse or related trauma is associated with increased health care utilization in functional bowel disorders (Biggs et al. 2003; Guthrie and Creed 2003; Leserman et al. 1998). The likely mechanisms appear to be general rather than specific to the pelvic or anal region, as has been suggested by some authors. Self-reported abuse is associated with complaints in adulthood of a greater number of bodily symptoms; this may be associated with a lower pain threshold and a tendency to be hypervigilant toward bodily symptoms (Salmon et al. 2003). Perhaps the mechanism most commonly involves mood, panic, and other anxiety disorders, which occur in those subjected to abuse during childhood (Blanchard et al. 2002). As we have seen, these psychiatric disorders are more common in functional bowel disorders than

organic GI diseases, and they are independently associated with higher health care utilization in IBS (Budauvri and Olden 2003).

In clinical practice, it is important for psychiatrists to assess possible childhood abuse as a routine in patients with functional GI disorders, especially those who have not responded to treatment. Whatever the type of disorder, patients will usually not have had the opportunity to speak to their gastroenterologist about such intimate aspects of their life (Drossman et al. 1990).

Other Functional Gastrointestinal Disorders

There is a wide array of other functional GI disorders other than IBS and functional dyspepsia—for example, gastroesophageal reflux, globus, functional abdominal pain, and cyclic vomiting. The characteristics of these disorders are described in the Rome book (Drossman et al. 2000a). They often coexist with other functional GI disorders, and their features are very similar to the two disorders described here; anxiety and depression are common. These functional GI disorders have been less well researched than IBS, and the abnormalities of GI physiology are not sufficiently consistent to be reliable. Clinical assessment and treatment follows the general pattern described in this chapter, with the exception that speech therapy may be helpful for globus (Khalil et al. 2003).

Liver Disease

A variety of liver diseases are important in psychosomatic medicine. We focus here primarily on HCV infection. Viral hepatitides are also discussed in Chapter 27, "Infectious Diseases." In the developed nations, alcohol is the most common cause of liver disease (see Chapter 18, "Substance-Related Disorders"), and alcohol is a frequent aggravating factor in other causes of liver disease. Most forms of chronic liver disease can result in cirrhosis, leading to hepatic encephalopathy, which may manifest with symptoms of psychosis, mania, depression, apathy, or confusion before becoming a frank delirium (Dieperink et al. 2000) (see Chapter 6, "Delirium," and Chapter 31, "Organ Transplantation"). Wilson's disease (see Chapter 32, "Neurology and Neurosurgery") and the porphyrias (see Chapter 23, "Endocrine and Metabolic Disorders") are rare diseases affecting the liver whose first symptoms may be psychiatric. Fatigue is a common symptom in liver disease in general and may be caused by the disease, its treatment, or a comorbid depression. In one study of patients with primary biliary cirrhosis, fatigue was more closely associated with depression than with liver disease (Cauch-Dudek et al. 1998). Depression is also common in people undergoing liver transplantation, and there is some evidence that the depression may improve following transplantation (see Chapter 31, "Organ Transplantation").

Chronic liver disease leads to significantly impaired health-related quality of life, and there is some evidence that successful treatment, either by transplant or by antiviral treatment, leads to improvement (De Bona et al. 2000; Dieperink et al. 2000). The severity of the hepatic disease is not necessarily the most important predictor of impaired health-related quality of life; one study suggests that comorbid conditions, including depression, are the major determinants of health-related quality of life (Fontana et al. 2001). Thus, treatment of depression in patients with chronic liver disease is important for three reasons: in its own right, to improve health-related quality of life, and to facilitate treatment of liver disease.

Chronic Hepatitis C Virus Infection

Chronic HCV (previously known as non-A, non-B hepatitis) has become epidemic; it has become the major cause of chronic liver disease in the United States, with a prevalence of 1.8% of the population. It is estimated that 4 million Americans are infected with HCV (Alter 1997).

HCV infection is not infrequently acquired through intravenous drug abuse, which is also a strong risk factor for other psychiatric disorders (Dwight et al. 2000). In a recent case–control study, individuals with HCV infection were found to be significantly more likely to have major depressive, posttraumatic stress disorder (PTSD), and anxiety disorders as well as alcohol- and drug-use disorders (El-Serag et al. 2002). This strong propensity for psychiatric comorbidity in individuals infected with HCV is bidirectional. First, the HCV-infected population (exclusive of individuals who acquired the infection through blood transfusions) represent a population that clearly is at higher risk for psychiatric disorders. Similarly, individuals infected with HCV are more likely to be depressed than are people with other forms of end-stage liver disease, such as hepatitis B or alcohol-induced cirrhosis. In addition, depressive disorder is seen more frequently in individuals undergoing liver transplantation who are infected with HCV as compared with those who do not carry the virus (Singh et al. 1997). Some studies of war veterans with HCV have recorded a very high prevalence of alcohol and drug abuse (80%) combined with current depression and PTSD, which occurred in 60% of the sample (Nguyen et al. 2002).

In contrast to HCV, hepatitis B virus (HBV) is acquired mainly through sexual contact and through maternal–fetal transmission. It is not commonly transmitted via intravenous drug use, and it is much less likely to induce depression or other psychiatric symptoms as compared

with HCV. This makes it less of an issue for the consultation psychiatrist. Moreover, with the advent of HBV vaccination, the overall prevalence of this disease in Western society is dropping quite significantly.

A major concern now lies in the increased chance of developing significant depression with interferon (antiviral) treatment of hepatitis C. Interferon treatment has significant side effects, including almost universal fatigue, common neurological and cognitive symptoms, and depression (fulfilling the criteria for major depression in approximately one-third of people) (Bonaccorso et al. 2002; Finkleman 2003; Horikawa et al. 2003; Kraus et al. 2003). Suicidal ideation occurs frequently and often has led to cessation of treatment. In a prospective trial, individuals who received interferon were significantly more likely to develop depression and elevated levels of anger and hostility during interferon-alfa therapy compared with a control group, which did not receive the therapy (Kraus et al. 2003). Pretreatment levels of major depressive disorder (15.5%) and anxiety disorder (13.1%) rose in the interferon group to 35% and 26%, respectively. Overall, 58% of the individuals receiving interferon had a diagnosable psychiatric illness after initiation of therapy (Kraus et al. 2003). These findings have been replicated by others (Ho et al. 2001). Although high levels of depression have been reported in patients with HCV infection who had not received interferon treatment (Hilsabeck et al. 2002), well-documented increases in depression level were noted several weeks after initiation of the interferon (Finkelman 2003; Kraus et al. 2003).

In patients with chronic HCV infection, the severity of depressive symptoms is highly correlated with fatigue severity. By contrast, measures of hepatic disease severity, interferon dosage, and the severity of comorbid medical illnesses are not correlated with the patient's overall level of fatigue and functional disability (Dwight et al. 2000). The importance of recognizing psychiatric illness in the HCV-infected patient here is clear. Patients' symptoms of listlessness, anhedonia, fatigue, and physical pain may be mistaken as manifestations of their liver disease; however, it is much more likely that these symptoms are the result of a comorbid psychiatric disorder, most likely major depressive disorder (Porcelli et al. 1996; Wessely and Pariante 2002). The ability to modulate these symptoms has implications not only for improving the patient's overall well-being but also for helping the physician to correctly interpret the patient's clinical condition.

Antidepressants, most often selective serotonin reuptake inhibitors (SSRIs), are useful in the treatment of depressive disorder during interferon-alfa treatment. Paroxetine (Kraus et al. 2001, 2002), sertraline (Schramm et al. 2000), and citalopram (Gleason 2002) have all been effective in clinical trials for the treatment of interferon-induced depression in patients infected with HCV. Psychopharmacology in patients with liver disease is discussed in depth in Chapter 37, "Psychopharmacology."

Diagnostic Issues

The diagnosis of psychiatric disorders in gastroenterology patients does not usually present great difficulties. Some GI symptoms, such as pain, anorexia, or constipation, may be ambiguous (i.e., resulting from either psychiatric or GI disorders), but there are usually a host of other somatic and psychological symptoms that enable the psychiatrist to diagnose anxiety or depressive disorders. Somatization and somatoform pain disorders may be more difficult to distinguish from GI disorders, because both present with physical symptoms; but the diagnosis will usually become apparent after a careful history and physical and psychiatric examinations.

In practice, the more common problem lies in persuading gastroenterologists and primary care doctors to recognize anxiety or depressive disorders early in their management of GI diseases. If this does not occur, the search for possible organic causes of symptoms such as abdominal pain and diarrhea can become very extensive, leading the patient to become increasingly concerned that the illness must be serious as well as elusive. The doctor's attention can be drawn to the possibility of a psychiatric disorder by the use of a simple screening questionnaire such as the Beck Depression Inventory (BDI) (Beck et al. 1961) or the Hospital Anxiety and Depression Scale (HADS) (Drossman et al. 2000a; Zigmond and Snaith 1983).

Rarely, but especially in older people, an undiagnosed depressive illness can lead to marked diarrhea (as a manifestation of accompanying anxiety), abdominal pain, and weight loss. These symptoms may lead to the suspicion of an underlying GI malignancy and numerous investigations. Psychiatrists should be prepared to treat such a person energetically with antidepressants and monitor closely both the depressive and GI symptoms. Of course, it is possible for there to be two disorders—a malignancy and depression—in which case sleep, pain, mood, and hopelessness might improve, but weight and diarrhea might not.

Patients with carcinoma of the pancreas has a reputation for presenting first with depression (Passik and Breitbart 1996) (see Chapter 24, "Oncology"). Gastroenterologists may encounter patients with unsuspected anorexia nervosa with chronic diarrhea, generalized weakness, and hypokalemia from laxative abuse, or chronic vomiting induced by self or ipecac abuse (see Chapter 15, "Eating

Disorders"). Psychiatric symptoms in patients with ostomies are discussed in Chapter 30, "Surgery."

Treatment

Clinical Assessment

The clinical psychiatric assessment of patients with GI disorders is similar to that in other medical disorders (see Chapter 1, "Psychiatric Assessment and Consultation"). In this section, we principally emphasize points that are relevant to patients seen by psychiatrists referred from gastroenterologists. Because the majority of relevant points concern functional GI disorders, these will be discussed first.

Accurate Dating of Symptom Onset

Because many patients may, rightly or wrongly, link their symptoms to stress, it is important to establish several dates: the date of onset and exacerbation of the GI symptoms and the date of onset of depressive or anxiety symptoms. These dates may be compared to the dates of any important life events to establish an accurate time course. Thus, for instance, the psychiatrist may be able to determine the sequence of a stressful life event, for example, discovery of spouse's extramarital affair, followed by the onset of anxiety symptoms, later marital separation, and subsequent simultaneous onset of depressive symptoms, abdominal pain, and diarrhea. This sequence suggests that the bowel symptoms are related to stress. It does *not*, however, prove that the symptoms are caused by a functional, as opposed to an organic, disorder, because symptoms of IBD may also get worse with stress and precipitate anxiety or depression. The time sequence allows the psychiatrist to evaluate any suggestion from the patent that the depression is unrelated or simply a reaction to the bowel disturbance. It also allows a full exploration of the patient's feelings about the life events.

Systems Review

It is also important to perform a thorough review of symptoms in other bodily systems, because many extraintestinal symptoms may accompany psychiatric disorders concurrent with a functional GI disorder. The patient may or may not have been asked about these symptoms as part of the gastroenterologist's assessment. By eliciting all of the patient's symptoms, the psychiatrist makes the patient *feel understood*, which is the first stage of management of patients with medically unexplained symptoms (Morriss et al. 1999). A thorough review of all systems may also aid in explaining the nature of functional

GI disorders and facilitate expanding beyond a limited discussion of bowel symptoms to a broad discussion of health and illness.

Health Anxiety

It is important to elicit fears of cancer or other serious illness. It is desirable for the gastroenterologist to take a psychosocial history and make a specific effort to address the patient's concerns about serious illness. If the consultation with a gastroenterologist is satisfactory, IBS patients will show reduction in overall anxiety, fear of cancer, and preoccupation and helplessness in relation to the pain; this result may lead to fewer subsequent visits to the clinic (van Dulmen et al. 1995). However, if these issues have not been addressed previously, the psychiatrist should address them. In addition, the psychiatrist should explore the reasons underlying fears of serious illness; one of the most common reasons is serious illness in the family. Depressive, panic, and other anxiety disorders and hypochondriacal personality traits may all be responsible for increased health anxiety (Colgan et al. 1988a).

Early Environmental Experiences

As noted earlier in this chapter, sexual abuse in childhood and related traumatic experiences may be common in some patients with functional GI disorders, especially those with high health care utilization.

Abnormal Attitudes to Illness and Treatment

In their extreme forms, the illness attitudes and behaviors in patients with functional GI disorders may amount to a psychiatric diagnosis of a somatoform disorder (see Chapter 12, "Anxiety Disorders") or a factitious disorder or malingering (see Chapter 14, "Deception Syndromes: Factitious Disorders and Malingering").

Measurement and Monitoring

Modern psychiatrists often use standardized instruments to measure the severity of depressive or anxiety disorders, particularly for screening and in research. Many common psychiatric instruments include GI symptoms, so it may be wise to consider the total score with and without these symptoms included, especially in borderline cases. For example, the BDI has items concerning aches and pains, upset stomach, constipation, and changes in appetite (Beck et al. 1961). The HADS (Zigmond and Snaith 1983) was designed for use in medical populations and may be particularly useful in GI patients because it specifically excludes items concerning bodily symptoms. The Rome committee has reviewed the instruments commonly used (Drossman et al. 1999, 2000a).

Pharmacological Treatment

Functional Gastrointestinal Syndromes

Pharmacological treatment of IBS has been recently reviewed (Talley 2003). There is clear evidence of the effectiveness of tricyclic antidepressants in IBS (Clouse 2003; Jackson et al. 2000). Systematic reviews of the existing literature show an odds ratio of 4.2 (95% CI: 2.3 to 7.9) for the efficacy of TCAs over placebo, mostly measured in terms of pain relief (Jackson et al. 2000). The mechanism of the benefit derived from TCAs in functional bowel disorders is not entirely clear. They are effective in low doses with rapid onset, suggesting the benefits may be the result of analgesic and anticholinergic effects. Imipramine was helpful in chest pain in one study (Cannon et al. 1994), but the mechanism(s) of action are also not clear.

Too few studies have examined the effect of SSRI antidepressants to be clear about their efficacy, but they are active in doses that are effective in clinical depression, and the onset of action is slower, suggesting that they act through a different mechanism from tricyclic antidepressants (TCAs) (Creed et al. 2003; Kirsch and Louie 2000; Masand et al. 2002).

In larger studies, the effectiveness of TCAs and SSRIs in improving abdominal pain is related to medication adherence (Creed et al. 2003; Drossman et al. 2003). Some patients with constipation-predominant IBS cannot tolerate TCAs, and some with diarrhea may experience an increase in diarrhea with SSRIs. Dropout rates are high for either class of drug unless special effort is made to promote adherence (Clouse 2003; Creed et al. 2003). Newer drugs developed for IBS have been agonists and antagonists of enteric serotonin receptors (e.g., alosetron, tegaserod), but they do not seem to interact adversely with SSRIs.

In clinical practice, it is important to decide why antidepressants are being used—for their analgesic properties in people who have severe pain or to treat a concurrent depressive illness—and to carefully explain this to the patient. On many occasions, doctors have prescribed low-dose antidepressants for patients' pain, only to be told later that these patients did not take (or stopped taking) the medication because they learned that the drug is an antidepressant and they did not consider themselves depressed.

The Rome committee has reviewed in detail the use of psychotropic drugs in treating functional GI disorders (Drossman et al. 2000a). Antidepressants have also been used with some degree of success for functional dyspepsia. In a placebo-controlled trial, Mertz and colleagues demonstrated the effectiveness of amitriptyline at low doses in improving both well-being and dyspeptic symptoms in patients with functional dyspepsia (Mertz et al. 1998). A number of other agents may also provide symptom relief (see Stanghellini et al. 2003).

Depression in People With Organic Gastrointestinal Disorders

Antidepressant treatment for interferon-induced depression was discussed earlier in this chapter (see subsection "Chronic Hepatitis C Virus Infection"). Psychopharmacology in patients with GI diseases is reviewed in detail in Chapter 37, "Psychopharmacology."

Psychological Treatment

Functional Gastrointestinal Disorders

There have been many studies of psychological treatments of functional bowel disorders, but the sample sizes have been small in some studies, and different therapies and different measures have been used (Talley et al. 1996). The quality of some studies is not high, with follow-up rates sometimes less than 50% (Talley et al. 1996). However, the overall evidence suggests that these treatments are helpful. In one recent review, 10 of 13 studies showed superiority of psychological therapies over conventional medical treatment (Drossman et al. 2000a, p. 215). This result held for five out of six studies that controlled for expectancy of treatment. There was no difference according to specific treatment—dynamic interpersonal therapy, cognitive-behavioral therapy, hypnosis, and relaxation training all appeared to be successful. It is not clear whether these therapies have a specific effect on gut function or whether they act in a general way by reducing tension or improving interpersonal relationships and assertiveness. Because of their time-consuming nature and associated expense, psychological treatments tend to be reserved for the more severe cases.

In clinical practice, there is good reason to try a combination of psychological treatments and antidepressants, though there have not been adequate studies to demonstrate the efficacy of combined treatment (Olden and Drossman 2000). Because psychotherapy and pharmacotherapy probably have different modes of action, it is reasonable to assume that they may have synergistic effects. A detailed clinical assessment might reveal that a patient has a depressive disorder, excessive concern about serious illness that cannot be entirely attributed to the depressive disorder, and a clear marital problem. Such a patient might well benefit from antidepressant treatment combined with cognitive-behavioral therapy for the health anxiety and marital counseling. In their original description of the "irritable colon syndrome," Chaudhury and Truelove (1962) described a man whose symptoms completely resolved once his marital dispute was ended and he was happily settled in a new relationship.

Peptic Ulcer and Inflammatory Bowel Disease

There is nearly always a need to provide proper education and support to patients with organic GI diseases (peptic ulcer and IBD). The provision of information can lead to decreasing patient anxiety, empowering patients to participate more fully in their care and to obviate unnecessary worries such as an undue fear of cancer and the like.

Both dynamic interpersonal therapy and hypnosis have been studied in patients with peptic ulcer. These studies are interesting because they employed the same treatment method for patients with peptic ulcer as they did for patients with IBS. One used dynamic psychotherapy (Sjodin et al. 1985), and the other used hypnotherapy (Colgan et al. 1988b). Both found a more pronounced positive result in IBS, but the psychological treatments had a clear beneficial effect on ulcer symptoms compared to the control condition. This is a reminder that psychological factors may play a part in the etiology or perpetuation of the symptoms of peptic ulcer disease.

Psychotherapy trials, both controlled and uncontrolled, have not shown a benefit in improving outcome in IBD (Jantschek et al. 1998; Maunder and Esplen 2001).

Conclusion

The detection and treatment of psychiatric disorders in patients presenting to gastroenterologists is an important aspect of clinical practice. Whereas anxiety and depression have a more prominent role in functional gastrointestinal disorders, they have important effects on treatment, outcome, and quality of life in patients with "organic" gastrointestinal disorders as well. Chronic hepatitis C infection is of particular concern, both because of its frequency in patients with serious mental illness and substance abuse and because of the psychiatric side effects associated with its treatment.

References

Acosta-Ramirez D, Pagan-Ocasio V, Torres EA: Profile of the inflammatory bowel disease patient with depressive disorders. P R Health Sci J 20:215–220, 2001

Alter MJ: Epidemiology of hepatitis C. Hepatology 26 (suppl): 62S–65S, 1997

American Psychiatric Association: Diagnostic and Statistical Manual of Mental Disorders, 3rd Edition. Washington, DC, American Psychiatric Association, 1980

American Psychiatric Association: Diagnostic and Statistical Manual of Mental Disorders, 4th Edition. Washington, DC, American Psychiatric Association, 1994

American Psychiatric Association: Diagnostic and Statistical Manual of Mental Disorders, 4th Edition, Text Revision. Washington, DC, American Psychiatric Association, 2000

Anda RF, Williamson DF, Escobedo LG, et al: Self-perceived stress and the risk of peptic ulcer disease. A longitudinal study of US adults. Arch Intern Med 152: 829–833, 1992

Andrews H, Barczak P, Allan RN: Psychiatric illness in patients with inflammatory bowel disease. Gut 28:1600–1604, 1987

Beck AT, Ward CH, Mendelson M, et al: An inventory for measuring depression. Arch Gen Psychiatry 14:561–571, 1961

Bennett EJ, Tennant CC, Piesse C, et al: Level of chronic life stress predicts clinical outcome in irritable bowel syndrome. Gut 43:256–262, 1998

Biggs AMA: Effect of childhood adversity on health related quality of life in patients with upper abdominal or chest pain. Gut 53:180–186, 2004

Biggs AM, Aziz Q, Tomenson B, et al: Do childhood adversity and recent social stress predict health care use in patients presenting with upper abdominal or chest pain? Psychosom Med 65:1020–1028, 2003

Blanchard EB, Keefer L, Payne A, et al: Early abuse, psychiatric diagnoses and irritable bowel syndrome. Behav Res Ther 40:289–298, 2002

Bonaccorso S, Marino V, Biondi M, et al: Depression induced by treatment with interferon-alpha in patients affected by hepatitis C virus. J Affect Disord 72:237–241, 2002

Budavari AI, Olden KW: Psychosocial aspects of functional gastrointestinal disorders. Gastroenterol Clin North Am 32: 477–506, 2003

Cannon RO, Quyyumi AA, Mincemoyer R, et al: Imipramine in patients with chest pain despite normal coronary angiograms. N Engl J Med 20:1411–1417, 1994

Casellas F, Lopez-Vivancos J, Badia X, et al: Influence of inflammatory bowel disease on different dimensions of quality of life. Eur J Gastroenterol Hepatol 13:567–572, 2001

Cauch-Dudek K, Abbey S, Stewart DE, et al: Fatigue in primary biliary cirrhosis. Gut 43:705–710, 1998

Chaudhury NA, Truelove SC: Irritable colon syndrome. A study of the clinical features, predisposing causes and prognosis in 130 cases. Q J Med 31:307–322, 1962

Clouse RE: Antidepressants for irritable bowel syndrome (therapy update). Gut 52:598–599, 2003

Colgan S, Creed F, Klass H: Symptom complaints, psychiatric disorder and abnormal illness behaviour in patients with upper abdominal pain. Psychol Med 18:887–892, 1988a

Colgan SM, Faragher EB, Whorwell PJ: Controlled trial of hypnotherapy in relapse prevention of duodenal ulceration. Lancet 1(8598):1299–1300, 1988b

Craig TKJ: Abdominal pain, in Life Events and Illness. Edited by Brown GW, Harris TO. New York, Guilford, 1989, pp 233–259

Creed F: The relationship between psychosocial parameters and outcome in irritable bowel syndrome. Am J Med 107:74S–80S, 1999

Creed F, Guthrie E: Techniques for interviewing the somatising patient. Br J Psychiatry 162:467–471, 1993

Creed F, Craig T, Farmer R: Functional abdominal pain, psychiatric illness, and life events. Gut 29:235–242, 1988

Creed F, Ratcliffe J, Fernandez L, et al: Health-related quality of life and health care costs in severe, refractory irritable bowel syndrome. Ann Intern Med 134:860–868, 2001

Creed F, Morgan R, Fiddler M, et al: Depression and anxiety impair health-related quality of life and are associated with increased costs in general medical inpatients. Psychosomatics 43:302–309, 2002

Creed F, Fernandes L, Guthrie E, et al: The cost-effectiveness of psychotherapy and paroxetine for severe irritable bowel syndrome. Gastroenterology 124:303–317, 2003

de Boer AG, Sprangers MA, Bartelsman JF, et al: Predictors of health care utilization in patients with inflammatory bowel disease: a longitudinal study. Eur J Gastroenterol Hepatol 10:783–789, 1998

De Bona M, Ponton P, Ermani M, et al: The impact of liver disease and medical complications on quality of life and psychological distress before and after liver transplantation. J Hepatol 33: 609–615, 2000

Delvaux M, Denis P, Allemand H: Sexual abuse is more frequently reported by IBS patients than by patients with organic digestive diseases or controls. Results of a multicentre inquiry. French Club of Digestive Motility. Eur J Gastroenterol Hepatol 9: 345–352, 1997

Dieperink E, Willenbring M, Ho SB: Neuropsychiatric symptoms associated with hepatitis C and interferon alpha: a review. Am J Psychiatry 157:867–876, 2000

Dimenas E, Glise H, Hallerback B, et al: Well-being and gastrointestinal symptoms among patients referred to endoscopy owing to suspected duodenal ulcer. Scand J Gastroenterol 30:1046–1052, 1995

Drossman DA: Presidential address: gastrointestinal illness and the biopsychosocial model. Psychosom Med 60:258–267, 1998

Drossman DA, McKee DC, Sandler RS, et al: Psychosocial factors in the irritable bowel syndrome. A multivariate study of patients and nonpatients with irritable bowel syndrome. Gastroenterology 95:701–708, 1988

Drossman DA, Patrick DL, Mitchell CM, et al: Health-related quality of life in inflammatory bowel disease: functional status and patient worries and concerns. Dig Dis Sci 34:1379–1386, 1989

Drossman DA, Leserman J, Nachman G, et al: Sexual and physical abuse in women with functional or organic gastrointestinal disorders. Ann Intern Med 113:828–833, 1990

Drossman DA, Leserman J, Mitchell CM, et al: Health status and health care use in persons with inflammatory bowel disease. A national sample. Dig Dis Sci 36:1746–1755, 1991

Drossman DA, Talley NJ, Leserman J, et al: Sexual and physical abuse and gastrointestinal illness. Review and recommendations. Ann Intern Med 123:782–794, 1995

Drossman DA, Creed FH, Olden KW, et al: Psychosocial aspects of the functional gastrointestinal disorders. Gut 45 (suppl 2):II25–II30, 1999

Drossman DA, Creed FH, Olden KW, et al: Psychosocial aspects of the functional gastrointestinal disorders, in Rome II: The Functional Gastrointestinal Disorders. Edited by Drossman DA, Corazziari E, Talley NJ, et al. McLean, VA, Degnon Associates, 2000a, pp 157–245

Drossman DA, Leserman J, Li Z, et al: Effects of coping on health outcome among women with gastrointestinal disorders. Psychosom Med 62:309–317, 2000b

Drossman DA, Whitehead WE, Toner BB, et al: What determines severity among patients with painful functional bowel disorders? Am J Gastroenterol 95:974–980, 2000c

Drossman DA, Camilleri M, Mayer EA, et al: AGA technical review on irritable bowel syndrome. Gastroenterology 123:2108–2131, 2002

Drossman DA, Toner BB, Whitehead WE, et al: Cognitive-behavioral therapy versus education and desipramine versus placebo for moderate to severe functional bowel disorders. Gastroenterology 125:19–31, 2003

Duffy LC, Zielezny MA, Marshall JR, et al: Lag time between stress events and risk of recurrent episodes of inflammatory bowel disease. Epidemiology 2:141–145, 1991

Dwight MM, Kowdley KV, Russo JE, et al: Depression, fatigue, and functional disability in patients with chronic hepatitis C. J Psychosom Res 49:311–317, 2000

Ellard K, Beaurepaire J, Jones M, et al: Acute chronic stress in duodenal ulcer disease. Gastroenterology 99:1628–1632, 1990

El-Serag HB, Kunik M, Richardson P, et al: Psychiatric disorders among veterans with hepatitis C infection. Gastroenterology 123:476–482, 2002

Finkleman D: High incidence of depression and sleep disturbances associated with PegIFN-aplha-2b/ribivirin therapy for hepatitis C in routine clinical practice. Am J Gastr 98 (suppl 1):S85–S86, 2003

Fontana RJ, Moyer CA, Sonnad S, et al: Comorbidities and quality of life in patients with interferon-refractory chronic hepatitis C. Am J Gastroenterol 96:170–178, 2001

Ford MJ, Miller PM, Eastwood J, et al: Life events, psychiatric illness and the irritable bowel syndrome. Gut 28:160–165, 1987

Gleason OC, Yates WR, Isbell MD, et al: An open-label trial of citalopram for major depression in patients with hepatitis C. J Clin Psychiatry 63:194–198, 2002

Gomborone J, Dewsnap P, Libby G, et al: Abnormal illness attitudes in patients with irritable bowel syndrome. J Psychosom Res 39:227–230, 1995

Goodwin RD, Stein MB: Generalized anxiety disorder and peptic ulcer disease among adults in the United States. Psychosom Med 64:862–866, 2002

Goodwin RD, Stein MB: peptic ulcer disease and neuroticism in the United States Adult Population. Psychother Psychosom 72:10–15, 2003

Guthrie E, Creed FH: Basic skills, in Seminars in Liaison Psychiatry. Edited by Guthrie E, Creed FH. London, Gaskell Press, 1996, pp 21–52

Guthrie E, Creed F: Cluster analysis of symptoms and health seeking behaviour differentiates subgroups of patients with severe irritable bowel syndrome. Gut 52:1616–1622, 2003

Guthrie E, Creed FH, Whorwell PJ: Severe sexual dysfunction in women with the irritable bowel syndrome: comparison with inflammatory bowel disease and duodenal ulceration. Br Med J (Clin Res Ed) 295:577–578, 1987

Guthrie E, Creed F, Dawson D, et al: A controlled trial of psychological treatment for the irritable bowel syndrome. Gastroenterology 100:450–457, 1991

Guthrie EA, Creed FH, Whorwell PJ, et al: Outpatients with irritable bowel syndrome: a comparison of first time and chronic attenders. Gut 33:361–363, 1992

Guthrie E, Jackson J, Shaffer J, et al: Psychological disorder and severity of inflammatory bowel disease predict health-related quality of life in ulcerative colitis and Crohn's disease. Am J Gastroenterol 97:1994–1999, 2002

Hamilton J, Guthrie E, Creed F, et al: A randomized controlled trial of psychotherapy in patients with chronic functional dyspepsia. Gastroenterology 119:661–669, 2000

Haug TT, Wilhelmsen I, Ursin H, et al: What are the real problems for patients with functional dyspepsia? Scand J Gastroenterol 30:97–100, 1995

Helzer JE, Stillings WA, Chammas S, et al: A controlled study of the association between ulcerative colitis and psychiatric diagnoses. Dig Dis Sci 27:513–518, 1982

Hilsabeck RC, Perry W, Hassanein TI: Neuropsychological impairment in patients with chronic hepatitis C. Hepatology 35:440–446, 2002

Ho SB, Nguyen H, Tetrick LL, et al: Influence of psychiatric diagnoses on interferon-alpha treatment for chronic hepatitis C in a veteran population. Am J Gastroenterol 96:157–164, 2001

Horikawa N, Yamazaki T, Izumi N, et al: Incidence and clinical course of major depression in patients with chronic hepatitis type C undergoing interferon-alpha therapy: a prospective study. Gen Hosp Psychiatry 25:34–38, 2003

Jackson JL, O'Malley PG, Tomkins G, et al: Treatment of functional gastrointestinal disorders with antidepressant medications: a meta-analysis. Am J Med 108:65–72, 2000

Jantschek G, Zeitz M, Pritsch M, et al: Effect of psychotherapy on the course of Crohn's disease. Results of the German prospective multicenter psychotherapy treatment study on Crohn's disease. German Study Group on Psychosocial Intervention in Crohn's Disease. Scand J Gastroenterol 33:1289–1296, 1998

Jess P, Von der Lieth L, Matzen P, et al: The personality pattern of duodenal ulcer patients in relation to spontaneous healing and relapse. J Int Med 226: 395–400, 1989

Katon W, Sullivan M, Walker E: Medical symptoms without identified pathology: relationship to psychiatric disorders, childhood and adult trauma, and personality traits. Ann Intern Med 134:917–925, 2001

Kettell J, Jones R, Lydiard S: Reasons for consultation in irritable bowel syndrome: symptoms and patient characteristics. Br J Gen Pract 42:459–461, 1992

Khalil HS, Bridger MW, Hilton-Pierce M, et al: The use of speech therapy in the treatment of globus pharyngeus patients. A randomised controlled trial. Rev Laryngol Otol Rhinol (Bord) 124:187–190, 2003

Kirsch MA, Louie AK: Paroxetine and irritable bowel syndrome. Am J Psychiatry 157:1523–1524, 2000

Koloski NA, Talley NJ, Boyce PM: Does psychological distress modulate functional gastrointestinal symptoms and health care seeking? A prospective, community Cohort study. Am J Gastroenterol 98:789–797, 2003

Kraus MR, Schafer A, Scheurlen M: Paroxetine for the prevention of depression induced by interferon alfa. N Engl J Med 345:375–376, 2001

Kraus MR, Schafer A, Faller H, et al: Paroxetine for the treatment interferon–induced depression in chronic hepatitis C. Aliment Pharmacol Ther 16:1091–1099, 2002

Kraus MR, Schafer A, Faller H, et al: Psychiatric symptoms in patients with chronic hepatitis C receiving interferon alfa-2b therapy. J Clin Psychiatry 64:708–714, 2003

Kurata JH, Nogawa AN, Noritake D: NSAIDs increase risk of gastrointestinal bleeding in primary care patients with dyspepsia. J Fam Pract 45:227–235, 1997

Kurina LM, Goldacre MJ, Yeates D, et al: Depression and anxiety in people with inflammatory bowel disease. J Epidemiol Community Health 55:716–720, 2001

Langeluddecke P, Goulston K, Tennant C: Type A behaviour and other psychological factors in peptic ulcer disease. J Psychosom Res 31:335–340, 1987

Leserman J, Drossman DA, Li Z, et al: Sexual and physical abuse history in gastroenterology practice: how types of abuse impact health status. Psychosom Med 58:4–15, 1996

Leserman J, Li Z, Drossman DA, et al: Selected symptoms associated with sexual and physical abuse history among female patients with gastrointestinal disorders: the impact on subsequent health care visits. Psychol Med 28:417–425, 1998

Levenstein S: Peptic ulcer at the end of the 20th century: biological and psychological risk factors. Can J Gastroenterol 13:753–759, 1999

Levenstein S: The very model of a modern etiology: a biopsychosocial view of peptic ulcer. Psychosom Med 62:176–185, 2000

Levenstein S, Prantera C, Varvo V, et al: Life events, personality, and physical risk factors in recent-onset duodenal ulcer. A preliminary study. J Clin Gastroenterol 14:203–210, 1992

Levenstein S, Prantera C, Scribano ML, et al: Psychologic predictors of duodenal ulcer healing has shown that persistence is related to psychological factors J Clin Gastroenterol 22:84–89, 1996

Levenstein S, Kaplan GA, Smith MW: Psychological predictors of peptic ulcer incidence in the Alameda County Study. J Clin Gastroenterol 24:140–146, 1997

Lewin J, Lewis S: Organic and psychosocial risk factors for duodenal ulcer. Psychosom Res 39:531–548, 1995

Longstreth GF, Wolde-Tsadik G: Irritable-bowel symptoms in HMO examinees. Prevalence, demographics and clinical correlates. Dig Dis Sci 38:1581–1589, 1993

Lucock MP, Morley S, White C, et al: Responses of consecutive patients to reassurance after gastroscopy: results of self-administered questionnaire survey. BMJ 315:572–575, 1997

Lydiard S, Jones R: Factors affecting the decision to consult with dyspepsia: comparison of consulters and nonconsulters. Br J Gen Pract 39:495–498, 1989

Lydiard RB, Fossey MD, Marsh W, et al: Prevalence of psychiatric disorders in patients with irritable bowel syndrome. Psychosomatics 34:229–234, 1993

Magni G, Salmi A, Paterlini A, et al: Psychological distress in duodenal ulcer and acute gastroduodenitis. A controlled study. Dig Dis Sci 27:1081–1084, 1982

Magni G, Bernasconi G, Mauro P, et al: Psychiatric diagnoses in ulcerative colitis. A controlled study. Br J Psychiatry 158:413–415, 1991

Masand PS, Gupta S, Schwartz TL, et al: Does a preexisting anxiety disorder predict response to paroxetine in irritable bowel syndrome? Psychosomatics 43:451–455, 2002

Matsushima Y, Aoyama N, Fukuda H, et al: Gastric ulcer formation after the Hanshin-Awaji earthquake: a case study of *Helicobacter pylori* infection and stress-induced gastric ulcers. Helicobacter 4:94–99, 1999

Maunder RG, Esplen MJ: Supportive-expressive group psychotherapy for persons with inflammatory bowel disease. Can J Psychiatry 46:622–626, 2001

Maunder RG, de Rooy EC, Toner BB, et al: Health-related concerns of people who receive psychological support for inflammatory bowel disease. Can J Gastroenterol 11:681–685, 1997

Mendeloff AI, Calkins BM: The epidemiology of idiopathic inflammatory bowel disease, in Inflammatory Bowel Disease, 4th edition. Edited by Kirsner JB, Shorter RG. Philadelphia, Lee & Febiger, 1995, p 31

Mertz H, Fass R, Kodner A, et al: Effect of amitriptyline on symptoms, sleep, and visceral perception in patients with functional dyspepsia. Am J Gastroenterol 93:160–165, 1998

Mittermaier C, Dejaco C, Waldhoer T, et al: Impact of depressive mood on relapse in patients with inflammatory bowel disease: a prospective 18-month follow-up study. Psychosom Med 66:79–84, 2004

Morriss RK, Gask L, Ronalds C, et al: Clinical and patient satisfaction outcomes of a new treatment for somatized mental disorder taught to general practitioners. Br J Gen Pract 49:263–267, 1999

Nguyen HA, Miller AI, Dieperink E, et al: Spectrum of disease in U.S. veteran patients with hepatitis C. Am J Gastroenterol 97:1813–1820, 2002

Nordin K, Pahlman L, Larsson K, et al: Health-related quality of life and psychological distress in a population-based sample of Swedish patients with inflammatory bowel disease. Scand J Gastroenterol 37:450–457, 2002

North CS, Alpers DH, Helzer JE, et al: Do life events or depression exacerbate inflammatory bowel disease? Ann Intern Med 114:381–386, 1991

Nunes GC, Ahlquist RE Jr: Increasing incidence of Crohn's disease. Am J Surg 145:578, 1983

Olden KW, Drossman DA: Psychologic and psychiatric aspects of gastrointestinal disease. Med Clin North Am 84:1313–1327, 2000

Parsonnet J: The incidence of *Helicobacter pylori* infection. Aliment Pharmacol Ther 9 (suppl 2):45–51, 1995

Passik SD, Breitbart WS: Depression in patients with pancreatic carcinoma. Diagnostic and treatment issues. Cancer 78:615–626, 1996

Porcelli P, Leoci C, Guerra V: A prospective study of the relationship between disease activity and psychologic distress in patients with inflammatory bowel disease. Scand J Gastroenterol 31:792–796, 1996

Quadri A, Vakil N: Health-related anxiety and the effect of open-access endoscopy in U.S. patients with dyspepsia. Aliment Pharmacol Ther 17:835–840, 2003

Quartero AO, Post MW, Numans ME, et al: What makes the dyspeptic patient feel ill? A cross sectional survey of functional health status, *Helicobacter pylori* infection, and psychological distress in dyspeptic patients in general practice. Gut 45:15–19, 1999

Rose M, Hildebrandt M, Fliege H, et al: T-cell immune parameters and depression in patients with Crohn's disease. J Clin Gastroenterol 34:40–48, 2002

Rosenstock SJ, Jorgensen T: Prevalence and incidence of peptic ulcer disease in a Danish County—a prospective cohort study. Gut 36:819–824, 1995

Rosenstock S, Jorgensen T, Bonnevie O, et al: Risk factors for peptic ulcer disease: a population based prospective cohort study comprising 2416 Danish adults. Gut 52:186–193, 2003

Salmon P, Skaife K, Rhodes J: Abuse, dissociation, and somatization in irritable bowel syndrome: towards an explanatory model. J Behav Med 26:1–18, 2003

Schramm TM, Lawford BR, Macdonald GA, et al: Sertraline treatment of interferon-alfa-induced depressive disorder. Med J Aust 173:359–361, 2000

Sewitch MJ, Abrahamowicz M, Bitton A, et al: Psychological distress, social support and disease activity in patients with inflammatory bowel disease. Am J Gastroenterol 96:1470–1479, 2001

Simren M, Axelsson J, Gillberg R, et al: Quality of life in inflammatory bowel disease in remission: the impact of IBS-like symptoms and associated psychological factors. Am J Gastroenterol 97:389–396, 2002

Singh N, Gayowski T, Wagener MM, et al: Vulnerability to psychologic distress and depression in patients with end-stage liver disease due to hepatitis C virus. Clin Transplant 11:406–411, 1997

Sjodin I, Svedlund J, Ottosson JO, et al: Controlled study of psychotherapy in chronic peptic ulcer disease. Psychosomatics 27:187–191, 1985

Sperber AD, Carmel S, Atzmon Y, et al: Use of the Functional Bowel Disorder Severity Index (FBDSI) in a study of patients with the irritable bowel syndrome and fibromyalgia. Am J Gastroenterol 95:995–998, 2000

Stanghellini V, De Ponti F, De Giorgio R, et al: New developments in the treatment of functional dyspepsia. Drugs 63:869–892, 2003

Talley NJ: Evaluation of drug treatment in irritable bowel syndrome. Br J Clin Pharmacol 56:362–369, 2003

Talley NJ, Fett SL, Zinsmeister AR: Self-reported abuse and gastrointestinal disease in outpatients: association with irritable bowel-type symptoms. Am J Gastroenterol 90:366–371, 1995a

Talley NJ, Weaver AL, Zinsmeister AR: Impact of functional dyspepsia on quality of life. Dig Dis Sci 40:584–589, 1995b

Talley NJ, Owen BK, Boyce P, et al: Psychological treatments for irritable bowel syndrome: a critique of controlled treatment trials. Am J Gastroenterol 91:277–283, 1996

Talley NJ, Boyce PM, Jones M: Is the association between irritable bowel syndrome and abuse explained by neuroticism? A population-based study. Gut 42: 47–53, 1998

Tarter RE, Switala J, Carra J, et al: Inflammatory bowel disease: psychiatric status of patients before and after disease onset. Int J Psychiatry Med 17:173–181, 1987

Tennant C, Goulston K, Langeluddecke P: Psychological correlates of gastric and duodenal ulcer disease. Psychol Med 16:365–371, 1986

Thompson WG, Longstreth G, Drossman DA, et al: Functional bowel disorders, in Rome II: The Functional Gastrointestinal Disorders. Edited by Drossman DA, Corazziari E, Talley NJ, et al. McLean, VA, Degnon Associates, 2000, p 355

Turnbull GK, Vallis TM: Quality of life in inflammatory bowel disease: the interaction of disease activity with psychosocial function. Am J Gastroenterol 90:1450–1454, 1995

van Dulmen AM, Fennis JFM, Mokkink HGA, et al: Doctor-dependent changes in complaint-related cognitions and anxiety during medical consultations in functional abdominal complaints. Psychol Med 25:1011–1018, 1995

Walker EA, Gelfand AN, Gelfand MD, et al: Psychiatric diagnoses, sexual and physical victimization and disability in patients with irritable bowel syndrome or inflammatory bowel disease. Psychol Med 25:1259–1267, 1995

Walker EA, Gelfand MD, Gelfand AN, et al: The relationship of current psychiatric disorder to functional disability and distress in patients with inflammatory bowel disease. Gen Hosp Psychiatry 18:220–229, 1996

Weiner H, Thaler M, Reiser MF, et al: Etiology of duodenal ulcer, I: relation of specific psychological characteristics to rate of gastric secretion (serum pepsinogen). Psychosom Med 19:1–10, 1957

Wells KB, Stewart CD, Hays RD, et al: The functioning and well-being of depressed patients: results from the Medical Outcomes Study. JAMA 262:914–919, 1989

Wessely S, Pariante C: Fatigue, depression and chronic hepatitis C infection. Psychol Med 32:1–10, 2002

Whitehead WE, Winget C, Fedoravicius AS, et al: Learned illness behavior in patients with irritable bowel syndrome and peptic ulcer. Dig Dis Sci 27:202–208, 1982

Whitehead WE, Burnett C, Cook E, et al: Impact of irritable bowel syndrome on quality of life. Dig Dis Sci 41:2248–2253, 1996

Whitehead WE, Palsson O, Jones KR: Systematic review of the comorbidity of irritable bowel syndrome with other disorders: what are the causes and implications? Gastroenterology 122:1140–1156, 2002

Xuan J, Kirchdoerfer LJ, Boyer JG, et al: Effects of comorbidity on health-related quality of life scores: an analysis of clinical trials data. Clin Ther 21: 383–403, 1999

Zigmond AS, Snaith RP: The hospital anxiety and depression scale. Acta Psychiatr Scand 67:361–370, 1983

22 Renal Disease

Lewis M. Cohen, M.D.

Norman B. Levy, M.D.

Edward G. Tessier, Pharm.D., M.P.H.

Michael J. Germain, M.D.

NEPHROLOGY HAS RECOGNIZED the need for psychiatric consultation since the initial development of kidney dialysis in the late 1960s and early 1970s. Nearly universal access to treatment followed passage of the 1972 End-Stage Renal Disease amendment to the Social Security Act, which provided government subsidy for dialysis. Subsequently, the population has steadily grown, aged, and become more severely ill (McBride 1990). Psychiatry's potential role in the collaborative care of patients with renal disease is increasing.

Each year, approximately 80,000 Americans develop end-stage renal disease (ESRD). More than 340,000 individuals are treated for kidney failure (U.S. Renal Data System 2002); 240,000 people are receiving maintenance dialysis, and 100,000 have a functioning kidney transplant. In 2001, the prevalent dialysis population was 292,215 patients (U.S. Renal Data System 2003). The number of patients starting renal replacement therapy in the United States continues to increase each year by 5%–7%. An additional 8 million individuals are estimated to have chronic renal insufficiency (Robertson et al. 2002). The current annual cost for treating ESRD in the United States is approximately $19 billion, and the average Medicare expenditure is $54,000 per hemodialysis patient and $17,000 per transplant patient. As of 2002, there were 3,600 dialysis facilities and 255 transplant programs in the United States (U.S. Renal Data System 2002).

Every year data have been collected, the average age of the ESRD incident population has increased. In 1986, the mean age was 56 years, and by 1995, it was 60 years (National Institutes of Health 2000). The fastest growth has occurred among the oldest age groups. In 1996, 46% of the incident patients were age 65 years or older, and 20% were over 75 years of age. By 1999, 58% of the newly diagnosed chronic ESRD patients in New England were 65 years or older, and 17% were 80 years and older (Network of New England 1999).

It is not an exaggeration to claim that even young patients with ESRD have old bodies and that geriatric issues are commonplace in this population (Cohen et al. 2003a). The causes of renal failure include diabetes; hypertension; generalized arteriosclerosis; lupus; AIDS; and primary renal diseases, such as chronic glomerulonephritis, chronic interstitial nephritis, polycystic kidney disease, and other hereditary and congenital disorders. In 1999, only 9% of dialysis patients were free of significant comorbid conditions. Of particular importance, diabetes is now found in almost half of ESRD incident cases, and because of its plethora of microvascular and macrovascular complications, patients are especially likely to have increased morbidity (Lea and Nicholas 2002).

In some surveys, almost two-thirds of ESRD patients rate quality of life as being less than "good" (Levy and Wynbrandt 1975; Roberts and Kjellstrand 1988). In a recent survey at nine New England dialysis clinics involving 619 patients, 57% of the sample reported that physical health problems during the previous 4 weeks forced them to cut down on the amount of time spent on work or other activities, 69% accomplished less than they would prefer, and 71% were limited in the kind of work or activities that they could pursue (Poppel et al. 2003). A study of 14,815 dialysis patients demonstrated a significant correlation between mortality and mental-health and physical-function scores on the SF-36 Health Survey (Knight 2003).

While the clinical challenges presented by the patient population steadily mount, there have been corresponding advances in the technology and treatments of renal transplantation and dialysis.

Renal transplantation (see also Chapter 31, "Organ Transplantation," and Chapter 34, "Pediatrics") is the treatment of choice for many patients, and if a transplant is successful, the patient's survival (U.S. Renal Data System 2002; Wolfe et al. 1999) and quality of life (Franke 2003; Laupacis 1996) are almost always better than they would be with dialysis. The major issue in transplantation is the shortage of donor organs. Transplanted kidneys may come from a living donor or through organ donation following death. During the past decade, the number of cadaveric transplants increased by only 16%, whereas living-related transplants have increased by 68% (U.S. Renal Data System 2003). Despite this, many more transplants are performed with cadaveric kidneys than with living-donor kidneys. More than 14,000 transplants were performed in 2000. Long-term kidney survival is greater with living donors. Most cadaveric kidneys are procured from brain-dead individuals following acute trauma, intracerebral bleeds, and cerebral vascular accidents. Commercially available organs from individuals who were willing to sell their kidneys are banned by federal statute in the United States and in many other countries. The critical shortage of cadaveric organs is leading many transplant programs to liberalize their requirements and to make use of kidneys from living, unrelated donors.

Peritoneal dialysis and *hemodialysis* are the two forms of dialysis. In peritoneal dialysis, dialysate fluid is introduced and then removed from the peritoneal space through an indwelling catheter. The peritoneum serves as a semipermeable membrane, and fluid and wastes are removed together with dialysate. Peritoneal dialysis may be performed by a machine in the home at night (continuous cycling peritoneal dialysis, or CCPD), or manually at home four to six times per day (continuous ambulatory peritoneal dialysis, or CAPD). Only 11% of ESRD patients use peritoneal dialysis as the initial mode of renal replacement therapy (U.S. Renal Data System 1997a). Hemodialysis may be conducted at the patient's home, but it usually takes place at dialysis units for 4-hour sessions held three times per week. Home dialysis requires the participation of another person, who must be available to assist with 12–15 hours of weekly treatment. There has been a great deal of recent interest in daily and nocturnal dialysis done at home or in a dialysis facility (Lockridge et al. 2001). Data suggest that this new approach may result in improved quality of life and health. Although patients have not been randomized to dialysis modalities, most studies continue to show that patients receiving peritoneal dialysis rate their care higher than do those receiving hemodialysis (Rubin et al. 2004).

Psychiatric Disorders in Renal Disease

In a review of psychiatric illness involving 200,000 U.S. dialysis patients, almost 10% had been hospitalized with a psychiatric diagnosis, and this was the primary reason for hospitalization of 25% of the subgroup (Kimmel et al. 1993). Depression and other affective disorders were the most common diagnoses, followed by delirium and dementia. Compared with other medical illnesses, the primary diagnosis of depression was higher in renal failure patients than in those with ischemic heart disease and cerebrovascular disease (Kimmel et al. 1993).

The diagnosis of major depressive disorder (MDD) was highlighted in the NIMH-NIDDK conference "Depression and Mental Disorders in Patients With Diabetes, Renal Disease, and Obesity/Eating Disorders" (Bethesda, MD; January 29–30, 2001). Although MDD is the second most common chronic disorder after hypertension encountered in general medical practice, surprisingly little is clear concerning something as basic as its prevalence among patients who receive hemodialysis. Studies of depression and ESRD have reported prevalence rates ranging from 0% to 100% (Cohen-Cole and Stoudemire 1987; Kimmel 2000; Kimmel 2002), reflecting widely variable definitions, criteria, and measurement methods.

Because depression frequently follows loss, its occurrence is understandable in the context of dialysis, where patients commonly lose strength, energy, sexual ability, employment, physical freedom, and independence. Another potential contributing factor to depression is survival guilt, when a fellow dialysis patient dies (Vamos 1997). A recent study highlighted the significance of comorbid disorders (e.g., diabetes) and job status in the etiology of clinical depression (Chen et al. 2003). Examination of the ESRD literature suggests that subsyndromal depressive syndromes are likely in about 25% of patients; and major depression is likely in 5%–22% of patients (O'Donnell and Chung 1997).

Our own diagnostic approach entails describing the criteria for major depression and eliciting the patient's opinion as to whether he or she believe himself or herself to be depressed, and then documenting the existence of associated factors, such as depressive episodes prior to the onset of renal failure, a family history of depression, and previous suicide attempts (Cohen 1998; Cohen et al. 2000). The presence of depressive affect and cognition, such as poor self-esteem, worthlessness, hopelessness, and helplessness, is valuable in arriving at the correct diagnosis.

Major depression appears to be frequently unrecognized and untreated (Finkelstein and Finkelstein 2000). In a recent study of Connecticut dialysis patients (*N* = 123) initiating dialysis treatment, almost half (44%) of the sample scored above the depressed range of the Beck Depression Inventory (score = 15), but only 16% of these patients were receiving antidepressant medications (Watnick et al. 2003).

Suicide, the ultimate complication of depression, is reportedly more common among dialysis patients than in the general population (Abram et al. 1971; Haenel et al. 1980; Kimmel 2001). ESRD suicide rates were originally calculated by combining ordinary clinical suicides with deaths following dialysis discontinuation and deaths caused by noncompliance (Abram et al. 1971). Kishi and Kathol (2002) observed that suicide in the context of terminal illness is increasing, and although suicide usually is a consequence of comorbid major depression or alcohol abuse, it also may occur in the absence of demonstrable psychiatric illness. These "philosophical" or "preemptive" suicides are a focus of interest in the psychiatric and palliative-care communities (Cohen 1998). In an intriguing observation, Kjellstrand (1992) pointed out that Western Europe has one-third the dialysis-withdrawal rate of the United States and three times the number of deliberate suicides among dialysis patients.

Anxiety and depression are the most common psychological symptoms seen in the physically ill (Lefebvre et al. 1972); this is also true in ESRD. Anxiety may be present during dialysis treatments, particularly in hemodialysis. Hemodialysis involves the continuous removal of blood into a machine and its return to the patient's body. The fear of a medical emergency, such as significant blood loss or a cardiac event, may cause understandable anxiety. Phobias of needles and the sight of blood are common in the general population (see Chapter 12, "Anxiety Disorders"). Rapid removal of fluid and electrolytes may also produce hypotension, nausea, vomiting, and muscular cramps. Anxiety is evident in the uncertainty many patients have about the future, fears about sexual performance, and apprehension over their ability to cope with the ongoing demands of dialysis and expectations of staff and family (Levy 1990).

Substance use disorders, such as cocaine or heroin dependence, can directly lead to ESRD (Norris et al. 2001). They may also result in HIV infection and, later, AIDS, which can secondarily cause renal failure.

Cognitive disorders are common in the ESRD patient population and may be related to uremia, a variety of medical comorbidities (e.g., electrolyte disturbances, severe malnutrition, impaired metabolism, cerebrovascular disease), or adverse effects of treatment. *Uremia* refers to the clinical syndrome resulting from profound loss of renal function. Signs and symptoms vary considerably, with severity depending on both the magnitude and the rapidity with which renal function is lost. Central nervous system symptoms may begin with mild cognitive dysfunction, fatigue, and headache, progressing to a usually hypoactive delirium and, if untreated, coma. Restless legs syndrome, muscle cramps, and sleep disorders are also common. Other common symptoms include pruritus, anorexia, nausea, and vomiting. Metabolic abnormalities may include hyperkalemia, hyperphosphatemia, metabolic acidosis, and of course azotemia (elevated BUN and creatinine levels). The specific cause of uremic encephalopathy remains unknown. Many patients will tend to note progressive impairment as their day for dialysis approaches (Levy and Cohen 2000). After dialysis, they may experience a short period of delirium lasting from minutes to hours that is termed "dysequilibrium syndrome," likely caused by the rapid changes in fluid and electrolytes during the dialysis session. Acute changes in mental status are not commonly seen in CAPD, because this procedure is slow, continuous, and without sudden fluxes of fluid and electrolytes. The presence of a transient metabolic encephalopathy can be confirmed by an electroencephalogram, demonstrating diffuse slowing. Single photon emission tomography has been used to compare hemodialysis patients with matched controls (Fazekas et al. 1996). Patients with ESRD appear to have reduced cerebral blood flow in the frontal cortex and thalamus, and even well-dialyzed patients have subtle abnormalities of cognitive function (Levy and Cohen 2001) Finally, cognitive dysfunction in a uremic patient could be the result of the uremia and associated comorbidities, including, for example, electrolyte disturbances, severe malnutrition, impaired metabolism, and cerebrovascular disease.

The usual types of dementia, such as vascular and Alzheimer's, are increasingly encountered as the ESRD population continues to age. Vascular dementia is especially common because of the high prevalence of diabetes, hypertension, and atherosclerosis in ESRD patients.

The most serious cognitive disorder seen in dialysis patients in the 1970s and 1980s was "dialysis encephalopathy" or "dialysis dementia" (Levy and Cohen 2000). This usually fatal syndrome occurred in patients who had been on hemodialysis for at least 2 years, and the early signs were memory impairment, dysarthria, stuttering speech, depression, and psychosis (O'Hare et al. 1983). Patients often displayed asterixis, bizarre limb movements, and generalized tremulousness. Magnetic resonance imaging of demented dialysis patients suggested that there was a toxic–metabolic etiology to their brain degeneration (Fazekas et al. 1995). The cause of this disorder is not fully understood, but aluminum was the most likely culprit, and it was found in phosphate-binding gels and in trace amounts in dialysate water (Alfrey 1986). There are conflicting data, however, concerning aluminum toxicity, because aluminum tends to be present in higher-than-normal quantities in the brain in other types of dementia, including Alzheimer's disease. Trace amounts of tin and zinc have also been blamed as a cause of this syndrome. In dialysis dementia, the EEG showed typical slow-wave bursts in the early stages (Alfrey 1986). This disorder markedly decreased in incidence following the general use of aluminum-free dialysates and the avoidance of aluminum phosphate binders.

Effects of Psychological Factors on Choice of Modality and Compliance

Many factors are involved in the choice of the treatment modality for renal failure. A parallel situation occurs in the treatment of localized prostate cancer; the treating physician must choose between radical prostatectomy, conformal radiation, and radioactive seed implantation. In renal failure, the choice involves center hemodialysis versus various methods of self-care, such as home hemodialysis, CAPD, and CCPD. As in the example of prostate disease, the physician's orientation and preferences are often the main factors that influence treatment choice; ideally, patient preferences should be paramount. In contrast with European nephrologists, most American nephrologists treat patients with hemodialysis. Nephrologists who work in medical centers where renal transplantation is the centerpiece of treatment and hemodialysis space is limited will tend, when feasible, to favor transplantation. Economic factors may also influence the recommended treatment, and proprietary dialysis centers provide the majority of care in this country.

Psychosocial factors significantly impact the choice of treatment modality (Maher et al. 1983). A medical history marked by noncompliance argues against modalities of self-care. This is especially true for transplantation, where nonadherence to immunosuppressant treatment will generally result in organ rejection (Surman 1989). Modality decisions must take into account the social support system of the individual patient. In order for home dialysis to take place, it is essential not only that the patient have a home but also that another individual be available to pro-

vide care. This individual is usually the spouse or significant other. In some cases, insurance will permit hiring of a nursing assistant. The character structure of patients is also an influence on modality choice. The very independent patient will tend to favor modalities of self-care, whereas the dependent person will tend to prefer being cared for.

Compliance is a common problem and is often a central issue in the management of patients. Compliance is a complex, multidimensional array of behaviors, and its relationship with health outcomes in dialysis patients is difficult to study. However, the widespread belief among physicians and nurses that noncompliance results in worse outcomes, including higher mortality in ESRD, is supported by a large multicenter study (Leggat et al. 1997). ESRD occurs more frequently in people who have had previous difficulty adhering to the treatment requirements of those illnesses that lead to renal failure, such as diabetes and hypertension. Chronic overuse of nonsteroidal anti-inflammatory agents and analgesics is recognized to be a fairly common contributing cause of chronic renal insufficiency (Fored et al. 2001). Nephropathies caused by addictive substances, such as heroin, result in greater representation of nonadherent patients. It is difficult enough for the dialysis patient to engage in a lifelong procedure that occurs daily in the case of CAPD, and three times weekly in the case of hemodialysis, but the burdens of dietary restrictions and required medications add major compliance chores. Hemodialysis patients in particular, and peritoneal patients to a lesser degree, need to restrict their intake of protein, sodium, potassium (fruit), phosphates (dairy), and, most difficult of all, fluids. Required medications often include antihypertensive agents, phosphate binders, antacids, and drugs to treat comorbid conditions (e.g., insulin, nitrates, antidepressants, and lipid-lowering agents).

There is no validated method to measure compliance, but clinical indices include dialysis attendance, interdialytic weight gain, serum potassium, and medication adherence. Lack of adherence to treatment regimens is believed to be a common cause for inadequate dialysis and poor outcome (Kaveh and Kimmel 2001). Common noncompliant behaviors include skipping or missing dialysis sessions, and dietary and medication indiscretions. According to self-report, one peritoneal dialysis exchange per week is missed by 12% of patients, and two to three exchanges per week are skipped by 5% of patients (U.S. Renal Data System 1997b). Noncompliance is more common in younger patients, those without diabetes, and black and Hispanic patients, as compared with white and Asian patients (Blake et al. 2000). Among the factors associated with noncompliance are depression, hostility toward authority, memory impairment, ethnic barriers, and financial problems (Anderson and Kirk 1982). The field of nephrology appreciates that appropriate patient and modality selection needs to be combined with a multidisciplinary approach to improve adherence (Raj 2002), with particular attention to patient education (Golper 2001).

Diagnostic Issues

Does the psychiatric disorder come first or the medical illness and its treatment? It is probably most accurate to say that each influences the other. The order of events is largely irrelevant, because both need to be treated, and treatment does not require that this issue be resolved, if indeed it can ever be (Levenson and Glocheski 1991).

Progressive uremia and its treatment modalities are associated with both physical and psychological symptoms, and it is often difficult to delineate the etiology, particularly when patients have comorbid systemic disorders, such as diabetes. It is important to understand that dialysis only partially corrects the uremic state equivalent to less than 10 cc/min glomerular filtration rate, and in three-times-per-week hemodialysis, this clearance is provided only intermittently. This limited amount of clearance of uremic toxins is enough to prevent death; however, patients may remain symptomatic. There has been relatively little research focused on identifying common symptoms and examining different treatment approaches (Weisbord et al. 2004).

In the nephrology literature, there is a lack of clarity around the term *depression* and whether it refers to the affective symptom or the psychiatric disorder (Cohen 1996). Most ESRD research studies have relied on instruments that determine the severity of the symptom (Craven et al. 1988; Kimmel et al. 1998; Smith et al. 1985). In contrast, psychiatric studies in the medically ill now more often rely on the combination of such measures with a structured diagnostic interview based on DSM-IV criteria (American Psychiatric Association 2000) (e.g., Chochinov et al. 1994; Sullivan et al. 1999). In addition, the evaluation of depression is complicated by the fact that the somatic signs and symptoms of ESRD may fulfill the criteria for MDD. Many patients have diminished appetite, loss of energy, dryness of the mouth, constipation, and diminished sexual interest. However, during interviews some individuals will adamantly maintain that they are not depressed, and it is likely that the vegetative symptoms are being produced by the kidney failure and renal replacement therapy. For a full discussion of the diagnosis of depression in the medically ill, see Chapter 9, "Depression."

Withholding or Withdrawing Dialysis: Renal Palliative Care

Psychiatrists have an opportunity to participate in the ongoing integration of palliative medicine and nephrology (Cohen and Germain 2003). Recent ESRD patient demographics reveal a robust increase in numbers, severity of comorbid illnesses, and age (Weisbord et al., in press). Consequently, it should be no surprise that despite continuing improvements in technology, more than 65,000 Americans with ESRD will die this year, and the annual mortality rate is around 23% (U.S. Renal Data System 2002). This mortality rate is comparable to that of non-Hodgkin's lymphoma and higher than that of prostate (0.2%), breast (2.4%), colorectal (17.4%), and ovarian (20.8%) cancer (Ries et al. 2002). The expected remaining lifetime of dialysis patients is one-quarter to one-fifth that of the age- and sex-matched general population (U.S. Renal Data System 2003). Although the figures are better for transplant patients, their expected remaining lifetime is still only 70%–80% that of the general population. To illustrate, a 60-year-old white, male dialysis patient would expect to have an average of around 3 remaining years of life, whereas his counterpart among the general population would have 19 more years. Despite the omnipresence of death, only a minority of ESRD patients complete formal advance directives or engage in ongoing discussions with staff about end-of-life treatment preferences (Cohen et al. 2001). Advance directives are more commonly used in dialysis patients in the United States compared with Germany and Japan (Sehgal et al. 1996). Multidisciplinary involvement is needed to lift the denial of death and improve the provision of end-of-life care and symptom management (Cohen et al. 1997).

Psychiatrists can play a crucial role in the complex determinations to withhold or withdraw renal replacement treatment. Treatment guidelines have been developed by a task force from the Renal Physician's Association, American Society of Nephrology, National Kidney Foundation, and other renal organizations (Moss et al. 2000). Guidelines also exist or are under development in other nations—for example, Japan (Sakaguchi and Akizawa 2002) and Italy (Buzzi 2001). The U.S. guidelines, which directed attention to the ethical and psychological issues in decisions to withhold or withdraw renal replacement treatment, were prompted by the finding that the percentage of patient deaths preceded by decisions to stop dialysis steadily increased during the 1990s. In the United States, between 1990 and 1995, more than 20,000 deaths were preceded by dialysis discontinuation (Leggat et al. 1997). During the same period of time, beginning in 1995, there were 36,000 withdrawal deaths in the incident sample of patients (U.S. Renal Data System 2002). Furthermore, an unknown number of patients die after they or their families decide to withhold or not initiate dialysis. All of these decisions are emotionally complex and stressful for patients, caregivers, and staff. Psychiatrists can assist with determinations of patient capacity and also the potential influence of depression or other psychosocial factors.

In providing better end-of-life care for this very ill population, attention should focus on the following issues:

1. *Early frank discussions concerning prognosis and goals of care.* Ideally, these discussions, which include the family, should start when the patient is first diagnosed with progressive renal disease. Options of care to be discussed and offered ought to include the possibility of not starting dialysis (see below), especially if the burdens of dialysis outweigh the benefits. Patients should also know they have the option of stopping dialysis if suffering is unrelieved. Written advance directives such as the "Five Wishes" (agingwithdignity.com) can help focus the discussion and provide the family with guidance when the patient can no longer make decisions. Do-not-resuscitate orders should be strongly considered when cardiopulmonary resuscitation is likely to be futile (Moss et al. 2000).
2. *Attention to symptoms at all stages of the disease process.* Patients with ESRD have a high burden of symptoms, related to dialysis and their comorbid conditions (Cohen et al. 2001).
3. *Early hospice referrals.* Such referrals can take place in the hospital, home, nursing home, or inpatient hospice unit. Dialysis need not be stopped to receive hospice services, as long as the patient has a nonrenal terminal diagnosis. However, because of the financial burden, most hospice programs are reticent to become involved with patients who continue to receive dialysis. Unquestionably, all patients who terminate dialysis should be offered referral to hospice.
4. *Maximal palliative care at the end of life.* This care includes aggressive pain control, spiritual and emotional support, and attention to the patient's terminal treatment preferences and goals.

The decision not to start dialysis is more common than withdrawal from dialysis. Patients who are already uremic at the time of decision to initiate dialysis may be encephalopathic and lack sufficient decision-making capacity. If dialysis is otherwise indicated, and the patient is refusing dialysis, it is appropriate to seek legal authorization to provide involuntary dialysis until the patient's mental status has improved enough to enable an informed decision (see Chapter 3, "Legal Issues," and Chapter 4, "Ethical Issues"). Utmost sensitivity is needed in making withholding or discontinuation decisions, and one needs to be alert to cultural biases, countertransference, and other complicating factors. In a survey of American nephrologists, nearly 90% reported withholding dialysis at least once in the previous year, and over 30% reported withholding it at least six times (Singer 1992). In a prospective Canadian study, about 25% of patients with advanced chronic kidney disease referred for initiation of hemodialysis were not offered dialysis (Hirsch et al. 1994). There are significant differences between countries in how often dialysis is offered and the relative factors affecting the decision, even among the English-speaking nations. American nephrologists offer dialysis more often and give more weight to patient or family wishes and fear of lawsuit than do British or Canadian nephrologists. British nephrologists more often consider their perception of patients' quality of life as a reason to provide or not provide dialysis than do their American counterparts (McKenzie et al. 1998). Primary care physicians can also withhold dialysis by not referring the patients to nephrologists for evaluation of their progressive renal failure. One study among physicians in West Virginia, for example, found that 20 of 76 primary care providers (26%) had effectively withheld dialysis for at least one patient through nonreferral to a nephrologist (Sekkarie and Moss 1998).

The conditions in the following patients are considered appropriate reasons to withhold dialysis based on recently published U.S. guidelines (Moss et al. 2000):

- Patients with severe and irreversible dementia
- Patients who are permanently unconscious (as in a persistent vegetative state)
- Patients with end-stage cancer or end-stage lung, liver, or heart disease who need considerable assistance with activities of daily living and may be confined to bed, chair, or involved in a hospice program
- Patients with severe mental disability who are uncooperative with the procedure of dialysis itself, are unable to interact with the environment or other people, or are persistently combative with family or staff
- Patients with severe, continued, and unrelenting pain, in whom dialysis may prolong life for a short period of time but will also prolong suffering
- Hospitalized patients (especially elderly) with multiple organ system failure that persists after 3 days of intensive therapy (The mortality rate in such patients is very high.)

Withdrawal from dialysis is often appropriate for the dying dialysis patient. It provides the patient and family with the blessing of a quick death (Cohen et al. 2003b).

The mean time to death after stopping dialysis is 8 days, and dialysis termination does not cause pain or discomfort (Cohen et al. 2001). It typically results in lethargy progressing to coma. Renal physicians' organizations, nephrology fellowship training directors, and dialysis corporations are all becoming more appreciative of the need to integrate palliative care in the treatment of this population. Psychiatrists have an important opportunity to assist in this effort.

Treatment Issues

Psychotherapy

There is a growing body of literature on this topic (Israel 1986; Sacks et al. 1990). In one of the earliest publications involving a 4-year intensive study of 25 patients on hemodialysis (Reichsman and Levy 1972), the sample was described as being among the biggest deniers of psychiatric illness in the experience of the authors. The subjects disowned personal factors as playing a role, and they invariably attributed problems to their physical illness. This observation is common among people with chronic medical disorders, and it complicates psychotherapeutic intervention. Nevertheless, there are data suggesting that a wide variety of forms of psychotherapy may be helpful. In a recent study of Japanese hemodialysis patients (Sagawa et al. 2003), cognitive-behavioral therapy (CBT) achieved a 65% reduction of fluid intake. In a study of five Boston patients (Surman and Tolkoff-Rubin 1984), hypnosis was successful in curtailing psychiatric symptoms. In a study of 116 patients, Cummings et al. (1981) demonstrated that behavioral contracting and weekly telephone contacts were effective in the short term in improving compliance with medical regimens. More recently, behavioral interventions were shown to improve compliance with fluid restriction in both a small quasi-experimental study (Sagawa et al. 2003) and a controlled trial (Christensen et al. 2002). A controlled trial of group therapy in Israeli dialysis patients showed a significant decrease in psychological distress and interdialytic weight gain in those who received group therapy (Auslander and Buchs 2002). A naturalistic nonrandomized study of group therapy in New York City found increased survival among participants in a patient support group compared with other patients, even after multiple psychosocial and psychological variables were controlled (Friend et al. 1986). In a novel study by Hener et al. (1996), patients were randomized with their spouses to a supportive couples group, a CBT couples group, or nonintervention controls. Both interventions improved patients' psychosocial adjustment.

Any form of psychotherapy stands the best chance of success if conducted during dialysis treatment sessions (Levy 1999). Patients with ESRD feel overdoctored and overburdened by the time requirements of treatment. Therefore, therapies should be piggybacked with medical treatment whenever feasible. Even group therapy can be performed while patients are being dialyzed. This necessitates an essential nonselection of participants, because an entire room or partially divided room of patients would be involved, some of whom may be resistant to anything called psychiatric. Groups that have been most successful are those that have a strong educational component. This component may comprise lectures from social workers, nutritionists, transplant surgeons, and nephrologists. Such sessions are especially valuable in the earliest phases of groups when patients may be most hesitant to talk about themselves. As time progresses, personal stories and problems usually emerge. Individual psychotherapy is mainly limited to those few patients who see themselves as having psychological problems and who are willing and able to engage in this form of treatment. The availability of psychoactive medications gives the psychiatrist an important "foot in the front door."

In respect to confidentiality, the psychiatrist must pay special attention to privacy issues in dialysis settings. Patients should always be offered the opportunity to meet in a private office. When patients are seen on dialysis units, curtains should be drawn, and the use of portable, white-noise machines may be helpful.

Miscellaneous Treatment Issues

Aggression, irritability, drug abuse, persistent insomnia, and noncompliance are frequent reasons for referral. During the past several years, the authors have also received increasing requests from nephrologists to assist in determinations of capacity, as well as issues related to dialysis discontinuation decisions. The general topic of capacity and competency are discussed in Chapter 3, "Legal Issues," and Chapter 4, "Ethical Issues," but it is important to make explicit here that most nephrologists feel justified in pressuring patients who resist initiating dialysis to at least enter into a trial of several weeks or months of treatment. The rationale is that this is a life-and-death situation, and the patient's insight and judgment may be impaired by renal encephalopathy, interfering with their decision to initiate dialysis. This topic is addressed in the previously mentioned task force guidelines (Moss et al. 2000).

When it comes to delirium and dementia, the basic treatment involves recognition and correction of the underlying pathology. Intensified dialysis, parathyroidectomy, and improved control of diabetes mellitus can each prove to be ameliorative. Neuroleptics or benzodiazepines may provide symptomatic treatment of agitation and delusions, and antidepressant medications can likewise be highly effective (Levy and Cohen 2001).

Sexual disorders and erectile dysfunction are common in the ESRD population, and these may sometimes result in consultations or requests for counseling. Many different behavioral and physical therapies offer the hope of some improvement. The latter include vacuum tumescence therapy, renal transplantation, use of recombinant human erythropoietin, and sildenafil (Rosas et al. 2001; see also Chapter 17, "Sexual Disorders").

Psychopharmacology

Although antidepressants are frequently prescribed for patients with ESRD, there is only one very small controlled clinical trial (Blumenfield 1997). There is interesting recent evidence that SSRIs may help control hypotension during dialysis (Yalcin 2002).

Most psychotropic medications are fat soluble with large volumes of distribution. With the exception of lithium, they are metabolized in the liver, and metabolites are eliminated in urine and bile. The majority of these drugs can be safely used in ESRD patients, but attention must be paid to medications with active metabolites, those that may be highly plasma-protein bound, and those with altered pharmacokinetics or pharmacodynamics.

When dose adjustments of psychiatric drugs in ESRD are required, it is usually because of comorbidities (e.g., diabetic autonomic neuropathy) and concurrent drug therapy (e.g., other agents metabolized by cytochrome P450 enzyme systems, and those with pharmacodynamic interactions), rather than the ESRD per se. Psychopharmacological management of transplant patients requires an appreciation of potential interactions with immunosuppressant medications (Robinson and Levenson 2001). Table 37–10 in Chapter 37, "Psychopharmacology," summarizes information about the use of individual psychotropic medications and the current knowledge of pharmacokinetic considerations. Given the size of the population, there has been a dearth of systematic investigations, and further psychopharmacological research is greatly needed.

Conclusion

In this chapter we have summarized the existing literature on psychiatric care of patients with end stage renal disease As the techniques of dialysis and transplantation have ad-

vanced, patients are living longer, including patients with more severe illness and more comorbidities. Because comorbid psychiatric disorders are widely prevalent among the dialysis and renal transplant populations, psychiatrists can play a vital role in management, including choice of treatment modality and promotion of compliance, as well as in palliative care for patients who wish to decline or discontinue dialysis. Finally, specific psychotherapeutic techniques and psychopharmacological interventions must be tailored to meet the special needs of patients with compromised renal function.

References

Abram HS, Moore GL, Westervelt BS Jr: Suicidal behavior in chronic dialysis patients. Am J Psychiatry 127:1199–1204, 1971

Alfrey A: Dialysis encephalopathy. Kidney Int 29 (suppl):S53–S57, 1986

American Psychiatric Association: Diagnostic and Statistical Manual of Mental Disorders, 4th Edition, Text Revision. Washington, DC, American Psychiatric Association, 2000

Anderson RJ, Kirk LM: Methods of improving compliance in chronic disease states. Arch Intern Med 142:1673–1675, 1982

Auslander GK, Buchs A: Evaluating an activity intervention with hemodialysis patients in Israel. Soc Work Health Care 35:407–423, 2002

Blake PG, Korbert SM, Blake R, et al: A multicenter study of noncompliance with continuous ambulatory peritoneal dialysis exchanges in U.S. and Canadian patients. Am J Kidney Dis 35:506–514, 2000

Blumenfield M, Levy NB, Spinowitz B, et al: Fluoxetine in depressed patients on dialysis. Int J Psychiatry Med 27:71–80, 1997

Buzzi F, Cecioni R, Di Paolo M, et al: Bioethics in nephrology: guidelines for decision-making in Italy. J Nephrol 14:93–97, 2001

Chen YS, Wu SC, Wang SY, et al: Depression in chronic haemodialysed patients. Nephrology (Carlton) 8:121–126, 2003

Chochinov HM, Wilson KG, Enns M, et al: Prevalence of depression in the terminally ill: Effects of diagnostic criteria and symptom threshold judgments. Am J Psychiatry 51:537–540, 1994

Christensen AJ, Moran PJ, Wiebe JS, et al: Effect of a behavioral self-regulation intervention on patient adherence in hemodialysis. Health Psychol 21:393–397, 2002

Cohen LM: Renal disease, in American Psychiatric Press Textbook of Consultation-Liaison Psychiatry. Edited by Rundell JR, Wise M. Washington, DC, American Psychiatric Press, 1996, pp 573–578

Cohen LM: Suicide, hastening death, and psychiatry. Arch Intern Med 158:1973–1976, 1998

Cohen LM, Germain MJ: Palliative and supportive care, in Therapy of Nephrology and Hypertension: A Companion to Brenner's The Kidney, 2nd Edition. Edited by Brady HR, Wilcox CS. Philadelphia, PA, Elsevier, 2003, pp 753–756

Cohen LM, McCue J, Germain M, et al: Denying the dying: advance directives and dialysis discontinuation. Psychosomatics 38:27–34, 1997

Cohen LM, Steinberg MD, Hails KC, et al: The psychiatric evaluation of death-hastening requests: lessons from dialysis discontinuation. Psychosomatics 41:195–203, 2000

Cohen LM, Reiter G, Poppel D, et al: Renal palliative care, in Palliative Care for Non-Cancer Patients. Edited by Addington-Hall J, Higginson I. London, Oxford University Press, 2001, pp 103–113

Cohen LM, Germain M, Brennan M: End-stage renal disease and discontinuation of dialysis, in Geriatric Palliative Care. Edited by Morrison RS, Meier DE, Capello CF. New York, Oxford University Press, 2003a, pp 192–202

Cohen LM, Germain MJ, Poppel DM: Practical considerations in dialysis withdrawal: "to have the option is a blessing." JAMA 289:2113–2119, 2003b

Cohen-Cole SA, Stoudemire A: Major depression and physical illness: special considerations in diagnosis and biologic treatment. Psychiatr Clin North Am 10:1–17, 1987

Craven JL, Rodin GM, Littlefield C: The Beck Depression Inventory as a screening device for major depression in renal dialysis patients. Int J Psychiatry Med 18:365–374, 1988

Cummings KB, Becker M, Kirscht JP, et al: Intervention strategies to improve compliance with medical regimens by ambulatory hemodialysis patients. J Behav Med 4:111–127, 1981

Fazekas G, Fazekas F, Schmidt R, et al: Brain MRI findings and cognitive impairment in patient undergoing chronic hemodialysis treatment. J Neurol Sci 134:83–88, 1995

Fazekas G, Fazekas F, Schmidt R, et al: Pattern of cerebral blood flow and cognition in patients undergoing chronic haemodialysis treatment. Nucl Med Commun 17:603–608, 1996

Finkelstein FO, Finkelstein SH: Depression in chronic dialysis patients: assessment and treatment. Nephrol Dial Transplant 15:191–192, 2000

Fored CM, Ejerblad E, Lindblad P, et al: Acetaminophen, aspirin and chronic renal failure. N Engl J Med 345:1801–1808, 2001

Franke GH, Reimer J, Philipp T, et al: Aspects of quality of life through end-stage renal disease. Qual Life Res 12:103–115, 2003

Friend R, Singletary Y, Mendell NR, et al: Group participation and survival among patients with end-stage renal disease. Am J Public Health 76:670–672, 1986

Golper T: Patient education: can it maximize the success of therapy? Nephrol Dial Transplant 16 (suppl 7):20–24, 2001

Haenel T, Brunner F, Battegay R: Renal dialysis and suicide: occurrence in Switzerland and Europe. Compr Psychiatry 21:140–145, 1980

Hener T, Weisenberg M, Har-Even D: Supportive versus cognitive-behavioral intervention programs in achieving adjustment to home peritoneal kidney dialysis. J Consult Clin Psychol 64:731–741, 1996

Hirsch DJ, West ML, Cohen AD, et al: Experience with not offering dialysis to patients with a poor prognosis. Am J Kidney Dis 23:463, 1994

Israel M: Depression in dialysis patients: a review of psychological factors. Can J Psychiatry 31:445–451, 1986

Kaveh K, Kimmel PL: Compliance in hemodialysis patients: multidimensional measures in search of a gold measure. Am J Kidney Dis 37:244–266, 2001

Kimmel PL: Just whose quality of life is it anyway? Kidney Int 57:S74, S113–S120, 2000

Kimmel PL: Nephrology forum. Psychosocial factors in dialysis patients. Kidney Int 59:1599–1613, 2001

Kimmel PL: Depression in patients with chronic renal disease: What we know and what we need to know. J Psychosom Res 53:951–956, 2002

Kimmel PL, Weihs K, Peterson RA: Survival in hemodialysis patients: the role of depression. J Am Soc Nephrol 3:12–27, 1993

Kimmel PL, Thamer M, Richard CM, et al: Psychiatric illness in patients with end-stage renal disease. Am J Med 105:214–221, 1998

Kishi Y, Kathol RG: Assessment of patients who attempt suicide. Prim Care Companion J Clin Psychiatry 4:132–136, 2002

Kjellstrand CM: Practical aspects of stopping dialysis and cultural differences, in Ethical Problems in Dialysis and Transplantation. Edited by Kjellstrand C. Dossetor, Dordrect, Kluwer, 1992, pp 103–116

Knight EL, Ofsthun N, Teng M, et al: The association between mental health, physical function, and hemodialysis mortality. Kidney Int 63:1843–1851, 2003

Laupacis A, Keown P, Pus N, et al: A study of the quality of life and cost-utility of renal transplantation. Kidney Int 50:235–42, 1996

Lea JP, Nicholas SB: Diabetes mellitus and hypertension: Key risk factors for kidney disease. J Natl Med Assoc 94:7S–15S, 2002

Lefebvre P, Nobert A, Crombez JC: Psychological and psychopathological reactions in relation to chronic hemodialysis. Can Psychiatr Assoc J 17:9–13, 1972

Leggat JE Jr, Bloembergen WE, Levine G, et al: An analysis of risk factors for withdrawal from dialysis before death. J Am Soc Nephrol 8:1755–1763, 1997

Levenson JL, Glocheski S: Psychological factors affecting end-stage renal disease. Psychosomatics 32:382–389, 1991

Levy NB: Renal failure, dialysis and transplantation, in Psychiatric Treatment of the Medically Ill. Edited by Robinson RG. New York, Marcel Dekker, 1999, pp 141–153

Levy NB, Cohen LM: End-stage renal disease and its treatment: dialysis and transplantation, in Psychiatric Care of the Medical Patient, 2nd Edition. Edited by Stoudemire A, Fogel BS, Greenberg D. London, Oxford University Press, 2000, pp 791–800

Levy NB, Cohen LM: Central and peripheral nervous systems in uremia, in Textbook of Nephrology, 4th Edition. Edited by Massry SG, Glassock R. Philadelphia, PA, Williams & Wilkins, 2001, pp 1279–1282

Levy NB, Wynbrandt GD: The quality of life on maintenance haemodialysis. Lancet 1:1328–30, 1975

Lockridge RS Jr, Spencer M, Craft V, et al: Nocturnal home hemodialysis in North America. Adv Ren Replace Ther 8: 250–256, 2001

Maher HS, Lamping DL, Dickinson CA, et al: Psychosocial aspects of hemodialysis. Kidney Int 23:S13, S50–S57, 1983

McBride P: The development of hemodialysis, in Clinical Dialysis, 2nd Edition. Edited by Nissenson AR, Fine RN, Gentile DE. Norwalk, CT, Appleton & Lang, 1990, p 20

McKenzie JK, Moss AH, Feest TG, et al: Dialysis decision making in Canada, the United Kingdom, and the United States. Am J Kidney Dis 31:12–18, 1998

Moss AH, Renal Physicians Association, American Society of Nephrology Working Group: A new clinical practice guideline on initiation and withdrawal of dialysis that makes explicit the role of palliative medicine. J Palliat Med 3:253–260, 2000

National Institutes of Health NIDDK/DKUHD: Excerpts from the United States Renal Data System 2000 Annual Data Report. Am J Kidney Dis 36 (suppl 2):S1–S239, 2000

Network of New England, Inc: End Stage Renal Disease 1999 Annual Report. New Haven, CT, Health Care Financing Administration, 1999, p 84

Norris KC, Thornhill-Joyner M, Robinson C, et al: Cocaine use, hypertension, and end-stage renal disease. Am J Kidney Dis 38:523–529, 2001

O'Donnell K, Chung Y: The diagnosis of major depression in end-stage renal disease. Psychother Psychosom 66:38–43, 1997

O'Hare JA, Callaghan NM, Murnaghan DJ: Dialysis encephalopathy. Medicine 62:129–141, 1983

Poppel D, Cohen L, Germain M: The renal palliative care initiative. J Palliat Med 6:321–326, 2003

Raj DSC: Role of APD in compliance with therapy. Semin Dial 15:434–436, 2002

Reichsman F, Levy NB: Adaptation to hemodialysis: A four-year study of 25 patients. Arch Intern Med 138:859–865, 1972

Ries LA, Eisner MP, Kosary CL, et al: SEER Cancer Statistics Review, 1973–1999. National Cancer Institute, Bethesda, MD, 2002. Available at: http://seer.cancer.gov/csr/1973_1999/. Accessed July 2, 2003.

Roberts JC, Kjellstrand CM: Choosing death: withdrawal from chronic dialysis without medical reason. Acta Med Scand 223:181–186, 1988

Robertson S, Newbigging K, Isles CG, et al: High incidence of renal failure requiring short-term dialysis: a prospective observational study. Q J Med 95:585–590, 2002

Robinson MJ, Levenson JL: Psychopharmacology in transplant patients, in Biopsychosocial Perspectives on Transplantation. Edited by Rodrigues JR. New York, NY, Kluwer Academic, 2001, pp 151–172

Rosas ES, Wasserstein A, Kobrin S, et al: Preliminary observations of sildenafil treatment for erectile dysfunction in dialysis patients. Am J Kidney Dis 37:134–137, 2001

Rubin HR, Fink NE, Plantinga LC, et al: Patients' ratings of dialysis care with peritoneal dialysis vs. hemodialysis. JAMA 291:697–703, 2004

Sacks CR, Peterson RA, Kimmel PL: Perception of illness and depression in chronic renal disease. Am J Kidney Dis 15:31–39, 1990

Sagawa M, Oka M, Chaboyer W: The utility of cognitive behavioural therapy on chronic haemodialysis patients' fluid intake: a preliminary examination. Int J Nurs Stud 40:367–373, 2003

Sakaguchi T, Akizawa T: Clinical guideline review: standards for initiation of chronic dialysis. Nippon Naika Gakkai Zasshi 91:1561–1569, 2002

Sehgal AR, Weisheit C, Miura Y, et al: Advance directives and withdrawal of dialysis in the United States, Germany, and Japan. JAMA 276:1652–1656, 1996

Sekkarie MA, Moss AH: Withholding and withdrawing dialysis: the role of physician specialty and education and patient functional status. Am J Kidney Dis 31:464–472, 1998

Singer PA: Nephrologists' experience with and attitudes towards decisions to forego dialysis. The End-Stage Renal Disease Network of New England. J Am Soc Nephrol 2:1235–1240, 1992

Smith MD, Hong BA, Robson AM: Diagnosis of depression in patients with end stage renal disease. Am J Med 79:160–166, 1985

Sullivan M, LaCroix A, Russo J, et al: Depression in coronary heart disease: what is the appropriate diagnostic threshold? Psychosomatics 40:286–292, 1999

Surman OS: Psychiatric aspects of organ transplantation. Am J Psychiatry 146:872–882, 1989

Surman OS, Tolkoff-Rubin N: Use of hypnosis in patients receiving hemodialysis for end stage renal disease. Gen Hosp Psychiatry 6(1):31–35, 1984

U.S. Renal Data System: Treatment modalities for ESRD patients. Am J Kidney Dis 30:S54–S66, 1997a

U.S. Renal Data System: USRDS 1997 Annual Data Report. Bethesda, MD, National Institutes of Health, National Institute of Diabetes and Digestive and Kidney Diseases, 1997b, pp 49–67

U.S. Renal Data System: USRDS 2002 Annual Data Report: Atlas of End-Stage Renal Disease in the United Status. Bethesda, MD, National Institutes of Health, National Institute of Diabetes and Digestive and Kidney Diseases, 2002

U.S. Renal Data System: Excerpts from the USRDS 2002 Annual Data Report: Atlas of End-Stage Renal Disease in the United States. Am J Kidney Dis 41 (suppl 2):S15–S28, S135–S150, 2003

U.S. Renal Data System: USRDS 2003 Annual Data Report. Bethesda, MD, National Institutes of Health, National Institute of Diabetes and Digestive and Kidney Diseases, 2003, p 48

Vamos M: Survivor guilt and chronic illness. Aust N Z J Psychiatry 31:592–596, 1997

Watnick S, Kirwin P, Mahnensmith R, et al: The prevalence and treatment of depression among patients starting dialysis. Am J Kidney Dis 41:105–110, 2003

Weisbord SD, Carmody SS, Bruns FJ, et al: Symptom burden, quality of life, advance care planning and the potential value of palliative care in severely ill haemodialysis patients. Nephrol Dial Transplant 18:1345–1352, 2003

Wolfe R, Ashley V, Milford E, et al: Comparison of mortality in all patients on dialysis, patients on dialysis awaiting transplantation, and recipients of a first cadaveric transplant. N Engl J Med 341:1725–1730, 1999

Yalcin AU, Sahin G, Erol M, Bal C: Sertraline hydrochloride treatment for patients with hemodialysis hypotension. Blood Purif 20:150–153, 2002

23 Endocrine and Metabolic Disorders

Ann Goebel-Fabbri, Ph.D.

Gail Musen, Ph.D.

Caitlin R. Sparks, B.A.

Judy A. Greene, M.D.

James L. Levenson, M.D.

Alan M. Jacobson, M.D.

THE ONSET, COURSE, and outcomes of endocrine disorders have traditionally been linked to psychological and social factors. A growing body of neuroendocrine research has begun to illuminate important biological mechanisms underlying the interplay of psyche and soma, and there are important clinical ramifications of these connections. This chapter focuses primarily on these latter pragmatic issues. Diabetes mellitus is the most common endocrine condition and is now growing in epidemic proportions, so it has been given major emphasis. Other topics covered include disturbances in thyroid, parathyroid, adrenal, growth, prolactin, and gonadal hormones; pheochromocytomas; and metabolic disorders including electrolyte and acid-base disturbances, vitamin deficiencies, and the porphyrias.

Diabetes

Type 1 Diabetes

Type 1 diabetes is a chronic, autoimmune disease that affects an estimated 500,000 to 1 million people in the United States. It is most commonly diagnosed in children and young adults, with peak onset occurring during puberty (i.e., ages 10–12 in girls and 12–14 in boys). (See also Chapter 34, "Pediatrics," for discussion of diabetes in pediatric populations.) The exact cause of type 1 diabetes is not known; however, it appears that genetic and environmental factors trigger an autoimmune response, which attacks the insulin-producing beta cells of the pancreas. Prolonged hyperglycemia can lead to the severe macro- and microvascular complications of diabetes, such as cardiovascular disease, retinopathy, nephropathy, and peripheral and autonomic neuropathy (Kahn and Weir 1994).

The Diabetes Control and Complications Trial (DCCT), a 9-year, multicenter intervention study in the United States, established that improvement in glycemic control delays the onset and slows the progression of diabetic complications (Diabetes Control and Complications Trial Research Group 1993). The DCCT's findings have informed and increased the complexity of what is now the standard treatment for type 1 diabetes. As such, treatment is aimed at lowering and stabilizing blood glucose to near normal levels through dietary control, exercise, blood glucose monitoring, and multiple daily insulin injections. Intensive blood glucose management for type 1 diabetes usually entails three or more insulin injections per day (or the use of a continuous insulin infusion pump)—with the goal of mirroring as closely as possible the physiological patterns of insulin release and near-normal blood glucose levels. Hemoglobin A_{1c} is a laboratory value reflective of average blood glucose concentrations over a 2- to 3-month period. It is used as the standard measure of diabetes self-care success and treatment effectiveness, with a typical target of as close to 7% as possible (normal range in people without diabetes is 4%–6%).

Type 2 Diabetes

Approximately 90%–95% (16 million in the United States) of all people with diabetes have type 2 diabetes, which encompasses a variety of abnormalities involving blood glucose metabolism. The hallmark of the disease is insulin resistance, in which the body requires progressively increased pancreatic insulin production to achieve normal glycemia. In patients with type 2 diabetes, the pancreas can no longer meet the need, and chronic hyperglycemia results. Risk factors for type 2 diabetes include obesity and sedentary lifestyle, because both lead to insulin resistance. Onset of type 2 diabetes is typically during middle age, but with growing rates of obesity at younger ages, children and adolescents are starting to develop the disease at higher rates. Because they decrease insulin resistance, prescribed weight loss and regular exercise are first-line treatments for type 2 diabetes (Beaser 2001).

The United Kingdom Prospective Diabetes Study (UKPDS), the largest and longest prospective study of type 2 diabetes to date, found that for every 1-point reduction in hemoglobin A_{1c}, there was a corresponding 35% reduction in risk of diabetes complications. Successfully treating hypertension led to similar or greater reduction in cardiovascular complications (Krentz 1999; Matthews 1999). Treatment for type 2 diabetes is aimed at lowering and stabilizing blood glucose levels through weight loss (when applicable), dietary control, exercise, blood glucose monitoring, oral hypoglycemic medication, and treatment with insulin injections if insulin resistance and hyperglycemia persist.

Stress and Diabetes

There is conflicting evidence whether stress directly affects the onset of diabetes or its course (Helz and Templeton 1990; Mooy et al. 2000; Wales 1995). Stress hormones are involved in the body's counterregulatory response to insulin, so it is likely that stress plays a role in increasing blood glucose. A number of studies have shown that glycemic control is poorer in people with diabetes who report more stress (Garay-Sevilla et al. 2000; Lloyd et al. 1999). However, it is not clear whether stress

directly influences metabolic regulation or whether people under stress change their self-care behaviors. In an effort to evaluate the effects of stress under controlled conditions, a few laboratory studies have been undertaken. Although some laboratory studies have suggested that psychological stress can impair glucose control in both type 1 (Moberg et al. 1994) and type 2 diabetes (Goetsch et al. 1993), other studies have not demonstrated this effect (Kemmer et al. 1986). Thus, it is not yet clear to what extent stressful events directly affect the physiology of glucose regulation.

Psychiatric Disorders and Diabetes Management

The publication of the DCCT and UKPDS studies demonstrated that intensive management of type 1 and type 2 diabetes improves long-term health outcomes in diabetes (Diabetes Control and Complications Trial Research Group 1993; Krentz 1999; Matthews 1999; UK Prospective Diabetes Study Group 1998a, 1998b). However, the goal of achieving near-normal blood glucose values requires a complex set of daily behaviors and problem solving. Many patients have difficulty sustaining the burden of self-care over time—the stress of coping with a chronic disease is a major risk factor for psychopathology and nonadherence to complex treatment recommendations. There is a growing literature examining the relationship of type 1 and type 2 diabetes and psychiatric disorders, especially depression, anxiety, and eating disorders. In both types of diabetes, psychiatric disorders have been linked to treatment nonadherence, worse blood glucose control, and ultimately greater prevalence of micro- and macrovascular complications. Because disease outcomes in diabetes are so dependent on patient behaviors, attitudes, and cognitions, optimal treatment is multidisciplinary, including psychiatrists and other mental health professionals, and takes into account the psychology of individual patients, their support systems, and doctor–patient relationships.

Depression and Diabetes

The prevalence of depression in diabetes is two to three times higher than that found in the general population (Anderson et al. 2001; Gavard et al. 1993). Several studies suggest that patients with depressive disorders appear to develop worse glycemic control and have a heightened risk of diabetes complications such as retinopathy, nephropathy, hypertension, cardiac disease, and sexual dysfunction (Ciechanowski et al. 2000; M. de Groot et al. 2001). However, it remains unclear if depression is a cause or an effect of poorer outcomes in diabetes. In a recent meta-analysis of 24 studies of depression, hyperglycemia, and diabetes, Lustman et al. (2000a) reported a consistently strong association between elevated hemoglobin A_{1c} values (indicating chronic hyperglycemia) and depression. However, they were unable to determine the direction of the association through their analyses, so it remains unclear if hyperglycemia causes depressed mood or if hyperglycemia is a consequence of depression. Further, Lustman et al. (2000a) noted that the relationship may be a reciprocal one, in which hyperglycemia is provoked by depression as well as independently contributes to the exacerbation of depression.

Until recently it was assumed that depression develops as a consequence of diabetes with both psychosocial and biological mechanisms suggested to account for this excess prevalence. Although depression may be a result of complications and disease duration, it has been found to occur relatively early in the course of illness before the onset of complications (Jacobson et al. 2002; Kovacs et al. 1997; Mayou et al. 1991). Therefore, it does not appear that the increased rate of depression in diabetes can be explained solely by emotional reactions to a chronic disease with complications. Another meta-analysis, by M. de Groot et al. (2001), of studies of depression and diabetes indicated that an increase in depressed symptoms was consistently associated with an increase in severity and number of diabetes complications. Depression may cause poorer outcomes in diabetes through biological and behavioral mechanisms because symptoms of depression such as decreased motivation, poor energy, and hopelessness likely interfere with adherence to diabetes treatment and lead to worse glycemic control (M. de Groot et al. 2001).

Studies of type 2 diabetes are less clear with regard to the development of psychiatric disorders (Talbot and Nouwen 2000). The increased rates of depression seen in patients with type 2 diabetes appear in some instances to precede the onset of illness, thereby raising an entirely different hypothesis about the etiological relationship— that is, that depressive disorders themselves may place patients at risk for developing type 2 diabetes. Support for this hypothesis derives in part from the fact that patients with depression can have alterations in the hypothalamic-pituitary axis, which lead to increased rates of cortisol production and other counterregulatory hormones leading to insulin resistance (Musselman et al. 2003). Other biological mechanisms include alterations in central glucose transporter function and increased inflammatory activation (Cameron et al. 1984; Geringer 1990; Hudson et al. 1984). Depressed patients also decrease physical activity and increase cardiovascular risk factors by smoking and eating high-caloric and fatty foods, which place them at higher risk for developing type 2 diabetes (Marcus et al. 1992).

Some investigators have suggested that the metabolic problems of diabetes (increased rates of hypoglycemia and hyperglycemia) could themselves play a causal role in the development of depression. There is increasing evidence that diabetes leads to changes in white matter in the brain (Dejgaard et al. 1991), and that these white matter abnormalities, if present in regions of the brain involved in affect regulation (e.g., the limbic system), may play a causal role in the development of depression (Jacobson et al. 2000). At this point, such white matter changes are of unknown etiology; however, they may be associated with accelerated vascular disease in diabetes.

Screening measures such as the Beck Depression Inventory (BDI) (Lustman et al. 1992, 2000b; Musselman et al. 2003) may be useful in identifying patients with diabetes and depression. In fact, the BDI has been found to accurately distinguish between depressed and nondepressed patients with diabetes even after elimination of neurovegetative symptoms that could otherwise be attributed to diabetes (Lustman et al. 1992). Diabetes-specific measures of quality of life, such as the Problem Areas in Diabetes Scale (PAID) (Polonsky et al. 1995; Welch et al. 1997, 2003) and the Diabetes Quality of Life Measure (DQOL) (Jacobson 1996; Jacobson et al. 1994), may also be useful in screening patients who are overburdened by the demands of self-care and risk of complications and may be at increased risk for depression.

There is now evidence that specific treatment of depression can lead to improvements in diabetes treatment adherence and improved glycemic control. No large-scale, randomized, controlled trials exist in the area of psychopharmacological treatment of depression in diabetes. However, two small controlled studies have demonstrated that nortriptyline and fluoxetine are effective treatments for depression in diabetes. However, nortriptyline improved mood but did not improve glucose regulation, whereas fluoxetine was associated with improvements in both (Lustman et al. 1997, 2000b). Compared with patients receiving diabetes education only, patients treated with cognitive-behavioral therapy (CBT) to address their depression symptoms showed significant improvements in hemoglobin A_{1c} levels (Lustman et al. 1998). It appears that standard treatments for depression not only lead to improvement in depressive symptoms but also can lead to better glycemic control. Thus, whatever the causal links between depression and diabetes, psychiatric treatment can improve psychological and biomedical outcomes (Jacobson and Weinger 1998; Lustman et al. 1998, 2000a).

In summary, the high prevalence of depression and its adverse effects in diabetes, combined with clinically proven treatments, argues for aggressive identification and treatment of depression as early as possible in diabetes. Depression should always be suspected in patients who are having difficulty adapting to diabetes and show poor or worsening glycemic control.

Bipolar Disorder and Diabetes

A number of studies have demonstrated a significantly increased prevalence of diabetes (mainly type 2) in patients with bipolar disorder: 10%–12% of bipolar outpatients (Cassidy et al. 1999; Ruzickova et al. 2003) and 26% of bipolar inpatients (Regenold et al. 2002) have diabetes. Much of the association appears to be related to more obesity in bipolar patients, which is associated with but not fully accounted for by weight gain–associated psychotropic drugs (McElroy et al. 2002). Several other explanations for the increased prevalence of diabetes in bipolar disorder have been considered, including lifestyle, psychiatric and medical comorbidities, shared genetic risk, and physiological ways either disorder might aggravate the other.

Schizophrenia and Diabetes

There is a growing literature suggesting that patients with schizophrenia have a risk two to four times greater than that in the general population of developing type 2 diabetes (Dixon et al. 2000). The reasons for this added risk are unclear. It may reflect the generally poor lifestyle choices of individuals with schizophrenia—that is, they are quite sedentary, frequently smoke, and tend to overeat high-carbohydrate and high-fat foods. However, attention has recently been focused on the role played by antipsychotic medications, most of which can cause weight gain, glucose intolerance, and hyperlipidemia (Buse 2002; Dixon et al. 2000; Geller and MacFadden 2003; Henderson 2002; Henderson and Ettinger 2002; Koro et al. 2002; Lindenmayer et al. 2003; Newcomer et al. 2002; Ryan and Thakore 2002; Sernyak et al. 2002) (see Chapter 37, "Psychopharmacology," for a full discussion). With several of the atypical antipsychotics, the onset of diabetes may occur suddenly and dramatically, with emergent ketoacidosis or hyperosmolar coma, in schizophrenic patients (Buse 2002; Dixon et al. 2000; Geller and MacFadden 2003; Henderson 2002; Henderson and Ettinger 2002; Koro et al. 2002; Lindenmayer et al. 2003; Newcomer et al. 2002; Ryan and Thakore 2002; Sernyak et al. 2002). It is believed that antagonism of serotonin 5-HT_{1A} receptors may play a role in decreasing levels of insulin and increasing hyperglycemia (Wirshing et al. 2003). The diabetes typically recedes once the antipsychotic medication is stopped, but it is likely that sudden emergence of symptoms occurs in patients who already had glucose intolerance, for the increased risk of diabetes among individuals with schizophrenia precedes the use of the atypical agents (Dixon et al. 2000).

Therefore, glucose intolerance should be assessed when treatment with antipsychotics is initiated and should be monitored regularly. Unfortunately, fasting blood glucose is a relatively insensitive method, so that when there is a high index of suspicion (e.g., history of gestational diabetes, family history of diabetes, presence of obesity), postprandial blood glucose testing may be warranted. In patients with known diabetes, antipsychotics least likely to cause weight gain and glucose intolerance should be favored (e.g., aripiprazole and ziprasidone) (see Chapter 37, "Psychopharmacology").

Eating Disorders and Diabetes

Despite its promise of reducing long-term complications of type 1 diabetes, a negative side of intensive diabetes management is weight gain (see also Chapter 15, "Eating Disorders"). For example, during the first 6 years of follow-up in the DCCT, patients in the intensively treated group gained an average of 10.45 pounds more than the patients in the standard treatment cohort (Diabetes Control and Complications Trial Research Group 1988). The most recent follow-up data, 9 years after completion of the DCCT, indicated that once patients on intensive treatment gained weight, this weight was difficult to lose (Diabetes Control and Complications Trial Research Group 2001). A survey of patients' responses to the recommendations of the DCCT study documented that women with type 1 diabetes were especially concerned about tight glucose control causing weight gain (Thompson et al. 1996). It has been argued that the heightened attention to food portions, blood sugars, and risk of weight gain in intensive diabetes management parallels the obsessional thinking about food and body image characteristic of women with eating disorders, and this might place women with diabetes at heightened risk for developing eating disorders. Women with type 1 diabetes may use insulin manipulation (i.e., administering reduced insulin doses or omitting necessary doses altogether) as a means of caloric purging. Intentionally induced glycosuria is a powerful weight loss behavior and a symptom of eating disorders unique to type 1 diabetes.

The most recent controlled studies suggest an increased risk of eating disorders among female patients with type 1 diabetes. For example, Jones et al. (2000) report that young women with type 1 diabetes had 2.4 times the risk of developing an eating disorder and 1.9 times the risk for subclinical eating disorders than age-matched women without diabetes. Intermittent insulin omission or dose reduction for weight loss purposes has been found to be a common practice among women with type 1 diabetes. For example, in a group of 341 women with type 1 diabetes between ages 13 and 60 years, Polonsky et al. (1994) found that 31% reported intentional insulin omission. Rates of omission peaked in late adolescence and early adulthood, with 40% of women between ages 15 and 30 years reporting intentional omission. This behavior, even at a subclinical level of severity, places women at heightened risk for medical complications of diabetes. Women reporting intentional insulin misuse had higher hemoglobin A_{1c} values, higher rates of hospital and emergency room visits, and higher rates of neuropathy and retinopathy than women who did not report insulin omission (Polonsky et al. 1994). In a longitudinal study, Rydall et al. (1997) reported that after 4 years, 86% of patients classified as having high levels of eating disorders had retinopathy, as compared with 43% and 24% of women with moderate or no reported eating disturbance, respectively. Women with diabetes and eating disorders are in poorer glycemic control, with hemoglobin A_{1c} values approximately 2 or more percentage points higher than those in similarly aged women without eating disorders (Rydall et al. 1997). The chronic hyperglycemia found in women with diabetes who intentionally omit or reduce their insulin doses places these women at much greater risk for frequent episodes of diabetic ketoacidosis and the long-term onset of macro- and microvascular complications of diabetes.

Because such patients may not use other means of purging (such as self-induced vomiting or laxative abuse), their eating disorders may go undiagnosed. Once established as a long-standing behavior pattern, the problem of frequent insulin omission can be particularly difficult to treat, pointing to the importance of early detection and intervention. Questions like "Do you ever change your insulin dose or skip insulin doses to influence your weight?" can be helpful in screening for insulin omission especially when patients present with persistently elevated hemoglobin A_{1c} levels or unexplained diabetic ketoacidosis.

Because obesity is a significant risk factor in type 2 diabetes, recurrent binge eating may increase the chances of developing it in part because of significantly higher body mass index (BMI) (Striegel-Moore et al. 2000). The literature on binge eating in type 2 diabetes is still in its infancy, with initial studies relying on small, nonrepresentative samples. Kenardy et al. (1994) found that 14% of the patients with newly diagnosed type 2 diabetes experienced problems with binge eating compared with 4% of the age-, sex-, and weight-matched control group. Recurrent binge eating can be expected to make it very difficult to control diabetes.

A multidisciplinary team approach, including an endocrinologist or diabetologist, nurse educator, nutritionist with eating disorder and diabetes training, and mental health practitioner, is ideal for the treatment of comorbid eating disorders and diabetes (Kahn and Weir 1994; Mitchell et al. 1997). Depending on the severity of the eating disorder and other comorbid psychopathology, a psychiatrist may also be needed for psychopharmacological evaluation and treatment. At this time, little research has examined treatment efficacy for eating disorders in the context of diabetes; however, a large research literature on treatment outcomes in bulimia nervosa supports the use of CBT in combination with antidepressant medications as the most effective treatment (Peterson and Mitchell 1999; B.T. Walsh and Devlin 1995). These approaches would need to be adapted slightly to directly address the role of insulin omission as the means of caloric purging.

Early on in treatment, intensive glycemic management of diabetes is not an appropriate target for a person with diabetes and an eating disorder. As noted earlier, overly intensive diabetes management may actually aggravate obsessional thinking about food and weight in patients with eating disorders. The first goal should focus on medical stabilization. Gradually, the team can build toward increasing doses of insulin, increases in food intake, greater flexibility of meal plan, regularity of eating routine, and more frequent blood glucose monitoring.

Diabetes and Sexual Function

For information on diabetes and sexual function, see Chapter 17, "Sexual Disorders."

Diabetes and Cognitive Functioning

Several researchers have studied the impact of diabetes on cognitive functioning. It has been shown that adolescents and children with onset of diabetes before age 6 experience some cognitive difficulties (Bjorgaas et al. 1997; Kaufman et al. 1999; Rovet and Ehrlich 1999; Rovet et al. 1987; Ryan et al. 1985). In a series of longitudinal studies, Northam and colleagues tested children with diabetes 2 and 6 years after diagnosis. They found that speed of processing, vocabulary, learning, and block design performance was worse in these patients as compared with a control group (Northam et al. 1998). In addition, they found that recurrent hypoglycemia predicted worse performance on measures of learning, attention, and short-term memory (Northam et al. 2001). Finally, Northam et al. (1999) found that chronic hyperglycemia led to problems with visual organization as measured by the Rey Complex Figure Test.

Equivocal results have been obtained as to the role of repeated hypoglycemic events on cognition in adults. Deary and colleagues observed mild IQ deficits and slowing of psychomotor speed using a cross-sectional design, whereas the longitudinal analyses from the DCCT suggested no deficits in cognition (Bale 1973; Deary et al. 1993; Langan et al. 1991). Long-term exposure to hyperglycemia and related micro- and macrovascular damage have also been posited to heighten risk of cognitive decline and dementia in diabetes. In fact, two studies report a 60%–100% increased risk for cognitive decline among patients with diabetes as compared with those without diabetes (Gregg and Brown 2003). This increased risk appears to be mediated primarily by an increase in vascular dementia rather than a heightened risk for Alzheimer's disease in diabetes (Gregg and Brown 2003).

Hypoglycemia in Diabetic and Nondiabetic Individuals

Hypoglycemia has been a popular explanation for anxiety symptoms, especially panic attacks, with past widespread use of 5-hour glucose tolerance tests for diagnosis and recommendations for dietary management with multiple small meals. This practice is no longer commonly recommended by physicians, but hypoglycemia is still a popular diagnosis among alternative medicine practitioners and many patients. Symptomatic hypoglycemia rarely occurs except in diabetic (mainly insulin-dependent) patients and patients with insulinomas. Although marked hypoglycemia does cause symptoms of adrenergic hyperactivity, they can be reliably distinguished by patients from panic attacks (Schweizer et al. 1986; Uhde et al. 1984).

However, insulin-induced hypoglycemia is an aversive experience, which has been reported to cause phobic anxiety—that is, a fear of hypoglycemia—in diabetic patients, leading to poorer diabetic control (Green et al. 2000).

Thyroid Disorders

Hyperthyroidism and hypothyroidism are accompanied by a variety of physiological, psychiatric, and cognitive symptoms. In this section, we focus on cognitive and psychiatric symptoms associated with thyroid problems.

Hyperthyroidism

Hyperthyroidism is accompanied by a host of physiological symptoms, including nervousness, sweating, fatigue, heat intolerance, weight loss, and muscle weakness (Kornstein et al. 2000). The most common cause of hyper-

thyroidism (or thyrotoxicosis) is Graves' disease. Graves' disease is an autoimmune disorder that results in hyperthyroidism when thyroid-stimulating immunoglobulins (TSIs) bind to thyroid-stimulating hormone (TSH) receptors and mimic TSH. TSIs thereby stimulate the synthesis of hormones (T_4 and T_3), while serum TSH levels are very low or undetectable (Porterfield 1997). The factors that trigger this immune response are unknown. Patients with type 1 diabetes are at increased risk for Graves' disease. There is some evidence that stress can precipitate Graves' disease (Santos et al. 2002; Yoshiuchi et al. 1998) and aggravate treated disease (Fukao et al. 2003).

Patients with Graves' disease often present with anxiety, hypomania, depression, and/or cognitive difficulties. Both physiological and psychiatric symptoms correlate poorly with thyroid hormone levels (Trzepacz et al. 1989). These symptoms typically resolve with antithyroid therapy (Alvarez et al. 1983; Kathmann et al. 1994) or with use of beta-blockers such as propranolol (Trzepacz et al. 1988b). Treatment options for Graves' disease include antithyroid medications, thyroidectomy, and radioactive iodine. Graves' disease patients have been reported to have difficulties with sustained attention and visuomotor speed tasks (Alvarez et al. 1983) and with memory and concentration (MacCrimmon et al. 1979). It is possible that the memory and concentration difficulties appear only after long-term thyroid dysregulation. We do know that without treatment for Graves' disease, psychiatric symptoms such as major depressive disorder, generalized anxiety disorder, and hypomania will persist (Trzepacz et al. 1988a). Affective psychosis (e.g., depression and mania) can also result from thyrotoxicosis (Brownlie et al. 2000).

Although thyroid disorders are known to affect behavior, the relationship between thyroid hormones per se and brain functions has not been well studied. To investigate the effect of T_3 (the biologically active thyroid hormone), Kathmann et al. (1994) conducted a study using only healthy subjects. They varied T_3 levels to note the effect on brain performance. They found that subjects made subjective overestimates of time intervals and were able to increase their word fluency, in the absence of more global cognitive problems (Kathmann et al. 1994).

Anxiety and irritability are common in Graves' disease prior to treatment. Only a few studies (Trzepacz et al. 1988b) have investigated the prevalence of psychiatric complaints in hyperthyroid patients and whether these complaints persist after treatment. R.A. Stern et al. (1996) conducted a survey of members of the National Graves' Disease Foundation to investigate patient self-report of psychiatric and cognitive symptoms. The most common symptoms reported were irritability (78%), shakiness

(77%), and anxiety (72%). Slowed thinking was reported by 40%.

In addition to anxiety and cognitive difficulties, some patients with hyperthyroidism experience depression secondary to their medical condition. When patients are given antithyroid therapy, depressive symptoms often disappear. Thus, antithyroid therapy should be the first course of action in treating depression in these patients (Kathol et al. 1986). However, treatment for depression may be indicated if the symptoms are sufficiently problematic or persistent. Hyperthyroidism may present differently depending on the age of the patient. In younger patients, hyperthyroidism typically presents as hyperactivity or anxious dysphoria (Bhatara and Sankar 1999), whereas in the elderly, it can present as apathy or depression (Bailes 1999).

Hypothyroidism

Hypothyroid patients often experience weakness, fatigue, somnolence, cold intolerance, weight gain, constipation, hair loss, hoarseness, stiffness, and muscle aches (Kornstein et al. 2000). The most common cause of hypothyroidism is autoimmune thyroiditis (Hashimoto's thyroiditis). Hypothyroidism can also be a side effect of lithium. Radioactive iodine, the most commonly used modality for treating hyperthyroidism (such as in Graves' disease), may cause hypothyroidism, which may go undiagnosed for several years after treatment for hyperthyroidism (New York Thyroid Center 2003).

The symptoms of hypothyroidism overlap with retarded depression and the diagnosis is easy to miss in patients already diagnosed as depressed. Physical signs of hypothyroidism include weakness, bradycardia, facial puffiness, weight gain, hair loss, hoarseness, and slowed speech (Kornstein et al. 2000). The best screening test for hypothyroidism is measurement of serum TSH concentration, but an elevated TSH should be followed by a free T_4 determination to confirm the diagnosis. A serum TSH determination will be misleading in the patient with secondary hypothyroidism caused by pituitary or hypothalamic disease. In such a patient, a free T_4 measurement will usually allow the clinician to make the appropriate diagnosis.

Severe hypothyroidism is relatively rare, although milder hypothyroidism is fairly common (Joffe and Levitt 1992). Hypothyroidism can be divided into three grades (Haggerty and Prange 1995). Grade 1 refers to patients with *overt* hypothyroidism who are usually symptomatic and have elevated serum TSH and low serum free T_4 concentrations. Patients with *subclinical* hypothyroidism are classified as having grade 2 or 3; these patients typically have either mild or no symptoms of thyroid hormone deficiency. The laboratory features of grade 2 hypothyroidism are an elevated serum TSH level and a serum free T_4 level within the normal range. Patients with grade 3 hypothyroidism have normal TSH and free T_4 levels, and the diagnosis can only be confirmed by an exaggerated serum TSH response to thyrotropin-releasing hormone (TRH). Subclinical hypothyroidism is fairly common, affecting 5%–10% of the population, mainly women, and occurs in 15%–20% of women over the age of 45. Subclinical hypothyroidism is particularly common in elderly women.

Cognitive Function

Hypothyroidism can impair memory function. It is not well understood whether this impairment is limited to memory or whether it extends to other cognitive skills such as attention, inhibition of irrelevant information, and task switching. One possibility is that cognitive inefficiency in hypothyroidism is a result of secondary depression. However, in some cases, cognitive problems are independent of depression. For example, Burmeister et al. (2001) found no relationship between cognitive ability and level of depression in a group of hypothyroid patients (although patients in this study scored within normal limits on most aspects of cognition). This study suggests that patient perceptions of cognitive difficulty (rather than actual cognitive dysfunction) may be a result of depression, fatigue, or response bias.

Patients with subclinical hypothyroidism often show subtle signs of cognitive dysfunction on tests of memory that may improve after treatment (Baldini et al. 1997; Capet et al. 2000; Jensovsky et al. 2002). Further, although most hypothyroid patients who receive treatment are prescribed thyroxine, administration of both thyroxine and triiodothyronine may improve cognitive performance more than thyroxine alone (Bunevicius et al. 1999). More recent studies, however, do not support this observation (Sawka et al. 2003; J.P. Walsh et al. 2003). Mennemeier et al. (1993) demonstrated that after thyroid treatment, some forms of cognition returned to normal levels (e.g., performance on the Object Assembly subtest of the Wechsler Adult Intelligence Scale and on the Peterson-Peterson task that assesses short-term memory), whereas other functions remained impaired (e.g., logical memory or paired-associate learning). Whether to treat subclinical hypothyroidism, however, remains controversial.

Depression

Hypothyroidism is a known cause of secondary depression. Almost all patients with hypothyroidism have some concurrent symptoms of depression (Haggerty and Prange 1995). In the early stages of hypothyroidism, circulating T_4 levels drop, while T_3 levels often remain in the normal range. The brain preferentially uses T_4, as compared with other body tissues, and is thus more sensitive than other areas of the body to lower levels of T_4 (J.J. Haggerty et al. 1990). This imbalance in thyroid hormones may contribute to mood disorder, and subclinical hypothyroidism is now recognized as a potential risk factor for depression (Haggerty and Prange 1995).

Patients with bipolar disorder with either rapid cycling or mixed episodes have particularly high rates of subclinical hypothyroidism. In one study, almost 40% of rapid or mixed episode bipolar patients were found to have subclinical hypothyroidism (although lithium-induced thyroid dysfunction could have contributed) (Joffe et al. 1988). Every patient with rapid-cycling bipolar disorder should be evaluated for (subclinical) hypothyroidism and receive thyroxine if TSH levels are elevated. Some patients may benefit even if they are euthyroid (Haggerty and Prange 1995).

Psychosis

Untreated hypothyroidism can result in psychosis, so-called myxedema madness. This condition was fairly common—reported in up to 5% of all hypothyroid patients (Kudrjavcev 1978)—before the widespread use of modern thyroid function tests, but it is now rare. Psychotic symptoms typically remit when TSH levels return to normal, although cognitive dysfunction may continue (J. J. Haggerty Jr. et al. 1986). The syndrome can be difficult to diagnose because of confusion between hypothyroidism and primary Axis I psychopathology (Darko et al. 1988). Another rare possibility in hypothyroid patients is Hashimoto's encephalopathy, a delirium with psychosis, seizures, and focal neurological signs, associated with high serum antithyroid antibody concentrations, responsive to corticosteroids, and thought to be an autoimmune disorder (Chong et al. 2003).

Congenital Hypothyroidism

Congenital hypothyroidism usually occurs as a result of thyroid agenesis or dysgenesis, although inherited defects in thyroid hormone synthesis may also play a role. From a global perspective, iodine deficiency is the most common cause of congenital hypothyroidism. Newborns with untreated hypothyroidism develop the syndrome of cretinism, characterized by mental retardation, short stature, poor motor development, and a characteristic puffiness of the face and hands. Because early treatment is essential to prevent permanent mental retardation, all infants born in the United States are screened for hypothyroidism at birth (Kooistra et al. 1996). Treatment with thyroid hormones before age 3 months can result in normal intellectual development in the majority of infants.

Parathyroidism

Hyperparathyroidism

Hyperparathyroidism can cause bone disease, kidney stones, and hypercalcemia via oversecretion of parathyroid hormone (PTH). Symptoms of hypercalcemia include anorexia, thirst, frequent urination, lethargy, fatigue, muscle weakness, joint pain, constipation, and, when severe, depression and eventually coma.

The prevalence of hyperparathyroidism is 0.1%. It is three times more common in women than in men, and its prevalence increases with age. Hyperparathyroidism may occur as a consequence of radiation therapy to head and neck or lithium therapy (Bendz et al. 1996). Prior to 1970, more than 90% of patients with hyperparathyroidism presented with renal disease or bone disease. However, after the introduction of routine calcium screening, fewer than 20% of patients present with renal or bone disease, and more than 50% of patients present with no symptoms at all.

With mild hypercalcemia, patients may show personality changes, lack of spontaneity, and lack of initiative. Moderate hypercalcemia (serum calcium concentration 10–14 mg/dL) may cause dysphoria, anhedonia, apathy, anxiety, irritability, and impairment of concentration and recent memory. In severe hypercalcemia (serum calcium concentration >14 mg/dL), confusion, disorientation, catatonia, agitation, paranoid ideation, delusions, auditory and visual hallucinations, and lethargy progressing to coma may occur (Kornstein et al. 2000). Verbal memory and logical abilities are also impaired (Reus 1986). After treatment of hypercalcemia, psychotic and cognitive symptoms disappear in most patients. However, psychosis has also been reported postparathyroidectomy, possibly because of the rapid decrease in serum calcium concentrations (Reus 1986).

Hypoparathyroidism

Patients with hypoparathyroidism present with hypocalcemia causing increased neuromuscular irritability. Typical symptoms include paresthesias, muscle cramps, carpopedal spasm, and rarely facial grimacing. Psychiatric symptoms may include anxiety and emotional irritability and lability (Kornstein et al. 2000). Severe hypocalcemia causes tetany and seizures. Hypoparathyroidism is caused by inadequate parathyroid hormone secretion, usually as a result of parathyroid or thyroid surgery.

Kowdley et al. showed that cognitive and neurological deficits are often present in patients with long-standing hypoparathyroidism (≥9 years). These deficits are thought to be related to the presence of intracranial calcification and thus irreversible (Kowdley et al. 1999).

Adrenal Gland Disorders

Cushing's Syndrome

Cushing's syndrome (CS) results from abnormally high levels of cortisol and other glucocorticoids. The most common cause is the pharmacological use of corticosteroids, followed by excessive adrenocorticotropic hormone (ACTH) secretion (most commonly by a pituitary tumor, referred to as Cushing's disease) and adrenal tumors (Porterfield 1997). Symptoms and signs of CS include truncal obesity and striae, diabetes, hypertension, hyperglycemia, muscle weakness, osteopenia, skin atrophy and bruising, increased susceptibility to infections, and gonadal dysfunction.

CS patients commonly experience a range of psychiatric symptoms (Kornstein et al. 2000), with rates varying widely across studies. Depression is the most prevalent psychiatric disturbance associated with CS. A full depressive syndrome has been reported in up to 50%–70% of cases (Sonino et al. 1998), accompanied by irritability, insomnia, crying, decreased energy and libido, poor concentration and memory, and suicidal ideation (Kornstein et al. 2000). The high prevalence suggests that there is a specific mechanism linking CS and depression. In the past, the depression was attributed to a psychological reaction to the physical symptoms; however, this hypothesis is unlikely because mental symptoms often precede physical changes (Fava 1994; Sonino and Fava 1998, 2001). There is support in the literature for two possible mechanisms linking CS and depression: 1) depression in patients with Cushing's disease may be caused by hypothalamic dysfunction (Sonino et al. 1998), and 2) elevated cortisol levels may directly cause depression in CS (Sonino et al. 1998).

Anxiety has been reported in 12%–79% of cases (Loosen et al. 1992; Starkman and Schteingart 1981; Starkman et al. 1981). Kelly et al. (1996) reported that 3% of CS patients experienced hypomania. Periods of hyperactivity subside as the disease progresses (Starkman and Schteingart 1981; Starkman et al. 1981). There are also case reports of CS patients presenting with a variety of psychotic symptoms, for example, mania (Kathol et al. 1985), schizophreniform psychosis (Hirsh et al. 2000), hallucinations, paranoia, and erotomania (Tadami et al. 1994). A misdi-

agnosis of bipolar disorder has particularly occurred in cyclical CS (Kathol et al. 1985).

Cognition may be impaired in patients with CS. For example, Starkman et al.(2001) found that, compared with a healthy control group, Cushing's disease patients scored poorly on Verbal and Performance IQ measures and had lower memory quotients, with verbal skills the most affected. The deficits in cognitive function were not explained by depression (Starkman et al. 2001). The neocortex and the hippocampus are rich in glucocorticoid receptors (Sapolsky 2000; Starkman et al. 2001), so it is not surprising that learning and memory are affected in CS. In fact, Cushing's disease causes reduction in hippocampal volume, reversible after cortisol levels return to normal. This effect is age-dependent, such that the older the individual, the less plastic is the hippocampus and the less susceptible the patient is to recovery (Starkman et al. 1999).

Cushing himself acknowledged that psychological "traumas" might play a role in the pathogenesis of adrenal disorders (Sonino 1997). Indeed, there is a small body of research suggesting that patients with Cushing's disease experience more stressful events in the year before diagnosis compared to patients with pituitary tumors secreting growth hormone and prolactin (Kelly et al. 1996; Sonino and Fava 2001). Furthermore, there is evidence that stressful events play a causal role in the development of Cushing's disease but not in other forms of CS (Mazet et al. 2003; Sonino and Fava 1998). Therefore, the relationship of stressful life events to the onset of Cushing's disease is comparable to the relationship of such events to the onset of depression in general (Fava et al. 1981).

Adrenal Insufficiency: Addison's Disease and ACTH Deficiency

Insufficient production of adrenal corticosteroids can be caused by a number of mechanisms. Primary adrenal insufficiency, or Addison's disease, results in deficient secretion of mineralocorticoids and glucocorticoids. The major causes of Addison's disease are autoimmune destruction of the adrenal cortex, tuberculosis, and HIV (Kornstein et al. 2000). The most common cause of secondary adrenal insufficiency is suppression of ACTH secretion by chronic glucocorticoid administration. Less common secondary causes include diseases that result in pituitary destruction. In secondary adrenal insufficiency, ACTH levels are low, whereas in Addison's disease, the deficiency in cortisol results in an increase in ACTH production. This increase in ACTH can cause hyperpigmentation, particularly in sun-exposed skin, scars, and mucous membranes.

The decrease in mineralocorticoid levels results in contraction of the extracellular volume, leading to postural hypotension. In addition to hypotension, individuals with adrenal insufficiency are prone to hypoglycemia when stressed or fasting. Although electrolytes can be normal in mild Addison's disease, hyponatremia and hyperkalemia are typical (Kornstein et al. 2000). Water intoxication with hyponatremia can occur if a water load is given, because cortisol deficiency impairs the ability to increase free water clearance. Other manifestations of adrenal insufficiency include anemia, anorexia, nausea, vomiting, diarrhea, abdominal pain, weight loss, and muscle weakness.

Although there has been no formal study, psychiatric symptoms such as apathy, social withdrawal, fatigue, anhedonia, poverty of thought, and negativism have been reported in up to 60%–90% of patients with Addison's disease (Popkin and Mackenzie 1980). Some form of depression has been observed in 30%–50% of patients (Kornstein et al. 2000). Nonspecific symptoms such as weakness, fatigue, and anorexia often appear before more specific findings, making it difficult to attribute the cause to adrenal insufficiency. Cognitive impairment, especially memory loss, is often present but ephemeral and varying in severity. During Addisonian crisis, patients may experience delirium, disorientation, confusion, and even psychosis (Kornstein et al. 2000). Adrenal insufficiency is particularly likely to be misdiagnosed as primary major depression in patients with chronic medical illness previously treated with high doses of corticosteroids, resulting in unrecognized secondary adrenal insufficiency.

Although the diagnosis of adrenal insufficiency may be suspected on the basis of a low serum cortisol in the morning, definitive diagnosis requires an ACTH stimulation test. This is typically performed using cosyntropin, a synthetic ACTH analogue. An increase in the serum cortisol concentration to greater than 20 ng/dL following cosyntropin injection excludes the diagnosis of adrenal insufficiency.

The cause of depression in patients with Addison's disease is not clear. Regardless of the etiology of adrenal insufficiency, urgent treatment is indicated. Both glucocorticoid and mineralocorticoid replacement are usually necessary in the treatment of Addison's disease, whereas glucocorticoid replacement alone is sufficient in secondary adrenal insufficiency.

Adrenal insufficiency is also a feature in adrenoleukodystrophy, a rare, X-linked inherited metabolic disease, which also leads to leukoencephalic myeloneuropathy. Adult onset is rare but commonly presents with psychiatric symptoms, including mania, psychosis, and cognitive dysfunction (Garside et al. 1999).

Acromegaly

Acromegaly is a disease of excess growth hormone (GH) secretion. Deficiency of growth hormone in children results in short stature, as discussed in Chapter 34, "Pediatrics." The most common cause of acromegaly is a GH-secreting adenoma of the anterior pituitary. These benign tumors account for 30% of all hormone secreting pituitary adenomas (L.J. DeGroot et al. 2001). Clinical manifestations of acromegaly include headache, cranial nerve palsies, acral enlargement (frontal bossing), increased hand and foot size, prognathism, soft tissue overgrowth (macroglossia), glucose intolerance, and hypertension (Melmed 2001). Suprasellar extension of the tumor may cause visual field defects.

Psychiatric disturbances associated with acromegaly, described in 1951 in a study of 28 patients, include mood lability and personality changes (Bleuler 1951). Cases of patients with acromegaly and depression (Avery 1973; Margo 1981), and less commonly psychosis (Schulte 1976), have been reported. Psychiatric symptoms in acromegaly have been attributed to the endocrine disorder itself and the psychosocial stress of disfigurement (Abed et al. 1987). Personality change, including loss of initiative and spontaneity with marked lability in mood, has been described in acromegalic patients (Pantanetti et al. 2002). However, one study of 60 acromegalic patients concluded that although psychiatric morbidity was higher in the women versus the men, there was no increase in psychiatric morbidity in general, nor was there an increased incidence of depression in comparison with the general population (Abed et al. 1987). Additionally, the authors found no relationship between GH levels and scores on the Present State Examination, a standard psychiatric interview. Thus, the literature to date does not conclusively support any particular increase in psychopathology in acromegaly.

Treatment of acromegaly may include surgery, medication, and radiation. Surgery is the primary treatment for GH-secreting pituitary adenomas and may enhance the effectiveness of subsequent medical therapy (L.J. DeGroot et al. 2001). Medical management includes somatostatin analogues (e.g., octreotide), dopamine agonists (e.g., bromocriptine), and radiation. High doses of bromocriptine are often necessary to reduce levels of GH, which increases the incidence of adverse effects. The treatment of acromegaly with bromocriptine has been associated with psychotic reactions (Boyd 1995; Le Feuvre et al. 1982; Turner et al. 1984). In a study of 600 patients with pituitary tumors treated with dopamine agonists, 1.3% experienced auditory hallucinations, delusions, and mood changes (Turner et al. 1984). A GH receptor antagonist, pegvisomant, has recently become available as another option for patients for whom surgery fails, and it has few adverse effects (Clemmons et al. 2003).

Pheochromocytoma

Pheochromocytomas are rare catecholamine-secreting tumors derived from the adrenal medulla and sympathetic ganglia. The clinical signs and symptoms result from the release of catecholamines, leading to increased heart rate, blood pressure, myocardial contractility, and vasoconstriction (Keiser 1991). Symptoms of pheochromocytoma can include headache, profuse sweating, palpitations, apprehension, and a sense of impending doom (Melmed 2001). Because these are nonspecific symptoms, pheochromocytomas may mimic anxiety disorders (especially panic), migraine or cluster headaches, amphetamine or cocaine abuse, alcohol withdrawal, brain tumors, subarachnoid hemorrhage, neuroblastoma in children, or temporal lobe seizures (L.J. DeGroot et al. 2001).

Cases of classic panic attacks in patients with pheochromocytoma have been reported in both adults and children (Carre 1996; Gokce et al. 1991; Prokhorova and Fritz 2002). Less commonly, depression has been observed (Gokce et al. 1991). Lambert (1992) described a patient with undiagnosed pheochromocytoma presenting as an exacerbation of PTSD and proposed that release of catecholamines from the tumor may have triggered dissociation.

Both tricyclic antidepressants (TCAs) and serotonin reuptake inhibitors have unmasked silent pheochromocytomas (Korzets et al. 1997; Lefebvre et al. 1995). The mechanism of action of TCAs is via inhibition of neuronal uptake of the high circulating levels of catecholamines (Korzets et al. 1997), and monoamine oxidase inhibitors (MAOIs) would be expected to be even more hazardous. The mechanism with selective serotonin reuptake inhibitors (SSRIs) is less clear (Seelen et al. 1997).

The diagnosis of pheochromocytoma is made by measurement of 24-hour urine to document increased excretion of catecholamines or catecholamine metabolites, including vanillylmandelic acid (VMA) and metanephrines. The availability of plasma metanephrine assays has greatly simplified the evaluation of the patient with a suspected pheochromocytoma. Plasma metanephrine determinations have an extremely high sensitivity, approaching 99%, and overall specificity in the 85%–90% range (Lenders et al. 2002). The finding of elevated urinary catecholamine levels is not specific for pheochromocytoma and can lead to misdiagnosis. A variety of psychological and physiological stressors can elevate levels of urinary catecholamines (Dimsdale and Ziegler 1991; Fukuda et al. 1996). Urinary VMA levels can be elevated with ingestion of foods high in vanillin, including vanilla extract, bananas, coffee, nuts, and citrus fruits (Sheps et al. 1990). Elevated urinary VMA levels are the least specific indicator of pheochromocytoma, whereas elevated metanephrines are the most sensitive (T.A. Stern and Cremens 1998). Misdiagnosis of pheochromocytoma has been reported in patients with hypertension and raised urinary catecholamines who were taking clozapine (Krentz et al. 2001; Li et al. 1997) or selegiline (Cook and Katritsis 1990; Lefebvre et al. 1995).

Multiple cases of factitious pheochromocytoma have been reported (Hyams et al. 1985; Kailasam et al. 1995; Keiser 1991; Spitzer et al. 1998; T.A. Stern and Cremens 1998. Case reports include intentional vanilla extract ingestion (T.A. Stern and Cremens 1998), phenylpropanolamine abuse (Hyams et al. 1985), surreptitious injection of catecholamines intravaginally (Spitzer et al. 1998), epinephrine injection (Keiser 1991), and conscious altering of autonomic function with Valsalva maneuvers (Kailasam et al. 1995).

The rare possibility of a pheochromocytoma should be considered in patients with panic attacks, headaches, and labile hypertension, particularly those who do not respond to treatment. It is not necessary to screen for pheochromocytoma in patients who only have psychiatric symptoms; elevated catecholamines are common and likely to be false positives. Some psychotropic drugs may cause hypertensive reactions that mimic pheochromocytoma, and in other cases, the drugs may be unmasking an unsuspected pheochromocytoma.

Hyperprolactinemia

Hyperprolactinemia is the most common pituitary hormone hypersecretion syndrome (Melmed 2001). The differential diagnosis of hyperprolactinemia includes pituitary adenomas, physiological causes (pregnancy and lactation), medication effects, chronic renal failure (via decreased peripheral PRL clearance), primary hypothyroidism, and lesions of the pituitary stalk and the hypothalamus (e.g., hypothalamic tumors). Clinical signs in women include galactorrhea, menstrual irregularities, infertility, and decreased libido. Men present with diminished libido and rarely with galactorrhea. The relationship between elevated prolactin and affective disorder was first described by Sachar et al. (1973).

Numerous studies and case reports demonstrate an association between hyperprolactinemia and depression and anxiety, as well as resolution of symptoms with treatment of hyperprolactinemia (Cohen 1995; Fava et al. 1983; Holroyd and Cohen 1990; Reavley et al. 1997; Thienhaus and Hartford 1986). Fava et al. (1982) found that hyperprolactinemic patients reported a significant increase in symptoms of depression, anxiety, and hostility compared with amenorrheic and healthy control subjects. However, the link between hyperprolactinemia and depression has been disputed because of small sample sizes and different inclusion criteria across studies (Merritt 1991). In a sample of 65 women with hyperprolactinemia, a surprisingly high prevalence of anxiety and a small increase in measures of hostility were found, yet no significant difference was seen in the prevalence or severity of depression (Reavley et al. 1997). The authors of this study subdivided subjects with hyperprolactinemia into those with pituitary adenomas on computed tomography (CT) versus those with normal CT scans. The subgroup of patients with normal CT scans had an increased prevalence of anxiety, which was thought to be secondary to "functional hyperprolactinemia." The authors proposed that this subgroup had a primary psychiatric disturbance with secondary increased prolactin.

Medication-induced hyperprolactinemia has been associated with antipsychotics and, to a lesser extent, antidepressants. Conventional antipsychotic drugs block dopamine D_2 receptors on lactotroph cells and thus remove the main inhibitory influence on prolactin secretion (Wieck and Haddad 2003). Prolactin levels between 10 and 100 ng/L are typical in drug-induced hyperprolactinemia (Melmed 2001). Serum prolactin levels in patients taking therapeutic doses of typical neuroleptics are increased six- to tenfold from mean baseline prolactin levels (Arvanitis and Miller 1997; Gruen et al. 1978; Kuruvilla et al. 1992; Meltzer and Fang 1976; Oseko et al. 1988).

Atypical antipsychotics vary with respect to their effects on prolactin. Clozapine, quetiapine, and olanzapine either cause no increase in prolactin secretion or increase prolactin transiently (Meltzer et al. 1979; AstraZeneca 1998; Small et al. 1997; Tollefson and Kuntz 1999), but sustained hyperprolactinemia can occur in patients taking risperidone (Becker et al. 2003). Haloperidol raises the serum prolactin concentration by an average of 17 ng/mL, whereas risperidone may raise it by 45–80 ng/mL, with larger increases in women than in men (David et al. 2000).

Antidepressants with serotonergic activity, including SSRIs, MAOIs, and some TCAs, can cause modest elevations of prolactin (Checkley 1991; Haddad et al. 2001) and may further elevate prolactin levels in patients also taking prolactin-elevating antipsychotics (Wieck and Haddad 2003).

Women taking psychiatric medications that chronically elevate prolactin levels are at risk for premature bone loss secondary to hypoestrogenism. Patients taking prolactin-elevating antipsychotics should be educated about—and regularly monitored for—signs and symptoms of hyperprolactinemia (David et al. 2000; Haddad et al. 2001).

In patients with affective disorders who are both unresponsive to treatment and have galactorrhea and/or amenorrhea, hyperprolactinemia should be considered as a causal factor (Holroyd and Cohen 1990).

Gonadal Disorders

Perimenstrual Disorders and Menopause

For information on perimenstrual disorders and menopause, refer to Chapter 33, "Obstetrics and Gynecology."

Polycystic Ovary Syndrome

Polycystic ovary syndrome (PCOS) is a common disorder, affecting 5%–10% of women of childbearing age. Clinical manifestations include amenorrhea or oligomenorrhea, infrequent or absent ovulation, increased levels of testosterone, infertility, truncal obesity or weight gain, alopecia, hirsutism, acanthosis nigricans, hypertension, and insulin resistance. The cause of the disorder is unknown. There is some evidence that valproate is associated with PCOS (McIntyre et al. 2003; O'Donovan et al. 2002).

There are adverse psychosocial consequences of PCOS. Women with PCOS may complain they feel "abnormal or freakish" (Kitzinger and Willmott 2002), related to hirsutism, obesity, and altered reproductive function (Eggers and Kirchengast 2001; Kitzinger and Willmott 2002). A study using standardized self-report measures found that social phobia, anxiety, and depression may occur in one-third to two-thirds of women with PCOS (Barth et al. 1993). Psychological problems have been commonly reported in women with hirsutism of any cause (Sonino et al. 1993). Although these physical abnormalities may affect feelings of self-worth and femininity, some research suggests that psychological morbidity, such as depression, may be caused by hormonal shifts in PCOS, not psychosocial factors (Derogatis et al. 1993). Rasgon et al. (2002) reported a patient with treatment-resistant depression and untreated PCOS whose depressive symptoms resolved when she was treated with metformin and spironolactone. In a sample of 32 women with PCOS, 16 had CES-D scores indicative of depression (Rasgon et al. 2003). Although the causal linkage between psychological symptoms and PCOS is not resolved, their frequency points to the importance of screening all PCOS patients for psychiatric syndromes, especially depression.

Testosterone Deficiency

Testosterone deficiency in men can result from diseases affecting the testes, pituitary gland, or hypothalamus. Consequences of testosterone deficiency vary depending on the stage of sexual development. Testosterone production declines naturally with age, so that a relative testosterone deficiency occurs in older males. Hypogonadal disorders of the testes (primary hypogonadism) are most commonly caused by Klinefelter's syndrome, mumps orchitis, trauma, tumor, cancer chemotherapy, or immune testicular failure (see Chapter 28, "HIV/AIDS," for a discussion of hypotestosteronism in HIV infection). Pituitary lesions caused by tumors, hemochromatosis, sarcoidism, or cranial irradiation can lead to secondary hypogonadism. The classic cause of hypothalamic hypogonadism is Kallmann's syndrome (hypogonadotropic hypogonadism with hyposmia, sensorineural hearing loss, oral clefts, micropenis, and cryptorchidism). Hypogonadism in childhood is characterized by failure of normal secondary sexual characteristics to develop and diminished muscle mass. In adult men, typical complaints are sexual dysfunction, diminished energy, decreased beard and body hair, muscle loss, and breast enlargement.

Although it has been suggested that decreasing testosterone levels as men age may be associated with changes in mood and cognition, there is no clear relationship between psychiatric syndromes and testosterone level (Sternbach 1998). However, a recent study found an adjusted hazard ratio for depression in hypogonadal men of 4.2 (95% CI=1.5–12.0, P=0.008) (Shores et al. 2004). The concept of a male climacteric and related mood, anxiety, and cognitive disorders is controversial (Sternbach 1998).

Patients with Klinefelter's syndrome (XYY) are reported to have higher rates of mental retardation and a wide variety of psychiatric and behavioral symptoms, but these are a consequence primarily of the chromosomal abnormality rather than hypogonadism (Swanson and Stipes 1969).

Questions remain about the value of testosterone replacement in age-related testosterone decline as well as in the treatment of depressive disorder in hypogonadal men. Testosterone appears to improve mood, as well as sexual dysfunction and muscle strength, in hypogonadal men (Wang et al. 2000). However, a placebo-controlled trial of intramuscular testosterone in hypogonadal men with major depressive disorder whose depression did not respond to SSRIs demonstrated no antidepressant benefits (Seidman and Rabkin 1998). The potential serious side effects of testosterone should be carefully considered before initiating replacement therapy in men with age-related low testosterone levels (Nolten 2000).

Testosterone deficiency in women can cause impaired sexual function, low energy, and depression, but what level represents deficiency and the indications, risks, and benefits of replacement are even less well defined than in men (Padero et al. 2002).

Other Metabolic Disorders

Electrolyte and Acid–Base Disturbances

Hyponatremia

Hyponatremia's principal manifestations are neuropsychiatric, and their severity is related both to the degree and rapidity with which it develops. Patients may have lethargy, stupor, confusion, psychosis, irritability, and seizures. There are many different causes, but those of particular psychiatric relevance include the syndrome of inappropriate antidiuretic hormone secretion (SIADH), which can be caused by many psychotropic drugs (especially carbamazepine), and psychogenic polydipsia. The signs of hypernatremia are also predominantly neuropsychiatric and include cognitive dysfunction, delirium, seizures, and lethargy progressing to stupor and coma. Similar symptoms are seen with any hyperosmolar state, for example, extreme hyperglycemia. Hypernatremia is usually caused by dehydration with significant total body water deficits.

Hypokalemia

Hypokalemia produces muscular weakness and fatigue and, if severe, may cause severe paralysis (hypokalemic periodic paralysis), but central nervous system functions are not typically affected. Nevertheless, patients with symptomatic hypokalemia are sometimes misdiagnosed as depressed. Hypokalemia is very common in eating disorders. (See Chapter 15, "Eating Disorders," for full discussion of the metabolic complications of eating disorders.) The adverse effects of hyperkalemia are mainly cardiac, but severe muscle weakness may also occur.

Hypocalcemia, Hypercalcemia, Hypomagnesemia, and Hypermagnesemia

Hypocalcemia and hypercalcemia were described earlier in this chapter under parathyroid disorders. Magnesium levels usually rise and fall in concert with calcium levels.

Hypomagnesemia can cause anxiety, irritability, tetany, and seizures. Low magnesium levels are very common in alcoholic patients and in refeeding starving patients (including those with anorexia nervosa and catatonia). Cyclosporine causes hypomagnesemia, which can contribute to its neuropsychiatric side effects (Craven 1991). Hypermagnesemia is much less common, but it causes central nervous system depression.

Hypophosphatemia

Hypophosphatemia causes anxiety, hyperventilation, irritability, weakness, delirium, and, if severe, seizures, coma, and death, in addition to symptoms in many other organ systems. Hypophosphatemia occurs in the same settings as hypomagnesemia.

Acidosis and Alkalosis

Metabolic acidosis results in compensatory hyperventilation. When the acidosis is severe and acute, as in diabetic ketoacidosis, fatigue and delirium are present and may progress to stupor and coma. Patients with chronic metabolic acidosis appear depressed, with prominent anorexia and fatigue. Patients with severe metabolic alkalosis present with apathy, confusion, and stupor. Respiratory acidosis results from ventilatory insufficiency; and respiratory alkalosis, from hyperventilation (see Chapter 20, "Lung Disease").

Vitamin Deficiencies

The clinical signs of vitamin B_{12} deficiency can include megaloblastic anemia, myelopathy (subacute combined degeneration), dementia, delirium, peripheral neuropathy, and a variety of psychiatric symptoms including psychosis, anxiety, mood disorder, catatonia, and personality change. Psychiatric symptoms may be the sole presenting complaint and can occur even in the absence of hematological changes. Vitamin B_{12} deficiency occurs most often in pernicious anemia, but it also should be suspected in chronic peptic ulcer disease, after gastrectomy or gastric bypass, in alcohol dependence, in inflammatory bowel disease, and in eating disorders, as well as in vegetarians and malnourished individuals. Vitamin B_{12} deficiency can be masked by folate supplementation or iron deficiency (Kunkel et al. 2000).

Folate deficiency causes cognitive dysfunction and depression. The hematological abnormalities are similar to those in B_{12} deficiency. Folate deficiency was common in pregnancy until supplementation became part of routine prenatal care. Folate deficiency occurs frequently in patients taking certain anticonvulsants, in the elderly, in al-

coholic persons, in patients with eating disorders, and in other malnourished populations.

Pellagra, originally thought to be a deficiency of niacin, is now recognized to be a complex deficiency of multiple vitamins and amino acids. The classic triad of symptoms is dermatitis, dementia, and diarrhea, but psychosis, apathy, insomnia, and delirium have all been reported. Pellagra is now rare in the developed nations, but cases are still reported in anorexia nervosa, inflammatory bowel disease, and alcoholism.

Thiamine deficiency (beriberi) causes cardiac and neuropsychiatric syndromes, including peripheral neuropathy and Wernicke-Korsakoff encephalopathy. Wernicke's consists of vomiting, nystagmus, ophthalmoplegia, fever, ataxia, and confusion that can progress to coma and death. Korsakoff's is a dementia with amnesia, impaired ability to learn, confabulation, and often psychosis. Improvement usually occurs with thiamine replacement but may be slow. Giving intravenous glucose to a thiamine-deficient patient without coadministering thiamine may precipitate acute beriberi. Thiamine deficiency is well known and most frequent in alcoholic patients, but it also occurs in patients undergoing chronic dialysis, patients refeeding after starvation (including patients with anorexia nervosa), and individuals on fad diets.

Pyridoxine (vitamin B_6) deficiency causes peripheral neuropathy and neuropsychiatric disorders, including reports of seizures, migraine, chronic pain, depression, and psychosis. Homocysteine is elevated in B_6 deficiency and may play a role in accelerating vascular disease and dementia. Pyridoxine deficiency is common because many drugs act as its antagonists. Clinical trials of B_6 supplementation in healthy elderly subjects to date have not shown improvements in mood or cognition, but there have been no controlled trials in the cognitively impaired (Malouf and Grimley 2003).

Vitamin E deficiency can cause areflexia, ataxia, and decreased vibratory and proprioceptive sensation. Although an association between low vitamin E levels and depressive symptoms has been reported, the data to date do not support this (Tiemeier et al. 2002).

Porphyrias

The porphyrias are a group of rare disorders of heme biosynthesis that can be inherited or acquired. Neuropsychiatric manifestations occur in the two neuroporphyrias (acute intermittent porphyria and plumboporphyria) and two neurocutaneous porphyrias (hereditary coproporphyria and variegate porphyria) (Gonzalez-Arriaza and Bostwick 2003). Acute intermittent porphyria is the most common. Recurrent acute attacks are typical in all four, with variable manifestations. In acute porphyria, the cardinal signs are abdominal pain, peripheral neuropathy, and mental disturbances (Regan et al. 1999). Psychiatric symptoms, including anxiety, depression, psychosis, and delirium, have been reported in 20%–58% of cases (Ibrahim and Carney 1995). Seizures, autonomic instability, dehydration, electrolyte imbalance, and dermatological changes may also occur. Symptoms may vary considerably among patients and in the same patient over a period of time, and they can mimic symptoms of other psychiatric and medical disorders, making diagnosis a challenge. The diagnosis is made by measuring porphyrins and their metabolites in stool and urine during an acute episode. Between episodes, porphyrin levels return to normal. Diagnosis is more likely to be made when there is a high index of suspicion. The diagnosis may be especially difficult because neuropsychiatric symptoms may continue well after the end of an acute episode. Therapy is primarily supportive and includes identifying precipitants. Although barbiturates clearly can trigger attacks, there is inadequate evidence regarding the role of other psychotropic drugs. Whether stress is a precipitant remains controversial (Gonzalez-Arriaza and Bostwick 2003; Holroyd and Seward 1999; Ibrahim and Carney 1995).

Conclusion

Endocrine and metabolic disorders frequently occur in conjunction with common psychiatric conditions. The causal linkages and mechanisms vary widely. In some situations, the endocrine state manifests in part as a psychiatric condition. In other instances, the psychiatric condition may be a complex biopsychosocial and/or biological response to the endocrine disorder. Psychiatric conditions and their treatment may also increase risk of endocrine disorders. Moreover, treatment with psychotropic drugs can induce endocrinopathies. Consequently, understanding the ways in which these disorders intersect represents an important facet of knowledge for the practitioners treating patients with psychiatric and/or endocrine disorders.

References

Abed RT, Clark J, Elbadawy MH, et al: Psychiatric morbidity in acromegaly. Acta Psychiatr Scand 75:635–639, 1987

Alvarez MA, Gomez A, Alavez E, et al: Attention disturbance in Graves' disease. Psychoneuroendocrinology 8:451–454, 1983

Anderson R, Freedland KE, Clouse RE, et al: The prevalence of comorbid depression in adults with diabetes. Diabetes Care 24:1069–1078, 2001

Arvanitis LA, Miller BG: Multiple fixed doses of "Seroquel" (quetiapine) in patients with acute exacerbation of schizophrenia: a comparison with haloperidol and placebo. The Seroquel Trial 13 Study Group. Biol Psychiatry 42:233–246, 1997

AstraZeneca: A literature review of prolactin in schizophrenia. Clear Perspectives 1(3):5–42, 1998

Avery TL: A case of acromegaly and gigantism with depression. Br J Psychiatry 122:599–600, 1973

Bailes BK: Hypothyroidism in elderly patients. AORN J 69: 1026–1030, 1999

Baldini IM, Vita A, Mauri MC, et al: Psychopathological and cognitive features in subclinical hypothyroidism. Prog Neuropsychopharmacol Biol Psychiatry 21:925–935, 1997

Bale RN: Brain damage in diabetes mellitus. Br J Psychiatry 122: 337–341, 1973

Barth JH, Catalan J, Cherry CA, et al: Psychological morbidity in women referred for treatment of hirsutism. J Psychosom Res 37:615–619, 1993

Beaser RS: Joslin Diabetes Deskbook: A Guide for Primary Care Providers. Boston, MA, Joslin Diabetes Center, 2001

Becker D, Liver O, Mester R, et al: Risperidone, but not olanzapine, decreases bone mineral density in female premenopausal schizophrenia patients. J Clin Psychiatry 64:761–766, 2003

Bendz H, Sjodin I, Toss G, et al: Hyperparathyroidism and long-term lithium therapy—a cross-sectional study and the effect of lithium withdrawal. J Intern Med 240:357–365, 1996

Bhatara VS, Sankar R: Neuropsychiatric aspects of pediatric thyrotoxicosis. Indian J Pediatr 66:277–284, 1999

Bjorgaas M, Gimse R, Vik T, et al: Cognitive function in type 1 diabetic children with and without episodes of hypoglycaemia. Acta Paediatr 86:148–153, 1997

Bleuler M: The psychopathology of acromegaly. J Nerv Ment Dis 113:497–511, 1951

Boyd A: Bromocriptine and psychosis: a literature review. Psychiatr Q 66:87–95, 1995

Brownlie BE, Rae AM, Walshe JW, et al: Psychoses associated with thyrotoxicosis—"thyrotoxic psychosis." A report of 18 cases, with statistical analysis of incidence. Eur J Endocrinol 142:438–444, 2000

Bunevicius R, Kazanavicius G, Zalinkevicius R, et al: Effects of thyroxine as compared with thyroxine plus triiodothyronine in patients with hypothyroidism. N Engl J Med 340:424–429, 1999

Burmeister LA, Ganguli M, Dodge HH, et al: Hypothyroidism and cognition: preliminary evidence for a specific defect in memory. Thyroid 11:1177–1185, 2001

Buse JB: Metabolic side effects of antipsychotics: focus on hyperglycemia and diabetes. J Clin Psychiatry 63 (suppl 4): 37–41, 2002

Cameron O, Kronfol Z, Greden J, et al: Hypothalamic-pituitary-adrenocortical activity in patients with diabetes mellitus. Arch Gen Psychiatry 41:1090–1095, 1984

Capet C, Jego A, Denis P, et al: Is cognitive change related to hypothyroidism reversible with replacement therapy? Rev Med Interne 21:672–678, 2000

Carre A: Panic attack: viewpoint of the internist. Encephale 22 (spec no 5):11–12, 1996

Cassidy F, Ahearn E, Carroll BJ: Elevated frequency of diabetes mellitus in hospitalized manic-depressive patients. Am J Psychiatry 156:1417–1420, 1999

Checkley S: Neuroendocrine effects of psychotropic drugs. Baillieres Clin Endocrinol Metab 5:15–33, 1991

Chong JY, Rowland LP, Utiger RD: Hashimoto encephalopathy: syndrome or myth? Arch Neurol 60:164–171, 2003

Ciechanowski PS, Katon WJ, Russo JE: Depression and diabetes: impact of depressive symptoms on adherence, function, and costs. Arch Intern Med 160:3278–3285, 2000

Clemmons DR, Chihara K, Freda PU, et al: Optimizing control of acromegaly: integrating a growth hormone receptor antagonist into the treatment algorithm. J Clin Endocrinol Metab 88:4759–4767, 2003

Cohen AJ: Bromocriptine for prolactinoma-related dissociative disorder and depression. J Clin Psychopharmacol 15:144–145, 1995

Cook RF, Katritsis D: Hypertensive crisis precipitated by a monoamine oxidase inhibitor in a patient with phaeochromocytoma. BMJ 300:614, 1990

Craven JL: Cyclosporine-associated organic mental disorders in liver transplant recipients. Psychosomatics 32:94–102, 1991

Darko DF, Krull A, Dickinson M, et al: The diagnostic dilemma of myxedema and madness, Axis I and Axis II: a longitudinal case report. Int J Psychiatry Med 18:263–270, 1988

David SR, Taylor CC, Kinon BJ, et al: The effects of olanzapine, risperidone, and haloperidol on plasma prolactin levels in patients with schizophrenia. Clin Ther 22:1085–1096, 2000

Deary I, Crawford J, Hepburn DA, et al: Severe hypoglycemia and intelligence in adult patients with insulin-treated diabetes. Diabetes 341–344, 1993

DeGroot LJ, Jameson JL, Burger, HG, et al: Endocrinology, 4th Edition. Philadelphia, PA, WB Saunders, 2001

de Groot M, Anderson RJ, Freedland KE, et al: Association of depression and diabetes complications: a meta-analysis. Psychosom Med 63:619–630, 2001

Dejgaard A, Gade A, Larsson H, et al: Evidence for diabetic encephalopathy. Diabet Med 8:162–167, 1991

Derogatis LR, Rose LI, Shulman LH, et al: Serum androgens and psychopathology in hirsute women. J Psychosom Obstet Gynaecol 14:269–282, 1993

Diabetes Control and Complications Trial Research Group: Weight gain associated with intensive therapy in the diabetes control and complications trial. Diabetes Care 11:567–573, 1988

Diabetes Control and Complications Trial Research Group: The effect of intensive treatment of diabetes on the development and progression of long-term complications in insulin-dependent diabetes mellitus. N Engl J Med 329:977–986, 1993

Diabetes Control and Complications Trial Research Group: Influence of intensive diabetes treatment on body weight and composition of adults with type 1 diabetes in the Diabetes Control and Complications Trial. Diabetes Care 24:1711–1721, 2001

Dimsdale JE, Ziegler MG: What do plasma and urinary measures of catecholamines tell us about human response to stressors? Circulation 83 (4 suppl):II36–II42, 1991

Dixon L, Weiden P, Delahanty J, et al: Prevalence and correlates of diabetes in national schizophrenia samples. Schizophr Bull 26:903–912, 2000

Eggers S, Kirchengast S: The polycystic ovary syndrome—a medical condition but also an important psychosocial problem. Coll Antropol 25:673–685, 2001

Fava GA: Affective disorders and endocrine disease. New insights from psychosomatic studies. Psychosomatics 35:341–353, 1994

Fava GA, Munari F, Pavan L, et al: Life events and depression. A replication. J Affect Disord 3:159–165, 1981

Fava M, Fava GA, Kellner R, et al: Depression and hostility in hyperprolactinemia. Prog Neuropsychopharmacol Biol Psychiatry 6:479–482, 1982

Fava M, Fava GA, Kellner R, et al: Psychosomatic aspects of hyperprolactinemia. Psychother Psychosom 40:257–262, 1983

Fukao A, Takamatsu J, Murakami Y, et al: The relationship of psychological factors to the prognosis of hyperthyroidism in antithyroid drug-treated patients with Graves' disease. Clin Endocrinol (Oxf) 58:550–555, 2003

Fukuda M, Hata A, Niwa S, et al: Plasma vanillylmandelic acid level as an index of psychological stress response in normal subjects. Psychiatry Res 63:7–16, 1996

Garay-Sevilla ME, Malacara JM, Gonzalez-Contreras E, et al: Perceived psychological stress in diabetes mellitus type 2. Rev Invest Clin 52:241–245, 2000

Garside S, Rosebush PI, Levinson AJ, et al: Late-onset adrenoleukodystrophy associated with long-standing psychiatric symptoms. J Clin Psychiatry 60:460–468, 1999

Gavard JA, Lustman PJ, Clouse RE: Prevalence of depression in adults with diabetes. An epidemiological evaluation. Diabetes Care 16:1167–1178, 1993

Geller WK, MacFadden W: Diabetes and atypical neuroleptics. Am J Psychiatry 160:388, 2003

Geringer ED: Affective disorders and diabetes mellitus, in Neuropsychological and Behavioral Aspects of Diabetes. Edited by Holmes CS. New York, Springer, 1990, pp 239–272

Goetsch VL, VanDorsten B, Pbert LA, et al: Acute effects of laboratory stress on blood glucose in noninsulin-dependent diabetes. Psychosom Med 55:492–496, 1993

Gokce O, Gokce C, Gunel S, et al: Pheochromocytoma presenting with headache, panic attacks and jaundice in a child. Headache 31:473–475, 1991

Gonzalez-Arriaza HL, Bostwick JM: Acute porphyrias: a case report and review. Am J Psychiatry 160:450–459, 2003

Green L, Feher M, Catalan J: Fears and phobias in people with diabetes. Diabetes Metab Res Rev 16:287–293, 2000

Gregg E, Brown A: Cognitive and physical disabilities and aging-related complications of diabetes. Clinical Diabetes 21:113–116, 2003

Gruen PG, Sachar EJ, Altman N, et al: Relation of plasma prolactin to clinical response in schizophrenic patients. Arch Gen Psychiatry 35:1222–1227, 1978

Haddad PM, Helleweil JS, Wieck A: Antipsychotic induced hyperprolactinaemia: a series of illustrative case reports. J Psychopharmacol 15:293–295, 2001

Haggerty JJ Jr, Prange AJ: Borderline hypothyroidism and depression. Annu Rev Med 46:37–46, 1995

Haggerty JJ Jr., Evans DL, Prange AJ Jr: Organic brain syndrome associated with marginal hypothyroidism. Am J Psychiatry 143:785–786, 1986

Haggerty JJ Jr, Garbutt JC, Evans DL, et al: Subclinical hypothyroidism: a review of neuropsychiatric aspects. Int J Psychiatry Med 20:193–208, 1990

Helz JW, Templeton B: Evidence of the role of psychosocial factors in diabetes mellitus: a review. Am J Psychiatry 147:1275–1282, 1990

Henderson DC: Diabetes mellitus and other metabolic disturbances induced by atypical antipsychotic agents. Curr Diab Rep 2:135–140, 2002

Henderson DC, Ettinger ER: Schizophrenia and diabetes. Int Rev Neurobiol 51:481–501, 2002

Hirsh D, Orr G, Kantarovich V, et al: Cushing's syndrome presenting as a schizophrenia-like psychotic state. Isr J Psychiatry Relat Sci 37:46–50, 2000

Holroyd S, Cohen MJ: Treatment of hyperprolactinemia in major depression. Am J Psychiatry 147:810, 1990

Holroyd S, Seward RL: Psychotropic drugs in acute intermittent porphyria. Clin Pharmacol Ther 66:323–325, 1999

Hudson J, Hudson M, Rothschild A, et al: Abnormal results of dexamethasone suppression test in non-depressed patients with diabetes mellitus. Arch Gen Psychiatry 41:1086–1089, 1984

Hyams JS, Leichtner AM, Breiner RG, et al: Pseudopheochromocytoma and cardiac arrest associated with phenylpropanolamine. JAMA 253:1609–1610, 1985

Ibrahim ZY, Carney MM: Safe use of haloperidol in acute intermittent porphyria. Ann Pharmacother 29:200, 1995

Jacobson AM: The psychological care of patients with insulin-dependent diabetes mellitus. N Engl J Med 334:1249–1253, 1996

Jacobson AM, Weinger K: Treating depression in diabetic patients: is there an alternative to medications? Ann Intern Med 129:656–657, 1998

Jacobson AM, de Groot M, Samson JA: The evaluation of two measures of quality of life in patients with type I and type II diabetes. Diabetes Care 17:267–274, 1994

Jacobson AM, Weinger K, Hill TC, et al: Brain functioning, cognition and psychiatric disorders in patients with type 1 diabetes. Diabetes 49 (suppl 1):537, 2000

Jacobson AM, Samson JA, Weinger K, et al: Diabetes, the brain, and behavior: is there a biological mechanism underlying the association between diabetes and depression? Int Rev Neurobiol 51:455–479, 2002

Jensovsky J, Ruzicka E, Spackova N, et al: Changes of event related potential and cognitive processes in patients with subclinical hypothyroidism after thyroxine treatment. Endocr Regul 36:115–122, 2002

Joffe RT, Levitt AJ: Major depression and subclinical (grade 2) hypothyroidism. Psychoneuroendocrinology 17:215–221, 1992

Joffe RT, Kutcher S, MacDonald C: Thyroid function and bipolar affective disorder. Psychiatry Res 25:117–121, 1988

Jones JM, Lawson ML, Daneman D, et al: Eating disorders in adolescent females with and without type 1 diabetes: cross sectional study. BMJ 320:1563–1566, 2000

Kahn CR, Weir GC: Joslin's Diabetes Mellitus. Malvern, PA: Lea & Febiger, 1994

Kailasam MT, Parmer RJ, Stone RA, et al: Factitious pheochromocytoma: novel mimicry by Valsalva maneuver and clues to diagnosis. Am J Hypertens 8:651–655, 1995

Kathmann N, Kuisle U, Bommer M, et al: Effects of elevated triiodothyronine levels on cognitive performance and mood in healthy subjects. Neuropsychobiology 29:136–142, 1994

Kathol RG, Delahunt JW, Hannah L: Transition from bipolar affective disorder to intermittent Cushing's syndrome: case report. J Clin Psychiatry 46:194–196, 1985

Kathol RG, Turner R, Delahunt J: Depression and anxiety associated with hyperthyroidism: response to antithyroid therapy. Psychosomatics 27:501–505, 1986

Kaufman FR, Epport K, Engilman R, et al: Neurocognitive functioning in children diagnosed with diabetes before age 10 years. J Diabetes Complications 13:31–38, 1999

Keiser HR: Surreptitious self-administration of epinephrine resulting in "pheochromocytoma." JAMA 266:1553–1555, 1991

Kelly WF, Kelly MJ, Faragher B: A prospective study of psychiatric and psychological aspects of Cushing's syndrome. Clin Endocrinol (Oxf) 45:715–720, 1996

Kemmer FW, Bisping R, Steingruber HJ, et al: Psychological stress and metabolic control in patients with type I diabetes mellitus. N Engl J Med 314:1078–1084, 1986

Kenardy J, Mensch M, Bowen K, et al: A comparison of eating behaviors in newly diagnosed NIDDM patients and case-matched control subjects. Diabetes Care 17:1197–1199, 1994

Kitzinger C, Willmott J: "The thief of womanhood": women's experience of polycystic ovarian syndrome. Soc Sci Med 54:349–361, 2002

Kooistra L, van de Meere JJ, Vulsma T, et al: Sustained attention problems in children with early treated congenital hypothyroidism. Acta Paediatr 85:425–429, 1996

Kornstein SG, Sholar EF, Gardner DG: Endocrine disorders, in Psychiatric Care of the Medical Patient, 2nd Edition. Edited by Stoudemire A, Fogel BS, Greenberg D. New York, Oxford University Press, 2000, pp 801–819

Koro CE, Fedder DO, L'Italien GJ, et al: Assessment of independent effect of olanzapine and risperidone on risk of diabetes among patients with schizophrenia: population based nested case-control study. BMJ 325:243, 2002

Korzets A, Floro S, Ori Y, et al: Clomipramine-induced pheochromocytoma crisis: a near fatal complication of a tricyclic antidepressant. J Clin Psychopharmacol 17:428–430, 1997

Kovacs M, Obrosky DS, Goldston D, et al: Major depressive disorder in youths with IDDM: a controlled prospective study of course and outcome. Diabetes Care 20:45–51, 1997

Kowdley KV, Coull BM, Orwoll ES: Cognitive impairment and intracranial calcification in chronic hypoparathyroidism. Am J Med Sci 317:273–277, 1999

Krentz AJ: UKPDS and beyond: into the next millennium. United Kingdom Prospective Diabetes Study. Diabetes Obes Metab 1:13–22, 1999

Krentz AJ, Mikhail S, Cantrell P, et al: Pseudophaeochromocytoma syndrome associated with clozapine. BMJ 322:1213, 2001

Kudrjavcev T: Neurologic complications of thyroid dysfunction. Adv Neurol 19:619–636, 1978

Kunkel EJS, Thompson TL, an Oyesanmi O: Hematologic disorders, in Psychiatric Care of the Medical Patient. Edited by Fogel BS, Greenberg D. Oxford, UK, Oxford University Press, 2000, pp 835–856

Kuruvilla A, Peedicayil J, Srikrishna G, et al: A study of serum prolactin levels in schizophrenia: comparison of males and females. Clin Exp Pharmacol Physiol 19:603–606, 1992

Lambert MT: Pheochromocytoma presenting as exacerbation of post traumatic stress disorder symptomology. Int J Psychiatry Med 22:265–268, 1992

Langan SJ, Deary IJ, Hepburn DA, et al: Cumulative cognitive impairment following recurrent severe hypoglycaemia in adult patients with insulin-treated diabetes mellitus. Diabetologia 34:337–344, 1991

Lefebvre H, Noblet C, Moore N, et al: Pseudo-phaeochromocytoma after multiple drug interactions involving the selective monoamine oxidase inhibitor selegiline. Clin Endocrinol (Oxf) 42:95–98, 1995

Le Feuvre CM, Isaacs AJ, Frank OS: Bromocriptine-induced psychosis in acromegaly. Br Med J (Clin Res Ed) 285:1315, 1982

Lenders JW, Pacak K, Walther MM, et al: Biochemical diagnosis of pheochromocytoma: which test is best? JAMA 287:1427–1434, 2002

Li JK, Yeung VT, Leung CM, et al: Clozapine: a mimicry of phaeochromocytoma. Aust N Z J Psychiatry 31:889–891, 1997

Lindenmayer JP, Czobor P, Volavka J, et al: Changes in glucose and cholesterol levels in patients with schizophrenia treated with typical or atypical antipsychotics. Am J Psychiatry 160:290–296, 2003

Lloyd CE, Dyer PH, Lancashire RJ, et al: Association between stress and glycemic control in adults with type 1 (insulin-dependent) diabetes. Diabetes Care 22:1278–1283, 1999

Loosen PT, Chambliss B, DeBold CR, et al: Psychiatric phenomenology in Cushing's disease. Pharmacopsychiatry 25:192–198, 1992

Lustman PJ, Griffith LS, Gavard JA, et al: Depression in adults with diabetes. Diabetes Care 15:1631–1639, 1992

Lustman PJ, Griffith LS, Clouse RE, et al: Effects of nortriptyline on depression and glycemic control in diabetes: results of a double-blind, placebo-controlled trial. Psychosom Med 59:241–250, 1997

Lustman PJ, Griffith LS, Freedland KE, et al: Cognitive behavior therapy for depression in type 2 diabetes mellitus: a randomized, controlled trial. Ann Intern Med 129:613–621, 1998

Lustman PJ, Anderson RJ, Freedland KE, et al: Depression and poor glycemic control: a meta-analytic review of the literature. Diabetes Care 23:934–942, 2000a

Lustman PJ, Freedland KE, Griffith LS, et al: Fluoxetine for depression in diabetes: a randomized double-blind placebo-controlled trial. Diabetes Care 23:618–623, 2000b

MacCrimmon DJ, Wallace JE, Goldberg WM, et al: Emotional disturbance and cognitive deficits in hyperthyroidism. Psychosom Med 41:331–340, 1979

Malouf R, Grimley EJ: The effect of vitamin B6 on cognition. Cochrane Database Syst Rev (4):CD004393, 2003

Marcus MD, Wing RR, Guare J, et al: Lifetime prevalence of major depression and its effect on treatment outcome in obese type II diabetic patients. Diabetes Care 15:253–255, 1992

Margo A: Acromegaly and depression. Br J Psychiatry 139:467–468, 1981

Matthews DR: The natural history of diabetes-related complications: the UKPDS experience. United Kingdom Prospective Diabetes Study. Diabetes Obes Metab 1 (suppl 2): S7–S13, 1999

Mayou R, Peveler R, Davies B, et al: Psychiatric morbidity in young adults with insulin-dependent diabetes mellitus. Psychol Med 21:639–645, 1991

Mazet P, Simon D, Luton J, et al: Syndrome de Cushing: Symptomatologie psychique et personalité de 50 malades. Nouv Presse Med 1988:2565–2570, 2003

McElroy SL, Frye MA, Suppes T, et al: Correlates of overweight and obesity in 644 patients with bipolar disorder. J Clin Psychiatry 63:207–213, 2002

McIntyre RS, Mancini DA, McCann S, et al: Valproate, bipolar disorder and polycystic ovarian syndrome. Bipolar Disord 5:28–35, 2003

Melmed S: Disorders of the anterior pituitary and hypothalamus, in Principles of Internal Medicine, 15th Edition. Edited by Braunwald E, Fauci AS, Kasper DL, et al. New York, McGraw-Hill, 2001, pp 2029–2051

Meltzer HY, Fang VS: The effect of neuroleptics on serum prolactin in schizophrenic patients. Arch Gen Psychiatry 33:279–286, 1976

Meltzer HY, Goode DJ, Schyve PM, et al: Effect of clozapine on human serum prolactin levels. Am J Psychiatry 136:1550–1555, 1979

Mennemeier M, Garner RD, Heilman KM: Memory, mood and measurement in hypothyroidism. J Clin Exp Neuropsychol 15:822–831, 1993

Merritt DF: Hyperprolactinemia and depression. JAMA 266:2004, 1991

Mitchell JE, Pomeroy C, Adson DE: Managing medical complications, in Handbook for Treatment of Eating Disorders. Editor by Garner D, Garfinkel P. New York, Guilford, 1997, pp 383–393

Moberg E, Kollind M, Lins PE, et al: Acute mental stress impairs insulin sensitivity in IDDM patients. Diabetologia 37:247–251, 1994

Mooy JM, de Vries H, Grootenhuis PA, et al: Major stressful life events in relation to prevalence of undetected type 2 diabetes: the Hoorn Study. Diabetes Care 23:197–201, 2000

Musselman DL, Betan E, Larsen H, et al: Relationship of depression to diabetes types 1 and 2: epidemiology, biology, and treatment. Biol Psychiatry 54:317–329, 2003

Newcomer JW, Haupt DW, Fucetola R, et al: Abnormalities in glucose regulation during antipsychotic treatment of schizophrenia. Arch Gen Psychiatry 59:337–345, 2002

New York Thyroid Center: Thyroid disorders—an overview. New York, 2003. Available at: http://cpmcnet.columbia.edu/dept/thyroid. Accessed August 2004.

Nolten WE: Androgen deficiency in the aging male: when to evaluate and when to treat. Curr Urol Rep 1:313–319, 2000

Northam EA, Anderson PJ, Werther GA, et al: Neuropsychological complications of IDDM in children 2 years after disease onset. Diabetes Care 21:379–384, 1998

Northam EA, Anderson PJ, Werther GA, et al: Predictors of change in the neuropsychological profiles of children with type 1 diabetes 2 years after disease onset. Diabetes Care 22:1438–1444, 1999

Northam EA, Anderson PJ, Jacobs R, et al: Neuropsychological profiles of children with type 1 diabetes 6 years after disease onset. Diabetes Care 24:1541–1546, 2001

O'Donovan C, Kusumakar V, Graves GR, et al: Menstrual abnormalities and polycystic ovary syndrome in women taking valproate for bipolar mood disorder. J Clin Psychiatry 63:322–330, 2002

Oseko F, Morikawa K, Motohashi T, et al: Effects of chronic sulpiride-induced hyperprolactinemia on menstrual cycles of normal women. Obstet Gynecol 72:267–271, 1988

Padero MC, Bhasin S, Friedman TC: Androgen supplementation in older women: too much hype, not enough data. J Am Geriatr Soc 50:1131–1140, 2002

Pantanetti P, Sonino N, Arnaldi G, et al: Self image and quality of life in acromegaly. Pituitary 5:17–19, 2002

Peterson CB, Mitchell JE: Psychosocial and pharmacological treatment of eating disorders: a review of research findings. J Clin Psychol 55:685–697, 1999

Polonsky WH, Anderson BJ, Lohrer PA, et al: Insulin omission in women with IDDM. Diabetes Care 17:1178–1185, 1994

Polonsky WH, Anderson BJ, Lohrer PA, et al: Assessment of diabetes-related distress. Diabetes Care 18:754–760, 1995

Popkin MK, Mackenzie TB: Psychiatric presentations of endocrine dysfunction, in Psychiatric Presentations of Medical Illness. Edited by Hall RCW. New York, Spectrum Publications, 1980, pp 139–156

Porterfield SP: Endocrine Physiology. St Louis, MO, Mosby-Year Book, 1997

Prokhorova M, Fritz S: Case of a 73-year-old man with dementia and a likely pheochromocytoma mistaken for an anxiety disorder. Psychosomatics 43:82, 2002

Rasgon NL, Carter MS, Elman S, et al: Common treatment of polycystic ovarian syndrome and major depressive disorder: case report and review. Curr Drug Targets Immune Endocr Metabol Disord 2:97–102, 2002

Rasgon NL, Rao RC, Hwang S, et al: Depression in women with polycystic ovary syndrome: clinical and biochemical correlates. J Affect Disord 74:299–304, 2003

Reavley A, Fisher AD, Owen D, et al: Psychological distress in patients with hyperprolactinaemia. Clin Endocrinol (Oxf) 47:343–348, 1997

Regan L, Gonsalves L, Tesar G. Acute intermittent porphyria. Psychosomatics 40:521–523, 1999

Regenold WT, Thapar RK, Marano C, et al: Increased prevalence of type 2 diabetes mellitus among psychiatric inpatients with bipolar I affective and schizoaffective disorders independent of psychotropic drug use. J Affect Disord 70:19–26, 2002

Reus VI: Behavioral disturbances associated with endocrine disorders. Annu Rev Med 37:205–214, 1986

Rovet JF, Ehrlich RM: The effect of hypoglycemic seizures on cognitive function in children with diabetes: A 7-year prospective study. J Pediatr 134:503–506, 1999

Rovet JF, Ehrlich RM, Hoppe M: Intellectual deficits associated with early onset of insulin-dependent diabetes mellitus in children. Diabetes Care 10:510–515, 1987

Ruzickova M, Slaney C, Garnham J, et al: Clinical features of bipolar disorder with and without comorbid diabetes mellitus. Can J Psychiatry 48:458–461, 2003

Ryan C, Vega A, Drash A: Cognitive deficits in adolescents who developed diabetes early in life. Pediatrics 75:921–927, 1985

Ryan MC, Thakore JH: Physical consequences of schizophrenia and its treatment: the metabolic syndrome. Life Sci 71:239–257, 2002

Rydall AC, Rodin GM, Olmsted MP, et al: Disordered eating behavior and microvascular complications in young women with insulin-dependent diabetes mellitus. N Engl J Med 336:1849–1854, 1997

Sachar EJ, Frantz AG, Altman N, et al: Growth hormone and prolactin in unipolar and bipolar depressed patients: responses to hypoglycemia and L-dopa. Am J Psychiatry 130:1362–1367, 1973

Santos AM, Nobre EL, Garcia e Costa, et al: Graves' disease and stress [in Portuguese]. Acta Med Port 15:423–427, 2002

Sapolsky RM: Glucocorticoids and hippocampal atrophy in neuropsychiatric disorders. Arch Gen Psychiatry 57:925–935, 2000

Sawka AM, Gerstein HC, Marriott MJ, et al: Does a combination regimen of thyroxine (T₄) and 3,5,3'-triiodothyronine improve depressive symptoms better than T₄ alone in patients with hypothyroidism? Results of a double-blind, randomized, controlled trial. J Clin Endocrinol Metab 88:4551–4555, 2003

Schulte DB: Paranoid-hallucinatory psychoses in acromegaly. Schweiz Arch Neurol Neurochir Psychiatr 118:357–377, 1976

Schweizer E, Winokur A, Rickels K: Insulin-induced hypoglycemia and panic attacks. Am J Psychiatry 143:654–655, 1986

Seelen MA, de Meijer PH, Meinders AE: Serotonin reuptake inhibitor unmasks a pheochromocytoma. Ann Intern Med 126:333, 1997

Seidman SN, Rabkin JG: Testosterone replacement therapy for hypogonadal men with SSRI-refractory depression. J Affect Disord 48:157–161, 1998

Sernyak MJ, Leslie DL, Alarcon RD, et al: Association of diabetes mellitus with use of atypical neuroleptics in the treatment of schizophrenia. Am J Psychiatry 159:561–566, 2002

Sheps SG, Jiang NS, Klee GG, et al: Recent developments in the diagnosis and treatment of pheochromocytoma. Mayo Clin Proc 65:88–95, 1990

Shores MM, Sloan KL, Matsumoto AM, et al: Increased incidence of diagnosed depressive illness in hypogonadal older men. Arch Gen Psychiatry 61:162–7, 2004

Small JG, Hirsch SR, Arvanitis LA, et al: Quetiapine in patients with schizophrenia. A high- and low-dose double-blind comparison with placebo. Seroquel Study Group. Arch Gen Psychiatry 54:549–557, 1997

Sonino N: From the lesson of Harvey Cushing to current knowledge: psychosocial aspects of endocrine disease. Psychother Psychosom 66:113–116, 1997

Sonino N, Fava GA: Psychosomatic aspects of Cushing's disease. Psychother Psychosom 67:140–146, 1998

Sonino N, Fava GA: Psychiatric disorders associated with Cushing's syndrome. Epidemiology, pathophysiology and treatment. CNS Drugs 15:361–373, 2001

Sonino N, Fava GA, Mani E, et al: Quality of life of hirsute women. Postgrad Med J 69:186–189, 1993

Sonino N, Fava GA, Raffi AR, et al: Clinical correlates of major depression in Cushing's disease. Psychopathology 31:302–306, 1998

Spitzer D, Bongartz D, Ittel TH, et al: Simulation of a pheochromocytoma—Munchausen syndrome. Eur J Med Res 3:549–553, 1998

Starkman MN, Schteingart DE: Neuropsychiatric manifestations of patients with Cushing's syndrome. Relationship to cortisol and adrenocorticotropic hormone levels. Arch Intern Med 141:215–219, 1981

Starkman MN, Schteingart DE, Schork MA: Depressed mood and other psychiatric manifestations of Cushing's syndrome: relationship to hormone levels. Psychosom Med 43:3–18, 1981

Starkman MN, Giordani B, Gebarski SS, et al: Decrease in cortisol reverses human hippocampal atrophy following treatment of Cushing's disease. Biol Psychiatry 46:1595–1602, 1999

Starkman MN, Giordani B, Berent S, et al: Elevated cortisol levels in Cushing's disease are associated with cognitive decrements. Psychosom Med 63:985–993, 2001

Stern RA, Robinson B, Thorner AR, et al: A Survey study of neuropsychiatric complaints in patients with Graves' disease. J Neuropsychiatry Clin Neurosci 8:181, 1996

Stern TA, Cremens CM: Factitious pheochromocytoma. Psychosomatics 39:283–287, 1998

Sternbach H: Age-associated testosterone decline in men: clinical issues for psychiatry. Am J Psychiatry 155:1310–1318, 1998

Striegel-Moore RH, Wilfley DE, Pike KM, et al: Recurrent binge eating in black American women. Arch Fam Med 9:83–87, 2000

Swanson DW, Stipes AL: Psychiatric aspects of Klinefelter's syndrome. Am J Psychiatry 126:82–90, 1969

Tadami S, Murata A, Wakabayashi T, et al: A case of Cushing's disease: hallucinatory paranoid state preceding physical symptoms. Seishin Shinkeigaku Zasshi 96:461–468, 1994

Talbot F, Nouwen A: A review of the relationship between depression and diabetes in adults: is there a link? Diabetes Care 23:1556–1562, 2000

Thienhaus OJ, Hartford JT: Depression in hyperprolactinemia. Psychosomatics 27:663–664, 1986

Thompson CJ, Cummings JF, Chalmers J, et al: How have patients reacted to the implications of the DCCT? Diabetes Care 19:876–879, 1996

Tiemeier H, Hofman A, Kiliaan AJ, et al: Vitamin E and depressive symptoms are not related. The Rotterdam Study. J Affect Disord 72:79–83, 2002

Tollefson GD, Kuntz AJ: Review of recent clinical studies with olanzapine. Br J Psychiatry 174 (suppl 37) 30–35, 1999

Trzepacz PT, McCue M, Klein I, et al: A psychiatric and neuropsychological study of patients with untreated Graves' disease. Gen Hosp Psychiatry 10:49–55, 1988a

Trzepacz PT, McCue M, Klein I, et al: Psychiatric and neuropsychological response to propranolol in Graves' disease. Biol Psychiatry 23:678–688, 1988b

Trzepacz PT, Klein I, Roberts M, et al: Graves' disease: an analysis of thyroid hormone levels and hyperthyroid signs and symptoms. Am J Med 87:558–561, 1989

Turner TH, Cookson JC, Wass JA, et al: Psychotic reactions during treatment of pituitary tumours with dopamine agonists. Br Med J (Clin Res Ed) 289:1101–1103, 1984

Uhde TW, Vittone BJ, Post RM: Glucose tolerance testing in panic disorder. Am J Psychiatry 141:1461–1463, 1984

UK Prospective Diabetes Study (UKPDS) Group: Effect of intensive blood-glucose control with metformin on complications in overweight patients with type 2 diabetes (UKPDS 34). Lancet 352:854–865, 1998a

UK Prospective Diabetes Study (UKPDS) Group: Intensive blood-glucose control with sulphonylureas or insulin compared with conventional treatment and risk of complications in patients with type 2 diabetes (UKPDS 33). Lancet 352:837–853, 1998b

Wales JK: Does psychological stress cause diabetes? Diabet Med 12:109–112, 1995

Walsh BT, Devlin MJ: Pharmacotherapy of bulimia nervosa and binge eating disorder. Addict Behav 20:757–764, 1995

Walsh JP, Shiels L, Lim EM, et al: Combined thyroxine/liothyronine treatment does not improve well-being, quality of life, or cognitive function compared to thyroxine alone: a randomized controlled trial in patients with primary hypothyroidism. J Clin Endocrinol Metab 88:4543–4550, 2003

Wang C, Swedloff R, Iranmanesh A, et al: Transdermal testosterone gel improves sexual function, mood, muscle strength, and body composition parameters in hypogonadal men. Testosterone Gel Study Group. J Clin Endocrinol Metab 2839–2853, 2000

Welch GW, Jacobson AM, Polonsky WH: The problem areas in diabetes scale. An evaluation of its clinical utility. Diabetes Care 20:760–766, 1997

Welch G, Weinger K, Anderson B, et al: Responsiveness of the Problem Areas in Diabetes (PAID) questionnaire. Diabet Med 20:69–72, 2003

Wieck A, Haddad PM: Antipsychotic-induced hyperprolactinaemia in women: pathophysiology, severity and consequences. Selective literature review. Br J Psychiatry 182:199–204, 2003

Wirshing DA, Pierre JM, Erhart SM, et al: Understanding the new and evolving profile of adverse drug effects in schizophrenia. Psychiatr Clin North Am 26:165–190, 2003

Yoshiuchi K, Kumano H, Nomura S, et al: Stressful life events and smoking were associated with Graves' disease in women, but not in men. Psychosom Med 60:182–185, 1998

24 Oncology

Mary Jane Massie, M.D.
Donna B. Greenberg, M.D.

CANCER IS A major public health problem in the United States and other developed nations. In 2004, more than 1.4 million new cases of cancer will be diagnosed and more than one-half million people will die of cancer in the United States (Jemal et al. 2004). Although one in four deaths is now caused by cancer, there has been a decline in death rates from many cancers, including those of the prostate, breast, colon, and rectum. However, as the death rate decreases and the population ages, there will be more people living with cancer, with an anticipated doubling from 1.3 million to 2.6 million between the years 2000 and 2050. Although only modest cancer-specific survival differences are evident for blacks and whites receiving comparable treatment for similar-stage cancer, African Americans still carry a higher burden because they are often diagnosed at a later stage and have poorer survival within each stage. Differences in access to treatment, stage at presentation, and mortality from other diseases represent the primary targets of research and interventions designed to reduce disparities in cancer outcomes (Bach et al. 2002).

In this chapter, we review psychological factors in cancer risk and progression, the most frequently encountered psychiatric disorders (depression, anxiety, and delirium) in adult cancer patients, psychiatric issues in specific cancers, psychiatric aspects of cancer treatments, psychiatric interventions in cancer patients, survivor issues, and cancer patients' use of complementary and alternative medicine treatments. See Chapter 34, "Pediatrics," for additional coverage of cancer in children.

Psychological Factors Affecting Cancer Risk and Progression

Although many people believe that psychological factors play a major role in cancer onset and progression, scientific evidence has not yet clarified these relationships, and the role of psychological factors remains controversial (Levenson and McDonald 2002).

The most active area has been the effort to link depression with the onset and course of cancer. Depressive symptoms were associated with a higher-than-normal frequency of cancer and twice as high a risk for death from cancer in an early large epidemiological study (Persky et al. 1987; Shekelle et al. 1981). Later epidemiological studies and a meta-analysis did not find statistically or clinically significant associations (Gallo et al. 2000; McGee et al. 1994; Vogt et al. 1994).

Others have wondered whether emotional states affect outcome in cancer patients. Emotional distress may predict lower survival with lung cancer (Faller et al. 1999), as may anger in metastatic melanoma patients (Butow et al. 1999). Other studies have found positive, negative, or mixed associations between depression and mortality in cancer patients (Garssen and Goodkin 1999; Watson et al. 1999). Depression may directly affect the course of illness in patients with cancer because it results in poorer pain control (Glover et al. 1995), poorer compliance (Ayres et al. 1994), and less desire for life-sustaining therapy (Lee and Ganzini 1992).

Dr. Massie gratefully acknowledges Theresa Carpenter's and Alex Pisani's assistance in the preparation of this chapter and the continued generous support of her work by William E. Pelton and Sylvia Rosenberg.

The finding that bereavement is associated with a decrement in immune function rekindled an interest in whether bereavement affects cancer risk (Schleifer et al. 1983), but neither cancer onset nor progression has been clearly shown to be influenced by bereavement (Helsing and Szklo 1981; Levav et al. 2000; McKenna et al. 1999).

Cancer patients' degree of emotional expressiveness and its possible effect on prognosis have been the subject of a large body of literature. Early descriptive case reports noted shorter survival in patients with a depressed, resigning attitude compared with patients who were able to express more negative emotions, such as anger. Using a variety of conceptualizations of the "expressive" versus "repressive" dichotomy in various cancer types, several investigators found reduced cancer risks in more expressive subjects (G.A. Kune et al. 1991; Temoshok et al. 1985). Other clinical and epidemiological studies have not supported such an influence in cancer risk or in cancer mortality (Buddeberg et al. 1991; Cassileth et al. 1985; Ragland et al. 1987; Shekelle et al. 1981). In separate studies, investigators found that patients with breast cancer (Greer et al. 1979) and those with leukemia (Tschushke et al. 2001) who had a "fighting spirit" had longer survival than those with stoic acceptance or those who were hopeless or helpless, but other outcome studies in cancer patients found no such association (Watson et al. 1999).

Social relations and social support are complex phenomena. How they affect cancer patients may vary with cancer site and extent of disease (Helgeson and Cohen 1996). Some research has tentatively linked life stressors with cancer recurrence or progression, although not unequivocally (Ramirez et al. 1989). More frequent stressful life events preceding the onset of cervical, pancreatic, gastric, lung, colorectal, and breast cancer have been shown in a number of human studies (Geyer 1991; S. Kune et al. 1991). Many other studies have failed to find any association between preceding stressful life events and cancer onset, relapse, or progression (Giraldi et al. 1997; Maunsell et al. 2001). Occupational stress might increase the risk of lung cancer (Jahn et al. 1995; Lynge and Anderson 1997) and colorectal cancer (Courtney et al. 1993).

Psychiatric Disorders in Cancer Patients

A person's ability to manage a cancer diagnosis and treatment commonly changes over the course of the illness and depends on medical, psychological, and social factors: the disease itself (i.e., site, symptoms, clinical course, prognosis, type of treatments required); prior level of adjustment; the threat that cancer poses to attaining age-appropriate developmental tasks and goals (i.e., adolescence, career, family, retirement); cultural, spiritual, and religious attitudes; the presence of emotionally supportive persons; the potential for physical and psychological rehabilitation; the patient's own personality and coping style; and prior experience with loss.

Depression

Depression has received the most attention in cancer patients and has been challenging to study because symptoms span the spectrum from sadness to major affective disorder, and mood change is difficult to evaluate when a patient experiences repeated threats to life, cancer treatments, fatigue, and pain. In other words, depressive symptoms may represent a normal reaction, a psychiatric disorder, or a somatic consequence of cancer or its treatment. Many depressed patients adhere poorly to treatment schedules and other recommendations; some may have reduced chance of survival (Faller and Bülzebruck 2002; Watson et al. 1999).

Cancer, exclusive of site, is associated with a rate of depression that is higher than that in the general population and at least as high as the rate associated with other serious medical illnesses (Massie 2004). Depression has been studied in patients with cancer using a range of assessment methods (Trask 2004), including self-report, brief screening instruments, and structured clinical interviews. In general, the more narrowly the term is defined, the lower the prevalence of depression that is reported. The clinical rule of thumb is that 25% of cancer patients are likely depressed enough at some point in the course of disease to warrant evaluation and treatment. Many research groups have assessed depression in cancer patients, with widely variable reported prevalence (major depression, 0%–38%; depression spectrum syndromes, 0%–58%) in more than 150 studies (Massie 2004). Cancer types highly associated with depression include oropharyngeal (22%–57%), pancreatic (33%–50%), breast (1.5%–46%), and lung (11%–44%). The prevalence of depression is reported to be less in patients with other cancers, such as colon cancer (13%–25%), gynecological cancer (12%–23%), and lymphoma (8%–19%) (Massie 2004). It is difficult to compare the prevalences reported in different studies because each study uses different definitions of depression, and because the time since diagnosis and the cancer type, stage, and treatments often vary. Whether high rates of depression associated with some cancers result from the pathophysiological effect of the tumor (e.g., pancreatic cancer) or from treatment effects (e.g., steroids) is not clear.

Depression in cancer patients results from 1) stress related to the cancer diagnosis and treatment; 2) medications; 3) underlying neurological or medical problems, such as nutritional deficiencies (e.g., folate, B_{12}), endocrine disturbances (e.g., thyroid abnormalities, adrenal insufficiency), brain metastases, and leptomeningeal disease; or 4) recurrence of a preexisting affective disorder. Whereas the diagnosis of depression in physically healthy patients depends heavily on the somatic symptoms of anorexia, fatigue, and weight loss, these indicators are of less value in the assessment of a cancer patient, because they are common to both cancer and depression. Clinical diagnosis rests on psychological symptoms: social withdrawal; anhedonia; dysphoric mood; feelings of hopelessness, helplessness, worthlessness, or guilt; poor self-esteem; or suicidality. Cancer patients likely at higher risk for depression are those in poor physical condition and in the advanced stages of illness who have inadequately controlled pain, a history of depression, or other significant life stresses or losses (Massie and Popkin 1998; Newport and Nemeroff 1998). An increased risk has also been associated with pancreatic, head and neck, and lung cancers (Ginsberg et al. 1995; Holland et al. 1986).

During acute anticancer treatment, the diagnosis of depression is often missed. Oncologists often underestimate the level of depressive symptoms and do not prescribe adequate treatment or assess the response (Passik et al. 1998). They tend to recognize low mood, pain, and anxiety, but they do not ask about suicidal ideation. When physicians are uncertain of the correct psychiatric treatment or its benefit, they are less apt to ask, and patients, not wanting to appear weak or to risk abandonment, are less apt to reveal their discouragement to oncologists (Greenberg 2004). Not infrequently, the psychiatric consultant is asked to evaluate a "depressed" cancer patient who really has a hypoactive delirium, poorly controlled pain, fatigue, or anorexia–cachexia syndrome.

Cancer-Related Suicide

Although few cancer patients commit suicide, they may be at a somewhat greater risk than the general population (Fox et al. 1982; Louhivuori and Hakama 1979; Massie and Popkin 1998). Passive suicidal thoughts are relatively common as patients battle a life-threatening illness, and these thoughts provide a sense of control in those overwhelmed by suffering, uncertainty, and helplessness. Both patients and doctors struggle to understand the degree to which noncompliance with or refusal of treatment represents a deliberate decision to end life (Nuland 1994).

An increased risk of suicide in cancer patients is associated with male gender, advanced stage of disease, poor prognosis, delirium with poor impulse control, inadequately controlled pain, depression, history of psychiatric illness, current or previous alcohol or substance abuse, previous suicide attempts, physical and emotional exhaustion, social isolation, and extreme need for control. Recognition of suicidal thoughts should lead to emergent psychiatric evaluation with frank discussion (see also Chapter 9, "Depression").

Anxiety

Anxiety is a normal response to threat, uncertainty, and loss of control. It is common as patients face the existential plight of cancer and the specific threats of deformity, abandonment, pain, or death. The diagnosis and treatment of cancer is stressful and often traumatic. After the initial shock and disbelief of diagnosis, patients typically feel anxious and irritable. They may experience anorexia, insomnia, and difficulty with concentration because they are distracted by intrusive thoughts about their prognosis. Often this acute anxiety dissipates as a treatment plan is established and prognosis clarified. Anxiety is common at crisis points such as the start of a new treatment or the diagnosis of recurrence or illness progression, but it also occurs before routine follow-up visits without evidence of disease. Cancer often changes body functions and appearance and disrupts personal relationships and social roles (Noyes et al. 1998). In a recent cross-sectional observational study of 178 patients with cancer, almost half had significant anxiety, but the rate of anxiety disorder and its subtypes was 18%, comparable to that in the normal population. Two cases were attributed to drugs like interferon, but none of the others were attributed to medical variables (Stark et al. 2002).

Specific syndromes of anxiety can prevent the patient from accepting appropriate medical treatment. Patients with claustrophobia have difficulty tolerating magnetic resonance imaging (MRI) scans, radiation therapy, or placement in isolation because of neutropenia. Needle phobia and other health-related phobias (see Chapter 12, "Anxiety Disorders") may interfere with chemotherapy and surgery. Radiation phobia makes some patients reluctant to accept radiation treatment. Anticipatory anxiety may prevent patients from following up with diagnostic or treatment visits.

In recent years, improved antiemetic treatments have reduced the number of patients who vomit with chemotherapy, but nausea is still common (Hickok et al. 2003). The nausea and vomiting with treatment are aversive stimuli that may condition anxious responses to reminders of treatment. Younger patients, patients with more emetic treatments, and those with trait anxiety are more prone to conditioning (Andrykowski 1990). Survivors of leukemia who had anticipatory nausea and vomiting during treatment are more apt to have a visceral reaction to reminders of treatment (Greenberg et al. 1997).

Evaluation of acute anxiety in cancer patients includes consideration of conditions that mimic anxiety disorders. Antiemetic phenothiazines (prochlorperazine, perphenazine, promethazine) or metoclopramide, especially when given intravenously, may cause restlessness or severe akathisia. The inner feeling of restlessness is frequently misdiagnosed as anxiety. The abrupt onset of anxiety and dyspnea may signal pulmonary emboli, which are common among cancer patients. The experience of severe, intermittent, or uncontrolled pain is associated with acute and chronic anxiety, and the patient's confidence that he or she has the analgesics to control pain alleviates anxiety. Furthermore, anxiety amplifies pain, and the momentum behind additional requests for analgesia may be anxiety rather than somatic pain (see also Chapter 12, "Anxiety Disorders").

Reminders of the traumas of cancer can provoke anxiety and physiological arousal. A sample of women 2 years after diagnosis of stages I to III breast cancer had heightened arousal (as measured by skin conductance, heart rate, and facial muscle electrical activity) during mental imagery of the traumatic event as they listened to their own narrative of their two most stressful experiences associated with breast cancer. Breast-specific posttraumatic stress symptoms were noted in 24%, but only 9% reported full posttraumatic stress disorder (PTSD). Those with the strongest responses had current PTSD, and the majority had comorbid major depressive disorder (Pitman et al. 2001).

The prevalence of cancer-related posttraumatic stress disorder (PTSD) in women treated for breast cancer varies from 3% to 10% (Green et al. 1998). Younger age, less education, and lower income are associated with more PTSD symptoms (Cordova et al. 1995) as well as more advanced disease and lengthier hospitalizations (Jacobsen et al. 1998). Medical sequelae of cancer treatment (e.g., paresthesias because of nerve injury) may act as a trigger for memories of treatment (Kornblith et al. 2004).

Treatment of Anxiety Disorders

The management of anxiety symptoms begins with the provision of emotional support and information for the patient and family. Patients are relieved to have their anxiety recognized, to understand the interplay of psychological and somatic symptoms, and to find that that severe distress is treatable.

Many patients are helped through behavioral techniques such as relaxation, distraction, and cognitive reframing (Fawzy et al. 1995). In addition to behavioral interventions, individual psychotherapy and group interventions can reduce anxiety in cancer patients. A group intervention that included education, emotional support, and behavioral training reduced tension and phobias in cancer patients (Spiegel et al. 1989).

Phobias related to medical procedures are common in children with cancer (and also some adults). Although careful preparation of children in advance of painful procedures (e.g., role-playing) may reduce anxiety, specific behavioral interventions, including relaxation training and distraction, may be indicated for some symptoms (Redd 1989). Self-hypnosis is a highly effective treatment for both generalized anxiety and specific phobias in children and adolescents.

Mania

In cancer patients, corticosteroid medications are the most common reason for hypomania or mania. Steroids are commonly given as a component of chemotherapy for lymphoma, as an antiemetic or to prevent hypersensitivity reactions with chemotherapy, or to prevent edema in the CNS during radiation therapy. Psychotic mania secondary to steroids may be misdiagnosed as delirium. Interferon has also been associated with mania and mixed affective syndromes (Greenberg et al. 2000). Diencephalic tumors are a rare cause of secondary mania (see also Chapter 11, "Mania, Catatonia, and Psychosis").

Delirium

Delirium is common in cancer as a result of metabolic sequelae of the disease and treatment, medications, metastatic tumors in the brain, and, more rarely, paraneoplastic syndromes. The prevalence of delirium in cancer patients has been reported as 5%–30% and is substantially higher (40%–85%) in terminal stages of illness (Fleishman et al. 1993). Delirium is associated with greater morbidity and mortality in patients and greater distress in patients, their families, and caregivers.

Early symptoms of delirium are often unrecognized or misdiagnosed by medical or nursing staff as depression or anxiety. Early recognition of delirium is essential because the etiology may be a treatable complication of cancer. In addition to the general causes of delirium (see Chapter 6, "Delirium"), there are particular considerations in cancer patients. Primary brain tumor and brain metastases (especially common with lung and breast cancer) can cause delirium. Immunosuppressed cancer patients, especially those with hematological malignancies, are at high risk for opportunistic infection. Head and neck cancer patients undergoing surgery are at high risk for delirium because of their older age and high prevalence of alcohol abuse and withdrawal. Several antineoplastic agents (e.g., cytarabine, methotrexate, ifosfamide, asparaginase, procarbazine, and fluorouracil) and immunotherapeutic agents (e.g., interferon and interleukins) can cause delirium and other changes in mental status (Table 24–1) (Brown and Stoudemire 1998). Some antibiotics (e.g., quinolones) and antifungals (e.g., amphotericin B), as well as opioids, anticholinergics, and nutritional deficiencies, can cause delirium. Hypercalcemia causes delirium in patients with bone metastases or ectopic hormone production. Hyperviscosity syndrome with lymphoma, Waldenström's macroglobulinemia, and myeloma are unusual causes of delirium. There are also rare autoimmune encephalopathies resulting from paraneoplastic syndromes (Lieberman and Schold 2002) that manifest with cognitive impairment and delirium. Limbic encephalopathy is a specific type of autoimmune encephalopathy (see Chapter 32, "Neurology and Neurosurgery") that presents with impaired memory, fluctuating mood, and seizures (Kung et al. 2002). (See Chapter 6, "Delirium," for the general management of delirium and Chapter 40, "Palliative Care," for terminal delirium.)

Pain and Psychiatric Symptoms in Cancer Patients

Depression and anxiety are very common in cancer patients suffering from severe pain. In one early study, 39% of patients with a psychiatric diagnosis (often depression) experienced significant pain, whereas only 19% of patients with no psychiatric diagnosis had significant pain (Derogatis et al. 1983). The psychiatric symptoms of patients who are in significant pain should initially be considered a consequence of uncontrolled pain. Acute anxiety, depression with despair (especially when the patient believes the pain means disease progression), agitation, irritability, lack of cooperation, anger, and insomnia all may accompany pain. Such symptoms should not be diagnosed as a psychiatric disorder unless they persist after pain is adequately controlled. Undertreatment of pain is a major problem in both adult and pediatric cancer patients. Long-term psychiatric sequelae of cancer are less frequent in children whose pain is well treated. There is no evidence of increased risk of abuse or addiction in cancer patients receiving opioids. In fact, many patients associate the narcotics with the unpleasant aspects of the illness and avoid them after their recovery. (The issues in pain management are discussed in full in Chapter 36, "Pain.")

TABLE 24–1. Neuropsychiatric side effects of common chemotherapeutic agents

Hormones
  Corticosteroids
    Mild to severe insomnia, hyperactivity, anxiety, depression, psychosis with prominent affective and manic-like features
  Tamoxifen
    Sleep disorder, irritability

Biologicals
  Cytokines
    Encephalopathy
  Interferon
    Depression, mania, psychosis
    Delirium, akathisia
  Interleukin-2
    Dysphoria, delirium, psychosis

Chemotherapy agents
  L-Asparaginase
    Somnolence, lethargy, delirium
  Cisplatin
    Encephalopathy (rare), sensory neuropathy
  Cytarabine
    Delirium
    Leukoencephalopathy: syndrome of personality change, drowsiness, dementia, psychomotor retardation, ataxia
  5-Fluorouracil
    Fatigue, rare seizure or confusion, cerebellar syndrome
  Gemcitabine
    Fatigue
  Ifosfamide
    Lethargy, seizures, drunkenness, cerebellar signs, delirium, hallucinations
  Methotrexate
    Intrathecal regimens can cause leukoencephalopathy (acute and delayed forms)
    High dose can cause transient delirium
  Procarbazine
    Somnolence, depression, delirium, psychosis
  Taxanes
    Sensory neuropathy, fatigue
  Thalidomide
    Fatigue
  Vincristine, vinblastine, vinorelbine
    Depression, fatigue, encephalopathy

Cancer-Related Fatigue

Fatigue is a sign of illness in patients who have certain tumors (e.g., lymphoma) or extensive liver metastases. Both chemotherapy and radiation treatment are associated with predictable periods of fatigue following treatment. Causes of cancer-related fatigue are listed in Table 24–2. Psychia-

TABLE 24–2. Causes of cancer-related fatigue

Cancer treatment
    Interferon
    Chemotherapy
    Irradiation
Pain
Anemia
Nutritional deficits
Hormonal imbalance
    Thyroid
    Estrogen
    Androgens
Immune response
Cytokine release
Drug effects
    Opioids
    Sedatives
Psychiatric disorders
    Sleep disruption
    Depression

TABLE 24–3. Causes of cancer anorexia–cachexia syndrome

Gastrointestinal dysfunction
    Mechanical obstruction from tumors of mouth, esophagus, stomach, gastrointestinal tract
    Extrinsic pressure from metastatic disease
Anticancer treatment
    Change in food smell or taste (food aversions): dysosmia, dysgensia
    Nausea, vomiting, mucositis
Altered (hyper) metabolism
    Carbohydrate
    Lipid
    Protein
Host response to cancer
    Cytokine production
        Tumor necrosis factor, interleukin-1, interleukin-6, interferon
Psychological
    Depression
    Anxiety
    Preexisting eating disorder
    Conditioned responses

trists play an important role in the treatment of depression and sleep disorders, and these common conditions may be more important as a cause of fatigue than the cancer or its treatment. Hypnotics and other psychotropic drugs may also contribute to fatigue. Patients who have persistent fatigue with progressive disease or cancer treatment may respond well to low-dose psychostimulants and do not increase the dose over time.

Anorexia–Cachexia Syndrome

Cachexia in cancer patients is debilitating and life-threatening. It is associated with anorexia, fat and muscle wasting, decreased quality of life, and psychological distress. The causes of cachexia are gastrointestinal dysfunction, altered metabolism and host response to cancer (cytokine production), hormone production by tumors, and anticancer treatments (Inui 2002) (see Table 24–3).

Anorexia may be the result of depression or anxiety. Preexisting eating disorders complicate nutritional management in cancer patients. Treatments of anorexia and cachexia in cancer patients are shown in Table 24–4.

Psychiatric Issues in Specific Cancers

Prostate Cancer

The prostate is the most common site of cancer in males in the United States, with more than 230,000 new cases diagnosed in 2004. Men over 65 account for 80% of these cancers (Jemal et al. 2004). In general, although the reaction of men with prostate cancer depends on age, marital status, recent losses, and social support, older men are less likely to seek or accept intervention for emotional distress.

The recent increased incidence of prostate cancer directly relates to improved detection with the serum prostate specific antigen test (PSA). The PSA has limitations as a broad screening tool (Garnick 1993) because of its lack of sensitivity and specificity. False-positive results can be seen with prostatitis and benign prostatic hypertrophy, as well as with manipulation of the prostate. Distress surrounding each PSA test has been dubbed "PSA anxiety" (Roth and Passik 1996) and may be even greater in spouses than in patients (Kornblith et al. 1994).

It is difficult to distinguish indolent forms of prostate cancer that will not impact the quality or quantity of a patient's survival from more lethal varieties. It is also difficult to assess the relative risk of treatment complications that may significantly impair quality of life. Controversy among clinicians about primary treatment (surgery vs. radiation) or "watchful waiting" creates uncertainty and makes treatment decisions difficult. Counseling assists patients with these choices, based on the extent of disease, age of patient, life expectancy, expense, and geography (Harlan et al. 1995), and the choices are often based on the potential side effects (e.g., impotence, urinary incon-

TABLE 24–4. Treatment of cancer anorexia–cachexia syndrome

Hypercaloric feeding (enteral and parenteral nutrition)
  Does not increase skeletal muscle mass
  Useful for nutritional support for patients with potentially therapy responsive cancer

Drugs
  Amino acids; ATP
  Corticosteroids
      Increase sense of well-being
      Useful adjunct for pain control
      Decrease nausea
      May cause osteoporosis, muscle weakness, immunosuppression, delirium
      No demonstrated effects on body weight
  Progestational
      Megestrol acetate
      • Increases body weight (fat) gain
      • Increases appetite and sense of well-being
      • Can cause thromboembolic phenomena, edema, hyperglycemia, hypertension, adrenal insufficiency (abrupt discontinuation)
      Medroxyprogesterone acetate
      • Increases appetite and body weight
      • Available in depot and oral suspension
  Antiserotonergic
      Cyproheptadine
      • Increases appetite; does not prevent weight loss
      Ondansetron
      • Does not prevent weight loss
  Prokinetic
      Metoclopramide
      • Treatment for chemotherapy-induced emesis
      • May relieve anorexia
      Cannabinoids
      • Dronabinol (Marinol)
      • May improve mood and appetite
      • Minimally effective in increasing body weight in cancer
      • Can cause euphoria, dizziness
  Emerging drugs
      Melatonin, thalidomide
      Nonsteroidal anti-inflammatory drugs (prostaglandin inhibitors)
      Testosterone

Educational and behavioral approaches

tinence, and bowel problems). In general, men undergoing surgery, older men, and men with less serious disease have less mental distress (Litwin et al. 2002).

A model of an effective psychiatric liaison to a genitourinary clinic at a cancer center, which includes a brief meeting of the patient with a psychiatrist at the initial clinic visit, has been described (Roth et al. 2000). Patients are screened for coping mechanisms; depressed mood; anxiety; and disturbances in concentration, sleep, daily functioning, and family life. They are introduced to the concept of a multidisciplinary team approach including the psychiatrist. Roth et al. (1998) found that a third of men screened on initial visit had high levels of anxiety, but a large proportion did not want further psychiatric evaluation or treatment. Men who are reluctant to participate in individual therapy may agree to participate in psycho-educational or support groups and use other sources of information about the illness and treatment options (e.g., interactive video program).

In prostate cancer patients, the most important risk factor for depression is a past history of depression (Ingram et al. 2003; Pirl et al. 2002). Androgen deprivation therapy (ADT) by orchiectomy or chronic administration of gonadotropin-releasing hormone agonists may cause hot flashes, loss of sexual interest, fatigue, anemia, decreased muscle mass, and osteoporosis. Men with prostate cancer who received ADT reported poorer quality of life compared with men who underwent any prostate cancer treatment without hormonal treatment (Wei et al. 2002).

Breast Cancer

Breast cancer is the most common cancer in women, second only to lung cancer in cancer deaths in women. More than 215,000 women in the United States will be diagnosed with breast cancer in 2004, and more than 40,000 women will die (Jemal et al. 2004). The number of women diagnosed with breast cancer has increased as a result of mammography screening, and the modest improvement in the death rate is probably attributable to successful treatment of cancers diagnosed at an early stage. More than 85% of women diagnosed with stage I (small cancers confined to the breast) cancers will be alive 5 years later. Survival drops dramatically when cancers are diagnosed at later stages.

Although only 5% of breast cancer occurs in women younger than 40 years, a disproportionately large number of younger women seek psychiatric consultation to consider treatment options; sexual side effects of treatments; fertility; self- and body image; prophylactic contralateral mastectomy; genetic testing; and the effects of cancer on relationships, children, and career.

The treatments of breast cancer are surgery, irradiation, chemotherapy, and antiestrogen therapy (tamoxifen, raloxifene, anastrazole, and exemestane). Local control is still critical; the size, location, and aggressiveness of the tumor usually dictate the initial surgery (mastectomy vs. limited resection). Use of sentinel-node mapping reduces, but does not eliminate, the risk of developing unsightly and disabling lymphedema. Although many women now have a choice between mastectomy and limited resection, mastectomy is preferred by some instead of daily irradiation treatment for 5–6 weeks. Natural tissue or silicone or saline implant breast-reconstruction techniques provide satisfactory to excellent results for women eligible for reconstruction. Involvement of the patient's husband or partner in preoperative medical appointments, in viewing the scar, and in discussions about resuming sexual activity is helpful for optimal recovery.

Chemotherapy with alkylating agents can cause alopecia, ovarian failure, premature menopause, and weight gain. Taxanes can cause painful and disabling peripheral neuropathy. Antiestrogen therapy is prescribed over a period of years and may cause insomnia, hot flashes, irritability, and depression in some women (Duffy et al. 1999). Many women undergoing chemotherapy report difficulty with concentration and memory, but these reports do not correlate consistently with persistent deficits on neuropsychological testing, and the difficulty may primarily be caused by the malaise of chemotherapy and concomitant symptoms.

Psychological distress is common at the conclusion of cancer treatment. Women feel vulnerable and less protected when not being seen regularly by their oncologist (Rowland and Massie 2004). Increased doctor visits and emotional support at this time are often beneficial. Ganz et al. (1996) found that survivors appear to attain maximum recovery from the physical and emotional trauma at 1 year after breast surgery. Sexual problems are important to address after acute treatment (see Chapter 17, "Sexual Disorders").

The emotional burden of breast cancer treatment is high, particularly for young women who hope to become pregnant. Although there is no evidence that pregnancy affects the outcome of breast cancer, continuation versus elective termination of pregnancy is a consideration for some who are diagnosed very early in a pregnancy and are unwilling to postpone treatment with teratogenic alkylating agents. Most young women, even women who are considered to have a good prognosis and are likely cured by initial treatments, ponder the ramifications of adoption or future child bearing, taking into account the unpredictability of disease recurrence or progression.

Genetics

The two most significant risk factors for breast cancer are increasing age and family history. The hereditary breast or ovarian cancer syndrome accounts for 5%–7% of all breast cancer cases and 10% of all ovarian cancer cases,

and is attributed to germ-line mutations in *BRCA1* and *BRCA2* genes (Robson et al. 2001). In the pre-gene-testing era, bilateral prophylactic mastectomy was a treatment option for women with strong family histories of breast cancer and extreme anxiety about their risk, and psychiatrists often were involved in preoperative assessment. Now that gene testing is available, women who likely have a hereditary predisposition are first referred for consultation with a clinical geneticist, which includes preparing a pedigree, documenting cancer diagnoses, estimating cancer risks, and discussing options for genetic testing and cancer screening and prevention (Robson and Offit 2002). The woman who tests positive for a gene mutation is advised to enroll in a high-risk surveillance clinic where she will receive information about chemoprevention and the potential effectiveness of risk-reducing surgery. Bilateral prophylactic mastectomy (PM) is associated with a greater than 90% reduction in the incidence of breast cancer in women with a family history of breast cancer (Hartmann et al. 1999). Prophylactic oophorectomy (PO), usually performed laparoscopically as an ambulatory procedure, reduces breast cancer risk by 50% in *BRCA1* mutation carriers and prevents most ovarian cancer in women with *BRCA1/BRCA2* mutations (Weber et al. 2000).

In some cancer centers, psychiatric consultation is an essential part of the evaluation process. The psychiatric evaluation of a woman who is considering prophylactic surgery includes a review of the woman's family and personal psychiatric history (e.g., body dysmorphic disorder, depressive disorder, personality disorder); family history of all cancers; perception of cancer risk and anxiety associated with perceptions; understanding of actual risk; satisfaction with previous plastic surgery(ies); litigation history; history of abuse, rape or assault; sexual, pregnancy, and breast-feeding history; desire to have (more) children and planned timing of PM and PO in relationship to future pregnancies; and the feasibility of child rearing with uncertainty about the future. A partner's role in considering the decision to have PM or PO is explored. Patients have an opportunity to clarify information, discuss decisions and the decision-making process, and obtain psychological understanding and support. Regardless of whether PM and PO will be selected as an option, strategies to reduce anxiety are discussed. Some women at high risk choose to have PM or PO in the absence of genetic testing. In this case, psychiatric evaluation should be a standard component of the surgical evaluation. The women who later express regret about having had prophylactic mastectomy are those who feel that the decision to have surgery was driven by their surgeon (Payne et al. 2000).

Colorectal Cancer

Although screening can detect precancerous polyps, more than 140,000 people in the United States will be newly diagnosed with colorectal cancer in 2004, and more than 56,000 will die (Jemal et al. 2004). Only 36% of colorectal cancers are diagnosed at an early stage, and surgical resection is the only curative therapy. A patient's adjustment is closely related to the type and extent of surgery, the presence or absence of a stoma and ostomy, and the partner's adjustment. Psychosocial adjustment to colon cancer can be complicated by anorexia, nausea and vomiting, weight loss, abdominal discomfort, diarrhea, and constipation. Concerns about body image, sexual functioning, fatigue, pain, and odor can lead to social withdrawal (Bernhard et al. 1999; Sahay et al. 2000). In patients with liver metastases, serum interleukin-2r, a cytokine, may be an independent predictor of depression (Allen-Mersh et al. 1998). Confusion occurs in 1% colon cancer patients in the last 6 months of life but in 28% in the last 3 days. Significant financial burden occurs in the 3–6 months before death (McCarthy et al. 2000).

A recent survey of colorectal cancer survivors demonstrated that they had a relatively uniform and high quality of life, irrespective of stage at and time from diagnosis. Noncancer comorbid disorders and low-income status had more influence on quality of life than stage or time since diagnosis. Compared with an age-matched population, long-term survivors reported higher quality-of-life scores, but they had higher rates of depression. Frequent bowel movements and chronic recurrent diarrhea were a problem for many (Ramsey et al. 2002) (see Chapter 30, "Surgery," for a discussion of ostomies). There are many self-help groups that provide vital education and coping skills for these patients and their families.

Lung Cancer

There will be an estimated 173,000 new cases of lung cancer diagnosed and 160,000 deaths in 2004 in the United States (Jemal et al. 2004). Lung cancer accounts for 25% of all cancer deaths. Although it is the most preventable of all cancers, with 87% of cases linked to cigarette smoking, lung cancer is difficult to diagnose early. About one-fifth of patients with non–small-cell lung cancer (NSCLC) have depressed mood at the time of diagnosis, and their depression tends to persist. In one study, depression following the diagnosis or resection of operable NSCLC predicted depression 1 year later (Uchitomi et al. 2003). At the time of diagnosis, many tumors are inoperable. In unresectable NSCLC, self-reported anxiety and depression at baseline was found to predict subsequent psychological distress (Akechi et al. 2001).

Depressive symptoms and difficulty concentrating are more common at diagnosis of small-cell lung cancer than NSCLC. Small-cell lung cancer, more than any other tumor, is associated with paraneoplastic syndromes such as Cushing's syndrome, hyponatremia, and autoimmune encephalopathy. Because pulmonary emboli are common during treatment, dyspnea and anxiety should be evaluated carefully. Hypoxia due to preexisting chronic obstructive pulmonary disease and postradiation hypothyroidism may contribute to cognitive dysfunction. Postthoracotomy neuralgic pain is common.

In lung cancer, there is a substantial risk of brain metastases. Isolated lesions may be removed surgically, but cranial radiation is common once the metastasis is noted. Patients with small-cell lung cancer often receive prophylactic cranial radiation because the risk of brain metastases is 50% over 2 years. Some cognitive deficits have been noted in long-term survivors of small-cell cancer whether or not they received cranial radiation. Leukoencephalopathy has occurred after treatment for small-cell cancer as a result of the combination of chemotherapy and radiation, but changes in chemotherapy have decreased this risk.

In one recent study of 145 survivors of NSCLC who were 5 or more years disease-free, most were hopeful. Half viewed the cancer experience as contributing to positive life changes (Sarna et al. 2002).

Many smokers with cancer experience guilt, but many continue to smoke. Continued smoking is associated with decreased survival, development of a secondary primary cancer, and increased risk of developing or exacerbating other medical conditions. Chemotherapy and radiation are likely to produce more complications and greater morbidity among smokers than among nonsmokers (Sanderson et al. 2002). Although some health care providers are hesitant to raise the issue of smoking cessation during the stress of initial diagnosis, the literature supports early antismoking intervention with patients and their family members (Sanderson et al. 2002). But in terminal lung cancer, if the patient derives pleasure from smoking, cessation interventions are not indicated. For further review of lung cancer, see Chapter 20, "Lung Disease."

Ovarian Cancer

The second most frequent gynecological cancer among women in the United States, ovarian cancer, is the fourth most frequent cause of cancer death and has the highest mortality rate of all gynecological cancers (Jemal et al. 2004). Annually, more than 25,000 new cases of ovarian cancer are diagnosed, and 16,000 deaths result. Ovarian cancer usually has an insidious onset and progression; 70% of cases are stages II to IV at time of diagnosis. The 5-year survival rate is only 37%, and of those who respond to treatment, nearly 90% will have a recurrence with a fatal outcome.

Because CA 125 levels often rise before symptoms appear, patients' emotions often rise and fall with the report of the CA 125 level (Fertig 1998). Kornblith and colleagues found that more than 60% of ovarian cancer patients were worried, tired, feeling sad, and in pain (Kornblith et al. 1995).

Patients report difficulties with sexual desire, response, and communication after gynecological cancer treatment (Schover 1997) (see Chapter 17, "Sexual Disorders"). Infertility concerns are vital for younger women, who require information about fertility and emotional support to make treatment decisions and to cope with those choices.

Melanoma

More than 55,000 Americans will be diagnosed with melanoma in 2004 (Jemal et al. 2004). Melanoma is a very variable tumor. Fawzy and associates reported that a short-term focused psychological treatment could diminish distress and prolong survival (Fawzy et al. 2003). The intervention was associated with survival benefit after 6 years, but the benefit weakened after 10 years.

Patients with advanced disease are currently treated with a 12-month protocol of interferon-alfa, the side effects of which include fatigue, anxiety, insomnia, depression, and rarely mania (Kirkwood et al. 2002). Paroxetine started at the time interferon-alfa is started has been shown to reduce the incidence of depression (Musselman et al. 2001). Brain metastases are always a consideration in advanced disease.

Head and Neck Cancers

Head and neck cancers carry the risks of facial deformity and loss of speech. These tumors are most frequent in patients with a history of alcohol abuse and smoking. Treatment is daunting and leads to mucositis, pain, dysphagia, and dry mouth or sticky saliva, all of which make eating difficult. Feeding tubes and tracheotomies are often necessary (List et al. 1997). Hypothyroidism is common following radiation treatment to the neck (Mercado et al. 2001). Because these tumors are more common among isolated men with a history of substance abuse, the risk of suicide has been thought to be high, but one study suggested that the rate of suicide remains low (Henderson and Ord 1997).

Pancreatic Cancer

Depression, anxiety, restlessness, and insomnia have been thought to be common first signs of pancreatic cancer, before physical signs appear, and physicians have wondered whether pancreatic hormones or neuropeptides might be responsible (Alter 1996; Fras et al. 1967; Green and Austin 1993; Joffe et al. 1986; Krech et al. 1991). One clinical study reported that depressive thoughts were more common in people with pancreatic cancer than in those with gastric cancer (Holland et al. 1986), and a recent epidemiological study found that depression preceded pancreatic cancer more often than other GI malignancies (odds ratio 4.6) (Carney et al. 2003). In a depressed patient, clues to the diagnosis of pancreatic cancer include abdominal symptoms and weight loss out of proportion to the degree of psychological symptoms. However, the symptoms of pancreatic cancer are typically vague and nonspecific. Symptoms of upper abdominal disease occur in 25% of patients 6 months before diagnosis. Anorexia, early satiety, and back pain are features of progressive disease. Diabetes may also be present (DiMagno 1999). One study of 130 patients presenting with pancreatic cancer found 38% had scores above 15 on the Beck Depression Inventory. Depression was more common in those who had pain (Kelsen et al. 1995).

Following diagnosis, patients come to surgical evaluation, but few have surgically treatable disease. Finding that the tumor is not resectable is an additional psychological blow. Management of pain and discomfort includes pancreatic enzymes to relieve the cramps of fat malabsorption, octreotide for diarrhea, prevention of constipation, narcotics, and sometimes celiac block, as well as antidepressants for depression.

Psychiatric Aspects of Cancer Treatments

Chemotherapy

The neuropsychiatric side effects of common chemotherapeutic agents are listed in Table 24–1. The effects of chemotherapy on cognition are under investigation, but there are no definitive findings thus far (Phillips and Bernhard 2003). For the most part, there are no significant clinical interactions between cancer drugs and antidepressant medications, antipsychotic medications, and benzodiazepines. Procarbazine, a weak monoamine oxidase (MAO) inhibitor, is an exception. Alcohol may lead to an Antabuse-like reaction, and antidepressant medications should be prescribed only with consideration of possible MAO inhibition in mind.

Radiation

Radiation treatment usually requires a patient to remain absolutely still on a flat table for 5–10 minutes daily, 5 days a week, so that a prescribed dose can be applied to a specific site over 2–9 weeks. Patients worry that they cannot remain still either because of claustrophobia or because of inadequate pain control. Fatigue continues to increase during the month following radiation treatment but then begins to diminish. Nausea and vomiting from radiation treatment, more severe when viscera are irradiated, is reduced by serotonin 5-HT$_3$ antagonists like ondansetron. Brain irradiation causes more profound fatigue than treatment of other sites. Concomitant dexamethasone reduces cerebral edema, but late sequelae of brain radiation may occur, including radiation necrosis in focal areas or leukoencephalopathy. Newer methods to reduce the volume of brain that requires radiation may reduce these risks.

Bone Marrow Transplantation

Bone marrow transplantation (BMT) is used to treat acute and chronic leukemia, aplastic anemia, lymphomas, some solid tumors, and immunological deficiency states. There is no correlation between type of transplant and psychological morbidity (Leigh et al. 1995). Wettergren and colleagues found that patients undergoing autologous BMT who had more functional limitations coped worse than did patients who were less functionally impaired (Wettergren et al. 1997).

The psychological stress of BMT begins when transplant is first considered. It offers a chance of cure but carries significant risk of morbidity and mortality. In one study of BMT candidates, one-third reported depression (Baker et al. 1997); in another study, two-thirds reported a high level of anxiety (Keogh et al. 1998).

An important part of the pretransplant planning is to evaluate and shore up the patient's social support. Parents making this decision for a child may show depressive symptoms pretransplant and develop mental and physical exhaustion as the process continues (Pot-Mees and Zeitlin 1987). Some family members have alterations in immune status at various phases of the transplant (Futterman et al. 1996) and overall report distress similar to that of patients (Siston et al. 2001).

During high-dose chemotherapy and irradiation, visitors are limited to avoid infection. Patients often experience nausea, vomiting, and fatigue. During this time, psychiatric disorders are extremely common, especially adjustment disorder with anxiety and depression. Graft-versus-host disease is not generally associated with occurrence of mental disorders (Sasaki et al. 2000), although when severe, it may result in delirium.

The transplant itself (a brief intravenous infusion of several packets of concentrated bone marrow) is anticlimactic compared to the pretransplant regimen and the anxious recovery period waiting for platelet and red and white blood cell counts to "come back," the evidence of hematological recovery. Hypervigilant patients keep charts of their cell counts, anticipating the day of "probable" recovery; others request medications to "sleep through the experience," a passive attitude antithetical to caregivers who want the patient to participate in self-care.

After a prolonged period of dependence, patients are often very fearful as they anticipate hospital discharge and must assume greater roles in self-care. Persistent fatigue is a major problem when patients resume normal activities at home and work (Hann et al. 1997). Chronic anxiety and depression are the most common psychiatric sequelae, and psychological adjustment is particularly difficult for those patients who have delayed or disrupted important developmental life tasks.

In general, successful adaptation to BMT is associated with the ability to use information about illness and treatment, coupled with the ability to delegate control and authority temporarily and to trust the staff (Lesko and Holland 1998). A study of adults undergoing allogeneic BMT for acute leukemia found three variables affected outcome: illness status, presence of depressed mood, and the extent of perceived social support (Colon et al. 1991). Depressed mood pretransplant is associated with poorer survival (Colon et al. 1991; Loberiza et al. 2002), perhaps suggesting the potential benefit of early psychiatric intervention.

Long-term survivors of BMT for acute leukemia show no difference in psychological and social functioning than those who received standard chemotherapy (Wellisch et al. 1996). A decrease in sexual frequency and satisfaction is seen in women (Mumma et al. 1992).

Bone marrow transplant recipients are at increased risk for developing central nervous system (CNS) toxicity such as neuropsychological impairment, including compromised motor and cognitive test performance (Tschuschke et al. 2001).

Surgery

See Chapter 30, "Surgery," for a full discussion of the emotional aspects of surgery.

Psychiatric Interventions in Cancer

Psychotherapy

Psychotherapy can often help patients to accept the diagnosis of cancer; sort out treatment options; overcome fear; depression, or denial; and enhance patients' ability to cope with cancer treatment (Weisman 1979). Suffering is intensified by lack of meaning, and some interventions for cancer patients have focused on the maintenance of morale and the search for meaning (Frankl 1946; Greenstein and Breitbart 2000; Weisman 1993). Chochinov (2002) has developed methods to support patients' desire for dignity at the end of life.

Psychosocial interventions can reduce distress, facilitate problem-solving strategies, and augment a sense of control. Cognitive and behavioral models can be tailored to the specific tumor type. Educational and behavioral training, either in group or individual psychotherapy, are the best-documented approaches to reducing distress in cancer patients (Fawzy et al. 1995; Newell et al. 2002).

Although some enthusiasts have advocated counseling for all cancer patients on the assumption that they can benefit from help and will take advantage of it, in one study, only two-thirds of the patients identified as high risk accepted counseling (Worden and Weisman 1984). Refusers had a positive outlook, minimized the implications of their diagnosis, and viewed the offer of therapy as a threat to their emotional equilibrium. Those who accepted counseling were less able to deny the diagnosis and its implications; they were less hopeful and were more apt to experience their situation in religious or existential terms. Thus, pushing too hard for group or individual psychotherapy is countertherapeutic for some patients. Because of the bond between families and the psychiatrist who took care of their relative over the course of a long illness, families often enter into bereavement counseling with this same psychiatrist after the patient's death to provide a healing conclusion to a long illness.

Group therapy and self-help groups allow cancer patients to receive support from others who are coping with similar problems. In a group setting, patients can glean practical tips and see the range of normal reactions to illness, as well as adaptive coping styles and strategies that make adjustment to illness easier. Group therapy helps to decrease the sense of isolation and alienation as the patient and family see that they are not alone adjusting to illness. Groups are often disease specific or targeted for patients at the same stage of illness. Past concerns about having dying patients in a group with those recently diagnosed or whose prognosis was good have been dispelled.

Spiegel et al. (1989) developed supportive expressive group psychotherapy led by trained professionals for women with breast cancer. The goal of supportive-expressive psychotherapy is to help patients with existential concerns and disease-related emotions as well as to deepen social support and physician relationships and provide symptom control. The therapist challenges patients' tendency to withdraw from the implications of having metastatic breast cancer. Such groups relieve distress while reducing avoidance of the implications of the diagnosis. This strategy improves mood and pain perception, especially in the most distressed (Goodwin et al. 2001).

Studies of psychosocial interventions in hopes of prolonging survival have had a mixed outcome. Spiegel and colleagues' report of greater longevity in a small number of women with advanced breast cancer undergoing group supportive-expressive psychotherapy was not replicated in larger studies (Goodwin et al. 2001; Spiegel et al. 1989). Fawzy and colleagues' study of a structured psychoeducational intervention for patients with early-stage melanoma showed a modest survival benefit at 6 years that weakened at 10-year follow-up (Fawzy et al. 1993, 2003). Patients can be told that group support contributes to living better, not necessarily longer.

Psychopharmacology

Patients commonly ask whether psychiatric drugs increase cancer risk or render antineoplastics ineffective. There is no evidence for either belief (Steingart and Cotterchio 1995; Theoharides and Konstantinidou 2003).

Depression

The selective serotonin reuptake inhibitors (SSRIs) are the first-line antidepressants prescribed in cancer settings because they are effective, have few sedative and autonomic side effects, and have few drug interactions. A small minority of cancer patients experience transient weight loss when starting an SSRI; however, weight usually returns to baseline level, and the anorectic properties of these drugs are usually not a limiting factor in those with cancer anorexia–cachexia. Ondansetron can be used to block initial serotonin-mediated nausea. Antidepressants like mirtazapine that can cause weight gain may be advantageous in anorexic–cachectic cancer patients but are not a good choice in those who are gaining weight from steroids or from chemotherapy (Theobald et al. 2002). If recurrent periods of inability to eat and drink tend to interrupt the antidepressant regimen, then fluoxetine, with its longer half-life, has an advantage. The SSRIs and venlafaxine reduce both the number and the intensity of hot flashes and night sweats in nondepressed women who become menopausal after chemotherapy for breast cancer or who have a recurrence of vasomotor symptoms when they discontinue hormone replacement therapy (Duffy et al. 1999; Loberiza et al. 2002; Stearns et al. 2000; Weitzner et al. 2002). Hot flashes are also an issue for men on androgen deprivation treatment regimens.

Bupropion's stimulating properties make it useful in lethargic patients, but because of its association with increased seizure risk, it should be used with caution in patients who are malnourished or who have a history of seizures or brain tumor. Bupropion may assist in smoking cessation, especially in patients with lung or head and neck cancers.

The tricyclic antidepressants (TCAs) are used to treat both depression and the neuropathic pain syndromes caused by chemotherapy and surgery. Nortriptyline and desipramine have more favorable side-effect profiles compared with amitriptyline, with fewer anticholinergic symptoms.

Psychostimulants (i.e., dextroamphetamine and pemoline), can promote a sense of well-being, treat depression, decrease fatigue, stimulate appetite, and improve cognitive function. Psychostimulants are used as an adjuvant to potentiate the analgesic effects of opioid analgesics and are commonly used to counteract opioid-induced sedation (Rozans et al. 2002). Psychostimulants offer clear benefits, especially in terminally ill patients, because there may be an improvement in symptoms within hours to days. See also Chapter 9, "Depression," for a full discussion of the pharmacological treatment of depression.

In patients with primary bipolar disorder, mood stabilizers and neuroleptics can be continued. Lithium tends to increase the patient's white blood count and usually can be continued during cancer treatment. However, complications of chemotherapy, including vomiting, diarrhea, dehydration, and renal insufficiency, may raise lithium levels, and symptoms of toxicity, nausea, diarrhea, and confusion may be misattributed to chemotherapy. See Chapter 11, "Mania, Catatonia, and Psychosis," for a full discussion of the pharmacological treatment of mania and psychosis.

Anxiety

Prior to treatment with a benzodiazepine, all patients should be screened for depressive symptoms as well as for specific anxiety disorders such as PTSD and obsessive-compulsive disorder. When anxiety is a manifestation of a primary depressive disorder, treatment should be an antidepressant with, or instead of, a benzodiazepine. The experience of cancer treatment may reawaken problems in patients who were the victims of earlier traumas, increasing their risk of anxiety and depressive symptoms (Baider et al. 2000).

Benzodiazepines are frequently given to patients for acute anxiety and are often prescribed to augment antiemetics during chemotherapy. Dosing depends on the patient's tolerance and the drug's duration of action. Lorazepam and alprazolam are favored in the acute setting because of their rapid onset of action and benefit on an "as-needed" basis. Buspirone and antidepressants are alternatives for longer treatment of anxiety. Low doses of neuroleptics are useful in patients who are unresponsive to or intolerant of benzodiazepines or in patients with severe anxiety and agitation. If patients have been taking a benzodiazepine chronically, they may suffer withdrawal if the dose is not tapered. See Chapter 12, "Anxiety Disorders," for a full discussion of the psychopharmacological treatment of anxiety.

Delirium

See Chapter 6, "Delirium," for a full discussion of the psychopharmacological treatment of delirium.

Electroconvulsive Therapy

Although the use of electroconvulsive therapy (ECT) in patients with brain tumor was once believed to be contraindicated because of the risk of brain herniation, there are numerous case reports describing safe and effective use of ECT in such patients (Patkar et al. 2000). See Chapter 39, "Electroconvulsive Therapy," for a full discussion of ECT.

Survivor Issues

Advances in cancer treatment over the past 30 years have led to a rapidly growing population of more than 9 million long-term survivors in the United States, many of them children and young adults. The long-term adjustment of many appears to be largely unimpaired (Kornblith et al. 2004). Some cured cancer patients have delayed medical complications (i.e., organ failure, CNS dysfunction, sterility, secondary malignancies, and decreased physical stamina) and psychiatric concerns, including fears of termination of treatment; preoccupation with the threat of disease recurrence (the Damocles syndrome) and a sense of greater vulnerability to illness; pervasive awareness of mortality and difficulty with reentry into normal life (the Lazarus syndrome); persistent guilt (the survivor syndrome); difficult adjustment to physical losses and handicaps that lead to problems with peer acceptance and social integration; diminished self-esteem or confidence; perceived loss of job mobility; and fear of job and insurance discrimination. Concerns about infertility, often understandably submerged at the time of diagnosis and treatment, reappear when treatment concludes. The survivor's intellectual functioning is also a major concern. Children and adults with brain tumors or

CNS involvement, and those undergoing bone marrow transplant, are at risk from both the disease and the treatment. Most have residual deficits, with neuropsychological impairment including compromised motor and cognitive test performance (Anderson et al. 2001; Bhatia 2003; Phipps et al. 2000).

Potential resources include the National Coalition of Cancer Survivorship, the Office of Cancer Survivorship of the National Cancer Institute, and the organizations whose Web sites are shown in Table 24–5.

Complementary and Alternative Medicine

Some 80% of cancer patients use complementary and alternative medicine (CAM) treatments. Some alternative treatments (acupuncture; relaxation; yoga; meditation; massage; tai chi; biofeedback; music, art, movement, and aroma therapies) are offered as adjuncts to traditional cancer care aimed at increasing quality of life and decreasing symptoms with no promise of cure. Other therapies such as shark cartilage, colonics, herbal remedies, and high-dose vitamin therapies do not improve quality of life and may be harmful. Some remedies are highly toxic (Markman 2002). Laetrile, now banned in the United States, contains cyanide; chaparral tea causes liver damage; and Ma huang contains ephedrine, a CNS stimulant. No CAM technique or preparation has been demonstrated to cause tumor regression. Memorial Sloan-Kettering Cancer Center has a Web site (http://www. mskcc.org/aboutherbs) on which it provides unbiased scientific reviews about potential drug interactions and adverse effects of some 135 herbal and botanical agents relevant to cancer patients (Mitka 2003).

In the United States, 83 million people use alternative therapies for malignant and nonmalignant disorders, and 70%–90% do not describe these treatments to their doctors (Gertz and Bauer 2001), in part because doctors often do not ask or provide negative remarks about CAM. A study of women with newly diagnosed early-stage breast cancer found that 28% used alternative medicine (Burstein et al. 1999). Interestingly, the use of alternative medicine was independently associated with depression, fear of recurrence of cancer, lower scores for mental health and sexual satisfaction, and more physical symptoms, suggesting that those who seek alternative medicine therapies may be experiencing more anxiety, depression, or physical symptoms. Those taking alternative medications may be more in need of but less open to psychiatric consultation.

Most patients who elect to use untried or unproven therapies do so in a desperate search for a cure or for a

TABLE 24–5. Organizations (and their Web sites) that provide accurate information for cancer patients and health professionals

- National Cancer Institute
  http://www.cancer.gov/cancer_information
- 1–800–4-CANCER
  Telephone number to get answers to cancer-related questions
- National Comprehensive Cancer Network
  http://www.nccn.com
- Memorial Sloan-Kettering Cancer Center
  About herbs, botanicals, and other products
  www.mskcc.org/aboutherbs
- American Cancer Society
  http://www.cancer.org
- American Society of Clinical Oncology
  http://www.asco.org
- People Living With Cancer
  http://www.plws.org

more acceptable quality of life. The clinician has to find a balance between condoning unproven or harmful treatment and preserving the patient's hope.

References

Akechi T, Okamura H, Nishiwaki Y, et al: Psychiatric disorder and associated and predictive facts in patients with unresectable nonsmall cell lung carcinoma: a longitudinal study. Cancer 92:2609–2622, 2001

Allen-Mersh TG, Glover C, Fordy C, et al: Relation between depression and circulating immune products in patients with advanced colorectal cancer. J R Soc Med 91:408–413, 1998

Alter C: Palliative and supportive care in patients with pancreatic cancer. Sem Oncol 23:229–240, 1996

Anderson DM, Rennie KM, Ziegler RS, et al: Medical and neurocognitive late effects among survivors of childhood center nervous system tumors. Cancer 92:2709–2719, 2001

Andrykowski MA: The role of anxiety in the development of anticipatory nausea in cancer chemotherapy: a review and synthesis. Psychosom Med 52:458–475, 1990

Ayres A, Hoon PW, Franzoni JB, et al: Influence of mood and adjustment to cancer on compliance with chemotherapy among breast cancer patients. J Psychosom Res 38:393–402, 1994

Bach PB, Schrag D, Brawley OW, et al: Survival of blacks and whites after a cancer diagnosis. JAMA 287:2106–2113, 2002

Baider L, Peretz R, Hadani Pe, et al: Transmission of response to trauma? Second-generation Holocaust survivors' reaction to cancer. Am J Psychiatry 157:904–910, 2000

Baker F, Marcellus D, Zabora J, et al: Psychological distress among adult patients being evaluated for bone marrow transplantation. Psychosomatics 38:10–19, 1997

Bernhard J, Hurny C, Maibach R, et al: Quality of life as subjective experience: reframing of perception in patients with colon cancer undergoing radical resection with or without adjuvant chemotherapy. Ann Oncol 10:775–782, 1999

Bhatia S: Late effects among survivors of leukemia during childhood and adolescence. Blood Cells Mol Dis 31:84–92, 2003

Brown TM, Stoudemire A: Antineoplastic agents, in Psychiatric Side Effects of Prescription and Over-the-Counter Medications. Edited by Brown TM, Stoudemire A. Washington DC, American Psychiatric Press, 1998, pp 239–261

Buddeberg C, Wolf C, Sieber M, et al: Coping strategies and course of disease of breast cancer patients. Results of a 3-year longitudinal study. Psychother Psychosom 55:151–157, 1991

Burstein HJ, Gelber S, Guadagnoli E, et al: Use of alternative medicine by women with early stage breast cancer. N Engl J Med 340:1733–1739, 1999

Butow PN, Coates AS, Dunna SM: Psychosocial predictors of survival in metastatic melanoma. J Clin Oncol 17:2256, 1999

Carney CP, Jones L, Woolson RF, et al: Relationship between depression and pancreatic cancer in the general population. Psychosom Med 65:884–888, 2003

Cassileth BR, Lusk EJ, Miller DS, et al: Psychological correlates of survival in advanced malignant disease. N Engl J Med 312:1551–1555, 1985

Chochinov HM: Dignity-conserving care—a new model for palliative care: helping the patient feel valued. JAMA 287:2253–2260, 2002

Colon EA, Callier AL, Popkin MJ, et al: Depressed mood and other variables related to bone marrow transplantation survival in acute leukemia. Psychosomatics 32:420–425, 1991

Cordova MJ, Andrykowski MA, Kenady DE, et al: Frequency and correlates of posttraumatic-stress-disorder-like symptoms after treatment for breast cancer. J Consult Clin Psychol 63:981–986, 1995

Courtney JG, Longnecker MP, Theorell T, et al: Stressful life events and the risk of colorectal cancer. Epidemiology 4:407–414, 1993

Derogatis LR, Morrow GR, Fetting JH, et al: The prevalence of psychiatric disorders among cancer patients. JAMA 249:751–757, 1983

DiMagno EP: Pancreatic cancer: clinical presentation, pitfalls and early clues. Ann Oncol 4:S140–S142, 1999

Duffy LS, Greenberg DB, Younger J, et al: Iatrogenic acute estrogen deficiency and psychiatric syndromes in breast cancer patients. Psychosomatics 40:304–308, 1999

Faller H, Bulzebruck H: Coping and survival in lung cancer: a 10-year follow-up. Am J Psychiatry 159:2105–2107, 2002

Faller H, Bulzebruck H, Drungs P, et al: Coping, distress, and survival among patients with lung cancer. Arch Gen Psychiatry 56:756–762, 1999

Fawzy FI, Fawzy N, Hun CS, et al: Malignant melanoma: effects of an early structured psychiatric intervention, coping and affective state on recurrence and survival 6 years later. Arch Gen Psychiatry 50:681–689, 1993

Fawzy FI, Fawzy NW, Arndt LA, et al: Critical review of psycho-social interventions in cancer care. Arch Gen Psychiatry 52:100–113, 1995

Fawzy FI, Canada AL, Fawzy NW: Effects of a brief, structured psychiatric intervention on survival and recurrence at 10-year follow-up. Arch Gen Psychiatry 60:100–103, 2003

Fertig DL, Hayes DF: Psychological responses to tumor markers, in Psycho-oncology. Edited by Holland, JC. New York, Oxford University Press, 1998, pp 1147–1160

Fleishman S, Lesko L, Breitbart WS: Treatment of organic mental disorders in cancer patients, in Psychiatric Aspects of Symptom Management in Cancer Patients. Edited by Breitbart WS, Holland JC. Washington DC, American Psychiatric Press, 1993, pp 23–47

Fox BH, Stanek EJ III, Boldy SC, et al: Suicide rates among cancer patients in Connecticut. J Chronic Dis 35:85–100, 1982

Frankl V: Man's Search for Meaning. Boston, MA, Beacon, 1946

Fras I, Litin EM, Pearson JS: Comparison of psychiatric symptoms in carcinoma of the pancreas with those in some other intra-abdominal neoplasms. Am J Psychiatry 123:1553–1562, 1967

Futterman AD, Wellisch DK, Zighelboim J, et al: Psychological and immunological reactions of family members to patients undergoing bone marrow transplantation. Psychom Med 58:472–480, 1996

Gallo JJ, Amernian HK, Ford DE, et al: Major depression and cancer: the 13-year follow-up of the Baltimore epidemiologic catchment area sample (United States). Cancer Causes Control 11:751–758, 2000

Ganz PA, Coscarelli A, Fred C, et al: Breast cancer survivors: Psychosocial concerns and quality of life. Breast Cancer Res Treat 38:183–199, 1996

Garnick, MB: Prostate cancer: screening, diagnosis, and management. Ann Intern Med 118:804–818, 1993

Garssen B, Goodkin K: On the role of immunological factors as mediators between psychosocial factors and cancer progression. Psychiatry Res 85:51–61, 1999

Gertz MA, Bauer BA: Caring (really) for patients who use alternative therapies for cancer. J Clin Oncol 19:4346–4349, 2001

Geyer S: Life events prior to manifestation of breast cancer: a limited prospective study covering eight years before diagnosis. J Psychosom Res 35:355–363, 1991

Ginsburg ML, Quirt C, Ginsburg AD, et al: Psychiatric illness and psychological concerns of patients with newly diagnosed lung cancer. CMAJ 1:152:701–708, 1995

Giraldi T, Rodani MG, Cartei G, et al: Psychosocial factors and breast cancer: a 6-year Italian follow-up study. Psychother Psychosom 66:229–236, 1997

Glover J, Dibble SL, Dood MJ, et al: Mood states of oncology outpatients: does pain make a difference? J Pain Symptom Manage 10:120–128, 1995

Goodwin PJ, Leszcz M, Ennis M, et al: The effects of group psychosocial support on survival in metastatic breast cancer. N Engl J Med 345:1719–1726, 2001

Green AI, Austin CP: Psychopathology of pancreatic cancer. A psychobiological probe (review). Psychosomatics 34:208–221, 1993

Green BL, Rowland JH, Krupnick JL, et al: Prevalence of posttraumatic stress disorder in women with breast cancer. Psychosomatics 39:102–111, 1998

Greenberg DB: Barriers to the treatment of depression in cancer patients. J Natl Cancer Inst Monogr 32:127–135, 2004

Greenberg DB, Kornblith AB, Herndon JE, et al: Quality of life of adult leukemia survivors treated on clinical trials of the Cancer and Leukemia Group B from 1971–1988: predictors for later psychological distress. Cancer 80:1936–1944, 1997

Greenberg DB, Jonasch E, Gadd MA, et al: Adjuvant therapy of melanoma with interferon alpha 2b associated with mania and bipolar syndromes. Cancer 89:356–362, 2000

Greenstein M, Breitbart WS: Cancer and the experience of meaning: a group psychotherapy program for people with cancer. Am J Psychother 54:486–500, 2000

Greer S, Morris T, Pettingale KW: Psychological response to breast cancer: effect on outcome. Lancet 2:785–787, 1979

Hann DM, Jacobsen PB, Martin SC, et al: Fatigue in women treated with bone marrow transplantation for breast cancer: a comparison with women with no history of cancer. Support Care Cancer 5:44–52, 1997

Harlan L, Brawley O, Pommerenke F, et al: Geographic, age, and racial variation in the treatment of local/regional carcinoma of the prostate. J Clin Oncol 13:93–100, 1995

Hartmann LC, Schaid DJ, Woods JE, et al: Efficacy of bilateral prophylactic mastectomy in women with a family history of breast cancer. N Engl J Med 340:77–84, 1999

Helgeson VS, Cohen S: Social support and adjustment to cancer: reconciling descriptive, correlational, and intervention research. Health Psychol 15:135–148, 1996

Helsing KJ, Szklo M: Mortality after bereavement. Am J Epidemiol 114:41–52, 1981

Henderson JM, Ord RA: Suicide in head and neck cancer patients. J Oral Maxillofac Surg 55:1217–1221; (discussion) 1221–1222, 1997

Hickok JT, Roscoe JA, Morrow GR, et al: Nausea and emesis remain significant problems of chemotherapy despite prophylaxis with 5-hydroxytryptamine-3 antiemetics. Cancer 97:2880–2886, 2003

Holland JC, Korzun AH, Tross S, et al: Comparative psychological disturbance in patients with pancreatic and gastric cancer. Am J Psychiatry 143:982–986, 1986

Ingram D, Browne G, Reyno L, et al: Prevalence, correlates and cost of anxiety and affective disorder in men with prostate cancer one year after initial assessment (abstract #523). Psychooncology 12:S1–S277, 2003

Inui A: Cancer Anorexia-cachexia syndrome. CA Cancer J Clin 52:72–91, 2002

Jacobson PB, Widows MR, Hann DM, et al: Posttraumatic stress disorder symptoms after bone marrow transplantation for breast cancer. Psychosom Med 62:366–371, 1998

Jahn I, Becker U, Jockel KH, et al: Occupational life course and lung cancer risk in men. Findings from a socio-epidemiological analysis of job-changing histories in a case-control study. Soc Sci Med 40:961–975, 1995

Jemal A, Tiwari RC, Murray T, et al: Cancer statistics, 2004. CA Cancer J Clin 54:8–29, 2004

Joffe RT, Rubinow DR, Denicoff KD, et al: Depression and carcinoma of the pancreas. Gen Hosp Psychiatry 8:241–245, 1986

Kelsen DP, Portenoy RK, Thaler HT, et al: Pain and depression in patients with newly diagnosed pancreas cancer. J Clin Oncol 13:748–755, 1995

Keogh F, O'Riordan J, McNamara C, et al: Psychosocial adaptation of patients and families following bone marrow transplantation: a prospective, longitudinal study. Bone Marrow Transplant 22:905–911, 1998

Kirkwood JM, Bender C, Agarwala S, et al: Mechanisms and management of toxicities associated with high-dose interferon alfa-2b therapy. J Clin Oncol 20:3703–3718, 2002

Kornblith AB, Herr HW, Ofman US, et al: Quality of life of patients with prostate cancer and their spouses. The value of a database in clinical care. Cancer 73:2791–2802, 1994

Kornblith AB, Thaler HT, Wong G, et al: Quality of life of women with ovarian cancer. Gynecol Oncol 59:231–242, 1995

Kornblith AB, Herndon JE II, Weiss RB, et al: Long-term adjustment of survivors of early stage breast carcinoma, 20 years after adjuvant chemotherapy. Cancer 98:679–689, 2004

Krech RL, Walsh D: Symptoms of pancreatic cancer. J Pain Symptom Manage 6:360–367, 1991

Kune GA, Kune S, Watson LF, et al: Personality as a risk factor in large bowel cancer: data from the Melbourne Colorectal Cancer Study. Psychol Med 21:29–41, 1991

Kune S, Kune GA, Watson LF, et al: Recent life change and large bowel cancer. data from the Melbourne Colorectal Cancer Study. J Clin Epidemiol 44:57–68, 1991

Kung S, Mueller PS, Yonas EG, et al: Delirium resulting from paraneoplastic limbic encephalitis caused by Hodgkin's disease. Psychosomatics 43:498–501, 2002

Lee MA, Ganzini L: Depression in the elderly: effect on patient attitudes toward life-sustaining therapy. J Am Geriatr Soc 40:983–988, 1992

Leigh S, Wilson KC, Burns R, et al: Psychosocial morbidity in bone marrow transplant recipients: a prospective study. Bone Marrow Transplant 16:635–640, 1995

Lesko LM, Holland JC: Psychosocial issues in patients with hematological malignancies, in Supportive Care in Cancer Patients (Vol. 108 in Recent Results in Cancer Research series). Edited by Senn HJ, Claus A, Schmid L. Berlin, Germany, Springer-Verlag, 1998, pp 109–243

Levav I, Kohn R, Iscovich J, et al: Cancer incidence and survival following bereavement. Am J Public Health 90:1601–1607, 2000

Levenson JL, McDonald MK: The role of psychological factors in cancer onset and progression: a critical appraisal, in The Psychoimmunology of Cancer, 2nd Edition. Edited by Lewis CE, O'Brien R, Barraclough J. New York, Oxford University Press, 2002, pp 149–163

Lieberman FS, Schold SC: Distant effects of cancer on the nervous system. Oncology 16:1539–1548, 2002

List MA, Mumby P, Haraf D, et al: Performance and quality of life outcome in patients completing concomitant chemoradiotherapy protocols for head and neck cancer. Qual Life Res 6:274–284, 1997

Litwin MS, Lubeck DP, Spitalny GM, et al: Mental health in men treated for early stage prostate carcinoma. Cancer 95:54–60, 2002

Loberiza FR Jr, Rizzo JD, Bredeson CN, et al: Association of depressive syndrome and early deaths among patients after stem-cell transplantation for malignant diseases. J Clin Oncol 20:2118–2126, 2002

Louhivuori KA, Hakama M: Risk of suicide among cancer patients. Am J Epidemiol 109:59–65, 1979

Lynge E, Andersen O: Unemployment and cancer in Denmark, 1970–1975 and 1986–1990. IARC Scientific Publications 138:353–359, 1997

Markman M: Safety issues in using complementary and alterative medicine. J Clin Oncol 20:S39–S41, 2002

Massie MJ: Prevalence of depression in patients with cancer. J Natl Cancer Inst Monogr 32:57–71, 2004

Massie MJ, Popkin M: Depressive disorders, in Psycho-Oncology. Edited by Holland JC. New York, Oxford University Press, 1998, pp 518–540

Maunsell E, Brisson J, Mondor M, et al: Stressful life events and survival after breast cancer. Psychosom Med 63:306–315, 2001

McCarthy EP, Phillips RS, Zhong Z, et al: Dying with cancer: patients' function, symptoms, and care preferences as death approaches. J Am Geriatr Soc 48:S110-S121, 2000

McGee R, Williams S, Elwood M: Depression and the development of cancer: a meta-analysis. Soc Sci Med 38:187–192, 1994

McKenna MC, Zevon MA, Corn B, et al: Psychosocial factors and the development of breast cancer: a meta-analysis. Health Psychol 18:520–531, 1999

Mercado G, Adelstein DJ, Saxton JP, et al: Hypothyroidism, a frequent event after radiotherapy and after radiotherapy with chemotherapy for patients with head and neck carcinoma. Cancer 92:2892–2897, 2001

Mitka M: Website showcases science-based information on herbs, other supplements. JAMA 289:829–830, 2003

Mumma GH, Mashberg D, Lesko LM: Long-term psychosexual adjustment of acute leukemia survivors: impact of marrow transplantation versus conventional chemotherapy. Gen Hosp Psychiatry 14:43–55, 1992

Musselman DL, Lawson DH, Gumnick JF, et al: Paroxetine for the prevention of depression induced by high-dose interferon alfa. N Engl J Med 344:961–966, 2001

Newell SA, Sanson-Fisher RW, Savolainen NJ: Systematic review of psychological therapies for cancer patients: overview and recommendations for future research. J Natl Cancer Inst 94:558–584, 2002

Newport DJ, Nemeroff CB: Assessment and treatment of depression in the cancer patient. J Psychosom Res 45:215–237, 1998

Noyes R, Holt CS, Massie MJ: Anxiety disorders, in Pyscho-Oncology. Edited by Holland JC. New York, Oxford University Press, 1998, pp 548–563

Nuland SB: How We Die: Reflections on Life's Final Chapter. New York, Knopf, 1994

Passik SD, Dugan W, McDonald MV, et al: Oncologists' recognition of depression in their patients with cancer. J Clin Oncol 16:1594–1600, 1998

Patkar AA, Hill KP, Weinstein SP, et al: ECT in the presence of brain tumor and increased intracranial pressure: evaluation and reduction of risk. J ECT 16:189–197, 2000

Payne DK, Biggs C, Tran KN, et al: Women's regrets after bilateral prophylactic mastectomy. Ann Surg Oncol 7:150–154, 2000

Persky VW, Kempthorne-Rawson J, Shekelle RB: Personality and risk of cancer: 20 year follow-up of the Western Electric Study. Psychosom Med 49: 435–449, 1987

Phillips K-A, Bernhard J: Adjuvant breast cancer treatment and cognitive function: current knowledge and research directions. J Natl Cancer Inst 95:190–197, 2003

Phipps S, Dunavant M, Srivastava DK, et al: Cognitive and academic functioning in survivors of pediatric bone marrow transplantation. J Clin Oncol 18:1004–1011, 2000

Pirl WF, Siegel GI, Goode MJ, et al: Depression in men receiving androgen deprivation therapy for prostate cancer: a pilot study. Psychooncology 11:518–523, 2002

Pitman RK, Lanes DM, Williston SK, et al: Psychophysiologic assessment of post-traumatic stress disorder in breast cancer patients. Psychosomatics 42:133–140, 2001

Pot-Mees CC, Zeitlin H: Psychosocial consequences of bone marrow transplantation in children: a preliminary communication. Journal of Psychosocial Oncology 5:73–78, 1987

Ragland DR, Brand RJ, Fox BH: Type A behavior and cancer mortality in the Western Collaborative Group Study (abstract). Psychosom Med 49:209, 1987

Ramirez AJ, Craig TK, Watson JP, et al: Stress and relapse of breast cancer. BMJ 298:291–293, 1989

Ramsey SD, Berry K, Moinpour C, et al: Quality of life in long term survivors of colorectal cancer. Am J Gastroenterol 97:1228–1234, 2002

Redd WH: Management of anticipatory nausea and vomiting, in Handbook of Psycho-Oncology. Edited by Holland JC, Rowland J. New York, Oxford University Press, 1989, pp 423–433

Robson ME, Offit K: Considerations in genetic counseling for inherited breast cancer predisposition. Semin Radiat Oncol 12:362–370, 2002

Robson ME, Boyd J, Borgen PI, et al: Hereditary breast cancer. Curr Probl Surg 38:377–480, 2001

Roth A, Passik SD: Anxiety in men with prostate cancer may interfere with effective management of the disease. Primary Care and Cancer 16:30, 1996

Roth AJ, Kornblith AB, Barel-Copel L, et al: Rapid screening for psychological distress in men with prostate carcinoma: a pilot study. Cancer 82:1904–1908, 1998

Roth AJ, McClear KZ, Massie MJ: Oncology, in Psychiatric Care of the Medical Patient. Edited by Stoudemire A, Fogel BS, Greenberg D. New York, Oxford University Press, 2000, pp 733–756

Rowland JR, Massie MJ: Psychosocial issues and interventions, in Diseases of the Breast, 3rd Edition. Edited by Harris JR, Lippman ME, Morrow M, et al. Philadelphia, PA, Lippincott Williams & Wilkens, 2004, pp 1419–1452

Rozans M, Dreisbach A, Lertora JJ, et al: Palliative uses of methylphenidate in patients with cancer: a review. J Clin Oncol 20:335–339, 2002

Sahay TB, Gray RE, Fitch M: A qualitative study of patient perspectives on colorectal cancer. Cancer Pract 8:38–44, 2000

Sanderson L, Patten CH, Ebbert JO: Tobacco use outcomes among patients with lung cancer treated for nicotine dependence. J Clin Oncol 20:3461–3469, 2002

Sarna L, Padilla G, Holmes C, et al: Quality of life of long-term survivors on non-small-cell lung cancer. J Clin Oncol 20:2920–2929, 2002

Sasaki T, Akaho R, Sakamaki H, et al: Mental disturbances during isolation in bone marrow transplant patients with leukemia. Bone Marrow Transplant 25:315–318, 2000

Schleifer SJ, Keller SE, Camerino M, et al: Suppression of lymphocyte stimulation following bereavement. JAMA 250:374–377, 1983

Schover LR: Sexuality and Fertility After Cancer. New York, Wiley, 1997

Shekelle RB, Raynor WJ, Ostfeld AM, et al: Psychological depression and 17-year risk of death from cancer. Psychosom Med 43:117–125, 1981

Siston AK, List MA, Daugherty CK, et al: Psychosocial adjustment of (40) patients and (39) caregivers prior to allogenic bone marrow transplant. Bone Marrow Transplant 27:1181–1188, 2001

Spiegel D, Bloom JR, Kramer HJC, et al: Effect of psychosocial treatment on survival of patients with metastatic breast cancer. Lancet 14:88–89, 1989

Stark D, Kiely M, Smith A, et al: Anxiety disorders in cancer patients: their nature, associations, and relation to quality of life. J Clin Oncol 20:3137–3148, 2002

Stearns V, Isaacs C, Rowland J, et al: A pilot trial assessing the efficacy of paroxetine hydrochloride (Paxil) in controlling hot flashes in breast cancer survivors. Ann Oncol 11:17–22, 2000

Steingart AB, Cotterchio M: Do antidepressants cause, promote, or inhibit cancers. J Clin Epidemiol 48:1407–1412, 1995

Temoshok L, Heller BW, Sageview RW, et al: The relationship of psychological factors of prognostic indicators in cutaneous malignant melanoma. J Psychosom Res 29:138–153, 1985

Theobald DE, Kirsh KL, Holtsclas E, et al: An open-label, crossover trial of mirtazapine (15 and 30 mg) in cancer patients with pain and other distressing symptoms. J Pain Symptom Manage 23:7–8, 2002

Theoharides T, Konstantinidou A: Antidepressants and risk of cancer: a case of misguided associations and priorities. J Clin Psychopharmacol 23:1–4, 2003

Trask PC: Assessment of depression in cancer patients. J Natl Cancer Inst Monogr 32:80–92, 2004

Tschuschke V, Hertenstein B, Arnold R, et al: Associations between coping and survival time of adult leukemia patients receiving allogeneic bone arrow transplantation: results of a prospective study. J Psychosom Res 50:277–285, 2001

Uchitomi Y, Mikami I, Nagai K, et al: Depression and psychological distress in patients during the year after curative resection of non-small-cell lung cancer. J Clin Oncol 21:69–77, 2003

Vogt T, Pope C, Mullooly J, et al: Mental health status as a predictor of morbidity and mortality: a 15-year follow-up of members of a health maintenance organization. Am J Public Health 84:227–231, 1994

Watson M, Haviland JS, Greer S, et al: Influence of psychological response on survival in breast cancer: a population-based cohort study. Lancet 354:1331–1336, 1999

Weber BL, Punzalan C, Eisen A, et al: Ovarian cancer risk reduction after bilateral prophylactic oophorectomy (BPO) in BRCA1 and BRCA2 mutation carriers (abstract). Am J Hum Genet 67 (suppl):59, 2000

Wei JT, Dunn RL, Sandler HM, et al: Comprehensive comparison of health related quality of life after contemporary therapies for localized prostate cancer. J Clin Oncol 20:557–566, 2002

Weisman AD: Coping with Cancer. New York, McGraw-Hill, 1979

Weisman AD: Vulnerable Self. New York, Plenum, 1993

Weitzner MA, Moncello J, Jacobsen PB, et al: A pilot trial of paroxetine for the treatment of hot flashes and associated symptoms in women with breast cancer. J Pain Symptom Manage 23:337–345, 2002

Wellisch DK, Centeno J, Guzman J, et al: Bone marrow transplantation vs. high-dose cytarabine-based consolidation chemotherapy for acute myelogenous leukemia. A long-term follow-up study of quality of life measures of survivors. Psychosomatics 37:144–154, 1996

Wettergren L, Langius A, Bjorkholm M, et al: Physical and psychosocial functioning in patients undergoing autologous bone marrow transplantation—a prospective study. Bone Marrow Transplant 20:497–502, 1997

Worden JW, Weisman AD: Preventive psychosocial intervention with newly diagnosed cancer patients. Gen Hosp Psychiatry 6:243–249, 1984

25 Rheumatology

Chris Dickens, M.B.B.S., Ph.D.

James L. Levenson, M.D.

Wendy Cohen, M.D.

RHEUMATOLOGICAL DISORDERS are an overlapping group of conditions that are characterized by chronic inflammation involving connective tissues and organs. The disorders arise as the result of autoimmune processes, and the various diseases are differentiated on the basis of the clinical presentation and the patterns of immune disturbance.

In the following chapter, we describe aspects of the rheumatological disorders that are likely to be relevant to a clinician working in the field of psychosomatic medicine. Most of the chapter is devoted to rheumatoid arthritis (RA) and systemic lupus erythematosus (SLE), because these disorders are likely to be encountered most commonly; other disorders, including osteoarthritis, Sjögren's syndrome, systemic sclerosis, temporal arteritis, polymyositis, polyarteritis nodosa, Behçet's disease, and Wegener's granulomatosis, are also discussed. Issues relating to the psychiatric problems resulting from treatments are dealt with at the end of the chapter because of the considerable degree of overlap between the different disease states. Fibromyalgia is covered in Chapter 26, "Chronic Fatigue and Fibromyalgia Syndromes."

General Principles of Diagnosis and Assessment

Detecting Central Nervous System Involvement in Rheumatological Disorders

Although many clinical signs and symptoms, as well as laboratory test results, are suggestive of neuropsychiatric involvement, none is diagnostic. Diagnosis is primarily based on a constellation of clinical findings, lab test results, and neuroimaging that are corroboratory and that exclude comorbid conditions and secondary causes of neuropsychiatric symptoms (Sibbitt et al. 1999).

Mental Status Examination and Neuropsychological Testing

The mental status examination is the most sensitive, available, and least expensive tool for detecting and tracking neuropsychiatric status in rheumatological disorders. Neuropsychological testing provides a more detailed, sensitive assessment of cognitive function, but it is not specific. Even in the absence of any rheumatological disorder, neuropsychiatric testing often reveals subtle cognitive abnormalities; consequently, such findings are not necessarily diagnostic of active neuropsychiatric rheumatological disease (Carbotte et al. 1995).

Laboratory Tests

No laboratory test, or set of tests, is considered diagnostic of neuropsychiatric involvement in rheumatological disorders. Nevertheless, laboratory studies serve two purposes. First, they help rule out infection, as well as other complications of rheumatological disorders or their treatment that can present with neuropsychiatric symptoms. Second, positive laboratory results confirm the presence of rheumatological disease activity. Although neuropsychiatric involvement can pursue a clinical course somewhat independent of flares in other organs, high disease activity increases the likelihood of primary central nervous system (CNS) involvement, because the pathogenesis is shared. However, the absence of systemic disease activity does not preclude CNS involvement. Moreover, systemic disease activity seems to have little, if any, correlation with certain neuropsychiatric symptoms, particularly fatigue and cognitive dysfunction (Carbotte et al. 1995; Waterloo et al. 2002).

Laboratory tests can also be useful in evaluating psychiatric symptoms in rheumatology patients with a history of a primary psychiatric illness such as schizophrenia or major depression. Primary psychiatric disorders do not cause elevations in erythrocyte sedimentation rate (ESR) or other markers of inflammation. Accordingly, if the psychiatric symptoms temporally coincide with a markedly increased ESR, then medical etiologies, particularly infection and CNS involvement, must be strongly considered.

When rheumatology patients have neuropsychiatric symptoms, lumbar puncture is indicated to rule out CNS infection and assess the degree of disease activity in the CNS. In patients without CNS infection, cerebrospinal fluid (CSF) pleocytosis and increased CSF protein are suggestive of CNS involvement by lupus or other rheumatological disease (West 1994). In addition, CSF studies should include oligoclonal bands, which are only present in a small number of disorders, including neurosyphilis, Lyme disease, multiple sclerosis, Sjögren's syndrome, and CNS SLE. A number of other CSF tests have been associated with neuropsychiatric SLE but are not widely available or timely (W. Cohen et al. 2004).

Electroencephalogram

In patients with rheumatological disorders who also have neuropsychiatric symptoms, the electroencephalogram (EEG) is often abnormal but seldom useful (Waterloo et al. 1999), except in diagnosing subclinical seizure activity or differentiating hypoactive delirium (diffuse slowing on EEG) from depression (normal EEG).

Neuroimaging

Although magnetic resonance imaging (MRI) is the best available imaging technique for identifying focal neurological lesions in patients with rheumatological disorders and neuropsychiatric symptoms, it is inherently limited because it detects only structural lesions, whereas the pathophysiology of the neuropsychiatric problems can be entirely functional. Also, MRI cannot reliably differentiate active from chronic lesions resulting from a previous neuropsychiatric insult (Sabbadini et al. 1999).

Detecting, Diagnosing, and Quantifying Psychiatric Symptoms and Disorders

Despite their high prevalence and significant impact on the patient's illness and overall quality of life, psychiatric disorders remain mostly unrecognized and undertreated in patients with rheumatological disorders. This under-recognition is partly attributable to a tendency to focus on the physical aspects of disease, coupled with limited resources in some health care systems. The problem of undertreatment of depression in rheumatological disorders is exacerbated by a misconception that because depression is understandable, occurring secondary to the pain and disability, treatment of the depression is not appropriate or necessary (Rifkin 1992). Furthermore, diagnosing depression in patients with rheumatological disorders is complicated because there is an overlap in symptoms of depression and rheumatological disorders (e.g., fatigue, weight loss, insomnia, and lack of appetite) such that the depression frequently goes unrecognized (Rifkin 1992).

Use of standardized psychiatric questionnaires (the Minnesota Multiphasic Personality Inventory, the Beck Depression Inventory [BDI], and the Center for Epidemiologic Studies Depression Scale) tends to overestimate the prevalence of depression, because many questionnaires include somatic symptoms that may be attributable to the rheumatological disorders (Callahan et al. 1991; Pincus et al. 1986). Scales that have little somatic content, such as the Geriatric Depression Scale (Sheikh and Yesavage 1989), the Hospital Anxiety and Depression Scale (HADS) (Zigmond and Snaith 1983), or disease-specific instruments (Smedstad et al. 1995) may aid accurate diagnosis of depression in such patients. These self-rated questionnaires may be used by rheumatologists or specialist nurses to identify probable cases of psychiatric disorder. With additional training in the use of follow-up questions to confirm cases of depression, rheumatologists can initiate antidepressant treatment where indicated, thus avoiding referrals to psychiatrists in uncomplicated cases.

Complex cases will require more detailed assessment by a psychosomatic medicine specialist. In addition to assessing the patient's current mental state, the specialist psychiatrist should explore the development of psychiatric symptoms and how these relate to the recent disease state and changes in management, availability of social support, psychosocial stresses resulting from pain and disability, and stresses independent of the illness. Inquiries about maladaptive coping strategies to physical symptoms (e.g., "I just lie down and wait for my symptoms to ease"; "I simply avoid activities that cause me pain") can identify fruitful targets for psychological interventions. Assessing past psychiatric history and family history will help identify which patients are most vulnerable to developing depression and other psychiatric disorders. Finally, investigating the patient's personal beliefs about the illness, such as the perceived causes, possible outcomes, and likelihood of controlling disease progression through treatment, can identify psychological mechanisms by which psychiatric problems have arisen.

General Principles of Treatment

Primary Neuropsychiatric Involvement

When rheumatological diseases affect the CNS, the primary treatment is *corticosteroids* when the pathophysiology is thought to be neuronal injury or inflammation resulting from autoantibodies, and *anticoagulants* when hypercoagulability is involved (e.g., the anticardiolipin antibody syndrome). When corticosteroids are ineffective, other immunosuppressive agents may be helpful.

Primary Psychiatric Disorders

Intervention studies have shown that psychological treatments, mostly cognitive and behavioral, are effective in reducing psychological distress and improving coping in subjects with rheumatological disorders (Bradley et al. 1987; Sharpe et al. 2001). In addition, such therapies may reduce pain and improve functioning, though it is unclear whether any of these effects is mediated by changes to the inflammatory state (Bradley et al. 1987; Sharpe et al. 2001).

Psychological interventions should always be considered in patients with rheumatological disorders who have psychiatric problems. Because of easier access, pharmacological interventions are more often used, with psychological therapies usually reserved for more complex cases. Cognitive-behavioral principles, however, can be employed by rheumatologists, specialist nurses, and physical or occupational therapists to optimize patients' care. As a matter of routine, newly diagnosed patients should be educated about the disease and its likely course—an approach that can facilitate adherence. Subjects with severe advanced disease might benefit from psychological adjuncts to physical management. Between these two extremes, maintaining an awareness of the importance of psychological processes in determining illness behavior might help the rheumatologist identify, treat, and make referrals for problems appropriately.

Lack of familiarity with antidepressant drugs among rheumatologists may also contribute to the undertreatment of depression. There is a wide choice of antidepressants currently available to clinicians, yet the majority of these drugs have not undergone assessment of efficacy in patients with physical illness. Current evidence from studies in psychiatric and other chronic pain patient populations indicates that various types of antidepressants, when given in appropriate psychotherapeutic doses, have roughly equal efficacy in the treatment of depression (Anderson et al. 2000). However, they do differ in their analgesic efficacy, tolerability, and profile of drug interactions.

Tricyclic antidepressants (TCAs) with the least specific receptor activity, such as amitriptyline, appear to have the greatest analgesic efficacy (Onghena and Van Houdenhove 1992), even at low doses (e.g., 25 mg of amitriptyline) and independent of whether depression is present or not (Bromm et al. 1986). In higher doses, tolerability and safety are poor, particularly in the elderly. Newer drugs have comparable antidepressant efficacy, although their analgesic efficacy has yet to be established, and they are more expensive. In general, selective serotonin reuptake inhibitors (SSRIs), such as fluoxetine or citalopram, in doses up to recommended maxima should be considered as first-line treatment for depression in RA (Anderson et al. 2000). Gradually introduced TCAs, such as amitriptyline or dothiepin (not available in United States), should be used in low doses (25–75 mg) for pain relief (Onghena and Van Houdenhove 1992). Combined use of TCAs and SSRIs greatly increases the risk of adverse events and should be avoided unless under expert guidance. Drug interactions may occur, although this is not a problem with first- and second-line treatments for RA.

Treatment of anxiety, mania, psychosis, delirium, and pain in rheumatological disorders is similar to their treatment in other medical diseases, following the principles reviewed in other chapters in this book (Chapter 6, "Delirium"; Chapter 11, "Mania, Catatonia, and Psychosis"; Chapter 12, "Anxiety Disorders"; Chapter 36, "Pain").

Rheumatoid Arthritis

Rheumatoid arthritis affects approximately 0.8% of the population (range=0.3% to 2.1%), with women being affected approximately three times more frequently than men. It is a chronic disorder characterized by persistent inflammatory synovitis. Though any synovial joint can be affected, the disease typically involves peripheral small joints in a symmetrical pattern. Inflammation of the synovium can result in destruction of joint cartilage and bony erosions, which can eventually result in destruction of the joint. Extra-articular manifestations are common, with some degree of extra-articular involvement being found in most patients. These extra-articular manifestations vary widely among patients but may include systemic symptoms (anorexia, weight loss, myalgia); more localized abnormalities such as rheumatoid nodules; or involvement of the cardiovascular system (vasculitis, peri-carditis), respiratory system (pleural effusions, pulmonary fibrosis), or CNS (spinal cord compression, peripheral neuropathy). The typical course of RA is prolonged, characterized by relapses and remissions. As the disease advances, progressive joint destruction results in limitations to joint movements, joint instability and deformities that increase pain, and functional disability.

The main aims of treatment of RA are 1) analgesia, 2) reduction of inflammation, 3) joint protection, 4) maintenance of functional ability, and 5) reduction of systemic manifestations. Pharmacological management involves a number of different types of drug treatment.

- Nonsteroidal anti-inflammatory drugs (NSAIDs) control symptoms and signs of local inflammation, although they do not appear to alter the eventual course of the disease.
- A number of drugs have been found that alter the course of the disease by reducing the inflammatory component of RA (e.g., methotrexate, antimalarials, minocycline, and sulfasalazine); gold and penicillamine are almost never used anymore.
- Corticosteroids can be used to reduce signs of inflammation by systemic administrations (oral or parenteral) or by local injection.
- Currently available biological response modifiers include the anti–TNF-alpha therapies—namely, etanercept (Enbrel), infliximab (Remicade), adalimumab (Humira), and an interleukin-1 (IL-1) receptor antagonist, anakinra (Kineret) (Olson et al. 2004).
- Immunosuppressive agents (azathioprine, leflunomide, cyclosporin, and cyclophosphamide) also reduce inflammation in RA, but because of toxicity, their use is limited to patients who are resistant to other treatments.

Neuropsychiatric Disorders in Rheumatological Disorders

Epidemiology

Neuropsychiatric disorders are common in patients with RA, as they are in most chronic illness populations. The wide variation in prevalence figures in the literature may be attributed to the use of self-rated questionnaire assessments to identify cases of psychiatric disorder (Creed 1990). More conservative figures, obtained by using standardized research interviews, indicate that about one-fifth of patients with RA have a psychiatric disorder. Using the Present State Examination, Murphy and colleagues (1988) interviewed a mixed group of inpatients and outpatients with definite or classic RA and found that 21% of subjects

had a psychiatric disorder: 12.5% were depressed, and the remainder were anxious. This study also revealed that a population of RA patients of approximately equal size (19%) had psychiatric symptoms, although they did not meet the criteria for a psychiatric disorder. These prevalence figures are consistent with those from other studies that used standardized research interviews (Frank et al. 1988).

Etiology

Neuropsychiatric manifestations in RA can arise through four processes: 1) direct CNS involvement, 2) secondary effects of the illness or its treatments, 3) emotional reactions to chronic illness, and 4) comorbid primary psychiatric illness.

Involvement of the Central Nervous System in Rheumatoid Arthritis

Despite its multisystem manifestations, neurological complications in RA are not common. When present, the most common is peripheral neuropathy due to entrapment resulting from synovial proliferation or vasculitis. Direct involvement of the CNS is rare. Atlanto-axial subluxation may occur, resulting in transverse myelitis, and is the most widely recognized CNS complication of RA.

Vasculitis in RA can involve cerebral vessels, resulting in cerebral ischemia or infarction, and has been associated with acute and chronic brain syndromes (Ando et al. 1995; Gobernado et al. 1984; Ohta et al. 1998; Singleton et al. 1995). Treatment with corticosteroids can usually alleviate vasculitis and edema, with resultant improvement in symptoms, but impairment from the infarction is permanent. Rarer CNS complications include transient ischemic attacks resulting from RA-associated thrombocytosis (Pines et al. 1982) and embolic phenomena as a consequence of RA-related granulomata in major arteries (Chatzis et al. 1999).

Psychiatric Disorders as a Reaction to Illness

The vast majority of psychiatric disorders in patients with RA are emotional reactions to having RA. Patients experience life stress because of the burden not only of chronic physical symptoms but also of personal losses resulting from RA and associated disability. Albers et al. (1999) found that in 89% of RA patients, the disease adversely affected at least one domain of socioeconomic functioning (work, income, required rest time during day, leisure activity, transport mobility, housing, and social dependency), with 58% experiencing adverse effects in at least three domains. Other social impacts to consider are loss of personal ambitions, loss of social role, loss of future financial security, relationship disturbances, and body image concerns. Social support that might help to offset the stress of RA may be less available because of limited mobility. Furthermore, RA patients may have fewer coping resources available to deal with comorbid illnesses and stresses unrelated to RA. The evidence for the associations of emotional reactions and the various aspects of RA are dealt with next.

Psychological Symptoms and Clinical State

A large number of studies have examined the associations of depression with the physical symptoms of RA. Cross-sectional studies using self-report measures have shown that levels of depressive symptoms are associated with the severity of the pain experienced (Frank et al. 1988; Hurwicz and Berkanovic 1993; Peck et al. 1989; Smedstad et al. 1995; Wolfe 1999), and the degree of functional disability (Brown et al. 1989; Hurwicz and Berkanovic 1993; Pow 1987; Smedstad et al. 1996; Wolfe 1999). Some of the associations observed might be attributable to the use of depression measures such as the BDI, in which physical symptoms associated with the RA itself—for example, disturbed sleep, fatigue, and loss of appetite—are rated as indicators of depression. Exclusion of these somatic items leaves smaller though still significant associations between depression and the physical symptoms of RA (Peck et al. 1989).

Few longitudinal studies have examined whether changes in depression correlate with changes in the severity of RA symptoms. Wolfe et al. found that changes in depression were associated with changes in pain and disability, although only 17% of the variance in depression was accounted for by these two variables, indicating that the degree of association was weak (Wolfe and Hawley 1993).

The literature just cited indicates that psychological symptoms, particularly depression, are most marked in patients with worse pain and disability, although the strength of this association is modest at best. However, it is possible that these studies underestimate the strength of the association of physical symptoms and psychological problems. The measures used to assess physical state are generic assessments of functional ability. If depression is related to loss of function, the value or meaning of the lost activity to the individual could be important. In other words, generic measures provide a broad overview of function but may not be sensitive to what is important to the individual. Katz and Yelin (1995) performed an extremely detailed prospective longitudinal study of women with RA. Subjects were followed for 4 years to identify aspects of function that predicted the development of depression in the final year of the study. Although generic measures of function predicted a fourfold increase in depression, a 10% loss in activities that the individuals had identified as being important to them resulted in a sevenfold increase in depression in the subsequent year.

Furthermore, the vast majority of the research performed in this area has focused on ambulatory outpatients, probably for a combination of ethical and convenience reasons. It is possible that the association between physical and psychiatric symptoms is weak because of the mild to moderate nature of the symptoms in many of the patients studied. Mindham et al. (1981) conducted a prospective study involving a small number of patients with RA. They confirmed the positive association between symptoms of RA and the development of psychiatric symptoms considered to be of "pathological severity," though this association was weak and nonspecific in the majority of their patients. Only in subjects with the most severe and disabling RA did they find an association between symptoms of RA and the development of several psychiatric symptoms together, indicating the development of a psychiatric disorder. Thus, the association between symptoms of RA and psychological symptoms may become more pronounced in subjects with the most severe disease.

Role of Cognitive Factors

The way RA patients think about their illness is crucial to understanding the association of depression with pain and disability. Depression is associated with increased worry about illness and conviction of severe disease (Pilowsky 1993). Depressed RA patients perceive their illness as being more serious and feel hopeless about a cure compared with nondepressed RA patients (Murphy et al. 1999). Furthermore, depressed patients are more likely to have cognitive distortions relating to the RA (Smith et al. 1988). These associations remain significant in RA patients even after the extent of disease and pain levels are controlled, indicating that the association between depression and negative appraisals of health status is not simply the result of depressed people having more severe illness.

The way people think about or understand their illness is also important, because it influences the way RA patients cope with the illness. According to Leventhal's model, individuals hold personal representations and beliefs about their health and any threat posed to it (Leventhal et al. 1997). These personal representations have both cognitive and emotional components, are based on a lay knowledge or understanding of health and illness, and thus may significantly differ from those of the consulting clinician. Patients' perceptions of a health threat initiate the use of coping strategies, the results of which are then appraised and may result in a change in the representations or a revision of the strategy. Coping strategies may be broadly described as adaptive if they result in normalization of a patient's life—that is, minimizing symptom impact—or maladaptive if they result in increased dependency. Depression is associated with impairment of general coping, especially at high levels of pain (Brown et al. 1989; Hurwicz and Berkanovic 1993).

Thus, psychiatric disorders, particularly depression, appear to be associated with a more negative appraisal of the illness and impairment in ability to cope with the illness. As such, these cognitive factors may act as mediators in the association between the physical symptoms of RA and psychiatric disorders. It should be recognized, however, that the amount of variance in depression accounted for by perceived control, coping ability, and cognitive distortions is small, with the majority being unexplained (Persson et al. 1999)

Other Psychosocial Factors

A number of other psychosocial factors that may predispose any RA patient toward psychiatric problems have been suggested.

Neuroticism

Some individuals are predisposed to experience and react to stress, including health stress, in a negative way. People with such negative affectivity, or *neuroticism*, have been shown to be more sensitive to physical sensations (Harkins et al. 1989; Larsen 1992), interpret physical sensations as threatening (Larsen 1992), experience more emotional distress regardless of the environment (Ormel and Wohlfart 1991), and choose less effective coping strategies (Bolger and Schilling 1991; Bolger and Zuckerman 1995). The importance of neuroticism has been confirmed in patients with RA. In a prospective study, RA patients completed daily reports on joint pain and mood for a period of 75 days. Those scoring higher on neuroticism experienced more chronic distress, regardless of their pain intensity (Affleck et al. 1992).

Social Support

It is recognized that social support is associated with health and good quality of life in the general population (S. Cohen and Wills 1985). A number of studies have demonstrated that social support benefits patients with RA (Goodenow et al. 1990). In patients with RA, social support, and its actual or perceived availability, have been

shown to be associated with use of more adaptive coping strategies (Manne and Zautra 1989), greater perception of ability to control the disease (Spitzer et al. 1995), and less psychological distress (Affleck et al. 1988; Doeglas et al. 1994; Evers et al. 1997, 1998; Revenson et al. 1991). Not all social contacts are supportive, however, and critical or punishing comments are associated with increased psychological distress (Griffin et al. 2001; Kraaimaat et al. 1995; Revenson et al. 1991).

Rheumatoid arthritis has an adverse effect on the availability of social support to its patients, however. Patients with RA have been shown to have reduced social networks and social support (Fitzpatrick et al. 1991; Fyrand et al. 2000, 2001). This disruption of social support appears to be greatest in those with disease of greatest duration with most severe functional disability, possibly caused by a significant reduction in the availability of important others to patients with RA (Murphy et al. 1988).

Social Stresses

Social stresses are recognized as being potent causes of depression in the general population. Particularly important in causing depression are those stresses in which the degree of threat to the individual is great—so-called severe events and marked difficulties (Brown and Harris 1979). As indicated previously, in addition to the burden of the symptoms, RA patients experience considerable hardship in association with their chronic illness. Social stresses independent of those of RA are also likely to contribute to the development of depression in RA patients, however. In fact, among ambulatory outpatients the stresses independent of RA may well have a greater importance in predicting depression than the RA-related stresses (Dickens et al. 2003). The findings of this study indicate that in patients with mild to moderate arthritis, RA-related life difficulties cause psychological distress that does not amount to a full-blown psychiatric disorder, perhaps because the degree of threat is not marked. The combination of RA-related and RA-independent stresses, however, is sufficient to cause a depressive disorder. Clearly, in subjects with the most severe, disabling arthritis, the situation is likely to be different, with RA-related difficulties alone being a sufficiently potent stress to result in depressive disorder (Mindham et al. 1981).

A number of studies have suggested that social stresses might play an important part in triggering the onset of RA in adults (G.H.B. Baker and Brewerton 1981; Hendrie et al. 1971; Rimon 1969; Shochet et al. 1969). All of these studies use unreliable retrospective measures that could be contaminated by the RA patients' effort to explain the onset of their disease by linking it spuriously with life events occurring around the time of the onset of the symptoms: Three studies used unstructured interviews, and one used a simple scale. In the most careful research in this area (Conway et al. 1994), 60 consecutive outpatients with RA were studied with the most reliable method of assessing life events, the Life Events and Difficulties Schedule (Brown and Harris 1979). This semi-standardized research interview allowed the researcher to ask questions in detail about the timing of any life stresses, and the severity of the stress was rated by a panel blinded to the details of the illness. In this study there was no evidence of an excess of stressful events in the 12 months preceding the onset of RA. However, there was no control group in this study, and the researchers' findings relied on comparisons with so-called normal populations. More research is needed in this area.

Impact of Mental Disorders

The mechanisms by which depression influences pain and disability are also poorly understood. Although depression and psychological stress have been shown to result in immune dysfunction (Herbert and Cohen 1993), there is no evidence to suggest that depression increases the pain and disability of RA by changing the underlying inflammatory activity. Studies suggesting that depression increases disease activity, or that psychological treatment reduces RA activity, have mostly relied on clinical assessments of disease activity such as counting tender joints (Bradley et al. 1987). Such clinical assessments rely on patient reports of tenderness and are vulnerable to the effects of depression, including pessimistic self-perception and the negative way patients react to their illness.

Few studies have shown that psychological interventions improve biological markers of disease activity in RA (e.g., ESR, C-reactive protein [CRP], or rheumatoid factors). In a recent blind, controlled trial of a cognitive-behavioral therapy (CBT) intervention for patients in an early stage of RA, those receiving adjunctive CBT versus standard treatment showed an improvement in CRP (but not ESR) immediately following therapy, but this effect was lost by 6 months (Sharpe et al. 2001). It remains unclear whether this was a direct effect of the CBT on inflammatory activity or a result of behavior-mediating factors, which seems more likely, such as improved compliance with treatment in the intensively followed-up group.

As mentioned previously, psychiatric disorders, particularly anxiety and depression, are associated with more negative illness cognitions in RA. As a result of these negative illness cognitions, health-seeking behaviors and health care utilization may increase as they do in other medical patients (Macfarlane et al. 1999; Manning and Wells 1992; Wells et al. 1989). Depressed RA patients are more likely to report physical symptoms (Murphy et al. 1999), less likely to be reassured by a doctor (Pilowsky 1993), and less likely to comply with medications (DiMatteo et al. 2000). We know there is an immense variation in the health care costs among subjects that is not directly related to the severity of RA (Lubeck et al. 1986; Simon et al. 1995). Depression is likely to contribute to these hitherto unexplained costs. The impact of depression on indirect (social) costs is likely to be even greater (Yelin et al. 1979).

Osteoarthritis

Osteoarthritis (OA) is the most common joint disease, with the idiopathic form being the most prevalent. Secondary OA arises most frequently as the result of trauma (acute or chronic), although it also may occur in a variety of metabolic and endocrine disorders. The prevalence of OA increases sharply with age: less than 2% of women younger than 45 years are affected, compared with 30% of those between 45 and 64 years of age and 68% of those older than 65 years.

The pattern of joint involvement varies with age and sex; OA involving the hip is more common in older men, whereas involvement of the interphalangeal joints and of the first metacarpophalangeal joint is more common in elderly women. Previous joint overload—in particular, repetitive incidences, as in vocational injuries—have a considerable influence on the distribution of joint involvement. Clinically affected joints are painful, especially on movement, and are stiff after a period of inactivity. In later stages of the disease, movements are limited, and joint instability may occur, which is exacerbated by atrophy of muscles adjacent to the affected joint.

There has been considerably less research interest in the causes, prevalence, and impact of psychological disorders in OA compared with those in other musculoskeletal disorders. Because direct involvement of the CNS is not a feature of primary OA, one can conclude that psychological disorders in patients with this disorder arise either as a reaction to the pain, disability, and life difficulties related to the OA or for reasons independent of the OA.

In regard to the prevalence of psychological disorders, depression was found to be no more common in a community sample of persons with OA than in the general population (Dexter et al. 1994). The extremely high prevalence of OA in the population means that a large proportion of those with the disease experience relatively minor pain and disability from their OA. These people are not troubled excessively by their OA, they do not seek medical care, and adverse psychological sequelae are not common. In a study of patients with a variety of musculoskeletal disorders who were attending a secondary care facility, patients with OA of the knee or hand tended to have slightly lower scores on an standardized assessment of depression compared with patients with other musculoskeletal disorders (Hawley et al. 1993). These results taken together indicate that OA is less closely associated with depression than is RA, although studies of patients with more advanced disease are required.

When depression does occur in patients with OA, it has been shown to be associated with a number of factors: younger age, less education, higher pain, and greater self-reported impact of the OA (Dexter et al. 1994; van Baar et al. 1998; Zautra et al. 2001). Other psychological factors such as anxiety and hopelessness have been shown to be associated with functional disability (Creamer et al. 2000).

Few intervention studies have examined the efficacy of antidepressants and psychological therapies in OA. Those that have been performed suggest that both antidepressants and cognitive-behavioral therapy are efficacious in the treatment of depression in patients with OA and that improvement in depression is associated with reduced pain and disability from the disease (Calfas et al. 1992; Lin et al. 2003).

Systemic Lupus Erythematosus

SLE is an autoimmune disorder of unknown cause characterized by immune dysregulation with tissue damage caused by pathogenic autoantibodies, immune complexes, and T lymphocytes. Approximately 90% of cases are in women, usually of childbearing age. The incidence is 2.4 per 100,000 across genders and race, 9.2 for black women and 3.5 for white women; and prevalence rates are 90 per 100,000 for white women and 280 for black women. Asians are also more often affected than whites. At onset, SLE may involve one or multiple organ systems. Common clinical manifestations include cutaneous lesions (photosensitivity, malar or discoid rash, oral ulcers), constitutional symptoms (fatigue, weight loss, fevers), arthralgias and frank arthritis, serositis (pericarditis or pleuritis), renal disease, neuropsychiatric disorders, and hematological disorders (anemia, leukopenia). Autoantibodies are detectable at presentation in most cases. The spectrum of treatment options in SLE is similar to that in RA: namely, NSAIDs, antimalarials (e.g., hydroxychloroquine), corticosteroids, and other immunosuppressants (e.g., azathioprine, mycophenolate mofetil, methotrexate, cyclophosphamide). The role of biological response modifiers is currently under investigation, but none is now approved for this indication.

In addition, anticoagulants are used in SLE patients who have antiphospholipid antibodies if there is a history of arterial or venous thrombosis. The rate of 20-year survival has been reported to be 50%–70% (Lahita 2004) but is improving with newer immunosuppressive treatments.

Psychiatric Manifestations

Neuropsychiatric symptoms of SLE were first reported in 1872 by Kaposi (1872). Depending on the diagnostic methodology used, neuropsychiatric manifestations have a prevalence of up to 75%–90% (Ainiala et al. 2001a; West 1994), ranging from stroke, seizures, headaches, neuropathy, transverse myelitis, and movement disorders, to cognitive deficits, depression, mania, anxiety, psychosis, and delirium. CNS involvement is a major cause of morbidity in SLE, second only to renal failure as a cause of mortality. The pathogenesis of neuropsychiatric syndromes in SLE is complex. For a more detailed review of psychiatric aspects of SLE, see W. Cohen et al. 2004.

Pathogenesis of Neuropsychiatric Manifestations

Psychiatric syndromes in SLE can be caused by 1) direct CNS involvement; 2) infection, other systemic illness, or drug-induced side effects; 3) reaction to chronic illness; or 4) comorbid primary psychiatric illness.

Direct Pathophysiological CNS Effects

Two major antibody-mediated mechanisms of CNS injury have been proposed: neuronal injury and microvasculopathy (Scolding and Joseph 2002). Autoantibodies may directly damage neurons by either causing cell death or transiently and reversibly impairing neuronal function. Antibody-mediated microvasculopathy seems to involve two processes: either endothelial damage (Wierzbicki 2000) or coagulation disturbances resulting from the prothrombotic effects of antiphospholipid (including anticardiolipin) antibodies (Gharavi 2001), both culminating in ischemia or infarction. These two pathogenic mechanisms may be mutually reinforcing, perpetuating the disease process. Microvascular endothelial injury in the CNS may increase the permeability of the blood-brain barrier, leading to influx of autoantibodies and further CNS damage.

Autoimmune antibodies seem to play a much larger role in direct CNS involvement (Jennekens and Kater 2002; Scolding and Joseph 2002) than does immune complex deposition. Antiribosomal-P antibodies have been associated with psychosis (Isshi and Hirohata 1998) and severe depression (Arnett et al. 1996), but not consistently (Gerli 2002). Antineuronal antibodies have been associated with psychosis, depression, delirium, coma, and cognitive dysfunction (West et al. 1995). In contrast, antiphospholipid antibodies (e.g., anticardiolipin) cause focal deficits (strokes) and cognitive dysfunction (Levine et al. 2002; Menon et al. 1999; West et al. 1995). Cytokines also appear to be involved in the pathogenesis of neuropsychiatric SLE, although their role remains unclear.

With the possible exception of cognitive dysfunction, all the major psychiatric manifestations of SLE (i.e., psychosis, depression, mania, anxiety, and delirium) exhibit a degree of reversibility, as does coma. Even the cognitive deficits sometimes respond to corticosteroids (Denburg et al. 1994; Hanly et al. 1997). Because psychiatric syndromes tend to resolve within 2–3 weeks with corticosteroid treatment (Denburget al. 1994), they are probably caused by reversible or transient mechanisms rather than irreversible neuronal death. The reversibility of psychiatric dysfunction stands in contrast to most focal neurological events, which often have no more reversibility than atherosclerotic stroke and are associated with fixed lesions on neuroimaging. Similarly, in some patients, the progressive nature of cognitive impairment (Hanly et al. 1997; Menon ct a1. 1999), often with cerebral atrophy, suggests cumulative irreversible CNS damage.

Risk factors for direct CNS involvement in SLE include cutaneous vasculitis and antiphospholipid syndrome and its manifestations, especially arterial thromboses (Karassa et al. 2000). Patients with mainly articular manifestations or discoid rash have a much lower risk of neuropsychiatric lupus, as do those few who are antinuclear antibody (ANA)–negative and those with drug-induced SLE. Antiphospholipid antibodies may be the single strongest marker of CNS risk, because they are associated with stroke, cognitive dysfunction, and epilepsy (Herranz 1994; Sabet et al. 1998).

Psychological Impact

Coping with SLE is particularly challenging because lupus is a chronic, often debilitating multisystem illness, and its course is unpredictable. Because SLE can involve almost any organ system or include vague systemic symptoms, the diagnosis is often elusive. The inability to make a diagnosis may erode the patient's confidence in the medical system, and when no etiology can be found, the physician may deem the illness psychogenic. Given that SLE can affect many organ systems, patients may worry that the illness pervades their entire body, even when the disease is limited. The diffuse nature of SLE distinguishes it from most other chronic, recurrent diseases, such as asthma or inflammatory bowel disease, which are primarily limited to one organ. SLE patients are often under the care of an entourage of specialists, which may frag-

ment care. One of the most stressful aspects of SLE is its unpredictable course, with sudden exacerbations, remissions, and variable prognoses, resulting in a profound loss of control, as well as a loss of ability to plan for the future.

Psychological reactions to having SLE are common and include grief, depression, anxiety, regression, denial, and invalidism. A feeling of isolation is reinforced by public ignorance about lupus. People with SLE may become socially withdrawn, especially if they are self-conscious about their appearance. Women with a malar rash or discoid lesions may feel branded as if by the "scarlet letter." (Perry and Miller 1992). The most prevalent fears of SLE patients are worsening disease, disability, and death. In particular, patients fear cognitive impairment, stroke, renal failure, and becoming a burden on their families (Liang et al. 1984). Although negative reactions to having SLE are common, at least 50% of patients experience positive reactions at some point during their illness (Liang et al. 1984).

Stress and SLE

Although stress may cause a lupus flare, it is also likely, if not inevitable, that lupus flares cause stress. Several studies have provided support for stress-induced immune dysregulation in SLE. In response to acoustic, psychological, and exercise-induced stress, the normal increase in B- and T-suppressor or cytotoxic lymphocytes and decrease in T-helper lymphocytes are blunted in SLE patients, relative to healthy control subjects, patients with sarcoidosis, and others receiving corticosteroids (Ferstl et al. 1992; Hinrichsen 1989). Stress (because of public speaking) was associated with a transient increase in interleukin-4 (IL-4)–producing cells in SLE patients, but not in healthy control subjects. This immune response might precipitate a flare because IL-4–producing cells cause proliferation of activated B cells and, consequently, increased autoantibody production (Jacobs et al. 2001). In a 6-month prospective study of 41 patients with SLE, daily stress correlated positively with ANAs and anti-double-stranded DNA antibodies (Pawlak et al. 2003).

Whether stress precipitates onset or exacerbation of SLE symptoms has received relatively little study. There is only one controlled study demonstrating that 20 patients hospitalized for SLE had significantly greater stress prior to the onset of their illness than did the seriously ill hospitalized controls (Otto and Mackay 1967). Retrospective uncontrolled studies link lupus flares to preceding stress (Hall et al. 1981; Ropes 1976). However, in a naturalistic study after a severe earthquake in Los Angeles, none of the rheumatology patients studied (10 with SLE and 13 with rheumatoid arthritis) residing near the epicenter developed a significant flare of illness (Wallace and Metzger 1994).

Classification of Psychiatric Disorders in Systemic Lupus Erythematosus

The literature on neuropsychiatric SLE has been plagued by terminology that has been imprecise and unstandardized. Terms such as "lupus cerebritis" have obfuscated our understanding because they imply a pathogenesis (inflammation) that remains unproven. Furthermore, because there is no gold standard for the diagnosis of neuropsychiatric SLE, ascertaining which conditions are direct CNS manifestations of SLE versus a reaction to illness has been controversial. To rectify these problems, the American College of Rheumatology (ACR) convened a committee to develop a standardized nomenclature for neuropsychiatric SLE, and guidelines were published in 1999 (American College of Rheumatology Ad Hoc Committee 1999). The guidelines defined neuropsychiatric lupus as "the neurological syndromes of the central, peripheral, and autonomic nervous systems, and the psychiatric syndromes observed in patients with SLE in which other causes have been excluded." Psychiatric disorders included psychosis, acute confusional state, cognitive dysfunction, anxiety disorder, and mood disorders. Overall, the ACR criteria significantly broadened the spectrum of syndromes that can be considered neuropsychiatric SLE (American College of Rheumatology Ad Hoc Committee 1999). The criteria have good sensitivity but low specificity (Ainiala et al. 2001b), making them better suited for identifying all possible cases of neuropsychiatric SLE. A more fundamental problem with the ACR classification system is that it is difficult to apply clinically. To diagnose neuropsychiatric SLE as the cause of the psychiatric symptoms, one must exclude a primary psychiatric disorder. In contrast, in DSM-IV and its text revision, DSM-IV-TR (American Psychiatric Association 1994, 2000), a primary psychiatric disorder cannot be diagnosed unless medical disorders and substance use are ruled out as etiologies. Whereas medical disorders and substance use can be easily excluded, there are no clinical criteria or laboratory tests for excluding primary psychiatric disorders. For example, if a patient with SLE becomes depressed, it is unclear how one would rule out primary depression as the cause.

Cognitive dysfunction is the most common neuropsychiatric disorder in patients with SLE, occurring in up to 80% of patients (Ainiala et al. 2001a; Denburg et al. 1994). On neuropsychological testing, even patients who have never had overt neuropsychiatric symptoms are often found to have cognitive impairment. Patients with anticardiolipin antibodies have a three- to fourfold increased risk of cognitive impairment, which is often progressive (Hanly et al. 1997; Menon et al. 1999). Cognitive impairment may be associated with lymphocytotoxic antibodies, CSF antineuronal antibodies, and pathological findings such as microinfarcts and cortical atrophy. Although cognitive dysfunction often fluctuates and is reversible (Hanly et al. 1997; Hay et al. 1994), presumably when attributable to edema and inflammation, it tends to be irreversible when secondary to multiple infarcts and may culminate in dementia.

Depression is the second most common neuropsychiatric disorder in SLE. The reported prevalence of depression has varied widely, depending on the diagnostic criteria, patient population, and study design. Using structured interviews, the prevalence of depression in SLE has been approximately 50% (Giang 1991). Depression may be a preexisting primary psychiatric disorder; an iatrogenically induced illness, particularly from corticosteroids; a reaction to having a chronic disease; and, possibly, a direct CNS manifestation of lupus. The question of whether depression is a direct manifestation of CNS SLE or a reaction to the stress and multiple losses associated with having a chronic debilitating illness remains unresolved (for a review of the evidence, see W. Cohen et al. 2004). Diagnosing depression in SLE is confounded by the overlap between depressive symptoms and those associated with SLE or its treatment. Hypothyroidism should be ruled out, because it can mimic depression and is more common in SLE than in the general population.

Anxiety is quite common in SLE patients, often as a reaction to the illness. The question of whether anxiety is attributable to direct CNS involvement in SLE or simply a reaction to chronic illness remains controversial, as with depression. In patients with SLE, the most common cause of mania is corticosteroid therapy. Psychosis in SLE patients can be a manifestation of direct CNS involvement, and in some but not all studies, it has been linked to antiribosomal P antibodies. Distinguishing psychosis caused by CNS lupus from corticosteroid-induced psychosis presents a major diagnostic challenge (see the following section). Delirium, referred to as "acute confusional state" in the ACR criteria, is common in severe SLE and is a result of CNS lupus, medication, or medical disorders, as shown in Table 25–1. Personality changes have been reported in SLE patients whose disease has damaged the frontal or temporal lobes, and symptoms are typical of those resulting from pathology in those brain regions.

Prevalence of Neuropsychiatric Disorders

Estimates of the prevalence of neuropsychiatric disorders in SLE have ranged from 17% to 91% (Ainiala et al. 2001b; Brey et al. 2002; W. Cohen et al. 2004). This variation is a

TABLE 25–1. Secondary medical and psychiatric causes of neuropsychiatric symptoms in systemic lupus erythematosus and other rheumatological disorders

CNS infections
Systemic infections
Renal failure (e.g., due to lupus nephritis or vasculitis involving the renal artery)
Fluid/electrolyte disturbance
Hypertensive encephalopathy
Hypoxemia
Fever
CNS tumor (e.g., cerebral lymphoma because of immunosuppression)
Medication side effects (see Tables 25–2 and 25–3)
Comorbid medical illness
Psychiatric symptoms in reaction to illness
Comorbid psychiatric illness

Note. CNS = central nervous system.

consequence of multiple factors: 1) lack of standardized terminology, 2) changing terminology over time, 3) differences in diagnostic methods, 4) variations in which disease entities are considered direct manifestations of CNS SLE versus a reaction to a chronic unpredictable illness, 5) differences in study population, 6) differences in specialty of investigator, 7) inclusion or exclusion of mild psychiatric symptoms, and 8) inclusion or exclusion of particular CNS neurological disorders, as well as the arbitrariness of separating them from psychiatric disorders.

Using the ACR nomenclature, two studies, a cross-sectional Finnish population-based study (Ainala et al. 2001b) and a cohort study of predominantly Mexican Americans (Brey et al. 2002), examined the prevalence of neuropsychiatric syndromes in outpatients with SLE. Overall, 80%–91% of patients had at least one neuropsychiatric disorder, and the prevalence rates in the two studies were similar for individual neuropsychiatric syndromes. Cognitive dysfunction was the most common neuropsychiatric condition, occurring in 79%–80% of patients; however, less than a third of those patients had moderate to severe impairment. Major depression occurred in 28%–39%; mania or mixed episodes, in 3%–4%; anxiety, in 13%–24%; and psychosis, in 0%–5%. Acute confusional state occurred in 7% of the Finnish patients with SLE; it was not reported in the Mexican American cohort. Although comparable prevalence studies have not been reported for acutely ill inpatients with neuropsychiatric SLE, the incidence of psychosis and delirium is likely to be substantially higher.

Detection of CNS Systemic Lupus Erythematosus

The general principles of treatment discussed earlier in this chapter are applicable to neuropsychiatric SLE, but there are also relevant laboratory tests specific to SLE. In SLE, complement levels (C3, C4, CH50) and anti-DNA antibodies are elevated during disease flares (West et al. 1995). Serum ANA titers need not be obtained in SLE because they do not seem to correlate with systemic or CNS lupus activity. Testing for antiphospholipid antibodies (including lupus anticoagulant and anticardiolipin) is crucial, particularly in patients with focal symptoms, because the results may determine treatment and prognosis (Gharavi 2001; Levine et al. 2002). Unlike antiphospholipid antibody–negative patients, those with antiphospholipid syndrome are treated primarily with anticoagulation rather than corticosteroid or cytotoxic therapy. Antiribosomal-P antibodies have been linked to psychosis, but their usefulness is limited by their low positive predictive value: 13%–16% for psychosis and depression (Arnett et al. 1996). Other serum autoantibodies, including antineuronal, antineurofilament, and antiganglioside antibodies, have not proven to be diagnostic markers for CNS lupus (Bruyn 1995; Hanly 2001; Sibbitt et al. 1999; West et al. 1995).

Corticosteroid-Induced Psychiatric Symptoms

Corticosteroids have been shown to cause a variety of psychiatric syndromes. However, such symptoms in SLE patients are usually not attributable to corticosteroids. First, severe psychiatric syndromes were reported historically in SLE prior to the introduction of corticosteroids and occur in SLE patients who have not received corticosteroids. Second, psychiatric symptoms in SLE are more frequent and severe than in other disorders treated with comparable doses of corticosteroids. Third, psychiatric symptoms in SLE are often ameliorated, not worsened, by maintenance or an increase in high-dose corticosteroids. In contrast, a reduction in steroid dosage often does not alleviate psychiatric symptoms and may exacerbate them. Finally, in SLE patients who have had a previous psychotic episode while taking corticosteroids, retreatment with steroids usually does not precipitate a recurrence of the psychosis (M. Baker 1973).

Distinguishing corticosteroid-induced psychiatric reactions from a flare of CNS lupus is one of the most challenging aspects of treating SLE. Helpful distinguishing features are summarized in Table 25–2 (Kohen et al. 1993). Given the risk of untreated CNS lupus, and the likelihood that corticosteroids will alleviate such flares

TABLE 25–2.   Differentiating CNS lupus flares from corticosteroid-induced psychiatric reactions

	Active primary CNS lupus	Corticosteroid-induced psychiatric reaction
Onset	After ↓ corticosteroid dosage or ongoing low-dose treatment	Generally <2 weeks after ↑ corticosteroid dosage (~90% within 6 weeks)
Corticosteroid dosage	Variable	Rare if <40 mg/day, common if >60 mg/day
Psychiatric symptoms	Psychosis, delirium > mood disorders, cognitive impairment (new onset)	Mania, mixed states, or depression (often with psychotic features) >> delirium, psychosis
SLE symptoms	Often present, may coincide with onset of psychiatric symptoms	Often present, but precede onset of psychiatric symptoms
Labs	↑ Indices of inflammation	No specific lab findings
Response to corticosteroids	Improvement	Exacerbation of symptoms
Response to ↓ corticosteroid dose	Exacerbation	Improvement

Note.   CNS = central nervous system; SLE = systemic lupus erythematosus.
Source.   Adapted from Kohen M, Asheron RA, Gharavi AE, et al.: "Lupus Psychosis: Differentiation From the Steroid-Induced State." *Clinical and Experimental Rheumatology* 11:323–326, 1993. Used with permission.

and only temporarily exacerbate corticosteroid-induced psychiatric reactions, an empirical initiation or increase of corticosteroids is often the most prudent intervention (Denburg et al. 1994; McCune 1988). (Corticosteroid-induced psychiatric reactions are discussed in-depth later in this chapter.)

Pregnancy in Women With Systemic Lupus Erythematosus

Women may be at increased risk of SLE flares (usually mild) during pregnancy, especially in the second and third trimesters, and during the postpartum period (Khamashta et al. 1997; Ruiz-Irastorza 1996). Some patients with antiphospholipid syndrome have been advised to forego reproduction because of the risk of thrombosis, preeclampsia, and fetal demise (now uncommon because of anticoagulation therapy). Family tension may escalate when a patient wants to (or her partner wants her to) risk jeopardizing her health by becoming pregnant, despite admonitions about possible worsening renal or heart failure, hypertension, or stroke.

Differential Diagnosis of Psychiatric Disorders

Other Medical Disorders

A wide variety of diseases can mimic neuropsychiatric SLE. One group of diseases, associated with a medium to high ANA titer (>1:160), includes Sjögren's syndrome and mixed or undifferentiated connective tissue disease. A second group of diseases, associated with a low ANA titer

(<1:160), includes multiple sclerosis and, less commonly, ANA-positive rheumatoid arthritis, sarcoidosis, and hepatitis C. A third group of diseases, characterized by a negative ANA, may also be mistaken for CNS lupus. This group includes polyarteritis nodosa, microscopic angiitis, Wegener's granulomatosis, chronic fatigue syndrome, fibromyalgia, temporal arteritis, and Behçet's disease.

Psychotropic Drug–Induced Positive ANA

Patients who are receiving antipsychotic drugs, particularly phenothiazines such as chlorpromazine, may have positive ANAs and antiphospholipid antibodies (Canoso et al. 1990; Yannitsi et al. 1990). Drug-induced lupus has also been reported with other psychotropic drugs, including carbamazepine, divalproex, other anticonvulsants, and lithium, (Wallach 2000). In drug-induced lupus, CNS manifestations are rare (Stratton 1985). If the offending drug is discontinued, the lupus symptoms typically resolve within weeks, although the ANA may remain positive for over a year.

Somatization Disorder ("Psychogenic Pseudolupus")

Systemic lupus erythematosus can be misdiagnosed in "somatizing" patients with multisystem complaints and mildly positive tests for ANAs, which are common in young women.

Factitious Systemic Lupus Erythematosus

Factitious SLE appears to be rare, but several cases have been reported (Tlacuilo–Parra et al. 2000). Patients have simulated hematuria by pricking their finger surreptitiously to add trace amounts of blood to urine specimens, injected themselves with feces or other contaminants to cause infections, or applied rouge to their cheeks to simulate a malar rash. One patient feigned proteinuria by inserting a packet of protein into her bladder. These patients had no serological evidence of an autoimmune disorder.

Sjögren's Syndrome

Sjögren's syndrome is characterized by lymphocytic infiltration of the exocrine glands. It can occur alone (primary Sjögren's) or in association with another autoimmune rheumatic disease. It is associated with a medium to high ANA titer (>1:160), and positive anti-double-stranded DNA antibodies. Although Sjögren's syndrome may be difficult to distinguish from CNS SLE (and the two syndromes may overlap), establishing a specific diagnosis is less crucial clinically, because the treatment is the same. While the most common symptoms result from drying of the eyes, mouth, and upper respiratory and urogenital tracts, systemic manifestations can occur in up to one-third of patients. In general these extraglandular manifestations are rare in secondary Sjögren's syndrome but are relatively common in primary Sjögren's syndrome. These extraglandular manifestations of primary Sjögren's syndrome have been shown to involve the CNS in approximately 25% of patients (Alexander et al. 1981, 1982, 1988a; Provost et al. 1987). Rates of CNS involvement are even greater in subjects with cutaneous vasculitic features (up to 70% showing CNS signs) (Alexander et al. 1988b). Unlike SLE, there is no clear association between the CNS involvement and titers of auto-antibodies (Moll et al. 1993; Spezialetti et al. 1993).

The nature of CNS involvement can be focal (cerebellar ataxia, vertigo, ophthalmoplegia, cranial nerve involvement) or diffuse (encephalopathy, aseptic meningoencephalitis, dementia or psychiatric manifestations). Focal lesions are visible on MRI scanning and most frequently involve the white matter (periventricular and subcortical) in the frontal and temporal lobes (Alexander et al. 1988a). Cognitive deficits were found to be common, with more than 80% of subjects with primary Sjögren's syndrome reporting subjective cognitive deficits (Alexander et al. 1988a). Objective cognitive deficits were confirmed in 85% of those with subjective problems: Impairment in attention and concentration were most common (63% of subjects with neuropsychiatric involvement), with deficits in short-term memory and verbal fluency also being detected. Of those with recognized neuropsychiatric manifestations, 25% had progressive dementia, although it should be recognized that the number of subjects was small, and subjects were recruited based on having neuropsychiatric symptoms.

Psychiatric manifestations do occur and usually take the form of affective disturbance (depression, hypomania, anxiety) and somatization (Alexander Et Al. 1988a). The exact prevalence of psychiatric complications is not clear because most studies have investigated small populations with unreliable questionnaire assessments.

Systemic Sclerosis (Scleroderma)

Systemic sclerosis is a chronic disorder of unknown etiology. The condition is characterized by thickening of the skin as a result of the accumulation of fibrotic connective tissue and damage to the microvasculature. Multiple body systems can be involved, including the gastrointestinal tract, heart, lungs, and kidneys. Of all the connective tissue disorders, systemic sclerosis is considered to be the least likely to cause CNS damage (Hietaharju et al. 1993). The exact prevalence of CNS involvement in systemic sclerosis is not clear because previous studies have mostly investigated small samples of nonrepresentative patients. In a recent study, all patients with a diagnosis of systemic sclerosis in an area of Finland over an 11-year period were traced, and 16% were found to have neurological involvement (Hietaharju et al. 1993).

Psychiatric symptoms are common, with up to half of patients reporting symptoms of depression, and about 20% scoring in the moderate to severe range on the BDI (Roca et al. 1996). Symptoms of anxiety, hostility, somatization, and sensitivity have been shown to be higher in those with systemic sclerosis than in healthy control subjects (Angelopoulos et al. 2001). Body image dissatisfaction is common in these patients and is likely to increase distress and psychosocial impairment in this group (Benrud-Larson et al. 2003).

There is no known treatment to prevent progression of scleroderma (although some medications alleviate symptoms), and the prognosis can be poor because of renal failure and pulmonary hypertension. Some patients have severe pain secondary to digital ischemia. Anxiety about prognosis and depression as a consequence of disfigurement (skin thickening, discoloration, and telangiectasias on face) and pain are common in patients with scleroderma.

Temporal (Giant-Cell) Arteritis

Temporal (giant-cell) arteritis, a granulomatous arteritis of unknown etiology, predominantly affects those over the age of 60. Although almost any large artery may be involved, most of the clinical features arise because of involvement of the carotid artery and its branches. Extradural arteries are most commonly involved, leading to the typical clinical picture of headache, superficial pain, or sensitivity in skin overlying inflamed vessels (e.g., pain on combing hair). Pain overlying the temporal artery with loss of pulsations is characteristic of temporal arteritis. Pain in the face, mouth, and jaw may occur, the latter characteristically being worse on eating (jaw claudication). Visual problems occur in 25% of untreated patients, and avoidable blindness may occur if treatment with corticosteroids is delayed. In 50% of patients, pain and tenderness occur in the proximal limb muscles without signs of joint effusion, which constitutes the diagnosis of polymyalgia rheumatica. Systemic features such as weight loss and malaise can occur.

Neuropsychiatric manifestations of temporal arteritis arise because of the involvement of arteries supplying blood to the CNS. The insults to the CNS in temporal arteritis can be ischemic (either permanent or transient) or hemorrhagic. The clinical characteristics of the presentation depend on the nature and extent of the brain areas affected. Resultant impairments can be focal (e.g., cerebrovascular accidents leading to specific motor or sensory deficit) or diffuse, resulting in impairment of consciousness. Other neuropsychiatric manifestations include affective symptoms (Johnson et al. 1997). Visual hallucinations have been reported as occurring in up to 80% of patients, who progress to develop permanent visual loss (Nesher et al. 2001).

Treatment with high-dose steroids is commenced as soon as the diagnosis is made on clinical grounds, before results of arterial biopsy are available, to prevent progression of the disease resulting in irreversible blindness or other serious CNS damage.

Polymyositis

Polymyositis is a disease of unknown etiology that results in inflammation of the muscles. The disease can occur on its own or as part of other rheumatological diseases. The clinical picture is typically that of symmetrical, proximal muscle weakness. Involvement of cardiac (arrhythmias, cardiac failure), gastrointestinal tract (dysphagia, reflux, constipation), and respiratory muscles (breathlessness and respiratory failure) can occur. Vasculitis can occur, affecting the CNS and resulting in neuropsychiatric manifestations. As with SLE and temporal arteritis, the clinical features of neuropsychiatric involvement secondary to vasculitis depend on the site and extent of the vasculitic le-

sions. In 20% of patients, an underlying malignancy is present (most commonly bronchus, breast, stomach, or ovary). Thus neuropsychiatric manifestations may occur as the result of secondary spread of malignancy to the CNS.

Polyarteritis Nodosa

Polyarteritis nodosa (PAN) is a systemic, necrotizing arteritis affecting small and medium-sized vessels, often related to hepatitis B virus infection. Although multiple organ systems can be damaged in this disease, direct involvement of the CNS is rare and usually occurs after the disease is well established. Small cerebral infarcts are the most common neuroradiological findings, although intracranial aneurysms and intracranial hemorrhage have been reported (Iaconetta et al. 1994; Oran et al. 1999).

Behçet's Disease

Behçet's disease (Sakane et al. 1999) is an idiopathic inflammatory disorder with incidence primarily in Asia and highest incidence in Turkey. In Europe, most cases are in Turkish immigrants. The most common symptoms include oral and genital ulcers, uveitis, and skin lesions. Behçet's can be life-threatening. Neuropsychiatric involvement occurs in 10%–20% of cases. Acutely, aseptic meningitis or meningoencephalitis may occur. Later manifestations include personality change, meningoencephalitis, and motor signs. Depression and anxiety are common (Calikoglu et al. 2001). In terminal Behçet's, one-third of patients have dementia (Kaklamani et al. 1998). Differential diagnosis includes other autoimmune disorders, multiple sclerosis, and herpes simplex infections. Brain imaging and CSF studies are abnormal but not specific. Acute neuropsychiatric symptoms respond to corticosteroids, but chronic progressive CNS disease does not.

Wegener's Granulomatosis

Wegener's granulomatosis, an uncommon disorder of unknown etiology, is characterized by a granulomatous vasculitis, predominantly affecting the upper and lower respiratory tracts together with glomerulonephritis. Necrotizing vasculitis is the hallmark of this disorder, involving both small arteries and veins. As the result of vasculitis and granuloma formation, virtually any organ in the body can be involved including the brain and CNS. Literature relating to the neuropsychiatric manifestations is sparse.

Secondary Causes of Neuropsychiatric Symptoms in Rheumatological Disorders

Infection, Other CNS or Systemic Illness, and Drug-Induced Side Effects

Neuropsychiatric symptoms are often secondary to complications of the rheumatological disorder or its treatment, especially infection. Because a number of the rheumatological disorders or their treatments can be associated with immune dysregulation or immunosuppression, these disorders predispose individuals to CNS and systemic infections. These infections can simulate direct involvement of the CNS by the primary disease process as in, for example, neuropsychiatric lupus (West et al. 1995). Infections causing these secondary neuropsychiatric complications include cryptococcal, tubercular, and meningococcal infections and Listeria meningitis; herpes encephalitis; neurosyphilis; CNS nocardiosis; toxoplasmosis; brain abscesses; and progressive multifocal leukoencephalopathy (see also Chapter 27, "Infectious Diseases"). Other etiologies of neuropsychiatric manifestations in rheumatological disorders include uremia, hypertensive encephalopathy, cerebral lymphoma, and medication side effects, as well as comorbid medical or psychiatric disorders and psychological reactions to illness (see Tables 25–1 and 25–3).

Corticosteroid-Induced Psychiatric Syndromes

Corticosteroids have psychiatric adverse effects, including mania, depression, mixed states, psychosis, anxiety, insomnia, and delirium. A previous psychiatric reaction to corticosteroids does not necessarily predict recurrent reactions with subsequent steroids. Mild psychiatric side effects include insomnia, hyperexcitability, mood lability, mild euphoria, irritability, anxiety, agitation, and racing thoughts. Mood disorders, including mania, are the most common psychiatric reaction to corticosteroids. Patients may experience both mania and depression during a single course of corticosteroid therapy. Affective symptoms are often accompanied by psychotic symptoms. The psychiatric symptoms induced by corticosteroids most often resemble those of bipolar disorder (Brown and Suppes 1998). Delirium and psychosis (without mood symptoms) are less common. Cognitive dysfunction also has been reported and may be attributable to corticosteroid-induced cortical atrophy and loss of hippocampal neurons (Sapolsky 2000; Wolkowitz 1997).

TABLE 25–3. Psychiatric side effects of medications used in treating systemic lupus erythematosus

Medication	Psychiatric side effects
NSAID (high dose)	Depression, anxiety, paranoia, hallucinations, hostility, confusion, delirium, ↓ concentration
Sulfasalazine	Insomnia, depression, hallucinations
Corticosteroids	Mood lability, euphoria, irritability, anxiety, insomnia, mania, depression, psychosis, delirium, cognitive disturbance
Gold	None reported
Penicillamine	None reported
Leflunomide	Anxiety
Azathioprine	Delirium
Mycophenolate mofetil	Anxiety, depression, sedation (all rare)
Cyclophosphamide	Delirium (at high doses) (rare)
Methotrexate	Delirium (at high doses) (rare)
Cyclosporine	Anxiety, delirium, visual hallucinations
Tacrolimus	Anxiety, delirium, insomnia, restlessness
Immunoglobulin (intravenous)	Delirium, agitation
LJP-394[a]	None reported
Hydroxychloroquine	Confusion, psychosis, mania, depression, nightmares, anxiety, aggression, delirium

Note. NSAID=nonsteroidal anti-inflammatory drug.
[a]B-cell tolerogen–anti-anti-double-stranded DNA antibodies.

The incidence of corticosteroid-induced psychiatric symptoms is dose-related: 1.3% in patients receiving less than 40 mg/day of prednisone, 4.6% in those receiving 41–80 mg/day, and 18.4% in those receiving greater than 80 mg/day (Boston Collaborative Drug Surveillance Program 1972). For the majority of patients, the onset of psychiatric symptoms is within the first 2 weeks (and in 90%, within the first 6 weeks) of initiating or increasing corticosteroid treatment.

The preferred treatment for corticosteroid-induced psychiatric reactions is tapering of corticosteroids, if possible, resulting in greater than 90% response rate. However, rapid tapering or discontinuation of corticosteroids can also induce psychiatric reactions by precipitating a flare of the rheumatological disease, iatrogenic adrenal insufficiency, or possibly corticosteroid-withdrawal syndrome. Corticosteroid-withdrawal syndrome is manifested by headache, fever, myalgias, arthralgias, weakness, anorexia, nausea, weight loss, and orthostatic hypotension and sometimes depression, anxiety, agitation, or psychosis (Wolkowitz 1989). Symptoms respond to an increase or resumption of corticosteroid dosage. Adjunctive treatment with antipsychotics, antidepressants, and mood stabilizers can be helpful, depending on the particular psychiatric symptom constellation.

Other drugs used in treating rheumatological disorders may also cause psychiatric side effects, especially hydroxychloroquine (see Table 25–3).

References

Affleck G, Pfeiffer C, Tennen H, et al: Social support and psychological adjustment to rheumatoid arthritis. Arthritis Care Res 1:927–931, 1988

Affleck G, Tennen H, Urrows S, et al: Neuroticism and the pain-mood relation in rheumatoid arthritis: insights from a prospective daily study. J Consult Clin Psychol 60:119–126, 1992

Ainiala H, Loukkola J, Peltola J, et al: The prevalence of neuropsychiatric syndromes in systemic lupus erythematosus. Neurology 57:496–500, 2001a

Ainiala H, Hietaharju A, Loukkola J, et al: Validity of the American College of Rheumatology criteria for neuropsychiatric lupus syndromes: a population-based evaluation. Arthritis Care Res 45:419–423, 2001b

Albers JM, Kuper HH, van Riel PL, et al: Socio-economic consequences of rheumatoid arthritis in the first years of the disease. Rheumatology (Oxf) 38:423–430, 1999

Alexander EL, Provost TT, Stevens MB, et al: Neurologic complications of primary Sjögren's syndrome. Medicine 61:247–257, 1982

Alexander EL, Beall SS, Gordon B, et al: Magnetic resonance imaging of cerebral lesions in patients with Sjögren's syndrome. Ann Intern Med 108:815–823, 1988a

Alexander EL, Provost TT, Sanders ME, et al: Serum complement activation in central nervous system disease in Sjögren's syndrome. Am J Med 85:513–515, 1988b

Alexander GE, Provost TT, Stevens MB, et al: Sjögren's syndrome: central nervous system manifestations. Neurology 5:405–426, 1981

American College of Rheumatology Ad Hoc Committee on Neuropsychiatric Lupus Nomenclature: Nomenclature and case definitions for neuropsychiatric lupus syndromes. Arthritis Rheum 42:599–608, 1999

American Psychiatric Association: Diagnostic and Statistical Manual of Mental Disorders, 4th Edition. Washington, DC, American Psychiatric Association, 1994

American Psychiatric Association: Diagnostic and Statistical Manual of Mental Disorders, 4th Edition, Test Revision. Washington, DC, American Psychiatric Association, 2000

Anderson IM, Nutt DJ, Deakin JF: Evidence-based guidelines for treating depressive disorders with antidepressants: a revision of the 1993 British Association for Psychopharmacology guidelines. J Psychopharmacol 14:3–20, 2000

Ando Y, Kai S, Uyama E, et al: Involvement of the central nervous system in rheumatoid arthritis: its clinical manifestations and analysis by magnetic resonance imaging. Intern Med 34:188–191, 1995

Angelopoulos NV, Drosos AA, Moutsopoulos HM: Psychiatric symptoms associated with scleroderma. Psychother Psychosom 70:145–150, 2001

Arnett FC, Reveille JD, Moutsopoulos HM, et al: Ribosomal P autoantibodies in systemic lupus erythematosus: frequencies in different ethnic groups and clinical and immunogenetic associations. Arthritis Rheum 39:1833–1839, 1996

Baker GHB, Brewerton DA: Rheumatoid arthritis: a psychiatric assessment. BMJ 282:2014, 1981

Baker M: Psychopathology in systemic lupus erythematosus, I: psychiatric observations. Semin Arthritis Rheum 3:95–110, 1973

Benrud-Larson LM, Heinburg LJ, Boling C, et al: Body image dissatisfaction among women with scleroderma and relationship to psychosocial function. Health Psychol 22:130–139, 2003

Bolger N, Schilling EA: Personality and the problems of everyday life: the role of neuroticism in exposure and reactivity to daily stressors. J Pers 59:355–386, 1991

Bolger N, Zuckerman A: A framework for studying personality in the stress process. J Pers Soc Psychol 69:890–902, 1995

Boston Collaborative Drug Surveillance Program: Acute adverse reactions to prednisone in relation to dosage. Clin Pharmacol Ther 13:694–698, 1972

Bradley LA, Young LD, Anderson KO, et al: Effects of psychological therapy on pain behavior of rheumatoid arthritis patients. Treatment outcome and six-month follow-up. Arthritis Rheum 30:1105–1114, 1987

Brey RL, Holliday SL, Saklad AR, et al: Neuropsychiatric syndromes in lupus: prevalence using standardized definitions. Neurology 58:1214–1220, 2002

Bromm B, Meier W, Scharein E: Imipramine reduces experimental pain. Pain 25:245–257, 1986

Brown ES, Suppes T: Mood symptoms during corticosteroid therapy: a review. Harv Rev Psychiatry 5:239–246, 1998

Brown GK, Nicassio PM, Wallston KA: Pain coping strategies and depression in rheumatoid arthritis. J Clin Psychol 57:652–657, 1989

Brown GW, Harris T: Social Origins of Depression: A Study of Psychiatric Disorder in Women. London, Tavistock, 1979

Bruyn GAW: Controversies in lupus: nervous system involvement. Ann Rheum Dis 54:159–167, 1995

Calfas KJ, Kaplan RM, Ingram RE: One year evaluation of cognitive behavioral intervention in osteoarthritis. Arthritis Care and Research 5:202–209, 1992

Calikoglu E, Onder M, Cosar B, et al: Depression, anxiety levels and general psychological profile in Behçet's disease. Dermatology 203:238–240, 2001

Callahan LF, Kaplan MR, Pincus T: The Beck Depression Inventory, Center for Epidemiological Studies Depression Scale (CES-D), and general Well-Being Schedule Depression Subscale in rheumatoid arthritis. Arthritis Care Res 4:3–11, 1991

Canoso RT, de Oliveira RM, Nixon RA: Neuroleptic-associated autoantibodies. A prevalence study. Biol Psychiatry 27:863–870, 1990

Carbotte RM, Denburg SD, Denburg JA: Cognitive dysfunction in SLE is independent of active disease. J Rheumatol 22:863–867, 1995

Chatzis A, Giannopoulos N, Baharakakis S, et al: Unusual cause of a stroke in a patient with seronegative rheumatoid arthritis. Cardiovasc Surg 7:659–660, 1999

Cohen S, Wills TA: Stress, social support and the buffering hypothesis. Psychol Bull 98:310–357, 1985

Cohen W, Roberts WN, Levenson JL: Psychiatric aspects of SLE, in Systemic Lupus Erythematosis. Edited by Lahita R. San Diego, CA, Elsevier, 2004, pp 785–825

Conway S, Creed FH, Symmons DPM: Life events and the onset of rheumatoid arthritis. J Psychosom Res 38:837–847, 1994

Creamer P, Lethbridge-Cejku M, Hochberg MC: Factors associated with functional impairment in symptomatic knee osteoarthritis. Rheumatology 39:490–496, 2000

Creed F: Psychological disorders in rheumatoid arthritis: a growing consensus? Ann Rheum Dis 49:808–812, 1990

Denburg SD, Carbotte RM, Denburg JA: Corticosteroids and neuropsychological functioning in patients with systemic lupus erythematosus. Arthritis Rheum 37:1311–1320, 1994

Dexter P, Brandt K: Distribution and predictors of depressive symptoms in osteoarthritis. Journal of Rheumatology 21: 279–286, 1994

Dickens C, Jackson J, Tomenson B, et al: Associations of depression in rheumatoid arthritis. Psychosomatics 44:209–215, 2003

DiMatteo MR, Lepper HS, Croghan TW: Depression is a risk factor for noncompliance with medical treatment: meta-analysis of the effects of anxiety and depression on patient adherence. Arch Intern Med 160:2101–2107, 2000

Doeglas D, Suurmeijer T, Krol B, et al: Social support, social disability, and psychological well-being in rheumatoid arthritis. Arthritis Care Res 7:10–15, 1994

Evers AW, Kraaimaat FW, Geenen R, et al: Determinants of psychological distress and its course in the first year after diagnosis in rheumatoid arthritis patients. J Behav Med 20: 489–504, 1997

Evers AW, Kraaimaat FW, Geenen R, et al: Psychosocial predictors of functional change in recently diagnosed rheumatoid arthritis patients. Behav Res Ther 36:179–193, 1998

Ferstl R, Niemann T, Biehl G, et al: Neuropsychological impairment in auto-immune disease. Eur J Clin Invest 20 (suppl 1):16–20, 1992

Fitzpatrick R, Newman S, Archer R, et al: Social support, disability and depression: a longitudinal study of rheumatoid arthritis. Soc Sci Med 33:605–611, 1991

Frank RG, Beck NC, Parker JC, et al: Depression in rheumatoid arthritis. J Rheumatol 15:920–925, 1988

Fyrand L, Moum T, Wichstrom L, et al: Social network size of female patients with rheumatoid arthritis compared to healthy controls. Scand J Rheumatol 29:38–43, 2000

Fyrand L, Moum T, Finset A, et al: Social support in female patients with rheumatoid arthritis compared with healthy controls. Psychol Health 6:429–439, 2001

Gerli R, Caponi L, Tincani A, et al: Clinical and serological associations of ribosomal P autoantibodies in systemic lupus erythematosus: prospective evaluation in a large cohort of Italian patients. Rheumatology (Oxf) 41:1357–1366, 2002

Gharavi AE: Anticardiolipin syndrome: antiphospholipid syndrome. Clin Med 1:14–17, 2001

Giang DW: Systemic lupus erythematosus and depression. Neuropsychiatry Neuropsychol Behav Neurol 4:78–82, 1991

Gobernado JM, Leiva C, Rabano J, et al: Recovery from rheumatoid cerebral vasculitis. J Neurol Neurosurg Psychiatry 47:410–413, 1984

Goodenow C, Reisine ST, Grady KE: Quality of social support and associated social and psychological functioning in women with rheumatoid arthritis. Health Psychol 9:266–284, 1990

Griffin KW, Friend R, Kaell AT, et al: Distress and disease status among patients with rheumatoid arthritis: roles of coping styles and perceived responses from support providers. Ann Behav Med 23:133–138, 2001

Hall RCW, Stickney SK, Gardner ER: Psychiatric symptoms in patients with systemic lupus erythematosus. Psychosomatics 22:15–24, 1981

Hanly JG: Neuropsychiatric lupus. Curr Rheumatol Rep 3:205–212, 2001

Hanly JG, Cassell K, Fisk JD: Cognitive function in systemic lupus erythematosus: results of a 5-year prospective study. Arthritis Rheum 40:1542–1543, 1997

Harkins SW, Price DD, Braith J: Effects of extraversion and neuroticism on experimental pain, clinical pain and illness behaviours. Pain 36:209–218, 1989

Hawley DJ, Wolfe F: Depression is not more common in RA: a 10 year longitudinal study of 6,153 patients with rheumatic disease. Journal of Rheumatology 20:2025–2031, 1993

Hay EM, Black D, Huddy A, et al: A prospective study of psychiatric disorder and cognitive function in systemic lupus erythematosus. Ann Rheum Dis 53:298–303, 1994

Hendrie HC, Paraskevas F, Baragar FD, et al: Stress, immunoglobulin levels and early polyarthritis. J Psychosom Res 15:337–343, 1971

Herbert TB, Cohen S: Stress and immunity in humans: a meta-analytic review. Psychosom Med 55:364–379, 1993

Herranz MT, Rivier G, Khamashta MA, et al: Association between antiphospholipid antibodies and epilepsy in patients with systemic lupus erythematosus. Arthritis Rheum 37:568–571, 1994

Hietaharju A, Jaaskelainen S, Hietarinta M, et al: Central nervous system involvement and psychiatric manifestations in systemic sclerosis: clinical and neurophysiological involvement. Acta Neurol Scand 87:382–387, 1993

Hinrichsen H, Barth J, Ferstl R, et al: Changes of immunoregulatory cells induced by acoustic stress in patients with systemic lupus erythematosus, sarcoidosis, and in healthy controls. Eur J Clin Invest 19:372–377, 1989

Hurwicz ML, Berkanovic E: The stress process in rheumatoid arthritis. J Rheumatol 20:1836–1844, 1993

Iaconetta G, Benvenuti D, Lamaida E, et al: Cerebral hemorrhagic complication in polyarteritis nodosa. Case report and review of the literature. Acta Neurol 16:64–69, 1994

Isshi K, Hirohata S: Differential roles of antiribosomal P antibody and antineuronal antibody in the pathogenesis of central nervous system involvement in systemic lupus erythematosus. Arthritis Rheum 41:1819–1827, 1998

Jacobs R, Pawlak CR, Mikeska E, et al: Systemic lupus erythematosus and rheumatoid arthritis patients differ from healthy controls in their cytokine pattern after stress exposure. Rheumatology 40:868–875, 2001

Jennekens FGI, Kater L: The central nervous system in systemic lupus erythematosus. Part 2. Pathogenic mechanisms of clinical syndromes: a literature investigation. Rheumatology 41:619–630, 2002

Johnson H, Bouman W, Pinner G: Psychiatric aspects of temporal arteritis: a case report and review of the literature. J Geriatr Pychiatry Neurol 10:142–145, 1997

Kaklamani VG, Vaiopoulos G, Kaklamanis PG: Behçet's disease. Semin Arthritis Rheum 27:197–217, 1998

Kaposi M: Neue beitrage zur Kenntnis des lupus erythematosus. Archiv fur Dermatologie und Syphilis 4:36–79, 1872

Karassa FB, Ioannidis JPA, Touloumi G, et al: Risk factors for central nervous system involvement in systemic lupus erythematosus. QJM 93:169–174, 2000

Katz PP, Yelin EH: The development of depressive symptoms among women with rheumatoid arthritis. The role of function. Arthritis Rheum 38:49–56, 1995

Khamashta MA, Ruiz-Irastorza G, Hughes GR: Systemic lupus erythematosus flares during pregnancy. Rheum Dis Clin North Am 23:15–30, 1997

Kohen M, Asheron RA, Gharavi AE, et al: Lupus psychosis: differentiation from the steroid-induced state. Clin Exp Rheumatol 11:323–326, 1993

Kraaimaat FW, Dam-Baggen RM, Bijlsma JW: Association of social support and the spouse's reaction with psychological distress in male and female patients with rheumatoid arthritis. J Rheumatol 22:644–648, 1995

Lahita R (ed): Systemic Lupus Erythematosus. San Diego, CA, Elsevier, 2004

Larsen RJ: Neuroticism and selective encoding and recall of symptoms: evidence from a combined concurrent retrospective study. J Pers Soc Psychol 62:480–488, 1992

Leventhal H, Benyamini Y, Brownlee S, et al: Illness representations: theory and measurement, in Perceptions of Health and Illness. Edited by Petrie KJ, Weinman JA. Amsterdam, Harwood Academic Publishers, 1997, pp 19–46

Levine JS, Branch DW, Rauch J: The antiphospholipid syndrome. N Engl J Med 346:752–763, 2002

Liang MH, Rogers M, Larson M, et al: The psychosocial impact of systemic lupus erythematosus and rheumatoid arthritis. Arthritis Rheum 27:13–19, 1984

Lin E, Katon, W, Von Korff M, et al: Effects of improving depression care on pain and functional outcomes among older adults with arthritis. JAMA 290:2428–2434, 2003

Lubeck DP, Spitz PW, Fries JF, et al: A multicenter study of annual health service utilization and costs in rheumatoid arthritis. Arthritis Rheum 29:488–493, 1986

Macfarlane GJ, Morris S, Hunt IM, et al: Chronic widespread pain in the community: the influence of psychological symptoms and mental disorder on health care seeking behavior. J Rheumatol 26:413–419, 1999

Manne SL, Zautra AJ: Spouse criticism and support: their association with coping and psychological adjustment among women with rheumatoid arthritis. J Pers Soc Psychol 56:608–617, 1989

Manning WG Jr, Wells KB: The effects of psychological distress and psychological well-being on use of medical services. Med Care 30:541–553, 1992

McCune WJ: Neuropsychiatric lupus. Rheum Dis Clin N Am 14:149–167, 1988

Menon S, Jameson-Shortall E, Newman SP, et al: A longitudinal study of anticardiolipin antibody levels and cognitive functioning in systemic lupus erythematosus. Arthritis Rheum 42:735–741, 1999

Mindham RH, Bagshaw A, James SA, et al: Factors associated with the appearance of psychiatric symptoms in rheumatoid arthritis. J Psychosom Res 25:429–435, 1981

Moll JWB, Markusse HM, Pijnenburg JJ, et al: Antineuronal antibodies in patients with neurologic complications of primary Sjögren's syndrome. Neurology 43:2574–2581, 1993

Murphy H, Dickens C, Creed F, et al: Depression, illness perception and coping in rheumatoid arthritis. J Psychosom Res 46:155–164, 1999

Murphy S, Creed F, Jayson MI: Psychiatric disorder and illness behaviour in rheumatoid arthritis. Br J Rheumatol 27:357–363, 1988

Nesher G, Nesher R, Rozenman Y, et al: Visual hallucinations in giant cell arteritis: association with visual loss. J Rheumatol 28:2046–2048, 2001

Ohta K, Tanaka M, Funaki M, et al: Multiple cerebral infarction associated with cerebral vasculitis in rheumatoid arthritis. Rinsho Shinkeigaku 38:423–429, 1998

Olsen NJ, Stein CM: New drugs for rheumatoid arthritis. N Engl J Med 350:2167–2179, 2004

Onghena P, Van Houdenhove B: Antidepressant-induced analgesia in chronic non-malignant pain: a meta-analysis of 39 placebo-controlled studies. Pain 49:205–219, 1992

Oran I, Memis A, Paridar M, et al: Multiple intracranial aneurysms in polyarteritis nodosa: MRI and angiography. Neuroradiology 41:436–439, 1999

Ormel J, Wohlfart T: How neuroticism, long-term difficulties and life situation change influence psychological distress: a longitudinal model. J Pers Soc Psychol 60:744–755, 1991

Otto R, Mackay IR: Psycho-social and emotional disturbance in systemic lupus erythematosus. Med J Aust 2:488–493, 1967

Pawlak C, Witte T, Heiken H, et al: Flares in patients with systemic lupus erythematosus are associated with daily psychological stress. Psychother Psychosom 72:159–165, 2003

Peck JR, Smith TW, Ward JR, et al: Disability and depression in rheumatoid arthritis. A multi-trait, multi-method investigation. Arthritis Rheum 32:1100–1106, 1989

Perry S, Miller F: Psychiatric aspects of systemic lupus erythematosus, in Systemic Lupus Erythematosus, 2nd Edition. Edited by Lahita R. New York, Churchill Livingstone, 1992, pp 845–863

Persson LO, Berglund K, Sahlberg D: Psychological factors in chronic rheumatic diseases—a review. The case of rheumatoid arthritis, current research and some problems. Scand J Rheumatol 28:137–144, 1999

Pilowsky I: Dimensions of illness behaviour as measured by the Illness Behaviour Questionnaire. J Psychosom Res 37:53–62, 1993

Pincus T, Callahan LF, Bradley L, et al: Elevated MMPI scores for hypochondriasis, depression and hysteria in patients with rheumatoid arthritis reflect disease rather than psychosocial status. Arthritis Rheum 29:1456–1466, 1986

Pines A, Kaplinsky N, Olchovsky D, et al: Recurrent transient ischemic attacks associated with thrombocytosis in rheumatoid arthritis. Clin Rheumatol 1:291–293, 1982

Pow J: The role of psychological influences in rheumatoid arthritis. J Psychosom Res 31:223–229, 1987

Provost TT, Vasily D, Alexander EL: Sjögren's syndrome: cutaneous, immunologic and central nervous system manifestations. Neurol Clin 5:405–426, 1987

Revenson TA, Schiaffino KM, Majerovitz SD, et al: Social support as a double-edged sword: the relation of positive and problematic support to depression among rheumatoid arthritis patients. Soc Sci Med 33:807–813, 1991

Rifkin A: Depression in physically ill patients. Postgrad Med 92:147–154, 1992

Rimon R: A psychosomatic approach to rheumatoid arthritis: a clinical study of 100 patients. Acta Psychiatr Scand 13:1–154, 1969

Roca RP, Wigley FM, White B: Depressive symptoms associated with scleroderma. Arthritis Rheum 39:1035–1040, 1996

Ropes MW: Systemic Lupus Erythematosus. Cambridge, MA, Harvard University Press, 1976

Ruiz-Irastorza G, Lima F, Alves J, et al: Increased rate of lupus flare during pregnancy and the puerperium: a prospective study of 78 pregnancies. Br J Rheumatol 35:133–138, 1996

Sabbadini MG, Manfredi AA, Bozzolo E, et al: Central nervous system involvement in systemic lupus erythematosus patients without overt neuropsychiatric manifestations. Lupus 8:1–2, 1999

Sabet A, Sibbitt WL, Stidley CA, et al: Neurometabolite markers of cerebral injury in the antiphospholipid antibody syndrome of SLE. Stroke 29:2254–2260, 1998

Sakane T, Takeno M, Suzuki N, et al: Behçet's disease. N Engl J Med 341:1284–1291, 1999

Sapolsky, RM: Glucocorticoids and hippocampal atrophy in neuropsychiatric disorders. Arch Gen Psychiatry 57:925–935, 2000

Scolding NJ, Joseph FG: The neuropathology and pathogenesis of systemic lupus erythematosus. Neuropathol Appl Neurobiol 28:173–189, 2002

Sharpe L, Sensky T, Timberlake N, et al: A blind, randomized, controlled trial of cognitive-behavioural intervention for patients with recent onset rheumatoid arthritis: preventing psychological and physical morbidity. Pain 89:275–283, 2001

Sheikh JI, Yesavage J: Geriatric Depression Scale (GDS): recent evidence and development of a shorter version. Clin Gerontol 9:37–43, 1989

Shochet BR, Lisansky ET, Schubart AF, et al: A medical-psychiatric assessment of patients with rheumatoid arthritis. Psychosomatics 10:271–279, 1969

Sibbitt WL, Jung RE, Brooks WM: Neuropsychiatric systemic lupus erythematosus. Compr Ther 25:198–208, 1999

Singleton JD, West SG, Reddy VV, et al: Cerebral vasculitis complicating rheumatoid arthritis. South Med J 88:470–474, 1995

Simon G, Von Korff M, Barlow W: Healthcare costs of primary care patients with recognised depression. Arch Gen Psychiatry 52:850–856, 1995

Smedstad LM, Vaglum P, Kvien TK, et al: The relationship between self-reported pain and sociodemographic variables, anxiety, and depressive symptoms in rheumatoid arthritis. J Rheumatol 22:514–520, 1995

Smedstad LM, Moum T, Vaglum P, et al: The impact of early rheumatoid arthritis on psychological distress. A comparison between 238 patients with RA and 116 matched controls. Scand J Rheumatol 25:377–382, 1996

Smith TW, Peck JR, Milano RA, et al: Cognitive distortion in rheumatoid arthritis: relation to depression and disability. J Consult Clin Psychol 56:412–416, 1988

Spezialetti R, Bluestein HG, Peter JB, et al: Neuropsychiatric disease in Sjögren's syndrome: anti-ribosomal P and anti-neuronal antibodies. Am J Med 95:153–160, 1993

Spitzer A, Bar-Tal Y, Golander H: Social support: how does it really work? J Adv Nurs 22:850–854, 1995

Stratton MA: Drug induced systemic lupus erythematosus. Clin Pharm 4:657–663, 1985

Tlacuilo-Parra JA, Guevara-Gutierrez E, Garcia-De La Torre I: Factitious disorders mimicking systemic lupus erythematosus. Clin Exp Rheumatol 18:89–93, 2000

van Baar ME, Dekker J, Lemmens JA, et al: Pain and disability in patients with osteoarthritis of the hip or knee: the relationship with articular, kinesiological and psychological characteristics. Journal of Rheumatology 25:125–133, 1998

Wallace DJ, Metzger AL: Can an earthquake cause flares of rheumatoid arthritis or lupus nephritis? Arthritis Rheum 37:1826–1828, 1994

Wallach J: Interpretation of Diagnostic Tests, 7th Edition. Baltimore, MD, Lippincott, 2000

Waterloo K, Omdal R, Jacobsen EA, et al: Cerebral computed tomography and electroencephalography compared with neuropsychological findings in systemic lupus erythematosus. J Neurol 246:706–711, 1999

Waterloo K, Omdal R, Husby G, et al: Neuropsychological function in systemic lupus erythematosus: a five-year longitudinal study. Rheumatology 41:411–415, 2002

Wells KB, Stewart A, Hays RD, et al: The functioning and well-being of depressed patients. Results from the Medical Outcomes Study. JAMA 262:914–919, 1989

West SG: Neuropsychiatric lupus. Rheum Dis Clin N Am 20:129–158, 1994

West SG, Emlen W, Wener MH, et al: Neuropsychiatric lupus erythematosus: a prospective study on the value of diagnostic tests. Am J Med 99:153–163, 1995

Wierzbicki AS: Lipids, cardiovascular disease and atherosclerosis in systemic lupus erythematosus. Lupus 9:194–201, 2000

Wolfe F: Psychological distress and rheumatic disease. Scand J Rheumatol 28:131–136, 1999

Wolfe F, Hawley DJ: The relationship between clinical activity and depression in rheumatoid arthritis. J Rheumatol 20: 2032–2037, 1993

Wolkowitz OM: Long-lasting behavioral changes following prednisolone withdrawal. JAMA 261:1731–1732, 1989

Wolkowitz OM, Reus VI, Canick J, et al: Glucocorticoid medication, memory, and steroid psychosis in medical illness. Ann N Y Acad Sci 823:81–96, 1997

Yannitsi SG, Manoussakis MN, Mavridis AK, et al: Factors related to the presence of autoantibodies in patients with chronic mental disorders. Biol Psychiatry 27:747–756, 1990

Yelin EH, Feshbach DM, Meenan RF, et al: Social problems, services and policy for persons with chronic disease: the case of rheumatoid arthritis. Soc Sci Med [Med Econ] 13C:13–20, 1979

Zautra AJ, Smith BW: Depression and reactivity to stress in older women with rheumatoid arthritis and osteoarthritis. Psychosom Med 63:687–696, 2001

Zigmond AS, Snaith RP: The Hospital Anxiety and Depression Scale. Acta Psychiatr Scand 67:361–370, 1983

26 Chronic Fatigue and Fibromyalgia Syndromes

Michael C. Sharpe, M.A., M.D., F.R.C.P., M.R.C.Psych.

Patrick G. O'Malley, M.D., M.P.H.

IN THIS CHAPTER, we review two symptom-defined somatic syndromes: chronic fatigue syndrome (CFS) and fibromyalgia syndrome (FMS). The central feature of CFS is the symptom of severe chronic, disabling fatigue that is typically exacerbated by exertion and unexplained by any other medical condition. The central feature of FMS is widespread pain with localized tenderness that similarly is unexplained by any other diagnosis. Although these syndromes have different historical origins, it is increasingly recognized that they have much in common (Sullivan et al. 2002). Therefore, in this chapter we consider them together.

CFS, FMS, and other symptom-defined somatic syndromes are conditions whose homes in medicine (as functional syndromes) and in psychiatry (as somatoform disorders) are both rather temporary structures located in unfashionable areas of their respective communities. These functional disorders (Wessely et al. 1999) are, however, of central concern to psychosomatic medicine. Other functional or medically unexplained syndromes are covered elsewhere in this volume, including noncardiac chest pain (see Chapter 19, "Heart Disease"), hyperventilation syndrome (see Chapter 20, "Lung Disease"), irritable bowel and functional upper gastrointestinal disorders (see Chapter 21, "Gastrointestinal Disorders"), idiopathic pruritus (see Chapter 29, "Dermatology"), migraine (see Chapter 32, "Neurology and Neurosurgery"), chronic pelvic pain and vulvodynia (see Chapter 33, "Ob-

stetrics and Gynecology"), and several other pain syndromes (see Chapter 36, "Pain"). Somatization is also discussed (see Chapter 13, "Somatization and Somatoform Disorders").

General Issues

Symptom or Disorder?

Although CFS and FMS are often regarded as discrete conditions, the severity of the symptoms of fatigue and pain is continuously distributed in the general population (Croft et al. 1996; Pawlikowska et al. 1994), and the case definitions also can be regarded as simply defining cutoff points on these continua.

Organic or Psychogenic?

The history of CFS and FMS has been notable for its vigorous disputes about whether these disorders are organic or psychogenic (Asbring and Narvanen 2003). The extreme organic position argues that they eventually will be found to be as firmly based in disease pathology as any other medical condition. Attempts to establish a conventional pathology (e.g., inflammation in muscles in fibromyalgia and chronic infection in CFS) have not yet succeeded, however. An extreme psychogenic view is that these syndromes are pseudodiseases, not rooted in biol-

We are grateful to the following for helpful comments on earlier versions of the chapter: Dr. Peter White, Dr. Leslie Arnold, Professor Simon Wessely, Professor Gijs Belijenberg, Professor Dan Clauw, and Dr. Robert Perry.

ogy but rather representing social constructions based on psychological amplification of normal somatic sensations such as tiredness and pain. Neither of these extreme positions is sustained by the evidence or helpful for patients. In clinical practice, an extreme organic position encourages patients to search for a doctor who will find the pathology and prescribe the right medication while they adapt themselves to a chronic disease. The extreme psychological view ignores the demonstrable physiological disturbances associated with these conditions and, if perceived as dismissive and rejecting, paradoxically can encourage the patients in a defensive entrenchment of the belief that they really do have an untreatable disease (Hadler 1996b). An etiologically neutral and integrated perspective that recognizes these functional disorders as real and that also acknowledges the likely contribution of biological, psychological, and social factors is the best basis for clinical practice (Engel 1977).

Medical or Psychiatric Diagnosis?

In parallel with the debate about etiology is an argument about whether these conditions are most appropriately regarded as medical or as psychiatric. For the same symptoms, the medical diagnosis is CFS (chronic fatigue and immune dysfunction syndrome; myalgic encephalomyelitis or encephalopathy—see "History" subsection in the following section "The Syndromes") or FMS, and the psychiatric diagnosis is often an anxiety, mood, or somatoform disorder. However, it can be argued that neither alone is adequate. Proper use of the DSM-IV-TR (American Psychiatric Association 2000) axes allows the patient to be given both a medical (Axis III) and a psychiatric (Axis I) diagnosis. The final diagnosis may be, for example, FMS and generalized anxiety disorder (GAD). Ultimately, a classification that avoids two diagnoses being given for the same symptoms is required. This is a task for the authors of the forthcoming DSM-V (Mayou et al. 2003).

The Syndromes

Chronic Fatigue Syndrome

History

It has been convincingly argued that CFS is not a new illness. A very similar, if not identical, condition was described as *neurasthenia* more than 100 years ago and probably much earlier (Wessely 1990). The term *chronic fatigue syndrome* was coined in 1988 to describe a condition characterized by chronic disabling fatigue, with many other somatic symptoms and strict psychiatric exclusions (Holmes et al. 1988). The authors of this early definition anticipated that a specific disease cause, possibly infectious, would be found, but this has never been established.

The term *chronic fatigue syndrome* subsumed a multitude of previous terms used to describe patients with similar symptoms. These include *chronic Epstein-Barr virus infection* (see Chapter 27, "Infectious Diseases"), *myalgic encephalomyelitis*, *neurasthenia* (still a specific diagnosis in ICD-10 [World Health Organization 1992]), and *postviral fatigue syndrome*. Arguments persist about the similarity of these conditions to CFS. Patient advocacy groups in particular have been very vocal and politically active in arguing that CFS is an inadequate description of their illness and that a name such as *myalgic encephalomyelitis or encephalopathy* or *chronic fatigue and immune dysfunction syndrome*, which emphasizes a biological pathology, is more appropriate. The new terminology of CFS did, however, have the important advantage for researchers of being clearly operationally defined and provided a basis for replicable scientific research.

Definition

Several operational diagnostic criteria for CFS have been published. The first (noted in the preceding subsection, "History") (Holmes et al. 1988) were in practice found to be excessively cumbersome and restrictive. Furthermore, it was found that requiring multiple somatic symptoms and fatigue selected patients more rather than less likely to have psychiatric diagnoses, which, combined with the strict psychiatric exclusions, made the condition very rare. Consequently, simpler and less exclusive Australian (Lloyd et al. 1988) and British (Oxford) (Sharpe et al. 1991) case definitions were published. The most recent criteria (shown in Table 26–1) were based on an international consensus and were published in 1994. These remain the most widely used (Fukuda et al. 1994), although they are likely to be clarified and revised (Reeves et al. 2003). The different definitions have been a source of confusion and dispute, but it should be remembered that all have been constructed by committees to aid research. Clinical practice therefore should not necessarily be bound by them.

Clinical Features

The clinical presentation of the individuals whose symptoms meet the criteria for CFS is heterogeneous, although the core symptoms of fatigue exacerbated by exercise, subjective cognitive impairment, and disrupted and unrefreshing sleep are almost universally described,

TABLE 26–1. Diagnostic criteria for chronic fatigue syndrome

Inclusion criteria

1. Clinically evaluated, medically unexplained fatigue of at least 6 months' duration that is
   - Of new onset (not lifelong)
   - Not the result of ongoing exertion
   - Not substantially alleviated by rest
   - Associated with a substantial reduction in previous level of activities

2. The occurrence of four or more of the following symptoms:
   - Subjective memory impairment
   - Sore throat
   - Tender lymph nodes
   - Muscle pain
   - Joint pain
   - Headache
   - Unrefreshing sleep
   - Postexertional malaise lasting more than 24 hours

Exclusion criteria

- Active, unresolved or suspected medical disease
- Psychotic, melancholic, or bipolar depression (but not uncomplicated major depression)
- Psychotic disorders
- Dementia; anorexia or bulimia nervosa
- Alcohol or other substance misuse
- Severe obesity

Source. Adapted from Fukuda et al. 1994.

and some degree of widespread pain is common. Patients often report marked fluctuations in fatigue that occur from week to week and even from day to day. Most patients are not so disabled that they cannot attend an outpatient consultation, although some describe difficulty walking or cannot attend an outpatient consultation without the aid of wheelchairs and other appliances. Other patients remain bedridden, unable to visit the clinic, and represent an important and neglected group.

The symptom of fatigue is subjective, and a poor correlation exists between the feeling of fatigue and objectively measured performance (Welford 1953). If patients with CFS are asked to perform exercise tests, they may not show the expected decrement but rather report greater effort and increased fatigue, both at the time of the test and over the following days. Similarly, standard neuropsychological testing usually has normal results but is often accompanied by complaints of greater effort (Vercoulen et al. 1998). Some evidence indicates that more complex cognitive tests do show deficits, although these usually appear less severe than that expected from the pa-

tient's subjective complaints and are difficult to distinguish from those associated with depression (Wearden and Appleby 1996). In summary, the core clinical features of CFS are physical and mental fatigue exacerbated by physical and mental effort. These are subjective phenomena, often less evident on objective testing. Although some may interpret this observation as evidence of exaggeration of disability, such findings also can be interpreted as indicating the essentially subjective and sensory nature of this condition.

Fibromyalgia

History

In 1904, Gowers first coined the term *fibrositis* to describe a chronic widespread pain thought to be caused by inflammation of muscles. However, as with CFS, specific disease pathology in muscle has not subsequently been confirmed. In 1990, the American College of Rheumatology (ACR) adopted the operationally defined and descriptive term *fibromyalgia* as an alternative to *fibrositis* (Wolfe et al. 1990). Other terms have been used, such as *chronic widespread pain* and *myofascial pain syndrome*. As with CFS, the new definition facilitated replicable research and has been widely adopted.

Definition

A variety of different diagnostic criteria for fibromyalgia have been proposed. The ACR criteria published in 1990 are the most widely accepted (Wolfe et al. 1990). These specify widespread pain of at least 3 months' duration and tenderness at 11 or more of 18 specific sites on the body. The ACR criteria are shown in Table 26–2.

TABLE 26–2. American College of Rheumatology 1990 criteria for fibromyalgia

1. History of widespread pain. Pain in the right and left side of the body, pain above and below the waist, axial skeletal pain (cervical spine or anterior chest or thoracic spine or low back). In this definition, shoulder and buttock pain is considered as pain for each involved side. "Low back" pain is considered lower-segment pain.

2. Pain, on digital palpation, must be present in at least 11 of 18 specified tender point sites. Digital palpation should be performed with an approximate force of 4 kg. For a tender point to be considered "positive," the patient must state that the palpation was painful. "Tender" is not to be considered "painful."

Source. Adapted from Wolfe et al. 1990.

A particular feature of the FMS criteria is the specification of examination findings as well as of symptoms. A standardized method of eliciting these "tender points" has been defined (i.e., the application of pressure with the thumb pad perpendicular to each defined site with increasing force by approximately 1 kg/second until 4 kg of pressure is achieved, which usually leads to whitening of the thumbnail bed). Despite the apparent precision of this clinical sign, both the specificity of the locations and the uniqueness of the proposed tender points to FMS have been questioned (Croft et al. 1996; Wolfe 1997).

Clinical Features

The core features of fibromyalgia are chronic widespread pain and musculoskeletal tenderness (muscle, ligaments, and tendons). Pain occurs typically in all four quadrants of the body and the axial skeleton but also can be regional. Fatigue, sleep disturbance, and subjective cognitive impairment (memory and concentration) are common associations. As with CFS, the report of pain is essentially a subjective phenomenon and may not be reflected in attempts to assess physical and mental performance objectively.

Patients have a range of associated disability, although most patients are able to attend outpatient services. The symptoms of FMS overlap considerably with those of other rheumatological conditions. Up to 25% of the patients with systemic inflammatory conditions (such as systemic lupus erythematosus and rheumatoid arthritis) can meet ACR criteria for fibromyalgia in the initial stages, thus creating a diagnostic dilemma for the clinician faced with a patient who has an undifferentiated constellation of chronic musculoskeletal symptoms (see subsection "Identifying Medical and Psychiatric Conditions" later in this chapter).

Primary or Secondary?

Both CFS and FMS are typically diagnosed when the patient has no evidence of another medical condition. This makes it easy to define the symptoms as unexplained by another condition. However, similar symptoms are often found in patients with other medical diagnoses. For example, symptoms of FMS have been reported in patients with systemic lupus erythematosus (Buskila et al. 2003) and rheumatoid arthritis (Wolfe et al. 1984), and symptoms of CFS have been reported in disease-free cancer patients (Servaes et al. 2002) and in patients with multiple sclerosis (Vercoulen et al. 1996a). The terms *primary* (occurring in the absence of another condition) and *secondary* (accompanying a medical condition) have been used to describe these findings. The terminology is, however, con-

fusing and arguably more a matter of differential diagnosis than of comorbidity (see subsection "Association With Other Symptom-Defined Syndromes" later in this section). It is best avoided.

Same or Different?

Many studies have shown an overlap in the symptoms of patients with a diagnosis of FMS and those with a diagnosis of CFS if these are specifically asked about. Put simply, CFS is fatigue with pain, and FMS is pain with fatigue. A latent class analysis of the symptoms of more than 600 patients failed to identify separate syndromes (Sullivan et al. 2002). Not only are the symptoms similar, but a patient who has received the diagnosis of one of these conditions is also likely to meet the diagnostic criteria for the other. Of 163 consecutive female patients with CFS enrolled at a tertiary care clinic, more than a third also met criteria for FMS (Ciccone and Natelson 2003). Consequently, most authorities now accept that important similarities exist between CFS and FMS (Aaron and Buchwald 2003; Wessely et al. 1999). One potential difference between FMS and CFS is the presence of so-called tender points in the former. However, tender points also are often found in patients with CFS. Whether they will be found ultimately to be distinct entities, overlapping conditions, or aspects of the same condition remains both unclear and controversial.

Association With Other Symptom-Defined Syndromes

Studies that have assessed the comorbidity of FMS and CFS with other symptom-defined syndromes (also known as medically unexplained symptoms or functional somatic syndromes) also have found high rates of migraine, irritable bowel syndrome, pelvic pain, and temporomandibular joint pain. These syndromes, like CFS and FMS, are also associated with high lifetime rates of comorbid mood and anxiety disorders (Hudson and Pope 1994). Other similarities are also seen between FMS, CFS, and these disorders, including a female predominance, association with childhood abuse, and response to similar treatments. This observation raises the possibility not only that CFS and FMS are similar but also that all the functional syndromes have more in common than previously thought by the specialists who diagnose each (Sullivan et al. 2002; Wessely et al. 1999). It has been further suggested that these syndromes, along with mood and anxiety disorders, share a common psychological and central nervous system (CNS) pathophysiology (Clauw and Chrousos 1997).

Association With Psychiatric Disorders

In clinical practice, many but not all patients with CFS and FMS can be given a psychiatric diagnosis. Most will meet criteria for a depression or an anxiety syndrome. Those who do not are likely to meet DSM criteria for a somatoform disorder or merit an ICD-10 diagnosis of neurasthenia (Sharpe 1996). The more somatic symptoms the patient has, the more likely a diagnosis of depression or anxiety is (Skapinakis et al. 2003). Precise prevalence rates of psychiatric disorder do, however, depend on the nature of the patient population studied and the diagnostic criteria used. Several factors may influence the estimates obtained. First, compared with a community sample, patients attending clinics are likely to be more disabled and distressed and therefore to have more depression and anxiety. Second, some symptoms (such as fatigue, sleep disturbance, and poor concentration) overlap with the symptoms of depression and anxiety, and the observed prevalence of psychiatric disorders will depend on whether all symptoms are counted toward a diagnosis of psychiatric disorder or whether those considered medically explained by CFS or FMS are excluded. Third, it has been argued that atypical presentations of depression (Van Hoof et al. 2003) and anxiety (Kushner and Beitman 1990) are common in these groups, adding further unreliability to the estimates quoted in the following subsections.

Depression

Fatigue is strongly associated with depression. The international World Health Organization (WHO) study of more than 5,000 primary care patients in several countries (Sartorius et al. 1993) found that 67% of the patients with CFS (defined from survey data) also had an ICD-10 depressive syndrome (Skapinakis 2000). Studies of clinic attenders with CFS reported that more than 25% have a current DSM major depression diagnosis, and 50%–75% have a lifetime diagnosis (Afari and Buchwald 2003). Population studies also find an elevated prevalence, although a lower rate than in some clinic studies (Taylor and Jason 2003).

Chronic pain is also strongly associated with depression in the general population (Ohayon and Schatzberg 2003) (see also Chapter 36, "Pain"). In FMS, a study of attenders at a specialist clinic reported that 32% had a depressive disorder (22% major depression) (Epstein et al. 1999). An increased prevalence of lifetime and family history of major depression also has been reported in FMS (Hudson and Pope 1996). As with CFS, the prevalence of depression is probably lower in patients with FMS in the general population (Clauw and Crofford 2003).

GAD, Panic Disorder, and Posttraumatic Stress Disorder

Anxiety disorders have been relatively neglected in association with CFS and FMS. One study reported GAD in as many as half of the clinic patients with CFS or FMS when the hierarchical rules that subsume it under major depression were suspended (Fischler et al. 1997).

Panic disorder is especially common in patients with medically unexplained symptoms. A prevalence of 7% has been reported in clinic patients with FMS (Epstein et al. 1999), and the prevalence was 13% in one study of CFS (Manu et al. 1991). Panic should be suspected when symptoms are markedly episodic.

The prevalence of posttraumatic stress disorder (PTSD) has been reported to be higher in patients with CFS (Taylor and Jason 2002) and FMS (Cohen et al. 2002) than in the general population, and PTSD is associated with a report of previous abuse (see "Abuse" subsection in the "Etiology" section later in this chapter).

Somatoform Disorders

Somatoform disorders are descriptive diagnoses primarily defined by somatic symptoms not explained by a medical condition. Hence, replacing a diagnosis of CFS or FMS with a somatoform one may simply be relabeling. Furthermore, the choice of diagnosis depends on one's beliefs about the nature of these conditions. If one regards CFS and FMS as medical conditions, then the symptoms will not be counted toward a diagnosis of a somatoform disorder, whereas if one regards CFS and FMS as medically unexplained syndromes, then they will be counted toward a diagnosis of a somatoform disorder (Johnson et al. 1996). Some patients will meet the criteria for hypochondriasis because of persistent anxious concern about the nature of their illness. Others may meet the criteria for somatization disorder because of a long history of multiple symptoms. Patients with FMS are likely to meet the criteria for somatoform pain disorder. Most patients with CFS and FMS who do not meet the criteria for anxiety, depression, or these more specific disorders will fit the undemanding criteria for a diagnosis of undifferentiated somatoform disorder.

Summary

Depressive and anxiety disorders are relatively common in patients with CFS and FMS. There is some suggestion that anxiety is associated more with pain, and depression with fatigue (Kurtze and Svebak 2001). This association with psychiatric disorders appears not to be explained simply by overlapping symptoms, because it remains high even when fatigue is excluded from the diagnostic criteria for major depression (Kruesi et al. 1989). The occurrence of depression or anxiety disorders in patients with CFS or FMS cannot be attributed entirely to referral bias because the rate is still elevated, although less so, in community cases. Also, it does not appear that depression can be explained entirely as a reaction to disability, because it has been found to be more common than in patients with disabling rheumatoid arthritis (Katon et al. 1991; Walker et al. 1997a). However, many patients with CFS and FMS do not have depressive and anxiety syndromes, even after detailed assessment (Henningsen et al. 2003). Whether these patients are given appropriate diagnoses of a somatoform disorder is controversial.

It has been proposed that depression, anxiety, CFS, and FMS have shared risk factors. These may include both genetics (Hudson et al. 2003) and adverse experiences such as abuse and victimization (Van Houdenhove et al. 2001b). The lack of acceptance by others of the suffering associated with these medically ambiguous conditions also may contribute to emotional distress (Lehman et al. 2002).

The relation between symptom syndromes defined by psychiatry and those of CFS and FMS is an intimate and complex one. It can be conceived of either as psychiatric comorbidity with a medical condition or as different perspectives on the same condition. Whichever view one takes, the importance of making the psychiatric diagnosis in patients with CFS and FMS is its implications for treatment.

Epidemiology

Prevalence of Fatigue and Chronic Fatigue Syndrome

Fatigue is common, but CFS as currently defined is relatively rare. A large survey of 90,000 residents in Wichita, Kansas, which used rigorous assessment and exclusion criteria, found that 6% of the population had fatigue of more than 1 month's duration, but only 235 per 100,000 (or 0.2%) had CFS (Reyes et al. 2003). It should be noted, however, that the application of current diagnostic criteria (Fukuda et al. 1994) excluded numerous patients, mainly because of diagnoses of rheumatoid arthritis and psychiatric disorder.

Prevalence of Pain and Fibromyalgia Syndrome

The studies of prevalence of pain and FMS have reported similar findings (Makela 1999). Chronic pain is common and has been reported in as many as 10% of the general population (Croft et al. 1993). However, FMS defined according to the ACR criteria has an estimated prevalence of only 2% (Wolfe et al. 1995) to 4% (K.P. White et al.

1999). The observation that FMS appears to be more common than CFS (Bazelmans et al. 1997) may indicate that chronic pain states are more common than chronic fatigue states but also may simply reflect the requirement in the CFS diagnostic criteria for a longer duration and greater disability from the condition (see Tables 26–1 and 26–2).

Associations

Gender

Both CFS and FMS are more common in women. The female-to-male ratio for CFS has been reported to be about 4:1 (Reyes et al. 2003) and for FMS, 8:1 (Wolfe et al. 1995), although this increased female preponderance in FMS may be primarily associated with tender points rather than with pain (Clauw and Crofford 2003).

Age

The most common age at onset for both CFS and FMS is between 30 and 50 years. However, patients who present with FMS are on average 10 years older (Reyes et al. 2003; K.P. White et al. 1999). These syndromes are also diagnosed, although controversially, in children. A recent epidemiological study from the United Kingdom found a prevalence of CFS of only 0.002% in 5- to 15-year-olds (Chalder et al. 2003). CFS and FMS are also diagnosed in the elderly, but the frequency of other chronic medical conditions complicates the differential diagnosis.

Socioeconomic Status

Both CFS and FMS are more prevalent in persons of lower socioeconomic status and in those who have received less education (Jason et al. 1999; K.P. White et al. 1999). CFS is 50% more common in semiskilled and unskilled workers than in professionals.

International and Cross-Cultural Studies

It is often noted that the diagnoses of CFS and FMS are almost entirely restricted to Western nations, whereas the symptoms of fatigue and pain are universal. It is unclear to what extent this reflects differing epidemiology or simply different diagnostic practice. For example, fatigue in France may be diagnosed as a condition called *spasmophilia*. In the Far East, neurasthenia remains a popular diagnosis and accordingly is still listed in the ICD-10 diagnostic classification. The WHO Collaborative Study of Psychological Problems in General Health Care conducted in 14 countries reported wide variations in the prevalence of both persistent pain (including both medically explained and medically unexplained pain) and fatigue (Gureje et al. 2001; World Health Organization 1995).

Disability and Work

FMS and CFS are both associated with substantial self-reported loss of function and substantial work disability (Assefi et al. 2003). Unemployment in patients with CFS and FMS attending specialist services in the United States is as high as 50% (Bombardier and Buchwald 1996).

Prognosis

The prognosis for patients with CFS or FMS is variable and typically has a chronic but fluctuating course. Rehabilitative therapy improves outcome (see subsection "Specialist Nonpharmacological Treatments" later in this chapter).

Prospective studies of CFS and FMS in the general population report that in about half the cases, the syndrome is in partial or complete remission at 2–3 years (Granges et al. 1994; Nisenbaum et al. 2003). Poor outcome in CFS and FMS is predicted by longer illness duration, more severe symptoms, older age, depression, and lack of social support (van der Werf et al. 2002), and in CFS, by a strong belief in physical causes (Joyce et al. 1997). Severely disabled patients attending specialist clinics have a particularly poor prognosis for recovery (Hill et al. 1999; Wolfe et al. 1997).

Etiology

The precise etiology of CFS and FMS remains unknown. A wide range of etiological factors have been proposed, but none has been unequivocally established. The available evidence may be summarized as suggesting that a combination of environmental factors and individual vulnerability initiates a series of biological, psychological, and social processes that lead to the development of CFS or FMS (see Table 26–3). These factors are discussed in the following subsections as predisposing factors, precipitating factors, and perpetuating factors. It is worth mentioning that, with notable exceptions, the preponderance of research in this area is based largely on small, case–control studies (typically 10–20 patients per case and control group) with insufficient power to control for confounding variables, thereby limiting the ability to draw strong causal inferences about any of the findings reported below.

Predisposing Factors

Biological Factors

Genetics. Modest evidence from family and twin studies suggests that genetic factors play a part in predisposing individuals to CFS and to FMS. In CFS, a small study found that individuals whose family member had CFS were more likely to have the condition (Walsh and Bennett 2001). In a study of 146 female–female twins, one of whom had CFS, the concordance was 55% in monozygotic and 20% in dizygotic twins (Buchwald et al. 2001), suggesting both moderate heritability and the importance of environmental factors. In FMS, a similar familial clustering was reported (Buskila and Neumann 1997), as well as a possible link with human leukocyte antigen types (Yunus et al. 1999).

TABLE 26–3. Possible etiological factors to consider in a formulation of chronic fatigue

	Predisposing	Precipitating	Perpetuating
Biological	Genetics	Acute infection, disease, or injury	Neuroendocrine changes Immunological changes Deconditioning Sleep disorder
Psychological	Personality	Perceived stress	Depression Fixed disease attribution Catastrophizing Low self-efficacy Avoidance of activity
Social	Lack of support	Life events	Information Lack of legitimacy of illness Social or work stress Occupational and financial factors

Psychological and Social Factors

Personality and activity.   Clinicians often claim a predisposing "obsessional" personality type, but this theory has been little studied. The clinical observation that CFS and FMS patients lead abnormally active lives before becoming ill has received limited empirical support (Van Houdenhove et al. 2001a).

Abuse.   Childhood and adult neglect, abuse, and maltreatment have been reported by some, but not all, studies to be more common in both FMS and CFS groups than in medical comparison groups (Van Houdenhove et al. 2001b). In FMS, a particular association with abuse in adulthood has been noted (Walker et al. 1997b). Both psychological and biological etiological mechanisms have been suggested, and particular association with comorbid posttraumatic stress disorder and anxiety has been noted (Taylor and Jason 2002).

Social status.   Low social status and lower levels of education are risk factors for both CFS and FMS (see subsection "Socioeconomic Status" in the "Epidemiology" section earlier in this chapter).

Precipitating Factors

Precipitating factors trigger the illness in vulnerable persons.

Biological Factors

Infection.   Some evidence indicates that infection can precipitate CFS, and some, but less, evidence indicates that infection also may trigger FMS (Rea et al. 1999). Specific infections have been found to be associated with the subsequent development of CFS in 10%–40% of patients. These infections are Epstein-Barr virus (P.D. White et al. 2001), Q fever (Ayres et al. 1998), viral meningitis (Hotopf et al. 1996), and viral hepatitis (Berelowitz et al. 1995). The etiological mechanism to explain this association remains unclear but may include both immunological factors and an acute reduction in activity (P.D. White et al. 2001) (see subsection "Perpetuating Factors" later in this section).

Injury.   The role of physical injury in the etiology of CFS and FMS has been controversial, in part because of the implications for legal liability and compensation. Limited evidence indicates that both conditions may be precipitated by injury, particularly to the neck. If a link exists, it is stronger for FMS (Al Allaf et al. 2002).

Psychological and Social Factors

Life stress.   Clinical experience indicated that patients often report the onset of CFS and FMS as occurring during or after a stressful period in their lives. The evidence for life stress or life events being a precipitant of FMS and CFS is, however, both limited and retrospective (Anderberg et al. 2000; Theorell et al. 1999). One of the best studies so far published examined 64 patients and a similar number of matched control subjects. An excess of severe life events and difficulties was found in the CFS patients for the year prior to onset. More specifically, a certain type of life event called a *dilemma* (defined as an event when the person had to choose between two equally undesirable responses to circumstances) was found in a third of the patients with CFS and none of the control subjects (Hatcher and House 2003).

Perpetuating Factors

Perpetuating factors are those that maintain a condition once it is established. They are clinically the most important because they are potential targets for treatment.

Biological Factors

Chronic infection.   There has been much interest in the potential role of ongoing infection and in associated immunological factors, especially in CFS. It was previously thought that chronic Epstein-Barr virus was a cause of CFS, but that hypothesis has been rejected. There have been numerous reports of evidence of chronic infection with other agents in both CFS and FMS, but none has been substantiated.

Immunological factors.   Immunological factors, especially cytokines, also have been much investigated in CFS and FMS, not only because of the possible triggering effect of infection but also because administration of immune active agents, such as interferons, is recognized as a cause of fatigue and myalgia (Vial and Descotes 1994) and because similar symptoms in conditions such as hepatitis C have been associated with changes in measured cytokines (Thompson and Barkhuizen 2003). Various minor immune abnormalities have been reported in patients with CFS and FMS. However, a recent systematic review found no evidence of any consistent immune abnormality in CFS (Lyall et al. 2003). The hypothesis that CFS is associated with immune activation therefore remains tantalizing but unproven.

Myopathic or biochemical abnormalities and physiological deconditioning.   The bulk of evidence indicates that there are no proven pathological or biochemical abnormalities of muscle or muscle metabolism, either at rest or with exercise, other than those associated with deconditioning. *Deconditioning* describes the physiological changes that lead to the loss of tolerance of activity after prolonged rest (e.g., as a result of pain). It has been found in many, but not all, patients with CFS (Bazelmans et al. 2001; Fulcher and White 2000) and also in FMS (Valim et al. 2002). Deconditioning offers a potential biological explanation for exercise-induced fatigue and worsening or persistent muscle pain in patients with CFS and FMS and also provides a rationale for treatment with graded activity (see subsection "Specialist Non-pharmacological Treatments" later in this chapter).

Sleep abnormalities. Patients with CFS and FMS typically complain of unrefreshing and broken sleep, a symptom that has been objectively confirmed with polysomnography. Abnormalities in sleep have been claimed to be of major etiological importance, especially in FMS. Early work (Moldofsky et al. 1975) reported a specific sleep electroencephalogram abnormality of alpha wave intrusion into slow wave sleep (so-called alpha-delta sleep) and suggested that this was a cause of the myalgia. However, attempts to replicate this finding in both FMS and CFS have produced inconsistent results, and its specificity to chronic pain remains unclear (Rains and Penzien 2003).

Neuroendocrine changes. One of the best-supported biological abnormalities reported to be associated with both CFS and FMS is changes in neuroendocrine stress hormones. A repeated observation has been of a tendency to low blood levels of cortisol and a poor cortisol response to stress (Parker et al. 2001). This finding differs from what would be expected in depression (in which blood levels of cortisol are typically elevated) but is similar to that reported in other stress-induced and anxiety states. It is not known whether this is a primary abnormality or merely a consequence of inactivity or sleep disruption, however.

Patients with FMS also have an elevated level of substance P in their cerebrospinal fluid (Russell et al. 1994). A similar finding has been made in patients with other chronic pain syndromes such as osteoarthritis. However, elevated substance P has not been found in CFS patients (Evengard et al. 1998).

Blood pressure regulation. Failure to maintain blood pressure when assuming erect posture (orthostatic intolerance), and particularly a pattern in which the heart rate increases abnormally (postural orthostatic tachycardia syndrome), have been reported in both CFS (Rowe et al. 1995) and FMS (Bou-Holaigah et al. 1997). These findings have been interpreted as indicating abnormal autonomic nervous system function. However, postural hypotension

occurs after prolong[...] 1986), and its specifi[...]

CNS structure. T[...] are probably str[...] malities have b[...] CFS (Cook e[...] imaging (MRI)[...] choline in CFS patien[...] subjects (Puri et al. 2002).

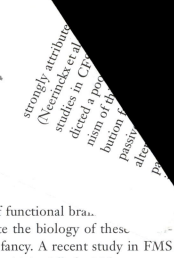

CNS function. The use of functional bra[...] great potential to elucidate the biology of thes[...] tions but remains in its infancy. A recent study in FMS examined abnormal pain sensitivity (allodynia) by comparing brain activation in 16 patients with FMS and 16 control subjects during the application of pressure to their thumbnail beds. Similar pressures resulted in more widespread activation in FMS. This finding was interpreted as supporting the hypothesis that a central augmentation of pain processing occurs in FMS (Gracely et al. 2002).

An early single photon emission computed tomography (SPECT) study (Costa et al. 1995) and a positron emission tomography (PET) study (Tirelli et al. 1998) reported reduced brain stem perfusion in patients with CFS. However, another study that found fewer differences when CFS patients were compared with depressed patients reminds us of the need for careful control for variables such as depression (Machale et al. 2000). As with pain, more widespread cerebral activation is seen in CFS patients than in control subjects when performing a fatiguing cognitive task (Schmaling et al. 2003).

Although tantalizing, these functional brain imaging findings must be regarded as preliminary. Furthermore, evidence of changes in brain activation or brain reorganization must not be taken to mean that the symptoms are necessarily based in fixed neurological pathology; behavioral rehabilitation and drug therapy can potentially reverse such changes (Flor 2003).

Psychological and Social Factors

There is good evidence that psychological and behavioral factors play a major role in perpetuating CFS and FMS.

Illness beliefs. Some of the striking aspects of CFS and FMS are the concern, and often strong beliefs, of many patients about the causes of such illnesses. Three categories of illness beliefs are considered here: 1) cause (attributions), 2) significance of symptoms (catastrophizing), and 3) what one can do despite symptoms (self-efficacy).

Although the cause of CFS and FMS is unknown, many patients, and especially those seen in specialist clinics,

their symptoms to a physical disease
2000). A systematic review of prognostic
found that such strong attributions pre-
er outcome (Joyce et al. 1997). The mecha-
s effect is unclear. It may be that such an attri-
avors a focusing of attention on symptoms, more
e coping, and greater inactivity (Heijmans 1998), or,
natively, that such an attribution leads to nonpartici-
tion in potentially effective psychological and behav-
oral treatment.

Catastrophizing is a tendency to make excessively negative predictions about symptoms, such as "If I do more,
my pain or fatigue will keep getting worse and worse."
Catastrophizing has been observed in patients with CFS
(Petrie et al. 1995) and FMS (Hassett et al. 2000) and is
associated with increased symptom vigilance, avoidance
of activity, and more severe disability. Furthermore, a reduction in the belief that activity is damaging is associated
with recovery during rehabilitative therapy (Deale et al.
1998), suggesting that it may be a critical psychological target for effective rehabilitation.

Self-efficacy—the belief that one can do something,
despite symptoms—has been found to be low and to be
associated with more severe disability in patients with
CFS (Findley et al. 1998), FMS (Buckelew et al. 1996),
and chronic pain (Asghari and Nicholas 2001). Achieving
an increase in self-efficacy is another potential target for
treatment that aims to improve function.

Behavioral factors.   Patients cope with their symptoms
in different ways. The way in which a patient copes will
be influenced by his or her illness beliefs (Silver et al.
2002). Of particular interest is coping by avoiding any activity that the patient fears will exacerbate symptoms.
This fear–avoidance phenomenon is well established in
chronic pain patients (Philips 1987) and also has been observed in CFS (Afari et al. 2000) and in FMS (Davis et al.
2001). Objective assessment also confirms that patients
with CFS and FMS show reduced overall activity, with
most patients oscillating between activity and rest, and a
quarter being more pervasively inactive. This reduced activity produces deconditioning; gradually increasing activity is a treatment task.

Another potentially important coping behavior is the
focusing of attention on symptoms—so-called symptom
focusing or symptom vigilance (Roelofs et al. 2003). This
behavior is, not surprisingly, associated with catastrophizing beliefs and greater perceived symptom intensity; it offers another target for treatment.

Social factors.   Patients' beliefs about their illness and associated coping behavior will be influenced by information received from others. A striking social aspect of CFS
and FMS is the high level of activity in patient support
and advocacy organizations mainly over the Internet
(Ross 1999). Studies from the United Kingdom have reported that patients who are members of a support group
have a poorer outcome, despite similar illness duration
and disability (Sharpe et al. 1992), and a poorer response
to rehabilitation (Bentall et al. 2002). It is now unknown
whether this reflects self-selection into such groups or the
effect of the group on patients' beliefs, coping, and willingness to engage in rehabilitation. Other social factors
include the experience of repeated questioning of the legitimacy of one's illness by doctors and others that probably serves to drive some patients to join advocacy organizations. Perhaps unsurprisingly, the acquisition of a
disability pension is also associated with a worse prognosis (Wigers 1996).

Summary

In summary, the evidence suggests that patients are predisposed to develop CFS and FMS by some combination
of genetics, previous experience, and possibly lack of social support. Many patients with CFS have a history of
preceding infection, and many patients with FMS point
to an accident, injury, or trauma as the triggering event.
Others can identify no precipitant. Most research has
been into factors associated with established illness, so-
called perpetuating factors, because these are both clearly
more accessible to study and more relevant to treatment
of established cases. Many biological factors have been investigated, with interest initially being directed at peripheral nerves and muscles and subsequently focusing on the
CNS and its neuroendocrine and autonomic outputs.
Also, some tantalizing findings have suggested but not yet
established the role of immune factors. The physiological
effects of inactivity seem to be important. Substantial evidence indicates the importance of psychological and behavioral factors, especially the fear of exacerbating symptoms and the associated avoidance of activity in both FMS
and CFS. Social factors are more difficult to study but often are of striking importance clinically.

Models of Chronic Fatigue and Fibromyalgia Syndromes

The findings discussed in the previous section can be
amalgamated into models. Three main models can be dis-
cerned that correspond approximately to biological, psychological, and social perspectives, although, in reality, all
three are probably relevant.

Biological Model

It is well known that the immune system and the CNS and endocrine system interact and also have reciprocal relations with sleep and activity. It is thus possible to construct a tentative biological model in which these systems interact to perpetuate the illness (Moldofsky 1995). There seems to be stronger evidence for the role of infection in triggering CFS and for the role of trauma and changes in central pain processing in FMS. However, it is unclear whether these represent real differences or simply differences in the hypotheses pursued by researchers.

Cognitive-Behavioral Model

Whatever the biological aspects of these conditions, cognitive-behavioral models assume that the symptoms and disability are perpetuated, at least in part, by psychological, behavioral, and social factors. Biological factors are assumed to be either only partially responsible for the illness or largely reversible (Surawy et al. 1995). The cognitive-behavioral models for chronic pain and CFS have much in common (Philips 1987). Both emphasize the importance of fear of symptoms leading to a focusing on the symptoms, helplessness, and avoidance of activity. This model provides the rationale for behavioral and cognitive-behavioral approaches to rehabilitation (see section "Management" later in this chapter).

Social Model

The social model emphasizes the role of social factors in shaping the illness. A fight for the legitimacy of the syndrome as a chronic medical condition is central (Banks and Prior 2001). Patient advocacy has been strongly hostile to psychological and psychiatric involvement, probably because it is seen as undermining legitimacy. The social model proposes that patient organizations, while providing valuable social support, can also shape patients' illness beliefs, medical care, and disability payment seeking in ways that are not conducive to recovery (Shorter 1997).

Diagnostic Evaluation

Effective management of patients with possible CFS or FMS requires that 1) alternative medical and psychiatric diagnoses are considered and 2) the patient receives a comprehensive assessment so that collaborative management may be planned.

Identifying Medical and Psychiatric Conditions

Medical Differential Diagnosis

The medical differential diagnosis for CFS and FMS is a long one because many diseases present with pain and/or fatigue (Sharpe and Wilks 2002; Yunus 2002) (Table 26–4). Both a physical and a mental status examination must be performed in every case to determine any alternative medical and psychiatric diagnoses. As with many chronic diseases, particularly rheumatological conditions, time is often the principal arbiter because the conditions evolve clinically. For symptoms in general, 75% of the patients presenting to primary care improve within 2–4 weeks (Kroenke 2003). Thus, it makes sense to rely on an initial 4- to 6-week wait to clarify whether the symptoms will persist (Kroenke and Jackson 1998). For persistent symptoms, most of the common medical disorders can be diagnosed from a standard history, physical examination, and basic laboratory studies.

Routine investigations.   Initial investigation depends on the clinical signs, symptoms, and temporal nature of symptoms. When symptoms exceed 4–6 weeks, an initial basic screening workup is appropriate. If there are no specific indications for special investigations, the following have been found to be adequate as screening tests: thyrotropin, erythrocyte sedimentation rate (sensitive for any condition with systemic inflammation), complete blood count, basic chemistries, and withdrawal of some medications (particularly statins or 3-hydroxy-3-methylglutaryl coenzyme A reductase inhibitors; typical resolution of symptoms in 4–6 weeks).

Special investigations.   Special investigations should be carried out only if clearly indicated by history or examination. Immunological and virological tests are generally unhelpful as routine investigations and remain research tools. Sleep studies can be useful in excluding other diagnoses, especially when the fatigue is characterized by sleepiness. Diagnoses include sleep apnea, narcolepsy, nocturnal myoclonus, and periodic leg movements during sleep (see Chapter 16, "Sleep Disorders"). Once symptoms become chronic (>3 months) and remain unexplained, the general approach is to avoid excessive testing, establish regular follow-up, screen for depressive and anxiety disorders, and focus on symptom management.

Medical misdiagnosis.   Those concerned about missing a serious medical diagnosis can be reassured that in most cases, the primary care physician's initial judgment in this

TABLE 26–4. Medical differential diagnosis for patients with chronic fatigue syndrome (CFS) and fibromyalgia syndrome (FMS)

Relative frequency	Diagnoses	Syndrome	Differentiating clinical features	Initial workup
Very common (~1 per 100)	Thyroid disorders	CFS, FMS	Hypothyroidism: cold intolerance, slowed relaxation phase of reflexes, weight gain, elevated cholesterol Hyperthyroidism: heat intolerance, tremor, weight loss	Thyrotropin
	Medications (statins)	CFS, FMS	Symptom resolution with withdrawal of medication	Creatine kinase, aldolase
	Sleep apnea	CFS, FMS	Daytime somnolence, motor vehicle accidents, witnessed nighttime apnea and snoring, hypertension	Sleep study
	Spinal stenosis	FMS	History of osteoarthritis, degenerative disc disease, back pain with radiculopathy, sensory and/or motor deficits, pseudoclaudication	Nerve conduction study, electromyogram, magnetic resonance imaging of spine if neurological deficits
	Anemia	CFS	Pallor	Complete blood cell count
Common (~1 per 1,000)	Chronic infection: HIV, hepatitis C, endocarditis, osteomyelitis, Lyme disease, occult abscess	CFS, FMS	Infection-specific risk factors and signs (e.g., sexual habits, diabetes, fevers, murmur)	Serology, erythrocyte sedimentation rate, liver function tests, serial blood cultures, bone scan, indium scan
	Polymyalgia rheumatica	FMS	>60 years old	Erythrocyte sedimentation rate
	Cancer	CFS	Pallor, anemia, anorexia, weight loss, cachexia	Complete blood cell count, albumin, age-appropriate cancer screening studies
	Pulmonary condition: asthma, obstructive lung disease, interstitial lung disease	CFS	Shortness of breath, prominent exertional symptoms, smoking history, hypoxia	Chest X ray, pulmonary function tests, oxygenation saturation with exercise
	Symptomatic hyperparathyroidism	CFS	Bone pain, nephrolithiasis, pancreatitis, renal insufficiency	Serum calcium and parathyroid hormone
Uncommon (~1 per 2,500–100,000)	Systemic lupus	FMS	Malar rash, joint pain	Antinuclear antibody, double–stranded DNA
	Rheumatoid arthritis	FMS	Symmetric synovitis, morning stiffness	Rheumatoid factor
	Polymyositis, dermatomyositis, myopathy	CFS, FMS	Proximal muscle weakness	Antinuclear antibody, creatine kinase, aldolase
	Myasthenia gravis, multiple sclerosis	CFS	Neurological findings: extinguishing strength with repetitive movements, ptosis, swallowing difficulties, optic neuritis, sensory deficits	Tensilon test, acetylcholine receptor antibodies, magnetic resonance imaging of brain
	Narcolepsy	CFS	Drop attacks, falling asleep during daily activities	Sleep study
	Inflammatory bowel disease (Crohn's)	CFS	Diarrhea, weight loss, fever, anemia	Serial fecal occult blood with endoscopy if positive

regard is likely to be accurate (Khan et al. 2003). However, some evidence shows that CFS and FMS may be overdiagnosed by primary care physicians (Fitzcharles and Boulos 2003), and psychiatrists should feel able to request second medical opinions.

Psychiatric Differential Diagnosis

Underdiagnosis of psychiatric disorders is particularly common (Torres-Harding et al. 2002), probably reflecting a focus of the initial medical assessment on somatic symptoms and a tendency to disregard mood changes as simply being a consequence of these symptoms. The most important psychiatric diagnoses to consider are depressive and anxiety disorders because of their frequency and their implications for treatment. Depression may be masked and require expert assessment if it is to be detected. Panic attacks with agoraphobia may cause intermittent severe fatigue and disability. Somatoform disorders are common but have fewer implications for management. A diagnosis of somatization disorder indicates a poorer prognosis, and hypochondriasis indicates special attention to repeated reassurance seeking, which may perpetuate fears of undiagnosed disease (Sharpe and Williams 2001).

Assessment of the Illness

Other than to make diagnoses, the aims of the assessment are to 1) establish a collaborative relationship with the patient, 2) elicit the patient's own understanding of his or her illness and how he or she copes with it, and 3) identify current family and social factors such as employment and litigation that may complicate management. It is important to inquire fully about the patient's understanding of his or her illness (e.g., "What do you think is wrong with you?" or "What do you think the cause is?"). Patients may be fearful that their symptoms indicate a progressive, as yet undiagnosed, disease or that exertion will cause a long-term worsening of their condition. A formulation that identifies potential predisposing, precipitating, and perpetuating factors (see Table 26–3) is valuable both in providing an individualized explanation to the patient and for targeting interventions.

Management

Diagnosis, Formulation, and Management Plan

Forming a Therapeutic Relationship With the Patient

The patient often will have seen many other doctors and will have experienced problematic interactions with them

(Asbring and Narvanen 2003). Other doctors may have offered overly biomedical or overly psychological explanations or even dismissed the patient completely.

Explaining Psychiatric Involvement

Psychiatrists' involvement in management may be interpreted by the patient as indicating that his or her condition is considered to be "all in his or her head." It is often best to begin with a somatic assessment and only then to introduce discussion of psychological factors. This can be done in a nonblaming and normalizing way. For example; "You have clearly had a terrible time made worse by not being believed. It is entirely understandable that this has gotten you down." It is generally unhelpful to force a psychiatric diagnosis on an unwilling patient. It is also important to explain how treatments commonly associated with psychiatry (particularly antidepressants and cognitive-behavioral therapy [CBT]) do not necessarily imply that the person is mentally ill. Rather, they can be explained as ways of normalizing brain and bodily function in conditions that are exacerbated by stress (Sharpe and Carson 2001).

Giving the Diagnosis

It is important to give the patient a positive diagnosis supplemented with an etiological formulation. Some controversy exists about whether giving patients a diagnosis of CFS or FMS is helpful or harmful (Finestone 1997). Some who believe that a diagnosis is helpful argue that it enables patients to both conceptualize their illness and communicate about it with others (Sharpe 1998). Others who are concerned about the potentially harmful effect of diagnosis argue that it medicalizes and pathologizes symptoms in a way that can exacerbate social and occupational disability (Hadler 1996a). It is our clinical experience that a positive diagnosis linked to an explanation of the potential reversibility of symptoms and a management plan to achieve this is an essential starting point for effective management.

Offering an Explanation

The explanation ideally should be scientifically accurate, acceptable to the patient, and congruent with the management plan. It can be explained that although the specific causes of CFS or FMS remain unknown, a combination of vulnerability and environmental stress likely to involve the brain and endocrine system is most likely. One such explanation is that the illness is a disorder of brain function rather than *structure*—that is, a functional nervous disorder (Stone et al. 2002).

Explaining the Management Plan

The management plan should be explained to the patient as following from the formulation, focusing on illness perpetuating factors and consisting of elements to 1) relieve symptoms such as depression, pain, and sleep disturbance with agents such as antidepressants; 2) assist the patient's efforts at coping by stabilizing activity and retraining the body to function effectively (graded exercise, CBT); and 3) assist the patient in managing the social and financial aspects of his or her illness and, when possible, remaining in or returning to employment (problem solving).

General Measures

Providing Advice on Symptom Management

One of the most important interventions the clinician can make is to encourage and guide patients in the active self-management of the illness. Such advice will include the importance of being realistic about what they are able to accomplish without giving up hope for improvement in the future. It should involve advice on the pros and cons of self-medication, particularly with analgesics, and also might require a discussion of the potential benefits and risks of iatrogenic harm associated with seeking treatment from other practitioners, both conventional and alternative. The overall aim is to encourage the patients to feel that they can do things to manage the condition themselves, to accept the reality of their illness while still planning positively for the future, and to be cautious about seeking potentially harmful and expensive treatments.

Managing Activity and Avoidance

Once activity is stabilized and large fluctuations between excessive rest and unsustainable activity are reduced, gradual increases in activity can be advised. It is critical, however, to distinguish between carefully graded increases carried out in collaboration with the patient and a forced or an overambitious exercise regimen.

Managing Occupational and Social Factors

Patients who continue working may be overstressed by the effort of doing this. Those who have left work may have become inactive and demoralized and may not wish to return to the same job. These situations require a problem-solving approach to consider how to manage work demands, achieve a graded return to work, or plan an alternative career. Ongoing litigation is potentially a complicating factor because it reinforces (and may reward) the patient for remaining symptomatic and disabled. A large trial in Canada that randomized patients either to litigation or to no-fault compensation for whiplash injury found that symptoms lasted longer in the former group (Cassidy et al. 2000).

Pharmacological Therapies

Most pharmacological treatment studies in CFS and FMS have focused on antidepressants, although various other agents have been advocated.

Antidepressants

Antidepressant drug treatment is indicated by the fact that 1) many patients with CFS or FMS have depressive and anxiety syndromes and 2) these agents reduce pain and improve sleep, even in the absence of depression. However, the evidence that antidepressants lead to an overall improvement in CFS and FMS is mixed, with the evidence being better for FMS (O'Malley et al. 2000) than for CFS (Reid et al. 2003).

The tricyclic antidepressants (TCAs) are probably more effective than the selective serotonin reuptake inhibitors (SSRIs) for relieving pain (Fishbain 2003) and for inducing sleep. Small doses (e.g., 25–50 mg of amitriptyline) are often adequate for these purposes (Arnold et al. 2000; O'Malley et al. 2000), but full doses are required to treat major depression.

Cyclobenzaprine, a tricyclic agent chemically similar to amitriptyline but used as a "muscle relaxant" rather than as an antidepressant, has been found to be effective in improving symptoms in FMS, especially pain and sleep disturbance (Tofferi et al. 2004).

SSRIs are generally better tolerated than TCAs. In CFS, fluoxetine was found in a large trial to be no more effective than placebo (Vercoulen et al. 1996b). In FMS, one recent study found that patients who received fluoxetine (mean dose=45 mg) experienced a greater reduction in pain, fatigue, and depressed mood than did those who received placebo (Arnold et al. 2002); however, in a small previous trial, fluoxetine at a dosage of 20 mg/day did not have the same effect (Wolfe et al. 1994).

Other antidepressant agents also have been tried. Venlafaxine, a dual serotonin-norepinephrine reuptake inhibitor (SNRI), is useful for pain and has been reported as showing initial promise in both FMS (Dwight et al. 1998) and CFS (Goodnick 1996). Moclobemide, a reversible inhibitor of monoamine oxidase A, has been reported to be of no benefit in FMS but of some value in increasing energy in CFS (Hickie et al. 2000).

Other Pharmacological Agents

Patients with FMS and CFS frequently use nonsteroidal anti-inflammatory drugs (NSAIDs) to relieve pain. No evidence from clinical trials indicates that NSAIDs are effective when used alone, although they may be of some benefit in FMS when combined with amitriptyline (Goldenberg et al. 1986).

Opiates are occasionally used for pain in FMS and CFS. However, no trials of their use have been done, and a major concern is the development of dependence.

As with opiates, great caution is required with benzodiazepines because of the risk of dependence in patients with chronic conditions. TCAs are probably preferable to benzodiazepines for treating insomnia, and the chronic use of benzodiazepines should be reserved for patients with intractable anxiety.

Given the finding of low serum levels of cortisol, it is not surprising that corticosteroids have been tried. Prednisone was found to be ineffective in FMS (Clark et al. 1985). Hydrocortisone was reported to produce some benefit in CFS but was not recommended because of the long-term risks of adrenal suppression (Cleare et al. 1999). In CFS, fludrocortisone has been used in patients with orthostatic hypotension but has not been found to be of value (Rowe et al. 2001).

Serotonin$_3$ receptor antagonists (e.g., ondansetron and tropisetron) have analgesic effects (Kranzler et al. 2002). A randomized, placebo-controlled, double-blind trial in FMS found short-term benefit only with the lowest dosage (5 mg/day) (Farber et al. 2001). Trials of longer duration are needed.

Gabapentin has substantial analgesic effects, but its mechanism of action is unknown. There are only anecdotal reports of its successful use in FMS. Pregabalin, a drug still in clinical development that has pharmacological properties similar to those of gabapentin, also may have potential efficacy.

Amphetamines have been used in CFS with some evidence of short-term efficacy (Olson et al. 2003) but are not widely used because of the risk of dependence.

Summary

It is wise to exercise caution when prescribing pharmacological therapy for CFS and FMS. The mainstay of therapy continues to be the so-called antidepressant drugs, which may be helpful for mood, pain, and sleep but have limited effect on overall outcome. TCAs are preferred for nighttime sedation and pain, but greater tolerability may mean that an SSRI or an SNRI is preferable as first-line treatment. In current clinical practice, although patients often receive low doses of antidepressants, higher doses may be required to achieve a therapeutic response. The increased interest in pharmacological treatment of functional syndromes in the past few years will likely expand treatment options, and several medications in clinical development show promise, including duloxetine, milna-

cipran, and pregabalin. However, the available evidence suggests that drug therapy has a limited role in the management of these conditions.

Specialist Nonpharmacological Treatments

If the patient does not respond to, or requires more active treatment than, the general and pharmacological management described above, referral for specialist therapy should be considered. For most patients, a rehabilitative outpatient program based on appropriately managed increases in activity, either as graded exercise therapy (GET) or as CBT, is indicated. Some patients may require inpatient multidisciplinary rehabilitation, although evidence of its efficacy is inadequate (Karjalainen et al. 2000).

Graded Exercise Therapy

Graded exercise therapy is a structured progressive exercise program administered and carefully monitored by an exercise therapist. It also may be given in individual or group form, but the evidence is best for individually administered treatment (Fulcher and White 1998).

Graded exercise therapy follows the basic principles of exercise prescription for healthy individuals, adapted to the patient's current capacity. The initial exercise intensity and duration are determined on an individual basis and may be done via heart rate monitoring. Most patients can begin at an intensity of 40% of their maximum aerobic capacity, which approximately equates to 50% of their estimated individual heart rate reserve added to their resting heart rate (e.g., if the maximum heart rate is 180 beats/minute [bpm] and the resting heart rate is 80 bpm, the heart rate reserve is 100 bpm, and the exercise target heart rate is $80 + (0.5 \times 100) = 130$ bpm). This heart rate should not be exceeded; if it is, the patient should stop exercising for 1–2 minutes and then resume. Patients who are very disabled, or who have extremely low exercise tolerance to begin with, should begin with 2 weeks of stretching alone without aerobic activity and then should adopt alternate-day aerobic exercise before building up frequency, duration, and then intensity. The important principle is to calculate exercise capacity conservatively to start with, as well as to ensure that the patient will try that which is proposed.

At each clinic visit, joint planning of the exercise prescription for the following 1–2 weeks is completed. The initial aim is to establish a regular pattern of exercise (usually walking), with exercise 5 days/week. Home exercise sessions should initially last between 5 and 15 minutes, depending on ability and exercise tolerance. The duration is increased by 1–2 minutes/week up to a maximum of 30 minutes per homework session. Then, the intensity of exercise can be increased to a target heart rate of 60% and then 70% of the patient's heart rate reserve added to his or her resting heart rate. Patients will respond differently; some will take a lot longer to adapt to each new level, whereas others will have to be held back, particularly those who have been active sports participants in the past. Those patients who are inclined to overexert themselves in an attempt to speed up the recovery process should be monitored carefully because this can be a contributing factor in nonrecovery or relapse.

Graded exercise therapy has been found in systematic review to be of benefit in both CFS and FMS. In FMS, four high-quality aerobic training studies (total 227 patients) reported significantly greater improvements in aerobic performance, tender point pain pressure threshold, and pain with exercise than with comparison treatments (Busch et al. 2002).

In CFS, three high-quality trials (total 340 patients) all found benefits over comparison treatments in symptoms and disability. However, the number of dropouts in one study was substantial (Whiting et al. 2001). Of particular interest is a trial of brief simple education about the physiology and rationale of exercise that found the education to be as effective as CBT (Powell et al. 2001).

Cognitive-Behavioral Therapy

There are a variety of types of CBT (Williams 2003). Here, we refer to a collaborative psychologically informed type of rehabilitation that aims to achieve both graded increases in activity and changes in unhelpful beliefs and concerns about symptoms. It also may include problem solving for life and occupational dilemmas. It can be given in an individual or a group form, although more evidence exists for the efficacy of individual therapy (Sharpe 1997).

The procedure is 1) to elicit nonjudgmentally the patient's own illness model, appraisal of his or her situation, and the ways in which he or she copes; 2) to introduce the possibility of alternatives; and 3) to help the patient select the beliefs and coping behaviors that are most helpful by conducting behavioral experiments. The key question for the behavioral experiment is "Is it possible for me to make changes in my behavior that will allow me to achieve my goals?" The patient is encouraged to think of the illness as real but reversible by his or her own efforts rather than (as many patients do) as a fixed, unalterable disease. The ability to make changes is a test of these alternative hypotheses. The aim of behavior change is to achieve specific goals. Problem solving is used to address relevant occupational and interpersonal difficulties. A typical therapy takes place over 14 sessions (the first 90 minutes, the rest 50 minutes), the first 4 sessions being weekly and thereafter biweekly over 5 months.

In CFS, individually administered CBT has now been found to be effective in two systematic reviews, with approximately two-thirds of the patients showing significant improvement. Three high-quality trials (total 164 patients) found improvement in both symptoms and disability and concluded that CBT appears to be an effective and acceptable treatment for adult outpatients with CFS (Price and Couper 2003; Whiting et al. 2001).

Although CBT is an established treatment for chronic pain (Morley et al. 1999) (see also Chapter 36, "Pain"), in FMS, only group CBT has been adequately evaluated in randomized trials. One trial reported no benefit (Vlaeyen et al. 1996), but a more recent study did find a clear advantage of group CBT over usual medical care (Williams et al. 2002). Further evaluation of the intensive individual CBT shown to be effective in CFS is required in FMS.

Patients Who Do Not Respond to Treatment

Most patients respond to some degree to rehabilitative therapies, but many will achieve only partial improvement, and some will fail to improve at all. In such cases, the management is the same as that for other chronic conditions—to maximize functioning and quality of life while minimizing the risk of iatrogenic harm. Although it is desirable that all patients should have a trial of rehabilitative treatment, a balance has to be struck between heroic efforts at therapy and acceptance of chronic illness. Many physicians are reluctant to accept chronic disability in these patients, perhaps because they do not regard these conditions as true diseases. Pushing patients beyond their capabilities may only demoralize them or cause them to retreat further into invalidism. For such patients, regular follow-up from a single physician is often the best form of management.

Conclusion

Although peripheral to both internal medicine and psychiatry, somatic syndromes such as chronic fatigue syndrome and fibromyalgia are core to the practice of psychosomatic medicine. A willingness and ability to integrate biological, psychological, and social factors is essential to both an adequate understanding of these syndromes' etiology and their effective management. The challenge that these syndromes present to the more narrow paradigms of the biomedical and psychopathological perspectives makes them an effective Trojan horse for those who seek to persuade others of the benefits of much greater integration of medical and psychiatric theory and practice.

References

Aaron LA, Buchwald D: Chronic diffuse musculoskeletal pain, fibromyalgia and co-morbid unexplained clinical conditions: Bailliere's best practice and research. Clin Rheumatol 17:563–574, 2003

Afari N, Buchwald D: Chronic fatigue syndrome: a review. Am J Psychiatry 160:221–236, 2003

Afari N, Schmaling KB, Herrell R, et al: Coping strategies in twins with chronic fatigue and chronic fatigue syndrome. J Psychosom Res 48:547–554, 2000

Al Allaf AW, Dunbar KL, Hallum NS, et al: A case-control study examining the role of physical trauma in the onset of fibromyalgia syndrome. Rheumatology (Oxford) 41:450–453, 2002

American Psychiatric Association: Diagnostic and Statistical Manual of Mental Disorders, 4th Edition, Text Revision. Washington, DC, American Psychiatric Association, 2000

Anderberg UM, Marteinsdottir I, Theorell T, et al: The impact of life events in female patients with fibromyalgia and in female healthy controls. Eur Psychiatry 15:295–301, 2000

Arnold LM, Keck PE Jr, Welge JA: Antidepressant treatment of fibromyalgia: a meta-analysis and review. Psychosomatics 41:104–113, 2000

Arnold LM, Hess EV, Hudson JI, et al: A randomized, placebo-controlled, double-blind, flexible-dose study of fluoxetine in the treatment of women with fibromyalgia. Am J Med 112:191–197, 2002

Asbring P, Narvanen AL: Ideal versus reality: physicians' perspectives on patients with chronic fatigue syndrome (CFS) and fibromyalgia. Soc Sci Med 57:711–720, 2003

Asghari A, Nicholas MK: Pain self-efficacy beliefs and pain behaviour: a prospective study. Pain 94:85–100, 2001

Assefi NP, Coy TV, Uslan D, et al: Financial, occupational, and personal consequences of disability in patients with chronic fatigue syndrome and fibromyalgia compared to other fatiguing conditions. J Rheumatol 30:804–808, 2003

Ayres JG, Flint N, Smith EG, et al: Post-infection fatigue syndrome following Q fever. Q J Med 91:105–123, 1998

Banks J, Prior L: Doing things with illness: the micro politics of the CFS clinic. Soc Sci Med 52:11–23, 2001

Bazelmans E, Vercoulen JH, Galama JMD, et al: Prevalence of chronic fatigue syndrome and primary fibromyalgia syndrome (PFS) in the Netherlands. Ned Tijdschr Geneeskd 141:1520–1523, 1997

Bazelmans E, Bleijenberg G, Van der Meer JW, et al: Is physical deconditioning a perpetuating factor in chronic fatigue syndrome? A controlled study on maximal exercise performance and relations with fatigue, impairment and physical activity. Psychol Med 31:107–114, 2001

Bentall RP, Powell P, Nye FJ, et al: Predictors of response to treatment for chronic fatigue syndrome. Br J Psychiatry 181:248–252, 2002

Berelowitz GJ, Burgess AP, Thanabalasingham T, et al: Post-hepatitis syndrome revisited. J Viral Hepat 2:133–138, 1995

Bombardier CH, Buchwald D: Chronic fatigue, chronic fatigue syndrome, and fibromyalgia: disability and health-care use. Med Care 34:924–930, 1996

Bou-Holaigah I, Calkins H, Flynn JA, et al: Provocation of hypotension and pain during upright tilt table testing in adults with fibromyalgia. Clin Exp Rheumatol 15:239–246, 1997

Buchwald D, Herrell R, Ashton S, et al: A twin study of chronic fatigue. Psychosom Med 63:936–943, 2001

Buckelew SP, Huyser B, Hewett JE, et al: Self-efficacy predicting outcome among fibromyalgia subjects. Arthritis Care Res 9:97–104, 1996

Busch A, Schachter CL, Peloso PM, et al: Exercise for treating fibromyalgia syndrome. Cochrane Database Syst Rev 3: CD003786, 2002

Buskila D, Neumann L: Fibromyalgia syndrome (FM) and nonarticular tenderness in relatives of patients with FM. J Rheumatol 24:941–944, 1997

Buskila D, Press J, Abu-Shakra M: Fibromyalgia in systemic lupus erythematosus: prevalence and clinical implications. Clin Rev Allergy Immunol 25:25–28, 2003

Cassidy JD, Carroll LJ, Cote P, et al: Effect of eliminating compensation for pain and suffering on the outcome of insurance claims for whiplash injury. N Engl J Med 342:1179–1186, 2000

Chalder T, Goodman R, Wessely S, et al: Epidemiology of chronic fatigue syndrome and self reported myalgic encephalomyelitis in 5–15 year olds: cross sectional study. BMJ 327:654–655, 2003

Ciccone DS, Natelson BH: Comorbid illness in women with chronic fatigue syndrome: a test of the single-syndrome hypothesis. Psychosom Med 65:268–275, 2003

Clark SR, Tindall E, Bennett RM: A double blind crossover trial of prednisone versus placebo in the treatment of fibrositis. J Rheumatol 12:980–983, 1985

Clauw DJ, Chrousos GP: Chronic pain and fatigue syndromes: overlapping clinical and neuroendocrine features and potential pathogenic mechanisms. Neuroimmunomodulation 4:134–153, 1997

Clauw DJ, Crofford LJ: Chronic widespread pain and fibromyalgia: what we know, and what we need to know. Bailliere's best practice and research. Clin Rheumatol 17:685–701, 2003

Cleare AJ, Heap E, Malhi GS, et al: Low-dose hydrocortisone in chronic fatigue syndrome: a randomised crossover trial. Lancet 353:455–458, 1999

Cohen H, Neumann L, Haiman Y, et al: Prevalence of posttraumatic stress disorder in fibromyalgia patients: overlapping syndromes or post-traumatic fibromyalgia syndrome? Semin Arthritis Rheum 32:38–50, 2002

Cook DB, Lange G, DeLuca J, et al: Relationship of brain MRI abnormalities and physical functional status in chronic fatigue syndrome. Int J Neurosci 107:1–6, 2001

Costa DC, Tannock C, Brostoff J: Brainstem perfusion is impaired in chronic fatigue syndrome. Q J Med 88:767–773, 1995

Croft P, Rigby AS, Boswell R, et al: The prevalence of chronic widespread pain in the general population. J Rheumatol 20: 710–713, 1993

Croft P, Burt J, Schollum J, et al: More pain, more tender points: is fibromyalgia just one end of a continuous spectrum? Ann Rheum Dis 55:482–485, 1996

Davis MC, Zautra AJ, Reich JW: Vulnerability to stress among women in chronic pain from fibromyalgia and osteoarthritis. Annals of Behavioural Medicine 23:215–226, 2001

Deale A, Chalder T, Wessely S: Illness beliefs and treatment outcome in chronic fatigue syndrome. J Psychosom Res 45: 77–83, 1998

Dwight MM, Arnold LM, O'Brien H, et al: An open clinical trial of venlafaxine treatment of fibromyalgia. Psychosomatics 39:14–17, 1998

Engel GL: The need for a new medical model: a challenge for biomedicine. Science 196:129–196, 1977

Epstein SA, Kay G, Clauw D, et al: Psychiatric disorders in patients with fibromyalgia: a multicenter investigation. Psychosomatics 40:57–63, 1999

Evengard B, Nilsson CG, Lindh G, et al: Chronic fatigue syndrome differs from fibromyalgia: no evidence for elevated substance P levels in cerebrospinal fluid of patients with chronic fatigue syndrome. Pain 78:153–155, 1998

Farber L, Stratz TH, Bruckle W, et al: Short-term treatment of primary fibromyalgia with the 5-HT3-receptor antagonist tropisetron: results of a randomized, double-blind, placebo-controlled multicenter trial in 418 patients. Int J Clin Pharmacol Res 21:1–13, 2001

Findley JC, Kerns R, Weinberg LD, et al: Self-efficacy as a psychological moderator of chronic fatigue syndrome. J Behav Med 21:351–362, 1998

Finestone AJ: A doctor's dilemma: is a diagnosis disabling or enabling? Arch Intern Med 157:491–492, 1997

Fischler B, Cluydts R, De Gucht Y, et al: Generalized anxiety disorder in chronic fatigue syndrome. Acta Psychiatr Scand 95:405–413, 1997

Fishbain DA: Analgesic effects of antidepressants. J Clin Psychiatry 64:96–97, 2003

Fitzcharles MA, Boulos P: Inaccuracy in the diagnosis of fibromyalgia syndrome: analysis of referrals. Rheumatology (Oxford) 42:263–267, 2003

Flor H: Cortical reorganisation and chronic pain: implications for rehabilitation. Journal of Rehabilitative Medicine 41 (suppl):66–72, 2003

Fukuda K, Straus SE, Hickie IB, et al: Chronic fatigue syndrome: a comprehensive approach to its definition and management. Ann Intern Med 121:953–959, 1994

Fulcher KY, White PD: Chronic fatigue syndrome: a description of graded exercise treatment. Physiotherapy 84:223–226, 1998

Fulcher KY, White PD: Strength and physiological response to exercise in patients with chronic fatigue syndrome. J Neurol Neurosurg Psychiatry 69:302–307, 2000

Goldenberg DL, Felson DT, Dinerman H: A randomized, controlled trial of amitriptyline and naproxen in the treatment of patients with fibromyalgia. Arthritis Rheum 29:1371–1377, 1986

Goodnick PJ: Treatment of chronic fatigue syndrome with venlafaxine (letter). Am J Psychiatry 153:294, 1996

Gowers WR: A lecture on lumbago: its lessons and analogues. BMJ 1:117–121, 1904

Gracely RH, Petzke F, Wolf JM, et al: Functional magnetic resonance imaging evidence of augmented pain processing in fibromyalgia. Arthritis Rheum 46:1333–1343, 2002

Granges G, Zilko P, Littlejohn GO: Fibromyalgia syndrome: assessment of the severity of the condition 2 years after diagnosis. J Rheumatol 21:523–529, 1994

Gureje O, Simon GE, Von Korff M: A cross-national study of the course of persistent pain in primary care. Pain 92:195–200, 2001

Hadler NM: Fibromyalgia, chronic fatigue, and other iatrogenic diagnostic algorithms: do some labels escalate illness in vulnerable patients? Postgrad Med 102:161–162, 1996a

Hadler NM: If you have to prove you are ill, you can't get well: the object lesson of fibromyalgia. Spine 21:2397–2400, 1996b

Hassett AL, Cone JD, Patella SJ, et al: The role of catastrophizing in the pain and depression of women with fibromyalgia syndrome. Arthritis Rheum 43:2493–2500, 2000

Hatcher S, House A: Life events, difficulties and dilemmas in the onset of chronic fatigue syndrome: a case-control study. Psychol Med 33:1185–1192, 2003

Heijmans MJ: Coping and adaptive outcome in chronic fatigue syndrome: importance of illness cognitions. J Psychosom Res 45:39–51, 1998

Henningsen P, Zimmermann T, Sattel H: Medically unexplained physical symptoms, anxiety, and depression: a meta-analytic review. Psychosom Med 65:528–533, 2003

Hickie IB, Wilson AJ, Wright JM, et al: A randomized, double-blind placebo-controlled trial of moclobemide in patients with chronic fatigue syndrome. J Clin Psychiatry 61:643–648, 2000

Hill NF, Tiersky LA, Scavalla VR, et al: Natural history of severe chronic fatigue syndrome. Arch Phys Med Rehabil 80:1090–1094, 1999

Holmes GP, Kaplan JE, Gantz NM, et al: Chronic fatigue syndrome: a working case definition. Ann Intern Med 108:387–389, 1988

Hotopf MH, Noah N, Wessely S: Chronic fatigue and minor psychiatric morbidity after viral meningitis: a controlled study. J Neurol Neurosurg Psychiatry 60:504–509, 1996

Hudson JI, Pope HG: The concept of affective spectrum disorder: relationship to fibromyalgia and other syndromes of chronic fatigue and chronic muscle pain. Baillieres Clin Rheumatol 8:839–856, 1994

Hudson JI, Pope HG Jr: The relationship between fibromyalgia and major depressive disorder. Rheum Dis Clin North Am 22:285–303, 1996

Hudson JI, Mangweth B, Pope HG Jr, et al: Family study of affective spectrum disorder. Arch Gen Psychiatry 60:170–177, 2003

Jason LA, Richman JA, Rademaker AW, et al: A community-based study of chronic fatigue syndrome. Arch Intern Med 159:2129–2137, 1999

Johnson SK, DeLuca J, Natelson BH: Assessing somatization disorder in the chronic fatigue syndrome. Psychosom Med 58:50–57, 1996

Joyce J, Hotopf M, Wessely S: The prognosis of chronic fatigue and chronic fatigue syndrome: a systematic review. Q J Med 90:223–233, 1997

Karjalainen K, Malmivaara A, van Tulder M, et al: Multidisciplinary rehabilitation for fibromyalgia and musculoskeletal pain in working age adults. Cochrane Database Syst Rev 2, 2000

Katon W, Buchwald DS, Simon GE, et al: Psychiatric illness in patients with chronic fatigue and rheumatoid arthritis. J Gen Intern Med 6:277–285, 1991

Khan AA, Khan A, Harezlak J, et al: Somatic symptoms in primary care: etiology and outcome. Psychosomatics 44:471–478, 2003

Kranzler JD, Gendreau JF, Rao SG: The psychopharmacology of fibromyalgia: a drug development perspective. Psychopharmacol Bull 36:165–213, 2002

Kroenke K: Patients presenting with somatic complaints: epidemiology, psychiatric comorbidity and management. Int J Methods Psychiatr Res 12:34–43, 2003

Kroenke K, Jackson JL: Outcome in general medical patients presenting with common symptoms: a prospective study with a 2-week and a 3-month follow-up. Fam Pract 15:398–403, 1998

Kruesi MJ, Dale JK, Straus SE: Psychiatric diagnoses in patients who have chronic fatigue syndrome. J Clin Psychiatry 50:53–56, 1989

Kurtze N, Svebak S: Fatigue and patterns of pain in fibromyalgia: correlations with anxiety, depression and co-morbidity in a female county sample. Br J Med Psychol 74:523–537, 2001

Kushner MG, Beitman BD: Panic attacks without fear: an overview. Behav Res Ther 28:469–479, 1990

Lehman AM, Lehman DR, Hemphill KJ, et al: Illness experience, depression, and anxiety in chronic fatigue syndrome. J Psychosom Res 52:461–465, 2002

Lloyd AR, Wakefield D, Boughton CR, et al: What is myalgic encephalomyelitis? Lancet i:1286–1287, 1988

Lyall M, Peakman M, Wessely S: A systematic review and critical evaluation of the immunology of chronic fatigue syndrome. J Psychosom Res 55:79–90, 2003

Machale SM, Lawrie SM, Cavanagh JT, et al: Cerebral perfusion in chronic fatigue syndrome and depression. Br J Psychiatry 176:550–556, 2000

Makela MO: Is fibromyalgia a distinct clinical entity? The epidemiologist's evidence. Baillieres Best Pract Res Clin Rheumatol 13:415–419, 1999

Manu P, Matthews DA, Lane TJ: Panic disorder among patients with chronic fatigue. South Med J 84:451–456, 1991

Mayou R, Levenson J, Sharpe M: Somatoform disorders in DSM-V. Psychosomatics 44:449–451, 2003

Moldofsky H: Sleep, neuroimmune and neuroendocrine functions in fibromyalgia and chronic fatigue syndrome. Adv Neuroimmunol 5:39–56, 1995

Moldofsky H, Scarisbrick P, England R, et al: Musculoskeletal symptoms and Non-REM sleep disturbances in patients with fibrositis syndrome and healthy subjects. Psychosom Med 37:341–351, 1975

Morley S, Eccleston C, Williams A: Systematic review and meta-analysis of randomized controlled trials of cognitive behaviour therapy and behaviour therapy for chronic pain in adults, excluding headache. Pain 80:1–13, 1999

Neerinckx E, Van Houdenhove B, Lysens R, et al: Attributions in chronic fatigue syndrome and fibromyalgia syndrome in tertiary care. J Rheumatol 27:1051–1055, 2000

Nisenbaum R, Jones JF, Unger ER, et al: A population-based study of the clinical course of chronic fatigue syndrome. Health Qual Life Outcomes 1:49, 2003

Ohayon MM, Schatzberg AF: Using chronic pain to predict depressive morbidity in the general population. Arch Gen Psychiatry 60:39–47, 2003

Olson LG, Ambrogetti A, Sutherland DC: A pilot randomized controlled trial of dexamphetamine in patients with chronic fatigue syndrome. Psychosomatics 44:38–43, 2003

O'Malley PG, Balden E, Tomkins G, et al: Treatment of fibromyalgia with antidepressants: a meta-analysis. J Gen Intern Med 15:659–666, 2000

Parker AJ, Wessely S, Cleare AJ: The neuroendocrinology of chronic fatigue syndrome and fibromyalgia. Psychol Med 31:1331–1345, 2001

Pawlikowska T, Chalder T, Hirsch SR, et al: Population based study of fatigue and psychological distress. BMJ 308:763–766, 1994

Petrie KJ, Moss-Morris R, Weinman J: The impact of catastrophic beliefs on functioning in chronic fatigue syndrome. J Psychosom Res 39:31–38, 1995

Philips HC: Avoidance behaviour and its role in sustaining chronic pain. Behav Res Ther 25:273–279, 1987

Powell P, Bentall RP, Nye FJ, et al: Randomised controlled trial of patient education to encourage graded exercise in chronic fatigue syndrome. BMJ 322:387–390, 2001

Price JR, Couper J: Cognitive behaviour therapy for chronic fatigue syndrome in adults. Cochrane Database Syst Rev 4, 2003

Puri BK, Counsell SJ, Zaman R, et al: Relative increase in choline in the occipital cortex in chronic fatigue syndrome. Acta Psychiatr Scand 106:224–226, 2002

Rains JC, Penzien DB: Sleep and chronic pain: challenges to the alpha-EEG sleep pattern as a pain specific sleep anomaly. J Psychosom Res 54:77–83, 2003

Rea T, Russo J, Katon W, et al: A prospective study of tender points and fibromyalgia during and after an acute viral infection. Arch Intern Med 159:865–870, 1999

Reeves WC, Lloyd A, Vernon SD, et al: Identification of ambiguities in the 1994 chronic fatigue syndrome research case definition and recommendations for resolution. BMC Health Serv Res 3:25, 2003

Reid S, Chalder T, Cleare A, et al: Chronic fatigue syndrome. Clin Evid 9:1172–1185, 2003

Reyes M, Nisenbaum R, Hoaglin DC, et al: Prevalence and incidence of chronic fatigue syndrome in Wichita, Kansas. Arch Intern Med 163:1530–1536, 2003

Roelofs J, Peters ML, McCracken L, et al: The pain vigilance and awareness questionnaire (PVAQ): further psychometric evaluation in fibromyalgia and other chronic pain syndromes. Pain 101:299–306, 2003

Ross SE: "Memes" as infectious agents in psychosomatic illness. Ann Intern Med 131:867–871, 1999

Rowe PC, Bou Holaigah I, Kan JS, et al: Is neurally mediated hypotension an unrecognised cause of chronic fatigue? Lancet 345:623–624, 1995

Rowe PC, Calkins H, DeBusk K, et al: Fludrocortisone acetate to treat neurally mediated hypotension in chronic fatigue syndrome: a randomized controlled trial. JAMA 285:52–59, 2001

Russell IJ, Orr MD, Littman B, et al: Elevated cerebrospinal fluid levels of substance P in patients with the fibromyalgia syndrome. Arthritis Rheum 37:1593–1601, 1994

Sandler H, Vernikos J: Inactivity: Physiological Effects. London, Academic Press, 1986

Sartorius N, Ustun TB, Costa e Silva JA, et al: An international study of psychological problems in primary care: preliminary report from the World Health Organization collaborative project on psychological problems in general health care. Arch Gen Psychiatry 50:819–824, 1993

Schmaling KB, Lewis DH, Fiedelak JI, et al: Single-photon emission computerized tomography and neurocognitive function in patients with chronic fatigue syndrome. Psychosom Med 65:129–136, 2003

Servaes P, Prins J, Verhagen S, et al: Fatigue after breast cancer and in chronic fatigue syndrome: similarities and differences. J Psychosom Res 52:453–459, 2002

Sharpe M: Chronic fatigue syndrome. Psychiatr Clin North Am 19:549–574, 1996

Sharpe M: Cognitive behavior therapy for functional somatic complaints: the example of chronic fatigue syndrome. Psychosomatics 38:356–362, 1997

Sharpe M: Doctors' diagnoses and patients' perceptions: lessons from chronic fatigue syndrome. Gen Hosp Psychiatry 20:335–338, 1998

Sharpe M, Carson A: "Unexplained" somatic symptoms, functional syndromes, and somatization: do we need a paradigm shift? Ann Intern Med 134(9 Pt 2):926–930, 2001

Sharpe M, Wilks D: ABC of psychological medicine: fatigue. BMJ 325:480–483, 2002

Sharpe M, Williams A: Treating patients with hypochondriasis and somatoform pain disorder, in Psychological Approaches to Pain Management. Edited by Turk DC, Gatchel RJ. New York, Guilford, 2001, pp 515–533

Sharpe M, Archard LC, Banatvala JE, et al: A report—chronic fatigue syndrome: guidelines for research. J R Soc Med 84:118–121, 1991

Sharpe M, Hawton KE, Seagroatt V, et al: Patients who present with fatigue: a follow up of referrals to an infectious diseases clinic. BMJ 305:147–152, 1992

Shorter E: Somatization and chronic pain in historic perspective. Clin Orthop 336:52–60, 1997

Silver A, Haeney M, Vijayadurai P, et al: The role of fear of physical movement and activity in chronic fatigue syndrome. J Psychosom Res 52:485–493, 2002

Skapinakis P: Clarifying the relationship between unexplained chronic fatigue and psychiatric morbidity: results from a community survey in Great Britain. Am J Psychiatry 157:1492–1498, 2000

Skapinakis P, Lewis G, Mavreas V: Unexplained fatigue syndromes in a multinational primary care sample: specificity of definition and prevalence and distinctiveness from depression and generalized anxiety. Am J Psychiatry 160:785–787, 2003

Stone J, Wojcik W, Durrance D, et al: What should we say to patients with symptoms unexplained by disease? The number needed to offend. BMJ 325:1449–1450, 2002

Sullivan PF, Smith W, Buchwald D: Latent class analysis of symptoms associated with chronic fatigue syndrome and fibromyalgia. Psychol Med 32:881–888, 2002

Surawy C, Hackmann A, Hawton KE, et al: Chronic fatigue syndrome: a cognitive approach. Behav Res Ther 33:535–544, 1995

Taylor RR, Jason LA: Chronic fatigue, abuse-related traumatization, and psychiatric disorders in a community-based sample. Soc Sci Med 55:247–256, 2002

Taylor RR, Jason LA: Chronic fatigue and sociodemographic characteristics as predictors of psychiatric disorders in a community-based sample. Psychosom Med 65:896–901, 2003

Theorell T, Blomkvist V, Lindh G, et al: Critical life events, infections, and symptoms during the year preceding chronic fatigue syndrome (CFS): an examination of CFS patients and subjects with a nonspecific life crisis. Psychosom Med 61:304–310, 1999

Thompson ME, Barkhuizen A: Fibromyalgia, hepatitis C infection, and the cytokine connection. Curr Pain Headache Rep 7:342–347, 2003

Tirelli U, Chierichetti F, Tavio M, et al: Brain positron emission tomography (PET) in chronic fatigue syndrome: preliminary data. Am J Med 105:54S–58S, 1998

Tofferi J, Jackson JL, O'Malley PG: Treatment of fibromyalgia with cyclobenzaprine: a meta-analysis. Arthritis Rheum 51:9–13, 2004

Torres-Harding SR, Jason LA, Cane V, et al: Physicians' diagnoses of psychiatric disorders for people with chronic fatigue syndrome. Int J Psychiatry Med 32:109–124, 2002

Valim V, Oliveira LM, Suda AL, et al: Peak oxygen uptake and ventilatory anaerobic threshold in fibromyalgia. J Rheumatol 29:353–357, 2002 van der Werf SP, de Vree B, Alberts M, et al: Natural course and predicting self-reported improvement in patients with chronic fatigue syndrome with a relatively short illness duration. J Psychosom Res 53:749–753, 2002

Van Hoof E, Cluydts R, De Meirleir K: Atypical depression as a secondary symptom in chronic fatigue syndrome. Med Hypotheses 61:52–55, 2003

Van Houdenhove B, Neerinckx E, Onghena P, et al: Premorbid overactive lifestyle in chronic fatigue syndrome and fibromyalgia: an etiological factor or proof of good citizenship? J Psychosom Res 51:571–576, 2001a

Van Houdenhove B, Neerinckx E, Lysens R, et al: Victimization in chronic fatigue syndrome and fibromyalgia in tertiary care: a controlled study on prevalence and characteristics. Psychosomatics 42:21–28, 2001b

Vercoulen JH, Hommes OR, Swanink CM, et al: The measurement of fatigue in patients with multiple sclerosis: a multidimensional comparison with patients with chronic fatigue syndrome and healthy subjects. Arch Neurol 53:642–649, 1996a

Vercoulen JH, Swanink CM, Zitman FG, et al: Randomized, double-blind, placebo-controlled study of fluoxetine in chronic fatigue syndrome. Lancet 347:858–861, 1996b

Vercoulen JH, Bazelmans E, Swanink CM, et al: Evaluating neuropsychological impairment in chronic fatigue syndrome. J Clin Exp Neuropsychol 20:144–156, 1998

Vial T, Descotes J: Clinical toxicity of the interferons. Drug Saf 10:115–150, 1994

Vlaeyen JW, Teeken-Gruben NJ, Goossens ME, et al: Cognitive-educational treatment of fibromyalgia: a randomized clinical trial, I: clinical effects. J Rheumatol 23:1237–1245, 1996

Walker EA, Keegan D, Gardner G, et al: Psychosocial factors in fibromyalgia compared with rheumatoid arthritis, I: sexual, physical, and emotional abuse and neglect. Psychosom Med 59:572–577, 1997a

Walker EA, Keegan D, Gardner G, et al: Psychosocial factors in fibromyalgia compared with rheumatoid arthritis, II: psychiatric diagnoses and functional disability. Psychosom Med 59:565–571, 1997b

Walsh K, Bennett G: Parkinson's disease and anxiety. Postgrad Med J 77:89–93, 2001

Wearden AJ, Appleby J: Research on cognitive complaints and cognitive functioning in patients with chronic fatigue syndrome (CFS): what conclusions can we draw? J Psychosom Res 41:197–211, 1996

Welford AT: The psychologist's problem in measuring fatigue, in Fatigue. Edited by Floyd WF, Welford AT. London, HK Lewis, 1953, pp 183–191

Wessely S: Old wine in new bottles: neurasthenia and M.E. Psychol Med 20:35–53, 1990

Wessely S, Nimnuan C, Sharpe M: Functional somatic syndromes: one or many? Lancet 354:936–939, 1999

White KP, Speechley M, Harth M, et al: The London Fibromyalgia Epidemiology Study: the prevalence of fibromyalgia syndrome in London, Ontario. J Rheumatol 26:1570–1576, 1999

White PD, Thomas JM, Kangro HO, et al: Predictions and associations of fatigue syndromes and mood disorders that occur after infectious mononucleosis. Lancet 358:1946–1954, 2001

Whiting P, Bagnall A, Sowden A, et al: Interventions for the treatment and management of chronic fatigue syndrome: a systematic review. JAMA 286:1360–1368, 2001

Wigers SH: Fibromyalgia outcome: the predictive values of symptom duration, physical activity, disability pension, and critical life events—a 4.5 year prospective study. J Psychosom Res 41:235–243, 1996

Williams DA: Psychological and behavioural therapies in fibromyalgia and related syndromes. Baillieres Best Pract Res Clin Rheumatol 17:649–665, 2003

Williams DA, Cary MA, Groner KH, et al: Improving physical functional status in patients with fibromyalgia: a brief cognitive behavioral intervention. J Rheumatol 29:1280–1286, 2002

Wolfe F: The relation between tender points and fibromyalgia symptom variables: evidence that fibromyalgia is not a discrete disorder in the clinic. Ann Rheum Dis 56:268–271, 1997

Wolfe F, Cathey MA, Kleinheksel SM: Fibrositis (fibromyalgia) in rheumatoid arthritis. J Rheumatol 11:814–818, 1984

Wolfe F, Smythe HA, Yunus MB, et al: The American College of Rheumatology 1990 criteria for the classification of fibromyalgia: report of the Multicenter Criteria Committee. Arthritis Rheum 33:160–172, 1990

Wolfe F, Cathey MA, Hawley DJ: A double-blind placebo controlled trial of fluoxetine in fibromyalgia. Scand J Rheumatol 23:255–259, 1994

Wolfe F, Ross K, Anderson JA, et al: The prevalence and characteristics of fibromyalgia in the general population. Arthritis Rheum 38:19–28, 1995

Wolfe F, Anderson J, Harkness D, et al: Health status and disease severity in fibromyalgia: results of a six-center longitudinal study. Arthritis Rheum 40:1571–1579, 1997

World Health Organization: International Statistical Classification of Diseases and Related Health Problems, 10th Revision. Geneva, World Health Organization, 1992

World Health Organization: Mental Illness in General Health Care: An International Study. Chichester, Wiley, 1995

Yunus MB: A comprehensive medical evaluation of patients with fibromyalgia syndrome. Rheum Dis Clin North Am 28:201–205, 2002

Yunus MB, Khan MA, Rawlings KK, et al: Genetic linkage analysis of multicase families with fibromyalgia syndrome. J Rheumatol 26:408–412, 1999

27

Infectious Diseases

James L. Levenson, M.D.

Robert K. Schneider, M.D.

PSYCHIATRIC SYMPTOMS ARE part of the clinical presentation of many systemic and central nervous system (CNS) infectious processes. Recently, several factors have combined to increase the prevalence and significance of infectious diseases. Rapid cultural and economic changes affecting regional and international mobility, sexuality, and other behaviors have led to worldwide spread of new epidemics (e.g., HIV, severe acute respiratory syndrome [SARS] [Cheng et al. 2004]) and more limited spread of previously geographically isolated diseases (e.g., cysticercosis). Infectious diseases have been considered as contributing to the pathogenesis of psychiatric disorders (e.g., viral antibodies in schizophrenia). Causal links between specific infections and a subset of psychiatric syndromes (e.g., pediatric autoimmune neuropsychiatric disorder associated with streptococcal infection [PANDAS]) provide intriguing models of etiology. Controversy surrounds some attributions of psychopathology to infectious pathophysiology (e.g., Lyme disease, Epstein-Barr virus [EBV]).

As a result of these developments, consulting psychiatrists should carefully consider relevant aspects of patients' histories, including immune status, regions of origin and residence, travel, high-risk sexual behaviors, occupation, and recreational activities. Physicians must consider which infectious diseases are endemic in the practice area and in the areas where the patient has traveled or resided. Similar psychiatric symptoms might suggest possible Lyme disease in a hiker in the northeastern United States and neurocysticercosis in an immigrant from Central America.

Many brain diseases or injuries, as well as the effects of aging, render patients more vulnerable to neuropsychiatric effects of even minor metabolic or toxic insults and similarly to adverse effects of even limited infectious dis-

eases. For example, a simple upper respiratory or bladder infection may cause only discomfort in an otherwise healthy individual but agitation, irritability, and frank delirium in the elderly, especially in patients who also have dementia. In a study of elderly patients admitted to a psychogeriatric inpatient unit with delirium and a coincident urinary tract infection, as well as underlying dementia in more than 70%, two-thirds had resolution of delirium with treatment of the urinary tract infection (Manepalli and Grossberg 1990). The reasons that older age and brain disease would make patients vulnerable to delirium with minor infections are not understood but may involve changes in immune function (Prio et al. 2002) and the blood-brain barrier.

Psychological factors may significantly affect the risk for and course of infectious diseases, with HIV as the most studied example (see Chapter 28, "HIV/AIDS"). Psychological factors have been shown to influence other infectious diseases as well, including the common cold (Takkouche et al. 2000), pneumonia (Mehr et al. 2001), genital herpes (Levenson et al. 1987), hepatitis B and C infection (Osher et al. 2003), and recurrent urinary tract infections (Hunt and Waller 1992). Several studies have convincingly shown that psychological stress suppresses the secondary (but not primary) antibody response to immunization (S. Cohen et al. 2001).

We divide this chapter into bacterial, viral, fungal, and parasitic infections, followed by psychiatric side effects of antimicrobial drugs and their interactions with psychotropic medications. We end the chapter by discussing fears of infectious disease and psychiatric aspects of immunization. HIV and AIDS are covered in Chapter 28. In the current chapter, we focus on psychiatric aspects of all other infectious diseases.

Occult Infections

Occult infections, irrespective of location, by definition are concealed or mysterious, often requiring diligent detective work. Such infections may occur essentially anywhere in the body (see Table 27–1). Psychiatric symptoms may result from even a small focus of chronic infection (e.g., Becarevici 1988; Yamasaki et al. 1997). The psychiatric symptoms most likely to be present are subtle cognitive dysfunction or mood change (e.g., irritability) consistent with a mild encephalopathy, but depression, psychosis, and delirium also may occur.

The diagnosis is suggested by secondary signs of infection, specifically temperature dysregulation, or increases in white blood cell count, granulocyte count, or sedimentation rate. A careful history and physical examination may identify overlooked clues to guide the search (e.g., chronic toothache or lymphadenopathy). If repeat history and physical examination are not fruitful, other studies may be needed (e.g., chest X rays, computed tomography [CT] scans, ultrasounds). Nuclear medicine studies may be useful in a "shotgun" search for a site of infection, but they have a high frequency of false-positive and false-negative results.

Bacterial Infections

Bacteremia and Sepsis

Bacteremia literally means entry of bacteria into the bloodstream, whereas *sepsis* refers to the systemic inflammatory response to bacteremia. Systemic symptoms of sepsis, including CNS symptoms, result from many different mechanisms, including bacterial toxins, release of cytokines, hyperthermia, shock (poor perfusion), acute renal insufficiency, pulmonary failure ("shock lung"), coagulopathy, disruption of the blood-brain barrier, and spread of the organism into the CNS and other organs. An acute change in mental status may be the first sign of impending sepsis and may precede the development of fever. Any patient who has an abrupt change in mental status in concert with a shaking chill should be presumed to have a high risk for impending sepsis. Diagnosis focuses on culturing the organism from blood or the primary site of infection.

Septic encephalopathy occurs more frequently than is generally assumed. Its severity is associated with the severity of overall illness, and it is often part of multiorgan failure (Zauner et al. 2002). Standard treatment is broad-spectrum antibiotics at first and is then tailored to the identified organism and its antimicrobial susceptibilities. Recent evidence suggests that the use of low-dose corti-

TABLE 27–1. Occult infections that may cause psychiatric symptoms

Sinusitis
Chronic otitis
Abscess (e.g., dental, lung, intra-abdominal, retroperitoneal, perirectal)
Bronchiectasis
Endocarditis
Cholecystitis
Parasitosis
Urinary tract infection
Pelvic inflammatory disease
Osteomyelitis
Subclinical systemic infections (e.g., HIV, tuberculosis)

costeroids may improve outcomes (Annane 2001; Schelling et al. 2001). Symptoms of posttraumatic stress disorder recently have been recognized as very common following septic shock (Schelling et al. 2001).

Toxic Shock Syndrome

Toxic shock syndrome (TSS) typically occurs in otherwise healthy people with intact immune systems. TSS is typically caused by either *Staphylococcus aureus* (Lowy 1998) or *Streptococcus pyogenes*, with the latter much more common currently. TSS generally manifests with rapid onset of fever, rash, and hypotension (shock) and is a multisystem disease with at least three organ systems involved, very often including the CNS. Most cases of TSS are associated with a wound and/or foreign body. Most staphylococcal TSS occurs in young menstruating white women (the proportion of menstrual cases has decreased following removal of superabsorbent tampons from the market) but can occur at any age, even in early childhood (Broome 1989; Van Lierde et al. 1997). Staphylococcal TSS is most likely caused by the production of a toxin (TSS toxin 1) that acts as a superantigen, a substance that rapidly initiates a multisystem inflammatory response (Stevens 1996). There is a great peril in missing this diagnosis because TSS often occurs in healthy, young women; the onset of the disease is fast; and early morbidity and mortality are high. TSS should be suspected in any patient with a recent wound who acutely develops unexplained pain, lethargy, and confusion and may occur even when a surgical wound appears not to be inflamed.

There may be a prodromal period of 2–3 days of malaise, myalgia, and chills followed by confusion and lethargy. Early CNS symptoms may include confusion, weakness, and headache. These early features rapidly progress to hypotension and shock. Following recovery, CNS sequelae may persist for years and include deficits in memory, computation, and concentration (Rosene et al. 1982). It is unclear to what extent these sequelae are a result of the toxin or the shock.

Clinical suspicion is necessary for early diagnosis of staphylococcal TSS. No tests are available for the antigen, and cultures of blood, cerebrospinal fluid (CSF), and throat usually have negative results. In contrast, blood cultures are positive in 60% of the cases of streptococcal TSS (Stevens 1989). Treatment includes aggressive supportive care, removal of the foreign body, drainage of the abscess, and antibiotics. Experimental antitoxin agents are being explored.

Pediatric Autoimmune Neuropsychiatric Disorder Associated With Streptococcal Infection

PANDAS is a fascinating etiological model of psychiatric illness (Swedo 2002). Sir William Osler (1894) had first noted "a certain perseverativeness of behavior" among patients with Sydenham's chorea (a complication of rheumatic fever). A century later, investigators at the National Institute of Mental Health found that approximately 70% of the children with Sydenham's chorea had obsessive-compulsive symptoms shortly before the chorea began (Swedo et al. 1998).

PANDAS is not a diagnosis but an acronym for the clinical characteristics of a subgroup of children whose obsessive-compulsive and tic disorders seem to have been triggered by an infection with group A beta-hemolytic streptococci (GABHS). The syndrome is defined by early childhood onset of symptoms; an episodic course characterized by abrupt onset of symptoms with frequent relapses and remissions; association with neurological signs, especially tics; and temporal association with GABHS infections (most commonly pharyngitis) (Swedo et al. 1997). The best way to show the association between recent GABHS infection and PANDAS symptoms is to document a rapid rise in antistreptococcal (ASO) titers associated with symptom onset or exacerbation and a decrease in titers associated with symptom resolution or improvement. Children with PANDAS also may have behavioral symptoms (e.g., attention deficits and hyperactivity) (Perlmutter et al. 1998; Schneider et al. 2002; Swedo et al. 1998). GABHS may play a role in Tourette's syndrome as well (Church et al. 2003). Adult onset of illness fulfilling criteria for PANDAS has been reported (Bodner et al. 2001), and obsessive-compulsive disorder (OCD) and tics are more common in first-degree relatives of PANDAS probands (Lougee et al. 2000).

In addition to ASO titers, a throat culture should be obtained, keeping in mind that some children who have GABHS infection may not have a sore throat (Swedo et al. 1998). Prompt antibiotic treatment may prevent the expected rise in ASO titers. Although PANDAS is conceptualized as an autoimmune disorder, antibiotics active against GABHS may be beneficial in reducing current symptoms (Murphy and Pichichero 2002) but have not been shown to have prophylactic value in PANDAS patients (Garvey et al. 1999). Randomized clinical trials of antibiotic treatment are under way, and immunomodulatory treatments are also being investigated (Perlmutter et al. 1999).

Bacterial Endocarditis

Bacterial endocarditis may cause neuropsychiatric symptoms at all stages of the disease, via focal, systemic, and CNS disease processes. Osler first described the triad of fever, heart murmur, and cerebral infarction in 1885. Endocardial infections are focal infections that usually occur on one of the valves of the heart. Rheumatic heart disease was originally the typical cause of the predisposing cardiac abnormality. Its incidence has decreased, while the incidence of senescent valvular disease, prosthetic valve placement, and intravenous drug use have increased, thus changing the risk factors in the developed world. Malaise and fatigue may represent early symptoms before progression of the infection is evident. CNS symptoms are related to 1) occlusion of cerebral arteries by septic emboli (Singhal et al. 2002); 2) expansion, leakage, or rupture of mycotic aneurysms; and 3) direct infection of meninges or brain abscess. Neuropsychiatric deficits resulting from septic emboli will reflect which cerebral vessels have been affected. The most common psychiatric symptoms are those of diffuse encephalopathy, which may occur at any stage of infection. Their onset may be insidious to acute, paralleling the course of the endocarditis (chronic, subacute, acute).

Diagnosis is based on clinical history and physical examination, particularly looking for new or changing heart murmurs, signs of microembolism (splinter hemorrhages, retinal hemorrhages, microscopic hematuria), plus positive blood cultures in a patient with fever. Cardiac echocardiography is important for evaluation of valvular abnormalities. Magnetic resonance imaging (MRI) scans are more sensitive than CT scans in detecting cerebral infarction. Treatment is based on blood culture results. The choice of antibiotics and length of parenteral treatment required vary according to the specific organism, its antibiotic susceptibilities, whether it is the first or a recurrent episode, whether a prosthetic heart valve is present, and other factors (Bertorini and Gelfand 1990; Lerner 1985).

Rocky Mountain Spotted Fever

The etiological agent for Rocky Mountain spotted fever (RMSF) is *Rickettsia rickettsii*. RMSF is a tickborne disease with a seasonal distribution paralleling human contact with ticks, peaking May through September. Its name is misleading because half of the United States cases are in the South Atlantic region, and rickettsial spotted fevers occur worldwide. After the tick bite, *R. rickettsii* enters vascular endothelial cells, proliferates, and disseminates, causing a diffuse vasculitis in many organs. RMSF typically (although not invariably) includes fever and a rash characterized by erythematous macules that later progress to maculopapular lesions with central petechiae. Initially appearing as a nonspecific severe febrile illness, the diagnosis is seldom suspected until the rash appears. CNS involvement occurs in 25% of cases, including lethargy, confusion, and occasionally fulminant delirium. Subtle changes such as irritability, personality changes, and apathy may occur before the rash, particularly in children. Abnormalities on CT or MRI of the brain may include infarctions, cerebral edema, meningeal enhancement, or prominent perivascular spaces, but 80% of RMSF patients with normal scans have symptoms of encephalopathy as well (Bonawitz et al. 1997). Cognitive dysfunction persisting months after resolution of the acute illness has been reported (Bergeron et al. 1997).

R. rickettsii may be detected by direct immunofluorescence of skin biopsies, but serology is the usual diagnostic method; confirmation requires convalescent titers. Because mortality is high in untreated patients, a provisional clinical diagnosis (e.g., fever, rash in the appropriate season, and geographic setting) is sufficient to initiate definitive antimicrobial therapy. Only half of these patients report exposure to ticks. Response to the treatment is quick and usually heralded by defervescence and mental clearing (Woodward 1992).

Typhus Fevers

Typhus fevers are caused by two species of *Rickettsia*. *R. prowazekii* is the cause of mouseborne and squirrelborne typhus. *R. typhi* is the cause of fleaborne typhus. Mouseborne typhus usually occurs in epidemics related to war or famine when communal hygiene deteriorates. Fleaborne typhus is associated with fleas found on rodents. The annual disease frequency in the United States was 2,000–5,000 cases in the 1940s. It is now fewer than 100, with most in Texas. This dramatic change is a result of the initiation of rat control programs. Clinical manifestations, diagnosis, and treatment of typhus are similar to those of RMSF. The psychiatric manifestations are confusion, lethargy, and particularly headache in a febrile illness with rash. Typhus has been implicated as a cause of febrile cerebrovasculitis in the United States (Hechemy et al. 1991). The delirium of typhus and typhoid has been classically described as having a peculiar preoccupied nature, with patients picking at the bedclothes and imaginary objects (Verghese 1985). In fact, the word *typhus* in Greek means "cloud" or "mist," a term Hippocrates used to describe clouded mental status in patients with unremitting fevers.

Typhoid Fever

Typhoid fever is an enteric fever caused by salmonellae. The incidence of typhoid fever has steadily declined in the United States over the last century primarily because of improved sanitation. Typhoid fever is still endemic in many places in the world. Sixty percent of the cases in the United States are acquired outside the country, most often in Mexico and India.

Abdominal pain, headache, and fever are the classic presentation. However, when typhoid fever is endemic or not treated promptly, psychiatric symptoms appear. *Salmonella typhi* enters a bacteremic phase, and the typhoid bacilli can localize in the CNS. The high fever and electrolyte imbalances also may cause encephalopathy, with delirium reported in up to 75% of the cases in some parts of the world (Aghanwa and Morakinyo 2001; Ali et al. 1997) and very infrequently (2%) in others (Parry et al. 2002). Mental symptoms such as indifference, listlessness, and dullness are common at presentation (Farmer and Graeme-Cook 1999), but psychosis remains a frequent complication (Parry et al. 2002). Published cases have described persistent psychiatric symptoms, including irritability, personality change, hallucinations, and even psychosis requiring electroconvulsive therapy, after definitive treatment (Breakey and Kala 1977). Most symptoms in survivors completely resolve following treatment. Diagnosis is made by isolation of the typhoid bacilli. The treatment of choice is a fluoroquinolone or ceftriaxone.

Tetanus

Tetanus is uncommon in the United States but remains internationally significant. *Clostridium tetani* produces a potent neurotoxin called *tetanospasmin*, which is the cause of tetanus. The greatest risk factor for tetanus remains lack of up-to-date immunization. In the United States, 60% of the cases occur in people older than 60 years, with older women especially at risk. The first mass vaccinations were offered during World War II, and many women never received vaccination then (Sreve and Spivack 1994).

Infections generally occur because an open wound comes into contact with soil contaminated with spores from *C. tetani*. After initial inoculation, tetanospasmin is disseminated via blood, lymph, and nerves and produces symptoms by binding to receptors at the neuromuscular junction.

The classic symptom is muscle stiffness, particularly in the muscles of mastication, thus the descriptive term *lockjaw*. If the muscle stiffness extends across the entire face, risus sardonicus occurs, an expression of continuous grimace. Also, stiffness may progress to the entire body if left untreated.

Tetanospasmin may enter the CNS, causing encephalopathic symptoms. Diagnosis is based on the clinical manifestations and a history of likely exposure. On initial presentation, patients with tetanus have been given misdiagnoses of an anxiety disorder or a conversion disorder (Treadway and Prange 1967), although more commonly, a conversion disorder is mistakenly thought to be possible tetanus (Barnes and Ware 1993). If the patient had received neuroleptics or antiemetics, one could easily mistake the symptoms as drug-induced acute dystonia. Treatment is aimed at reducing exposure to the neurotoxin and includes tetanus immunoglobulin, debridement of the wound, and administration of high-dose penicillin G. Infection does not always result in immunity, so active immunization is needed following treatment for the infection (Gray 1997).

Brucellosis

Brucellosis is a worldwide zoonosis caused by species of *Brucella*, gram-negative intracellular coccobacilli. They infect many animals, but most human cases are acquired from consumption of unpasteurized dairy products from sheep or goats. It has become rare in developed countries (about 100 cases per year in the United States) but is likely underdiagnosed because of the nonspecificity of symptoms. Brucellosis occurs at any age, with insidious or abrupt onset, affecting any organ system, and hence is notorious for mimicking other diseases. Signs of acute brucellosis include fever, diaphoresis, headache, and myalgia. Chronic brucellosis is not always preceded by acute symptoms. Its manifestations include fatigue, depression, and multiple chronic pains, so it is not surprising that patients' symptoms are frequently misdiagnosed as primary psychiatric illness (Sacks and Van Rensbueg 1976). Protean complications in many different organs have been reported. CNS involvement occurs in about 5% of cases and may present as meningitis, psychosis, or cranial nerve dysfunction (Bodur et al. 2003; Mousa et al. 1986). Diagnosis is confirmed by isolation of the organism or sero-

logical testing. Treatment regimens usually include multiple antibiotics.

Syphilis

Syphilis is a chronic systemic disease caused by the spirochetal bacterium *Treponema pallidum*. Although *T. pallidum* was not identified until 1905, syphilis was described in the medical literature before the sixteenth century. A hundred years ago, syphilis was the leading diagnosis in psychiatric inpatients; the incidence declined as the antibiotic era began. The rates of syphilis increased in the 1990s, exceeding the rates in the previous 40 years, probably linked to the global pandemic of HIV infection. With the current trend, psychiatrists must relearn this disease.

The clinical manifestations are varied and mimic those of other diseases. Syphilis was the original "great imitator." In adults, syphilis passes through several stages. *Primary syphilis* develops first as a small papule at the site of inoculation that develops into an ulcer called a chancre. If left untreated, the chancre will disappear, but about 6–24 weeks after the initial infection, *secondary syphilis* occurs with a variety of symptoms. During this stage, multiple organ systems, including the CNS, may become involved. Most symptoms are constitutional (malaise, fatigue, anorexia, and weight loss). Skin, gastrointestinal tract, lymphatics, bones, kidneys, and eyes all may be affected. Most syphilitic meningitis occurs within the first year of infection. Symptoms of headache, stiff neck, nausea, and vomiting prevail, and focal neurological findings may be present. Often, signs and symptoms of secondary syphilis disappear, and the infection becomes latent.

Tertiary syphilis refers to infection years to decades after initial infection. It has been divided into three types: late benign (gummatous), cardiovascular syphilis, and neurosyphilis. Gummatous and cardiovascular forms were very prevalent before antibiotics; neurosyphilis is now the predominant form of tertiary syphilis (Gliatto and Caroff 2001). A recent resurgence of neurosyphilis has occurred in persons with HIV infection, although during the period 1985 to 1992 in San Francisco, California, neurosyphilis in AIDS was a rare event (Flood et al. 1998).

Neurosyphilis is divided into asymptomatic, meningeal, meningovascular, and parenchymatous forms. Meningeal syphilis may occur early in the course (as noted earlier in this subsection) or late. Meningovascular syphilis typically occurs 4–7 years after infection. Presenting symptoms of neurosyphilis include changes in memory and personality, dizziness, and other encephalopathic symptoms that can mimic atherosclerotic disease (e.g., transient ischemic attack, multi-infarct dementia). Parenchymatous neurosyphilis syndromes are tabes dorsalis and general paresis. Tabes dorsalis occurs 20–25 years after infection and results from demyelination of the posterior columns and dorsal roots. Paresthesias, Argyll Robertson pupils (pupils that accommodate but do not react to light), impotence, incontinence, and truncal ataxia may develop. General paresis is an insidious dementia that can include seizures and personality deterioration. This form of syphilis presents 15–20 years after infection and if untreated may be fatal. In our clinical experience, the infection has "burned out" in some patients; they manifest dementia, have positive CSF and serum serology, and yet show no clinical response to penicillin G.

Diagnosis relies on serological testing because *T. pallidum* cannot be cultivated on artificial media. However, in primary and secondary syphilis, dark-field microscopy of material from chancres, condylomata, and mucous patches usually identifies a large number of organisms.

Except in populations where syphilis is common, it is not cost-effective to screen all new psychiatric patients for syphilis (Banger et al. 1995; Roberts et al. 1992); screening should focus on patients with unexplained cognitive dysfunction or other neurological symptoms accompanying the psychopathology. The most frequently used tests and their sensitivities are shown in Table 27–2.

Serological testing is based on two types of antibody response to the syphilitic infection: nontreponemal antibodies and antitreponemal antibodies. The Venereal Disease Research Laboratory (VDRL) and the rapid plasma reagin (RPR) are the most commonly used tests that detect nontreponemal (nonspecific) antibodies. The reactivity of these tests depends on the stage of the disease. In secondary syphilis and early latent syphilis, the nontreponemal tests show reactivity 95%–100% of the time. However, the reactivity in primary syphilis and tertiary syphilis is 76% and 70%, respectively. The fluorescent treponemal antibody absorption (FTA-ABS) test is more sensitive and more specific. This test is used to confirm the diagnosis when syphilis is suspected and a nontreponemal test was nonreactive and to confirm a positive nontreponemal test result. The FTA-ABS test is not used as a screening test because its false-positive rate is as high as 1%. Another treponemal test is the microhemagglutination assay of *T. pallidum* (MHA-TP). This assay is used as a confirmatory test, typically after a positive RPR test result (Hicks 2004).

False-positive nontreponemal tests (i.e., positive VDRL or RPR and negative FTA-ABS and no clinical evidence of disease) are divided into acute (those that revert to normal in less than 6 months) and chronic (those that persist for longer than 6 months). Acute false-positive results occur after some immunizations, during acute infections, and during pregnancy. Chronic false-positive results occur in individuals with autoimmune disease (e.g., lupus), in narcotic-addicted persons, in persons with leprosy, and in the elderly (Relman and Swartz 1998).

Treatment requires penicillin at varying dosages depending on the stage. If a definitive diagnosis cannot be made, it is prudent to treat presumptively.

Lyme Disease

Lyme disease is caused by the spirochete *Borrelia burgdorferi*, which is transmitted by deer ticks. The risk of contracting Lyme disease from a single tick bite is 3% (Nadelman et al. 2001). Lyme disease occurs worldwide; it is the most common tickborne disease in the United States, with four times as many cases as reported in Europe. Disease onset is marked by erythema migrans, a characteristic (more than 90% of cases) large, spreading rash with central clearing. Acute disseminated disease includes fatigue, arthralgia, headache, fever, and stiff neck. If untreated, Lyme disease may disseminate to other organs and produce subacute or chronic disease. Neurological symptoms occur in about 15% and may include

---

TABLE 27–2.   Sensitivity (%) of diagnostic tests of serum[a] in different stages of syphilis

| | Screening[b] | | Confirmatory[c] | |
Stage of disease	RPR or VDRL	FTA-ABS	TPI	MHA-TP
Primary	75	85	40	80
Secondary and early latent	95–100	100	98	100
Late latent and tertiary	70	99	95	98

Note.   RPR=rapid plasma reagin; VDRL=Venereal Disease Research Laboratory; FTA-ABS=fluorescent treponemal antibody absorption; TPI = *Treponema pallidum* immunofluorescence assay; MHA-TP=microhemagglutination assay of *Treponema pallidum*.
[a]Sensitivity and specificity cannot be determined on cerebrospinal fluid because no gold standard exists.
[b]Detects nontreponemal antibodies.
[c]Detects treponemal antibodies. Typically, a laboratory performs one of these tests when a screening test result is positive.

cranial neuropathies (most often, the facial nerve), meningitis, or painful radiculopathy (Rahn and Evans 1998). If still untreated, patients may develop chronic neuroborreliosis, including a mild sensory radiculopathy, cognitive dysfunction, or depression. Typical symptoms of chronic Lyme encephalopathy include difficulty with concentration and memory, fatigue, daytime hypersomnolence, irritability, and depression. Rarely, Lyme disease has included chronic encephalomyelitis. While these chronic syndromes are not distinctive, they are almost always preceded by the classic early symptoms of Lyme disease, such as erythema migrans, arthritis, cranial neuropathy, or radiculopathy (Rahn and Evans 1998).

The clear relation between another spirochetal disease, syphilis, and psychopathology makes the possibility of *B. burgdorferi* causing psychiatric syndromes an area of interest and controversy. Many different psychiatric symptoms have been reported to be associated with Lyme disease, including depression, mania, delirium, dementia, psychosis, obsessions or compulsions, panic attacks, catatonia, and personality change (Tager and Fallon 2001). However, association does not allow one to infer causation by Lyme. Evaluation of patients with Lyme disease at 10- to 20-year follow-up showed no significant differences in symptoms or neuropsychological testing compared with control subjects without Lyme disease. Although symptoms such as pain, fatigue, and difficulty with daily activities are common in patients who received treatment for Lyme disease years earlier, the frequencies of such symptoms are similar in control subjects without Lyme disease (Seltzer et al. 2000).

The differential diagnosis of neuroborreliosis in a patient presenting with fatigue, depression, and/or impaired cognition includes fibromyalgia, chronic fatigue syndrome, other infections (e.g., babesiosis or ehrlichiosis), somatoform disorders, depression, autoimmune diseases, and multiple sclerosis (Schneider et al. 2002; Tager and Fallon 2001).

Unfortunately, Lyme disease has been grossly overdiagnosed in patients with nonspecific cognitive, affective, or other psychiatric symptoms. As noted earlier in this section, numerous reports in the literature attribute a wide variety of psychiatric symptoms to neuroborreliosis on the basis of positive serological testing. As explained later in this section, this is inappropriate. Adverse consequences of overdiagnosis include reinforcement of somatization and the creation of invalidism. Overdiagnosis leads to overtreatment. The diagnosis of an infection that can be treated with antibiotics can be very appealing to patients for whom depression or somatoform disorder is an unacceptable diagnosis, but this leads to inappropriate diagnostic procedures and inappropriate extended prescription of antibiotics for a putative chronic CNS infection. Chronic antibiotic prescription is not benign and may lead to secondary infections, antibiotic resistance, and drug toxicity (Rahn and Evans 1998). Even in patients with classic symptomatic Lyme disease confirmed by serological testing, persisting symptoms are usually explained by some illness other than chronic borreliosis if these patients have received adequate antibiotic therapy (Kalish et al. 2001; Seltzer et al. 2000).

Diagnosis is based on the characteristic clinical features. Serological testing (enzyme-linked immunosorbent assay followed by Western blot) can support the diagnosis but should never be the primary basis (Rahn and Evans 1998). False-negative and false-positive results are common with serological testing. Even a true-positive test result simply indicates that the patient has had Lyme disease at some point in life, but no conclusion about current disease activity or extent of infection can be drawn. In chronic neuroborreliosis, increased CSF protein and antibody to the organism occur in more than 50% of the patients. Electroencephalograms (EEGs) are typically normal, whereas MRI shows nonspecific white matter lesions in about 25%. Neuropsychological assessment is useful in measuring cognitive dysfunction, but the findings are not specific (Ravdin et al. 1996).

Treatment is straightforward for acute Lyme disease (see Wormser et al. 2000). Neither serological testing nor antibiotic treatment is cost-effective in patients who have a low probability of having the disease (i.e., nonspecific symptoms, low incidence region) (Nichol et al. 1998). Two controlled trials found no benefit of extended intravenous or oral antibiotics in patients with well-documented, previously treated Lyme disease who had persistent pain, neurocognitive symptoms, or dysesthesia, often with fatigue (Klempner et al. 2001). A vaccine was developed that provided some protection (Steere et al. 1998) but was removed from the market in 2002.

Leptospirosis

Leptospirosis is another protean spirochetal disease. It was previously thought of as a rural, tropical disease, but it occurs globally in rural and urban areas (Vinetz 2001), even in the American inner city (Vinetz et al. 1996). The organism is spread through the urine of many species of mammals. Most infections resemble influenza and are relatively benign. The more severe form of leptospirosis is a multiorgan disease affecting liver, kidneys, lung, and brain (meningoencephalitis, aseptic meningitis). Confusion and delirium are common, and mental status changes are the strongest predictor of mortality (Ko et al. 1999).

Bacterial Meningitis

Bacterial meningitis is an acute illness associated with significant morbidity and mortality. Psychiatric symptoms play an important role in its presentation. Irrespective of the organism, most cases of bacterial meningitis result from hematogenous spread of bacteria from a primary site to the subarachnoid space. Once the organism crosses the blood-brain barrier at the choroid plexus and enters the subarachnoid space, host defenses become activated. Psychiatric symptoms may result by several mechanisms, including toxic effects of the organism, mediators of inflammation, cerebral edema, and hypoxia.

The classic sign of meningeal inflammation is nuchal rigidity. Headache, nausea, vomiting, confusion, lethargy, and apathy also may occur. Psychiatric symptoms are the result of encephalopathy. As in other infections, encephalopathy may present subtle changes in personality, mood, motivation, or mentation. Symptom severity generally correlates with the magnitude of the host's immune response (Weinstein 1985). When the patient cannot mount a full inflammatory response, the classic symptoms may not occur. In infants, the elderly, or immunocompromised patients, the only clinical signs may be irritability or minor changes in mentation or personality (Segreti and Harris 1996).

Once clinically suspected, the diagnosis is usually confirmed by examination of the CSF, which typically shows pleocytosis, low glucose, high protein, and evidence of the offending organism on appropriate staining. Although neuroimaging is routinely performed to rule out other CNS processes, it rarely establishes the diagnosis of bacterial meningitis. Morbidity and mortality of bacterial meningitis increase with delay in the initiation of effective antibiotic treatment (Gray 1997).

Initially, antibiotics are chosen to cover a broad range of organisms common to the population to which the patient belongs (e.g., age and immune status). Recent developments affect medication choice. The *Haemophilus influenzae* type B and the pneumococcal conjugate vaccines have greatly reduced cases of meningitis caused by these agents (Schuchat et al. 1997; Whitney et al. 2003), and penicillin resistance has emerged in *Streptococcus pneumoniae* infections.

Cat-Scratch Disease

Cat-scratch disease (CSD), which is caused by *Bartonella henselae*, usually presents as self-limiting lymphadenopathy in young people following a cat scratch or bite. Encephalopathy is one of the common complications, with almost all cases reported in children. Patients with CSD encephalopathy present with combative behavior, lethargy, and seizures, and significant fever may be absent. Diagnosis is made by serology and/or biopsy of skin or lymph node. Antibiotic treatment is indicated in CSD with encephalopathy, although most CSD cases resolve spontaneously without it (Carithers and Margileth 1991; Windsor 2001).

Bacterial Brain Abscess

The portals of entry for organisms causing brain abscesses are similar to those in bacterial meningitis. In fact, brain abscesses frequently occur as a complication of bacterial meningitis, although they also are a frequent complication of infective endocarditis. The classic triad of headache, fever, and focal neurological deficits has been described for the diagnosis of brain abscess, but these symptoms occur in fewer than half of the patients who have a brain abscess. Seizures are common. Various psychiatric symptoms may occur, depending on the size and location of the abscess(es), how irritating the organism is, and the extent of the inflammatory response. Disordered mood, cognitive dysfunction, psychosis, and aggression are the most common psychiatric complications (Chang et al. 1997; Douen and Bourque 1997).

Mortality rates have markedly declined as a result of improved neuroimaging and antimicrobials, but morbidity remains high. Early detection and aggressive treatment are necessary to further reduce morbidity and mortality. Neuroimaging can be very helpful in the diagnosis of brain abscess, unlike in bacterial meningitis. Neuroimaging can show focal abscesses in the CNS with very good sensitivity. Effective treatment includes empirical antibiotics that cross the blood-brain barrier, with primary excision or aspiration of the abscess usually required. After successful treatment of the infection, psychiatric symptoms may persist.

Tuberculous Meningitis

Tuberculosis remains a major world health problem, endemic in many developing countries. Where AIDS is prevalent, the epidemiology of tuberculosis has markedly changed. Tuberculosis now represents the most common serious HIV-related complication worldwide. Where tuberculosis is not endemic, the diagnosis of tuberculous meningitis is often not considered because the clinical manifestations are often nonspecific. Early diagnosis of tuberculous meningitis is essential because delay in treatment is associated with high morbidity and mortality. Tuberculous meningitis is caused by bacilli discharged from small tuberculous lesions adjacent to the meninges. These small tuberculous lesions arise early via hematogenous spread following a primary pulmonary infection or as a consequence of reactivation.

Early symptoms of tuberculous meningitis are nonspecific and include low-grade fever, generalized malaise, fatigue, and mild headache. Over the course of a week, there is progression to high-grade fever, severe nuchal rigidity, confusion, and delirium. Persons with HIV, the elderly, substance abusers, and others with impaired immunity are more likely to present without nuchal rigidity and headache. In such patients, the symptoms will tend to be most nonspecific, with a higher risk of missing the correct diagnosis while attributing the symptoms to more common diagnoses such as alcohol withdrawal.

Confirming the diagnosis can be difficult. The organisms are difficult to detect in the CSF, so diligent search is needed to identify them when present. Early in the course when symptoms are mild, CSF glucose may be unchanged and protein only marginally elevated. As the disease progresses, glucose declines drastically, and protein becomes markedly elevated, with white blood cell counts typically between 50 and 200 per cubic millimeter (predominantly lymphocytes). Later complications include cerebral vasculitis and cranial nerve involvement. Diffuse meningeal involvement by tuberculosis may be seen on MRI (Gray 1997).

Strong suspicion of tuberculous meningitis calls for early multidrug treatment because it is better to have temporarily treated a few patients needlessly than to miss prompt treatment in those who really have the disease. Regimens of multiple antitubercular drugs should be used until sensitivities are determined after cultures. In many parts of the world today, including the United States, multidrug-resistant tuberculosis is present, requiring different drug combinations.

Viral Infections

The overwhelming majority of viral infections are asymptomatic or mild and do not receive medical attention. Many viruses are difficult to detect, most infections are difficult to treat, and none are cured by treatment. Viruses can produce psychiatric symptoms by primary CNS involvement, from secondary effects of immune activation, or indirectly from systemic effects. One serious sequela of several viral infections is acute disseminated encephalomyelitis; patients with this condition can present with encephalopathy, acute psychosis, seizures, and other CNS dysfunction. Active demyelination is widespread, and the disease may be difficult to distinguish from multiple sclerosis (Nasr et al. 2000). Despite viral syndromes' ubiquity and frequent nonspecificity, it is important for psychiatrists to know particular viral syndromes.

Epstein-Barr Virus

EBV, one of the herpesviruses, causes an acute lymphoproliferative disease called *infectious mononucleosis* ("mono"), common in children and young adults. The prodromal stage of infectious mononucleosis is characterized by headache, fatigue, and malaise, with progression to fever, sore throat, and lymphadenopathy. Diagnosis is based on the combination of typical clinical symptoms and a positive heterophil antibody test (Monospot) result. Because the Monospot test is an antibody measure, it may have false-negative results in immunosuppressed patients. Therapy is supportive, and most cases completely resolve, although some may take several months. Fatigue commonly persists for a few months, but this can occur with other viral infections as well (White et al. 1998). In the rare, more severe form of infectious mononucleosis, anemia, leukopenia, eosinophilia, thrombocytopenia, pneumonitis, heptosplenomegaly, uveitis, and an abnormal pattern of serum globulins occur.

In patients with chronic fatigue and malaise, the differential diagnosis may include depression or chronic EBV infection. Because EBV may persist lifelong in a latent state following acute infection, periodic reactivation may occur. Patients with latent EBV infection typically report overwhelming fatigue, malaise, depression, low-grade fever, lymphadenopathy, and other nonspecific symptoms. Often, there are no other findings with these patients. This picture is essentially that of chronic fatigue syndrome, even though only a small fraction of chronic fatigue symptoms are attributable to EBV infection. In the past, patients with chronic fatigue caused by depression or somatoform disorder who resisted considering a psychiatric diagnosis (and sometimes their physicians) often pursued an explanation in chronic EBV infection. They found (erroneous) confirmation in a positive Monospot test result; it is erroneous because the test result remains positive long after complete resolution of uncomplicated infectious mononucleosis in youth, often for life. With wider recognition of the limitations of Monospot testing, this misdiagnosis is now very infrequent (but see earlier discussion in "Lyme Disease" subsection).

The role of the psychiatrist is to help the infectious disease clinician or primary care provider distinguish which patients have a primary psychiatric diagnosis (mood, anxiety, or somatoform disorders). Chronic EBV infection should never be diagnosed solely on the basis of a positive Monospot test result. The absence of any objective findings (e.g., significant lymphadenopathy, atypical lymphocytes, lymphocytosis, elevated sedimentation rate, fever, hepatosplenomegaly) increases the likelihood of a primary psychiatric diagnosis, but the diagnosis should be based on positive criteria, never made only by exclusion of an identifiable diagnosis such as EBV. As in other postviral syndromes, antidepressant therapy is often helpful if depression exists in the recovery phase of infectious mononucleosis.

Cytomegalovirus

Like EBV, cytomegalovirus (CMV) is a common herpesvirus, and most infections are subclinical. CMV infection occurs in a broader age group than does EBV. Seroprevalence in adults older than 35 years has ranged from 38% in Rochester, New York, to 99% in Tanzania (Hoeprich et al. 1994). In adults, CMV can produce a syndrome identical to infectious mononucleosis, except that heterophil antibody testing is negative in CMV, and a sore throat is usually absent. CMV also may cause hepatitis, retinitis, colonitis, and pneumonitis. In immunocompromised patients, CMV has been implicated as a cause of depression or dementia. CMV should always be considered in the differential diagnosis of acute depression or cognitive dysfunction in the first few months after organ transplantation. CMV is referred to as the "most important pathogen affecting transplant recipients," potentially causing immunosuppression or allograft rejection (Fishman and Rubin 1998). Diagnosis is most accurate when CMV can be recovered in body fluids. Antiviral agents (e.g., acyclovir, ganciclovir) are helpful, but significant side effects can occur (Hibberd et al. 1995). Antidepressant therapy may be needed if the patient develops a postviral mood disorder.

Viral Meningoencephalitis

Most viruses that cause encephalitis cause meningitis as well. Enteroviruses, mumps, and lymphocytic choriomeningitis primarily affect the meninges, with enteroviruses responsible for most identifiable cases. Patients with viral meningitis (often referred to as *aseptic meningitis*) present with headache, fever, nuchal rigidity, malaise, drowsiness, nausea, and photophobia. Typically, the CSF shows pleocytosis, elevated protein, and no evidence of an organism. Treatment is generally supportive. Antiviral drugs such as acyclovir are being increasingly used, most effectively for herpes encephalitis. Correct early diagnosis is critical to a successful outcome (Deresiewicz et al. 1997).

Arboviruses

Arboviruses (short for arthropod-borne viruses) are the most common cause of viral encephalitis worldwide (Solomon 2004). Of the arbovirus diseases, Japanese encephalitis is the most common worldwide and annually causes 10,000 deaths in Asia. In the United States, the four major types are St. Louis encephalitis, eastern equine encephalomyelitis, western equine encephalomyelitis, and California encephalitis. Recently, West Nile virus has appeared in the United States. West Nile virus is a flavivirus like the virus in Japanese encephalitis and has a similar clinical course (Solomon 2003). Most arboviruses are mosquito-borne. Arboviral encephalitis typically appears in the summer or fall in children (Japanese encephalitis) or young adults (West Nile virus and St. Louis encephalitis), with abrupt onset of fever, headache, nausea, photophobia, and vomiting, and may be fatal. Reduced level of consciousness, flaccid paralysis resembling poliomyelitis, parkinsonism, and seizures are common (Solomon 2004). Occasionally, patients with viral encephalitis may present initially with psychopathology without neurological symptoms. Caroff et al. (2001) reviewed 108 published cases of psychiatric presentation, classified as psychosis (35%), catatonia (33%), psychotic depression (16%), or mania (11%). Patients in such cases often receive misdiagnosis and inappropriate treatment, and Caroff et al. (2001) noted that patients with viral encephalitis are more vulnerable to adverse effects of neuroleptics, including extrapyramidal side effects, catatonia, and neuroleptic malignant syndrome. Although no specific treatment is available for arboviral encephalitis, rapid diagnosis is important for public health measures, mosquito control, and, ideally, vaccines. Although a vaccine exists for Japanese encephalitis, access is limited (Monath 2002). For those who survive, outcomes vary from complete recovery to serious neuropsychiatric sequelae.

Dengue

Dengue, another disease caused by an arbovirus, is transmitted by mosquitoes, endemic in 100 countries, and encountered in temperate developed countries mainly in travelers and new immigrants (Castleberry and Mahon 2003). The virus causes three syndromes: 1) the relatively more benign dengue fever, which is a painful influenza-like illness, and the serious forms, 2) hemorrhagic dengue and 3) dengue shock syndrome; the latter two are rare in travelers. However, neuropsychiatric symptoms were noted in 14% of the tourists who returned to France with dengue (Badiaga et al. 1999). In the more serious endemic dengue infections, meningoencephalitis is common, with confusion, delirium, and seizures (Pancharoen and Thisyakorn 2001).

Herpes Simplex Virus

Herpes encephalitis is caused by invasion of the brain by herpes simplex type 1 virus in 90% of herpes encephalitis cases. Symptoms may include personality change, dysphasia, seizures, autonomic dysfunction, ataxia, delirium, psychosis, and focal neurological symptoms. Herpes simplex virus (HSV) encephalitis differs from arboviral encephalitis by causing more unilateral and focal findings, with a predilection for temporoparietal areas of the brain. HSV encephalitis is more likely to cause focal seizures, olfactory hallucinations, and personality change (Whitley et al. 1982). HSV is the most common identified cause of viral encephalitis simulating a primary psychiatric disorder (Caroff et al. 2001). CSF typically shows pleocytosis, red blood cells (because of the hemorrhagic nature of HSV encephalitis), and elevated protein. Glucose is usually normal. EEG is a sensitive (but not specific) diagnostic test, showing periodic temporal spikes and slow waves as opposed to more diffuse changes usually seen in other forms of viral encephalitis (Smith et al. 1975). MRI may show diffuse inflammation, particularly in the temporoparietal areas. Serological evaluation is helpful only retrospectively. Brain biopsy is reliable and has a high yield and low complication rate. Diagnosis based on symptoms and signs alone misses 50% of the cases. Rapid diagnosis is essential because only early treatment improves outcome. Acyclovir is the drug of choice. One possible sequela of HSV encephalitis is the Klüver-Bucy syndrome, which includes oral touching compulsions, hypersexuality, amnesia, placidity, agnosia, and hyperphagia (Hart et al. 1986).

Varicella/Herpes Zoster

The varicella/herpes zoster virus causes chickenpox in children and herpes zoster in adults. Most cases of encephalopathy in children with varicella infection have been due to Reye's syndrome, although the virus itself can cause encephalitis. The most common neurological sequela of herpes zoster is postherpetic neuralgia (see Chapter 36, "Pain") (Gnann and Whitley 2002). Comorbid psychopathology is common in postherpetic neuralgia, especially depression (Clark et al. 2000), and may influence the choice of treatment for the neuropathic pain (e.g., tricyclic antidepressant vs. anticonvulsant). Weeks or months after recovery from herpes zoster, encephalitis or arteritis may appear. In immunocompetent hosts, it is usually a granulomatous arteritis affecting large vessels, producing strokelike symptoms. In immunosuppressed patients, the vasculitis mostly affects small vessels, producing headache, altered mental status, fever, seizures, and focal deficits (Gilden et al. 2000).

Postencephalitis Syndromes

Following recovery from acute viral encephalitis, psychiatric sequelae are common and constitute a major cause of disability, especially mood disorders. Depression, hypomania, irritability, and disinhibition of anger, aggression, or sexuality have been frequently noted months after recovery, and psychosis occurs rarely (Caparros-Lefebvre et al. 1996). Depressive symptoms may respond to treatment with antidepressants or stimulants. Hypomania, irritability, and disinhibition have benefited from mood stabilizers, and behavior modification also may be helpful for aggressive and sexual behaviors (Boulais et al. 1976; Vallini and Burns 1987).

The global pandemic encephalitis in 1917–1929 known as *encephalitis lethargica* (von Economo's disease) had an acute encephalitic phase during which lethargy, psychosis, and catatonia were common. This period was followed by a chronic postencephalitic syndrome, including parkinsonism, mania, depression, and apathy in adults (Cummings et al. 2001; Dolan and Kamil 1992) and conduct disorder, emotional lability, and tics in children, with relatively little cognitive impairment (Cummings et al. 2001; Hokkanen and Launes 1997).

Viral Hepatitis

Some viruses—including hepatitis A, B, and C; EBV; and CM—cause acute or chronic hepatitis. Hepatitis C infection is very common in the chronically mentally ill (Dinwiddie et al. 2003; Osher et al. 2003; Rosenberg et al. 2003). Fatigue, malaise, and anorexia are usually prominent in viral hepatitis and may lead to a misdiagnosis of depression. However, fatigue in chronic hepatitis is more closely correlated with depression and other psychological factors than is severity of hepatitis (McDonald et al. 2002). Depression is frequently comorbid, especially in the chronic forms of hepatitis B infection (Kunkel et al. 2000) and C (Gallegos-Orozco et al. 2003), but whether the etiology of depression in hepatitis C infection is really viral has been questioned (Wessely and Pariante 2002). Subtle cognitive dysfunction not attributable to depression, substance abuse, or hepatic encephalopathy has been documented in hepatitis C infection, and the virus has been identified in brain, suggesting that cerebral infection also may occur (Forton et al. 2002). Complicating the diagnostic picture further, treatment with interferon causes depression itself in 20%–40% of patients (Bonaccorso et al. 2002; Dieperink et al. 2003). Depression has been the most common adverse effect leading to cessation of interferon treatment. Depression associated with hepatitis or interferon is amenable to treatment with antidepressants (Kraus et al. 2002; Levenson and Fallon 1993), allowing continuation of interferon in most patients (Schaefer et al. 2003). Therefore, depression should not be considered a contraindication to interferon therapy.

Dosing should be adjusted downward if the patient has impaired liver function.

Rabies

Rabies is a viral infection of mammals transmitted by bite. In the United States, nondomesticated animals (i.e., bats, raccoons) account for most cases of rabies because domesticated animals are vaccinated (Kauffman and Goldmann 1986). In contrast, India has no vaccination program, and 15,000 deaths each year have been attributed to rabies infection (Miller and Nathanson 1977). Transmission to humans is rare but has been misdiagnosed as an anxiety disorder (Centers for Disease Control 1991) or alcohol withdrawal (Centers for Disease Control and Prevention 1998).

Initial symptoms are nonspecific and include generalized anxiety, fever, depression, hyperesthesia, and dysesthesia, especially at the site of inoculation. In the most recent United States case, "mild personality changes" preceded more suggestive symptoms such as unsteady gait and slurred speech by more than a week (Centers for Disease Control and Prevention 2003). The rabies virus has a proclivity for attacking the limbic system; thus, delusions may result. The initial phase is followed by an excitatory phase, when the classic symptom of hydrophobia may occur. Hydrophobia is an aversion to swallowing liquids (not a phobia of water) secondary to the spasmodic contractions of the muscles of swallowing and respiration, resulting in pain and aspiration. The final phase is a progressive, general, flaccid paralysis that progresses relentlessly to death. Both rabies and the rabies vaccine may cause delirium (Leung et al. 2003).

No effective treatment exists for rabies once symptoms are evident (Fishbein and Robinson 1993). After a bite by an infected animal, the rabies vaccine should be given as soon as possible because outcome is related to the proximity in time to the bite.

Prion Diseases

Prions are proteinaceous agents that cause spongiform changes in the brain. Prion diseases are rare and universally fatal, with an incubation period of months to years—hence, the term *slow viruses* (see also Chapter 32, "Neurology and Neurosurgery"). Kuru occurs only in Papua, New Guinea. It is spread by the cannibalistic consumption of dead relatives during mourning rituals. Scrapie is a spongiform encephalopathy found in sheep. Although known to have been present in Great Britain for almost three centuries, scrapie has never been shown to cause disease in humans.

Bovine spongiform encephalopathy ("mad cow disease") appears to have been transmitted to cattle by the practice of feeding cattle recycled sheep by-products.

Creutzfeldt-Jakob disease (CJD) occurs sporadically and sometimes familially in humans. It also has been transmitted by intracerebral electrodes, grafts of dura mater, corneal transplants, human growth hormone, and gonadotropin, but iatrogenic transmission is now rare (Ironside 1996; Tyler 2003). CJD is a severe dementia accompanied by psychosis, affective lability, and dramatic myoclonus that rapidly progresses to rigid mutism and then death. In the last few years, mainly in Great Britain, there have been 139 cases of "new-variant" CJD (nvCJD) with distinct differences from CJD.

nvCJD patients are younger than CJD patients (average age=26 vs. 60 years). In most cases of nvCJD, psychiatric symptoms appear several months before any neurological symptoms, including depression, irritability, anxiety, and apathy (Spencer et al. 2002; Tyler 2003). Although bovine spongiform encephalopathy and nvCJD are temporally and geographically associated, a causative link has not been proven. The EEG is usually abnormal in both forms of CJD, but definitive diagnosis requires brain biopsy.

Fatal familial insomnia is an even rarer prion disease in which progressive insomnia (and sometimes behavior change) appears months before any cognitive, autonomic, or motor symptoms develop. Despite its name, the disease also occurs through sporadic mutation. Patients with this disorder may be given misdiagnoses of mood, anxiety, or somatoform disorders (Mastrianni et al. 1999; Tabernero et al. 2000).

Fungal Infections

The frequency of fungal infection has steadily increased over the last three decades, coincident with the growing number of immunosuppressed patients who are surviving longer than in the past. An aging population, an increased number of malignancies, the spread of AIDS, the use of immunosuppressive and cytotoxic drugs, the use of intravenous catheters, hyperalimentation, illicit drug use, extensive surgery, and the development of burn units also have contributed to the increased frequency of fungal infection (Hawkins and Armstrong 1984). CNS symptom development depends on the size and shape of the fungi. The smallest fungi have access to the cerebral microcirculation and infect the subarachnoid space. Large hyphae obstruct large and intermediate arteries, giving rise to extensive infarcts (e.g., aspergillosis). Fungi with pseudohyphae occlude small blood vessels, producing small infarctions and microabscesses (e.g., *Candida*). Most fungi are opportunistic (as in aspergillosis, mucormycosis, and candidiasis), whereas others are pathogenic (as in coccidioidomycosis and cryptococcosis) irrespective of the host's defenses (Chimelli and Mahler-Araújo 1997).

Aspergillosis

Aspergillus, an opportunistic organism, infects only debilitated patients. *Aspergillus* genus is commonly found in soil. CNS involvement usually follows infection of the lungs or gastrointestinal tract. Symptoms of confusion, headache, and lethargy often accompany focal neurological signs.

Cryptococcosis

Cryptococcosis is an infection caused by *Cryptococcus* species, a pathogen distributed worldwide, found in bird excreta, the soil, and other animals. *Cryptococcus* may act as a solo pathogen, but in up to 85% of cases, it is associated with another illness, especially AIDS. The portal of entry is usually the respiratory tract from which hematogenous spread occurs, although at the time of presentation, pulmonary infection may not be evident. This pathogen has a predilection for the subarachnoid space (Sabetta and Andriole 1985).

Cryptococcus is the most common form of fungal meningitis. It is typically insidious in onset and slowly progressive. Headache is present in up to 75% of the cases, varying from mild and episodic to progressively incapacitating and constant. Other signs include cerebellar, cranial nerve, and motor deficits; irritability; psychosis; and lethargy, which may progress to coma. Remission and relapse are common in untreated patients. Isolation of the fungi provides definitive diagnosis. Serological testing of patients with cryptococcal meningitis identifies cryptococcal antigen in serum, CSF, or both 90% of the time. Treatment is typically a prolonged course of an antifungal agent.

Coccidioidomycosis

Coccidioidomycosis is restricted to warm, dry areas such as the southwestern United States, Mexico, and parts of South America (particularly Argentina and Paraguay). Its spores are inhaled in infected dust. Initial infection produces a mild febrile illness, often followed by pulmonary symptoms (Chimelli and Mahler-Araújo 1997). Dissemination beyond the lung is relatively rare, and the CNS is not the most common extrapulmonary site. When it does occur, CNS infection is typically insidious in onset, 1–3

months after initial infection (Castleman and McNeely 1971), with severe headache associated with confusion, restlessness, hallucinations, lethargy, and transient focal signs (Bañuelos et al. 1996). Neuroimaging and serological testing of the CSF confirm the diagnosis. Amphotericin is the treatment of choice.

Histoplasmosis

Histoplasmosis is a common respiratory infection found throughout the world and is especially common in the central United States. *Histoplasma capsulatum* is inhaled with dust contaminated with chicken, bird, or bat excreta. Most infections are asymptomatic and involve the lungs or the reticuloendothelial system. Two peaks of increased incidence occur—in infancy and in the fifth and sixth decades. CNS involvement is rare but is of insidious onset. After a few weeks of irregular fever and persistent cough, extreme nervousness and irritability progress to marked lethargy and, if untreated, coma (Tan et al. 1992).

Blastomycosis

Blastomyces dermatitidis is an uncommon mycotic infection that rarely causes CNS infections. Blastomycosis is coendemic with histoplasmosis in the central United States. The most common CNS manifestations are stiff neck and headache, eventually progressing to confusion and lethargy.

Mucormycosis

Mucormycosis refers to any infection caused by a member of the family Mucoraceae, opportunistic fungi found in common bread and fruit molds. Mucormycosis is notorious for causing an acute fulminant infection in diabetic patients and patients with neutropenia. *Mucor* directly invades tissue and disseminates by attacking contiguous structures. Any diabetic patient with a purulent, febrile infection of the face or nose should be emergently evaluated for mucormycosis, because it may rapidly erode into the orbit and cerebrum in a matter of hours. Early mild encephalopathy (Crowley and Wilcox 1996) may quickly progress to severe delirium. Aggressive debridement and intravenous antifungal medication are required.

Candidiasis

Candida causes limited local infections (cutaneous, vaginal, oral) in immune-competent hosts, typically after broad-spectrum antibiotics. Disseminated candidiasis occurs only in immunocompromised patients. Psychiatric symptoms occur from the toxic effects of fungemia or from direct invasion of the CNS. Cerebral lesions generally occur late in the course of disseminated candidiasis. *Candida* may cause meningitis, microabscesses, macroabscesses, or vasculitis in the CNS. The nonspecific signs include confusion, drowsiness, lethargy, and headache. Sometimes *Candida* can be cultured from blood or CSF, but most cases of CNS candidiasis are not discovered until autopsy. Suggestive neuroimaging findings and isolation of *Candida* from a non-CNS site in an immunocompromised patient should prompt treatment with appropriate antifungal agents.

An alternative medicine belief is that occult systemic *Candida* infection is the cause of a wide array of somatic and psychological symptoms. There is no scientific support for this theory or its advocated treatments.

Parasitic Infections

Neurocysticercosis

One of the world's most common parasitic infections—neurocysticercosis—is an infection of the CNS by the larval form (cysticerci) of *Taenia solium*, also known as the pork tapeworm. For neurocysticercosis to occur, a human must ingest the tapeworm's eggs, from contact with infected swine or humans. Once ingested, the eggs hematogenously spread to the CNS and other sites. Cysticercosis is endemic in the developing nations. In the United States, it is usually reported in immigrants from Latin America and recently has been reportedly found in 10% of the patients with seizures presenting to an emergency department in Los Angeles, California, and in 6% in an emergency department in New Mexico (Ong et al. 2002). However, infected food handlers may transmit it to people who have no contact with pork or other contaminated foods (e.g., an Orthodox Jewish community in New York City) (Schantz et al. 1992).

A high percentage of neurocysticercosis infections remain asymptomatic. Cerebral involvement may produce seizures, stroke, or hydrocephalus; neurocysticercosis is the leading cause of seizures in adults in endemic areas. Psychiatric symptoms are frequently reported, including depression, psychosis, and cognitive decline (Forlenza et al. 1997; Shandera et al. 1994).

Between clinical history, neuroimaging, and serology, a presumptive diagnosis of neurocysticercosis usually can be made (Pittella 1997a). Definitive diagnosis of neurocysticercosis is through biopsy, but this is usually impractical. Treatment of neurocysticercosis has involved anticonvulsants, steroids, antihelminthics, and shunting for

hydrocephalus. However, antihelminthic drugs in neurocysticercosis may actually aggravate neuropsychiatric symptoms, and their use in some forms of the disease is controversial (Garcia et al. 2004; Salinas and Prasad 2000).

Toxoplasmosis

Toxoplasmosis refers to the disease caused by *Toxoplasma gondii*, a parasite ubiquitously affecting all mammals, some birds, and probably some reptiles (Yermakov et al. 1982). Latent infection is common, but in immunosuppressed individuals, particularly those with AIDS, it may preferentially infect the CNS, resulting in a wide range of clinical presentations. Mass lesions mimicking tumor or abscess are most common, but psychosis has been reported as a presenting symptom (Donnet et al. 1991). Effective antibiotic therapy can produce rapid remission of active infection but must be continued throughout life to prevent recurrence (B.A. Cohen 1999).

Trypanosomiasis

The family of protozoa Trypanosomatidae causes two different syndromes: African trypanosomiasis (sleeping sickness) and American trypanosomiasis (Chagas' disease). African trypanosomiasis, which occurs in several sub-Saharan African countries, is caused by a subspecies of *Trypanosoma brucei* and is transmitted to humans and animals by the bite of the blood-sucking tsetse fly. The illness begins with a lesion at the site of the fly bite, headache, fever, malaise, weight loss, and myalgia and is often misdiagnosed as malaria. Patients with African trypanosomiasis often report excruciating pain after minor injuries (Kerandel's hyperesthesia) (Chimelli and Scaravilli 1997). Meningoencephalitis may develop with prominent somnolence—hence the name *sleeping sickness* (Villanueva 1993). Posterior cervical lymphadenopathy in Africans is considered highly suggestive of CNS infection by *T. brucei* (Chimelli and Scaravilli 1997). Africans living in other countries have received misdiagnoses of primary psychiatric disorder (Bedat-Millet et al. 2000). The drug used to treat late-stage disease is very toxic, with an often-fatal encephalopathy the most feared complication of treatment (Blum et al. 2001); for this reason, early detection—permitting less toxic treatment—is important (Hoeprich et al. 1994).

American trypanosomiasis, or Chagas' disease, is caused by *Trypanosoma cruzi*, which is carried by insects ("kissing bugs" or "assassin bugs") in Latin America. Transmission is so inefficient that years of exposure are required to acquire the infection, and most infections are quiescent.

Following immunosuppression, reactivated disease may present as meningoencephalitis.

On brain imaging, the lesions are indistinguishable from those of toxoplasmosis, and the organism is often not identifiable in blood. Reactivated Chagas' disease should be suspected in immunosuppressed immigrants from endemic areas of Latin America, especially in presumed cases of toxoplasmosis not responsive to chemotherapy (Chimelli and Scaravilli 1997; Villanueva 1993).

Malaria

Malaria remains a major cause of morbidity in tropical nations, especially in young children and pregnant women. In other parts of the world, cases occur in immigrants and travelers to malarial areas. *Plasmodium* species are transmitted to humans by the bite of mosquitoes. The complete life cycle of the parasite is described elsewhere (Hoeprich et al. 1994).

Relapsing fever typifies malaria, and with temperatures commonly in excess of 41°C (105°F), delirium is common. *Plasmodium falciparum* causes cerebral malaria, the most catastrophic complication of malaria, which begins with disorientation, mild stupor, or even psychosis and rapidly progresses to seizures and coma with decerebrate posturing. The severity of the symptoms is correlated with the amount of sequestered parasitized red blood cells in the CNS (Turner 1997). Despite the severity and high fatality of cerebral malaria, those who recover appear to have little or no persisting cognitive dysfunction (Dugbartey et al. 1998), although one case–control study in U.S. Vietnam veterans three decades after they had had cerebral malaria found subtle affective and cognitive abnormalities (Varney et al. 1997). Anxiety and depression do appear to be common after recovery (Dugbartey et al. 1998), but they are more likely a result of psychological and social stress associated with severe illness (Weiss 1985). More severe neuropsychiatric signs, including psychosis in fully recovered (aparasitemic) cerebral malaria, are most likely attributable to pharmacotherapy (Nguyen et al. 1996). Antimalarial drugs commonly cause psychiatric side effects (see Table 27–3 later in this chapter).

Schistosomiasis

Schistosomiasis is an infection caused by blood flukes (trematodes) of the genus *Schistosoma*. Infection by the larval stage usually occurs while the individual is swimming in infected fresh water. The infection affects about 200 million people in 74 countries (*Schistosoma japonicum* in the Far East; *Schistosoma mansoni* and *Schistosoma hae-*

matobium in Africa). Most infections are asymptomatic. CNS symptoms are uncommon, but once the worms mature and the eggs have been laid, CNS involvement may be observed with any of the clinical forms of schistosomal infection. Eggs in the CNS may induce a granulomatous reaction, leading to symptoms of increased intracranial pressure (e.g., headache, confusion, nausea, and papilledema) (Pittella 1997b). Focal lesions in brain or spinal cord reflect location of the granulomas. However, in most cases, eggs in the CNS are clinically silent. In advanced disease with *S. mansoni* or *S. haematobium*, portal hypertension is a serious complication, with hepatic encephalopathy.

Trichinosis

Trichinosis is a worldwide disease caused by the ingestion of *Trichinella* larvae encysted in the muscles of infected animals. They are most commonly found in pork in the United States and Europe, but 150 species of mammals from all latitudes may acquire the infection. Trichinosis has become rare in developed nations but still occurs in ethnic groups that prefer raw or undercooked pork or wild animals, such as polar bear or walrus. Typical symptoms of infection include a febrile illness with myalgias and diarrhea, accompanied by marked eosinophilia. CNS involvement occurs in 10%–20% through a variety of mechanisms, including obstruction, toxicity, inflammation, vasculitis, and allergic reactions, such as headache, delirium, insomnia, meningoencephalitis, and seizures (Nikolic et al. 1998; Taratuto and Venturiello 1997). CT scan shows multiple small hypodense lesions with ringlike enhancement with contrast. A muscle biopsy is usually diagnostic. Treatment in severe cases requires corticosteroids for the inflammation and antihelminthic drugs to kill *Trichinella*. Residual cognitive dysfunction may occur (Harms et al. 1993).

Amebiasis

Several amebas cause human disease, and all are ubiquitous in the environment worldwide. CNS infection with amebas is rare in the United States, but it is increasing. Primary amebic meningoencephalitis is produced by *Naegleria fowleri* in healthy, young individuals engaged in water sports. Its course is acute and fulminant, with headache, nausea, confusion, and stiff neck followed by coma and death within days. Granulomatous amebic encephalitis, caused by *Balamuthia mandrillaris* and some species of *Acanthamoeba*, usually occurs in debilitated, immunosuppressed (especially in cases of AIDS) or malnourished individuals. The course is more chronic, with personality changes, confusion, and irritability, eventually progressing to seizures and death (Martinez and Visvesvara 1997).

Other Organisms

Pfiesteria

Pfiesteria piscicida is a dinoflagellate, a microorganism difficult to classify as a plant or an animal, that can release a toxin capable of killing large numbers of fish. It occurs along the eastern coast of the United States from the Gulf of Mexico to Delaware Bay. A similar species has been identified in northern Europe. There have been reports of neurotoxic effects in humans in Maryland and North Carolina, primarily in waterpersons exposed to large-scale fish kills and in researchers who cultured *Pfiesteria*. Prominent symptoms included headache, skin lesions, burning sensation on contact with water, and reversible difficulties with learning and other higher cognitive func-

tions, improving months after cessation of exposure (Grattan et al. 1998). However, a multistate prospective cohort study has not yet detected adverse human effects (Moe et al. 2001).

Drugs for Infectious Diseases: Adverse Psychiatric Effects and Drug Interactions

That antibiotics can cause delirium and other psychiatric symptoms is not well appreciated. The best-documented psychiatric side effects of drugs for infectious diseases are listed in Table 27–3. Delirium and psychosis have been particularly associated with quinolones (e.g., ciprofloxacin), procaine penicillin, antimalarial and other antiparasitic drugs, and the antituberculous drug cycloserine. The most common adverse effect causing discontinuation of interferon is depression. More detailed review is available elsewhere (Brown and Stoudemire 1998).

TABLE 27–3.   Psychiatric side effects of drugs for infectious diseases (excluding antiretroviral drugs)

Drug	Side effects
Antibacterial	
Cephalosporins	Euphoria, delusions, depersonalization, illusions
Dapsone	Insomnia, agitation, hallucinations, mania, depression
Procaine penicillin[a]	Agitation, depersonalization, fear of imminent death, hallucinations (probably due to procaine)
Quinolones[a]	Psychosis, paranoia, mania, agitation, Tourette-like syndrome
Trimethoprim–sulfamethoxazole	Delirium, psychosis
Gentamicin	Delirium, psychosis
Clarithromycin	Delirium, mania
Antituberculous	
Cycloserine[a]	Agitation, depression, psychosis, anxiety
Isoniazid	Psychosis, mania
Ethionamide	Depression, hallucinations
Antiviral	
Acyclovir, ganciclovir	Psychosis, delirium, depression, anxiety
Amantadine[a]	Psychosis, delirium
Interferon-alfa[a]	Irritability, depression, agitation, paranoia
Interleukin-2	Psychosis, delirium
Antiparasitic	
Antimalarials[a]	Confusion, psychosis, mania, depression, anxiety, aggression, delirium
Metronidazole	Depression, delirium
Thiabendazole	Psychosis
Antifungal	
Amphotericin	Delirium, psychosis, depression

Note.   See also Brown and Stoudemire 1998.
[a]More significant (more frequent and/or better established) effects.
Source.   Adapted from Abouesh A, Stone C, Hobbs WR: "Antimicrobial-Induced Mania (Antiomania): A Review of Spontaneous Reports." *Journal of Clinical Psychopharmacology* 22:71–81, 2002; "Drugs That May Cause Psychiatric Symptoms." *Medical Letter* 44:59–62, 2002.

Table 27–4 shows selected well-established interactions between antimicrobial and psychotropic drugs. Drug interactions between antibiotics and nonpsychiatric drugs also may present risk in psychiatric practice. Erythromycin (and similar antibiotics like clarithromycin) and ketaconazole (and similar antifungals) may cause QT interval prolongation and ventricular arrhythmias when given to a patient taking other QT-prolonging drugs, including tricyclic antidepressants and many antipsychotics.

TABLE 27–4. Selected antimicrobial–psychotropic drug interactions

Antimicrobial	Effect on psychiatric drug
Antimalarials	Increase phenothiazine level
Azoles	Increase alprazolam, midazolam levels
	Increase buspirone level
Clarithromycin, erythromycin	Increase alprazolam, midazolam levels
	Increase carbamazepine level
	Increase buspirone level
	Increase clozapine level
Quinolones	Increase clozapine level
	Increase benzodiazepine level
	Decrease benzodiazepine effect via GABA receptor
Isoniazid	Increase haloperidol level
	Increase carbamazepine level
	With disulfiram, causes ataxia

Note. GABA=gamma-aminobutyric acid.
Source. Adapted from Cozza KL, Armstrong SC, Oesterheld JR: *Concise Guide to Drug Interaction Principles for Medical Practice,* 2nd Edition. Washington, DC, American Psychiatric Publishing, 2003; Hansten PD, Horn JR: *Drug Interactions and Management.* Vancouver, WA, Applied Therapeutics, 1997.

Fears of Infectious Disease

Infectious diseases historically have been, and remain, frightening. In the recent epidemic of SARS, both affected patients and health care workers experienced fears of the illness and fears of contagion to family and friends. Quarantined patients struggle with loneliness, isolation, and stigmatization, and they fear the effect of their absence on those who depend on them (Maunder et al. 2003). Both individual and group reactions to real or imagined threats of infectious diseases also may include hysterical and phobic behaviors. Anxiety about acquiring a feared disease may lead to conversion symptoms, hypochondriacal preoccupation, and unnecessary avoidance behaviors. Contamination obsessions and washing compulsions are among the most frequent symptoms in OCD. Delusional fears or beliefs that one is infected also occur in psychotic disorders, including schizophrenia, psychotic depression, and delusional disorder, somatic type (e.g., delusions of intestinal parasitosis) (Ford et al. 2001; Podoll et al. 1993); however, it is important to consider that a patient with a delusion of infection may actually be infected (Chigusa et al. 2000). Unrealistic fears of infection are especially likely with venereal diseases (particularly HIV), serious outbreaks (e.g., meningococcal meningitis on campus), and infectious threats given heavy media coverage (e.g., bacterial food contamination, bovine spongiform encephalopathy, SARS, anthrax, smallpox) (Logsdail et al. 1991; McEvedy and Basquille 1997; Vuorio et al. 1990; Weir 2001). Of course, how much vigilance and which precautions are optimal may be uncertain even among experts, but the early years of the AIDS epidemic were a clear example of the potential for widespread, irrational behaviors among the public, health care professionals, and officials.

At times, mass outbreaks of symptoms occur, falsely attributed to a supposed toxic exposure (e.g., bacterial food poisoning or toxic fumes) or infectious disease. There have been hundreds of reports in the literature of such outbreaks of "mass psychogenic" or "mass sociogenic" illness, and they tend to follow trends in societal concerns (e.g., bioterrorism) (Bartholomew and Wessely 2002). They are most likely to occur in groups of young people in close quarters, such as students at schools (Jones et al. 2000) or military recruits (Struewing and Gray 1990). Some aspects of "germ panic" have become socially normative (Tomes 2000)—for example, inappropriate use of antibiotics such as ciprofloxacin during the anthrax scare, and the widespread overuse of antiseptic soaps, mouthwashes, sprays, and cleaning agents. A related phobia of fever in their children remains prevalent among parents (Crocetti et al. 2001).

Psychiatric Aspects of Immunizations

Mass outbreaks of psychogenic symptoms similar to those described earlier in this chapter have been reported several times following vaccinations (Kharabsheh et al. 2001; Peiro et al. 1996). In developed countries, the public's fears of vaccine-preventable diseases have waned, and awareness of potential adverse effects of the vaccines has increased, which is threatening vaccine acceptance (Wilson and Marcuse 2001). The media and Web sites have disseminated much disinformation about vaccination risks, adding to the tendency toward phobic avoidance of immunization. Rare, serious CNS adverse effects, including acute disseminated encephalomyelitis (see section "Viral Infections" earlier in this chapter; see also Nasr et al. 2000), can occur after a variety of vaccinations. However, recent studies have found no basis for the widely publicized fears that measles-mumps-rubella vaccination causes encephalitis, aseptic meningitis, or autism (Chen et al. 2004; Madsen et al. 2002; Makela et al. 2002).

Finally, it should be kept in mind that the chronically mentally ill often do not receive basic preventive medical care (Folsom et al. 2002). Psychiatrists can help ensure that their patients receive important immunizations.

References

Aghanwa HS, Morakinyo O: Correlates of psychiatric morbidity in typhoid fever in a Nigerian general hospital setting. Gen Hosp Psychiatry 23:158–162, 2001

Ali G, Rashid S, Kamli MA, et al: Spectrum of neuropsychiatric complications in 791 cases of typhoid fever. Trop Med Int Health 2:314–318, 1997

Annane D: Corticosteroids for septic shock. Crit Care Med 29:S117–S120, 2001

Badiaga S, Delmont J, Brouqui P, et al: Imported dengue: study of 44 cases observed from 1994 to 1997 in 9 university hospital centers. Infectio-Sud-France group [in French]. Pathol Biol (Paris) 47:539–542, 1999

Banger M, Olbrich HM, Fuchs S, et al: Cost-effectiveness of syphilis screening in a clinic for general psychiatry [in German]. Nervenarzt 66:49–53, 1995

Bañuelos AF, Williams PL, Johnson RH, et al: Central nervous system abscesses due to coccidioides species. Clin Infect Dis 22:240–250, 1996

Barnes V, Ware MR: Tetanus, pseudotetanus, or conversion disorder: a diagnostic dilemma? South Med J 86:591–592, 1993

Bartholomew RE, Wessely S: Protean nature of mass sociogenic illness: from possessed nuns to chemical and biological terrorism fears. Br J Psychiatry 180:300–306, 2002

Becarevici V: Acute delusion psychosis (acute delusion crisis) secondary to a dental infection. Rev Med Suisse Romande 108:257–262, 1988

Bedat-Millet AL, Charpentier S, Monge-Strauss MF, et al: Psychiatric presentation of human African trypanosomiasis: overview of diagnostic pitfalls, interest of difluoromethylornithine treatment and contribution of magnetic resonance imaging. Rev Neurol (Paris) 156:505–509, 2000

Bergeron JW, Braddom RL, Kaelin DL: Persisting impairment following Rocky Mountain spotted fever: a case report. Arch Phys Med Rehabil 78:1277–1280, 1997

Bertorini TE, Gelfand M: Neurological complications of bacterial endocarditis. Compr Ther 6:47–55, 1990

Blum J, Nkunku S, Burri C: Clinical description of encephalopathic syndromes and risk factors for their occurrence and outcome during melarsoprol treatment of human African trypanosomiasis. Trop Med Int Health 6:390–400, 2001

Bodner SM, Morshed SA, Peterson BS: The question of PANDAS in adults. Biol Psychiatry 49:807–810, 2001

Bodur H, Erbay A, Akinci E, et al: Neurobrucellosis in an endemic area of brucellosis. Scand J Infect Dis 35:94–97, 2003

Bonaccorso S, Marino V, Biondi M, et al: Depression induced by treatment with interferon-alpha in patients affected by hepatitis C virus. J Affect Disord 72:237–241, 2002

Bonawitz C, Castillo M, Mukherji SK: Comparison of CT and MR features with clinical outcome in patients with Rocky Mountain spotted fever. Am J Neuroradiol 18:459–464, 1997

Boulais P, Delcros J, Signoret JL, et al: Subacute excitation caused by probable herpetic encephalitis: favorable effects of lithium. Ann Med Interne (Paris) 127:345–352, 1976

Breakey WR, Kala AK: Typhoid catatonia responsive to ECT. BMJ 2:357–359, 1977

Broome CV: Epidemiology of toxic shock syndrome in the United States: overview. Rev Infect Dis 11:S14–S21, 1989

Brown TM, Stoudemire A: Antibiotics, in Psychiatric Side Effects of Prescription and Over-the-Counter Medications: Recognition and Management. Washington, DC, American Psychiatric Press, 1998, pp 173–208

Caparros-Lefebvre D, Girard-Buttaz I, Reboul S, et al: Cognitive and psychiatric impairment in herpes simplex virus encephalitis suggest involvement of the amygdalo-frontal pathways. J Neurol 243:248–256, 1996

Carithers HA, Margileth AM: Cat-scratch disease: acute encephalopathy and other neurologic manifestations. Am J Dis Child 145:98–101, 1991

Caroff SN, Mann SC, Glittoo MF, et al: Psychiatric manifestations of acute viral encephalitis. Psychiatr Ann 31:193–204, 2001

Castleberry JS, Mahon CR: Dengue fever in the Western Hemisphere. Clin Lab Sci 16:34–38, 2003

Castleman B, McNeely B (eds): Case records of the Massachusetts General Hospital: case 36–1971. N Engl J Med 285:621–630, 1971

Centers for Disease Control: Human rabies—Texas, Arkansas, and Georgia, 1991. MMWR Morb Mortal Wkly Rep 40:765–769, 1991

Centers for Disease Control and Prevention: Human rabies: Texas and New Jersey, 1997. MMWR Morb Mortal Wkly Rep 47:1–5, 1998

Centers for Disease Control and Prevention: First human death associated with raccoon rabies—Virginia, 2003. MMWR Morb Mortal Wkly Rep 52:1102–1103, 2003

Chang CZ, Wang CJ, Howng SL: Epidural abscess presented with psychiatric symptoms. Kaohsiung J Med Sci 13:578–582, 1997

Chen W, Landau S, Sham P, et al: No evidence for links between autism, MMR and measles virus. Psychol Med 34:543–553, 2004

Cheng SK, Tsang JS, Ku KH, et al: Psychiatric complications in patients with severe acute respiratory syndrome (SARS) during the acute treatment phase: a series of 10 cases. Br J Psychiatry 184:359–360, 2004

Chigusa Y, Shinonaga S, Koyama Y, et al: Suspected intestinal myiasis due to Dryomyza formosa in a Japanese schizophrenic patient with symptoms of delusional parasitosis. Med Vet Entomol 14:453–457, 2000

Chimelli L, Mahler-Araújo B: Fungal infections. Brain Pathol 7:613–627, 1997

Chimelli L, Scaravilli F: Trypanosomiasis. Brain Pathol 7:599–611, 1997

Church AJ, Dale RC, Lees AJ, et al: Tourette's syndrome: a cross sectional study to examine the PANDAS hypothesis. J Neurol Neurosurg Psychiatry 74:602–607, 2003

Clark MR, Heinberg LJ, Haythornthwaite JA, et al: Psychiatric symptoms and distress differ between patients with post-herpetic neuralgia and peripheral vestibular disease. J Psychosom Res 48:51–57, 2000

Cohen BA: Neurologic manifestations of toxoplasmosis in AIDS. Semin Neurol 19:201–211, 1999

Cohen S, Miller GE, Rabin BS: Psychological stress and antibody response to immunization: a critical review of the human literature. Psychosom Med 63:7–18, 2001

Crocetti M, Moghbeli N, Serwint J: Fever phobia revisited: have parental misconceptions about fever changed in 20 years? Pediatrics 107:1241–1246, 2001

Crowley P, Wilcox JA: Cerebral mucormycosis presenting as psychiatric distress. Psychosomatics 37:164–165, 1996

Cummings JL, Chow T, Masterman D: Encephalitis lethargica: lessons for neuropsychiatry. Psychiatr Ann 31:165–169, 2001

Deresiewicz RL, Thaler SJ, Hsu L, et al: Clinical and neuro-radiographic manifestations of eastern equine encephalitis. N Engl J Med 336:1867–1874, 1997

Dieperink E, Ho SB, Thuras P, et al: A prospective study of neuropsychiatric symptoms associated with interferon-alpha-2b and ribavirin therapy for patients with chronic hepatitis C. Psychosomatics 44:104–112, 2003

Dinwiddie SH, Shicker L, Newman T: Prevalence of hepatitis C among psychiatric patients in the public sector. Am J Psychiatry 160:172–174, 2003

Dolan JD, Kamil R: Atypical affective disorder with episodic dyscontrol: a case of von Economo's disease (encephalitis lethargica). Can J Psychiatry 37:140–142, 1992

Donnet A, Harle JR, Cherif AA, et al: Acute psychiatric pathology disclosing subcortical lesion in neuro-AIDS. Encephale 17:79–81, 1991

Douen AG, Bourque PR: Musical auditory hallucinosis from Listeria rhombencephalitis. Can J Neurol Sci 24:70–72, 1997

Dugbartey AT, Dugbartey MT, Apedo MY: Delayed neuropsychiatric effects of malaria in Ghana. J Nerv Ment Dis 186:183–186, 1998

Farmer PE, Graeme-Cook FM: Case records of the Massachusetts General Hospital. Weekly clinicopathological exercises. Case 8—1999. A 28-year-old man with gram-negative sepsis of uncertain cause. N Engl J Med 340:869–876, 1999

Fishbein DB, Robinson LE: Rabies. N Engl J Med 329:1632, 1993

Fishman JA, Rubin RH: Infection in organ-transplant recipients. N Engl J Med 338:1741–1751, 1998

Flood JM, Weinstoack HS, Guroy ME, et al: Neurosyphilis during the AIDS epidemic, San Francisco, 1985–1992. J Infect Dis 177:931–940, 1998

Folsom DP, McCahill M, Bartels SJ, et al: Medical comorbidity and receipt of medical care by older homeless people with schizophrenia or depression. Psychiatr Serv 53:1456–1460, 2002

Ford EB, Calfee DP, Pearson RD: Delusions of intestinal parasitosis. South Med J 94:545–547, 2001

Forlenza OV, Filho AHGV, Nobrega JPS, et al: A study of 38 patients from a neurology clinic in Brazil. J Neurol Neurosurg Psychiatry 62:612–616, 1997

Forton DM, Wright M, Knapp S, et al: New insights into hepatitis C. Clin Med 2:554–559, 2002

Gallegos-Orozco JF, Fuentes AP, Gerardo AJ, et al: Health-related quality of life and depression in patients with chronic hepatitis C. Arch Med Res 34:124–129, 2003

Garcia HH, Pretell EJ, Gilman RH, et al: A trial of antiparasitic treatment to reduce the rate of seizures due to cerebral cysticercosis. N Engl J Med 350:249–258, 2004

Garvey MA, Perlmutter SJ, Allen AJ, et al: A pilot study of penicillin prophylaxis for neuropsychiatric exacerbations triggered by streptococcal infections. Biol Psychiatry 45:1564–1571, 1999

Gilden DH, Klienschmidt-DeMasters BK, LaGuardia JJ, et al: Neurologic complications of the reactivation of varicella-zoster virus. N Engl J Med 342:635–645, 2000

Gliatto MF, Caroff SN: Neurosyphilis: a history and clinical review. Psychiatr Ann 31:153–161, 2001

Gnann JW, Whitley RJ: Herpes zoster. N Engl J Med 347:340–346, 2002

Grattan LM, Oldach D, Perl TM, et al: Learning and memory difficulties after environmental exposure to waterways containing toxin-producing Pfiesteria or Pfiesteria-like dinoflagellates. Lancet 352:532–539, 1998

Gray F: Bacterial infections. Brain Pathol 7:629–647, 1997

Harms G, Binz P, Feldmeier H, et al: Trichinosis: a prospective controlled study of patients ten years after acute infection. Clin Infect Dis 17:637–643, 1993

Hart RP, Kwentus JA, Frazier RB, et al: Natural history of Kluver-Bucy syndrome after the treatment of herpes encephalitis. South Med J 79:1376–1378, 1986

Hawkins C, Armstrong D: Fungal infections in the immunocompromised host. Clin Haematol 13:599–630, 1984

Hechemy KE, Fox JA, Groschel DH, et al: Immunoblot studies to analyze antibody to the Rickettsia typhi group antigen in sera from patients with acute febrile cerebrovasculitis. J Clin Microbiol 29:2559–2565, 1991

Hibberd PL, Surman OS, Bass M, et al: Psychiatric disease and cytomegalovirus viremia in renal transplant recipients. Psychosomatics 36:561–563, 1995

Hicks CB: Serologic testing for syphilis. UpToDate Online 12.2, 2004. Available at: http://patients.uptodate.com. Accessed July 2004

Hoeprich PD, Jordan CM, Ronald AR: Infectious Diseases: A Treatise of Infectious Processes, 5th Edition. Philadelphia, PA, JB Lippincott, 1994

Hokkanen L, Launes J: Cognitive recovery instead of decline after acute encephalitis: a prospective follow up study. J Neurol Neurosurg Psychiatry 63:222–227, 1997

Hunt JC, Waller G: Psychological factors in recurrent uncomplicated urinary tract infection. Br J Urol 69:460–464, 1992

Ironside JW: Review: Creutzfeldt-Jakob disease. Brain Pathol 6:379–388, 1996

Jones TF, Craig AS, Hoy D, et al: Mass psychogenic illness attributed to toxic exposure at a high school. N Engl J Med 342:96–100, 2000

Kalish RA, Kaplan RF, Taylor E, et al: Evaluation of study patients with Lyme disease: 10–20 year follow-up. J Infect Dis 183:453–460, 2001

Kauffman FH, Goldmann BJ: Rabies. Am J Emerg Med 4:525–531, 1986

Kharabsheh S, Al-Otoum H, Clements J, et al: Mass psychogenic illness following tetanus-diphtheria toxoid vaccination in Jordan. Bull World Health Organ 79:764–770, 2001

Klempner MS, Hu LT, Evans J, et al: Two controlled trials of antibiotic treatment in patients with persistent symptoms and a history of Lyme disease. N Engl J Med 344:85–92, 2001

Ko AI, Galvao RM, Ribeiro D, et al: Urban epidemic of severe leptospirosis in Brazil. Salvador Leptospirosis Study Group. Lancet 354:820–825, 1999

Kraus MR, Schafer A, Faller H, et al: Paroxetine for the treatment of interferon-alpha-induced depression in chronic hepatitis C. Aliment Pharmacol Ther 16:1091–1099, 2002

Kunkel EJ, Kim JS, Hann HW, et al: Depression in Korean immigrants with hepatitis B and related liver diseases. Psychosomatics 41:472–480, 2000

Lerner PI: Neurologic complications of infective endocarditis. Med Clin North Am 69:385–398, 1985

Leung AM, Kennedy R, Levenson JL: Rabies exposure and psychosis. Psychosomatics 44:336–338, 2003

Levenson JL, Fallon HJ: Fluoxetine treatment of depression caused by interferon. Am J Gastroenterol 88:760–761, 1993

Levenson JL, Hamer RM, Myers T, et al: Psychological factors predict symptoms of severe recurrent genital herpes infection. J Psychosom Res 31:153–159, 1987

Logsdail S, Lovell K, Warwick H, et al: Behavioural treatment of AIDS-focused illness phobia. Br J Psychiatry 159:422–425, 1991

Lougee L, Perlmutter SJ, Nicolson R, et al: Psychiatric disorders in first-degree relatives of children with pediatric autoimmune neuropsychiatric disorders associated with streptococcal infections (PANDAS). J Am Acad Child Adolesc Psychiatry 39:1120–1126, 2000

Lowy FD: Staphylococcus aureus infections. N Engl J Med 339:520–532, 1998

Madsen KM, Hviid A, Vestergaard M, et al: A population-based study of measles, mumps, and rubella vaccination and autism. N Engl J Med 347:1477–1482, 2002

Makela A, Nuorti JP, Peltola H: Neurologic disorders after measles-mumps-rubella vaccination. Pediatrics 110:957–963, 2002

Manepalli J, Grossberg GT, Mueller C: Prevalence of delirium and urinary tract infection in a psychogeriatric unit. J Geriatr Psychiatry Neurol 3:198–202, 1990

Martinez AJ, Visvesvara G: Free-living, amphizoic and opportunistic amebas. Brain Pathol 7:583–598, 1997

Mastrianni JA, Nixon R, Layzer R, et al: Prion protein conformation in a patient with sporadic fatal insomnia. N Engl J Med 340:1630–1638, 1999

Maunder R, Hunter J, Vincent L, et al: The immediate psychological and occupational impact of the 2003 SARS outbreak in a teaching hospital. CMAJ 168:1245–1251, 2003

McDonald J, Jayasuriya J, Bindley P, et al: Fatigue and psychological disorders in chronic hepatitis C. J Gastroenterol Hepatol 17:171–176, 2002

McEvedy CJ, Basquille J: BSE, public anxiety and private neurosis. J Psychosom Res 42:485–486, 1997

Mehr DR, Binder EF, Kruse RL, et al: Predicting mortality in nursing home residents with lower respiratory tract infection: the Missouri LRI Study. JAMA 286:2427–2436, 2001

Miller A, Nathanson R: Rabies: recent advances in pathogenesis and control. Ann Neurol 2:511–519, 1977

Moe CL, Turf E, Oldach D, et al: Cohort studies of health effects among people exposed to estuarine waters: North Carolina, Virginia, and Maryland. Environ Health Perspect 109 (suppl 5):781–786, 2001

Monath TP: Japanese encephalitis vaccines: current vaccines and future prospects. Curr Top Microbiol Immunol 267:105–138, 2002

Mousa AR, Koshy TS, Araj GF, et al: Brucella meningitis: presentation, diagnosis and treatment—a prospective study of ten cases. Q J Med 60:873–885, 1986

Murphy ML, Pichichero ME: Prospective identification and treatment of children with pediatric autoimmune neuropsychiatric disorder associated with group A streptococcal infection (PANDAS). Arch Pediatr Adolesc Med 156:356–361, 2002

Nadelman RB, Nowakowski J, Fish D, et al: Prophylaxis with single-dose doxycycline for the prevention of Lyme disease after an Ixodes scapularis tick bite. N Engl J Med 345:79–84, 2001

Nasr JT, Andriola MR, Coyle PK: ADEM: literature review and case report of acute psychosis presentation. Pediatr Neurol 22:8–18, 2000

Nguyen TH, Day NP, Ly VC, et al: Post-malaria neurological syndrome. Lancet 348:917–921, 1996

Nichol G, Dennis DT, Steere AC, et al: Test-treatment strategies for patients suspected of having Lyme disease: a cost-effectiveness analysis. Ann Intern Med 128:37–48, 1998

Nikolic S, Vujosevic M, Sasic M, et al: Neurologic manifestations in trichinosis. Srp Arh Celok Lek 126:209–213, 1998

Ong S, Talan DA, Moran GJ, et al: Neurocysticercosis in radiographically imaged seizure patients in U.S. emergency departments. Emerg Infect Dis 8:608–613, 2002

Osher FC, Goldberg RW, McNary SW, et al: Substance abuse and the transmission of hepatitis C among persons with severe mental illness. Psychiatr Serv 54:842–847, 2003

Osler W: On Chorea and Choreiform Affections. Philadelphia, PA, HK Lewis, 1894

Pancharoen C, Thisyakorn U: Neurological manifestations in dengue patients. Southeast Asian J Trop Med Public Health 32:341–345, 2001

Parry CM, Hien TT, Dougan G, et al: Typhoid fever. N Engl J Med 347:1770–1782, 2002

Peiro EF, Yanez JL, Carraminana I, et al: Study of an outbreak of hysteria after hepatitis B vaccination. Med Clin (Barc) 107:1–3, 1996

Perlmutter SJ, Garvey M, Castellanos X, et al: A case of pediatric autoimmune neuropsychiatric disorders associated with streptococcal infections. Am J Psychiatry 155:1592–1598, 1998

Perlmutter SJ, Leitman SF, Garvey MA, et al: Therapeutic plasma exchange and intravenous immunoglobulin for obsessive-compulsive disorder and tic disorders in childhood. Lancet 354:1153–1158, 1999

Pittella JEH: Neurocysticercosis. Brain Pathol 7:681–693, 1997a

Pittella JEH: Neuroschistosomiasis. Brain Pathol 7:649–662, 1997b

Podoll K, Bofinger F, von der Stein B, et al: Delusional parasitosis in a patient with endogenous depression [in German]. Fortschr Neurol Psychiatr 61:62–66, 1993

Prio TK, Bruunsgaard H, Roge B, et al: Asymptomatic bacteriuria in elderly humans is associated with increased levels of circulating TNF receptors and elevated numbers of neutrophils. Exp Gerontol 37:693–699, 2002

Rahn DW, Evans J (eds): Lyme Disease. Philadelphia, PA, American College of Physicians, 1998

Ravdin LD, Hilton E, Primeau M, et al: Memory functioning in Lyme borreliosis. J Clin Psychiatry 57:281–286, 1996

Relman DA, Swartz MN: Syphilis and nonvenereal treponematoses, in SAM-CD Annual 1998 (Chapter 4). New York, Scientific American Medicine, 1998

Roberts MC, Emsley RA, Jordaan GP: Screening for syphilis and neurosyphilis in acute psychiatric admissions. S Afr Med J 82:16–18, 1992

Rosenberg SD, Swanson JW, Wolford GL, et al: The five-site health and risk study of blood-borne infections among persons with severe mental illness. Psychiatr Serv 54:827–835, 2003

Rosene KA, Copass MK, Kastner LS, et al: Persistent neuropsychological sequelae of toxic shock syndrome. Ann Intern Med 96:865–870, 1982

Sabetta JR, Andriole VT: Cryptococcal infection of the central nervous system. Med Clin North Am 68:333–344, 1985

Sacks N, Van Rensbueg AJ: Clinical aspects of chronic brucellosis. S Afr Med J 50:725–728, 1976

Salinas R, Prasad K: Drugs for treating neurocysticercosis (tapeworm infection of the brain). Cochrane Database Syst Rev 2:CD000215, 2000

Schaefer M, Schmidt F, Folwaczny C, et al: Adherence and mental side effects during hepatitis C treatment with interferon alfa and ribavirin in psychiatric risk groups. Hepatology 37:443–451, 2003

Schantz PM, Moore AC, Munoz JL, et al: Neurocysticercosis in an orthodox Jewish community in New York City. N Engl J Med 327:692–695, 1992

Schelling G, Briegel J, Roozendaal B, et al: The effect of stress doses of hydrocortisone during septic shock on posttraumatic stress disorder in survivors. Biol Psychiatry 50:978–985, 2001

Schneider RK, Robinson MJ, Levenson JL: Psychiatric presentations of non-HIV infectious diseases: neurocysticercosis, Lyme disease, and pediatric autoimmune neuropsychiatric disorder associated with streptococcal infection. Psychiatr Clin North Am 25:1–15, 2002

Schuchat A, Robinson K, Wenger JD, et al: Bacterial meningitis in the United States in 1995. N Engl J Med 337:970–976, 1997

Segreti J, Harris AA: Acute bacterial meningitis. Infect Dis Clin North Am 10:797–809, 1996

Seltzer EG, Gerber MA, Cartter ML, et al: Long-term outcomes of persons with Lyme disease. JAMA 283:609–616, 2000

Shandera WX, White AC Jr, Chen JC, et al: Neurocysticercosis in Houston, Texas. Medicine 73:37–52, 1994

Singhal AB, Topcuoglu MA, Buonanno FS: Acute ischemic stroke patterns in infective and nonbacterial thrombotic endocarditis: a diffusion-weighted magnetic resonance imaging study. Stroke 33:1267–1273, 2002

Smith JB, Westmoreland BF, Reagan TJ, et al: A distinctive clinical EEG profile in herpes simplex encephalitis. Mayo Clin Proc 50:469, 1975

Solomon T: Recent advances in Japanese encephalitis. J Neurovirol 9:274–283, 2003

Solomon T: Flavivirus encephalitis. N Engl J Med 351:370–378, 2004

Spencer MD, Knight RS, Will RG: First hundred cases of variant Creutzfeldt-Jakob disease: retrospective case note review of early psychiatric and neurological features. BMJ 324:1479–1482, 2002

Sreve ST, Spivack B: Tetanus in a 74-year-old woman. J Am Geriatr Soc 42:424–425, 1994

Steere AC, Sikand VK, Meurice F, et al: Vaccination against Lyme disease with recombinant *Borrelia burgdorferi* outer-surface lipoprotein A with adjuvant. N Engl J Med 339:209–215, 1998

Stevens DL: Severe group A streptococcal infections associated with a toxic shock-like syndrome and scarlet fever toxin A. N Engl J Med 321:1–7, 1989

Stevens DL: The toxic shock syndrome. Infect Dis Clin North Am 10:727–746, 1996

Struewing JP, Gray GC: An epidemic of respiratory complaints exacerbated by mass psychogenic illness in a military recruit population. Am J Epidemiol 132:1120–1129, 1990

Swedo SE: Pediatric autoimmune neuropsychiatric disorders associated with streptococcal infections (PANDAS). Mol Psychiatry 7 (suppl 2):S24–S25, 2002

Swedo SE, Leonard HL, Mittleman BB, et al: Identification of children with pediatric autoimmune neuropsychiatric disorders associated with streptococcal infections by a marker associated with rheumatic fever. Am J Psychiatry 154:110–112, 1997

Swedo SE, Susan E, Leonard HL, et al: Pediatric autoimmune neuropsychiatric disorders associated with streptococcal infections: clinical description of the first 50 cases. Am J Psychiatry 155:264–271, 1998

Tabernero C, Polo JM, Sevillano MD, et al: Fatal familial insomnia: clinical, neuropathological, and genetic description of a Spanish family. J Neurol Neurosurg Psychiatry 68:774–777, 2000

Tager FA, Fallon BA: Psychiatric and cognitive features of Lyme disease. Psychiatr Ann 31:172–181, 2001

Takkouche B, Regueira C, Gestal-Otero JJ: A cohort study of stress and the common cold. Epidemiology 12:345–349, 2001

Tan V, Wilkins P, Badve S, et al: Histoplasmosis of the central nervous system. J Neurol Neurosurg Psychiatry 55:619–622, 1992

Taratuto AL, Venturiello SM: Trichinosis. Brain Pathol 7:663–672, 1997

Tomes N: The making of a germ panic, then and now. Am J Public Health 90:191–198, 2000

Treadway CR, Prange AJ Jr: Tetanus mimicking psychophysiologic reaction: occurrence after dental extraction. JAMA 200:891–892, 1967

Turner G: Cerebral malaria. Brain Pathol 7:569–582, 1997

Tyler KL: Creutzfeldt-Jakob disease. N Engl J Med 348:681–682, 2003

Vallini AD, Burns RL: Carbamazepine as therapy for psychiatric sequelae of herpes simplex encephalitis. South Med J 80:1590–1592, 1987

Van Lierde S, van Leeuwen WJ, Ceuppens J, et al: Toxic shock syndrome without rash in a young child: link with syndrome of hemorrhagic shock and encephalopathy? Pediatrics 13:130–134, 1997

Varney NR, Roberts RJ, Springer JA, et al: Neuropsychiatric sequelae of cerebral malaria in Vietnam veterans. J Nerv Ment Dis 185:695–703, 1997

Verghese A: The "typhoid state" revisited. Am J Med 79:370–372, 1985

Villanueva MS: Trypanosomiasis of the central nervous system. Semin Neurol 13:209–218, 1993

Vinetz JM: Leptospirosis. Curr Opin Infect Dis 14:527–538, 2001

Vinetz JM, Glass GE, Flexner CE, et al: Sporadic urban leptospirosis. Ann Intern Med 125:794–798, 1996

Vuorio KA, Aarela E, Lehtinen V: Eight cases of patients with unfounded fear of AIDS. Int J Psychiatry Med 20:405–411, 1990

Weinstein L: Bacterial meningitis. Specific etiologic diagnosis on the basis of distinctive epidemiologic, pathogenetic, and clinical features. Med Clin North Am 69:219–229, 1985

Weir E: Anthrax: walking the fine line between precaution and panic. CMAJ 165:1528, 2001

Weiss MG: The interrelationship of tropical disease and mental disorder: conceptual framework and literature review (Part I: malaria). Cult Med Psychiatry 9:121–200, 1985

Wessely S, Pariante C: Fatigue, depression and chronic hepatitis C infection. Psychol Med 32:1–10, 2002

White PD, Thomas JM, Amess J, et al: Incidence, risk and prognosis of acute and chronic fatigue syndromes and psychiatric disorders after glandular fever. Br J Psychiatry 173:475–481, 1998

Whitley RJ, Soong SJ, Linneman C Jr, et al: Herpes simplex encephalitis: clinical assessment. JAMA 247:317–320, 1982

Whitney CG, Farley MM, Hadler J, et al: Decline in invasive pneumococcal disease after the introduction of protein-polysaccharide conjugate vaccine. N Engl J Med 348:1737–1746, 2003

Wilson CB, Marcuse EK: Vaccine safety, vaccine benefits: science and the public's perception. Nat Rev Immunol 1:160–165, 2001

Windsor JJ: Cat-scratch disease: epidemiology, aetiology and treatment. Br J Biomed Sci 58:101–110, 2001

Woodward TE: Rocky Mountain spotted fever: a present day perspective (classics in medicine: commentary). Medicine 71:255–259, 1992

Wormser GP, Nadelman RB, Dattwyler RJ, et al: Practice guidelines for the treatment of Lyme disease. The Infectious Diseases Society of America. Clin Infect Dis 31 (suppl 1):1–14, 2000

Yamasaki K, Morimoto N, Gion T, et al: Delirium and a subclavian abscess. Lancet 350:1294, 1997

Yermakov V, Rashid RK, Vuletin JC, et al: Disseminated toxoplasmosis. Arch Pathol Lab Med 106:524–528, 1982

Zauner C, Gendo A, Kramer L, et al: Impaired subcortical and cortical sensory evoked potential pathways in septic patients. Crit Care Med 30:1136–1139, 2002

28 HIV/AIDS

Niccolo D. Della Penna, M.D.

Glenn J. Treisman, M.D., Ph.D.

SOON AFTER THE human immunodeficiency virus (HIV) epidemic began in the early 1980s, neurologists described several HIV-related central nervous system (CNS) syndromes. Psychiatrists and other mental health professionals initially focused on grief, loss, and supportive psychotherapy but soon recognized some specific psychiatric conditions, including acquired immunodeficiency syndrome (AIDS) dementia; AIDS mania; increased rates of major depression; and psychiatric consequences of CNS involvement with HIV, opportunistic infections, and neoplasms.

Two decades later, it is apparent that psychiatric issues play a central role in the HIV epidemic. HIV is transmitted almost entirely by specific risk behaviors and in high-risk populations targeted for education and prevention since the mid-1980s. Because of this, HIV, at least in the developed countries, has become a condition predominantly of vulnerable people with certain risk factors. Transfusion recipients and homosexual men who were unaware of the risk of HIV were the early patients, whereas many current individuals are aware of the risks but are at increased risk because of addictions, personality vulnerabilities, mood disorders, impulse-control disorders, cognitive impairment, social isolation and disenfranchisement, or other barriers to behavior change. HIV-infected patients with psychiatric illness may have great difficulty in modifying risk behaviors. Psychiatric disorders also can adversely affect the treatment of HIV infection primarily through undermining adherence, and taking medications as prescribed is critical to successful treatment. Thus, the same psychiatric disorders that prevented patients from reducing their risk prevent them from obtaining benefit from their treatment. Untreated patients with high viral loads are more infectious, leading to an increased potential for spread of the HIV epidemic.

In this chapter, we address those conditions commonly seen in HIV, including those that increase risk for HIV or are barriers to HIV treatment. The introductory part of the chapter is a medical overview of HIV disease. The second part considers neuropsychiatric and medical complications associated with HIV, and the third part includes psychiatric conditions associated with HIV. Additional details regarding psychiatric disorders and treatment issues can be found in the American Psychiatric Association's "Practice Guideline for the Treatment of Patients With HIV/AIDS" (American Psychiatric Association 2000b).

Overview of HIV Infection and AIDS

HIV was originally recognized through a series of cases of young homosexual men with *Pneumocystis carinii* pneumonia in the early 1980s in California. It later became clear that these patients had severe immune system compromise and were vulnerable to infections commonly seen in other immunocompromised individuals. Current global statistics suggest that 750,000 infants are born each year with HIV infection, and some estimate that 16,000 new infections occur each day, with one individual being infected about every 10 seconds (UNAIDS Joint United Nations Programme on HIV/AIDS Update 2000).

In the United States, as of December 31, 2001, 807,075 adults and adolescents had been reported as having AIDS, with current estimates suggested around 1 million. Of these, 462,653 (57%) have died. As of the end of 2002, 42 million people were estimated to be living with HIV/AIDS worldwide, with an estimated 5 million people acquiring the infection in 2002 (Centers for Disease Control and Prevention 2001). An estimated 20 million individuals have died from HIV worldwide.

Some populations within the United States are at increased risk for infection. Homosexual men have reduced their risk substantially but as a group continue to have high seroprevalence. Blood product screening has made transfusion risk negligible. Vertical transmission risk from mother to fetus, which occurs in up to 25%–30% of live births without intervention, is influenced by delivery type, severity of HIV disease, and the availability of preventive antiviral treatment. The frequency of vertical transmission in the developed countries has decreased dramatically in the last decade but remains a significant problem in many other parts of the world and in some subpopulations in the United States and other developed countries. Unfortunately, psychiatric disorders continue to make many vulnerable patients unable to access or benefit from prevention efforts. For example, intravenous drug users and their sexual partners are currently the population with the greatest risk for infection.

Patients who are likely to have poor adherence and therefore fail treatment may be excluded from treatment. The primary reason for excluding them from antiretroviral drug treatment is that inconsistent adherence breeds viral resistance, rendering treatment ineffective and increasing public health risk. Additionally, resources are often scarce in HIV clinics, and patients who are less likely to remain adherent are the least likely to receive effective treatment. These patients include intravenous drug users, mentally ill patients, and other patients at high risk for poor outcomes. Therefore, the ability to provide adequate psychiatric care to HIV-infected patients is critical for effective treatment of HIV. Psychiatric disorders compromise the ability to take medications, adhere to treatment, practice safer sexual behaviors, and stop using intravenous drugs.

Neuropsychiatric and Medical Complications of HIV Infection

Opportunistic infections are covered in Chapter 27, "Infectious Diseases," but here we review some specifics related to HIV infection.

Toxoplasmosis

Infection with *Toxoplasma gondii* generally occurs in patients with fewer than 200 CD4 cells/mm^3. In AIDS patients, toxoplasmosis is the most common reason for intracranial masses, affecting between 2% and 4% of the AIDS population. Symptoms of CNS infection are fever, change in level of alertness, headache, focal neurological signs (approximately 80% of cases), and partial or generalized seizures (approximately 30% of cases). Computed tomography (CT) and magnetic resonance imaging (MRI) scans usually show multiple ring-enhancing lesions in the basal ganglia or at the gray–white matter junction.

Treatment is usually empirical, based on clinical and imaging findings, and consists of pyrimethamine and leucovorin plus sulfadiazine or clindamycin. Clinical and radiological improvement is seen in more than 85% of the patients by day 7 (Luft et al. 1993). Acute treatment (6 weeks) must be followed by continuous prophylaxis to prevent relapse. The use of trimethoprim–sulfamethoxazole as prophylaxis has reduced the incidence of *Toxoplasma* infection in HIV. Patients with hypersensitivity to sulfa drugs may use pyrimethamine plus dapsone.

Cytomegalovirus

Cytomegalovirus (CMV) infection is found at autopsy in about 30% of brains from HIV-infected patients. However, the development of clinically evident CMV encephalitis is fairly rare and most often occurs in patients with CD4 cell counts less than 50 cells/mm^3. CMV infection of another organ, such as retina, blood, adrenal glands, or gastrointestinal tract, is often found at the time of encephalitis diagnosis. CMV encephalitis in AIDS may progress gradually as a dementia with focal deficits (Holland et al. 1994) or rapidly as a fatal delirium (Kalayjian et al. 1993).

Treatment is mostly supportive. Ganciclovir and foscarnet may be prescribed but are of questionable benefit. Trials of a promising new medication, cidofovir, are under way.

Cryptococcal Meningitis

Although meningitis caused by *Cryptococcus neoformans* is rare in immunocompetent persons, it occurs in approximately 8%–10% of AIDS patients and may be devastating. Patients generally present with fever and delirium. Meningeal signs are not universally seen. Seizures and focal neurological deficits occur in about 10% of patients, and intracranial pressure is elevated in about 50% of patients.

Treatment of cryptococcal meningitis in HIV requires amphotericin B. Patients who survive must receive prophylaxis against recurrence. Prophylaxis can be prescribed as oral fluconazole or intermittent intravenous amphotericin B. Some authors suggest that patients who receive highly active antiretroviral therapy (HAART) for 6 months with a rise in CD4 cell count to greater than 100 cells/mm^3 may terminate secondary prophylaxis (E. Martinez et al. 2000). Primary prophylaxis for *C. neoformans* is not recommended.

Progressive Multifocal Leukoencephalopathy

Progressive multifocal leukoencephalopathy (PML) is a demyelinating disease of white matter in immunocompromised patients. First described in cancer patients, the causative agent is a polyomavirus, named JC virus after a patient. Its transmission route is unclear but may be respiratory, and there is no clear clinical syndrome of acute infection. The prevalence of PML in AIDS is between 1% and 10%, and AIDS patients account for almost three-quarters of PML cases reported in the United States. Typically, PML affects AIDS patients with fewer than 100 CD4 cells/mm^3.

The clinical syndrome consists of multiple focal neurological deficits, such as mono- or hemiparetic limb weakness, dysarthria, gait disturbances, sensory deficits, and progressive dementia, with eventual coma and death. Occasionally, seizures or visual losses may occur. Usually, no fever or headache occurs.

The pathology of PML consists of demyelination and death of astrocytes and oligodendroglia. MRI is more useful than CT in diagnosis; multiple areas of attenuated signal are seen on T2 images, primarily in the white matter of brain, although gray matter, brain stem, cerebellar, and spinal cord lesions are possible. Cerebrospinal fluid (CSF) studies are generally unhelpful, except for polymerase chain reaction evaluation for the presence of JC virus, which is sensitive and specific. Brain biopsy provides the definitive diagnosis but is rarely used. Trials of antiviral agents for the treatment of PML are under way but have been largely unsuccessful, probably because the acute infection with JC virus occurs many years before PML develops.

Central Nervous System Neoplasms

Lymphoma is the most common neoplasm seen in AIDS patients, affecting between 0.6% and 3%. AIDS is the most common condition associated with primary CNS lymphoma. The patient is generally afebrile; may develop a single lesion with focal neurological signs or small, multifocal lesions; and most commonly presents with mental status change. Seizures occur in about 15% of these patients.

CNS lymphoma is at times misdiagnosed as toxoplasmosis, HIV dementia, or other encephalopathy. CT scan of the brain may be normal or show multiple hypodense or patchy, nodular enhancing lesions. MRI generally shows enhanced lesions that may be difficult to differentiate from CNS toxoplasmosis, but thallium single photon emission computed tomography (SPECT) scanning

may help differentiate the two disorders. CSF studies may be normal or show a moderate monocytosis; cytology studies report lymphoma cells in fewer than 5% of patients. Brain biopsy is required for confirmation of the diagnosis of CNS lymphoma. Because this procedure carries some morbidity, clinicians should strongly consider the possibility of lymphoma in afebrile patients with a negative toxoplasma immunoglobulin G (IgG) screening test result, patients with a single lesion, and patients who fail to respond to empirical therapy for toxoplasmosis as indicated by clinical examination and repeat MRI. The differential diagnosis of CNS neoplasm also includes metastatic Kaposi's sarcoma and primary glial tumors.

Lymphoma may respond in part to radiation therapy, thus alleviating high intracranial pressure and its associated symptoms. Chemotherapy is generally adjunctive for lymphoma. CNS lymphoma had a grim prognosis with an average survival of 3–5 months prior to the advent of HAART, but the prognosis is now dependent on the HAART response, with considerable improvement possible in patients who respond.

Fatigue in HIV

Fatigue is a very common symptom in HIV-infected patients, which is often overlooked, improperly assessed, or inadequately investigated. It is associated with poor quality of life and impaired physical functioning (Breitbart et al. 1998; Darko et al. 1992; Hoover et al. 1993; Longo et al. 1990; Vlahov et al. 1994). Estimates of prevalence of fatigue in patients infected with HIV range from 10% to 30% in early cases to 40% to 50% in AIDS cases (Anderson and Grady 1994; Crocker 1989; Miller et al. 1991; Revicki et al. 1994; Richman et al. 1987). Fatigue may be mild and annoying, or it may be severe enough to impair function. Several scales have been published to assess fatigue symptoms and severity (Portenoy et al. 1992, 1994). Fatigue is a nonspecific symptom and may have a single or multifactorial etiology. In a sample of ambulatory AIDS patients, fatigue significantly correlated with anemia and pain (Breitbart et al. 1998). In addition to disease causes, fatigue may be a side effect of medications, including HAART. Fatigue is one of the most common side effects of protease inhibitors and may be a reason for nonadherence (Duran et al. 2001).

Fatigue also may be the result of substance abuse, depression, or other psychiatric disorders. HIV patients with major depression are much more likely to complain of fatigue than are patients without depression (Ferrando et al. 1998a; Perkins et al. 1995). HIV wasting syndrome, chronic diarrhea, and testosterone deficiency are all associated with fatigue. Low serum testosterone has been found among symptomatic AIDS patients, especially those with HIV wasting syndrome (Berger et al. 1998; Dobs et al. 1996; Grinspoon et al. 1998; Laudat et al. 1995; Muurahainen and Mulligan 1998). Hypotestosteronism is most likely in advanced AIDS (Kopicko et al. 1999) but also may be due to medications (e.g., fluconazole, ketoconazole, or ganciclovir) (Wagner et al. 1995).

In many HIV patients, the fatigue has no clear etiology, and empirical treatment is reasonable. Testosterone may be a successful treatment for fatigue in HIV-infected men, even when depressive symptoms are present (Wagner et al. 1998). More activating antidepressants may be better tolerated by fatigued depressed patients. Some authors have reported that stimulants may be useful in treating fatigue and depression in HIV, as discussed later in this chapter. Care must be exercised in using stimulants in patients with histories of substance abuse, although risk of abuse loses relevance in terminal AIDS.

Psychiatric Conditions Associated With HIV

Delirium

Delirium occurs frequently in patients with advanced HIV infection (Bialer et al. 1991; Fernandez et al. 1989). One study found that 46% of the AIDS patients at a skilled nursing facility had at least one episode of delirium (Uldall and Berghuis 1997). More subtle delirium is common in compromised patients, although assessment can be difficult. In addition, delirium has been shown to be a marker for decreased survival in patients with AIDS (Uldall et al. 2000b). Hospitalized patients with AIDS also were found to have increased mortality if delirium complicated their hospital course (Uldall et al. 2000a).

The clinical presentation of delirium in HIV patients is the same as in non-HIV-infected individuals and is characterized by inattention, disorganized thinking or confusion, and fluctuations in level of consciousness. Emotional changes are common and often unpredictable, and hallucinations and delusions are frequently seen. The syndrome has an acute or a subacute onset and remits fairly rapidly once the underlying etiology is treated. If untreated, patients have a marked increased risk of mortality, with estimates of about 20% in hospitalized patients.

Aside from general risk factors such as older age, multiple medical problems, multiple medications, impaired visual acuity, and previous episodes of delirium, patients with HIV-associated dementia are at increased risk to develop delirium. The differential diagnosis of delirium includes HIV-associated dementia (especially with AIDS mania), minor cognitive-motor disorder, major depression, bipolar disorder, panic disorder, and schizophrenia. Delirium usually can be differentiated on the basis of its rapid onset, fluctuating level of consciousness, and link to medical etiology.

The cause of delirium should be aggressively sought. The approach to determining cause is similar to that for delirium in general (see Chapter 6, "Delirium"). Particular considerations in HIV patients include hypoxia with *Pneumocystis* pneumonia, malnutrition, CNS infections and neoplasms, systemic infections (e.g., mycobacteria, CMV, bacterial sepsis), HIV nephropathy, substance intoxication and withdrawal, medication toxicity, and polypharmacy. Variations in hydration or electrolyte status also may profoundly affect patients with HIV who already have cerebral compromise. HIV infection itself also may produce an acute encephalopathy similar to that reported with CMV (Bialer et al. 2000).

Treatment

Management of delirium in HIV is very similar to that for delirium in general (see Chapter 6, "Delirium"), including identification and removal of the underlying cause (when possible), nonpharmacological reorientation and environmental interventions, and pharmacotherapy. Low doses of high-potency antipsychotic agents usually are effective. Newer, atypical antipsychotics are currently being used with some success, but those with more anticholinergic activity may worsen the condition. Benzodiazepines should be used with caution because they may contribute to delirium in some patients but are of particular use in alcohol or benzodiazepine withdrawal deliria. Physical restraint may be necessary if the patient becomes violent but should be used only when alternatives are inadequate, because restraint may worsen delirium.

Treatment with antipsychotic medication requires awareness of the higher susceptibility of patients with HIV to neuroleptic-induced extrapyramidal symptoms (EPS), even with exposure to drugs with low potential for inducing EPS (Edelstein and Knight 1987; Hollander et al. 1985; Hriso et al. 1991). This susceptibility is a result of HIV-induced damage to the basal ganglia (American Psychiatric Association 2000b; Ferrando and Wapenyi 2002). Increased susceptibility to EPS has been particularly notable with use of conventional neuroleptic medications and has limited the dosage that can be used to treat patients (Maj 1990; Sewell et al. 1994b). Patients with AIDS-related psychosis are more sensitive to EPS and respond to lower than standard doses of antipsychotics (M. Harris et al. 1991; Sewell et al. 1994b; A. Singh et al. 1997). Extreme sensitivity to EPS is encountered in patients with HIV dementia (Fernandez et al. 1989). Marked neuronal degeneration in the basal ganglia of patients with HIV (Itoh et al. 2000), with accompanying dopaminergic neuron destruction and/or alteration, may explain these findings.

To date, only one randomized controlled trial in delirious patients with AIDS has documented efficacy of low-dose haloperidol and chlorpromazine. Lorazepam was ineffective and was associated with significant adverse effects (Breitbart et al. 1996). Lorazepam was reported to be useful in cases of AIDS-associated psychosis with catatonia, however (Scamvougeras and Rosebush 1992). Case reports indicate that molindone is of benefit for HIV-associated psychosis and has minimal EPS (Fernandez and Levy 1993).

If indicated, typical neuroleptic medications should be used at the lowest dosage and for the briefest duration possible. Atypical antipsychotics are generally preferred because of lower risk for EPS. Terminal delirium in HIV, as in other terminal diseases, is much more refractory to treatment.

Dementia

Prevalence

Early in the AIDS epidemic, some patients presented with rapidly progressing neurocognitive disturbances, which led to an intensive search for etiology. Several CNS opportunistic conditions were identified, including CMV encephalitis, PML, cerebral toxoplasmosis, cryptococcal meningitis, and CNS lymphoma. However, a subset of patients remained for which no identifiable pathogen could be found, and it was deduced that HIV itself was the causative factor behind the dementia. Autopsy studies of AIDS patients with dementia found characteristic white matter changes and demyelinization, microglial nodules, multinucleated giant cells, and perivascular infiltrates but a marked absence of HIV within neurons. This has led to the current theories of neuronal loss through the action of macrophages and microglial cells and/or through activation of cytokines and chemokines that trigger abnormal neuronal pruning. It appears that basal ganglia and nigrostriatal structures are affected early in the dementia process, with diffuse neuronal losses following. Typical late findings show an approximate 40% reduction in frontal and temporal neurons. Analyses of CSF (Gallo et al. 1989; Laverda et al. 1994) and autopsy material (Tyor et al. 1992; Wesselingh et al. 1994) also have shown aberrant production of specific cytokines in patients with HIV-associated dementia.

In 1986, HIV-associated dementia was reported in up to two-thirds of AIDS patients (Navia et al. 1986), but it is less frequent now in patients receiving HAART. It has become one of the leading causes of dementia in persons younger than 60 (McArthur et al. 1993). However, its frequency among patients with otherwise asymptomatic HIV infection or CD4 cell count greater than 500 cells/mm^3 is probably less than 5% in a community sample (Handelsman et al. 1992; Krikorian et al. 1990; Maj et al. 1994; McKegney et al. 1990; Wilkie et al. 1990). For hospitalized HIV-infected patients seen in psychiatric consultation, the rate of HIV-associated dementia has been measured at 7%–25%. In a study in a general hospital, HIV-associated dementia was diagnosed in 17% of the patients with HIV for whom psychiatric consultation was requested (Buhrich and Cooper 1987; Dilley et al. 1985). In the Multicenter AIDS Cohort Study (Sacktor et al. 1999a), the incidence of HIV-associated dementia declined 50% from 1990–1992 to 1996–1998, a period during which effective antiretroviral therapy was used (Sacktor et al. 1999a). HIV-associated dementia is generally seen in late stages of HIV illness, usually in patients who have had a CD4 cell count nadir of less than $200/mm^3$.

Risk factors associated with eventual development of HIV dementia include higher HIV RNA viral load, lower educational level, older age, anemia, illicit drug use, and female sex. High CSF HIV RNA levels may be present in patients with relatively low serum HIV RNA levels and may correlate more directly with severity of neurological deficits (McArthur et al. 1997).

Pathophysiology

Mechanisms of neuronal death in HIV-associated dementia are unclear (McArthur et al. 1989; Wiley et al. 1991). Neurotoxic proteins, such as gp120 and Tat, have been associated with overstimulation of glutamate receptors, which can be blocked by N-methyl-D-aspartate (NMDA) and non-NMDA antagonists (Magnuson et al. 1995; Nath et al. 2000). Patients with HIV-associated dementia have been found to have increased CSF levels of glutamate compared with nondemented control subjects (Ferrarese et al. 1997) and patients with other neurological diseases or Alzheimer's dementia (Ferrarese et al. 2001). Atrophy of the caudate nuclei was particularly notable in those patients with HIV-associated dementia, supporting other reports of basal ganglia sensitivity to excitotoxicity (Bernal et al. 2000). Known HIV-associated dementia markers include CSF HIV RNA (Brew et al. 1997; McArthur et al. 1997; Sei et al. 1996), CSF beta$_2$-microglobulin, neopterin, quinolinic acid, prostaglandins, and matrix metalloproteinases (Brew 2001). Recent evidence also suggests axonal injury with presence of beta-amyloid precursor protein in brains of patients with HIV-associated dementia (Nebuloni et al. 2001).

Assessment

Clinically, HIV dementia presents with the typical triad of symptoms seen in other subcortical dementias—memory and psychomotor speed impairments, depressive symptoms, and movement disorders. Initially, patients may notice slight problems with reading, comprehension, memory, and mathematical skills, but these symptoms are subtle, so they may be overlooked or discounted as being caused by fatigue and illness. Patients with early dementia usually will show impairments in timed trials, such as a timed oral Trail-Making Test or grooved pegboard. The Modified HIV Dementia Scale is a very useful bedside screen and can be administered serially to document disease progression (Davis et al. 2002). Later, patients develop more global dementia, with marked impairments in naming, language, and praxis.

Motor symptoms are also often subtle in the early stages and include occasional stumbling while walking or running; slowing of fine repetitive movements, such as playing the piano or typing; and slight tremor. On examination, patients will have impaired saccadic eye movements, dysdiadochokinesia, hyperreflexia, and, especially in later stages, frontal release signs. In late stages, motor symptoms may be quite severe, with marked difficulty in smooth limb movements, especially in the lower extremities. Impairments on tests of psychomotor speed in patients at the time of AIDS diagnosis with no memory complaints have been shown to predict development of HIV-associated dementia up to 2 years later (Dunlop et al. 2002). Rate of progression is variable and may cause mild dysfunction over a long period or rapid progression with severe impairment (Price and Brew 1988). Parkinsonian features are common in HIV-associated dementia, and clinical correlates between HIV and parkinsonism have been identified (Koutsilieri et al. 2002; Mirsattari et al. 1998). Parkinsonian features may be provoked by dopamine antagonists (Hriso et al. 1991), opportunistic infections including toxoplasmosis (P. Maggi et al. 2000), or CNS infection with HIV itself (Mirsattari et al. 1998).

Apathy is a common early symptom of HIV-associated dementia, often causing noticeable withdrawal by the patient from social activity. A frank depressive syndrome also commonly develops, typically with irritable mood and anhedonia instead of sadness and crying spells. Sleep disturbances and weight loss are common. Restlessness and anxiety may occur. Psychosis develops in a significant number of patients, typically with paranoid thoughts and hallucinations. In about 5%–8% of patients, a syndrome known as AIDS mania develops (see subsection "Bipolar Disorder in HIV" later in this chapter). Overall, HIV-associated dementia is rapidly progressive, usually ending in death within 2 years. Because of impulsive behavior and emotional lability, HIV-associated dementia has been suggested as a strong risk factor for suicide (Alfonso and Cohen 1994).

Diagnosis

Typical findings on MRI of patients with advanced HIV-associated dementia include significant white matter lesions, as well as cortical and subcortical atrophy (Dal Pan et al. 1992; Jarvik et al. 1988; Stout et al. 1998). These abnormalities may appear as discreet foci, as patchy regions of confluent involvement, or as diffuse parenchymal involvement (Broderick et al. 1993; M.P. Grassi et al. 1997; Hawkins et al. 1993; Olsen et al. 1988). Partial improvement of MRI signal abnormalities (Olsen et al. 1988) and worsening of atrophy and white matter lesions (Post et al. 1992) have been reported in small reviews of patients taking zidovudine. MRI also has been suggested to be of utility in monitoring HIV-associated dementia treatment with HAART (Thurnher et al. 2000).

Various functional neuroimaging techniques, including positron-emission tomography (PET) (Rottenberg et al. 1996), SPECT (G.J. Harris et al. 1994; Rosci et al. 1996), and magnetic resonance spectroscopy (MRS) (Barker et al. 1995; Chang et al. 1999; Lopez-Villegas et al. 1997), have shown alterations in cerebral blood flow and metabolic patterns in the brains of individuals infected with HIV. Most of these studies were done in patients with dementia or other cognitive impairment, but other MRS investigations showed abnormalities in patients with no cognitive deficit (Chang et al. 1999; Meyerhoff et al. 1999; Suwanwelaa et al. 2000). Increased brain activation on functional MRI during working memory was found in patients with early HIV cognitive disturbance (Chang et al. 2001). Further studies showed increased activation on functional MRI in HIV-positive patients that predated clinical signs or deficits on cognitive tests (Ernst et al. 2002).

Recent evidence suggests that HIV-associated dementia may develop in the presence of milder immunosuppression (Dore et al. 1999). The rates of HIV-associated dementia have declined but not to the same extent that other AIDS-defining illnesses have declined, suggesting that CNS eradication of HIV is becoming more challenging with current antiretroviral regimens. It has been proposed that increasing resistance to HAART regimens may be linked to this possible evolution. In the Multicenter AIDS Cohort Study (1990–1998; Sacktor et al. 2001), the proportion of cases of HIV-associated dementia in patients with CD4 cell counts between 201 and 350 cells/mm^3 was higher in 1996–1998 compared with the early 1990s. This suggests that screening for HIV-associated dementia should be extended to patients with CD4 cell counts less than 350 cells/mm^3 (Sacktor et al. 1999b, 2001).

The extended survival that antiretroviral regimens have offered patients also may increase their vulnerability to developing dementia rather than dying secondary to other fulminant complications (Lopez et al. 1999).

Treatment

Controlled trials for HIV-associated dementia through 2000 have been reviewed elsewhere (Clifford 2000). The addition of protease inhibitors to antiviral regimens improves cognitive outcomes in comparison with regimens with less intensive antiretroviral therapy (Ferrando et al. 1998b). Intensification of antiretroviral therapy and associated control of viral load are associated with significantly lower risk for progression to HIV-associated dementia (Childs et al. 1999). Initial open-label studies of zidovudine showed promising results, with patients improving on neuropsychological tests (Fischl et al. 1987). The AIDS Clinical Trial Groups trial compared high doses of zidovudine with placebo but was stopped prematurely after preliminary data showed dramatic cognitive improvement in those receiving zidovudine (Sidtis et al. 1993). A sharp decline in the incidence of HIV-associated dementia was observed following widespread use of zidovudine (Chiesi et al. 1990, 1996; Portegies et al. 1989), and HIV-associated dementia became rare in patients receiving continued zidovudine treatment (Portegies et al. 1989). Zidovudine might produce improvement in patients already affected by dementia (Tozzi et al. 1993; Vion-Dury et al. 1995). More recent studies have shown efficacy of HAART in improving cognitive impairment in patients with HIV-associated dementia (Ferrando et al. 1998b; Giesen et al. 2000; Halman and Rourke 2000; Letendre et al. 2000; Price et al. 1999; Tozzi et al. 1999, 2001).

Controversy exists regarding the duration of treatment and outcome of dementia. Some studies suggest a dose–response relationship between duration of exposure to zidovudine and dementia-related morbidity (Cornelisse et al. 2000; Portegies 1994; Vago et al. 1993). Other evidence shows a temporary relation between zidovudine and stability of improvement of cognitive function (Vago et al. 1993). The long-term effect of HAART on the course of HIV-associated dementia remains undetermined, with some evidence of ongoing HIV-related cognitive damage despite more than 3 years of potent antiretroviral treatment (Tozzi et al. 2001). The only other controlled trial of antiretroviral drugs compared effective antiviral therapy with and without added high-dose abacavir (Brew et al. 1998), but the study did not detect further cognitive improvement.

At first, it was believed that only antiretroviral agents with good penetration into the CNS would be useful in treating HIV-associated dementia with associated reduction of CSF HIV RNA levels (Halman and Rourke 2000), but later efforts indicated that HAART in many different combinations, including those with poor CNS levels, could provide some relief. Drugs that cross well into CSF include nucleoside reverse transcriptase inhibitors (zidovudine, stavudine, and abacavir) and the nonnucleoside nevirapine. Despite these theoretical considerations, little evidence suggests an improved outcome for any particular antiretroviral regimen (Clifford 2000). However, the observation of increased proportions of patients with HIV-associated dementia compared with other AIDS-defining illnesses (Dore et al. 1999; Masliah et al. 2000) suggests that HAART may not be as effective for treating HIV-associated dementia.

Various clinical trials have evaluated neuroprotective medications for HIV-associated dementia. Nimodipine was found to be tolerable but not efficacious (Navia et al. 1998). Other trials assessing tolerability have been performed with antioxidants (The Dana Consortium on the Therapy of HIV Dementia and Related Cognitive Disorders 1998, 1999), a platelet-activating factor antagonist (Schifitto et al. 1999), and peptide T (Heseltine et al. 1998). Memantine, an NMDA antagonist, is currently being studied (Clifford 2000) for use in AIDS dementia but has been approved for use in other dementia syndromes.

Use of dopamine receptor agonists in pediatric patients with HIV and parkinsonian features has led to improvement in motor function (Mintz et al. 1996), yet results of similar medications in adults have been less fruitful (Kieburtz et al. 1991a). Psychostimulants have been shown to improve cognitive performance in patients with HIV (Brown 1995; Hinkin et al. 2001), but others have noted apparent acceleration of HIV-associated dementia following psychostimulant use (Czub et al. 2001; Nath et al. 2001).

Risperidone and clozapine have been described in case reports of HIV-associated dementia with psychosis, with significant improvement in psychotic symptoms and few EPS (Dettling et al. 1998; Zilikis et al. 1998).

Quality care for patients with HIV-associated dementia is to ensure an optimal HAART regimen and to treat associated symptoms aggressively. Depression can be treated with standard antidepressants, and, in some cases, methylphenidate or other stimulants may be useful in treatment of apathy.

Minor Cognitive-Motor Disorder

HIV-associated dementia is a late-stage disorder, whereas minor cognitive-motor disorder (or mild neurocognitive disorder) is a less severe syndrome seen in earlier HIV infection. The symptoms of minor cognitive-motor disorder are often overlooked because they may be very subtle, but they are essentially mild manifestations of the same symptoms seen in HIV-associated dementia (cognitive and motor slowing). Patients with this disorder may present with a singular minor complaint, such as taking longer to read a novel, dysfunction when performing fine motor tasks such as playing the piano, an increased tendency to stumble or trip, or making more mistakes when balancing the checkbook. Minor cognitive-motor disorder is now regarded as part of the spectrum of HIV-associated dementia, and its description in the literature has fallen out of use.

Prevalence data for minor cognitive-motor disorder are variable, often suggesting up to 60% prevalence by late-stage AIDS. Prevalence in earlier stages is not well defined. Whether minor cognitive-motor disorder inevitably leads to HIV-associated dementia is uncertain. It appears that some patients may continue to have minor problems, whereas others will progress to frank dementia. This question is now confounded by the effects of HAART; data from earlier in the epidemic cannot be reasonably compared with current data.

Treatment

No controlled treatment data are available specifically for minor cognitive-motor disorder.

Major Depression

Depression is a significant problem among persons with HIV and AIDS. The question of whether the incidence or prevalence of major depression is increased in HIV-infected patients has been a controversial topic (Ciesla and Roberts 2001). Several factors complicate this issue. First, identification of major depressive disorder rather than depressive symptoms is a methodological barrier to cross-sample comparison. Additionally, populations at risk for HIV infection, including homosexual men and patients with substance use disorders, have elevated rates of major depression. A recent meta-analysis of 10 studies comparing HIV-positive and at-risk HIV-negative patients found a twofold increase in the prevalence of major depression in patients infected with HIV (Ciesla and Roberts 2001). Studies have shown that depression has a negative effect on patient adherence (Dimatteo et al. 2000), quality of life (Lenz and Demal 2000; Meltzer-Brody and Davidson 2000), and treatment outcome (J. Holmes and House 2000).

Lyketsos and Treisman reported an association between depression and HIV infection as early as 1993 and speculated that major depression was a risk factor for developing HIV (Lyketsos et al. 1993a). Studies have shown prevalence rates of major depression among individuals with HIV of 15%–40%, depending on the setting and risk group studied (American Psychiatric Association 2000b; Atkinson et al. 1988; Perkins et al. 1994; Treisman et al. 1998). However, the prevalence exceeds 50% in persons with HIV seeking psychiatric treatment (American Psychiatric Association 2000b). Major depression is a risk factor for HIV infection (McDermott et al. 1994) by virtue of its effect on behavior, intensification of substance abuse, exacerbation of self-destructive behaviors, and promotion of poor partner choice in relationships. HIV-negative persons with higher scores on screening instruments for general psychological distress were found to have increased risk behaviors for HIV acquisition (Hartgers et al. 1992). Distress symptoms in AIDS patients have been found to correlate with poor performance, decreased global quality of life, and presence of HIV-related medical conditions but not with CD4 cell count (Vogl et al. 1999). A sevenfold increase was found in the lifetime prevalence of mood disorders among patients without substance use disorders presenting for HIV screening (Perry et al. 1990).

Major depression also is a risk factor for various behavioral disturbances that may increase exposure to HIV infection (Regier et al. 1990). In this way, depression can be seen as a vector of HIV transmission (Angelino and Treisman 2001; Treisman et al. 1998). Depression not only serves as a risk for perpetuation of the HIV epidemic (Morrill et al. 1996; Nyamathi 1992; Orr et al. 1994) but also is a complication preventing effective treatment. It has been clearly shown to hinder effective treatment of HIV infection (van Servellen et al. 2002). Patients with major depression are at increased risk for disease progression and mortality (Ickovics et al. 2001).

HIV increases the risk of developing major depression through a variety of mechanisms, including direct injury to subcortical areas of brain, chronic stress, worsening social isolation, and intense demoralization. Direct evidence for a relation between worsening HIV disease and the development of major depression is limited, but several studies support this link, particularly the Multicenter AIDS Cohort Study. This study showed that rates of depression increased 2.5-fold as CD4 cells declined to fewer than 200/mm^3 just before patients developed AIDS (Lyketsos et al. 1996a), suggesting that lower CD4 cell counts predict increased rates of depression.

Patients with AIDS have been recognized as a group with a high risk for psychological distress (Lyketsos et al. 1996b). High prevalence rates of suicide have been reported among HIV-infected patients (Cournos et al. 1991;

L. Grassi 1996; Pugh et al. 1993; Sacks et al. 1992; Weinhardt and Carey 1995). Factors associated with HIV and suicide include depression, hopelessness, alcohol abuse, poor social support, low self-esteem, and history of psychiatric disorder (Fawcett 1992; Murphy 1977). Recent diagnosis of HIV or presence of pain also is associated with increased suicidal thoughts (Louhivuori and Hakama 1979; Steer et al. 1994). The course of HIV has been purported to affect the prevalence of suicidal thoughts and behavior (Rabkin et al. 1993), and stage of HIV infection also may alter the potential for suicidal behavior and other psychiatric symptoms (Lyketsos et al. 1994) (see also Chapter 10, "Suicidality").

Taken together, these lines of evidence indicate that HIV is a risk factor for depression and that depression is a risk factor for HIV and its morbidity, underlining the importance of recognition and treatment of depression in HIV-infected patients.

Differential Diagnosis

The diagnosis of major depression in the HIV clinic is complicated by the high frequency of depressive symptoms that are associated with these other problems. Despite this, studies of HIV-positive patients with major depression have shown that its response to treatment is similar to that expected in other populations.

The differential diagnosis of depression in HIV includes nonpathological states of grief and mourning (sometimes made quite severe by the vulnerabilities of the person) and a variety of psychological and physiological disturbances. Patients with complaints of depressive syndromes can have dysthymia, dementia, delirium, demoralization, intoxication, withdrawal, CNS injury or infection, malnutrition, wasting syndromes, medication side effects, and a variety of other conditions. HIV-associated dementia and other HIV-related CNS conditions can produce a flat, apathetic state that is often misdiagnosed as depression. Cocaine withdrawal produces a depressive syndrome, and hypoactive delirium can be mistaken for depression. CNS syphilis, a condition that had become quite rare prior to the HIV epidemic, has been reappearing and remains "the great imitator," as it was originally described.

HIV-infected patients with major depression frequently present to internists and family practitioners with multiple somatic symptoms. These include, but are not limited to, headache, gastrointestinal disturbances, inexplicable musculoskeletal or visceral pain, cardiac symptoms, dizziness, tinnitus, weakness, and anesthesia. Neurovegetative symptoms are especially common. Patients report slowed thought processes, with impairments in concentration and short-term memory and occasionally generalized confusion. Given the burdens of HIV, the medical problems associated with the disease, and the side effects of medications, depression may be very low on the list of considered causes of the patient's complaints. Even patients complaining of depressive symptoms may have their depression overlooked or discounted because of the presence of a plethora of other diagnoses. Nonspecific somatic symptoms are often the result of depression rather than HIV infection in patients whose infection is early and asymptomatic. Depression is most likely to be missed when symptoms are attributed to HIV-associated dementia, fatigue, demoralization and disenfranchisement, wasting syndrome, or substance abuse. Care should be taken in distinguishing between major depression and demoralization (i.e., adjustment disorder) in patients with HIV. Approximately one-half of the patients presenting to an urban HIV clinic with depressive complaints were found to have demoralization alone (Lyketsos et al. 1994). The ability to report feeling fairly normal when distracted from thinking about the precipitating event or circumstance causing distress is a hallmark of demoralization.

As an example, fatigue has been found to be more associated with depression than with HIV disease progression. Worsening of fatigue and insomnia at 6-month follow-up was highly correlated with worsening depression but not with CD4 cell count, change in CD4 cell count, or disease progression by Centers for Disease Control and Prevention category (Perkins et al. 1995). These findings support the notion that somatic symptoms generally suggestive of depression should trigger a full psychiatric evaluation. In later-stage HIV infection, various illnesses are common, often moving depression down on the differential diagnosis list. Somatic symptoms always should be evaluated carefully and considered in context (i.e., either with other indicators of progression of HIV disease or with other indicators of depression).

Certain HIV-related medical conditions and medications can cause depressive symptoms. These include CNS infections, such as toxoplasmosis, cryptococcal meningitis, lymphoma, and syphilis. Some investigators have found significant rates of depressive symptoms, including low mood, poor appetite with loss of weight, decreased libido, and fatigue, among male HIV-positive patients with low testosterone levels (Rabkin et al. 1999b). Several drugs used in patients with HIV, including efavirenz, interferon, metoclopramide, clonidine, propranolol, sulfonamides, anabolic steroids, and corticosteroids, have been reported to produce depression. These depressive symptoms often respond to withdrawal of the offending drug; when they do not respond to withdrawal of the drug or when the drug must be continued, the symptoms should be treated as major depression with appropriate antidepressant medication.

Routine screening for psychiatric disease in HIV clinic patients can effectively preempt urgent referrals for rapidly progressing disorders. In one study that specifically examined HIV-infected patients, the combination of two brief self-administered questionnaires, the Beck Depression Inventory and the General Health Questionnaire, prospectively predicted a psychiatric disorder (depression in most cases) other than substance abuse with a sensitivity of 81%, a specificity of 61%, and a positive predictive value of 71% (Lyketsos et al. 1994).

Treatment

Treatment with HAART was associated with significant improvement in symptoms of depression but did not necessarily have a causal relationship (Brechtl et al. 2001). Several studies reported efficacy of various antidepressants in HIV-infected patients, but no single antidepressant has been found superior in treating HIV-infected patients as a group. As with all depressed patients, nonadherence is the most common reason for ineffective drug treatment, and adverse effects are the most common reason for nonadherence. Because HIV-infected patients are likely to be more sensitive to side effects, antidepressants should be started at subtherapeutic dosage and raised slowly.

For a detailed review of the pharmacological treatment of major depression in HIV, see the article by Ferrando and Wapenyi (2002). There are methodological limitations in interpreting these clinical trial outcomes, including variable stage of infection, wide-ranging durations of treatment, overrepresentation of gay and bisexual males, and underrepresentation of intravenous drug users and women. Inclusion and outcome criteria also have been variable, and high placebo response rates have been seen (up to 50%).

One early double-blind study reported a favorable response to imipramine; 74% of the patients responded, compared with 30% taking placebo (Rabkin et al. 1994a). Another study found a favorable response to imipramine but showed a slightly higher placebo response (Manning et al. 1990). Attrition from the imipramine group was significant; 30% discontinued it by 6 months, most often because of side effects. Open-label trials of fluoxetine, sertraline, and paroxetine in various stages of HIV illness reported response rates (including affective and somatic depressive symptoms) between 70% and 90%, and all the medications were well tolerated (Ferrando et al. 1997; Rabkin et al. 1994a, 1994b). One double-blind, placebo-controlled study of fluoxetine found significant response (Rabkin et al. 1999a). Another similarly designed trial in HIV-infected users of intravenous cocaine and opioids showed significant reduction in depressive symptoms with fluoxetine compared with placebo (Batki et al. 1993).

Supportive group psychotherapy and fluoxetine were found to be superior to placebo plus group therapy for a population of homosexual or bisexual men with HIV, and patients with more severe symptoms tended to achieve greater benefits from medication (Zisook et al. 1998). In a comparison of paroxetine and imipramine, both drugs were superior to placebo in patients with HIV and major depression (Elliott et al. 1998). Small open-label trials of venlafaxine, mirtazapine, and nefazodone in patients with major depression and HIV found that response rates were higher than 70% and there were few side effects (Elliott and Roy-Byrne 2000; Elliott et al. 1999; Fernandez and Levy 1997).

Few specific studies of the treatment of major depression in HIV-positive women have been done. In a comparison between fluoxetine and desipramine in women with AIDS, rates of response were 53% and 75%, respectively (Schwartz and McDaniel 1999). A separate trial comparing women taking fluoxetine and sertraline showed response rates of 78% and 75%, respectively (Ferrando et al. 1999).

Major depression in HIV-positive men with testosterone deficiency has been effectively treated with intramuscular testosterone in an open trial (with 79% response in mood symptoms) (Rabkin et al. 1999b) and was replicated in a double-blind, controlled trial (Rabkin et al. 2000b). Dehydroepiandrosterone, a precursor to testosterone, improved mood symptoms during an open-label phase but not during a placebo-controlled discontinuation phase (Rabkin et al. 2000a).

Psychostimulants also have been evaluated for treatment of fatigue, cognitive impairment, and depression in patients with HIV. Open-label trials report an 85% mood response rate in patients with HIV-associated dementia taking methylphenidate (V.F. Holmes et al. 1989) and a 95% mood response rate in men with AIDS taking dextroamphetamine (Wagner et al. 1997). A double-blind trial showed a significant response to dextroamphetamine compared with placebo in patients with AIDS and major depression, subthreshold major depression, or dysthymia (Wagner and Rabkin 2000). Double-blind comparison of methylphenidate, pemoline, and placebo in patients with HIV (most with AIDS) found improvement in both depressive symptoms and fatigue (Breitbart et al. 2001). Others have reported similar outcomes in treating fatigue and depression in HIV (Fernandez et al. 1995; Masand and Tesar 1996; White et al. 1992). No known reports document abuse of prescription stimulants in patients with HIV (Ferrando and Wapenyi 2002).

St. John's wort is often used by patients as alternative antidepressant treatment, but it may lower serum levels of protease inhibitors ("St. John's Wort and HAART" 2000) (see also Chapter 37, "Psychopharmacology"), and patients receiving any HIV treatment should be advised not to take it. *S*-Adenosylmethionine also has been studied in patients with HIV and major depression, with preliminary suggestion of antidepressant efficacy (Cerngul et al. 2001).

The side effects of certain antidepressants can render them advantageous or disadvantageous in particular patients with HIV. For example, selective serotonin reuptake inhibitors are best avoided in patients with chronic diarrhea. Sedating antidepressants should be avoided in patients with weakness, lethargy, orthostasis, or other risk for falls. Tricyclic antidepressants should be avoided with oral candidiasis because of the aggravating effect of dry mouth on thrush. In cases of anorexia or cachexia, antidepressants with appetite-stimulating effects are best selected.

An important issue is the interaction of antidepressants and HAART medications. Potential interactions are designated in Table 37–2 in Chapter 37, "Psychopharmacology." Two points deserve emphasis. First, particularly because depression is associated with reductions in adherence to HAART, the risks of untreated depression must be measured against those of potential medication interactions. Second, clinical significance of these drug–drug interactions has not yet been clearly established (i.e., dose adjustments are probably not required). This is likely because both antidepressants and HAART, unlike drugs such as warfarin or digoxin, have wide therapeutic indices. Finally, no evidence indicates that antidepressants cause fluctuations in CD4 cell counts (Wagner et al. 1996).

Psychotherapy. The literature on the use of psychotherapy for treatment of depression in HIV-infected patients is extensive, but clinical trial data are sparse. One study showed that interpersonal psychotherapy and supportive psychotherapy with adjunctive use of imipramine were superior to cognitive-behavioral therapy (CBT) or supportive psychotherapy without antidepressants in treating symptoms of depression and improving Karnofsky performance scores (Markowitz et al. 1998). Group CBT used alone or in combination with medication also has shown efficacy for HIV-infected patients. Improvements have been reported as well for HIV-positive patients receiving group CBT either as a single treatment modality or combined with medication (Antoni et al. 1991; Chesney et al. 1996; Kelly 1998; Lutgendorf et al. 1997a). Quality of life in women with AIDS also improved after group-based cognitive-behavioral interventions (Lechner et al. 2003).

A wide range of intrapsychic or interpersonal issues may be the focus of psychotherapy. Supportive psychotherapy can help patients with major depression who interpret their suffering to be a sign of weakness in the face of adversity. These patients often believe that they should pull themselves out of depression and get frustrated when they fail. Education about the disease and nature of their depression, encouragement, and therapeutic optimism all may be helpful. Other issues that arise in psychotherapy include guilt over acquiring HIV; guilt over infecting others; and anger at the source of disease, at oneself, or at God. The diagnosis of HIV infection may lead to precipitous revelation of hidden sexual or drug abuse behavior, eliciting shame and self-loathing. The stigma of HIV may lead to rejection or abandonment by loved ones, and shunning by wider society, making patients feel like lepers. Despite the development of HAART, some patients become hopeless and nihilistic and forgo HIV treatment.

Bipolar Disorder

Patients with preexisting bipolar disorder may experience exacerbations because of the stresses of HIV illness. Perhaps the additional presence of CNS inflammation or degeneration secondary to HIV may also worsen underlying bipolar disorder, and new-onset mania could be a result of the organic insult itself. The first report of mania associated with HIV was in 1984; a 31-year-old man with Kaposi's sarcoma and recent diagnosis of *P. carinii* pneumonia developed an acute brain syndrome during antibiotic treatment. After a seizure, symptoms of mania with psychotic features were noted, along with confusion, and treatment with haloperidol effected resolution (Hoffman 1984). Numerous case reports and case series since then have described mania in HIV-infected patients (Boccellari et al. 1988; Halman et al. 1993; Kieburtz et al. 1991b; Lyketsos et al. 1993b, 1997).

The prevalence of mania has been found to be increased in patients with AIDS when compared with the general population (Halman et al. 1993; Kieburtz et al. 1991b). One report indicated a 17-month prevalence of 1.4% in those with HIV and 8.0% in patients with AIDS, which was 10 times the expected 6-month prevalence in the general population (Lyketsos et al. 1993b). In this group, late-onset patients were less likely to have a personal or family history of mood disorder. Another study among inpatients reported a 29-month prevalence of secondary mania of 1.2% in patients with HIV and 4.3% in those with AIDS (Ellen et al. 1999).

Some have suggested that mania should be subdivided into primary and secondary types, with patients who have the secondary type showing close temporal proximity to an organic insult, no history of illness, essentially negative family history, and late age at onset (Krauthammer and Klerman 1978). Secondary mania includes those cases due to HIV brain disease itself (Gabel et al. 1986; Kermani et al. 1985; Perry and Jacobsen 1986; Schmidt and Miller 1988), those due to antiretroviral drugs (Brouillette et al. 1994; Maxwell et al. 1988; O'Dowd and McKegney 1988; Wright et al. 1989), and those due to other HIV-related conditions (e.g., cryptococcal meningitis) or medications (Fichtner and Braun 1992; V. F. Holmes and Ficchione 1989; Johannessen and Wilson 1988; Nightingale et al. 1995; Pickles and Spelman 1996). Concurrent or subsequent cognitive impairment has been reported among cases of HIV-related mania (Kermani et al. 1985; Lyketsos et al. 1997; Perry and Jacobsen 1986; Schmidt and Miller 1988); however, cases without such deficits also have been reported (Buhrich et al. 1988; Ellen et al. 1999; Schmidt and Miller 1988). An increased risk of HIV-associated dementia and cognitive slowing was found in one group of patients with secondary HIV mania, with cognitive decline prior to onset of mania (Lyketsos et al. 1997). In addition, the secondary mania associated with HIV was found to be associated with low CD4 cell count (Ellen et al. 1999; Lyketsos et al. 1993b), often lower than 100 cells/mm^3. The incidence of secondary mania, like that of HIV-associated dementia, appears to have declined since the widespread use of HAART (Ferrando and Wapenyi 2002).

AIDS mania seems to have a clinical profile somewhat different from that of primary mania (Ellen et al. 1999; Lyketsos et al. 1993b, 1997). Irritable mood is often a prominent feature, but elevated mood can be observed. Sometimes prominent psychomotor slowing accompanying the cognitive slowing of AIDS dementia will replace the expected hyperactivity of mania, which complicates the differential diagnosis. AIDS mania is usually quite severe in its presentation and malignant in its course. In one series, late-onset patients (presumed to have AIDS mania) had a greater total number of manic symptoms than did early-onset patients. Late-onset patients also were more commonly irritable and less commonly hyperverbal. AIDS mania seems to be more chronic than episodic, with infrequent spontaneous remissions, and usually relapses with cessation of treatment. Because of their cognitive deficits, patients have little functional reserve to begin with and are less able to pursue treatment independently or consistently.

One presentation of mania, either early or late, is the delusional belief that one has discovered a cure for HIV or has been cured. Although this belief may serve to cheer otherwise demoralized patients, it also may result in the resumption of high-risk behavior and lead to the spread of HIV and exposure to other infections. When euphoria is a prominent symptom in otherwise debilitated late-stage patients, caregivers may question whether to deprive patients of the illusion of happiness. It is the often-devastating effects of the other symptoms of mania that tip the balance toward treatment.

Neuroradiological correlates of secondary HIV mania have been attempted, but the results have been conflicting. Some studies indicate that findings on neuroimaging are not of any clinical significance (Ellen et al. 1999). Abnormal MRI scans have been reported, however (Kieburtz et al. 1991b).

Treatment

Treatment of secondary HIV or AIDS mania has not been systematically studied to date, and the optimal treatment remains unclear. Reports often have indicated a particular resistance of manic symptoms to treatment. Others have noted few differences in response in the treatment of secondary HIV mania compared with bipolar disorder (Ellen et al. 1999). The treatment of mania in early-stage HIV infection is not substantially different from the standard treatment of bipolar disorder with mood stabilizers and antipsychotics. As HIV infection advances, with lower CD4 cell counts, more medical complications, more CNS involvement, and greater overall physiological vulnerability, changes in treatment may be required. Treatment with traditional antimanic agents can be very difficult in patients with advanced disease. AIDS mania patients may respond to monotherapy with antipsychotic agents, as was shown in case reports (Ellen et al. 1999). Late-stage patients are sensitive to side effects of antipsychotics, especially EPS, as noted earlier in this chapter (see "Treatment" subsection of "Delirium" section). As such, the dose of antipsychotic required may be much lower than that customarily used for mania. The more advanced these patients' HIV and/or dementia, the more sensitive they are to small dosage changes. These patients are also very sensitive to anticholinergic side effects, including delirium.

There has been considerable experience with traditional mood-stabilizing agents in selected AIDS mania patients, but with relatively little published literature. One case report of lithium use in secondary HIV mania showed control of symptoms at a dose of 1,200 mg/day (Tanquary 1993). Lithium use has been problematic for several reasons, including side effects of cognitive slowing, nausea, diarrhea, and polyuria resulting in dehydration, all of which may already plague HIV-infected patients. The major problem with lithium in AIDS patients has been rapid fluctuations in blood level, especially in the hospital despite previously stable doses. Anecdotal reports describe problems with administering lithium and valproic acid because of subsequent delirium (Angelino and Treisman 2001).

Valproic acid has been used with success, titrated to the usual therapeutic serum levels of 50–100 µg/L. Enteric-coated valproic acid is better tolerated in many patients. A study of valproic acid in the treatment of HIV-associated mania reported that it was well tolerated and led to significant improvement in manic symptoms, with doses up to 1,750 mg/day and serum levels greater than 50 µg/L (Halman et al. 1993). Another report documented reduction in symptoms with levels of 93 and 110 µg/L (RachBeisel and Weintraub 1997). Concern has been raised over hepatotoxicity in patients with HIV taking valproic acid (Cozza et al. 2000). In cases of severe hepatic insufficiency (e.g., *Mycobacterium avium* complex [MAC] infiltration with portal hypertension), valproic acid probably should be avoided, but this has not been studied. Valproic acid also can affect hematopoietic function, so white blood cell and platelet counts must be monitored. In addition, sodium valproate has been reported to increase HIV replication in vitro (Jennings and Romanelli 1999; Moog et al. 1996; Simon et al. 1994; Witvrouw et al. 1997), as well as increase CMV replication (Jennings and Romanelli 1999). However, retrospective case series reports of divalproex sodium in patients with secondary HIV mania found no increase in HIV-1 viral load in the presence of antiretroviral medications (J.D. Maggi and Halman 2001). Prospective studies of in vivo increases in HIV viral load have not been reported (Ferrando and Wapenyi 2002), but trials are under way.

Carbamazepine also may be effective, but concerns exist regarding the potential for synergistic bone marrow suppression in combination with antiviral medications and HIV itself. It also may lower serum levels of protease inhibitors (Ferrando and Wapenyi 2002). No reports are available for newer anticonvulsants such as gabapentin and lamotrigine in HIV mania. Potential drug interactions between anticonvulsant mood stabilizers and HAART are shown in Chapter 37, "Psychopharmacology."

The treatment of psychosis in HIV-related mania with risperidone has shown significant improvement (A. Singh et al. 1997). No evidence of notable drug interactions, drug-induced leukopenia, or extrapyramidal signs was found. Olanzapine has been anecdotally reported to be effective in HIV-associated mania (Ferrando and Wapenyi 2002). Remoxipride was found to be effective in HIV-related mania but was subsequently withdrawn because of reports of aplastic anemia (Scurlock et al. 1995). Atypical antipsychotics have the advantage of lower risk of tardive dyskinesia, but this is not an important issue for patients with end-stage AIDS. Reduction of the risk of EPS is a noteworthy consideration in selecting an antipsychotic, in addition to other factors including affordability. The common side effect of significant weight gain with some atypical antipsychotics is less problematic for patients with HIV who are cachectic.

One case report showed rapid clinical improvement of HIV-associated manic symptoms with clonazepam, allowing reduction of antipsychotic dosage (Budman and Vandersall 1990). No unacceptable side effects were reported, but treatment with benzodiazepines is less useful in maintenance treatment because of tolerance, abuse liability, and cognitive impairment.

Schizophrenia

The literature on patients with severe and chronic mental illnesses, primarily schizophrenia and bipolar disorder, reports HIV prevalence rates of between 2% and 20% in both inpatient and outpatient samples (Ayuso-Mateos et al. 1997; Blank et al. 2002; Empfield et al. 1993; Meyer et al. 1993; Naber et al. 1994; Silberstein et al. 1994; Volavka et al. 1991; Walkup et al. 1999). Investigators have noted that clinicians working with patients with schizophrenia were often unaware of their increased risk for acquiring HIV and made little effort to screen for seropositivity (Cournos et al. 1991). Perhaps this is because schizophrenic patients have been traditionally seen as markedly hyposexual because of the illness itself (Akhtar and Thomson 1980; Gray et al. 2002) and antipsychotic drugs (Gray 1999). However, many schizophrenic patients are sexually active (Cournos et al. 1994), often with higher risk partners (Kalichman et al. 1994); seldom use condoms (Cournos et al. 1994); and do not otherwise practice safe sex. Substance abuse is very common in schizophrenic patients, including during sexual activity (Cournos et al. 1994). Patients with schizophrenia have significantly less knowledge about HIV infection and transmission than do persons without schizophrenia (Kalichman et al. 1994; Kelly et al. 1992). Even increased knowledge about HIV in schizophrenic patients may not lead to decreased risk behaviors (McKinnon et al. 1996). Cumulatively, these factors help explain the increased risk of HIV infection in schizophrenic patients (Cournos et al. 1991). Suicidality is increased in patients with both schizophrenia and HIV infection. For all these reasons, clinicians should evaluate schizophrenic patients for risk behaviors and for their knowledge about HIV. A validated screening tool—the Risk Behaviors Questionnaire—is available (Volavka et al. 1992).

Treatment

Treatment of schizophrenia in HIV-infected patients follows the same basic principles as for other patients with schizophrenia—namely, control of symptoms with medications and psychosocial support and rehabilitation. Close collaboration with HIV providers is strongly suggested, so that HIV treatment can be coordinated and monitored. Schizophrenic patients are very likely to have difficulties accessing care, affording medication, and adhering to complex HAART regimens. Educational interventions have promoted safer sexual practices (Baer et al. 1988; Jacobs and Bobek 1991) and may decrease risk behaviors (Carmen and Brady 1990; Kalichman et al. 1995).

Haloperidol was found to be effective in treating psychotic symptoms of schizophrenia in patients with HIV (Mauri et al. 1997; Sewell et al. 1994a, 1994b). Patients with HIV may be highly sensitive to the EPS of antipsychotic medications, as already noted. Treatment with thioridazine was reported to be efficacious without EPS (Sewell et al. 1994b). Molindone was reported to be of benefit for psychosis and agitation with few EPS in patients with HIV (Fernandez and Levy 1993). Clozapine also has shown efficacy in treating HIV-associated psychosis in patients with drug-induced parkinsonism (Lera and Zirulnik 1999). Risperidone also has been reported to be effective (A. Singh et al. 1997). Drug interactions between antipsychotics and HAART are discussed in Chapter 37, "Psychopharmacology."

Substance Abuse and Addiction

Substance abuse is a primary vector for the spread of HIV for those who use intravenous drugs and their sexual partners and those who are disinhibited by intoxication or driven by addiction to unsafe sexual practices. Patients with substance use disorders may not seek health care or may be excluded from or discriminated against in health care. In addition, intoxication and the behaviors necessary to obtain drugs interfere with access to, and effectiveness of, health care.

Triple diagnosis refers to a patient with a dual diagnosis (substance abuse and psychiatric disorder) who also has HIV, and such patients are overrepresented in HIV treatment. One study found that as many as 44% of the new entrants to the HIV medical clinic at the Johns Hopkins Hospital had an active substance use disorder. Of these patients, 24% had both a current substance use disorder and another nonsubstance-related Axis I diagnosis (Lyketsos et al. 1994).

In the United States at the end of 2001, the proportion of injection drug users with AIDS was 24% (Centers for Disease Control and Prevention 2001). Even among non–injection drug users, substance abuse plays a major, albeit more subtle, role in HIV transmission. Addiction and high-risk sexual behavior have been linked across a wide range of settings. For example, crack cocaine abusers are more likely to engage in prostitution to obtain money for drugs (Astemborski et al. 1994; Edlin et al. 1994). Men who use crack cocaine are more likely to engage in unprotected anal sex with casual male contacts (de Souza et al. 2002). Alcohol intoxication also can lead to risky sexual behaviors by way of cognitive impairment and disinhibition (Rees et al. 2001; Stein et al. 2000).

Neuropsychological testing of drug abusers with and without HIV indicates that substance use can contribute to the cognitive decline of HIV-associated dementia (Pakesch et al. 1992). Substance use may augment HIV replication in the CNS and increase HIV encephalopathy in early AIDS (Kibayashi et al. 1996). For example, cocaine abuse augments HIV replication in vitro (Peterson et al. 1991) and also increases permeability of the blood-brain barrier to HIV (Nottet et al. 1996; Zhang et al. 1998).

Substance abuse can be successfully treated in those at risk for HIV. One of the most extensively studied interventions in risk reduction is methadone maintenance, which resulted in sustained reductions in HIV risk and lower incidence of HIV infection (Metzger et al. 1991, 1998).

Substance Use Disorders and Interaction With HIV Treatment

The medical sequelae of chronic substance abuse accelerate the process of immunocompromise and amplify the burdens of HIV infection. Injection drug users are at higher risk for developing bacterial infections such as pneumonia, sepsis, and endocarditis. Tuberculosis, sexually transmitted diseases (STDs), viral hepatitis, coinfection with human CD4 cell lymphotrophic virus, and lymphomas also occur more commonly in injection drug users with HIV than in other patients with HIV. HIV-infected injection drug users are at higher risk for fungal or bacterial infections of the CNS. Alcohol abuse is immunosuppressive and increases risk for bacterial infections, tuberculosis, and dementia. Heroin may worsen HIV-associated nephropathy.

Important drug interactions occur between abused substances and antiretroviral and antibiotic drugs. Rifampin increases the elimination of methadone and may result in withdrawal symptoms. Decreased plasma levels of methadone also occur with concurrent administration of ritonavir, nelfinavir, efavirenz, and nevirapine (Gourevitch and Friedland 2000). Patients in a methadone program will be unlikely to take medications that have caused withdrawal.

Posttraumatic Stress Disorder

Posttraumatic stress disorder (PTSD) and its symptoms occur at greatly increased rates in HIV-infected patients

(A. Martinez et al. 2002). Of the HIV-infected women attending county medical clinics, 42% met diagnostic criteria for PTSD (Cottler et al. 2001). Minority women (Bassuk et al. 1998) and women prisoners (Hutton et al. 2001) are particularly at risk for both PTSD and HIV. Male veterans with a diagnosis of PTSD are at increased risk for HIV infection, especially if they are substance abusers (Hoff et al. 1997). PTSD symptoms are associated with high-risk behaviors, including prostitution, choosing other high-risk sexual partners, injection drug use, and unsafe sexual practices (Stiffman et al. 1992). Among the HIV-infected female partners of male drug users, those who had a history of rape or being assaulted were more likely to engage in high-risk HIV behaviors (He et al. 1998). These studies are cross-sectional and cannot determine causality. PTSD from early life trauma may predispose an individual to engage in high-risk sexual or drug behavior. On the other hand, risk behaviors such as prostitution and drug abuse increase exposure to trauma and thus the likelihood of developing PTSD. Finally, HIV infection itself may be the cause of PTSD. Rates of PTSD in response to HIV infection are higher than those in response to other debilitating illnesses (Fauerbach et al. 1997; Perez-Jimenez et al. 1994; van Driel and Op den Velde 1995), including cancer (Alter et al. 1996; Cordova et al. 1995). In one study, about 30% of persons recently diagnosed with HIV subsequently developed PTSD, with half of the cases appearing within 1 month of HIV diagnosis (Kelly et al. 1998). Prior PTSD increased the risk for PTSD in response to HIV diagnosis. Even asymptomatic HIV-infected individuals have high levels of PTSD symptoms (Botha 1996).

PTSD in at-risk or HIV-infected individuals is significant for several reasons. PTSD has high rates of psychiatric comorbidity (up to 80%), most often depression (Kelly et al. 1998) and cocaine and opioid abuse (Kessler et al. 1995), which are also risks for HIV (Lyketsos and Federman 1995). HIV-infected persons with PTSD have higher levels of pain (Smith et al. 2002). PTSD symptoms in HIV-positive patients in one study predicted lower CD4 cell counts (Lutgendorf et al. 1997b) and in another study, lower CD4 to CD8 T-cell ratios (Kimerling et al. 1999). This may represent faster HIV disease progression, generally associated with stressful life events (Evans et al. 1997; Leserman et al. 2000; Moss et al. 1988).

Persons at risk for HIV and HIV-infected individuals should be routinely screened for PTSD and psychiatric comorbidities, with treatment targeted accordingly. Failure to do so in this very high-risk population has serious consequences, both for this population's welfare and for public health.

Issues of Personality in Patients Infected With HIV

A disturbing trend in the HIV epidemic has been the persistence of modifiable risk factors among persons who are HIV infected. Such individuals, who report high rates of sexual and/or drug risk behaviors, include HIV-infected drug users (Avants et al. 2000; Novotna et al. 1999), patients presenting at HIV primary care clinics for medical treatment (Erbelding et al. 2000), and HIV-infected men who have sex with other men (Kohl et al. 1999). The fact that knowledge of HIV and its transmission is insufficient to deter these individuals from engaging in HIV risk behaviors suggests that certain personality characteristics may enhance a person's tendency to engage in such behaviors.

Traditional approaches in risk reduction counseling emphasize the avoidance of negative consequences in the future, such as condom use during sexual intercourse to prevent STDs. Such educational approaches have proved ineffective for individuals with certain personality characteristics (Kalichman et al. 1996; Trobst et al. 2000). Effective prevention and treatment programs for HIV-infected individuals must consider specific personality factors. In this section, we outline the role of personality characteristics and personality disorders in the risk of acquiring HIV and highlight specific interventions to reduce the risk of HIV that are formulated for individuals whose personality characteristics place them at increased risk.

Implications for HIV Risk Behavior

Our clinical experience suggests that unstable extroverts are the most prone to engage in practices that place them at risk for HIV. We estimate that in the psychiatry service of the Johns Hopkins AIDS clinic (a referral-biased sample), about 60% of our patients present with this blend of extroversion and emotional instability. These individuals are preoccupied by, and act on, their feelings, which are labile, leading to unpredictable and inconsistent behavior. Most striking is the inconsistency between thought and action. Regardless of intellectual ability or knowledge of HIV, unstable extroverts can engage in extremely risky behavior. Past experience and future consequences have little importance in decision making for the individual who is ruled by feeling; the present is paramount. Their primary goal is to achieve immediate pleasure or removal of pain, regardless of circumstances. As part of their emotional instability, they experience intense fluctuations in mood. It is difficult for them to tolerate painful affects; they want to escape or avoid feelings as quickly as possible. They are motivated to pursue pleasurable experiences, however risky, to eliminate negative moods.

Unstable extroverts are more likely to engage in behavior that places them at risk for HIV infection and are more likely to pursue sex promiscuously. They are less likely to plan and carry condoms and more likely to have unprotected vaginal or anal sex. They are more fixed on the reward of sex and remarkably inattentive to the STD they may acquire if they do not use a condom. Unstable extroverts are also less likely to accept the diminution of pleasure associated with the use of condoms or, once aroused, to interrupt the "heat of the moment" to use condoms. Similarly, unstable extroverts are more vulnerable to alcohol and drug abuse. They are drawn to alcohol and drugs as a quick route to pleasure. They are more likely to experiment with different kinds of drugs and to use greater quantities. Unstable extroverts are also more likely to become injection drug users.

The second most common personality type that we have observed, which may represent about 25% of our patients, is that of the stable extrovert. Stable extroverts are also present oriented and pleasure seeking; however, their emotions are not as intense, as easily provoked, or as mercurial. Hence, they are not as strongly driven to achieve pleasure. Stable extroverts may be at risk because they are too optimistic or sanguine to believe that they will become infected with HIV.

Introverted personalities appear to be less common among our psychiatric patients. Their focus on the future, avoidance of negative consequences, and preference for cognition over feeling render them more likely to engage in protective and preventive behaviors. HIV risk for introverts is determined by the dimension of emotional instability–stability. About 14% of our patients present with a blend of introversion and instability. Unstable introverts are anxious, moody, and pessimistic. Typically, these patients seek drugs and/or sex not for pleasure, but for relief or distraction from pain. They are concerned about the future and adverse outcomes but believe that they have little control over their fates. Stable introverts constitute the remaining 1% of patients. These patients, with their controlled, even-tempered personalities, are least likely to engage in risky or hedonistic behaviors. Typically, these individuals are HIV positive as a result of a blood transfusion or an occupational needle stick. These percentages of personality styles are illustrative of one center's experience and may not be generalizable.

Personality Disorder in HIV

Prevalence rates of personality disorders among HIV-infected patients (19%–36%) and individuals at risk for HIV (15%–20%) (Jacobsberg et al. 1995; J.G. Johnson et al. 1995; Perkins et al. 1993) are high and significantly exceed rates found in the general population (10%) (J.G. Johnson et al. 1995). The most common personality disorders among HIV-infected patients are antisocial and borderline types (Golding and Perkins 1996). Antisocial personality disorder is the most common (Perkins et al. 1993) and is a risk factor for HIV infection (Weissman 1993). Individuals with personality disorder, particularly antisocial personality disorder, have high rates of substance abuse and are more likely to inject drugs and share needles compared with those without an Axis II diagnosis (Brooner et al. 1993; Dinwiddie et al. 1996; Golding and Perkins 1996). Approximately half of drug abusers may meet criteria for a diagnosis of antisocial personality disorder. Individuals with antisocial personality disorder are also more likely to have higher numbers of lifetime sexual partners, engage in unprotected anal sex, and contract STDs compared with individuals without antisocial personality disorder (Brooner et al. 1993; Hudgins et al. 1995; Kleinman et al. 1994).

In our AIDS clinic, patients are characterized along the dimensions of extraversion–introversion and emotional stability–instability rather than in the discrete categories provided by DSM's Axis II for several reasons. First, it is easier for staff to determine where a patient falls along two dimensions than to evaluate the many criteria for personality disorders. Second, it is simpler to design intervention strategies for two dimensions. Third, a diagnosis of antisocial or borderline personality disorder can be stigmatizing, particularly in a general medical clinic. Finally, a classification system based on a continuum approach may be a better predictor of HIV risk behavior than are DSM-IV-TR (American Psychiatric Association 2000a) Axis II categories (Tourian et al. 1997).

Implications for Medication Adherence

Identifying factors that influence adherence in HIV disease is important in improving overall health outcomes (Eldred et al. 1998). Adherence is especially challenging in HIV, which carries all of the components of low adherence—long duration of treatment, preventive rather than curative treatment, asymptomatic periods, and frequent and complex medication dosing (Blackwell 1996; Haynes 1979; Kruse et al. 1991). In patients with HIV, estimates of zidovudine adherence vary widely from 26% to 94% (Wagner et al. 1996).

Our clinical experience suggests that nonadherence is more common among our extraverted or unstable patients. The same personality characteristics that place them at risk for HIV also reduce their ability to adhere to demanding drug regimens. Specifically, their present-time orientation, combined with reward-seeking behavior, makes it more difficult to tolerate side effects from drugs whose benefits may not be immediately apparent. It is also difficult for feeling-driven individuals to maintain consistent, well-ordered routines, so following frequent, rigid dosing schedules is problematic. Our unstable, extroverted patients usually intend to follow the schedule, but their chaotic and mercurial emotions interfere and disrupt daily routines. For example, a patient may report that he felt very upset and nihilistic after a fight with a family member and missed several doses of his antiretroviral medicines. Missing doses of HAART can increase the chance of HIV resistance developing.

Treatment Implications

We have found that a cognitive-behavioral approach is most effective in treating patients who present with extroverted and/or emotionally unstable personalities. Five principles guide our care:

1. *Focus on thoughts, not feelings.* Individuals with unstable, extroverted personalities often do not recognize the extent to which their actions are driven by feelings of the moment.
2. *Use a behavioral contract for all patients to build consistency.* The contract outlines goals for treatment and responsibilities and expectations of both the patient and the providers.
3. *Emphasize constructive rewards.* Positive outcomes, not adverse consequences, are salient to extroverts. Most of the patients have already experienced negative consequences from their behavior. Exhortations to use condoms to avoid STDs are unpersuasive. More success has been achieved with extroverts by eroticizing the use of condoms (Tanner and Pollack 1988) or by incorporating novel techniques into sexual repertoires (Abramson and Pinkerton 1995). Similarly, the rewards of abstaining from drugs or alcohol are emphasized, such as having money to buy clothing, having a stable home, or maintaining positive relationships with children. In building adherence to antiretroviral therapies, the focus is on the rewards of an increased CD4 cell count and reduced viral load rather than on avoidance of illness. Use of the viral load as a strategy to build adherence can increase acceptance in all patients but is especially effective in reward-driven extroverts.
4. *Use relapse prevention techniques.* The relapse prevention model, originally developed for treatment of substance abuse behavior, is an effective method for changing habitual ways of behaving.
5. *Develop a coordinated treatment plan.* The mental health professional coordinates with the medical care provider, supplying information about a patient's personality and how it influences behavior. Both professionals work in tandem to develop behavioral contracts to reduce HIV risk behaviors and build medication adherence.

Psychosocial Interventions to Prevent HIV Transmission

In intervention studies of men who have sex with other men (still the largest subgroup in terms of new HIV infections in the United States), many psychosocial interventions have shown a decrease in either risk behaviors or infection (Dilley et al. 2002; W.D. Johnson et al. 2002). A meta-analysis examining the effect of HIV prevention strategies found that psychosocial interventions can lead to sexual risk reduction among drug users (Semaan et al. 2002), as did a separate large study of cocaine-dependent patients (Woody et al. 2003). Studied interventions have included stress management and relaxation techniques, group counseling, education, cognitive training, negotiation skills training, psychotherapy directed at emotional distress reduction, relapse prevention models of high-risk behavior reduction, education directed at eroticizing safer sex, assertiveness training, and peer education in bars. All of these interventions showed a modest effect on either risk behavior or HIV infection. Although most studies focused on men who have sex with other men, the results have been similar in heterosexually transmitted HIV, women, and injection drug users. It is unclear from the data what the best intervention is and how to stratify the interventions.

Adherence Counseling

The single most important factor regarding outcome of HIV treatment is the patient's ability to adhere to a prescribed regimen. A recent study of HIV-infected prisoners reported that under directly observed therapy in a prison setting, 85% of the individuals developed undetectable viral loads with prisoners taking approximately 93% of doses (Kirkland et al. 2002). In contrast, British community studies found that only 42% of treatment-naive patients taking antiretroviral medications attained undetectable viral loads (Lee and Monteiro 2003). Antiretroviral adherence rates between 54% and 76% have been reported in other general clinic or community samples (Liu et al. 2001; McNabb et al. 2001; Paterson et al. 2000; Wagner and Ghosh-Dastidar 2002), including a group of patients with serious mental illness (Wagner et al. 2003).

The literature on adherence indicates that four groups of factors affect adherence: environmental factors, treatment factors, illness factors, and patient factors. Environmental factors include medication cost, work schedules, transportation, housing issues, and lack of supportive relationships. Missed appointments are a strong predictor of treatment failure, suggesting that any factor that interferes with patients coming for treatment will interfere with adherence (Lucas et al. 1999). Patient survey data indicate that the patient–provider relationship has a strong effect on adherence (Altice et al. 2001; Stone et al. 1998). These factors should be assessed when discussing a patient's readiness to start treatment, and identified barriers must be targeted.

Treatment factors include the type of medication and amount of pill burden. Once-a-day medications are easier to remember to take regularly than twice-a-day medications, but both are markedly better for adherence than three- or four-times-a-day medications (Kleeberger et al. 2001). However, some studies have not found any effect of pill burden on adherence (Gifford et al. 2000). Perceived side effects also correlate with poor adherence and can prevent patients from taking all required doses in an attempt to prevent adverse consequences. Patients are less likely to adhere to regimens if they believe that they are ineffective. These barriers should be assessed before treatment and at every follow-up visit, and treatment must be tailored accordingly.

Illness chronicity, symptoms, and curability also affect adherence. Lifelong illnesses have the highest degree of nonadherence, as do illnesses that are asymptomatic, because the patient is unable to feel any benefit or effect from taking a medication. Similarly, illnesses that cause symptoms that are unrelieved by treatment are often associated with poor adherence. Diseases with no potential cure may make patients nihilistic about treatment and unable to perceive the potential benefits. Providers who practice therapeutic optimism and are willing to explore patients' feelings about these issues, remain supportive, and emphasize positive aspects of treatment will find improved adherence in their patients.

Patient factors associated with nonadherence, including dementia, depression, psychosis, personality factors, and substance use, are detailed elsewhere in this chapter. Many studies have shown decreased adherence to HAART attributable to depression (Catz et al. 2000; Chesney et al. 2000; N. Singh et al. 1996). Depressed patients feel hopeless and may see no purpose in taking further medications. Psychotic patients may refuse medications, deny their illness, or be too disorganized to manage adherence.

Patients with dementia may forget doses and appointments. Personality vulnerabilities also have strong effects on adherence. Constant and consistent coaching of patients at each visit is imperative, including clarifying goals of treatment (both short-term and long-term) and anticipating misunderstandings. It is also useful over time to show rewards of adherence to treatment, no matter how small.

More subtle factors affecting adherence include psychosocial support networks, individual coping skills, life structure, access to resources, and behavioral control. Interventions such as cognitive-behavioral psychotherapy, structured psychoeducational psychotherapy, supportive psychotherapy, and group interventions all have been used to improve patient adherence to medication regimens. The current literature on HIV medication adherence focuses on technical interventions, such as pillbox and timer reminders, less complex pharmacological interventions, decreased pill burdens, and increased access to care. A growing literature examines psychosocial interventions, relationship with care providers, case management, and psychiatric disorders as barriers to adherence. In this arena, mental health care can have an enormous effect on outcome.

Mental Health Care for Patients With HIV Infection

Patients with HIV infection are underserved with regard to mental health. This is critical because psychiatric disorders increase the risk for HIV and have a negative effect on HIV treatment. Although model clinics exist, in which treatment for HIV, substance abuse, and psychiatric illness is integrated, these clinics are exceptional. Psychiatric disorders are underrecognized and undertreated in patients with many chronic medical conditions, but HIV-infected patients are especially likely to be impoverished, disenfranchised, vulnerable, and members of underserved minorities, all of which further decrease the likelihood that they will receive adequate treatment. Integrated expert care by psychiatrists and other mental health professionals should be a high priority both to promote effective treatment of HIV infection and to stem the tide of an epidemic that spreads through modifiable behaviors.

Conclusion

The interrelationships between HIV/AIDS and psychiatry are myriad and complex. In a sense, psychiatric disorders can be seen as vectors of HIV transmission, through associated high-risk behaviors. They also complicate the treatment of HIV infection. HIV causes a number of psychiatric conditions and exacerbates many others. Comorbid psychopathology—including major depression, schizophrenia, addictions, personality vulnerabilities such as unstable extraversion, and the effects of traumatic life experiences—is highly prevalent in patients with HIV/AIDS. Each of these problems has the potential to sabotage treatment for HIV infection and its many complications. Yet there is a profound shortage of funding and availability of psychiatric care in HIV clinics. Our experience in caring for HIV patients is that by developing a comprehensive diagnostic formulation on which to base treatment, even many of the most difficult patients can be successfully treated.

With the advent of HAART, we have seen terminal patients who have undergone nearly miraculous recoveries only to find themselves unprepared to meet the challenges of facing life again—of pressing on in the face of the daily burdens of ongoing treatment, side effects, stigma, and continuing injury. To assist them with this monumental task is a great challenge, but we have the lessons from the field of psychiatry that have helped patients shoulder similar burdens from chronic mental illness. At the heart of our work we try to impart hope for the future, therapeutic optimism, advocacy, sanctuary, and rehabilitation.

References

Abramson PR, Pinkerton SD: With Pleasure: Thought on the Nature of Human Sexuality. New York, Oxford University Press, 1995

Akhtar S, Thomson JA: Schizophrenia and sexuality: a review and a report of twelve unusual cases, part II. J Clin Psychiatry 41:166–174, 1980

Alfonso CA, Cohen MA: HIV-dementia and suicide. Gen Hosp Psychiatry 16:45–46, 1994

Alter CL, Pelcovitz D, Axelrod A, et al: Identification of PTSD in cancer survivors. Psychosomatics 37:137–143, 1996

Altice FL, Mostashari F, Friedland GH: Trust and the acceptance of and adherence to antiretroviral therapy. J Acquir Immune Defic Syndr 28:47–58, 2001

American Psychiatric Association: Diagnostic and Statistical Manual of Mental Disorders, 4th Edition, Text Revision. Washington, DC, American Psychiatric Association, 2000a

American Psychiatric Association, Work Group on HIV/AIDS: Practice guideline for the treatment of patients with HIV/AIDS. Am J Psychiatry 157 (11 suppl):1–62, 2000b

Anderson R, Grady C: Symptoms reported by "asymptomatic" HIV-infected subjects (abstract). Proceedings of the 7th Annual Association of Nurses in AIDS Care. Nashville, TN, November 10–12, 1994

Angelino AF, Treisman GJ: Management of psychiatric disorders in patients infected with human immunodeficiency virus. Clin Infect Dis 33:847–856, 2001

Antoni MH, Baggett L, Ironson G, et al: Cognitive-behavioral stress management buffers distress responses and immunologic changes following notification of HIV-1 seropositivity. J Consult Clin Psychol 59:906–915, 1991

Astemborski J, Vlahov D, Warren D, et al: The trading of sex for drugs or money and HIV seropositivity among female intravenous drug users. Am J Public Health 84:382–387, 1994

Atkinson JH Jr, Grant I, Kennedy CJ, et al: Prevalence of psychiatric disorders among men infected with human immunodeficiency virus: a controlled study. Arch Gen Psychiatry 45:859–864, 1988

Avants SK, Warburton LA, Hawkins KA, et al: Continuation of high-risk behavior by HIV-positive drug users. J Subst Abuse Treat 19:15–22, 2000

Ayuso-Mateos JL, Montanes-Lastra L, De La Garza PJ, et al: HIV infection in psychiatric patients: an unlinked anonymous study. Br J Psychiatry 170:181–185, 1997

Baer JW, Dwyer PC, Lewitter-Koehler S: Knowledge about AIDS among psychiatric inpatients. Hosp Community Psychiatry 39:986–988, 1988

Barker PB, Lee RR, McArthur JC: AIDS dementia complex: evaluation with proton MR spectroscopic imaging. Radiology 195:58–64, 1995

Bassuk EL, Buckner JC, Perloff JN, et al: Prevalence of mental health and substance use disorders among homeless and low-income housed mothers. Am J Psychiatry 155:1561–1564, 1998

Batki SL, Manfredi LB, Murphy JM, et al: Randomized, placebo-controlled trial of paroxetine versus imipramine in depression in HIV-infected injection drug users (abstract PO-B16–1685). Berlin, Germany, International Conference on AIDS, June 1993

Berger D, Muurahainen N, Wittert H, et al: Hypogonadism and wasting in the era of HAART in HIV-infected patients (32174). Geneva, Switzerland, World AIDS Conference, June 1998

Bernal F, Saura J, Ojuel J, et al: Differential vulnerability of hippocampus, basal ganglia, and prefrontal cortex to long-term NMDA excitotoxicity. Exp Neurol 161:686–695, 2000

Bialer PA, Wallack JJ, Snyder SL: Psychiatric diagnosis in HIV-spectrum disorders. Psychiatr Med 9:361–375, 1991

Bialer PA, Wallack JJ, McDaniel S: Human immunodeficiency virus and AIDS, in Psychiatric Care of the Medical Patient, 2nd Edition. Edited by Stoudemire A, Fogel B, Greenberg D. New York, Oxford University Press, 2000, pp 871–887

Blackwell B: From compliance to alliance: a quarter century of research. Neth J Med 48:140–149, 1996

Blank MB, Mandell DS, Aiken L, et al: Co-occurrence of HIV and serious mental illness among Medicaid recipients. Psychiatr Serv 53:868–873, 2002

Boccellari A, Dilley JW, Shore MD: Neuropsychiatric aspects of AIDS dementia complex: a report on a clinical series. Neurotoxicology 9:381–390, 1988

Botha KIT: Posttraumatic stress disorder and illness behaviour in HIV+ patients. Psychol Rep 79:843–845, 1996

Brechtl JR, Breitbart W, Galietta M, et al: The use of highly active antiretroviral therapy (HAART) in patients with advanced HIV infection: impact on medical, palliative care, and quality of life outcomes. J Pain Symptom Manage 21:41–51, 2001

Breitbart W, Marotta R, Platt M, et al: A double-blind trial of haloperidol, chlorpromazine and lorazepam in the treatment of delirium in hospitalized AIDS patients. Am J Psychiatry 153:231–237, 1996

Breitbart W, McDonald MV, Rosenfeld B, et al: Fatigue in ambulatory AIDS patients. J Pain Symptom Manage 15:159–167, 1998

Breitbart W, Rosenfeld B, Kaim M, et al: A randomized, double-blind, placebo-controlled trial of psychostimulants for the treatment of fatigue in ambulatory patients with human immunodeficiency virus disease. Arch Intern Med 161:411–420, 2001

Brew BJ: AIDS dementia complex, in HIV Neurology (Contemporary Neurology Series, Vol 61). Edited by Brew B. New York, Oxford University Press, 2001, pp 62–81

Brew BJ, Pemberton L, Cunningham P, et al: Levels of human immunodeficiency virus type 1 RNA in cerebrospinal fluid correlate with AIDS dementia stage. J Infect Dis 175:963–966, 1997

Brew BJ, Brown SJ, Catalan J, et al: Phase III, randomized, double-blind, placebo-controlled, multicentre study to evaluate the safety and efficacy of abacavir (ABC, 1592) in HIV-1 infected subjects with AIDS dementia complex (CNA3001), in Abstracts of the 12th World AIDS Conference. Geneva, Switzerland, June 29–July 2, 1998

Broderick DF, Wippold FJ II, Clifford DB, et al: White matter lesions and cerebral atrophy on MR images in patients with and without AIDS dementia complex. Am J Roentgenol 161:177–181, 1993

Brooner RK, Greenfield L, Schmidt CW, et al: Antisocial personality disorder and HIV infection among intravenous drug users. Am J Psychiatry 150:53–58, 1993

Brouillette M-J, Chouinard G, Lalonde R: Didanosine-induced mania in HIV infection (letter). Am J Psychiatry 151:1839–1840, 1994

Brown GR: The use of methylphenidate for cognitive decline associated with HIV disease. Int J Psychiatry 25:21–37, 1995

Budman CL, Vandersall TA: Clonazepam treatment of acute mania in an AIDS patient. J Clin Psychiatry 51:212, 1990

Buhrich N, Cooper DA: Requests for psychiatric consultation concerning 22 patients with AIDS and ARC. Aust N Z J Psychiatry 21:346–353, 1987

Buhrich N, Cooper DA, Freed E: HIV infection associated with symptoms indistinguishable from functional psychosis. Br J Psychiatry 152:649–653, 1988

Carmen E, Brady SM: AIDS risk and prevention in the chronic mentally ill. Hosp Community Psychiatry 41:652–657, 1990

Catz SL, Kelly JA, Bogart LM, et al: Patterns, correlates and barriers to medication adherence among persons prescribed new treatments for HIV disease. Health Psychol 19:124–133, 2000

Centers for Disease Control and Prevention: HIV/AIDS Surveillance Report, 2001. Available at: http://www.cdc.gov. Accessed March 2004

Cerngul I, Jones K, Ernst J: S-Adenosylmethionine (SAM-e) in the treatment of depressive disorders in HIV-positive individuals: interim results. AMFAR 13th International HIV/AIDS Update Conference, San Francisco, CA, March 20–23, 2001

Chang L, Ernst T, Leonido-Yee M, et al: Cerebral metabolite abnormalities correlate with clinical severity of HIV-1 cognitive motor complex. Neurology 52:100–108, 1999

Chang L, Speck O, Miller E, et al: Neural correlates of attention and working memory deficits in HIV patients. Neurology 57:1001–1007, 2001

Chesney MA, Folkman S, Chambers D: Coping effectiveness training for men living with HIV: preliminary findings. Int J STD AIDS 7:75–82, 1996

Chesney MA, Ickovics JR, Chambers DB, et al: Self-reported adherence to antiretroviral medications among participants in HIV clinical trials: the AACTG adherence instruments. AIDS Care 12:255–266, 2000

Chiesi A, Agresti MG, Dally LG, et al: Decrease in notifications of AIDS dementia complex in 1989–1990 in Italy: possible role of the early treatment with zidovudine. Medicina (Firenze) 10:415–416, 1990

Chiesi A, Vella S, Dally LG, et al: Epidemiology of AIDS dementia complex in Europe. AIDS in Europe Study Group. J Acquir Immune Defic Syndr Hum Retrovirol 11:39–44, 1996

Childs EA, Lyles RH, Selnes OA, et al: Plasma viral load and CD4 lymphocytes predict HIV-associated dementia and sensory neuropathy. Neurology 52:607–613, 1999

Ciesla JA, Roberts JE: Meta-analysis of the relationship between HIV infection and risk for depressive disorders. Am J Psychiatry 158:725–730, 2001

Clifford DB: Human immunodeficiency virus-associated dementia. Arch Neurol 57:321–324, 2000

Cordova MJ, Andrykowski MA, Kenady DE, et al: Frequency and correlates of posttraumatic-stress-disorder-like symptoms after treatment for breast cancer. J Consult Clin Psychol 63:981–986, 1995

Cornelisse PGA, Montessori V, Yip B, et al: The impact of zidovudine on dementia-free survival in a population of HIV-positive men and women on antiretroviral therapy. Int J STD AIDS 11:52–56, 2000

Cottler LB, Nishith P, Compton WM III: Gender differences in risk factors for trauma exposure and post-traumatic stress disorder among inner-city drug abusers in and out of treatment. Compr Psychiatry 42:111–117, 2001

Cournos F, Empfield M, Horwath E, et al: HIV seroprevalence among patients admitted to two psychiatric hospitals. Am J Psychiatry 48:1225–1230, 1991

Cournos F, Guido JR, Coomaraswamy S, et al: Sexual activity and risk of HIV infection among patients with schizophrenia. Am J Psychiatry 151:228–232, 1994

Cozza KL, Swanton EJ, Humphreys CW: Hepatotoxicity with combination of valproic acid, ritonavir, and nevirapine: a case report. Psychosomatics 41:452–453, 2000

Crocker KS: Gastrointestinal manifestations of the acquired immunodeficiency syndrome. Nurs Clin North Am 24:395–406, 1989

Czub S, Koutsilieri E, Sopper S, et al: Enhancement of CNS pathology in early simian immunodeficiency virus infection by dopaminergic drugs. Acta Neuropathol 101:85–91, 2001

Dal Pan GJ, McArthur JH, Aylward E, et al: Patterns of cerebral atrophy in HIV-1-infected individuals: results of a quantitative MRI analysis. Neurology 42:2125–2130, 1992

The Dana Consortium on the Therapy of HIV Dementia and Related Cognitive Disorders: A randomized, double-blind, placebo-controlled trial of deprenyl and thioctic acid in HIV-associated cognitive impairment. Neurology 50:645–651, 1998

The Dana Consortium on the Therapy of HIV Dementia and Related Cognitive Disorders: Safety and tolerability of the antioxidant OPC-14,117 in HIV associated cognitive impairment. Neurology 49:142–146, 1999

Darko DF, McCutchan JA, Kripke DF, et al: Fatigue, sleep disturbance, disability and indices of progression of HIV infection. Am J Psychiatry 149:514–520, 1992

Davis HF, Skolasky RL Jr, Selnes OA, et al: Assessing HIV-associated dementia: modified HIV Dementia Scale versus the grooved pegboard. AIDS Reader 12:29–31, 38, 2002

de Souza CT, Diaz T, Sutmoller F, et al: The association of socioeconomic status and use of crack/cocaine with unprotected anal sex in a cohort of men who have sex with men in Rio de Janeiro, Brazil. J Acquir Immune Defic Syndr 29:95–100, 2002

Dettling M, Muller-Oerlinghausen B, Britsch P: Clozapine treatment of HIV-associated psychosis: too much bone marrow toxicity? Pharmacopsychiatry 31:156–157, 1998

Dilley JW, Ochitill HN, Perl M, et al: Findings in psychiatric consultations with patients with acquired immune deficiency syndrome. Am J Psychiatry 142:82–86, 1985

Dilley JW, Woods WJ, Sabatino J, et al: Changing sexual behavior among gay male repeat testers for HIV: a randomized, controlled trial of a single-session intervention. J Acquir Immune Defic Syndr 30:177–186, 2002

Dimatteo MR, Lepper HS, Croghan TW: Depression is a risk factor for noncompliance with medical treatment. Arch Intern Med 160:2101–2107, 2000

Dinwiddie SH, Cottler L, Compton W, et al: Psychopathology and HIV risk behaviors among injection drug users in and out of treatment. Drug Alcohol Depend 43:1–11, 1996

Dobs A, Few W III, Blackman M, et al: Serum hormones in men with human immunodeficiency virus associated wasting. J Clin Endocrinol Metab 81:4108–4112, 1996

Dore GJ, Correll PK, Li Y, et al: Changes to AIDS dementia complex in the era of highly active antiretroviral therapy. AIDS 13:1249–1253, 1999

Dunlop O, Bjørklund R, Bruun JN, et al: Early psychomotor slowing predicts the development of HIV dementia and autopsy-verified HIV encephalitis. Acta Neurol Scand 105:270–275, 2002

Duran S, Spire B, Raffi F, et al: Self-reported symptoms after initiation of a protease inhibitor in HIV-infected patients and their impact on adherence to HAART. HIV Clin Trials 2:38–45, 2001

Edelstein H, Knight RT: Severe parkinsonism in two AIDS patients taking prochlorperazine. Lancet 2(8554):341–342, 1987

Edlin BR, Irwin KL, Faruque S, et al: Multicenter Crack Cocaine and HIV Infection Study Team. Intersecting epidemics: crack cocaine use and HIV infection among inner-city young adults. N Engl J Med 331:1422–1427, 1994

Eldred LJ, Wu AW, Chaisson RE, et al: Adherence to antiretroviral and pneumocystis prophylaxis in HIV disease. J Acquir Immune Defic Syndr Hum Retrovirol 18:117–125, 1998

Ellen SR, Judd FK, Mijch AM, et al: Secondary mania in patients with HIV infection. Aust N Z J Psychiatry 33:353–360, 1999

Elliott AJ, Roy-Byrne PP: Mirtazapine for depression in patients with human immunodeficiency virus (letter). J Clin Psychopharmacol 20:265–267, 2000

Elliott AJ, Uldall KK, Bergam K, et al: Randomized, placebo-controlled trial of paroxetine versus imipramine in depressed HIV-positive outpatients. Am J Psychiatry 155:367–372, 1998

Elliott AJ, Russo J, Bergam K, et al: Antidepressant efficacy in HIV-seropositive outpatients with major depressive disorder: an open trial of nefazodone. J Clin Psychiatry 60:226–231, 1999

Empfield M, Cournos F, Meyer I, et al: HIV seroprevalence among homeless patients admitted to a psychiatric inpatient unit. Am J Psychiatry 150:47–52, 1993

Erbelding EJ, Stanton D, Quinn TC, et al: Behavioral and biologic evidence of persistent high-risk behavior in an HIV primary care population. AIDS 14:297–301, 2000

Ernst T, Chang L, Jovicich J, et al: Abnormal brain activation on functional MRI in cognitively asymptomatic HIV patients. Neurology 59:1343–1349, 2002

Evans DL, Leserman J, Perkins DO, et al: Severe life stress as a predictor of early disease progression in HIV infection. Am J Psychiatry 154:630–634, 1997

Fauerbach JA, Lawrence J, Haythornthwaite J, et al: Preburn psychiatric history affects post-trauma morbidity. Psychosomatics 38:374–385, 1997

Fawcett J: Suicide risk factors in depressive disorders and in panic disorder. J Clin Psychiatry 53 (suppl):93–95, 1992

Fernandez F, Levy JK: The use of molindone in the treatment of psychotic and delirious patients infected with the human immunodeficiency virus: case reports. Gen Hosp Psychiatry 15:31–35, 1993

Fernandez F, Levy J: Efficacy of venlafaxine in HIV-depressive disorders. Psychosomatics 38:173–174, 1997

Fernandez F, Levy JK, Mansell PW: Management of delirium in terminally ill AIDS patients. Int J Psychiatry Med 19:165–172, 1989

Fernandez F, Levy JK, Samley HR, et al: Effects of methylphenidate in HIV-related depression: a comparative trial with desipramine. Int J Psychiatry Med 25:53–67, 1995

Ferrando S, Wapenyi K: Psychopharmacological treatment of patients with HIV and AIDS. Psychiatr Q 73:33–49, 2002

Ferrando SJ, Goldman JG, Charness W: SSRI treatment of depression in symptomatic HIV infection and AIDS: improvements in affective and somatic symptoms. Gen Hosp Psychiatry 19:89–97, 1997

Ferrando S, Evans S, Goggin K, et al: Fatigue in HIV illness: relationship to depression, physical limitations, and disability. Psychosom Med 60:759–764, 1998a

Ferrando S, van Gorp W, McElhiney M, et al: Highly active antiretroviral treatment in HIV infection: benefits for neuropsychological function. AIDS 12 (suppl):F65–F70, 1998b

Ferrando SJ, Rabkin JG, de Moore G, et al: Antidepressant treatment of depression in HIV+ women. J Clin Psychiatry 60:741–746, 1999

Ferrarese C, Riva R, Dolara A, et al: Elevated glutamate in cerebrospinal fluid of patients with HIV dementia (letter). JAMA 277:630, 1997

Ferrarese C, Aliprandi A, Tremolizzo L, et al: Increased glutamate in CSF and plasma of patients with HIV dementia. Neurology 57:671–675, 2001

Fichtner CG, Braun BG: Bupropion-associated mania in a patient with HIV infection (letter). J Clin Psychopharmacol 12:366–367, 1992

Fischl MA, Daikos GL, Uttamchandani RB, et al: The efficacy of azidothymidine (AZT) in the treatment of patients with AIDS and AIDS-related complex. N Engl J Med 317:185–191, 1987

Gabel RM, Barnard M, Norko M, et al: AIDS presenting as mania. Compr Psychiatry 27:251–254, 1986

Gallo P, Piccinno MG, Krzalic L, et al: Tumor necrosis factor alpha (TNF alpha) and neurological diseases: failure in detecting TNF alpha in the cerebrospinal fluid from patients with multiple sclerosis, AIDS dementia complex, and brain tumours. J Neuroimmunol 23:41–44, 1989

Giesen HJV, Hefter H, Jablonowski H, et al: HAART is neuroprophylactic in HIV-1 infection. J Acquir Immune Defic Syndr 23:380–385, 2000

Gifford AL, Bormann JE, Shively MJ, et al: Predictors of self-reported adherence and plasma HIV concentrations in patients on multidrug antiretroviral regimens. J Acquir Immune Defic Syndr 23:386–395, 2000

Golding M, Perkins DO: Personality disorder in HIV infection. Int Rev Psychiatry 8:253–258, 1996

Gourevitch MN, Friedland GH: Interactions between methadone and medications used to treat HIV infection: a review. Mt Sinai J Med 67:429–436, 2000

Grassi L: Risk of HIV infection in psychiatrically ill patients. AIDS Care 8:103–116, 1996

Grassi MP, Clerici F, Boldorini R, et al: HIV encephalitis and HIV leukoencephalopathy are associated with distinct clinical and radiological subtypes of the AIDS dementia complex. AIDS 11:690–691, 1997

Gray R: Antipsychotics, side effects and effective management. Mental Health Practice 2:14–20, 1999

Gray R, Brewin E, Noak J, et al: A review of the literature on HIV infection and schizophrenia: implications for research, policy and clinical practice. J Psychiatr Ment Health Nurs 9:405–409, 2002

Grinspoon S, Anderson C, Schoenfeld D, et al: Long-term effects of androgen administration in men with AIDS wasting (32176). Geneva, Switzerland, World AIDS Conference, June 1998

Halman M, Rourke SB: HAART and neuropsychological impairment: neuroscience in HIV infection, Edinburgh 22–24 June 2000 (abstract 03). J Neurovirol 6:246, 2000

Halman MM, Worth JL, Sanders KM, et al: Anticonvulsant use in the treatment of manic syndromes in patients with HIV-1 infection. J Clin Neuropsychiatry Clin Neurosci 5:430–434, 1993

Handelsman L, Aronson M, Maurer G, et al: Neuropsychological and neurological manifestations of HIV-1 dementia in drug users. J Neuropsychiatry Clin Neurosci 4:21–28, 1992

Harris GJ, Pearlson GD, McArthur JC, et al: Altered cortical blood flow in HIV-seropositive individuals with and without dementia: a single photon emission computed tomography study. AIDS 8:495–499, 1994

Harris M, Jeste D, Gleghorn A, et al: New-onset psychosis in HIV-infected patients. J Clin Psychiatry 52:369–376, 1991

Hartgers C, Van Den Hoek JAR, Coutinho RA, et al: Psychopathology, stress and HIV-risk injecting behaviour among drug users. Br J Addict 87:857–865, 1992

Hawkins CP, McLaughlin JE, Kendall BE, et al: Pathological findings correlated with MRI in HIV infection. Neuroradiology 35:264–268, 1993

Haynes RB: Determinants of compliance: the disease and the mechanics of treatment, in Compliance in Health Care. Edited by Haynes RB, Taylor DW, Sackett DL. Baltimore, MD, Johns Hopkins University Press, 1979, pp 46–62

He H, McCoy HV, Stevens SJ, et al: Violence and HIV sexual risk behaviors among female sex partners of male drug users. Women Health 27:161–175, 1998

Heseltine PNR, Goodkin K, Atkinson JH, et al: Randomized double-blind placebo-controlled trial of peptide T for HIV-associated cognitive impairment. Arch Neurol 55:41–51, 1998

Hinkin CH, Castellon SA, Hardy DJ, et al: Methylphenidate improves HIV-1-associated cognitive slowing. J Neuropsychiatry Clin Neurosci 13:248–254, 2001

Hoff RA, Beam-Goulet J, Rosenheck RA: Mental disorder as a risk factor for human immunodeficiency virus infection in a sample of veterans. J Nerv Ment Dis 185:556–560, 1997

Hoffman RS: Neuropsychiatric complications of AIDS. Psychosomatics 25:393–400, 1984

Holland NR, Power C, Mathews VP, et al: Cytomegalovirus encephalitis in acquired immunodeficiency syndrome (AIDS). Neurology 44:507–514, 1994

Hollander H, Golden J, Mendelson T, et al: Extrapyramidal symptoms in AIDS patients given low-dose metoclopramide or chlorpromazine (letter). Lancet 2(8465):1186, 1985

Holmes J, House A: Psychiatric illness predicts poor outcome after surgery for hip fracture: a prospective cohort study. Psychol Med 30:921–929, 2000

Holmes VF, Ficchione GL: Hypomania in an AIDS patient receiving amitriptyline for neuropathic pain. Neurology 39:305, 1989

Holmes VF, Fernandez F, Levy JK: Psychostimulant response in AIDS-related complex patients. J Clin Psychiatry 50:5–8, 1989

Hoover DR, Saah AJ, Bacellar H, et al: Signs and symptoms of "asymptomatic" HIV-1 infection in homosexual men. J Acquir Immune Defic Syndr 6:66–71, 1993

Hriso E, Kuhn T, Masdeu JC, et al: Extrapyramidal symptoms due to dopamine-blocking agents in patients with AIDS encephalopathy. Am J Psychiatry 148:1558–1561, 1991

Hudgins R, McCusker J, Stoddard A: Cocaine use and risky injection and sexual behaviors. Drug Alcohol Depend 37:7–14, 1995

Hutton HE, Treisman GJ, Hunt WR, et al: HIV risk behaviors and their relationship to posttraumatic stress disorder among women prisoners. Psychiatr Serv 52:508–513, 2001

Ickovics JR, Hamburger ME, Vlahov D, et al: Mortality, CD4 cell count decline, and depressive symptoms among HIV-seropositive women: longitudinal analysis from the HIV epidemiology research study. JAMA 285:1466–1474, 2001

Itoh K, Mehraein P, Weis S: Neuronal damage of the substantia nigra in HIV-1 infected brains. Acta Neuropathol (Berl) 99:376–384, 2000

Jacobs P, Bobek SC: Sexual needs of the schizophrenic client. Perspect Psychiatr Care 27:15–20, 1991

Jacobsberg L, Frances A, Perry S: Axis II diagnoses among volunteers for HIV testing and counseling. Am J Psychiatry 152:1222–1224, 1995

Jarvik JG, Hesselink JR, Kennedy C, et al: Acquired immunodeficiency syndrome: magnetic resonance patterns of brain involvement with pathologic correlation. Arch Neurol 45:731–736, 1988

Jennings HR, Romanelli F: The use of valproic acid in HIV-positive patients. Ann Pharmacol 33:1113–1116, 1999

Johannessen DJ, Wilson LG: Mania with cryptococcal meningitis in two AIDS patients. J Clin Psychiatry 49:200–201, 1988

Johnson JG, Williams JBW, Rabkin JG, et al: Axis I psychiatric symptomatology associated with HIV infection and personality disorder. Am J Psychiatry 152:551–554, 1995

Johnson WD, Hedges LV, Ramirez G, et al: HIV prevention research for men who have sex with men: a systematic review and meta-analysis. J Acquir Immune Defic Syndr 30 (suppl 1): S118–S129, 2002

Kalayjian RC, Cohen ML, Bonomo RA, et al: Cytomegalovirus ventriculoencephalitis in AIDS: a syndrome with distinct clinical and pathologic features. Medicine (Baltimore) 72:67–77, 1993

Kalichman SC, Sikkema KJ, Kelly JA, et al: Factors associated with risk for HIV infection among chronic mentally ill adults. Am J Psychiatry 15:221–227, 1994

Kalichman SC, Sikkema KJ, Kelly JA, et al: Use of a brief behavioral skills intervention to prevent HIV infection among chronic mentally ill adults. Psychiatr Serv 46:275–280, 1995

Kalichman SC, Heckkman T, Kelly JA: Sensation-seeking as an explanation for the association between substance use and HIV-related risky sexual behavior. Arch Sex Behav 25:141–154, 1996

Kelly B, Raphael B, Judd F, et al: Posttraumatic stress disorder in response to HIV infection. Gen Hosp Psychiatry 20:345–352, 1998

Kelly J: Group psychotherapy for persons with HIV and AIDS-related illnesses. Int J Group Psychother 98:143–162, 1998

Kelly JA, Murphy DA, Bahn GR, et al: AIDS/HIV risk behaviour among the chronic mentally ill. Am J Psychiatry 149:886–889, 1992

Kermani EJ, Borod JC, Brown PH, et al: New psychopathologic findings in AIDS: case report. J Clin Psychiatry 46:240–241, 1985

Kessler RC, Sonega A, Bromer E: Posttraumatic stress disorder in the national comorbidity survey. Arch Gen Psychiatry 52:1048–1060, 1995

Kibayashi K, Mastri AR, Hirsch CS: Neuropathology of human immunodeficiency virus infection at different disease stages. Hum Pathol 27:637–642, 1996

Kieburtz KD, Epstein LG, Gelbard HA, et al: Excitotoxicity and dopaminergic dysfunction in the acquired immunodeficiency syndrome dementia complex: therapeutic implications. Arch Neurol 48:1281–1284, 1991a

Kieburtz K, Zettelmaier AE, Ketonen L, et al: Manic syndromes in AIDS. Am J Psychiatry 148:1068–1070, 1991b

Kimerling R, Calhoun KS, Forehand R, et al: Traumatic stress in HIV-infected women. AIDS Educ Prev 11:321–330, 1999

Kirkland LR, Fischl MA, Tashima KT, et al: Response to lamivudine-zidovudine plus abacavir twice daily in antiretroviral-naive, incarcerated patients with HIV infection taking directly observed treatment. Clin Infect Dis 34:511–518, 2002

Kleeberger CA, Phair JP, Strathdee SA, et al: Determinants of heterogeneous adherence to HIV-antiretroviral therapies in the Multicenter AIDS Cohort Study. J Acquir Immune Defic Syndr 26:82–92, 2001

Kleinman PH, Millman RB, Robinson H, et al: Lifetime needle sharing: a predictive analysis. J Subst Abuse Treat 11:449–455, 1994

Kohl KD, Wendell D, Farley T: Sexual risk behavior in men who have sex with men: statewide gay bar survey, Louisiana, 1995–1998 (abstract no. 335). Atlanta, GA, National HIV Prevention Conference, August 1999

Kopicko JJ, Momodu I, Adedokun A, et al: Characteristics of HIV-infected men with low serum testosterone levels. Int J STD AIDS 10:817–820, 1999

Koutsilieri E, Sopper S, Scheller C, et al: Parkinsonism in HIV dementia. J Neural Transm 109:767–775, 2002

Krauthammer C, Klerman GL: Secondary mania: manic syndromes associated with antecedent physical illness or drugs. Arch Gen Psychiatry 35:1333–1339, 1978

Krikorian R, Wrobel AJ, Meinecke C, et al: Cognitive deficits associated with human immunodeficiency virus encephalopathy. J Neuropsychiatry Clin Neurosci 2:256–260, 1990

Kruse W, Eggert-Kruse W, Rampmaier J, et al: Dosage frequency and drug-compliance behavior: a comparative study on compliance with a medication to be taken twice or four times daily. Eur J Clin Pharmacol 41:589–592, 1991

Laudat A, Blum L, Guechot J, et al: Changes in systemic gonadal and adrenal steroids in symptomatic human immunodeficiency virus infected men: relationship with CD4 cell counts. Eur J Endocrinol 133:418–424, 1995

Laverda AM, Gallo P, De Rossi A, et al: Cerebrospinal fluid analysis in HIV-1-infected children: immunological and virological findings before and after AZT therapy. Acta Paediatr 83:1038–1042, 1994

Lechner SC, Antoni MH, Lydston D, et al: Cognitive-behavioral interventions improve quality of life in women with AIDS. J Psychosom Res 54:253–261, 2003

Lee R, Monteiro EF: Third regional audit of antiretroviral prescribing in HIV patients. International Journal of Studies in AIDS 14:58–60, 2003

Lenz G, Demal U: Quality of life in depression and anxiety disorders: an exploratory follow-up after intensive cognitive-behavior therapy. Psychopathology 33:297–302, 2000

Lera G, Zirulnik J: Pilot study with clozapine in patients with HIV-associated psychosis and drug-induced parkinsonism. Mov Disord 14:128–131, 1999

Leserman J, Petitto JM, Golden RN, et al: Impact of stressful life events, depression, social support, coping, and cortisol on progression to AIDS. Am J Psychiatry 157:1221–1228, 2000

Letendre S, Ellis R, Rippeth J, et al: Reduction of HIV RNA levels correlates with reversal of HIV-induced cognitive dysfunction: neuroscience in HIV infection. Edinburgh 22–24 June 2000 (abstract 04). J Neurovirol 6:246, 2000

Liu H, Golin CE, Miller LG, et al: A comparison study of multiple measures of adherence to HIV protease inhibitors. Ann Intern Med 134:968–977, 2001

Longo MB, Spross JA, Locke AM: Identifying major concerns of persons with acquired immunodeficiency syndrome: a replication. Clin Nurse Spec 4:21–26, 1990

Lopez OL, Smith G, Meltzer CC, et al: Dopamine systems in human immunodeficiency virus-associated dementia. Neuropsychiatry Neuropsychol Behav Neurol 12:184–192, 1999

Lopez-Villegas D, Lenkinski RE, Frank I: Biochemical changes in the frontal lobe of HIV-infected individuals detected by magnetic resonance spectroscopy. Proc Natl Acad Sci U S A 94:9854–9859, 1997

Louhivuori KA, Hakama M: Risk of suicide among cancer patients. Am J Epidemiol 109:50–65, 1979

Lucas GM, Chaisson RE, Moore RD: Highly active antiretroviral therapy in a large urban clinic: risk factors for virologic failure and adverse drug reactions. Ann Intern Med 131:81–87, 1999

Luft BJ, Hafner R, Korzun AH, et al: Toxoplasmic encephalitis in patients with the acquired immunodeficiency syndrome. N Engl J Med 329:995–1000, 1993

Lutgendorf S, Antoni MH, Ironson G, et al: Cognitive-behavioral stress management decreases dysphoric mood and herpes simplex virus-type 2 antibody titers in symptomatic HIV-seropositive gay men. J Consult Clin Psychol 65:31–43, 1997a

Lutgendorf SK, Antoni MH, Ironson G, et al: Cognitive processing style, mood, and immune function following HIV seropositivity notification. Cognit Ther Res 21:157–184, 1997b

Lyketsos CG, Federman EB: Psychiatric disorders and HIV infection: impact on one another. Epidemiol Rev 17:152–164, 1995

Lyketsos CG, Hoover DR, Guccione M, et al: Depressive symptoms as predictors of medical outcomes in HIV infection. Multicenter AIDS Cohort Study. JAMA 270:2563–2567, 1993a

Lyketsos CG, Hanson AL, Fishman M, et al: Manic syndrome early and late in the course of HIV. Am J Psychiatry 150:326–327, 1993b

Lyketsos CG, Hanson A, Fishman M, et al: Screening for psychiatric morbidity in a medical outpatient clinic for HIV infection: the need for a psychiatric presence. Int J Psychiatry Med 24:103–113, 1994

Lyketsos CG, Hoover DR, Guccione M, et al: Changes in depressive symptoms as AIDS develops. Am J Psychiatry 153:1430–1437, 1996a

Lyketsos CG, Hutton H, Fishman M, et al: Psychiatric morbidity on entry to an HIV primary care clinic. AIDS 10:1033–1039, 1996b

Lyketsos CG, Schwartz J, Fishman M, et al: AIDS mania. J Neuropsychiatry Clin Neurosci 9:277–279, 1997

Maggi JD, Halman MH: The effect of divalproex sodium on viral load: a retrospective review of HIV-positive patients with manic syndromes. Can J Psychiatry 46:359–362, 2001

Maggi P, de Mari M, Moramarco A, et al: Parkinsonism in a patient with AIDS and cerebral opportunistic granulomatous lesions. Neurol Sci 21:173–176, 2000

Magnuson DS, Knudsen BE, Geiger JD, et al: Human immunodeficiency virus type 1 tat activates non-N-methyl-D-aspartate excitatory amino acid receptors and causes neurotoxicity. Ann Neurol 37:373–380, 1995

Maj M: Psychiatric aspects of HIV-1 infection and AIDS. Psychol Med 20:547–563, 1990

Maj M, Satz P, Janssen R, et al: WHO Neuropsychiatric AIDS Study, cross-sectional phase II: neuropsychological and neurological findings. Arch Gen Psychiatry 51:51–61, 1994

Manning D, Jacobsberg L, Erhart S, et al: The efficacy of imipramine in the treatment of HIV-related depression (abstract no. Th.B.32). International Conference on AIDS, San Francisco, CA, June 20–23, 1990

Markowitz JC, Kocsis JH, Fishman B, et al: Treatment of depressive symptoms in human immunodeficiency virus-positive patients. Arch Gen Psychiatry 55:452–457, 1998

Martinez A, Israelski D, Walker C, et al: Posttraumatic stress disorder in women attending human immunodeficiency virus outpatient clinics. AIDS Patient Care STDS 16:283–291, 2002

Martinez E, Garcia-Viejo MA, Marcos MA, et al: Discontinuation of secondary prophylaxis for cryptococcal meningitis in HIV-infected patients responding to highly active antiretroviral therapy. AIDS 14:2615–2617, 2000

Masand PS, Tesar GE: Use of stimulants in the medically ill. Psychiatr Clin North Am 19:515–547, 1996

Masliah E, De Teresa RM, Mallory RE, et al: Changes in pathological findings at autopsy in AIDS cases for the last 15 years. AIDS 14:69–74, 2000

Mauri MC, Fabiano L, Bravin S, et al: Schizophrenic patients before and after HIV infection: a case-control study. Encephale 23:437–441, 1997

Maxwell S, Scheftner WA, Kessler MA, et al: Manic syndromes associated with zidovudine therapy (letter). JAMA 259:3406–3407, 1988

McArthur JC, Becker PS, Parisi JE, et al: Neuropathological changes in early HIV dementia. Ann Neurol 26:681–684, 1989

McArthur JC, Hoover DR, Bacellar H, et al: Dementia in AIDS patients: incidence and risk factors. Multicenter AIDS Cohort Study. Neurology 43:2245–2252, 1993

McArthur JC, McClernon DR, Cronin MR, et al: Relationship between human immunodeficiency virus-associated dementia and viral load in cerebrospinal fluid and brain. Ann Neurol 42:689–698, 1997

McDermott BE, Sautter FJ, Winstead DK, et al: Diagnosis, health beliefs, and risk of HIV infection in psychiatric patients. Hosp Community Psychiatry 45:580–585, 1994

McKegney FP, O'Dowd MA, Feiner C, et al: A prospective comparison of neuropsychologic function in HIV-seropositive and seronegative methadone-maintained patients. AIDS 4:565–569, 1990

McKinnon K, Cournos F, Sugden R, et al: The relative contributions of psychiatric symptoms and AIDS knowledge to HIV risk behaviors among people with severe mental illness. J Clin Psychiatry 57:506–513, 1996

McNabb J, Ross JW, Abriola K, et al: Adherence to highly active antiretroviral therapy predicts outcome at an inner-city human immunodeficiency virus clinic. Clin Infect Dis 33:700–705, 2001

Meltzer-Brody S, Davidson JR: Completeness of response and quality of life in mood and anxiety disorders. Depress Anxiety 12 (suppl 1):95–101, 2000

Metzger DS, Woody GE, DePhillipis D, et al: Risk factors for needle sharing among methadone patients. Am J Psychiatry 148:636–640, 1991

Metzger DS, Navaline H, Woody GE: Drug abuse treatment as AIDS prevention. Public Health Rep 113 (suppl 1):97–106, 1998

Meyer I, McKinnon K, Cournos F, et al: HIV seroprevalence among long-stay patients in a state psychiatric hospital. Hosp Community Psychiatry 44:282–284, 1993

Meyerhoff DJ, Bloomer C, Cardenas V, et al: Elevated subcortical choline metabolites in cognitively and clinically asymptomatic HIV+ patients. Neurology 52:995–1003, 1999

Miller RG, Carson PJ, Moussavi RS, et al: Fatigue and myalgia in AIDS patients. Neurology 41:1603–1607, 1991

Mintz M, Tardieu M, Hoyt L, et al: Levodopa therapy improves motor function in HIV-infected children with extrapyramidal syndromes. Neurology 47:1583–1585, 1996

Mirsattari SM, Power C, Nath A: Parkinsonism with HIV infection. Mov Disord 13:684–689, 1998

Moog C, Kuntz-Simon G, Caussin-Schwemling C, et al: Sodium valproate, an anticonvulsant drug, stimulates human immunodeficiency virus type 1 replication independently of glutathione levels. J Gen Virol 77:1993–1999, 1996

Morrill AC, Ickovics JR, Golubchikov VV, et al: Safer sex: social and psychological predictors of behavioral maintenance and change among heterosexual women. J Consult Clin Psychol 64:819–828, 1996

Moss AR, Bacchetti P, Osmond D, et al: Seropositive for HIV and the development of AIDS or AIDS related condition: three year follow up of the San Francisco General Hospital cohort. BMJ 296:745–750, 1988

Murphy GE: Suicide and attempted suicide. Hosp Pract 12:78–81, 1977

Muurahainen N, Mulligan K: Clinical trial updates in human immunodeficiency virus wasting. Semin Oncol 25:104–111, 1998

Naber D, Pajonk FG, Perro C, et al: Human immunodeficiency virus antibody test and seroprevalence in psychiatric patients. Acta Psychiatr Scand 89:358–361, 1994

Nath A, Haughey NJ, Jones M, et al: Synergistic neurotoxicity by human immunodeficiency virus proteins tat and gp120: protection by memantine. Ann Neurol 47:186–194, 2000

Nath A, Maragos WF, Avison MJ, et al: Acceleration of HIV dementia with methamphetamine and cocaine. J Neurovirol 7:66–71, 2001

Navia BA, Jordan BD, Price RW: The AIDS dementia complex, I: clinical features. Ann Neurol 19:517–524, 1986

Navia BA, Dafni U, Simpson D, et al (for the AIDS Clinical Trials Group): A phase I/II trial of nimodipine for HIV-related neurologic complications. Neurology 51:221–228, 1998

Nebuloni M, Pellegrinelli A, Ferri A, et al: Beta amyloid precursor protein and patterns of HIV p24 immunohistochemistry in different brain areas of AIDS patients. AIDS 15:571–575, 2001

Nightingale SD, Kosto FT, Mertz CJ, et al: Clarithromycin-induced mania in two patients with AIDS. Clin Infect Dis 20:1563–1564, 1995

Nottet HS, Persidsky Y, Sasseville VG, et al: Mechanisms for the transendothelial migration of HIV-1-infected monocytes into brain. J Immunol 156:1284–1295, 1996

Novotna L, Wilson TE, Minkoff HL, et al: Predictors and risk-taking consequences of drug use among HIV-infected women. J Acquir Immune Defic Syndr Hum Retrovirol 20:502–507, 1999

Nyamathi A: Comparative study of factors relating to HIV risk level of black homeless women. J Acquir Immune Defic Syndr 5:222–228, 1992

O'Dowd MA, McKegney FP: Manic syndrome associated with zidovudine (letter). JAMA 260:3587, 1988

Olsen WL, Longo FM, Mills CM, et al: White matter disease in AIDS: findings at MR imaging. Radiology 169:445–448, 1988

Orr S, Celentano DD, Santelli J, et al: Depressive symptoms and risk factors for HIV acquisition among black women attending urban health centers in Baltimore. AIDS Educ Prev 6:230–236, 1994

Pakesch G, Loimer N, Grunberger J, et al: Neuropsychological findings and psychiatric symptoms in HIV-1 infected and non-infected drug users. Psychiatry Res 41:163–177, 1992

Paterson DL, Swindells S, Mohn J, et al: Adherence to protease inhibitor therapy and outcomes in patients with HIV infection. Ann Intern Med 133:21–30, 2000

Perez-Jimenez JP, Gomez-Bajo GJ, Lopez-Castillo JJ, et al: Psychiatric consultation and post-traumatic stress disorder in burned patients. Burns 20:532–536, 1994

Perkins DO, Davidson EJ, Leserman J, et al: Personality disorder in patients infected with HIV: a controlled study with implications for clinical care. Am J Psychiatry 150:309–315, 1993

Perkins DO, Stern RA, Golden RN, et al: Mood disorders in HIV infection: prevalence and risk factors in a nonepicenter of the AIDS epidemic. Am J Psychiatry 151:233–236, 1994

Perkins DO, Leserman J, Stern RA, et al: Somatic symptoms and HIV infection: relationship to depressive symptoms and indicators of HIV disease. Am J Psychiatry 152:1776–1781, 1995

Perry S, Jacobsen P: Neuropsychiatric manifestations of AIDS-spectrum disorders. Hosp Community Psychiatry 37:135–142, 1986

Perry S, Jacobsberg LD, Fishman B, et al: Psychiatric diagnosis before serological testing for the human immunodeficiency virus. Am J Psychiatry 147:89–93, 1990

Peterson PK, Gekker G, Chao CC, et al: Cocaine potentiates HIV-1 replication in human peripheral blood mononuclear cell cocultures: involvement of transforming growth factor-beta. J Immunol 146:81–84, 1991

Pickles RW, Spelman DW: Suspected ethambutol-induced mania. Med J Aust 164:445–446, 1996

Portegies P: AIDS dementia complex: a review. J Acquir Immune Defic Syndr Hum Retrovirol 7:S48–S49, 1994

Portegies P, De Gans J, Lange JM, et al: Declining incidence of AIDS dementia complex after introduction of zidovudine treatment. BMJ 299:819–821, 1989 (published erratum appears in BMJ 299:1141, 1989)

Portenoy R, Miransky J, Thaler HT, et al: Pain in ambulatory patients with lung or colon cancer: prevalence, characteristics, and impact. Cancer 70:1616–1624, 1992

Portenoy RK, Thaler HT, Kornblith AB, et al: The Memorial Symptom Assessment Scale: an instrument for the evaluation of symptom prevalence, characteristics and distress. Eur J Cancer 30A:1326–1336, 1994

Post MJD, Levin BE, Berger JR, et al: Sequential cranial MR findings of asymptomatic and neurologically symptomatic HIV+ subjects. Am J Neuroradiol 13:359–370, 1992

Price RW, Brew BJ: The AIDS dementia complex. J Infect Dis 158:1079–1083, 1988

Price RW, Yiannoutsos CT, Cliffort DB, et al: Neurological outcomes in late HIV infection: adverse impact of neurological impairment on survival and protective effect of antiviral therapy. AIDS 13:1677–1685, 1999

Pugh K, O'Donnell I, Catalan J: Suicide and HIV disease. AIDS Care 4:391–400, 1993

Rabkin JG, Remien R, Katoff L, et al: Suicidality in AIDS long-term survivors: what is the evidence? AIDS Care 5:401–411, 1993

Rabkin JG, Rabkin R, Harrison W, et al: Effect of imipramine on mood and enumerative measures of immune status in depressed patients with HIV illness. Am J Psychiatry 151:516–523, 1994a

Rabkin JG, Rabkin R, Wagner G: Effects of fluoxetine on mood and immune status in depressed patients with HIV illness. J Clin Psychiatry 55:92–97, 1994b

Rabkin JG, Wagner GJ, Rabkin R: Fluoxetine treatment for depression in patients with HIV and AIDS: a randomized, placebo-controlled trial. Am J Psychiatry 156:101–107, 1999a

Rabkin JG, Wagner GJ, Rabkin R: Testosterone therapy for human immunodeficiency virus-positive men with and without hypogonadism. J Clin Psychopharmacol 19:19–27, 1999b

Rabkin JG, Ferrando SJ, Wagner G, et al: DHEA treatment of men and women with HIV infection. Psychoneuroendocrinology 25:53–68, 2000a

Rabkin JG, Wagner GJ, Rabkin R: A double-blind, placebo-controlled trial of testosterone therapy for HIV-positive men with hypogonadal symptoms. Arch Gen Psychiatry 57:141–147, 2000b

RachBeisel JA, Weintraub E: Valproic acid treatment of AIDS-related mania. J Clin Psychiatry 58:406–407, 1997

Rees V, Saitz R, Horton NJ, et al: Association of alcohol consumption with HIV sex- and drug-risk behaviors among drug users. J Subst Abuse Treat 21:129–134, 2001

Regier DA, Farmer ME, Rae DS, et al: Comorbidity of mental disorders with alcohol and other drug abuse. JAMA 264:2511–2518, 1990

Revicki DA, Brown RE, Henry DH, et al: Recombinant human erythropoietin and health-related quality of life of AIDS patients with anemia. J Acquir Immune Defic Syndr 7:474–484, 1994

Richman DD, Fischl MA, Grieco MH, et al: The toxicity of azidothymidine (AZT) in the treatment of patients with AIDS and AIDS-related complex. N Engl J Med 317:192–197, 1987

Rosci MA, Pignorini F, Bernabei A, et al: Methods for detecting early signs of AIDS dementia complex in asymptomatic subjects: a quantitative tomography study of 18 cases. AIDS 6:1309–1316, 1996

Rottenberg DA, Sidtis JJ, Strother SC, et al: Abnormal cerebral glucose metabolism in HIV-1 seropositive subjects with and without dementia. J Nucl Med 37:1133–1141, 1996

Sacks M, Dermatis H, Looser-Ott S, et al: Undetected HIV infection among acutely ill psychiatric inpatients. Am J Psychiatry 149:544–545, 1992

Sacktor NC, Lyles RH, McFarlane G, et al (for the Multicenter AIDS Cohort Study): The changing incidence of HIV-1 related neurologic diseases (abstract 145), in Abstracts of the 6th Conference on Retroviruses and Opportunistic Infections. Chicago, IL, January 31–February 4, 1999a

Sacktor NC, Lyles RH, McFarlane G, et al: HIV-1-related neurological disease incidence changes in the era of highly active antiretroviral therapy. Neurology 52:A252–A253, 1999b

Sacktor N, Lyles RH, Skolasky R, et al: HIV-associated neurologic disease incidence changes: Multicenter AIDS Cohort Study, 1990–1998. Neurology 56:257–260, 2001

Scamvougeras A, Rosebush PI: AIDS-related psychosis with catatonia responding to low-dose lorazepam. J Clin Psychiatry 53:414–415, 1992

Schifitto G, Sacktor N, Marder K, et al. (for the Neurological AIDS Research Consortium): Randomized, placebo-controlled trial of the PAF antagonist lexipafant in HIV-associated cognitive impairment. Neurology 53:391–396, 1999

Schmidt U, Miller D: Two cases of hypomania in AIDS. Br J Psychiatry 152:839–842, 1988

Schwartz JAJ, McDaniel JS: Double-blind comparison of fluoxetine and desipramine in the treatment of depressed women with advanced HIV disease: a pilot study. Depress Anxiety 9:70–74, 1999

Scurlock H, Singh A, Catalan J: Atypical antipsychotic drugs in the treatment of manic syndromes in patients with HIV-1 infection. J Psychopharmacol 9:151–154, 1995

Sei S, Stewart SK, Farley M, et al: Evaluation of human immunodeficiency virus (HIV) type 1 RNA levels in cerebrospinal fluid and viral resistance to zidovudine in children with HIV encephalopathy. J Infect Dis 174:1200–1206, 1996

Semaan S, Des Jarlais DC, Sogolow E, et al: A meta-analysis of the effect of HIV prevention interventions on the sex behaviors of drug users in the United States. J Acquir Immune Defic Syndr 30 (suppl 1):S73–S93, 2002

Sewell D, Jeste D, Atkinson J, et al: HIV-associated psychosis: a study of 20 cases. Am J Psychiatry 151:237–242, 1994a

Sewell DD, Jeste DV, McAdams LA, et al: Neuroleptic treatment of HIV-associated psychosis. HNRC group. Neuropsychopharmacology 10:223–229, 1994b

Sidtis JJ, Gatsonis C, Price RW, et al (for the AIDS Clinical Trials Group): Zidovudine treatment of the AIDS dementia complex: results of a placebo-controlled trial. Ann Neurol 33:343–349, 1993

Silberstein C, Galanter M, Marmor M, et al: HIV-1 among inner city dually diagnosed inpatients. Am J Drug Alcohol Abuse 20:201–213, 1994

Simon G, Moog C, Obert G: Valproic acid reduces the intracellular level of glutathione and stimulates human immunodeficiency virus. Chem Biol Interact 91:111–121, 1994

Singh A, Golledge H, Catalan J: Treatment of HIV-related psychotic disorders with risperidone: a series of 21 cases. J Psychosom Res 42:489–493, 1997

Singh N, Squier C, Sivek C, et al: Determinants of compliance with antiretroviral therapy in patients with human immunodeficiency virus: prospective assessment with implications for enhancing compliance. AIDS Care 8:261–269, 1996

Smith MY, Egert J, Winkel G, et al: The impact of PTSD on pain experience in persons with HIV/AIDS. Pain 98:9–17, 2002

St. John's wort and HAART. AIDS Patient Care STDS 14:281–283, 2000

Steer RA, Iguchi MY, Platt JJ: Hopelessness in IV drug users not in treatment and seeking HIV testing and counseling. Drug Alcohol Depend 34:99–103, 1994

Stein MD, Hanna L, Natarajan R, et al: Alcohol use patterns predict high-risk HIV behaviors among active injection drug users. J Subst Abuse Treat 18:359–363, 2000

Stiffman AR, Dore P, Earls F, et al: The influence of mental health problems on AIDS-related risk behaviors in young adults. J Nerv Ment Dis 180:314–320, 1992

Stone VE, Clarke J, Lovell J, et al: HIV/AIDS patients' perspectives on adhering to regimens containing protease inhibitors. J Gen Intern Med 13:586–593, 1998

Stout JC, Ellis RJ, Jernigan TL, et al: Progressive cerebral volume loss in human immunodeficiency virus infection: a longitudinal volumetric magnetic resonance imaging study. HIV Neurobehavioral Research Center Group. Arch Neurol 55:161–168, 1998

Suwanwelaa N, Phanuphak P, Phanthumchinda K, et al: Magnetic resonance spectroscopy of the brain in neurologically asymptomatic HIV-infected patients. Magn Reson Imaging 18:859–865, 2000

Tanner WM, Pollack RH: The effect of condom use and erotic instructions on attitudes towards condoms. J Sex Res 25:537–541, 1988

Tanquary J: Lithium-induced neurotoxicity at therapeutic levels in an AIDS patient. J Nerv Ment Dis 181:519–520, 1993

Thurnher MM, Schindler EG, Thurnher SA, et al: Highly active antiretroviral therapy for patients with AIDS dementia complex: effect on MR imaging findings and clinical course. Am J Neuroradiol 21:670–678, 2000

Tourian K, Alterman A, Metzger D, et al: Validity of three measures of antisociality in predicting HIV risk behaviors in methadone-maintenance patients. Drug Alcohol Depend 47:99–107, 1997

Tozzi V, Narciso P, Galgani S, et al: Effects of zidovudine in 30 patients with mild to end-stage AIDS dementia complex. AIDS 7:683–692, 1993

Tozzi V, Balestra P, Galgani S, et al: Positive and sustained effects of highly active anti-retroviral therapy on HIV associated neurocognitive impairment. AIDS 13:1889–1897, 1999

Tozzi V, Balestra P, Galgani S, et al: Changes in neurocognitive performance in a cohort of patients treated with HAART for 3 years. J Acquir Immune Defic Syndr Hum Retrovirol 28:19–27, 2001

Treisman GJ, Fishman M, Schwartz J, et al: Mood disorders in HIV infection. Depress Anxiety 7:178–187, 1998

Trobst KK, Wiggins JS, Costa PT Jr, et al: Personality psychology and problem behaviors: HIV risk and the five-factor model. J Pers 68:1232–1252, 2000

Tyor WR, Glass JD, Griffin JW, et al: Cytokine expression in the brain during the acquired immunodeficiency syndrome. Ann Neurol 31:349–360, 1992

Uldall KK, Berghuis JP: Delirium in AIDS patients: recognition and medication factors. AIDS Patient Care STDS 11:435–441, 1997

Uldall KK, Harris VL, Lalonde B: Outcomes associated with delirium in acutely hospitalized acquired immune deficiency syndrome patients. Compr Psychiatry 41:88–91, 2000a

Uldall KK, Ryan R, Berghuis JP, et al: Association between delirium and death in AIDS patients. AIDS Patient Care STDS 14:95–100, 2000b

UNAIDS Joint United Nations Programme on HIV/AIDS. AIDS Epidemic Update: December 2000. Available at: http://www.thebody.com/unaids/update/contents.html. Accessed March 2004

Vago L, Castagna A, Lazzarin A, et al: Reduced frequency of HIV-induced brain lesions in AIDS patients treated with zidovudine. J Acquir Immune Defic Syndr Hum Retrovirol 6:42–45, 1993

van Driel RC, Op den Velde W: Myocardial infarction and posttraumatic stress disorder. J Trauma Stress 8:151–159, 1995

van Servellen G, Chang B, Garcia L, et al: Individual and system level factors associated with treatment nonadherence in human immunodeficiency virus-infected men and women. AIDS Patient Care STDS 16:269–281, 2002

Vion-Dury J, Nicoli F, Salvan AM, et al: Reversal of brain metabolic alterations with zidovudine detected by proton localized magnetic resonance spectroscopy (letter). Lancet 345:60–61, 1995

Vlahov D, Munow A, Solomon L, et al: Comparison of clinical manifestations of HIV infection between male and female injecting drug users. AIDS 8:819–823, 1994

Vogl D, Rosenfeld B, Breitbart W, et al: Symptom prevalence, characteristics, and distress in AIDS outpatients. J Pain Symptom Manage 18:253–262, 1999

Volavka J, Convit A, Czobor P, et al: HIV seroprevalence and risk behaviours in psychiatric inpatients. Psychiatry Res 39:109–114, 1991

Volavka J, Convit A, O'Donnell J, et al: Assessment of risk behaviors for HIV infection among psychiatric inpatients. Hosp Community Psychiatry 43:482–485, 1992

Wagner GJ, Ghosh-Dastidar B: Electronic monitoring: adherence assessment or intervention? HIV Clin Trials 3:45–51, 2002

Wagner GJ, Rabkin R: Effects of dextroamphetamine on depression and fatigue in men with HIV: a double-blind, placebo-controlled trial. J Clin Psychiatry 61:436–440, 2000

Wagner G, Rabkin J, Rabkin R: Illness stage, concurrent medications, and other correlates of low testosterone in men with HIV illness. J Acquir Immune Defic Syndr Hum Retrovirol 8:204–207, 1995

Wagner GJ, Rabkin JG, Rabkin R: A comparative analysis of standard and alternative antidepressants in the treatment of human immunodeficiency virus patients. Compr Psychiatry 37:402–408, 1996

Wagner GJ, Rabkin JG, Rabkin R: Dextroamphetamine as a treatment for depression and low energy in AIDS patients: a pilot study. J Psychosom Res 42:407–411, 1997

Wagner GJ, Rabkin JG, Rabkin R: Testosterone as a treatment for fatigue in HIV+ men. Gen Hosp Psychiatry 20:209–213, 1998

Wagner GJ, Kanouse DE, Koegel P, et al: Adherence to HIV antiretrovirals among persons with serious mental illness. AIDS Patient Care STDS 17:179–186, 2003

Walkup J, Crystal S, Sambamoorthri U: Schizophrenia and major affective disorder among Medicaid recipients with HIV/AIDS in New Jersey. Am J Public Health 89:1101–1103, 1999

Weinhardt LS, Carey KB: Prevalence of infection with HIV among the seriously mentally ill: review of research and implications for practice. Prof Psychol 26:262–268, 1995

Weissman MM: The epidemiology of personality disorders: a 1990 update. J Personal Disord 7 (suppl):44–62, 1993

Wesselingh SL, Glass J, McArthur JC, et al: Cytokine dysregulation in HIV-associated neurological disease. Adv Neuroimmunol 4:199–206, 1994

White JC, Christensen JF, Singer CM: Methylphenidate as a treatment for depression in acquired immunodeficiency syndrome: an n-of-1 trial. J Clin Psychiatry 53:153–156, 1992

Wiley CA, Masliah E, Morey M, et al: Neocortical damage during HIV infection. Ann Neurol 29:651–657, 1991

Wilkie FL, Eisdorfer C, Morgan R, et al: Cognition in early human immunodeficiency virus infection. Arch Neurol 41:433–440, 1990

Witvrouw M, Schmit JC, Van Remoortel B, et al: Cell type-dependent effect of sodium valproate on human immunodeficiency virus type 1 replication in vitro. AIDS Res Hum Retroviruses 13:87–92, 1997

Woody GE, Gallop R, Luborsky L, et al: HIV risk reduction in the National Institute on Drug Abuse Cocaine Collaborative Treatment Study. J Acquir Immune Defic Syndr 33:82–87, 2003

Wright JM, Sachder PS, Perkins RJ, et al: Zidovudine-related mania. Med J Aust 150:334–341, 1989

Zhang L, Looney D, Taub D, et al: Cocaine opens the blood-brain barrier to HIV-1 invasion. J Neurovirol 4:619–626, 1998

Zilikis N, Nimatoudis I, Kiosses V, et al: Treatment with risperidone of an acute psychotic episode in a patient with AIDS. Gen Hosp Psychiatry 20:384–385, 1998

Zisook S, Peterkin J, Goggin KJ, et al: Treatment of major depression in HIV-seropositive men. J Clin Psychiatry 59:217–224, 1998

29 Dermatology

Lesley M. Arnold, M.D.

PSYCHOCUTANEOUS DISORDERS include dermatological diseases that are affected by psychological factors and psychiatric illnesses in which the skin is the target of disordered thinking, behavior, or perception. Emerging evidence of the role of the nervous system in skin pathophysiology provides clues into possible links between stress and dermatological diseases. In this chapter, I review the pathophysiology of these dermatological diseases, emphasizing the involvement of the central nervous system (CNS), and examine recent developments in the management of psychocutaneous disorders.

Classification

Table 29–1 shows the classification of psychocutaneous disorders in DSM-IV-TR (American Psychiatric Association 2000) categories. Psychological factors affecting medical condition includes dermatological diseases that are commonly affected by psychiatric factors. Somatoform disorders include disorders of the skin that are not fully explained by a known dermatological disease. Delusional disorder, somatic type, is the most common diagnosis in patients with delusional parasitosis, but the differential diagnosis of delusions of parasitosis includes major depressive disorder, bipolar disorder, schizophrenia, psychotic disorder due to a general medical condition, and substance-induced psychotic disorder. A preoccupation with a defect in appearance (body dysmorphic disorder) has a delusional variant, classified as a delusional disorder, somatic type. Trichotillomania is classified under the impulse-control disorders. Psychogenic excoriation and onychophagia are not currently included in DSM-IV-TR but could probably be classified under the category of impulse-control disorder not otherwise specified. Trichotillomania, psychogenic excoriation, and onychophagia frequently have symptoms that overlap with

obsessive-compulsive disorder. Factitious disorders include factitious dermatitis (also called dermatitis artefacta) and psychogenic purpura.

Psychological Factors Affecting Medical Condition

Atopic Dermatitis

Atopic dermatitis, a chronic skin disorder characterized by pruritus and inflammation (eczema), often begins as an erythematous, pruritic, maculopapular eruption (Ehlers et al. 1995; Gil et al. 1987; Lammintausta et al. 1991). Lichenification, excoriations, and infections frequently occur in response to excessive scratching (Gil et al. 1987). Atopic dermatitis typically begins in early infancy, childhood, or adolescence and is frequently associated with a personal or family history of atopic dermatitis, allergic rhinitis, or asthma (Ginsburg et al. 1993). Atopic dermatitis is a common disorder, with a female-to-male ratio of 1.2:1.0 (M.L. Johnson 1977; Rajka 1989). The prevalence of atopic dermatitis has increased to greater than 10% in the past decade, possibly as a result of greater exposure to provocative factors such as outdoor pollution, reagents in highly insulated buildings, house mites, food additives, and increased parental and physician awareness of atopic dermatitis (Leung et al. 1999; Rothe and Grant-Kels 1996; Williams 1992, 1995).

Mild cases of atopic dermatitis may spontaneously resolve, but most patients experience persistent or relapsing symptoms. In one study of 47 patients diagnosed with atopic dermatitis by age 2 years and followed up for 20 years, 72% continued to have signs of atopic dermatitis (Kissling and Wuthrich 1994). In another study, symptoms persisted or recurred in 77%–91% of the adult patients who had moderate or severe symptoms as teenagers

TABLE 29–1.   Classification of psychocutaneous disorders by DSM-IV-TR categories

I. **Psychological factors affecting medical condition**
Atopic dermatitis
Psoriasis
Alopecia areata
Urticaria and angioedema
Acne vulgaris

II. **Somatoform disorders**
Chronic idiopathic pruritus
Idiopathic pruritus ani, vulvae, and scroti
Body dysmorphic disorder

III. **Delusional disorder, somatic type**
Delusional parasitosis
Delusions of a defect in appearance
Delusions of a foul body odor

IV. **Impulse-control disorders**
Psychogenic excoriation
Trichotillomania
Onychophagia

V. **Factitious disorders**
Factitious dermatitis (dermatitis artefacta)
Psychogenic purpura

(Lammintausta et al. 1991). In general, comorbid asthma or allergic rhinitis, early age at onset, severe dermatitis, female sex, and a family history of Alzheimer's disease positively correlate with disease chronicity (Leung et al. 1999).

Although genetic factors are probably involved in the pathophysiology of atopic dermatitis (Schultz Larson 1993; Uehara and Kimura 1993), environmental factors frequently trigger or exacerbate the disease (Ehlers et al. 1995). Environmental triggers include food allergy or intolerance, contact irritants and allergens, aeroallergens (house dust mite, pollen, molds, human and animal dander), microbial organisms, hormones, climate, sweating, and stress (Morren et al. 1994). Affected patients seem to have a lower response threshold and more prolonged reaction than control subjects to pruritic stimuli (Morren et al. 1994). A vicious cycle of itching, scratching, and lesion aggravation frequently develops and contributes to symptom chronicity (Gil et al. 1987; Gupta and Gupta 1996; Morren et al. 1994).

Stressful life events often precede the onset or exacerbation of atopic dermatitis (Kodama et al. 1999; Morren et al. 1994; Picardi and Abeni 2001). Stress may have an effect on atopic dermatitis through an interaction between the CNS and the immune system. The CNS appears to regulate immune function through the neuroendocrine system and through direct efferent autonomic

nervous system connections. Stress-related fluctuations in the neuroendocrine system or autonomic nervous system might contribute to the development of altered immunological reactivity and subsequent increased vulnerability to allergic inflammation (Buske-Kirshbaum et al. 2001).

Controlled studies have found that adult patients with atopic dermatitis are more anxious and depressed compared with clinical and disease-free control groups (Ehlers et al. 1995; Hashiro and Okumura 1997). Anxiety or depression might exacerbate atopic dermatitis by eliciting the scratching behavior. In another study of pruritus associated with atopic dermatitis and other dermatological conditions, depressive symptoms appeared to amplify the itch perception (Gupta et al. 1994). Furthermore, emotional distress aggravates pruritus in many patients with Alzheimer's disease (Heyer et al. 1995). Distress appears to perturb the epidermal permeability barrier homeostasis, resulting in inflammation and pruritus. The stress-induced deterioration of the barrier function may be mediated by glucocorticoids or by neuropeptides released within the epidermis (Garg et al. 2001).

In a study of children with atopic dermatitis, about a third of the children with severe atopic dermatitis symptoms had significantly higher morbidity levels on behavioral screening questionnaires. The emotional state in children with atopic dermatitis was closely related to the severity of the illness (Daud et al. 1993). In another study, children with moderate to severe atopic dermatitis were significantly more likely to be distressed than a control group with minor skin problems (Absolon et al. 1997). Certain dimensions of family environment, such as independence and organization, correlated with less severe symptoms of atopic dermatitis, whereas parental responses of attention or physical contact reinforced scratching (Gil and Sampson 1989).

Because increased distress, anxiety, and depression occur in many patients with atopic dermatitis, a psychiatric evaluation should be included in the overall management of patients with atopic dermatitis, especially in those with moderate to severe symptoms. Psychiatric treatment also might help to improve health-related quality of life, which is adversely affected by atopic dermatitis, particularly in social functioning and psychological well-being (Kiebert et al. 2002).

Treatment of atopic dermatitis strives to interrupt the vicious cycle of itching and scratching. Psychiatric treatment modalities include psychological or behavioral therapies and psychotropic medications. In controlled studies, relaxation training, habit reversal training, cognitive-behavioral techniques, and stress management training resulted in significant and stable adjunctive treatment responses to standard medical care and reduction in anxiety and depression (Ehlers et al. 1995). Topical 5% doxepin cream, which has potent histamine antagonism, was effective in reducing pruritus in patients with atopic dermatitis in controlled trials (Drake et al. 1994, 1995). Another antidepressant with histamine receptor antagonism, trimipramine (50 mg/day), decreased the fragmentation of sleep and reduced the time spent in stage I sleep, which reduced the amount of scratching during the night in atopic dermatitis patients (Savin et al. 1979).

Psoriasis

Psoriasis is a chronic, relapsing disease of the skin with characteristic lesions that involve both the vasculature and the epidermis and have clear-cut borders and noncoherent silvery scales over a glossy, homogeneous erythema. The lesions vary from pinpoint plaques to extensive (erythrodermic) skin involvement, nail dystrophy, and arthritis (Christophers and Mrowietz 1999). Psoriasis affects about 2% of the United States general population and is equally common in women and men. Most develop initial lesions in the third decade of life (Christophers and Mrowietz 1999). Early onset (before age 15 years), commonly associated with a family history of psoriasis, predicts greater disease severity, with a higher percentage of body surface involvement and a worse treatment response (Christophers and Mrowietz 1999). Although spontaneous remissions have been reported and have lasted between 1 and 54 years (Farber and Nall 1974), most patients with psoriasis experience unpredictable exacerbations throughout life.

The pathogenesis of psoriasis appears to involve skin repair systems, inflammatory defense mechanisms, and immunity. Both genetic (Christophers and Mrowietz 1999) and environmental factors probably contribute to the liability to psoriasis. Common triggers of psoriasis include cold weather, physical trauma, acute bacterial and viral infections, corticosteroid withdrawal, beta-adrenergic blockers, and lithium (Christophers and Mrowietz 1999). Lithium-induced psoriasis typically occurs within the first few years of treatment, is resistant to treatment, and resolves after discontinuation of lithium (Krahn and Goldberg 1994). In patients with comorbid psoriasis and bipolar disorder, alternatives to lithium that are less likely to exacerbate psoriasis include valproate and carbamazepine (Gerner and Stanton 1992).

Psoriasis is associated with substantial impairment of health-related quality of life, with a negative effect on psychological, vocational, social, and physical function (McKenna and Stern 1997; Rapp et al. 1999). In a survey of psoriatic patients, 46% reported daily problems secondary to psoriasis (Gupta et al. 1990b). More than any other medical or health status variable, the best predictor of disability in patients with psoriasis in one study was the amount of stress that resulted from the anticipation of others' reaction to their psoriasis lesions (Fortune et al. 1997b). Other studies also have found that psychological factors, including perceived health, perceptions of stigmatization, and depression, are stronger determinants of disability in patients with psoriasis than are disease severity, location, and duration (Rapp et al. 1997; Richards et al. 2001).

Stress has been reported to trigger psoriasis (Al'Abadie et al. 1994; Farber and Nall 1993; Gaston et al. 1987). Most patients who report episodes of psoriasis triggered by stress describe disease-related stress, resulting from the cosmetic disfigurement and social stigma of psoriasis, rather than stressful major life events or general levels of distress (Ginsburg 1995; Gupta et al. 1989, 1990b; Richards et al. 2001). Psoriasis-related stress appears to result from psychosocial difficulties inherent in the interpersonal relationships of patients with psoriasis rather than the severity or chronicity of psoriasis activity (Fortune et al. 1997a). The mechanism of stress-induced exacerbations may involve the nervous, endocrine, and immune systems. For example, descending autonomic information from the CNS might be transmitted to sensory nerves in the skin, resulting in release of neuropeptides such as substance P, which could initiate and maintain the inflammatory response in psoriatic lesions (Farber 1995; Harvima et al. 1993; Raychaudhuri et al. 1995).

In controlled studies, patients with psoriasis had high levels of anxiety and depression and significant comorbidity with several personality disorders, including schizoid, avoidant, passive-aggressive, and compulsive personality disorders (Devrimci-Ozguven et al. 2000; Fried et al. 1995; Gupta and Gupta 1998; Richards et al. 2001; Rubino et al. 1995). A direct correlation was found between patients' self-report of psoriasis severity and depression and suicidal ideation. Furthermore, comorbid depression reduced the threshold for pruritus in psoriatic patients (Gupta et al. 1993b, 1994). Heavy alcohol drinking (>80 g/day of ethanol) in male psoriatic patients predicts a poor treatment outcome (Gupta et al. 1993a).

Evidence of psychological morbidity associated with psoriasis has led to the development of psychosocial interventions as part of its treatment. Meditation, hypnosis, relaxation training, cognitive-behavioral stress management, and symptom control imagery training were effective in reducing psoriasis activity in controlled studies (Fortune et al. 2002; Gaston et al. 1991; Kabat-Zinn et al. 1998; Zachariae et al. 1996). Controlled trials of psychopharmacological treatment of psoriasis are needed to determine whether treatment of depressive or anxiety symptoms has an effect on psoriasis activity (Griffiths and Richards 2001).

Alopecia Areata

Alopecia areata is characterized by nonscarring hair loss in patches of typically well-demarcated smooth skin. Breakage of the hair shaft results in characteristic "exclamation-mark hairs." Hair loss often occurs on the scalp but also can affect the eyebrows, eyelashes, beard, and body hair and varies from a single patch to multiple patches or total hair loss (Koblenzer 1987). Alopecia areata accounts for about 2% of new dermatological outpatient visits in the United States. An estimated 1% of the U.S. population will have at least one episode by age 50 years (V. Price 1991). The incidence is equal in men and women and peaks during the third to fifth decades (Olsen 1999). Of the patients with alopecia areata, 30% completely recover, but 20%–30% never recover from the first episode (Koblenzer 1987). Factors associated with poor prognosis include rapid evolution, prepubertal onset, ophiasis (loss of hair along the scalp margins), multiple episodes, associated atopy, severe nail changes, and loss of eyebrows and eyelashes (Olsen 1999). The pathogenesis of alopecia areata probably involves immunological and genetic factors (Olsen 1999).

Debate continues about the role of psychiatric factors in the development of alopecia areata (Picardi and Abeni 2001). Controlled studies have yielded contradictory findings regarding the rates of psychopathology and the role of psychosocial events or stress in the onset of alopecia areata. In one controlled study, patients with alopecia areata reported significantly more life events with a substantial effect, including exits from social fields (e.g., death, divorce), uncontrolled events, and socially desirable and undesirable events in the 6 months preceding the onset of symptoms than did control subjects (Perini et al. 1984). In uncontrolled studies of lifetime comorbid psychiatric disorders in adults with alopecia areata, many patients reported lifetime psychiatric diagnoses, particularly major depression, generalized anxiety disorder, and paranoid disorder (Colón et al. 1991; Koo et al. 1994). Patients with highly stress-reactive alopecia areata reported more depressive symptoms than did patients without stress-reactive alopecia areata (Gupta et al. 1997). Finally, children with alopecia areata reported more symptoms of depression and anxiety than did control subjects (Liakopoulou et al. 1997).

Recent studies suggest ways in which stress might precipitate alopecia areata. Substance P, a neuropeptide that induces neurogenic inflammation, has been found to be endogenously released by dermal nerve fibers around hair follicles and may be involved in the pathogenesis of alopecia areata (Toyoda et al. 2001). Locally released corticotropin-releasing hormone in the skin from dorsal root ganglia or immune cells in response to stress also might contribute to the intense local inflammation around hair follicles and symptoms of alopecia areata (Katsarou-Katsari et al. 2001).

Few studies of the psychiatric treatment of patients with alopecia areata have been done. In a double-blind, placebo-controlled trial, patients taking imipramine (75 mg/day) had significantly more hair regrowth than did control subjects, an effect that was independent of a reduction in anxiety or depression (Perini et al. 1994). Patients with alopecia areata and comorbid depressive and anxiety disorders who received selective serotonin reuptake inhibitors (SSRIs) in open trials and a small controlled study also experienced improvement in the symptoms of alopecia areata (Cipriani et al. 2001; Ruiz-Doblado et al. 1999). Uncontrolled studies of psychotherapy and relaxation training have been promising in the treatment of alopecia areata, but more study is needed (Garcia-Hernandez et al. 1999).

Urticaria and Angioedema

Urticaria (hives) is characterized by circumscribed, raised, erythematous, usually pruritic areas of edema that involve the superficial dermis. Angioedema occurs when the edema extends into the deep dermis, subcutaneous, or submucosal layers (Soter 1999). About 15%–20% of the general population develops urticaria, with a peak incidence between ages 20 and 40 (Koblenzer 1987). The male-to-female ratio is equal in children, but more women than men develop urticaria in adulthood (Koblenzer 1987). Most patients with acute urticaria (duration of less than 6 weeks) readily respond to treatment of the underlying cause, usually infection or intolerance to specific drugs or food. However, the cause of chronic urticaria or angioedema (duration of greater than 6 weeks) in about 70% of patients is unknown. Chronic idiopathic urticaria often responds poorly to usual dermatological treatment. The prognosis is better in patients with mild severity, relatively short duration of the episode, and positive response to antihistamines (Champion et al. 1969). About 20% of the patients with chronic idiopathic urticaria have persistent symptoms after 10 years (Champion et al. 1969). Chronic idiopathic urticaria adversely affects quality of life to an extent comparable to that of patients with chronic heart disease (O'Donnell et al. 1997).

The manifestations of urticaria are a result of the release of vasoactive mediators in the skin, primarily histamine from mast cells or basophils (Soter 1999). The etiology of chronic idiopathic urticaria is unknown, but studies have found an association with autoantibodies against the high-affinity immunoglobulin E receptor on mast cells, suggesting an autoimmune pathogenesis in some patients (Demera et al. 2001). One form of angioedema is caused by a hereditary deficiency of C1-esterase inhibitor function (Goring et al. 1998).

Psychiatric factors are involved in the development of adrenergic urticaria. The typical "halo-hives" (papules surrounded by a white halo) that develop after acute emotional stress are associated with increased levels of plasma noradrenaline and adrenaline, are reproduced with intradermal injection of noradrenaline, and resolve after treatment with the beta-adrenoreceptor blocker propranolol (Haustein 1990; Shelley and Shelley 1985).

The relation between chronic idiopathic urticaria or angioedema and psychiatric factors is less clear. Controlled studies have found that patients, particularly females, with chronic idiopathic urticaria are frequently depressed and anxious (Badoux and Levy 1994; Hashiro and Okumura 1994; Sheehan-Dare et al. 1990; Sperber et al. 1989). Controlled studies also demonstrated an association between stressful life events and the onset of urticaria (Fava et al. 1980; Lyketsos et al. 1985). Clinically, stress so often seemed a precipitant to angioedema that for many years it was referred to as *angioneurotic edema*. The connection between stress and urticaria and angioedema might have a physiological basis. For example, stress may lead to the secretion of neuropeptides, such as vasoactive intestinal peptide and substance P, that can cause vasodilation and contribute to the development of urticarial wheals (see Koblenzer 1987).

In a controlled study of psychological treatment of chronic idiopathic urticaria, hypnosis with relaxation reduced pruritus but not the number of hives (Shertzer and Lookingbill 1987). Controlled trials indicated that antidepressant medications were effective in the management of chronic idiopathic urticaria. Doxepin (10 mg three times a day) was more effective than diphenhydramine (25 mg three times a day) for the control of chronic idiopathic urticaria (Greene et al. 1985), and nortriptyline (25 mg three times a day) was significantly better than placebo in the treatment of pruritus and wheals (Morley 1969). In two case reports, both comorbid panic disorder and urticaria responded to treatment with the SSRI fluoxetine (40 mg/day) or sertraline (100 mg/day), suggesting a possible role for serotonergic mechanisms (Gupta and Gupta 1995).

Acne Vulgaris

Acne vulgaris, a common sebaceous gland disease, is characterized by a variety of lesions, including comedones, papules, pustules, and nodules. Possible complications from the lesions include development of pitted or hypertrophic scars. Most cases of acne vulgaris develop between the middle and late teenage years. The course of acne vulgaris is usually self-limited, with spontaneous remission after several years, but it may persist through the third decade and later. Although women are more likely than men to have persistent acne, it tends to be more severe in men (Strauss and Thiboutot 1999).

Although the cause of acne vulgaris is unknown, many factors are probably involved in its pathogenesis, including stress. Stress-induced aggravation of acne might be caused by the release of adrenal steroids, which affect the sebaceous glands (Koo and Smith 1991; Strauss and Thiboutot 1999).

Severe acne is associated with increased anxiety and poor self-image (Koo and Smith 1991). Acne can substantially interfere with social and occupational functioning. Patients with even mild to moderate acne may experience significant psychological distress and body image concerns (Gupta et al. 1990a). Successful treatment of acne with isotretinoin led to a reduction in both anxiety and depressive symptoms and a significant improvement in self-image (Kellet and Gawkrodger 1999; Rubinow et al. 1987). Also, case reports have shown improvement in acne after treatment of depression with paroxetine (Moussavian 2001). In another study, biofeedback-assisted relaxation and cognitive imagery added to usual dermatological treatment resulted in significant reduction in acne severity compared with medical control groups (Hughes et al. 1983).

The use of isotretinoin for treatment of acne vulgaris has been associated with depression, suicidal ideation, suicide attempts, and suicide in anecdotal reports that received extensive media attention (Jick et al. 2000). The U.S. Food and Drug Administration (FDA) MedWatch system reports of psychiatric disorders linked to use of isotretinoin led to additional label warnings in 1998. Recently, the FDA and isotretinoin's manufacturer added the possible development of aggressive and/or violent behavior to the psychiatric disorder warning section of the package insert (Enders and Enders 2003). However, a large population-based cohort study comparing the prevalence of psychiatric disorders, suicide, and attempted suicide in isotretinoin and antibiotic users found no evidence for an increased risk of depression, suicide, or other psychiatric disorders with the use of isotretinoin (Jick et al. 2000). Other studies also found no causal connection between isotretinoin and depression or suicide (Hersom et al. 2003; Jacobs et al. 2001). Design limitations of these studies preclude firm conclusions about a possible causal relation between isotretinoin and psychiatric disorders

(Enders and Enders 2003). Furthermore, many patients with acne vulgaris present with psychiatric comorbidity. Therefore, it is important to educate patients about the risk of major depressive disorder, suicide, and other psychiatric disorders and to monitor each patient carefully (Gupta and Gupta 2001).

Somatoform Disorders

Chronic Idiopathic Pruritus

Pruritus, or itchiness, is a common symptom of dermatological diseases and of several systemic diseases, including chronic renal disease, hepatic disease, hematopoietic disorders, endocrine disorders, malignant neoplasms, drug toxicity, neurological syndromes (e.g., multiple sclerosis), infections with parasites, and viremia. Advanced age is also associated with pruritus (Gilchrest 1982). The pathophysiology of pruritus is not completely understood (Greaves and Wall 1996). Chronic idiopathic pruritus and idiopathic pruritus ani (itching in the anal area), vulvae (itching in the vaginal area), and scroti (itching in the scrotum) may be the result of central nervous mechanisms.

In a study of histamine-induced pruritus, psychic trauma lowered itch threshold, aggravated itch intensity, and prolonged itch duration. Furthermore, the duration of the pruritus was more pronounced in subjects reporting "moodiness" during stressor exposure (Fjellner and Arnetz 1985; Fjellner et al. 1985). Recent stressful life events also have been correlated with an increased ability to detect itch. A study of pruritus in psoriasis, atopic dermatitis, and chronic idiopathic urticaria found a direct correlation between pruritus severity and the degree of depressive symptoms, possibly a result of a reduced itch threshold (Gupta et al. 1994).

Antidepressant medications, particularly the tricyclic antidepressants, can relieve chronic idiopathic pruritus. Behavioral treatment, such as habit reversal training and cognitive-behavior therapy (Rosenbaum and Ayllon 1981; Welkowitz et al. 1989), aimed at interrupting the itch-scratch cycle may help to prevent complications of long-term scratching, such as lichen simplex chronicus, a condition of prominent skin markings and thickening of the tissue.

Body Dysmorphic Disorder

Body dysmorphic disorder is a preoccupation with an imagined defect in appearance (Phillips et al. 1993). Body dysmorphic disorder is common in dermatology practice. Approximately 12% of the patients seeking dermatologi-

cal treatment for concerns about the skin or hair had positive screening test results for body dysmorphic disorder, and it was equally common in men and women (Phillips et al. 2000). Patients with body dysmorphic disorder in cosmetic dermatology practice may have more severe symptoms than those in general dermatology practice (Phillips et al. 2000). Some patients with body dysmorphic disorder pick their skin in an attempt to improve their appearance, as discussed later in this chapter in the "Psychogenic Excoriation" subsection (Phillips and Taub 1995). Although body dysmorphic disorder is classified as a somatoform disorder, it has phenomenological similarities to obsessive-compulsive disorder (Phillips et al. 1995). Dermatological treatment alone is not effective for body dysmorphic disorder, which often responds to treatment with SSRIs and cognitive-behavioral therapy (Phillips et al. 2002).

Delusional Disorder, Somatic Type

Delusional Parasitosis

Delusional parasitosis is characterized by a fixed, false conviction that one is infested with living organisms (G.C. Johnson and Anton 1985). Patients with delusional parasitosis seek treatment from dermatologists because the delusions often involve a cutaneous invasion. There are also cases of delusional oral, ocular, and intestinal parasitosis (Ford et al. 2001; Maeda et al. 1998; Sherman et al. 1998). Delusional parasitosis typically occurs as a single somatic delusion with no other impairment of thought or thought process. It was previously called *monosymptomatic hypochondriacal psychosis* (Munro 1978) and is classified under delusional disorder, somatic type, in DSM-IV-TR. Occasionally, patients describe tactile sensations of crawling, biting, or stinging and other perceptual abnormalities such as buzzing or other sounds. Delusional parasitosis appears to be uncommon, with an equal sex distribution in patients younger than 50 years and a female-to-male ratio of 3:1 in patients ages 50 years and older (Lyell 1983).

The differential diagnosis of delusions of parasitosis includes numerous medical disorders, such as tuberculosis, syphilis, chronic lymphocytic leukemia, polycythemia vera, malignant lymphoma, congestive heart failure, arteriosclerosis, diabetes mellitus, vitamin B_{12} deficiency, pellagra, renal failure, hypothyroidism, hepatic disease, and the dermatological disorders stasis dermatitis and vitiligo (G.C. Johnson and Anton 1985; Wykoff 1987). Neurological conditions associated with delusions of parasitosis include dementia, multiple sclerosis, Parkinson's disease, Huntington's disease, cerebral infarction, and CNS tumors (G.C. Johnson and Anton 1985; Morris 1991). Patients with other psychiatric disorders, including major depressive disorder, bipolar disorder, and schizophrenia, also may have delusions of parasitosis (Freinhar 1984; G.C. Johnson and Anton 1985). Finally, delusions of parasitosis are associated with long-term use of amphetamines, methylphenidate, cocaine, alcohol, phenelzine, pargyline, or corticosteroids. The delusions usually resolve with discontinuation of the drug (G.C. Johnson and Anton 1985; Morris 1991; Wykoff 1987).

Characteristic features of delusional parasitosis include a specific precipitant, a history of potential or actual exposure to contagious organisms or actual infestation, and a history of multiple consultations with physicians and other professionals such as entomologists and exterminators (Lyell 1983). Many patients are reluctant to accept psychiatric evaluation for fear of being told the infestation is not real (Morris 1991). Patients make multiple attempts at treatment, including repetitive washing, checking, and cleaning; excoriation of the skin with needles, knives, or fingernails; discarding or destroying possessions; and excessive use of insect repellents and insecticides (Lyell 1983; Wykoff 1987). Other individuals may share the delusion (folie à deux), and the fear of contaminating others is often present (Lyell 1983; Morris 1991). Also, cases of delusional parasitosis by proxy involve children or pets (Nel et al. 2001). Patients may bring in specimens of inanimate material, nonharmful insects, or bits of hair and skin for examination by the physician in an attempt to provide evidence of infestation (Lyell 1983). Descriptions of the offending parasite vary from the imprecise "things" or "bugs" to detailed explanations of the organism's (usually insects, spiders, or worms) appearance, behavior, and life cycle (Lyell 1983; Morris 1991; Wykoff 1987). The mistaken worries about infestation span a spectrum from nondelusional to delusional thinking (Wykoff 1987). Sometimes the preoccupation with infestation resembles obsessions in that it is distressing, anxiety-provoking, persistent, recurrent, and difficult to resist or control. The repetitive behaviors accompanying the preoccupation are often compulsive in nature. Patients frequently report social isolation and loss of employment as a result of the delusions (Wykoff 1987), and rarely patients have been reported to commit suicide (Monk and Rao 1994).

Patients with delusional parasitosis respond to treatment with the potent neuroleptic pimozide. Only one controlled study of the treatment of delusional parasitosis with pimozide has been done, in which 10 of 11 patients improved after 6 weeks of 1–5 mg/day (Hamann and Avnstorp 1982). A follow-up study indicated that many patients taking pimozide could discontinue the medication

after a mean treatment duration of 5 months without recurrence of the delusions (Lindskov and Baadsgaard 1985). In other anecdotal reports, pimozide doses of up to 12 mg/day have been used in delusional parasitosis (G.C. Johnson and Anton 1985). Full remission of delusional parasitosis has been reported in 50% of the patients receiving pimozide (Trabert 1995). There are uncontrolled reports of efficacy with other antipsychotic medications, including chlorpromazine, trifluoperazine, haloperidol, risperidone, and fluphenazine decanoate (DeLeon et al. 1997; Freinhar 1984; Gallucci and Beard 1995; Kitamura 1997; Morris 1991; Songer and Roman 1996). Although pimozide is most commonly advocated for the treatment of delusional parasitosis, no conclusive evidence indicates that pimozide is superior to other antipsychotics. However, pimozide is the only neuroleptic used in the treatment of delusional parasitosis that is a potent opiate antagonist (Creese et al. 1976). Pimozide may be antipruritic as a result of its opiate antagonism, and the relief of pruritus or paresthesias could contribute to improvement in delusional parasitosis (G.C. Johnson and Anton 1983). The cardiovascular side effect of QT prolongation associated with pimozide precludes its use in patients with cardiac dysrhythmias and prolonged congenital QT syndrome because of the risk of life-threatening arrhythmias. Patients without a significant cardiac history whose treatment with pimozide is initiated at low doses and increased slowly are at minimal risk for cardiac complications (Opler and Feinberg 1991).

Case reports show successful treatment of delusional parasitosis with tricyclic antidepressants, SSRIs, and electroconvulsive therapy (Bhatia et al. 2000; Morris 1991; Pylko and Sicignan 1985; Slaughter et al. 1998). Because of the obsessive-compulsive symptoms in many patients with delusional parasitosis, controlled studies with the SSRIs are needed.

Psychotherapy has minimal efficacy in the treatment of delusional parasitosis (Freinhar 1984). Dermatologists have advocated an approach to patients with delusional parasitosis that allows for the development of a therapeutic relationship. This is accomplished by listening to patients' stories, asking how the condition affects their lives, being alert to any area in which patients will accept help, and trying to reduce the patients' sense of isolation (Gould and Gragg 1976).

Other Delusional Disorders, Somatic Type

In the delusional variant of body dysmorphic disorder, the preoccupations with a defect in appearance are of delusional intensity, although the distinction between an obsessive concern and delusions is not always clear (see

McElroy et al. 1993; Phillips et al. 1994). Delusional body dysmorphic disorder may respond preferentially to SSRIs, and if a patient's symptoms do not completely respond to an SSRI, the addition of an antipsychotic, such as pimozide, may be helpful (Phillips 1996; Phillips et al. 2002).

The delusion of a foul body odor is another encapsulated somatic delusion that a dermatologist may encounter in patients. Treatment data are limited, but pimozide and other antipsychotic medications may be effective (Manschreck 1996).

Impulse-Control Disorders

Psychogenic Excoriation

Psychogenic excoriation (neurotic excoriation, acne excoriée, pathological or compulsive skin picking, or dermatotillomania) is a disorder characterized by self-induced skin lesions from excoriating the skin in response to skin sensations or an urge to remove an irregularity on the skin (Gupta et al. 1987). Lesions are found in areas that the patient can easily reach, such as the face, upper back, and upper and lower extremities. Typical lesions are a few millimeters in diameter and weeping, crusted, or scarred with occasional postinflammatory hypo- or hyperpigmentation (Koblenzer 1987). Psychogenic excoriation occurs in about 2% of dermatology outpatients and is more common in women (Gupta et al. 1986). Most studies report a mean age at onset between 30 and 45 years, although the disorder can begin in adolescence. The mean duration of symptoms is 5 years, with a better prognosis for patients who have had the symptoms for less than 1 year (Gupta et al. 1986).

The behavior associated with psychogenic excoriation is heterogeneous. Some patients exhibit behavior that resembles obsessive-compulsive disorder in that it is repetitive, ritualistic, and tension reducing, and patients attempt, often unsuccessfully, to resist excoriating, a behavior they find ego-dystonic (Stein and Hollander 1992a). Patients sometimes describe obsessions about an irregularity on the skin or preoccupations with having smooth skin and may excoriate in response to such thoughts. The preoccupation with appearance can be severe enough to meet criteria for body dysmorphic disorder, a disorder possibly related to obsessive-compulsive disorder (Phillips and Taub 1995). Patients also may describe symptoms of impulse-control disorders, such as an increase in tension before the behavior and transient pleasure or relief immediately afterward (Arnold et al. 1998). As in other impulse-control disorders, patients with psychogenic ex-

coriation often find themselves acting automatically. Thus, behaviors can span a "compulsivity–impulsivity" continuum from purely obsessive-compulsive to purely impulsive, with mixed symptoms between these poles (McElroy et al. 1994). Preliminary operational criteria that take into account the heterogeneity of the behaviors and allow for subtyping along a "compulsivity–impulsivity" spectrum have been proposed for the diagnosis of psychogenic excoriation (Arnold et al. 2001) (Table 29–2).

Depressive and anxiety disorders are common in patients with psychogenic excoriation (Arnold et al. 1998; Gupta et al. 1987; Simeon et al. 1997). In one study, patients with impulsive excoriative behavior had a high rate of comorbid bipolar disorder, particularly bipolar II disorder, consistent with studies of other impulse-control disorders in which bipolar disorder is frequently comorbid (Arnold et al. 1998).

Case reports and open trials suggest that psychogenic excoriation responds to treatment with oral doxepin (Harris et al. 1987) and the serotonin reuptake inhibitors fluoxetine (Gupta and Gupta 1993; Phillips and Taub 1995; Stein et al. 1993; Stout 1990; Vittorio and Phillips 1997), sertraline (Kalivas et al. 1996), clomipramine (Gupta et al. 1986), paroxetine (Biondi et al. 2000; Ravindran et al. 1999), and fluvoxamine (Arnold et al. 1999). There are also case reports of successful treatment of psychogenic excoriation with olanzapine (Garnis-Jones et al. 2000; Gupta and Gupta 2000), pimozide (Duke 1983), and naltrexone (Lienemann and Walker 1989). A 10-week double-blind, placebo-controlled trial found that fluoxetine, at a mean dose of 55 mg/day, was significantly better than placebo in reducing psychogenic excoriation (Simeon et al. 1997). A study of open-label fluoxetine, at a mean dose of 41 mg/day for 6 weeks followed by a 6-week double-blind, placebo-controlled phase, also reported that fluoxetine significantly reduced skin excoriation (Block et al. 2000). Studies of the behavioral treatment of psychogenic excoriation are limited to case reports, which showed promising results (Deckersbach et al. 2002; Kent and Drummond 1988; Welkowitz et al. 1989).

Trichotillomania

Trichotillomania is a disorder of chronic pulling out of one's hair. Trichotillomania is classified as an impulse-control disorder in DSM-IV-TR but, like psychogenic excoriation, has both impulsive and compulsive features (Stein et al. 1995a, 1995b). Trichotillomania causes substantial distress and impairment in functioning and leads to alopecia, most commonly involving the scalp hair but also eyelashes, eyebrows, pubic hair, and other body hair

TABLE 29–2.   Proposed diagnostic criteria for psychogenic excoriation

A. Maladaptive skin excoriation (e.g., scratching, picking, gouging, lancing, digging, rubbing, or squeezing skin) or maladaptive preoccupation with skin excoriation as indicated by at least one of the following:
   1. Preoccupation with skin excoriation and/or recurrent impulses to excoriate the skin that is/are experienced as irresistible, intrusive, and/or senseless.
   2. Recurrent excoriation of the skin resulting in noticeable skin damage.
B. The preoccupation, impulses, or behaviors associated with skin excoriation cause marked distress, are time-consuming, significantly interfere with social or occupational activities, or result in medical problems (e.g., infections).
C. The disturbance is not better accounted for by another mental disorder and is not due to a general medical condition.

Subtypes:

Compulsive type:
1. Skin excoriation is performed to avoid increased anxiety or to prevent a dreaded event or situation and/or is elicited by an obsession (e.g., obsession about contamination of the skin).
2. It is performed in full awareness.
3. It is associated with some resistance to performing the behavior.
4. There is some insight into its senselessness or harmfulness.

Impulsive type:
1. Skin excoriation is associated with arousal, pleasure, or reduction of tension.
2. It is performed at times with minimal awareness (e.g., automatically).
3. It is associated with little resistance to performing the behavior.
4. There is little insight into its senselessness or harmfulness.

Mixed type:
Skin excoriation has both compulsive and impulsive features.

Source.   Reprinted from Arnold LM, Auchenbach MB, McElroy SL: "Psychogenic Excoriation: Clinical Features, Proposed Diagnostic Criteria, Epidemiology, and Approaches to Treatment." *CNS Drugs* 15:351–359, 2001. Used with permission. Adis International Ltd., Auckland, New Zealand.

(Christenson et al. 1991a). The extracted hair is sometimes chewed or swallowed, resulting in the development of trichobezoars (Christenson and Crow 1996). Patients may develop infections at the site of hair pulling, change in texture or color of the hair, or carpal tunnel syndrome from pulling (Christenson and Crow 1996).

In a survey of college freshmen, the lifetime prevalence of trichotillomania (by strict criteria) was 0.6% for both men and women but rose to 3.4% for women and 1.5% for men if all hair pulling with noticeable hair loss was included (Christenson et al. 1991b). The condition typically persists for years, with a mean age at onset of 13 years (Christenson et al. 1991a). The prognosis appears to be better with hair pulling of 6 months' duration or less. Most patients do not seek treatment (Christenson and Crow 1996).

There are two types of hair pulling (Christenson and Crow 1996). In the "focused style," patients focus solely on the pulling without attention to other thoughts and activities. Symptoms resemble obsessive-compulsive disorder in that the patient resists the pulling and feels relief with pulling. However, most patients engage in an "automatic style" of pulling that occurs during situations described as sedentary or contemplative, such as reading or watching television, which is consistent with impulse-

control disorders. Many patients have a combination of these two styles (Christenson et al. 1993).

Comorbid psychiatric disorders in patients with trichotillomania include anxiety, mood, substance abuse or dependence, and eating disorders (Christenson et al. 1991a; Cohen et al. 1995; Schlosser et al. 1994; Swedo and Leonard 1992). The most frequent comorbid personality disorders include Cluster B (histrionic, borderline) and Cluster C (obsessive-compulsive, avoidant, dependent) disorders (Schlosser et al. 1994; Swedo and Leonard 1992). One particular personality disorder is not characteristic of patients with trichotillomania (Christenson et al. 1992). Patients with trichotillomania frequently have first-degree relatives with obsessive-compulsive disorder and trichotillomania (Swedo and Leonard 1992) and family histories of mood disorders, substance use disorders, anxiety disorders, and schizophrenia (Cohen et al. 1995).

In a double-blind crossover study, trichotillomania responded preferentially to the antiobsessional agent clomipramine, at a mean dose of 180 mg/day, over desipramine, at a mean dose of 173 mg/day (Swedo et al. 1989). In another report, response to clomipramine negatively correlated with anterior cingulate and orbital frontal metabolism on positron emission tomography (PET) examination, a finding also characteristic of obsessive-compulsive disorder (Swedo et al. 1991). Open studies of the SSRI fluoxetine reported positive short- and long-term results (Koran et al. 1992; Winchel et al. 1992); however, controlled studies have yielded mixed findings. Two placebo-controlled studies found that fluoxetine was not superior to placebo in the treatment of trichotillomania (Christenson et al. 1991c; Streichenwein and Thornby 1995), but in a double-blind crossover study of clomipramine and fluoxetine, both medications had positive treatment effects on trichotillomania (Pigott et al. 1992). Case reports and open trials reported positive responses to treatment with other drugs, including fluvoxamine (Christenson et al. 1998; Stanley et al. 1997), paroxetine (Reid 1994), sertraline (Bradford and Gratzer 1995; Rahman and Gregory 1995), citalopram (Stein et al. 1997), venlafaxine (Ninan et al. 1998), other antidepressants (Christenson and Crow 1996), lithium (Christenson et al. 1991d), and buspirone (Reid 1992). Pimozide augmentation of clomipramine or fluoxetine also has proved useful in a small case series (Stein and Hollander 1992b). A case series of olanzapine augmentation of citalopram was effective in three of four patients (Ashton 2001). Finally, there are case reports of successful treatment of resistant trichotillomania with a combination of risperidone and fluvoxamine (Gabriel 2001) and with risperidone alone (Sentürk and Tanrtverdi 2002).

The behavioral treatment of habit reversal has been reported to be effective in trichotillomania and involves increasing awareness of situations or stressors associated with hair pulling, relaxation training, and competing response training (Azrin et al. 1980). A small 9-week controlled study examining the efficacy of cognitive-behavior therapy and clomipramine compared with placebo found that cognitive-behavior therapy substantially reduced the symptoms of trichotillomania and was significantly more effective than clomipramine or placebo. Clomipramine treatment resulted in symptom reduction greater than that of placebo, but the difference was not statistically significant (Ninan et al. 2000). A 12-week controlled study compared fluoxetine with behavioral treatment that consisted of six individual 45-minute sessions aimed at self-control, which relied on self-report and self-monitoring. The behavioral treatment resulted in significantly greater reduction in trichotillomania symptoms compared with the fluoxetine or a waiting-list control condition (van Minnen et al. 2003). Hypnosis and other behavioral treatments also have been useful according to case reports (Peterson et al. 1994).

For many patients with trichotillomania, the initial response to treatment is followed by a plateau in improvement and, for up to one-third, a loss of beneficial medication effect (Keuthen et al. 2001). Preliminary evidence suggests that concurrent use of behavioral therapies and medication treatment for trichotillomania may be more effective than either treatment alone, but more study is needed (Keuthen et al. 1998).

Onychophagia

Onychophagia, or repetitive nail biting, is a common behavior that can begin as early as age 4 years, with a peak between ages 10 and 18 years, and that appears to be familial (Leonard et al. 1991). Severe onychophagia can lead to significant medical and dental problems, such as hand infection (Zook 1986) and craniomandibular disorders (Westling 1988). Onychotillomania, the picking or tearing of the nail, may be a variant of the behavior. Like trichotillomania and psychogenic excoriation, onychophagia has the phenomenological features of repetition, resistance, and relief (Leonard et al. 1991).

A double-blind crossover study reported that onychophagia responded preferentially to clomipramine, at a mean dosage of 120 mg/day, over desipramine, at a mean dosage of 135 mg/day (Leonard et al. 1991). Many forms of behavior therapy, including habit reversal, have been efficacious (Peterson et al. 1994). In a recent controlled study of chronic nail biting, habit reversal training (a total of 2 hours spread over three sessions) was compared with a placebo treatment in which patients simply discussed their nail biting. The habit reversal intervention produced a greater increase in nail length compared with the placebo (Twohig et al. 2003).

Factitious Disorders

Factitious Dermatitis

Factitious dermatitis (dermatitis artefacta) is a disorder in which patients intentionally produce skin lesions in order to assume the sick role. Patients typically deny the self-inflicted nature of the disorder (Gupta et al. 1987).

Factitious dermatitis can present with a wide variety of lesions depending on the methods used by the patient. Patients may either simulate actual medical dermatoses or aggravate a preexisting dermatological condition (Koblenzer 1987). Lesions include excoriations, blisters, purpura, ulcers, erythema, edema, sinuses, and nodules (Gupta et al. 1987). Methods used by patients include rubbing; scratching; picking; cutting; puncturing; sucking; biting; applying suction cups; occluding; applying dye, heat, or caustic substances onto the skin; or injecting caustics, infected material, blood, feces, or other substances into the skin (Gupta et al. 1987; Koblenzer 1987; Lyell 1979; Spraker 1983).

Skin damage can be extensive, with full-thickness skin loss and severe scarring requiring plastic surgery or even amputation (Hollender and Abram 1973). Affected sites tend to be easily accessible to the patient and are more prominent on one side of the body, depending on the handedness of the patient (Hollender and Abram 1973). Excoriated lesions frequently have sharp, geometric borders with normal surrounding skin or lines at the margin if a caustic was used and some liquid dripped out of the site (Hollender and Abram 1973; Spraker 1983). The natural progression of the lesions through the different stages of development is not evident (Spraker 1983). The history is often vague and "hollow" (Lyell 1979), and patients are often very suggestive as to the site of the next lesion (Hollender and Abram 1973). The use of an occlusive dressing such as an Unna's paste boot (a dressing that hardens to form a protective covering) can help make the diagnosis because the lesions heal when the patients are unable to reach them (Hollender and Abram 1973; Koblenzer 1987).

Factitious dermatitis occurs in about 0.3% of dermatology patients (Gupta et al. 1987), with a female-to-male ratio between 3:1 and 8:1 and the greatest frequency in adolescents and young adults (Koblenzer 1987). It reportedly begins after severe psychosocial stress, usually involving loss, threatened loss, or isolation (Stein and Hollander 1992a). As in other factitious disorders, the patient often has experience in medicine as a result of either prior exposure to illness or employment in a health care field. The prognosis varies; some cases resolve after a brief episode, whereas others become lifelong problems (Lyell 1979). In a classic long-term study, 30% of the patients continued to produce lesions more than 12 years after the onset of their symptoms (Sneddon and Sneddon 1975).

The differential diagnosis of factitious dermatitis includes other forms of self-inflicted dermatoses described in the earlier sections. Although borderline personality disorder is commonly comorbid with factitious dermatitis, some patients with borderline personality disorder readily acknowledge that they damage their skin in an impulsive act that resembles obsessive-compulsive spectrum disorders. Self-mutilation in impulsive patients may be a result of low serotonergic function and may respond to the SSRI fluoxetine (Stein and Hollander 1992a). Other self-mutilating patients with psychosis or mental retardation do not have the other characteristics of a factitious disorder (Hollender and Abram 1973).

No controlled trials of the treatment of factitious dermatitis have been published, and treatment recommendations are based on anecdotal experience. An empathic, therapeutic relationship between the dermatologist and the patient is essential in the management of these patients. Because the patients deny the self-inflicted nature of the lesions, they usually do not immediately accept a referral to a psychiatrist, and direct confrontation may disrupt the doctor–patient relationship. However, once a therapeutic relationship has been established, some patients will accept a psychotherapeutic approach (Koblenzer 1987; Spraker 1983) (see also Chapter 14, "Deception Syndromes: Factitious Disorders and Malingering").

Psychogenic Purpura

The spontaneous appearance of recurrent bruising (purpura) is a rare dermatological disorder that often follows an injury or a surgical procedure and typically is initiated by pain, burning, or stinging, followed by warmth, erythema, swelling, and sometimes pruritus and, after hours or days, by ecchymosis (Gardner and Diamond 1955). Blood coagulation and hemostatic tests, however, have normal results (Koblenzer 1987; Stocker et al. 1977). The incidence is unknown, but it affects women more frequently than men, with a female-to-male ratio of 20:1. The age at onset varies from 9 to 53 years, with most cases occurring between ages 14 and 40 (Koblenzer 1987). Three different proposed mechanisms currently exist: autoerythrocyte sensitization, conversion reaction, and factitious disorder.

Autoerythrocyte sensitization (Gardner-Diamond syndrome) is thought to result from sensitization to the stroma of extravasated erythrocytes after trauma (Gardner and Diamond 1955). Some, but not all, patients' bruises have been reproduced by intracutaneous injection of washed red blood cells or erythrocyte stroma. However, there is no evidence for circulating antibodies to red blood cell components or abnormalities in immunological function. Attempts to use immunosuppressive treatment and desensitization with autologous blood products also have been unsuccessful (Koblenzer 1987). Therefore, the evidence for autoerythrocyte sensitization is very limited.

In support of a psychogenic cause of the purpura, studies have found that it often begins after significant psychosocial stressors. Most patients present with several other unexplained somatic symptoms and have significant comorbid psychiatric symptoms, including depression, anxiety, and personality disorders, particularly borderline and histrionic personality disorders (Ratnoff 1989). The differentiation between conversion and factitious purpura is unclear because patients thought to have conversion symptoms and those found to have factitious disorder share many common features (Stocker et al. 1977). In addition, physicians can identify no mechanism for a conversion reaction or convincingly disprove factitious causation in many cases (Stocker et al. 1977). Although more study is needed, it appears that factitious disorder is the most likely cause of psychogenic purpura.

Cutaneous Side Effects of Psychiatric Medications

Selected cutaneous side effects of psychiatric medications are summarized in Table 29–3.

TABLE 29–3.   Selected cutaneous side effects of psychotropic medications

Agent	Cutaneous side effects
Anticonvulsants	Allergic rashes, alopecia, Stevens-Johnson syndrome and toxic epidermal necrolysis (especially lamotrigine), lupuslike syndrome
Antidepressants	Allergic rashes, photosensitivity (tricyclic antidepressants), hyperhidrosis
Antipsychotics	Skin pigmentation (especially thioridazine and chlorpromazine), photosensitivity (especially phenothiazines), lupuslike syndrome (phenothiazines), contact dermatitis, depot injection site reactions
Lithium	Urticaria; rash; alopecia; folliculitis; exacerbation of acne, warts, psoriasis

Conclusion

Patients with psychocutaneous disorders are a diverse group who frequently present to dermatologists for evaluation and treatment. Included in this group are patients who have dermatological diseases (e.g., psoriasis), in which the course may be affected by psychological factors, such as stress or comorbid mood and anxiety disorders. Patients who have primary psychiatric disorders with skin-related symptoms (e.g., delusional parasitosis) are also included under the broad category of psychocutaneous disorders. Psychocutaneous disorders can be particularly challenging for dermatologists because patients with these disorders are often reluctant to seek psychiatric treatment. Furthermore, the understanding of the pathophysiology of these disorders is limited, and relatively few treatment studies are available to guide the management of these disorders.

Patients may be more willing to accept a psychiatric evaluation if a psychiatrist is working within the dermatology clinic. In a study of a dermatology-liaison clinic, most of the psychiatric workload involved the treatment of comorbid depressive and anxiety disorders. Furthermore, most of the patients who were seen in the liaison clinic responded well to psychiatric treatment (Woodruff et al. 1997). However, many communities do not have psychiatrists available to perform a liaison function within dermatology settings. As an alternative, psychiatrists with an interest in psychocutaneous disorders could develop working relationships with dermatologists to improve the access to psychiatric evaluation and treatment. Collaboration between the psychiatrist and dermatologist is likely to positively affect the treatment outcome of patients with psychocutaneous disorders.

References

Absolon CM, Cottrell D, Eldridge SM, et al: Psychological disturbance in atopic eczema: the extent of the problem in school aged children. Br J Dermatol 137:241–245, 1997

Al'Abadie MS, Kent GG, Gawkrodger DJ: The relationship between stress and the onset and exacerbation of psoriasis and other skin conditions. Br J Dermatol 130:199–203, 1994

American Psychiatric Association: Diagnostic and Statistical Manual of Mental Disorders, 4th Edition, Text Revision. Washington, DC, American Psychiatric Association, 2000

Arnold LM, McElroy SL, Mutasim DF, et al: Characteristics of 34 adults with psychogenic excoriation. J Clin Psychiatry 59:509–514, 1998

Arnold LM, Mutasim DF, Dwight MM, et al: An open clinical trial of fluvoxamine treatment of psychogenic excoriation. J Clin Psychopharmacol 19:15–18, 1999

Arnold LM, Auchenbach MB, McElroy SL: Psychogenic excoriation: clinical features, proposed diagnostic criteria, epidemiology and approaches to treatment. CNS Drugs 15:351–359, 2001

Ashton AK: Olanzapine augmentation for trichotillomania. Am J Psychiatry 158:1929–1930, 2001

Azrin NH, Nunn RG, Frantz SE: Treatment of hairpulling (trichotillomania): a comparative study of habit reversal and negative practice training. J Behav Ther Exp Psychiatry 11:13–20, 1980

Badoux A, Levy DA: Psychologic symptoms in asthma and chronic urticaria. Ann Allergy 72:229–234, 1994

Bhatia MS, Jagawat T, Choudhary S: Delusional parasitosis: a clinical profile. Int J Psychiatry Med 30:83–91, 2000

Biondi M, Arcangeli T, Petrucci RM: Paroxetine in a case of psychogenic pruritus and neurotic excoriations. Psychother Psychosom 69:165–166, 2000

Block MR, Elliott MA, Thompson H, et al: Fluoxetine for skin picking. Abstracts of the New Clinical Drug Evaluation Unit Annual Meeting. Boca Raton, FL, May 30–June 2, 2000

Bradford JMW, Gratzer TG: A treatment for impulse control disorders and paraphilia: a case report. Can J Psychiatry 40:4–5, 1995

Buske-Kirschbaum A, Geiben A, Hellhammer D: Psychobiological aspects of atopic dermatitis: an overview. Psychother Psychosom 70:6–16, 2001

Champion RH, Roberts SOB, Carpenter RG, et al: Urticaria and angio-oedema: a review of 554 patients. Br J Dermatol 81:588–597, 1969

Christenson GA, Crow SJ: The characterization and treatment of trichotillomania. J Clin Psychiatry 57:42–49, 1996

Christenson GA, Mackenzie TB, Mitchell JE: Characteristics of 60 adult chronic hair pullers. Am J Psychiatry 148:365–370, 1991a

Christenson GA, Pyle RL, Mitchell JE: Estimated lifetime prevalence of trichotillomania in college students. J Clin Psychiatry 52:415–417, 1991b

Christenson GA, Mackenzie TB, Mitchell JE, et al: A placebo-controlled, double-blind crossover study of fluoxetine in trichotillomania. Am J Psychiatry 148:1566–1571, 1991c

Christenson GA, Popkin MK, Mackenzie TB, et al: Lithium treatment of chronic hair pulling. J Clin Psychiatry 52:116–120, 1991d

Christenson GA, Chernoff-Clementz E, Clementz BA: Personality and clinical characteristics in patients with trichotillomania. J Clin Psychiatry 53:407–413, 1992

Christenson GA, Ristvedt SL, Mackenzie TB: Identification of trichotillomania cue profiles. Behav Res Ther 31:315–320, 1993

Christenson GA, Crow SJ, Mitchell JE, et al: Fluvoxamine in the treatment of trichotillomania: an 8-week, open-label study. CNS Spectr 3:64–71, 1998

Christophers E, Mrowietz U: Epidermis: disorders of persistent inflammation, cell kinetics and differentiation, in Fitzpatrick's Dermatology in General Medicine, 5th Edition. Edited by Freedberg IM, Eisen AZ, Wolff K, et al. New York, McGraw-Hill, 1999, pp 495–521

Cipriani R, Perini GI, Rampinelli S: Paroxetine in alopecia areata. Int J Dermatol 40:600–601, 2001

Cohen LJ, Stein DJ, Simeon D, et al: Clinical profile, comorbidity, and treatment history in 123 hair pullers: a survey study. J Clin Psychiatry 56:319–326, 1995

Colón EA, Popkin MK, Callies AL, et al: Lifetime prevalence of psychiatric disorders in patients with alopecia areata. Compr Psychiatry 32:245–251, 1991

Creese I, Feinberg AP, Snyder SH: Butyrophenone influences on the opiate receptor. Eur J Pharmacol 36:231–235, 1976

Daud IR, Garralda ME, David TJ: Psychosocial adjustment in preschool children with atopic eczema. Arch Dis Child 69:670–676, 1993

Deckersbach T, Wilhelm S, Keuthen NJ, et al: Cognitive-behavior therapy for self-injurious skin picking. Behav Modif 26:361–377, 2002

De Leon OA, Furmaga KM, Canterbury AL, et al: Risperidone in the treatment of delusions of infestation. Int J Psychiatry Med 27:403–409, 1997

Demera RS, Ryhal B, Gershwin ME: Chronic idiopathic urticaria. Compr Ther 27:213–217, 2001

Devrimci-Ozguven H, Kundakci N, Kumbasar H, et al: The depression, anxiety, life satisfaction and affective expression levels in psoriasis patients. J Eur Acad Dermatol Venereol 14:267–271, 2000

Drake LA, Millikan LE: The Doxepin Study Group: the antipruritic effect of 5% doxepin cream in patients with eczematous dermatitis. Arch Dermatol 131:1403–1408, 1995

Drake LA, Fallon JD, Sober A, et al: Relief of pruritus in patients with atopic dermatitis after treatment with topical doxepin cream. J Am Acad Dermatol 31:613–616, 1994

Duke EE: Clinical experience with pimozide: emphasis on its use in postherpetic neuralgia. J Am Acad Dermatol 8:845–850, 1983

Ehlers A, Stangier U, Gieler U: Treatment of atopic dermatitis: a comparison of psychological and dermatological approaches to relapse prevention. J Consult Clin Psychol 63:624–635, 1995

Enders SJ, Enders JM: Isotretinoin and psychiatric illness in adolescents and young adults. Ann Pharmacother 37:1124–1127, 2003

Farber EM: Therapeutic perspectives in psoriasis. Int J Dermatol 34:456–460, 1995

Farber EM, Nall ML: The natural history of psoriasis in 5600 patients. Dermatologica 148:1–18, 1974

Farber EM, Nall L: Psoriasis: a stress-related disease. Cutis 51:322–326, 1993

Fava GA, Perini GI, Santonastaso P, et al: Life events and psychological distress in dermatologic disorders: psoriasis, chronic urticaria and fungal infections. Br J Med Psychol 53:277–282, 1980

Fjellner B, Arnetz BB: Psychological predictors of pruritus during mental stress. Acta Derm Venereol 65:504–508, 1985

Fjellner B, Arnetz BB, Eneroth P, et al: Pruritus during standardized mental stress: relationship to psychoneuroendocrine and metabolic parameters. Acta Derm Venereol 65:199–205, 1985

Ford EB, Calfee DP, Pearson RD: Delusions of intestinal parasitosis. South Med J 94:545–547, 2001

Fortune DG, Main CJ, O'Sullivan TM, et al: Assessing illness-related stress in psoriasis: the psychometric properties of the psoriasis life stress inventory. J Psychosom Res 42:467–475, 1997a

Fortune DG, Main CJ, O'Sullivan TM, et al: Quality of life in patients with psoriasis: the contribution of clinical variables and psoriasis-specific stress. Br J Dermatol 137:755–760, 1997b

Fortune DG, Richards HL, Kirby B, et al: A cognitive-behavioural symptom management programme as an adjunct in psoriasis therapy. Br J Dermatol 146:458–465, 2002

Freinhar JP: Delusions of parasitosis. Psychosomatics 25:47–53, 1984

Fried RG, Friedman S, Paradis C, et al: Trivial or terrible? The psychosocial impact of psoriasis. Int J Dermatol 34:101–105, 1995

Gabriel A: A case of resistant trichotillomania treated with risperidone-augmented fluvoxamine (letter). Can J Psychiatry 46:285–286, 2001

Gallucci G, Beard G: Risperidone and the treatment of delusions of parasitosis in an elderly patient. Psychosomatics 36:578–580, 1995

García-Hernández MJ, Ruiz-Doblado S, Rodriguez-Pichardo A, et al: Alopecia areata, stress and psychiatric disorders: a review. J Dermatol 26:625–632, 1999

Gardner FH, Diamond LK: Autoerythrocyte sensitization: a form of purpura, producing painful bruising following autosensitization to red blood cells in certain women. Blood 10:675–690, 1955

Garg A, Chren MM, Sands LP, et al: Psychological stress perturbs epidermal permeability barrier homeostasis. Arch Dermatol 137:53–59, 2001

Garnis-Jones S, Collins S, Rosenthal D: Treatment of self-mutilation with olanzapine. J Cutan Med Surg 4:161–163, 2000

Gaston L, Lassonde M, Bernier-Buzzanga J, et al: Psoriasis and stress: a prospective study. J Am Acad Dermatol 17:82–86, 1987

Gaston L, Crombez J, Lassonde M, et al: Psychological stress and psoriasis: experimental and prospective correlational studies. Acta Derm Venereol 156:37–43, 1991

Gerner RH, Stanton A: Algorithm for patient management of acute manic states: lithium, valproate, or carbamazepine? J Clin Psychopharmacol 12:57S–63S, 1992

Gil KM, Sampson HA: Psychological and social factors of atopic dermatitis. Allergy 44:84–89, 1989

Gil KM, Keefe FJ, Sampson HA, et al: The relation of stress and family environment to atopic dermatitis symptoms in children. J Psychosom Res 31:673–684, 1987

Gilchrest BA: Pruritus: pathogenesis, therapy, and significance in systemic disease states. Arch Intern Med 142:101–105, 1982

Ginsburg IH: Psychological and psychophysiological aspects of psoriasis. Dermatol Clin 13:793–804, 1995

Ginsburg IH, Prystowsky JH, Kornfeld DS, et al: Role of emotional factors in adults with atopic dermatitis. Int J Dermatol 32:656–660, 1993

Goring HD, Bork K, Spath PJ, et al: Hereditary angioedema in the German-speaking region. Hautarzt 49:114–122, 1998

Gould WM, Gragg TM: Delusions of parasitosis: an approach to the problem. Arch Dermatol 112:1745–1748, 1976

Greaves MW, Wall PD: Pathophysiology of itching. Lancet 348:938–940, 1996

Greene SL, Reed CE, Schroeter AL: Double-blind crossover study comparing doxepin with diphenhydramine for the treatment of chronic urticaria. J Am Acad Dermatol 12:669–675, 1985

Griffiths CEM, Richards HL: Psychological influences in psoriasis. Clin Exp Dermatol 26:338–342, 2001

Gupta MA, Gupta AK: Fluoxetine is an effective treatment for neurotic excoriations: case report. Cutis 51:386–387, 1993

Gupta MA, Gupta AK: Chronic idiopathic urticaria associated with panic disorder: a syndrome responsive to selective serotonin reuptake inhibitor antidepressants? Cutis 56:53–54, 1995

Gupta MA, Gupta AK: Psychodermatology: an update. J Am Acad Dermatol 34:1030–1046, 1996

Gupta MA, Gupta AK: Depression and suicidal ideation in dermatology patients with acne, alopecia areata, atopic dermatitis and psoriasis. Br J Dermatol 139:846–850, 1998

Gupta MA, Gupta AK: Olanzapine is effective in the management of some self-induced dermatoses: three case reports. Cutis 66:143–146, 2000

Gupta MA, Gupta AK: The psychological comorbidity in acne. Clin Dermatol 19:360–363, 2001

Gupta MA, Gupta AK, Haberman HF: Neurotic excoriations: a review and some new perspectives. Compr Psychiatry 27:381–386, 1986

Gupta MA, Gupta AK, Haberman HF: The self-inflicted dermatoses: a critical review. Gen Hosp Psychiatry 9:45–52, 1987

Gupta MA, Gupta AK, Kirkby S, et al: A psychocutaneous profile of psoriasis patients who are stress reactors: a study of 127 patients. Gen Hosp Psychiatry 11:166–173, 1989

Gupta MA, Gupta AK, Schork NJ, et al: Psychiatric aspects of the treatment of mild to moderate facial acne; some preliminary observations. Int J Dermatol 29:719–721, 1990a

Gupta MA, Gupta AK, Ellis CN, et al: Some psychosomatic aspects of psoriasis. Adv Dermatol 5:21–32, 1990b

Gupta MA, Schork NJ, Gupta AK, et al: Alcohol intake and treatment responsiveness of psoriasis: a prospective study. J Am Acad Dermatol 28:730–732, 1993a

Gupta MA, Schork NJ, Gupta AK, et al: Suicidal ideation in psoriasis. Int J Dermatol 32:188–190, 1993b

Gupta MA, Gupta AK, Schork NJ, et al: Depression modulates pruritus perception: a study of pruritus in psoriasis, atopic dermatitis, and chronic idiopathic urticaria. Psychosom Med 56:36–40, 1994

Gupta MA, Gupta AK, Watteel GN: Stress and alopecia areata: a psychodermatologic study. Acta Derm Venereol 77:296–298, 1997

Hamann K, Avnstorp C: Delusions of infestation treated by pimozide: a double-blind crossover clinical study. Acta Derm Venereol 62:55–58, 1982

Harris BA, Sherertz EF, Flowers FP: Improvement of chronic neurotic excoriations with oral doxepin therapy. Int J Dermatol 26:541–543, 1987

Harvima IT, Viinamäki H, Naukkarinen A, et al: Association of cutaneous mast cells and sensory nerves with psychic stress in psoriasis. Psychother Psychosom 60:168–176, 1993

Hashiro M, Okumura M: Anxiety, depression, psychosomatic symptoms and autonomic nervous function in patients with chronic urticaria. J Dermatol Sci 8:129–135, 1994

Hashiro M, Okumura M: Anxiety, depression and psychosomatic symptoms in patients with atopic dermatitis: comparison with normal controls and among groups of different degrees of severity. J Dermatol Sci 14:63–67, 1997

Haustein U: Adrenergic urticaria and adrenergic pruritus. Acta Derm Venereol 70:82–84, 1990

Hersom K, Neary MP, Levaux HP, et al: Isotretinoin and antidepressant pharmacotherapy: a prescription sequence symmetry analysis. J Am Acad Dermatol 49:424–432, 2003

Heyer G, Ulmer FJ, Schmitz J, et al: Histamine-induced itch and allokinesis (itchy skin) in atopic eczema patients and controls. Acta Derm Venereol 75:348–352, 1995

Hollender MH, Abram HS: Dermatitis factitia. South Med J 66:1279–1285, 1973

Hughes H, Brown BW, Lawlis GF, et al: Treatment of acne vulgaris by biofeedback relaxation and cognitive imagery. J Psychosom Res 27:185–191, 1983

Jacobs DG, Deutsch NL, Brewer M: Suicide, depression, and isotretinoin: is there a causal link? J Am Acad Dermatol 45:S168–S175, 2001

Jick SS, Kremers HM, Vasilakis-Scaramozza C: Isotretinoin use and risk of depression, psychotic symptoms, suicide, and attempted suicide. Arch Dermatol 136:1231–1236, 2000

Johnson GC, Anton RF: Pimozide in delusions of parasitosis (letter). J Clin Psychiatry 44:233, 1983

Johnson GC, Anton RF: Delusions of parasitosis: differential diagnosis and treatment. South Med J 78:914–918, 1985

Johnson ML: Prevalence of dermatologic disease among persons 1–74 years of age: United States, in Advance Data from Vital and Health Statistics of the National Center for Health Statistics, no 4. Washington, DC, U.S. Department of Healthm Education, and Welfare, U.S. Government Printing Office, January 26, 1977

Kabat-Zinn J, Wheeler E, Light T, et al: Influence of a mindfulness meditation-based stress reduction intervention on rates of skin clearing in patients with moderate to severe psoriasis undergoing phototherapy (UVB) and photochemotherapy (PUVA). Psychosom Med 60:625–632, 1998

Kalivas J, Kalivas L, Gilman D, et al: Sertraline in the treatment of neurotic excoriations and related disorders. Arch Dermatol 132:589–590, 1996

Katsarou-Katsari A, Singh LK, Theoharides TC: Alopecia areata and affected skin CRH receptor upregulation induced by acute emotional stress. Dermatology 203:157–161, 2001

Kellett SC, Gawkrodger DJ: The psychological and emotional impact of acne and the effect of treatment with isotretinoin. Br J Dermatol 140:273–282, 1999

Kent A, Drummond LM: Acne excoriée—a case report of treatment using habit reversal. Clin Exp Dermatol 14:163–164, 1988

Keuthen NJ, O'Sullivan RI, Goodchild P, et al: Behavior therapy and pharmacotherapy for trichotillomania: choice of treatment, patient acceptance, and long-term outcome. CNS Spectr 3:72–78, 1998

Keuthen NJ, Fraim C, Deckersbach T, et al: Longitudinal follow-up of naturalistic treatment outcome in patients with trichotillomania. J Clin Psychiatry 62:101–107, 2001

Kiebert G, Sorensen SV, Revicki D, et al: Atopic dermatitis is associated with a decrement in health-related quality of life. Int J Dermatol 41:151–158, 2002

Kissling S, Wuthrich B: Dermatitis in young adults: personal follow-up 20 years after diagnosis in childhood. Hautarzt 45:368–371, 1994

Kitamura H: A case of somatic delusional disorder that responded to treatment with risperidone (letter). Psychiatry Clin Neurosci 51:337, 1997

Koblenzer CS: Psychocutaneous Disease. Orlando, FL, Grune & Stratton, 1987

Kodama A, Horikawa T, Suzuki T, et al: Effect of stress on atopic dermatitis: investigation in patients after the Great Hanshin Earthquake. J Allergy Clin Immunol 104:173–176, 1999

Koo JYM, Smith LL: Psychologic aspects of acne. Pediatr Dermatol 8:185–188, 1991

Koo JYM, Shellow WVR, Hallman CP, et al: Alopecia areata and increased prevalence of psychiatric disorders. Int J Dermatol 33:849–850, 1994

Koran LM, Ringold A, Hewlett W: Fluoxetine for trichotillomania: an open clinical trial. Psychopharmacol Bull 28:145–149, 1992

Krahn LE, Goldberg RL: Psychotropic medications and the skin, in Psychotropic Drug Use in the Medically Ill. Edited by Silver PA. Basel, Switzerland, S Karger AG, 1994, pp 90–106

Lammintausta K, Kalimo K, Raitala R, et al: Prognosis of atopic dermatitis, a prospective study in early adulthood. Int J Dermatol 30:563–568, 1991

Leonard HL, Lenane MC, Swedo SE, et al: A double-blind comparison of clomipramine and desipramine treatment of severe onychophagia (nail biting). Arch Gen Psychiatry 48:821–827, 1991

Leung DYM, Tharp M, Boguniewicz M: Atopic dermatitis, in Fitzpatrick's Dermatology in General Medicine, 5th Edition. Edited by Freedberg IM, Eisen AZ, Wolff K, et al. New York, McGraw-Hill, 1999, pp 1464–1480

Liakopoulou M, Alifieraki T, Katideniou A, et al: Children with alopecia areata: psychiatric symptomatology and life events. J Am Acad Child Adolesc Psychiatry 36:678–684, 1997

Lienemann J, Walker FD: Reversal of self-abusive behavior with naltrexone (letter). J Clin Psychopharmacol 9:448–449, 1989

Lindskov R, Baadsgaard O: Delusions of infestation treated with pimozide: a follow-up study. Acta Derm Venereol 65:267–270, 1985

Lyell A: Cutaneous artifactual disease: a review amplified by personal experience. J Am Acad Child Adolesc Psychiatry 1:391–407, 1979

Lyell A: Delusions of parasitosis. Br J Dermatol 108:485–499, 1983

Lyketsos GC, Stratigos J, Tawil G, et al: Hostile personality characteristics, dysthymic states and neurotic symptoms in urticaria, psoriasis and alopecia. Psychother Psychosom 44:122–131, 1985

Maeda K, Yamamoto Y, Yasuda M, et al: Delusions of oral parasitosis. Prog Neuropsychopharmacol Biol Psychiatry 22:243–248, 1998

Manschreck TC: Delusional disorder: the recognition and management of paranoia. J Clin Psychiatry 57:32–38, 1996

McElroy SL, Phillips KA, Keck PE, et al: Body dysmorphic disorder: does it have a psychotic subtype? J Clin Psychiatry 54:389–395, 1993

McElroy SL, Phillips KA, Keck PE: Obsessive compulsive spectrum disorder. J Clin Psychiatry 55:33–51, 1994

McKenna KE, Stern RS: The impact of psoriasis on the quality of life of patients from the 16-center PUVA follow-up cohort. J Am Acad Dermatol 36:388–394, 1997

Monk BE, Rao YJ: Delusions of parasitosis with fatal outcome. Clin Exp Dermatol 19:341–342, 1994

Morley WN: Nortriptyline in the treatment of chronic urticaria. Br J Clin Pract 23:305–306, 1969

Morren MA, Przybilla B, Bamelis M, et al: Atopic dermatitis: triggering factors. J Am Acad Dermatol 31:467–473, 1994

Morris M: Delusional infestation. Br J Psychiatry 159:83–87, 1991

Moussavian H: Improvement of acne in depressed patients treated with paroxetine. J Am Acad Child Adolesc Psychiatry 40:505–506, 2001

Munro A: Monosymptomatic hypochondriacal psychosis manifesting as delusions of parasitosis: a description of four cases treated with pimozide. Arch Dermatol 114:940–943, 1978

Nel M, Schoeman JP, Lobetti RG: Delusions of parasitosis in clients presenting pets for veterinary care. J S Afr Vet Assoc 72:167–169, 2001

Ninan PT, Knight B, Kirk L, et al: A controlled trial of venlafaxine in trichotillomania: interim phase I results. Psychopharmacol Bull 34:221–224, 1998

Ninan PT, Rothbaum BO, Marsteller FA, et al: A placebo-controlled trial of cognitive-behavioral therapy and clomipramine in trichotillomania. J Clin Psychiatry 61:47–50, 2000

O'Donnell BF, Lawlor F, Simpson J, et al: The impact of chronic urticaria on the quality of life. Br J Dermatol 136:197–201, 1997

Olsen EA: Disorders of epidermal appendages and related disorders, in Fitzpatrick's Dermatology in General Medicine, 5th Edition. Edited by Freedberg IM, Eisen AZ, Wolff K, et al. New York, McGraw-Hill, 1999, pp 729–751

Opler LA, Feinberg SS: The role of pimozide in clinical psychiatry. J Clin Psychiatry 52:221–233, 1991

Perini GI, Fornasa CV, Cipriani R, et al: Life events and alopecia areata. Psychother Psychosom 41:48–52, 1984

Perini G, Zara M, Cipriani R, et al: Imipramine in alopecia areata: a double-blind, placebo-controlled study. Psychother Psychosom 61:195–198, 1994

Peterson AL, Campise RL, Azrin NH: Behavioral and pharmacological treatments for tic and habit disorders: a review. J Dev Behav Pediatr 15:430–441, 1994

Phillips KA: Body dysmorphic disorder: diagnosis and treatment of imagined ugliness. J Clin Psychiatry 57:61–65, 1996

Phillips KA, Taub SL: Skin picking as a symptom of body dysmorphic disorder. Psychopharmacol Bull 31:279–288, 1995

Phillips KA, McElroy SL, Keck PE, et al: Body dysmorphic disorder: 30 cases of imagined ugliness. Am J Psychiatry 150:302–308, 1993

Phillips KA, McElroy SL, Keck PE, et al: A comparison of delusional and nondelusional body dysmorphic disorder in 100 cases. Psychopharmacol Bull 30:179–186, 1994

Phillips KA, McElroy SL, Hudson JI, et al: Body dysmorphic disorder: an obsessive-compulsive spectrum disorder, a form of affective spectrum disorder, or both? J Clin Psychiatry 56:41–51, 1995

Phillips KA, Dufresne RG, Wilkel CS, et al: Rate of body dysmorphic disorder in dermatology patients. J Am Acad Dermatol 42:436–441, 2000

Phillips KA, Albertini RS, Rasmussen SA: A randomized placebo-controlled trial of fluoxetine in body dysmorphic disorder. Arch Gen Psychiatry 59:381–388, 2002

Picardi A, Abeni D: Stressful life events and skin diseases: disentangling evidence from myth. Psychother Psychosom 70:118–136, 2001

Pigott TA, L'Heueux F, Grady TA, et al: Controlled comparison of clomipramine and fluoxetine in trichotillomania, in Abstracts of Panels and Posters of the 31st Annual Meeting of the American College of Neuropsychopharmacology, San Juan, Puerto Rico, December 1992

Price V: Alopecia areata: clinical aspects. J Invest Dermatol 96:68, 1991

Pylko T, Sicignan J: Nortriptyline in the treatment of a monosymptomatic delusion (letter). Am J Psychiatry 142:1223, 1985

Rahman MA, Gregory R: Trichotillomania associated with HIV infection and response to sertraline (letter). Psychosomatics 36:417–418, 1995

Rajka G: Essential Aspects of Atopic Dermatitis. Berlin, Germany, Springer, 1989

Rapp SR, Lyn Exum M, Reboussin DM, et al: The physical, psychological and social impact of psoriasis. Br J Health Psychol 2:525–537, 1997

Rapp SR, Feldman SR, Exum ML, et al: Psoriasis causes as much disability as other major medical diseases. Am Acad Dermatol 41:401–407, 1999

Ratnoff OD: Psychogenic purpura (autoerythrocyte sensitization): an unsolved dilemma. Am J Med 87:16–21, 1989

Ravindran AV, Lapierre YD, Anisman H: Obsessive-compulsive spectrum disorders: effective treatment with paroxetine. Can J Psychiatry 44:805–807, 1999

Raychaudhuri SP, Rein G, Farber EM: Neuropathogenesis and neuropharmacology of psoriasis. Int J Dermatol 34:685–693, 1995

Reid TL: Treatment of generalized anxiety disorder and trichotillomania with buspirone (letter). Am J Psychiatry 149:573–574, 1992

Reid TL: Treatment of resistant trichotillomania with paroxetine (letter). Am J Psychiatry 151:290, 1994

Richards HL, Fortune DG, Griffiths CEM, et al: The contribution of perceptions of stigmatization to disability in patients with psoriasis. J Psychosom Res 50:11–15, 2001

Rosenbaum MS, Ayllon T: The behavioral treatment of neurodermatitis through habit-reversal. Behav Res Ther 19:313–318, 1981

Rothe MJ, Grant-Kels JM: Atopic dermatitis: an update. J Am Acad Dermatol 35:1–13, 1996

Rubino IA, Sonnino A, Pezzarossa B, et al: Personality disorders and psychiatric symptoms in psoriasis. Psychol Rep 77:547–553, 1995

Rubinow DR, Peck GL, Squillace KM, et al: Reduced anxiety and depression in cystic acne patients after successful treatment with oral isotretinoin. J Am Acad Dermatol 17:25–32, 1987

Ruiz-Doblado S, Carrizosa A, Garcia-Hernandez MJ, et al: Selective serotonin re-uptake inhibitors (SSRIs) and alopecia areata. Int J Dermatol 10:798–799, 1999

Savin JA, Paterson WD, Adam K, et al: Effects of trimeprazine and trimipramine on nocturnal scratching in patients with atopic eczema. Arch Dermatol 115:313–315, 1979

Schlosser S, Black DW, Blum N, et al: The demography, phenomenology, and family history of 22 persons with compulsive hair pulling. Ann Clin Psychiatry 6:147–152, 1994

Schultz Larson F: Atopic dermatitis: a genetic-epidemiologic study in a population-based twin sample. J Am Acad Dermatol 28:719–723, 1993

Sentürk V, Tanrtverdi N: Resistant trichotillomania and risperidone (letter). Psychosomatics 43:429–430, 2002

Sheehan-Dare RA, Henderson MJ, Cotterill JA: Anxiety and depression in patients with chronic urticaria and generalized pruritus. Br J Dermatol 123:769–774, 1990

Shelley WB, Shelley ED: Adrenergic urticaria: a new form of stress-induced hives. Lancet 2:1031–1033, 1985

Sherman MD, Holland GN, Holsclaw DS, et al: Delusions of ocular parasitosis. Am J Ophthalmol 125:852–856, 1998

Shertzer CL, Lookingbill DP: Effects of relaxation therapy and hypnotizability in chronic urticaria. Arch Dermatol 123:913–916, 1987

Simeon D, Stein DJ, Gross S, et al: A double-blind trial of fluoxetine in pathologic skin picking. J Clin Psychiatry 58:341–347, 1997

Slaughter JR, Zanol K, Rezvani H, et al: Psychogenic parasitosis. Psychosomatics 39:491–500, 1998

Sneddon I, Sneddon J: Self-inflicted injury: a follow-up study of 43 patients. BMJ 2:527–530, 1975

Songer DA, Roman B: Treatment of somatic delusional disorder with atypical antipsychotic agents. Am J Psychiatry 153:578–579, 1996

Soter NA: Urticaria and angioedema, in Fitzpatrick's Dermatology in General Medicine, 5th Edition. Edited by Freedberg IM, Eisen AZ, Wolff K, et al. New York, McGraw-Hill, 1999, pp 1409–1418

Sperber J, Shaw J, Bruce S: Psychological components and the role of adjunct interventions in chronic idiopathic urticaria. Psychother Psychosom 51:135–141, 1989

Spraker MK: Cutaneous artifactual disease: an appeal for help. Pediatr Clin North Am 30:659–668, 1983

Stanley MA, Breckenridge JK, Swann AC, et al: Fluvoxamine treatment of trichotillomania. J Clin Psychopharmacol 17:278–283, 1997

Stein DJ, Hollander E: Dermatology and conditions related to obsessive-compulsive disorder. J Am Acad Dermatol 26:237–242, 1992a

Stein DJ, Hollander E: Low-dose pimozide augmentation of serotonin reuptake blockers in the treatment of trichotillomania. J Clin Psychiatry 53:123–126, 1992b

Stein DJ, Hutt CS, Spitz JL, et al: Compulsive picking and obsessive-compulsive disorder. Psychosomatics 34:177–181, 1993

Stein DJ, Mullen L, Islam MN, et al: Compulsive and impulsive symptomatology in trichotillomania. Psychopathology 28:208–213, 1995a

Stein DJ, Simeon D, Cohen LJ, et al: Trichotillomania and obsessive-compulsive disorder. J Clin Psychiatry 56:28–34, 1995b

Stein DJ, Bouwer C, Maud CM: Use of the selective serotonin reuptake inhibitor citalopram in treatment of trichotillomania. Eur Arch Psychiatry Clin Neurosci 247:234–236, 1997

Stocker WW, McIntyre OR, Clendenning WE: Psychogenic purpura. Arch Dermatol 113:606–609, 1977

Stout RJ: Fluoxetine for the treatment of compulsive facial picking (letter). Am J Psychiatry 147:370, 1990

Strauss JS, Thiboutot DM: Diseases of the sebaceous glands, in Fitzpatrick's Dermatology in General Medicine, 5th Edition. Edited by Freedberg IM, Eisen AZ, Wolff K, et al. New York, McGraw-Hill, 1999, pp 769–784

Streichenwein SM, Thornby JI: A long-term, double-blind, placebo-controlled crossover trial of the efficacy of fluoxetine for trichotillomania. Am J Psychiatry 152:1192–1196, 1995

Swedo SE, Leonard HL: Trichotillomania: an obsessive compulsive spectrum disorder? Psychiatr Clin North Am 15:777–790, 1992

Swedo SE, Leonard HL, Rapoport JL, et al: A double-blind comparison of clomipramine and desipramine in the treatment of trichotillomania (hair pulling). N Engl J Med 321:497–501, 1989

Swedo SE, Rapoport JL, Leonard HL, et al: Regional cerebral glucose metabolism of women with trichotillomania. Arch Gen Psychiatry 48:828–833, 1991

Toyoda M, Makino T, Kagoura M, et al: Expression of neuropeptide-degrading enzymes in alopecia areata: an immunohistochemical study. Br J Dermatol 144:46–54, 2001

Trabert W: 100 years of delusional parasitosis: meta-analysis of 1,223 case reports. Psychopathology 28:238–246, 1995

Twohig MP, Woods DW, Marcks BA, et al: Evaluating the efficacy of habit reversal: comparison with a placebo control. J Clin Psychiatry 64:40–48, 2003

Uehara M, Kimura C: Descendant family history of atopic dermatitis. Acta Derm Venereol 73:62–63, 1993

van Minnen A, Hoogduin KAL, Keijsers GPJ, et al: Treatment of trichotillomania with behavioral therapy or fluoxetine. Arch Gen Psychiatry 60:517–522, 2003

Vittorio CC, Phillips KA: Treatment of habit-tic deformity with fluoxetine. Arch Dermatol 133:1203–1204, 1997

Welkowitz LA, Held JL, Held AL: Management of neurotic scratching with behavioral therapy. J Am Acad Dermatol 21: 802–804, 1989

Westling L: Fingernail biting. Cranio 6:182–187, 1988

Williams HC: Is the prevalence of atopic dermatitis increasing? Clin Exp Dermatol 17:385–391, 1992

Williams HC: On the definition and epidemiology of atopic dermatitis. Dermatol Clin 13:649–657, 1995

Winchel RM, Jones JS, Stanley B, et al: Clinical characteristics of trichotillomania and its response to fluoxetine. J Clin Psychiatry 53:304–308, 1992

Woodruff PWR, Higgins EM, du Vivier AWP, et al: Psychiatric illness in patients referred to a dermatology-psychiatry clinic. Gen Hosp Psychiatry 19:29–35, 1997

Wykoff RF: Delusions of parasitosis: a review. Rev Infect Dis 9:433–437, 1987

Zachariae R, Øster H, Bjerring P, et al: Effects of psychologic intervention on psoriasis: a preliminary report. J Am Acad Dermatol 34:1008–1015, 1996

Zook F: Complications of the perionychium. Hand Clin 2:407–442, 1986

30 Surgery

Pauline S. Powers, M.D.

Carlos A. Santana, M.D.

SURGICAL PATIENTS OFTEN have preexisting psychiatric disorders, and a range of psychosocial problems may become evident after surgery. Estimates of the prevalence of psychiatric problems in surgical patients range from 15% to 50% (Kain et al. 2002; Strain 1982). Although surgeons report lower-than-actual frequencies of various psychiatric disorders in their patients than do other nonpsychiatric physicians, the difference between the medical and the surgical specialties is low (Chadda 2001). Surgeons are also less likely to refer patients to psychiatrists than are other physicians, who themselves generally underestimate the prevalence of psychiatric disorders among their patients. Thus, a large proportion of psychopathology in surgical patients is either undiagnosed or misdiagnosed.

In the hospital, psychiatrists provide consultations for patients on general surgical floors, but they are more likely to provide liaison services to specialized surgical units such as burn units or organ transplant programs. Consultations for general surgical patients often involve preoperative issues such as consent for surgery, fear of anesthesia or surgery, or management of preexisting psychiatric disorders during hospitalization. Postoperative hospital consultations are often initiated for assessment and treatment of delirium or behavior problems. On specialized surgical units, the psychiatrist is likely to provide classic liaison services, including teaching other members of an interdisciplinary team to recognize and manage various psychiatric and psychological problems unique to the unit.

General Issues

Open, Closed, and Random Systems

The general surgical unit and specialized units often have significant differences in operational style. Systems theory can be helpful in understanding these differences (Luhmann and Knodt 1995). An *open system* has regular members who belong to the system and flexible rules about entering and leaving the system. In the *closed system*, only certain individuals can come into and go out of the system, and "outsiders" are excluded from the system. In *random systems*, individuals move into and out of the system at random, with few rules about how entry and exit occur.

Most general surgical units are open systems, and some poorly functioning ones are random systems. Specialized units, such as burn units, are often closed systems with very rigid rules about entering or leaving the system. Because hospital consultations are usually one to three sessions, it is important that the consultant be able to move easily into and out of the system. This is possible in the open systems typically present on general surgical floors. However, communication with the consultee may require significant effort on the part of the consultant, who may have to track down the consulting surgeon (who may be in the operating room all day); this problem is accentuated on a ward that tends toward randomness. In contrast, the psychiatrist who provides liaison to a closed specialized unit will need to be well known to the team and be a regular attendee at team meetings. Communication within the closed system may be easier because all members are likely to accept recommendations from another member of the team.

Outpatient Consultation-Liaison Services

In the outpatient department, the psychiatrist may be an integral part of a specialized team. For example, bariatric surgery teams typically rely on a presurgical psychiatric assessment of patients to determine whether the patient is an appropriate candidate for surgery; the psychiatrist also may participate in the long-term follow-up of the patient after bariatric surgery. This type of psychiatry requires detailed knowledge of the unique risks and benefits of the proposed surgery.

Other consultations from surgery in the outpatient department are often related to complex problems in which the patient has multiple comorbid psychiatric, surgical, and medical problems. Outpatient consultations sometimes relate to transferential or countertransferential problems between the surgeon and the patient.

Transference and Countertransference

Transference is defined as the set of emotional reactions that a patient has toward the surgeon: these reactions are shaped by previous relationships with important people in the life of the patient and may facilitate or inhibit the relationship with the surgeon. Relationships with parents and others in authority typically influence current reactions to the surgeon. For example, a surgical candidate who has had a trusting relationship with parents and positive experiences with physicians is likely to approach surgery calmly and to be able to discuss options openly with the surgeon. However, a patient who grew up with harsh, controlling, and demanding parents, and who also has had negative interactions with physicians, is more likely to be suspicious of the surgeon and fearful of the surgery. Recognition of the likely source of the patient's reactions to the surgeon is the key to managing these reactions. For example, if a new patient is suspicious and unduly fearful of a usually safe surgical procedure, it may be helpful to give the patient time to discuss the procedure with a trusted partner or friend and then offer to explain the procedure to this person while the patient is present.

Surgeons, like other physicians, may have countertransference reactions to their patients. Clues to negative countertransferential reactions to the patient include feelings of anger, irritability, sadness, or boredom. In these situations, it is often helpful for the surgeon to ask him- or herself: "Why am I (angry, sad, or bored or overly involved with this patient)?" The answer may be that the patient has elicited feelings related to another situation in the surgeon's life. Recognition of this fact usually allows the surgeon to refocus on the patient. An example might be an overly solicitous response to a woman shot by an abusive husband; it might be that in this situation, the surgeon was reminded of his own abusive father. Another example is the surgeon who is angry because a patient fails to improve after multiple back surgeries. This reaction may relate to the surgeon's un-

recognized and unrealistic grandiose belief that she can conquer any problem.

Staff Coping Mechanisms

Certain surgical situations, such as traumas and burns, particularly among children, elicit powerful emotional responses from the surgeons and nurses working with these patients and their families (Wetzel and Burns 2002). A. Jones (2001) poignantly described the reaction of a patient and her husband to life-threatening surgery and commented that the "impact of physical illness is such that there is potential for the seriously ill to saturate health workers in anxiety and raw feelings" (p. 459). To protect themselves emotionally, the surgeon or nurse may ignore the emotional needs of the patient (and family) and focus solely on the physical aspects of care.

To be able to function effectively, the surgeon must be able to maintain defense mechanisms, including, when appropriate, isolation of affect, denial, humor, and suppression. Treatment team members, including psychiatrists, psychologists, and chaplains, may be able to cope more effectively with the feelings emanating from the patient because they do not have to perform surgery. Although surgeons are often blamed for not attending to the emotional needs of their patients, it may be that it is not usually possible both to fully empathize with the feelings of the patient and to maintain the objectivity needed to perform surgery. Thus, the emotional needs of both the surgeon and the patient must be respected.

Role of the Family

The effect of the family on the patient's experience with surgery and on long-term recovery is known to be very important.

Qualitative research methods including narratives have been evaluated to understand the experience of the perioperative phase of treatment (Angus 2001; Wyness et al. 2002). A consistent theme from these reports is that for the patient and the family, knowing is better than not knowing. Another consistent theme is that specific information about various surgical strategies and their possible outcomes is important but should be delivered in a way that recognizes the time needed for assimilation (Bunch 2000). Patients and their families are now able to access information in a variety of ways, notably the Internet, and many know details of various surgical critical care pathways. If the patient does not improve as expected on the critical pathway, the family may experience significant stress. Family support groups may be helpful in such situations (Micik and Borbasi 2002).

General Conceptual Model

To conceptualize the problems requiring psychiatric intervention, the perioperative period can be divided into preoperative, intraoperative, and postoperative periods. Although these periods are considered separately because special strategies and different personnel may be required in each, the connection between preoperatively identified psychiatric problems and outcome of surgery has been a topic widely studied. For example, in a study of patients with severe low back pain who underwent surgery, low presurgical neuroticism scores were associated with better postoperative functional improvement (Hagg et al. 2003). In another study of patients with gastroesophageal reflux disorder undergoing laparoscopic antireflux surgery (Kamolz et al. 2003), all the patients had normalized physiological findings after surgery, but the patients with comorbid major depression had significantly more symptoms of postoperative dysphagia and had less improvement in quality of life than did the patients without depression.

Psychiatry is often consulted in the preoperative period around the issues of consent for treatment or refusal of surgery and may be consulted at any time when the patient threatens to sign out against medical advice (AMA). Preexisting psychiatric disorders and their management often are also the reason for psychiatric consultation. Fear of surgery, anesthesia, needles, or machines may result in preoperative panic and necessitate urgent psychiatric intervention.

With the emergence of outpatient surgery and use of drugs that induce a lighter stage of anesthesia, some patients may recall events from the intraoperative period. Psychiatric consultation may be needed to assist the patient in coping with these memories.

In the postoperative period, delirium (including withdrawal from various substances) is a very common cause for consultation. Agitation and management problems are also common. Patients who were admitted because of trauma (including burns) may begin to develop symptoms of posttraumatic stress disorder (PTSD). Other issues in this period include ventilator weaning and the "intensive care unit (ICU) syndrome."

General Preoperative Issues

Capacity and Consent

The ethical practice of surgery requires a patient's voluntary informed consent. In some instances, however, direct consent is impossible, and surgeons seek permission from surrogates or guidance from written advance directives. Informed consent and decision making are at the core of the preoperative period. The communication of factual information understandable to the patient is the responsibility of the surgeon. It should include diagnosis, reasons that the operation is thought to be the treatment of choice, and expected risks and benefits and their probabilities. Alternatives and their consequences, as well as financial costs, also should be discussed. Competent patients have a right to decide whether to accept or reject proposed surgery. A psychiatric consultant cannot legally declare a patient incompetent, but he or she can evaluate the medical-legal elements of the decision-making capacity of the patient. Examiners must be aware of the legal standards governing determination of competence in their jurisdiction.

The assessment also includes a determination of the cause of the patient's limitation (i.e., the nature of the mental disorder) and the recommendations for treatment, if treatment is possible. The general principles regarding legal and ethical aspects of capacity and consent are discussed in Chapter 3, "Legal Issues," and Chapter 4, "Ethical Issues."

Preoperative Psychiatric Evaluation

The preoperative period is the time to obtain a psychiatric history. Patients with a history of anxiety disorder, depression, bipolar disorder, or psychosis are at risk for experiencing symptoms of these disorders during the postoperative period. Knowing what medications have been effective or not tolerated in the past is obviously valuable. Certain personality disorders and traits are known to predispose to behavior problems during the postoperative period.

When a surgeon requests a psychiatric consultation, the consultant should establish the urgency. Surgical patients seldom initiate or request a psychiatric consultation and may even assume an adversarial attitude toward the consultant.

However, one of the most common reasons for the underreferral of surgical inpatients is lack of recognition (or dismissal) of psychological distress by the surgical team. In some cases, surgical inpatients have felt the need to refer themselves for psychiatric evaluation of anxiety, although the surgical staff did not consider their anxiety sufficient to warrant a consultation (Fulop and Strain 1985). On the other hand, inappropriate or premature psychiatric consultation sometimes occurs when a patient expresses normal feelings (e.g., starts to cry) that the surgeon finds uncomfortable. One of the psychiatrist's major tasks is establishing a relationship with the referring surgeon, who may or may not be knowledgeable about psychiatric issues.

Psychiatric Disorders in the Perioperative Period

Depression

The proportion of patients taking antidepressants who undergo surgery is reported to be 35% (Scher and Anwar 1999). In the past, when monoamine oxidase inhibitors (MAOIs) were more frequently prescribed, it was common to discontinue antidepressants prior to general anesthesia. This is no longer the case. In their study of 80 depressed patients who were scheduled to undergo orthopedic surgery under general anesthesia, Kudoh and colleagues (2002) determined that antidepressants administered to depressed patients should be continued. Their group concluded that discontinuation of antidepressants did not increase the incidence of hypotension or arrhythmias during anesthesia, but discontinuation increased the symptoms of depression and delirium.

Schizophrenia

The management of schizophrenic patients requiring surgery can be difficult. Bizarre behavior and expression by schizophrenic patients can confuse and upset surgeons, nurses, and other patients, eliciting fear, anger, and nontherapeutic responses. Patients with paranoid delusions may refuse surgery because of psychotic misperception of the surgeon's intentions. Schizophrenic patients also often have deficits in the processing of cognitive or sensory information and concrete reasoning. These deficits may complicate the consent process and the patient's ability to cooperate with treatment, requiring the staff to make changes in management (Adler and Griffith 1991).

Bipolar Disorder

The stress of surgery may psychologically and physiologically destabilize bipolar disorder, and acute relapse into mania in the postoperative period can be extremely disruptive to care, even life-threatening. Periods without oral intake in the perioperative period preclude the use of lithium, anticonvulsants, antidepressants, and most antipsychotics, during which parenteral haloperidol serves as the primary substitute for mood stabilization. Abrupt discontinuation of anticonvulsant mood stabilizers risks causing seizures. Lithium is difficult to use safely during periods of rapid fluid shifts (e.g., after cardiac surgery and acute burns).

Preoperative Fears

An emerging literature has begun to systematically assess the nature and etiology of common fears, including fears of surgery, anesthesia, needles, and medical machines. The treatments that are likely to be effective are being studied, but current recommendations are based primarily on case reports or consensus rather than clinical trials (see also Chapter 12, "Anxiety Disorders").

Fear of Surgery and Anesthesia

Nearly 20 years ago, Regal and colleagues (1985) systematically assessed 150 patients before surgery and found that 54% were anxious or very anxious. Many patients were anxious about the anesthesia: patients often feared that the anesthetic would prematurely wear off or that they would not wake up from the anesthesia. Nearly one-third of patients are afraid of anesthesia, as distinct from the operation itself (vanWijk and Smalhout 1990).

It has been consistently shown that appropriate provision of information in an empathic relationship can reduce preoperative anxiety, postoperative pain, and length of hospital stay (Klafta and Roizen 1996; Koivula et al. 2002; Nelson 1996). Timing the delivery of information is important and may vary depending on the surgery. For example, among patients undergoing elective coronary artery bypass grafting, fear is highest during the waiting period prior to hospital admission. Providing support and information during this period produces the greatest benefit. Nurses have been in the forefront of devising methods for delivering these services, and the results of their investigations also can inform psychiatric practice.

Treatment of Preoperative Anxiety

Preoperative anxiety has been treated with antianxiety medications, particularly benzodiazepines. Although the Cochrane Database reviewers concluded that the use of benzodiazepines does not delay discharge after adult outpatient surgery, less is known about the actual clinical benefit of these medications for preoperative anxiety (Smith and Pittaway 2003). For example, in an outpatient surgery program, preoperative benzodiazepines were shown to decrease levels of stress hormones, but the actual effect on clinical anxiety was equivocal (Duggan et al. 2002). However, pediatric dental and oral surgery patients have been the most thoroughly studied, and most of these patients seem to benefit from use of benzodiazepines (see Erlandsson et al. 2001; Marshall et al. 1999). The difference in these findings may relate to differences in the subject populations (age, type of surgery), as well as the relatively greater sophistication of dental anxiety evaluation methods.

Although providing information and social support may be more time-consuming than prescribing an anti-anxiety agent, it may be more effective than medication in reducing preoperative anxiety and is likely to have postoperative benefits as well.

Children and Preoperative Anxiety

It is estimated that as many as 3 million children undergo anesthesia and surgery annually in the United States. Many children (40%–60%) experience significant anxiety before surgery. It has been postulated that postoperative outcome may be influenced by preoperative anxiety. Kain and colleagues (1996, 2002) emphasized the importance of educating parents about the possible negative behavioral responses that children may have after surgery. Figure 30–1 illustrates changes in the number of negative behavioral responses after surgery as a function of time. At 2 weeks postoperatively, most children had one to three negative behavioral responses, but only 7.6% had seven or more negative responses. By 1 year, only 7.3% of children had one to three negative responses, and no subjects had more than four negative responses. These authors describe preoperative preparation programs for parents and children but note that research is needed to validate their effectiveness in improving postoperative outcomes.

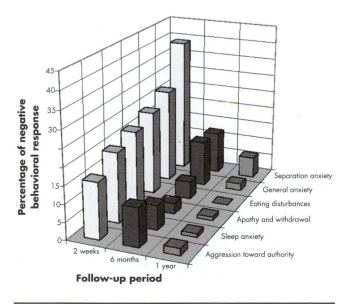

FIGURE 30–1. **Decreases in postoperative negative behavioral symptoms in children shown as a function of time.**

Source.   Reprinted from Kain ZN, Mayes LC, O'Connor TZ, et al.: "Preoperative Anxiety in Children: Predictors and Outcomes." *Archives of Pediatrics and Adolescent Medicine* 150:1238–1245, 1996. Used with permission.

Fear of Needles, Blood, and Medical Equipment

Fear of needles is common and may first arise in the preoperative period. Estimates of the prevalence of needle phobia have ranged from 10% to 21% (Hamilton 1995; Nir et al. 2003), but probably about 8%–10% of adults have unreasonable fears of needles that interfere with treatment. Needle phobia appears to be partly inherited (especially the vasovagal response that may result in fainting) and partly learned from conditioned responses, including past fainting spells when injected or after watching others be vaccinated (Hamilton 1995; Neale et al. 1994; Nir et al. 2003). Individuals who experience disgust in response to needles may be more likely to faint (Page 2002). Treatments for needle phobia have been primarily described in case reports and include behavioral strategies (exposure techniques and participant modeling), empathy from treating professionals, and anesthesia.

Fear of blood is closely related to fear of needles. There may be a genetic component to these fears as well. In a study of 541 monozygotic twins and 388 dizygotic twins in the Virginia Twin Registry, unreasonable fears of blood, needles, hospitals, and illness were correlated and showed family aggregation (Neale et al. 1994). Some patients are fearful of contracting HIV or hepatitis virus from blood transfusions (now a very rare occurrence) or from needles contaminated with blood (although this should never occur, except in very poor countries); correcting misconceptions and providing accurate information can be reassuring.

Blood refusal is common and is usually related to religious beliefs or fear of bloodborne infections. Because Jehovah's Witnesses and others have refused blood transfusions, there has been a rigorous pursuit of alternatives. Many surgeries previously thought to require transfusions are now routinely done without them. A recent study (Carson et al. 2002) of more than 2,000 postsurgical patients who refused blood found that the risk of death was low when the hemoglobin level was between 7.1 and 8.0 g/dL, but if postoperative levels fell below this range, the risk of death increased dramatically.

If the patient refuses blood, a careful psychiatric assessment may be needed to determine why the patient is refusing and whether the patient is competent to refuse treatment. For anxious patients, cognitive-behavioral interventions and benzodiazepines are helpful. If the patient is a child and the parents refuse transfusion on the basis of the parents' beliefs, legal and ethical consultation should be obtained, but the decision is usually to transfuse the child.

Fear of medical equipment is also common. Claustrophobia in a closed magnetic resonance imaging (MRI) device is the best described and may result in inability to obtain a scan. Use of an open MRI was shown to result in successful scans in 94% of 50 patients with claustrophobia who had been unable to tolerate the closed MRI (Spouse and Gedroyc 2000). Various coping strategies for the claustrophobia, including patient education and various relaxation techniques, are often helpful but have not been systematically investigated.

Intraoperative Issues— Anesthesia and Intraoperative Recall

The prospect of anesthesia can be frightening for many reasons, and some people envision anesthesia as a "death-like" state. Although patients expect to be amnestic for surgery, at the same time, they may fear the loss of control involved, or they may be afraid that they will not wake up from the anesthesia. Some fear that the anesthesia will wear off while the surgery is still under way. Patients also may fear that they will reveal secrets during anesthesia (Blacker 1987), even though this has not been shown during general anesthesia.

In 1992, Ghoneim and Block stated: "It is a sobering commentary that after 145 years it is not always possible to determine with certainty whether an anesthetized patient is conscious during surgery" (p. 296). This is still true more than a decade later despite multiple efforts to determine whether the patient is conscious. During the last decade, several studies have concluded that a small percentage of patients (perhaps 0.5%–2.5%) can explicitly recall events that occurred during surgery (Ranta et al. 2002). Although this is a small percentage, it has been estimated that 40,000 incidents occur per year (Maye and Smith 2001). Several factors are known to influence the likelihood of intraoperative recall, including type of anesthesia, type of preanesthetic, and depth of anesthesia.

Although relatively uncommon, intraoperative recall can be associated with marked psychiatric disability, including PTSD symptoms, especially flashbacks, nightmares, and preoccupation with the surgery. One traumatic component is the experience of total paralysis while aware. In a small series of 18 consecutive, prospectively identified cases of intraoperative awareness with recall, 9 patients were located 2 years later; 4 of the 9 were still severely psychiatrically disabled, and 2 had milder symptoms (Lennmarken et al. 2002). Furthermore, in a study of the American Society of Anesthesiologists Closed Claims Project (Domino et al. 1999), intraoperative awareness claims accounted for 1.9% of the 4,183 claims. Among

these, 18 claims were for the inadvertent paralysis of an aware patient, and the remaining 61 claims were for recall during general anesthesia.

It may not be possible to prevent all cases of intraoperative awareness because outpatient surgery is common and drugs that induce a lighter stage of anesthesia are often indicated. It is always prudent for the surgical team to avoid inappropriate comments that may be remembered by the patient. In addition, preparation of the patient for the unlikely possibility of intraoperative awareness may be helpful.

General Postoperative Issues

Alcohol Dependence

Chronic alcohol misuse is more common in surgical patients than in psychiatric or neurological patients. More than 50% of the patients with carcinoma of the gastrointestinal tract have alcohol dependence (Seitz and Simanowski 1986). Almost half of all trauma beds are occupied by patients who were injured while under the influence of alcohol (Gentilello et al. 1995; Spies et al. 1996). In addition to the life-threatening complications of the alcohol withdrawal syndrome, the rate of morbidity and mortality resulting from infections, cardiopulmonary insufficiency, and bleeding disorders is two to four times greater in patients with chronic alcoholism (Spies et al. 1997). The development of an alcohol withdrawal syndrome can change a normal postoperative course into a life-threatening situation in which the patient requires ICU treatment.

An alcohol-related history is frequently unobtainable in trauma patients because of their injuries (which may include closed head injury) and subsequent endotracheal intubation. Laboratory tests with sufficient sensitivity and specificity may assist in the diagnosis and possible prevention of complications (Sillanaukee 1996). If an ordinary alcohol history is not obtainable, the biological marker known as carbohydrate-deficient transferrin is a useful alternative. The carbohydrate-deficient transferrin correlates with alcohol consumption in surgical patients (Tønnesen et al. 1999).

Chronic alcohol intake may produce either enhanced or reduced sensitivity to anesthetics. The net effect varies with the amount of alcohol used, the relative affinity of alcohol and other drugs for the microsomal enzymes, and the severity of any underlying liver injury (Lieber 1995).

Alcohol dependence is often complicated by disorders such as cirrhosis, seizures, pancreatitis, polyneuropathy, or cardiomyopathy. It seems obvious that surgical interventions in an alcoholic patient with one or more of these disorders may be associated with increased morbidity and mortality. Increased risk of complications is seen after both minor and major surgery, as well as after elective and emergency procedures. In general, the risk of postoperative infections is related to decreased immune function and enhanced stress response to surgical trauma. This enhanced stress response is characterized by a greater release of stress hormones and catecholamines in patients with alcoholism compared with control subjects (Moesgaard and Lykkegaard-Nielsen 1989; Tønnesen et al. 1992). Alcoholic patients are at risk for excessive surgical blood loss secondary to coagulopathy from liver disease and platelet dysfunction. Many alcoholic patients are chronically malnourished, which retards wound healing.

Opioid Dependence

No evidence indicates that provision of appropriate doses of opiates for postoperative pain in the hospital creates addiction, yet some patients who fear becoming dependent decline or underuse postoperative opiates. If a surgical patient is receiving methadone maintenance, the dose used for maintenance should be continued throughout the surgical hospitalization. If the opioid-dependent patient does not have an established maintenance regimen, control of withdrawal can, in most cases, be achieved with methadone dosages of 10–30 mg/day. Once-daily dosing is usually sufficient to prevent withdrawal, but the total daily dose can be split into two or three doses to prevent breakthrough symptoms. If anesthesia is necessary, the anesthesiologist obviously should be provided with the history of the patient's opioid dependence. Pentazocine or other mixed agonist–antagonists such as buprenorphine are contraindicated for analgesia, because they might cause or worsen withdrawal because they compete with other opiates and block their effect.

Postoperative opiate-dependent patients require higher doses of opiates to control surgical pain because of tolerance. When such patients are given only "normal" doses, they complain of not receiving enough and often are considered to be inappropriately "drug-seeking" when in fact they are being undermedicated.

Postoperative Delirium

Postoperative delirium is very common, particularly in elderly patients undergoing certain types of surgery such as emergency repair of hip fractures, major gastrointestinal surgery, coronary bypass graft surgery, or lung transplant. Elderly orthopedic surgery patients have been the best studied, with rates of delirium higher than 40% documented

(Galanakis et al. 2001). Estimates of prevalence among post–cardiac surgery patients range from 2% to more than 30%, depending on several factors, including age, type of surgery, and whether the patient was on heart-lung bypass (Bayindir et al. 2000; Segatore et al. 1998). Delirium may be even more common and severe after certain procedures such as lung transplant (Craven 1990).

Risk Factors and Diagnosis

Multiple preoperative risk factors for postoperative delirium have been identified and include older age, alcohol use, cognitive impairment (especially the dementias), chronic comorbid illnesses and medications used to treat these illnesses, the severity of the acute illness, and the type of surgery (Flacker and Marcantonio 1998; Williams-Russo et al. 1992). Postoperative changes in the sleep–wake cycle (Kaneko et al. 1997), inadequately treated pain, and use of medications such as benzodiazepines increase the likelihood of delirium.

The diagnosis of delirium is discussed in detail in Chapter 6, "Delirium," and includes acute onset of changes in mental status, a fluctuating course, the presence of inattention, and an altered level of consciousness or disorganized thinking precipitated by a medical cause. Postoperative delirium usually is identified 2–5 days after surgery and typically, although certainly not always, resolves in about a week. Despite reliable methods for detecting delirium, it is often not diagnosed, or is misdiagnosed, particularly in the postoperative period.

Treatment

Psychiatrists are often consulted on an emergency basis for patients with postoperative delirium. Management is the same as that for other deliria, starting with an attempt to identify a remediable course. Although there is a general consensus on drug treatment of postoperative and other deliria, few controlled clinical trials have been done (see Chapter 6, "Delirium").

Recent controlled trials have examined interventions that might prevent postoperative delirium. In a Japanese study (Aizawa et al. 2002), half the patients were given diazepam for 3 days immediately following surgery to try to prevent disruption of their sleep–wake cycle; only 5% of the treated patients developed delirium compared with 35% of the nontreated group. This study contradicts the usual wisdom that benzodiazepines are contraindicated in delirium, but the diazepam was given at a particular time with the specific goal of maintaining a normal sleep–wake pattern after surgery. Tokita et al. (2001) found that better pain control through patient-controlled analgesia (compared with a fixed continuous regimen) reduced the incidence of delirium following hepatectomy. Spanish investigators studied the procholinergic drug citicoline for prevention of delirium after hip fracture but found no benefits (Diaz et al. 2001).

Controlled trials of nonpharmacological interventions also have been done. Geriatric consults, compared with usual care, for elderly patients admitted for hip fracture surgery were associated with less postoperative delirium (32% vs. 50%) and even greater improvement in cases of severe delirium (12% vs. 29%) (Marcantonio et al. 2001). A Dutch study found that a nurse-led interdisciplinary psychosocial intervention program for delirium in elderly patients with hip fractures reduced the length and severity, but not the incidence, of postoperative delirium, compared with usual care (Milisen et al. 2001).

Intensive Care Unit Psychosis

The concept of ICU psychosis emerged after Kornfeld and colleagues (1965) described a delirium that occurred in 38% of the patients in the recovery room after open-heart surgery. Their report noted several organic factors that they thought contributed to the delirium. Patients also were interviewed soon after they left the recovery room. Patients complained of lack of sleep and "the frightening environment, unusual sounds and sense of being chained" (p. 287). This article was very influential and resulted in many positive changes in the ICU environment, including adding windows (so that patients could determine whether it was day or night) and clocks within sight of the patients. It also became standard practice for the ICU staff to reorient patients and help them to understand ongoing procedures.

Despite the fact that the original authors emphasized that this was an acute organic psychosis influenced by environmental factors, the term *ICU psychosis* has come to imply that environmental factors are capable of inducing psychosis. It seems likely that environmental factors can worsen delirium caused by any of a variety of physiological factors, but psychosis resulting from solely a frightening environment occurs rarely, if ever. The danger of invoking the term *ICU psychosis* is that the underlying physiological cause of the postoperative delirium will be unrecognized and untreated. Thus, the psychiatric consultant to surgery may need to educate other medical personnel to diagnose and treat the underlying physiological cause of the delirium.

Discontinuation of Ventilator Support

A common problem in the surgical ICU is associated with discontinuation of ventilator support (ventilator weaning).

McCartney and Boland (1994) commented, "to be in respiratory distress is to be anxious. To be mechanically ventilated is to be grossly uncomfortable at best. To undergo weaning in the presence of possible severe respiratory compromise, again, inevitably is anxiety provoking" (p. 679). The objective clinical parameters for determining physiological readiness for ventilator weaning are well known (MacIntyre et al. 2001), but much less is known about psychological readiness for ventilator weaning.

Commonsense guidelines for determining psychological readiness for weaning from mechanical ventilation have been proposed (Blackwood 2000). These parameters include ensuring that the patient is oriented to person, place, date, and circumstances; is at mental ease; and has a positive mental attitude. An experienced ICU nurse who knows the patient may be able to determine when ventilator weaning is likely to progress successfully, and the nurse also may be able to recognize early signs of anxiety that will interfere with weaning. Multiple treatments have been proposed, including relaxation techniques, biofeedback, patient education, positive reinforcement, improvement of sleep–wake cycle, and incorporation of the family into the treatment team. A promising single case report described the successful use of several of these techniques (Jacavone and Young 1998), but only one randomized clinical trial has been completed (Holliday and Hyers 1990). In that trial, a control group receiving daily visits consisting of reassurance and attention was compared with the intervention group receiving daily relaxation biofeedback. The intervention group had statistically significantly fewer days from the start of ventilator weaning to completion than did the control group (17 vs. 20 days, $P=0.01$).

The effects of two drugs—midazolam (a short-acting benzodiazepine) and propofol (a sedative-hypnotic agent)—on ventilator weaning time have been widely studied. A recent meta-analysis found that among postoperative patients who had required sedation for less than 36 hours, ventilator weaning was faster with propofol (Walder et al. 2001). However, propofol was associated with an increased likelihood of hypotension and hypertriglyceridemia. An open-label study found that intravenous haloperidol might facilitate ventilator weaning, but several complications were associated with its use (Riker et al. 1994). In an open-label study of patients with DSM-IV–diagnosed depression (American Psychiatric Association 1994), methylphenidate (up to 15 mg/day) improved mood, and ventilator weaning was successful in five of seven patients treated (Rothenhausler et al. 2000). Methylphenidate was chosen because it has much faster onset of action and a shorter half-life compared with traditional antidepressants.

Posttraumatic Stress Disorder in the Postoperative Period

In the surgical arena, PTSD has been best studied in trauma patients (especially burn patients) and motor vehicle accident victims (Klein et al. 2003), but several recent studies have shown that a significant percentage of patients also develop PTSD following cardiac surgery or neurosurgery (Powell et al. 2002; Stoll et al. 2000). Although full syndromal PTSD develops in 18%–40% of adult patients after trauma, many more develop some of the symptoms of PTSD. Children who experience traumatic disfiguring injuries seem to be at particular risk, with up to 82% having some symptoms of PTSD 1 month after the trauma (Rusch et al. 2002). Quality of life is significantly impaired in patients who develop PTSD posttrauma or postsurgery compared with patients who do not develop PTSD (Zatzick et al. 2002).

Several studies have tried to identify factors that predict the emergence of PTSD (for review, see Tedstone and Tarrier 2003). As expected, better prior emotional adjustment and social support are relatively protective. However, contrary to expectation, the severity of the injury, or the severity of the illness requiring surgery, is not clearly correlated with the emergence of PTSD. Also, alcohol intoxication or concussion at the time of the trauma seems to decrease the likelihood of PTSD (perhaps because memory for the event is impaired). Furthermore, some patients with no apparent predisposing factors develop PTSD. The course of PTSD is not completely clear, but symptoms usually appear within the first week after a trauma and increase in intensity over the next 3 months. Perhaps the best predictor of PTSD at 1 year is the presence of symptoms during the acute hospitalization after a trauma (Zatzick et al. 2002). Although most studies show that symptoms decrease by 1 year, many patients continue to meet full criteria, and many more still have symptoms.

Diagnosis of acute stress disorder, PTSD's predecessor, can be difficult in surgical trauma or postoperative patients who manifest symptoms of delirium. For the diagnosis of PTSD, the duration criterion is often not met in hospitalized patients because of relatively brief hospital stays. Almost all patients who meet full criteria will have nightmares, but among patients with only some symptoms, the cluster of symptoms likely to be affected varies. For example, female burn victims with facial burns have been reported to have predominantly avoidance and emotional numbness symptoms (Fukunishi 1999), whereas reexperiencing and startle symptoms are more likely in other burn patients (Ehde et al. 1999).

Treatment of PTSD in medical settings is covered in Chapter 12, "Anxiety Disorders." Few studies of treatment of PTSD have been done specifically in surgical patients, but general principles appear applicable. Cognitive-behavioral therapy (CBT) has been shown to be more effective than a waiting-list control condition or supportive psychotherapy for PTSD among motor vehicle accident survivors (Blanchard et al. 2003). There is general agreement (although not much evidence) that psychotherapy should be the primary treatment of trauma-related PTSD in children and that the selective serotonin reuptake inhibitors should be adjunctive (Putnam and Hulsmann 2002).

Postoperative Pain

Unrelieved postoperative pain is still reported to be a common clinical problem, which may be related to inadequate routines for pain assessment (Sjostrom et al. 1997). Postoperative pain management remains suboptimal on surgical wards in many countries despite the availability of effective analgesics. New technologies for drug administration and clinical practice guidelines for pain management are now available (Stomberg et al. 2003). The appropriate and optimal use of analgesics is essential for the adequate management of postoperative pain. Greer and colleagues (2001) concluded that fear of addiction is not prevalent among postoperative patients, yet clinician education can further decrease the proportion of surgical patients who fear addiction to pain medication.

During the 1990s, the Joint Commission on Accreditation of Health Care Organizations (JCAHO) studied patterns of pain assessment and management and found that pain often was not recognized and was inadequately treated when it was diagnosed. Multiple reasons for this were identified, including an inappropriate fear of addiction. It was repeatedly documented that many doctors and nurses based clinical practice on myths and misconceptions about pain medications rather than on evidence-based research. Education was attempted to ensure that pain medication was used appropriately, but prescribing patterns did not change (see Summers 2001 for review of the development of these guidelines); consequently, the 1999–2000 JCAHO standards of pain management practice were modified (Curtiss 2001) (see also Chapter 36, "Pain").

Body Image and Surgery

Body image is the inner mental experience of one's body, with a neurological substrate, also influenced by prior life events and interactions with important people. All of the senses contribute to body image, but touch and kinesthesia are probably the most important. Whereas body image develops throughout life, the changes that occur during childhood, and particularly during adolescence, are relatively enduring. Nonetheless, there can be wide fluctuations in the experiencing of one's body, even over a few minutes. Adaptations to the new realities of the body (including aging, trauma, and surgical alteration) can occur, but a host of factors influence how readily these changes are incorporated. In three important surgical areas, body image is key to patient outcome: 1) amputation and the phenomenon of phantom limb pain; 2) change in body image that may occur after trauma or surgery, including cosmetic surgery; and 3) body image concerns in bariatric surgery patients.

Phantom limb is the experience of feeling as if an amputated part is still present. It was first described by Ambrose Paré (1649), a seventeenth-century surgeon. In the United States, more than 200,000 surgical amputations occur each year. Up to 70% of these patients experience phantom limb pain immediately after the amputation, and 50% still experience it 5 years later (Bloomquist 2001). The general agreement is that avoiding as much pain as possible prior to amputation decreases the likelihood of phantom limb pain, but other factors contribute as well. For example, phantom limb pain in burned children is more common after electrical injuries than after thermal injuries (Thomas et al. 2003). The exact etiology of both phantom limb and the pain that often accompanies it is complex and poorly understood. The body is schematically represented in the sensory motor cortex of the brain as a homunculus in which the hands and feet (among the most common body parts amputated) have more neural connections than do other body parts. Although investigations are studying the relation between phantom limb pain and various neural pathways, much remains to be understood. The occurrence of phantom limb pain has been shown to be associated with poorer health-related quality of life (van der Schans et al. 2002).

Body image can change after trauma or surgery. Trauma, as in the case of burn injures, may cause dramatic changes in the body that require significant adaptation and integration of the changes into a new body image. However, the ease with which this integration occurs is influenced more by premorbid adjustment and stage of development than by the actual total body surface area burned. Among changes that occur following surgery, recent work has shown that the type of surgery may influence body image outcome. For example, total abdominal hysterectomy is associated with greater body image dissatisfaction than is vaginal hysterectomy because of the abdominal scar (Gutl et al. 2002).

The literature on body image in obesity is extensive. Stunkard and Burt (1967) studied body image in obese in-dividuals who had lost significant weight. They found that these patients often misperceived themselves as still large and frequently had negative attitudes toward this misperception. The definition of body image in patients with eating disorders has evolved to divide body image into perceptual and attitudinal aspects. Most current studies of body image following bariatric surgery focus on one part of the attitudinal aspect of body image called *body satisfaction*.

General Determinants of Functional Outcome

Functional outcome includes the ability to carry out the activities of daily living, the ability to function in one's usual role, and satisfaction with life. These areas are currently being explored under the category of quality of life. Perhaps the most interesting finding is that the actual severity of the underlying trauma or surgery does not necessarily determine quality of life. For example, the total body surface area burned does not directly correlate with the likelihood of PTSD nor does the size of a scar necessarily correlate with posttrauma adjustment. It has been repeatedly reported that an adequate social support system is positively correlated with postsurgical and posttrauma adaptation.

A confluence of factors determines functional outcome. These factors include the condition requiring surgical intervention, presurgical psychiatric status, and surgical strategy. Other factors that may improve outcome include preparation of the patient and family for surgery, detection and management of preoperative fears, respectful attitude of the surgeon and operating room personnel during surgery, detection and appropriate treatment of pain, and detection and management of various psychiatric problems following surgery, including delirium and PTSD.

Specific Topics in Surgery

Burn Trauma

The experience of being seriously burned and the treatment that follows for the survivors is one of the most frightening and painful known to humanity. Perhaps because of this, several important concepts in psychiatry and medicine have been learned from the study of burn victims. For example, Erich Lindemann (1944/1994) described the evaluation and treatment of survivors, friends, and relatives of people who died in the Coconut Grove fire. He identified five major symptoms of normal grief: somatic distress, preoccupation with the image of the deceased, guilt, hostile reactions, and loss of patterns of conduct. These concepts continue to guide the detection and management of normal and pathological acute grief in burn units and elsewhere.

Imbus and Zawacki (1977) opened an ethical debate over prolongation of life that continues today. An unusual aspect of burns is that even mortally burned patients often have a lucid period that lasts for a few hours during which patients can participate in making decisions about their own care. For every severely burned patient, these investigators searched the literature to determine whether cases of survival had been reported, and, if not, they offered the patients a choice between a full therapeutic regimen and palliative care. They concluded that the mortality rate did not change but that this strategy increased the autonomy of patients and increased the empathy that they received. This report ignited a controversy that has grown to encompass all critical care: when is treatment futile, and who should decide?

In the United States, annually, thermal burns result in 1 million injuries, 4,500 deaths, 700,000 emergency department visits, and 45,000 general hospital admissions, half of which are to specialized burn centers (American Burn Association 2003). Patients with major burns should be treated in burn centers (Heimbach 2002). At present, the American Burn Association (1999) lists 139 burn care facilities in the United States and 17 in Canada. During the past 40 years, interdisciplinary burn centers have emerged, staffed by physicians, nurses, physical and occupational therapists, pain specialists, mental health professionals, social workers, and chaplains. Typically, the burn center is directed by either a general surgeon or a plastic surgeon.

Psychiatric Disorders Among Burn Patients

Many burn patients have preexisting psychiatric disorders, the most common of which are substance use disorders and mood disorders. The classic studies of adults by Andreasen and colleagues (1972) and of children by N.R. Bernstein (1976) led to the recognition that psychiatric problems are very common among burn patients. It is now known that about 35% of patients have an Axis I psychiatric disorder prior to the burn injury (Powers et al. 2000) and that 20%–30% of patients (many of whom do not have preexisting psychiatric disorders) develop full syndromal PTSD while in the hospital or after discharge (Powers et al. 1994b; Yu et al. 1999). In addition, many patients have preexisting maladaptive coping mechanisms or dysfunctional families, and these factors are known to contribute to poor functional outcomes.

The best-studied psychiatric topics in burn care include substance use disorders (particularly alcohol use), self-immolation, and PTSD. The neuropsychiatric consequences of electrical burn injuries also have been studied (Kelley et al. 1999). There are a few reports on the long-term psychiatric and functional consequences of burns in both children and adults. Several studies have tried to compare preburn adjustment and/or immediate postburn psychiatric status with outcome. The meaning and psychological importance of burn scars (particularly of the face, hands, and genital area) have been studied as well. Equally important in burn care is the delirium that frequently occurs during the acute-care phase. Psychiatric consultants also have described effective methods for the management of pain in burn patients (N.R. Bernstein 1976; Watkins et al. 1992).

One method of conceptualizing the psychiatric problems seen in burn patients is to envision a time sequence from preexisting psychiatric problems to problems that develop after the patient leaves the hospital. Thus, there are preexisting psychiatric disorders and psychosocial problems (including those that have resolved but may be rekindled by the trauma), problems that occur at the time of the injury, problems that emerge during acute hospitalization, and psychiatric disorders that develop after discharge from the hospital. The most common psychiatric problems at each time point are illustrated in Table 30–1.

Burns and substance use disorders.   Preinjury substance use disorders are common among burn victims. One study found that among 727 deaths from fires, blood alcohol assays were positive in 29%, with a mean blood-ethanol level of 193.9 mg/dL; 14.6% of the victims studied had positive results for other substances of abuse (Barillo and Goode 1996). Although 40% of the fatalities were in people younger than 11 or older than 70, 75% of the drug-positive and 58% of the ethanol-positive fatalities were in people between ages 21 and 50. The authors concluded that substance use disorders are a particular risk factor for death from fires in the middle-aged sector of the population.

Among patients who survive to be treated, several studies have attempted to identify the prevalence of alcohol intoxication, alcohol abuse, or alcohol dependence. One study (J.D. Jones et al. 1991) found that 27% were intoxicated at the time of the burn, and 90% of these were then identified as having an alcohol abuse diagnosis compared with 11% of the nonintoxicated burn patients. Other reports estimated the prevalence of alcohol abuse and dependence in patients with burn injuries between 6% and 11% (Powers et al. 1994a; Tabares and Peck 1997). However, L. Bernstein and colleagues (1992) reported

TABLE 30–1.   Phase of injury

	Resuscitative	Acute	Convalescent
Setting	Emergency department, intensive care unit, burn unit	Intensive care unit, burn unit	Hospital ward, home, rehabilitation facility
Surgical care	Fluid resuscitation, maintenance of vital signs, urine output, debridement of necrotic tissue, antibiotic therapy	Debridement, skin grafting and reconstructive surgery, physical therapy	Skin grafting and reconstructive surgery, physical therapy, occupational therapy
Patient response			
Physiological	Shock, initial decrease in renal function and increase in hepatic metabolism, varied acute serum protein changes with net decrease	Stabilization of vital signs with persistent hypermetabolism, increase in renal clearance, and decrease in hepatic oxidative metabolism; variable presence of bone marrow suppression	Hypermetabolic response present up to 1–2 years
Endocrine	Dramatic increase in endorphins, corticosteroids, and catecholamines	Persistent elevation in corticosteroids, decrease in endorphins	Unknown
Psychological	Denial, projection	Regression, mourning, coping	Coping, adjustment, transition to home
Psychiatric	Substance withdrawal, delirium, cognitive disorders, posttraumatic stress disorder	Pain syndromes, posttraumatic stress disorder, secondary mood disorders, adjustment disorders, delirium	Adjustment reactions, mood disorders, posttraumatic stress disorder, marital/family/work problems, alcohol abuse
Family response	Shock, denial, anticipatory mourning	Mourning, coping, anger, emotional support of patient	Adjustment and acceptance, transition to home and work
Psychiatric interventions	Pharmacotherapy, liaison with family and burn team	Psychotherapy, pharmacotherapy, behavior therapy	Psychotherapy, pharmacotherapy, marital and group therapies

Source.   Adapted from Bernstein LF: "Burn Trauma," in *Psychiatric Care of the Medical Patient*, Second Edition. Edited by Stoudemire A, Fogel B. New York, New York, Oxford University Press, 1993. Copyright 1993 by Oxford University Press, Inc. Used by permission of Oxford University Press, Inc.

that screening for alcohol problems with the usual blood screen or physician evaluation missed 70% of the patients who had positive test results for alcoholism on the CAGE questionnaire. Steenkamp and colleagues (1994) found that 57% of the patients had evidence of alcohol problems on the Michigan Alcoholism Screening Test, and of these patients, 57% thought that the use of alcohol had contributed to the accident.

Among burn patients who are identified as having alcohol or drug problems, referral for treatment occurs in fewer than half of the patients (Powers et al. 1994a), and among those who are referred, fewer than half accept treatment (Tabares and Peck 1997). Denial is a key defense mechanism in patients with substance use disorders, but the crisis of a burn trauma may be an opportunity to broach this defense. Psychiatrists (and other mental health consultants) on the burn unit are often in a unique posi-

tion to help burn patients relinquish the denial that prevents appropriate treatment. Alcohol use has been found to be associated with increased total body surface area burned, an increased likelihood of death, longer length of hospital stay, and, consequently, increased medical costs (J.D. Jones et al. 1991; Powers et al. 1994a).

Withdrawal symptoms from alcohol dependence are probably common during the acute-care phase but may be difficult to distinguish from other causes of delirium. The few available studies on this topic are case reports or case series. The best approach in a burn unit may be a standard withdrawal protocol with a relatively long-acting benzodiazepine (e.g., chlordiazepoxide). Because 90% of intoxicated burn patients abuse alcohol, and because the development of alcohol withdrawal can be particularly dangerous in a burn patient, a liberal approach to prescribing the withdrawal regimen among patients suspected of alcohol dependence is probably the safest course of treatment. Although intermittent administration of benzodiazepines, especially the short-acting types such as lorazepam, has been advocated, so many problems in the acute phase of burn care may obscure the presence of withdrawal symptoms that this may not be wise. Haloperidol is frequently added to the regimen for psychotic symptoms during withdrawal but should not be used alone.

Even though burn patients have a high rate of preexisting drug abuse, withdrawal from narcotics is less likely because most patients require narcotic treatment for pain. However, it is helpful to remember that these patients may require a larger dose of narcotics to suppress pain, and this larger dose should be provided.

Self-inflicted burn injuries.   The frequency of self-immolation varies widely from nation to nation. In India, for example, ritual self-immolation is a common problem (32% of married women with lethal burn injuries have self-inflicted the burn). Multiple sociopolitical problems (Kumar 2003) contribute to this high rate of self-immolation among married women in India. In Zimbabwe, 22% of the adult burn patients have been reported to have self-immolated; most of these patients are married women, and the most common reason for self-immolation is conflict in a love relationship (Mzezewa et al. 2000).

In the United States, the frequency of self-inflicted injuries among patients who are admitted to a burn center ranges from 0.067% to 9% (Daniels et al. 1991; Scully and Hutcherson 1983). Although political and cultural motivations for self-immolation may predominate in some cultures, in the United States, most severely burned patients admitted to burn centers have a preexisting Axis I psychiatric disorder, including major depression or schizophrenia. Substance abuse appears to increase the likelihood of a severe self-inflicted injury. Not all of these patients are actually suicidal. Patients with schizophrenia may be responding to command hallucinations.

Among patients who have inflicted less severe burns, personality disorders are common (Cameron et al. 1997), especially borderline personality disorder. The patient may continue to self-injure in the hospital and thereby pose a difficult management problem. The psychiatric consultant is often able to defuse these problems with judicious use of behavioral strategies known to be helpful for patients with borderline personality disorder (Wiechman et al. 2000). Close supervision may be required to prevent further self-harm when the patient moves from an ICU to a unit with less nursing supervision.

Patients who have self-inflicted their burn injuries often elicit intense countertransference reactions from the entire staff, including the psychiatric team. It is helpful to remember that most patients seen in the burn center who have self-inflicted their injuries have a chronic mental illness and that many patients cannot access appropriate psychiatric care. Burn center teams understand chronic medical illness and the need for expert treatment, and this "medical model" analogy may help them better understand and empathize with a patient who has chronic mental illness and who has self-inflicted a burn injury.

PTSD in burn patients.   PTSD occurs in a significant minority of patients who have been burned. Estimates range from 21% to 43% (Ehde et al. 2000; Powers et al. 1994b). The difficulties in estimating frequency were discussed earlier and are related to the confounding effects of delirium and the duration criterion requirement of 1 month. Many patients have been discharged from the hospital before a month elapses, and less severely injured patients may not be seen again, and thus a formal diagnosis is not made. Nonetheless, many patients do develop the full syndrome of PTSD, and many more have symptoms in the reexperiencing cluster even though they do not meet the other criteria. Some patients also have PTSD symptoms related to their treatment, especially the extreme pain inflicted during debridement and dressing changes. Some patients also remember psychotic experiences during the delirium that often occurs during the initial acute phase of treatment, and these memories may elicit symptoms of PTSD.

Several attempts have been made to identify factors that predispose to the emergence of PTSD in burn patients, but researchers have been unable to show an association between preinjury Axis I diagnoses and the emergence of PTSD. Fauerbach and colleagues (2000) found that the personality characteristic of neuroticism increased risk and that high extroversion was protective. Six independent risk and protective factors for PTSD were identified from assessments of 127 burn victims trapped in a ballroom fire (Maes et al. 2001). The odds of developing PTSD were increased with the number of previous traumas, a history of simple phobia, and a sense of loss of control. In contrast, odds were decreased with a sense of control, alcohol consumption, and alcohol intoxication. The duration of PTSD symptoms appears to be lengthy. For example, Taal and Faber (1998) found that 33% of 428 burn patients in the Netherlands continued to have PTSD symptoms 14–24 months after their injury.

Treatment of PTSD in burn patients is similar to treatment of PTSD in other patients and includes psychotherapeutic techniques and medication. Increasing a sense of control and alleviating pain in patients when they are being treated at the burn center also may prevent some PTSD symptoms.

Delirium and psychosis in burn patients.   Delirium during the acute care of severely burned patients is common, although this topic has not been thoroughly studied. In one unpublished report, one-fourth of the burn patients were noted to be psychotic during their initial acute hospitalization. Most of these patients had delirium related to sepsis, pain medication, or other organic factors (Powers 1996). Other causes of delirium in burn patients include hypoxia from smoke inhalation and massive fluid shifts and electrolyte imbalance, especially hyponatremia and hypophosphatemia. The psychotic symptoms that occur most often include hallucinations (often visual and not always distressing) and delusions. The delusions are often paranoid and frequently involve nursing care personnel. Because patients with delirium are disoriented, they frequently misinterpret events and then suspect treatment personnel of malevolent intent. It is often difficult to distinguish between pain, agitation, anxiety, and confusion in the ICU, and the psychiatric consultant is invaluable in this differentiation. The principles of treatment of delirium in the burn unit are the same as described earlier for postoperative delirium (see subsection "Postoperative Delirium").

Burn Pain Management

Pain in burn care arises from both the pain from various procedures, including dressing changes and burn wound debridement, and the background pain of the injury itself. The key concept in managing pain on the burn unit is to recognize that it is often undertreated, and this can result in worsening delirium, anxiety, and other management problems. Pain is undertreated for many reasons, but the most important reasons are an unrealistic fear of addiction (both by the patient and by the physician) and fear of respiratory compromise (which, at least in the intensive care portion of most burn centers, can be adequately managed by a knowledgeable, alert nursing staff). Burn wound debridement (in which the eschar is removed) is an excruciatingly painful procedure, and various techniques are now available to alleviate much of the pain. When sharp debridement (involving use of a scalpel) is needed, general anesthesia offers the greatest relief of pain and also may facilitate a more thorough debridement (Powers et al. 1993). Parenteral narcotics, especially intravenous morphine, is often preferable for blunt debridement (in which scalpels are not used) and dressing changes. A common error is not waiting the 10–15 minutes required for adequate distribution after intravenous injection before beginning blunt debridement. Intramuscular injections are often contraindicated because they may add to the pain, and sufficient injection sites may not be available.

The background pain of burn injuries is best managed with oral narcotics whenever possible. Fentanyl is often helpful for intermittent pain because it is short acting and will allow the patient to be awake to participate in various rehabilitation activities. Meperidine is usually contraindicated because it is relatively ineffective orally and may aggravate delirium. Benzodiazepines are often used to promote sedation and reduce anxiety, but the optimal dose is not known. They are often used inappropriately to treat pain. If pain is adequately managed and the patient has anticipatory anxiety, use of benzodiazepines is then very helpful.

Treatment of Burns in Children

Several psychosocial research teams have been particularly interested in the treatment of burned children (Martin-Herz et al. 2003; Stoddard et al. 2002). These groups have emphasized the importance of the developmental stage of the burned child and the need for careful age-appropriate assessment and treatment of pain and anxiety. Emerging studies indicate that appropriate management of pain partially predicts the long-term outcome for the child. For example, one study found that receiving higher levels of morphine in the hospital was associated with fewer PTSD symptoms at follow-up 6 months later (Saxe et al. 2001).

A guideline has been proposed for the management of pain and anxiety in children (Stoddard et al. 2002). It is based on intensity of care, whether the pain is background or procedural pain, and stage in the hospital (see Table 30–2). In designing this guideline, the focus was on safe, effective medications; a limited formulary; and nursing strategies to assess pain (with age-appropriate ratings). The guideline also was designed to contain explicit recommendations. This guideline has been used in a series of 125 pediatric patients and was associated with excellent to adequate control of both pain and anxiety in most patients most of the time. One major advantage of the guideline is that the most-recommended drugs (morphine and lorazepam) are well known to most physicians. Only the use of intravenous infusion of midazolam for background anxiety in mechanically ventilated acutely ill pediatric patients would require an anesthesiologist or a critical care specialist.

Although many psychological treatments may ultimately prove to be effective for children, several are not. For example, imagery-based interventions do not seem to help, and having a parent in the room during procedures seems to make the experience worse for the child (and probably for the parent) (Foertsch et al. 1998).

Several studies have attempted to assess outcome in burned children. On the basis of rather brief follow-ups of

TABLE 30–2. Guidelines for pain and anxiety management in children with burns

Patient category	Background pain	Background anxiety	Procedural pain	Procedural anxiety	Transition to next clinical state
Category 1: mechanically ventilated acute	Morphine sulfate intravenous infusion	Midazolam intravenous infusion	Morphine sulfate intravenous bolus	Midazolam intravenous bolus	Wean infusions 10%–20% per day and substitute nonmechanically ventilated guideline
Category 2: nonmechanically ventilated acute	Scheduled enteral morphine sulfate	Scheduled enteral lorazepam	Morphine sulfate enteral or intravenous bolus	Lorazepam intravenous or enteral bolus	Wean scheduled drugs 10%–20% per day and substitute chronic guideline
Category 3: chronic acute patient	Scheduled enteral morphine sulfate	Scheduled enteral lorazepam	Morphine sulfate enteral bolus	Lorazepam enteral bolus	Wean scheduled and bolus drugs 10%–20% per day to outpatient requirements and pruritus medications
Category 4: reconstructive surgical patient	Scheduled enteral morphine sulfate	Scheduled enteral lorazepam	Morphine sulfate enteral bolus	Lorazepam enteral bolus	Wean scheduled and bolus drugs to outpatient requirement

Source. Reprinted from Stoddard FJ, Sheridan RL, Saxe GN, et al.: "Treatment of Pain in Acutely Burned Children." *Journal of Burn Care and Rehabilitation* 23:135–156, 2002. Used with permission.

small groups of children, some have concluded that children do not develop significant long-term psychological or behavioral problems (e.g., Kent et al. 2000). However, in the thoughtful report by Stoddard et al. (1992), the rate of long-term depression in children appeared to be high. One important confounding factor is that many children who are burned have preexisting psychosocial problems that influence long-term outcome. Other factors accounting for the discrepancy in findings include differences in patient populations and the hypotheses and study methodologies. A better understanding of the long-term course of burned children will require multisite studies with larger numbers of children sharing similar characteristics.

Psychiatric Practice Guideline for Adults With Acute Burns

Although the evidence base is sparse, consensus guidelines have been developed for several areas of burn care, and a practice guideline has been proposed for the management of adult psychiatric disorders in burn patients during their initial hospitalization (Powers 2002). Figure 30–2 is an algorithm designed to guide the clinician in assessment and management of the burn patient with psychiatric problems.

Facial Disfigurement and Scars

The adaptation to facial disfigurement depends, in part, on the age at which the disfigurement occurs. Children with congenital disfigurement often encounter significant developmental difficulties and are frequently stigmatized by peers, adults, and health care personnel. These problems may be incorporated into an enduring negative sense of self. If the child has a strong social support system and receives well-informed physiological and psychological care, these problems can be mitigated.

The adjustment to facial disfigurement also depends on the patient's preexisting personality and mental defense mechanisms. In his classic book, N.R. Bernstein (1976) described variables critical to adaptation, including adaptive versus maladaptive defenses; active coping versus passive surrender; loving exchange versus rage; leading and comanaging treatment versus resisting treatment; and denial versus overawareness. For example, a patient who participates in managing his or her own care; who has a flexible, extensive repertoire of mental defense mechanisms; and who has loving exchanges with friends and family is likely to make a successful adjustment to facial disfigurement.

Irrespective of the cause of facial disfigurement, the objective nature of the disfigurement usually is not correlated with the patient's self-perception. For example, among

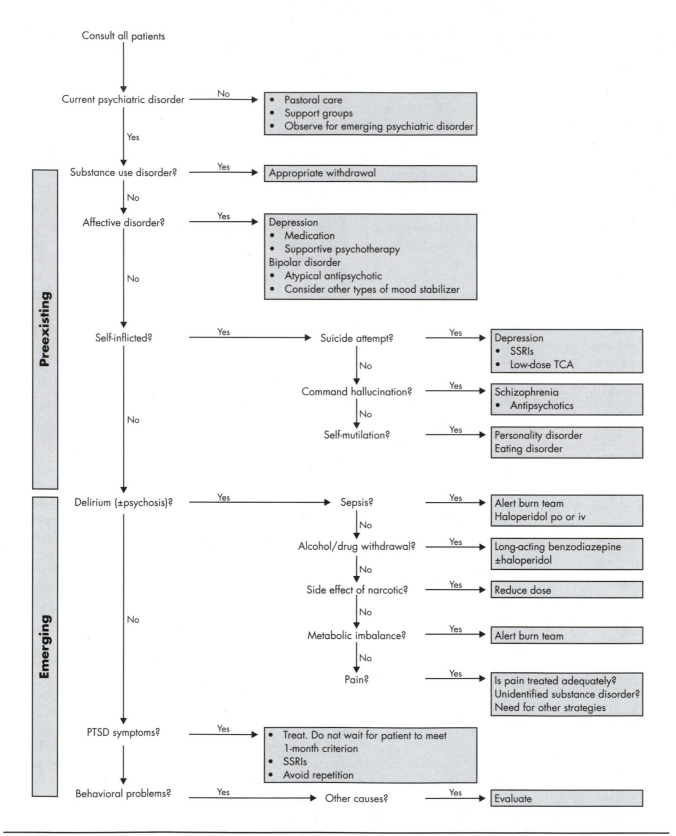

FIGURE 30–2.   Algorithm for the initial psychiatric assessment of the burn patient during the initial acute hospitalization.

Note.   PTSD=posttraumatic stress disorder; SSRI=selective serotonin reuptake inhibitor; TCA=tricyclic antidepressant.

50 patients who received extensive multidisciplinary treatment from birth to age 18 years for cleft palate, no correlation was found between the objective measure of the residual deformities and the patient's subjective judgment of the remaining deformity (Vegter and Hage 2001). Thus, the subjective assessment of the deformity is probably more important than the actual nature of the deformity in determining quality of life. Other factors that are important include proneness to shame, body image, and self-esteem (Van Loey and Van Son 2003).

Scars that develop after burn injuries can be very extensive. Scar tissue is different from normal skin and has an aberrant color, a rough surface texture, increased thickness, and decreased pliability and may be associated with pain or pruritus. Assessment of the various treatments for scars (including surgical treatments) has been limited by the difficulty in scar measurement. Developments in computer imaging may eventually permit the objective measurement of scars (Powers et al. 1999b; Tsap et al. 1998). However, even when better physiological treatments of scars are available, the subjective experience of the scar appears to be more important than the actual physical characteristics of the scar. Sarwer and colleagues (1998) reported that a subset of patients who underwent surgical revision of their scars had a level of dissatisfaction consistent with body dysmorphic disorder.

Despite the recognition that the *emotional* experience of the facial disfigurement is one of the primary determinants of quality of life, little research is available on possible interventions. An interesting pilot study titled "Changing Faces: The Way You Face Disfigurement" was conducted by a lay group (available at: http://www.changingfaces.co.uk). They found that among a group of nurses managing patients with burns or with head and neck cancer, a 1-day skills training course improved their confidence so that they could provide psychosocial rehabilitation care to these patients (Clarke and Cooper 2001). These researchers also sent a self-help leaflet to half of a group of patients who had facial disfigurement and found that, compared with a group of control subjects who did not receive the leaflet, the intervention group reported decreased anxiety and depression.

Trauma Victims of Terrorist Attacks

The psychological consequences of trauma or disaster may include a variety of clinical symptoms, including a disruption of homeostasis, a shattering of ego integrity, and a feeling of fright and being overwhelmed (Figley 1978; Wilkinson 1983).

The federal disaster mental health approach in the United States was developed largely out of experiences with natural disasters. The 1995 Oklahoma City, Oklahoma, bombing and the events of September 11, 2001, highlighted how little we know about the provision of services in the aftermath of mass trauma caused by humans.

The United States federal approach emphasizes crisis intervention, support services, triage, referral, outreach, and public education for affected individuals (Center for Mental Health Services 1994; Myers 1994). The federal program concluded that although many individuals may have psychological reactions to a natural disaster, few actually develop diagnosable mental disorders significant enough to warrant more than crisis intervention, brief treatment, or supportive therapy (Flynn and Nelson 1998; Myers 1994). However, in the Oklahoma City bombing, 6 months after the incident, 45% of the sample had an active psychiatric disorder, and one-third had PTSD (North et al. 1999).

Experiences in Oklahoma City suggest that large-scale disasters caused by humans may result in greater psychiatric impairment of direct victims than do natural disasters (North et al. 1999). In a developing field like disaster mental health, in which experience is expanding faster than research and in which we are faced with events for which models were not designed, the learning curve is both steep and incomplete.

Consulting psychiatrists will be most effective directing their efforts toward disaster victims in their hospital's emergency department, medical-surgical units, and ICUs. The psychiatry consultation-liaison service at Walter Reed Hospital Army Medical Center provided an immediate mental health response to hospitalized victims of the Pentagon attack on September 11, 2001, and at follow-up, some patients remembered this intervention better than other aspects of their burn care (Wain et al. 2002). The practice of "critical incident stress management" has become widespread despite empirical studies that have raised concerns about both efficacy in preventing PTSD symptoms and the possibility of worsening such symptoms.

Pelvic Surgery

Hysterectomy

In patients who have undergone hysterectomy, four stages in the experience have been described (Krouse 1990):

1. The recognition/exploration stage centers on the discovery of symptoms and diagnosis.
2. The crisis/climax stage occurs when treatment is initiated.
3. The adaptation stage occurs after treatment.
4. The resolution/disorganization stage concerns the long-term sequelae.

Guilt, embarrassment, anxiety, isolation, fear, and denial of the disease are hallmarks of the first stage of the hysterectomy experience, whereas anxiety, depression, altered body image, and concerns about changing relationships characterize the second stage. Many women associate the uterus with femininity, the sex drive, sexual attractiveness, and status as a wife or mother. Thus, for some women, a hysterectomy leads to impaired self-image and self-esteem. If concerns about the quality of the marital relationship and the deleterious effect of surgery on sexual functioning arise, they must be addressed. Anxiety and depression are common and should be addressed (see also Chapter 33, "Obstetrics and Gynecology").

Gynecological Cancer

Gynecological cancer treatment leads to deterioration of sexual functioning in 30%–35% of patients in terms of sexual motivation, arousal, and orgasm. Prognostic variables include previous sexual behavior, partner-related factors, availability of education and counseling, dyspareunia, postcoital bleeding, estrogen deprivation, and vaginal stenosis or shortening. The magnitude of the surgery and psychosocial factors (including presurgical body image, pretreatment libidinal level, anxiety, attitude toward sex role, and age) contribute to postsurgical adjustment (Weigman-Schultz and van de Wiel 1992) (see also Chapter 17, "Sexual Disorders").

Prostatectomy

In prostatectomy, the frequency of postsurgical impotence and incontinence dramatically affects quality of life. Libman and colleagues (1991) reported that prostatectomy often has a negative effect on erectile function, particularly in older men. Rossignol et al. (1991) evaluated the effect of radical prostatectomy on 429 patients and found that those who were satisfied with their postsurgical sexual life were younger and had normal sexual function prior to the surgery. Braslis et al. (1995) concluded that despite fairly drastic complications (incontinence and impotence) and associated distress, radical prostatectomy is a well-accepted procedure (see also Chapter 17, "Sexual Disorders").

Ostomies

Patients with stomas face many problems, both physical and psychosocial. Anxiety and embarrassment over a stoma may lead to an alteration in lifestyle and overall self-image (Nugent et al. 1999). Successful adjustment to colostomy depends on education for ostomy self-care, psychosocial support to help accept the changes in body image, and a social support network (Piwonka and Merino 1999).

In colostomy patients, Wade (1990) reported that physical symptoms such as fatigue, nausea, diarrhea, flatulence, urinary incontinence, and stoma complications were associated with higher levels of distress. Unmarried men were more likely to enjoy better emotional health than married men and women, and this may be related to pressure to perform sexually among married men. A study by Kelly (1991) found that malfunction of the stoma, skin damage, and poor healing of the perianal wound add their toll to an already trying situation and interfere with functioning and, sometimes, identity. Accidental leakage, or the fear thereof, may limit activity or travel. Anger, depression, and anxiety are common.

Several bothersome aspects of caring for ostomies, with resulting changes in daily routines, troublesome side effects, and embarrassing accidental leakage, further stress the patient's resilience and coping skills (Thomas et al. 1988). The studies of psychosocial complications are limited by retrospective designs, small sample sizes, variable lengths of postoperative follow-up, high proportions of nonrespondents, and untested validity and reliability of the assessment tools used.

Management Strategies After Pelvic Surgery

Pelvic surgery is often associated with pain, changes in body image, self-image distortions, and fear of becoming dependent or abandoned. Patients also fear possible sexual and reproductive changes. Patients undergoing these types of surgery are at risk for poor psychosocial outcome in terms of psychological distress, limitation of activities, and sexual adjustment. Patients and physicians may feel uncomfortable discussing sexual matters, and concerns about sexual functioning may be minimized. This may create severe distress postoperatively. Patients should be fully informed about the sexual effects of surgery, provided ample opportunity to ask questions, and provided assistance in coping with the aftermath of the surgery (see also Chapter 17, "Sexual Disorders").

Bariatric Surgery

The National Heart, Lung, and Blood Institute (1998) clinical guidelines define *extreme obesity* as a body mass index (BMI) greater than 40 kg/m^2. BMI is a calculated number attained by dividing weight in kilograms by height in meters squared. Extreme obesity is also called *morbid obesity* because it is associated with high premature morbidity and mortality, most commonly as a result of complications of type 2 diabetes mellitus, hypertension, hyperlipidemia, or sleep apnea. Multiple treatments have been tried for morbid obesity, but clearly the most effective is bariatric surgery (Fisher and Schauer 2002). The current weight criterion for bariatric (or obesity) surgery is a BMI greater than 40 or a BMI greater than 35 with life-threatening comorbidities. Fifteen million people in the United States, or 1 out of 20 people, have a BMI of 35 kg/m^2 or greater (Buchwald and Buchwald 2002).

Bariatric surgery works in one of two ways: 1) by restricting a patient's ability to eat (restrictive procedures) and 2) by interfering with absorption of ingested food (malabsorptive procedures). Although more than five bariatric procedures are currently performed, the Roux-en-Y gastric bypass (RYGBP) and the laparoscopic adjustable gastric banding (LAGB) with the LAP-BAND system (INAMED Health, Santa Barbara, CA) are the most widely used. The RYGBP combines restriction and malabsorption principles and results in greater weight loss than the previously popular vertical banded gastroplasty (so-called stomach stapling) that was purely a restrictive procedure. The restrictive element of the RYGBP involves creation of a small gastric pouch with a small outlet; the malabsorptive element involves bypass of the distal stomach, the entire duodenum, and about 20–40 cm of the proximal jejunum. The LAGB is a purely restrictive procedure and involves placement of a silicone band around the upper stomach. The two procedures are illustrated in Figures 30–3 and 30–4.

In the bariatric surgery field, there has been a strong effort to standardize reports of weight loss following surgery by using either percent initial excess weight loss or percent initial BMI loss. Both the RYGBP and the LAGB result in approximately 33%–34% initial BMI loss at 1 year (Buchwald 2002; Fox et al. 2003). Weight loss continues during the next year, but not all weight loss is maintained during the next 5–10 years. These results mean that the average patient has a meaningful weight loss but does not achieve ideal body weight; that is, morbid obesity is exchanged for moderate obesity. Perhaps the most important question is whether bariatric surgery results in improvement in the usual physiological complications of morbid obesity. The evidence for significant and sustained improvement in type 2 diabetes mellitus is strong (Greenway et al. 2002), and, although less impressive, reduction in hypertension and improvement in lipid metabolism usually occur.

Psychosocial Aspects

Multiple studies have attempted to identify psychosocial predictors of outcome after bariatric surgery. Early studies of the vertical banded gastroplasty procedure found no relation between presurgical psychiatric diagnoses or presurgical eating pathology and degree of weight loss at follow-up (Powers et al. 1997, 1999a). This does not allow one to conclude that psychopathology will have no influ-

ence on postoperative adherence and outcome because 1) published studies are not large enough to examine the effect of each specific psychiatric disorder, and 2) patients with severe psychiatric disorders tend not to be referred by their physicians to bariatric surgeons.

More recent studies have convincingly shown that many measures of psychopathology and quality of life improve after bariatric surgery (Bocchieri et al. 2002; Guisado et al. 2002). In addition, one study showed that patients who received preoperative brief strategic therapy (average six sessions) had a greater weight loss at 1 year after LAGB than did patients who did not receive this therapy (Caniato and Skorjanec 2002).

Despite these very encouraging findings, it is worth remembering that some patients who might benefit substantially from the surgery (in terms of both weight loss and quality of life) do not receive it. Examples include patients with schizophrenia or bipolar disorder, whose obesity may have been caused by psychotropic medications. Many surgeons exclude these patients because of early reports in the literature of negative outcomes and concerns about whether they would comply with postoperative requirements. Finally, some health insurers refuse to cover, or make access difficult to, bariatric surgery.

Eating Disorders and Bariatric Surgery

Presurgical binge-eating disorder occurs among 16%–33% of the patients who have bariatric surgery, and an even greater percentage binge eat (i.e., they have subsyndromal binge-eating disorder) (Powers et al. 1999a; Saunders 1999). These figures are significantly higher than those reported in the general population. Presurgical night-eating syndrome also appears to be more common among bariatric surgery patients than in the general population (Kuldau and Rand 1986). Although binge eating is usually absent after surgery, vomiting is frequent after vertical banded gastroplasty, and this may result from failed attempts to binge (Powers et al. 1999a). In other cases, such vomiting may represent a continuation of conditioned vomiting in patients who had frequently purged before surgery. However, before postgastroplasty vomiting is attributed to a behavior, a mechanical cause (i.e., overly restrictive anatomy) should be ruled out.

Ophthalmological Surgery

Cataract Surgery

Early reports by psychiatric consultants of "black patch" psychosis following cataract surgery ushered in studies of complications following eye surgery (Weisman and Hackett 1958). The initial reports focused on the sensory deprivation that occurred after bilateral cataract removal

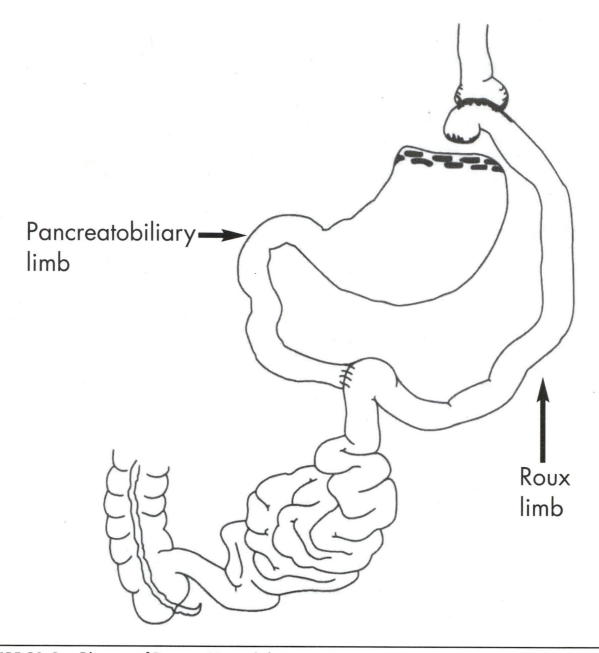

FIGURE 30–3. **Diagram of Roux-en-Y gastric bypass.**

Source. Reprinted from Neven K, Dymek M, leGrange D, et al.: "The Effects of Roux-en-Y Gastric Bypass Surgery on Body Image." *Obesity Surgery* 12:265–269, 2002. Used with permission.

and initially led to recommendations that only one eye be operated on at a time. Subsequently, "black patch" psychosis was identified as a postoperative delirium that was relatively uncommon. Milstein and colleagues (2002) found that following cataract surgery, 4.4% of 296 patients had an immediate postoperative delirium according to the Confusion Assessment Method (Inouye 1998), a standardized measure of delirium. Factors found to be statistically associated with postoperative delirium included very old age (82 years compared with 73 years) and frequent preoperative use of benzodiazepines.

Although cataract surgery is commonplace, relatively little is known about whether expectations of the surgery are fulfilled. One study (Tielsch et al. 1995) found that only 61% of the patients achieved or surpassed their preoperative expectations of visual function after cataract surgery. Those patients least likely to achieve their preoperative expectations were older (older than 75 years) and more likely to have ocular comorbidities. Preoperative counseling about realistic visual functional outcome is likely to be helpful in decreasing disappointment after surgery.

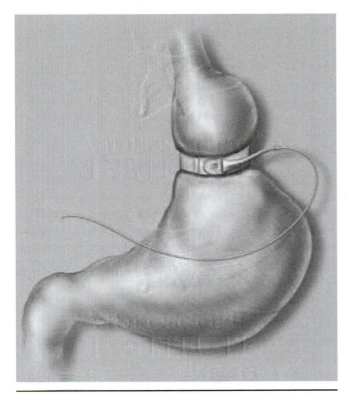

FIGURE 30–4. **Diagram of laparoscopic adjustable gastric banding (LAGB) with the LAP-BAND system (INAMED Health, Santa Barbara, CA).**

Cataract surgery usually is performed in an outpatient setting, and typically either topical or regional anesthesia is used. These anesthetic approaches usually result in the patient being aware during the surgery, and patients often have visual experiences. In the last few years, these experiences have been studied, and the nature of the visual experiences probably depends on the varying degrees of optic nerve blockade that result from the different anesthetics (Tranos et al. 2003). Visual experiences during cataract surgery are the norm: most patients see light; some see various colors (especially red and yellow); and a minority see vague movements, instruments, and the surgeon's hands (Au Eong et al. 1999). Almost all patients (93%) find these visual experiences acceptable, but 4% find them unpleasant, and 3% are frightened by the experiences (Prasad et al. 2003). Preoperative counseling and inclusion of the possibility of these experiences in the written informed consent for surgery have been recommended. A controlled study (Moon and Cho 2001) found that handholding during cataract surgery decreased both anxiety and epinephrine levels.

Stigma and Eye Abnormalities

Facial expression and eye contact are critically important in interpersonal relationships. Thus, abnormalities are likely to significantly influence quality of life. Several recent studies have confirmed this. For example, Bullock and colleagues (2001) showed pictures of patients with blepharoptosis and dermatochalasis to subjects without such abnormalities and asked them to rate the person in the picture on several dimensions, including friendliness, trustworthiness, mental illness, and happiness. After surgical correction of these eye abnormalities, the ratings of the pictures by the healthy subjects improved significantly.

In another study, patients with serious childhood-onset strabismus (before age 5 years) were evaluated at ages 15–25 years prior to corrective surgery (Menon et al. 2002). Eighty-five percent of the males and 75% of the females reported social problems caused by their continuous squint; they had been ridiculed at school and work, they had greater difficulty obtaining employment, and many avoided social activities. After corrective surgery, more than 90% reported improved self-confidence and self-esteem.

Eye Removal

Self-removal of the eye (autoenucleation) is a form of self-mutilation that occurs very uncommonly (Shiwach 1998). When it does, the patient is usually psychotic and often has religious preoccupations associated with a literal interpretation of the Bible ("and if thy right eye offend thee, pluck it out, and cast it from thee"; Matthew 5:28–30). Conjoint management of the patient by ophthalmologists and psychiatrists is crucial, especially because some patients reinjure themselves later.

Eye gouging, an assaultive eye injury, also has been reported in a series of 10 patients (Bukhanovsky et al. 1999). Among the perpetrators, 4 were psychotic, 1 was mentally retarded, and 5 committed the act during extreme sexual violence.

Cosmetic Surgery

In an age and a culture in which people have increased interest in physical attractiveness, cosmetic surgery has dramatically increased. In 1998, more than 132,000 women had breast augmentation procedures in the United States (Sarwer et al. 2000). Early studies of cosmetic surgery found that patients with psychiatric problems were common among cosmetic surgery candidates. Findings from more recent studies suggest that because more people consider cosmetic surgery a reasonable choice, the percentage of applicants with psychiatric disorders may be relatively lower. Most patients do well with cosmetic surgery, although it is thought that so-called type changes (e.g., rhinoplasty) require more extensive psychological adjustments than do restorative changes (e.g., face-lifts) (Castle et al. 2002).

Age at the time of cosmetic surgery is also important; it may be easier to incorporate changes into body image during childhood or adolescence. Cosmetic surgery is usually helpful in adolescents with a true defect if they are selected carefully and if genuine informed consent is obtained before surgery (McGrath and Mukerji 2000).

Because quality of life is significantly influenced by body image, a philosophical question raised by the increased number of aesthetic surgeries is whether cosmetic surgery should be considered medically necessary. The focus on possible negative body image changes after life-saving surgeries for illnesses such as breast cancer has resulted in trials comparing the effectiveness (in terms of survival) of less disfiguring surgeries with that of more radical approaches. A persuasive argument can be made that improvements in body image and self-esteem may dramatically improve quality of life.

Preoperative Assessment

Even though the percentage of patients with psychiatric disorders may be lower among patients seeking aesthetic surgery than in previous decades, the percentage is probably still higher than among most other surgical candidates. Several research groups have attempted to determine which patients should not have cosmetic surgery at all and which patients should have psychiatric treatment before aesthetic surgery. A series of questions designed to detect psychiatric problems has been proposed (Grossbart and Sarwer 1999). One problem in determining who is likely to benefit from cosmetic surgery is that no widespread accepted method is available for determining patient satisfaction with the surgical results. Ching and colleagues (2003) reviewed the literature and suggested specific measures of body image and quality of life likely to provide valid evidence concerning the question of who should receive surgery.

Body Dysmorphic Disorder

Body dysmorphic disorder also has been called the *disorder of imagined ugliness*. Patients with body dysmorphic disorder frequently consult plastic surgeons for correction of trivial or nonexistent defects. The diagnostic criteria include impairment in functioning, in addition to preoccupation with an imagined defect in appearance not accounted for by another mental disorder. The prevalence of body dysmorphic disorder is unknown but in clinical mental health settings is under 5% (American Psychiatric Association 2000). Phillips and her colleagues (Phillips 1991; Phillips and Dufresne 2002) have been in-

strumental in showing that body dysmorphic disorder is relatively common and that treatment should be psychiatric, not surgical. There are case reports of patients with body dysmorphic disorder becoming violent toward surgeons or committing suicide in a dermatology setting (Cotterill and Cunliffe 1997). Current promising nonsurgical treatments include selective serotonin reuptake inhibitors in addition to cognitive-behavioral strategies (Hollander et al. 1999; Phillips and Dufresne 2002) (see also Chapter 13, "Somatization and Somatoform Disorders").

Conclusion

Psychiatric problems occur in a significant minority of surgical patients. We have discussed common problems that occur during the preoperative, intraoperative, and postoperative periods. Preoperatively, issues around capacity and consent are important, as well as planning for the surgical and postoperative management of psychiatric disorders known to be present. Preoperative anxiety is common, and appropriate treatment can improve postoperative recovery. Psychiatric reactions to intraoperative recall can often be ameliorated through careful preparation for surgery. Postoperatively, delirium is a key issue, often related to alcohol or drug withdrawal syndromes. Postoperative pain, problems related to discontinuation of ventilator support, and PTSD are common reasons for psychiatric intervention. An awareness of specific issues that can arise in burn care, pelvic surgery, bariatric surgery, ophthalmological surgery, and cosmetic surgery is also important.

References

Adler LE, Griffith JM: Concurrent medical illness in the schizophrenic patient: epidemiology, diagnosis, and management. Schizophr Res 4:91–107, 1991

Aizawa KI, Kanai T, Saikawa Y, et al: A novel approach to the prevention of postoperative delirium in the elderly after gastrointestinal surgery. Surgery Today 32:310–314, 2002

American Burn Association: Burn Care Facilities in the United States, in Burn Care Resources in North America, 1999–2000 Edition. Chicago, IL, American Burn Association, 1999, pp 1–26

American Burn Association: Burn Incidence Fact Sheet. Available at: http://www.ameriburn.org. Accessed July 2, 2004.

American Psychiatric Association: Diagnostic and Statistical Manual of Mental Disorders, 4th Edition. Washington, DC, American Psychiatric Association, 1994

American Psychiatric Association: Diagnostic and Statistical Manual of Mental Disorders, 4th Edition, Text Revision. Washington, DC, American Psychiatric Association, 2000

Andreasen NJ, Noyes R Jr, Hartford CE, et al: Management of emotional reactions in seriously burned adults. N Engl J Med 286:65–69, 1972

Angus J: The material and social predicaments of home: women's experiences after aortocoronary bypass surgery. Can J Nurs Res 33:27–42, 2001

Au Eong KG, Lee HM, Lim AT, et al: Subjective visual experience during extracapsular cataract extraction and intraocular lens implantation under retrobulbar anaesthesia. Eye 13(Pt 3a):325–328, 1999

Barillo DJ, Goode R: Substance abuse in victims of fire. J Burn Care Rehabil 17:71–76, 1996

Bayindir O, Akpinar B, Can E, et al: The use of the 5-HT$_3$-receptor antagonist ondansetron for the treatment of postcardiotomy delirium. J Cardiothorac Vasc Anesth 14:288–292, 2000

Bernstein LF: Burn trauma, in Psychiatric Care of the Medical Patient, 2nd Edition. Edited by Stoudemire A. Fogel B. New York, Oxford University Press, 1993

Bernstein L, Jacobsberg L, Ashman T, et al: Detection of alcoholism among burn patients. Hosp Community Psychiatry 43:255–256, 1992

Bernstein NR: Emotional Care of the Facially Burned and Disfigured. Boston, MA, Little, Brown, 1976

Blacker RS: General Surgery and Anesthesia: The Emotional Experience. New York, Wiley, 1987, pp 1–26

Blackwood B: The art and science of predicting patient readiness for weaning from mechanical ventilation. Int J Nurs Stud 37:145–151, 2000

Blanchard EB, Hickling EJ, Devineni T, et al: A controlled evaluation of cognitive behavioural therapy for posttraumatic stress in motor vehicle accident survivors. Behav Res Ther 41:79–96, 2003

Bloomquist T: Amputation and phantom limb pain: a pain-prevention model. AANA J 69:211–217, 2001

Bocchieri LE, Meana M, Fisher BL: A review of psychosocial outcomes of surgery for morbid obesity. J Psychosom Res 52:155–165, 2002

Braslis KG, Santa-Cruz C, Brickman AL, et al: Quality of life 12 months after radical prostatectomy. Br J Urol 75:48–53, 1995

Buchwald H: A bariatric surgery algorithm. Obes Surg 12:733–746, 2002

Buchwald H, Buchwald JN: Evolution of operative procedures for the management of morbid obesity 1950–2000. Obes Surg 12:705–717, 2002

Bukhanovsky AO, Hempel A, Ahmed W, et al: Assaultive eye injury and enucleation. J Am Acad Psychiatry Law 27:590–602, 1999

Bullock JD, Warwar RE, Bienenfeld DG, et al: Psychosocial implications of blepharoptosis and dermatochalasis. Trans Am Ophthalmol Soc 99:65–71, 2001

Bunch EH: Delayed clarification: information, clarification and ethical decisions in critical care in Norway. J Adv Nurs 32:1485–1491, 2000

Cameron DR, Pegg SP, Muller M: Self-inflicted burns. Burns 23:519–521, 1997

Caniato D, Skorjanec B: The role of brief strategic therapy on the outcome of gastric banding. Obes Surg 12:666–671, 2002

Carson JL, Noveck H, Berlin JA, et al: Mortality and morbidity in patients with very low postoperative Hb levels who decline blood transfusion. Transfusion 42:812–818, 2002

Castle DJ, Honigman RJ, Phillips KA: Does cosmetic surgery improve psychosocial wellbeing? Med J Aust 176:601–604, 2002

Center for Mental Health Services Program Guidance: Crisis Counseling and Mental Health Treatment Similarities and Differences. Rockville, MD, Center for Mental Health Services, 1994

Chadda RK: Psychiatry in non-psychiatric setting: a comparative study of physicians and surgeons. J Indian Med Assoc 99:24, 26–27, 62, 2001

Ching S, Thoma A, McCabe RE, et al: Measuring outcomes in aesthetic surgery: a comprehensive review of the literature. Plast Reconstr Surg 111:469–480, 2003

Clarke A, Cooper C: Psychological rehabilitation after disfiguring injury or disease: investigating the training needs of specialist nurses. J Adv Nurs 34:18–26, 2001

Cotterill JA, Cunliffe WJ: Suicide in dermatological patients. Br J Dermatol 137:246–250, 1997

Craven J: Psychiatric aspects of lung transplant. The Toronto Lung Transplant Group. Can J Psychiatry 35:759–764, 1990

Curtiss CP: JCAHO: meeting the standards for pain management. Orthop Nurs 20:27–30, 41, 2001

Daniels SM, Fenley JD, Powers PS, et al: Self-inflicted burns: a ten-year retrospective study. J Burn Care Rehabil 12:144–147, 1991

Diaz V, Rodriguez J, Barrientos P, et al: Use of procholinergics in the prevention of postoperative delirium in hip fracture surgery in the elderly: a randomized controlled trial. Rev Neurol 33:716–719, 2001

Domino KB, Posner KL, Caplan RA, et al: Awareness during anesthesia: a closed claims analysis. Anesthesiology 90:1053–1061, 1999

Duggan M, Dowd N, O'Mara D, et al: Benzodiazepine premedication may attenuate the stress response in daycase anesthesia: a pilot study. Can J Anaesth 49:932–935, 2002

Ehde DM, Patterson DR, Wiechman SA, et al: Post-traumatic stress symptoms and distress following acute burn injury. Burns 25:587–592, 1999

Ehde DM, Patterson DR, Wiechman SA, et al: Post-traumatic stress symptoms and distress 1 year after burn injury. J Burn Care Rehabil 21:105–111, 2000

Erlandsson AL, Backman B, Stenstrom A, et al: Conscious sedation by oral administration of midazolam in paediatric dental treatment. Swed Dent J 25:97–104, 2001

Fauerbach JA, Lawrence JW, Schmidt CW Jr, et al: Personality predictors of injury-related posttraumatic stress disorder. J Nerv Ment Dis 188:510–517, 2000

Figley CR: Stress Disorder Among Vietnam Veterans: Theory, Research and Treatment. New York, Brunner/Mazel, 1978

Fisher BL, Schauer P: Medical and surgical options in the treatment of severe obesity. Am J Surg 184:9S–16S, 2002

Flacker JM, Marcantonio ER: Delirium in the elderly: optimal management. Drugs Aging 13:119–130, 1998

Flynn BW, Nelson ME: Understanding the needs of children following large-scale disasters and the role of government. Child Adolesc Psychiatr Clin North Am 7:211–227, 1998

Foertsch CE, O'Hara MW, Stoddard FJ, et al: Treatment-resistant pain and distress during pediatric burn-dressing changes. J Burn Care Rehabil 19:219–224, 1998

Fox SR, Fox KM, Srikanth MS, et al: The lap-band system in a North American population. Obes Surg 13:275–280, 2003

Fukunishi I: Relationship of cosmetic disfigurement to the severity of posttraumatic stress disorder in burn injury or digital amputation. Psychother Psychosom 68:82–86, 1999

Fulop G, Strain JJ: Medical and surgical inpatients who referred themselves for psychiatric consultation. Gen Hosp Psychiatry 7:267–271, 1985

Galanakis P, Bickel H, Gradinger R, et al: Acute confusional state in the elderly following hip surgery: incidence, risk factors and complications. Int J Geriatr Psychiatry 16:349–355, 2001

Gentilello LM, Donovan DM, Dunn CW, et al: Alcohol interventions in trauma centers: current practice and future directions. JAMA 274:1043–1048, 1995

Ghoneim MM, Block RI: Learning and consciousness during general anesthesia. Anesthesiology 76:279–305, 1992

Greenway SE, Greenway FL, III, Klein S: Effects of obesity surgery on non-insulin-dependent diabetes mellitus. Arch Surg 137:1109–1117, 2002

Greer SM, Dalton JA, Carlson J, et al: Surgical patients' fear of addiction to pain medication: the effect of an educational program for clinicians. Clin J Pain 17:157–164, 2001

Grossbart TA, Sarwer DB: Cosmetic surgery: surgical tools—psychosocial goals. Semin Cutan Med Surg 18:101–111, 1999

Guisado JA, Vaz FJ, Alarcon J, et al: Psychopathological status and interpersonal functioning following weight loss in morbidly obese patients undergoing bariatric surgery. Obes Surg 12:835–840, 2002

Gutl P, Greimel ER, Roth R, et al: Women's sexual behavior, body image and satisfaction with surgical outcomes after hysterectomy: a comparison of vaginal and abdominal surgery. J Psychosom Obstet Gynaecol 23:51–59, 2002

Hagg O, Fritzell P, Ekselius L, et al: Predictors of outcome in fusion surgery for chronic low back pain: a report from the Swedish Lumbar Spine Study. Eur Spine J 12:22–33, 2003

Hamilton JG: Needle phobia: a neglected diagnosis. J Fam Pract 41:169–175, 1995

Heimbach D: What's new in general surgery: burns and metabolism. J Am Coll Surg 194:156–164, 2002

Hollander E, Allen A, Kwon J, et al: Clomipramine vs desipramine crossover trial in body dysmorphic disorder: selective efficacy of a serotonin reuptake inhibitor in imagined ugliness. Arch Gen Psychiatry 56:1033–1039, 1999

Holliday JE, Hyers TM: The reduction of weaning time from mechanical ventilation using tidal volume and relaxation biofeedback. Am Rev Respir Dis 141(5 pt 1):1214–1220, 1990

Imbus SH, Zawacki BE: Autonomy for burned patients when survival is unprecedented. N Engl J Med 297:308–311, 1977

Inouye SK: Delirium in hospitalized older patients: recognition and risk factors. J Geriatr Psychiatry Neurol 11:118–125, 1998

Jacavone J, Young J: Use of pulmonary rehabilitation strategies to wean a difficult-to-wean patient: case study. Crit Care Nurs 18:29–37, 1998

Jones A: A psychoanalytically informed conversation with a woman and her husband following major surgery for cancer of her neck and torso. J Adv Nurs 35:459–467, 2001

Jones JD, Barber B, Engrav L, et al: Alcohol use and burn injury. J Burn Care Rehabil 12:148–152, 1991

Kain ZN, Mayes LC, O'Connor TZ, et al: Preoperative anxiety in children: predictors and outcomes. Arch Pediatr Adolesc Med 150:1238–1245, 1996

Kain ZN, Caldwell-Andrews A, Wang SM: Psychological preparation of the parent and pediatric surgical patient. Anesthesiol Clin North Am 20:29–44, 2002

Kamolz T, Granderath FA, Pointner R: Does major depression in patients with gastroesophageal reflux disease affect the outcome of laparoscopic antireflux surgery? Surg Endosc 17:55–60, 2003

Kaneko T, Takahashi S, Naka T, et al: Postoperative delirium following gastrointestinal surgery in elderly patients. Surg Today 27:107–111, 1997

Kelley KM, Tkachenko TA, Pliskin NH, et al: Life after electrical injury: risk factors for psychiatric sequelae. Ann N Y Acad Sci 888:356–363, 1999

Kelly MP: Coping with an ileostomy. Soc Sci Med 33:115–125, 1991

Kent L, King H, Cochrane R: Maternal and child psychological sequelae in paediatric burn injuries. Burns 26:317–322, 2000

Klafta JM, Roizen MF: Current understanding of patients' attitudes toward and preparation for anesthesia: a review. Anesth Analg 83:1314–1321, 1996

Klein E, Koren D, Arnon I, et al: Sleep complaints are not corroborated by objective sleep measures in post-traumatic stress disorder: a 1-year prospective study in survivors of motor vehicle crashes. J Sleep Res 12:35–41, 2003

Koivula M, Tarkka MT, Tarkka M, et al: Fear and in-hospital social support for coronary artery bypass grafting patients on the day before surgery. Int J Nurs Stud 39:415–427, 2002

Kornfeld DS, Zimberg S, Malm JR: Psychiatric complications of open-heart surgery. N Engl J Med 273:287–292, 1965

Krouse HJ: Psychological adjustment of women to gynecologic cancers. NAACOGS Clin Issu Perinat Womens Health Nurs 1:495–512, 1990

Kudoh A, Katagai H, Takazawa T: Antidepressant treatment for chronic depressed patients should not be discontinued prior to anesthesia. Can J Anaesth 49:132–136, 2002

Kuldau JM, Rand CSW: The night eating syndrome and bulimia in the morbidly obese. Int J Eat Disord 5:143–148, 1986

Kumar V: Burnt wives: a study of suicides. Burns 29:31–35, 2003

Lennmarken C, Bildfors K, Enlund G, et al: Victims of awareness. Acta Anaesthesiol Scand 46:229–231, 2002

Libman E, Fichten CS, Rothenberg P, et al: Prostatectomy and inguinal hernia repair: a comparison of the sexual consequences. J Sex Marital Ther 17:27–34, 1991

Lieber CS: Medical disorders of alcoholism. N Engl J Med 333:1058–1065, 1995

Lindemann E: Symptomatology and management of acute grief (1944). Am J Psychiatry 151 (suppl 6):155–160, 1994

Luhmann N, Knodt EM: Social Systems (Writing Science). Translated by Bedrara J, Baeder D. Stanford, CA, Stanford University Press, 1995

MacIntyre NR, Cook DJ, Ely EW Jr, et al: Evidence-based guidelines for weaning and discontinuing ventilatory support: a collective task force facilitated by the American College of Chest Physicians, the American Association for Respiratory Care, and the American College of Critical Care Medicine. Chest 120 (suppl):375S–395S, 2001

Maes M, Delmeire L, Mylle J, et al: Risk and preventive factors of post-traumatic stress disorder (PTSD): alcohol consumption and intoxication prior to a traumatic event diminishes the relative risk to develop PTSD in response to that trauma. J Affect Disord 63:113–121, 2001

Marcantonio ER, Flacker JM, Wright RJ, et al: Reducing delirium after hip fracture: a randomized trial. J Am Geriatr Soc 49:516–522, 2001

Marshall WR, Weaver BD, McCutcheon P: A study of the effectiveness of oral midazolam as a dental pre-operative sedative and hypnotic. Spec Care Dentist 19:259–266, 1999

Martin-Herz SP, Patterson DR, Honari S, et al: Pediatric pain control practices of North American Burn Centers. J Burn Care Rehabil 24:26–36, 2003

Maye JP, Smith TL: Evaluation of word associations as a reliable postoperative indicator of implicit memory formation during the intraoperative period. AANA J 69:27–30, 2001

McCartney JR, Boland RJ: Anxiety and delirium in the intensive care unit. Crit Care Clin 10:673–680, 1994

McGrath MH, Mukerji S: Plastic surgery and the teenage patient. J Pediatr Adolesc Gynecol 13:105–118, 2000

Menon V, Saha J, Tandon R, et al: Study of the psychosocial aspects of strabismus. J Pediatr Ophthalmol Strabismus 39:203–208, 2002

Micik S, Borbasi S: Effect of support programme to reduce stress in spouses whose partners "fall off" clinical pathways post cardiac surgery. Aust Crit Care 15:33–40, 2002

Milisen K, Foreman MD, Abraham IL, et al: A nurse-led interdisciplinary intervention program for delirium in elderly hip-fracture patients. J Am Geriatr Soc 49:523–532, 2001

Milstein A, Pollack A, Kleinman G, et al: Confusion/delirium following cataract surgery: an incidence study of 1-year duration. Int Psychogeriatr 14:301–306, 2002

Moesgaard F, Lykkegaard-Nielsen M: Preoperative cell-mediated immunity and duration of antibiotic prophylaxis in relation to postoperative infectious complications: a controlled trial in biliary, gastroduodenal and colorectal surgery. Acta Chir Scand 155:281–286, 1989

Moon JS, Cho KS: The effects of handholding on anxiety in cataract surgery patients under local anaesthesia. J Adv Nurs 35:407–415, 2001

Myers D: Disaster Response and Recovery: A Handbook for Mental Health Professionals (DHHS Publ No SMA 94-3010). Menlo Park, CA, Center for Mental Health Services, 1994

Mzezewa S, Jonsson K, Aberg M, et al: A prospective study of suicidal burns admitted to the Harare burns unit. Burns 26:460–464, 2000

National Heart, Lung, and Blood Institute: Clinical Guidelines on the Identification, Evaluation, and Treatment of Overweight and Obesity in Adults. Bethesda, MD, National Institutes of Health, National Heart, Lung, and Blood Institute, June 1998

Neale MC, Walters EE, Eaves LJ, et al: Genetics of blood-injury fears and phobias: a population-based twin study. Am J Med Genet 54:326–334, 1994

Nelson S: Pre-admission education for patients undergoing cardiac surgery. Br J Nurs 5:335–340, 1996

Nir Y, Paz A, Sabo E, et al: Fear of injections in young adults: prevalence and associations. Am J Trop Med Hyg 68:341–344, 2003

North CS, Nixon SJ, Shariat S, et al: Psychiatric disorders among survivors of the Oklahoma City bombing. JAMA 282:755–762, 1999

Nugent KP, Daniels P, Stewart B, et al: Quality of life in stoma patients. Dis Colon Rectum 42:1569–1574, 1999

Page AC: The role of disgust in faintness elicited by blood and injection stimuli. J Anxiety Disord 17:45–58, 2002

Paré A: The Works of that Famous Chirurgion, Ambrose Parey, translated out of the Latin and compared with the French by T. Johnson. London, England, Cotes, 1649

Phillips KA: Body dysmorphic disorder: the distress of imagined ugliness. Am J Psychiatry 148:1138–1149, 1991

Phillips KA, Dufresne RG Jr: Body dysmorphic disorder: a guide for primary care physicians. Prim Care 29:99–111, vii, 2002

Piwonka MA, Merino JM: A multidimensional modeling of predictors influencing the adjustment to a colostomy. J Wound Ostomy Continence Nurs 26:298–305, 1999

Powell J, Kitchen N, Heslin J, et al: Psychosocial outcomes at three and nine months after good neurological recovery from aneurysmal subarachnoid haemorrhage: predictors and prognosis. J Neurol Neurosurg Psychiatry 72:772–781, 2002

Powers PS: Psychosis in hospitalized burn patients: a two year prospective study. Ninth Annual Regional Burn Seminar, Charleston, SC, December 1996

Powers PS: Practice Guideline for Psychiatric Disorders. 15th Regional Burn Meeting, Lexington, KY, December 2002

Powers PS, Cruse CW, Daniels S, et al: Safety and efficacy of debridement under anesthesia in patients with burns. J Burn Care Rehabil 14(2 Pt 1):176–180, 1993

Powers PS, Stevens B, Arias F, et al: Alcohol disorders among patients with burns: crisis and opportunity. J Burn Care Rehabil 15:386–391, 1994a

Powers PS, Cruse CW, Daniels S, et al: Posttraumatic stress disorder in patients with burns. J Burn Care Rehabil 15:147–153, 1994b

Powers PS, Rosemurgy A, Boyd F, et al: Outcome of gastric restriction procedures: weight, psychiatric diagnoses, and satisfaction. Obes Surg 7:471–477, 1997

Powers PS, Perez A, Boyd F, et al: Eating pathology before and after bariatric surgery: a prospective study. Int J Eat Disord 25:293–300, 1999a

Powers PS, Sarkar S, Goldgof DB, et al: Scar assessment: current problems and future solutions. J Burn Care Rehabil 20 (1 Pt 1):54–60, 1999b

Powers PS, Cruse CW, Boyd F: Psychiatric status, prevention, and outcome in patients with burns: a prospective study. J Burn Care Rehabil 21(1 Pt 1):85–88, 2000

Prasad N, Kumar CM, Patil BB, et al: Subjective visual experience during phacoemulsification cataract surgery under sub-Tenon's block. Eye 17:407–409, 2003

Putnam FW, Hulsmann JE: Pharmacotherapy for survivors of childhood trauma. Semin Clin Neuropsychiatry 7:129–136, 2002

Ranta SO, Herranen P, Hynynen M: Patients' conscious recollections from cardiac anesthesia. J Cardiothorac Vasc Anesth 16:426–430, 2002

Regal H, Rose W, Hahnel S, et al: Evaluation of psychological stress before general anesthesia. Psychiatr Neurol Med Psychol (Leipz) 37:151–155, 1985

Riker RR, Fraser GL, Cox PM: Continuous infusion of haloperidol controls agitation in critically ill patients. Crit Care Med 22:433–440, 1994

Rossignol G, Leandri P, Gautier JR, et al: Radical retropubic prostatectomy: complications and quality of life (429 cases, 1983–1989). Eur Urol 19:186–191, 1991

Rothenhausler HB, Ehrentraut S, von Degenfeld G, et al: Treatment of depression with methylphenidate in patients difficult to wean from mechanical ventilation in the intensive care unit. J Clin Psychiatry 61:750–755, 2000

Rusch MD, Gould LJ, Dzwierzynski WW, et al: Psychological impact of traumatic injuries: what the surgeon can do. Plast Reconstr Surg 109:18–24, 2002

Sarwer DB, Whitaker LA, Pertschuk MJ, et al: Body image concerns of reconstructive surgery patients: an underrecognized problem. Ann Plast Surg 40:403–407, 1998

Sarwer DB, Nordmann JE, Herbert JD: Cosmetic breast augmentation surgery: a critical overview. J Womens Health Gend Based Med 9:843–856, 2000

Saunders R: Binge eating in gastric bypass patients before surgery. Obes Surg 9:72–76, 1999

Saxe G, Stoddard F, Courtney D, et al: Relationship between acute morphine and the course of PTSD in children with burns. J Am Acad Child Adolesc Psychiatry 40:915–921, 2001

Scher CS, Anwar M: The self-reporting of psychiatric medications in patients scheduled for elective surgery. J Clin Anesth 11:619–621, 1999

Scully JH, Hutcherson R: Suicide by burning. Am J Psychiatry 140:905–906, 1983

Segatore M, Dutkiewicz M, Adams D: The delirious cardiac surgical patient: theoretical aspects and principles of management. J Cardiovasc Nurs 12:32–48, 1998

Seitz HK, Simanowski UA: Ethanol and carcinogenesis of the alimentary tract. Alcohol Clin Exp Res 10 (suppl):33S–40S, 1986

Shiwach RS: Autoenucleation—a culture-specific phenomenon: a case series and review. Compr Psychiatry 39:318–322, 1998

Sillanaukee P: Laboratory markers of alcohol abuse. Alcohol Alcohol 31:613–616, 1996

Sjostrom B, Haljamae H, Dahlgren LO, et al: Assessment of postoperative pain: impact of clinical experience and professional role. Acta Anaesthesiol Scand 41:339–344, 1997

Smith AF, Pittaway AJ: Premedication for anxiety in adult day surgery. Cochrane Database Syst Rev 1:CD002192, 2003

Spies CD, Neuner B, Neumann T, et al: Intercurrent complications in chronic alcoholic men admitted to the intensive care unit following trauma. Intensive Care Med 22:286–293, 1996

Spies CD, Spies KP, Zinke S, et al: Alcoholism and carcinoma change the intracellular pH and activate platelet Na+/H+-exchange in men. Alcohol Clin Exp Res 21:1653–1660, 1997

Spouse E, Gedroyc WM: MRI of the claustrophobic patient: interventionally configured magnets. Br J Radiol 73:146–151, 2000

Steenkamp WC, Botha NJ, Van der Merwe AE: The prevalence of alcohol dependence in burned adult patients. Burns 20:522–525, 1994

Stoddard FJ, Stroud L, Murphy JM: Depression in children after recovery from severe burns. J Burn Care Rehabil 13:340–347, 1992

Stoddard FJ, Sheridan RL, Saxe GN, et al: Treatment of pain in acutely burned children. J Burn Care Rehabil 23:135–156, 2002

Stoll C, Schelling G, Goetz AE, et al: Health-related quality of life and post-traumatic stress disorder in patients after cardiac surgery and intensive care treatment. J Thorac Cardiovasc Surg 120:505–512, 2000

Stomberg MW, Wickstrom K, Joelsson H, et al: Postoperative pain management on surgical wards—do quality assurance strategies result in long-term effects on staff member attitudes and clinical outcomes? Pain Manag Nurs 4:11–22, 2003

Strain JJ: Needs for psychiatry in the general hospital. Hosp Community Psychiatry 33:996–1001, 1982

Stunkard A, Burt V: Obesity and the body image, II: age at onset of disturbances in the body image. Am J Psychiatry 123:1443–1447, 1967

Summers S: Evidence-based practice, part 3: acute pain management of the perianesthesia patient. J Perianesth Nurs 16:112–120, 2001

Taal LA, Faber AW: Posttraumatic stress and maladjustment among adult burn survivors 1–2 years postburn. Burns 24:285–292, 1998

Tabares R, Peck MD: Chemical dependency in patients with burn injuries: a fortress of denial. J Burn Care Rehabil 18:283–286, 1997

Tedstone JE, Tarrier N: Posttraumatic stress disorder following medical illness and treatment. Clin Psychol Rev 23:409–448, 2003

Thomas C, Turner P, Madden F: Coping and the outcome of stoma surgery. J Psychosom Res 32:457–467, 1988

Thomas CR, Brazeal BA, Rosenberg L, et al: Phantom limb pain in pediatric burn survivors. Burns 29:139–142, 2003

Tielsch JM, Steinberg EP, Cassard SD, et al: Preoperative functional expectations and postoperative outcomes among patients undergoing first eye cataract surgery. Arch Ophthalmol 113:1312–1318, 1995

Tokita K, Tanaka H, Kawamoto M, et al: Patient-controlled epidural analgesia with bupivacaine and fentanyl suppresses postoperative delirium following hepatectomy. Masui 50:742–746, 2001

Tønnesen H, Petersen KR, Hojgaard L, et al: Postoperative morbidity among symptom-free alcohol misusers. Lancet 340:334–337, 1992

Tønnesen H, Carstensen M, Maina P: Is carbohydrate deficient transferrin a useful marker of harmful alcohol intake among surgical patients? Eur J Surg 165:522–527, 1999

Tranos PG, Wickremasinghe SS, Sinclair N, et al: Visual perception during phacoemulsification cataract surgery under topical and regional anaesthesia. Acta Ophthalmol Scand 81:118–122, 2003

Tsap LV, Goldgof DB, Sarkar S, et al: A vision-based technique for objective assessment of burn scars. IEEE Trans Med Imaging 17:620–633, 1998

van der Schans CP, Geertzen JH, Schoppen T, et al: Phantom pain and health-related quality of life in lower limb amputees. J Pain Symptom Manage 24:429–436, 2002

Van Loey N, Van Son M: Psychopathology and psychological problems in patients with burn scars: epidemiology and management. Am J Clin Dermatol 4:245–272, 2003

van Wijk MG, Smalhout B: A postoperative analysis of the patient's view of anaesthesia in a Netherlands' teaching hospital. Anaesthesia 45:679–682, 1990

Vegter F, Hage JJ: Lack of correlation between objective and subjective evaluation of residual stigmata in cleft patients. Ann Plast Surg 46:625–629, 2001

Wade BE: Colostomy patients: psychological adjustment at 10 weeks and 1 year after surgery in districts which employed stoma-care nurses and districts which did not. J Adv Nurs 15:1297–1304, 1990

Wain HJ, Grammer GG, Stasinos JJ, et al: Meeting the patients where they are: consultation-liaison response to trauma victims of the Pentagon attack. Mil Med 167 (suppl):19–21, 2002

Walder B, Elia N, Henzi I, et al: A lack of evidence of superiority of propofol versus midazolam for sedation in mechanically ventilated critically ill patients: a qualitative and quantitative systematic review. Anesth Analg 92:975–983, 2001

Watkins PN, Cook EL, May SR, et al: The role of the psychiatrist in the team treatment of the adult patient with burns. J Burn Care Rehabil 13:19–27, 1992

Weigman-Schultz WCM, van de Wiel HBM: Sexual rehabilitation after gynecological cancer. J Educ Ther 18:286–293, 1992

Weisman AD, Hackett TP: Psychosis after eye surgery: establishment of a specific doctor–patient relation in the prevention and treatment of "black-patch delirium." N Engl J Med 258:1284–1289, 1958

Wetzel RC, Burns RC: Multiple trauma in children: critical care overview. Crit Care Med 30 (suppl):S468–S477, 2002

Wiechman SA, Ehde DM, Wilson BL, et al: The management of self-inflicted burn injuries and disruptive behavior for patients with borderline personality disorder. J Burn Care Rehabil 21:310–317, 2000

Wilkinson CB: Aftermath of a disaster: the collapse of the Hyatt Regency Hotel skywalks. Am J Psychiatry 140:1134–1139, 1983

Williams-Russo P, Urquhart BL, Sharrock NE, et al: Postoperative delirium: predictors and prognosis in elderly orthopedic patients. J Am Geriatr Soc 40:759–767, 1992

Wyness MA, Durity MB, Durity F: Narratives of patients with skull base tumors and their family members: lessons for nursing practice. Axone 24:18–35, 2002

Yu BH, Dimsdale JE: Posttraumatic stress disorder in patients with burn injuries. J Burn Care Rehabil 20:426–433, 1999

Zatzick DF, Jurkovich GJ, Gentilello L, et al: Posttraumatic stress, problem drinking, and functional outcomes after injury. Arch Surg 137:200–205, 2002

31

Organ Transplantation

Andrea F. DiMartini, M.D.

Mary Amanda Dew, Ph.D.

Paula T. Trzepacz, M.D.

THE BENEFIT OF solid organ transplantation was realized in 1954 when Dr. Joseph E. Murray performed the first successful kidney transplant, with the patient's identical twin as donor. However, for most patients an identical-twin donor was not an option, and more than a decade passed before immunosuppressive medications were available to conquer the immunological barrier. In 1967, the first successful liver transplant was performed, followed a year later by the first successful heart transplant. Yet despite the fact that the surgical challenges of solid organ transplantation had been overcome, it was not until the early 1980s, with the advent of improved immunosuppression, that organ transplantation changed from an experimental procedure to a standard of care for many types of end-stage organ disease.

In that decade, the National Organ Transplant Act established the framework for a national system of organ transplantation, and the United Network of Organ Sharing (UNOS) was contracted by the U.S. Congress to administer the nation's only Organ Procurement and Transplantation Network (OPTN) (United Network of Organ Sharing 2004). Currently, UNOS administers the OPTN under contract with the U.S. Department of Health and Human Services. In addition to facilitating organ matching and placement, UNOS collects data about every transplant performed in the United States and maintains information on every organ type (e.g., wait-list counts, survival rates) in an extensive database available on the OPTN Web site (http://www.OPTN.org) (United Network of Organ Sharing 2004).

Although immunological barriers still exist for transplant recipients, the greatest obstacle to receiving a transplant is the shortage of donated organs. The number of wait-listed individuals is increasing far beyond the avail-

ability of donated organs. As illustrated in Figure 31–1, the numbers of wait-listed patients for kidney (the most frequent) and liver transplants increased steadily between 1995 and 2001 (United Network of Organ Sharing 2004). By contrast, the numbers of patients waiting for heart, lung, and pancreas transplants increased only marginally during the same period. The median wait-listed time depends on the organ type, the blood type of the recipient, and the severity of the recipient's illness at the time of listing. For example, as of 2001, the median wait time for a heart transplant candidate initially listed as a category heart status 2 was 374 days, whereas that for a liver transplant candidate listed as a UNOS 2B was 282 days (United Network of Organ Sharing 2004). Figure 31–2 shows the numbers of transplant recipients in 2001 for each solid organ type (United Network of Organ Sharing 2004), which ranged from a low of 924 for lung to a high of 11,502 for kidney. These numbers are much lower than the 2001 wait-listed values, and ratios of transplant recipients to wait-listed patients are lowest for kidney, liver, and lung (about 1:4 to 1:5). Each year, 10%–15% of liver, heart, and lung transplant candidates will die while on the waiting list (United Network of Organ Sharing 2004). Additionally, posttransplantation graft survival rates can be significantly lower (e.g., 36.4% kidney and 45% liver graft survival after 10 years) than patient survival rates, which means that many transplant recipients will have to face a second transplant 5–10 years after their first (Figure 31–3) (United Network of Organ Sharing 2004).

These stark facts highlight the enormous stresses facing transplant candidates, transplant recipients, and their caregivers. These issues have also created a particular environment in which hospitals must evaluate, treat, and se-

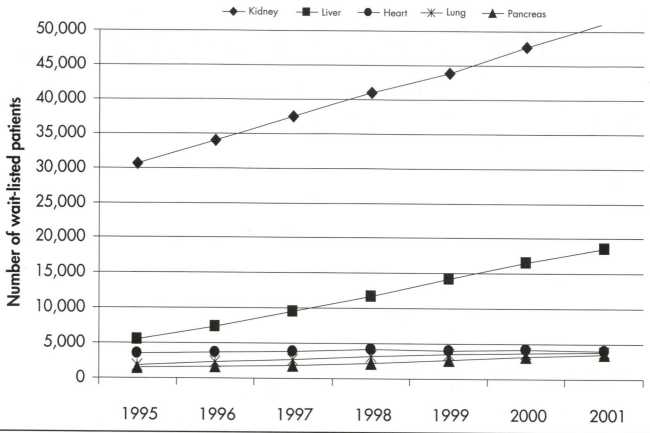

FIGURE 31–1.   **Year-end numbers of wait-listed patients, by organ type: 1995 to 2001.**

Source.   United Network of Organ Sharing (UNOS; http://www.optn.org).

lect patients for organ transplantation. The scarcity of donated organs has driven efforts to select candidates believed to have the best chance for optimal posttransplant outcomes. Additionally, the organ shortage has increasingly led to the consideration of living kidney donors and, more recently, living liver donors (and, more rarely, living lung donors) as transplantation options.

Pretransplant psychosocial evaluations are commonly requested to assist in candidate and donor selection, and psychiatric consultation is often needed for clinical input during the pre- and posttransplant phases. Although a wide body of knowledge has been developed in the clinical care of transplant candidates and recipients, little longitudinal research is available to answer questions about long-term outcomes or the impact of psychiatric factors (assessed pretransplant and/or in the early years posttransplantation) on outcomes. Research primarily has focused on kidney, heart, and liver transplantation, which in combination currently account for almost 90% of transplants performed in the United States.

In this chapter, we outline the essential areas of the field for psychosomatic medicine specialists and other mental health clinicians involved in the care of transplant pa-

tients—pretransplant assessment and candidate selection, emotional and psychological aspects of the transplant process, therapeutic issues, patients with complex or controversial features, psychopharmacological treatment, and neuropsychiatric side effects of immunosuppressive medications. Special pretransplantation topics of emerging importance to psychosomatic medicine specialists are also discussed (i.e., hepatic encephalopathy, ventricular assist devices in heart transplantation, tobacco use, and living donors). The neuropsychiatric sequelae of end-stage organ disease are not covered in this chapter, because those aspects are addressed in the respective chapters on each organ system. Specific transplant issues are also discussed in Chapter 19, "Heart Disease"; Chapter 20, "Lung Disease"; Chapter 22, "Renal Disease"; and Chapter 34, "Pediatrics."

Pretransplantation Issues

Psychosocial/Psychiatric Assessment

Pretransplant psychosocial evaluations have been a traditional role of the psychiatric consultation team in the

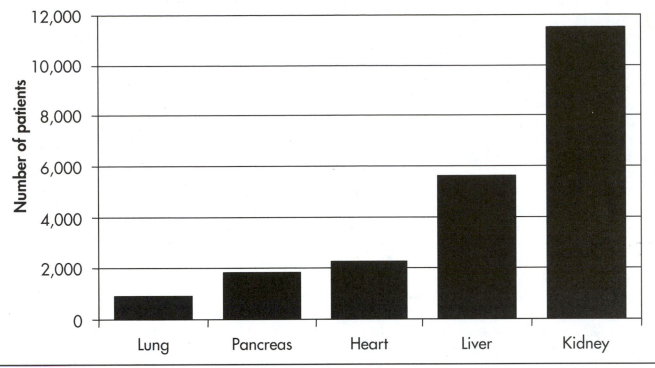

FIGURE 31–2. Numbers of transplant recipients in 2001, by organ type.

Source. United Network of Organ Sharing (UNOS; http://www.OPTN.org).

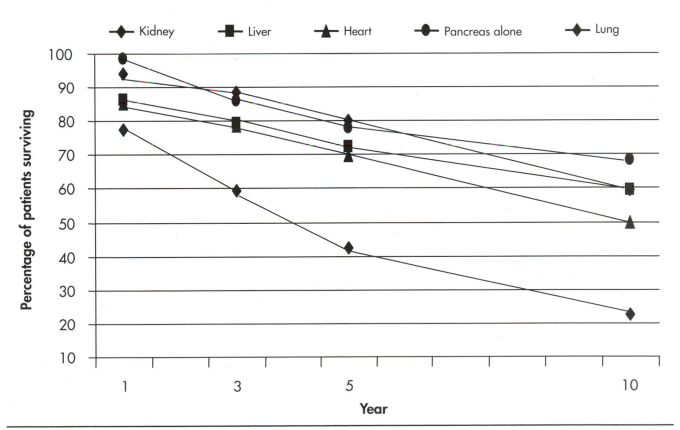

FIGURE 31–3. Survival rates of transplant recipients, by organ type.

Source. United Network of Organ Sharing (UNOS; http://www.optn.org).

transplantation process. These evaluations are frequently used to assist in the determination of a candidate's eligibility for transplantation, to identify psychiatric/psychosocial problems that may need to be addressed to prepare the candidate and family for transplantation, and to identify pre- and posttransplant psychiatric and/or psychosocial needs of the candidate. These evaluations are also critical for the identification of psychiatric, behavioral, and psychosocial risk factors that may portend poor transplant outcomes (Crone and Wise 1999; Dew et al. 2000b).

Transplant programs will often refer for evaluation candidates with a known history of psychiatric problems or those who are identified during the initial clinical interviews with the transplant team as having such problems. Pretransplant psychosocial evaluations are also usually requested for patients with substance use disorders (including tobacco) and other poor health behaviors (e.g., obesity, noncompliance).

Although a truly comprehensive assessment of a potential transplant candidate would require a full psychiatric consultation, the current high numbers of candidates preclude this. To handle the increasing volume of evaluations, some centers employ screening batteries of patient-rated measures to identify candidates with elevated levels of psychological distress, who then undergo a full psychiatric evaluation. Screening instruments can provide baseline cognitive, affective, and psychosocial ratings for candidates; use of these instruments maximizes staff resources and minimizes costs. For example, using this strategy, Jowsy et al. (2002) identified 20%–44% of liver transplant candidates who had mild to severe symptoms on a range of measures, which prompted a higher level of evaluation.

Emerging evidence shows that preoperatively assessed psychosocial variables can predict posttransplantation psychiatric adjustment among recipients of most organ types (Dew et al. 2000b). These variables are increasingly being investigated as contributing to medical outcomes as well, although a consistent predictive effect has not yet been demonstrated (Dew et al. 2000b). Thus, psychosocial assessment of transplant candidates provides an opportunity to identify potential problems and intervene prior to transplantation, with the goal of improving posttransplant outcomes. Transplant programs vary considerably in their psychosocial assessment criteria and procedures (see Olbrisch and Levenson 1995 for a review of methodological and philosophical issues); in general, however, psychosocial evaluations have 10 objectives (although a given assessment may not include all 10), as enumerated in Table 31–1 (see Levenson and Olbrisch 2000).

TABLE 31–1. Goals of psychosocial screening

1. Assess coping skills; disqualify or intervene with patients who appear to be unable to cope effectively.
2. Diagnose comorbid psychiatric conditions; provide for pre- and posttransplant monitoring and treatment.
3. Determine the candidate's capacity to understand the transplant process and to provide informed consent.
4. Evaluate the candidate's ability to collaborate with the transplant team and to adhere to treatment.
5. Assess substance use/abuse history, recovery, and ability to maintain long-term abstinence.
6. Identify health behaviors that may influence posttransplant morbidity and mortality (i.e., tobacco use, poor eating or exercise habits) and evaluate the candidate's ability to modify these behaviors over the long term.
7. Help the transplant team to understand the patient better as a person.
8. Evaluate the level of social support available to the candidate for pre- and posttransplant phases (including stable family/others committed to assisting the candidate, adequate insurance and financial resources, and logistical support).
9. Determine the psychosocial needs of the patient and family and plan for services during the waiting, recovery, and rehabilitation phases of the transplant process.
10. Establish baseline measures of mental functioning in order to be able to monitor postoperative changes.

Source. Adapted from Levenson J, Olbrisch ME: "Psychosocial Screening and Selection of Candidates for Organ Transplantation," in *The Transplant Patient.* Cambridge, UK, Cambridge University Press, 2000, p. 23. Used with permission.

Because information on all of these domains may not be obtainable during a single clinical interview, a follow-up reassessment may be necessary to clarify relevant issues, solidify a working relationship with the patient and family, and resolve problems. A multidisciplinary approach is often used with input from psychiatrists, psychologists, psychiatric nurse clinical specialists, addiction specialists, social workers, transplant surgeons, and transplant coordinators to construct a comprehensive picture of the patient and develop a coordinated treatment plan. As with any psychiatric evaluation, verbal feedback provided to the patient and family will serve to solidify the expectations of the transplant team and the requirements of the patient for listing if indicated. Some centers also use written "contracts" to formalize these recommendations (Cupples and Steslowe 2001; Stowe and Kotz 2001). In difficult cases, these contracts serve to document expectations, thereby minimizing misinterpretation. Written contracts outline a treatment plan that can be referred to with each follow-up appointment. These contracts are particularly useful with transplant candidates who have alcohol or substance abuse/dependence problems, specifying the transplant program's requirements for addiction treatment, monitoring of compliance (e.g., documented random negative blood alcohol levels), and length of abstinence (see subsection "Alcohol and Other Substance Use Disorders" later in this chapter).

Psychosocial Instruments and Measures

Transplant-specific (e.g., Psychosocial Assessment of Candidates for Transplant [Olbrisch et al. 1989], Transplant Evaluation Rating Scale [Twillman et al. 1993]), disease-specific (e.g., Miller Health Attitude Scale for cardiac disease [Miller et al. 1981], Quality of Life Questionnaire—Chronic Lung Disease [Guyatt et al. 1987]), and disorder-specific (e.g., High Risk Alcohol Relapse Scale for alcoholism [Yates et al. 1993]) instruments have been used to evaluate transplant candidates and monitor their posttransplant recovery. These instruments have been used in conjunction with general instruments for rating behavior, coping, cognitive and affective states, and quality of life. Psychosocial instruments can be used to identify individuals who require further assessment (as described earlier) or to pursue evaluation of patients already identified as requiring additional screening. The evaluator's purpose for using such instruments will determine the type and specificity of the instruments chosen; for instance, in the subsection "Hepatic Encephalopathy" later in this chapter, we discuss the use of neuropsychiatric tests to aid in the identification of cognitive impairment. Some instruments are more applicable to transplant populations than others. For example, although there are many instruments and measures for assessing alcoholism, none of these instruments are tailored to transplant candidates; they are focused on general issues of detection and treatment of addiction rather than on issues important in evaluating appropriateness for transplantation.

Because psychosocial selection criteria differ significantly by program and organ type, development and use of structured evaluation instruments may help to direct and standardize the transplant selection protocols used nationally. The two instruments most commonly used to assess candidates for transplantation are the Psychosocial Assessment of Candidates for Transplantation and the Transplant Evaluation Rating Scale.

The Psychosocial Assessment of Candidates for Transplantation (PACT) was the first published psychosocial structured instrument specifically designed for screening transplant candidates (Olbrisch et al. 1989). It provides an overall score and subscale scores for psychological health (psychopathology, risk for psychopathology, stable personality factors), lifestyle factors (healthy lifestyle, ability to sustain change in lifestyle, compliance, drug and alcohol use), social support (support system stability and availability), and patient educability and understanding of the transplant process. The PACT can be completed in only a few minutes by the consultant following the evaluation but requires scoring by a skilled clinician, without which the instrument's predictive power could be diminished (Presberg et al. 1995). The final rating for candidate acceptability is made by the clinician, with the freedom to weigh individual item ratings variably (Presberg et al. 1995). Thus, a single area, such as alcohol abuse, could be assigned greater weight and thus could disproportionately influence the final rating.

The PACT has been used to predict mortality in bone marrow recipients (independent of age, gender, or diagnosis), as well as to predict hospital lengths of stay following liver transplantation (Levenson et al. 1994). Its "risk for psychopathology" subscale identifies psychopathology that may require referral and treatment after liver, heart, and bone marrow transplantation (Levenson et al. 1994).

The Transplant Evaluation Rating Scale (TERS) is used to rate patients' level of adjustment in 10 areas of psychosocial functioning: prior psychiatric history, DSM-III-R Axis I and Axis II diagnoses, substance use/abuse, compliance, health behaviors, quality of family support, prior history of coping, coping with disease and treatment, quality of affect, and mental status (Twillman et al. 1993). In one study, the TERS was significantly correlated with several clinician-reported outcome variables (compliance, health behaviors, substance use), with particularly high correlations between pretransplant TERS scores and posttransplant substance use ($r = 0.64$) (Twillman et al. 1993). The instrument requires administration by a skilled clinician to maintain accuracy (Presberg et al. 1995). The TERS summary score is derived from a mathematical formula in which individual item scores are multiplied by theoretical, predetermined weightings.

Although individual candidates do not always easily fit within one of the three categories of each item on the TERS, the TERS has more items than the PACT, a feature that may prove useful in future research (Presberg et al. 1995). However, the PACT is the more flexible of the two instruments, both in the range of rating individual items and in the manner in which the summary score is determined (Presberg et al. 1995). Together, these instruments are useful in the organization of patient information and can be helpful both as tools for increasing the evaluator's understanding of the candidate and for research purposes.

The Unique Role of the Psychiatric Consultant

Unlike in most psychiatric interviews, the psychiatrist performing the pretransplant assessment primarily serves the needs of the transplant team rather than those of the patient (a possible exception is the evaluation of living organ donors; see subsection "Living Donor Transplantation" later in this chapter). The psychiatric consultant must be candid with the patient about this role. Careful delineation of specific transplant-related expectations, explanation of the importance of these requirements to the success of transplantation, and exploration of the implications of these criteria for the individual candidate serve to establish a meaningful dialogue with the patient from which the therapeutic alliance necessary for future intervention can develop.

For the clinician, the seemingly reverse nature of this role can be uncomfortable or even anxiety provoking. This is especially true if the clinician is not recommending the candidate for transplantation. Fortunately, many programs do not reject patients outright for psychosocial reasons; rather, they offer such patients the opportunity to work to bring their problematic areas into compliance with the recommendations (i.e., through addiction counseling, behavioral changes, psychiatric treatment, identification of appropriate social supports) and then undergo reevaluation for candidacy. In these cases, the psychiatric consultant can often function as an advocate for the patient and assist in referral for appropriate treatment if indicated. Nevertheless, some patients will be unable to comply with the specified transplant requirements or will not survive to complete their efforts to meet candidacy requirements.

Philosophical, moral, ethical, legal, and therapeutic dilemmas are inherent in the role of transplant psychiatrist, as conflicting team opinions present themselves in the course of work with potential transplant candidates. Team discussions and consultation with other colleagues are the rule in complicated cases. In these instances, team discussions not only aid in resolving candidacy quandaries but also can help alleviate team members' anxiety and discomfort over declining a patient for transplantation. Group or team debriefing may also be desirable, and occasionally consultation with risk management and the legal department of the hospital is needed (e.g., when a candidate is challenging candidacy requirements or the candidacy decision of the transplant team). Thorough documentation is essential in order to delineate the issues involved, the expectations of the team for transplantation candidacy, and the efforts to work with the patient.

Psychological and Psychiatric Issues in Organ Transplantation

Psychiatric Symptoms and Disorders in Transplant Patients

Similar to other medically ill populations, transplant candidates and recipients experience a significant amount of psychological distress and are at heightened risk of developing psychiatric disorders. The prevalence rates of major depression range from 4% to 28% in liver transplant patients, 0% to 58% in heart transplant patients, and 0.4% to 20% in kidney transplant patients (Dew 2003; Dew et al. 2000b). The range of rates for anxiety disorders appears to be 3% to 33% (Dew 2003; Dew et al. 2000b), but there are not enough studies to identify specific types of anxiety disorders. One study found that 10% of a cohort of heart or lung transplant recipients experienced posttraumatic stress disorder (PTSD) related to their transplant experience (Köllner et al. 2002). In a prospective study of 191 heart transplant recipients, the cumulative prevalence rates for psychiatric disorders during the 3 years posttransplantation were 38% for any disorder, including 25% with major depression, 21% with adjustment disorders, and 17% with PTSD (Dew et al. 2001a). Factors that increased the cumulative risk for psychiatric disorders included a pretransplant psychiatric history, a longer period of hospitalization, female gender, greater impairments in physical functioning, and fewer social supports (Dew et al. 2001a).

Several studies have suggested an association between psychiatric disorders and transplant health outcomes, although the results have been mixed. A study of wait-listed liver transplant candidates found that candidates with Beck Depression Inventory (BDI) scores higher than 10 (64% of patients) were significantly more likely than nondepressed candidates to die while awaiting transplantation (Singh et al. 1997). The higher BDI scores were due more to psychological distress than to somatic symptoms. However, for candidates who reached transplantation, pretransplant depression was not associated with poorer posttransplant survival (Singh et al. 1997). These results were not affected by the severity of and complications from liver disease, or by patients' social support, employment, or education (Singh et al. 1997). A study of lung transplant recipients found that those with a pretransplant psychiatric history (anxiety and/or depressive disorders) were more likely than those without such a history to be alive 1 year after transplantation (Woodman et al. 1999). However, in a study of 191 heart transplant recipients, a DSM-III-R diagnosis of PTSD (with the traumatic event being transplant related) was associated with higher mortality (odds ratio=13.74) (Dew and Kormos 1999). Another study of heart transplant recipients found that patients with ischemic cardiomyopathy and high self-rated depression scores pretransplant had significantly higher posttransplant mortality compared with the low-depression group after adjustment for sociodemographic and somatic symptoms (Zipfel et al. 2002). Although causal directions cannot be inferred from these data, studies in other medically ill populations have demonstrated the substantial contribution of depression and anxiety to health outcomes (see Chapter 9, "Depression," and Chapter 12, "Anxiety Disorders"). Whether treating these disorders will affect patient outcomes is unclear. However, the role of the psychiatrist in evaluating, diagnosing, and treating psychiatric disorders both pre- and posttransplantation is critical.

Adaptation to Transplantation

Transplant candidates typically experience a series of adaptive challenges as they proceed through evaluation, waiting, perioperative management, postoperative recuperation, and long-term adaptation to life with a transplant (Olbrisch et al. 2002). With chronic illness, there can be progressive debility and gradual loss of vitality and of physical and social functioning. Adapting to these changes can elicit anxiety, depression, avoidance, and denial and requires working through of grief (Olbrisch et al. 2002). Patients who are wait-listed may develop contraindications to transplantation (i.e., infection, serious stroke, progressive organ dysfunction), and both patients and families should be made aware that a candidate's eligibility can change over time for many reasons (Stevenson 2002). During this phase, psychiatrists may provide counseling to patients and families to help them prepare for either transplantation or death.

The summons for transplantation can evoke a mixture of elation and great fear. Many programs use electronic pagers to contact recipients, and some patients can develop anxiety related to anticipation of the pager's ring. Patients may experience a panic attack when they are called for transplantation, and some may even decline the offer of an organ.

Much of illness behavior depends on the coping strategies and personality style of the individual. In our experience, the adaptive styles of adult transplant recipients often depend on whether patients' pretransplant illness experience was chronic or acute, as delineated in the following broadly generalized profiles.

Patients who have dealt with chronic illness for years may adapt psychologically to the sick role and can develop coping strategies that perpetuate a dependency on being ill (Olbrisch et al. 2002). For these patients, transplantation may psychologically represent a transition from one state of illness to another, and such patients can have difficulty adjusting to or transitioning into a "state of health." They often complain that the transplant team is expecting too fast a recovery from them, and they may describe feeling pressured to get better. Some patients may develop unexplained chronic pain or other somatic complaints or may begin to evidence noncompliance with transplant team directives.

For patients with good premorbid functioning who become acutely ill, with only a short period of pretransplant infirmity, the transplant can be an unwelcome event. These patients can experience a heightened sense of vulnerability, and they may deny the seriousness of their medical situation (Olbrisch et al. 2002). These patients often wish to return to normal functioning as quickly as possible posttransplantation, and they may in fact recover more rapidly than the transplant team expects; however, they may suffer later as the result of pushing themselves too much (e.g., returning to work before they are physically ready). They may resent being a transplant recipient, with all of the restrictions and regimens inherent in that role, and may act out their anger or denial in episodes of noncompliance (Olbrisch et al. 2002).

Treatment Modalities

A prospective study of kidney transplant recipients demonstrated that individual psychotherapy was effective in resolving transplant-related emotional problems, with significant reductions in BDI scores after therapy (Baines et al. 2002). Three recurring psychological themes were expressed by patients in this study: 1) fear of organ rejection, 2) feelings of paradoxical loss after surgery despite successful transplantation, and 3) psychological adaptation to the new kidney (Baines et al. 2002).

In addition to traditional therapies and pharmacotherapy (see section "Psychopharmacological Treatment in End-Stage Organ Disease" later in this chapter), various innovative strategies have been employed to deal with specific issues of transplantation and also to address logistical and staffing resource issues. At the University of Toronto, a mentoring program was developed for heart transplant recipients. Mentorship by an already transplanted recipient augmented patient care by providing information and support from a peer perspective (Wright et al. 2001). The four topics most commonly discussed between mentors and mentees were postoperative complications (70%), medications (70%), wait on the transplant list (70%), and the surgery itself (50%) (Wright et al.

2001). Participants less frequently discussed psychiatric topics such as anxiety (40%) and depression (10%) and personal topics such as sexual relations (20%) and marital problems (10%). The program was well received, and patients were very satisfied with the experience. To increase patient satisfaction with the mentor program, Wright and colleagues recommend early introduction of a mentor and matching of mentors with mentees according to demographics and clinical course (Wright et al. 2001).

Group therapy for organ transplantation patients and family members has also been successfully used. At the Toronto Hospital Multi-Organ Transplantation Program, group psychotherapy is organized along three dimensions: course of illness (pre- vs. posttransplantation), homogeneous versus heterogeneous group membership (e.g., separate groups for patients and caregivers vs. integrated groups, organ-specific groups vs. cross-organ groups), and group focus (issue-specific vs. unstructured) (Abbey and Farrow 1998). Increasing levels of group therapy intensity are used, depending on the needs of the patient. Educational groups are mandatory for pretransplant candidates to prepare them for transplantation. From these groups, candidates at risk for psychosocial problems are referred to supportive and psychoeducational groups. Interpersonal and supportive–expressive psychotherapy groups are available to those who require them and have the psychological capacity to benefit from them. Group therapy participants report decreases in negative affect, increases in positive affect and happiness, less illness intrusiveness, and improved quality of life (Abbey and Farrow 1998). Transplant coordinators also report that patients in group therapy require less contact, both in clinic and by telephone for social support (Abbey and Farrow 1998).

Dew and colleagues (2004) have developed an innovative strategy for managing the logistical problem of recipients living at a distance from the transplant program. These researchers designed and evaluated an Internet-based psychosocial intervention for heart transplant recipients and their families. This multifaceted Web-based intervention included stress and medical regimen management workshops, monitored discussion groups, access to electronic communication with the transplant team, and information on transplant-related health issues (Dew et al. 2004). Compared with heart recipients without access to the Web site, intervention patients reported significant reductions in depressive and anxiety symptoms and improved quality of life in the social functioning domain; in addition, caregivers of intervention patients reported significant declines in anxiety and hostility symptoms ($P<0.05$). Mental health and quality-of-life benefits were greater among more-frequent users of the Web site. The subgroup using the Web site's medical regimen workshop showed significantly better compliance at follow-up than did all other patients in attending clinic appointments, completing blood work, and following diet (Dew et al. 2004). Dew and colleagues concluded that a Web-based intervention could improve follow-up care, compliance, and mental health in patients and families as they adjust to heart transplantation.

Patients With Complex or Controversial Psychosocial and Psychiatric Issues

The stringency of selection criteria for transplantation appears to depend on the type of organ transplant being considered, and transplant programs often have strongly formed beliefs about the suitability of candidates with certain types of mental illness. Cardiac transplant programs are more likely than liver transplant programs to consider psychosocial issues as contraindications, and liver transplant programs in turn are more stringent than kidney transplant programs (Corley et al. 1998; Levenson and Olbrisch 1993). These differences may be attributable to the relative availability of specific types of organs (Yates et al. 1993); alternatively, the extent of experience with specific organ transplants allowing programs to feel more comfortable with less stringent criteria (e.g., kidney transplantation, with more than three decades of experience and nearly 300,000 kidney transplants performed in the United States) (United Network of Organ Sharing 2004). In addition, for kidney transplantation, cost-effectiveness research has clearly demonstrated the long-term cost savings of kidney transplantation relative to dialysis (Eggers 1992). With such unequivocal evidence, insurance payers have a strong financial incentive to refer patients early for preemptive transplantation, before the high costs of dialysis begin to accumulate (Eggers 1992). In such a setting, psychosocial factors may have less impact on transplantation candidacy. Other issues influencing the selection process include moral and ethical beliefs, societal views, personal beliefs, and even financial constraints.

Although increasing numbers of poor prognostic indicators during the perioperative period may increase risk for noncompliance posttransplantation (Dew et al. 1996; see subsection "Posttransplant Compliance" below), it should be emphasized that candidates with any one of these features are not categorically poor recipients or that patients without any of these features do not categorically make the best candidates. What little research is available provides some support for clinical assumptions that patients with certain personality disorders, substance disorders, poor coping skills, poor compliance, and poor social supports can have worse posttransplant outcomes. Nevertheless, case reports have demonstrated that even some patients who might seem inappropriate for transplant (e.g., patients with active psychosis or with severe personality disorders) (Carlson et al. 2000; DiMartini and Twillman 1994) can undergo transplantation and maintain adequate compliance after the procedure. Such patients should be carefully assessed pretransplant with optimization of their pretransplant condition and ongoing psychiatric monitoring and treatment posttransplantation. Prospective longitudinal studies are needed to clarify pretransplant factors that contribute to increased risk of poor outcomes (both psychological and medical) and the contribution of posttransplant factors on outcomes as well.

Posttransplant Compliance

Lifelong immunosuppression is a prerequisite for good graft function, and noncompliance with immunosuppressive medication is often associated with late acute rejection episodes, chronic rejection, graft loss, and death. It might be assumed that transplant patients, in general, constitute a highly motivated group and that their compliance would be high. Unfortunately, overall posttransplant medical noncompliance rates of all organ types range from 20% to 50% (see Laederach-Hofmann and Bunzel 2000 for a complete review). With organ transplantation, noncompliance impairs both life quality and life span, as it is a major risk factor for graft-rejection episodes and may be responsible for up to 25% of deaths after the initial recovery period (Bunzel and Laederach-Hofmann 2000). Noncompliance leads to waste, as it reduces the potential benefits of therapy and adds to the costs of treating avoidable consequent morbidity. Graft loss from noncompliance is also tragic, given the large numbers of patients on the waiting lists. The global assessment of transplant patient compliance is difficult, and patients can manifest varying degrees of adherence to medical recommendations. For transplant recipients, compliance is commonly conceptualized as adherence to immunosuppressive medications. Yet the occurrence of clinically measurable events such as rejection episodes, organ loss, or death underrepresents the true amount of noncompliance, as some patients who are only partially compliant have not yet experienced a clinically adverse event (see Bunzel and Laederach-Hofmann 2000; De Geest et al. 1995). Although such "subclinical" noncompliance is undetectable as a medical event, it is important as an indicator of those patients having difficulty following their medical regimens (Feinstein 1990).

De Geest et al. (1995) reported a medication noncompliance rate of 22.3% in kidney transplant patients, whereas Paris et al. (1994) found a rate of 47% among heart transplant recipients. Shapiro et al. (1995) observed that of 93 heart transplant recipients, about one-third (34.4%) were noncompliant in at least some areas over the course of long-term follow-up. Dew and colleagues (1996) examined compliance in eight domains of posttransplant care in a cohort of 101 heart recipients. During the first postoperative year, the degree of noncompliance varied across time. However, they found persistent noncompliance in the domains of exercise (37%), blood pressure monitoring (34%), immunosuppressive medication (20%), smoking (19%), diet (18%), blood work completion (15%), clinic attendance (9%), and heavy drinking (6%). These studies also identified associations between noncompliance and increased risk of morbidity and mortality in transplant recipients (De Geest et al. 1995; Dew and Kormos 1999; Dew et al. 1996; Paris et al. 1994).

Dew et al. (1996) carried out a "dose–response" analysis of specific factors found to contribute to noncompliance in a preliminary regression analysis. A "dose" variable was created by determining how many of these six psychosocial risk factors—anxiety, anxiety–hostility, poor support from caregivers, poor support from friends, failure to use active cognitive coping strategies, and use of avoidance coping strategies—a recipient possessed. The logistic regression model showed a strong dose effect, in that if 0 to 1 psychosocial risk factor was present, the probability of having postoperative compliance difficulties was less than 30%. With 2 to 3 factors present, the probability rose to about 50%, and if 4 or more risk factors were present, more than 80% of patients encountered significant compliance difficulties. This means that if predictors cumulate, compliance problems are likely to rise dramatically.

Other studies have determined that psychiatric problems that persist after transplantation are highly associated with noncompliance (Paris et al. 1994; Phipps et al. 1997). In an extensive literature review of posttransplant compliance for all organ types, Bunzel and Laederach-Hofmann (2000) found that anxiety disorders—and, in particular, untreated major depression—were significantly associated with noncompliance. In a study of 125 heart transplant recipients (Shapiro et al. 1995), compliance problems were associated with a history of substance abuse ($P=0.0007$).

Alcohol and Other Substance Use Disorders

Compared with other solid organ transplant candidates, liver transplant (LTX) candidates more often require psychiatric consultation for substance addiction assessment, due to the prevalence of alcoholic liver disease (ALD) and viral hepatitis transmitted through contaminated needles. An estimated 50% of LTX recipients have a pre-LTX history of alcohol and/or drug abuse/dependence (DiMartini et al. 2002). A survey of 69 U.S. liver transplant programs found that 83% of programs have a psychiatrist or addiction medicine specialist routinely see each patient with ALD during the evaluation phase (Everhart and Beresford 1997). In the optimal situation, the psychiatric clinician is an integral member of the transplant clinical care team and can integrate the addiction treatment plan into the patient's pre-and posttransplant care. The Cleveland Clinic Foundation has formed a chemical-dependence transplant team to assess, treat, and monitor transplant patients with addictive disorders (Stowe and Kotz 2001). This program is a model for the integration of such services.

Psychiatric consultation provides a thorough evaluation of the candidate's addiction history; their understanding of their addiction (especially in the context of their health and need for transplantation, their stability in recovery, and their need for further or ongoing addiction treatment), and the presence of other psychiatric disorders. Family and social support for the candidate's continued abstinence both pre- and posttransplantation must also be evaluated. In one study of LTX candidates, those with a history of substance abuse revealed significantly more distress, less adaptive coping styles, and more character pathology than their counterparts (Stilley et al. 1999). Because these features may heighten the potential for relapse, periodic reassessment by the psychiatric consultant provides follow-up on the candidate's progress in recovery, including verifying ongoing participation in rehabilitation as well as monitoring for psychological and affective distress and poor coping styles with therapeutic interventions targeting these problems as they arise. Documentation of treatment participation is desirable, as is random toxicological screening for alcohol and other substances. These measures are especially important for patients early in recovery and for those with a short period of abstinence, denial over their problem, resistance to seeking treatment, or poor social support for continuing abstinence. One study of pretransplant wait-listed ALD candidates found that 15% of candidates had used alcohol at some point after the initial transplant evaluation (Weinrieb 2003).

One-year post-LTX drinking rates (i.e., the percentage who used any alcohol by 1 year post-LTX) range from 8% to 37% (DiMartini 2000b; Everson et al. 1997), with cumulative rates estimated at 30%–40% by 5 years post-LTX (Lucey 1999). Rates of pathological drinking, defined as drinking that results in physical injury or alcohol dependence, are 10%–15% (Everson et al. 1997; Fireman 2000). Although the rate of alcohol use appears to attenuate with the passage of time, post-LTX (Berlakovich et al. 1994; Campbell et al. 1993), dependent drinking can occur years post-LTX (DiMartini 2000a). In one study, 15% of LTX recipients had their first drink within the first 6 months post-LTX, a finding that highlights the importance of early and intensive clinical follow-up to identify alcohol use at its onset (DiMartini et al. 2001).

Consistent predictors of posttransplant alcohol use have been difficult to identify. This may be due to the heterogeneity of the ALD transplant population and the potential selection bias whereby the most stable candidates are chosen, making this population different from the general alcohol-abusing/dependent populations (DiMartini et al. 2002). For example, a pretransplant history of illicit drug use has not been consistently associated with increased risk for posttransplant alcohol relapse in ALD recipients (Coffman et al. 1997; DiMartini et al. 2002; Fireman 2000; Foster et al. 1997; Newton 1999), possibly because many ALD recipients had discontinued their drug use many years prior to transplantation (Coffman et al. 1997). In one of the few prospective studies to examine posttransplant alcohol use, a pretransplant history of alcohol dependence, a family history of alcoholism, and prior rehabilitation experience (thought to be a marker for those with more severe addiction) were all found to be associated with posttransplant alcohol use ($P<0.05$). A prior history of other substance use was associated with a higher (but non–statistically significant) risk of posttransplant drinking (DiMartini 2000b).

Compared with LTX candidates with alcohol dependence, LTX candidates with polysubstance dependence are more likely to have multiple prior addiction treatments; more likely to be diagnosed with personality disorders, especially cluster B type (antisocial, narcissistic, histrionic, borderline); and less likely to have stable housing, a consistent work history, or stable social support (Fireman 2000). Yet despite evidence that this specific population could be at higher risk for relapse, there are few published outcome studies addressing the issue of posttransplant nonalcohol substance use. Most studies have investigated the rates of relapse only in ALD recipients who also had a nonalcohol other substance use disorder. One of the few studies to investigate all patients with a pre-LTX addiction history found not only that patients with a pre-LTX history of polysubstance use disorders had a higher relapse rate compared with those with alcohol dependence alone (38% vs. 20%), but also that the majority of polysubstance users demonstrated ongoing post-LTX substance use (Fireman 2000). Studies investigating all transplant recipients are needed to identify the true posttransplant rates of other substance use.

After transplantation, maintaining an open, nonjudgmental dialogue with transplant recipients appears to be the most effective way to identify alcohol and/or other substance use in the posttransplant period, and most recipients are open to discussing their substance use habits with the transplant team (DiMartini et al. 2001; Weinrieb et al. 2000). A review of liver enzymes and biopsy results and a candid discussion of the damage caused by alcohol and other substances provide an opportunity to explore the patient's denial of the consequences of their use. Even in the most difficult cases, patients wish to maintain their health and are willing to listen to advice and recommendations on addiction treatment. In our experience, the transplant team has established a powerful emotional bond with the recipient. Many patients who have resumed substance use were relieved to learn that the transplant team would not abandon them. On the other hand, it is important not to condone or dismiss small amounts of alcohol or other substance use. What may seem supportive can be distorted by the patient with an addiction and become an excuse to use more regularly. In the case of alcohol use, we have found that few patients with alcoholism can drink "socially" posttransplantation (Tringali et al. 1996) and that those who take their first drink often consume moderate to heavy amounts of alcohol (DiMartini et al. 2002). Therefore, total alcohol abstinence is recommended for these patients.

Medications that may reduce cravings and potentially diminish relapse risk for alcohol (e.g., acamprosate, ondansetron, naltrexone) or opioids (naltrexone) have not been studied in transplant patients. One study that attempted to use naltrexone in actively alcohol-relapsing LTX recipients found that patients were reluctant to use naltrexone as a result of its potential, albeit small, risk of hepatotoxicity (Weinrieb et al. 2001). Naltrexone can be a direct hepatotoxin at dosages higher than recommended (>300 mg/day) and is not recommended for patients with active hepatitis or liver failure. Disulfiram has been used in nontransplant populations to provide a negative reinforcement to drinking alcohol. This agent blocks the oxidation of alcohol at the acetaldehyde stage and can create severe nausea, vomiting, and hemodynamic instability. It requires hepatic metabolism for conversion into an active drug. A metabolite of disulfiram is an inhibitor of cytochrome P450 3A4 (Madan et al. 1998), and posttransplantation may cause immunosuppressive medication toxicity. Use of disulfiram in transplant recipients could place these individuals at risk for serious harm and is not recommended. In nontransplant patients, selective serotonin reuptake inhibitors (SSRIs) and tricyclic antidepressants

(TCAs) can stabilize mood and improve abstinence rates in depressed relapsing alcoholic individuals (Cornelius et al. 2003) and may be the most appropriate pharmacological interventions for transplant recipients if concurrent mood symptoms are present.

Methadone-Maintained Candidates

Transplant program acceptance of opioid-dependent patients receiving methadone maintenance treatment (MMT) is a controversial issue. Recent studies have examined candidate selection processes and posttransplant outcomes for this population.

In a recent survey of U.S. liver transplant programs (Koch and Banys 2001), of the 56% of programs that reported accepting patients for evaluation who were taking methadone, a surprising 32% required patients to discontinue their methadone use prior to transplantation. Of even more concern was the overall lack of experience with such patients (i.e., only 10% of the programs had treated more than five MMT patients). Although there are no studies of pretransplant methadone cessation in liver transplant patients, there exists an abundance of evidence showing that tapering methadone in stable methadone-maintained patients results in relapse to illicit opiate use in up to 82% of these individuals (Ball and Ross 1991). In our opinion, an attempt to taper a recovering opiate addict from methadone should not be made at a time when the patient is struggling with the stresses and pain associated with end-stage liver disease. Until data to the contrary emerge, requiring methadone tapering in stable opiate-dependent patients as a prerequisite for transplant candidacy could be considered unethical. This strategy potentially heightens the risk for relapse, and those that relapse would be denied transplantation.

In regard to posttransplant outcomes of MMT patients, Koch and Banys (2001) found that of the approximately 180 transplant patients on methadone maintenance at the time of the survey, relapse to illicit opiate use was reported for less than 10% of patients. Similar to other reports of noncompliance in transplant patients (see subsection "Posttransplant Compliance" earlier in this chapter), approximately 26% of MMT patients had compliance difficulties with immunosuppressive medications (Koch and Banys 2001). However, it was not reported whether those who used illicit drugs were also among those who had problems with compliance. In general, the transplant programs did not consider that the noncompliance necessarily affected outcomes, and the transplant coordinator's impressions were that only 7 of 180 patients had poor outcomes (Koch and Banys 2001). In two small series of MMT LTX recipients (5 in each), overall long-term patient and graft survival were found to be comparable to those of other LTX recipients at the transplant centers, with none of the MMT patients evidencing posttransplant noncompliance or illicit drug use (Hails and Kanchana 2000; Kanchana et al. 2002). Liu et al. (2003), in a study of the largest single cohort (*N*=36) of MMT LTX recipients to date, concluded that patient and graft survival were comparable to national averages (they did not use a control group, however). Although four patients (11%) reported isolated episodes of heroin use posttransplantation, relapses were not considered to have resulted in poorer outcomes.

These descriptive studies demonstrate that MMT transplant recipients can successfully undergo transplantation and do well; however, the lack of control groups makes it difficult to prove that MMT patients' rates of complications and survival are no different from those of transplant recipients in general. Although the small numbers of MMT candidates and recipients preclude large-scale prospective studies, a case–control study conducted by Gordon et al. (1986) found that posttransplant patient and graft survival rates in the 20 heroin-addicted kidney recipients were similar to those in the control group. The leading cause of death (infection) was the same in both groups. In the study group, only one patient returned to heroin use. Two other study patients who were not suspected of using heroin lost their grafts as a result of medication noncompliance, whereas no patient in the control group lost a graft as a result of noncompliance (Gordon et al. 1986). In summary, the data to date justify neither automatic exclusion of MMT patients from transplantation nor any requirement that such patients be tapered off methadone prior to transplant.

Personality Disorders

Personality disorders are characterized by persisting and inflexible maladaptive patterns of subjective experience and behavior that may create emotional distress and interfere with the individual's interpersonal relationships and social functioning. The requirements of successful transplantation can be too difficult for such an individual, as the process requires a series of adaptations to changes in physical and social functioning and significant ability to work constructively with both caregivers and the transplant team. By identifying personality traits and disorders, the psychiatrist can potentially predict patterns of behavior, recommend treatment, develop a behavioral plan with the team to work constructively with the patient, and render an opinion as to the candidate's ability to proceed with transplantation. Patients with personality disorders can require excessive amounts of time from the

transplant team, which raises the issue of resource allocation as a potential selection criterion (Carlson et al. 2000). Not surprisingly, a majority of programs (50%–60% across organ types) consider personality disorders to be a relative contraindication to transplantation (Levenson and Olbrisch 1993). Yet all personality disorders should not be viewed similarly, as the behavioral and coping styles of different personality disorders can present varying degrees of concordance with the needs of transplantation. For example, the need for structure and orderliness of a candidate with obsessive-compulsive personality disorder would be more adaptive to the demands of transplantation than the coping style of a patient with borderline personality disorder.

The incidence of personality disorders in transplant populations is similar to that in the general population, ranging from 10% to 26% (Chacko et al. 1996; Dobbels et al. 2000), although in some cohorts estimates have been as high as 57% (Stilley et al. 1997). However, the identification of personality disorders depends on the definition and measurement methods used. Unfortunately, studies investigating personality disorders and transplantation outcomes have not distinguished among the various personality disorder types (perhaps because of the low prevalence of each type), which makes generalizations difficult. Nevertheless, case reports of patients with severe character pathology demonstrate the extent of compliance problems that can arise from these disorders, resulting in significant morbidity and recipient death (Surman and Purtilo 1992; Weitzner et al. 1999). The disturbances in interpersonal relationships that can occur with personality disorders also can decrease the likelihood that patients will have stable and reliable social supports during the pre- and posttransplant phases (Yates et al. 1998). Of the personality disorders, borderline personality disorder is considered to represent the highest risk for posttransplant noncompliance (Bunzel and Laederach-Hofmann 2000).

Whereas sociopathy has not consistently been associated with substance relapse in the addiction literature (Vaillant 1997), a survey of transplant programs in the United States revealed that 4 of 14 programs (29%) would reject a candidate with comorbid antisocial personality disorder and alcohol dependence (Snyder et al. 1996). In a study of 73 ALD transplant candidates, patients with severe personality disorders had higher rates of divorce, higher rates of comorbid drug abuse/dependence, lower IQs, higher scores on indicators of emotional impairment, and were more likely, although not significantly so, to return to drug use during the pretransplant follow-up period (Yates et al. 1998). However, of this cohort, 3 patients with serious personality disorders underwent liver transplantation and did not relapse or become noncompliant in the early postoperative phase (Yates et al. 1998). In contrast, another study of 91 patients transplanted for ALD and followed for up to 3 years identified 18 patients exhibiting antisocial behavior (Coffman et al. 1997). Of those with antisocial behavior, 50% returned to either alcohol (n=6) or prescription narcotic addiction (n=3) posttransplantation, which was significantly higher than the 19.8% alcohol use by the total group (Coffman et al. 1997). In a prospective study of 125 heart transplant recipients, personality disorders were associated with posttransplant compliance problems (P=0.007) (Shapiro et al. 1995). Although personality disorders were not associated with survival, those individuals with personality disorders tended to have more graft rejection (P=0.06) (Shapiro et al. 1995).

Although not identified as specific personality disorder styles, various coping and behavioral styles have also been shown to influence survival. A study by Chacko et al. (1996) of survival post–heart transplant found that whereas the presence of clinician-rated Axis II disorders (26% of the group) was not associated with survival time, some of the strongest predictors of survival were health behaviors, maladjustment, and coping styles. Using the same measure of health behavior and coping (Millon Behavioral Health Inventory [Millon et al. 1982]), Coffman and Brandwin (1999) found that wait-listed heart transplant candidates with high scores on the Life Threat Reactivity subscale had significantly higher mortality before transplantation (42% vs. 18%; P=0.0001) but not after transplantation. These investigators suggested that one possible explanation was that the detrimental psychological traits of the high-risk group were ameliorated by surviving to be transplanted (Coffman and Brandwin 1999).

Patients with personality disorders do best with ongoing pre- and posttransplant psychotherapy, specifically cognitive and behavioral interventions to promote compliance with the care regimen and to establish a working alliance with transplant team members (Dobbels et al. 2000). These patients should be given clear and consistent instructions on rules and requirements of transplantation, reinforced by regular outpatient appointments. A limited number of transplant center staff should maintain contact with the patient, and staff should communicate regularly among themselves and the outpatient psychiatric team (Carlson et al. 2000) to coordinate care and to reduce opportunities for cognitive distortions and splitting by the patient. A formal written contract can document the expectations of the transplant team and serve as a therapeutic treatment plan whereby the patient and team agree to work together toward common goals for the transplant recipient's health (Dobbels et al. 2000).

Psychotic Disorders

Although chronic and active psychosis is thought by many to be incompatible with successful transplantation, case reports of carefully selected patients with psychosis demonstrate that such patients can successfully undergo transplantation and survive after the procedure (DiMartini and Twillman 1994; Krahn et al. 1998). A recent survey of transplant psychiatrists at national and international transplant programs identified only 35 cases of pretransplant psychotic disorders in transplant recipients from 12 transplant centers (Coffman and Crone 2002), suggesting that such patients are highly underrepresented among transplant recipients. Results of this survey confirmed previously expressed stipulations that patients with psychotic disorders be carefully screened before acceptance. Candidates should have demonstrated good compliance with both medical and psychiatric follow-up; possess adequate social supports, especially in-residence support; and be capable of establishing a working relationship with the transplant team. In this survey (Coffman and Crone 2002), risk factors for problems with compliance after transplantation included antisocial or borderline personality disorder features, a history of assault, living alone, positive psychotic symptoms, and a family history of schizophrenia. Posttransplant noncompliance with nonpsychiatric medications was found in 20% of patients (7 of 35), and noncompliance with laboratory tests was found in 17% (6 of 35 patients) (Coffman and Crone 2002); however, these numbers are similar to percentages of medication and laboratory testing noncompliance in general transplant populations. Overall, noncompliance resulted in rejection episodes in 5 patients (14%) and in reduced graft function or loss in 4 patients (12%) (Coffman and Crone 2002). Thirty-seven percent of patients experienced psychotic or manic episodes posttransplantation (not necessarily associated with immunosuppression), 20% attempted suicide (with two completed suicides), 20% experienced severe depression or catatonia, 5.7% committed assaults, 5.7% were arrested for disorderly conduct, and 8.6% required psychiatric commitment (Coffman and Crone 2002).

Although concerns have been raised in regard to the potential of immunosuppressive medications to produce or exacerbate psychotic symptoms, patients with a prior psychiatric history are not necessarily more susceptible to "steroid psychosis" than are patients without such a history (Hall et al. 1979), and appropriate use of antipsychotic medication is usually adequate to manage these symptoms if they emerge. Because transplant teams often overlook the early postoperative reinstitution of antipsychotic medications, it is essential that the psychiatrist devote careful attention to this issue during the immediate postoperative phase. If quick reintegration of the patient into his or her pretransplant outpatient psychiatric treatment regimen is not possible because of infirmity, interim in-home psychiatric follow-up care should be instituted.

Special Issues During the Pretransplant Phase

Hepatic Encephalopathy

Hepatic encephalopathy (HE), a neuropsychiatric syndrome commonly encountered in liver transplant candidates, is characterized by a constellation of signs and symptoms, such as alteration of consciousness (including stupor or coma), cognitive impairment, confusion/disorientation, affective/emotional dysregulation, psychosis, behavioral disturbances, bioregulatory disturbances, and physical signs such as asterixis. Identification of HE is important, because its symptoms directly affect patient quality and quantity of life; fulminant HE is associated with intracranial hypertension, cerebral edema, and death pretransplant (Ferenci et al. 2002). It is also critical to differentiate between the fluctuating course of HE and more persistent cognitive deficits that may indicate a preexisting dementia rather than delirium. Recent efforts to define HE have emphasized that it reflects a continuum of symptoms, with subclinical HE lying at the minimal end of the spectrum. Even subclinical HE is clinically important, because it can impair patient safety (Schomerus et al. 1981) and is associated with persistent cognitive deficits post-LTX (Tarter et al. 1990). In one study, 85% of patients with subclinical HE were found to be either of questionable fitness or unfit to drive on psychometric testing of driving capacity (Schomerus et al. 1981). By definition, subclinical HE is not identifiable on a typical clinical examination; detection may require additional neuropsychological tests of psychomotor speed, praxis, concentration, and attention. The Trail Making Test (A and B) and the Digit Symbol and Block Design tests from the Wechsler Adult Intelligence Scale—Revised are commonly used to identify subclinical HE impairment. Whereas the prognostic significance of HE is well known, the long-term impact of subclinical encephalopathy on cognitive functioning requires further investigation.

The predominant strategy for treating HE involves reducing the production and absorption of ammonia from the intestinal tract, although a variety of compounds and metabolites (e.g., mercaptans, false neurotransmitters, manganese, endogenous benzodiazepines, increased concentrations of central nervous system [CNS] gamma-aminobutyric acid [GABA]) have also been implicated in HE (Chung and Podolsky 2003; Riordan and Williams 1997). Psychiatric consultants should be familiar with ammonia-reducing strategies, because they are often the ones who must recognize and monitor HE symptoms, identify whether patients are being treated for HE, and make recommendations regarding the need for initiating or improving treatment. HE can be precipitated by gastrointestinal hemorrhage, uremia, use of some psychoactive medications or diuretics, dietary indiscretions, dehydration, or electrolyte imbalance (Chung and Podolsky 2003; Riordan and Williams 1997), and these problems should be corrected first. Treatment should strive to normalize ammonia levels, despite the fact that blood ammonia levels are not well correlated with symptoms of HE (Riordan and Williams 1997). Treatment strategies include administration of a nonabsorbable disaccharide, lactulose, that acts as an osmotic laxative to flush out ammonia; adherence to a protein-restricted diet to decrease the production of ammonia from protein; and prescription of nonabsorbable antibiotics to reduce intestinal bacteria that convert protein to ammonia. Some patients require all three treatments simultaneously. Medications that can contribute to symptoms of HE—anticholinergic drugs, tranquilizers, and sedatives—should be avoided.

Ventricular Assist Devices in Heart Transplantation

Progress in the development of implantable left ventricular assist devices (LVADs) has dramatically improved both the physical and the psychological health of potential cardiac transplant candidates. The new LVADs consist of a mechanical pump implanted in the abdomen with conduits from the apex of the left ventricle to the ascending aorta. Blood returning from the lungs to the left side of the heart exits through the left ventricular apex into the LVAD pumping chamber. Blood is then actively pumped through the LVAD outflow valve into the ascending aorta. One transcutaneous line carries an electrical cable to an external battery pack and electronic controls, which are worn on a shoulder holster or belt.

Prior to the use of LVADs, the need for prolonged inotrope infusions before transplantation could lead to very lengthy hospitalizations for cardiac transplant candidates. These patients would become deconditioned and were at risk for deep vein thrombosis, pulmonary emboli, multiple organ dysfunction, and sudden cardiac death. However, recent experience with newer LVADs reveals improvement in mechanical/electrical failure rates and lessened risks for thromboembolism (Rose et al. 2001a, 2001b). Patients on LVADs can achieve better hepatic, renal, cerebral, and peripheral perfusion, leading to improvement in overall physical function, exercise tolerance, and well-being (Goldstein et al. 1998; Morrone et al. 1996). These devices are now portable, permitting discharge from the hospital before transplantation and a generally acceptable quality of life (Dew et al. 2000a; Frazier 1993; Loisance et al. 1994). Patients on LVADs can undergo physical and physiological rehabilitation, develop exercise tolerance, and rebuild muscle mass, thus stabilizing their cardiac condition (Goldstein et al. 1998; McCarthy 2002; Morrone et al. 1996). The lack of mobility restriction means that patients often can return to work and engage in activities such as dancing and driving (Catanese et al. 1996). With the urgency for transplantation diminished, the transplant team can wait for an optimal donor organ.

On the downside, however, the logistics of arranging outpatient care require a well-trained medical team whose members are available at all times, resulting in significant patient, caregiver, and medical system burden. All persons involved in the patient's care must receive extensive training, arrangements for outpatient housing or maintenance at home must be coordinated, and local emergency paramedical personnel must also be trained. Infection can occur in more than 60% of LVAD recipients (Gordon et al. 2001); in one study of patients with permanent LVADs, 41% of deaths were related to infection (Rose et al. 2001b). Not surprisingly, in a study of recipients of ventricular assist devices (including both LVADs and biventricular assist devices), the most common concern was risk of infection (52%) (Dew et al. 2000a). In addition, 52% had difficulty sleeping because of the driveline, 46% had pain at the driveline site, 40% worried about device malfunction, and 32% were bothered by the noise (Dew et al. 2000a). In posttransplantation comparisons with heart recipients who did not receive a ventricular assist device (VAD), patients who were bridged to transplantation with a VAD showed similar improvements in physical functioning and emotional well-being, significantly lower rates of anxiety, but poorer cognitive status (Dew et al. 2001b). The cognitive impairments observed in the VAD recipients were believed to be attributable to neurological events that occurred during the period of VAD support and were higher than that of non-VAD patients during the waiting period before transplantation. Although mild, these impairments appeared to persist during the first year following transplantation and were associated with less likelihood of returning to employment (Dew et al. 2001b). In the future, as the technology continues to improve, selected patients may receive LVADs as permanent implants rather than as bridges to transplantation (Rose et al. 2001a, 2001b).

Tobacco Use and Transplantation

Tobacco use by transplant candidates and recipients has received surprisingly little attention. Even in lung and heart transplantation, tobacco use is not routinely reported. Tobacco use coupled with immunosuppressive therapy, which also increases cancer risk (Nabel 1999), may result in higher rates of cancer posttransplantation. For ALD liver transplant recipients in one study, the rates of oropharyngeal cancer and lung cancer were 25 and 3.7 times higher, respectively, than rates in the general nontransplant population matched for age and gender (Jain et al. 2000), presumably as a result of tobacco use.

One study of heart transplant recipients found that 26%–50% of smokers resumed smoking posttransplantation (Bell and Van Triget 1991; Nagele et al. 1997). Compared with nonsmokers, smokers had higher rates of vasculopathy and of malignancies (Nagele et al. 1997); they also had significantly worse survival, with none of the smokers surviving 11.5 years posttransplantation (vs. 80% of the nonsmokers surviving). When patients were grouped by carboxy-hemoglobin level, investigators found that no patients with a level higher than 2.5% were surviving 4 years after transplantation (Nagele et al. 1997). In this cohort, smoking appeared to be much more important than other classical risk factors (Nagele et al. 1997). Similarly, a study of liver transplant recipients found a higher rate of vascular complications in patients with a history of smoking (17.8% vs. 8% in patients without such a history; $P=0.02$); furthermore, having quit smoking 2 years prior to transplantation reduced the incidence of vascular complications by 58% (Pungpapong et al. 2002). In a prospective study of ALD liver transplant recipients, 53% were found to be using tobacco posttransplantation (DiMartini et al. 2002). A study of 60 heart transplant recipients reported that 3 patients had resumed smoking within 6 months following transplantation and that all 3 had also relapsed to drug or alcohol abuse (Paris et al. 1994). Another study of heart transplant recipients found that elevated posttransplant anxiety was associated with a higher risk of resuming smoking (Dew et al. 1996).

The cessation of tobacco use (both smoked and smokeless) prior to transplantation is strongly recommended, given that many pretransplant users resume use posttransplantation. Treatments for smoking cessation include bupropion, nicotine replacement (patches, gum, lozenges, and aerosolized formulations), and behavioral therapies (Hurt et al. 1997; Jorenby et al. 1999). Because of its association with seizure risk, bupropion should be used with caution in transplant recipients, who are already at increased risk from immunosuppressive medications, particularly during the early posttransplant period, when immunosuppressive levels are higher. A good alternative would be nortriptyline, which in combination with cognitive-behavioral therapy in general-population studies has been demonstrated to have a smoking cessation success rate similar to that of bupropion (Hall et al. 1998). Notwithstanding, the anticholinergic side effects of nortriptyline could be problematic in candidates or recipients at risk for delirium, and although the drug's α-adrenergic, antiarrhythmic, and negative inotropic effects are tolerated post–heart transplant (Kay et al. 1991; Shapiro 1991), these effects should be carefully monitored in heart transplant candidates.

Living Donor Transplantation

Despite the physical risks, discomfort and pain, expense and inconvenience, and potential psychological consequences of donating an organ, increasing numbers of people are becoming donors, and transplant programs are considering living donation as one solution to the organ shortage. In fact, in 2001 the number of living donors exceeded the number of cadaveric donors (6,526 vs. 6,081) for the first time, with the majority from kidney donors, although an increasing number are coming from living liver donors in the form of a partial hepatectomy (United Network of Organ Sharing 2004). Currently, more than 50% of kidney transplants come from living donors (United Network of Organ Sharing 2004). Kidneys and portions of the liver, lung, pancreas, intestine, and even the heart (through a domino procedure in which a heart-lung recipient donates their heart) are donated for transplantation (Oaks et al. 1994; Rodrigue et al. 2001; Taguchi and Suita 2002).

Donation of an organ—putting one's life at risk to help another—is an incredibly generous and altruistic gift. Yet the evaluation of such donors is complex process requiring assessment of the circumstances and motives of the donor, the dynamics of the relationship between donor and recipient, the severity of the recipient's illness, and family and societal forces. Current practice guidelines require a psychosocial evaluation for each potential donor to thoroughly examine these and other issues (Table 31–2) (Olbrisch et al. 2001; Surman 2002). Donors must be fully willing, independently motivated, and completely informed about the surgery. Yet for liver donors in particular, long-term sequelae that may affect the donor's future health, functioning, and even ability to obtain health insurance (due to the presence of a preexisting condition) are not known.

Living liver donation is a much more surgically complex, invasive, and potentially more dangerous procedure than kidney donation. Although mortality rates have been

---

TABLE 31–2.   Areas of assessment for living donor evaluation

Reasons for donation
Relationship between donor and recipient
Donor's knowledge about the surgery
Motivation
Ambivalence
Evidence of coercion/inducement
Attitudes of significant others toward the donation
Availability of support
Financial resources
Work- and/or school-related issues (if applicable)
Donor's psychological health, including the following:
    Psychiatric disorders
    Personality disorders
    Coping resources/style
    Pain syndromes
    Prior psychological trauma/abuse
    Substance use

---

less than 1% for both kidney and liver donors (Brown et al. 2003; Najarian et al. 1992), about one-third of liver donors have complications, with serious complications occurring in 14% of donors (Brown et al. 2003; Grewal et al. 1998). There have been consensus recommendations that all potential live liver donors be evaluated by an independent physician advocate (i.e., not a member of the transplant team responsible for the recipient's care) as part of the informed consent process (Abecassis et al. 2000; Conti et al. 2002) to avoid conflicts of interest. However, in only 50% of programs does a physician who is not part of the transplant team evaluate the potential donor (Brown et al. 2003). Kidney donors should expect to miss 4–6 weeks of work and liver donors 8–12 weeks of work, especially if the job involves heavy lifting. Since the late 1990s, laparoscopic donor nephrectomy has been increasingly used, a procedure that results in less postoperative pain, shorter hospital stays, overall quicker recovery times, and more favorable cosmetic results. Future research may also show this approach has psychosocial benefits as well.

Adult-to-adult living donor liver transplantation (LDLT) is a relatively new procedure in the United States, preceded by adult-to-child transplants. Whereas only 9 such procedures had been performed in the United States prior to 1998, in 2001 more than 400 adult-to-adult LDLTs were performed. Unfortunately, too few procedures are performed at any one center—and approaches to recipients and donors are too diverse across centers—to provide reliable and generalizable information about donor and recipient outcomes. In one study that examined outcomes of parent-to-child liver donation, psychological testing was found to be useful in identifying families that were more likely to experience problems postdonation (Goldman 1993). Although donor outcomes were reported as good, with donors experiencing increased self-esteem and satisfaction, marital dissolution occurred in 2 of the 20 families following donation (Goldman 1993). In another study, one donor committed suicide 2 years after donation, and although this event was deemed by the transplantation center to be unrelated to the donation, the details were not known (Brown et al. 2003).

A U.S. live organ donor consensus group recommended the development of a living donor registry to collect demographic, clinical, and outcome information on all living organ donors. The rationale for the development of such a registry includes concern for donor well-being, limitations of current knowledge regarding the long-term consequences of donation, the potential to evaluate the impact of changes in criteria for donor eligibility on the outcome of donors, and the need within the transplant community to develop mechanisms to provide for quality assurance assessments (Abecassis et al. 2000). In the near future, a multicenter study of adult-to-adult living liver donor outcomes commissioned by the National Institute of Diabetes and Digestive and Kidney Diseases should help provide answers to these questions (see "Adult-to-Adult Living Donor Liver Transplantation Cohort Study [A2ALL]" 2003).

In contrast with the United States, Japan has extensive experience with living liver donation as a result of cultural beliefs (lack of acceptance of brain death criteria) that hamper cadaveric donation. This created an environment in which living liver donation was necessary for LTX. More than 1,500 adult-to-adult LDLTs have been performed in Japan, with no reported donor mortality (Surman 2002). Fukunishi et al. (2001) first reported on psychiatric outcomes in LDLT donors and recipients, identifying post-LTX psychiatric disorders (excluding delirium) in 37% of LDLT recipients and "paradoxical reactions" (including guilt over receiving donation, avoidant coping behaviors, and psychological distress) in 34% of recipients, despite favorable medical outcomes for both recipient and donor. Ten percent of liver donors experienced major depression within the first month after donation. Fukunishi and colleagues speculated that predonation, the stronger sense of duty of adult children donating to their parents masked their true concerns and fears. Following donation, these concerns manifested as anxiety, fear, and pain (Fukunishi et al. 2003). The prevalence of psychiatric disorders was higher in LDLT recipients than in a comparison group of living donor kidney recipients, suggesting a potential greater need for psychiatric evaluation and care of LDLT patients.

Altruistic donors—those donating to an unknown recipient—pose one of the most complex challenges to transplant evaluation. In these cases, the psychosocial evaluation has particular importance in determining the suitability of the donor, and some believe that the medical standards for such donors should be higher (Friedman 2002). Altruistic donors are commonly viewed with some skepticism and are evaluated with greater caution than related donors. A detailed evaluation is critical, both to understand the motives and psychological meaning of the donation to the donor and to identify any financial or other types of compensation expected for the donation. A recent study of nondirected donors reported that 21% were excluded for psychological reasons (Matas et al. 2000). Psychological outcomes of altruistic liver donors are unknown.

Psychopharmacology in End-Stage Organ Disease

Given the high prevalence of psychiatric disorders in transplant candidates and recipients, pharmacological treatment is often required. Unfortunately, psychotropic medications are often not provided because of concerns about patients' medical fragility and the potential risks of psychotropic medications. The fact that psychiatric symptoms may evolve from complex, intertwined psychological and physiological processes should not preclude treatment. Although the treatment of transplant candidates and recipients can be complicated, a thorough knowledge of psychotropic pharmacokinetics in specific types of end-stage organ failure, coupled with careful attention to medication dosing, side effects, and drug interactions, can provide the necessary foundation for pharmacological management (see also Chapter 37, "Psychopharmacology"; Robinson and Levenson 2001; Trzepacz et al. 2000).

Liver Disease

Liver failure affects many key steps of medication pharmacokinetics, from absorption to metabolism, distribution, and elimination, causing changes in drug levels, duration of action, and efficacy. As the liver becomes cirrhotic, collateral blood vessels develop that circumvent the liver. Intrahepatic and extrahepatic physiological (and, in many patients, surgical) shunts create portal–systemic diversion that reduces liver perfusion and particularly affects first-pass metabolism as less drug is delivered to hepatic enzymes. Loss of functional parenchyma and hepatic enzymes decreases phase I metabolism (such as the cytochrome P450 enzyme system) or phase II metabolism (conjugation enzymes). Most psychotropic medications require hepatic metabolism and are highly bound to plasma proteins. The liver's production of plasma proteins is reduced, with a resulting increase of the free and pharmacologically active fraction of highly protein-bound drugs. These processes will raise effective drug levels, increasing the risk of drug side effects or toxicity (Leipzig 1990; Levy 1990; Pond and Tozer 1984). Increased volume of distribution resulting from fluid retention (ascites, peripheral edema) can lower effective levels of both water-soluble and highly protein-bound drugs (because more will be in the unbound state due to hypoproteinemia) (Klotz 1976).

The etiology and severity of liver disease will determine changes in drug pharmacokinetics, including changes in enzymatic activity that affect drug metabolism. In addition, the type of disease (e.g., cholestatic vs. noncholestatic liver disease), the type of disease process (e.g., periportal [affecting phase II enzymes] vs. pericentral [affecting phase I cytochrome P450 enzymes] disease processes), and the type of drug (high-clearance or flow-dependent vs. low-clearance or enzyme-saturating drugs) all play an important role in pharmacokinetics.

One semiquantitative measure of liver functioning, the Child-Pugh Score (CPS), uses commonly available clinical and biochemical indices to rate the severity of end-stage liver disease. The CPS provides a readily reproducible and standardized method for assessing the degree of liver failure and is generalizable to patients with liver disease regardless of its etiology (Albers et al. 1989). Although the categories of the CPS may overgeneralize the complexities of drug pharmacokinetics, the indices used identify impairment in pharmacokinetic functions (i.e., protein production, portal–systemic shunting, ascites), making the CPS total rating a useful guideline for psychotropic medication dosing (see Table 31–3). Nevertheless, for the newer medications the pharmaceutical companies typically publish detailed information on drug absorption, metabolism, and elimination, with suggested guidelines for patients with hepatic disease (often using the CPS), and these documents should be referred to for specific medication dosing. In our clinical experience, we have found that patients rated as having CPS class A liver failure are early in the disease process and can usually tolerate 75%–100% of a standard dosage. Those with CPS class B should be dosed more cautiously, starting with a 50%–75% reduction in the normal starting dose. As a result of the prolongation of the elimination half-life and the subsequent delay in reaching steady state, more gradual increments in dosing are required. Patients with CPS class B liver failure can often obtain relief or remission of symptoms with 50% of a typical psychotropic medication dosage. Those with CPS class C commonly have some degree of hepatic encephalopathy, and medication usage must be cautiously monitored to avoid worsening of the hepatic encephalopathy symptoms. Sometimes distinguishing whether depressive symptoms represent primary depression or the affective dysregulation of hepatic encephalopathy may not be possible, in which case a cautious empirical trial of medication may be warranted.

Renal Disease

Reduced renal clearance of drugs can occur in renal insufficiency due to primary renal disease or from hypoperfusion in hepatorenal syndrome (McLean and Morgan 1991) or severe heart failure (Shammas and Dickstein 1988). Reduced renal clearance is especially important for psychotropic medications that are predominantly excreted by the kidneys (e.g., lithium, gabapentin, topiramate, methylphenidate) and also for psychotropic drugs for which renal excretion of active metabolites is the primary route of elimination (e.g., venlafaxine and its active metabolite *O*-desmethylvenlafaxine). In uremia, drug oxidation is normal or accelerated, reduction and hydrolysis are slowed, glucuronide and glycine conjugations are normal-

TABLE 31–3.   Grading of liver disease severity using the Child-Pugh Score (CPS)

	1 Point	2 Points	3 Points
Bilirubin (mg/dL)	<2.0	2–3	>3.0
Albumin (g/dL)	>3.5	2.8–3.4	<2.7
Protime (INR)	<1.5	1.6–2.4	>2.5
Ascites	None	Mild	Moderate
Encephalopathy	None	Stage 1–2	Stage 3–4

Note.   Grading: A = 5–6 points; B = 7–9 points; C = 10–15 points.
Source.   Adapted from Albers et al. 1989.

and acetylation may be slowed (Reidenberg 1977). Excess urea may cause gastric alkalinizing effects, decreasing intestinal absorption of some medications (Levy 1990). In renal failure, hypoalbuminemia, coupled with the inhibition of drug–protein binding from uremia and the accumulation of endogenous protein-binding inhibitors (Wilkinson 1983), can increase free drug concentrations, especially for drugs with protein binding greater than 80% (i.e., most psychotropics). The effect of diminished renal clearance was demonstrated in a study of TCAs in which inactive metabolites reached 500% to 1,500% of normal levels (Lieberman et al. 1985). Although these metabolites are thought to be clinically inert, they can alter disposition of the active drug by displacing it from protein binding, competing for active transport mechanisms, and inhibiting drug metabolism (Lieberman et al. 1985). For patients in severe renal failure, dosing can be complicated (see Chapter 37, "Psychopharmacology"), and renally excreted psychotropic medications should be used very cautiously.

Heart Disease

In cardiac insufficiency and congestive heart failure, organ hypoperfusion (especially the liver and kidneys) and increased volume of distribution of drugs due to "third spacing" into interstitial tissues result in decreased drug metabolism and clearance (Shammas and Dickstein 1988). In one study of patients with congestive heart failure, the half-life of midazolam was prolonged by 50% and the plasma clearance was reduced by 32% (Patel et al. 1990). Right-sided heart failure can lead to intestinal and hepatic venous congestion, which can impair drug absorption and metabolism, respectively (Shammas and Dickstein 1988). Acute hypoxia can change blood flow dynamics. Splanchnic blood flow is reduced in the liver, decreasing metabolism, and renal blood flow is also reduced (du Souich and Erill 1978). Hepatically cleared drugs are more affected than renally cleared drugs in congestive heart failure (Woosley 1987). Patients with severe right-sided heart failure with passive congestion of the liver should be treated as patients with hepatic insufficiency and dosages initially reduced by 50%.

Lung Disease

In pulmonary disease, the binding of some drugs to plasma proteins may be increased, resulting in a lengthened time course of the drug effect, increased drug distribution, and more rapid hepatic and renal clearance (du Souich and Erill 1978). As with heart disease, acute hypoxia can reduce splanchnic blood flow to the liver,

decreasing drug metabolism, and can reduce renal blood flow (du Souich and Erill 1978). Increased pulmonary vascular resistance, leading to decreased cardiac output (cor pulmonale), causes increased systemic venous pressures, which in turn decrease perfusion of the liver and kidneys. The lungs also contain cytochrome P450 isoenzymes, which may play a minor role in first-pass and overall drug metabolism (Pond and Tozer 1984). Additionally, high-affinity binding sites for both imipramine and SSRIs have been identified in the lungs, perhaps reflecting the high affinity of these drugs for the serotonin transporter (Suhara et al. 1998). The significance of these findings in heart and lung disease patients is unknown, although it is speculated that the lungs act as a reservoir for medications with a high affinity to the serotonin transporter (Suhara et al. 1998).

Neuropsychiatric Side Effects of Immunosuppressive Agents

Recent advances in our understanding of immunology and the development of newer strategies for immunosuppression may significantly reduce the need for—if not obviate completely—long-term maintenance immunosuppression. In the future, transplant recipients of all organ types may require immunosuppressive medication dosages only one or two times a week, or not at all (Starzl 2002). This achievement would remove the final obstacle to long-term successful outcomes for transplant recipients, given that the majority of long-term morbidity and mortality is due to chronic immunosuppression (e.g., infections, renal failure, cancer). Additionally, reduced requirements for immunosuppressive medication would aid in medication compliance and relieve some of the financial burden of long-term immunosuppression. However, for now, transplant recipients will continue to require immunosuppressive therapy and to be subject to their potential neurotoxic and neuropsychiatric side effects. Psychiatrists should be familiar with the signs, symptoms, differential diagnosis, neuroimaging findings, and management of immunosuppressive neurotoxicity and secondary psychiatric disorders in solid organ recipients (Strouse et al. 1998).

Cyclosporine

Cyclosporine (Gengraf, Neoral, Sandimmune), a lipophilic polypeptide derived from the fungus *Tolypocladium inflatum Goma*, is used as a primary immunosuppressive agent. Side effects are usually mild and include tremor, restlessness, and headache (Wijdicks et al. 1999). A smaller proportion of patients (12%) experience more serious neurotoxicity characterized by acute confusional states, psychosis, seizures, speech apraxia, cortical blindness, and coma (deGroen 1987; Wijdicks et al. 1995, 1996; Wilson et al. 1988). A higher incidence (33%) of serious neurotoxic side effects was reported in one study of 52 liver transplant recipients. Seizures were experienced by 25%; less commonly reported effects included central pontine myelinolysis, delirium, cerebral abscess, and psychosis (Adams et al. 1987).

More recent evidence suggests that earlier reports of serious neurological side effects may have been attributable to intravenous administration and higher dosages (Wijdicks et al. 1999). The use of the oral form of cyclosporine (Neoral) results in fewer serious neurological side effects (Wijdicks et al. 1999). Cyclosporine trough levels correlate poorly with cyclosporine neurotoxicity (Wijdicks et al. 1999), although in most studies symptoms resolved when the cyclosporine was discontinued and subsequently reinstated at a lower dosage (Wijdicks et al. 1999). Anticonvulsants can successfully treat cyclosporine-induced seizures but are not required long-term (Wijdicks et al. 1996), and seizures may cease with reduction or discontinuation of cyclosporine. A few patients with serious clinical neurotoxic side effects have been found to have diffuse white matter abnormalities, predominantly in the occipitoparietal region, on computed tomography (CT) scanning (deGroen et al. 1987; Gijtenbeek et al. 1999; Wijdicks et al. 1995). In one case, symptoms of cyclosporine-induced cortical blindness resolved with drug discontinuation, although pathological evidence of CNS demyelination persisted for months afterward (Wilson et al. 1988).

Several mechanisms may contribute to the CNS neurotoxicity of cyclosporine. Hypocholesterolemia has been found in a high percentage of patients with serious neurotoxicity (deGroen et al. 1987; Wijdicks et al. 1995). Access may be particularly high in the white matter, with a relatively high density of low-density lipoprotein receptors (Wijdicks et al. 1995). In addition to hypocholesterolemia, hypertension, hypomagnesemia, and the vasoactive agent endothelin may play a role in the pathogenesis of cyclosporine neurotoxicity (Gijtenbeek et al. 1999).

Tacrolimus

Tacrolimus (FK506, Prograft), a macrolide produced by *Streptomyces tsukubaensis*, is used as primary immunosuppressive therapy, as rescue therapy for patients who fail to respond to cyclosporine, and as treatment for graft-versus-host disease. It is more potent and possibly less toxic than cyclosporine, although the neuropsychiatric side effects appear to be similar (DiMartini et al. 1991; Freise et al. 1991). As with cyclosporine, neuropsychiatric side effects are more common with intravenous administration and diminish with oral administration and dosage reduction. Common symptoms include tremulousness, headache, restlessness, insomnia, vivid dreams, hyperesthesias, anxiety, and agitation (Fung et al. 1991). Cognitive impairment, coma, seizures, dysarthria, and delirium occur less often (8.4%) and are associated with higher plasma levels (DiMartini et al. 1997; Fung et al. 1991). FK506 can produce symptoms of akathisia (Bernstein and Daviss 1992). However, a prospective study of 25 renal transplant recipients found no correlation between FK506 plasma levels and scores on an akathisia rating scale, although higher plasma levels were associated with higher levels of subjective restlessness, tension, and autonomic and cognitive symptoms of anxiety (DiMartini et al. 1996).

FK506 has low aqueous solubility and cannot be detected in the cerebrospinal fluid of patients with suspected neurotoxicity (Venkataramanan et al. 1991). However, because FK506 has been identified in the brain tissue of animals, it is believed to cross the blood–brain barrier in humans. In addition, more serious neurotoxic side effects (focal neurological abnormalities, speech disturbances, hemiplegia, and cortical blindness) may occur from higher CNS levels in patients who have a disrupted blood–brain barrier (Eidelman et al. 1991). In a study of 294 consecutive transplant recipients on FK506, those with preexisting CNS damage (e.g., from stroke, multiple sclerosis) were at higher risk for neurotoxic side effects (Eidelman et al. 1991). A rare syndrome of immunosuppression-induced leukoencephalopathy, involving demyelination (particularly in the parieto-occipital region and centrum semiovale), has been described in transplant recipients receiving FK506 (Small et al. 1996). The clinical presentation includes generalized seizures without a clear metabolic etiology and radiographic abnormalities in the cerebral white matter of the parietal/occipital lobes. Like other serious neurotoxic side effects, this syndrome is not associated with the absolute serum level of FK506 but does resolve on discontinuation of FK506 (Small et al. 1996). The mechanism of FK506 neurotoxicity is unclear but may include direct activity at the CNS neuronal level (Dawson and Dawson 1994) or an immune-mediated cause (Wilson et al. 1994).

Corticosteroids

Although chronic corticosteroid use has become less essential in immunosuppression for most patients post-transplantation, high dosages of corticosteroids are still employed in the early postoperative phase and also as "pulsed" dosages to treat acute rejection. Behavioral and psychiatric side effects are common, but conclusions regarding the incidence or characteristics of these effects—or the specific dosages required to cause such effects—are not well established. Serious psychiatric side effects have a reported incidence of 5%–6% (Kershner and Wang-Cheng 1989; Lewis and Smith 1983) and include a wide range of cognitive, affective, psychotic, and behavioral symptoms (Hall et al. 1979; Kershner and Wang-Cheng 1989; Lewis and Smith 1983; Varney et al. 1984). These side effects are reviewed elsewhere in this book, particularly in Chapter 9, "Depression"; Chapter 11, "Mania, Catatonia, and Psychosis"; Chapter 23, "Endocrine and Metabolic Disorders"; and Chapter 25, "Rheumatology."

Sirolimus

Sirolimus (SRL, rapamycin, Rapamune), a macrocyclic lactone isolated from *Streptomyces hygroscopicus*, is a recent addition to the posttransplant immunosuppressive armamentarium. The side-effect profile of sirolimus so far does not include neurotoxicity (Watson et al. 1999), perhaps because sirolimus does not block calcineurin (Sindhi et al. 2001). However, a systematic evaluation of sirolimus neurotoxicity has yet to be conducted.

Azathioprine

Azathioprine (Imuran) is a purine analog first used in organ transplantation in 1968. It is primarily used as an adjunctive immunosuppressive agent and is less widely used today because of the availability of alternative agents. Specific neuropsychiatric side effects have not been reported for this agent, although CNS complications of immunosuppression are a mechanism to keep in mind. Several reports of depressive symptoms in patients receiving azathioprine have been complicated by the concurrent use of other medications (specifically cyclosporine and prednisone) that may have contributed to mood disturbance. Nevertheless, caution is recommended when using azathioprine in patients with a history of depression.

Mycophenolate Mofetil

Few neuropsychiatric symptoms have been reported with mycophenolate mofetil (CellCept), a relatively new immunosuppressant promoted as an improvement over azathioprine. Adverse CNS events (>3% to <20% incidence) included anxiety, depression, delirium, seizures, agitation, hypertonia, paresthesias, neuropathy, psychosis, and somnolence (Roche Pharmaceuticals 2003); however, because the patients in whom these symptoms occurred were being treated with mycophenolate in combination with cyclosporine and corticosteroids, the precise contribution of mycophenolate to the symptoms is difficult to interpret.

Drug Interactions Between Psychotropic and Immunosuppressive Medications

Many of the immunosuppressive medications (i.e., tacrolimus, cyclosporine, and mycophenolate) are metabolized by cytochrome P450 3A4; thus, concurrent use of psychotropic medications that strongly inhibit 3A4 should be avoided. Specific cytochrome P450 3A4 inhibitors capable of interacting adversely with immunosuppressive medications, in decreasing order of inhibition, are as follows: fluvoxamine, nefazodone > fluoxetine > sertraline, TCAs, paroxetine > venlafaxine (see also Table 37–1 in Chapter 37, "Psychopharmacology"). There are case reports in which nefazodone has caused toxic tacrolimus levels (Campo et al. 1998) and a 70% increase in the trough plasma level of cyclosporine (Helms-Smith et al. 1996). In a study in which fluoxetine and TCAs were used to treat depressed transplant recipients, no difference in cyclosporine blood level–to–dosage ratios and dose–response relationships was found between those treated and those not treated with antidepressants (Strouse et al. 1996). This finding suggests that antidepressants with less cytochrome P450 3A4 inhibition may not have clinically meaningful drug interactions with these immunosuppressive medications.

Psychotropic medications theoretically may alter immune function. Some psychotropic medications induce a variety of neuroendocrine and cellular actions that could have immunological effects, yet this area has not been well investigated (Surman 1993). For example, lithium has been shown to enhance neutrophil migration, increase phagocytosis by macrophages, and amplify mitogen stimulation of lymphocytes (Surman 1993). Although the role of these effects in allograft function is not known, lithium has been used to increase the number of peripheral neutrophils (Ballin et al. 1998) to reduce neutropenia. The modulatory effects of psychotropic drugs on the immune system are largely unexplored but may provide valuable information for the future care of transplant patients (see Kradin and Surman 2000 for a complete review).

References

Abbey S, Farrow S: Group therapy and organ transplantation. Int J Group Psychother 48:163–185, 1998

Abecassis M, Adams M, Adams P, et al: The Live Organ Donor Consensus Group: consensus statement on the live organ donor. JAMA 284:2919–2926, 2000

Adams DH, Ponsford S, Gunson B, et al: Neurological complications following liver transplantation. Lancet 1(8539): 949–951, 1987

Adult-to-adult living donor liver transplantation cohort study (A2ALL). Hepatology 38:792, 2003

Albers I, Hartmann H, Bircher J, et al: Superiority of the Child-Pugh classification to quantitative liver function tests for assessing prognosis of liver cirrhosis. Scand J Gastroenterol 24:269–276, 1989

Baines LS, Joseph JT, Jindal RM: Emotional issues after kidney transplantation: a prospective psychotherapeutic study. Clin Transplant 16:455–460, 2002

Ball J, Ross A: The Effectiveness of Methadone Maintenance Treatment. New York, Springer-Verlag, 1991

Ballin A, Lehman D, Sirota P, et al: Increased number of peripheral blood CD34+ cells in lithium-treated patients. Br J Haematol 100:219–221, 1998

Bell M, Van Triget P: Addictive behavior patterns in cardiac transplant patients (abstract). J Heart Lung Transplant 10: 158, 1991

Berlakovich G, Steininger R, Herbst F: Efficacy of liver transplantation for alcoholic cirrhosis with respect to recidivism and compliance. Transplantation 58:560–565, 1994

Bernstein L, Daviss S: Organic anxiety disorder with symptoms of akathisia in a patient treated with the immunosuppressant FK506. Gen Hosp Psychiatry 14:210–211, 1992

Brown RS Jr, Russo MW, Lai M: A survey of liver transplantation from living adult donors in the United States. N Engl J Med 348:818–825, 2003

Bunzel B, Laederach-Hofmann K: Solid organ transplantation: are there predictors for posttransplant noncompliance? A literature overview. Transplantation 70:711–716, 2000

Campbell D, Beresford T, Merion R, et al: Alcohol relapse following liver transplantation for alcoholic cirrhosis: long term follow-up. Proceedings of the American Society of Transplant Surgeons (May):A131, 1993

Campo JV, Smith C, Perel JM: Tacrolimus toxic reaction associated with the use of nefazodone: paroxetine as an alternative agent. Arch Gen Psychiatry 55:1050–1052, 1998

Carlson J, Potter L, Pennington S, et al: Liver transplantation in a patient at psychosocial risk. Prog Transplant 10:209–214, 2000

Catanese KA, Goldstein DJ, Williams DL, et al: Outpatient left ventricular assist device support: a new destination rather than a bridge. Ann Thorac Surg 62:646–652, 1996

Chacko RC, Harper RG, Gotto J, et al: Psychiatric interview and psychometric predictors of cardiac transplant survival. Am J Psychiatry 153:1607–1612, 1996

Chung RT, Podolsky DK: Cirrhosis and its complications, in Harrison's Principles of Internal Medicine. Edited by Braunwald E, Fauci AS, Isselbacher KJ, et al. New York, McGraw-Hill, 2003

Coffman KL, Brandwin M: The Millon Behavioral Health Inventory Life Threat Reactivity Scale as a predictor of mortality in patients awaiting heart transplantation. Psychosomatics 40:44–49, 1999

Coffman K, Crone C: Rational guidelines for transplantation in patients with psychotic disorders. Current Opinion in Organ Transplantation 7:385–388, 2002

Coffman KL, Hoffman A, Sher L, et al: Treatment of the postoperative alcoholic liver transplant recipient with other addictions. Liver Transpl Surg 3:322–327, 1997

Conti DJ, Delmonico FL, Dubler N, et al: New York State Committee on Quality Improvement in Living Liver Donation: A Report to New York State Transplant Council and New York State Department of Health, December 2002. Available at: www.health.state.ny.us. Accessed January 14, 2004

Corley MC, Westerberg N, Elswick RK Jr, et al: Rationing organs using psychosocial and lifestyle criteria. Res Nurs Health 21:327–337, 1998

Cornelius JR, Bukstein O, Salloum I, et al: Alcohol and psychiatric comorbidity. Recent Dev Alcohol 16:361–374, 2003

Crone CC, Wise TN: Psychiatric aspects of transplantation: evaluation and selection of candidates. Crit Care Nurse 19:79–87, 1999

Cupples SA, Steslowe B: Use of behavioral contingency contracting with heart transplant candidates. Prog Transplant 11:137–144, 2001

Dawson TM, Dawson VL: Nitric oxide: actions and pathologic roles. Neuroscience (preview issue):9–20, 1994

De Geest S, Borgermans L, Gemoets H: Incidence, determinants, and consequences of subclinical noncompliance with immunosuppressive therapy in renal transplant recipients. Transplantation 59:340–347, 1995

deGroen PC, Aksamit AJ, Rakela J, et al: Central nervous system toxicity after liver transplantation: the role of cyclosporine and cholesterol. N Engl J Med 317:861–866, 1987

Dew MA: Anxiety and depression following transplantation. Presented at the Contemporary Forums Conference on Advances in Transplantation, Chicago, IL, September 2003

Dew M, Kormos R: Early posttransplant medical compliance and mental health predict physical morbidity and mortality one to three years after heart transplantation. J Heart Lung Transplant 18:549–562, 1999

Dew MA, Roth LH, Thompson ME, et al: Medical compliance and its predictors in the first year after heart transplantation. J Heart Lung Transplant 15:631–645, 1996

Dew MA, Kormos RL, Winowich S, et al: Human factors issues in ventricular assist device recipients and their family caregivers. ASAIO J 46:367–373, 2000a

Dew MA, Switzer GE, DiMartini AF, et al: Psychosocial assessments and outcomes in organ transplantation. Prog Transplant 10:239–259, 2000b

Dew MA, Kormos RL, DiMartini AF, et al: Prevalence and risk of depression and anxiety-related disorders during the first three years after heart transplantation. Psychosomatics 42: 300–313, 2001a

Dew MA, Kormos RL, Winowich S, et al: Quality of life outcomes after heart transplantation in individuals bridged to transplant with ventricular assist devices. J Heart Lung Transplant 20:1199–1212, 2001b

Dew MA, Goycoolea JM, Harris RC, et al: An Internet-based intervention to improve psychosocial outcomes in heart transplant recipients and family caregivers: development and evaluation. J Heart Lung Transplant 23:745–758, 2004

DiMartini A: Monitoring alcohol use following liver transplantation. Presented at the Research Society on Alcoholism, Symposium on Liver Transplantation for the Alcohol Dependent Patient. Denver, CO, June 2000a

DiMartini A: Psychosocial variables for predicting outcomes after liver transplantation for alcoholic liver disease. Presented at the Alcohol Induced Liver Disease: The Role of Transplantation conference, University of Massachusetts Medical Center, October 20, 2000b

DiMartini A, Twillman R: Organ transplantation in paranoid schizophrenia: two case studies. Psychosomatics 35:159–161, 1994

DiMartini A, Pajer K, Trzepacz P, et al: Psychiatric morbidity in liver transplant patients. Transplant Proc 23:3179–3180, 1991

DiMartini AF, Trzepacz PT, Daviss SR: Prospective study of FK506 side effects: anxiety or akathisia? Biol Psychiatry 40:407–411, 1996

DiMartini AF, Trzepacz PT, Pager K, et al: Neuropsychiatric side effects of FK506 vs. cyclosporine A: first-week postoperative findings. Psychosomatics 38:565–569, 1997

DiMartini A, Day N, Dew M, et al: Alcohol use following liver transplantation: a comparison of follow-up methods. Psychosomatics 42:55–62, 2001

DiMartini A, Weinreib R, Fireman M: Liver transplantation in patients with alcohol and other substance use disorders. Psychiatr Clin North Am 25:195–209, 2002

Dobbels F, Put C, Vanhaecke J: Personality disorders: a challenge for transplantation. Prog Transplant 10:226–232, 2000

du Souich P, Erill S: Metabolism of procainamide in patients with chronic heart failure, chronic respiratory failure and chronic renal failure. Eur J Clin Pharmacol 14:21–27, 1978

Eggers P: Comparison of treatment costs between dialysis and transplantation. Semin Nephrol 12:284–289, 1992

Eidelman BH, Abu-Elmagd K, Wilson J, et al: Neurologic complications of FK 506. Transplant Proc 23:3175–3178, 1991

Everhart JE, Beresford TP: Liver transplantation for alcoholic liver disease: a survey of transplantation programs in the United States. Liver Transpl Surg 3:220–226, 1997

Everson G, Bharadhwaj G, House R, et al: Long-term follow-up of patients with alcoholic liver disease who underwent hepatic transplantation. Liver Transpl Surg 3:263–274, 1997

Feinstein AR: On white-coat effects and the electronic monitoring of compliance. Arch Intern Med 150:1377–1378, 1990

Ferenci P, Lockwood A, Mullen K, et al: Hepatic encephalopathy—definition, nomenclature, diagnosis, and quantification: final report of the working party at the 11th World Congresses of Gastroenterology, Vienna, 1998. Hepatology 35:716–721, 2002

Fireman M: Outcome of liver transplantation in patients with alcohol and polysubstance dependence. Presented at Research Society on Alcoholism: Symposium on Liver Transplantation for the Alcohol Dependent Patient. Denver, CO, June 2000

Foster P, Fabrega F, Karademir S, et al: Prediction of abstinence from ethanol in alcoholic recipients following liver transplantation. Hepatology 25:1469–1477, 1997

Frazier OH: Chronic left ventricular support with a vented electric assist device. Ann Thorac Surg 55:273–275, 1993

Freise CE, Rowley H, Lake J, et al: Similar clinical presentation of neurotoxicity following FK506 and cyclosporine in a liver transplant recipient. Transplant Proc 23:3173–3174, 1991

Friedman L: All donations should not be treated equally. Journal of Law, Medicine, and Ethics 30:448–451, 2002

Fukunishi I, Sugawara Y, Takayama T, et al: Psychiatric disorders before and after living-related transplantation. Psychosomatics 42:337–343, 2001

Fukunishi I, Sugawara Y, Makuuchi M, et al: Pain in liver donors. Psychosomatics 44:172–173, 2003

Fung JJ, Alessiani M, Abu-Elmagd K, et al: Adverse effects associated with the use of FK506. Transplant Proc 23:3105–3108, 1991

Gijtenbeek HJ, van den Bent MJ, Vecht CJ: Cyclosporine neurotoxicity: a review. J Neurol 246:339–346, 1999

Goldman LS: Liver transplantation using living donors: preliminary donor psychiatric outcomes. Psychosomatics 34:235–240, 1993

Goldstein DJ, Oz MC, Rose EA: Implantable left ventricular assist devices. N Engl J Med 339:1522–1533, 1998

Gordon MJ, White R, Matas AJ, et al: Renal transplantation in patients with a history of heroin abuse. Transplantation 42:556–557, 1986

Gordon SM, Schmitt SK, Jacobs M, et al: Nosocomial bloodstream infections in patients with implantable left ventricular assist devices. Ann Thorac Surg 72:725–730, 2001

Grewal HP, Thistlewaite JR Jr, Loss GE, et al: Complications in 100 living-liver donors. Ann Surg 228:214–219, 1998

Guyatt GH, Berman LB, Townsend M, et al: A measure of quality of life for clinical trials in chronic lung disease. Thorax 42:773–778, 1987

Hails KC, Kanchana T: Outcome of liver transplants for patients on methadone. Poster presentation, American Psychiatric Association Annual Meeting, Chicago, IL, May 2000

Hall RC, Popkin MK, Stickney SK, et al: Presentation of the steroid psychoses. J Nerv Ment Dis 167:229–236, 1979

Hall SM, Reus VI, Munoz RF, et al: Nortriptyline and cognitive-behavioral therapy in the treatment of cigarette smoking. Arch Gen Psychiatry 55:683–690, 1998

Helms-Smith KM, Curtis SL, Hatton RC: Apparent interaction between nefazodone and cyclosporine (letter). Ann Intern Med 125:424, 1996

Hurt RD, Sachs DP, Glover ED, et al: A comparison of sustained-release bupropion and placebo for smoking cessation. N Engl J Med 337:1195–1202, 1997

Jain A, DiMartini A, Kashyap R, et al: Long-term follow-up after liver transplantation for alcoholic liver disease under tacrolimus. Transplantation 70:1335–1342, 2000

Jorenby DE, Leischow SJ, Nides MA, et al: A controlled trial of sustained-release bupropion, a nicotine patch, or both for smoking cessation. N Engl J Med 340:685–691, 1999

Jowsy SG, Taylor M, Trenerry MR: Special topics in transplantation: psychometric screening of transplant candidates. Oral presentation at the annual Academy of Psychosomatic Medicine meeting, Tucson, AZ, November 2002

Kanchana T, Kaul V, Manzarbeitia C, et al: Transplantation for patients on methadone maintenance. Liver Transplant 8:778–782, 2002

Kay J, Bienenfeld D, Slomowitz M, et al: Use of tricyclic antidepressants in recipients of heart transplants. Psychosomatics 32:165–170, 1991

Kershner P, Wang-Cheng R: Psychiatric side effects of steroid therapy. Psychosomatics 30:135–139, 1989

Klotz U: Pathophysiological and disease-induced changes in drug distribution volume: pharmacokinetic implications. Clin Pharmacokinet 1:204–218, 1976

Koch M, Banys P: Liver transplantation and opioid dependence. JAMA 285:1056–1058, 2001

Köllner V, Schade I, Maulhardt T, et al: Posttraumatic stress disorder and quality of life after heart or lung transplantation. Transplant Proc 34:2192–2193, 2002

Kradin R, Surman O: Psychoneuroimmunology and organ transplantation: theory and practice, in The Transplant Patient. Edited by Trzepacz P, DiMartini A. Cambridge, England, Cambridge University Press, 2000, pp 255–274

Krahn LE, Santoscoy G, Van Loon JA: A schizophrenic patient's attempt to resume dialysis following renal transplantation. Psychosomatics 39:470–473, 1998

Laederach-Hofmann K, Bunzel B: Noncompliance in organ transplant recipients: a literature review. Gen Hosp Psychiatry 22:412–424, 2000

Leipzig RM: Psychopharmacology in patients with hepatic and gastrointestinal disease. Int J Psychiatry Medicine 20:109–139, 1990

Levenson JL, Olbrisch ME: Psychosocial evaluation of organ transplant candidates: a comparative survey of process, criteria, and outcomes in heart, liver and kidney transplantation. Psychosomatics 34:314–323, 1993

Levenson J, Olbrisch ME: Psychosocial screening and selection of candidates for organ transplantation, in The Transplant Patient. Edited by Trzepacz PT, DiMartini AF. Cambridge, England, Cambridge University Press, 2000, pp 21–41

Levenson JL, Best A, Presberg B, et al: Psychosocial Assessment of Candidates for Transplantation (PACT) as a predictor of transplant outcome. Oral presentation at the 41st Annual Meeting of the Academy of Psychosomatic Medicine. Phoenix, AZ, November 19, 1994

Levy NB: Psychopharmacology in patients with renal failure. Int J Psychiatry Med 20:325–334, 1990

Lewis DA, Smith RE: Steroid-induced psychiatric syndromes: a report of 14 cases and a review of the literature. J Affect Disord 5:319–332, 1983

Lieberman JA, Cooper TB, Suckow RF, et al: Tricyclic antidepressant and metabolite levels in chronic renal failure. Clin Pharmacol Ther 37:301–307, 1985

Liu L, Schiano T, Lau N, et al: Survival and risk of recidivism in methadone-dependent patients undergoing liver transplantation. Am J Transplant 3:1273–1277, 2003

Loisance DY, Deleuze PH, Mazzucotelli JP, et al: Clinical implantation of the wearable Baxter Novacor ventricular assist system. Ann Thorac Surg 58:551–554, 1994

Lucey M: Liver transplantation for alcoholic liver disease: a progress report. Graft 2:S73–S79, 1999

Madan A, Parkinson A, Faiman MD: Identification of the human P-450 enzymes responsible for the sulfoxidation and thiono-oxidation of diethyldithiocarbamate methyl ester: role of P-450 enzymes in disulfiram bioactivation. Alcohol Clin Exp Res 22:1212–1219, 1998

Matas AJ, Garvey CA, Jacobs CL, et al: Nondirected donation of kidneys from living donors. N Engl J Med 343:433–436, 2000

McCarthy PM: Implantable left ventricular assist device bridge-to-transplantation: natural selection, or is this the natural selection? J Am Coll Cardiol 39:1255–1237, 2002

McLean AJ, Morgan DJ: Clinical pharmacokinetics in patients with liver disease. Clin Pharmacokinet 21:42–69, 1991

Miller P, Wikoff R, McMahon M, et al: Development of a health attitude scale. Nurs Res 31:132–136, 1981

Millon T, Green C, Meagher R: Millon Behavioral Health Inventory Manual, 3rd Edition. Minneapolis, MN, National Computer Systems, 1982

Morrone TM, Buck LA, Catanese KA, et al: Early progressive mobilization of patients with left ventricular assist devices is safe and optimizes recovery before heart transplantation. J Heart Lung Transplant 15:423–429, 1996

Nabel GJ: A transformed view of cyclosporine. Nature 397:471–472, 1999

Nagele H, Kalmar P, Rodiger W: Smoking after heart transplantation: an underestimated hazard? Eur J Cardiothorac Surg 12:70–74, 1997

Najarian JS, Chavers BM, McHugh LE: 20 years or more of follow-up of living kidney donors. Lancet 340:807–810, 1992

Newton SE: Recidivism and return to work posttransplant. J Subst Abuse Treat 17:103–108, 1999

Oaks TE, Aravot D, Dennis C, et al: Domino heart transplantation: the Papworth experience. J Heart Lung Transplant 13:433–437, 1994

Olbrisch ME, Levenson J: Psychosocial assessment of organ transplant candidates: current status of methodological and philosophical issues. Psychosomatics 36:236–243, 1995

Olbrisch ME, Levenson JL, Hamer R: The PACT: a rating scale for the study of clinical decision making in psychosocial screening of organ transplant candidates. Clin Transplant 3:164–169, 1989

Olbrisch ME, Benedict SM, Haller DL, et al: Psychosocial assessment of living organ donors: clinical and ethical considerations. Prog Transplant 11:40–49, 2001

Olbrisch ME, Benedict SM, Ashe K, et al: Psychological assessment and care of organ transplant patients. J Consult Clin Psychol 70:771–783, 2002

Paris W, Muchmore J, Pribil A, et al: Study of the relative incidences of psychosocial factors before and after heart transplantation and the influence of posttransplantation psychosocial factors on heart transplantation outcome. J Heart Lung Transplant 13:424–432, 1994

Patel IH, Soni PP, Fukuda EK, et al: The pharmacokinetics of midazolam in patients with congestive heart failure. Br J Clin Pharmacol 29:565–569, 1990

Phipps L: Psychiatric evaluation and outcomes in candidates for heart transplantation. Clin Invest Med 20:388–395, 1997

Pond SM, Tozer TN: First-pass elimination: basic concepts and clinical consequences. Clin Pharmacokinet 9:1–25, 1984

Presberg BA, Levenson JL, Olbrisch ME, et al: Rating scales for the psychosocial evaluation of organ transplant candidates: comparison of the PACT and TERS with bone marrow transplant patients. Psychosomatics 36:458–461, 1995

Pungpapong S, Manzarbeitia C, Ortiz J, et al: Cigarette smoking is associated with an increased incidence of vascular complications after liver transplantation. Liver Transplant 8:582–587, 2002

Reidenberg MM: The biotransformation of drugs in renal failure. Am J Med 62:482–485, 1977

Riordan SM, Williams R: Treatment of hepatic encephalopathy. N Engl J Med 337:473–479, 1997

Robinson MJ, Levenson JL: Psychopharmacology in transplant patients, in Biopsychosocial Perspectives on Transplantation. Edited by Rodrigue JR. New York, Kluwer Academic/Plenum Publishers, 2001, pp 151–172

Roche Pharmaceuticals: CellCept® (mycophenolate mofetil) Product Information. Nutley, NJ, Roche Laboratories, 2003

Rodrigue JR, Bonk V, Jackson S: Psychological considerations of living organ donation, in Biopsychosocial Perspectives on Transplantation. Edited by Rodrigue JR. New York, Kluwer Academic/Plenum Publishers, 2001, pp 59–70

Rose EA, Gelijns AC, Moskowitz AJ, et al: Long-term use of a left ventricular assist device for end-stage heart failure. N Engl J Med 345:1435–1493, 2001a

Rose EA, Gelijns AC, Moskowitz AJ, et al: Randomized Evaluation of Mechanical Assistance for the Treatment of Congestive Heart Failure (REMATCH) Study Group: long-term mechanical left ventricular assistance for end-stage heart failure. N Engl J Med 345:1435–1443, 2001b

Schomerus H, Hamster W, Blunck H, et al: Latent portasystemic encephalopathy, I: nature of cerebral functional defects and their effect on fitness to drive. Dig Dis Sci 26:622–630, 1981

Shammas FV, Dickstein K: Clinical pharmacokinetics in heart failure: an updated review. Clin Pharmacokinet 15:94–113, 1988

Shapiro PA: Nortriptyline treatment of depressed cardiac transplant recipients. Am J Psychiatry 148:371–373, 1991

Shapiro PA, Williams DL, Foray AT, et al: Psychosocial evaluation and prediction of compliance problems and morbidity after heart transplantation. Transplantation 60:1462–1466, 1995

Sindhi R, Webber S, Venkataramanan R, et al: Sirolimus for rescue and primary immunosuppression in transplanted children receiving tacrolimus. Transplantation 72:851–855, 2001

Singh N, Gayowski T, Wagener MM, et al: Depression in patients with cirrhosis: impact on outcome. Dig Dis Sci 42:1421–1427, 1997

Small S, Fukui M, Bramblett G, et al: Immunosuppression-induced leukoencephalopathy from tacrolimus. Ann Neurol 40:575–580, 1996

Snyder SL, Drooker M, Strain JJ: A survey estimate of academic liver transplant teams' selection practices for alcohol-dependent applicants. Psychosomatics 37:432–437, 1996

Starzl TE: The saga of liver replacement, with particular reference to the reciprocal influence of liver and kidney transplantation (1955–1967). J Am Coll Surg 195:587–610, 2002

Stevenson LW: Indications for listing and de-listing patients for cardiac transplantation (Chapter 233 [Cardiac Transplantation], reviews and editorials), in Harrison's Online. Available at: http://harrisons.accessmedicine.com. Accessed August 3, 2004

Stilley CS, Miller DJ, Tarter RE: Measuring psychological distress in candidates of liver transplantation: a pilot study. J Clin Psychol 53:459–464, 1997

Stilley CS, Miller DJ, Gayowski T, et al: Psychological characteristics of candidates for liver transplantation: differences according to history of substance abuse and UNOS listing. United Network for Organ Sharing. J Clin Psychol 55:1287–1297, 1999

Stowe J, Kotz M: Addiction medicine in organ transplantation. Prog Transplant 11:50–57, 2001

Strouse TB, Fairbanks LA, Skotzko CE, et al: Fluoxetine and cyclosporine in organ transplantation: failure to detect significant drug interactions or adverse clinical events in depressed organ recipients. Psychosomatics 37:23–30, 1996

Strouse TB, el-Saden SM, Glaser NE, et al: Immunosuppressant neurotoxicity in liver transplant recipients: clinical challenges for the consultation-liaison psychiatrist. Psychosomatics 39:124–133, 1998

Suhara T, Sudo Y, Yoshida K, et al: Lung as reservoir for antidepressants in pharmacokinetic drug interactions. Lancet 351:332–335, 1998

Surman OS: Possible immunological effects of psychotropic medication. Psychosomatics 34:139–143, 1993

Surman OS: The ethics of partial-liver donation (comment). N Engl J Med 346:1038, 2002

Surman OS, Purtilo R: Reevaluation of organ transplantation criteria: allocation of scarce resources to borderline candidates. Psychosomatics 33:202–212, 1992

Taguchi T, Suita S: Segmental small-intestinal transplantation: a comparison of jejunal and ileal grafts. Surgery 131:S294–S300, 2002

Tarter RE, Switala JA, Arria A, et al: Subclinical hepatic encephalopathy: comparison before and after orthotopic liver transplantation. Transplantation 50:632–637, 1990

Tringali RA, Trzepacz PT, DiMartini A, et al: Assessment and follow-up of alcohol-dependent liver transplantation patients: a clinical cohort. Gen Hosp Psychiatry 18 (suppl): 70S–77S, 1996

Trzepacz PT, DiMartini AF, Gupta B: Psychopharmacologic issues in transplantation, in The Transplant Patient. Edited by Trzepacz P, DiMartini A. Cambridge, England, Cambridge University Press, 2000, pp 187–213

Twillman RK, Manetto C, Wellisch DK, et al: The Transplant Evaluation Rating Scale: a revision of the psychosocial levels system for evaluating organ transplant candidates. Psychosomatics 34:144–153, 1993

United Network of Organ Sharing (UNOS) Web site. Available at: http://www.OPTN.org. Accessed January 14, 2004

Vaillant GE: The natural history of alcoholism and its relationship to liver transplantation. Liver Transpl Surg 3:304–310, 1997

Varney NR, Alexander B, MacIndoe JH: Reversible steroid dementia in patients without steroid psychosis. Am J Psychiatry 141:369–372, 1984

Venkataramanan R, Jain A, Warty VS, et al: Pharmacokinetics of FK 506 in transplant patients. Transplant Proc 23:2736–2740, 1991

Watson CJ, Friend PJ, Jamieson NV, et al: Sirolimus: a potent new immunosuppressant for liver transplantation. Transplantation 67:505–509, 1999

Weinrieb RM: A matched comparison of medical/psychiatric complication and anesthesia/analgesia requirements in methadone maintained liver transplant patients. Poster presented at the Academy of Psychosomatic Medicine annual meeting, San Diego, CA, November 20, 2003

Weinrieb RM, Van Horn DH, McLellan AT, et al: Interpreting the significance of drinking by alcohol-dependent liver transplant patients: fostering candor is the key to recovery. Liver Transplant 6:769–776, 2000

Weinrieb RM, Van Horn DH, McLellan AT, et al: Alcoholism treatment after liver transplantation: lessons learned from a clinical trial that failed. Psychosomatics 42:111–115, 2001

Weitzner MA, Lehninger F, Sullivan D, et al: Borderline personality disorder and bone marrow transplantation: ethical considerations and review. Psycho-Oncology 8:46–54, 1999

Wijdicks EF, Wiesner RH, Krom RA: Neurotoxicity in liver transplant recipients with cyclosporine immunosuppression. Neurology 45:1962–1964, 1995

Wijdicks EF, Eelco FM, Plevak DJ, et al: Causes and outcome of seizures in liver transplant recipients. Neurology 47:1523–1525, 1996

Wijdicks EF, Dahlke LJ, Wiesner RH: Oral cyclosporine decreases severity of neurotoxicity in liver transplant recipients. Neurology 52:1708–1710, 1999

Wilkinson GR: Plasma and tissue binding considerations in drug disposition. Drug Metab Rev 14:427–465, 1983

Wilson JR, Conwit RA, Eidelman BH, et al: Sensorimotor neuropathy resembling CIDP in patients receiving FK506. Muscle Nerve 17:528–532, 1994

Wilson SE, deGroen PC, Aksamit AJ, et al: Cyclosporin A–induced reversible cortical blindness. J Clin Neuro-Ophthalmol 8:215–220, 1988

Woodman CL, Geist LJ, Vance S, et al: Psychiatric disorders and survival after lung transplantation. Psychosomatics 40:293–297, 1999

Woosley RL: Pharmacokinetics and pharmacodynamics of antiarrhythmic agents in patients with congestive heart failure. Am Heart J 114:1280–1291, 1987

Wright L, Pennington JJ, Abbey S, et al: Evaluation of a mentorship program for heart transplant patients. J Heart Lung Transplant 20:1030–1033, 2001

Yates WR, Booth BM, Reed DA, et al: Descriptive and predictive validity of a high-risk alcoholism relapse model. J Stud Alcohol 54:645–651, 1993

Yates WR, LaBrecque DR, Pfab D: Personality disorder as a contraindication for liver transplantation in alcoholic cirrhosis. Psychosomatics 39:501–511, 1998

Zipfel S, Schneider A, Wild B, et al: Effect of depressive symptoms on survival after heart transplantation. Psychosom Med 64:740–747, 2002

32 Neurology and Neurosurgery

Alan J. Carson, M.Phil., M.D., M.R.C.Psych.

Adam Zeman, M.A., D.M., M.R.C.P.

Lynn Myles, B.Sc., M.D., F.R.C.S.Ed.

Michael C. Sharpe, M.A., M.D., F.R.C.P., M.R.C.Psych.

THE DIVIDE BETWEEN neurology and psychiatry is viewed by many as a historical artifact (Baker et al. 2002). Psychiatrists have taken on primary responsibility for caring for brain injury, epilepsy, early-onset dementias, and sleep and movement disorders while retaining their more traditional role of diagnosing and treating "psychiatric" disorders in patients with neurological disease. Some neurologists have developed interests in cognitive and behavioral neurology and have focused on disorders traditionally considered to be psychiatric. New developments in neuroscience are bringing an understanding of the mechanisms of interaction between biological, psychological and social aspects of illness, making this one of the most intellectually fascinating areas of work for a psychiatrist.

Psychiatrists working in a clinical neurosciences center are likely to be required to address four main categories of clinical problems:

1. Cognitive impairment—either as a primary presentation or as a secondary complication of a known condition such as multiple sclerosis.
2. Neurological disease accompanied by emotional disturbance in excess of the clinical norm.
3. Physical symptoms that do not correspond to any recognized pattern of neurological disease.
4. Postneurosurgery complications—usually involving behavioral, cognitive, or emotional disturbance.

In this chapter, we concentrate on commonly encountered neurological conditions—stroke, Parkinson's disease, multiple sclerosis, amnestic syndromes, dementias with additional prominent neurological signs, epilepsy, headache, movement disorders, and conversion disorder—as well as on selected psychiatric aspects of neurosurgery. The principles of assessment applicable to these disorders are also relevant to other, rarer neurological conditions. Psychopharmacological and psychological treatments are not discussed in detail here because they are covered in other chapters. Although we refer to drug therapies, we wish to remind the reader that for many neuropsychiatric conditions, behavioral management and environmental manipulation are of equal importance.

Neuropsychiatric topics covered elsewhere in this book include the mental status examination (Chapter 1, "Psychiatric Assessment and Consultation"), neuropsychological testing (Chapter 2, "Neuropsychological and Psychological Evaluation"), delirium (Chapter 6, "Delirium"), dementia (Chapter 7, "Dementia"), traumatic brain and spinal cord injuries (Chapter 35, "Physical Medicine and Rehabilitation"), pain syndromes (Chapter 36, "Pain"), and psychopharmacological interventions in neurological disease (Chapter 37, "Psychopharmacology").

Stroke

A cerebrovascular accident, or stroke, is a rapidly developed clinical sign of a focal disturbance of cerebral function of presumed vascular origin and of more than 24 hours' duration. One of two main pathological processes is responsible: cerebral infarction or hemorrhage. *Infarction* may result from thrombosis of vessels or emboli lodged within them. *Hemorrhage* can be either into brain tissue directly or into the subarachnoid space. Infarctions are four times more common than hemorrhages and, as a result of a lower immediate fatality rate, are a much greater source of enduring disability, with approximately 75% survival, compared with 33% survival at 1 year after hemorrhage. Strokes are the third most common cause of death in the Western world. The Oxfordshire Community Stroke Project reported a population incidence of 2 per 1,000 for first-ever stroke (Bamford et al. 1988). Age is the major risk factor, although one-quarter of persons affected are younger than 65 years. Stroke occurs more commonly in men.

Psychiatrists are not usually involved in the diagnosis of acute stroke but occasionally are consulted when alterations in cognition, affect, or behavior dominate the clinical picture.

Clinical Features

The classical presentation of *middle cerebral artery* infarction is contralateral hemiparesis and sensory loss of a cortical type. These are often accompanied by hemianopsia if the optic radiation is affected. If the lesion is in the dominant hemisphere, then aphasia may be expected, whereas a lesion in the nondominant hemisphere may be accompanied by neglect or perceptual disturbance.

Infarctions affecting the distribution of the *anterior cerebral artery* will lead to contralateral hemiparesis affecting the leg more severely than the arm. A grasp reflex and motor dysphasia may be present. Cognitive changes resembling a global dementia may occur, with incontinence. Residual personality changes (apathy and/or dysexecutive function) of a frontal type can also result.

Posterior cerebral artery infarction presents with a contralateral hemianopsia sometimes accompanied by visual hallucinations, visual agnosias, or spatial disorientation. Transient confusion may obscure the detection of hemianopsia. Vital memory structures are supplied from the posterior cerebral artery, and in some neurologically normal individuals both medial thalamic areas are supplied by a single penetrating artery. Dense amnestic symptoms occur if the hippocampus and other limbic structures are involved bilaterally. Diagnosis may be difficult, because early computed tomography (CT) scan findings are often negative; however, magnetic resonance imaging (MRI) will show the bilateral lesions.

Internal carotid artery occlusion can be entirely asymptomatic, but much depends on the collateral circulation.

The clinical picture is often that of middle cerebral artery infarction. However, in some situations, cognitive and behavioral symptoms are predominant, with general slowing, decreased spontaneous activity, and dyspraxia.

Vertebrobasilar strokes can be extremely diverse in their manifestations. Total occlusion of the basilar artery is usually rapidly fatal. Partial occlusions typically affect the brain stem, with a combination of uni- or bilateral pyramidal signs and ipsilateral cranial nerve palsies. One variant of brain-stem stroke is the "locked in" syndrome, in which total paralysis is accompanied by full alertness and awareness. Occlusions of the rostral branches of the basilar artery can result in infarction of the midbrain, thalamus, and portions of the temporal and occipital lobes. A striking example of basilar artery occlusion is peduncular hallucinosis, in which patients have vivid, well-formed hallucinations that they recognize as unreal. One patient described seeing his wife growing a full and bushy black beard! States of bizarre disorientation can also occur and can be mistaken for confabulation or even deliberate playacting.

Cognitive Impairment and Delirium

Delirium affects 30%–40% of patients during the first week after a stroke, especially after a hemorrhagic stroke (Gustafson et al. 1993; Langhorne et al. 2000; Rahkonen et al. 2000). It is important to distinguish delirium from focal cognitive deficits affecting declarative memory. The presence of delirium after stroke is associated with poorer prognosis, longer duration of hospitalization, and increased risk of dementia (see Gustafson et al. 1991; Henon et al. 1999).

Dementia following stroke is common, occurring in approximately one-quarter of patients at 3 months after stroke (Desmond et al. 2000; Tatimichi et al. 1994a, 1994b). This figure rises significantly if focal impairments also are considered. *Vascular dementia* is an imprecise term referring to a heterogeneous group of dementing disorders caused by impairment of the brain's blood supply. These disorders fall into three principal categories: subcortical ischemic dementia, multi-infarct dementia, and dementia due to focal "strategic" infarction. Several sets of diagnostic criteria (e.g., the National Institute of Neurological Disorders and Stroke–Association Internationale pour la Recherche et l'Enseignement en Neurosciences [NINDS-AIREN] criteria) are available, with high specificity but low sensitivity for pathologically defined vascular dementia (Chui et al. 1992; Hachinski et al. 1974; Roman et al. 1993). The common occurrence of relatively subtle cognitive decline, falling short of frank dementia, in the context of cerebrovascular disease has given rise to the broader concept of "vascular cognitive impairment." Subcortical ischemic dementia and multi-infarct dementia are described in more detail in Chapter 7 ("Dementia"). The term *strategic infarction* describes the occurrence of unexpectedly severe cognitive impairment following limited infarction, often in the absence of classic signs such as hemiplegia. Sites at which infarctions can have such an effect include the thalamus, especially the medial thalamus; the inferior genu of the internal capsule; the basal ganglia; the left angular gyrus (causing Gerstmann's syndrome of agraphia, acalculia, left–right disorientation, and finger agnosia); the basal forebrain; and the territory of the posterior cerebral arteries (Clark et al. 1994; Kumral et al. 1999; Rockwood et al. 1999; Tatimichi et al. 1992, 1995).

Behavioral Changes

The diverse behavioral changes following stroke are not unique to this condition and can therefore serve as a helpful model for understanding the clinical consequences of focal cerebral lesions of other causes (Bogousslavsky and Cummings 2000).

Aphasia

Global aphasia leads to the abolition of all linguistic faculties. Consequently, the physician must draw inferences about mental state from the patient's behavior and nonverbal communication. Some accounts associate Broca's aphasia with intense emotional frustration that may be secondary to problems in social interaction (Carota et al. 2000). Wernicke's aphasia has been characterized as lack of insight accompanied by irritability and rage, with recovered patients reporting that they believed the examiner was being deliberately incomprehensible (Lazar et al. 2000).

Anosognosia

Anosognosia refers to partial or complete unawareness of a deficit. It may coexist with depression (Starkstein et al. 1990), a finding that both implicates separate neural systems for different aspects of emotions (Damasio 1994) and suggests that depression after stroke cannot be explained solely as a psychological reaction to disability (Ramasubbu 1994). Anosognosia for hemiplegia is perhaps the most often described form of the condition, but anosognosia can occur with reference to any function and is commonly associated with visual and language dysfunction. Patients with anosognosia for hemiplegia have no spontaneous complaints and may indeed claim normal movements in the paralyzed limb. Behavioral correlates include attempting to walk normally despite the hemiplegia and paradoxical acceptance of a wheelchair while simultaneously maintaining that one has normal function. In extreme cases, ownership of the limb is denied or, exceptionally, phantom limb sensations can occur. Anosognosia occurs more frequently with right-sided lesions, particularly those in the region of the middle cerebral artery (Breier et al. 1995; Jehkonen et al. 2000; Meador et al. 2000).

Affective Dysprosodia

Affective dysprosodia is impairment of the production and comprehension of those language components that communicate inner emotional states in speech. These components include stresses, pauses, cadence, accent, melody, and intonation. Affective dysprosodia is not associated with an actual deficit in the ability to *experience* emotions; rather, it is associated with a deficit in the ability to *communicate* or *recognize emotions in the speech of others*. Affective dysprosodia is particularly associated with right-sided lesions. A depressed patient with dysprosodia will appear depressed and say that he is depressed, but he or she will not "sound" depressed. This is in contrast to a patient with anosognosia, who will both appear and sound depressed but may deny that he or she is depressed.

Apathy

Patients with apathy show little spontaneous action or speech; their responses may be delayed, short, slow, or absent (Fisher 1995). Apathy is frequently associated with hypophonia, perseveration, grasp reflex, compulsive motor manipulations, cognitive and functional impairment, and older age. Hypoactivity of the frontal and anterior temporal regions has been observed (Starkstein et al. 1993a).

Depression

Although depression following stroke is commonly defined according to DSM-IV-TR (American Psychiatric Association 2000) or ICD-10 criteria (Starkstein and Robinson 1989), the imposition of these categorical diagnoses on patients who have suffered a stroke is problematic, because it is often unclear which symptoms are attributable to the stroke and which are attributable to depression (Gainotti et al. 1997, 1999). One solution is to focus on symptoms other than somatic ones, and scales such as the Hospital Anxiety and Depression Scale have been designed to do this. However, this is not an adequate solution, because the neurobehavioral consequences of cerebral lesions—such as aphasia, indifference, denial, cognitive impairment, and dissociation of subjective from displayed emotion—can obscure and complicate the diagnosis of depression. Most clinicians take a pragmatic approach, treating depression if the patient has symptoms suggestive of low mood or anhedonia accompanied by some somatic symptoms (e.g., insomnia, anorexia) as well as signs of lack of engagement with the environment (e.g., poor participation in physiotherapy).

Most epidemiological studies have suggested an association between depression and increased disability (Andersen et al. 1994b; Herrmann et al. 1995; Parikh et al. 1990; Pohjasvaara et al. 2001) and possibly mortality (House et al. 2001; Morris et al. 1993a). However, the direction of causality is unclear and is most probably circular. Some, but not all, pharmacological treatment studies have suggested that effective treatment of the depression leads to a reduction in overall disability (Andersen et al. 1994a; Lipsey et al. 1984).

There has been much speculation over the etiological mechanisms of depression after stroke, and emphasis has been placed on the site of the stroke lesion. One hypothesis put forward is that left frontal lesions are associated with an increased rate of depressive illness (Starkstein and Robinson 1989). There are, however, several limitations to this theory. First, it has been consistently found that patients with a premorbid history of depression are at higher risk of developing depression after stroke (Andersen et al. 1995). Second, it has proved impossible to clinically distinguish left frontal depression from depression associated with lesions in other brain regions (Gainotti et al. 1997). Finally, a recent meta-analysis reported that the available scientific literature does not support the left frontal hypothesis (Carson et al. 2000a).

It is generally recommended—but has not been conclusively demonstrated—that treatment for depression should be started early, in order to maximize functional outcome. However, disappointingly few randomized, controlled trials have tested this recommendation. Most studies suggest an improved outcome in mood with early treatment, but findings on measures of function have been contradictory (Andersen et al. 1994a; Chemerinski et al. 2001; Gainotti et al. 2001; Lipsey et al. 1984; Robinson et al. 2000; Wiart et al. 2000). Although both selective serotonin reuptake inhibitors (SSRIs) and tricyclic antidepressants (TCAs) have been reported to be effective, the SSRIs are probably preferable because of fewer adverse effects, particularly if cognitive or cardiac function is compromised. Nonetheless, this greater tolerability must be balanced against the finding that nortriptyline was more effective than fluoxetine in the only trial that compared these agents (Robinson et al. 2000). What is clear is that all stroke patients receiving antidepressants should be closely monitored for both treatment effectiveness and adverse drug effects. Psychological treatment—in particular, cognitive-behavioral therapy (CBT)—potentially offers a solution for cases in which pharmacotherapy is ineffective or contraindicated, but thus far psychological approaches have received only limited evaluation (Kneebone and Dunmore 2000; Lincoln and Flannagan 2003). It is likely that only a minority of patients with poststroke depression are suitable for such treatment (Lincoln et al. 1997).

Anxiety

Anxiety disorders are common after stroke and probably share the same risk factors as depression (Astrom 1996). Estimates of prevalence have varied markedly, depending on whether the investigators subsumed anxiety symptoms within the construct of major depressive disorder. Thus, the reported prevalence of generalized anxiety disorder ranges from 4% to 28% (Astrom 1996). However, the percentage of patients experiencing anxiety symptoms appears to be 25%–30% (Burvill et al. 1995).

Stroke is a sudden and unpredictable life-threatening stressor and, not surprisingly, a highly aversive experience (McEwen 1996). Poststroke anxiety states may include posttraumatic stress symptoms, with compulsive and intrusive revisiting of the event, as well as health worries, with checking and reassurance seeking about the risk of recurrence (Lyndsay 1991). These worries can be associated with agoraphobia and the misinterpretation of somatic anxiety symptoms, especially headache and dizziness, as evidence of recurrence. Phobic states have a prevalence of 5%–10%, with an excess found in women (Burvill et al. 1995). Although there is a paucity of controlled-trial evidence, it is our experience that these symptoms respond to standard drug and behavioral therapies.

Emotional Lability

Emotionalism, or emotional lability, is an increase in laughing or crying that occurs with little or no warning. It is frequent in acute stroke but can also occur with delayed onset (Berthier et al. 1996). The displayed emotions are not related to the patient's internal emotional state. Whether emotional lability is associated with depression is a moot point; both conditions can exist independently (House et al. 1989; Robinson et al. 1993).

It has been suggested that the neurological basis is in serotonergic systems and that there is a specific response to SSRIs (Andersen et al. 1994a). In practice, the evidence is contradictory, with reports of response to TCAs as well (Robinson et al. 1993). There is no consistently reported associated lesion location: pontine, subcortical, and frontal lesions have all been found (Andersen et al. 1994a; Derex et al. 1997; Morris et al. 1993b).

Catastrophic Reactions

Catastrophic reactions manifest as disruptive emotional behavior precipitated when a patient finds a task unsolvable (Goldstein 1939). The sudden, dramatic appearance of such marked self-directed and stereotypical anger or frustration can be startling for both staff and relatives. This symptom is often associated with aphasia, and it has been suggested that damage to language areas is a critical part of the etiology (Carota et al. 2001). Catastrophic reactions generally occur independently of depression in acute stroke; however, many patients who show early catastrophic reactions go on to develop depression (Starkstein et al. 1993b).

Psychosis

Psychosis—and, in particular, mania—has been observed following acute stroke. Its true incidence is unknown, although a rate of 1% has been reported (Starkstein et al. 1987). Psychotic symptoms have generally been associated with right-sided lesions (Cummings and Mendez 1984), although the failure to substantiate the proposed association of lesion location with depression should lead to caution in evaluating such claims. Old age and preexisting degenerative disease seem to increase the risk (Starkstein 1998) (see Chapter 11, "Mania, Catatonia, and Psychosis," for further details and treatment considerations). Reduplicative paramnesias can occur: One memorable patient believed he was being treated on a cruise liner; on looking out of the window and seeing hospital porters delivering goods, he surmised that the ship must be in "dry dock." Such paramnesias are usually short-lived, although a small number of chronic cases have been reported (Vighetto et al. 1980).

Obsessive-Compulsive Disorder

Obsessive-compulsive disorder has been reported after cerebral infarctions, particularly those affecting the basal ganglia (Maraganore et al. 1991; Rodrigo et al. 1997).

Hyposexuality

Hyposexuality is a common complaint after stroke in both men and women (see also Chapter 17, "Sexual Disorders"). The symptoms generally are nonspecific, although health worries concerning body image and fear of recurrence may also be relevant. A relationship between reduced libido and emotionalism has also been proposed, suggesting a common serotonergic dysfunction (Kim and Choi-Kwon 2000).

Executive Function Impairment

Executive function is regulated by complex systems that are relatively resistant to damage after stroke (Carota et al. 2002), although executive function is commonly impaired as part of a general dementia.

Inhibition Dyscontrol

Deficit of inhibition control occurs with impulsive behavior. The most striking examples of inhibition dyscontrol are grasp reflexes, but utilization behavior (a tendency to use objects present in the environment automatically), hyperphasia, and hypergraphia have all been described. Such behavior tends to improve during the first few months after stroke (Carota et al. 2002).

Loss of Empathy

Loss of empathy has been reported after bilateral orbitofrontal lesions (Stone et al. 1998). It has been suggested that this difficulty in understanding and adapting to the needs of others may underlie many of the personality changes associated with frontal lesions. These changes include lack of tact, inappropriate familiarity, loss of initiative and spontaneity, childish behavior, sexual disinhibition, and poverty of emotional expression (Carota et al. 2002).

Parkinson's Disease

Parkinson's disease (PD) is a degenerative condition characterized by tremor, rigidity, and bradykinesis.

Incidence

Two recent incidence studies of PD, one from Minnesota (Bower et al. 1999) and one from Finland (Kupio et al. 1999), estimated 10.8 cases per 100,000 person-years and 17.2 per 100,000 population, respectively. Both studies found a slight excess in men and confirmed that incidence increases with age. The Finnish study also suggested that PD was more common in rural areas.

Etiology

The cause of PD remains unknown. Genetic forms of the disease have been described, but the implicated genes are not identified in most patients. Similarly, environmental causes have been suggested, but no single exposure has been consistently replicated, with the exception of cases associated with MPTP (1-methyl-4-phenyl-1,2,3,6-tetrahydropyridine) (Tanner and Aston 2000). Cigarette smoking appears to decrease risk (Gorell et al. 1999).

Clinical Features

The core feature of PD is the triad of tremor, rigidity, and bradykinesia (Sethi 2002). Bradykinesia—usually of insidious onset and easily misdiagnosed as depression or boredom—is the most common first sign and ultimately is the most disabling symptom. Resting tremor is the most characteristic feature of PD, affecting more than 70% of patients. In the early stages of the disease, the tremor is described as "pill-rolling." The rigidity manifests as fixed abnormalities of posture and resistance to passive movement throughout the range of motion. Concurrent tremor creates a "cogwheel" sensation. Postural instability is a common additional feature, giving rise to an increasing liability to falls as the disorder progresses. Abnormal involuntary movements are a result both of the disease process and of dopaminergic therapy. Freezing of gait is particularly distressing to patients, but it is one of the most poorly understood features of PD. Because such freezing may occur in response to visual cues (especially freezing during "off" periods), it can be misdiagnosed as willful behavior.

Nonmotor manifestations are common in PD and include autonomic (in particular, orthostatic hypotension and bladder and gastrointestinal dysfunction), sensory (pain), cognitive, and other psychiatric symptoms.

Cognitive Features

Dementia with Lewy bodies (DLB), PD, and PD with dementia share common features, motor symptoms, and responses to treatment. The boundaries between these disorders may be less distinct than originally thought. Hallucinations and delusions occur in 57%–76% of DLB cases, in 29%–54% of cases of PD with dementia, and in 7%–14% of cases of PD without dementia (Aarsland et al. 2001). Delusions are often paranoid in type and mainly involve persecution and jealousy. Hallucinations usually occur in the presence of intact insight and frequently are visual and phenomenologically similar to those of Charles Bonnet syndrome (Diederich et al. 2000).

In the early days of levodopa (L-dopa) treatment, adverse psychiatric reactions were reported in 10%–50% of patients (Goodwin 1971). Psychosis occurred in about 10% of patients initially, but this percentage rose to 60% after 6 years of treatment (Sweet et al. 1976). The addition of carbidopa to L-dopa made this adverse effect less common. More recent studies have suggested that dopaminomimetic medication is a significant risk factor for psychosis (Aarsland et al. 1999). Other studies have shown correlations between psychotic symptoms and higher rates of cognitive dysfunction and depression, but no association

with dosage or length of exposure to dopaminomimetic medication has been found (Giladi et al. 2000). The most likely etiology of psychosis in PD is a combination of cortical PD pathology and age-related loss of central cholinergic function. This is corroborated by the fact that psychotic symptoms in PD are often part of nondopaminomimetic medication–induced toxic (i.e., delirious) states and that psychosis was commonly reported in the pre-levodopa era (Wolters and Berendse 2001). Cognitive impairment and sleep disruption are predictive of the development of psychosis (Arnulf et al. 2000).

Clinically, one should distinguish a delirium of acute onset with disorientation, impaired attention, perceptive and cognitive disturbance, and alterations in the sleep–wake cycle from true dopaminomimetic psychosis, which is a subacute, gradually progressive psychotic state unaccompanied by a primary deficit of attention. The former may be induced by drugs used in the treatment of PD, such as selegiline and anticholinergic medication. For the latter, active treatment is recommended only if symptoms begin to interfere with daily functioning. Dose reduction of dopaminomimetic drugs is seldom effective, and antipsychotic drugs are often required (Wolters and Berendse 2001). The atypical antipsychotic drugs clozapine and quetiapine are preferred (Cummings 1999; Rabinstein and Shulman 2000), and high-potency typical antipsychotics should be avoided (see Chapter 11, "Mania, Catatonia, and Psychosis"). There is also increasing interest in the role of cholinesterase inhibitors in the treatment of dementia in PD, with early studies showing promising results (McKeith et al. 2000).

Emotional Symptoms

Depression is a common symptom in PD, with a prevalence of around 40%–50%. Timing of onset shows a bimodal distribution, with peaks during early and late stages of the disease (Cummings and Masterman 1999). Several large-scale studies have demonstrated that depression is one of the major determinants of quality of life in PD (Findlay 2002; Peto et al. 1995). The extent to which depression is caused by brain pathology as opposed to a psychological reaction to disability is unknown.

The diagnosis of depression in PD is difficult, because many depressive symptoms overlap with the core features of PD—motor retardation, attention deficit, sleep disturbance, hypophonia, impotence, weight loss, fatigue, preoccupation with health, and reduced facial expression. However, anhedonia and sustained sadness are important diagnostic features, particularly if they are out of proportion to the severity of motor symptoms (Brooks and Doder 2001).

Mood changes can accompany the late-stage fluctuations in response to levodopa (known as "on–off" phenomena), and some patients fulfill criteria for major depressive disorder during the "off" phase but not during the "on" phase (Cantello et al. 1986; Menza et al. 1990). Bipolar mood changes reflecting the on–off phases have also been described (Keshavan et al. 1986). There is currently insufficient evidence to offer definitive recommendations for treatment of depression in PD (Olanow et al. 2001). Although SSRIs are popular, there have been case reports of exacerbation of motor symptoms with fluoxetine, citalopram, and paroxetine (Ceravolo et al. 2000; Chuinard and Sultan 1992; Jansen Steur 1993; Leo 1996; Tessei et al. 2000). In recent small-scale trials, TCAs have led to better motor outcomes than have SSRIs; however, TCAs with marked anticholinergic activity (e.g., amitriptyline) should be used with caution because of their potential adverse effects on cognition and autonomic function (Olanow et al. 2001). It may be that newer drugs such as mirtazapine will offer a compromise. The non-ergot dopamine agonist pramipexole has been found to improve both mood and motivation in PD (Armin et al. 1997). Case report data suggest that both electroconvulsive therapy (ECT) and transcranial magnetic stimulation (TMS) can be used to treat depression in PD, although TMS is associated with short-lived adverse effects and seizures (George et al. 1996; Olanow et al. 2001). The use of ECT in PD is reviewed at length in Chapter 39, "Electroconvulsive Therapy."

Anxiety phenomena are common in PD; they tend to occur later in the disease process than depression and are more closely associated with severity of motor symptoms (Witjas et al. 2002). In particular, marked anticipatory anxiety related to freezing of gait is common. Treatment with antidepressant drugs (Olanow et al. 2001) and CBT, particularly if delivered in conjunction with an active physiotherapy program, can be helpful. Occasionally, benzodiazepines may be required.

Multiple Sclerosis

Multiple sclerosis (MS) is a demyelinating disorder of the central nervous system (CNS) that causes some degree of cognitive impairment in almost half of cases and that can present with unexplained subcortical dementia. It can also be accompanied by affective disorders. The presence of high signal abnormalities on T2-weighted MRI and of oligoclonal bands of immunoglobulin in the cerebrospinal fluid (CSF) helps to confirm the diagnosis.

Demyelinating diseases are the most common non-traumatic cause of chronic neurological disability in young adults. Although a number of inflammatory demyelinating diseases can affect the CNS after vaccinations or systemic viral infection (collectively referred to as acute disseminated encephalomyelitis [ADEM]), MS is by far the most common of these.

MS can occur at any age, but the median age at onset is 24 years, with a tendency for relapsing–remitting disease to present earlier than primary progressive MS. MS is more common in women. Epidemiological studies suggest that an exogenous or environmental factor, possibly viral infection, plays a part, although its nature remains unclear. The prevalence of the disorder rises with increasing distance from the equator. Genetic factors appear to influence susceptibility. A family history in a first-degree relative increases the risk some 30- to 50-fold: the risk for siblings is usually estimated to be 3%–5%, with that for children slightly lower (Franklin and Nelson 2003).

Common neurological syndromes occurring at or close to the onset of MS include optic neuritis (unilateral visual impairment, usually painful), ascending sensory loss, and upper-motor-neuron or cerebellar disorders of the limbs and gait. These deficits typically develop and remit over the course of weeks and result from conduction block in regions of inflammation. Transient worsening of function, lasting for minutes, can occur in partially demyelinated axons as a result of physiological changes (e.g., increase in body temperature). Positive symptoms, including L'hermitte's phenomena (electric shock–like sensations on flexing the neck) and trigeminal neuralgia, can also occur. Over time, the remissions and relapses of MS tend to give way to a progressive worsening of disability. A minority of patients present with a primary progressive form of the disease, with gradual worsening from onset without remissions (McDonald et al. 2001).

Pathologically, MS is characterized by multifocal areas of demyelination with relative preservation of axons, loss of oligodendrocytes, and astroglial scarring. Although axons are relatively spared, axonal loss and cortical atrophy occur, and their development probably contributes to the permanent disability, including cognitive dysfunction, caused by the disorder (Lucchinetti et al. 2001).

Patients with unsuspected MS may first present to psychiatrists with changes in cognitive function, mood, or personality. More often, however, psychiatrists are involved in the treatment of established cases. MS demonstrates the interactive nature of many of the common symptoms of diffuse neurological disease, in particular the "vicious cycle" of mood symptoms, pain, and fatigue, necessitating intervention across the spectrum of complaints in order to improve outcome.

Cognitive Impairment

Cognitive impairment affects at least half of all patients with MS (Beatty et al. 1989a; Heaton et al. 1985; Rao 1986; Rao et al. 1991). The impairment is generally described as a subcortical dementia characterized by problems with memory, speed of processing, and executive functions (Beatty et al. 1989b; Litvan et al. 1988b; Rao et al. 1984, 1989). Cortical syndromes such as aphasia, apraxia, and agnosia are relatively rare. It has been suggested that greater impairments may occur in secondary progressive MS, although this has been disputed (Rao 1986; Rao et al. 1991). Disorders of working memory may be prominent, particularly verbal but sometimes visuospatial memory (Litvan et al. 1988a; Rao et al. 1993). It is important to bear in mind that depression, anxiety, and fatigue all may affect cognitive function; thus, neuropsychological testing can be helpful in determining whether true deficits are present.

Mood Disorders

Mood disorders are common in MS, with more than half of patients reporting depressive symptoms. Mania and emotional lability are also frequently reported (Joffe et al. 1987; Sadovnick et al. 1996) (see also Chapter 9, "Depression," and Chapter 11, "Mania, Catatonia, and Psychosis").

It is important to distinguish depression from the fatigue and pain that are commonly associated with MS (see subsections "Fatigue" and "Pain" below). As in stroke, there has been an attempt to separate out a "biological" depression from a "psychological reactive" depression (Patten and Metz 1997) and to link symptoms to the site of the brain lesions (Fassbender et al. 1998; Honer et al. 1987; Pujol et al. 1997). However, supporting evidence has been inconsistent and hampered by small study samples; for this reason, it appears to be more productive to consider depression in MS as multifactorial. There are few randomized, controlled trials of antidepressant drug therapy in MS, but those available suggest modest efficacy for these agents (Feinstein 1997), similar to their efficacy for depression associated with neurological illness in general (Schiffer and Wineman 1990).

Interferon-beta therapy was reported to cause depression (and fatigue) in 40% of MS patients in an open-label trial (Neilley et al. 1996). However, depression is highly prevalent in untreated MS, and more recent studies have found no increase in depression following interferon-beta therapy (Patten and Metz 2001; Zephir et al. 2003). In one prospective study, the rate of depression actually fell with interferon-beta treatment (Feinstein et al. 2002).

Fatigue

Fatigue is the most common single symptom in MS, affecting 80% of those with the disease (Fisk et al. 1994; Freal et al. 1984). It is generally a disabling and aversive experience and affects motivation as well as physical strength. It is important to differentiate fatigue from depression, adverse medication side effects, or pure physical exhaustion secondary to gait abnormalities, because management may differ (Multiple Sclerosis Council for Practice Guidelines 1998). The mechanism of fatigue is poorly understood and almost certainly multifactorial. Amantadine 100 mg twice daily has been reported to be of some benefit (Krupp et al. 1995), and pemoline has also been suggested as useful (Krupp et al. 1995). A number of other agents, including 4-aminopyridine (Polman et al. 1994), 3,4-diaminopyridine (Sheean et al. 1997), and modafinil (Rammohan et al. 2002), have been advocated, but results of studies with these drugs have been inconclusive. Some patients respond to SSRIs, and cognitive-behavioral treatments have also been used (Mohr et al. 2003).

Pain

Pain, both acute and chronic, is a common and disabling complication of MS. A recent study found that one-quarter of MS patients in a large community-based sample had severe chronic pain (Ehde et al. 2003). Mechanisms may include dysesthesia, altered cognitive function, and other MS complications such as spasticity. Of the acute pain syndromes, trigeminal neuralgia is the most common and usually responds to carbamazepine (Thompson 1998). Widespread chronic pain is more frequent and harder to manage. Dysesthetic limb pain is particularly troublesome; treatment is usually with amitriptyline or gabapentin (Samkoff et al. 1997). Pain in the lumbar area, by contrast, usually tends to respond better to physiotherapy than to analgesia (Thompson 1998; see also Chapter 36, "Pain").

Amnestic Syndromes

The amnestic or amnesic syndrome is an abnormal mental state in which learning and memory are affected out of proportion to other cognitive functions in an otherwise alert and responsive patient (Victor et al. 1971). The most common cause of amnestic states is Wernicke-Korsakoff syndrome, which results from nutritional depletion, particularly thiamine deficiency. Other causes include carbon monoxide poisoning, herpes simplex encephalitis and other CNS infections, hypoxic and other acquired brain injuries, stroke, deep midline cerebral tumors, and surgical resections, particularly for epilepsy. In the majority of cases, the pathology lies in midline or medial temporal structures, but there are also case reports of amnestic disorder following frontal lobe lesions.

Wernicke-Korsakoff Syndrome

Wernicke-Korsakoff syndrome results from thiamine depletion, and any cause of such depletion can lead to the syndrome. However, the overwhelming majority of cases are associated with chronic alcohol abuse, which results in both decreased intake and decreased absorption of thiamine. A genetic defect for thiamine metabolism has been described in a small proportion of patients (Blass and Gibson 1977).

The syndrome presents acutely with Wernicke's encephalopathy, which is characterized by confusion, ataxia, nystagmus, and ophthalmoplegia. Peripheral neuropathy can also be present. Parenteral administration of high-dose B vitamins is required as *emergency* treatment if the chronic state of Korsakoff's syndrome is to be avoided. The majority of cases of Korsakoff's syndrome occur following Wernicke's encephalopathy.

On clinical examination, patients with Korsakoff's syndrome may perform well on standard tasks of attention and working memory (serial sevens and reverse digit span) (Kopelman 1985) but may struggle on more complex tasks involving shifting and dividing attention. A severe memory impairment involving both anterograde and retrograde deficits is present (Kopelman et al. 1999). The defective encoding of new information is the core component of this memory disorder (Meudell and Mayes 1982). This results in a dense anterograde amnesia affecting declarative functions, and inconsistent, poorly organized retrieval of retrograde memories with a temporal gradient (more impairment for relatively recent than for more remote memories). The retrograde amnesia is more pronounced in diencephalic amnestic syndromes such as Korsakoff's than in amnestic syndromes of hippocampal origin, in which retrograde amnesia is present but with a deficit measured in months rather than years (Kopelman et al. 1999). A limited degree of new learning may be possible, particularly if patients are given a strategy to follow. Confabulation commonly occurs, particularly early in the disorder. Procedural memory remains relatively intact (Schacter 1987).

Other cognitive impairments and behavioral changes may accompany the amnesia. Executive functions are commonly mildly affected, but this impairment may be secondary to chronic alcoholism rather than representing a specific deficit. Disorientation and apathy, often with lack of curiosity about the past, are common, yet such disengaged patients frequently demonstrate labile irritability.

The pathological process is neuronal loss, microhemorrhages, and gliosis in the paraventricular and periaqueductal gray matter (Victor et al. 1971). The mammillary bodies, mammillothalamic tract, and the anterior thalamus are the main structures affected (Mair et al. 1979; Mayes et al. 1988). There is often a degree of generalized cortical atrophy, more marked in the frontal lobes (Jacobson and Lishman 1990). The atrophy may, however, be nonspecific and secondary to alcohol abuse. MRI indicates specific atrophy in diencephalic structures (Colchester et al. 2001).

With vitamin replacement and abstinence from alcohol, the prognosis is fair: one-quarter of patients will recover, half will improve but with some persistent impairment, and one-quarter will show no change (Victor et al. 1971). High-dose B vitamins should be given to all patients acutely and probably continued, but it is unclear how long this therapy should be maintained.

Transient Amnestic Syndromes

Transient amnesia can occur in several contexts. Transient global amnesia (TGA) is a distinctive benign disorder affecting middle-aged or elderly persons, who become amnestic for recent events and unable to lay down new memories for a period of around 4 hours (Hodges and Ward 1989). Repetitive questioning by patients of their companions is a characteristic feature. Episodes can be provoked by physical or emotional stress and are usually isolated; the medium-term recurrence rate is 3% per year (Hodges 1991). There is good evidence that TGA results from reversible medial temporal lobe dysfunction, but the etiological mechanism is uncertain (Stillhard et al. 1990). Although temporal lobe epilepsy occasionally mimics TGA ("transient epileptic amnesia"), episodes are typically briefer (lasting less than an hour), recurrent (several per year), and tend to occur on waking (Zeman et al. 1998). Other causes of transient amnesia include transient cerebral ischemia (usually accompanied by other neurological symptoms and signs), migraine, drug ingestion, and head injury.

Dementias Accompanied by Neurological Signs

Dementia refers to a deterioration of intellectual faculties, such as memory, concentration, and judgment, that is sometimes accompanied by emotional disturbance and personality changes. An approach to management of dementing conditions (including Alzheimer's disease, vascular dementia, Lewy body dementia, frontotemporal dementia, Huntington's disease, Parkinson's disease, and normal-pressure hydrocephalus, among others) is described in detail in Chapter 7, "Dementia." In this section, we concentrate on those disorders that are particularly likely to present with other neurological symptoms, often a movement disorder. Other causes of dementia are also discussed elsewhere in this volume: HIV (see Chapter 28, "HIV/ AIDS"), other infections (see Chapter 27, "Infectious Diseases"), alcohol and other substance use (see Chapter 18, "Substance-Related Disorders"), toxic and metabolic conditions (see Chapter 23, "Endocrine and Metabolic Disorders"), rheumatological and inflammatory conditions (see Chapter 25, "Rheumatology"), and traumatic and brain injury (see Chapter 35, "Physical Medicine and Rehabilitation").

Huntington's Disease

Huntington's disease (HD), also known as Huntington's chorea, was first described in Long Island in 1872 by George Huntington. This dominantly inherited disorder, which causes a combination of progressive motor, cognitive, psychiatric, and behavioral dysfunction, results from an abnormality in the *IT15* gene on chromosome 4 encoding the protein huntingtin.

Epidemiology

HD occurs at a prevalence of 5–7 per 100,000 population in the United States, with wide regional variations (Chua and Chiu 1994). The sexes are affected equally. Onset can be at any age but most commonly is in young or middle adulthood (Adams et al. 1988; Farrer and Conneally 1985). The disorder exhibits the phenomenon of *anticipation*, in which the age at onset tends to decrease over the generations, especially with paternal transmission (Brinkman et al. 1997) (see subsection "Pathology and Etiology" below).

Clinical Features

Chorea—involuntary fidgety movements of the face and limbs—is the characteristic motor disorder. As the disease progresses, other extrapyramidal features can develop, including rigidity, dystonia, and bradykinesia, as well as dysphagia, dysarthria, and pyramidal signs (Harper 1991). Childhood-onset HD tends to be dominated by rigidity and myoclonus (the "Westphal variant"). Epilepsy can occur. Cognitive dysfunction goes hand in hand with the motor disorder. The dementia of HD is predominantly

"subcortical," with impairment of attention, executive function, speed of processing, and memory (Zakzanis 1998). Psychiatric symptoms and behavioral changes are the norm (Mendez 1994; Zappacosta et al. 1996), with depression, apathy, and aggressiveness present in most cases (Burns et al. 1990; Levy et al. 1998) and psychosis, obsessional behavior, and suicide in a significant minority (Almqvist et al. 1999; Cummings and Cunningham 1992; Folstein et al. 1979). Progression to a state of immobility and dementia typically occurs over a period of 15–20 years (Feigin et al. 1995). Cognitive and behavioral changes may predate the clear-cut emergence of symptomatic HD (Kirkwood et al. 1999).

Pathology and Etiology

The key pathological processes of HD occur in the striatum, caudate, and putamen. The loss of small neurons in the striatum is accompanied by neuronal loss in the cerebral cortex, cerebral atrophy, ventricular dilatation, and, eventually, neuronal depletion throughout the basal ganglia (De la Monte et al. 1988; Vonsattel and DiFiglia 1998).

The underlying genetic abnormality is expansion of a "base triplet repeat" within the huntingtin gene. The normal gene contains 10–35 CAG (cytosine–adenine–guanine) repeats; repeat lengths beyond 39 give rise to symptomatic HD over the course of a normal life span (Duyao et al. 1993). Repeat lengths between 36 and 39 can cause disease. Repeats in the 27–35 range appear to be unstable and liable to increase into the pathological range in the next generation. The tendency for pathologically expanded repeats to increase in length between generations, especially in paternal transmission, underlies the clinical phenomenon of *anticipation*. The function of huntingtin remains uncertain.

Investigation and Differential Diagnosis

A number of disorders can cause the combination of chorea and cognitive change seen in HD, including other inherited disorders such as neuroacanthocytosis and dentato-rubro-pallido-luysian atrophy (DRPLA) and acquired disorders such as systemic lupus erythematosus. However, the diagnosis of HD can now be made with confidence by DNA analysis. Counseling by a clinical geneticist is mandatory before presymptomatic testing and should be considered in other circumstances as well (Codori et al. 1997).

Management

Chorea may require treatment. However, given the cognitive and extrapyramidal side effects of the agents used (neuroleptics, dopamine depletors such as tetrabenazine or benzodiazepines), this is often best avoided (Rosenblatt et al. 1999). Other psychiatric symptoms should be treated along standard lines (Leroi and Michalon 1998).

Wilson's Disease (Hepatolenticular Degeneration)

First described by Wilson in 1912, Wilson's disease is a very rare, autosomal recessive, progressive degenerative brain disease caused by a disorder of copper metabolism, producing personality change, cognitive decline, extrapyramidal signs, and cirrhosis of the liver.

Clinical Features

The onset of Wilson's disease most commonly occurs in childhood or adolescence but can occur as late as the fifth decade (Bearn 1957). Patients may present to psychiatrists with personality change, behavioral disturbance (including psychosis), or dementia (Akil and Brewer 1995; Dening and Berrios 1989) or to neurologists with a variety of extrapyramidal signs, including tremor, dysarthria and drooling, rigidity, bradykinesia, and dystonia (Walsh 1986; Walsh and Yelland 1992). Careful examination reveals these features and also, in virtually all symptomatic cases, the presence of *Kayser-Fleischer rings*—rings of greenish-brown copper pigment at the edge of the cornea (Wiebers et al. 1997). (In suspected cases, an ophthalmologist should be asked to look for this feature with a slit lamp.). The liver failure and the neuropsychiatric syndrome can occur together or independently.

Pathology and Etiology

The causative genetic mutation is in the copper-transporting P-type ATPase coded on chromosome 13 (Bull et al. 1993). The result is excessive copper deposition in the brain, cornea, liver, and kidneys and increased copper excretion in urine. The caudate and putamen are the brain regions most severely affected, but other parts of the basal ganglia and the cerebral cortex are also involved (Mochizuki et al. 1997; Starosta-Rubinstein et al. 1987).

Investigation and Differential Diagnosis

Ninety-five percent of patients with Wilson's disease have low serum levels of the copper-binding protein ceruloplasmin. Normal ceruloplasmin levels and an absence of Kayser-Fleischer rings render the diagnosis very unlikely in cases with neuropsychiatric features (Ferenci 1998). Uncertain cases may require measurement of urinary copper excretion and liver biopsy for measurement of copper content (Pfeil and Lynn 1999). DNA analysis

is becoming increasingly available. The differential diagnosis varies with the type of presentation. The combination of psychological disturbance and unusual neurological features has led to misdiagnosis as conversion disorder.

Management

Several copper-chelating agents (penicillamine, tetraethylene tetramine, zinc acetate) are available to treat patients with Wilson's disease, but the risk of significant side effects mandates care by a specialist (Pfeil and Lynn 1999).

Leukodystrophies

Leukodystrophies—recessively inherited or X-linked disorders of myelination—can be accompanied by neuropsychiatric syndromes, usually with associated neurological features. Metachromatic leukodystrophy, caused by a deficiency of the enzyme arylsulfatase A (Hyde et al. 1992), and adrenoleukodystrophy (see also Chapter 23, "Endocrine and Metabolic Disorders"), an X-linked disorder associated with abnormalities of very-long-chain fatty acids (James et al. 1984), are the most commonly encountered types.

Progressive Supranuclear Palsy

Progressive supranuclear palsy is characterized by supranuclear gaze palsy (an inability to direct eye movements voluntarily, especially vertical eye movements, in the presence of normal reflex eye movements); truncal rigidity, akinesia, postural instability, and early falls; bulbar features, with dysarthria and dysphagia; subcortical dementia; and alteration of mood (including pathological crying and laughing), personality, and behavior (De Bruin and Lees 1992). Neurofibrillary tangles, consisting of tau protein, are found in neurons of the basal ganglia and brain stem. Midbrain atrophy may be apparent on MRI.

Corticobasal Degeneration

Corticobasal degeneration typically manifests as a combination of limb apraxia, usually asymmetric at onset, alien limb phenomena, limb myoclonus, parkinsonism, and cognitive decline (Rinne et al. 1994). The pathology involves neuronal loss in both the basal ganglia and the frontal and parietal cortex, with intraneuronal accumulations of tau protein resembling that seen in progressive supranuclear palsy. MRI usually reveals frontoparietal atrophy.

Transmissible Spongiform Encephalopathies (Prion Dementias)

The transmissible spongiform encephalopathies are a group of rare dementias caused by an accumulation of abnormal prion protein within the brain. Related illnesses occur in animals: indeed, one recently described disorder, variant Creutzfeldt-Jakob disease, is thought to result from infection of humans by consumption of beef products from cattle with bovine spongiform encephalopathy (BSE) (Will et al. 1996). The term *prion*, coined by Stanley Prusiner, stands for "proteinaceous infectious pathogen" (Prusiner 1994, 2001).

Epidemiology

All of the transmissible spongiform encephalopathies are rare. Sporadic Creutzfeldt-Jakob disease, the most common human transmissible spongiform encephalopathy, occurs with an annual incidence of one per million, usually affecting people between the ages of 55 and 70 years (P. Brown et al. 1987). At the time of this writing, variant Creutzfeldt-Jakob disease has been diagnosed in some 150 individuals, almost all of them in the United Kingdom. Variant Creutzfeldt-Jakob disease more often develops in younger subjects than does sporadic Creutzfeldt-Jakob disease: most cases have occurred during the second through fourth decades of life (Will et al. 1996).

Clinical Features

Sporadic Creutzfeldt-Jakob disease typically causes a rapidly progressive dementia, with early changes in behavior, visual symptoms, and cerebellar signs. Within weeks to months, marked cognitive impairment develops, often progressing to mutism, with pyramidal, extrapyramidal, and cerebellar signs and myoclonus (P. Brown et al. 1994). The median duration of symptom onset to death is only 4 months, although in rare cases the disorder evolves over several years. Iatrogenic cases of Creutzfeldt-Jakob disease have occurred when CNS tissue from patients with sporadic Creutzfeldt-Jakob disease has unwittingly been transferred from patient to patient by surgical instruments or used in medical procedures as a source of growth hormone, gonadotropins, dura mater, or corneal grafts (P. Brown et al. 2000).

Variant Creutzfeldt-Jakob disease differs markedly from sporadic Creutzfeldt-Jakob disease (Spencer et al. 2002). The initial symptoms are usually psychiatric, most commonly anxiety or depression, and often of sufficient severity to lead to psychiatric referral. Limb pain or tingling is common early in the course of the illness. After

some months, cognitive symptoms typically develop, causing difficulty at school or work, together with varied neurological features including pyramidal, extrapyramidal, and cerebellar signs and myoclonus. The disorder evolves more slowly than does sporadic Creutzfeldt-Jakob disease, with an average duration of 14 months from symptom onset to death.

Three other varieties of human transmissible spongiform encephalopathy have been described. *Kuru*, now extremely rare, causes a cerebellar syndrome with progression to dementia. It is confined to the Fore Indians of Papua New Guinea and was caused by cannibalism of CNS tissues from affected relatives (Gajdusek 1977). *Gerstmann-Straussler-Scheinker syndrome* is an autosomal dominant prion dementia characterized primarily by cerebellar dysfunction and dementia with a protracted clinical course (Piccardo et al. 1998). *Fatal familial insomnia* is a very rare autosomal dominant prion disorder with severe insomnia and autonomic disturbance manifesting early in the course of the disease (Gambetti et al. 1995).

Pathology and Etiology

The light microscope reveals "spongiform change" in the brains of patients with transmissible spongiform encephalopathies; this change is associated with neuronal loss, gliosis, and deposition of "amyloid." Immunocytochemistry and direct biochemical analysis indicate that the amyloid is composed of a protease-resistant form of prion protein (PrP) (Prusiner 2001).

Investigation and Differential Diagnosis

In sporadic Creutzfeldt-Jakob disease, the electroencephalogram (EEG) shows 1- to 2-per-second triphasic waves in 80% of cases at some time during the course of the illness (Steinhoff et al. 1996). Detection of 14–3–3 protein in CSF has a sensitivity and specificity of approximately 90% for sporadic Creutzfeldt-Jakob disease (Hsich et al. 1996). Brain biopsy is usually diagnostic but is rarely performed. In variant Creutzfeldt-Jakob disease, the EEG and CSF examination are less useful, but characteristic MRI abnormalities (especially high signal in the pulvinar nucleus) are found in a substantial proportion of cases, with a reported sensitivity of 78% and a specificity of 100% (Zeidler et al. 2000). Tonsillar biopsy has also been used as a confirmatory test, because prion protein scrapie (PrP^{SC}) is found in lymphoid tissue in variant Creutzfeldt-Jakob disease (Hill et al. 1999). In suspected cases of familial transmissible spongiform encephalopathy, sequencing of the PrP gene will identify the causative mutation.

Management

At present, there is no proven remedy for the disease.

Whipple's Disease

Whipple's disease is rare but important, because it is treatable. Infection with *Tropheryma whippelii* typically causes a multisystem disorder with prominent steatorrhea, weight loss, and abdominal pain (Fleming et al. 1988). CNS involvement is common, and neurological and psychiatric symptoms and signs occur in the absence of systemic features (A.P. Brown et al. 1990; Louis et al. 1996). Small-bowel biopsy, lymph node biopsy, brain MRI, and CSF examination, including polymerase chain reaction studies to identify the causative organism, can all be helpful in diagnosis (Louis et al. 1996). Antibiotic treatment can be effective.

Subacute Sclerosing Panencephalitis

Subacute sclerosing panencephalitis (SSPE) is a rare complication of childhood measles in which intraneuronal persistence of a defective form of the virus in the CNS results in a continuing immune response, with high levels of measles antibody in the CSF. Neurological signs, including myoclonus, accompany the dementia (Lishman 1997; Risk et al. 1978). Average life expectancy from onset is 1–2 years.

Progressive Multifocal Leukodystrophy

Progressive multifocal leukodystrophy is caused by activation of JC papovavirus within the CNS in an immunocompromised patient. The resulting demyelination gives rise to pyramidal signs, visual impairment, and a subcortical dementia, usually with progression to death within months (Lishman 1997; Richardson 1961).

Paraneoplastic Syndromes

Paraneoplastic "limbic encephalitis" results from an immunological cross-reaction between tumor antigens and antigens present within the CNS. It can cause a range of psychiatric presentations, including cognitive deficits, confusional states, a pure amnestic syndrome, and affective symptoms. There are also paraneoplastic syndromes that affect the cerebellum, spinal cord, and peripheral nerves (Darnell and Posner 2003). Small-cell lung cancer is the most common cause of paraneoplastic syndromes, but breast, ovarian, renal, and testicular carcinoma and lymphoma can also be responsible. The tumor may be small and sometimes initially undetectable by imaging. The diagnosis is supported by detection of antineuronal antibodies in serum or CSF, most commonly "anti-Hu"; the CSF often contains oligoclonal bands of immunoglobulin.

CNS Tumors, Hydrocephalus, and Subdural Hematoma

CNS tumors, hydrocephalus, and subdural hematoma are discussed in the section "Neurosurgical Issues" later in this chapter.

Epilepsy

Epileptic seizures are transient cerebral dysfunctions resulting from an excessive and abnormal electrical discharge of neurons. The clinical manifestations are numerous. As a result, psychiatrists commonly encounter epilepsy, both when considering whether epilepsy is the primary cause of paroxysmal psychiatric symptoms and when treating its significant psychiatric complications.

Epidemiology

Problems with case definition and ascertainment complicate epidemiological estimates. However, incidence rates of 40–70 per 100,000 population in developed countries and 100–190 per 100,000 in developing countries are generally accepted. The prevalence of active epilepsy is around 7 per 1,000 population in the developed world (Bell and Sander 2001; Kotsopoulos et al. 2002; Sander and Shorvon 1996). Reasons for the higher incidence in developing nations are believed to include increased rates of birth trauma and head injury and lack of health services to manage them, and poor sanitation leading to high rates of CNS infection (e.g., cysticercosis; see Chapter 27, "Infectious Diseases"). Most studies show a bimodal distribution for age of incidence, with increased rates in persons younger than 10 years and older than 60 years. Epilepsy is more common in men and may be more common in black Africans (Sandler and Shorvon 1996).

A specific etiological mechanism is identified in less than one-third of cases. These mechanisms include perinatal disorders, learning disabilities, cerebral palsy, head trauma, CNS infection, cerebrovascular disease, brain tumors, Alzheimer's disease, and substance misuse. In addition, many so-called idiopathic seizures are likely to have a genetic basis.

Estimates of seizure recurrence after a first event are widely varied and depend on the population being studied (Cockerell et al. 1997; Sander 1993). However, if seizures are going to recur, they usually do so within 6 months of the first event; the prognosis improves as the seizure-free period lengthens. In patients with established epilepsy, the prognosis is extremely variable. In some benign childhood epilepsies, anticonvulsant medication is unnecessary and remission the rule. In the majority of patients with epilepsy, remission occurs with treatment, and it may be possible to withdraw treatment in the long term. In some epilepsy syndromes, such as juvenile myoclonic epilepsy, treatment is effective but must be continued indefinitely. In around one-third of patients with epilepsy, anticonvulsants fail to provide adequate control of seizures. This is particularly likely in patients with aggressive pediatric epilepsy syndromes (e.g., infantile spasms, Lennox-Gastaut syndrome) or in patients whose epilepsy has a defined structural or congenital cause.

Clinical Features

Epilepsy constitutes a heterogeneous group of disorders with multiple causes, and its clinical features reflect this diversity. The key clinical distinction is between seizures with a focal and seizures with a generalized cerebral origin. The former are more likely to be associated with a detectable and potentially remediable cerebral lesion, whereas the latter are more likely to start in childhood or adolescence and to be familial. Despite the wide variety of possible seizure manifestations, an individual patient's seizures are usually stereotyped. Their clinical features result from a recurrent pattern of cortical hyperactivity during the ictal event followed by hypoactivity in the same area postictally.

Documentation of the clinical features of the seizure is the key to diagnosis. Because firsthand observation is seldom possible unless seizures are very frequent, the history of the episode, including an eyewitness account (or a home video), is of paramount importance.

Tonic-Clonic Seizures

Tonic-clonic seizures are the most dramatic manifestation of epilepsy and are characterized by motor activity and sudden loss of consciousness. In a typical seizure, a patient has no warning (with the possible exception of a couple of myoclonic jerks) of its onset. The seizure begins with sudden loss of consciousness and a tonic phase during which there are sustained muscle contractions lasting 10–20 seconds. This is followed by a clonic phase of repetitive muscle contractions that last approximately 30 seconds. A number of autonomic changes, including increase in blood pressure and pulse rate, apnea, mydriasis, incontinence, piloerection, cyanosis, and perspiration, may also occur. In the postictal period, the patient is drowsy and confused. Abnormal neurological signs are often elicited.

Partial Seizures

Partial seizures are categorized according to whether they are simple (without impairment in consciousness) or complex (with impairment of consciousness). This classification may be difficult to apply in practice, however.

Simple partial seizures. The clinical features of simple partial seizures depend on the brain region activated. Although the initial area is relatively localized, it is common for the abnormal activity to spread to adjacent areas, producing a progression of seizure pattern. If the activity originates in the motor cortex, there will be jerking movements in the contralateral body part. This can cause progressive jerking in contiguous regions (known as "Jacksonian march"). Activity in the supplementary motor cortex causes head turning with arm extension on the same side—the classic "fencer's posture."

Seizures originating in the *parietal lobe* can cause tingling or numbness in a bodily region or more complex sensory experiences such as a sense of absence on one side of the body, asomatognosia. Seizures in the inferior regions of the parietal lobe can cause severe vertigo and disorientation in space. Dominant-hemisphere parietal lobe seizures can cause language disturbance.

Seizures of the *occipital lobe* are associated with visual symptoms, which are usually elementary (e.g., simple flashing lights). However, if the seizure occurs at the border with the temporal lobe, more complex experiences can occur, including micropsia, macropsia, and metamorphosia, as well as visual hallucinations of previously experienced imagery.

Seizures affecting the *temporal lobe* can be the most difficult to diagnose, but this lobe is also the most common site of onset, accounting for 80% of partial seizures. Symptoms may include auditory hallucinations, ranging from simple sounds to complex language. Olfactory hallucinations, usually involving unpleasant odors, follow discharge in the mesial temporal lobe. Seizures in the Sylvian fissure or operculum will cause gustatory sensations; ictal epigastric sensations such as nausea or emptiness generally have a temporal lobe origin. The well-known emotional and psychic phenomena of temporal lobe seizure activity can occur in simple seizures but are more common in complex partial seizures.

Complex partial seizures. In a complex partial seizure, the patient frequently experiences an aura at the onset of the seizure. The aura is a simple partial seizure lasting seconds to minutes. It should be distinguished from a prodrome, which is not an ictal event and which can last for hours or even days before a seizure. Prodromes usually consist of a sense of nervousness or irritability. The content of the aura will depend on the location of the abnormal discharge within the brain. Thus, it may contain motor, sensory, visceral, or psychic elements. These can include hallucinations; intense affective symptoms such as fear, depression, panic, or depersonalization; and cognitive symptoms such as aphasia. Distortions of memory can include dreamy states, flashbacks, and distortions of familiarity with events (déjà vu or jamais vu). Occasionally, rapid recollection of episodes from earlier life experiences occurs (panoramic vision). Rage is rare; when it does occur, it is characterized by lack of provocation and abrupt abatement. This phase is followed by impairment of consciousness and a seizure usually lasting 60–90 seconds, which may generalize into a tonic-clonic seizure. Automatisms may occur and can involve an extension of the patient's actions prior to seizure onset. Common facial automatisms include chewing or swallowing, lip smacking, and grimacing; automatisms in the extremities include fumbling with objects, walking, or trying to stand up. Postictal confusion is usually significant and typically lasts 10 minutes or longer.

Complex partial seizures of frontal lobe origin tend to begin and end abruptly, with minimal postictal confusion. They often occur in clusters. The attacks are usually bizarre, with motor automatisms such as bicycling or with sexual automatisms and vocalizations.

Absence Seizures

Absence seizures are well-defined clinical and EEG events. The essential feature is an abrupt, brief episode of decreased awareness that occurs without any warning, aura, or postictal symptoms. At the onset there is a disruption of activity.

A *simple* absence seizure is characterized by only an alteration in consciousness. The patient remains mobile, breathing is unaffected, and there is no cyanosis or pallor and no loss of postural tone or motor activity. The ending is abrupt, and the patient resumes previous activity immediately, often unaware that a seizure has taken place. An attack usually lasts around 15 seconds. A *complex* absence seizure involves additional symptoms such as loss or increase of postural tone, minor clonic movements of the face or extremities, minor automatisms, or autonomic symptoms such as pallor, flushing, tachycardia, piloerection, mydriasis, and urinary incontinence.

Violent Behavior

Epilepsy, in particular epilepsy involving the temporal lobe, may cause emotional symptoms and very occasionally can result in undirected violent behavior (Kotagal 1997). However, in the majority of cases of epilepsy-related violence, the behavior occurs in response to being restrained during a seizure. One should be very cautious in attributing other violent assaults to a seizure. This issue is discussed in more detail in Chapter 8, "Aggression and Violence," which includes criteria for determining whether a violent act resulted from an epileptic seizure.

Differential Diagnosis

Differentiating epilepsy from nonepileptic attack disorder (psychogenic epilepsy, or pseudoseizures) and syncope can be difficult (Roberts 1998). Other paroxysmal disorders should also be considered; these include transient ischemic attacks, hypoglycemia, migraine, transient global amnesia, cataplexy, paroxysmal movement disorders, and paroxysmal symptoms in multiple sclerosis. Attacks during sleep can pose particular difficulties, as informant reports are less useful.

Nonepileptic Attack Disorder

Nonepileptic attack disorder (NEAD), also referred to as "pseudoseizures" or "psychogenic epilepsy," is the most common alternative diagnosis, accounting for about 30% of patients presenting to clinics with suspected epilepsy (Reuber and Elger 2003), and with a reported community prevalence of 33 per 100,000 population (Benbadis and Allen 2000). The terminology is confused, and it is unclear whether NEAD is a specific diagnosis or a collective term for a number of psychiatric diagnoses or symptoms that may cause seizurelike spells, including conversion, panic attacks, hyperventilation syndrome (see Chapter 20, "Lung Disease"), posttraumatic stress disorder (PTSD), and catatonia. We personally favor the view that NEAD is a variant of panic disorder without the expression of fear (Vein et al. 1994). Some patients have both epilepsy and nonepileptic attacks, but probably only around 10% of individuals with NEAD fall into this category (Benbadis et al. 2001; Reuber et al. 2002). Many of these patients are learning disabled and at increased risk of both epilepsy and psychiatric disorders.

The diagnosis of NEAD can often be made on the basis of a careful history and examination. Clinical clues include the presence of prior or current psychiatric disorders, including somatoform disorders; atypical varieties of seizure, especially the occurrence of frequent and prolonged seizures in the face of normal interictal intellectual function and EEG; a preponderance of seizures in public places, especially in clinics and hospitals; and behavior during an apparent generalized seizure that suggests preservation of awareness (e.g., resistance to attempted eye opening, persistent aversion of gaze from the examiner). Previous childhood sexual abuse is very common but not universal among those with the diagnosis (Binzer et al. 2004). When doubt remains after careful clinical assessment and standard investigations, the gold standard for diagnosis is observation of attacks during videotelemetry. A normal EEG during or immediately following an apparent generalized seizure also provides strong evidence for NEAD.

The diagnosis of NEAD is regarded as distinct from deliberate falsification of attacks (i.e., malingering or factitious disorder). The majority of patients will be cooperative with investigation and diagnosis, even when they know in advance that the purpose is to confirm NEAD and refute epilepsy (McGonigal et al. 2002).

Syncope

Syncope, usually due to temporary interruption of the blood supply to the brain, is often accompanied by myoclonic jerks that are frequently regarded as epileptic by lay and medical onlookers (Lempert et al. 1994). The occurrence of more complex movements, eye deviation, eyelid flicker, or vocalizations can confuse the diagnosis further, as can aura symptoms, which are recalled by the majority of subjects and which include epigastric, vertiginous, visual, and somatosensory experiences (Benke et al. 1997).

Sleep Disorders

Sleep disorders—including sleepwalking, night terrors, and confusional arousals, all of which occur during slow-wave sleep; rapid eye movement (REM) sleep behavior disorder; and a variety of other parasomnias, including bruxism, rhythmic movement disorder, and periodic limb movements—must all be distinguished from epilepsy (see Chapter 16, "Sleep Disorders").

Investigation of Seizures

Epilepsy is above all a clinical diagnosis, and the use and interpretation of tests should reflect this. Routine blood tests should include a complete blood count and routine chemistries, including serum calcium and magnesium. An electrocardiogram (ECG) should always be performed. An EEG is helpful in confirming the diagnosis and in clarifying the type of epilepsy (i.e., generalized versus focal, a distinction particularly relevant for children and adolescents). However, the EEG is insensitive: a single interictal EEG will detect clearly epileptiform abnormalities in only about 30% of patients with epilepsy. Therefore, a normal EEG does not exclude epilepsy, just as minor nonspecific abnormalities do not confirm it. Serial recordings, including sleep-deprived recordings, increase the diagnostic yield to around 80% (Chabolla and Cascino 1997). EEG can be supplemented with video recording to allow

examination of the correlation between the clinical symptoms and the EEG abnormalities (videotelemetry). Twenty-four-hour ambulatory monitoring is sometimes helpful.

Some form of neuroimaging should be performed in all patients with epilepsy, unless EEG has clearly demonstrated a syndrome of primary generalized epilepsy in a young patient. CT is adequate to exclude tumors and major structural abnormalities and has the benefit of ease of access in most developed countries; however, CT may miss subtle pathologies. MRI is undoubtedly the imaging modality of choice, capable of detecting pathological abnormalities in up to 90% of patients with intractable epilepsy, including mesial temporal sclerosis (Spencer 1994). It can, however, be difficult to access in some countries.

Measurement of serum prolactin after seizures has a limited role in the diagnosis of NEAD. Prolactin will rise after a generalized seizure but not, as a rule, after a nonepileptic attack. However, interpretation of the test requires knowledge of the basal prolactin and concurrent drug treatment (e.g., antipsychotics). Partial seizures and syncope can also elevate prolactin (Oribe et al. 1996; Pohlmann-Eden et al. 1997).

Additional cardiac investigations that may be helpful in selected cases include 24-hour ambulatory ECG to identify cardiac dysrhythmias; echocardiography, to identify structural cardiac abnormalities; and tilt-table testing, to help confirm orthostatic syncope.

Psychiatric Complications

Recent record-linkage studies (Bredkjaer et al. 1998; Jalava and Sillanpaa 1996) have reported an increase in psychotic symptoms, particularly schizophreniform and paranoid psychoses, in men but not women with epilepsy. Studies have also shown a fourfold increase in overall rates of psychiatric disorder in both men and woman with epilepsy compared with individuals in the general population, but not compared with patients with other medical diagnoses.

Psychosis

Psychotic symptoms may be categorized as transient postictal psychosis and chronic interictal psychosis. Patients with transient postictal psychosis often present with manic grandiosity with religious and mystical features (Kanemoto et al. 1996a). A number of small studies have suggested that such patients are more likely than other epilepsy patients to have psychic auras, bilateral interictal spikes, and nocturnal secondarily generalized seizures (Devinsky et al. 1995). In general, psychotic episodes do not start immediately after a seizure, but instead occur after a lucid interval of 2–72 hours. In one study, patients with chronic interictal psychosis had a higher frequency of perceptual delusions and auditory hallucinations than did patients with postictal psychoses (Kanemoto et al. 1996b).

Transient psychosis was reported in 1% of patients following temporal lobotomy for epilepsy. Men with right-sided foci who were not seizure free after surgery appeared to be at particular risk for this symptom (Manchanda et al. 1993). There may be an increased risk of postictal psychoses in patients with temporal lobe epilepsy and hippocampal sclerosis (in comparison with those with temporal lobe epilepsy and no sclerosis) (Kanemoto et al. 1996a). How mesial temporal sclerosis relates to psychosis is unclear.

The work of Landolt in the 1950s drew attention to the occurrence of psychosis in some patients in whom epileptiform EEG abnormalities were normalized by treatment ("forced normalization") (Krishnamoorthy and Trimble 1999; Landolt 1958). The concept remains controversial.

Antiepileptic drugs may contribute to the development of psychotic symptoms. Several of the newer drugs have significant psychiatric side effects. Vigabatrin, an irreversible inhibitor of gamma-aminobutyric acid (GABA) transaminase, has been shown to precipitate psychotic and affective symptoms in 3%–10% of patients (Levinson and Devinsky 1999). This effect occurs more commonly in patients with a history of psychiatric illness.

Depressive and Anxiety Disorders

Depressive and anxiety disorders affect approximately one-third of patients with epilepsy (Jalava and Sillanpaa 1996; Kanner and Balabanov 2002; Stefansson et al. 1998). Neurobiological, psychological, social, and iatrogenic factors have all been proposed and probably all are relevant (Lambert and Robertson 1999; Weigartz et al. 1999). Links have been suggested between complex partial seizures and concomitant frontal lobe dysregulation in the genesis of depression; however, study samples have been small and the possibility of confounding variables large (Weigartz et al. 1999). Depression arising from learned helplessness may occur in patients with epilepsy as a consequence of repeatedly experiencing unpredictable and unavoidable seizures (Weigartz et al. 1999). The stress of having to live with a stigmatized chronic illness may also be relevant. Finally, the antiepileptic drugs used in the treatment of epilepsy can themselves be a cause of depression. The relationship between depression and epilepsy is bidirectional (i.e., each is a risk factor for the

other). Depression is an independent risk factor for unprovoked seizures (Hesdorffer et al. 2000). This effect seems to be particularly marked for partial seizures.

Similarly, anxiety in epilepsy may have a complex etiology (Goldstein and Harden 2000). Anticipatory anxiety about having a seizure without warning can lead to agoraphobic-like symptoms and behavior.

The treatment of depressive and anxiety disorders in epilepsy is the same as that of anxiety and depression in the medically ill (Hermann et al. 2000; see also Chapter 9, "Depression," and Chapter 12, "Anxiety Disorders"). Increased seizure risks associated with specific psychiatric drugs are reviewed in Chapter 37, "Psychopharmacology."

Treatment

The basic principles of epilepsy treatment are as follows:

1. Use a single drug whenever possible.
2. Increase the dose slowly until either the seizures are controlled or toxicity occurs.
3. If a single drug does not control seizures without toxicity, then switch initially to another drug used alone.
4. Drug-level monitoring is generally unnecessary except in the case of phenytoin and is sometimes misleading: some patients do well with drug levels below or above the "therapeutic range."
5. Consider using two drugs only when monotherapy is unsuccessful.
6. Be aware that the metabolism of drugs may be different in the young, the elderly, pregnant women, and patients with chronic disease, particularly hepatic and renal chronic disease, and be on the lookout for drug interactions.

Approximately 20%–30% of patients do not achieve seizure control with drug therapy. In carefully selected cases, surgery can be effective (Engel 1993; Vickrey et al. 1993). The criteria for selection generally include the presence of a focal lesion on neuroimaging, evidence from videotelemetry that the lesion is the source of the habitual seizures, and neuropsychological evidence that resection of the lesion should not cause major cognitive deficits (Sperling 1994). Psychological factors are also often relevant to the decision to perform surgery (see section "Neurosurgical Issues" later in this chapter).

Vagal nerve stimulation has been shown to reduce seizure frequency in some patients with refractory epilepsy (Schachter 2002), but it probably is no more effective than the addition of the newer anticonvulsants to established therapy.

Tic Disorders

Tics are habitual spasmodic muscular movements or contractions, usually of the face or extremities that are associated with a variety of disorders.

Gilles de la Tourette's syndrome (GTS) is characterized by a combination of multiple waxing and waning motor and vocal tics. These vary from simple twitches and grunts to complex stereotypies. Premonitory sensory sensations in body parts that "need to tic" are a common feature and complicate the picture, because their temporary suppressibility lends them a voluntary component. Other features are echolalia and coprolalia, particularly in severe cases. GTS is strongly associated with obsessive-compulsive disorder (OCD) (Eapen et al. 1997; Miguel et al. 1997; Muller et al. 1997; Zohar et al. 1997), but many claim that it is qualitatively different from pure OCD, with greater concern with symmetry, aggressive thoughts, forced touching, and fear of harming oneself in OCD-GTS compared with a more frequent focus on hygiene and cleanliness in pure OCD. Depressive symptoms are common (Wodrich et al. 1997). The prevalence of GTS is about 5 per 10 000 population, with a male:female ratio of 4:1 (Staley et al. 1997). A debate exists as to whether OCD in itself constitutes a specific psychopathological entity comorbid with GTS or whether diverse pathological disorders—including attention-deficit/hyperactivity disorder (ADHD), eating disorders, anxiety, and substance misuse—should also be considered part of the phenotype (Blum et al. 1997; Pauls et al. 1994). This issue clearly has implications for genetic studies, which have suggested a strong hereditary component in the disorder. Similarly, the neurobiology of GTS remains elusive, with evidence supporting dysfunctions in dopaminergic basal ganglia circuitry receiving the most attention. Structural imaging findings in GTS are usually normal; functional imaging data are contradictory at present (Robertson and Stern 1998).

A syndrome known as pediatric autoimmune neuropsychiatric disorders associated with streptococcal infection (PANDAS) has been defined, consisting of OCD accompanied by tics with abrupt onset or exacerbation associated with beta-hemolytic streptococcal infection (see Chapter 27, "Infectious Diseases"). PANDAS may lie on the same clinical spectrum as Sydenham's chorea, in which OCD and vocal tics have also been reported (Mercadante et al. 1997; Swedo et al. 1998), and may cast light on the etiology of GTS. Some preliminary studies have suggested that B-cell antigen D8/17, an immunological marker of susceptibility to rheumatic fever, may be associated with both PANDAS and GTS (Murphy et al. 1997; Swedo et al. 1997). This offers the attractive possibility of immune-mediated treatments as well as an explanation for the occurrence and subsequent successful treatment of GTS as a complication of both Lyme disease (Riedel et al. 1998) and oral herpes simplex (Budman et al. 1997).

Management of GTS is multidisciplinary, with clear need to address the educational, social, and family consequences of the disorder. Dopamine antagonists remain the mainstay of pharmacological management. Haloperidol has been the most widely used antipsychotic, but many authors advocate use of newer antipsychotic agents on the basis of fewer side effects (Jimenez-Jimenez and Garcia Ruiz 2001; Robertson and Stern 2000). Pimozide was shown to be superior to haloperidol in one of the few randomized, controlled trials conducted, but potential cardiac side effects generally prohibit its use (Sallee et al. 1997). The dopamine D_2 selective agent sulpiride (not available in the United States) is potentially useful. Of the newer antipsychotic agents, risperidone has attracted interest but thus far has appeared to be more effective in the treatment of related OCD phenomena than in the treatment of the tics themselves (Robertson et al. 1996; Stein et al. 1997). Tetrabenazine, a presynaptic monoamine depletor with postsynaptic blockade, has shown considerable efficacy in case series studies (Jankovic and Beach 1997), without a risk of dystonia or tardive dyskinesia but with a high risk of depression. In patients with comorbid restless legs syndrome, the dopamine agonist pergolide was effective in alleviating Tourette's symptoms, despite the fact that one might have predicted the opposite effect (Lipinski et al. 1997). Clonidine is used widely in the United States, but in the United Kingdom its use is generally restricted to patients with comorbid ADHD symptoms (Leckman et al. 1991). In establishing treatment priorities, one should bear in mind that the associated OCD and ADHD symptoms probably cause more functional and educational disability than the tics themselves (Abwender et al. 1996; De Groot et al. 1997).

Dystonias

The dystonias are a group of disorders characterized by involuntary twisting and repetitive movements and abnormal postures. The traditional clinical categorization is based on age at onset, distribution of symptoms, and site. Early-onset dystonia often starts in one limb, tends to generalize, and frequently has a genetic origin. By contrast, adult-onset dystonias usually spare the lower limbs, frequently involve the cervical or cranial muscles, and have a tendency to remain focal. They appear sporadic in most cases. Dystonias tend to improve with relaxation, hypnosis, and sleep. With the exception of cervical dystonia, pain is uncommon. Erroneous attribution of dystonia to a psychogenic cause is common because of the fluctuating nature of the symptoms, their often dramatic appearance, the ability of patients to use "tricks" to suppress them, and their association with task-specific symptoms (e.g., writer's cramp) (Eldridge et al. 1969). Dystonia may, however, occur as the presentation of a conversion disorder, although this is rare (Marjama et al. 1995; Verdugo and Ochoa 2000).

Primary torsion dystonia has autosomal dominant inheritance with reduced penetrance. It usually begins in childhood in one limb and then generalizes to other body parts.

Focal dystonia is the most prevalent form. It starts in adulthood and usually remains localized (e.g., as an isolated torticollis). The majority of cases are sporadic, although some family pedigree studies have shown an increased risk of focal dystonias in other family members (Waddy et al. 1991).

Dopa-responsive dystonia is characterized by childhood onset, diurnal fluctuation of symptoms, and a dramatic response to L-dopa therapy. It generally has autosomal dominant inheritance, although recessive forms associated with mutations in the tyrosine hydroxylase gene have been described (Knappskog et al. 1995).

It is important to remember the role of exposure to medications (antipsychotics, antiemetics) in the development of both acute and tardive dystonias (Sweet et al. 1995).

Medical treatment involves oral drugs and botulinum injections (Bentivoglio and Albanese 1999; Klein and Ozelius 2002). Botulinum therapy is the most effective treatment for focal dystonias such as torticollis. In generalized dystonia, a trial of L-dopa should be considered in all early-onset cases, given the possibility of dopa-responsive dystonia. Thereafter, the first-line treatment is usually anticholinergics, followed by baclofen and possibly benzodiazepines and dopamine depletors such as tetrabenazine. Surgical treatment can involve selective peripheral denervation or functional brain surgery. Comorbid psychiatric disorders are commonly associated with dystonias, particularly OCD, panic disorder, and depression (Wenzel et al. 1997). Their presence does not necessarily indicate that the dystonia is psychogenic, and they should be actively treated in their own right (Muller et al. 2002).

Headache

Acute Headache

Headache of abrupt onset that is very severe and prolonged can be due to *subarachnoid hemorrhage*, usually from a ruptured aneurysm, or to migraine, meningitis, or other cranial infection such as otitis media or sinusitis. The diagnosis of subarachnoid hemorrhage is suggested by the rapidity of onset ("thunderclap" headache, at its worst within 1 minute or so) and associated loss of consciousness, photophobia, vomiting, and neck stiffness. A headache with these features requires immediate neurological referral for assessment with CT scan (which reveals subarachnoid blood in the majority of cases) and lumbar puncture, when CT is negative, to examine for xanthochromia (which is present reliably from 12 hours after subarachnoid hemorrhage). Psychiatrists are predominantly involved in the management of the associated brain injury following subarachnoid hemorrhage. (For a further discussion of these management principles, see the section "Stroke" earlier in this chapter and Chapter 35, "Physical Medicine and Rehabilitation.")

Migraine can mimic subarachnoid hemorrhage. The diagnosis is usually suggested by a history of more typical migrainous headaches with prodromal visual (or other focal neurologic) disturbance and a gradually evolving hemicranial throbbing headache with photophobia and nausea or vomiting. *Meningitis* is suggested by a severe headache, usually worsening over hours, with photophobia, nausea, and neck stiffness in association with fever and other features of infection.

Chronic Headache

Headache is common. *Tension-type headache* is familiar to most of us as a global headache, usually of mild to moderate severity, sometimes with a "bandlike" or pressing quality. It often worsens as the day goes on or following stress and has few associated symptoms. *Chronic daily headache* (CDH) is usually of the tension type (Welch and Goadsby 2002) and has been associated with depression and persisting stressors (Holroyd et al. 1993; Mitsikostas and Thomas 1999; Rasmussen 1992), although this association does not necessarily indicate the causal mechanism. CDH is indicative of the need for more sophistication in our approach to understanding the complex interactions between brain biology, psychological processes, and behavioral responses. The majority of cases of CDH involve a prior history of migraine (Bahra et al. 2000; Lance et al. 1988). It appears that prolonged exposure to analgesics (e.g., opiates, ergotamine derivatives, nonsteroidal anti-inflammatory drugs) may be necessary for transformation to CDH to take place. Certainly, failure to withdraw from such analgesics usually results in failed treatment (Kudrow 1982). Treatment of comorbid mood disorders (Gill and Hatcher 1999) and CBT can also be helpful (Kroenke and Swindle 2000).

Classical *migraine* has the features described above; common migraine causes "migrainous" throbbing hemicranial headache, nausea, and photophobia in the absence of focal neurological symptoms such as visual disturbance (Cutrer 2003). Patients with chronic migraine headaches have often been described as having a "typical" personality characterized by conscientiousness, perfectionism, ambitiousness, rigidity, tenseness, and resentfulness; however, controlled studies have not consistently supported this profile. Specific personality traits in migraine appear more likely to be a consequence rather than a cause of suffering from recurrent headaches (Stronks et al. 1999) A community-based survey found more personality disturbance and 2.5 times more psychological distress in migraine sufferers than in matched control subjects, but there was no relationship between headache frequency and the severity of psychological distress or personality abnormality (Brandt et al. 1990; Breslau et al. 2003; Glover et al. 1993). An association with both depression and bipolar disorder is recognized (Lipton et al. 2000; Merikangas 1994), and there are interesting genetic studies linking migraine with the dopamine *DRD2* gene (Peroutka et al. 1997). Psychiatric management is as for CDH.

Cervicogenic headache is headache originating in the neck, usually associated with neck pain and limitation of movement, radiating forward from the neck or occiput. *Temporal arteritis* is a disorder of older people (it is very rare in persons younger than 55 years) that causes scalp pain and tenderness, jaw claudication, malaise, and an elevated erythrocyte sedimentation rate (usually of more than 50 mm/hour). Treatment with corticosteroids should be started immediately and arrangements made for confirmatory temporal artery biopsy. *Raised intracranial pressure* typically causes a headache that is worse on lying down (and can be relieved by standing), disturbing sleep and present in the mornings. The pressure eventually causes nausea and vomiting and, if brain stem compression occurs, a progressive reduction of consciousness. The raised pressure can result from space-occupying lesions (e.g., tumors, subdural hematomas), hydrocephalus, or idiopathic intracranial hypertension. The typical features of raised intracranial pressure (i.e., headache, ataxia, drowsiness, confusion, coma) are not always present. If they are, or if headache is associated with papilledema or focal neurological signs, a CT scan should be obtained urgently. *Low CSF volume headache* is an increasingly well-recognized syndrome with features inverse to those of the headache of raised intracranial pressure: the headache comes on after getting up and is relieved by lying down. This type of headache is often iatrogenic (e.g., following lumbar puncture), but it can also occur as a result of spontaneous CSF leaks.

Certain "headaches" are felt mainly in the face. *Cluster headache*, a rare type of headache that is more common in young men, gives rise to severe retro-orbital pain occurring in bursts lasting an hour or so that recur over a period of days to weeks (the "cluster"). The headache often wakes the sufferer in the middle of the night and usually makes him or her extremely restless (in contrast to migraine, which sends sufferers to their beds) (May and Goadsby 1998). *Trigeminal neuralgia* causes stabs of lancinating pain in the one of the three divisions of the trigeminal nerve (Graff-Radford 2000). *Atypical facial pain* is a diagnosis of exclusion, the facial equivalent of chronic daily headache.

Somatoform and Conversion Disorders in Neurology

Somatic symptoms unexplained by neurological disease are commonly encountered in neurological practice and may be diagnosed as somatoform disorders. Other names include medically unexplained symptoms, psychogenic disorders, and functional disorders. DSM-IV, and its text revision, DSM-IV-TR, use the term *somatoform disorders*, although patients may prefer the term "functional disorders" (Stone et al. 2002).

Conversion disorder is regarded as a subgroup of somatoform disorders. The term is reserved to describe patients with motor or sensory symptoms or deficits that suggest a neurological or other general medical condition but in whom no such condition is found by appropriate examination and investigation. DSM-IV-TR also requires that the psychological factors be judged to be associated with the symptoms because their initiation or exacerbation is *preceded by* conflicts or other stressors. This requirement is controversial, as its theoretical basis is unconfirmed. Furthermore, because psychological factors are common in all neurological presentations, the requirement is nonspecific and likely to be unreliable. Common conversion symptoms include paralysis, weakness, seizures, anesthesia, aphonia, blindness, amnesia, and stupor. Conversion disorder is also discussed in Chapter 13, "Somatization and Somatoform Disorders."

Epidemiology

Neurological symptoms in the absence of neurological disease or grossly disproportionate to disease are observed in approximately one-third of patients attending neurological clinics (Carson et al. 2000b). Functional weakness and paralysis, a subgroup of neurological symptoms occurring in the absence of disease, have an incidence of at least 4 per 100,000 (Binzer and Kullgren 1998), a rate similar to that of multiple sclerosis. In less than half of patients do the symptoms remit spontaneously (Carson et al. 2003).

Clinical Features

A careful history is essential to diagnosis, first concentrating on the somatic symptoms, and only then exploring psychological and social factors. Pain is the most common symptom (Carson et al. 2000b). In considering the diagnosis, particular attention should be paid to the presence of multiple somatic symptoms (multiple symptoms make a somatoform disorder more likely), depression or anxiety (particularly panic), and a history of previous functional symptoms or of multiple surgical operations in the absence of organic pathology (Barsky and Borus 1999). Childhood abuse and neglect, personality factors, recent stressful life events, secondary gain (financial or otherwise), and illness beliefs may all be relevant to management, but their presence does not allow one to infer a diagnosis of conversion disorder (Stone et al. 2002).

The history of the onset of the symptoms can be particularly useful in diagnosis. Patients with conversion weakness will often describe symptoms suggestive of depersonalization or derealization at the time of onset. These symptoms may have been associated with a panic attack, physical trauma (often minor), or unexpected physiological events (e.g., postmicturitional syncope, sleep paralysis). In this context, a patient might report that "the leg felt as if it was not connected to me," "I felt far away," or "I was in a place of my own" (Stone et al. 2002).

The neurological examination has an important role in diagnosis of conversion disorder. Helpful signs include inconsistency, Hoover's sign (Ziv et al. 1998), collapsing ("giveaway") weakness (Gould et al. 1986), and co-contraction (Knutsson and Martensson 1985). Muscle tone and reflexes should be normal but may be mildly asymmetrical. Mild temperature and color changes in the affected limb are common in conversion disorder (Stone et al. 2002). These signs should be demonstrated to patients in a collaborative, rather than confrontational, manner.

Pathology and Etiology

The etiology of conversion disorder remains unknown, and there is value in remaining neutral about the relative contributions of biological, psychological, and social factors (Kroenke 2002). In particular, one should be aware that although Freudian theory portrays conversion disorder as a mechanism for dealing with unconscious conflict and traumatic experience, this model fits only some pa-

tients. Early functional imaging studies have yielded intriguing results (Vuilleumier et al. 2001), and numerous, although often inconsistent, biochemical abnormalities have been described (Clauw and Chrousos 1997). The psychological and social risk factors for conversion disorder are similar to those for other somatoform disorders, as described in Chapter 13, "Somatization and Somatoform Disorders."

Investigation and Differential Diagnosis

Diagnostic accuracy is high, with an error rate between 5% and 10%, which compares favorably with diagnostic error rates for most common neurological conditions (Carson et al. 2003). Misdiagnosis may be more common in the presence of known psychiatric comorbidity such as schizophrenia or learning disability, particularly when the illness interferes with history taking. Further imaging or neurophysiological testing may be required, depending on the symptoms present. As a general rule, further investigations tend to rule out putative "organic" diagnoses rather than overturn the diagnosis of conversion disorder (Crimlisk et al. 1998). Although clinicians tend to worry about missing "organic" disease and therefore are often very conservative in making a diagnosis of conversion disorder, available evidence suggests that the reverse is more of a problem, leading to iatrogenic complications of unneeded treatment and invalidism (Fink 1992; Nimnuan et al. 2000).

Management

Patients are best managed by a psychologically sophisticated medical approach (Sharpe and Carson 2000). Key steps are first, an explicit acceptance of the reality of the symptoms; second, a nonstigmatizing, positive explanation of the diagnosis; and third, appropriate reassurance (Thomas 1987). Such reassurance communicates to the patient that a full, but gradual, recovery may be possible and that dreaded diseases, such as stroke and multiple sclerosis, have been ruled out. Dismissing the symptoms as "nothing wrong" risks antagonizing or humiliating the patient and is rarely a good basis for collaborative management.

There is evidence for moderate effectiveness of antidepressant drugs, particularly TCAs, in conversion disorder, with an odds ratio for improvement of 3.4 compared with placebo (O'Malley et al. 1999). Interestingly, this effectiveness does not depend on the presence of depressive symptoms. Clinical experience suggests a role for gabapentin, particularly when pain symptoms are prominent; however, controlled trials are lacking. CBT may be effective in up to 70% of cases (Kroenke and Swindle 2000). We have found that physical therapy, especially physiotherapy, can be helpful in aiding a return to full function, and in some patients with long-standing disuse due to conversion disorder, physical therapy is necessary to restore normal function (see Chapter 13, "Somatization and Somatoform Disorders," for further discussion).

Neurosurgical Issues

Many of the psychiatric issues arising in neurosurgical settings are described in other chapters in this book. Of particular relevance are Chapter 6, "Delirium"; Chapter 35, "Physical Medicine and Rehabilitation"; and Chapter 36, "Pain." High doses of corticosteroids are used by neurosurgeons to reduce elevated intracranial pressure; the psychiatric adverse effects of corticosteroids are reviewed in Chapter 25, "Rheumatology." Mood disorders are frequent after neurosurgery, and their assessment should be guided by the discussion in the earlier sections of this chapter, particularly the section on stroke.

Central Nervous System Tumors

Psychiatric aspects of cancer are reviewed in Chapter 24, "Oncology." Psychiatrists generally become involved in neuro-oncology cases after tumor diagnosis, when the clinical issues are adjustment, mood disorder, or cognitive impairment. Patients with primary and metastatic CNS tumors typically present with headache, focal neurological signs, or seizures, but these tumors can also cause cognitive impairment, and occasionally their presentation mimics a dementing illness (Lishman 1997). Some brain tumors present with predominantly psychiatric symptoms. CT scanning should reveal their presence, although diffusely infiltrating tumors are sometimes missed in the early stages.

Hydrocephalus

Hydrocephalus is caused by dilatation of the ventricles within the brain resulting from elevation of CSF pressure. Hydrocephalus is termed *communicating* when the blockage to CSF flow is outside the ventricular system, *noncommunicating* when the blockage is within the ventricles. In "compensated" hydrocephalus, the clinical signs and CSF dynamics stabilize at an elevated level of CSF pressure. In normal-pressure hydrocephalus (NPH), the ventricles enlarge despite apparently normal CSF pressure, possibly as the result of persistent elevation or intermittent surges of high pressure.

Clinical Features

Hydrocephalus can cause a wide range of psychiatric symptoms and signs. These include enlargement of the head (if present in infancy), depression, headache, sudden death due to "hydrocephalic attacks" with acute elevation of intracranial pressure, progressive visual failure, gait disturbance (often "gait apraxia"), incontinence, and subcortical cognitive impairment progressing to dementia (Hebb and Cusimano 2001). NPH in older individuals is classically associated with the triad of gait apraxia, incontinence, and cognitive decline (Hebb and Cusimano 2001).

Diagnosis

In younger persons, the radiological signs of hydrocephalus are usually clear-cut on CT scanning. This may also be the case in some elderly patients, but in other older patients apparent hydrocephalus is sometimes due to atrophy of the brain. When enlargement of the ventricles raises a suspicion of communicating hydrocephalus in an older person, determination of whether the scan appearance is relevant to the clinical problem requires specialized studies—usually either serial lumbar punctures with observation of the clinical effects or neurosurgical studies of CSF pressure (Hebb and Cusimano 2001).

Management

Shunting of hydrocephalus—diversion of CSF from a CSF space to the venous system or peritoneum—can be beneficial or even lifesaving. However, the procedure is prone to complications, including subdural hematoma and shunt infection, and should not be undertaken lightly (Hebb and Cusimano 2001).

Subdural Hematoma

Subdural hematoma is caused by accumulations of blood and blood products in the space between the fibrous dura mater and the more delicate arachnoid membrane that encloses the brain. Acute subdural hematomas accumulate rapidly following head injury; chronic hematomas can often (although not always) be traced back to a head injury.

Clinical Features

Acute subdural hematomas are, by definition, diagnosed close to the time of trauma, as a result of symptoms present at the time—headache, depressed level of consciousness, focal neurological signs—or seen on CT scan. Chronic subdural hematomas give rise to more gradually evolving symptoms and signs. Although they also can cause headache, depressed consciousness, and focal signs, chronic subdural hematomas sometimes result in predominantly cognitive features, including confusion and dementia (Black 1984; Lishman 1997). Marked variability of the mental state, and sometimes also of the neurological features, is often a clue to the diagnosis. Seizures can occur. Both acute and chronic subdural hematomas are especially common in alcoholic individuals, who frequently do not recall having experienced head trauma (Selecki 1965).

Pathology

The variability of the clinical features is explained by the tendency of the size of a chronic subdural hematoma to wax and wane as a result of alternating phases of bleeding and of breakdown of the contents of the hematoma (McIntosh et al. 1996). Subdural hematomas exert their effects both by local compression and irritation of adjacent cortical tissue and by global "brain shift" (with the risk of brain herniation and secondary brain stem compression).

Investigation and Differential Diagnosis

Subdural hematomas can generally be diagnosed on CT scanning. They are occasionally "isodense" with brain and therefore easily missed, especially if bilateral (Davenport et al. 1994). It is important to recognize that a small subdural hematoma can be an incidental finding; for example, cerebral atrophy occurring in the course of a dementing illness predisposes to subdural hematoma as vulnerable bridging veins are stretched between the dura and the arachnoid. In these circumstances, treatment of the subdural hematoma is unlikely to be helpful.

Management

Management requires liaison with a neurosurgical team. Small subdural hematomas often resorb spontaneously. If a subdural hematoma is considered to be relevant to a patient's problems and drainage is required, several surgical approaches are available. However, there is always a risk that the hematoma will reaccumulate after surgery (Bullock and Teasdale 1990).

Subarachnoid Hemorrhage

Severe, prolonged headache of abrupt onset can be due to a subarachnoid hemorrhage, usually arising from a ruptured Berry aneurysm. A diagnosis of subarachnoid hemorrhage is suggested by the rapidity of onset ("thunderclap" headache, at its worst within a minute or so) and associated loss of consciousness, photophobia, vomiting, and neck stiffness. Psychiatrists are rarely involved in the diagnosis of subarachnoid hemorrhage but are frequently asked to evaluate patients in the postacute phase, as for stroke (symptoms of irritability and anxiety may be more common after subarachnoid hemorrhage than after stroke) (Lishman 1997).

Fitness for Surgery

Psychiatrists may be requested to assess patients for fitness for neurosurgery. Such requests occur most commonly for patients with epilepsy and with Parkinson's disease. A general assessment of capacity (see Chapter 3, "Legal Issues") and consideration of specific issues relevant to the operation in question are required, necessitating special attention when the operation is considered investigational.

Epilepsy Surgery

A psychiatric opinion should be sought prior to surgery if there are significant associated behavioral or social problems. Such problems include anticipated noncompliance with medication, severe personality disturbance, psychosis, mood disorder, unrealistic expectations of surgery, and an absence of social support. The presence of mental retardation is not an absolute contraindication to surgery but can complicate postsurgical care (Sperling 1994). The most commonly performed procedures are temporal lobectomy and amygdalohippocampectomy. Other procedures include extratemporal cortical resections, hemispherectomy, and white matter transactions, including corpus callosotomy (Engel 1993). It is noteworthy that poor psychological outcomes occasionally accompany good postoperative seizure control, and some patients need considerable psychological help in adjusting to life without seizures (Vickrey 1993).

Parkinson's Disease Surgery

Neurosurgery for Parkinson's disease is an evolving field in which a number of different surgical interventions have been suggested (Olanow 2002). Psychiatric complications can follow surgery (e.g., corticobulbar syndromes and psychic akinesia after bilateral pallidotomy) (de Bie et al. 2002; Merello et al. 2001). However, there is little in the way of guidance available for the psychiatrist asked to assess a patient's fitness for neurosurgery. It is generally agreed that patients with dementia tend to have poor outcomes; otherwise, the same principles would apply as for epilepsy surgery.

Conclusion

The practice of psychiatry in a neurological or neurosurgical setting is both challenging and rewarding. One of the challenges is the often complex task of determining the relationship between comorbid neurological and psychiatric symptoms. In this chapter we have outlined general principles of assessment and management in relation to the more commonly encountered conditions. These same principles apply to the more rarely encountered problems. Working closely with colleagues who share an interest in disorders of the brain can be very rewarding, and new developments in neuroscience are providing a greater understanding of the mechanisms by which biological, psychological, and social factors interact to cause both neurological and psychiatric illness. Consequently, the interface between these specialties is rapidly becoming one of the most intellectually fascinating areas of work for the specialist in psychosomatic medicine.

References

Aarsland D, Larsen JP, Cummins JL, et al: Prevalence and clinical correlates of psychotic symptoms in Parkinson disease: a community-based study. Arch Neurol 56:595–601, 1999

Aarsland D, Ballard C, Larsen JP, et al: A comparative study of psychiatric symptoms in dementia with Lewy bodies and Parkinson's disease with and without dementia. Int J Geriatr Psychiatry 16:528–536, 2001

Abwender DA, Como PG, Kurlan R, et al: School problems in Tourette's syndrome. Arch Neurol 53:509–511, 1996

Adams P, Falek A, Arnold J: Huntington's disease in Georgia: age at onset. Am J Hum Genet 43:695–704, 1988

Akil M, Brewer GJ: Psychiatric and behavioural abnormalities in Wilson's disease. Adv Neurol 65:171–178, 1995

Almqvist EW, Bloch M, Brinkman R, et al: A worldwide assessment of the frequency of suicide, suicide attempts and psychiatric hospitalizations following predictive testing of Huntington disease. Am J Hum Genet 64:1293–1304, 1999

American Psychiatric Association: Diagnostic and Statistical Manual of Mental Disorders, 4th Edition, Text Revision. Washington, DC, American Psychiatric Association, 2000

Andersen G, Vestergaard K, Lauritzen L: Effective treatment of post-stroke depression with the selective reuptake inhibitor citalopram. Stroke 25:1099–1104, 1994a

Andersen G, Vestergaard K, Riis J, et al: Incidence of post-stroke depression during the first year in a large unselected stroke population determined using a valid standardized rating scale. Acta Psychiatr Scand 90:190–195, 1994b

Andersen G, Ingemann-Nielsen M, Vestergaard K, et al: Patho-anatomic correlation between poststroke pathological crying and damage to brain areas involved in serotoninergic neurotransmission. Stroke 25:1050–1052, 1994c

Andersen G, Vestergaard K, Ingemann-Nielsen M, et al: Risk factors for post-stoke depression. Acta Psychiatr Scand 92:193–198, 1995

Armin S, Andreas H, Hermann W, et al: Pramipexole, a dopamine agonist, in major depression: antidepressant effects and tolerability in an open-label study with multiple doses. Clin Neuropharmacol 20:S36–S45, 1997

Arnulf I, Bonnet AM, Damier P, et al: Hallucinations, REM sleep and Parkinson's disease: a medical hypothesis. Neurology 55:281–288, 2000

Astrom M: Generalised anxiety disorder in stroke patients: a 3-year longitudinal study. Stroke 27:270–275, 1996

Bahra A, Walsh M, Menon S, et al: Does chronic daily headache arise de novo in association with regular analgesic use? Cephalagia 20:294, 2000

Baker MG, Kale R, Menken M: The wall between neurology and psychiatry: advances in neuroscience indicate it's time to tear it down. BMJ 324:1468–1469, 2002

Bamford J, Sandercock P, Dennis M, et al: A prospective study of acute cerebrovascular disease in the community: the Oxfordshire Community Stroke Project 1981–86, I: methodology, demography and incident cases of first-ever stroke. J Neurol Neurosurg Psychiatry 51:1373–1380, 1988

Barsky AJ, Borus JF: Functional somatic syndromes. Ann Intern Med 130:910–921, 1999

Bearn AG: Wilson's disease: an unborn error of metabolism with multiple manifestations. Am J Med 22:747–757, 1957

Beatty WW, Goodkin DE, Monson N, et al: Cognitive disturbances in patients with relapsing-remitting multiple sclerosis. Arch Neurol 46:1113–1119, 1989a

Beatty WW, Goodkin DE, Beatty PA, et al: Frontal lobe dysfunction and memory in patients with chronic progressive multiple sclerosis. Brain Cogn 11:73–86, 1989b

Bell GS, Sander JW: The epidemiology of epilepsy: the size of the problem. Seizure 10:306–314, 2001

Benbadis SR, Allen HW: An estimate of the prevalence of psychogenic non-epileptic seizures. Seizure 9:280–281, 2000

Benbadis SR, Agrawal V, Tatum WO: How many patients with psychogenic non-epileptic seizures also have epilepsy? Neurology 57:915–917, 2001

Benke TH, Hockleitner M, Bauer G: Aura phenomena during syncope. Eur Neurol 37:28–32, 1997

Bentivoglio AR, Albanese A: Botulinum toxin in motor disorders. Curr Opin Neurol 12:447–456, 1999

Berthier ML, Kulisevsky J, Gironell A, et al: Poststroke bipolar affective disorder: clinical subtypes, concurrent movement disorders, and anatomical correlates. J Neuropsychiatry Clin Neurosci 8:160–170, 1996

Binzer M, Kullgren G: Motor conversion disorder: a prospective 2–5 year follow-up study. Psychosomatics 39:519–527, 1998

Binzer M, Stone J, Sharpe M: Recent onset pseudoseizures: clues to aetiology. Seizure 13:146–155, 2004

Black DW: Mental changes resulting from subdural haematoma. Br J Psychiatry 145:200–203, 1984

Blass JP, Gibson GE: Abnormality of a thiamine-requiring enzyme in patients with Wernicke-Korsakoff syndrome. N Engl J Med 297:1367–1370, 1977

Blum K, Braverman ER, Wu S, et al: Association of polymorphisms of dopamine D2 receptor (DRD2) and dopamine transporter (DAT1) genes with schizoid/avoidant behaviours (SAB). Mol Psychiatry 2:239–246, 1997

Bogousslavsky J, Cummings JL: Behavior and Mood Disorders in Focal Brain Lesions. New York, Cambridge University Press, 2000

Bower JH, Maraganore DM, McDonnell SK, et al: Incidence and distribution of parkinsonism in Olmsted County, Minnesota 1976–1990. Neurology 52:1214–1220, 1999

Brandt J, Celentano D, Stewart W, et al: Personality and emotional disorder in a community sample of migraine headache patients. Cephalagia 19:566–574, 1990

Bredkjaer SR, Mortensen PB, Parnas J: Epilepsy and non-organic non-affective psychosis: National Epidemiological Study. Br J Psychiatry 172:235–238, 1998

Breier JI, Adair JC, Gold M, et al: Dissociation of anosognosia for hemiplegia and aphasia during left-hemisphere anaesthesia. Neurology 45:65–67, 1995

Breslau N, Lipton RB, Stewart WF, et al: Comorbidity of migraine and depression: investigating potentiology and prognosis. Neurology 60:1308–1312, 2003

Brinkman RR, Mezei MM, Theilmann J, et al: The likelihood of being affected with Huntington's disease by a particular age, for a specific CAG size. Am J Hum Genet 60:1202–1210, 1997

Brooks DJ, Doder M: Depression in Parkinson's disease. Curr Opin Neurol 14:465–470, 2001

Brown AP, Lane JC, Murayama S, et al: Whipple's disease presenting with isolated neurological symptoms: case report. J Neurosurg 73:623–627, 1990

Brown P, Cathala F, Raubertas RF, et al: The epidemiology of Creutzfeldt-Jakob disease: conclusion of a 15-year investigation in France and review of the world literature. Neurology 37:895–904, 1987

Brown P, Gibbs CJ Jr, Rodgers-Johnson P, et al: Human spongiform encephalopathy: the National Institutes of Health series of 300 cases of experimentally transmitted disease. Ann Neurol 35:513–529, 1994

Brown P, Preece M, Brandel J-P, et al: Iatrogenic Creutzfeldt-Jakob disease at the millennium. Neurology 55:1075–1081, 2000

Brown R: Prion diseases, in Early Onset Dementia. Edited by Hodges JR. Oxford, England, Oxford University Press, 2001, pp 367–384

Budman CL, Kerjakovic M, Bruun R: Viral infection and tic exacerbation (letter). J Am Acad Child Adolesc Psychiatry 26:162–165, 1997

Bull PC, Thomas GR, Rommens JM, et al: Wilson's disease gene is a putative copper transporting P-type ATPase similar to the Menkes gene. Nat Genet 5:327–337, 1993

Bullock R, Teasdale G: Surgical management of traumatic intracranial haematomas, in Handbook of Clinical Neurology, Vol 15. Edited by Braakman R. Amsterdam, The Netherlands, Elsevier, 1990, pp 249–298

Burns A, Folstein S, Brandt J, et al: Clinical assessment of irritability, aggression and apathy in Huntington and Alzheimer disease. J Nerv Ment Dis 178:20–26, 1990

Burvill PW, Johnson GA, Jamrozik KD, et al: Anxiety disorders after stroke: results from the Perth Community Stroke Study. Br J Psychiatry 166:328–332, 1995

Cantello R, Gilli M, Ricco A, et al: Mood changes associated with "end of dose deterioration" in Parkinson's disease: a controlled study. J Neurol Neurosurg Psychiatry 49:1182–1190, 1986

Carota A, Nicola A, Aybek S, et al: Aphasia-related emotional behaviours in acute stroke. Neurology 54:A244, 2000

Carota A, Rossetti OA, Karapanayiotides T, et al: Catastrophic reaction in acute stroke: a reflex behaviour in aphasic patients. Neurology 57:1902–1906, 2001

Carota A, Staub F, Bogousslavsky J: Emotions, behaviours and mood changes in stroke. Curr Opin Neurol 15:57–59, 2002

Carson AJ, Machale S, Allen K, et al: Depression after stroke and lesion location: a systematic review. Lancet 356:122–126, 2000a

Carson AJ, Ringbauer B, Stone J, et al: Do medically unexplained symptoms matter? A study of 300 consecutive new referrals to neurology outpatient clinics. J Neurol Neurosurg Psychiatry 68:207–210, 2000b

Carson AJ, Postmas K, Stone J, et al: The outcome of neurology patients with medically unexplained symptoms: a prospective cohort study. J Neurol Neurosurg Psychiatry 74:897–900, 2003

Ceravolo R, Nuti A, Piccini A, et al: Paroxetine in Parkinson's disease: effects on motor and depressive symptoms. Neurology 55:1216–1218, 2000

Chabolla DR, Cascino GD: Interpretation of extracranial EEG, in The Treatment of Epilepsy: Principles and Practice, 2nd Edition. Edited by Wylie E. Baltimore, MD, Williams & Wilkins, 1997, pp 264–279

Chemerinski E, Robinson RG, Kosier JT: Improved recovery in activities of daily living associated with remission of PSD. Stroke 32:113–117, 2001

Chua P, Chiu E: Huntington's disease, in Dementia. Edited by Burns A, Levy R. London, Chapman & Hall, 1994, pp 827–844

Chui HC, Victoroff JI, Margolin D: Criteria for the diagnosis of ischemic vascular dementia proposed by the State of California Alzheimer Disease Diagnostic and Treatment Centers (ADDTC). Neurology 42:473–480, 1992

Chuinard G, Sultan S: A case of Parkinson's disease exacerbated by fluoxetine. Hum Psychopharmacol 7:63–66, 1992

Clark S, Assal G, Bogousslavsky J, et al: Pure amnesia after unilateral left polar thalamic infarct: tomographic and sequential neuropsychological and metabolic (PET) correlations. J Neurol Neurosurg Psychiatry 57:27–34, 1994

Clauw DJ, Chrousos GP: Chronic pain and fatigue syndromes: overlapping clinical and neuroendocrine features and potential pathogenic mechanisms. Neuroimmunomodulation 4:134–153, 1997

Cockerell OC, Johnson AL, Sander JW, et al: Prognosis of epilepsy: a review and further analysis of the first nine years of the British National General Practice Study of Epilepsy, a prospective population-based study. Epilepsy 38:31–46, 1997

Codori A-M, Slavney PR, Young C, et al: Predictors of psychological adjustment to genetic testing for Huntington's disease. Health Psychol 16:36–50, 1997

Colchester A, Kingsley D, Lasserson D, et al: Structural MRI volumetric analysis in patients with organic amnesia, I: methods and comparative findings across diagnostic groups. J Neurol Neurosurg Psychiatry 71:13–22, 2001

Crimlisk H, Bhatia K, Cope H, et al: Slater revisited: 6 year follow up study of patients with medically unexplained motor symptoms. BMJ 316:582–586, 1998

Cummings JL: Managing psychosis in patients with Parkinson's disease. N Engl J Med 340:801–803, 1999

Cummings JL, Cunningham K: Obsessive-compulsive disorder in Huntington's disease. Biol Psychiatry 31:263–270, 1992

Cummings JL, Masterman DL: Depression in patients with Parkinson's disease. Int J Geriatr Psychiatry 14:711–718, 1999

Cummings JL, Mendez MF: Secondary mania with focal cerebrovascular lesions. Am J Psychiatry 141:1084–1087, 1984

Cutrer FM: Migraine: does one size fit all? Curr Opin Neurol 16:315–317, 2003

Damasio AR: Emotion, Reason and the Human Brain. New York, GP Putman & Sons, 1994

Darnell RB, Posner JB: Paraneoplastic syndromes involving the nervous system. N Engl J Med 349:1543–1554, 2003

Davenport RJ, Statham PFX, Warlow CP: Detection of bilateral isodense subdural haematomas. BMJ 309:792–794, 1994

de Bie R, de Haan RJ, Schuurman PR, et al: Morbidity and mortality following pallidotomy in Parkinson's disease: a systematic review. Neurology 58:1008–1012, 2002

De Bruin VMS, Lees AJ: The clinical features of 67 patients with clinically definite Steele-Richardson-Olszeweski syndrome. Behav Neurol 5:229–232, 1992

De Groot CM, Yeates KP, Baker GB, et al: Impaired neuropsychological functioning in Tourette's syndrome subjects with co-occurring obsessive and attention deficit symptoms. J Neuropsychiatry Clin Neurosci 9:267–272, 1997

De la Monte SM, Vonsattel JP, Richardson EP: Morphometric demonstration of atrophic changes in the cerebral cortex, white matter and neostriatum in Huntington's disease. J Neuropathol Exp Neurol 47:516–525, 1988

Dening TR, Berrios GE: Wilson's disease: psychiatric symptoms in 195 cases. Arch Gen Psychiatry 46:1126–1134, 1989

Derex L, Ostrowsky K, Nighoghossian N, et al: Severe pathological crying after left anterior choroidal artery infarct: reversibility with paroxetine treatment. Stroke 28:1464–1469, 1997

Desmond DW, Moroney JT, Paik MC, et al: Frequency and clinical determinants of dementia after ischemic stroke. Neurology 54:1124–1131, 2000

Devinsky O, Abramson H, Alper K, et al: Postictal psychosis: a case control series of 20 patients and 150 controls. Epilepsy Res 20:247–253, 1995

Diederich NJ, Pieri V, Goetz CG: Visual hallucinations in Parkinson and Charles Bonnet syndrome patients: a phenomenological and pathogenetic comparison. Fortschr Neurol Psychiatr 68:129–136, 2000

Duyao M, Ambrose C, Myers R, et al: Trinucleotide repeat length: instability and age of onset of Huntington's disease. Nat Genet 4:387–392, 1993

Eapen V, Robertson MM, Alsobrook JP, et al: Obsessive-compulsive symptoms in Gilles de la Tourette syndrome and obsessive-compulsive disorder: differences by diagnosis and family history. Am J Med Genet 74:432–438, 1997

Ehde DM, Gibbons LE, Chwastiak L, et al: Chronic pain in a large community sample of persons with multiple sclerosis. Mult Scler 9:605–611, 2003

Eldridge R, Riklan M, Cooper IS: The limited role of psychotherapy in torsion dystonia: experience with 44 cases. JAMA 210:705–708, 1969

Engel JJ: Update on surgical treatment of the epilepsies: summary of the Second International Palm Desert Conference on the Surgical Treatment of Epilepsies, 1992. Neurology 43:1612–1617, 1993

Farrer LA, Conneally PM: A genetic model for age at onset in Huntington's disease. Am J Hum Genet 37:350–357, 1985

Fassbender K, Schmidt R, Mossner R, et al: Mood disorders and dysfunction of the hypothalamic-pituitary-adrenal axis in multiple sclerosis: association with cerebral inflammation. Arch Neurol 55:66–72, 1998

Feigin A, Kieburtz K, Bordwell K, et al: Functional decline in Huntington's disease. Mov Disord 10:211–214, 1995

Feinstein A: Multiple sclerosis, depression and suicide: clinicians should pay more attention to psychology. BMJ 315:691–692, 1997

Feinstein A, O'Connor P, Feinstein K: Multiple sclerosis, interferon beta-1b and depression: a prospective investigation. J Neurol 249:815–820, 2002

Ferenci P: Wilson's disease. Clin Liver Dis 2:31–49, 1998

Findlay LJ (for Global Parkinson's Disease Steering Committee): Factors impacting on quality of life in Parkinson's disease: results from an international survey. Mov Disord 17: 60–67, 2002

Fink P: Surgery and medical treatment in persistent somatizing patients. J Psychosom Res 36:439–447, 1992

Fisher CM: Abulia, in Stroke Syndromes. Edited by Bogousslavsky J, Caplan L. Cambridge, England, Cambridge University Press, 1995, pp 182–187

Fisk JD, Pontefract A, Ritvo PG, et al: The impact of fatigue on patients with multiple sclerosis. Can J Neurol Sci 21:9–14, 1994

Fleming JL, Wiesner RH, Shorter RG: Whipple's disease: clinical, biochemical and histopathological features and assessment of treatment in 29 patients. Mayo Clin Proc 63:539–551, 1988

Folstein SE, Folstein MF, McHugh PR: Psychiatric syndromes in Huntington's disease. Adv Neurol 23:281–290, 1979

Franklin GM, Nelson MPH: Environmental risk factors in multiple sclerosis. Neurology 61:1032–1034, 2003

Freal JE, Kraft GH, Coryell JK: Symptomatic fatigue in multiple sclerosis. Arch Phys Med Rehabil 65:135–138, 1984

Gajdusek DC: Unconventional viruses and the origin and disappearance of kuru. Science 197:943–960, 1977

Gainotti G, Azzoni A, Razzano C, et al: The Post-Stoke Depression Scale: a test specifically devised to investigate affective disorders of stroke patients. J Clin Exp Neuropsychol 19:340–356, 1997

Gainotti G, Azzoni A, Marra C: Frequency, phenomenology and anatomical-clinical correlates of major post-stroke depression. Br J Psychiatry 175:163–167, 1999

Gainotti G, Antonucci G, Marra C, et al: The relation between poststroke depression, antidepressant, therapy and rehabilitation outcome. J Neurol Neurosurg Psychiatry 71:258–261, 2001

Gambetti P, Parchi P, Peterson RB, et al: Fatal familial insomnia and familial Creutzfeldt-Jakob disease: clinical, pathological, and molecular genetic features. Brain Pathol 5:43–51, 1995

George MS, Wassermann EM, Post RM: Transcranial magnetic stimulation: a neuropsychiatric tool for the 21st century. J Neuropsychiatry Clin Neurosci 8:373–382, 1996

Giladi N, Treves TA, Paleacu D, et al: Risk factors for dementia, depression and psychosis in long standing Parkinson's disease. J Neurol Transm 107:59–71, 2000

Gill D, Hatcher S: A systematic review of the treatment of depression with antidepressant drugs in patients who also have a physical illness. J Psychosom Res 47:131–143, 1999

Glover V, Jarman J, Sandler M: Migraine and depression: biological aspects. J Psychiatr Res 27:223–231, 1993

Goldstein K: The Organism: A Holistic Approach to Biology Derived From Pathological Data in Man. New York, American Books, 1939

Goldstein MA, Harden CL: Epilepsy and anxiety. Epilepsy Behav 1:228–234, 2000

Goodwin FK: Behavioral effects of L-dopa in man. Semin Psychiatry 3:477–492, 1971

Gorell JM, Rybicki BA, Johnson CC, et al: Smoking and Parkinson's disease: a dose–response relationship. Neurology 52:115–119, 1999

Gould R, Miller BL, Goldberg MA, et al: The validity of hysterical signs and symptoms. J Nerv Ment Dis 174:593–597, 1986

Graff-Radford SB: Facial pain. Curr Opin Neurol 13:291–296, 2000

Gustafson Y, Olsson T, Erikkson S, et al: Acute confusional states (delirium) in stroke patients. Cerebrovasc Dis 1:257–264, 1991

Gustafson Y, Olsson T, Asplund K, et al: Acute confusional state (delirium) soon after stroke is associated with hypercortisolism. Cerebrovasc Dis 3:33–38, 1993

Hachinski VC, Lassen NA, Marshall J: Multi-infarct dementia: a cause of mental deterioration in the elderly. Lancet 2(7874):207–210, 1974

Harper PS: Huntington's Disease. London, England, WB Saunders, 1991

Heaton RK, Nelson LM, Thompson DS, et al: Neuropsychological findings in relapsing-remitting and chronic progressive multiple sclerosis. J Consult Clin Psychol 53:103–110, 1985

Hebb AO, Cusimano MD: Idiopathic normal pressure hydrocephalus: a systematic review of diagnosis and outcome. Neurosurgery 49:1166–1186, 2001

Henon H, Lebert F, Durieu I, et al: Confusional state in stroke: relation to pre-existing dementia, patient characteristics and outcome. Stroke 30:773–779, 1999

Hermann BP, Seidenburg M, Bell B: Psychiatric comorbidity in chronic epilepsy: identification, consequences and treatment of major depression. Epilepsia 41:S31–S41, 2000

Herrmann M, Bartels C, Schumacher M, et al: Poststroke depression: is there a pathoanatomic correlate for depression in the postacute stage of stroke? Stroke 26:850–856, 1995

Hesdorffer DC, Hauser WA, Annegers JF, et al: Major depression is a risk factor for seizures in older adults. Ann Neurol 47:246–249, 2000

Hill AF, Butterworth RJ, Joiner S, et al: Investigation of variant Creutzfeldt-Jakob disease and other human prion diseases with tonsil biopsy samples. Lancet 353:183–189, 1999

Hodges JR: Transient Amnesia: Clinical and Neuropsychological Aspects. London, WB Saunders, 1991

Hodges JR, Ward CD: Observations during transient global amnesia: a behavioural and neuropsychological study of five cases. Brain 112:595–620, 1989

Holroyd KA, France JL, Nash JM, et al: Pain state as artifact in the psychological assessment of recurrent headache sufferers. Pain 53:229–235, 1993

Honer WG, Hurwitz T, Li DKB, et al: Temporal lobe involvement in multiple sclerosis patients with psychiatric disorders. Arch Neurol 44:187–190, 1987

House A, Dennis M, Molyneux A, et al: Emotionalism after stroke. BMJ 298:991–994, 1989

House A, Knapp P, Bamford J, et al: Mortality at 12 and 24 months after stroke may be associated with depressive symptoms at 1 month. Stroke 32:696–701, 2001

Hsich G, Kenney K, Gibbs CJ Jr, et al: The 14–3–3 brain protein in cerebrospinal fluid as a marker for spongiform encephalopathies. N Engl J Med 335:924–930, 1996

Hyde TM, Ziegler JC, Weinberger DR: Psychiatric disturbances in metachromatic leukodystrophy: insights into the neurobiology of psychosis. Arch Neurol 49:401–406, 1992

Jacobson RR, Lishman WA: Cortical and diencephalic lesions in Korsakoff's syndrome: a clinical and CT scan study. Psychol Med 20:63–75, 1990

Jalava M, Sillanpaa M: Concurrent illnesses in adults with childhood-onset epilepsy: a population based 35-year follow up study. Epilepsia 37:1155–1163, 1996

James AC, Kaplan P, Lees A, et al: Schizophreniform psychosis and adrenomyeloneuropathy. J R Soc Med 77:882–884, 1984

Jankovic J, Beach J: Long-term effects of tetrabenazine in hyperkinetic movement disorders. Neurology 48:358–362, 1997

Jansen Steur ENH: Increase in Parkinson disability after fluoxetine medication. Neurology 43:211–213, 1993

Jehkonen M, Ahonen JP, Dastidar P, et al: Unawareness of deficits after right hemisphere stroke: double-dissociations of anosognosias. Acta Neurol Scand 102:378–384, 2000

Jimenez-Jimenez FJ, Garcia Ruiz PJ: Pharmacological options for the treatment of Tourette's disorder. Drugs 61:2207–2220, 2001

Joffe RT, Lippert GP, Gray TA, et al: Mood disorders and multiple sclerosis. Arch Neurol 44:376–378, 1987

Kanemoto K, Takeuchi J, Kawasaki J, et al: Characteristics of temporal lobe epilepsy with mesial temporal sclerosis, with special reference to psychotic episodes. Neurology 47:1199–1203, 1996a

Kanemoto K, Kawasaki J, Kawai I: Postictal psychosis: a comparison with acute interictal and chronic psychoses. Epilepsia 37:551–556, 1996b

Kanner AM, Balabanov A: Depression and epilepsy: how closely related are they? Neurology 58:S27–S39, 2002

Keshavan MS, David AS, Narayanen HS, et al: "On-off" phenomena and manic-depressive mood shifts: case report. J Clin Psychiatry 47:93–94, 1986

Kim JS, Choi-Kwon S: Poststroke depression and emotional incontinence: correlation with lesion location. Neurology 54:1805–1810, 2000

Kirkwood SC, Siemers E, Stout JC, et al: Longitudinal cognitive and motor changes among presymptomatic Huntington disease gene carriers. Arch Neurol 56:563–568, 1999

Klein C, Ozelius LJ: Dystonia: clinical features, genetics and treatment. Curr Opin Neurol 15:491–497, 2002

Knappskog PM, Flatmark T, Mallet J, et al: Recessively inherited L-dopa responsive dystonia caused by a point mutation (Q381K) in the tyrosine hydroxylase gene. Hum Mol Genet 4:1209–1212, 1995

Kneebone II, Dunmore E: Psychological management of post-stroke depression. Br J Clin Psychol 39:53–65, 2000

Knutsson E, Martensson A: Isokinetic measurements of muscle strength in hysterical paresis. Electroencephalogr Clin Neurophysiol 61:370–374, 1985

Kopelman MD: Rates of forgetting in Alzheimer-type dementia and Korsakoff's syndrome. Neuropsychologia 23:623–638, 1985

Kopelman MD, Stanhope N, Kingsley DEP: Retrograde amnesia in patients with diencephalic temporal lobe or frontal lesions. Neuropsychologia 37:939–958, 1999

Kotagal P: Complex partial seizures with automatisms, in The Treatment of Epilepsy: Principles and Practice, 2nd Edition. Edited by Wylie E. Baltimore, MD, Williams & Wilkins, 1997, pp 385–400

Kotsopoulos IA, Merode T, Kessels FG, et al: Systematic review and meta-analysis of incidence studies of epilepsy and unprovoked seizures. Epilepsia 43:1402–1409, 2002

Krishnamoorthy ES, Trimble MR: Forced normalization: clinical and therapeutic relevance. Epilepsia 40:S57–S64, 1999

Kroenke K: Integrating psychological care into general medical practice. BMJ 324:1536–1537, 2002

Kroenke K, Swindle R: Cognitive behavioural therapy for somatization and symptom syndromes: a critical review of controlled clinical trials. Psychother Psychosom 69:205–215, 2000

Krupp LB, Coyle PK, Doscher C, et al: Fatigue therapy in multiple sclerosis: results of a double-blind, randomized, parallel trial of amantadine, permoline and placebo. Neurology 45:1956–1961, 1995

Kudrow L: Paradoxical effects of frequent analgesic use. Adv Neurol 33:335–341, 1982

Kumral E, Evyapan D, Balkir K: Acute caudate vascular lesions. Stroke 30:100–108, 1999

Kupio AM, Marttila RJ, Helenius H, et al: Changing epidemiology of Parkinson's disease in southwestern Finland. Neurology 52:302–308, 1999

Lambert M, Robertson MM: Depression in epilepsy: etiology, phenomenology, and treatment. Epilepsia 40:S21–S47, 1999

Lance F, Parkes C, Wilkinson M: Does analgesic abuse cause headaches de novo? Headache 28:61–62, 1988

Landolt H: Serial electroencephalographic investigations during psychotic episodes in epileptic patients and during schizophrenic attacks, in Lectures on Epilepsy. Edited by Lorenz de Haas AM. Amsterdam, Elsevier, 1958, pp 256–284

Langhorne P, Stott DJ, Robertson L, et al: Medical complications after stroke: a multicenter study. Stroke 31:1223–1229, 2000

Lazar RM, Marshall RS, Prell GD, et al: The experience of Wernicke's aphasia. Neurology 55:1222–1224, 2000

Leckman JF, Hardin MT, Riddle MA, et al: Clonidine treatment of Gilles de la Tourette's syndrome. Arch Gen Psychiatry 48:324–328, 1991

Lempert T, Bauer M, Schmidt D: Syncope: a video metric analysis of 56 episodes of transient cerebral hypoxia. Ann Neurol 36:233–237, 1994

Leo RJ: Movement disorders associated with the serotonin selective reuptake inhibitors. J Clin Psychol 57:449–454, 1996

Leroi I, Michalon M: Treatment of the psychiatric manifestations of Huntington's disease: a review of the literature. Can J Psychiatry 43:933–940, 1998

Levinson DF, Devinsky O: Psychiatric adverse events during vigabatrin therapy. Neurology 53:1503–1511, 1999

Levy ML, Cummings JL, Fairbanks LA, et al: Apathy is not depression. J Neuropsychiatry Clin Neurosci 10:314–319, 1998

Lincoln NB, Flannagan T: Cognitive behavioural psychotherapy for depression after stroke: a randomised controlled trial. Stroke 34:111–115, 2003

Lincoln NB, Flannagan T, Sutcliff L, et al: Evaluation of cognitive behavioural treatment for depression after stroke: a pilot study. Clin Rehabil 11:114–122, 1997

Lipinski JF, Sallee FR, Jackson C, et al: Dopamine agonist treatment of Tourette disorder in children: results of an open-label trial of pergolide. Mov Disord 12:402–407, 1997

Lipsey JR, Robinson RG, Pearlson GD, et al: Nortriptyline treatment of post-stroke depression: a double blind treatment trial. Lancet S2:297–300, 1984

Lipton RB, Hamelsky SW, Kolodner KB, et al: Migraine, quality of life, and depression: a population-based case-control study. Neurology 55:629–635, 2000

Lishman WA: Organic Psychiatry: The Psychological Consequences of Cerebral Disorder, 3rd Edition. Oxford, UK, Blackwell Science, 1997

Litvan I, Grafman J, Vendrell P, et al: Multiple memory deficits in patients with multiple sclerosis. Exploring the working memory system. Arch Neurol 45:607–610, 1988a

Litvan I, Grafman J, Vendrell P, et al: Slowed information processing in multiple sclerosis. Arch Neurol 45:281–285, 1988b

Louis ED, Lynch T, Kaufmann P, et al: Diagnostic guidelines in central nervous system Whipple's disease. Ann Neurol 40: 561–568, 1996

Lucchinetti C, Bruck W, Noseworthy J: Multiple sclerosis: recent developments in neuropathology, pathogenesis, magnetic resonance imaging studies and treatment. Curr Opin Neurol 14:259–269, 2001

Lyndsay J: Phobic disorders in the elderly. Br J Psychiatry 159: 531–541, 1991

Mair WGP, Warrington EK, Weiskrantz L: Memory disorder in Korsakoff's psychosis: a neuropathological and neuropsychological investigation of two cases. Brain 102:749–783, 1979

Manchanda R, Miller H, McLachlan RS: Postictal psychosis after right temporal lobectomy. J Neurol Neurosurg Psychiatry 56:277–279, 1993

Maraganore DM, Lees AJ, Marsden CD: Complex stereotypies after right putaminal infarction: a case report. Mov Disord 6:358–361, 1991

Marjama J, Troster AI, Koller WC: Psychogenic movement disorders. Neurol Clin 13:283–297, 1995

May A, Goadsby PJ: Cluster headache: imaging and other developments. Headache 11:199–203, 1998

Mayes AR, Meudell PR, Mann D, et al: Location of lesions in Korsakoff's syndrome: neuropsychological and neuropathological data on two patients. Cortex 24:367–388, 1988

McDonald WI, Compston A, Edan G, et al: Recommended diagnostic criteria for multiple sclerosis guidelines from the International Panel on the Diagnosis of Multiple Sclerosis. Ann Neurol 50:121–127, 2001

McEwen B: Stressful experience, brain and emotions: developmental genetic and hormonal influences, in The Cognitive Neurosciences. Edited by Gazzaniga MS. Cambridge, MA, MIT Press, 1996, pp 1117–1135

McGonigal A, Oto M, Russell AJ, et al: Outpatient video EEG recording in the diagnosis of non-epileptic seizures: a randomised controlled trial of simple suggestion techniques. J Neurol Neurosurg Psychiatry 72:549–551, 2002

McIntosh TK, Smith DH, Meaney DF, et al: Neuropathological sequelae of traumatic brain injury: relationship to neurochemical and biomechanical mechanisms. Lab Invest 74: 315–342, 1996

McKeith IG, Grace JB, Walker Z, et al: Rivastigmine in the treatment of dementia with Lewy bodies: preliminary findings from an open trial. Int J Geriatr Psychiatry 15:387–392, 2000

Meador KJ, Loring DW, Feinburgh TE, et al: Anosognosia and asomatognosia during intracarotid amobarbital inactivation. Neurology 55:816–820, 2000

Mendez MF: Huntington's disease: update and review of neuropsychiatric aspects. Int J Psychiatry Med 24:189–208, 1994

Menza MA, Sage J, Marshall E, et al: Mood changes and "on-off" phenomena in Parkinson's disease. Mov Disord 5:148–151, 1990

Mercadante MT, Do Roasario Campos MC, Marques-Dias MJ, et al: Vocal tics in Sydenham's chorea (letter). J Am Acad Child Adolesc Psychiatry 36:305, 1997

Merello M, Starkstein S, Nouzeilles M, et al: Bilateral pallidotomy for treatment of Parkinson's disease induced corticobulbar syndrome and psychic akinesia avoidable by globus pallidus lesion combined with contralateral stimulation. J Neurol Neurosurg Psychiatry 71:611–614, 2001

Merikangas KR: Psychopathology and headache syndromes in the community. Headache 34:S17–S22, 1994

Meudell P, Mayes AR: Normal and abnormal forgetting: some comments on the human amnesic syndrome, in Normality and Pathology in Cognitive Functions. Edited by Willis AW. London, Academic Press, 1982, pp 203–238

Miguel EC, Bauer L, Coffey BJ, et al: Phenomenological differences appearing with repetitive behaviours in obsessive-compulsive disorder and Gilles de la Tourette disorder. Br J Psychiatry 170:140–145, 1997

Mitsikostas DD, Thomas AM: Comorbidity of headache and depressive disorders. Cephalagia 19:211–217, 1999

Mochizuki H, Kamakura K, Mazaki T, et al: Atypical MRI features of Wilson's disease: high signal in globus pallidus on T1 weighted images. Neuroradiology 39:171–174, 1997

Mohr DC, Hart SL, Goldberg A: Effects of treatment for depression on fatigue in multiple sclerosis. Psychosom Med 65:542–547, 2003

Morris PL, Robinson RG, Andrzejewski P, et al: Association of depression with 10-year poststroke mortality. Am J Psychiatry 150:124–129, 1993a

Morris PL, Robinson RG, Raphael B: Emotional lability after stroke. Aust NZ J Psychiatry 27:601–605, 1993b

Muller J, Kemmler G, Wissel J, et al: The impact of blepharospasm and cervical dystonia on health related quality of life and depression. J Neurol 249:842–846, 2002

Muller N, Putz A, Kathman N, et al: Characteristics of obsessive-compulsive disorder and Parkinson's disease. Psychiatry Res 70:105–114, 1997

Multiple Sclerosis Council for Practice Guidelines: Fatigue and multiple sclerosis: evidence-based management strategies for fatigue in multiple sclerosis. Washington, DC, Paralyzed Veterans of America, 1998

Murphy TK, Goodman WK, Fudge MW, et al: B lymphocyte antigen DB/17: a peripheral marker for childhood-onset obsessive-compulsive disorder and Tourette's syndrome. Am J Psychiatry 154:402–407, 1997

Neilley LK, Goodin DS, Goodkin DE, et al: Side effect profile of interferon beta-1b in multiple sclerosis: results of an open label trial. Neurology 46:552–554, 1996

Nimnuan C, Hotopf M, Wessely S: Medically unexplained symptoms: how often and why are they missed? Q J Med 93:21–28, 2000

Olanow CW: Surgical therapy for Parkinson's disease. Eur J Neurol 9:31–39, 2002

Olanow CW, Watts RL, Koller WC: An algorithm (decision tree) for the management of Parkinson's disease: treatment guidelines. Neurology 56:S1–S88, 2001

O'Malley PG, Jackson JL, Santoro J, et al: Antidepressant therapy for unexplained symptoms and symptom syndromes. J Fam Pract 48:980–990, 1999

Oribe E, Amini R, Nissenbaum E, et al: Serum prolactin concentrations are elevated after syncope. Neurology 47:60–62, 1996

Parikh RM, Robinson RG, Lipsey JR, et al: The impact of poststroke depression on recovery in activities of daily living over a 2-year follow-up. Arch Neurol 47:785–789, 1990

Patten SB, Metz LM: Depression in multiple sclerosis. Psychother Psychosom 66:286–292, 1997

Patten SB, Metz LM: Interferon beta-1 and depression in relapsing-remitting multiple sclerosis: an analysis of depression data from the PRISMS clinical trial. Mult Scler 7:243–248, 2001

Pauls DL, Leckman JF, Cohen DJ: Evidence against a genetic relationship between Tourette's syndrome and anxiety, depression, panic and phobic disorders. Br J Psychiatry 164:215–221, 1994

Peroutka SJ, Wilhoit T, Jones K: Clinical susceptibility to migraine with aura is modified by dopamine D2 receptor (DRD2) NcoI alleles. Neurology 49:201–206, 1997

Peto V, Jenkinson C, Fitzpatrick R, et al: The development and validation of a short measure of functioning and well being for individuals with Parkinson's disease. Qual Life Res 4:241–248, 1995

Pfeil SA, Lynn JD: Wilson's disease: copper unfettered. J Clin Gastroenterol 29:22–31, 1999

Piccardo P, Dlouhy SR, Lievens PJM: Phenotypic variability of Gerstmann-Straussler-Scheinker disease is associated with prion protein heterogeneity. J Neuropathol Exp Neurol 57:979–988, 1998

Pohjasvaara T, Vataja R, Leppavuori A, et al: Depression is an independent predictor of poor long-term functional outcome poststroke. Eur J Neurol 8:315–319, 2001

Pohlmann-Eden B, Stefanou A, Wellhausser H: Serum prolactin in syncope. Neurology 48:1477–1478, 1997

Polman CH, Bertelsmann EW, Van Loenen AC, et al: 4-Aminopyridine in the treatment of patients with multiple sclerosis: long-term efficacy and safety. Arch Neurol 51:292–296, 1994

Prusiner SB: Prion disease of humans and animals. J R Coll Phys Lond 28:1–30, 1994

Prusiner SB: Neurodegenerative disorders and prions. N Engl J Med 344:1516–1526, 2001

Pujol J, Bello J, Deus J, et al: Lesions in the left arcuate fasciculus region and depressive symptoms in multiple sclerosis. Neurology 49:1105–1110, 1997

Rabinstein AA, Shulman LM: Management of behavioural and psychiatric problems in Parkinson's disease. Parkinsonism Relat Disord 7:41–50, 2000

Rahkonen T, Makela H, Paanila S, et al: Delirium in elderly people without severe predisposing disorders: aetiology and 1-year prognosis after discharge. Int Psychogeriatr 12:473–481, 2000

Ramasubbu R: Denial of illness and depression in stroke (letter). Stroke 25:226–227, 1994

Rammohan KW, Rosenburgh JH, Lynn DJ, et al: Efficacy and safety of modafinil (Provigil) for the treatment of fatigue in multiple sclerosis: a two centre phase 2 study. J Neurol Neurosurg Psychiatry 72:179–183, 2002

Rao SM: Neuropsychology of multiple sclerosis. J Clin Exp Neuropsychol 8:503–542, 1986

Rao SM, Hammeke TA, McQuillen MP, et al: Memory disturbance in chronic progressive multiple sclerosis. Arch Neurol 41:625–631, 1984

Rao SM, St Aubin-Faubert P, Leo GJ: Information processing speed in patients with multiple sclerosis. J Clin Exp Neuropsychol 11:471–477, 1989

Rao SM, Leo GJ, Bernardin L, et al: Cognitive dysfunction in multiple sclerosis, I: frequency, patterns and prediction. Neurology 41:685–691, 1991

Rao SM, Grafman J, DiGiulio D, et al: Memory dysfunction in multiple sclerosis: its relation to working memory, semantic encoding and implicit learning. Neuropsychology 7:364–374, 1993

Rasmussen BK: Migraine and tension-type headache in a general population: psychosocial factors. Int J Epidemiol 21:1138–1143, 1992

Reuber M, Elger C: Psychogenic nonepileptic seizures: review and update. Epilepsy Behav 4:205–216, 2003

Reuber M, Fernandez G, Bauer J, et al: Diagnostic delay in psychogenic non-epileptic seizures. Neurology 58:493–495, 2002

Richardson EP: Progressive multifocal leukoencephalopathy. N Engl J Med 265:815–823, 1961

Riedel M, Straube A, Schwartz MJ, et al: Lyme disease presenting as Tourette's syndrome (letter). Lancet 351:418–419, 1998

Rinne JO, Lee MS, Thompson PD, et al: Corticobasal degeneration. A clinical study of 36 cases. Brain 117(pt 5):1183–1196, 1994

Risk WS, Haddad FS, Chemali P: Substantial spontaneous long-term improvement in subacute sclerosing panencephalitis: six cases from the Middle East and a review of the literature. Arch Neurol 35:494–502, 1978

Roberts R: Differential diagnosis of sleep disorders, non-epileptic attacks and epileptic seizures. Curr Opin Neurol 11:135–139, 1998

Robertson MM, Stern JS: Tic disorders: new developments in Tourette syndrome and related disorders. Curr Opin Neurol 11:373–380, 1998

Robertson MM, Stern JS: Gilles de la Tourette syndrome: symptomatic treatment based on evidence. Eur Child Adolesc Psychiatry 9:60–75, 2000

Robertson MM, Schull DA, Eapen V, et al: Risperidone in the treatment of Tourette syndrome: a retrospective case note study. J Psychopharmacol 10:317–320, 1996

Robinson RG, Parikh RM, Lipsey JR, et al: Pathological laughing and crying following stroke: validation of a measurement scale and a double-blind treatment study. Am J Psychiatry 150:286–293, 1993

Robinson RG, Schultz SK, Castillo C, et al: Nortriptyline versus fluoxetine in the treatment of depression and in short-term recovery after stroke: a placebo-controlled, double-blind investigation. Am J Psychiatry 157:351–359, 2000

Rockwood K, Bowler J, Erkinjuntti T, et al: Subtypes of vascular dementia. Alzheimer Dis Assoc Disord 13 (suppl 3):S59–S65, 1999

Rodrigo EP, Adair JC, Roberts BB, et al: Obsessive-compulsive disorder following bilateral globus pallidus infarction. Biol Psychiatry 42:410–412, 1997

Roman GC, Tatimichi TK, Erkinjuntti T: Vascular dementia: diagnostic criteria for research studies. Report of the NINDS-AIREN International Workshop. Neurology 43:250–260, 1993

Rosenblatt A, Ranen NG, Nance MA, et al: A Physician's Guide to the Management of Huntington's Disease, 2nd Edition. New York, Huntington's Disease Society of America, 1999

Sadovnick AD, Remick RA, Allen J, et al: Depression and multiple sclerosis. Neurology 46:628–632, 1996

Sallee FR, Nesbitt L, Jackson C, et al: Relative efficacy of haloperidol and pimozide in children and adolescents. Am J Psychiatry 154:1057–1062, 1997

Samkoff LM, Daras M, Tuchman AJ, et al: Amelioration of refractory dysesthetic limb pain in multiple sclerosis by gabapentin. Neurology 49:304–305, 1997

Sander JW: Some aspects of prognosis in the epilepsies: a review. Epilepsia 34:1007–1016, 1993

Sander JW, Shorvon SD: Epidemiology of the epilepsies. J Neurol Neurosurg Psychiatry 61:433–443, 1996

Schacter DL: Implicit memory: history and current status. J Exp Psychol Learn Mem Cogn 13:501–518, 1987

Schachter SC: Vagus nerve stimulation: where are we? Curr Opin Neurol 15:201–206, 2002

Schiffer RB, Wineman NM: Antidepressant pharmacotherapy of depression associated with multiple sclerosis. Am J Psychiatry 147:1493–1497, 1990

Selecki BR: Intracranial space-occupying lesions among patients admitted to mental hospitals. Med J Aust 1:383–390, 1965

Sethi KD: Clinical aspects of Parkinson disease. Curr Opin Neurol 15:457–460, 2002

Sharpe M, Carson A: Unexplained somatic symptoms, functional syndromes and somatization: do we need a paradigm shift? Ann Intern Med 134:926–930, 2000

Sheean GL, Murray NM, Rothwell JC, et al: An electrophysiological study of the mechanism of fatigue in multiple sclerosis. Brain 120:299–315, 1997

Spencer MD, Knight RSG, Will RG: First hundred cases of variant Creutzfeldt-Jakob disease: retrospective case note review of early psychiatric and neurological features. BMJ 324:1479–1482, 2002

Spencer SS: The relative contributions of MRI, SPECT and PET imaging in epilepsy. Epilepsia 35:S72–S89, 1994

Sperling MR: Who should consider epilepsy surgery? Medical failure in the treatment of epilepsy, in The Surgical Management of Epilepsy. Edited by Wyler AR, Herman BR. Boston, MA, Butterworth-Heinemann, 1994, pp 26–31

Staley D, Wand R, Shady G: Tourette's disorder: a cultural review. Compr Psychiatry 38:6–16, 1997

Starkstein SE: Mood disorders after stroke, in Cerebrovascular Disease. Edited by Grinsberg M, Bogousslavsky J. Oxford, England, Blackwell Science, 1998, pp 131–138

Starkstein SE, Robinson RG: Affective disorders and cerebral vascular disease. Br J Psychiatry 154:170–182, 1989

Starkstein SE, Pearlson GD, Boston J, et al: Mania after brain injury: a controlled study of causative factors. Arch Neurol 44:1069–1073, 1987

Starkstein SE, Berthier MI, Fedoroff P, et al: Anosognosia and major depression in 2 patients with cerebrovascular lesions. Neurology 40:1380–1382, 1990

Starkstein SE, Fedoroff JP, Price TR, et al: Apathy following cerebrovascular lesions. Stroke 24:1625–1630, 1993a

Starkstein SE, Fedoroff JP, Price TR, et al: Catastrophic reaction after cerebrovascular lesions: frequency, correlates, and validation of a scale. J Neuropsychiatry Clin Neurosci 5:189–194, 1993b

Starosta-Rubinstein S, Young AB, Kluin K, et al: Clinical assessment of 31 patients with Wilson's disease: correlations with structural changes on magnetic reasoning imaging. Arch Neurol 44:365–370, 1987

Stefansson SB, Olafsson E, Hauser WA: Psychiatric morbidity in epilepsy: a case controlled study of adults receiving disability benefits. J Neurol Neurosurg Psychiatry 64:238–241, 1998

Stein DJ, Bouwer C, Hawkridge S, et al: Risperidone augmentation of serotonin reuptake inhibitors in obsessive-compulsive and related disorders. J Clin Psychiatry 58:119–122, 1997

Steinhoff BJ, Racker S, Herrendorf G, et al: Accuracy and reliability of periodic sharp wave complexes in Creutzfeldt-Jakob disease. Arch Neurol 53:162–166, 1996

Stillhard G, Landis T, Schiess R, et al: Bitemporal hypoperfusion in transient global amnesia: 99m-Tc-HM-PAO SPECT and neuropsychological findings during and after an attack. J Neurol Neurosurg Psychiatry 53:339–342, 1990

Stone J, Zeman A, Sharpe M: Physical signs: functional weakness and sensory disturbance. J Neurol Neurosurg Psychiatry 73:241–245, 2002

Stone VE, Baron-Cohen S, Knight RT: Frontal lobe contributions to theory of mind. J Cogn Neurosci 10:640–656, 1998

Stronks DL, Tulen JH, Pepplinkhuizen L, et al: Personality sufferers. Am J Psychiatry 147:303–308, 1999

Swedo SE, Leonard HL, Garvey M, et al: Identification of children with pediatric autoimmune neuropsychiatric disorders associated with streptococcal infections by a marker associated with rheumatic fever. Am J Psychiatry 154:110–112, 1997

Swedo SE, Leonard HL, Garvey M, et al: Pediatric autoimmune neuropsychiatric disorders associated with streptococcal infections: clinical description of the first 50 cases. Am J Psychiatry 155:264–271, 1998

Sweet RA, Mulsant BH, Gupta B, et al: Duration of neuroleptic treatment and prevalence of tardive dyskinesia in late life. Arch Gen Psychiatry 52:478–486, 1995

Sweet RD, McDowell FH, Feigenson JS, et al: Mental symptoms in Parkinson's disease during chronic treatment with levodopa. Neurology 26:305–310, 1976

Tanner CM, Aston DA: Epidemiology of Parkinson's disease and akinetic syndromes. Curr Opin Neurol 13:427–430, 2000

Tatimichi TK, Desmond DW, Prohovnik I, et al: Confusion and memory loss from capsular genu infarction: a thalamocortical disconnection syndrome? Neurology 42:1966–1979, 1992

Tatimichi TK, Desmon DW, Stern Y, et al: Cognitive impairment after stroke: frequency, patterns and relationship to functional abilities. J Neurol Neurosurg Psychiatry 57:202–207, 1994a

Tatimichi TK, Paik M, Begiella E, et al: Risk of dementia after stroke in a hospitalised cohort: results of a longitudinal study. Neurology 44:1885–1891, 1994b

Tatimichi TK, Desmond DW, Prohovnik I: Strategic infarcts in vascular dementia: a clinical and brain imaging experience. Arzneimittelforschung 54:371–385, 1995

Tessei S, Antonin A, Canesi M, et al: Tolerability of paroxetine in Parkinson's disease: a prospective study. Mov Disord 15:986–989, 2000

Thomas KB: General practice consultations: is there any point in being positive? BMJ 294:1200–1202, 1987

Thompson AJ: Symptomatic treatment in multiple sclerosis. Curr Opin Neurol 11:305–309, 1998

Vein AM, Djukova GM, Vorobieva OV: Is panic attack a mask of psychogenic seizures? A comparative analysis of phenomenology of psychogenic seizures and panic attacks. Funct Neurol 9:153–159, 1994

Verdugo RJ, Ochoa JL: Abnormal movements in complex regional pain syndrome: assessment of their nature. Muscle Nerve 23:198–205, 2000

Vickrey BG, Hays RD, Hermann BP, et al: Outcomes with respect to quality of life, in Surgical Treatment of Epilepsies, 2nd Edition. New York, Raven, 1993, pp 623–635

Victor M, Adams RD, Collins GH: The Wernicke-Korsakoff syndrome. Philadelphia, PA, FA Davis, 1971

Vighetto A, Aimard G, Confavreux C, et al: Anatomo-clinical study of a case of topographic confabulation (or delusion) (in French). Cortex 16:501–507, 1980

Vonsattel JPG, DiFiglia M: Huntington disease. J Neuropathol Exp Neurol, 57:369–384, 1998

Vuilleumier P, Chicherio C, Assal F, et al: Functional neuroanatomical correlates of hysterical sensorimotor loss. Brain 124:1077–1090, 2001

Waddy HM, Fletcher NA, Harding AE, et al: A genetic study of idiopathic focal dystonias. Ann Neurol 29:320–324, 1991

Walsh JM: Wilson's disease, in Handbook of Clinical Neurology. Edited by Vinken PJ, Bruyn GW, Klawans HL. New York, Elsevier, 1986, pp 223–238

Walsh JM, Yealland M: Wilson's disease: the problem of delayed diagnosis. J Neurol Neurosurg Psychiatry 55:692–696, 1992

Weigartz P, Seidenberg M, Woodard A, et al: Comorbid psychiatric disorder in chronic epilepsy: recognition and etiology of depression. Neurology 53:S3–S8, 1999

Welch MKA, Goadsby PJ: Chronic daily headache: nosology and pathophysiology. Curr Opin Neurol 15:287–295, 2002

Wenzel T, Schnider P, Wimmer A, et al: Psychiatric comorbidity in patients with spasmodic torticollis. J Psychosom Res 44:687–690, 1997

Wiart L, Petit H, Joseph PA, et al: Fluoxetine in early poststroke depression: a double-blind placebo-controlled study. Stroke 31:1829–1832, 2000

Wiebers DO, Hollenhorst RW, Goldstein NP: The ophthalmologic manifestations of Wilson's disease. Mayo Clin Proc 52:409–416, 1997

Will RG, Ironside JW, Zeidler M, et al: A new variant of Creutzfeldt-Jakob disease in the UK. Lancet 347:921–925, 1996

Witjas T, Kaphan E, Azulay JP, et al: Nonmotor fluctuations in Parkinson's disease: frequent and disabling. Neurology 59:408–413, 2002

Wodrich DL, Benjamin E, Lachar D: Tourette's syndrome and psychopathology in a child psychiatry setting. J Am Acad Child Adolesc Psychiatry 26:1618–1624, 1997

Wolters ECH, Berendse HW: Management of psychosis in Parkinson's disease. Curr Opin Neurol 14:499–504, 2001

Zakzanis KK: The subcortical dementia of Huntington's disease. J Clin Exp Neuropsychol 20:565–578, 1998

Zappacosta B, Monza D, Meoni C, et al: Psychiatric symptoms do not correlate with cognitive decline, motor symptoms or CAG repeat length in Huntington's disease. Arch Neurol 53:493–497, 1996

Zeidler M, Sellar RJ, Collie DA, et al: The pulvinar sign on magnetic resonance imaging in variant CJD. Lancet 355:1412–1418, 2000

Zeman AZ, Boniface SJ, Hodges JR: Transient epileptic amnesia: a description of the clinical and neuropsychological features in 10 cases and a review of the literature. J Neurol Neurosurg Psychiatry 64:435–443, 1998

Zephir H, De Seze J, Stojkovic T, et al: Multiple sclerosis and depression: influence of interferon beta therapy. Mult Scler 9:284–288, 2003

Ziv I, Djaldetti R, Zoldan Y, et al: Diagnosis of "nonorganic" limb paresis by a novel objective motor assessment: the quantitative Hoover's test. J Neurol 245:797–802, 1998

Zohar AH, Pauls DL, Ratzoni G, et al: Obsessive-compulsive disorder with and without tics in an epidemiological sample of adolescents. Am J Psychiatry 154:274–276, 1997

33

Obstetrics and Gynecology

Nada L. Stotland, M.D., M.P.H.

Donna E. Stewart, M.D., F.R.C.P.C.

Sarah E. Munce, B.Sc.

Danielle E. Rolfe, B.P.H.E.

REPRODUCTIVE EXPERIENCES AND behavior are fraught with intense feelings: joy, pride, and passion, as well as shame, guilt, and fear. The ability to reproduce can be, or be perceived as, a requisite for a permanent relationship, a family, a place in society, or admission to the eternal afterlife. Therefore, interactions between obstetrics and gynecology and psychiatry are particularly important. Up-to-date information about obstetrics and gynecology is essential for the psychiatrist, and information about psychiatric issues is essential for the obstetrician/gynecologist. Each also needs to know something about the realities of practice for the other.

Tradition or regulations sometimes separate a patient's obstetrics and gynecology care from her mental health care and may divide her mental health care among two or more practitioners (Fugh-Berman and Kronenberg 2003). Obstetricians and gynecologists must master new technical developments, may provide primary care, and usually have little training in mental health. The fear of malpractice claims is especially onerous for obstetricians and gynecologists.

Since Hippocrates and the notion of the unmoored uterus causing "hysteria," physicians have linked women's reproductive functions to mental illness (Hirshbein 2003). The care of female patients requires an understanding of the anatomical and physiological substrates of reproduction, its social contexts, and the nature of obstetric and gynecological diseases and treatments. This understanding is also valuable in the care of male patients, whose mothers, sisters, (most) intimate partners, and daughters are female.

In this chapter, we cover gender identity, infertility, contraception, sterilization, hysterectomy, abortion (both spontaneous and induced), chronic pelvic pain, psychiatric disorders during pregnancy and postpartum and their treatment, menopause, and urinary incontinence. Eating disorders are covered in Chapter 15, "Eating Disorders," and female oncology is discussed in Chapter 24, "Oncology."

Note that some of the phenomena described in this chapter vary by culture and sexual orientation and that most findings are generally derived from research on presumably heterosexual women in North America and Europe. An often-overlooked minority group is lesbian women. Many lesbians experience or fear disapprobation and misunderstanding in most health care settings, are reluctant to seek care, and therefore experience adverse health outcomes. Psychiatrists can help gynecologists and other primary care physicians to phrase questions about sexual orientation and activity in nonjudgmental terms and become familiar with the range of lesbian sexual practices.

Gender Identity

The first question about a newborn (or fetus) is whether it is a boy or girl, a determination made on the basis of the external genitalia. Ambiguous genitalia cause consternation; physicians and parents must decide whether to live with the ambiguity or assign the child to one gender or the other. Some believe that gender assignment should be made and carried out as early as possible, so that the child can grow up with a clear gender, and others think that the child should be left as nature intended and allowed to make a personal gender assignment when of age. (Gender identity disorders are discussed in Chapter 17, "Sexual Disorders.") Reproductive organs are the first defining feature of each human being, and gender remains a core aspect of identity throughout life. Sex hormones influence not only physical development and a host of physiological functions but also brain structure and activity. Environmental factors influence developing anatomy and ongoing physiology. A lifelong, active interplay occurs among anatomy, physiology, social influences, and individual psychology.

The term *sex* refers to narrowly defined biological characteristics. The term *gender* includes social roles and an individual's sense of femininity or masculinity. Some evidence indicates that girls are aware of their sexual organs and identity as early as toddlerhood. As puberty approaches in females, the sense of gender identity is powerfully reinforced and reshaped by physical changes: the development of breasts and pubic hair and the onset of menstruation. In some cultures, girls are told at menarche that they are now women. With menarche come fertility and the possibility that sexual activity will lead to pregnancy. Although girls can be sexually abused at any age, the possibility of rape is more overt after puberty, and vulnerability to attack becomes part of gender identity. The possibility of pregnancy can be at once a worry and a wish. A young woman may feel that she is not truly a woman until she has had heterosexual intercourse or until she has borne a child. Girls who feel sexual attraction for other girls face a crisis in gender identity because society increasingly expects them to date, form relationships, and engage in sexual activity with males. Medical problems that interfere with any of these functions threaten core gender identity.

Infertility

Infertility is commonly defined as 12 months of appropriately timed unprotected intercourse that does not result in conception. Approximately 40% of infertility problems are attributable to the female, and 60% are attributable to the male or are of unknown etiology (Klock 1998). The World Health Organization has reported that between 8% and 12% of couples, or approximately 50–80 million people worldwide, experience some type of fertility problem during their reproductive lives (World Health Organization Programme of Maternal and Child Health and Family Planning Unit 1991). Within the United States, it

has been estimated that 7.1% of married couples, or 2.3 million married women of childbearing age, have a fertility problem (Abma et al. 1997). Although the popular impression is that the prevalence of infertility has risen over the past few decades, the rate of infertility has remained relatively stable since 1965 (Keye 1999). Rather, the use and availability of medical services, as well as willingness to disclose and public awareness of infertility treatment options, have increased (Burns and Covington 1999; Keye 1999). Although much of the public attention has centered on advances in medical treatment and technology, both organic and psychological factors may be involved in infertility (American Psychological Association 1996; Kainz 2001).

Psychological Factors Associated With Infertility

There has been increasing understanding of the psychosocial aspects of infertility. Early publications suggested that infertility without a detectable organic cause was "psychogenic." More recent studies have used a biopsychosocial approach and have examined the stresses of investigation and treatment, as well as psychiatric morbidity, influencing fertility and the outcomes of infertility treatments (Burns and Greenfield 1991). For example, in a study that used a nationally representative sample of 11,000 American women, generalized anxiety disorder was associated with lower fecundity, independent of treatment status (King 2003). A prospective study that investigated the effect of chronic stress levels (trait anxiety) on conception rates in normally fertile women found that a higher initial trait anxiety level significantly predicted a lower pregnancy rate (Demyttenaere et al. 1988). Similarly, these investigators found that increased depressive symptoms were associated with lower pregnancy rates after in vitro fertilization in infertile women (Demyttenaere et al. 1998). Eating disorders (anorexia nervosa, bulimia nervosa, and obesity) are all associated with infertility (Stewart et al. 1990). Restrictive or purging eating behaviors are often undisclosed and result in both subfecundity and poor pregnancy outcomes (Stewart and Robinson 2001a).

Studies on gender differences in psychological reactions to infertility have shown that women report a higher degree of anxiety, depression, and loss of self-esteem compared with their partners. What is unclear is whether this plays an etiological role or is reactive to infertility labeling, investigation, or treatment. Infertile women are also significantly more depressed than their fertile counterparts, with depression and anxiety levels equivalent to those in women with heart disease, cancer, or HIV-positive status (Kainz 2001). Women tend to report that the diagnosis and treatment of infertility are the most psychologically painful and challenging experiences they have ever had. Furthermore, infertile women report poorer sexual and marital adjustment; more sexual dysfunction; and more feelings of guilt, inferiority, and isolation compared with infertile men (Weaver et al. 1997). Finally, the negative effects of infertility on quality of life have been shown to be stronger for infertile women compared with infertile men (Hjelmstedt et al. 1999; Kainz 2001).

Psychosocial Assessment in Infertility Patients

Some have suggested that current levels of distress and coping strategies should be assessed in couples before initiating infertility treatment to provide the opportunity to learn and practice new adaptive behaviors that could enhance their ability to cope with infertility and the associated medical investigations and procedures (Lukse and Vacc 1999). Counseling is sometimes recommended in couples considering donor eggs or sperm or surrogacy.

The process of infertility diagnosis and treatment is grueling. Normally intimate and private behaviors are asked about, subjected to strict timing, and brought into the clinical situation. The psychological effects, particularly mood alterations, of fertility-enhancing drugs are underappreciated. Careful attention should be paid to recent changes in drug regimens and their potential contribution to recent-onset psychiatric symptoms such as depression, anxiety, mania, or psychosis (Lukse and Vacc 1999).

The goal of mental health evaluation is to identify and treat any comorbid psychiatric disorders, to prepare the couple for infertility treatments, to raise emotional and ethical treatment issues that the couple may not have considered, and to offer support and coping strategies. Group interventions are often helpful in providing mutual support, information, and coping techniques (Kainz 2001).

Contraception

Contraceptive information and care are widely available in the Western world. Nevertheless, half of the pregnancies in North America each year are unintended. Contraceptive choices and use are affected by knowledge and misinformation, by women's comfort with their own genitalia, by the preferences of sexual partners, by social custom, and by access to physicians for hormonal methods. Many women are ill-informed about the advantages of hormonal contraception (Picardo et al. 2003).

Gender and relationship power differentials play major roles in the use of contraception (Harvey et al. 2002). A psychological study of 132 heterosexual college men reported that condom users were more independent, clever, and uninhibited. Those who had not used condoms at last intercourse stated that they had not planned on sex and had no condoms available (Franzini and Sideman 1994). In another study of students, the attitudes of men and women toward male and female contraceptive pills were compared. Of the women, 71% expressed willingness to take an oral contraceptive; for men, the figure was 20%. Hesitancy about female pill use among women centered on "bother"; men were concerned about the safety of the female pill. Men thought that a male oral contraceptive would be more unnatural, bothersome, harmful, and opposed to their beliefs than would a female oral contraceptive. The authors concluded that, despite their level of education, these men were not willing to assume responsibility for contraception (Laird 1994). Women who do not discuss sexual decisions with their male partners are at increased risk for contraceptive failure (Zlokovich and Snell 1997). Ethnicity plays a role as well; Hispanic women may be less likely, and African American women more likely, to use condoms than are white women (Castaneda and Collins 1998; Upchurch et al. 2003).

Psychodynamics and psychiatric conditions can interfere with a woman's use of a contraceptive technique. Pregnancy may be sought, consciously or unconsciously, as proof of fertility and womanhood. Contraception requires the acknowledgment of future sexual activity. Unmarried women who do not approve of extramarital sexual intercourse may be able to engage in it only when "swept away" by a romantic situation and thus be unprepared to prevent pregnancy. Some women feel uncomfortable touching their own genitalia, as some contraceptive methods require. Many women have limited knowledge about their own anatomy, are too anxious to absorb the information in a hurried office or clinic visit, and are too embarrassed to ask that information be repeated (Sanders et al. 2003). Homeless women, among whom are many with psychiatric illnesses, have little access to information or care (Gelberg et al. 2002). Women who grow up in foster care are at increased risk for early coitus and unprotected sexual intercourse (Crocker and Carlin 2002; Koniak-Griffin et al. 2003).

Unplanned pregnancy is by no means always the result of unconscious conflict. Contraceptives do fail. Some women are sexually assaulted, bullied, and cajoled into unprotected sexual intercourse (Rickert et al. 2002). Some are threatened with abandonment if they do not keep their male partners sexually satisfied. Some trade sex for drugs. Some are members of religious groups requiring that they obey their husbands. However, the myth of female control over sexuality and female seduction, as reflected in the biblical story of Adam and Eve, persists. Women are blamed and looked down on, in general and in the medical context, for becoming pregnant at the wrong time or with the wrong partner. Their sense of shame can exacerbate whatever psychiatric symptoms they have and, paradoxically, leave them more vulnerable to future unplanned pregnancies.

New developments in contraception have important psychosocial implications (Fraser and Kovacs 2003). Emergency contraception consists of doses of oral contraceptives taken after unprotected intercourse. Although it was believed at first that the hormones had to be ingested within 24 hours, it now appears that they can be effective within at least 3, and possibly 5, days. In England, some parts of the United States and Canada, and some other countries, emergency contraceptives can be obtained without a prescription. In other areas, they can be obtained at family planning clinics, hospital emergency departments, or pharmacies by prescription. However, several barriers exist to the use of this highly effective contraceptive technique (DelBanco et al. 1997). Women who are young, especially those who are poor, may be uninformed, embarrassed, unaware of their level of risk for pregnancy, worried about side effects, and concerned about negative responses from others (Free et al. 2002). Pharmacies may decline to stock the medication, because of either moral objections, lack of demand, or disagreement over patient access without a physician prescription (N. Cooper et al. 2000).

Another new development is the use of hormonal contraceptives on a continuous, rather than intermittent, basis. Women can receive long-lasting hormone implants, use a contraceptive patch, or take contraceptive pills every day with breaks for withdrawal bleeding, which is easier to remember than the usual regimen. Continuous hormonal contraception causes months of amenorrhea. Women who experience menstrual periods as painful and inconvenient welcome amenorrhea, whereas others hold personal or cultural beliefs that bleeding is necessary to clean the uterus or confirm femininity (Glasier et al. 2003). Clinicians need to elicit and deal with patients' feelings and preferences.

Patients may be so accustomed to their birth control pills or injections that they fail to report them when asked what medications they are taking. Clinicians must ask about these contraceptives specifically. Hormonal contraceptives interact with some psychotropic medications. Implanted levonorgestrel metabolism is enhanced by phenobarbital, possibly resulting in a pregnancy (Shane-McWhorter et al. 1998). Modafinil, carbamazepine, and oxcarbazepine enhance the metabolism of oral contraceptives, decreasing their effectiveness; the oxidation of benzodiazepines and tricyclic antidepressants (TCAs) in the liver is inhibited, and their blood levels increased, by oral contraceptives (Schatzberg et al. 2003).

Inquiries about sexual behavior and protection from unwanted consequences should be part of every medical, including psychiatric, history and treatment. Some physicians ensure that all their female patients of reproductive age who are not intending to become pregnant are supplied with either emergency contraceptive prescriptions or the pills themselves. Because some psychiatric illnesses increase vulnerability to unprotected sexual intercourse, psychiatrists should be prepared to provide relevant information.

Sterilization

Sterilization is a permanent solution to unwanted fertility. A psychiatrist may be asked to consult when a young, nulliparous woman, or a patient with a mental illness, desires to be sterilized. The question of informed consent in the latter circumstance has been highlighted by state laws enacted in the wake of the involuntary sterilization of mental "defectives" in the past. The situation is paradoxical. Guardians may have difficulty obtaining sterilization procedures for severely cognitively impaired or developmentally delayed adult women who are unable to cope with the hygienic aspects of menstruation, are victimized by male predators, become pregnant, and are entirely unable to cope with the stresses of birth and parenting. Women may have psychotic symptoms, or a history of them, that interfere with capacity, but they also may make well-informed decisions not to have children, or more children, precisely because they recognize that their illness would interfere with their parenting. One way to approach this situation is to ask the patient to return in 3–6 months. If she is mature, not acutely psychotic, and persistent in her desire for sterilization, she may be as appropriate a candidate for the procedure as a woman without diagnosed psychiatric illness.

Recent studies of psychological aspects of sterilization in North America have focused almost entirely on the incidence of postsurgical regret. The occurrence of regret ranges from 5% to 20% (Hillis et al. 1999; Newton and McCormack 1990). Risk factors include youth, marital conflict over the procedure, and subsequent changes in marital partnerships (Jamieson et al. 2002). Studies of the effect of parity on postsurgical regret have been inconclusive. Sexual satisfaction does not appear to be affected (Pati and Cullins 2000). The provision of clear information about the nature, effectiveness, risks, and benefits of the procedure is a crucial factor in patient satisfaction.

Hysterectomy

Epidemiology and Indications

Hysterectomy (the surgical removal of the uterus) is one of the most common surgical procedures performed on North American women, with rates of approximately 500 of every 100,000 women (Farquhar and Steiner 2002; Stewart et al. 2002) (see also the "Pelvic Surgery" section in Chapter 30, "Surgery"). Hysterectomy rates in the United States and Canada are more than double those in many European countries, but small area rate variations are widespread in most countries and appear to depend on women's socioeconomic class, race/ethnicity, education level, religion, physician practice, reimbursement schedules, and availability of new technology (Stewart et al. 2002). Hysterectomy may be complete or incomplete (the cervix is left intact) and also may be combined with removal of the fallopian tubes and ovaries (salpingo-oophorectomy). Although vaginal hysterectomy is associated with lower mortality and shorter length of stay, abdominal hysterectomy remains the most common hysterectomy procedure.

A small proportion of hysterectomies are performed to treat malignancies or catastrophic hemorrhage, but the vast majority are elective procedures performed primarily to improve quality of life in women with abnormal uterine bleeding, fibroids, uterine prolapse, chronic pelvic pain, or endometriosis. The mean age of most women undergoing hysterectomy is the mid-40s, or an average of 6–7 years before the mean age of natural menopause, when some of these problems (abnormal uterine bleeding, fibroids) spontaneously resolve. However, hysterectomy is the treatment of choice for certain gynecological conditions, and the predicted advantage must be carefully weighed against the risks of surgery and other treatment alternatives such as hormonal therapy, and endometrial ablation (Lefebvre et al. 2002).

Psychosocial Issues

Information Needs and Decision-Making Preferences

Well-informed women who have been involved in decision making about hysterectomy have the best outcomes (Stewart et al. 2002). Various studies and expert panels have concluded that women and their family physicians should be provided with an adequate level of knowledge to make a fully informed decision of whether hysterectomy, less invasive procedures, medical management, or watchful waiting is the best option (Galavotti and Richter 2000; Mingo et al. 2000; Stewart et al. 2002; Uskul et al. 2003; Vigod and Stewart 2002; Williams and Clark 2000). Similarly, the options for retention or removal of the cervix and ovaries and route of hysterectomy (vaginal vs. abdominal) should be discussed. Women's decision making regarding, and response to, hysterectomy is influenced by their age, socioeconomic status, education, desire for fertility, sexual orientation, and ethnicity and by the role of their family, friends, and partners (Galavotti and Richter 2000; Groff et al. 2000; Richter et al. 2000) and the severity of their symptoms. Women who require hysterectomy for the treatment of malignancies are understandably focused more on the cancer, its treatment, and its outcome.

Variations With Ethnic, Socioeconomic, and Sexual Diversity

Several articles have explored ethnic differences and indications for hysterectomy (Farquhar and Steiner 2002; Groff et al. 2000; Lewis et al. 2000). Qualitative analyses with Hispanic, African American, and lesbian women (Groff et al. 2000) have explored their capacity to acquire a second opinion about hysterectomy and available alternatives that may be limited by education, ethnicity, economics, and access. African American women undergo hysterectomy at a younger age for most diagnostic categories, including leiomyomas, genital prolapse, and endometriosis. They are also more likely to have an abdominal hysterectomy, extended hospital stays, and higher in-hospital mortality (Lewis et al. 2000).

Psychological and Sexual Outcomes of Hysterectomy

Women with substantiated diagnoses and clear indication for hysterectomy have better physical and psychological outcomes than do women with less-defined symptoms and indicators such as chronic pelvic pain. A recent prospective study (Kjerulff et al. 2000) in more than 1,000 women with benign conditions at 28 Maryland hospitals collected and reported data for 2 years after hysterectomy. Although symptom severity, depression, and anxiety decreased significantly after hysterectomy and quality of life improved for most women, 8% of the women reported symptoms that were at least as severe 1–2 years after hysterectomy as before. Presurgical characteristics that predicted lack of symptom relief included previous therapy for psychological problems, history of depression, and household income less than $35,000. Bilateral oophorectomy also predicted lack of symptom relief at 2 years after hysterectomy (Kjerulff et al. 2000). A small study of 48 Chinese women undergoing elective hysterectomy found that a psychoeducational intervention resulted in lower postoperative anxiety, less pain, and higher levels of satisfaction than in women in the control group (Cheung et al. 2003).

A systematic review of English- and German-language literature on sexual outcomes after hysterectomy located 18 studies, 8 of which were prospective. The methodological quality of all the studies was poor, but most studies found no change in or an enhancement of sexuality in the women after hysterectomy (Farrell and Kieser 2000). The Maryland study discussed in the previous paragraph reported increased rates of sexual intercourse and decreased rates of dyspareunia, anorgasmia, low libido, and vaginal dryness at 1 and 2 years after hysterectomy. Prehysterectomy depression was notably associated with continuing dyspareunia, vaginal dryness, low libido, and anorgasmia after hysterectomy (Rhodes et al. 1999). Similar negative outcomes have been described in women seeking hysterectomy for poorly defined chronic pelvic pain. Studies exploring psychological outcomes of hysterectomy in diverse groups of women are rare (Galavotti and Richter 2000; Mingo et al. 2000).

Women undergoing hysterectomy with oophorectomy have to confront the onset of sudden surgical menopause if estrogen therapy is not begun shortly after surgery. This sudden hormonal change may result in vasomotor symptoms, sleep loss, and depression, especially in vulnerable women with a history of depression associated with reproductive events (Stewart and Boydell 1993). Even women whose ovaries were left intact sometimes enter premature menopause if the blood supply to the ovaries has been disrupted.

Role of the Psychiatrist

There may be a role for psychiatrists in assessing mood, anxiety, understanding, and feelings about sexuality and fertility in vulnerable women undergoing hysterectomy. For the informed, psychologically healthy woman who has failed to respond to other treatment options and who has a significantly impaired quality of life because of a specific gynecological condition, hysterectomy may offer an improved quality of life. However, for women with premorbid depression, anxiety, or personality disorders, especially if accompanied by ambivalence about sexuality, fertility, or the procedure, hysterectomy may fail to ameliorate, or may even exacerbate, preexisting symptoms

(Stoppe and Doren 2002). Psychiatrists should ascertain the hormonal status of women with sudden mood changes following hysterectomy and consider short-term hormonal treatment as well as antidepressants.

Psychiatrists who assess women after hysterectomy should evaluate their understanding of the procedure, attitudes toward fertility and sexuality, and experience and expectations of surgery, as well as psychiatric history. The appropriate treatment, whether psychotherapy, hormones, or psychotropics, will, as always, depend on the individual woman.

Abortion

Spontaneous Abortion

Abortion can be spontaneous (miscarriage) or induced (usually just termed *abortion*). Spontaneous abortion generally evokes feelings of failure and loss. A woman's body has failed to perform one of its basic functions; she has failed to produce a child for her partner and parents; she has expelled her own potential child; and she may have conceived an embryo with genetic anomalies (Friedman and Gath 1989). Decades ago, miscarriage was sometimes attributed to the woman's unconscious rejection of motherhood, but this theory has never been validated by empirical research. Spontaneous abortion, like a stillbirth or neonatal death, may precipitate pathological grief, postpartum depression, or posttraumatic stress (Beutel et al. 1995; Engelhard et al. 2003). Women report that the failure of society in general and of friends and family to acknowledge the loss is painful and complicates the grieving process. People often say, "There must have been something wrong with the baby," "This is God's way of correcting mistakes," or "You can just get pregnant again." There are no ceremonies to mark the occasion. Friends and co-workers tend to avoid the subject and to expect the woman to recover within days or weeks, but grief may last for months.

Health care providers also may fail to recognize the emotional effect of spontaneous abortion. They feel helpless to prevent it, and it is generally not associated with serious medical or obstetrical complications. Psychiatrists can help them to understand and tolerate how their patients are feeling and to appreciate the benefits of simply allowing patients to express those feelings. Health care providers should be aware that emotional recovery, depending on the circumstances, can take months, and they need to know when and how to make the diagnosis of pathological grief. It is often helpful for them to meet with the patient some weeks after the event to go over the medical findings, if any; the prognosis; and the state of the woman's recovery.

The loss of pregnancy through miscarriage or stillbirth is associated with an increase in anxiety during a subsequent pregnancy and sometimes with overprotectiveness toward children subsequently born (Bourne and Lewis 1984). Although patients are frequently counseled to wait 6 months or a year after such a loss, they often conceive as soon as possible, especially if they feel that the clock is ticking. The obstetrician must be prepared to offer them enhanced support.

Induced Abortion

Psychiatric Sequelae

Approximately 1 million abortions are performed every year in the United States; approximately one in four women will have an abortion in her lifetime (Ventura et al. 2000). Psychiatrists are seldom consulted about abortion and abortion decisions, and no evidence shows that formal mental health consultation is routinely necessary. The psychiatric ramifications of abortion are a matter of some debate, but the findings are clear once methodological confounds are taken into account. Unbiased reviews of the literature indicate that self-limited feelings of guilt and sadness are common after abortion, although the predominant reaction is one of relief, and new episodes of psychiatric illness are rare (Adler et al. 1990; Dagg 1991; Koop 1989; Torres and Forrest 1988). A recent study corroborated findings that women's quality of life improves in the period from before to after an early abortion (Garg et al. 2001; Westhoff et al. 2003). The best outcomes prevail when women are able to make autonomous, supported choices about their pregnancies. When women seek, but are denied, abortion, the resulting children have significantly poorer mental health than their siblings or matched control subjects (Kubicka et al. 2002).

Antiabortion groups and writers claim that abortion is associated with a higher risk of serious psychiatric disorders and suicide than is childbirth (Pro-Life Action Ministries, undated; Reardon et al. 2003; Thorp et al. 2003). These publications fail to address the circumstances of and reasons for abortion. Sometimes they confound common, self-limited feelings of loss and guilt with diagnosable depression (Dagg 1991). Women have abortions because they have been abandoned by the men who impregnated them, because those men threaten to leave if they continue the pregnancy, because the pregnancy is the result of rape or incest, because they are poor and overburdened with other responsibilities, or because they do not have the resources—educational, financial, emotional, or social—to provide adequate parenting. They may simply not want to be a parent. Preexisting serious psychiatric illness makes some women more vulnerable to unwanted pregnancy and less able to parent.

Risk Factors

Not surprisingly, coercion, lack of social support, poverty, rape, incest, and preexisting psychiatric illness are associated with increased risk for psychological difficulties following, but not causally related to, abortion. Women who belong to religious faiths opposed to abortion choose abortion as often as or more often than those who do not. Efforts have been made to reach out to this population, both to enlist them in antiabortion advocacy and to offer them spiritual support (Gay and Lynxwiler 1999; Jeal and West 2003; Ventura et al. 2000). Demonstrators or fear of terrorism at an abortion facility may exacerbate stress, and the attitudes and behaviors of medical personnel during the abortion procedure have a significant influence on patients' experience (Slade et al. 2001).

The delay of abortion into the second trimester, or later, is most often secondary to denial of pregnancy, difficulties with access, or diagnosis of a serious fetal defect, each of which increases the risk for postabortion reactions. The discovery of a fetal defect in a wanted pregnancy, or the need to abort because of serious illness in the mother, arouses the same sense of failure and loss as a miscarriage, with the added concern that one is carrying a genetic anomaly or is physically unable to bear a child. Consultation may be sought when a woman or family cannot decide, or manifests overwhelming anxiety, when making an abortion decision under these circumstances (Zlotogora 2002). Continuing a pregnancy and relinquishing the child for adoption pose a psychological burden as well (Cushman et al. 1993; Deykin et al. 1984; Rynearson 1982).

Minors and Abortion

The effect of abortion on minors, and their ability to make decisions about abortion, is another area of controversy. The vast majority of pregnant minors choose to involve their parents in the abortion decision. No evidence shows that those who think it is not safe or wise to inform their parents derive benefit from being forced to do so. Term pregnancy and delivery pose greater medical and psychological risks for adolescents than does abortion. Arguments that minors are too immature to elect abortion overlook the fact that these same minors, if their pregnancies are not terminated, will soon be mothers with responsibility for infants. In Zabin's classic study of inner-city girls who obtained pregnancy tests at a school clinic, those who had abortions had better outcomes than did those who carried to term and even than did those whose pregnancy test results were negative. This does not imply that the abortion improved their mental health; it may imply that the inability to tell whether one is pregnant is associated with other psychosocial problems. Marriage of the pregnant teenager to the father of the baby does not improve outcome and may worsen it (Zabin et al. 1989).

Chronic Pelvic Pain

Chronic pelvic pain is nonmenstrual pelvic pain of 6 or more months' duration that is severe enough to cause functional disability or require medical or surgical treatment (Howard 2003). It is a relatively common and significant disorder of women, with an estimated prevalence of 3.8% in adult women, similar to that of asthma or back pain (Zondervan et al. 1999). Chronic pelvic pain is one of the most common gynecological complaints and accounts for 2%–10% of outpatient gynecological referrals (Howard 2003; Savidge and Slade 1997). In the United States, indirect total costs for chronic pelvic pain may be more than $2 billion per year (Mathias et al. 1996). At the individual level, chronic pelvic pain may lead to disability and suffering, with loss of employment, marital discord and divorce, and an overall decline in quality of life (Howard 2003).

Etiology of Chronic Pelvic Pain

Despite the severity and frequency of chronic pelvic pain, its etiology is often difficult to discern. Disorders of the reproductive, gastrointestinal, urological, musculoskeletal, and neurological systems may be associated with chronic pelvic pain. In many cases, however, the pain is related to a combination of physical and psychological factors, such as endometriosis, adhesions, urological problems, irritable bowel syndrome, myofascial pain, depression, anxiety, somatization, and past abusive experiences (Howard 2003; Moore and Kennedy 2001). Endometriosis and pelvic adhesive disease are responsible for most cases of chronic pelvic pain with organic findings, but a significant number of patients have no obvious etiology for their pain at the time of laparoscopy (Gelbaya and El-Halwagy 2001; Savidge and Slade 1997). As with other chronic syndromes, especially those with ambiguous etiology, the biopsychosocial model offers the best way of integrating physical causes of pain with psychological and social factors. One model, the gate-control theory of pain, proposes that peripheral nociceptive signals can be modified by neurotransmitters, such as serotonin and endorphins, that

control mood states, and accordingly, the gateway to chronic pain can be opened by depression and by direct tissue irritation. Because interacting psychological and physical factors are likely to be present early in the course of pain, attempts to separate chronic pain into a simple cause-and-effect relation are usually unrewarding. An alternative theory, the diathesis stress model, proposes that some patients are at increased risk for chronic pain because of preexisting acquired vulnerability. This might explain why a disproportionate number of patients with chronic pelvic pain report histories of physical and sexual abuse (Gelbaya and El-Halwagy 2001).

Psychological Factors Associated With Chronic Pelvic Pain

The relation of chronic pelvic pain to psychological state or personality style has received great attention. A comprehensive review in *PsychLit* and *MEDLINE* (1966–1997) of psychosocial factors in chronic pelvic pain identified 43 articles considered to be salient in exploring this link. Early studies tried to separate the pain into psychogenic and organic etiologies, but this has been largely unhelpful. Most studies have reported more depression, somatic symptoms, substance abuse, sexual dysfunction, and physical and sexual abuse in patients with chronic pelvic pain than in comparison groups (Fry et al. 1997). The reviewers, however, pointed out the numerous limitations in sample size, methodology, and comparison groups inherent in most of these studies. In general, the concept of psychogenic pain (emotional pain displaced onto the body) has been largely superseded. Cognitive-behavioral and psychophysiological theories have moved increasingly toward supporting more complex, multicausal views of chronic pelvic pain. Chronic pelvic pain is likely to be the outcome of several somatic, social, and psychological influences acting together in varying degrees, but more recent work has questioned the specificity of some of these, such as child sexual abuse.

A subsequent review of chronic pelvic pain (Reiter 1998) described predisposing psychosocial variables in chronic pelvic pain to be familial pain models, mood and anxiety disorders, marital adjustment problems, spousal responses, abuse history, and somatization. The author reported that psychological diagnoses were apparent in 60% of the women referred for chronic pelvic pain, with major depressive disorder the most common.

Management of Chronic Pelvic Pain

A comprehensive evidence-based management review of chronic pelvic pain (Reiter 1998) recommended a multidisciplinary, multifocal approach to chronic pelvic pain, individualized for each woman. Management might include medical therapies (oral analgesics, antidepressants, drugs for dysmotility disorders, management of musculoskeletal pain, ovarian cycle suppression, and antibiotics) and cognitive-behavioral or other psychotherapeutic approaches. Focused psychotherapy may be useful to address issues such as pain management, current conflicts, past sexual and physical abuse, current domestic violence, substance abuse problems, and sexual and marital dysfunction. Phases of treatment include education, skills acquisition, behavior modification, and maintenance. Special techniques may increase the patient's coping ability and sense of control; such techniques include muscle relaxation, deep breathing and imagery, and cognitive-behavioral techniques to identify and address maladaptive thoughts. Because patients with chronic pelvic pain frequently limit their activity to avoid possible pain, activity programs can be initiated to decrease disability behaviors. Several studies have reported that multidisciplinary management of chronic pelvic pain has significantly better outcomes than does traditional medical management (Price and Blake 1999; Reiter 1998; Savidge and Slade 1997).

Endometriosis

Endometriosis is a common gynecological complaint caused by the presence of hormonally responsive endometrial tissue outside the uterine cavity. The precise pathogenesis is not clearly established but likely involves retrograde menstruation with seeding of endometrial glands in the dependent part of the pelvis and in or on the ovary, posterior cul-de-sac, broad ligament, uterosacral ligament, rectosigmoidal colon, bladder, and distal ureter. It has been proposed that retrograde menstruation occurs to some degree in all women, but that only those who are unable to clear the menstrual debris because of immune dysfunction will go on to develop endometriosis (Cramer and Missmer 2002). Family history is a risk factor for endometriosis, and current efforts are being made to investigate genetic factors. The mean age of women at diagnosis of endometriosis ranges from 25 to 30 years. This condition is often asymptomatic but is also found in association with dysmenorrhea, dyspareunia, infertility, chronic pelvic or back pain, and rectal discomfort. The pain from the disorder is often cyclic, although it can be constant. The gold standard for diagnosis and staging of endometriosis depends on laparoscopy; however, the intensity of pain and discomfort does not correlate well with the severity of the disease at laparoscopy (Lu and Ory 1995).

Management

Endometriosis can be treated by watchful waiting or medical or surgical management. Current medical regimens to treat this condition with gonadotropin-releasing hormone agonists and other drugs attempt to create states of pseudopregnancy, pseudomenopause, or chronic anovulation. Surgical treatments vary from conservative removal and destroying of endometrial implants by excision, electrocautery, or laser. However, implants have been shown to recur in up to 28% of patients within 18 months and 40% after 9 years of follow-up. Although surgical conservative treatment is widely used to enhance fertility, its efficacy for endometriosis-associated infertility has not yet been shown. The definitive treatment for endometriosis is total abdominal hysterectomy with bilateral salpingo-oophorectomy, although an ovarian-sparing procedure is reasonable for mild to moderate endometriosis in young women who wish to retain their fertility (Lu and Ory 1995).

Role of the Psychiatrist

Because endometriosis is often chronic, and its contribution to chronic pelvic pain is sometimes uncertain, psychiatric opinion may be sought. Women with endometriosis also experience a range of problems for which they may not be adequately supported. In fact, some women report that their worst experience is their encounter with health professionals and the way in which their symptoms are trivialized and dismissed (Cox et al. 2003). Depression is a common accompaniment of endometriosis that is accompanied by chronic pain, dyspareunia, or infertility. In addition, gonadotropin-releasing hormone agonists are often used to treat endometriosis, and depressive symptoms may be associated with this treatment. Selective serotonin reuptake inhibitor (SSRI) antidepressants appear to be significantly helpful in the treatment of mood symptoms during the course of gonadotropin-releasing hormone agonists (Warnock et al. 1998). Psychotherapy and antidepressants also may be helpful in addressing other psychological issues and symptoms in women with endometriosis.

Vulvodynia

Vulvodynia is chronic burning, stinging, or pain in the vulva in the absence of objective clinical or laboratory findings. Vulvodynia is divided into two classes: 1) vulvar vestibulitis, which is restricted burning and pain in the vestibular region that is solicited by touch, and 2) dysesthetic vulvodynia, which is burning or pain not limited to the vestibule, which may occur without touch or pressure. A population-based National Institutes of Health study found that approximately 16% of women reported lower genital tract discomfort persisting for 3 months or longer (Edwards 2003).

The etiology of vulvodynia is unknown, and previously suspect agents such as subclinical yeast infections and human papillomavirus have largely been discounted.

More recently, neuropathic pain has been invoked, particularly because TCAs, SSRIs, and gabapentin have shown some promise in treating this disorder. Many women with vulvodynia also have comorbid disorders, such as interstitial cystitis, headaches, fibromyalgia, and irritable bowel syndrome, as well as clinical depression. Depression and anxiety are common accompaniments to vulvodynia (Stewart et al. 1994).

Psychiatrists may be asked to assess the role of psychosexual factors and depression in women with vulvodynia. Given the efficacy recently shown by dual-action antidepressants (serotonin and norepinephrine reuptake inhibitors) in treating depression and chronic painful conditions, these antidepressants may be a promising treatment for vulvodynia. However, to date, no randomized, controlled trials with these medications have been published.

Pregnancy

The entire range of psychiatric disorders occurs during pregnancy, and some conditions are unique to pregnancy. Treatment of these disorders is discussed later in this chapter.

Psychiatric Disorders Occurring During Pregnancy

Depression

The incidence of depression during pregnancy is approximately the same as that for matched populations who are not pregnant. The signs and symptoms of depression must be carefully distinguished from the sleep, appetite, and energy changes often characteristic of pregnancy and from the signs and symptoms of thyroid dysfunction, anemia, or other diseases of pregnancy. Discontinuation of maintenance medication for women who have had recurrent depressions carries a high risk of relapse. Mild cases can be effectively treated with interpersonal or cognitive-behavioral psychotherapy (Grote and Frank 2003; Spinelli and Endicott 2003).

Bipolar Disorder

There is a growing literature on bipolar disorders during pregnancy (Cohen et al. 1995; Viguera et al. 2002). Some pregnant patients can forgo mood stabilizers, but a substantial proportion (up to 50%) may relapse. Serious episodes of mania pose a threat to the pregnancy, necessitating especially careful risk–benefit analysis with regard to psychotropic medication.

Anxiety Disorders

Panic disorder may remit or recur during pregnancy. Patients with panic disorder who wish to discontinue medication should be tapered off gradually and treated with cognitive-behavioral therapy. More than 10% of female patients with panic disorder report that their first episode occurred postpartum. Panic disorder during pregnancy may recur with subsequent pregnancies. Obsessive-compulsive disorder is likely to worsen pre- and postpartum, and withdrawal of medication is very likely to result in recurrence. Some centers report that as many as 50% of cases of obsessive-compulsive disorder in women begin during their first pregnancy; others disagree (Neziroglu et al. 1992). Patients with moderate to severe symptoms may require maintenance medication during pregnancy; patients with milder cases can be treated with cognitive-behavioral therapy.

Psychotic Disorders

Because almost all women with psychotic disorders have been deinstitutionalized, their rate of fertility approximates that of the general population. Pregnancy does not ameliorate, and may exacerbate, psychotic symptoms (Davies et al. 1995). Psychotic episodes during pregnancy may be characterized by delusions that the fetus is evil or dangerous, leading the pregnant woman to stab herself in the abdomen or engage in other self-destructive behaviors. Electroconvulsive therapy (ECT) for acute affective psychotic episodes can be effective and is relatively safe for the fetus. Psychotic illness can impair a woman's ability to recognize and react appropriately to the signs and symptoms of labor (L.J. Miller and Finnerty 1996). Hospitalization toward the end of pregnancy is not completely protective against these concerns. Psychiatric inpatient staff are not obstetrically trained and are often uncomfortable assuming responsibility for the safety of mother and child. Obstetrical staff are not comfortable with psychotic patients. The consulting psychiatrist can facilitate collaboration between the departments in these difficult cases (Muqtadar et al. 1986).

Prenatal assessment and treatment can mitigate wrenching custody disputes after the infant is born. Serious psychiatric illness, if treated, is not always incompatible with successful mothering. The psychiatrist and obstetrician, working together with the patient and family, can plan and make provision for the infant's needs. Psychiatrists may be called on to assist in the assessment of competency to parent an infant. When it is clear that the mother will not be able to care for the child, such as when her other children have been taken into state custody for their protection, the psychiatrist can help her come to terms with the painful separation that will occur.

Alcohol and Substance Abuse

Alcohol and substance abuse arouse heightened concern in a pregnant patient. Standing by while a woman's behavior puts her fetus at risk is a painful situation for prenatal care professionals. The most serious and well-documented result of alcohol abuse during pregnancy is fetal alcohol syndrome. A pregnant woman who drinks the equivalent of 10 beers per day has a one-third risk of delivering a child with fetal alcohol syndrome and a similar risk of delivering a child who is retarded but does not have the full syndrome. The perinatal mortality in these circumstances is 17% (Greenfield and Sugarman 2001). More recent studies have not substantiated early fears of an epidemic of "crack babies." It appears that most or all of the negative cognitive and behavioral findings in these children are a result of the environment in which they grow up rather than intrauterine exposure to cocaine (Chiriboga 1998). However, misinformation and rage at pregnant women who abuse substances has led to instances in which women have been imprisoned, either for the protection of the fetus or as punishment for harming the fetus. Many or most pregnant women who abuse drugs or alcohol will accept treatment if it is practical (e.g., providing child care) and humane. Evidence indicates that the threat of coercion and punishment leads women to avoid seeking prenatal care altogether, obviating any opportunity to treat her and improve the fetus's intrauterine environment (see also Chapter 3, "Legal Issues," for discussion of legal aspects).

Situational Anxiety

Some pregnant patients are referred for psychiatric consultation for evaluation of what seems to the primary care clinician to be an inordinate level of anxiety. A careful history often shows that the patient either has been frightened by the experiences of a close family member or has had a traumatic obstetrical or general medical care experience herself (Saisto and Halmesmaki 2003). The degree of pain a woman experiences in labor is related to many factors, including her expectations of pain (Chang et al. 2002). When the source of the anxiety is identified, it can be addressed by reviewing the past experience and making plans to avoid the frightening aspects of care in the com-

ing delivery, providing prenatal education about delivery, or using relaxation techniques or hypnosis. Domestic violence is another cause of prenatal anxiety. Literature about the effect of pregnancy on domestic violence is contradictory; in some reports, violence is increased, and in others, it is not (Johnson et al. 2003; Saltzman et al. 2003).

Issues Unique to Pregnancy

Denial of Pregnancy

Some women go into full-term labor without having recognized, or their families having recognized, that they are pregnant. Many such patients are not psychotic, but some are women with schizophrenia who are delusional in denying pregnancy (L.J. Miller 1990). Older patients may report that they thought pregnancy was impossible at their age and attributed their amenorrhea to menopause and the sensations of fetal movement to digestive problems. Younger patients in this situation are typically passive daughters isolated in very strict families without much knowledge about reproduction. Their preconscious or unconscious fears of the consequences of pregnancy are so terrifying that they keep its signs and symptoms out of awareness (Spielvogel and Hohener 1995). They wear loose-fitting clothing and go about their usual activities (Finnegan et al. 1982). These cases generally come to psychiatric attention only when the new mother kills the infant after birth (Brozovsky and Falit 1971). Therefore, these young women end up in the penal—rather than the mental health care—system, and there has been relatively little opportunity to work with them and their families to learn more about the dynamics of these situations. A recent epidemiological study in Germany, perhaps the first of its kind, reported an incidence of up to 1 case of pregnancy denial per 475 births (Wessel et al. 2002).

Pseudocyesis

At the other end of the spectrum from the patient who does not realize she is pregnant is the patient who is convinced she is pregnant when she is not. This condition, referred to as *pseudocyesis*, is a fascinating example of psychobiological interplay. The patient ceases to have menstrual periods. Her abdomen grows, and her cervix may show signs of pregnancy. Some patients with the delusion that they are pregnant are psychotic, but that is not the case in classical pseudocyesis. Patients with pseudocyesis are a heterogeneous group, and they have no other signs or symptoms of frank psychiatric disorder (Rosch et al. 2002). They declare an expected date of delivery and move the date forward when delivery does not ensue. Their conviction may or may not be swayed by ultrasonographic evidence or physical examination. For unknown reasons, the incidence of this condition is decreasing. Frequent antecedents are pregnancy loss, infertility, isolation, naiveté, and a belief that childbearing is a woman's crucial role. These individuals have no interest in psychiatric care, and little is known about how the condition eventually resolves (Whelan and Stewart 1990).

Hyperemesis

Pernicious vomiting in pregnancy was once thought to be the result of unconscious rejection of the pregnancy (Majerus et al. 1960). Hyperemesis, which can result in dehydration and electrolyte imbalance and may require hospitalization and intravenous treatment, certainly could induce ambivalence about a pregnancy in a woman who had been very pleased at the prospect of becoming a mother, but no scientific evidence indicates that ambivalence induces the vomiting (O'Brien and Newton 1991). Hyperemesis is no longer considered a psychiatric disorder. Mental health intervention can, however, help the patient and family cope until the condition resolves (Deuchar 1995).

Routine Psychiatric Screening

Psychiatrists may advise obstetricians that including psychiatric screening in routine antenatal care will decrease the frequency and intensity of noncompliance with antenatal care and of psychiatric emergencies during pregnancy and labor. Psychiatric illnesses can be identified and treated. Patients who might not otherwise recognize that they are in labor, and their families, can receive special education so that infants are not delivered into the toilet or in some other less-than-ideal environment. Prenatal education can prepare them for labor and delivery, so that they can best cooperate and communicate with medical staff when the time comes.

Postpartum Psychiatric Issues

Perinatal Death

Stillbirth and neonatal death provoke much the same reactions as do losses earlier in pregnancy, which are discussed earlier in this chapter, with the added stresses of full-term labor and delivery and the probability that many practical provisions for the expected infant have been made. Clinical practice in dealing with the bereaved and disappointed parents has varied over time. It is probably best to offer parents the opportunity to see or not to see the stillborn infant and to allow them to decide. Many bereaved parents report that their grief is exacerbated by the failure of friends and relatives to acknowledge the loss. For some, naming the baby and having a funeral service, with or without a burial, is a helpful ritual. A religious leader of the parents' choice also can help them reconcile their rage at God for depriving them of their child with their need to derive support from their faith in God.

When the cause of fetal or neonatal death is not clear, an autopsy or other tests may be performed. The results will not be immediately available. The obstetrician, pathologist, geneticist, and psychiatrist may want to meet with the parents some weeks later to convey the results, answer questions, observe the grieving process, and determine whether additional supports are necessary. As with miscarriage, stillbirth increases the risk of posttraumatic stress, anxiety, and depression in a subsequent pregnancy (Bourne and Lewis 1984; Hughes et al. 1999). These sequelae generally resolve within 1 year after the birth of a subsequent healthy child (Turton et al. 2001). Premature birth or the stress of complicated, or even normal, labor can precipitate posttraumatic stress symptoms as well, especially in women with preexisting psychiatric symptoms and poor social supports (Czarnocka and Slade 2000; Holditch-Davis et al. 2003).

Postpartum Psychiatric Disorders

"Baby Blues"

Within days after birth, 25%–75% of newly delivered women experience significantly heightened emotional lability. After a few days, the symptoms abate. The phenomenon has been reported in a wide variety of cultures and is not related to demographic variables (Sakumoto et al. 2002). Although the patient may be moved to tears from time to time, none of the other signs or symptoms of depression are present nor do they develop as an exacerbation of this condition. The mother also experiences moments of joy. This self-limited state may be caused by prolactin or other hormones. An interesting hypothesis is that "baby blues" may be related to the effects of oxytocin and other hormones involved in the initiation of mother–infant attachment and maternal behavior (L.J. Miller and Rukstalis 1999). Clinicians should offer reassurance. This is especially important because media reports of postpartum depression leading to the murder of children have frightened so many families.

Postpartum Depression

Postpartum depression occurs in up to 10%–20% of mothers in North America. Some cases of postpartum depression are simply continuations of prepartum depression. As noted earlier, depression during pregnancy is common. Symptoms can begin any time from days to months after birth but generally later than "baby blues" and ranging from 4 weeks to 12 months postpartum. The diagnostic process can be complicated by the similarity of symptoms of the aftermath of delivery and the stresses of caring for a newborn and the signs and symptoms of depression. New mothers are often tired, sleepless, distracted, and preoccupied with infant care rather than the enjoyment of previous pursuits. Their meal schedules and sleep are disrupted. It is useful to ask whether the mother can sleep when the baby sleeps.

Risk factors include previous depression, especially postpartum depression; complications of birth; and poor social supports. There appears to be some cross-cultural variation in the incidence of postpartum depression; this may be related to contrasting patterns of prepartum and postpartum care and social support. In many cultures, the newly delivered woman is traditionally provided with rest, warmth, and enriched nutrition (Kaewsarn et al. 2003). In North America, medical attention decreases drastically after an infant is delivered; few medical and social resources are available to the new family. Some evidence shows that postpartum calls and visits from health care professionals decrease the incidence of postpartum depression (Chabrol et al. 2002). Endocrine factors also play a major role; some women are particularly vulnerable to rapid changes in hormone levels. Estradiol and progesterone are strongly implicated (Bloch et al. 2003). Women with thyroid autoantibodies have an increased risk for postpartum depression, but thyroxine administration does not appear to reduce that risk (Harris et al. 2002; Oretti et al. 2003).

Anxiety accompanies pre- and postpartum depression in up to 50% of cases (Ross et al. 2003). In a recent Australian study of 408 primigravidas, the inclusion of panic disorder and acute adjustment disorder with anxiety doubled the cases of postpartum psychiatric illness identified. Antecedent anxiety disorders were a more important risk factor for postpartum depression than was antecedent depression (Matthey et al. 2003a).

The thought content of a woman with postpartum depression centers on mothering (e.g., ruminating that she is not a good mother and that her infant is suffering as a result). Sometimes the woman becomes obsessed with thoughts of harm coming to the infant and vividly imagines his or her injury or death. These thoughts are profoundly upsetting to the mother; they are thoughts, not intentions, and should be distinguished from the delusionally driven infanticidal impulses of postpartum psychosis.

Reassurance of eventual recovery is crucial to patient care. One of the fears of women with postpartum depression, and their families, is that the depression is the first sign of a condition that will result in self-harm or infanticide. Relatives may be tempted to take over care of the infant of a depressed mother to allow her to rest and recuperate. This can be counterproductive, exacerbating her sense of failure and deprivation. It is preferable for them to help the mother with household tasks, allow her to care for the infant, and reinforce her sense of maternal adequacy.

Although obstetricians have become more aware of and responsive to postpartum depression as a result of the notorious cases in the media and educational initiatives by a variety of professional and advocacy organizations, they may not be in the optimal position to identify it. Women are discharged from the hospital within a day or two after delivery, with a rather cursory office follow-up visit 4–6 weeks later. Obstetric clinicians should be encouraged to increase their contacts with and availability to new mothers, both for screening and for prevention. Several validated scales are available for screening; the Edinburgh Postnatal Depression Scale (Matthey et al. 2003b) is the best known. However, a simple query about depressed mood is often successful in identifying cases (Wisner et al. 2002b). After the birth, the specialist women see most is the pediatrician. There have been attempts, with mixed success, to convince pediatricians to screen mothers for postpartum depression. Efforts are under way to develop screening instruments for use in non-Western populations (Mantle 2003). Researchers in Hong Kong determined that screening should be delayed for several days after delivery in order to be accurate (Lee et al. 2003), although earlier assessment has been found accurate in North America (Dennis 2003). Screening in an inner-city population in New York uncovered far more cases than were anticipated (Morris-Rush et al. 2003).

Postpartum Psychosis

Many experts believe that most episodes of postpartum psychosis are bipolar (Attia et al. 1999; Chaudron and Pies 2003). The risk of postpartum relapse of bipolar disorder is 30%–50%; these relapses can be acute and severe. If pregnant women with bipolar disorder discontinue medication, there should be a plan for immediate medication resumption at delivery. Third trimester or immediate postpartum treatment significantly lowers the risk of recurrence (Cohen et al. 1995).

Postpartum psychosis is characterized by extreme agitation, delirium, confusion, sleeplessness, and hallucinations and/or delusions. Onset can be sudden and usually occurs between days 3 and 14 postpartum. The overall incidence of postpartum psychosis is estimated at 0.1%–0.2% and appears to have been stable for more than a century and among cultures. The risk of psychiatric hospitalization postpartum has been reported to be 18 times that prepartum (Paffenbarger 1982), although these findings have been questioned more recently by a Danish study (Terp and Mortensen 1998). Only a fraction of these women will go on to attempt suicide or infanticide, but the risk and the stakes are high enough to warrant considering postpartum psychosis as a medical emergency and hospitalizing the patient, at least for a period of observation. Women who have schizophrenic episodes may have more difficulty parenting their children after recovery from the acute episode than do women with other kinds of postpartum psychosis (Riordan et al. 1999).

Trials and media coverage of cases of infanticide disclose major misunderstandings about the state and motivation of the perpetrators. Most often, the mother in these cases has command hallucinations or delusions and/or is suicidal and does not wish to leave the child behind, but wants to be reunited with him or her in Heaven. Gibson (1982) reported that 62% of the mothers in his series who committed infanticide committed suicide as well. Appleby et al. (1998) reported that the risk of suicide in the first postnatal year is "increased 70-fold."

Custody

Psychiatric illness in and of itself does not rule out the possibility of adequate mothering. For general evaluation, and the legal and medical records, when the question of custody arises, it is useful to perform a regular mental status examination. What are most important, however, are the parenting knowledge, attitudes, and behaviors of the newly delivered patient. Has she been able to arrange adequate accommodations for herself and the infant? How does she plan to feed the infant? Does she know approximately how often a newborn must be fed and changed? Does she have delusions about the infant?

Observation of mother–infant interaction is key. It is very difficult to predict how a person will behave with an infant in the absence of the infant. The postpartum staff should allow the mother as much observed time with the infant as possible and note how the mother responds to the infant's cries and other needs, whether she can feed the infant and change his or her diapers, and how she relates to the infant overall. New mothers without psychiatric disorders can be tired and overwhelmed; expectations should be realistic.

Custody decisions can be life-or-death decisions. Removing a child from his or her mother, unless a well-disposed and capable relative can take over his or her care, exposes the child to the possibility of a lifetime in transient foster care situations. Allowing a severely ill mother to retain custody exposes the child to possible abuse and neglect. Interactions with child protective services can be problematic. Depending on current resources and recent scandals, child protective services may take a child into custody without giving the mother a chance to show her ability to parent, or they may refuse to intervene with a dangerously psychotic mother because the infant has not yet been damaged. Often, the most appropriate approach, when available, is the provision of home help and/or visiting nurse services, which provide both support and further opportunities for observation of the parenting and the condition of the infant. Having a mental illness does not diminish, and may exacerbate, the grief and rage of a mother whose child is taken away.

Legal aspects of maternal competency are discussed in Chapter 3, "Legal Issues."

Psychotropic Drugs, Psychotherapy, and Electroconvulsive Therapy in Pregnancy and Lactation

No perfect solution exists for treating mental illness during pregnancy and lactation, and a risk–benefit decision must be made in the face of imprecise data. For example, untreated clinical depression can result in problems with maternal nutrition, sleeping, exercise, and adherence to prenatal care. Infants born to mothers with depression are more likely to have low birth weight for gestational age and be born prematurely (Stewart and Robinson 2001b). Although mental illness of mild to moderate severity may be treated with psychotherapy, support, or environmental changes, more severe illness usually requires psychotropic medications, which carry variable and sometimes unknown risks (Hendrick et al. 2003).

Three types of adverse fetal effects may occur when psychotropics are taken during pregnancy. *Teratogenic effects* may be incurred from first trimester exposure, *neonatal toxicity and withdrawal syndromes* are related to third trimester exposure, and *behavioral or developmental effects* may manifest later in childhood (Marcus et al. 2001; Wisner et al. 2002a). Note that changes in drug metabolism and extracellular fluid volume during pregnancy may require dose adjustment for several drugs. For example, approximately twice the usual dose of lithium carbonate is required in the second and third trimesters to achieve therapeutic serum levels (Stewart and Robinson 2001b). (See also Chapter 37, "Psychopharmacology," for a discussion of pharmacotherapy during pregnancy.)

Classification of Drugs

Current U.S. Food and Drug Administration (FDA) (2003) risk assignments of drugs in pregnancy range from A (no risk) through B, C, D, and X (contraindicated). This classification is primarily based on concerns about teratogenicity and neonatal toxicity, because few or no data exist for later child behavior or development. The FDA classification lags behind current data and experience. At present, bupropion, clozapine, and buspirone have a B designation (absence of human risk) with a caveat of limited data. Most SSRI antidepressants, some TCAs (including desipramine), newer antidepressants (such as mirtazapine, nefazodone, and venlafaxine), clonazepam, and most conventional and atypical antipsychotics have received a C designation (human risk should not be eliminated because of inadequate human clinical trials and no or some risk in animals). Lithium, carbamazepine, sodium valproate, most TCAs, and some benzodiazepines (other than clonazepam) have received a D designation, indicating evidence of fetal risk without an absolute contraindication during pregnancy. A long-standing debate has existed, with contradictory data from several studies, on whether diazepam in pregnancy is associated with cleft lip or cleft palate. Some benzodiazepines, such as triazolam, temazepam, and flurazepam, have received an X designation, indicating complete contraindication in pregnancy (Marcus et al. 2001). Although the strength of evidence for safety of all psychotropics in pregnancy is fair to poor, expert consensus guidelines have been developed on the basis of current information and recent use (Altshuler et al. 2001). Insufficient data are available to ensure safety for most novel antipsychotics; however, high-potency antipsychotics, such as haloperidol, appear to be relatively safer in pregnancy (Patton et al. 2002).

Early reports warned of congenital heart disease in infants exposed in utero to lithium carbonate, but subsequent analyses have shown these risks to be only slightly greater than those of the general population (Altshuler et al. 1996). Other mood stabilizers such as carbamazepine and valproic acid are associated with greater teratogenicity than lithium (Stewart and Robinson 2001b). For women with unstable bipolar disorder, it is reasonable to continue lithium throughout pregnancy, while carefully monitoring serum levels. Divided doses may be safer than once-daily dosing. An ultrasound during the first trimester may be used to identify possible congenital cardiac malformations. Dosage should be reduced after delivery to avoid lithium toxicity in the early postpartum period. Lithium is contraindicated while breast-feeding (Stewart and Robinson 2001b).

Because the FDA is currently revising its method of classifying drug risk in pregnancy, physicians should consult the most recent classification, as well as other new literature. As this chapter was going to press, new data were published showing that infants exposed in utero to SSRI antidepressants had a shorter mean gestational age, were more active and tremulous, had more startles and sudden arousals, showed lower heart rate variability and lower peak behavioral status (Zeskind et al. 2004).

Disruptions in the wide range of neurobehavioral outcomes as well as seizures, respiratory and feeding problems prompted regulatory authorities in Canada to issue an advisory suggesting increased awareness of potential complications of all SSRIs in infants who were exposed during the third trimester of pregnancy. The FDA is currently considering a similar warning based on the advice of its Pediatric Advisory Committee.

Adverse Effects

Only a few long-term studies of behavioral teratogenicity following exposure to psychotropic drugs have been done. More studies of fluoxetine have been published compared with other SSRIs following its use in pregnancy (Goldstein et al. 1997) and its effects on child development and behavior. Nulman et al. (2002) found no difference in social, cognitive, or motor development in children up to 86 months whose mothers had taken a variety of TCAs or fluoxetine in pregnancy. In several studies, sertraline, paroxetine, fluvoxamine, citalopram, and venlafaxine were shown as relatively safe in pregnancy when infants were assessed in the early postnatal period (Altshuler et al. 2001; Einarson et al. 2003; Heikkinen et al. 2002; Wisner et al. 2002a), but none of these studies provided longer-term follow-up. In one report, acute withdrawal effects occurred in infants whose mothers took paroxetine during the third trimester (Stiskal et al. 2001). Longer-term follow-up studies of infants exposed to antipsychotics in the uterus have relied on imprecise measures of intelligence compared with siblings or the general population (Kris 1965).

Breast-Feeding and Psychotropic Drugs

The use of psychotropic drugs by breast-feeding women remains controversial. The amount of drug present in breast milk is small but extremely variable over time, even in the same woman. No controlled studies of the effects of psychotropic medication during breast-feeding exist, but several reviews provide further guidance (Altshuler et al. 1995, 2001; American Academy of Pediatrics Committee on Drugs 2001; Hendrick et al. 2001; Ilett et al. 2002; Stewart 2001; Wisner et al. 2001). In general, it appears relatively safe for depressed women to take antidepressants and typical antipsychotics while breast-feeding full-term and healthy babies. Fewer data are available for premature infants or newer antidepressants and atypical antipsychotics. Chaudron and Jefferson (2000) reviewed the literature on the use of mood stabilizers during lactation. They concluded that lithium is generally not recommended during lactation and that although carbamazepine and valproate may be considered acceptable, decisions about the care of women with a history of bipolar illness must be made on a case-by-case basis. The risk of recurrence is considerable, with significant implications for mother and child (Chaudron and Jefferson 2000).

Because new information on the use of drugs during pregnancy and lactation is frequently published, the reader is advised to consult the most recent reference in making risk–benefit decisions. The expert consensus guidelines (Altshuler et al. 2001) provide useful guidance on practice at that time. The clinician must be cognizant that untreated mental illness in pregnancy and postpartum also has risks to the woman and the developing fetus and newborn child. Decisions should be made in consultation with the woman (and partner, if appropriate) and other health care providers (such as obstetricians and pediatricians), and discussions should be carefully documented in the patient's chart.

Psychotherapy in Pregnancy and Postpartum

Spinelli (1997) found interpersonal psychotherapy to be effective in the treatment of depressed pregnant women. Appleby et al. (1997) compared the effects of antidepressant treatment and six sessions of cognitive-behavioral counseling for postnatal depression and found both treatments to be effective. More recent work by P. Cooper and colleagues (2003) has shown that psychotherapy has only short-term benefits for maternal mood that are not superior to spontaneous remission in the long term. Murray and colleagues (2003) showed that early psychotherapy intervention was beneficial for short-term mother–infant relationships but had no effect on infant behavior problems, secure attachment, cognitive development, or any child outcome at 5 years. O'Hara and colleagues (2000) established the efficacy of interpersonal psychotherapy for postpartum depression. In general, interpersonal and cognitive-behavioral psychotherapy appear to be efficacious for mild to moderate depression. Because many women refuse to take medication while pregnant or breastfeeding, psychotherapy is often a viable alternative. However, its efficacy for severe depression in unproven.

Electroconvulsive Therapy

ECT is generally regarded as a safe and effective treatment for severe depression, affective psychosis, and cata-

tonia in pregnancy and the puerperium. ECT is underused and should be considered in emergency situations in which the safety of the mother, fetus, or child is jeopardized; to avoid first-trimester exposure to teratogenic drugs; and in patients who are refractory to psychotropics or who have previously had successful treatment with ECT (Stewart and Robinson 2001b) (see also Chapter 39, "Electroconvulsive Therapy").

Premenstrual Psychiatric Symptoms: Premenstrual Syndrome and Premenstrual Dysphoric Disorder

Background

The study of premenstrual symptoms poses unique methodological challenges. Most women in North America, if asked, report premenstrual mood, behavior, and somatic changes. There is a strong cultural belief that the menstrual cycle is associated with such negative changes. This may be strong circumstantial evidence that such changes exist and are significant. However, it is also clear that both women and men attribute unpleasant or problematic feelings and behaviors to the menstrual cycle regardless of whether they are related. Many more than half of the women presenting for care of premenstrual symptoms, when assessed with prospective ratings and careful diagnostic interviews, have symptoms completely unrelated to their menstrual cycles. Investigators in this area tread between accusations that medical science has too long ignored women's cyclical suffering and allegations that reifying cultural beliefs about women's hormonal frailties does women a disservice. There has been virtually no investigation of the possibility that negative mood changes at one point in the cycle are counterbalanced by positive changes at another point. Strong feelings and methodological difficulties have made the diagnosis of premenstrual psychiatric syndromes controversial (Sveinsdottir et al. 2002).

Etiology

Many attempts have been made, over decades, to identify circulating levels of reproductive hormones to account for mood symptoms occurring in concert with reproductive events and cycles and to treat those symptoms with hormones. By and large, these efforts have been unsuccessful. The reality is probably more complex than linear effects of hormone levels on mood. It would seem that some women are particularly sensitive, not to specific levels, but to changes in the levels of reproductive hormones.

Women who report premenstrual symptoms are more likely to experience postpartum depression and may be predisposed to mood symptoms around perimenopause as well (Stewart and Boydell 1993). Women report that their premenstrual symptoms first appeared, on average, when they were in their early 20s but that they did not seek medical care for as many as 10 years. Premenstrual symptoms persist into the perimenopause, when they become difficult to distinguish from symptoms of perimenopause (Grady-Weliky 2003).

Diagnosis

Currently, premenstrual psychiatric symptoms are conceptualized and treated as part of the mood disorder spectrum. Experts, and the framers of DSM, have attempted to distinguish normative mood variations from symptoms worthy of medical attention by publishing research criteria for premenstrual dysphoric disorder (PMDD). For many years, the study of premenstrual psychiatric symptoms was complicated by the lack of a specific and uniform definition. More than 100 physical, emotional, and cognitive signs and symptoms have been attributed to premenstrual syndrome (PMS) (Janowsky et al. 2002). PMDD is listed in DSM-IV-TR as an example of a depressive disorder not otherwise specified (NOS) and is described as follows:

> In most menstrual cycles during the past year, five (or more) of the following symptoms (e.g., markedly depressed mood, marked anxiety, marked affective lability, decreased interest in activities) were present for most of the time during the last week of the luteal phase, began to remit within a few days after the onset of the follicular phase, and were absent in the week postmenses....The disturbance markedly interferes with work or school or with usual social activities and relationships with others. (American Psychiatric Association 2000, p. 774)

PMDD, as distinguished from PMS, is said to affect up to 8% of cycling women. Given the tendency to retrospectively overattribute symptoms to the menstrual cycle, prospective daily ratings and careful evaluation for other psychiatric disorders are essential (Landen and Eriksson 2003; Lane and Francis 2003; M.N. Miller and Miller 2001).

Psychosocial Effects

Another controversial aspect of PMDD is the severity or effect of the symptoms. The DSM definition specifies a significant negative effect on life function. It has been difficult to specify the distinction between PMS and PMDD in this regard (Smith et al. 2003). Preexisting beliefs about

work effect may color the findings in studies that use self-reports (Steiner et al. 2003). A large study of randomly selected members of a health maintenance organization found that women with PMDD reported decreased work productivity as compared with women with milder premenstrual symptoms, but the women with PMDD also reported lower productivity than the others in the follicular phase after the onset of menses, when their PMDD symptoms, according to the definition, should have been absent. This study did not produce significant evidence that premenstrual symptoms, regardless of their level of severity, caused women to stay in bed, reduce their hours at work, or decrease their activities at home or school (Chawla et al. 2002).

Management

No specific, empirically supported treatments for PMS are available, but several approaches have proved helpful for both the symptoms and the patients' general health. These include taking vitamins (especially B vitamins), reducing or eliminating caffeine and nicotine, exercising, and using stress reduction techniques. As stated earlier, exogenous hormones are not effective treatments for PMS or PMDD. Many women with premenstrual symptoms attempt complementary or alternative approaches (Domoney et al. 2003). Recent publications claim effectiveness for fish oil and for acupuncture, among others (Habek et al. 2002; Sampalis et al. 2003). (See Girman et al. 2003 for a comprehensive review of this literature.) In one study, cognitive-behavioral therapy was found to be equally effective as fluoxetine; fluoxetine produced more rapid results, and cognitive-behavioral therapy produced more lasting results (Hunter et al. 2002). Calcium carbonate also has produced promising results (Thys-Jacobs et al. 1998).

Like other disorders in the mood spectrum, PMDD is best treated with SSRIs (Freeman 2002; Wyatt et al. 2002). As of this writing, fluoxetine, sertraline, and paroxetine have received FDA indications for PMDD. For reasons still poorly understood, although SSRIs generally require 2–4 weeks for therapeutic effectiveness in depression, they are apparently effective for PMDD when used only in the premenstrual phase (Halbreich et al. 2002). Evidence also indicates that symptoms recur rapidly when luteal-phase treatment is discontinued (Pearlstein et al. 2003).

The possibility of cyclical changes in symptoms and/ or treatment response in all diagnostic categories should be considered in all menstruating women or at least in those whose diagnoses or treatment responses are puzzling or unsatisfactory (Lande and Karamchandani 2002).

Perimenopause and Menopause

The average age at menopause in North American and European women is 51 years, although the entire period of transition may extend over several years. By definition, menopause is said to have occurred after 12 months of amenorrhea, and perimenopause is that period of time leading up to menopause but before 12 consecutive months of amenorrhea. During the perimenopause, the ovarian follicles gradually decline with age, estradiol and inhibin production by the ovary decreases, and follicle-stimulating hormone and luteinizing hormone levels rise (through loss of feedback inhibition). These changes are orchestrated through the hypothalamic-pituitary-ovarian axis, and cyclic variability often occurs throughout the transitional period (Baram 1997).

The perimenopause may be asymptomatic, but 70%–90% of women will experience some vasomotor symptoms consisting of hot flashes and night sweats. In addition, some women will experience palpitations, dizziness, fatigue, headaches, insomnia, joint pains, and paresthesias. Women also may complain of lack of concentration and loss of memory during the transitional period, but because men also complain of these symptoms, distinguishing them from normal aging is difficult (Baram 1997).

The association of psychiatric symptoms with the perimenopause is controversial. Large community surveys in the United States (Avis and McKinlay 1995), Europe, and Canada (Kaufert et al. 1992) show no increase in psychopathology with menopause; however, increases in depression and anxiety prevalence have been reported over the perimenopausal years (Avis and McKinlay 1995; Freeman et al. 2004). Whether these symptoms are caused by hormonal changes, sociocultural factors, or psychological factors remains uncertain (Avis 2003). Biological factors include the reduction of estradiol production by the ovaries, hypothalamic age-related changes, increase in the proportion of estrone compared with estradiol, and decrease in the production of ovarian androgens (Baram 1997). Sociocultural theories focus on the importance of role changes in parenting, marriage, sex, and work. In addition, attitudes toward aging and female roles vary by culture. A consistent finding is that women with lower socioeconomic class and education report more perimenopausal symptoms. Psychological theories focus on stress during the perimenopausal years as a result of diminished personal and family health, socioeconomic status, family and work changes, other losses, retirement, illness, and deaths (Avis 2003). In addition, recent work also has shown that a lifetime history of major depression may be associated with an early decline in ovarian function and earlier menopause (Harlow et al. 2003).

Although epidemiological surveys show no increase in rates of depression over the climacteric, women seeking treatment for physical symptoms in menopause clinics report a high prevalence of depression, irritability, mood lability, anxiety, lack of concentration, short-term memory loss, and decreased libido (Stewart and Boydell 1993). New-onset depressive symptoms have been found to be moderately associated with perimenopause and are related to the length and intensity of symptoms (Avis and McKinlay 1995). Investigators also have reported that subgroups of women appear to be more vulnerable to physiological hormonal changes associated with the premenstruum, postpartum, and perimenopause (Stewart and Boydell 1993). Other investigators have shown that prior depression is a risk factor for depression at perimenopause and that poor physical health, social circumstances, divorce, widowhood, and interpersonal stress are closely correlated with depression in menopausal women (Hunter 1990; Kaufert et al. 1992; Stewart and Boydell 1993).

The incidence of depression in women mirrors estrogen shifts across the life cycle, at puberty, premenopause, postpartum, and perimenopause (Stahl 2001). Estrogen receptors are present throughout the body and are particularly dense in the limbic system, which mediates emotion. Estrogen performs an organizational role during fetal life, resulting in trophic and permanent modifications in sex-specific brain differentiation. It increases again in adult life and contributes to sex-differentiated brain function. Estrogen is known to influence serotonin through inhibiting monoamine oxidase at high doses and displacing tryptophan from plasma albumin–binding sites, influencing serotonin receptor–binding downregulation and increasing endogenous catecholamine release. It is not surprising that the actions of estrogen in the central nervous system may affect mood and cognition (Stahl 2001).

The above biological findings have led to studies to determine whether estrogen therapy in perimenopause can alleviate symptoms of clinical depression. A study by Schmidt et al. (2000) randomized 34 women to estradiol-17-beta patches or placebo for 3 weeks, then crossed over the women in the placebo group to the estrogen condition. They found that the women with both major depression ($n=8$) and minor depression ($n=26$) taking estrogen reported significantly improved mood (as measured by the Center for Epidemiologic Studies Depression Scale), whereas those receiving placebo reported no improvement. Notably, 80% of the women receiving estradiol reported improved mood, despite no improvement in hot flashes or sleep function. In a more recent study, 50 perimenopausal women with major depression ($n=26$), dysthymia ($n=11$), and minor depression ($n=13$) were treated by randomizing them to transdermal patches of estradiol-17-beta 100 mg for 12 weeks. Of the women receiving estradiol, 68% showed improvement on the Montgomery-Åsberg Rating Scale for Depression and the Blatt-Kupperman Menopause Index, compared with 20% of those taking placebo ($P=0.001$) (Soares et al. 2001). The improvement persisted after a 4-week washout, and the authors concluded that estradiol was a well-tolerated and effective treatment for perimenopausal depression.

Although estrogen appears to have a salutary effect on depression in some perimenopausal women, in contrast, progesterone and progestins are known to cause dizziness, drowsiness, and sedation in many women and may be associated with negative moods (Bjorn et al. 2000). Progestins are primarily used in women with an intact uterus to prevent an increase in endometrial cancer caused by unopposed estrogen therapy.

Studies also have been conducted on the role of estrogen as an augmentation agent with antidepressants. Women were given fluoxetine, with or without estrogen therapy. Women who were concurrently treated with estrogen had a threefold increased chance of responding to fluoxetine (Schneider et al. 1997). Further studies of estrogen and selective estrogen receptor modulators as psychotropic augmentation agents are needed.

Moreover, the role of estrogen in psychiatric disorders is not limited to depression. Work by Kulkarni et al. (2001), Seeman (2002), and others have shown a worsening in preexisting schizophrenic illness and other psychoses associated with decreases in estradiol during perimenopause and beyond. Interestingly, some patients appear to respond to estrogen therapy combined with antipsychotic drugs.

Of concern, however, are results from the Women's Health Initiative (WHI), which have indicated that estrogen–progesterone therapy is associated with an increased risk of breast cancer, cardiovascular disease (Writing Group for the Women's Health Initiative Investigators 2002), cognitive dysfunction, and dementia (Rapp et al. 2003; Shumaker et al. 2003). The estrogen-only arm of the WHI was also prematurely terminated in 2004 when estrogen monotherapy was found to be associated with increased rates of stroke, dementia, and mild cognitive impairment (but not breast cancer) (Women's Health Initiative Steering Committee 2004).

Emerging evidence may affect current use, but at present, estrogen is useful to control severe vasomotor symptoms and vaginal dryness, with current FDA guidelines recommending the smallest dosage for the shortest time possible. Antidepressants such as fluoxetine, venlafaxine, and paroxetine are also known to decrease hot flashes (Loprinzi et al. 2000, 2002; Stearns et al. 2000). Phytoestrogens (soy) and black cohosh have been shown

to have contradictory results in diminishing hot flashes in perimenopausal women (Kronenberg and Fugh-Berman 2002). A study published in the *Journal of the American Medical Association* in 2003 compared placebo with two dietary phytoestrogen supplements and found no significant difference in the frequency of hot flashes at 12 weeks (Tice et al. 2003).

In conclusion, the many estrogen effects on brain function are complex. The role of estrogen in treating mood, cognition, and psychosis, and as a psychotropic augmentation agent, requires further adequately powered, randomized controlled trials. Personal, social, and physical factors always should be considered in assessing the individual woman, and psychotherapy may be helpful in navigating the many transitions at midlife.

Urinary Incontinence

Urinary incontinence, the involuntary loss of urine, affects up to 23% of adults (Roe et al. 1999), with a prevalence in women that is twice that in men (Melville et al. 2002). Urinary incontinence affects the physical, psychological, social, and economic well-being of individuals and their families and imposes a considerable economic burden on health and social services. Many people are reluctant to seek help because they are embarrassed, are ashamed, or believe that the problem is a part of normal aging (Roe et al. 1999).

Etiology and Classification

The etiology of urinary incontinence is multifactorial and may be caused by impairment of the lower urinary tract or the nervous system or by various external factors. There are several subtypes of incontinence, but the most common are 1) stress incontinence (the involuntary loss of urine due to an increase in intraabdominal pressure, such as coughing, laughing, or exercise); 2) urge incontinence (the involuntary loss of urine preceded by a strong urge to void whether or not the bladder is full); and 3) mixed incontinence (Melville et al. 2002).

Psychosocial Effects

Urinary incontinence may affect quality of life, sexual function, and mood. Recent studies have found that incontinence has a major negative effect on quality of life (Melville et al. 2002). A recent population-based, cross-sectional study of nearly 6,000 American women between ages 50 and 69 found that 16% reported mild, moderate, or severe incontinence. After adjustment for medical morbidity, functional status, and demographic variables, women with severe and mild-to-moderate incontinence were 80% and 40%, respectively, more likely to have depression than were continent women (Nygaard et al. 2003).

A study of more than 200 consecutive women with urinary incontinence found an overall prevalence of 16% for major depression and 7% for panic disorder. Patients with urge and mixed urinary incontinence were significantly more likely than those with stress incontinence to have a coexisting psychiatric illness. Comorbid major depression also has been found to have a significant effect on patients' urinary incontinence symptom reporting, incontinent-specific quality of life, and functional status (Melville et al. 2002).

A systematic review of the literature on sexual function in women with urinary incontinence (Shaw 2002) found that most studies were of poor quality. They concluded that further research in which standard definitions and measures of sexual impairment are used is needed to establish reliable information and prevalence estimates.

Role of the Psychiatrist

Given the high prevalence of incontinence, particularly in middle-aged and older women, and their frequent reluctance to disclose their symptoms, psychiatrists may wish to tactfully ask about urinary problems, as well as comorbid psychiatric conditions and adjustment problems.

TCAs and duloxetine, the new dual serotonin-norepinephrine reuptake inhibitor, are useful treatments for stress urinary incontinence, particularly in women who have concurrent depression (Norton et al. 2002). Treatments that have been used for urinary incontinence include behavioral training with or without biofeedback, pelvic floor exercises, other drug therapies, and surgery (Hendrix 2002).

Psychosomatic Obstetrics/Gynecology and Men

A woman's significant other may be female or male, but published studies of relationships' effects on obstetric and gynecological events have been performed on heterosexual couples. Virtually every study of the psychosocial aspects of an obstetric and gynecological event or treatment indicates that the attitude of the male partner is a (or the) major determinant of outcome. Women turn to their significant others for reaffirmation of their worthiness if infertile, for reaffirmation of their femininity after hysterectomy, and for help deciding whether to take psychotropic medications while pregnant and whether to breastfeed or bottle-feed. Failure to achieve consensus on such

decisions can cause serious long-term repercussions, as when a child is born with problems after (although not necessarily because of) the use of psychotropic medication during the mother's pregnancy, and the child's father blames the mother.

Fathers, brothers, sons, male partners, and husbands can be deeply affected by the obstetrical and gynecological experiences of the women they care about, but they often feel uncomfortable, ignored, and excluded when their female loved ones are receiving care (Abboud and Liamputtong 2003; Buist et al. 2003). As mentioned in the section on infertility, men and women may manifest their feelings differently. Women are more likely to show emotion and to want to talk to friends and relatives. Men are more likely to keep their emotions to themselves and to withdraw into work or other activities. Women can mistake this behavior for a failure to care. Men can feel that their presence only makes their loved ones cry. Sometimes, one of the most useful interventions a psychiatric consultant can perform is to facilitate communication within the family.

Conclusion

Obstetricians and gynecologists are busy practitioners, challenged to deal with both specialized technological developments and primary care, and burdened by the likelihood of lawsuits. Despite the intense emotional aspects of much of their clinical work, obstetricians and gynecologists have relatively little training or time for psychiatric problems. The scope of psychosomatic medicine in the area of obstetrics and gynecology includes psychopathological aspects of normal reproductive events, psychiatric aspects of obstetrical and gynecological diseases and treatments, and psychiatric conditions specific to women's reproductive health. Gender-based medicine, which intersects psychosomatic obstetrics and gynecology at many points, is one of the most exciting and promising areas of research and clinical practice. Myriad opportunities exist for providing practical assistance to obstetricians and gynecologists and the women who are their patients, for educating fellow psychiatrists about developments in obstetrics and gynecology, and for basic and clinical research.

References

Abboud LN, Liamputtong P: Pregnancy loss: what it means to women who miscarry and their partners. Soc Work Health Care 36:37–62, 2003

Abma JC, Chandra A, Mosher WD, et al: Fertility, family planning, and women's health: new data from the 1995 National Survey of Family Growth. Vital Health Stat 23(19):1–114, 1997

Adler NE, David HP, Major BN, et al: Psychological responses after abortion. Science 248:41–44, 1990

Altshuler L, Burt V, McMullen M, et al: Breastfeeding and sertraline: a 24-hour analysis. J Clin Psychiatry 56:243–245, 1995

Altshuler L, Cohen L, Szuba M, et al: Pharmacologic management of psychiatric illness during pregnancy: dilemmas and guidelines. Am J Psychiatry 153:592–606, 1996

Altshuler LL, Cohen LS, Moline ML, et al: The Expert Consensus Guideline Series. Treatment of depression in women. Postgrad Med (Spec No):1–107, 2001

American Academy of Pediatrics Committee on Drugs: Transfer of drugs and other chemicals into human milk. Pediatrics 108:776–789, 2001

American Psychiatric Association: Diagnostic and Statistical Manual of Mental Disorders, 4th Edition, Text Revision. Washington, DC, American Psychiatric Association, 2000

American Psychological Association: Research agenda for psychosocial and behavioral factors in women's health. Washington, DC, American Psychological Association, 1996

Appleby L, Warner R, Whitton A, et al: A controlled study of fluoxetine and cognitive-behavioral counseling in the treatment of postnatal depression. BMJ 314:932–936, 1997

Appleby L, Mortensen PB, Faragher EB: Suicide and other causes of mortality after post-partum psychiatric admission. Br J Psychiatry 173:209–211, 1998

Attia A, Downey J, Oberman M: Postpartum psychoses, in Postpartum Mood Disorders. Edited by Miller L. Washington, DC, American Psychiatric Press, 1999, pp 99–117

Avis NE: Depression during the menopausal transition. Psychol Women Q 27:91–100, 2003

Avis NE, McKinlay SM: The Massachusetts Women's Health Study: an epidemiologic investigation of the menopause. J Am Med Womens Assoc 50:45–49, 1995

Baram DA: Physiology and symptoms of menopause, in A Clinician's Guide to Menopause. Edited by Stewart DE, Robinson GE. Washington, DC, American Psychiatric Press, 1997, pp 9–27

Beutel M, Deckardt R, von Rad M, et al: Grief and depression after miscarriage: their separation, antecedents, and course. Psychosom Med 57:517–526, 1995

Bjorn I, Bixo M, Nojd K, et al: Negative mood changes during hormone replacement therapy: a comparison between two progestogens. Am J Obstet Gynecol 183:1419–1426, 2000

Bloch M, Daly RC, Rubinow DR: Endocrine factors in the etiology of postpartum depression. Compr Psychiatry 44:234–246, 2003

Bourne S, Lewis E: Delayed psychological effects of perinatal deaths: the next pregnancy and the next generation. BMJ 289:209–210, 1984

Brozovsky M, Falit H: Neonaticide: clinical and psychodynamic consideration. J Am Acad Child Psychiatry 10:673–683, 1971

Buist A, Morse CA, Durkin S: Men's adjustment to fatherhood: implications for obstetric health care. J Obstet Gynecol Neonatal Nurs 32:172–180, 2003

Burns L, Covington S: Psychology of infertility, in Infertility Counseling. Edited by Burns LH, Covington SN. Pearl River, NY, Parthenon, 1999, pp 3–25

Burns L, Greenfield D: Comprehensive psychosocial history for infertility (CPHI), in Clinical Handbook of Health Psychology. Edited by Camic P, Knight S. Seattle, WA, Hogrefe & Huber, 1991, pp 374–375

Castaneda DM, Collins BE: The effects of gender, ethnicity, and a close relationship theme on perceptions of persons introducing a condom. Sex Roles 39:369–390, 1998

Chabrol H, Teissedre F, Saint-Jean M, et al: Prevention and treatment of post-partum depression: a controlled randomized study of women at risk. Psychol Med 32:1039–1047, 2002

Chang MY, Chen SH, Chen CH: Factors related to perceived labor pain in primiparas. Kaohsiung J Med Sci 18:604–609, 2002

Chaudron LH, Jefferson JW: Mood stabilizers during breastfeeding: a review. J Clin Psychiatry 61:79–90, 2000

Chaudron LH, Pies RW: The relationship between postpartum psychosis and bipolar disorder: a review. J Clin Psychiatry 64:1284–1292, 2003

Chawla A, Swindle R, Long S, et al: Premenstrual dysphoric disorder: is there an economic burden of illness? Med Care 40:1101–1112, 2002

Cheung LH, Callaghan P, Chang AM: A controlled trial of psycho-educational interventions in preparing Chinese women for elective hysterectomy. Int J Nurs Stud 40:207–216, 2003

Chiriboga CA: Neurological correlates of fetal cocaine exposure. Ann N Y Acad Sci 846:109–125, 1998

Cohen LS, Sichel DA, Robertson LM, et al: Postpartum prophylaxis for women with bipolar disorder. Am J Psychiatry 152:1641–1645, 1995

Cooper N, Blackwell D, Taylor G, et al: Pharmacist's perceptions of nurse prescribing of emergency contraception. Br J Community Nurs 5:126–131, 2000

Cooper P, Murray L, Wilson A, et al: Controlled trial of the short- and long-term effect of psychological treatment of post-partum depression, I: impact on maternal mood. Br J Psychiatry 182:412–419, 2003

Cox H, Henderson L, Andersen N, et al: Focus group study of endometriosis: struggle, loss and the medical merry-go-round. Int J Nurs Pract 9:2–9, 2003

Cramer DW, Missmer SA: The epidemiology of endometriosis. Ann N Y Acad Sci 955:11–22, 2002

Crocker AR, Carlin EM: Coitarche and care: does experience of the "looked after" system affect timing of a woman's sexual debut? Int J STD AIDS 13:812–814, 2002

Cushman LF, Kalmuss K, Namerow PB: Placing an infant for adoption: the experience of young birth mothers. Soc Work 38:264–272, 1993

Czarnocka J, Slade P: Prevalence and predictors of posttraumatic stress symptoms following childbirth. Br J Clin Psychol 39:35–51, 2000

Dagg PKB: The psychological sequelae of therapeutic abortion: denied and completed. Am J Psychiatry 148:578–585, 1991

Davies A, McIvor RJ, Kumar C: Impact of childbirth on a series of schizophrenic mothers: a comment on the possible influence of oestrogen on schizophrenia. Schizophr Res 16:25–31, 1995

DelBanco SF, Mauldon J, Smith MD: Little knowledge and limited practice: emergency contraceptive pills, the public, and the obstetrician-gynecologist. Obstet Gynecol 89:1006–1011, 1997

Demyttenaere K, Nijs P, Steeno O, et al: Anxiety and conception rates in donor insemination. J Psychosom Obstet Gynaecol 8:175–181, 1988

Demyttenaere K, Bonte L, Gheldof M, et al: Coping style and depression level influence outcome in vitro fertilization. Fertil Steril 69:1026–1033, 1998

Dennis CL: The effect of peer support on postpartum depression: a pilot randomized controlled trial. Can J Psychiatry 48:115–124, 2003

Deuchar N: Nausea and vomiting in pregnancy: a review of the problem with particular regard to psychological and social aspects. Br J Obstet Gynecol 102:6–8, 1995

Deykin E, Campbell L, Patti P: The postadoptive experience of surrendering parents. Am J Orthopsychiatry 54:271–280, 1984

Domoney CL, Vashisht A, Studd JW: Use of complementary therapies by women attending a specialist premenstrual syndrome clinic. Gynecol Endocrinol 17:13–18, 2003

Edwards L: New concepts in vulvodynia. Am J Obstet Gynecol 189:S24–S30, 2003

Einarson A, Bonari L, Voyer-Lavigne S, et al: A multicentre prospective controlled study to determine the safety of trazodone and nefazodone use during pregnancy. Can J Psychiatry 48:106–110, 2003

Engelhard IM, van den Hout MA, Kindt M, et al: Peritraumatic dissociation and posttraumatic stress after pregnancy loss: a prospective study. Behav Res Ther 41:67–78, 2003

Farquhar CM, Steiner CA: Hysterectomy rates in the United States: 1990–1997. Obstet Gynecol 99:229–234, 2002

Farrell SA, Kieser K: Sexuality after hysterectomy. Obstet Gynecol 95:1045–1051, 2000

Finnegan P, McKinstry E, Robinsons GE: Denial of pregnancy and childbirth. Can J Psychiatry 27:672–674, 1982

Franzini LR, Sideman LM: Personality characteristics of condom users. J Sex Educ Ther 20:110–118, 1994

Fraser IS, Kovacs GT: The efficacy of non-contraceptive uses for hormonal contraceptives. Med J Aust 178:621–623, 2003

Free C, Lee RM, Ogden J: Young women's accounts of factors influencing their use and non-use of emergency contraception: in-depth interview study. BMJ 325:1393–1396, 2002

Freeman EW: Current update of hormonal and psychotropic drug treatment of premenstrual dysphoric disorder. Curr Psychiatry Rep 4:435–440, 2002

Freeman EW, Sammel MD, Liu L, et al: Hormones and menopausal status as predictors of depression in women in transition to menopause. Arch Gen Psychiatry 61:62–70, 2004

Friedman T, Gath D: The psychiatric consequences of spontaneous abortion. Br J Psychiatry 155:810–813, 1989

Fry R, Crisp A, Beard R: Sociopsychological factors in chronic pelvic pain: a review. J Psychosom Res 42:1–15, 1997

Fugh-Berman A, Kronenberg F: Complementary and alternative medicine (CAM) in reproductive-age women: a review of randomized controlled trials. Reprod Toxicol 17:137–152, 2003

Galavotti C, Richter DL: Talking about hysterectomy: the experiences of women from four cultural groups. J Womens Health Gend Based Med 9:S63–S67, 2000

Garg M, Singh M, Mansour D: Peri-abortion contraceptive care: can we reduce the incidence of repeat abortions? J Fam Plann Reprod Health Care 27:77–80, 2001

Gay D, Lynxwiler J: The impact of religiosity on race variations in abortion attitudes. Sociol Spectr 19:359–377, 1999

Gelbaya T, El-Halwagy E: Focus on primary care: chronic pelvic pain in women. Obstet Gynecol Surv 56:757–764, 2001

Gelberg L, Leake B, Lu MC, et al: Chronically homeless women's perceived deterrents to contraception. Perspect Sex Reprod Health 34:278–285, 2002

Gibson E: Homicide in England and Wales, 1967–1971. London, Pitman, 1982

Girman A, Lee R, Kligler B: An integrative medicine approach to premenstrual syndrome. Am J Obstet Gynecol 188 (suppl):S56–S65, 2003

Glasier AF, Smith KB, van der Spuy ZM, et al: Amenorrhea associated with contraception--an international study on acceptability. Contraception 67:1–8, 2003

Goldstein D, Corbin L, Sundell K: Effects of first-trimester fluoxetine exposure on the newborn. Obstet Gynecol 89:713–718, 1997

Grady-Weliky TA: Clinical practice: premenstrual dysphoric disorder. N Engl J Med 348:433–438, 2003

Greenfield SF, Sugarman DE: Treatment and consequences of alcohol abuse and dependence during pregnancy, in Management of Psychiatric Disorders During Pregnancy. Edited by Yonkers KA, Little B. London, Edward Arnold, 2001, pp 213–227

Groff JY, Mullen PD, Byrd T, et al: Decision making, beliefs, and attitudes toward hysterectomy: a focus group study with medically underserved women in Texas. J Womens Health Gend Based Med 9:S39–S50, 2000

Grote NK, Frank E: Difficult-to-treat depression: the role of contexts and comorbidities. Biol Psychiatry 53:660–670, 2003

Habek D, Habek JC, Barbir A: Using acupuncture to treat premenstrual syndrome. Arch Gynecol Obstet 267:23–26, 2002

Halbreich U, Bergeron R, Yonkers KA, et al: Efficacy of intermittent, luteal phase sertraline treatment of premenstrual dysphoric disorder. Obstet Gynecol 100:1219–1229, 2002

Harlow BL, Wise LA, Otto MW, et al: Depression and its influence on reproductive endocrine and menstrual cycle markers associated with perimenopause: the Harvard Study of Moods and Cycles. Arch Gen Psychiatry 60:29–36, 2003

Harris B, Oretti R, Lazarus J, et al: Randomised trial of thyroxine to prevent postnatal depression in thyroid-antibody-positive women. Br J Psychiatry 180:327–330, 2002

Harvey SM, Bird ST, Galavotti C, et al: Relationship power, sexual decision making and condom use among women at risk for HIV/STDS. Womens Health 36:69–84, 2002

Heikkinen T, Ekblad U, Kero P, et al: Citalopram in pregnancy and lactation. Clin Pharmacol Ther 72:184–191, 2002

Hendrick V, Altshuler L, Wertheimer A, et al: Venlafaxine and breast-feeding. Am J Psychiatry 158:2089–2090, 2001

Hendrick V, Smith L, Suri R, et al: Birth outcomes after prenatal exposure to antidepressant medication. Am J Obstet Gynecol 188:812–815, 2003

Hendrix S: Urinary incontinence and menopause: an evidence-based treatment approach. Dis Mon 48:622–636, 2002

Hillis SD, Marchbanks PA, Tylor LR, et al: Poststerilization regret: findings from the United States Collaborative Review of Sterilization. Obstet Gynecol 93:889–895, 1999

Hirshbein LD: Biology and mental illness: a historical perspective. J Am Med Womens Assoc 58:89–94, 2003

Hjelmstedt A, Andersson L, Skoog-Svanberg A, et al: Gender differences in psychological reactions to infertility among couples seeking IVF- and ICSI-treatment. Acta Obstet Gynecol Scand 78:42–48, 1999

Holditch-Davis D, Bartlett TR, Blickman AL, et al: Posttraumatic stress symptoms in mothers of premature infants. J Obstet Gynecol Neonatal Nurs 32:161–171, 2003

Howard F: Chronic pelvic pain. Obstet Gynecol 101:594–611, 2003

Hughes PM, Turton P, Evans CD: Stillbirth as risk factor for depression and anxiety in the subsequent pregnancy: cohort study. BMJ 318:1721–1724, 1999

Hunter MS: Somatic experience of the menopause: a prospective study. Psychosom Med 52:357–367, 1990

Hunter MS, Ussher JM, Browne SJ, et al: A randomized comparison of psychological (cognitive behavior therapy), medical (fluoxetine) and combined treatment for women with premenstrual dysphoric disorder. J Psychosom Obstet Gynaecol 23:193–199, 2002

Ilett K, Kristensen J, Hackett L, et al: Distribution of venlafaxine and its O-desmethyl metabolite in human milk and their effects in breastfed infants. Br J Clin Pharmacol 53:17–22, 2002

Jamieson DJ, Kaufman SC, Costello C, et al: U.S. Collaborative Review of Sterilization Working Group: a comparison of women's regret after vasectomy versus tubal sterilization. Obstet Gynecol 99:1073–1079, 2002

Janowsky DS, Rausch JL, Davis JM: Historical studies of premenstrual tension up to 30 years ago: implications for future research. Curr Psychiatry Rep 4:411–418, 2002

Jeal RR, West LA: Rolling away the stone: post-abortion women in the Christian community. J Pastoral Care Counsel 57:53–64, 2003

Johnson JK, Haider F, Ellis K, et al: The prevalence of domestic violence in pregnant women. BJOG 110:272–275, 2003

Kaewsarn P, Moyle W, Creedy D: Traditional postpartum practices among Thai women. J Adv Nurs 41:358–366, 2003

Kainz K: The role of the psychologist in the evaluation and treatment of infertility. Womens Health Issues 11:481–485, 2001

Kariminia A, Saunders DM, Chamberlain M: Risk factors for strong regret and subsequent IVF request after having tubal ligation. Aust N Z J Obstet Gynaecol 42:526–529, 2002

Kaufert PA, Gilbert P, Tate R: The Manitoba Project: a re-examination of the link between menopause and depression. Maturitas 14:143–155, 1992

Keye W: Medical aspects of infertility for the counselor, in Infertility Counseling. Edited by Burns LH, Covington SN. Pearl River, NY, Parthenon, 1999, pp 27–46

King R: Subfecundity and anxiety in a nationally representative sample. Soc Sci Med 56:739–751, 2003

Kjerulff KH, Langenberg PW, Rhodes JC, et al: Effectiveness of hysterectomy. Obstet Gynecol 95:319–326, 2000

Klock S: Obstetric and gynecological conditions, in Clinical Handbook of Health Psychology. Edited by Camic P, Knight S. Seattle, WA, Hogrefe & Huber, 1998, pp 349–388

Koniak-Griffin D, Lesser J, Uman G, et al: Teen pregnancy, motherhood, and unprotected sexual activity. Res Nurs Health 26:4–19, 2003

Koop CE: Surgeon General's report: the public health effects of abortion, 101st Cong., 1st sess. Congressional Record (March 21, 1989): E906–909

Kris E: Children of mothers maintained on pharmacotherapy during pregnancy and postpartum. Curr Ther Res Clin Exp 7:785–789, 1965

Kronenberg F, Fugh-Berman A: Complementary and alternative medicine for menopausal symptoms: a review of randomized, controlled trials. Ann Intern Med 137:805–813, 2002

Kubicka L, Roth Z, Dytrych Z, et al: The mental health of adults born of unwanted pregnancies, their siblings, and matched controls: a 35-year follow-up study from Prague, Czech Republic. J Nerv Ment Dis 190:653–662, 2002

Kulkarni J, Riedel A, de Castella AR, et al: Estrogen: a potential treatment for schizophrenia. Schizophr Res 48:137–144, 2001

Laird J: A male pill? Gender discrepancies in contraceptive commitment. Fem Psychol 4:458–468, 1994

Lande RG, Karamchandani V: Chronic mental illness and the menstrual cycle. J Am Osteopath Assoc 102:655–659, 2002

Landen M, Eriksson E: How does premenstrual dysphoric disorder relate to depression and anxiety disorders? Depress Anxiety 17:122–129, 2003

Lane T, Francis A: Premenstrual symptomatology, locus of control, anxiety and depression in women with normal menstrual cycles. Arch Women Ment Health 6:127–138, 2003

Lee DT, Yip AS, Chan SS, et al: Postdelivery screening for postpartum depression. Psychosom Med 65:357–361, 2003

Lefebvre G, Allaire C, Jeffrey J, et al: SOGC clinical guidelines: hysterectomy. J Obstet Gynaecol Can 24:37–61, 2002

Lewis CL, Groff JY, Herman CJ, et al: Overview of women's decision making regarding elective hysterectomy, oophorectomy, and hormone replacement therapy. J Womens Health Gend Based Med 9:S5–S14, 2000

Loprinzi CL, Kugler JW, Sloan JA, et al: Venlafaxine in management of hot flashes in survivors of breast cancer: a randomised controlled trial. Lancet 356:2059–2063, 2000

Loprinzi CL, Sloan JA, Perez EA, et al: Phase III evaluation of fluoxetine for treatment of hot flashes. J Clin Oncol 20:1578–1583, 2002

Lu PY, Ory SJ: Endometriosis: current management. Mayo Clin Proc 70:453–463, 1995

Lukse M, Vacc N: Grief, depression, and coping in women undergoing fertility treatment. Obstet Gynecol 93:245–251, 1999

Majerus PW, Guze SB, Delong WB, et al: Psychologic factors and psychiatric disease in hyperemesis gravidarum: a follow-up study of 69 vomiters and 66 controls. Am J Psychiatry 117:421–428, 1960

Mantle F: Developing a culture-specific tool to assess postnatal depression in the Indian community. Br J Community Nurs 8:176–180, 2003

Marcus S, Barry K, Flynn H, et al: Treatment guidelines for depression in pregnancy. Int J Obstet Gynecol 71:61–70, 2001

Mathias S, Kuppermann M, Liberman R, et al: Chronic pelvic pain: prevalence, health-related quality of life, and economic correlates. Obstet Gynecol 87:321–327, 1996

Matthey S, Barnett B, Howie P, et al: Diagnosing postpartum depression in mothers and fathers: whatever happened to anxiety? J Affect Disord 74:139–147, 2003a

Matthey S, Barnett B, White T: The Edinburgh Postnatal Depression Scale. Br J Psychiatry 182:368–370, 2003b

Melville J, Walker E, Katon W, et al: Prevalence of comorbid psychiatric illness and its impact on symptom perception, quality of life, and functional status in women with urinary incontinence Am J Obstet Gynecol 187:80–87, 2002

Miller LJ: Psychotic denial of pregnancy: phenomenology and clinical management. Hosp Community Psychiatry 41:1233–1237, 1990

Miller LJ, Finnerty J: Sexuality, pregnancy and childrearing among women with schizophrenia-spectrum disorders. Psychiatr Serv 47:502–506, 1996

Miller LJ, Rukstalis M: Beyond the "blues": hypotheses about postpartum reactivity, in Postpartum Mood Disorders. Edited by Miller LJ. Washington, DC, American Psychiatric Press, 1999, pp 3–19

Miller MN, Miller BE: Premenstrual exacerbations of mood disorders. Psychopharmacol Bull 35:135–149, 2001

Mingo C, Herman CJ, Jasperse M: Women's stories: ethnic variations in women's attitudes and experiences of menopause, hysterectomy, and hormone replacement therapy. J Womens Health Gend Based Med 9:S27–S38, 2000

Moore J, Kennedy S: Causes of chronic pelvic pain. Baillieres Best Pract Res Clin Obstet Gynaecol 14:389–402, 2001

Morris-Rush JK, Freda MC, Bernstein PS: Screening for postpartum depression in an inner-city population. Am J Obstet Gynecol 188:1217–1219, 2003

Muqtadar S, Hamann MW, Molnar G: Management of psychotic pregnant patients in a medical-psychiatric unit. Psychosomatics 27:31–33, 1986

Murray L, Cooper P, Wilson A, et al: Controlled trial of the short- and long-term effect of psychological treatment of post-partum depression, 2: impact on the mother-child relationship and child outcome. Br J Psychiatry 182:420–427, 2003

Newton J, McCormack J: Female sterilization: a review of methods, morbidity, failure rates and medicolegal aspects. Contemp Rev Obstet Gynaecol 2:176–182, 1990

Neziroglu F, Anemone R, Yaryura-Tobias JA: Onset of obsessive-compulsive disorder in pregnancy. Am J Psychiatry 149:947–950, 1992

Norton P, Zinner N, Yalcin, I, et al: Duloxetine versus placebo in the treatment of stress urinary incontinence. Am J Obstet Gynecol 187:40–48, 2002

Nulman I, Rovet J, Stewart D, et al: Child development following exposure to tricyclic antidepressants or fluoxetine throughout fetal life: a prospective, controlled study. Am J Psychiatry 159:1889–1895, 2002

Nygaard I, Turvey C, Burns T, et al: Urinary incontinence and depression in middle-aged United States women. Obstet Gynecol 101:149–156, 2003

O'Brien B, Newton N: Psyche versus soma: historical evolution of beliefs about nausea and vomiting during pregnancy. J Psychosom Obstet Gynaecol 12:91–120, 1991

O'Hara MW, Stuart S, Gorman LL, et al: Efficacy of interpersonal psychotherapy for postpartum depression. Arch Gen Psychiatry 57:1039–1045, 2000

Oretti RG, Harris B, Lazarus JH, et al: Is there an association between life events, postnatal depression and thyroid dysfunction in thyroid antibody positive women? Int J Soc Psychiatry 49:70–76, 2003

Paffenbarger RS: Epidemiological aspects of mental illness associated with childbearing, in Motherhood and Mental Illness. Edited by Brockington IF, Kumar R. London, Academic Press, 1982, pp 19–36

Pati S, Cullins V: Female sterilization: evidence. Obstet Gynecol Clin North Am 27:859–899, 2000

Patton S, Misri S, Corral M, et al: Antipsychotic medication during pregnancy and lactation in women with schizophrenia: evaluating the risk. Can J Psychiatry 47:959–965, 2002

Pearlstein T, Joliat MJ, Brown EB, et al: Recurrence of symptoms of premenstrual dysphoric disorder after the cessation of luteal-phase fluoxetine treatment. Am J Obstet Gynecol 188:887–895, 2003

Picardo CM, Nichols M, Edelman A, et al: Women's knowledge and sources of information on the risks and benefits of oral contraception. J Am Med Womens Assoc 58:112–116, 2003

Price J, Blake F: Chronic pelvic pain: the assessment as therapy. J Psychosom Res 46:7–14, 1999

Pro-Life Action Ministries: What They Won't Tell You at the Abortion Clinic (flyer). St. Paul, MN, Pro-Life Action Ministries, undated

Rapp SR, Espeland MA, Shumaker SA, et al: Effect of estrogen plus progestin on global cognitive function in postmenopausal women. The Women's Health Initiative Memory Study: a randomized controlled trial. JAMA 289:2663–2672, 2003

Reardon DC, Cougle JR, Rue VM, et al: Psychiatric admissions of low-income women following abortion and childbirth. CMAJ 168:1253–1256, 2003

Reiter R: Evidence-based management of chronic pelvic pain. Clin Obstet Gynecol 41:422–435, 1998

Rhodes JC, Kjerulff KH, Langenberg PW, et al: Hysterectomy and sexual functioning. JAMA 282:1934–1941, 1999

Richter DL, McKeown RE, Corwin SJ, et al: The role of male partners in women's decision making regarding hysterectomy. J Womens Health Gend Based Med 9:S51–S61, 2000

Rickert VI, Wiemann CM, Harrykissoon SD, et al: The relationship among demographics, reproductive characteristics, and intimate partner violence. Am J Obstet Gynecol 187:1002–1007, 2002

Riordan D, Appleby L, Faragher B: Mother-infant interaction in post-partum women with schizophrenia and affective disorders. J Psychol Med 29:991–995, 1999

Roe B, Doll H, Wilson K: Help seeking behaviour and health and social services utilization by people suffering from urinary incontinence. Int J Nurs Stud 36:245–253, 1999

Rosch DS, Sajatovic M, Sivec H: Behavioral characteristics in delusional pregnancy: a matched control group study. Int J Psychiatry Med 32:295–303, 2002

Ross LE, Gilbert Evans SE, Sellers EM, et al: Measurement issues in postpartum depression part 1: anxiety as a feature of postpartum depression. Arch Womens Ment Health 6:51–57, 2003

Rynearson E: Relinquishment and its maternal complications: a preliminary study. Am J Psychiatry 139:338–340, 1982

Saisto T, Halmesmaki E: Fear of childbirth: a neglected dilemma. Acta Obstet Gynecol Scand 82:201–208, 2003

Sakumoto K, Masamoto H, Kanazawa K: Post-partum maternity "blues" as a reflection of newborn nursing care in Japan. Int J Gynaecol Obstet 78:25–30, 2002

Saltzman LE, Johnson CH, Gilbert BC, et al: Physical abuse around the time of pregnancy: an examination of prevalence and risk factors in 16 states. Matern Child Health J 7:31–43, 2003

Sampalis F, Bunea R, Pelland MF, et al: Evaluation of the effects of Neptune Krill Oil on the management of premenstrual syndrome and dysmenorrhea. Altern Med Rev 8:171–179, 2003

Sanders SA, Graham CA, Yarber WL, et al: Condom use errors and problems among young women who put condoms on their male partners. J Am Med Womens Assoc 58:95–98, 2003

Savidge C, Slade P: Psychological aspects of chronic pelvic pain. J Psychosom Res 42:433–444, 1997

Schatzberg AF, Cole JO, DeBattista C: Manual of Clinical Psychology, 4th Edition. Washington, DC, American Psychiatric Publishing, 2003

Schmidt P, Nieman L, Danaceau M, et al: Estrogen replacement in perimenopause-related depression: a preliminary report. Am J Obstet Gynecol 183:414–420, 2000

Schneider LS, Small GW, Hamilton SH, et al: Estrogen replacement and response to fluoxetine in a multicenter geriatric depression trial: Fluoxetine Collaborative Study Group. Am J Geriatr Psychiatry 5:97–106, 1997

Seeman MV: Does menopause intensify symptoms in schizophrenia? in Psychiatric Illness in Women: Emerging Treatments and Research. Edited by Lewis-Hall F, Williams TS, Panetta J, et al. Washington, DC, American Psychiatric Publishing, 2002, pp 239–248

Shane-McWhorter L, Cerveny JD, MacFarlane LL, et al: Enhanced metabolism of levonorgestrel during phenobarbital treatment and resultant pregnancy. Pharmacotherapy 18:1360–1365, 1998

Shaw C: A systematic review of the literature on the prevalence of sexual impairment in women with urinary incontinence and the prevalence of urinary leakage during sexual activity. Eur Urol 42:432–440, 2002

Shumaker SA, Legault C, Rapp SR, et al: Estrogen plus progestin and the incidence of dementia and mild cognitive impairment in postmenopausal women. The Women's Health Initiative Memory Study: a randomized controlled trial. JAMA 289:2651–2662, 2003

Slade P, Heke S, Fletcher J, et al: Termination of pregnancy: patients' perceptions of care. J Fam Plann Reprod Health Care 27:72–77, 2001

Smith MJ, Schmidt PJ, Rubinow DR: Operationalizing DSM-IV criteria for PMDD: selecting symptomatic and asymptomatic cycles for research. J Psychiatr Res 37:75–83, 2003

Soares CN, Almeida OP, Joffe H, et al: Efficacy of estradiol for the treatment of depressive disorders in perimenopausal women: a double-blind, randomized, placebo-controlled trial. Arch Gen Psychiatry 58:529–534, 2001

Spielvogel AM, Hohener HC: Denial of pregnancy: a review and case reports. Birth 22:220–226, 1995

Spinelli M: Interpersonal psychotherapy for depressed antepartum women: a pilot study. Am J Psychiatry 154:1028–1030, 1997

Spinelli MG, Endicott J: Controlled clinical trial of interpersonal psychotherapy versus parenting education program for depressed pregnant women. Am J Psychiatry 160:555–562, 2003

Stahl SM: Effects of estrogen on the central nervous system. J Clin Psychiatry 62:317–318, 2001

Stearns V, Isaacs C, Rowland J, et al: A pilot trial assessing the efficacy of paroxetine hydrochloride (Paxil) in controlling hot flashes in breast cancer survivors. Ann Oncol 11:17–22, 2000

Steiner M, Brown E, Trzepacz P, et al: Fluoxetine improves functional work capacity in women with premenstrual dysphoric disorder. Arch Womens Ment Health 6:71–77, 2003

Stewart DE: Antidepressant drugs during pregnancy and lactation. Int Clin Psychopharmacol 15 (suppl 3):S19–S24, 2001

Stewart DE, Boydell KM: Psychologic distress during menopause: associations across the reproductive life cycle. Int J Psychiatry Med 23:157–162, 1993

Stewart DE, Robinson G: Eating disorders and reproduction, in Psychological Aspects of Women's Health Care: The Interface Between Psychiatry and Obstetrics and Gynecology, 2nd Edition. Edited by Stotland N, Stewart D. Washington, DC, American Psychiatric Press, 2001a, pp 441–456

Stewart DE, Robinson G: Psychotropic drugs and electroconvulsive therapy during pregnancy and lactation, in Psychological Aspects of Women's Health Care: The Interface Between Psychiatry and Obstetrics and Gynecology, 2nd Edition. Edited by Stotland N, Stewart D. Washington, DC, American Psychiatric Press, 2001b, pp 67–93

Stewart DE, Robinson G, Goldbloom D, et al: Infertility and eating disorders. Am J Obstet Gynecol 163:1196–1199, 1990

Stewart DE, Reicher AE, Gerulath AH, et al: Vulvodynia and psychological distress. Obstet Gynecol 84:587–590, 1994

Stewart DE, Leyland NA, Shime J, et al: Achieving Best Practices in the Use of Hysterectomy: Report of Ontario's Expert Panel on Best Practices in the Use of Hysterectomy. Ontario, Canada, Ontario Women's Health Council, 2002

Stiskal J, Kulin N, Koren G, et al: Neonatal paroxetine withdrawal syndrome. Arch Dis Child Fetal Neonatal Ed 84: F134–F135, 2001

Stoppe G, Doren M: Critical appraisal of effects of estrogen replacement therapy on symptoms of depressed mood. Arch Womens Ment Health 5:39–47, 2002

Sveinsdottir H, Lundman B, Norberg A: Whose voice? Whose experiences? Women's qualitative accounts of general and private discussion of premenstrual syndrome. Scand J Caring Sci 16:414–423, 2002

Terp IM, Mortensen PB: Post-partum psychoses: clinical diagnoses and relative risk of admission after parturition. Br J Psychiatry 172:521–526, 1998

Thorp JM Jr, Hartmann KE, Shadigian E: Long-term physical and psychological health consequences of induced abortion: review of the evidence. Obstet Gynecol Surv 58:67–79, 2003

Thys-Jacobs S, Starkey P, Bernstein D, et al: Calcium carbonate and the premenstrual syndrome: effects on premenstrual and menstrual symptoms. Premenstrual Syndrome Study Group. Am J Obstet Gynecol 179:444–452, 1998

Tice JA, Ettinger B, Ensrud K, et al: Phytoestrogen supplements for the treatment of hot flashes: the Isoflavone Clover Extract (ICE) Study: a randomized controlled trial. JAMA 290:207–214, 2003

Torres A, Forrest JD: Why do women have abortions? Fam Plann Perspect 20:169–176, 1988

Turton P, Hughes P, Evans CD, et al: Incidence, correlates and predictors of post-traumatic stress disorder in the pregnancy after stillbirth. Br J Psychiatry 178:556–560, 2001

Upchurch DM, Kusunoki Y, Simon P, et al: Sexual behavior and condom practices among Los Angeles women. Womens Health Issues 13:8–15, 2003

U.S. Food and Drug Administration: Current categories for drug use in pregnancy. Available at: http://www.fda.gov/fdac/features/2001/301_preg.html. Accessed September 3, 2003

Uskul AK, Ahmad F, Leyland NA, et al: Women's hysterectomy experiences and decision-making. Women Health 38:53–67, 2003

Ventura SJ, Mosher WD, Curtin SC, et al: Trends in pregnancies and pregnancy rates by outcome: estimates for the United States 1976–96. Vital Health Stat 21:1–47, 2000

Vigod SN, Stewart DE: The management of abnormal uterine bleeding by northern, rural and isolated primary care physicians, part II: what do we need? BMC Womens Health 2:11, 2002

Viguera AC, Cohen LS, Baldessarini RJ, et al: Managing bipolar disorder during pregnancy: weighing the risks and benefits. Can J Psychiatry 47:426–436, 2002

Warnock JK, Bundren JC, Morris DW: Sertraline in the treatment of depression associated with gonadotropin-releasing hormone agonist therapy. Biol Psychiatry 43:464–465, 1998

Weaver S, Clifford E, Hay D, et al: Psychosocial adjustment to unsuccessful IVF and GFT treatment. Patient Educ Couns 31:7–18, 1997

Wessel J, Endrikat J, Buscher U: Frequency of denial of pregnancy: results and epidemiological significance of a 1-year prospective study in Berlin. Acta Obstet Gynecol Scand 81:1021–1027, 2002

Westhoff C, Picardo L, Morrow E: Quality of life following early medical or surgical abortion. Contraception 67:41–47, 2003

Whelan CI, Stewart DE: Pseudocyesis: a review and report of six cases. Int J Psychiatry Med 20:97–108, 1990

Williams RD, Clark AJ: A qualitative study of women's hysterectomy experience. J Womens Health Gend Based Med 9:S15–S25, 2000

Wisner K, Findling R, Perel J: Paroxetine in breast milk. Am J Psychiatry 158:144–145, 2001

Wisner K, Gelenberg A, Leonard H, et al: Pharmacologic treatment of depression during pregnancy. JAMA 282:1264–1269, 2002a

Wisner KL, Parry BL, Piontek CM: Postpartum depression. N Engl J Med 347:194–199, 2002b

Women's Health Initiative Steering Committee: Effects of conjugated equine estrogen in postmenopausal women with hysterectomy: the Women's Health Initiative randomized controlled trial. JAMA 291:1701–1712, 2004

World Health Organization Programme of Maternal and Child Health and Family Planning Unit: Infertility: a tabulation of available data on prevalence of primary and secondary infertility (WHO/MCM/91.9). 1991. Available at: http://www.who.int/reproductive-health/publications/Abstracts/infertility.html

Writing Group for the Women's Health Initiative Investigators: Risks and benefits of estrogen plus progestin in healthy post-menopausal women: principal results from the Women's Health Initiative randomized controlled trial. JAMA 288: 321–333, 2002

Wyatt KM, Dimmock PW, O'Brien PM: Selective serotonin reuptake inhibitors for premenstrual syndrome. Cochrane Database Syst Rev 4:CD001396, 2002

Zabin LS, Hirsch MB, Emerson MR: When urban adolescents choose abortion: effects on education, psychological status, and subsequent pregnancy. Fam Plann Perspect 21:248–255, 1989

Zeskind PS, Stephens LE: Maternal selective serotonin reuptake inhibitor use during pregnancy and newborn neuro-behavior. Pediatrics 113:368–375, 2004

Zlokovich MS, Snell WE Jr: Contraceptive behavior and efficacy: the influence of illusion of fertility control and adult attachment tendencies. J Psychol Human Sex 9:39–55, 1997

Zlotogora J: Parental decisions to abort or continue a pregnancy with an abnormal finding after an invasive prenatal test. Prenat Diagn 22:1102–1106, 2002

Zondervan K, Yudkin P, Vessey M, et al: Patterns of diagnosis and referral in women consulting for chronic pelvic pain in UK primary care. Br J Obstet Gynecol 106:1149–1155, 1999

34 Pediatrics

Brenda Bursch, Ph.D.

Margaret Stuber, M.D.

IN THIS CHAPTER, we provide a brief overview of the major issues in psychiatric or psychological consultation to pediatrics. (For pediatric topics discussed elsewhere in this book, see Chapter 14, "Deception Syndromes: Factitious Disorders and Malingering"; Chapter 15, "Eating Disorders"; Chapter 29, "Dermatology"; and Chapter 30, "Surgery"). Many of the issues addressed in pediatrics are similar to those seen with adults. However, because the relative importance of development and of the family is sufficiently different in pediatrics as opposed to working with adults, these issues should be considered at the start of any evaluation, and they infuse every intervention and recommendation.

General Principles in Evaluation and Management

Children's Developmental Understanding of Illness and Their Bodies

Children's conceptions of their bodies vary widely and are obviously influenced by experiences with illness. However, in general, children appear to follow a developmental path of understanding their bodies that roughly corresponds to Piaget's stages of cognitive development. *Sensorimotor children* (birth to approximately 2 years) are largely preverbal and do not have the capacity to create narratives to explain their experiences. Their perception of their bodies and of illness is therefore primarily built on sensory experiences and does not involve any formal reasoning. *Preoperational children* (approximately 2–7 years) also understand through perception, but they are able to use words and some very basic concepts of cause and effect. They tend to be most aware of parts of the body that they can directly sense, such as bones and heart (which

they can feel), and blood (which they have seen come out of their bodies). However, they do not have a clear sense of cause and effect and are therefore inclined to see events that are temporally related as causally related. They also have no real sense of organs, but conceptualize blood and food as going into or coming out of their bodies as though the body were itself the container. This leads to many humorous but confusing assumptions and misunderstandings. *Concrete operational children* (approximately 7–11 years) are able to apply logic to their perceptions in a more integrative manner. However, the logic is quite literal or concrete and allows for only one cause for an effect. They tend to be eager to learn factual information about the body and illness at this age, but will have difficulty with any concepts that require abstract reasoning. *Formal operational children* (11+ years) are able to use a level of abstract reasoning that allows discussion of systems rather than simple organs and can incorporate multiple causation of illness. It should not be assumed, however, that all adolescents approach the understanding of illness and their bodies at this level of cognition. In fact, most adults function at this level of thought only in areas of their own expertise, if at all.

As with all areas of cognition, education and experience make a difference. Children who have a medical problem (or who have a friend or family member with a medical history) may know more about the body and its function than other children. However, children will also often be able to repeat what has been said to them without any real understanding of what it means. It is always important to assess children's level of understanding by asking them to explain in their own words or give their own version of why something is happening. This can alert you and the treating team to gross misunderstandings or fears that could influence adherence to the treatment plan.

761

Family Systems

No pediatric patient can be considered in isolation from his or her family. Parents are the ones to whom children look to understand the world. It is from their reactions to the illness and the treatment that the child determines how dangerous this is and how to respond. Parents are also the legal decision makers for the child, and thus are involved in all aspects of his or her care. Parental helplessness, anger, or withdrawal is important to address. In the sections that follow, we review the role and impact of the parent as an integral aspect of care of the pediatric patient.

Psychiatric Issues

Psychological Responses to Illness

Psychological distress in response to serious pediatric illness has been a focus of many disease-specific and noncategorical studies over the years. Often symptoms of depression, anxiety, and behavioral problems are grouped together. For example, a recent review of empirical studies of pediatric heart transplant recipients found that 20%–24% of these children experienced significant problems of psychological distress (Todaro et al. 2000). A study of children with epilepsy, using the State Trait Anxiety Inventory and the Children's Depression Inventory (Oguz et al. 2002), found that the epileptic children reported significantly more depressed and anxious symptoms than a control group. Even in children undergoing a surgical procedure as minor as a tonsillectomy, 17% of 89 children followed prospectively had temporary symptoms consistent with a depressive episode (Papakostas et al. 2003). In some cases, the effects can be longer lasting, as was found in a study of 5,736 childhood cancer survivors, studied as young adults, who reported significantly more symptoms of depression than their sibling controls (Zebrack et al. 2002). The symptoms assessed in most of these cases would not necessarily meet criteria for a DSM diagnosis. However, these symptoms do appear to be associated with decrease in function. For example, the type of depression that is seen in association with chronic pain of various etiologies has been found to be strongly associated with functional disability (Kashikar-Zuck et al. 2001).

Social support appears to be a key element in psychological adjustment to illness. Social support was found to negatively correlate with problem behavior in adolescents with HIV over a period of 3 years (Battles and Wiener 2002). In a study of 160 pediatric rheumatology patients, children with higher classmate support had lower levels of depression (von Weiss et al. 2002). Depressed parents of chronically ill children have been found to have depressed children (Williamson et al. 2002). Social support has medical implications as well. For example, families that are less caring or are in more conflict are associated with poorer metabolic control of children with juvenile-onset diabetes (Schiffrin 2001). Recent studies have shown that serious pediatric illness or treatment may also lead to chronic as well as acute symptoms of emotional distress in the parents, which may interfere with their ability to provide support for the children. This has been found with pediatric cancer patients (Kazak et al. 1997) and pediatric transplant recipients (Young et al. 2003).

In some cases, psychological distress and behavioral problems can be directly caused by physical manifestations of the illness or the treatment. For example, mood disorders and anxiety are relatively common manifestations of involvement of the central nervous system (CNS) in pediatric systemic lupus erythematosus (Sibbitt et al. 2002). Depression, anxiety, aggression, and school problems are observed as side effects of tacrolimus, given to prevent rejection of a transplanted kidney (Kemper et al. 2003). Use of steroids for inflammatory conditions, such as rheumatoid arthritis, can have significant impact on mood (Klein-Gitelman and Pachman 1998). Treatment of behavioral distress, depression, or anxiety in juvenile-onset diabetes mellitus must always consider the agitation that is symptomatic of hypoglycemia or the confusion associated with hyperglycemia (Goodnick et al. 1995).

Because psychological adjustment problems appear to be relatively common, it is recommended that children who are chronically ill, acutely ill, or injured be screened by pediatricians for depression, anxiety, and behavioral disturbance (Borowsky et al. 2003). Preventive programs are indicated for some pediatric inpatient services in which anxiety and depression are common. For example, in chronic, painful treatment situations, such as pediatric burns, where significant emotional distress is the norm, anxiety treatment programs are best built-in along with pain management programs (Sheridan et al. 1997; Stoddard and Saxe 2001). There is some evidence that this may help prevent development of posttraumatic stress disorder (PTSD) (see Saxe et al. 1998; Stoddard and Saxe 2001). In treatments with high mortality, such as bone marrow transplantation, in which different phases of treatment appear to have varying levels of depression or anxiety associated with them (Robb and Ebberts, 2003), consistent psychosocial support should be available from the start.

Effective treatment for anxiety that persists after normal adjustment and comfort issues are addressed is similar to that provided in general psychiatric practice: cognitive-behavioral therapy (Kendall 1994; Ollendick and King 1998) and the use of selective serotonin reuptake inhibitors (SSRIs) (The Research Unit on Pediatric Psychopharmacology Anxiety Study Group 2001). Individual behavioral techniques, such as exposure and systematic desensitization, can be effective for patients with simple phobias such as needle phobia or food aversion. More extensive cognitive-behavioral treatment packages that address anxiety across many dimensions (including somatic, cognitive, and behavioral problems) are indicated for children with more complex anxiety disorders (Piacentini and Bergman 2001).

Pediatricians are familiar with the use of stimulants and some antidepressants in their practice (Efron et al. 2003), but there is yet a limited literature on the use of these medications in medically ill children. The strongest research effort in child psychiatry on effective medication treatments for depression and anxiety has been with SSRIs. In a five-center trial, fluvoxamine was superior to placebo in treating patients with separation anxiety disorder, social anxiety disorder, or generalized anxiety disorder (The Research Unit on Pediatric Psychopharmacology Anxiety Study Group 2001). Additionally, fluoxetine has been found to be effective for childhood obsessive-compulsive disorder (Liebowitz et al. 2002). Strong evidence does not exist to support the use of tricyclic antidepressants or benzodiazepines as a first-line treatment for child anxiety disorders (Riddle et al. 1999). Despite a lack of supporting data, low doses of benzodiazepines are frequently prescribed by pediatricians for acute anxiety or agitation in the hospital because they can have a more immediate effect than SSRIs. Therefore, it is important to note that some anxious children have agitated reactions to benzodiazepines. Psychiatric consultants can offer alternatives, including neuroleptics in cases where immediate response is necessary.

Because hospitalized and chronically ill children often experience many of the symptoms seen in depression, making a decision as to whether a pediatric patient should be treated for depression can be difficult. A depressed or irritable mood, diminished interest or pleasure in activities, significant weight loss or change in appetite, insomnia or hypersomnia, psychomotor agitation or retardation, and fatigue or loss of energy may be secondary to the medical condition or to prolonged separation from friends and family. Although medication may be indicated, often supportive and behavioral interventions can lead to significant improvements for such symptoms. Less common, and thus more concerning, are feelings of worthlessness or inappropriate guilt, diminished ability to think or concentrate, or thoughts of suicide (Goldston 1994). A care-

ful assessment is necessary, including suicidal fantasies or actions, concepts of what the child thinks would happen if suicide was attempted or achieved, previous experiences with suicidal behavior, circumstances at the time of the suicidal behavior, motivations for suicide, concepts and experiences of death, family situations, and environmental situations (Pfeffer 1986). Adolescents with suicidal intent and plan, family history of suicide, a comorbid psychiatric disorder, intractable pain, persistent insomnia, lack of social support, inadequate coping skills, a recent improvement in depressive symptoms, or impulsivity are at particular risk for suicide. Antidepressant medication should be started carefully in such cases. For some adolescents, the idea of suicide is an important source of control in the face of an unknown and uncontrollable illness course. Addressing a lack of perceived control, isolation, and distressing physical symptoms should be a high priority.

Adherence

The term *adherence* is generally used to describe the extent to which a patient's health behavior is consistent with medical recommendations. Defined as such, adherence would include not only the taking of medications and attendance at clinical appointments but also diet, exercise, and other lifestyle issues such as smoking and use of sunscreen (Lemanek et al. 2001). Adherence is measured using blood levels, pill counts, and self-report, all of which are problematic (Du Pasquier-Fediaevsky and Tubiana-Rufi 1999; Shemesh et al. 2004). With such a wide definition, and different assessment strategies, the estimates vary as to the number of pediatric patients who adhere to medical regimens for chronic conditions (Rapoff 1999; Steele and Grauer 2003). Despite these problems, there is general agreement that nonadherence with medication regimens is a serious problem in pediatric patients with both acute and chronic conditions, resulting in significant clinical morbidity (Bauman et al. 2002; DiMatteo et al. 2002; Phipps and DeCuir-Whalley 1990; Serrano-Ikkos 1998).

Many variables have been cited as potential predictors of nonadherence. Increasing age of the child is correlated with increased nonadherence, as is longer time on treatment and lack of appropriate family support in most studies across a variety of illnesses (Griffin and Elkin 2001; Lurie et al. 2000; Rapoff et al. 2002; Strunk et al. 2002). The patient's health beliefs regarding barriers to care, severity of the illness, and susceptibility to problems have been found to be related to nonadherence in some studies (Soliday and Hoeksel 2000), whereas other studies have found that parental health beliefs did not predict adherence (Steele et al. 2001). Some investigations have suggested that cultural beliefs may be equally or more important (Tucker et al. 2002; Snodgrass et al. 2001). Although lack of knowledge would seem to be an important predictor, this has proven more difficult to measure than might be expected (Ho et al. 2003; McQuaid 2003). Although one study actually found that mild anxiety was associated with better adherence (Strunk et al. 2002), others suggest that psychological distress is associated with nonadherence (Simoni et al. 1997)

Interventions to increase adherence have fallen under the general categories of educational (written and verbal instructions), organizational (simplification of regimens, improving access, increased supervision), and behavioral (reminders, incentives, and self-monitoring). A recent review of published studies of interventions to improve adherence found that different strategies appear to be more effective than others for specific illnesses. Although cognitive-behavioral approaches appear promising, no interventions have been found to meet criteria to be considered "well-established" for improving adherence in asthma, juvenile rheumatoid arthritis, or type 1 diabetes (Lemanek et al. 2001). A provocative pilot study found that treating liver transplant recipients for PTSD improved adherence to medication (Shemesh et al. 2000).

Death, Dying, and Bereavement

One of the most difficult issues for anyone to cope with is the death of a child (Field et al. 2003). Because of the tremendous advances in medicine over the past 20 years and the seeming unfairness of death in childhood, pediatricians and families often resist making the transition from an emphasis on cure to a focus on comfort care. The psychiatric consultant is often called when there is disagreement within the team or between the team and the family about whether this point has been reached or about how this transition is to be approached. Sometimes these differences are the result of cultural or philosophical differences. Physicians who believe that life is to be pursued at all costs may have trouble understanding the feelings of nurses who feel that the child is being needlessly subjected to painful interventions. Families who are deeply religious and remain hopeful for a miracle may lead the medical team to request a psychiatric consult to address the family's "denial." Family members who wish to protect the child may feel that it is best to withhold information about disease prognosis or other potentially upsetting information. The psychiatric consultant can serve as the interpreter and facilitate these often highly emotionally charged discussions to allow the individuals to understand one another well enough to plan together for the care of the child.

Although depression, withdrawal, and anxiety may be expected, a variety of emotional responses may be seen in terminally ill children and should be anticipated in conversations with parents. Children and adolescents may manifest their confusion and loss by negative, oppositional, aggressive, or emotional acting out, as well as with apathy and withdrawal from family and friends. They may frighten the medical staff or family as they talk about death or carry on conversations with someone who has died or with God. They may seem to know when they are going to die or "take a trip." What may initially appear to be confusion or delirium may actually be an attempt to communicate through a metaphor (Callanan and Kelley 1992). The approach of the consultant should be to allow such conversations to occur, and to support the staff and parents to tolerate these attempts of the child to cope with the process of dying. Play therapy or art therapy may be particularly helpful for younger children and for older children who prefer these modalities. In some cases, children will choose to specifically address unfinished business, such as saying good-bye, making amends, being absolved of perceived transgressions, planning their memorial service, or deciding who gets particular belongings (Gyulay 1989). Environmental interventions can relieve many physical discomforts. Interventions to improve communication and understanding can relieve many emotional discomforts and fears. If such interventions are not sufficient to resolve distressing symptoms, medications should be considered. It is important to recognize that children and parents vary in their preferences for sedation versus symptoms. It is important to understand these preferences when choosing medications. For a more thorough review of emotional and physical symptom management, see the article by Stuber and Bursch (2000) and the book by Behrman et al. (2004). For a more thorough review on the topic of talking to children about death, refer to the article by Stuber and Mesrkhani (2001).

Finally, consultants should be aware of community hospice services and be able to advocate for this approach to optimizing quality of life when indicated. Careful preparation and support are necessary if a family is to take a child home for the dying process. Parents typically need emotional and technical support as well as respite. Siblings will need age-appropriate information and emotional support. While it is often best for the child to be allowed to die at home, some families do not feel they can cope well with this plan. It is also important to consider that many palliative care treatment approaches can be used for symptom management well before a transition to hospice care is indicated or decided.

Psychiatric Disorders

Delirium

Although pediatric delirium (see Chapter 6, "Delirium") has received little research attention (Turkel et al. 2003) and appears to be less often diagnosed in pediatrics than on the adult units (Manos and Wu 1997), it is still a relatively common reason for psychiatric consultation. As in adults, it sometimes may present with what are interpreted to be psychotic symptoms (Webster and Holroyd 2000). The consultation request may also be put in terms of a request for an assessment of unexplained lethargy, depression, or confusion.

In adults, delirium has been found to be the strongest predictor of length of stay in the hospital, after controlling for severity of illness, age, gender, race, and medication (Ely et al. 2001). A recent evaluation of the widely used Delirium Rating Scale found that it does appear to be applicable to children, with scores comparable to those of adults. However, the scores or diagnosis of delirium in a child may not have the same implications that it has in adults. The scores for children, unlike those for adults, did not predict length of hospital stay or mortality (Turkel et al. 2003). Similarly, the Glasgow Coma Scale appears to be less effective in predicting prognosis for children than adults (Lieh-Lai et al. 1992).

Common causes of delirium include infections, metabolic disturbances, and toxicity of medications. These can often be determined with a careful chart review. Other potentially severe or life-threatening causes of confusion include stroke (Kothare et al. 1998), confusional migraine (Shaabat 1996), neuropsychiatric symptoms of systemic lupus erythematosus (Turkel et al. 2001), or inflammatory encephalopathy (Vasconcellos et al. 1999). Less common causes of acute confusional state in children would be multiple sclerosis (Gadoth 2003) or thiamine deficiency (Hahn et al. 1998). Conventional and quantitative electroencephalography (EEG) have been used to evaluate the etiology of delirium in adults, particularly elderly adults (S.A. Jacobson et al. 1993). In acute pediatric confusional states, EEG appears to be useful in differentiation of hepatic encephalopathy and convulsive pathology from other causes. Certain patterns had strong prognostic value (Navelet et al. 1998) Magnetic resonance imaging (MRI) and single photon emission computed tomography have been found to be useful in used in differentiation of inflammatory encephalopathy (Hahn et al. 1998) and systemic lupus erythematosus (Turkel et al. 2001), respectively.

Even after correction or treatment of the underlying etiology, the symptoms of delirium can last 1–2 weeks (Manos and Wu 1997). Therefore, symptomatic treatment is essential. Support and orienting cues can be very helpful in reducing the fear and confusion. These include the presence of familiar objects, photographs, and people who can reassure and orient the child, as well as age-appropriate clocks, calendars, or signs. Education can help the parents understand what is happening, reduce their distress, and help them to provide support for the child rather than irritation or fear.

Pharmacological intervention is indicated only if the child is distressed by the delirium or is becoming dangerous because of his or her lack of cooperation with care. Because the research into pharmacological approaches to pediatric delirium is almost nonexistent, the general guidelines are pragmatic, based on the adult literature and the pediatric anesthesia literature. Intravenous haloperidol or droperidol are titrated with careful monitoring, avoiding or weaning off benzodiazepines, which appear to compound the confusion with sedation (Breitbart et al. 1996).

Factitious Disorders and Malingering

Illness Falsification

The difference between factitious behavior and malingering is the primary motivation. *Factitious disorder* is defined as the intentional production or feigning (falsification) of physical or psychological signs or symptoms to assume the sick role. *Malingering* is the intentional falsification of physical or psychological signs or symptoms to achieve external gain or to avoid unwanted responsibilities or outcomes.

Little research has been conducted on the topic of illness falsification in children and adolescents. More is known about illness falsification in adults and in child victims of adults (see Chapter 14, "Deception Syndromes: Factitious Disorders and Malingering"). The literature suggests that adult factitious disorder may have origins in childhood for some individuals (Libow 2002), and that some children and adolescents falsifying illness in themselves may have had earlier experiences as a victim of illness falsification or as a recipient of caregiver reinforcement for illness falsification. The child victim experience, including feelings of powerlessness, chronic lack of control, and disappointment in the medical care system are possible dynamics in the future development of illness falsification.

Libow (2000) conducted the only literature review to date for cases of child and adolescent patients for illness falsification. She identified 42 published cases with a mean age of 13.9 (range 8–18 years). Most patients were female (71%), with the gender imbalance greater among older children. Patients engaged in false symptom reporting and induction, including active injections, bruising, and ingestions. The most commonly falsified or induced conditions were fevers, ketoacidosis, purpura, and infections. The average duration of the falsifications before detection was about 16 months. Many admitted to their deceptions when confronted, and some had positive outcomes at follow-up. The children were described as bland, depressed, and fascinated with health care. See Chapter 14, "Deception Syndromes: Factitious Disorders and Malingering," for assessment information.

Child Victims of Illness Falsification

Child victims of illness falsification (called *Munchausen syndrome by proxy* when the abuser's behavior is due to factitious disorder not otherwise specified [NOS]) experience significant psychological problems during childhood, including feelings of helplessness, self-doubt, and poor self-esteem; self-destructive ideation; eating disorders; behavioral growth problems; nightmares; and school concentration problems (Bools et al. 1993; Porter et al. 1994; Libow 1995). Adult survivors describe emotional difficulties, including suicidal feelings, anxiety, depression, low self-esteem, intense rage reactions, and PTSD symptoms (Libow 1995). Ayoub (2002) presented longitudinal data on a sample of 40 children found by courts to be victims of illness falsification. The findings revealed that child victims frequently develop serious psychiatric symptoms that vary depending on the child's developmental age, the length and intensity of his or her exposure, and the current degree of protection and support. PTSD and oppositional disorders are significant sequelae, as are patterns of reality distortion, poor self-esteem, and attachment difficulties.

Although these children can superficially appear socially skilled and well-adjusted, they often struggle with basic relationships. Lying is common, as is manipulative illness behavior and sadistic behavior toward other children. Many remain trauma-reactive and experience cyclical anger, depression, and oppositionality. Children who fared best were separated from their biological parents and remained in a single protected placement, or had an abuser who admitted to the abuse and worked over a period of years toward reunification.

Feeding Disorders

Food Refusal, Selectivity, and Phobias

Feeding problems and eating disturbances in toddlers and young school-age children (see also Chapter 15, "Eating Disorders") occur in 25%–40% of the population (Mayes et al. 1993). Most are transient and can be easily addressed

with parent training, education about nutrition or normal child development, child–caregiver interaction advice, and suggestions for food preparation and presentation. However, severe eating disturbances requiring more aggressive treatment occur in 3%–10% of young children and are most common in children with other physical or developmental problems (Ahearn et al. 2001; Kerwin 1999). These children are at risk for aspiration, malnutrition, invasive medical procedures, hospitalizations, limitations in normal functioning and development, liver failure, and death.

Some physical factors that can impair normal eating include anatomical abnormalities, sensory perceptual impairments, oral motor dysfunctions, and chronic medical problems (such as reflux, short-gut syndrome, inflammatory bowel disease, hepatic or pancreatic disease, or cancer). Other contributing factors can include the pairing of eating with an aversive experience, inadvertent caregiver reinforcement of progressively more selective food choices, or a lack of normal early feeding experiences.

Munk and Repp (1994) developed methods for assessing feeding problems in individuals with cognitive and physical disabilities that allow categorization of individual feeding patterns based on responses to repeated presentations of food. Complete food refusal or food selectivity can occur with or without an associated phobia and can be assessed by observing for fear and anxiety behaviors on food presentation (Kerwin 1999).

Food aversion and oral motor dysfunction is often treated by a speech pathologist and/or an occupational therapist. Effective behavioral interventions include contingency management with positive reinforcement for appropriate feeding and ignoring or guiding inappropriate responses. Desensitization techniques can be effectively used to address phobias or altered sensory processing. Although no research has directly examined the use of psychotropic medication in treating food refusal, selectivity, or phobias, it may be valuable to consider for use with children with associated anxiety disorders.

Failure to Thrive

It is helpful to think of failure to thrive (FTT) as a presenting symptom with varied and potentially multiple causes (Wren and Tarbell 1998). Parents might have a poor understanding of feeding techniques or might improperly prepare formula, or the mother may have an inadequate supply of breast milk. Biological contributors to failure to thrive include defects in food assimilation, excessive loss of ingested calories, increased energy requirements, and prenatal insults; environmental contributors include economic or emotional deprivation.

Research examining the role of the child–parent attachment reveals that feeding problems and growth deficiencies can occur within the context of organized and secure attachments; however, insecure attachment relationships may intensify feeding problems and lead to more severe malnutrition (Chatoor et al. 1998). In one study of FTT children (who had no identifiable biological contributors), 80% of the mothers reported they had a history of being victims of physical abuse (Weston et al. 1993).

Classic teaching has been that etiology can be determined by the child's ability to gain weight in the hospital, with a psychosocial etiology presumed if the child gains weight under these conditions. However, it is important to note that conclusions about likely FTT contributors cannot always be made on the basis of the child's ability to gain weight in the hospital. For example, some FTT children who have an inadequate caregiver will still lose weight in the hospital simply because they are separated from the caregiver. Former FTT children have been found to be smaller, less cognitively able, and more behaviorally disturbed than those children without a history of FTT, especially if their mothers are poorly educated (Drewett et al. 1999; Dykman et al. 2001).

The goal of treatment is to provide the medical, psychiatric, social, and environmental resources needed to promote satisfactory growth. Psychosocial treatment interventions need to be targeted at the likely contributors. Children with feeding skills deficits or maladaptive behavior related to food are likely to benefit from behavioral interventions. Primary caregivers with a history of abuse or with current psychopathology might require specific psychiatric assessment and treatment. Interventions targeting the child–parent relationship, sometimes including in-home intervention, might be effective for selected families (Black et al. 1995; Steward 2001). Interventions targeting the social–economic burdens of the family can be critical. In some cases of inadequate parenting, foster care is required while the parent receives needed parent training and psychiatric care. In such cases, the return to home should be closely monitored and based on the parents' demonstrated ability and resources to adequately care for their child.

Psychosocial Short Stature

Short stature can typically be attributed to defects in the growing tissues, abnormalities of the environment of the growing tissues (e.g., nutritional insufficiency or organ disease), or endocrine abnormalities. Psychosocial short stature is relatively rare, often confused with FTT, and not well studied (Wren and Tarbell 1998). It is distinguished from FTT in that it is considered a direct result of adverse social–environmental factors on endocrine functioning (suppression of normal pulsatile growth hormone [GH] secretion) that results in a failure to make expected gains in *height* or *length*, as opposed to weight. Examples of adverse social–environmental factors include physical abuse, extreme deprivation, or a seriously disturbed child–parent relationship. Other behavioral and emotional disturbances, also induced by the adverse social–environmental issues, are common. One diagnostic feature is that it is reversible, with rapid acceleration in growth and development often observed, when the child is removed from the environment.

Consequently, the primary intervention is often placement in a safe, structured, stimulating environment with ample opportunity to develop new attachments (Green et al. 1984). Distress related to separation is less likely to temporarily hinder progress in psychosocial short stature (when compared with FTT), because of the severity of the adverse social–environmental factors endured before separation. Other treatments should be geared toward the specific symptoms and experiences of the child, but may include individual psychotherapy, family therapy, school assessment and intervention, and psychotropic medication. Case reports suggest that attempts at in-home intervention must be intensive and comprehensive to be effective. The involvement of child protective services is often essential.

Pica

Pica is defined as eating nonnutritious substances on a continued basis over a period of at least 1 month (Wren and Tarbell 1998). It is most frequently found in children with mental retardation or a pervasive developmental disorder. Pica also has a high prevalence in children with sickle cell disease, with preliminary studies suggesting that over 30% are affected (Bond et al. 1994; Ivascu et al. 2001). Mouthing and occasional eating of nonnutritious substances is considered normal in children under 3 years. Young children with pica are most likely to eat sand, bugs, paint, plaster, paper, or other items within reach. Adolescents are more likely to eat clay, soil, paper, or similar substances. Pica can be a conditioned behavior, an indication of distress or environmental neglect, or evidence of a vitamin or mineral deficiency. One study (Singhi et al. 1981) in children with iron deficiency anemia (50 with pica and 50 without pica, individually matched for age, sex, socioeconomic class, and degree of anemia) found that stress factors significantly associated with pica included maternal deprivation, caretaker other than the mother, parental separation, parental neglect, joint family, child beating, and too little parent–child interaction (mother or father). Medical assessment includes screening for ingestion of toxic substances and evaluation for possible nutritional deficits. An evaluation and treatment plan to reduce psychosocial stress are also clearly important. Behavioral interventions have been shown to be effective in targeting the pica behavior, including food-versus-nonfood discrimination training, response interruption and positive practice overcorrection, habit reversal, and brief-duration physical restraint (Fisher et al. 1994; Johnson et al. 1994; Paniagua et al. 1986; Woods et al. 1996; Winton and Singh 1983). Psychiatric medications are not generally used to treat pica unless it is comorbid with another psychiatric disorder.

Rumination

Rumination syndrome is the effortless regurgitation into the mouth of recently ingested food followed by rechewing and reswallowing or expulsion (Clouse et al. 1999; Malcolm et al. 1997). Associated behavioral signs can include aversive posturing or gaze avoidance (Berkowitz 1999). Rumination can be conditioned after an illness, a sign of general distress, or a form of self-stimulation or self-soothing that appears to be associated with pleasure. It is most commonly seen in infants and the developmentally disabled, but also occurs in children and adolescents with normal intelligence (O'Brien et al. 1985; Soykan et al. 1997).

Patients with rumination syndrome can be misdiagnosed as having bulimia nervosa, gastroesophageal reflux disease, or upper gastrointestinal motility disorders (such as gastroparesis or chronic intestinal pseudo-obstruction). They might undergo extensive, costly, and invasive medical testing before diagnosis. Complications can include weight loss, fatal malnutrition, dental erosions, halitosis, dehydration, school absenteeism, hospitalizations, and iatrogenic problems from the extensive diagnostic testing (O'Brien et al. 1995).

Rumination syndrome is a clinical diagnosis based on symptoms and the absence of structural disease. However, the Rome II diagnostic groups include only "infant rumination syndrome," and criteria for older children have not been defined (Rasquin-Weber et al. 1999). Evaluation for gastroesophageal reflux disease is warranted if the rumination is accompanied by apnea, reactive airway disease, hematemesis, or food refusal.

In cases of rumination because of environmental neglect, the primary caretaker–child relationship and possible psychiatric disturbance in the primary caretaker should be evaluated and addressed. Operant behavioral methods can be used for conditioned rumination. Postmeal chewing gum has been used successfully to treat adolescents with rumination (Weakley et al. 1997). Habit reversal using diaphragmatic breathing as the competing re-

sponse can also be effective in older children and adolescents (Wagaman et al. 1998; Chial et al. 2003; Kerwin 1999). Rumination in the presence of other psychosocial problems or psychiatric disorders in the child or primary caretaker may require additional therapeutic interventions. Later experiences of stress, loss, or isolation can trigger a relapse, requiring the reinstitution of the previously effective intervention (Berkowitz 1999).

Chronic Somatic Symptoms

Children and adolescents often report persistent physical concerns that are not clearly accounted for by identifiable medical illness (Campo and Fritsch 1994; Garber et al. 1991). In fact, the most common reason for a pediatric psychiatry consultation is for evaluation of unexplained physical symptoms (Simonds 1977; Tsai et al. 1995). Somatoform disorders can be considered the severe end of a continuum that includes functional somatic symptoms in the middle and minor transient symptoms at the other end (Fritz et al. 1997). Examples of disorders on this continuum include atypical migraines, cyclic vomiting, chronic nausea, dizziness, fibromyalgia, chronic fatigue, functional abdominal pain, irritable bowel syndrome, myofascial pain, palpitations, conversion paralysis, and pseudoseizures (Caplan 1998; Heruti et al. 2002; Krilov et al. 1998; Li and Balint 2000; Schanberg et al. 1998; Volkmar et al. 1984). Disabling somatic symptoms can occur in the presence or absence of an identifiable etiology and in the presence or absence of other medical or psychiatric disorders.

It is helpful to remember that experiences of somatic symptoms are the result of an integration of biological processes, psychological and developmental factors, and social context (Bennett 1999; Li and Balint 2000; Mailis-Gagnon et al. 2003; Peyron et al. 2000; Terre and Ghiselli 1997; Zeltzer et al. 1997). Traditionally, disability and symptoms in excess of what would be expected given the amount of tissue pathology has been considered psychogenic. Children and families are informed that the symptom has no physiological basis, with the intended or unintended suggestion that the child is fabricating the symptom. It is misleading and often confusing to families to dichotomize symptoms as organic versus nonorganic because all symptoms are associated with neurosensory changes and influenced by psychosocial factors. Maintaining the organic versus nonorganic dichotomy can lead to unnecessary tests and treatments, or to an unhelpful lack of empathy.

Psychiatric assessment is geared toward identifying psychiatric symptoms, behavioral reinforcements, and psychosocial stressors that could be exacerbating the symptoms. Common comorbid findings include anxiety disorders, alexithymia, depression, unsuspected learning disorders (in high-achieving children), developmental or communication disorders, social problems, physical or emotional trauma, family illness, and family distress (Bursch and Zeltzer 2002; Campo et al. 1999, 2002; Egger et al. 1998; Fritz et al. 1997; Garber et al. 1990; Hodges et al. 1985a; Hodges et al. 1985b; Hyman et al. 2002; Lester et al. 2003; Livingston 1993; Livingston et al. 1995; Schanberg et al. 1998; Stuart and Noyes 1999; Zuckerman et al. 1987).

The family and treatment team often worry about missing a life-threatening problem or a diagnosis that could be easily remedied. This fear is particularly strong when the patient exhibits significant distress about the symptoms. The treatment team must feel that a reasonable evaluation has been completed so that they can clearly communicate to the family that no further evaluation is indicated to understand and treat the problem. A rehabilitation approach can improve independent and normal functioning, enhance coping and self-efficacy, and serve to prevent secondary disabilities (Bursch et al. 1998; Campo and Fritz 2001; Heruti et al. 2002). Functioning, rather than symptoms, should be tracked to determine whether progress is being made. As functioning, coping skills, and self-efficacy improve, symptoms and the distress related to the symptoms often remit.

Specific treatment plans target the biological, psychological, and social factors that are exacerbating or maintaining the symptoms and disability. Treatment techniques designed to target underlying sensory signaling mechanisms and specific symptoms can include cognitive-behavioral strategies (e.g., psychotherapy, hypnosis, biofeedback, or meditation), behavioral techniques, family interventions, physical interventions (e.g., massage, yoga, acupuncture, transcutaneous electrical nerve stimulation (TENS), physical therapy, heat or cold therapies, occupational therapy), sleep hygiene, and pharmacological interventions (Fritz et al. 1997; Minuchin et al. 1978; Sanders et al. 1989, 1994; Zeltzer and Bursch 2002). In general, interventions that promote active coping are preferred over those that require passive dependency.

Most of the currently employed pharmacological strategies are extrapolated from adult trials without evidence of efficacy in children. Classes of medications to consider include tricyclic antidepressants or anticonvulsants for neuropathic pain or irritable bowel syndrome, SSRIs for symptoms of anxiety or depression, muscle relaxants for myofascial pain, and low-dose antipsychotics (especially those with low potency) for acute anxiety, multiple somatic symptoms with significant distress, and chronic nausea. Benzodiazepines sometimes elicit para-

doxical reactions in those children who are hypervigilant to their bodies and concerned about losing control. Blocks, trigger point injections, epidurals, and other invasive assessments and treatments that further stimulate the CNS can sometimes exacerbate the problem. Evidence-based treatments should be used whenever available. For example, in adolescent migraine headache, cognitive-behavioral interventions have better evidence for efficacy than triptans, and ibuprofen appears to be more effective than acetaminophen.

Specific Medical Disorders

Oncology

Pediatric cancer presents a number of challenges to patients and their families. Despite the numerous stressors, pediatric oncology patients report relatively few depressive symptoms during the time of active treatment. Children with cancer report fewer symptoms of depression than healthy school children or children with asthma, and self-esteem concerns and somatic symptoms do not differentiate between depressed and nondepressed children with cancer (Worchel et al. 1988; Gizynski and Shapiro 1990). In fact, pediatric cancer patients report so few symptoms that clinical researchers have hypothesized that these children use an avoidant coping style to deal with their emotional response to cancer (Phipps and Srivastava 1997, 1999) or that their emotional response is shaped by traumatic avoidance (Erickson and Steiner 2000). Interventions that address the contextual issues that are precipitating distress are generally sufficient for the depressive symptoms seen during active treatment (Kazak et al. 2002).

One area of intervention that has been extensively researched is preparation for the many invasive procedures children experience during cancer treatment. Cognitive-behavioral techniques, including imagery, relaxation, distraction, modeling, desensitization, and positive reinforcement, are well established as effective (Powers 1999). This is consistent with the literature that suggests depressive attributional style and avoidance coping are major predictors of anxiety and depression in pediatric oncology patients (Frank et al. 1997). Although all children have some distress with painful procedures, some appear to be more sensitive to pain and have differential responses to psychological interventions for procedural distress (Chen et al. 2000). In cases of children with severe distress, integration of pharmacological interventions has proven useful (Jay et al. 1991; Kazak et al. 1998). Topical anesthetic cream has been used with some success to alleviate the pain of venipuncture or the topical pain of other invasive procedures with pediatric oncology patients (Robieux et al. 1990). In comparisons of conscious sedation and general anesthesia for lumbar punctures, the outcomes were similar, and the conscious sedation was generally preferred, as well as less expensive. However, for some children, the procedure could only be performed under general anesthesia because they were too distressed to cooperate (Ljungman et al. 2001). For conscious sedation, the amnestic effect of midazolam, as well as the ability to administer it nasally, rectally, or orally, has made it popular with anesthesiologists and intensivists. In a double-blind study, midazolam was shown to significantly reduce children's procedural anxiety, discomfort, and pain (Ljungman et al. 2000). For brief, general anesthesia, a combination of midazolam and ketamine has been found effective (Parker et al. 1997).

With increasing survival of childhood cancer patients, the long-term impact of cancer has become a major focus of psycho-oncology research over the past 20 years. Here again, depression does not seem to be a problem (Zebrack et al. 2002). However, a rapidly growing area is investigations of PTSD. A study of 309 childhood cancer survivors (ages 8–20), an average of almost 6 years after cancer treatment, found similar rates of PTSD symptoms in the cancer and comparison groups (219 healthy children) (Kazak et al. 1997). However, in a study of 78 young-adult (ages 18–37) survivors of childhood cancer, approximately 20% of the young adult survivors reported symptoms meeting diagnostic criteria for PTSD (Hobbie et al. 2000). Furthermore, PTSD in the young adults appeared predictive of adverse consequences. The young adult survivors who met criteria for PTSD were less likely to be married (none, compared with 23% of the non-PTSD group) and reported more psychological distress and poorer quality of life across all domains. The greatest differences reported were in social functioning, emotional well-being, and role limitations caused by emotional health and pain. Survivors without PTSD did not differ from population norms (Meeske et al. 2001). These findings indicate a need to prevent and intervene with children during the time of acute treatment, to prevent long-term consequences in much the same way that medical treatments are being adapted in light of the late effects of radiation and chemotherapy.

Parents report significant distress both during and after their children's cancer treatment (Best et al. 2002). Specific problem-solving therapy has been found to be effective in helping mothers deal with the stresses of treatment (Sahler et al. 2002), as have brief stress reduction techniques (Streisand et al. 2001). Rates of PTSD in parents of children off treatment appear comparable to those of adult cancer survivors (Manne et al. 1998). In a large study of pediatric cancer survivors' parents, 3% of the survivors' mothers reported severe, and 18.2% reported moderate, symptoms of PTSD; whereas 7% of the survivors' fathers reported severe, and 28.3% reported moderate, PTSD symptoms (Kazak et al. 1997).

Cystic Fibrosis

Cystic fibrosis (CF) affects approximately 30,000 children and adults in the United States and is the most common hereditary disease in white children. A defective gene causes the body to produce a thick, sticky mucus that clogs the lungs and leads to life-threatening lung infections. These secretions also obstruct the pancreas, preventing digestive enzymes from reaching the intestines. CF occurs in approximately one of every 3,200 live Caucasian births, with about 1,000 new cases diagnosed each year. More than 80% of patients are diagnosed by age 3; however, almost 10% are diagnosed at age 18 or older. The median age of survival is 33.4 years, and nearly 40% of those with CF are adults.

People with CF have a variety of symptoms that vary from person to person but include very salty-tasting skin; persistent coughing; wheezing or shortness of breath; an excessive appetite but poor weight gain; and greasy, bulky stools. Malnutrition can lead to poor growth, delayed puberty, impaired respiratory function, reduced exercise tolerance, and increased risk of infection. CF patients with end-stage pulmonary disease show marked nutritional failure. There is evidence that improving nutritional status may halt the decline in pulmonary function (Dalzell et al. 1992). Progressive respiratory failure is the most common cause of death.

The treatment of CF depends on the stage of the disease and the organs involved. Clearing mucus from the lungs is part of the daily CF treatment regimen; this entails vigorous clapping on the back and chest to dislodge the mucus from the lungs. Other types of treatments include antibiotics to treat lung infections and mucus-thinning drugs. A high-energy diet (a high-fat diet with significant amounts of carbohydrate and protein) aiming at 120% of the recommended daily intake for age has been linked to superior nutritional status. However, research has demonstrated that dietary adherence is poor, with up to 84% of CF children not reaching dietary goals. Both adherence and health status in children with CF are partially predicted by parental psychosocial variables, including knowledge specific to CF (Anthony et al. 1999; Patterson et al. 1993). More and more individuals with CF have received gene therapy or a lung, liver, and/or bowel transplant.

Many people with CF lead remarkably normal lives and maintain hope with the possibilities of gene therapy and organ transplantation in case of severe deterioration. Although early research suggested that eating disorders may be more prevalent in those with CF, recent work has suggested that this is not true. Similarly, rates of other psychiatric disorders among those with CF do not appear to be greater than the prevalence reported in the general population (Kashani et al. 1988a; Raymond et al. 2000). In one study of CF adolescents' health values, it was revealed that they are willing to trade very little of their life expectancy or take more than a small risk of death to obtain perfect health (Yi et al. 2003). Although there is little research on this topic, there are no apparent contraindications for standard assessment and treatments approaches for psychiatric disorders in those with CF. There is some data to suggest that family interventions can be successfully used to improve maternal mental health and treatment adherence among those at high risk (Goldbeck and Babka 2001; Ireys et al. 2001).

Asthma

Asthma is the most common pediatric chronic illness, and both prevalence and morbidity are rising, despite better pharmacological treatments. Comorbid psychiatric problems and increased levels of stress are cited as possible factors for the increases (Wamboldt and Gavin 1998). Comorbid psychiatric disorders may reduce asthma treatment compliance, impair daily functioning, or have a direct effect on autonomic reactions and pulmonary function (Norrish et al. 1977). While the literature contains some contradictory findings about the prevalence and type of comorbid psychiatric problems, it appears that internalizing disorders are more common and that over one-third of asthmatic children have anxiety disorders. Additionally, those with moderate to severe asthma appear to be at a higher risk for anxiety disorders compared to those with mild disease. Although depression has been less consistently identified as a comorbid psychiatric disorder among pediatric asthma patients, the literature suggests that depression, along with other psychosocial problems, may be a risk factor for death in children with asthma. Consequently, the presence of depression in a child with uncontrolled or severe asthma requires serious attention (Bussing et al. 1996; Butz and Alexander 1993; Graham et al. 1967; Kashani et al. 1988b; MacLean et al. 1988; McNichol et al. 1973; Mrazek et al. 1985; Steinhausen et al. 1983; Strunk et al. 1985; Vila et al. 1999).

Twin studies suggest that there may be a genetic relationship between atopic disorders and internalizing disorders (Wamboldt et al. 1998). One possible explanation is

that panic anxiety acts as an asphyxia alarm system that is triggered by central chemoreceptors monitoring $PaCO_2$. Children with a genetic vulnerability for panic disorder who also have periodic increased $PaCO_2$ from asthma exacerbations may thus have panic anxiety triggered by their asthma attacks. Left undiagnosed and untreated, this anxiety can develop into panic disorder. Indeed, recent prospective epidemiological studies indicate the primary risk factor for development of panic disorder in young adulthood is history of asthma as a child (Goodwin et al. 2003). Other reasons for increased comorbidity include the fact that most asthma medications (for example, steroids and beta-agonists) are known to cause symptoms that appear psychiatric in nature. An inflammatory allergic response may release cytokines and other mediators that cause fatigue, trouble concentrating, and irritability that could also be interpreted as depression. The physiological response accompanying strong emotions can trigger wheezing in some patients. Recent research indicates that not only can stress lead to increased asthma exacerbations, but those children with atopic illnesses have a reduced cortisol response to stress (Wamboldt et al. 2003). Stressors may thus have a direct effect on increased inflammation, leading to asthma symptoms or an increase in upper respiratory infections, which also exacerbate asthma. Depression and anxiety may indirectly influence asthma because distressed asthmatics tend to misperceive anxiety symptoms as asthma symptoms, often leading to unnecessary medication usage.

Vocal cord dysfunction (VCD) can mimic asthma and commonly occurs comorbidly with asthma. It is a condition of involuntary paradoxical adduction of the vocal cords during the inspiratory phase of the respiratory cycle (Wamboldt and Gavin 1998). It is often associated with anxiety or chronic stress; however, sexual abuse in this population is not as prevalent as previously believed (Brugman 1994; Gavin et al. 1998). Patients with VCD frequently present with stridulous breathing, experience tightness in their throats, and feel short of breath. It can be quite anxiety provoking that their symptoms are unrelieved by asthma medications.

Clinicians should assess for 1) psychosocial disruption and psychiatric symptoms, especially symptoms of anxiety and depression (including medical trauma); 2) the likelihood of nonadherence; 3) ability to perceive symptoms; and 4) presence of VCD. Asthma can increase family burden, and having depressed primary caretakers increases the risk of poorer treatment adherence. New electronic monitoring of adherence with inhaled medications helps determine how much nonadherence is undermining outcome. Having patients guess their peak flow or rate their symptoms before spirometry or after a methacholine challenge is one way to assess if the patient is an accurate perceiver or not. Patients who have difficulty with symptom perception (either under- or overperceiving symptoms) can be trained to use objective assessment methods, such as peak flow meters. Clinicians can assess for VCD by asking patients where they feel short of breath and if there is throat tightness. A flow volume loop can be helpful in showing VCD, especially on the inspiratory part of the loop. Definitive diagnosis of VCD is made by visualization of adducted cords during an acute episode using laryngoscopy. Provocation of symptoms during laryngoscopy has been achieved using methacholine, histamine, or exercise challenges.

Pharmacological and psychological treatments with efficacy to treat anxiety and depression in children are largely applicable to those with asthma. Focused family therapy to improve asthma management skills has been shown to be effective and efficient (Godding et al. 1997; Gustafsson et al 1986; Lask and Matthew 1979; Panton and Barley 2004). The primary treatment for VCD is speech therapy or hypnotherapy geared toward increasing awareness and control of breathing and throat muscles (Wamboldt and Gavin 1998). Although some concern has been raised about the concurrent use of tricyclic antidepressants with medicines used in treating asthma, they appear to be safe, and the anticholinergic effects can sometimes be helpful (Wamboldt et al. 1997). Beta-receptor agonists are often used to treat asthma, which makes beta-blockers potentially dangerous. There is no contraindication for using neuroleptics, and they may be particularly indicated for steroid-induced psychosis. Lithium increases theophylline clearance, requiring that levels of both drugs be monitored (Wamboldt and Gavin 1998). Some children with asthma have difficulty tolerating stimulants. Bupropion has shown efficacy in the treatment of attention-deficit/hyperactivity disorder in young patients in controlled trials (Barrickman et al 1995; Conners et al 1996) and does not interact with asthma medications.

Childhood Obesity

There has been a disturbing increase during the past 20 years in the prevalence of obesity in children and adolescents in the United States. Children and adolescents are considered obese if they have a body mass index (BMI) of greater than or equal to the 95th percentile for age and gender, and they are considered overweight if their BMI is between the 85th and the 95th percentiles (Dietz and Bellizzi 1999). Data from the third National Health and Nutrition Examination Survey, conducted from 1988 to 1994, indicated that approximately 11% of children were obese, and another 14% were overweight. These findings can be compared with the 5% obesity reported in a similar study conducted between 1976 and 1980 (Troiano et al 1995). This dramatic increase in obesity has been attributed to the proliferation of inexpensive, calorie-rich foods that are quickly and readily available in this country and the increased number of hours children spend in sedentary activities, such as watching television and playing computer games (Ebbeling et al. 2002). Similar increases in childhood obesity have been documented in Europe and Asia (Chinn et al. 2001; Chunming 2000) and in developing societies (de Onis and Blossner 2000).

The impact of obesity is both immediate and long-lasting. Children and adolescents with a BMI at or above the 95th percentile for age and sex have been found to have significantly reduced health-related quality of life compared with healthy children and adolescents. In a study of 106 children, ages 5–18 years, the obese subjects were more than five times more likely to have significant impairment of physical functioning and almost six times as likely to have impaired psychosocial health. These findings are similar to those for children with cancer (Schwimmer et al. 2003). A survey of approximately 10,000 women, ages 16–24 years, found that obese adolescents were less likely to complete college than non-overweight adolescents with similar educational backgrounds. The obese young adults were much less likely to marry than nonobese young adults, after controlling for IQ and parents' education or income level. Those obese women who did marry were more often married to men in a lower socioeconomic class (Stunkard and Sabal 1995; Gortmaker 1993).

The immediate health consequences of childhood obesity are serious and include slipped capital femoral epiphysis, pseudotumor cerebri, asthma, sleep apnea, gallstones, insulin resistance, early puberty, dyslipidemia, and hypertension (see Morgan et al. 2002 for review). Although obese children are likely to become obese adults (Guo et al. 1994), the long-term health risks also include increased likelihood of atherosclerotic cardiovascular disease, gout, and colorectal cancer in men and arthritis and menstrual abnormalities in women, even after adult body mass is taken into account (Mossberg 1989; Must et al. 1999).

Genetic factors may account for as much as 70% of the variability in human body weight (Stunkard et al. 1990; Allison et al 1996). The recent discovery of leptin opens the door for future interventions through what appears to be the body's approach to energy balance (Segal and Sanchez 2001). However, the behavioral contribution is sufficient to make lifestyle interventions a priority for pediatricians and the psychologists and psychiatrists who work with pediatric patients. A review of 42 randomized studies involving non-school-based programs found strong evidence for the efficacy of multicomponent behavioral treatments for children to decrease weight both short- and long-term when compared with placebo or education-only treatments. The smaller numbers of studies and shorter follow-up do not allow as much confidence about the effectiveness of such interventions with adolescents (Jelalian and Saelens 1999). Unfortunately, although the weight loss was significant, the majority of these children remained obese, and there is little evidence that behavioral interventions were effective with children who were morbidly obese. These results have led to recent investigations of the application of medication or surgery to treat serious obesity in adolescents.

There are currently no weight loss medications that have been approved for use in children and adolescents. Fenfluramine and phentermine, appetite suppressants that act by stimulating the release of serotonin and dopamine and selectively inhibiting their reuptake, were tested separately and jointly with children and adolescents but were not found to be consistently effective. Fenfluramine was later withdrawn from the market because of safety concerns (see Yanovski 2001 for review). However, sibutramine, an inhibitor of norepinephrine, serotonin, and dopamine reuptake, has proven useful and safe in adults and is now being tested with adolescents. Sibutramine appears to act by increasing satiety, rather than by decreasing appetite (Heal et al. 1998). A randomized, double-blind, placebo-controlled trial of 82 adolescents ages 13 to 17 years with a BMI of 32 to 44 studied the use of behavior therapy coupled with either sibutramine or placebo. Study participants were all given a 1200- to 1500-kilocalorie diet and followed for a year. The sibutramine group had significantly more weight loss than those who had placebo paired with the same diet and behavioral program, with a mean loss of 7 kg and reduction of 8.5% of BMI, compared with 3.2 kg and 4.0% for the control group. Hunger reported was also significantly reduced ($P = .002$) in those receiving the sibutramine (Berkowitz et al. 2003). Although safety has not been fully studied, in this study there were clinically significant side effects of the medication. Doses of the medication were reduced in 23 subjects and discontinued in 10 to manage increases in blood pressure, pulse rate, or other symptoms. Such interventions are therefore still reserved for those who are dangerously obese, where the benefit may outweigh the cost.

There have been some initial studies of the feasibility of doing surgery to induce weight loss in adolescents with severe obesity, given the high levels of morbidity and mortality associated with this condition. However, bariatric surgery is viewed as "a last resort option for severely obese adolescents" (Strauss et al. 2001, p. 503). Bariatric surgical interventions for adults are used only after behavioral approaches have failed and when medical complications of obesity outweigh the potential complications of the surgery (Fisher and Schauer 2002) (see also Chapter 30, "Surgery"). Restrictive approaches use gastric staples, bands, or bypasses to reduce the capacity of the stomach, decreasing the volume of food which can be consumed at one sitting, and increasing a sense of satiety. Mean loss of excess weight with the most popular method, the Roux-en-Y, ranges from 65% to 75% in adults. Morbidity is reported at 10% and includes deep venous thrombosis or pulmonary embolism, anastomotic leaks, and wound infection. Iron and vitamin B_{12} deficiency occur in more than 30% of patients. Mortality rates are less than 1%. Malabsorptive operations bypass parts or all of the duodenum or jejunum, reducing intestinal absorption of nutrients. Mean loss of excess weight is 75%–80% with excellent weight maintenance, and immediate mortality and morbidity is similar to that after restrictive procedures. However, 30% of the patients develop anemia, 30%–50% develop fat-soluble vitamin deficiencies, and diarrhea and foul-smelling stools are common (see Brolin 2002 for review). Given the likelihood of adolescents to be nonadherent with diet and other instructions, the potential interference with growth, and the lack of information on long-term consequences, surgical interventions should be reserved for those who have not responded to more conventional intervention and have significant complications of their obesity (Yanovski 2001).

Sickle Cell Anemia

The sickle cell gene for hemoglobin S is the most common inherited blood condition in the United States, with an estimated 72,000 people affected. Symptoms do not usually appear until late in the first year of life and may include fever; swelling of the hands and feet; pain in the chest, abdomen, limbs, and joints; nosebleeds; and frequent upper respiratory infections. Pain is the most common complaint after infancy, as are the added problems of anemia, fatigue, irritability, and jaundice. Children and adolescents may experience delayed puberty, severe joint pain, progressive anemia, leg sores, gum disease, long-term damage to major organs, stroke, and acute chest syndrome. A compromised spleen can cause increased susceptibility to infections. Current treatments for sickle cell disease are prolonging and improving quality of life. Although most people with sickle cell anemia were not previously expected to survive childhood, the majority now live into adulthood with about half living beyond 50 years (Platt et al. 1994).

Sickle cell crises are acute pain episodes that are usually followed by periods of remission and a relatively normal life. Some patients have few crises, others need to be frequently hospitalized, and some have clusters of severe attacks with long intermittent remissions. Crises become less frequent with age for some. The risk for a crisis is increased by anything that boosts the body's oxygen requirement (including illness, physical stress, or being at high altitudes). The first day of the crisis is usually the worst, with sharp, intense, and throbbing pain in the arms, legs, and back. Shortness of breath, bone pain, and abdominal pain are also common. The liver can become enlarged, causing pain, nausea, low-grade fever, and jaundice. Males may experience priapism. Acute chest syndrome can be life threatening.

Stroke is a common cause of death for sickle cell patients over 3 years (Kinney et al. 1999; Ohene-Frempong 1991; Ohene-Frempong et al. 1998;). Although transfusions may be preventive, 8%–11% of those affected suffer strokes. One study comparing sickle cell children with and without a history of stroke revealed relative deficits on measures of attention and executive functioning. Rodgers et al. (1984) provided positron emission tomography evidence of altered frontal lobe metabolism. Another study examined social information processing, social skills, and adjustment difficulties in children with sickle cell disease and learning and behavior problems, with or without CNS pathology on MRI. Children with CNS pathology displayed more errors on tasks of facial and vocal emotional decoding than did the control children (Boni et al. 2001).

Although children and adolescents with sickle cell disease do not appear to have a greater risk for psychiatric disorders than those in the same-race outpatient clinic control group, children attending outpatient medical clinics are at a higher risk for mental disorders than nonmedical populations (Cepeda 1997; Yang et al. 1994). Most well-designed studies report a prevalence rate of 25%–30% for psychiatric disorders among pediatric sickle cell patients, with internalizing disorders being most prevalent (Cepeda et al. 1997), similar to other pediatric outpatients (Costello and Shugart 1992; Costello et al. 1988). Psychosocial factors have accounted for more variability than biomedical ones in both depressive symptoms and anxiety, with social assertion, self-esteem, use of social support, and family factors accounting for a significant amount of the variability in adaptation (Burlew et al. 2000; Telfair 1994). Two studies suggest that pica (not often assessed) has a relatively high prevalence (up to 30%) in children with sickle cell disease (Bond et al. 1994; Ivascu et al. 2001).

Psychiatric assessment should look for 1) psychosocial disruption or psychiatric symptoms, especially related to pica, anxiety and depression; 2) school or social problems that could reflect subtle neurocognitive problems; and 3) chronic pain problems. Pharmacological and psychological treatments with efficacy to treat psychiatric disorders in children are applicable to those with sickle cell anemia. Problems with academic or social functioning might be assessed via neurocognitive testing and addressed within the school system with an Individualized Educational Program (IEP). Pain in sickle cell patients is most commonly medically managed pharmacologically with nonsteroidal anti-inflammatory drugs (NSAIDs), opioids, and adjuvant medications (American Pain Society 1999). Chronic as well as acute pediatric pain can also be reduced with behavioral, psychological, or physical interventions (American Pain Society 1999). Behavioral interventions might include relaxation, deep breathing, biofeedback, behavioral modification, or exercise. Psychological intervention might include cognitive therapies, hypnotherapy, imagery, distraction, or social support. Physical interventions might include hydration, heat, massage, hydrotherapy, ultrasound, acupuncture, TENS, or physical therapy. Successful treatment of anxiety symptoms can reduce pain and pain-related distress. Although there are no contraindications for the use of psychotropic medications with this population, it is important to remember that phenothiazines may antagonize the analgesic effects of opiate agonists; and tricyclic antidepressants, MAOIs, and other CNS depressants may potentiate adverse effects of opioids. It is important to note, however, that these agents may also serve to successfully augment pain control efforts and should be considered if needed.

Renal Disease

Each year 20,000 children are born with kidney abnormalities, and 4,500 children require dialysis for renal failure. Hemodialysis (at a center or at home) and peritoneal dialysis are used in children. The basic principles of treatment of end-stage renal disease (ESRD) are similar in adults and children (see Chapter 22, "Renal Disease"). However, attention to dialysis adequacy, control of osteodystrophy, nutrition, and correction of anemia are crucial because these factors can influence growth, cognitive development, and school performance (Warady et al. 1999).

Pediatric patients with chronic renal failure exhibit more problems in psychiatric adjustment than do healthy children, with a trend toward more psychological difficulties in those with higher illness severity (Garralda et al. 1988). However, even less severely physically ill children appear to have increased difficulties in school adjustment and feelings of loneliness (Garralda et al. 1988). Separation anxiety disorder in particular may be a relatively common disorder (up to 65.4%) among children on continuous ambulatory peritoneal dialysis (Fukunishi and Kudo 1995). This may be due to the forced dependence on parents for daily renal care. The burden for families caring for children with ESRD can be significant, especially when it involves dialysis. Disruption of family life, marital strain, and a tendency for more mental health problems in the parents also appear to be related to the severity of the child's renal illness and its associated care burdens (Reynolds et al. 1988). Children with ESRD (with or without transplant) have been shown to have lower-than-expected IQs and achievement scores. Lower achievement test scores were predicted by younger age at the time of renal disease diagnosis, increased time on dialysis, and caregiver's lower achievement (Brouhard et al. 2000; Fennell et al. 1984; Qvist et al. 2002). Overall, former pediatric ESRD adults appear to have a long-term favorable adjustment, with lower self-esteem related to early onset of the disease and to educational and social dysfunction (Morton et al. 1994).

According to the latest statistics (May 30, 2003) from The United Network for Organ Sharing (UNOS), 749 children were waiting for a kidney transplant in the United States, including 3 under 1 year, 79 in the 1- to 5-years age group, 121 in the 6- to 10-years age group, and 546 in the 11- to 17-years age group. The majority of transplanted kidneys come from cadavers. However, family members or unrelated individuals who are a good match may be able to donate one of their kidneys and live healthy lives with the kidney that remains. Pediatric kidney transplantation is associated with improved physical health, emotional health, and family functioning; however, poor peer relationships, school maladjustment, and other adjustment problems (as well as adherence problems) can remain after transplant (Fukunishi and Kudo 1995; Reynolds et al. 1991). Living with a transplant is a lifelong process requiring daily medications and monitoring for rejection. Medication nonadherence rates for pediatric renal transplant patients can be as high as 64% (Ettenger et al. 1991). Adverse consequences of nonadherence include medical complications and hospitalizations, higher health care costs and family stress, and increased risks for loss of the organ (Arbus et al. 1993; Bittar et al. 1992; Fukunishi and Honda 1995; Salvatierra et al. 1997; Swanson et al. 1992).

Those conducting mental health evaluations of children with renal disease should consider the impact of possible cognitive deficits, adaptation difficulties, and family strain on social and academic functioning, as well as adherence. The level of family stress and distress, as with all pediatric patients, is essential to evaluate and address as part of a larger treatment approach. Recommendations related to the use of psychotropic medication must be extrapolated from adult studies (see Chapter 22, "Renal Disease") because these data are not available for children.

Diabetes

Juvenile-onset diabetes mellitus affects 1.9 of every 1,000 school-age children in the United States (Sperling 2000). Type 1 diabetes mellitus is caused by autoimmune destruction of insulin-producing pancreatic beta cells and must be treated with exogenous insulin. Type 2 diabetes mellitus is the result of resistance to insulin rather than deficiency, can often be treated with diet or hypoglycemic agents, and is generally later in onset than type 1. There are genetic predispositions to both type 1 and type 2 diabetes mellitus (Drash 1993). Obesity and atypical antipsychotic medications appear to contribute to the development of type 2. Both can contribute to mortality and may cause significant morbidity, including retinopathy, nephropathy, peripheral neuropathy, and cardiovascular disease. Injected insulin may also precipitate potentially life-threatening episodes of hypoglycemia (DCCT Research Group 1993, 1994).

The complexity of the management of type 1 diabetes mellitus leads to frequent problems with adherence to medical instructions. Patients on Humalog (or regular) and NPH (neutral protamine Hagedorn) regimens must inject themselves with insulin and test their blood glucose at least three times a day to maintain "tight" control, decreasing the incidence or delaying the onset of complications. Patients on Lantus must take a shot every day and another every time they eat more than 15 grams of carbohydrates (e.g., an apple). Even on an insulin pump, blood glucose must be tested at least four times a day. Diet and exercise must be regulated, as both have significant impact on the need for exogenous insulin.

The physiological changes of puberty can lead to increased insulin resistance. In addition, the importance of peer acceptance and the withdrawal of parental supervision with the normal developmental focus on identity and autonomy lead to significant adherence problems during adolescence (Hauser et al. 1990). Poor control of diabetes has been repeatedly demonstrated using HBA1c (glycosylated hemoglobin), which allows one to get an estimate of glycemic control over past 3 months. The medical consequences of such poor control were demonstrated in a study of 78 adolescents with type 1 diabetes, ages 11–18 years, followed for 8 years. Their mean HbA1c peaked in late adolescence. Serious diabetic complications were seen in 38% of the females and 25% of the males (Bryden et al. 2001).

Studies of the utility of intervention with pediatric diabetic patients have found that interventions to enhance adherence must be intense and early to make a significant difference in long-term outcome. A study of 1,441 patients, ages 13–39 years, followed for a mean of 6.5 years demonstrated a decrease in long-term complications with intensive treatment. Retinopathy developed in 47% of the intensive intervention group, versus 76% in the comparison group, and neuropathy in 57% versus 69%. The price, however, was a two- to threefold increase in severe hypoglycemic events. A study of primary versus secondary intervention followed 195 patients, ages 13–17 years, for a mean of 7.4 years and found that the HBA1c values separated significantly by 6–12 months and were maintained throughout the study. Retinopathy and nephropathy were significantly reduced, although there was no statistical difference in neuropathy between the groups. Again, there was a two- to fourfold increase in severe hypoglycemia, as well as a twofold increase in becoming overweight in the intensive treatment group (DCCT Research Group 1993, 1994).

Psychiatric comorbidity in diabetic individuals is also a major issue for psychiatric consultants to pediatrics. Some moodiness and feelings of isolation and of loss or grief, as well as mild anxiety about the future, are to be expected as normal responses to diabetes. However, assessment for possible intervention is indicated if patients demonstrate aggression, school absences, hopelessness, or nonadherence to the insulin regimen (A.M. Jacobson 1996). In a study of 92 pediatric patients, ages 8–13 years, followed over 9 years, 42% developed at least one psychiatric disorder, and 26% developed two or more disorders. Of these, the most common were depression in 26% and anxiety in 20%, with various behavioral disorders in 16%. Children who were at higher risk of developing psychiatric comorbidity were those in the first year after diagnosis and those who had preexisting anxiety or mothers with psychopathology (Kovacs et al. 1997). Eating disorders are also relatively common. A study of 91 adolescent girls, ages 12–18 years, followed for 5 years found highly or moderately disordered eating in 29% at baseline and in 33% at follow-up (Rydall et al. 1997).

Treatment of comorbid psychiatric disorders with medications requires careful monitoring because most antidepressant, mood stabilizer, and atypical antipsychotic medications may stimulate appetite or affect glucose tolerance, inducing hypoglycemia or hyperglycemia. Beta-blockers should be avoided, as they mask the early warning signs of hypoglycemia, eliminating the window of opportunity for patients to address the problem themselves before requiring the assistance of others (Goodnick et al. 1995).

Effective behavioral interventions for children with diabetes and their parents include identifying readiness for change and improving self-efficacy, the belief that one can maintain behavior change despite regular challenges (Anderson et al. 1996, 1999). In 110 young adults (ages 18–35) with insulin-dependent diabetes mellitus, self-efficacy was more predictive than self-esteem of self-care and metabolic control. Factoring in previous adherence, self-efficacy continues to be predictive of self-care and HbA1c (Johnston-Brooks et al. 2002). A growing area of research is the application of motivational interviewing to work with adolescents with diabetes mellitus (Berg-Smith et al. 1999; Dunn et al. 2001; Williams et al. 1998).

Cardiac Disease

Congenital Heart Defects and Disease

Congenital heart defects and disease include patent ductus arteriosus, atrial septal defects, and ventricular septal defects. About 40,000 children are born with a heart defect each year, and most can benefit from surgery. It appears that heart defects are multidetermined by factors that include genetics as well as exposure during pregnancy by the mother to certain viruses (such as rubella, or German measles) or drugs (such as alcohol, anticonvulsants, or lithium). Acquired heart diseases that develop during childhood include Kawasaki disease, rheumatic fever, and infective endocarditis. Van Horn et al. (2001) studied concerns expressed by mothers of children with congenital heart disease during hospitalization and again 2–4 weeks after discharge. During hospitalization, mothers were most concerned about medical prognosis. Mothers' concerns, anxiety, and depressed mood decreased after discharge. At follow-up, mothers' perceptions of medical severity were related to distress about psychosocial issues. Overall, it appears that children with heart disease psychiatrically resemble a normal population without elevations in anxiety, depression, or behavioral problems (Connolly et al. 2002; DeMaso et al. 2000; Visconti et al. 2002). However, similar to the case in healthy or other chronically ill children, socioeconomic factors, medical severity, and family distress appear to be related to symptoms of depression, anxiety, or behavioral problems (Alden et al. 1998; Visconti et al. 2002; Yildiz et al. 2001). DeMaso et al. (2000) studied pediatric patients with recurrent cardiac arrhythmias who underwent radiofrequency catheter ablation of ectopic myocardial foci. Although these patients psychiatrically resembled a normal population before the procedure, they demonstrated reductions in their "fear of their heart problem" and increases in "the things that they enjoy" after the ablation (DeMaso et al. 2000, p. 134). Those who experienced a curative ablation had better functioning than those who did not experience improvement.

Heart Transplant Recipients

Serrano-Ikkos et al. (1999) compared the psychosocial outcome of pediatric heart and heart-lung transplant recipients with children and adolescents who underwent conventional cardiac surgery. Preoperatively, rates of psychiatric disorders (including anxiety and phobic states, depression and adjustment reaction) were relatively the same in all groups (26%–28.5%). The prevalence of psychiatric disorder was unchanged after transplant in the transplant groups but decreased in the conventional cardiac surgery group. DeMaso et al. (1995) similarly found that the majority of pediatric heart transplant patients studied (78.3%) had good psychological functioning after their heart transplantation. It was further noted that patients with psychological difficulties before and after transplantation had more hospitalizations after transplantation. Finally, Uzark et al. (1992) found that pediatric heart transplant recipients did not differ from peers on measures of self-concept and anxiety but demonstrated less social competence and more behavior problems than a normative population. Behavior problems were frequently suggestive of depression and related to greater family stress and diminished family resources for managing stress. Relaxation and imagery techniques have been successfully used for routine endomyocardial biopsies after heart transplantation (Bullock and Shaddy 1993). A review of the literature related to cognition revealed that children and adolescents generally function normally on measures of cognitive functioning posttransplant, but a complicated transplant course (caused by infections or rejections) may increase risk for cognitive difficulties (Todaro et al. 2000). Serrano-Ikkos et al. (1998) found medication adherence to be relatively high, with 91% adherence confirmed by cyclosporine levels; however, adherence to medical diary keeping was lower, at about 70%. Variables associated with poor adherence to medication were heart-lung as opposed to heart transplantation, one-parent or blended families, and family adjustment.

Chest Pain

Chest pain as a presenting symptom in a previously healthy child is not as ominous a symptom as in an adult because it is rarely a sign of underlying cardiac disease (Driscoll et al. 1976; Tunaoglu et al. 1995). Idiopathic chest pain is the most common diagnosis made, followed by functional pain associated with anxiety, and musculoskeletal pain (Selbst 1985). Laboratory tests are not typically helpful in establishing the etiology of chest pain. This topic is more fully discussed in the section on "Chronic Somatic Symptoms."

Psychotropic Medication

The American Heart Association (Gutgesell et al. 1999) has published recommendations for the use of psychotropic medications in children. Briefly, stimulants cause clinically insignificant increases in heart rate and blood pressure. Tricyclic antidepressant (TCA) treatment of pediatric patients is associated with cardiovascular changes that are likely of minor clinical significance (Wilens et al. 1996). The electrocardiographic effects of TCA administration include an increase in heart rate (by 20%–25%), PR interval (by 5%–10%), QRS duration (by 7%–25%), and QT interval (by 3%–10%). Malignant arrhythmias have not been documented except for the ventricular fibrillation observed in one pediatric patient with a family history of sudden death. To date, deaths in children on TCAs have not been conclusively linked to the medication and have not been demonstrated to be more frequent than expected in the population base. SSRIs have minimal cardiovascular effects. Clonidine has been associated with two deaths (in patients who also received methylphenidate), but the mechanism for these deaths is unknown and may have been sudden cessation of treatment. Adverse effects have occurred when the P450 system was inhibited, leading to elevated levels of medications that prolong the QT interval and produce ventricular tachycardia. Most notable have been deaths related to nonsedating histamine-blocking agents, now off the market. Other medications that inhibit or are metabolized by the P450 cytochrome system include antidepressants, calcium channel blockers, histamine blockers, gastrointestinal motility agents, and steroids. Antiarrhythmic drugs of class IA and class III prolong the QT interval, and therefore use of psychotropic medications with these drugs is not recommended.

Recommendations include taking a careful history, obtaining an electrocardiogram (ECG) at baseline before TCA or phenothiazine therapy is begun (primarily to detect unsuspected instances of long-QT syndrome) and another when steady state is achieved, careful monitoring of all prescribed medications along with heart rate and blood pressure, and avoiding use of psychotropic medications with medications that are metabolized by or inhibit the P450 enzyme system (Gutgesell et al. 1999). History that should be obtained includes past history of syncope, near syncope, or palpitations; family history of deafness, sudden unexpected cardiac death, syncope, or tachydysrhythmias; and a medication history to document all medications that may have direct or indirect effects on the cytochrome P450 system or ECG intervals. Some cardiologists argue that ECG screening in children with no symptoms of cardiovascular disease is less efficient and helpful than simply asking about patient and family history of syncope or sudden death. However, there are no data to clearly settle this question. The American Academy of Child and Adolescent Psychiatry does not specifically address this issue in its policy statement related to prescribing. Nevertheless, the recommendation to conduct ECG screens was recently reiterated (Francis 2002; Labellarte et al. 2003).

Fetal Alcohol Syndrome and Alcohol-Related Neurological Disorder

Prenatal alcohol exposure represents one of the leading preventable causes of congenital neurological impairment, affecting as many as 1 in 100 children born in the United States yearly (May and Gossage 2001), with severe, lifelong consequences for affected individuals. Fetal alcohol syndrome (FAS) is defined by a characteristic pattern of facial anomalies, growth retardation, and CNS dysfunction in one or more of the following areas: decreased cranial size at birth, structural brain abnormalities, and neurological hard or soft signs (Stratton et al. 1996). However, alcohol exposure to the fetus can result in neurocognitive changes even when none of the characteristic facial anomalies are present (Streissguth and O'Malley 2000).

The facial characteristics most frequently described in individuals with FAS include short palpebral fissures and abnormalities in the premaxillary zone, including a thin upper lip and flattened philtrum (Astley and Clarren 2001; Stratton et al. 1996). Neurocognitive changes include structural changes in the brain (Roebuck et al. 1998); verbal learning and memory problems; attention deficits; problems in executive functioning characterized by difficulties in planning, organizing, and sequencing behavior; and problems in abstract and practical reasoning (Adnams et al. 2001), complex nonverbal problem solving (Goodman et al. 1999), flexible thinking (Schonfeld et al. 2001), and behavioral inhibition (Mattson et al. 1999). These changes appear to last into adulthood (Streissguth and O'Malley 2000). Secondary disabilities include high levels of psychiatric illness, school failure, social problems, delinquency, and trouble with the law. No safe level of prenatal alcohol consumption has been established, making abstinence the best policy for those who are hoping to conceive. Because many women are often not aware of when they conceived and may continue to drink alcohol at least until pregnancy recognition, preconception counseling is suggested for all women of child-bearing age who consume alcohol.

References

Adnams CM, Kodituwakku PW, Hay A, et al: Patterns of cognitive-motor development in children with fetal alcohol syndrome from a community in South Africa. Alcohol Clin Exp Res 25:557–562, 2001

Ahearn WH, Castine T, Nault K, et al: An assessment of food acceptance in children with autism or pervasive developmental disorder–not otherwise specified. J Autism Dev Disord 31:505–511, 2001

Alden B, Gilljam T, Gillberg C: Long-term psychological outcome of children after surgery for transposition of the great arteries. Acta Paediatr 87:405–410, 1998

Allison DB, Kaprio J, Korkeil M, et al: The heritability of body mass index among an international sample of monozygotic twins reared apart. Int J Obes Relat Metab Disord 20:501–506, 1996

American Pain Society: Guideline for the management of acute and chronic pain in sickle-cell disease. Glenview, IL, American Pain Society, 1999

Anderson B, Ho J, Brackett J, et al: Parental involvement in diabetes management tasks: relationships to blood glucose monitoring adherence and metabolic control in young adolescents with insulin-dependent diabetes mellitus. J Pediatr 130:257–265, 1996

Anderson BJ, Bracett J, Ho J, et al: An office-based intervention to maintain parent-adolescent teamwork in diabetes management: impact on parent involvement, family conflict, and subsequent glycemic control. Diabetes Care 22:713–721, 1999

Anthony H, Paxton S, Bines J, et al: Psychosocial predictors of adherence to nutritional recommendations and growth outcomes in children with cystic fibrosis. J Psychosom Res 47:623–634, 1999

Arbus GS, Sullivan EK, Tejani A: Hospitalization in children during the first year after kidney transplantation. Kidney Int Suppl 43:83–86, 1993

Astley SJ, Clarren SK: Measuring the facial phenotype of individuals with prenatal alcohol exposure: correlations with brain dysfunction. Alcohol Alcohol 36:147–159, 2001

Ayoub CC: Munchausen by Proxy: Child Placement and Emotional Health. Denver, CO, The 14th International Congress for the Prevention of Child Abuse and Neglect, 2002

Barrickman LL, Perry PJ, Allen AJ, et al: Bupropion versus methylphenidate in the treatment of attention-deficit hyperactivity disorder. J Am Acad Child Adolesc Psychiatry 34:649–657, 1995

Battles HB, Wiener LS: From adolescence through young adulthood: psychosocial adjustment associated with long-term survival of HIV. J Adolesc Health 30:161–168, 2002

Bauman LJ, Wright E, Leickly FE, et al: Relationship of adherence to pediatric asthma morbidity among inner-city children. Pediatrics 110(1 pt 1):e6, 2002

Behrman RE, Kliegman RM, Jenson HB (eds): Nelson Textbook of Pediatrics, 17th Edition. Philadelphia, PA, JB Saunders, 2004

Bennett RM: Emerging concepts in the neurobiology of chronic pain: Evidence of abnormal sensory processing in fibromyalgia. Mayo Clin Proc 74:385–398, 1999

Berg-Smith SM, Stevens VJ, Brown KM, et al: A brief motivational intervention to improve dietary adherence in adolescents. Health Educ Res 14:339–410, 1999

Berkowitz C: Nonorganic failure to thrive and infant rumination syndrome, in Pediatric Functional Bowel Disorders. Edited by Hyman P. New York, Academy of Professional Information Services, 1999, pp 4.1–4.9

Berkowitz RI, Wadden TA, Tershakovec AM, et al: Behavior therapy and sibutramine for the treatment of adolescent obesity: a randomized controlled trial. JAMA 289:1805–1812, 2003

Best M, Streisand R, Catania L, et al: Parental distress during pediatric leukemia and parental posttraumatic stress symptoms after treatment ends. J Pediatr Psychol 26:299–307, 2002

Bittar AE, Keitel E, Garcia CD, et al: Patient noncompliance as a cause of late renal graft failure. Transplant Proc 24:2720–2721, 1992

Black MM, Dubowitz H, Hutcheson J, et al: A randomized clinical trial of home intervention for children with failure to thrive. Pediatrics 95:807–814, 1995

Bond S, Conner-Warren R, Sarnaik SA: Prevalence of pica in children with sickle cell disease. Paper presented at the 19th Annual Meeting of the National Sickle Cell Disease Program, New York, NY, March 25, 1994

Boni LC, Brown RT, Davis PC, et al: Social information processing and magnetic resonance imaging in children with sickle cell disease. J Pediatr Psychol 26(5):309–319, 2001

Bools CN, Neale BA, Meadow SR: Follow up of victims of fabricated illness (Munchausen syndrome by proxy). Arch Dis Child 69:625–630, 1993

Borowsky IW, Mozayeny S, Ireland M: Brief psychosocial screening at health supervision and acute care visits. Pediatrics 112(1 Pt 1):129–133, 2003

Breitbart W, Marotta R, Platt MM, et al: A double-blind trial of haloperidol, chlorpromazine, and lorazepam in the treatment of delirium in hospitalized AIDS patients. Am J Psychiatry 153:231–237, 1996

Brolin RE: Bariatric surgery and long-term control of morbid obesity. JAMA 288:2793–2796, 2002

Brouhard BH, Donaldson LA, Lawry KW, et al: Cognitive functioning in children on dialysis and post-transplantation. Pediatr Transplant 4:261–267, 2000

Brugman SM, Howell JH, Mahler JL, et al: The spectrum of pediatric vocal cord dysfunction. Am Rev Respir Dis 149:A353, 1994

Bryden KS, Peveler RC, Stein A, et al: Clinical and psychological course of diabetes from adolescence to young adulthood. Diabetes Care 24:1536–1540, 2001

Bullock EA, Shaddy RE: Relaxation and imagery techniques without sedation during right ventricular endomyocardial biopsy in pediatric heart transplant patients. J Heart Lung Transplant 12(1 Pt 1):59–62, 1993

Burlew K, Telfair J, Colangelo L, et al: Factors that influence adolescent adaptation to sickle cell disease. J Pediatr Psychol 25:287–299, 2000

Bursch B, Walco G, Zeltzer LK: Clinical assessment and management of chronic pain and pain-associated disability syndrome (PADS). J Dev Behav Pediatr 19:44–52, 1998

Bursch B, Zeltzer LK: Autism spectrum disorders presenting as chronic pain syndromes: case presentations and discussion. Journal of Developmental and Learning Disorders 6:41–48, 2002

Bussing R, Burket RC, Kelleher ET: Prevalence of anxiety disorders in a clinic-based sample of pediatric asthma patients. Psychosomatics 37:108–115, 1996

Butz AM, Alexander C: Anxiety in children with asthma. J Asthma 30:199–209, 1993

Callanan M, Kelley P: Final Gifts: Understanding the Special Awareness, Needs, and Communications of the Dying. New York, NY, Bantam, 1992

Campo JV, Comer DM, Jansen-McWilliams L, et al: Recurrent pain, emotional distress, and health service use in childhood. J Pediatr 141:76–83, 2002

Campo JV, Fritsch SL: Somatization in children and adolescents. J Am Acad Child Adolesc Psychiatry 33:1223–1235, 1994

Campo JV, Fritz G: A management model for pediatric somatization. Psychosomatics 42:467–476, 2001

Campo JV, Jansen-McWilliams L, Comer DM, et al: Somatization in pediatric primary care: association with psychopathology, functional impairment and use of services. J Am Acad Child Adolesc Psychiatry 38:1093–1101, 1999

Caplan R: Epilepsy syndromes in childhood, in Textbook of Pediatric Neuropsychiatry. Edited by Coffey CE, Brumback RA. Washington, DC, American Psychiatric Association, 1998, pp 977–1010

Cepeda ML, Yang YM, Price CC, et al: Mental disorders in children and adolescents with sickle cell disease. South Med J 90:284–287, 1997

Chatoor I, Ganiban J, Colin V, et al: Attachment and feeding problems: a reexamination of nonorganic failure to thrive and attachment insecurity. J Am Acad Child Adolesc Psychiatry 37:1217–1224, 1998

Chen E, Craske MG, Katz ER, et al: Pain-sensitive temperament: does it predict procedural distress and response to psychological treatment among children with cancer? J Pediatr Psychol 25:269–278, 2000

Chial HJ, Camilleri M, Williams DE, et al: Rumination syndrome in children and adolescents: diagnosis, treatment, and prognosis. Pediatrics 111:158–162, 2003

Chinn S, Rona RJ: Prevalence and trends in overweight and obesity in three cross-sectional studies of British children, 1974–1994. BMJ 322:24–26, 2001

Chunming C: Fat intake and nutritional status in children in China. Am J Clin Nutr 72:1368S–1372S, 2000

Clouse RE, Richter JE, Heading RC, et al: Functional esophageal disorders. Gut 45 (suppl 2):II31–II36, 1999

Conners CK, Casat CD, Gualtieri CT, et al: Bupropion hydrochloride in attention deficit disorder with hyperactivity. J Am Acad Child Adolesc Psychiatry 35:1314–1321, 1996

Connolly D, Rutkowski M, Auslender M, et al: Measuring health-related quality of life in children with heart disease. Appl Nurs Res 15:74–80, 2002

Costello EJ, Costello AJ, Edelbrock C, et al: Psychiatric disorders in pediatric primary care. Prevalence and risk factors. Arch Gen Psychiatry 45:1107–1116, 1988

Costello EJ, Shugart MA: Above and below the threshold: severity of psychiatric symptoms and functional impairment in a pediatric sample. Pediatrics 90:359–368, 1992

Dalzell AM, Shepherd RW, Dean B, et al: Nutritional rehabilitation in cystic fibrosis: a 5 year follow-up study. J Pediatr Gastroenterol Nutr 15:141–145, 1992

DCCT Research Group: The effects of intensive treatment of diabetes on the development and progression of long-term complications in insulin-dependent diabetes mellitus. N Engl J Med 329:977–986, 1993

DCCT Research Group: Effects of intensive diabetes treatment on the development and progression of long-term complications in adolescents with insulin-dependent diabetes mellitus: Diabetes Control and Complications Trial. J Pediatr 125:177–188, 1994

de Onis M, Blossner M: Prevalence and trends of overweight among preschool children in developing countries. Am J Clin Nutr 72:1032–1039, 2000

DeMaso DR, Spratt EG, Vaughan BL, et al: Psychological functioning in children and adolescents undergoing radiofrequency catheter ablation. Psychosomatics 41:134–139, 2000

DeMaso DR, Twente AW, Spratt EG, et al: Impact of psychologic functioning, medical severity, and family functioning in pediatric heart transplantation. J Heart Lung Transplant 14(6 Pt 1): 1102–1108, 1995

Dietz WH, Bellizzi MC: Introduction: the use of body mass index to assess obesity in children. Am J Clin Nutr 70:123S–125S, 1999

DiMatteo MR, Giordani PJ, Lepper HS, et al: Patient adherence and medical treatment outcomes: a meta-analysis. Med Care 40:794–811, 2002

Drash AL: The child, the adolescent, and the diabetes control and complications trial. Diabetes Care 16:1515–1516, 1993

Drewett RF, Corbett SS, Wright CM: Cognitive and educational attainments at school age of children who failed to thrive in infancy: a population-based study. J Child Psychol Psychiatry 40:551–561, 1999

Driscoll DJ, Glicklich LB, Gallen WJ: Chest pain in children: a prospective study. Pediatrics 57:648–651, 1976

Du Pasquier-Fediaevsky L, Tubiana-Rufi N: Discordance between physician and adolescent assessments of adherence to treatment: influence of HbA1c level. The PEDIAB Collaborative Group. Diabetes Care 22:1445–1449, 1999

Dunn C, Deroo L, Rivara F: The use of brief interventions adapted from motivational interviewing across behavioral domains: a systemic review. Addiction 96:1725–1742, 2001

Dykman RA, Casey PH, Ackerman PT, et al: Behavioral and cognitive status in school-aged children with a history of failure to thrive during early childhood. Clin Pediatr (Phila) 40:63–70, 2001

Ebbeling CA, Pawlak DB, Ludwig DS: Childhood obesity: public-health crisis, common sense cure. Lancet 360:473–482, 2002

Efron D, Hiscock H, Sewell JR, et al: Prescribing of psychotropic medications for children by Australian pediatricians and child psychiatrists. Pediatrics 111:372–375, 2003

Egger HL, Angold A, Costello EJ: Headaches and psychopathology in children and adolescents. J Am Acad Child Adolesc Psychiatry 37:951–958, 1998

Ely EW, Gautam S, Margolin R, et al: The impact of delirium in the intensive care unit on hospital length of stay. Intensive Care Med 27:1892–1900, 2001

Erickson SJ, Steiner H: Trauma spectrum adaptation: somatic symptoms in long-term pediatric cancer survivors. Psychosomatics 41:339–346, 2000

Ettenger RB, Rosenthal JT, Marik JL, et al: Improved cadaveric renal transplant outcome in children. Pediatr Nephrol 5:137–142, 1991

Fennell RS 3rd, Rasbury WC, Fennell EB, et al: Effects of kidney transplantation on cognitive performance in a pediatric population. Pediatrics 74:273–278, 1984

Field MJ, Institute of Medicine, Behrman RE: When Children Die: Improving Palliative and End-of-Life Care for Children and their Families. Washingtonm DC, National Academies Press, 2003

Fisher BL, Schauer P: Medical and surgical options in the treatment of severe obesity. Am J Surg 184(6, suppl 2):S9–S16, 2002

Fisher WW, Piazza CC, Bowman LG, et al: A preliminary evaluation of empirically derived consequences for the treatment of pica. J Appl Behav Anal 27:447–457, 1994

Francis PD: Effects of psychotropic medications on the pediatric electrocardiogram and recommendations for monitoring. Curr Opin Pediatr 14:224–230, 2002

Frank NC, Blount RL, Brown RT: Attributions, coping, and adjustment in children with cancer. J Pediatr Psychol 22:563–576, 1997

Fritz GK, Fritsch S, Hagino O. Somatoform disorders in children and adolescents: a review of the past 10 years. J Am Acad Child Adolesc Psychiatry 36:1329–1338, 1997

Fukunishi I, Honda M: School adjustment of children with end-stage renal disease. Pediatr Nephrol 9:553–557, 1995

Fukunishi I, Kudo H: Psychiatric problems of pediatric end-stage renal failure. Gen Hosp Psychiatry 17:32–36, 1995

Gadoth N: Multiple sclerosis in children. Brain Dev 25:229–232, 2003

Garber J, Zeman J, Walker L: Recurrent abdominal pain in children: psychiatric diagnoses and parental psychopathology. J Am Acad Child Adolesc Psychiatry 29:648–656, 1990

Garber J, Walker LS, Zeman J: Somatization symptoms in a community sample of children and adolescents: further validation of the children's somatization inventory. J Consult Clin Psychol 3:588–595, 1991

Garralda ME, Jameson RA, Reynolds JM, et al: Psychiatric adjustment in children with chronic renal failure. J Child Psychol Psychiatry 29:79–90, 1988

Gavin LA, Wamboldt M, Brugman S, et al: Psychological and family characteristics of adolescents with vocal cord dysfunction. J Asthma 35:409–417, 1998

Gizynski M, Shapiro V: Depression and childhood illness. Child Adolesc Social Work J 7:179–197, 1990

Godding V, Kruth M, Jamart J: Joint consultation for high-risk asthmatic children and their families, with pediatrician and child psychiatrist as co-therapists: model and evaluation. Fam Process 36:265–280, 1997

Goldbeck L, Babka C: Development and evaluation of a multifamily psychoeducational program for cystic fibrosis. Patient Educ Couns 44:187–192, 2001

Goldston DB, Kovacs M, Ho VY, et al: Suicidal ideation and suicide attempts among youth with insulin-dependent diabetes mellitus. J Am Acad Child Adolesc Psychiatry 33:240, 1994

Goodman AM, Mattson SN, Lang AR, et al: Concept formation and problem solving in children with heavy prenatal alcohol exposure. Alcohol Clin Exp Res 23 (suppl 5):32A, 1999

Goodnick PJ, Henry JH, Buki VM: Treatment of depression in patients with diabetes mellitus. J Clin Psychiatry 56:128–136, 1995

Goodwin RD, Pine DS, Hoven CW: Asthma and panic attacks among youth in the community. J Asthma 40:139–145, 2003

Gortmaker SL, Must A, Perrin JM, et al: Social and economic consequences of overweight in adolescence and young adulthood. N Engl J Med 329:1008–1012, 1993

Graham PJ, Rutter ML, Pless IB: Childhood asthma: a psychosomatic disorder? Some epidemiological considerations. Br J Prev Soc Med 2:78–85, 1967

Green WH, Campbell M, David R: Psychosocial dwarfism: a critical review of the evidence. J Am Acad Child Psychiatry 23:39–48, 1984

Griffin KJ, Elkin TD: Non-adherence in pediatric transplantation: a review of the existing literature. Pediatr Transplant 5:246–249, 2001

Guo SS, Roche AF, Chumlea WC, et al: The predictive value of childhood body mass index values for overweight at age 35 years. Am J Clin Nutr 59:810–819, 1994

Gustafsson PA, Kjellman NI, Cederblad M: Family therapy in the treatment of severe childhood asthma. J Psychosom Res 30:369–374, 1986

Gutgesell H, Atkins D, Barst R, et al: AHA Scientific Statement: cardiovascular monitoring of children and adolescents receiving psychotropic drugs. J Am Acad Child Adolesc Psychiatry 38:1047–1050, 1999

Gyulay JE: Home care for the dying child. Issues Compr Pediatr Nurs 12:33–69, 1989

Hahn JS, Berquist W, Alcorn DM, et al: Wernicke encephalopathy and beriberi during total parenteral nutrition attributable to multivitamin infusion shortage. Pediatrics 101:E10, 1998

Hauser ST, Jacobson AM, Lavori P, et al: Adherence among children and adolescents with insulin-dependent diabetes mellitus over a four-year longitudinal follow-up, II: immediate and long-term linkages with the family milieu. J Pediatr Psychol 15:527–542, 1990

Heal DJ, Aspley S, Prow MR, et al: Sibutramine: a novel antiobesity drug. A review of the pharmacological evidence to differentiate it from d-amphetamine and d-fenfluramine. Int J Obes Relat Metab Disord 22:S19–S29, 1998

Heruti RJ, Levy A, Adunski A, et al: Conversion motor paralysis disorder: overview and rehabilitation model. Spinal Cord 40:327–334, 2002

Ho J, Bender BG, Gavin LA, et al: Relations among asthma knowledge, treatment adherence, and outcome. J Allergy Clin Immunol 111:498–502, 2003

Hobbie W, Stuber M, Meeske K, et al: Symptoms of posttraumatic stress in young adult survivors of childhood cancer. J Clin Onc 18:4060–4066, 2000

Hodges K, Kline JJ, Barbero G, et al: Depressive symptoms in children with recurrent abdominal pain and in their families. J Pediatr 107:622–626, 1985a

Hodges K, Kline JJ, Barbero G, et al: Anxiety in children with recurrent abdominal pain and their parents. Psychosomatics 26:859, 862–866, 1985b

Hyman PE, Bursch B, Lopez E, et al: Visceral pain-associated disability syndrome: A descriptive analysis. J Pediatr Gastroenterol Nutr 35(5):663–668, 2002

Ireys HT, Chernoff R, DeVet KA, et al: Maternal outcomes of a randomized controlled trial of a community-based support program for families of children with chronic illnesses. Arch Pediatr Adolesc Med 155:771–777, 2001

Ivascu NS, Sarnaik S, McCrae J, et al: Characterization of pica prevalence among patients with sickle cell disease. Arch Pediatr Adolesc Med 155:1243–1247, 2001

Jacobson AM: The psychological care of patients with insulin-dependent diabetes mellitus. N Engl J Med 334:1249–1253, 1996

Jacobson SA, Leuchter AF, Walter DO: Conventional and quantitative EEG in the diagnosis of delirium among the elderly. J Neurol Neurosurg Psychiatry 56:153–158, 1993

Jay SM, Elliott CH, Woody PD, et al: An investigation of cognitive–behavioral therapy combined with oral Valium for children undergoing painful medical procedures. Health Psychol 10:317–322, 1991

Jelalian E, Saelens BE: Empirically supported treatments in pediatric psychology: pediatric obesity. J Pediatr Psychol 24:223–248, 1999

Johnson CR, Hunt FM, Siebert MJ: Discrimination training in the treatment of pica and food scavenging. Behav Modif 18:214–229, 1994

Johnston-Brooks CH, Lewis MA, Garg S: Self-efficacy impacts self-care and HbA1c in young adults with type 1 diabetes. Psychosom Med 64:43–51, 2002

Kashani JH, Barbero GJ, Wilfley DE, et al: Psychological concomitants of cystic fibrosis in children and adolescents. Adolescence 23:873–880, 1988a

Kashani JH, König P, Shepperd JA, et al: Psychopathology and self-concept in asthmatic children. J Pediatr Psychol 13: 509–520, 1988b

Kashikar-Zuck S, Goldschneider KR, Powers SW, et al: Depression and functional disability in chronic pediatric pain. Clin J Pain 17:341–349, 2001

Kazak A, Penati B, Brophy P, et al: Pharmacological and psychological interventions for procedural pain. Pediatrics 102: 59–66, 1998

Kazak A, Simms S, Rourke M: Family systems practice in pediatric psychology. J Pediatr Psychol 27:133–143, 2002

Kazak AE, Barakat LP, Meeske K, et al: Posttraumatic stress symptoms, family functioning, and social support in survivors of childhood leukemia and their mothers and fathers. J Consult Clin Psychol 65:120–129, 1997

Kemper MJ, Sparta G, Laube GF, et al: Neuropsychologic side-effects of tacrolimus in pediatric renal transplantation. Clin Transplant 17:130–134, 2003

Kendall P: Treating anxiety disorders in children: results of a randomized clinical trial. J Consult Clin Psychol 62:100–110, 1994

Kerwin ME: Empirically supported treatments in pediatric psychology: severe feeding problems. J Pediatr Psychol 24: 193–214, 1999

Kinney TR, Sleeper LA, Wang WC, et al: Silent cerebral infarcts in sickle cell anemia: a risk factor analysis. Pediatrics 103:640–645, 1999

Klein-Gitelman MS, Pachman LM: Intravenous corticosteroids: adverse reactions are more variable than expected in children. J Rheumatol 25:1995–2002, 1998

Kothare SV, Ebb DH, Rosenberger PB, et al: Acute confusion and mutism as a presentation of thalamic strokes secondary to deep cerebral venous thrombosis. J Child Neurol 13:300–303, 1998

Kovacs M, Goldston D, Obrosky DS, et al: Psychiatric disorders in youth with IDDM: rates and risk factors. Diabetes Care 20:36–44, 1997

Krilov LR, Fisher M, Friedman SB, et al: Course and outcome of chronic fatigue in children and adolescents. Pediatrics 102(2 Pt 1):360–366, 1998

Labellarte MJ, Crosson JE, Riddle MA: The relevance of prolonged QTc measurement to pediatric psychopharmacology. J Am Acad Child Adolesc Psychiatry 42:642–650, 2003

Lask B, Matthew D: Childhood asthma. A controlled trial of family psychotherapy. Arch Dis Child 54:116–119, 1979

Lemanek KL, Kamps J, Chung MB: Empirical supported treatments in pediatric psychology: regimen adherence. J Pediatr Psychol 26:253–275, 2001

Lester P, Stein JA, Bursch B: Developmental predictors of somatic symptoms in adolescents of parents with HIV: a 12-month follow-up. J Dev Behav Pediatr 24:242–250, 2003

Li B, Balint JP: Cyclic vomiting syndrome: the evolution of understanding of a brain-gut disorder. Adv Pediatr 47:117–160, 2000

Libow JA: Beyond collusion: active illness falsification. Child Abuse Negl 26:525–536, 2002

Libow JA: Child and adolescent illness falsification. Pediatrics 105:336–342, 2000

Libow JA: Munchausen by proxy victims in adulthood: a first look. Child Abuse Negl 19:1131–1142, 1995

Liebowitz MR, Turner SM, Piacentini J, et al: Fluoxetine in children and adolescents with OCD: a placebo-controlled trial. J Am Acad Child Adolesc Psychiatry 41:1431–1438, 2002

Lieh-Lai MW, Theodorou AA, Sarnaik AP, et al: Limitations of the Glasgow Coma Scale in predicting outcome in children with traumatic brain injury. J Pediatr 120(2 pt 1):195–199, 1992

Livingston R, Witt A, Smith GR: Families who somatize. J Dev Behav Pediatr 16:42–46, 1995

Livingston R: Children of people with somatization disorder. J Am Acad Child Adolesc Psychiatry 3:36–544, 1993

Ljungman G, Gordh T, Sorensen S, et al: Lumbar puncture in pediatric oncology: conscious sedation vs. general anesthesia. Med Pediatr Oncol 36:372–379, 2001

Ljungman G, Kreuger A, Andreasson S, et al: Midazolam nasal spray reduces procedural anxiety in children. Pediatrics 105(1 pt 1):73–78, 2000

Lurie S, Shemesh E, Sheiner PA, et al: Non-adherence in pediatric liver transplant recipients—an assessment of risk factors and natural history. Pediatr Transplant 4:200–206, 2000

MacLean W Jr, Perrin J, Gortmarkers S, et al: Psychological adjustment of children with asthma: effects of illness severity and recent stressful life events. J Pediatr Psychol 17:159–171, 1988

Mailis-Gagnon A, Giannoylis I, Downar J, et al: Altered central somatosensory processing in chronic pain patients with "hysterical" anesthesia. Neurology 60:1501–1507, 2003

Malcolm A, Thumshirn MB, Camilleri M, et al: Rumination syndrome. Mayo Clin Proc 72:646–652, 1997

Manne SL, Du Hamel K, Gallelli K, et al: Posttraumatic stress disorder among mothers of pediatric cancer survivors: diagnosis, comorbidity, and utility of the PTSD checklist as a screening instrument. J Pediatr Psychol 23:357–366, 1998

Manos PJ, Wu R: The duration of delirium in medical and post-operative patients referred for psychiatric consultation. Ann Clin Psychiatry 9:219–226, 1997

Mattson SN, Goodman AM, Caine C, et al: Executive functioning in children with heavy prenatal alcohol exposure. Alcohol Clin Exp Res 23:1808–1815, 1999

May PA , Gossage JP: Estimating the prevalence of fetal alcohol syndrome. Alcohol Health Res World 25:159–167, 2001

Mayes L, Volkmar F, Hooks M, et al: Differentiating pervasive developmental disorder not otherwise specified from autism and language disorders. J Autism Dev Disord 23:79–90, 1993

McNichol K, Williams H, Allan J, et al: Spectrum of asthma in children, III: psychological and social components. BMJ 4:16–20, 1973

McQuaid EL, Kopel SJ, Klein RB, et al: Medication adherence in pediatric asthma: reasoning, responsibility, and behavior. J Pediatr Psychol 28:323–333, 2003

Meeske K, Stuber ML: PTSD, Quality of life and psychological outcome in young adult survivors of pediatric cancer. Oncol Nurs Forum 28:481–489, 2001

Minuchin S, Rosman B, Baker L: Psychosomatic Families. Boston, MA, Harvard University Press, 1978

Morgan CM, Tanofsky-Kraff M, Wilfley DE, et al: Childhood obesity. Child Adolesc Psychiatr Clin N Am 11:257–278, 2002

Morton MJ, Reynolds JM, Garralda ME, et al: Psychiatric adjustment in end-stage renal disease: a follow up study of former paediatric patients. J Psychosom Res 38:293–303, 1994

Mossberg HO: Forty year follow-up of overweight children. Lancet 2(8661):491–493, 1989

Mrazek DA, Anderson IS, Strunk RC: Disturbed emotional development of severely asthmatic preschool children. J Child Psychol Psychiatry 4:81–94, 1985

Munk DD, Repp AC: Behavioral assessment of feeding problems of individuals with severe disabilities. J Appl Behav Anal 27:241–250, 1994

Must A, Spandano J, Coakley EH, et al: The disease burden associated with overweight and obesity. JAMA 282:1523–1529, 1999

Navelet Y, Nedelcoux H, Teszner D, et al: Emergency pediatric EEG in mental confusion, behavioral disorders and vigilance disorders: a retrospective study. Neurophysiol Clin 28:435–443, 1998

Norrish M, Tooley M, Godfry S: Clinical, physiological, and psychological study of asthmatic children attending a hospital clinic. Arch Dis Child 52:912–917, 1977

O'Brien MD, Bruce BK, Camilleri M: The rumination syndrome: clinical features rather than manometric diagnosis. Gastroenterology 108:1024–1029, 1995

Oguz A, Kurul S, Dirik E: Relationship of epilepsy-related factors to anxiety and depression scores in epileptic children. J Child Neurol 17:37–40, 2002

Ohene-Frempong K: Stroke in sickle cell disease: demographic, clinical, and therapeutic considerations. Semin Hematol 28:213–219, 1991

Ohene-Frempong K, Weiner SJ, Sleeper LA, et al: Cerebrovascular accidents in sickle cell disease: rates and risk factors. Blood 91:288–294, 1998

Ollendick TH, King NJ: Empirically supported treatments for children with phobic and anxiety disorders: current status. J Clin Child Psychol 27:156–167, 1998

Paniagua FA, Braverman C, Capriotti RM: Use of a treatment package in the management of a profoundly mentally retarded girl's pica and self-stimulation. Am J Ment Defic 90:550–557, 1986

Panton J, Barley EA: Family therapy for asthma in children. Cochrane Database Syst Rev (2):CD000089, 2000

Papakostas K, Moraitis D, Lancaster J, et al: Depressive symptoms in children after tonsillectomy. Int J Pediatr Otorhinolaryngol 67:127–132, 2003

Parker RI, Mahan RA, Giugliano D, et al: Efficacy and safety of intravenous midazolam and ketamine as sedation for therapeutic and diagnostic procedures in children. Pediatrics 99:427–431, 1997

Patterson JM, Budd J, Goetz D, et al: Family correlates of a 10-year pulmonary health trend in cystic fibrosis. Pediatrics 91:383–389, 1993

Peyron R, Laurent B, Garcia-Larrea L: Functional imaging of brain responses to pain. A review and meta-analysis 2000. Neurophysiol Clin 30:263–288, 2000

Pfeffer CR: Suicide prevention. Current efficacy and future promise. Ann N Y Acad Sci 487:341–350, 1986

Phipps S, DeCuir-Whalley S: Adherence issues in pediatric bone marrow transplantation. J Pediatr Psychol 15:459–475, 1990

Phipps S, Srivastava DK: Repressive adaptation in children with cancer. Health Psychol 16:521–528, 1997

Phipps S, Srivastava DK: Approaches to the measurement of depressive symptomatology in children with cancer: attempting to circumvent the effects of defensiveness. Development and Behavioral Pediatrics 20:150–156, 1999

Piacentini J, Bergman RL: Developmental issues in cognitive therapy for childhood anxiety disorders. Journal of Cognitive Psychotherapy 15:165–182, 2001

Platt OS, Brambilla DJ, Rosse WF, et al: Mortality in sickle cell disease. Life expectancy and risk factors for early death. N Engl J Med 330:1639–1644, 1994

Porter GE, Heitsch GM, Miller MD: Munchausen syndrome by proxy: unusual manifestations and disturbing sequelae. Child Abuse Negl 18:789–794, 1994

Powers SW. Empirically supported treatments in pediatric psychology: Procedure-related pain. J Pediatr Psychol 24:131–145, 1999

Qvist E, Pihko H, Fagerudd P, Valanne L, et al: Neurodevelopmental outcome in high-risk patients after renal transplantation in early childhood. Pediatr Transplant 6:53–62, 2002

Rapoff MA: Adherence to Pediatric Medical Regimens. New York, Kluwer/Plenum, 1999

Rapoff MA, Belmont J, Lindsley C, et al: Prevention of nonadherence to nonsteroidal anti-inflammatory medications for newly diagnosed patients with juvenile rheumatoid arthritis. Health Psychol 21:620–623, 2002

Rasquin-Weber A, Hyman PE, Cucchiara S, et al: Childhood functional gastrointestinal disorders. Gut 45 (suppl 2):II60–II68, 1999

Raymond NC, Chang PN, Crow SJ, et al: Eating disorders in patients with cystic fibrosis. J Adolesc 23:359–363, 2000

Reynolds JM, Garralda ME, Jameson RA, et al: How parents and families cope with chronic renal failure. Arch Dis Child 63:821–826, 1988

Reynolds JM, Garralda ME, Postlethwaite RJ, et al: Changes in psychosocial adjustment after renal transplantation. Arch Dis Child 66:508–513, 1991

Riddle MA, Bernstein GA, Cook EH, et al: Anxiolytics, adrenergic agents, and naltrexone. J Am Acad Child Adolesc Psychiatry 38:546–556, 1999

Robb SL, Ebberts AG: Songwriting and digital video production interventions for pediatric patients undergoing bone marrow transplantation, part I: an analysis of depression and anxiety levels according to phase of treatment. J Pediatr Oncol Nurs 20:2–15, 2003

Robieux IC, Kumar R, Rhadakrishnan S, et al: The feasibility of using EMLA (eutectic mixture of local anaesthetics) cream in pediatric outpatient clinics. Can J Hosp Pharm 43:235–236, xxxii, 1990

Rodgers GP, Clark CM, Kessler RM: Regional alterations in brain metabolism in neurologically normal sickle cell patients. J Am Med Assoc 256:1692–1700, 1984

Roebuck RM, Mattson SN, Riley EP: Behavioral and psychosocial profiles of alcohol-exposed children. Alcohol Clin Exp Res 22:339–344, 1998

Rydall AC, Rodin GM, Olmsted MP, et al: Disordered eating behavior and microvascular complications in young women with insulin-dependent diabetes mellitus. N Engl J Med 336:1849–1854, 1997

Sahler OJ, Varni JW, Fairclough DL, et al: Problem-solving skills training for mothers of children with newly diagnosed cancer: a randomized trial. J Dev Behav Pediatr 23:77–86, 2002

Salvatierra O, Alfrey E, Tanne, DC, et al: Superior outcomes in pediatric renal transplantation. Arch Surg 132:842–847, 1997

Sanders MR, Rebyetz M, Morrison M, et al: Cognitive-behavioral treatment of recurrent nonspecific abdominal pain in children: an analysis of generalization, maintenance and side effects. J Consult Clin Psychol 57:294–300, 1989

Sanders MR, Shepherd RW, Cleghorn G, et al: The treatment of recurrent abdominal pain in children: a controlled comparison of cognitive-behavioral family intervention and standard pediatric care. J Consult Clin Psychol 62:306–314, 1994

Saxe GN, Stoddard FJ, Sheridan RL: PTSD in children with burns: a longitudinal study. J Burn Care Rehabil 19(1 pt 2): S206, 1998

Schanberg LE, Keefe FJ, Lefebvre JC, et al: Social context of pain in children with Juvenile Primary Fibromyalgia Syndrome: parental pain history and family environment. Clin J Pain 14:107–115, 1998

Schiffrin A: Psychosocial issues in pediatric diabetes. Curr Diab Rep 1:33–40, 2001

Schonfeld A, Mattson SN, Lang A, Delis DC, Riley EP: Verbal and nonverbal fluency in children with heavy prenatal alcohol exposure. J Stud Alcohol 62:239–246, 2001

Schwimmer JB, Burwinkle TM, Varni JW: Health-related quality of life of severely obese children and adolescents. JAMA 289:1813–1819, 2003

Segal DG, Sanchez JC: Childhood obesity in the year 2001. Endocrinologist 11:296–306, 2001

Selbst SM: Chest pain in children. Pediatrics 75:1068–1070, 1985

Serrano-Ikkos E, Lask B, Whitehead B, et al: Incomplete adherence after pediatric heart and heart-lung transplantation. J Heart Lung Transplant 17:1177–1183, 1998

Serrano-Ikkos E, Lask B, Whitehead B, et al: Heart or heart-lung transplantation: psychosocial outcome. Pediatr Transplant 3:301–308, 1999

Shaabat A: Confusional migraine in childhood. Pediatr Neurol 15:23–25, 1996

Shemesh E, Lurie S, Stuber ML, et al: A pilot study of posttraumatic stress and nonadherence in pediatric liver transplant recipients. Pediatrics 105:E29, 2000

Shemesh E, Shneider BL, Savitzky JK, et al: Medication adherence in pediatric and adolescent liver transplant recipients. Pediatrics 113:825–832, 2004

Sheridan RL, Hinson M, Nackel A, et al: Development of a pediatric burn pain and anxiety management program. J Burn Care Rehabil 18:455–459, 1997

Sibbitt WL Jr, Brandt JR, Johnson CR, et al: The incidence and prevalence of neuropsychiatric syndromes in pediatric onset systemic lupus erythematosus. J Rheumatol 29:1536–1542, 2002

Simonds JF: Psychiatric consultations for 112 pediatric inpatients. South Med J 70:980–984, 1977

Simoni JM, Asarnow JR, Munford PR, et al: Psychological distress and treatment adherence among children on dialysis. Pediatr Nephrol 11:604–606, 1997

Singhi S, Singhi P, Adwani GB: Role of psychosocial stress in the cause of pica. Clin Pediatr (Phila) 20:783–785, 1981

Snodgrass SR, Vedanarayanan VV, Parker CC, et al: Pediatric patients with undetectable anticonvulsant blood levels: comparison with compliant patients. J Child Neurol 16:164–168, 2001

Soliday E, Hoeksel R: Health beliefs and pediatric emergency department after-care adherence. Ann Behav Med 22:299–306, 2000

Soykan I, Chen J, Kendall BJ, et al: The rumination syndrome: clinical and manometric profile, therapy, and long-term outcome. Dig Dis Sci 42:1866–1872, 1997

Sperling MA: Diabetes mellitus, in Nelson Textbook of Pediatrics. Edited by Behrman RE, Kliegman RM, Arvin AM. Philadelphia: Saunders, 2000, p 1768

Steele RG, Grauer D: Adherence to antiretroviral therapy for pediatric HIV infection: review of the literature and recommendations for research. Clin Child Fam Psychol Rev 6:17–30, 2003

Steele RG, Anderson B, Rindel B, et al: Adherence to antiretroviral therapy among HIV-positive children: examination of the role of caregiver health beliefs. AIDS Care 13:617–630, 2001

Steinhausen HC, Schindler HP, Stephan H: Comparative psychiatric studies on children and adolescents suffering from cystic fibrosis and bronchial asthma. Child Psychiatry Hum Dev 14:117–130, 1983

Steward DK: Behavioral characteristics of infants with nonorganic failure to thrive during a play interaction. MCN Am J Matern Child Nurs 26:79–85, 2001

Stoddard FJ, Saxe G: Ten-year research review of physical injuries. J Am Acad Child Adolesc Psychiatry. 40:1128–1145, 2001

Stratton K, Howe C, Battaglia F (eds): Fetal Alcohol Syndrome: Diagnosis, Prevention, and Treatment. Washington, DC, National Academy Press, 1996

Strauss RS, Bradley LJ, Brolin RE: Gastric bypass surgery in adolescents with morbid obesity. J Pediatr 138:499–504, 2001

Streisand R, Braniecki S, Tercyak KP, et al: Childhood illness-related parenting stress: the pediatric inventory for parents. J Pediatr Psychol 26:155–162, 2001

Streissguth AP, O'Malley K: Neuropsychiatric implications and long-term consequences of fetal alcohol spectrum disorders. Semin Clin Neuropsychiatry 5:177–190, 2000

Strunk RC, Mrazek DA, Wolfson Fuhrmann GS, et al: Psychologic and psychological characteristics associated with death due to asthma in childhood. A case-controlled study. JAMA 254:1193–1198, 1985

Strunk RC, Bender B, Young DA, et al: Predictors of protocol adherence in a pediatric asthma clinical trial. J Allergy Clin Immunol 110:596–602, 2002

Stuart S, Noyes R: Attachment and interpersonal communication in somatization. Psychosomatics 40:34–43, 1999

Stuber ML, Bursch B: Psychiatric care of the terminally ill child, in Psychiatric Dimensions of Palliative Medicine. Edited by Chochinov HM, Breitbart W. New York, NY, Oxford University Press, 2000, pp 225–264

Stuber ML, Mesrkhani VH: "What do we tell the children?": understanding childhood grief. West J Med 174:187–191, 2001

Stunkard A, Sabal J: Psychosocial consequences of obesity, in Eating Disorders and Obesity. Edited by Brownell KD, Fairburn CG. New York: Guilford, 1995, pp 417–421

Stunkard AJ, Harris JR, Pederson NL, et al: The body-mass index of twins who have been reared apart. N Engl J Med 322:1483–1487, 1990

Swanson M, Hall D, Bartas S, et al: Economic impact of noncompliance in kidney transplant recipients. Transplant Proc 24:2723–2724, 1992

Telfair J: Factors in the long term adjustment of children and adolescents with sickle cell disease: conceptualizations and review of the literature. J Health Soc Policy 5:69–96, 1994

Terre L, Ghiselli W: A developmental perspective on family risk factors in somatization. J Psychosom Res 42:197–208, 1997

The Research Unit on Pediatric Psychopharmacology Anxiety Study Group: Fluvoxamine for the treatment of anxiety disorders in children and adolescents. N Engl J Med 344:1279–1285, 2001

Todaro JF, Fennell EB, Sears SF, et al: Review: cognitive and psychological outcomes in pediatric heart transplantation. J Pediatr Psychol 25:567–576, 2000

Troiano RP, Flegal KM, Kuczmarski RJ, et al: Overweight prevalence and trends for children and adolescents: the national health and nutrition examination surveys, 1963 to 1991. Arch Pediatr Adolesc Med 149:1085–1091, 1995

Tsai SJ, Lee YC, Chang K, et al: Psychiatric consultations in pediatric inpatients. Zhonghua Min Guo Xiao Er Ke Yi Xue Hui Za Zhi 36:411–414, 1995

Tucker CM, Fennell RS, Pedersen T, et al: Associations with medication adherence among ethnically different pediatric patients with renal transplants. Pediatr Nephrol 17:251–256, 2002

Tunaoglu FS, Olgunturk R, Akcabay S, et al: Chest pain in children referred to a cardiology clinic. Pediatr Cardiol 16:69–72, 1995

Turkel SB, Miller JH, Reiff A: Case series: neuropsychiatric symptoms with pediatric systemic lupus erythematosus. J Am Acad Child Adolesc Psychiatry 40:482–485, 2001

Turkel SB, Braslow K, Tavare CJ, et al: The delirium rating scale in children and adolescents. Psychosomatics 44:126–129, 2003

Uzark KC, Sauer SN, Lawrence KS, et al: The psychosocial impact of pediatric heart transplantation. J Heart Lung Transplant 11:1160, 1992

Van Horn M, DeMaso DR, Gonzalez-Heydrich J, et al: Illness-related concerns of mothers of children with congenital heart disease. J Am Acad Child Adolesc Psychiatry 40:847–854, 2001

Vasconcellos E, Pina-Garza JE, Fakhoury T, et al: Pediatric manifestations of Hashimoto's encephalopathy. Pediatr Neurol 20:394–398, 1999

Vila G, Nollet-Clemencon C, Vera M, Robert JJ, et al: Prevalence of DSM-IV disorders in children and adolescents with asthma versus diabetes. Can J Psychiatry 44:562–569, 1999

Visconti KJ, Saudino KJ, Rappaport LA, et al: Influence of parental stress and social support on the behavioral adjustment of children with transposition of the great arteries. J Dev Behav Pediatr 23:314–321, 2002

Volkmar FR, Poll J, Lewis M: Conversion reactions in childhood and adolescence. J Am Acad Child Adolesc Psychiatry 23:424–430, 1984

von Weiss RT, Rapoff MA, Varni JW, et al: Daily hassles and social support as predictors of adjustment in children with pediatric rheumatic disease. J Pediatr Psychol 27:155–165, 2002

Wagaman JR, Williams DE, Camilleri M: Behavioral intervention for the treatment of rumination. J Pediatr Gastroenterol Nutr 27:596–598, 1998

Wamboldt MZ, Gavin L: Pulmonary disorders, in Handbook of Pediatric Psychology and Psychiatry, Vol I: Disease, Injury and Illness. Edited by Ammerman R, Campo J. Needham Heights, MA, Allyn & Bacon, 1998, pp 266–297

Wamboldt MZ, Laudenslager M, Wamboldt FS, et al: Adolescents with atopic disorders have an attenuated cortisol response to laboratory stress. J Allergy Clin Immunol 111:509–514, 2003

Wamboldt MZ, Schmitz S, Mrazek D: Genetic association between atopy and behavioral symptoms in middle childhood. J Child Psychol Psychiatry 39:1007–1016, 1998

Wamboldt MZ, Yancey AG Jr, Roesler TA: Cardiovascular effects of tricyclic antidepressants in childhood asthma: a case series and review. J Child Adolesc Psychopharmacol 7:45–64, 1997

Warady BA, Alexander SR, Watkins S, et al: Optimal care of the pediatric end-stage renal disease patient on dialysis. Am J Kidney Dis 33:567–583, 1999

Weakley MM, Petti TA, Karwisch G: Case study: chewing gum treatment of rumination in an adolescent with an eating disorder. J Am Acad Child Adolesc Psychiatry 36:1124–1127, 1997

Webster R, Holroyd S: Prevalence of psychotic symptoms in delirium. Psychosomatics 41:519–522, 2000

Weston JA, Colloton M, Halsey S, et al: A legacy of violence in nonorganic failure to thrive. Child Abuse Negl 17:709–714, 1993

Wilens TE, Biederman J, Baldessarini RJ, et al: Cardiovascular effects of therapeutic doses of tricyclic antidepressants in children and adolescents. J Am Acad Child Adolesc Psychiatry 35:1491–1501, 1996

Williams GC, Freedman ZR, Deci EL: Supporting autonomy to motivate patients with diabetes for glucose control. Diabetes Care 21:1644–1651, 1998

Williamson GM, Walters AS, Shaffer DR: Caregiver models of self and others, coping, and depression: predictors of depression in children with chronic pain. Health Psychol 21:405–410, 2002

Winton AS, Singh NN: Suppression of pica using brief-duration physical restraint. J Ment Defic Res 27(pt 2):93–103, 1983

Woods DW, Miltenberger RG, Lumley VA: A simplified habit reversal treatment for pica-related chewing. J Behav Ther Exp Psychiatry 27:257–262, 1996

Worchel FF, Nolan BF, Wilson VL, et al: Assessment of depression in children with cancer. J Pediatr Psychol 13:101–112, 1988

Wren F, Tarbell S: Feeding and growth disorders, in Handbook of Pediatric Psychology and Psychiatry, Vol I: Disease, Injury and Illness. Edited by Ammerman R, Campo J. Needham Heights, MA, Allyn & Bacon, 1998, pp 133–165

Yang YM, Cepeda M, Price C, et al: Depression in children and adolescents with sickle-cell disease. Arch Pediatr Adolesc Med 148:457–460, 1994

Yanovski JA: Intensive therapies for pediatric obesity. Pediatr Clin North Am 48:1041–1053, 2001

Yi MS, Britto MT, Wilmott RW, et al: Health values of adolescents with cystic fibrosis. J Pediatr 142:133–140, 2003

Yildiz S, Savaser S, Tatlioglu GS: Evaluation of internal behaviors of children with congenital heart disease. J Pediatr Nurs 16:449–452, 2001

Young GS, Mintzer LL, Seacord D, et al: Symptoms of posttraumatic stress disorder in parents of transplant recipients: incidence, severity, and related factors. Pediatrics 111(6 pt 1):e725–e731, 2003

Zebrack B, Zeltzer L, Whitton J, et al: Psychological outcomes in long-term survivors of childhood leukemia, Hodgkin's disease, and non-Hodgkin's lymphoma: a report from the childhood cancer survivors study. Pediatrics 110:42–52, 2002

Zeltzer LK, Bursch B: Psychological management strategies for functional disorders. J Pediatr Gastroenterol Nutr 32:S40–S41, 2002

Zeltzer LK, Bursch B, Walco GA: Pain responsiveness and chronic pain: a psychobiological perspective. J Dev Behav Pediatr 18:413–422, 1997

Zuckerman B, Stevenson J, Bailey V: Stomachaches and headaches in a community sample of preschool children. Pediatrics 79:677–682, 1987

35

Physical Medicine and Rehabilitation

Jesse R. Fann, M.D., M.P.H.

Richard Kennedy, M.D.

Charles H. Bombardier, Ph.D.

PHYSICAL MEDICINE AND rehabilitation, or *rehabilitation medicine*, is concerned with helping people reach the fullest physical, psychological, social, vocational, and educational potential consistent with their physiological or anatomic impairment, environmental limitations, and desires and life plans (DeLisa et al. 1998). The patients encountered in the rehabilitation setting are highly diverse, and their problems include those listed in Table 35–1. As can be seen, the medical and surgical issues range from acute to chronic and can involve nearly any organ system. Rehabilitation can take place in outpatient, inpatient, and extended-care programs and includes both prevention and treatment of disorders. Striving for maximum independence is central to the goal of maximizing quality of life.

Rehabilitation is generally a multi- or interdisciplinary effort. Rehabilitation medicine physicians (physiatrists) usually lead the team of other specialized professionals, including physical therapists, occupational therapists, speech pathologists, clinical and neuropsychologists, vocational rehabilitation counselors, recreation therapists, social workers, and nurses. Rehabilitation programs often have a dedicated psychologist on staff whose job is to conduct psychological and neuropsychological assessments; provide counseling to patients and families; oversee behavioral programs; and generally assist staff in the management of cognitive, behavioral, affective, and social aspects of rehabilitation.

Psychiatrists have an increasing role in the care of patients in the rehabilitation setting. As advances in medical care have increased survival in many medical and trau-

matic conditions that previously were fatal—the so-called epidemic of survival—opportunities and challenges have emerged that did not previously exist in the rehabilitation of thousands of individuals each year. Data from the 2000 National Health Interview Survey suggest that 12% of the United States population has a physical limitation in one or more activities (Schoenborn et al. 2003). For the first time, *Healthy People 2010: Understanding and Improving Health* (U.S. Department of Health and Human Services 2001), the national agenda for improving the health of Americans, includes a chapter on "Disability and Secondary Conditions," acknowledging that disability is a critical risk factor for many other health-related conditions.

The World Health Organization has shifted its framework for classifying functioning, health, and health-related states from an emphasis on "consequences of disease" found in the previous *International Classification of Impairments, Disabilities and Handicaps* (ICIDH) (World Health Organization 1980) to an emphasis on "components of health" in the current *International Classification of Functioning, Disability and Health* (ICF) (World Health Organization 2001). The ICF conceptually differentiates health and health-related components of the disabling process at the levels of 1) *body structures* (anatomic parts of the body, such as organs, limbs, and their components) and *functions* (physiological functions of body systems, including psychological functions), and 2) *activities* (execution of a task or an action by an individual) and *participation* (involvement in a life situation). The ICF defines *impairments* as problems in body function or structure,

TABLE 35–1. Problems treated in rehabilitation medicine

Stroke
Traumatic brain injury
Multiple sclerosis
Spinal cord injury
Degenerative movement disorders
Cancer
Human immunodeficiency virus and acquired
  immunodeficiency syndrome
Cardiac disease
Respiratory dysfunction
Chronic pain
Spinal and muscle pain
Osteoporosis
Rheumatological disorders
Peripheral vascular disease
Peripheral neuropathy and myopathy
Motor neuron diseases
Burn injury
Organ transplantation
Sports injuries
Occupational disorders
Cumulative trauma disorders
Total hip and knee replacements
Hand trauma and disorders
Visual impairment
Hearing impairment
Vestibular disorders

such as a significant deviation or loss, and focuses on *activity limitations* rather than disabilities and *participation limitations* rather than handicaps. A further change has been the inclusion of a section on *environmental factors* as part of the classification, with the recognition of the important role of environment in either facilitating functioning or creating barriers for people with disabilities. Environmental factors interact with a health condition to restore functioning or create a disability, depending on whether the environmental factor is a facilitator or barrier. Figure 35–1 illustrates the interactive and dynamic dimensions of this model. The ICF puts the burden of all diseases and health conditions, including mental illness, on an equal footing. Psychosocial factors can cause impairment and limit activities and participation in many ways, thus affording opportunities for multifaceted psychosocial interventions in the rehabilitation setting.

In this chapter, we focus on the psychiatric issues encountered in the treatment of traumatic brain injury (TBI) and spinal cord injury (SCI), two common and highly complex rehabilitation problems with aspects that may require psychiatric intervention. Although many of the other disorders encountered in the rehabilitation setting are covered in other chapters of this text, many of the principles discussed in this chapter also apply to them.

Traumatic Brain Injury

Epidemiology

TBI is a significant problem from both an individual and a public health perspective. An estimated 1.5 million Americans sustain TBI each year; of these, approximately 230,000 are hospitalized and survive, 50,000 die, and 80,000–90,000 experience the onset of long-term disability (Centers for Disease Control and Prevention 1999). According to data from hospitalized individuals, at least 5.3 million persons in the United States, or about 2% of the population, live with disabilities resulting from TBI (Thurman et al. 1999). Although about 80% of TBIs are mild in severity, many of these individuals experience long-term somatic and psychiatric problems that may lead to disability (Brown et al. 1994; Guerrero et al. 2000). TBI is often referred to as the *invisible epidemic* because TBI-related disabilities are not readily visible to the general public.

With improved medical care, TBI mortality and hospitalizations have declined 20% and 50%, respectively, since 1980 (Thurman et al. 1999), leading to more long-term morbidity and disability. The peak incidence of TBI is in 15- to 24-year-olds (mostly from motor vehicle accidents), with a secondary peak among those 60 years and older (mostly from falls) (J.F. Kraus and McArthur 1999). Because TBI affects a predominantly younger population, the effects of disability are much greater than for illnesses occurring later in life. Approximately one in four adults with TBI is unable to return to work 1 year after injury (Centers for Disease Control and Prevention 1999). In the United States in 1995, direct and indirect costs of TBI totaled an estimated $56.3 billion (Thurman 2001). Recent figures show that the total acute care and rehabilitation costs of TBI are $9–$10 billion per year (National Institutes of Health Consensus Development Panel on Rehabilitation of Persons With Traumatic Brain Injury 1999), and about $13.5 billion is necessary for continuing care of those who experienced TBI in previous years (J.F. Kraus and McArthur 1999). About 65% of TBI-related costs are accrued among survivors. Statistics from 1985 estimate that TBI-related work loss and disability cost approximately $20.6 billion (Max et al. 1991); this figure would be much higher today because of the rapid increase in the number of individuals with TBI surviving their injury but requiring supportive care (J.F. Kraus and McArthur

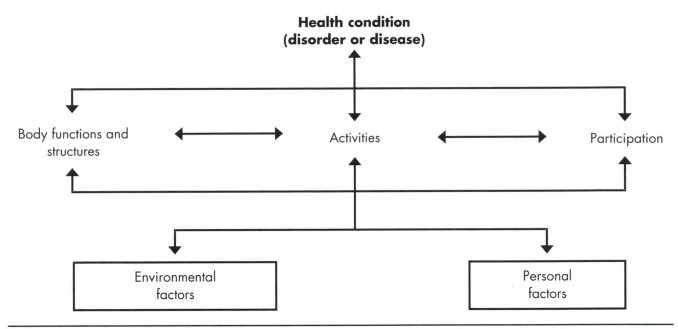

FIGURE 35–1. **Interactions between components of health as defined in the *International Classification of Functioning, Disability and Health.***

Source. Reprinted from World Health Organization: *International Classification of Functioning, Disability and Health: ICF.* Geneva, Switzerland, World Health Organization, 2001. Used with permission.

1999). Long-term disability has primarily been attributed to neurobehavioral factors (Sander et al. 1997; Witol et al. 1996). Thus, many psychiatrists will be involved a some level in the care of individuals with TBI.

Severity and Classification

Original severity classifications for TBI focused on the Glasgow Coma Scale (GCS) (Jennett and Bond 1975) because of its widespread use. A TBI with a lowest postresuscitation GCS score of 3–8 is considered severe, 9–12 is moderate, and 13–15 is mild. However, although the GCS is useful for predicting mortality after TBI, it has less utility in predicting level of disability and neurobehavioral outcome, particularly at the upper end of the scale. It is recognized that the group of individuals with GCS scores of 13–15 are quite heterogeneous in levels of impairment and outcome (Dikmen et al. 2001; Williams et al. 1990). Durations of coma and of posttraumatic amnesia are also used to describe TBI severity.

The American Congress of Rehabilitation Medicine has put forth a definition of mild TBI that is widely used, requiring loss of consciousness (LOC) of 30 minutes or less, posttraumatic amnesia of 24 hours or less, and any alteration of mental state at the time of the injury (including feeling dazed, disoriented, or confused) or a focal neurological deficit, in addition to a GCS score of 13–15 (Kay et al. 1993). Patients with a GCS score of 13–15 who have

imaging evidence of intracranial pathology have outcomes more similar to those of moderate TBI and are often classified as "complicated mild" injuries (see Williams et al. 1990).

Functional Pathophysiology

There has been considerable progress in understanding the pathophysiological mechanisms of TBI in recent years. The physical forces in TBI initiate mechanical and chemical changes that lead to neurological dysfunction. These are divided into *primary damage*, which occurs at the moment of injury, and *secondary damage*, which is initiated at injury but evolves over time. The latter is subdivided into direct injury, occurring within the neuron itself, and indirect injury, occurring outside the neuron but affecting its function.

Primary damage consists of injuries such as skull fractures, brain contusions and lacerations, and intracranial hemorrhage (McIntosh et al. 1996). Because these occur at the time of injury, the key treatment is prevention. Diffuse axonal injury is the predominant mechanism of injury in most cases of TBI (Meythaler et al. 2001), with shearing forces resulting in temporary or permanent disruption of axonal function. Diffuse axonal injury can evolve over a period of 24–72 hours after injury (Povlishock et al. 1983), making it potentially amenable to pharmacological intervention; however, no current therapeutic modality is known to influence its progression (Doppenberg and Bullock 1997).

Direct secondary injury occurs via neurochemical changes evolving over time after the mechanical disruption of neuronal pathways (McIntosh et al. 1996). The acute phase of this process has been well described, with a global increase in cerebral metabolism after injury (Bergsneider et al. 2001; Yoshino et al. 1991). This is accompanied by a period of excessive activity of neurotransmitters, including acetylcholine, glutamate, dopamine, norepinephrine, and various growth factors (Hayes et al. 1992; McIntosh et al. 1996). This may lead to abnormal activation of receptors, causing changes in intracellular signaling that lead to long-lasting modifications of cell function (Hamm et al. 2000). In addition, excessive transmitter activity may have direct neurotoxic effects, leading to apoptosis and permanent dysfunction. A key event in the early phase of injury is excessive influx of calcium (Gennarelli and Graham 1998), which may lead to gene activation, triggering preprogrammed cell death and enzyme activation, leading to damage to the cellular cytoskeleton and free radical generation.

The neurochemical changes in the subacute phase of TBI have been less intensively investigated, but current evidence indicates that this phase is associated with a dramatic reversal of acute processes. Cerebral metabolism and function of many neurotransmitters, including glutamate, acetylcholine, dopamine, and norepinephrine, become depressed (Hamm et al. 2000; Hayes and Dixon 1994); given the prominence of these neurotransmitters in psychiatric disorders, these alterations would potentially account for cognitive and neurobehavioral deficits in TBI. Research in animal models of TBI has successfully identified pharmacotherapies to reduce behavioral and histological complications (McIntosh et al. 1998). However, clinical investigations of such agents have been disappointing (Povlishock 2000). Interventions explored include anticholinergics, cholinomimetics, anti-inflammatory agents, calcium channel blockers, free radical scavengers, glutamate antagonists, and hypothermia (Bullock et al. 1999; McIntosh et al. 1998).

Psychiatric Disorders in Traumatic Brain Injury

Although useful data have been collected in recent years regarding the epidemiology of psychiatric disorders after TBI, the numbers of studies and subjects for each disorder remain small. Other limitations of many studies include selection bias (examining only hospitalized subjects or those referred for psychiatric evaluation), varying assessment periods, use of unstructured psychiatric interviews, and limited assessment of premorbid psychiatric history (Van Reekum et al. 2000). Such factors lead to wide variation in the estimates of incidence and prevalence of psychiatric disorders after TBI. Other complex disturbances seen after TBI are not adequately captured by current diagnostic systems such as DSM-IV-TR (American Psychiatric Association 2000). Some symptoms, such as fatigue or impulsivity, may cause significant impairment but may not fit into a specific diagnosis. Also, individuals with TBI may lack insight into, and not report, their deficits. Psychiatrists may give greater weight to the reports of family and treating clinicians for this reason. However, family ratings may be influenced by other factors, including caregiver personality characteristics (McKinlay and Brooks 1984). Similarly, the clinician's emotional response to the patient may interfere with accurate assessment of deficits (Heilbronner et al. 1989). In addition to these general concerns, there may be differences in the presentation and phenomenology of specific disorders in the context of TBI.

The development of psychiatric disorders involves a complex interplay between premorbid biological and psychological factors, postinjury biological changes, and psychosocial and environmental factors. The role of many risk factors has yet to be well elucidated, and many are specific to a given disorder. A recent review (Rao and Lyketsos 2002) compiled risk factors for the development of psychiatric sequelae in general (shown in Table 35–2). These are divided into highly significant risk factors (sufficient evidence exists for their role in psychiatric disorders) and less significant risk factors (evidence is still controversial). In a large unselected primary care population, Fann et al. (2004) found psychiatric history to be a highly significant risk factor for psychiatric illness in the 3 years following TBI. Their data suggested that moderate to severe TBI may be associated with higher initial risk for psychiatric problems, whereas mild TBI and prior psychiatric illness may increase the risk for more persistent psychiatric problems. The authors hypothesized that psychiatric symptoms that arise immediately after TBI may be etiologically related to the neurophysiological effects of the injury, consistent with the early relation between TBI severity and psychiatric risk, whereas other factors, such as psychological vulnerability, self-awareness of deficits, social influences, and secondary gain, may play roles over time, particularly in individuals with prior psychiatric illness and prior injury.

The role of TBI in the etiology of psychiatric disorders after TBI may have significant implications for prognosis and treatment, as well as medicolegal ramifications (Van Reekum et al. 2001). Although several psychiatric disorders are common after TBI, establishing a causal link between these remains difficult. Van Reekum and

TABLE 35–2.   Risk factors for psychiatric illness after traumatic brain injury

Highly significant risk factors
Preinjury psychiatric history
Preinjury social impairments
Increased age
Alcohol abuse
Arteriosclerosis

Less significant risk factors
More severe injury
Poor neuropsychological functioning
Marital discord
Financial instability
Poor interpersonal relationships
Low preinjury level of education
Compensation claims
Female gender
Short time since injury
Lesion location (especially left prefrontal)

Source.   Adapted from Rao and Lyketsos 2002.

colleagues (2000, 2001) noted that there is some evidence for causality, in that studies (particularly in experimental animals) have shown that TBI disrupts neuronal systems involved in mood and behavior. However, other lines of evidence are inconclusive. The following suggestive findings point to other possible associations: 1) the psychiatric disorder increases the risk for TBI (Fann et al. 2002); 2) the risk for both TBI and the psychiatric disorder is due to a common third factor, such as substance abuse; and 3) a postinjury condition, such as pain or change in family status, contributes to the psychiatric disorder. Evidence for a biological gradient, in which more severe injuries are associated with higher risk for psychiatric disorders, is mixed. There is also a lack of specificity: TBI has been postulated to cause a variety of psychiatric disorders and conditions rather than a single specific syndrome. Assigning TBI as the definitive cause of psychiatric disturbances in most instances is not possible under current evidence.

Depression

Varney (1987) noted that 77% of 120 outpatients with TBI who were referred for evaluation were depressed according to DSM-III (American Psychiatric Association 1980) criteria. Studies that used structured interviews noted lower rates. Fann and colleagues (1995) used the National Institute of Mental Health Diagnostic Interview Schedule (DIS) to assess 50 consecutive outpatients presenting to a rehabilitation clinic for evaluation of TBI. Of these, 26% were given the diagnosis of major depression, and another 28% had had major depression with onset af-

ter injury that had since resolved. Hibbard and colleagues (1998) administered the Structured Clinical Interview for DSM-IV (SCID) to 100 patients with TBI who were randomly selected from a larger quality-of-life study. Depression was found in 61%, with the onset of depression after injury in 48%. Deb and colleagues (1999) examined 164 outpatients previously admitted to the emergency department with a diagnosis of TBI. Assessment based on the Schedules for Clinical Assessment in Neuropsychiatry (SCAN) indicated that the rate of depression was 18%. Ashman et al. (2004) administered the SCID to 188 outpatients 3 months to 4 years after injury as part of a longitudinal follow-up of TBI. Major depression was present in 20% of patients before injury and in 24%–35% of patients during the first year of follow-up.

In a systematic examination of depression after TBI, Federoff and colleagues (1992) examined 66 consecutive trauma center admissions with the Present State Examination (PSE), a forerunner of the SCAN. Approximately 1 month after injury, 26% had symptoms that met criteria for major depression. Jorge and colleagues (1993a, 1993b) carried out follow-up examinations on this cohort. At 3 months after injury, 12 of 54 patients (22%) had major depression; at 6 months, 10 of 43 (23%) had major depression; and at 12 months, 8 of 43 (19%) had major depression. Although the prevalence of depression remained fairly stable, some individuals had resolution of depression during the course of the year, whereas others had onset of depression. Of the 41 patients without depression seen for follow-up, 11 (27%) developed depression during the study: 4 (10%) at 3 months, 4 (10%) at 6 months, and 3 (7%) at 12 months. Jorge et al. (2004) subsequently replicated these results in another cohort of 91 consecutive hospital admissions for TBI, showing 33% of the patients developing major depression during the first year after injury: 17% at initial evaluation, 10% at 3 months, and 6% at 6 months.

Kreutzer and colleagues (2001) examined the scores of 722 outpatient referrals for neuropsychological evaluation with the Neurobehavioral Functioning Inventory (NFI), which assesses a wide range of functions after TBI. By mapping 37 of the NFI items to DSM-IV diagnostic criteria, the authors reported that the prevalence of depression was 42%. A subsequent study (Seel et al. 2003) that used the same methodology in 666 patients at 17 TBI Model Systems centers found a rate of 27%. These studies had large sample sizes, but it remains unclear how the authors' mapping of NFI items corresponds with the diagnosis of depression on the basis of DSM-IV criteria in a clinical interview.

In their cohort, Jorge and colleagues (1993b) noted no difference between depressed and nondepressed patients with respect to demographic variables, type or severity of

TBI, family history of psychiatric disorder, or degree of physical or cognitive impairment. Those with depression were significantly more likely to have a premorbid history of psychiatric disorders, including substance abuse. Subjects with depression had significantly poorer social functioning prior to injury, and poor social functioning was the strongest and most consistent correlate of depression on follow-up. Findings from their later cohort were generally consistent with these observations, except that individuals with depression were not more likely than individuals without depression to have a history of substance abuse (Jorge et al. 2004). In their original study (Federoff et al. 1992), depression at 1 month was strongly associated with lesions in the left dorsolateral frontal and/or left basal ganglia regions on computed tomography scanning. Right parieto-occipital lesions were associated with depression to a lesser extent. Pure cortical lesions were associated with a decreased probability of depression. However, no relation was found between lesion location and depression in subsequent follow-ups (Jorge et al. 1993a). In their later study (Jorge et al. 2004), major depression was associated with reduced volume in the left prefrontal cortex at 3-month follow-up. Replication is needed to confirm these correlations.

Fann et al. (2004) found that patients with mild TBI had a higher risk for affective disorders (including depressive and anxiety disorders) than did patients with moderate to severe TBI (e.g., relative risk 2.7 vs. 1.0 in the first 6 months following TBI) among 939 health maintenance organization enrollees with TBI. This finding is consistent with other reports that more severe TBI is not necessarily associated with a higher risk of depression (Fann et al. 1995; Hibbard et al. 1998).

Early studies of major depression showed high rates of vegetative symptoms among individuals with TBI that exceeded the reported rate of depression in these patients. These symptoms include psychomotor slowing, reported at 67%–74% (Cavallo et al. 1992; McKinlay et al. 1981); difficulty concentrating, 38%–88% (Cavallo et al. 1992; Oddy et al. 1978b); fatigue, 33%–71% (Cavallo et al. 1992; Oddy et al. 1978b); insomnia, 27%–56% (Fictenberg et al. 2001); and decreased interest, 21%–55% (Oddy et al. 1978b; Thomsen 1984). Although these investigations did not include a structured psychiatric assessment, the findings raised concern about the validity of using physical symptoms in the diagnosis of depression after TBI. The "inclusive," "etiological," "substitutive," and "exclusive" approaches used in the medically ill have similar advantages and disadvantages in the TBI population. Although no studies have compared these approaches per se in TBI, Jorge et al. (1993a) did use a similar methodology to explore this issue. They found that TBI patients who reported depressed mood had higher rates of both physical and psychological symptoms of depression (as assessed with the PSE) than did those without depressed mood. The group with depressed mood also endorsed more DSM-III-R (American Psychiatric Association 1987) symptoms of major depression than did those without depressed mood. The symptoms of suicidal ideation, inappropriate guilt, anergia, psychomotor agitation, and weight loss or poor appetite occurred with significantly greater frequency in the depressed group. Studies from patients with other forms of brain injury are similarly encouraging for the use of DSM diagnostic criteria. Paradiso et al. (1997) examined patients with acute stroke; the frequency of major depression was 18% by the inclusive strategy and 22% by the substitutive strategy. Thus, it appears that the diagnosis of major depression can be accurately made with DSM criteria in brain-injured patients.

The course of major depression is the best described of disorders that develop after TBI. Jorge and colleagues found that the mean duration of depression was 4.7 months. Subjects with anxious depression had a significantly longer duration of symptoms than did those with depression and no anxiety (7.5 months vs. 1.5 months). In their follow-up study, 33% of the patients met criteria for major depression during the year after injury. In half of these patients, the depression developed acutely; in the other half, the depression was of delayed onset. The mean duration of depression was 4.7 months for those who received antidepressants and 5.8 months for those who did not. Collectively, these data show that the onset of depression is not immediately linked to the occurrence of TBI in a significant number of individuals.

Mania

The prevalence of bipolar disorder after TBI is difficult to determine because most reports have been single cases or small case series. Varney et al. (1987) noted that 5% of their sample met the criteria for manic episodes, although it is unclear how many of these cases of mania predated the injury. A prevalence of 2% was reported by Hibbard et al. (1998), with all occurring after TBI; and Jorge et al. (1993c) reported that 9% of their subjects met the criteria for mania at some point during the year after injury. In contrast, none of the subjects developed bipolar disorder in the study by Fann et al. (1995). Thus, although TBI may increase the risk for developing bipolar disorder, it still appears to be a relatively rare consequence of injury.

Phenomenologically, all forms of bipolar disorder, including bipolar I, bipolar II, and rapid-cycling variants, have been reported (McAllister 1992). The largest study addressing this topic suggested that patients are more likely to present with irritable than with euphoric mood

(Shukla et al. 1987). Shukla and colleagues (1987) observed that mania after TBI was associated with posttraumatic seizures but not with family history of bipolar disorder. Jorge and colleagues (1993c) noted that mania after TBI was significantly related to basopolar temporal lesions but was not associated with type or severity of TBI, degree of physical or intellectual impairment, family or personal history of psychiatric illness, or posttraumatic epilepsy. They also reported on the course of mania occurring in their subjects. Of the six cases of subjects developing mania after TBI, five occurred within 3 months after injury and one within 6 months after injury. The duration of the manic episode was only 2 months, but elevated or expansive mood persisted for a mean of 5.7 months. These limited data suggest that episodes of bipolar disorder may occur soon after TBI. Its duration is relatively brief, although patients may have subsyndromal disturbances present after mania resolves.

Anxiety

A recent area of interest and controversy has been the development of acute stress disorder and posttraumatic stress disorder (PTSD) after TBI. Early opinion was that PTSD could not develop after TBI; investigators argued that LOC or posttraumatic amnesia would prevent patients from having reexperiencing and avoidance because memories were not encoded (Harvey et al. 2003). This was supported by the studies of Mayou et al. (1993), Sbordone and Liter (1995), and Warden et al. (1997), each noting that none of their sample that had LOC during injury went on to develop PTSD. However, the first two studies relied on clinical interviews to determine PTSD; and the last used a modified version of the PSE, which assessed only two of the five criterion B (reexperiencing) symptoms. Thus, some experts have raised legitimate concerns that these studies did not adequately assess for PTSD.

Studies with more detailed, structured assessments of PTSD have yielded different results. Hibbard et al. (1998) noted that 19% of their subjects had symptoms that met criteria for PTSD. Mayou and colleagues (2000) examined consecutive admissions to an emergency department with the PTSD Symptom Scale, another structured interview providing DSM-IV diagnosis. Ten of the 21 subjects (48%) with definite LOC met the criteria for PTSD at 3 months, compared with 9 of 39 (23%) with probable LOC, and 179 of 796 (22%) without LOC. At 1-year follow-up, the rates of PTSD were 33%, 14%, and 17%, respectively. Levin and colleagues (2001) interviewed a sample of 69 patients with mild to moderate TBI drawn from admissions to a major trauma center. Twelve percent of the patients received diagnoses of PTSD at 3 months according to the SCID, which was identical to the rate in general

trauma control subjects. Ashman et al. (2004) found that 10% of their subjects met criteria for PTSD prior to injury, with 18%–30% meeting criteria during the first year of follow-up.

A series of studies by Bryant and Harvey represents the most extensive exploration of the topic. Bryant and Harvey (1995) examined 38 hospital admissions with mild TBI with the PTSD Interview, a structured interview for DSM-III-R symptoms of PTSD. Approximately 27% of the subjects met the criteria for diagnosis, although these were not consecutive admissions. In another study, Harvey and Bryant (1998) reported on 79 consecutive hospital admissions with mild TBI. According to the Acute Stress Disorder Interview, a structured clinical interview based on DSM-IV symptoms of acute stress disorder, 14% fulfilled diagnostic criteria. Seventy-one of these subjects participated in follow-up at 6 months (Bryant and Harvey 1998), undergoing assessment with the PTSD module of the Composite International Diagnostic Interview, with 50 following up at 2 years (Harvey and Bryant 2000). Rates of PTSD were 25% at 6 months and 22% at 2 years. Bryant and colleagues (2000) also examined 96 subjects drawn from admissions to a brain injury rehabilitation unit with severe TBI. Approximately 27% of the subjects met the criteria for PTSD on the basis of the PTSD Interview; however, again, subjects were not consecutive admissions, and these data cannot be used to estimate overall prevalence of PTSD after TBI.

Several of these studies also examined risk factors for, and the phenomenology of, PTSD. Bryant and Harvey (1998) noted that 82% of the mild TBI patients who met criteria for acute stress disorder went on to develop PTSD, whereas only 11% of those without acute stress disorder eventually developed PTSD. It is not entirely clear whether memory of the traumatic event is necessary for the development of PTSD. In some cases, those who are "amnestic" for the event will actually have "islands" of traumatic memories that are involved in PTSD. In other cases, patients who do not recall their injury may develop PTSD around traumatic experiences involved in hospitalization, which they do recall. However, patients with mild TBI initially may have low rates of posttraumatic symptoms such as intrusive memories, but these may increase over time to meet criteria for PTSD (Bryant and Harvey 1999). Among those with severe TBI, Bryant and colleagues (2000) noted that the overwhelming majority of patients with PTSD did not have nightmares or intrusive memories but met reexperiencing criteria on the basis of marked psychological distress in response to reminders of the trauma. This area clearly warrants further investigation to determine the appropriateness of a PTSD diagnosis for such individuals.

It seems rather certain that those who do have memories of traumatic events are at increased risk for developing PTSD and should be monitored accordingly (Hiott and Labbate 2002). This is particularly important in light of research suggesting that PTSD occurring after TBI may be less likely to spontaneously remit, with more than 80% of the patients meeting criteria for acute stress disorder having PTSD on reassessment 2 years later (Harvey and Bryant 2000).

Other anxiety disorders also may be fairly common, although the number of investigations into this topic remains quite small. Fann et al. (1995) found that 24% of subjects met the criteria for generalized anxiety disorder (GAD) and 4% had panic disorder after TBI. In the study by Jorge et al. (1993b), 7 subjects (11%) met the criteria for GAD, with all 7 also having major depression. In the follow-up study (Jorge et al. (1993b), 23 (76.7%) of the patients with major depression also met criteria for comorbid anxiety disorder, compared with 9 (20.4%) of the patients without major depression. Hibbard et al. (1998) reported rates of 14% for obsessive-compulsive disorder (OCD), 11% for panic disorder, 7% for phobias, and 8% for GAD after injury. Deb et al. (1999) noted that 9% of their subjects had panic disorder, 3% had GAD, 2% had OCD, and 1% had phobias. Finally, Ashman et al. (2004) found that 16% of their subjects met criteria for other anxiety disorders besides PTSD prior to injury, with 19%–27% having other anxiety disorders during the first year of follow-up. The paucity of studies precludes any firm statements about risk factors for development of anxiety disorders other than PTSD.

Psychosis

Relatively few studies have examined psychosis after TBI. Davison and Bagley (1969) reviewed eight studies before 1960, showing between 0.7% and 9.8% of the patients with TBI having a schizophrenia-like psychosis (but diagnosis was not based on structured criteria). In a different approach, Wilcox and Nasrallah (1987) performed a retrospective review of 659 hospital admissions, finding a significantly higher rate of prior head trauma in patients with schizophrenia compared with control subjects admitted for depression, mania, or general surgery. However, this study would not allow causal inferences to be made. Malaspina and colleagues (2001) examined 1,830 individuals who were first-degree relatives of patients with schizophrenia or bipolar disorder. Compared with other first-degree relatives, those individuals with a history of TBI were significantly more likely to develop schizophrenia. This suggested a synergistic relation between schizophrenia and TBI, in which familial factors among schizophrenic patients and their relatives increased the risk of TBI, and TBI further increased the risk of schizophrenia in those with genetic vulnerability.

Only a few studies have examined other forms of psychosis. Violon and DeMol (1987) performed a retrospective review of 530 patients with TBI admitted to a neurosurgical unit, noting that 3% had delusions during follow-up. Koponen and colleagues (2002) noted that 3 patients (5%) in their sample met criteria for delusional disorder, and 1 (2%) met criteria for psychotic disorder not otherwise specified. Fann et al. (2004) also found a higher rate of psychotic disorders among persons with TBI, compared with matched non-TBI control subjects, especially in those with moderate to severe TBI and with prior psychiatric illness.

Risk factors and phenomenology are similarly understudied. Sachdev and colleagues (2001) compared symptoms of 45 patients with TBI and psychosis with symptoms of 45 patients with TBI but no psychosis. They noted that auditory hallucinations and paranoid delusions were more common than negative symptoms. Fujii and Ahmed (2002) reviewed descriptions of psychosis after TBI in 69 patients from 39 publications, with particular emphasis on studies that used neuroimaging or neurophysiological measures. Delusions, most commonly persecutory, were much more common than hallucinations, and hallucinations were more likely to be observed in delayed-onset psychosis. Negative symptoms seen in schizophrenia were relatively uncommon.

In their review, Davison and Bagley (1969) identified several risk factors for psychosis, including left hemisphere and temporal lobe lesions, closed head injury, and increasing severity of TBI. Others have noted that more extensive brain injury, greater cognitive impairment, male gender, and having TBI in childhood are associated with psychosis (Fujii and Ahmed 2002; Sachdev et al. 2001).

Electroencephalogram abnormalities (especially in the temporal lobe) were common, and the rates for seizure disorder among individuals with psychosis after TBI were much higher than estimates for the rate of seizures after TBI in general (Fujii and Ahmed 2002). Neuroimaging lesions (predominantly in the frontal and temporal lobes) were also frequent. Finally, the severity and duration of psychosis occurring after TBI may be less than that of idiopathic psychotic disorders, with only about one-third having a chronic course similar to schizophrenia in the studies examining this issue (Hillbom 1960; Violon and DeMol 1987). The onset of psychotic symptoms is typically gradual and delayed, often occurring more than a year after injury (Fann et al. 2004; Fujii and Ahmed 2002; Sachdev et al. 2001).

Anger, Aggression, and Agitation

Many patients with TBI have difficulty modulating emotional reactions and controlling impulses (Rao and Lyketsos 2002), often described in the TBI literature as *post-traumatic agitation* (Sandel and Mysiw 1996). However, as noted by Yudofsky et al. (1997), *agitation* is a poorly defined term encompassing behaviors ranging from "constant unwarranted requests" to assaultiveness. Although measures such as the Agitated Behavior Scale (ABS) (Corrigan 1989) have been well validated for TBI, they are rarely used in clinical practice (Fugate et al. 1997). Brooke and colleagues (1992b) used the Overt Aggression Scale (Yudofsky et al. 1986) to measure agitation in 100 patients with severe TBI. Only 11% of the patients had agitation; an additional 35% were classified as "restless" but not severely enough to be labeled "agitated." Bogner and Corrigan (1995) examined 100 consecutive patients admitted to an inpatient TBI unit. Of these, 42% had agitation (as measured by the Agitated Behavior Scale) during at least one shift. Episodes of anger or aggression are also common (Auerbach 1989).

Although aggression may be a symptom of many disorders, several features are characteristic of aggression after TBI (Yudofsky et al. 1990). Such behavior is typically *nonreflective*, occurring without any premeditation or planning, and *nonpurposeful*, achieving no particular goals for the individual. It is also *reactive*, triggered by a stimulus, but often a stimulus that would not normally provoke a strong reaction. Aggression after TBI is *periodic*, occurring at intervals with relatively calm behavior in between, and *explosive*, occurring without a prodromal buildup. Finally, it is *ego-dystonic*, creating a great deal of distress for the patient.

The lack of precise definitions of agitation and aggression in the literature makes identification of risk factors difficult, although some have been reported. Agitation is more likely to occur with frontotemporal injuries (Van der Naalt et al. 1999). Disorientation, comorbid medical illness, and use of anticonvulsant medications are also associated with agitation (Galski et al. 1994). Risk of aggression is increased with a premorbid history of impulsive aggression (Greve et al. 2001), arrest (Kreutzer et al. 1995), or substance abuse (Dunlop et al. 1991). For these risk factors, it is often difficult to ascertain whether the aggression is a direct result of TBI, premorbid character pathology, or both (Kim 2002). Little is known about the course of agitation or aggression after TBI. However, in their review of the literature, Silver and Yudofsky (1994a) noted that 31%–71% of the individuals had these behaviors in long-term follow-up ranging from 1 to 15 years. Thus, it appears that agitation and aggression may be chronic problems not confined to the early stage of recovery. This would be expected for such behaviors that predate the injury; it is currently unclear whether agitation and aggression directly resulting from TBI follow this chronic course.

Substance Use Disorders

Substance abuse and dependence are of great concern in the TBI population, at the time of injury and afterward. Substance use disorders not only are highly prevalent and often the underlying cause of injury but also adversely affect outcomes, including agitation, length of coma, post-acute neuropsychological functioning, risk of reinjury, and the ability to reintegrate into the community (Bombardier 2000). Literature reviews have shown that in higher-quality studies, 44%–66% of the patients with TBI have a history of significant alcohol-related problems before injury and that 36%–51% are intoxicated at the time of injury (Bombardier 2000; Corrigan 1995). Those with a history of significant alcohol-related problems before injury are 11 times more likely to have alcohol problems after injury compared with those without alcohol problems before injury (Bombardier et al. 2003). Studies that used informal interviews and screening measures found that 21%–37% report a history of illicit drug use (Bombardier et al. 2002; Kolakowsky-Hayner et al. 1999; Kreutzer et al. 1991, 1996; Ruff et al. 1990). In one study, 37.7% had a positive toxicology screen at the time of injury for one or more illicit drugs (marijuana 23.7%, cocaine 13.2%, amphetamine 8.8%; Bombardier et al. 2002).

Substance abuse declines after TBI but remains significant. Longitudinal data indicate that, depending on the criteria used, rates of remission from alcohol problems range from 31% to 56% during the first year after injury (Bombardier et al. 2003). Data on post–acute heavy drinking and alcohol problems are relatively consistent in that 22%–29% of patients were moderate to heavy drinkers (Bombardier et al. 2002; Kreutzer et al. 1996) or met the criteria for substance abuse or dependence (Hibbard et al. 1998). However, some studies report much lower rates of substance abuse or dependence—8% by Fann and colleagues (1995), 4% by Deb and colleagues (1999), and 10%–14% by Ashman and colleagues (2004). Research in which less formal measures were used has shown that 14%–43% of individuals report significant alcohol or drug use after their injury (Kolakowsky-Hayner et al. 2002; Kreutzer et al. 1990, 1991). Timing of assessment, sensitivity of screening measures, and whether patients were unselected or from referral populations may play critical roles in explaining some of these variations. Risk factors for postinjury substance abuse include history of legal problems related to substance abuse, substance abuse problems among family and/or friends, age younger than 25 years, and less severe injuries (Taylor et al. 2003).

Brain injury rehabilitation may represent a window of opportunity for intervening in substance abuse disorders (Bombardier et al. 1997). More than 75% of TBI patients considered to be "at-risk" drinkers indicated that they were intending to reduce or were contemplating reductions in their alcohol use during inpatient rehabilitation (Bombardier et al. 2002). Of these patients, 17%–20% reported wanting to enter treatment or try Alcoholics Anonymous, and about 70% wanted to try changing on their own. Several potentially effective interventions, including TBI-specific education, physician advice to cut down or abstain, and brief motivational interventions, should be considered within rehabilitation (Bombardier 2000). Referral to outside substance abuse treatment programs also may be considered, especially when staff at available programs are comfortable with the cognitive and physical disabilities associated with TBI. If such specialized programs are not available, professionals with expertise in TBI should consider educating the program staff about the consequences of injury and assisting with treatment planning (Taylor et al. 2003).

Cognitive Impairment

Much effort has been devoted to characterizing the cognitive deficits that occur after TBI. Some have suggested that deficits can be divided into four time periods (Rao and Lyketsos 2000). The first is the period of LOC that results from the injury. After emerging from unconsciousness, many individuals enter a phase consisting of multiple cognitive and behavioral deficits, which some have described as posttraumatic delirium (Kwentus et al. 1985; Trzepacz 1994). The third period is a rapid recovery of cognitive function, which plateaus over time. This leads to the fourth period of permanent cognitive deficits. TBI is associated with deficits in multiple domains, including impaired memory, language deficits, reduced attention and concentration, slowed information processing, and executive dysfunction (Capruso and Levin 1996).

Although TBI is associated with an acute decrement in cognitive function that typically improves over time, recovery is very individualized, and there is no universally applicable description of the recovery process. Rao and Lyketsos (2000) offer the following general timeline: the first two periods of recovery will last from a few days to a month, the third period will last 6–12 months, and the fourth period will last 12–24 months. Such guidelines are more characteristic of moderate to severe injuries. By definition, individuals with mild TBI will have LOC of less

than 30 minutes, with many having none at all (Kay et al. 1993). It is also estimated that about 95% of patients with mild TBI will recover to baseline status within 3–6 months and not enter the fourth phase of permanent deficits (Binder et al. 1997). Even among individuals with moderate to severe TBI, some recovery of cognitive function may occur 2 years or more after injury, although the gains are typically small (Millis et al. 2001). A few patients may experience decline late in the course of recovery, perhaps caused by depression (Millis et al. 2001). Thus, these time frames must be considered general approximations only.

Descriptions of the period of recovery from TBI vary in the rehabilitation literature. One classical term is *posttraumatic amnesia*, which occurs "from injury until recovery of full consciousness and the return of ongoing memory" (Grant and Alves 1987). This would include the first two periods described above and potentially extend into the third. However, characterization of the deficits after TBI as purely amnestic is an oversimplification because multiple cognitive deficits occur (D.I. Katz 1992). Stuss and colleagues (1999) advocated discarding *posttraumatic amnesia* for the concept of *posttraumatic confusion*, although this has not gained widespread use in the TBI literature. Another common term for the period of recovery after TBI is *posttraumatic agitation*, characterized by "excesses of behavior that include some combination of aggression, akathisia, disinhibition, and/or emotional lability" (Sandel and Mysiw 1996, p. 619). This would correspond closely to the second period described earlier.

Unfortunately, the terminology used in the rehabilitation literature does not correspond exactly to DSM-IV psychiatric diagnoses. Most definitions of posttraumatic amnesia would be consistent with a period of delirium followed by an amnestic phase (Trzepacz and Kennedy 2005). The term *posttraumatic confusion* more closely resembles the diagnosis of delirium yet still omits features such as mood and perceptual disturbances. Posttraumatic agitation is defined by some experts as a subtype of delirium (Sandel and Mysiw 1996), yet others have noted that agitation may resolve while the confusional state persists (Van der Naalt et al. 1999). A recent study (Thompson et al. 2001) examined this issue in detail by concurrently rating inpatients with TBI on the Delirium Rating Scale (DRS) (Trzepacz et al. 1988), a standardized measure for delirium; the Galveston Orientation and Amnesia Test (GOAT) (Levin et al. 1979), a measure of posttraumatic amnesia; and the Agitated Behavior Scale (ABS) (Corrigan 1989), a measure of posttraumatic agitation. Of those with a diagnosis of delirium, 22.5% had normal scores on the ABS, and 7.5% had normal scores on the GOAT. Among those without delirium, 7.5% had abnormal scores on the ABS, and 27.5% had abnormal scores on the GOAT. A combination of GOAT and ABS scores classified the delirium diagnosis with 77.5% accuracy. Thus, although the terms *delirium*, *posttraumatic amnesia*, and *posttraumatic agitation* describe conditions that share many common features, they are not synonymous.

The long-term, diffuse cognitive deficits seen after TBI would be categorized as dementia due to head trauma or cognitive disorder not otherwise specified under DSM-IV-TR. This would include the fourth period described earlier and potentially the third period when the recovery process is slow. Rehabilitation experts have expressed concern with use of the term *dementia* in the TBI population (Leon-Carrion 2002). The impairments seen after TBI, unlike those seen in most dementias, tend to be either static or improving over time. Experts also have expressed concern that application of DSM criteria would lead to diagnoses of dementia in the vast majority of individuals with moderate and severe TBI, with potential legal and social ramifications. Clearly, these implications should be further studied and addressed, but the DSM framework provides a useful, standardized approach to diagnosis in this population that might otherwise be lacking.

Preliminary studies suggest that delirium after TBI shows phenomenological similarities to other types of delirium (Sherer et al. 2003b), with both hypo- and hyperactive subtypes noted in other patient populations. The hyperactive subtype appears more common and is associated with agitation and high frequency of hallucinations or delusions. Several risk factors for delirium in the medical-surgical population would likely apply to individuals with TBI (Trzepacz and Kennedy 2005), who are at increased risk for several medical illnesses (Kalisky et al. 1985; Shavelle et al. 2001). Risk factors for prolonged posttraumatic amnesia include older age, low initial GCS score, nonreactive pupils, coma duration, higher number of lesions detected by neuroimaging, and use of phenytoin (Ellenberg et al. 1996; Wilson et al. 1994). These would likely be risk factors for delirium as well. Unfortunately, patients who are traditionally considered to have a higher risk for delirium—especially alcoholic patients, elderly patients, those with psychiatric and neurological histories, and those with prior brain injury—are nearly always excluded from posttraumatic amnesia studies (Trzepacz and Kennedy 2005).

For dementia, severity of injury is consistently associated with the degree and duration of cognitive impairments. The extent of impairment is also influenced by premorbid intellectual abilities and the time after injury at which the patient is assessed (Dikmen et al. 1995). As with other dementias, the cognitive domains affected will vary from patient to patient (Kreutzer et al. 1993). Pa-

tients with TBI also may be at increased risk for developing dementia from other causes, such as Alzheimer's disease (Amaducci et al. 1986; Graves et al. 1990).

Postconcussive Syndrome

The diagnosis of postconcussive syndrome has been a source of wide controversy. It is important to differentiate postconcussive *symptoms* from postconcussive *syndrome*. The *symptoms* of postconcussive syndrome are very nonspecific and include disturbances such as headache, dizziness, irritability, fatigue, and insomnia. Indeed, several studies have documented high base rates of postconcussive *symptoms* among subjects without TBI, often at rates similar to those in individuals with mild TBI (Caveness 1966; Gouvier et al. 1988; McLean et al. 1983; Tuohimaa 1978). There is disagreement as to the number and types of symptoms required for postconcussive *syndrome*. Most experts concur that the diagnosis of postconcussive syndrome requires the presence of multiple concurrent symptoms (Brown et al. 1994; Mittenberg and Strauman 2000), although disagreement may remain over which specific symptoms are required. More recently, standardized diagnostic criteria for postconcussive syndrome have been developed. DSM-IV-TR lists provisional criteria for postconcussional disorder (Table 35–3), indicating that the diagnosis may still undergo refinement.

The most widely published criteria are those in ICD-10 (World Health Organization 1992), listed in Table 35–4. Unfortunately, few studies have used either of these criteria sets (Mittenberg and Strauman 2000). The adoption of such standard definitions will be a necessary step in advancing the study and treatment of postconcussive syndrome.

Because postconcussive symptoms are not specific to TBI, it is important to consider their differential diagnosis. Alexander (1995) and Mittenberg and Strauman (2000) noted that postconcussive syndrome has significant overlap with psychiatric disorders. Both major depression and postconcussive syndrome have symptoms of depressed mood, irritability, sleep disturbance, fatigue, and difficulty with concentration. However, unlike major depression, postconcussive syndrome does not include symptoms of changes in appetite, psychomotor changes, or suicidal ideation. PTSD and postconcussive syndrome have common symptoms of anxious mood, difficulty sleeping, irritability, poor concentration, and difficulty recalling the injury. Postconcussive syndrome is not associated with persistent reexperiencing of the event or with numbing of responsiveness, and PTSD is not associated with the headaches, dizziness, or general memory disturbance that characterize postconcussive syndrome. Symptoms such as headache, fatigue, dizziness, blurred vision,

TABLE 35–3. DSM-IV-TR research criteria for postconcussional disorder

A. A history of head trauma that has caused significant cerebral concussion.

Note: The manifestations of concussion include loss of consciousness, posttraumatic amnesia, and, less commonly, posttraumatic onset of seizures. The specific method of defining this criterion needs to be established by further research.

B. Evidence from neuropsychological testing or quantified cognitive assessment of difficulty in attention (concentrating, shifting focus of attention, performing simultaneous cognitive tasks) or memory (learning or recalling information).

C. Three (or more) of the following occur shortly after the trauma and last at least 3 months:
   (1) becoming fatigued easily
   (2) disordered sleep
   (3) headache
   (4) vertigo or dizziness
   (5) irritability or aggression on little or no provocation
   (6) anxiety, depression, or affective lability
   (7) changes in personality (e.g., social or sexual inappropriateness)
   (8) apathy or lack of spontaneity

D. The symptoms in criteria B and C have their onset following head trauma or else represent a substantial worsening of preexisting symptoms.

E. The disturbance causes significant impairment in social or occupational functioning and represents a significant decline from a previous level of functioning. In school-age children, the impairment may be manifested by a significant worsening in school or academic performance dating from the trauma.

F. The symptoms do not meet criteria for dementia due to head trauma and are not better accounted for by another mental disorder (e.g., amnestic disorder due to head trauma, personality change due to head trauma).

Source. Reprinted from American Psychiatric Association: *Diagnostic and Statistical Manual of Mental Disorders*, 4th Edition, Text Revision. Washington, DC, American Psychiatric Association, 2000, pp. 761–762. Used with permission.

TABLE 35–4. ICD-10 criteria for postconcussive syndrome

A. History of head trauma with loss of consciousness precedes symptom onset by maximum of 4 weeks.

B. Three or more symptom categories
   1. Headache, dizziness, malaise, fatigue, noise intolerance
   2. Irritability, depression, anxiety, emotional lability
   3. Subjective concentration, memory, or intellectual difficulties without neuropsychological evidence of marked impairment
   4. Insomnia
   5. Reduced alcohol tolerance
   6. Preoccupation with above symptoms and fear of brain damage with hypochondriacal concern and adoption of sick role

Source. Reprinted from World Health Organization: *International Statistical Classification of Diseases and Related Health Problems*, 10th Edition. Geneva, Switzerland, World Health Organization, 1992. Used with permission.

Thus, the presence of psychiatric disorders may lead to high rates of reporting of postconcussive symptoms, regardless of TBI history (Fox et al. 1995; Suhr and Gunstad 2002; Trahan et al. 2001). Careful history taking and diagnosis are needed to avoid mislabeling these patients as having postconcussive syndrome. The clinician also must keep in mind that individuals may have both postconcussive syndrome and a psychiatric disorder, which may blur the boundaries between the two.

Studies have examined risk factors and time course for the development of postconcussive syndrome. However, failure to use standardized diagnostic criteria for postconcussive syndrome in most studies makes generalization difficult. Most studies of postconcussive syndrome have focused on individuals with mild TBI, although postconcussive syndrome can occur with more severe injuries as well. The symptoms of postconcussive syndrome are extremely common after mild TBI, with 80%–100% of patients experiencing one or more symptoms in the immediate postinjury period (Levin et al. 1987a). Several studies have shown that such symptoms resolve completely within 3 months in most patients (Alves et al. 1986; R.W. Evans 1996; Leininger et al. 1990). However, other prospective studies have shown that 20%–66% of patients have persistent symptoms at 3 months (Alves et al. 1986; Englander et al. 1992) and that 1%–50% have persistent symptoms at 1 year (Middleboe et al. 1992; Rutherford et al. 1979). Alves and colleagues (1993) followed up the resolution of these symptoms in 587 consecutive adult hospital admissions with mild TBI, with assess-

memory disturbance, and hypochondriacal preoccupation with health may be part of postconcussive syndrome or of a somatoform disorder. Postconcussive syndrome is not associated with the gastrointestinal symptoms often seen in somatization disorder, and it is also not associated with marked motor or sensory deficits or nonepileptic seizures often seen in conversion disorder. Patients with chronic pain also may have symptoms of headaches, fatigue, poor sleep, poor concentration, depressed mood, and dizziness that overlap with postconcussive syndrome.

ments at baseline and at 3, 6, and 12 months. Approximately two-thirds of the patients had symptoms of postconcussive syndrome at discharge, with progressive decline in prevalence during recovery. At 3 months, 40%–60% experienced such symptoms; at 6 months, 25%–45%; and at 12 months, 10%–40%. Most of these subjects reported only one or two postconcussive symptoms and would not qualify for a diagnosis of postconcussive syndrome under DSM or ICD. Subjects with multiple symptoms consistent with a diagnosis of postconcussive syndrome were rare—between 1.9% and 5.8% of those studied. For this and many other studies, the lack of an appropriate control group makes it difficult to determine how many of these symptoms could be attributed to the TBI itself.

Because the symptoms of postconcussive syndrome are nonspecific, some have questioned whether it constitutes a true disorder or syndrome (King 1997, 2003). There also is a long-standing debate as to whether postconcussive syndrome constitutes a neurological or a psychiatric syndrome (King 2003; Mittenberg et al. 1996). Currently, the acute syndrome is thought to be related to neurological factors, whereas chronic symptoms are more likely to persist because of psychological factors (Larrabee 1997; Mittenberg and Strauman 2000). Complaints of poor sleep, difficulty concentrating, and memory disturbances that arise shortly after TBI may be caused by direct neuronal injury (Alexander 1997). Dizziness may be due to central or peripheral vestibular injury, and pain complaints may be due to musculoskeletal or scalp injury (Alexander 1997). It is not known how these putative neurological injuries, which should resolve quickly, transition into chronic postconcussive syndrome. Symptom expectations, in which patients fear that their symptoms will not resolve, may play a role (King 2003; Mittenberg and Strauman 2000; Mittenberg et al. 1996). However, the precise role of psychological factors in persistent postconcussive syndrome is far from clear (Dikmen et al. 1989). Thus, the risk factors for postconcussive syndrome are a mixture of biological and psychological.

The more commonly reported risk factors are female gender (Bazarian et al. 1999; Fenton et al. 1993; McCauley et al. 2001; McClelland et al. 1994), older age (Alexander 1997; McCauley et al. 2001), history of previous TBI (Alexander 1997; McCauley et al. 2001), psychosocial stress (Fenton et al. 1993; Moss et al. 1994; Radanov et al. 1991), and poor social support (Fenton et al. 1993; McCauley et al. 2001). Low socioeconomic status and ongoing litigation also increase risk (Alexander 1997; Binder and Rohling 1996; McCauley et al. 2001). However, for the latter, it should be noted that few individuals involved in litigation have improvement in postconcussive syn-

drome after settlement (King 2003). Finally, in examining postconcussive symptoms among individuals without TBI, Gouvier and colleagues noted that females had higher rates of symptom reporting, and rates of reporting increased with levels of psychosocial stress (Gouvier et al. 1992; Santa Maria et al. 2001).

A significant association is seen between depression and postconcussive symptoms, including those postconcussive symptoms that do not overlap with depression (Fann et al. 1995; King 2003), and severity of depressive symptoms predicts risk for postconcussive syndrome (McCauley et al. 2001). McCauley and colleagues (2001) used portions of the SCID to identify major depression and PTSD as significant moderators of postconcussive syndrome. It appears that psychiatric disorders, particularly depression, may significantly amplify the presentation of postconcussive symptoms.

Although the vast majority of the persons with mild TBI experience good recovery (Binder et al. 1997), Ruff (1999) identified a "miserable minority" of 10%–20% of mild TBI patients with poor outcome, and Malec (1999) noted that 20%–40% of mild TBI patients have residual long-term symptoms or disability. In many cases, such individuals complain of symptoms of postconcussive syndrome, indicating that ongoing postconcussive syndrome may be an important source of disability. Studies of such patients also have found significant deficits on a variety of neuropsychological tests (Bohnen et al. 1992; Guilmette and Rasile 1995; Leininger et al. 1990), although it remains unclear how these difficulties develop during the course of postconcussive syndrome. The severity of postconcussive symptoms is consistently correlated with severity of impairment in information-processing speed, but correlations with other cognitive domains (such as verbal and visuospatial abilities) are equivocal (King 2003). In particular, Larrabee (1999) commented on two of these studies, which consisted of patients experiencing postconcussive symptoms after TBI with LOC of less than 30 minutes. The effects on neuropsychological testing seen in these patients were equivalent to the effects observed in patients with 1–4 weeks of coma in other studies (Dikmen et al. 1995). These data suggest that individuals with persistent postconcussive syndrome differ in significant respects from most individuals with TBI, although the reasons for these differences remain unexplained. Investigators also have found that high rates of postconcussive symptoms were better predictors of neuropsychological test performance than was actual history of mild TBI (Hanna-Pladdy et al. 1997; Pinkston et al. 2000). These results cast further doubt on the contention that the cognitive impairment in persistent postconcussive syndrome is due to TBI.

Psychological Aspects

In addition to the defined DSM-IV-TR psychiatric disorders, TBI is associated with psychological challenges that may not fit into specific diagnostic categories. Four areas of importance are the neurological disorder and resultant cognitive deficits, the psychological meaning of deficits and effect on the patient, psychological factors that exist independently of TBI, and the broader social context (Lewis 1991).

Deficits due to neurological impairment may have a direct effect on psychological functioning. Impaired self-awareness is common after TBI, with 76%–97% of TBI patients showing some degree of impairment (Sherer et al. 1998c, 2003a). Many individuals with TBI also have deficits in awareness of their behavioral limitations (Prigatano and Altman 1990), which may be one of their most troubling problems (Ben-Yishay et al. 1985; Prigatano and Fordyce 1986). Awareness of cognitive and emotional changes tends to be worse than awareness of physical dysfunction (Sherer et al. 1998c). There is little agreement on the most appropriate way to measure lack of awareness (Sherer et al. 1998b, 2003a). Comparisons of patient reports with those of family members (D.J. Fordyce and Roueche 1986; Hendryx 1989; McKinlay and Brooks 1984; Prigatano 1996; Prigatano and Altman 1990; Prigatano et al. 1990; Walker et al. 1987) or rehabilitation providers (D.J. Fordyce and Roueche 1986; Gasquione 1992; Gasquione and Gibbons 1994; Heilbronner et al. 1989; Ranseen et al. 1990) may be biased by respondent characteristics. Comparing patient reports with neuropsychological test results can eliminate much of this subjectivity but may not allow the consultant to gauge the accuracy of patient self-reports of real-world functioning (Allen and Ruff 1990; Anderson and Tranel 1989; Heaton and Pendleton 1981). The method of questioning is also important, because studies have shown that patients are much less likely to report deficits when asked general questions rather than specific ones (Gasquione 1992; Sherer et al. 1998b).

Impaired awareness has both neurological and psychological dimensions. At one extreme is anosognosia, wherein the person has no awareness of neurological impairments (Prigatano 1999). At the other extreme is "defensive denial," which represents the person's attempt to cope with overwhelming anxiety associated with neurological impairment by minimizing the implications. Apparent impaired awareness also can be the result of moderate to severe memory impairment that prevents the person from consolidating and acting on new information about his or her condition. The neuroanatomic underpinnings of impaired self-awareness are not well documented, but hypoarousal associated with subcortical damage and various types of cortical damage are thought to contribute (Prigatano 1999). Few studies have attempted to separate neurological from psychological causes of decreased awareness (Boake et al. 1995; McGlynn and Schacter 1989). Phenomenologically, decreased awareness might appear the same regardless of cause but has significant treatment implications. Interventions designed to address denial and other forms of decreased awareness resulting from psychological causes may be ineffective when the decreased awareness is due to neurological dysfunction that cannot be reversed.

Finally, most studies of awareness have focused on individuals who overestimate their abilities compared with the reports of others. However, some patients underestimate their abilities; the deficits that these individuals have in awareness have not been well studied (Prigatano and Altman 1990). Although more than a half-dozen instruments have been developed for measurement of awareness in the TBI population, there has been little work on the psychometric properties or factor structures of these instruments (Seel et al. 1997; Sherer et al. 1998b). Currently, the most systematically studied are the Patient Competency Rating Scale (PCRS; Prigatano and Fordyce 1986) and the Awareness Questionnaire (Sherer et al. 1998a). The available literature suggests that such deficits are common immediately after TBI, with gradual improvement over time (C. Evans et al. 2003).

The patient's psychological state and the perceived meaning of physical and cognitive deficits may be strongly linked. Patients with depression or anxiety appear to perceive their injury and associated cognitive problems as more severe (Fann et al. 1995, 2000). Many patients with TBI experience grief in reaction to their disability and loss of their "former self." For many years, rehabilitation researchers have relied on bereavement concepts to explain the adjustment-to-disability process (Stewart and Shields 1985; Vargo 1978). However, long-held assumptions about the symptoms and process of normal bereavement have not withstood empirical testing (Marwit 1996; Stroebe et al. 2001; Wortman and Silver 1989). For example, the 2-month time limit placed on a "normal" grieving process in DSM-IV has been called into question (Parkes and Weiss 1983; Wortman and Silver 1989). Also, contrary to the belief that a person must make a "show" of grief, some support exists for the benefits of focusing on positive emotions (Bonanno and Kaltman 1999). Finally, advances in the understanding of grief following loss of a loved one, with few exceptions (Niemeier and Burnett 2001), have not yet been applied to the emotional experience of individuals with functional and cognitive losses due to illness or injury.

Psychological defenses and adaptations used by the patient prior to TBI are also important. In many cases, patients will continue to use previously learned defenses. However, in some instances, coping mechanisms used before the injury may no longer be available because of the degree of neurocognitive impairment; this can cause considerable distress for the patient. Evidence indicates that many behavioral traits are exacerbated by TBI rather than developing *de novo* after injury (Prigatano 1991). Such alterations would be diagnosed as personality change due to TBI in DSM-IV-TR.

Finally, as with many other chronic illnesses, TBI has a significant effect on family and social functioning. Patients with TBI may be unable to return to their former roles as breadwinner, parent, or spouse, placing significant demands on other members of the family system (Kay and Cavallo 1994). In general, neurobehavioral disturbances are the most important source of stress for the family, but this effect can be mediated by good social support (Ergh et al. 2002; Groom et al. 1998). Family members are at significantly increased risk for psychiatric disorders, particularly anxiety and depression, and for increased substance use (Hall et al. 1994; Kreutzer et al. 1994; Livingston et al. 1985). Caregivers may experience problems such as unemployment or financial loss, placing additional stresses on the patient and family (Hall et al. 1994). Sexual dysfunction after TBI stresses intimate relationships (Hibbard et al. 2000a), and partners may be uncomfortable with the dual role of caregiver (parentlike) and sexual partner (spouse) (Gosling and Oddy 1999). Rates of separation and divorce are also elevated for individuals with TBI (Webster et al. 1999).

Spinal Cord Injury

Epidemiology

SCI results from trauma to the spinal cord and may cause changes in motor, sensory, or autonomic functioning. SCI is an uncommon but often catastrophic injury with an annual incidence of 30–40 per million and a point prevalence of 183,000–230,000 in the United States (Go et al. 1995). Those that sustain spinal cord injuries are predominantly males (80%), young (half are aged 16–30), and Caucasian (89%). At the time that they are injured, those sustaining SCI are less likely to be married, twice as likely to be divorced, and slightly less educated than the general population. The most common causes of SCI are motor vehicle crashes (44.5%), falls (18.1%), sports activities (12.7%), and violence (16.6%).

Early survival and overall life expectancy rates for persons with SCI have improved dramatically over the last 30 years. However, life expectancy with SCI remains below that of the general population, especially among those that are ventilator-dependent (DeVivo et al. 1999). Leading causes of death are heart disease (19%); external causes such as accidents, suicide, and violence (18%); respiratory illness, especially pneumonia (18%); and septicemia (10%) (DeVivo et al. 1999). Death from suicide is approximately five times more common in people with SCI than in the general population (59.2 per 100,000) and represents about 9% of deaths. Most suicides occur within 5 years of injury (Charlifue and Gerhart 1991).

Severity and Classification

Tetraplegia (or quadriplegia) denotes SCI that affects all four limbs, whereas *paraplegia* denotes injuries affecting only the lower extremities. SCI usually is described in terms of the level and the completeness of injury. The level of injury refers to the most caudal segment with normal motor or sensory function. Neurological level of injury may vary on the right and the left side, and segments also may be partially innervated. More than half of all injuries (54%) result in tetraplegia, whereas 46% are classified as resulting in paraplegia. The midcervical region is the most common site of injury. Injury severity is most commonly described according to the American Spinal Injury Association (ASIA) Impairment Scale (Table 35–5). Approximately half of all injuries are considered ASIA-A or "complete." Of those admitted with an ASIA-A SCI, only about 2% are expected to improve to the point of having functional motor recovery below the level of their injury. In contrast, those admitted with an ASIA-B injury have about a 35% chance of regaining functional motor abilities below the level of their lesion. Those admitted with an ASIA-C injury have a 71% chance of regaining functional motor ability below the level of their injury (Marino et al. 1999).

Acute Management and Management of Secondary Complications

Emergency management of SCI involves immobilization of the spine as well as ensuring an open airway, breathing, and circulation. In many settings, standard practice is to administer a large intravenous bolus of methylprednisolone within 8 hours of injury to minimize secondary injury due to swelling within the spinal canal. Unstable spine fractures may require surgical decompression and stabilization. Various orthoses are used to maintain external spinal stabilization after surgery, typically for 3 months.

TABLE 35–5.   American Spinal Injury Association (ASIA) Impairment Scale

A **Complete**—No sensory or motor function is preserved in the sacral segments S4/5.

B **Sensory Incomplete**—Sensory but no motor function is preserved below the neurological level and includes the sacral segments S4/5.

C **Motor Incomplete**—Motor function is preserved below the neurological level, and more than half of the key muscles below the neurological level have muscle grade less than 3 (active movement against gravity). There must be some sparing of sensory and/or motor function in the sacral segments S4/5.

D **Motor Incomplete**—Motor function is preserved below the neurological level, and at least half of the key muscles below the neurological level have a muscle grade greater than or equal to 3. There must be some sparing of sensory and/or motor function in the sacral segments S4/5.

E **Normal**—Sensory and motor functions are normal. Patient may have abnormalities of reflex examination.

Source.   Reprinted from American Spinal Injury Association: *International Standards for Neurological and Functional Classification of Spinal Cord Injury.* Chicago, IL, American Spinal Injury Association, 1996. Used with permission.

Key aspects of postsurgical care include respiratory management and prevention of pneumonia, management of orthostatic hypotension associated with blood pooling in the lower extremities, and prevention of deep venous thrombosis and pulmonary embolus from venous stasis and hypercoagulability. Neurogenic bladder and bowel management begins with indwelling or intermittent catheterization and establishment of a regular bowel regimen. After injury, heterotopic ossification, the deposition of new bone in and around joints, may cause loss of range of motion. Spinal reflexes are initially depressed during the period of "spinal shock" but then become hyperactive during the first 6 months after injury. Daily range of motion and static muscle stretch are used to reduce spasticity and prevent contractures, along with medication such as baclofen, diazepam, and clonidine. Pain is a common problem; 25% complain of severe pain, and 44% report that pain interferes with daily activities (Staas et al. 1998). Several different types of pain are noted, including radicular pain, central or diffuse pain, visceral pain, musculoskeletal pain, and "psychogenic" pain (Staas et al. 1998). Of the patients with recent SCI, 10%–60% may have cognitive impairment (Davidoff et al. 1992). Cognitive deficits may be attributable to a variety of factors, including preinjury learning disabilities and substance abuse as well as traumatic or hypoxic brain injury sustained at the time of SCI. Behavior problems such as noncompliance, anger,

and agitation may be attributable to premorbid traits or undetected brain injury. A severe complication for people with midthoracic or higher spinal cord injuries is autonomic dysreflexia. Autonomic dysreflexia is often triggered by a noxious stimulus below the level of lesion that leads to sympathetic discharge uninhibited by descending neural control. Immediate steps must be taken to control hypertension and to identify and reverse the triggering stimulus. The most common secondary medical complication during the first year postinjury is pressure ulcers (McKinley et al. 1999).

Acute Rehabilitation

Patients are usually transferred to specialized rehabilitation programs once they are medically stable and can participate in therapies for at least 3 hours per day. Inpatient rehabilitation typically focuses on education, physical training, strengthening, and basic skills building needed to return to maximal functional independence for living in the community. People with paraplegia are usually expected to be able to function and live independently once their rehabilitation is complete. Those with low cervical lesions (C7–8) should be independent in most functional tasks. Depending on their neurological level, people with higher cervical lesions require different degrees of assistance for activities of daily living, such as managing bowel and bladder, bathing, dressing, eating, and transferring to and from a wheelchair. Whatever his or her level of injury, the person with SCI is expected to be independent in guiding others to care for him or her in areas the person cannot perform on his or her own.

Adjustment to Spinal Cord Injury

Following discharge from acute rehabilitation, 91% of the people with SCI are discharged to a home environment (Eastwood et al. 1999). Estimates of employment rates after SCI have varied from 13% to 69%. Recent data show that, overall, 27% were employed, with 14% employed within 1 year and 35% employed within 10 years postinjury (Krause et al. 1999). Subjective well-being and quality of life are somewhat controversial, especially with regard to patients with high tetraplegia. The controversy relates to the tendency of health care workers to overestimate depressed mood and underestimate potential quality of life in survivors of SCI (Caplan 1983; Gerhart et al. 1994; Trieschmann 1988). In sharp contrast with what health care workers predict, more than 90% of the people living in the community with high tetraplegia, including those with ventilator dependence, report that they are "glad to be alive" (Gerhart et al. 1994). Nevertheless, people with SCI tend to report lower subjective quality of life compared with nondisabled persons (Gerhart et al. 1994). It is somewhat surprising that quality of life is generally unrelated to level of injury or injury severity, weakly related to physical impairment, and more strongly related to one's ability to carry out day-to-day tasks and participate in school, work, or other community activities (Dijkers 1997). Therefore, factors such as environmental and psychosocial variables may play major roles in quality of life after SCI. Quality of life is higher among those with a longer time since injury, those who are working, and those with few or no medical problems, especially pain (Westgren and Levi 1998).

Common biased expectations among rehabilitation staff and their misapplication of stage models have interfered with appropriate understanding and intervention to promote psychological adjustment to SCI (Elliott and Frank 1996; Trieschmann 1988). In numerous studies, rehabilitation staff, primarily nurses and therapists, have been found to regularly overestimate depressed mood in SCI patients (Trieschmann 1988). Rehabilitation staff also tend to view signs of depression as a normal, even necessary, stage of grief. An SCI patient wrote that the most depressing part of his rehabilitation program was that staff expected him to be depressed, an expectation dubbed "the requirement of mourning" (Trieschmann 1988). Empirical data contradict popular conceptualizations of grief. Most people who sustain significant losses (including SCI) do not become depressed and do not go through traditional "stages of grief" (Bonanno et al. 2002; Wortman and Silver 1989). In a study that used the Beck Depression Inventory to measure depressive symptoms weekly during inpatient rehabilitation, about 60% of the SCI patients never scored in the depressed range, 20% endorsed significant depressive symptoms only once, and 20% reported significant depressive symptoms at multiple time points requiring treatment with antidepressants (Judd et al. 1989). Viewing persisting depression as a normal or even healing part of the grief process may interfere with appropriate recognition and treatment of major depression. Conversely, staff may judge the absence of depression to be pathological, a sign of denial or poor adjustment and an indication that the staff should confront the patient more forcefully with the implications of his or her impairments.

In the absence of empirically supported approaches to manage grief and poor adjustment, the consultant is advised to "do no harm" by eschewing confrontational approaches that may only damage relatively healthy defenses or increase patient resistance. We recommend tolerance of adjustment patterns that are not interfering with rehabilitation. We also attempt to educate staff and family members about countertherapeutic myths of coping with loss, such as the belief that it is necessary to "work through" the loss, that patients should reach a state of "acceptance," and that the absence of grief is pathological (Wortman and Silver 1989).

Psychiatric Disorders in Spinal Cord Injury

Depression

Major depressive disorder is probably the most common psychiatric disorder after SCI (Fullerton et al. 1981). The prevalence of major depression after SCI ranges from 23% to more than 30% in 12 separate studies (see Elliott and Frank 1996 for review). There is reasonable consistency across studies on rates of major depression based on diagnostic interviews and self-report measures. Some studies suggest that depression may be more common soon after injury but may remit after several months (Kishi et al. 1994, 1995). In unselected cases, mood tends to improve over the first year after injury (Richards et al. 1986). However, other studies suggest that a subgroup of about 30% of patients develop significant depressive and anxiety symptoms soon after injury and remain highly depressed and anxious through at least 2 years after injury (Craig et al. 1994).

Depression is a significant and disabling problem for persons with SCI. Depression is associated with longer lengths of hospital stay and fewer functional improvements (Malec and Neimeyer 1983) as well as less functional independence and mobility at discharge (Umlauf and Frank 1983). Depression is associated with the occurrence of pressure sores and urinary tract infections (Herrick et al. 1994), poorer self-appraised health (Schulz and Decker 1985), less leisure activity (Elliott and Shewchuck 1995), poorer community mobility and social integration, and fewer meaningful social pursuits (Furher et al. 1993; MacDonald et al. 1987). Persons with SCI and significant depression spend more days in bed and fewer days outside the home, require greater use of paid personal care, and incur greater medical expenses (Tate et al. 1994). Moreover, symptoms consistent with depression, such as documented expressions of despondency, hopelessness, shame, and apathy, are the variables most predictive of suicide 1–9 years after SCI (Charlifue and Gerhart 1991).

Anxiety

Relatively few studies have examined PTSD or other anxiety disorders in this population. Rates of current PTSD have been found in 14%–22% of the patients with SCI (Kennedy and Evans 2001; Radnitz et al. 1998). Rates of PTSD appear to vary as a function of level of injury, with lower rates found among those with tetraplegia (2%)

compared with those with paraplegia (22%; Radnitz et al. 1998). This variability has been attributed to diminished experience of psychophysiological arousal, which may occur in higher-level injuries (Kennedy and Duff 2001). Current PTSD appears to be no more prevalent in persons with SCI than in other trauma survivors. People with SCI who are war theater veterans, have prior exposure to violence, or have limited social support may be at higher risk for PTSD (Kennedy and Duff 2001). Elevated levels of general anxiety also have been found in people with SCI (Craig et al. 1994; Kennedy and Rogers 2000), particularly in a subgroup of patients with chronic comorbid depression.

PTSD symptoms are also common in families of persons with SCI. Boyer and colleagues (1998) found that 25% of pediatric SCI survivors reported significant current PTSD symptoms, but 41% of mothers and 36% of fathers also endorsed significant PTSD symptoms on self-report measures.

Substance Use Disorders

High rates of alcohol and drug abuse problems are found among trauma patients generally and SCI patients specifically (Bombardier 2000). Preinjury alcohol problems are common (35%–49%) (Bombardier and Rimmele 1998; Heinemann et al. 1988). Rates of alcohol intoxication at the time of injury range from 36% to 40% (Heinemann et al. 1988; Kiwerski and Krauski 1992). After SCI, substance abuse appears to decline but remains somewhat higher than in the general population and, importantly, may be more harmful because of its association with poorer health maintenance behaviors (Krause 1992). Acute SCI rehabilitation is a potential "teachable moment" for patients with a history of alcohol abuse or dependence to initiate changes in their drinking behavior (Bombardier and Rimmele 1998). Most do not have severe dependence and, depending on the person's history, may benefit from advice, brief motivational interventions, relapse prevention skills, or referral to specialist treatment (Turner et al. 2003).

Sexual Dysfunction

SCI affects erectile functioning, ejaculation, and emission in males and lubrication in females as a function of level (upper motor neuron vs. lower motor neuron) and completeness of injury (Table 35–6). Clinicians must test the integrity of the sacral reflex arc to determine whether injury at the level of sacral roots is upper motor neuron or lower motor neuron. This examination involves testing of the bulbocavernosis or "anal wink" reflex. Reflex erection ability is dependent on sacral stimulation and the parasympathetic nervous system, whereas psychogenic erection is dependent on the integrity of the hypogastric plexus, which includes both the T11–L2 segments and the sacral plexus (Sipski and Alexander 1997).

Recent laboratory research confirms that women with complete upper motor lesions affecting the sacral segments are likely to have vaginal lubrication from reflexive but not psychogenic mechanisms. Incomplete upper motor lesions affecting the sacral segments retain the capacity for reflex lubrication but will have psychogenic lubrication only if they have intact pinprick sensation in the T11–L2 dermatomes. Women with incomplete lower motor lesions affecting the sacral segments are expected to achieve psychogenic lubrication in 25% of cases and no reflex lubrication.

By contrast, achieving orgasm is less well studied but appears to be relatively independent of level and completeness of injury. Among males with SCI, 38%–47% report achieving orgasm, which may be experienced as similar to or different from preinjury experiences. In a laboratory study, about 50% of the women with SCI reported experiencing orgasm, with longer stimulation, greater sexual knowledge, and higher sexual drive associated with higher rates of orgasm (Sipski et al. 1995). Sexual desire, activity, and pleasure tend to decrease after SCI for both women and men, but most remain interested in sexual activity. Erogenous zones and preferences for type of sexual activity may change.

Numerous treatments are available for sexual dysfunction related to SCI (see also Chapter 17, "Sexual Disorder").

TABLE 35–6.   Male sexual functioning by level and type of lesion

Male sexual functioning	Psychogenic erection (%)	Reflex erection (%)	Anterograde ejaculation (%)
Upper motor neuron—complete	0	70–93	4
Upper motor neuron—incomplete	19	80	32
Lower motor neuron—complete	26–50	0	18
Lower motor neuron—incomplete	67–95		70

Source.   Adapted from Sipski and Alexander 1997.

Erectile dysfunction can be managed with sildenafil and other selective phosphodiesterase inhibitors, vacuum erection devices, pharmacological penile injections, and penile implants. Ejaculatory dysfunction and related infertility are treated with vibratory or electroejaculation procedures in conjunction with intrauterine insemination, in vitro fertilization, or intracytoplasmic sperm injection, depending on sperm quality and motility. A free on-line manual of resources for male infertility related to SCI is available at www.scifertility.com (Amador et al. 2000). Decreased lubrication in females can be managed by water-based lubricants. Regarding sexual enjoyment, patients can benefit from many standard counseling strategies adapted for people with SCI, such as communication skills, sensate focus exercises, addressing performance anxiety, and generally dispelling common counterproductive beliefs about sexual relationships (Zilbergeld 1978). It is important to broach the subjects of sexuality and fertility while the person is undergoing acute rehabilitation, but studies indicate that during this time many patients rate other rehabilitation concerns as more important and may prefer to discuss sexual concerns in more detail after the acute rehabilitation phase (Hanson and Franklin 1976).

The PLISSIT sexual counseling model is a useful framework when offering sexually related counseling to patients in a rehabilitation setting (Anon and Robinson 1980). First, one asks for **P**ermission to discuss sexuality during acute rehabilitation with all patients. If permitted, the clinician should provide **L**imited **I**nformation, generally educational in nature, about sexual functioning. The clinician should give **S**pecific **S**uggestions about how to manage sexuality or fertility problems and refer the patient to a sexual counseling specialist for **I**ntensive **T**herapy when indicated.

Personality and Psychological Testing

Personality assessment among persons with SCI has received justifiable criticism. Critics allege that clinicians are guilty of a negative bias, of overreliance on measures designed only to detect pathology, and of attributing behavior patterns only to intrapsychic and not to situational or environmental factors (Elliott and Umlauf 1995). Measures such as the Minnesota Multiphasic Personality Inventory (MMPI) and the Hopkins Symptom Checklist–90 (SCL-90) should be interpreted cautiously and with the aid of norms correcting for disability-related factors (Barncord and Wanlass 2000). Nonpathological measures such as the NEO Personality Inventory (NEO-PI), the 16 Personality Factor Questionnaire (16PFQ), and the Meyers-Briggs Type Indicator may be more appropriate

tests of personality functioning in this population (Elliott and Shewchuck 1995). Yet, evidence indicates that certain premorbid personality characteristics are more prominent among individuals with SCI than in the uninjured population. Nearly two-thirds of the patients with SCI have personality characteristics suggesting a strong physical orientation, difficulty expressing emotion, a preference for working with things rather than people, and a dislike of intellectual or academic interests (Rohe and Krause 1998). Neuropsychological evaluation that documents areas of cognitive impairment and strength can be critical in guiding treatment and vocational rehabilitation, especially when comorbid TBI is suspected (see Chapter 2, "Neuropsychological and Psychological Evaluation").

Treatment of Psychiatric Disorders in Traumatic Brain Injury and Spinal Cord Injury

General Principles

A patient's specific physical (e.g., spasticity) and cognitive impairments (e.g., defects in executive functions) must be considered in designing a treatment plan for psychiatric disorders in the rehabilitation setting. A detailed understanding of the patient's physical and psychological stage in rehabilitation and functional goals will help in choosing the most appropriate psychopharmacological or psychotherapeutic treatment modality. Consulting with other members of the multidisciplinary rehabilitation team will provide clues as to the patient's motivation and treatment limitations. Knowledge of the patient's current functional, social, and vocational status is required to tailor the psychiatric treatment to specific practical needs and limitations. For example, initial treatment with an activating antidepressant in a fatigued, cognitively impaired, depressed TBI patient who is not participating optimally in physical therapy may be more appropriate than attempting to engage the patient in cognitive-behavioral therapy (CBT).

Once rapport has been established, it is helpful to discuss the events that led up to the patient's impairment (e.g., the circumstances of the car accident that led to the TBI, the stroke that led to the left-sided hemiparesis) in order to explore the psychodynamic significance of these events. For example, patients will often blame themselves for their predicament, with such self-attribution leading to guilt and depression. In contrast, the patient may not associate his or her psychiatric symptoms with his or her physical impairment, which may affect readiness for psychotherapy.

Interviewing the patient's family, friends, and caregivers can provide critical information about the patient's past and present mental state. How patients handled prior losses and health problems can provide clues as to how resilient they will be during rehabilitation. Moreover, patients may report different symptoms from those observed by those close to them. For example, a patient often focuses on physical and cognitive deficits, whereas family members may consider the patient's emotional changes as more disabling (Hendryx 1989; Oddy et al. 1978a; Sherer et al. 1998b). Patients often report significantly less frequent symptoms of depression, aggression, and memory and attention problems on self-rating compared with ratings by their significant others (Hart et al. 2003). Close communication with family and other caregivers and acquaintances can provide critical longitudinal information about the progress of psychiatric treatment.

Because SCI may result in marked weight loss, alterations in appetite and sleep, and reduced energy and activity, diagnosing depression can be complicated. However, vegetative symptoms should not be dismissed because altered psychomotor activity, appetite change, and sleep disturbance are predictive of major depression (Clay et al. 1995). Core symptoms of depression in people with physical disabilities such as arthritis and SCI are worthlessness or self-blame, depressed mood, and suicidal ideation (Frank et al. 1992). The patient's own experience and interpretation of the vegetative symptoms can aid the diagnostic process (Elliott and Frank 1996).

As discussed earlier with TBI and SCI, the phenomenological presentation of psychiatric symptoms in rehabilitation patients may differ from symptoms that arise *de novo* or in other medical settings. Although psychopathology based on DSM-IV-TR criteria should be thoroughly explored, psychiatric symptoms that do not meet DSM diagnostic criteria but that still lead to significant functional impairment are common in the rehabilitation setting (e.g., the depressed TBI patient who has four depressive symptoms but shows apathy that affects his or her level of functioning, or the severely anxious SCI patient with few autonomic symptoms). These syndromes, or symptom clusters, still may warrant close monitoring and treatment to maximize functioning. Therefore, in addition to monitoring and documenting psychiatric signs and symptoms, functional status (e.g., activities of daily living, progress in physical and occupational therapy, role functioning) should be monitored closely as an indicator of overall progress. Consistent with the rehabilitation process's basic tenet of working toward realistic and measurable goals, psychiatric intervention should begin with defining treatment end points according to measurable outcomes. Examples of useful measures include the Patient Health Questionnaire (PHQ) (Spitzer et al. 1999) for depression and anxiety, the Neurobehavioral Rating Scale (NBRS) (Levin et al. 1987b) for behavior and cognition, and the Rivermead Postconcussion Questionnaire (King et al. 1995) or the Overt Aggression Scale (OAS) (Yudofsky et al. 1986) for severe agitation.

Realistic expectations, including the possibility of incomplete remission of symptoms, must be conveyed at the outset so that the patient, who is already frustrated with the often slow and arduous rehabilitation process, does not become even more hopeless or overwhelmed if some symptoms persist (Roy-Byrne and Fann 1997). A recent survey of 16,403 community-dwelling elderly and disabled Medicare beneficiaries found that persons with disabilities reported poor communication and lack of thorough care as negative aspects of their care (Iezzoni et al. 2003). Collaboration with rehabilitation psychologists and counselors can provide significant depth of assessment and breadth of intervention. Attending rehabilitation team meetings is often a valuable and efficient way of communicating and coordinating needs and treatment. Because the patient is likely already feeling overwhelmed about his or her situation, framing the psychiatric consultation and intervention as another modality, similar to, for example, occupational or speech therapy, that can help him or her achieve the rehabilitation goals during a period of intense stress and adaptation can quickly put the patient at ease. Often, appropriately applied treatments may not have been given ample time to work. This problem may be exacerbated by recently imposed pressures on rehabilitation centers to work within predetermined payment structures and lengths of stay on the basis of medical diagnoses (Carter et al. 2000).

Treatment of psychiatric problems in the rehabilitation setting typically warrants a combination of pharmacological and psychosocial interventions. Because treatments for most chronic diseases are covered in other chapters, the following treatment recommendations focus on TBI and SCI.

Psychopharmacology

Several common physiological changes in SCI (Table 35–7), often more pronounced in tetraplegia than in paraplegia, can have an effect on the pharmacokinetics and tolerability of many psychotropic medications. The goals and potential side effects of pharmacotherapy should be explained thoroughly to the patient and caregivers because unanticipated symptoms caused by medications may be viewed as a sign that the underlying condition is worsening. For example, urinary retention from an anticholinergic psychotropic drug may signal to the patient with SCI

TABLE 35–7. Common physiological changes associated with spinal cord injury

Increased body fat and glucose intolerance
Decreased gastrointestinal motility
Reduced cardiac output
Anemia
Orthostatic hypotension
Bradyarrhythmia
Decreased blood flow to skeletal muscle
Venous thrombosis
Osteoporosis

that the spinal lesion is progressing. Medications that can cause weight gain, constipation, dry mouth, orthostatic hypotension, or sexual dysfunction also may exacerbate already present pathophysiology. Medications that are sedating are of particular concern in TBI and SCI because they may impair mobility and cognition, increase risk for pressure sores, and interfere with rehabilitation. Sedation is a frequent problem because many patients with TBI and SCI are taking multiple central nervous system (CNS) depressants, such as anticonvulsants, muscle relaxants, and opioid analgesics (for discussion of interactions between neurological and psychiatric drugs, see Chapter 32, "Neurology and Neurosurgery," and Chapter 37, "Psychopharmacology").

Because patients with TBI or SCI are often more susceptible to sedative, extrapyramidal, anticholinergic, epileptogenic, and spasticity effects (Fann 2002), psychotropic dosages should be started at lower-than-standard levels and be titrated slowly. Despite this need for caution, some patients still may ultimately need full standard doses (Silver and Yudofsky 1994b).

Neuropsychiatric polypharmacy is common in TBI patients and should be critically examined. When multiple psychotropics are needed, they should be initiated one at a time, when possible, to accurately determine the therapeutic and adverse effects of each medication. This practice may become difficult to follow if patients' behavior endangers them or staff or significantly impairs rehabilitation, but it usually will prove beneficial in the long term.

Because few randomized, placebo-controlled studies exist that tested pharmacotherapy for psychiatric conditions in TBI and SCI populations, many of the following recommendations are based on case series or are extrapolated from other neurological populations. Heterogeneous study populations, including those varying in time elapsed since injury, confound the interpretation of study results. When TBI or SCI occurs in the context of a preexisting psychiatric illness, it is logical to continue a previously effective medication regimen, but previously ab-

sent side effects may emerge that require changes in dosages and/or drugs. Electroconvulsive therapy for refractory depression (Crow et al. 1996), mania (Clark and Davison 1987), and prolonged posttraumatic delirium and agitation (Kant et al. 1995) may be considered. However, efforts should be made to lessen cognitive dysfunction in TBI patients (e.g., by using high-dose unilateral electrode placement or twice-weekly treatment frequency), and caution should be exercised in treating patients with SCI who may have unstable spinal columns (see also Chapter 39, "Electroconvulsive Therapy").

Depression, Apathy, and Fatigue

The existing literature on the efficacy of pharmacological treatment of depression after TBI is limited to small studies varying widely in design, diagnostic and outcome assessment, severity of brain injury, and time after injury.

Because of a favorable side-effect profile, a selective serotonin reuptake inhibitor (SSRI) usually is the first-line antidepressant for patients with TBI. A single-blind, placebo run-in study of 15 patients (Fann et al. 2000) and a case series of 9 patients (Cassidy 1989) suggested that SSRIs are efficacious and well tolerated in TBI populations. The study by Fann et al. found that 67% had remission of their major depression after 8 weeks of sertraline and that treatment also was associated with improvements in postconcussive symptoms, neuropsychological functioning, functional status, and self-ratings of injury severity and distress. The areas of cognitive functioning that improved included short-term memory, mental flexibility, cognitive efficiency, and psychomotor speed. Perino et al. (2001) assessed 20 depressed post-TBI patients before and after administration of citalopram and carbamazepine and found that depression, anxiety, inappropriate and labile affect, and somatic overconcern improved significantly. SSRIs should be started at about half of their usual starting dose and titrated slowly. SSRI-induced akathisia sometimes can be mistaken for TBI-related agitation (Hensley and Reeve 2001). Escitalopram, citalopram, and sertraline all have low potential for significant drug–drug interactions. For patients at high risk for noncompliance (e.g., because of cognitive impairment), fluoxetine should be considered because of its lower risk for withdrawal symptoms.

No clinical trials of antidepressants in persons with SCI are available to help guide pharmacotherapy. The Paralyzed Veterans of America and their partners in the Consortium for Spinal Cord Medicine (1998) have published a clinical practice guideline for depression for primary care physicians, extrapolated from research conducted in the general population or among other disability groups. Although SSRIs are likely efficacious in patients with SCI, the risk for spasticity is increased (Stolp-Smith and Wainberg 1999).

The data on the efficacy and tolerability of tricyclic antidepressants (TCAs) and monoamine oxidase inhibitors (MAOIs) after TBI are more inconsistent (Dinan and Mobayed 1992; Saran 1985; Wroblewski et al. 1996). Because of the potentially problematic adverse effects of TCAs and MAOIs (e.g., sedation, hypotension, and anticholinergic effects) in patients with CNS impairment and their narrow therapeutic index (which can lead to inadvertent overdose in patients with cognitive impairment), these medications should be used with extreme caution in TBI patients. Autonomic dysfunction in patients with SCI makes them more vulnerable to TCA-related anticholinergic and orthostatic side effects. If a TCA is chosen, nortriptyline or desipramine may cause the fewest side effects.

Although not yet systematically studied, venlafaxine is likely safe and effective in patients with TBI. Mirtazapine, nefazodone, and trazodone may prove to be too sedating for some patients, particularly if they have cognitive impairment or gait instability, but if insomnia is a major problem, these drugs may be helpful. Venlafaxine and mirtazapine have low drug–drug interaction potential. Moclobemide, a reversible inhibitor of monoamine oxidase A, showed efficacy in an open subgroup analysis of 26 depressed patients with TBI (Newburn et al. 1999).

Some data suggest that antidepressants, especially TCAs and bupropion, are associated with an increased risk of seizures (Davidson 1989), a particular concern following severe TBI (Wroblewski et al. 1990); however, if the drugs are titrated cautiously, most patients will not experience increased seizures, particularly if they are taking an anticonvulsant (Ojemann et al. 1987).

The symptoms of apathy and fatigue, often associated with CNS impairment, can occur concomitantly with or independently of depression and are often mistaken for primary depression (Marin 1991). For apathy and fatigue, medications that augment dopaminergic activity appear to be the most useful (Marin et al. 1995). Methylphenidate and dextroamphetamine are generally safe at standard dosages (e.g., methylphenidate 10–30 mg/day in divided doses) and have been used successfully to enhance participation in rehabilitation (Gualtieri and Evans 1988). Methylphenidate and dextroamphetamine also have been shown in case series and double-blind studies to be effective in improving some aspects of mood, mental speed, attention, and behavior, although improvement was not always sustained long term (Bleiberg et al. 1993; R.W. Evans et al. 1987; Gualtieri and Evans 1988; Kaelin et al. 1996; Mooney and Haas 1993; Plenger et al. 1996; Speech et al. 1993; Whyte et al. 1997). Dextroamphetamine may exacerbate dystonia and dyskinesia in some cases.

Therapeutic use of these oral psychostimulants in the medically ill rarely leads to abuse in patients without a personal or family history of substance abuse (Masand and Tesar 1996), but substance abuse is overrepresented in the TBI and SCI populations.

Modafinil has been efficacious in treating fatigue in patients with multiple sclerosis (Rammahan et al. 2000; Terzoudi et al. 2000; Zifko et al. 2002) and excessive daytime sleepiness in patients with TBI (Teitelman 2001). Bupropion (Marin et al. 1995) and dopamine agonists, such as amantadine (Cowell and Cohen 1995; Gualtieri et al. 1989; M.F. Kraus and Maki 1997; Nickels et al. 1994), bromocriptine (Catsman-Berrevoets and Harskamp 1988; Eames 1989; Gupta and Mlcoch 1992), and levodopa/carbidopa (Lal et al. 1988), have been used for apathy states, fatigue, and cognitive impairment. Bupropion's stimulating properties may be of particular benefit in the fatigued or apathetic depressed patient. Stimulants and dopamine agonists can increase the risk for delirium and psychosis and thus should be used with caution in more vulnerable patients. Amantadine has been associated with an increased risk of seizures (Gualtieri et al. 1989), but methylphenidate, dextroamphetamine, and bromocriptine do not appear to lower seizure threshold at typical doses. The TCA protriptyline also has been used to improve arousal and behavior (Wroblewski et al. 1993).

There is great interest in pharmacological agents that could improve not only arousal and attention following TBI but also memory; however, data are lacking. Preliminary evidence indicates that the acetylcholinesterase inhibitor donepezil may improve memory and global functioning (Taverni et al. 1998; Whelan et al. 2000; Whitlock 1999).

Another secondary benefit of some antidepressants in TBI and SCI patients is their analgesic properties (Onghena and Van Houdenhove 1992) (see also Chapter 36, "Pain"). TCAs have been shown to be effective for the treatment of chronic nonmalignant pain, including neuropathic pain (McQuay et al. 1996). SSRIs have not been shown to be effective in neuropathic pain (Jung et al. 1997). Venlafaxine and duloxetine may be effective in treating a variety of pain syndromes, including neuropathic pain (Diamond 1995; Lang et al. 1996; Schreiber et al. 1999).

Mania

For mania following TBI, the mood stabilizers lithium carbonate (Oyewumi and Lapierre 1981; Stewart and Nemsath 1988), valproic acid (Pope et al. 1988), and carbamazepine (Stewart and Nemsath 1988) all have been used successfully. Clonidine (Bakchine et al. 1989) and electroconvulsive therapy (Clark and Davison 1987) also can be used as second-line modalities. Dikmen et al. (2000)

have shown that valproic acid is well tolerated following TBI, but lithium and carbamazepine have been associated with neurocognitive adverse effects (Hornstein and Seliger 1989; Schiff et al. 1982). Lithium has a narrow therapeutic window and also can lower the seizure threshold; thus, caution is required when lithium is used in TBI patients whose cognitive impairment may lead to poor adherence or inadvertent overdosage. Although serum blood levels of valproic acid and carbamazepine help in monitoring adherence and absorption, dosing should be guided primarily by therapeutic response and side effects. The possible roles for other anticonvulsants in secondary mania are reviewed in Chapter 11 ("Mania, Catatonia, and Psychosis"). Carbamazepine, gabapentin, and clonazepam also can be effective for the treatment of neuropathic pain.

Anxiety

Benzodiazepines are the treatment of choice for acute anxiety in TBI, but they should be used initially at lower doses because of their propensity to exacerbate or cause cognitive impairment and oversedation. The high prevalence of substance abuse in patients with TBI and SCI adds to the risk of benzodiazepine use and precludes their use in some patients. Although few studies exist in TBI patients, antidepressants also appear to be effective for anxiety, particularly in the context of depression. SSRIs also have been found to be effective in decreasing mood lability after brain injury (Nahas et al. 1998; Sloan et al. 1992), although this effect may take as long as their antidepressant effects. Valproic acid and gabapentin may be of benefit, especially in patients with concomitant mood lability or seizures (Pande et al. 1999, 2000). Buspirone is another option for generalized anxiety symptoms; however, it has been associated, albeit rarely, with seizures and movement disorders (Levitt et al. 1993).

Sleep Disorders

Treatment of sleep problems in patients with TBI and SCI ideally should be based on diagnosis of a specific sleep disorder. Sleep apnea is fairly common in TBI (Castriotta and Lai 2001; Masel et al. 2001) and SCI (Burns et al. 2000), and nocturnal periodic leg movements are frequent in SCI (Dickel et al. 1994). Fichtenberg et al. (2000) found that insomnia often appeared to be associated with depression in post–acute TBI patients. No specific data exist on treating insomnia or other sleep disorders in TBI or SCI, but trazodone is widely used in these patients for middle or late insomnia. Trazodone-associated orthostatic hypotension may be particularly problematic in the rehabilitation setting, however. Antihistamines such as diphenhydramine should be avoided because of their anticholinergic properties (see Chapter 16, "Sleep Disorders," for general diagnosis and treatment of sleep disorders).

Anger, Aggression, and Agitation

Anger, aggression, and agitation are common following TBI and can occur in isolation or as part of delirium or other psychiatric disorders (see Chapter 8, "Aggression and Violence," for a full review of agitation and aggression in the medically ill). The published literature regarding their treatment is often not diagnostically specific and consists of largely case reports, case series, and reviews (e.g., Burnett et al. 1999; Krieger et al. 2003; Maryniak et al. 2001; McAllister and Ferrell 2002; Stanislav and Childs 2000).

Treatment can be divided into acute treatment, in which the goal is timely management of behavior to prevent injury to self or others, and chronic treatment, in which the goal is long-term management and prevention (Silver et al. 2002). Many agents take from 2 to 8 weeks to gain full effectiveness. It is important to keep in mind that medications that worsen cognition or sedation can actually worsen confusion and may, therefore, worsen agitation during the confusional state of posttraumatic amnesia after TBI. Because the effects of medications on the patient with TBI can be unpredictable, and their side effects actually may potentiate the behavior problem (e.g., akathisia from antipsychotics), systematically eliminating certain medications, including those that were initially prescribed to treat the behavioral dyscontrol, can prove beneficial. A rationale for such an approach is the clinical observation that some patients have a natural course of recovery and that some medication efficacy may decrease over time.

A survey published in 1997 (Fugate et al. 1997) showed that physiatrist experts in TBI most often treated agitation with carbamazepine, TCAs, trazodone, amantadine, and beta-blockers. Psychiatrists appear more likely than physiatrists to use atypical antipsychotics (Burnett et al. 1999) and SSRIs.

The atypical antipsychotics afford the clinician many more options in the acute setting than were available a decade ago (Battaglia et al. 2003; Currier and Simpson 2001; Lesem et al. 2001). The efficacy of the atypical antipsychotics in treating aggression and agitation in TBI patients is undocumented; however, evidence is mounting to support their efficacy in treating other agitated states associated with neurological syndromes (Lee et al. 2001; Meehan et al. 2002). The typical antipsychotics given orally or intramuscularly also may be useful in the acute setting (Stanislav and Childs 2000), but the elevated risks of extrapyramidal and anticholinergic effects in TBI patients must be considered. Studies have suggested that haloperidol may impede neuronal recovery in animals (Feeney et al. 1982), but this finding has not been supported in humans with TBI.

Antipsychotic use for chronic agitation should be reserved for situations when aggression occurs in the context of psychotic symptoms. Risperidone (Cohen et al. 1998; De Deyn et al. 1999; I.R. Katz et al. 1999; McDougle et al. 1998) and olanzapine (Street et al. 2000) show promise in neuropsychiatric patients, although efficacy data are lacking in TBI patients for these and the other atypical antipsychotics. Clozapine use in TBI patients is limited by its seizure risk, although it has been found to be effective for chronic aggression (Duffy and Kant 1996; Michals et al. 1993).

The benzodiazepines offer rapid sedation that may be useful in the acute setting; however, they also have a high potential for neurocognitive effects, such as mental slowing, amnesia, disinhibition, and impaired balance, in patients with TBI. As a result, low doses of a short-acting agent, such as lorazepam 1–2 mg orally or parenterally, should be used initially and titrated as needed. If agitation is frequent, a longer-acting agent, such as clonazepam 0.5–1.0 mg two or three times a day, may be used for short durations. The combination of haloperidol and low-dose lorazepam (e.g., 0.5–1.0 mg) may offer a synergistic calming effect for some acutely agitated patients.

Serotonergic antidepressants, such as the SSRIs, trazodone, and amitriptyline, have been used to treat agitation and aggression in TBI populations (Mysiw et al. 1988; Rowland et al. 1992). In 8-week, nonrandomized trials with sertraline, Fann et al. (2000) showed that improved depression was associated with improved anger and aggression scores in patients with mild TBI, whereas Kant et al. (1998) found improved aggression independent of depression scores. One rationale for the use of antidepressants is the observation that serotonin and norepinephrine levels are reduced in the cerebrospinal fluid of agitated patients with brain injury (van Workeom et al. 1977). SSRIs are also effective in treating emotional incontinence, such as pathological crying or laughter (Muller et al. 1999; Nahas et al. 1998; Sloan et al. 1992).

Buspirone also has shown some efficacy for agitation in TBI and other neurological patients (Gualtieri 1991; Silver and Yudofsky 1994a; Stanislav et al. 1994) and can be particularly useful when anxiety also is present. Although one 6-week placebo-controlled trial found that methylphenidate significantly reduced anger an average of 27 months after severe TBI (Mooney and Haas 1993), stimulants should be used with caution in the agitated TBI patient because of the risks of exacerbating agitation and psychosis and of abuse.

Among the anticonvulsants, carbamazepine (Azouvi et al. 1999; Chatham-Showalter 1996) and valproic acid (Chatham Showalter and Kimmel 2000; Lindenmayer and Kotsaftis 2000; Wroblewski et al. 1997) have been studied the most for treatment of behavioral dyscontrol in TBI populations. Although evidence of seizures or epileptiform activity on electroencephalogram is a strong indication for anticonvulsant use in the agitated patient, these agents also have shown efficacy in those without electroencephalographic abnormalities. Oxcarbazepine, gabapentin, lamotrigine, and topiramate also may be efficacious, although data are more limited. Some TBI patients may experience paradoxical agitation with gabapentin (Childers and Holland 1997). Lamotrigine should be monitored for possible exacerbation of aggression, as is seen in some reports in mentally retarded patients with epilepsy (Beran and Gibson 1998; Ettinger et al. 1998). Evidence indicates that cognitive functioning may worsen with topiramate in some cases (Martin et al. 1999; Shorvon 1996; Tatum et al. 2001). Some patients may need to achieve serum levels of anticonvulsants that exceed therapeutic levels used for seizure prophylaxis to ensure adequate behavioral control. Lithium is also an effective mood stabilizer and has antiaggressive properties in TBI patients, according to case reports; however, its narrow therapeutic window and high potential for neurotoxicity limit its routine use, particularly in those with significant cognitive impairment or history of seizures.

When anger, aggression, or agitation occurs without signs of other psychiatric syndromes, beta-blockers such as propranolol, pindolol, and nadolol should be considered. Placebo-controlled studies have shown their efficacy in treating agitation in TBI patients (Brooke et al. 1992a; Greendyke and Kanter 1996; Greendyke et al. 1996). A Cochrane review (Fleminger et al. 2003) concluded that among the drugs used to treat agitation and aggression in TBI, beta-blockers have the best evidence for efficacy. Although dosages of propranolol in the range of 160–320 mg/day have been effective, Yudofsky et al. (1987) proposed titrating the dosage as high as 12 mg/kg or 800 mg/day. Bradycardia and hypotension are potential side effects; contraindications include asthma, chronic obstructive pulmonary disease, type 1 diabetes mellitus, congestive heart failure, persistent angina, significant peripheral vascular disease, and hyperthyroidism (Yudofsky et al. 1987). Pindolol is less likely to cause bradycardia.

Psychosis

Because of the increased susceptibility of patients with TBI to experience anticholinergic and extrapyramidal side effects and patients with SCI to experience problematic anticholinergic sequelae, the newer-generation atypical antipsychotics are the drugs of first choice for psychotic symptoms that emerge after TBI or SCI (Burnett et al. 1999) (see also earlier discussion of antipsychotics for agitation in "Anger, Aggression, and Agitation" subsection and Chapter 11, "Mania, Catatonia, and Psychosis"). Clozapine carries a risk of seizures and should be used with extreme caution in TBI patients, particularly when compliance is in question.

Cognitive Impairment

Little evidence is available to guide pharmacological treatments to enhance cognitive recovery following TBI; most data are derived from theoretical or animal models or case reports. Medications targeting the dopaminergic, cholinergic, and noradrenergic neurotransmitter systems have been tried (McElligott et al. 2003). Dopaminergic agents include levodopa/carbidopa, bromocriptine, amantadine, pergolide, the newer dopamine agonists (ropinirole, pramipexole), catecholamine-*O*-methyltransferase (COMT) inhibitors (entacapone, tolcapone), and the monoamine oxidase–B (MAO-B) inhibitor selegiline (Meythaler et al. 2002; Zafonte et al. 2001). The SSRI sertraline, which has some dopaminergic activity, may have a cognition-enhancing effect in addition to its antidepressant effect (Fann et al. 2001), although larger, controlled studies are needed to confirm this finding and to determine whether this effect is independent of its influence on depression. Medications that enhance cholinergic activity include cholinergic precursors such as lecithin and acetylcholinesterase inhibitors such as physostigmine (Cardenas et al. 1994) and donepezil (Taverni et al. 1998; Whelan et al. 2000; Whitlock 1999). The noradrenergic agents most commonly used to enhance cognition, perhaps by improving arousal and awareness, are the psychostimulants methylphenidate and dextroamphetamine, which also have dopaminergic effects. Modafinil, a treatment for narcolepsy whose mechanism of action is unclear, also may show some benefit. The opioid antagonist naltrexone helped improve TBI-associated memory impairment in a case series (Tennant and Wild 1987). None of these agents has yet been proven effective in controlled studies in improving cognition in TBI patients, and all would also require further study to better delineate appropriate indications, dosages, and treatment durations.

Psychological Treatment

Traumatic Brain Injury

A widely accepted model of psychological effects of TBI distinguishes among symptoms that are reactions to the effects of TBI (e.g., depression, anxiety, irritability, anger, hopelessness, helplessness, social withdrawal, distrust, and phobias), symptoms that are neurologically based (e.g., affective lability, impulsivity, agitation, paranoia, unawareness), and symptoms that reflect long-standing personality traits (e.g., obsessiveness, antisocial behavior, work attitude, social connectedness, dependence, entitlement) (Prigatano 1986). Although the genesis of symptoms can be multifactorial, it is useful to consider the potential contributions of all three factors to observed problem behaviors. Prigatano (1986) argued that reactive problems may be most amenable to psychotherapeutic interventions, whereas neurologically mediated symptoms may require multimodal interventions that also target underlying cognitive impairment. Characterological problems may require making coordinated changes in important environmental contingencies as well as working with families or caregivers.

Although psychotherapy is considered an important aspect of brain injury rehabilitation (National Institutes of Health Consensus Development Panel 1999), there are as yet no controlled studies of psychotherapeutic interventions in persons with TBI and little guidance on the indications for psychotherapeutic interventions. Empirically supported psychotherapies have been adapted for use in brain injured individuals (e.g., modified CBT for anxiety [Hibbard et al. 2000b] and depression [Hibbard et al. 1992]). Psychological interventions are more likely to require involvement of family members or caregivers to help cue follow-through and generalization to real-world situations. Psychotherapy has been used with selected patients to foster insight in comprehensive post–acute neurorehabilitation programs (Prigatano and Ben-Yishay 1999). Insight-focused psychotherapy often begins with providing the patient with a simple model to explain what has happened. These explanations and coping strategies must be rehearsed repeatedly until they are automatic. Group therapy may be used to foster more insight through feedback from peers.

When insight and self-management approaches are not feasible, applied behavioral analysis can be used to manage a wide variety of brain injury–related behavioral deficits or excesses, such as emotional lability, anger management, and impulsivity. Mostly case studies have shown the efficacy of contingency management for enhancing appropriate social behavior, improving participation in rehabilitation, and increasing independent functioning (Horton and Howe 1981). In some cases, such as anger management, both self-control and environmental control strategies can be combined to achieve better outcomes (Uomoto and Brockway 1992).

Therapy for impaired awareness is in its infancy but has included several different strategies. Mildly impaired patients may benefit from information about the effects of brain injury coupled with test data and observations about the specific ways they have been affected, including limited awareness. Basic cognitive compensatory strategies should be used to help patients attend to, understand, and recall this information. Family, friends, or caregivers should be included in these educational processes. With more severe or persistent problems, treatment may include more comprehensive, coordinated, and real-time feedback about impairments, such as via videotaping. Experiential learning paradigms can be used in which the person is asked to predict how well he or she will perform on a given test and is reinforced for successively improving the accuracy of his or her predictions. Failure experiences may be permitted, although staff should minimize the potential for shame or humiliation that may occur with failures. Improvements may be made in safety behaviors without corresponding changes in verbal awareness, so at times it may be therapeutic to ignore verbal denial and work strictly on the level of behavior. With intractable unawareness, it may be essential to enlist relatives and friends to create a protective environment by ensuring 24-hour supervision, removing access to cars or other dangerous equipment, contacting employers, and providing a written letter signed by the physician that lists all the behavioral restrictions to support caregivers when the restrictions are challenged. When adaptive denial is present, staff may benefit from information about how the denial helps the person psychologically. Staff may be inclined to confront the denial, not realizing the value of defensive denial in managing anxiety and maintaining a sense of self-efficacy.

Cognitive rehabilitation.   The science of cognitive rehabilitation has grown tremendously in the past 15 years to the point that evidence-based guidelines have been derived from significant efficacy and effectiveness trials (Cicerone et al. 2000). Empirically validated approaches are available for remediation of visuoperceptual deficits, language deficits, and impaired pragmatic communication and for memory compensation in patients with mild memory impairment (Cicerone et al. 2000). Some evidence suggests that attention training, including computer-based training modules, is effective (Park and Ingles 2001). Effective strategies are available to train patients to improve visual scanning, reading comprehension, language formation, and problem solving (Cicerone et al. 2000). Optional rehabilitation strategies that may be effective include the use of memory books for persons with moderate-to-severe impairment, verbal self-instructional training, and self-questioning and self-monitoring to address deficits in executive functioning. Isolated use of computer-based training procedures is not recommended for any form of impairment (Cicerone et al. 2000).

Controlled trials of comprehensive rehabilitation programs are rare for post–acute rehabilitation and absent for acute rehabilitation, primarily because of cost and ethical issues associated with withholding usual care. In one of the best controlled studies of post–acute rehabilitation, Ruff and colleagues (1989) compared outcomes resulting from an 8-week structured cognitively oriented day treatment program and a less structured psychosocially oriented day treatment program (control condition). The group receiving structured cognitively oriented treatment had improvement that was only marginally better than in the psychosocial group, whereas both groups improved significantly compared with stable pretreatment baselines. The data suggested that treatment in a structured setting that includes professional attention, psychosocial group therapy, TBI-relevant education, or cognitive remediation has positive benefits on neurobehavioral functioning. A current synthesis of the available evidence on comprehensive rehabilitation concludes that the greatest benefits accrue to those patients who receive individualized and integrated treatment oriented toward both cognitive and interpersonal areas of function (Cicerone et al. 2000).

Spinal Cord Injury

Three types of problems may require psychological interventions in the context of SCI: 1) primary psychiatric disorders, 2) problems with adjustment to disability, and 3) problems with adherence to medical and rehabilitation therapies. With the caveat that there may be significant time constraints on implementing psychotherapy during a relatively short rehabilitation stay, abbreviated forms of standard empirically supported psychotherapies can be used in many cases if cognition is intact. Additionally, if a rehabilitation psychologist is on staff, responsibilities for therapeutic interventions can be negotiated between the psychiatrist and the psychologist.

For depression and anxiety disorders, brief CBT is often indicated in conjunction with initiating pharmacotherapy. Rehabilitation activities should afford the patient numerous opportunities to practice CBT skills, such as identification of irrational thoughts and positive reframing within a supportive context. The consultant also can work within the rehabilitation team to accomplish additional therapy goals by proxy. For example, the recreation therapist can carry out graded exposure to being in a motor vehicle for a patient with acute PTSD–related anxiety and avoidance of cars.

Cognitive-behavioral therapies have been adapted to, and studied to a limited degree in, the SCI population.

Craig and colleagues (1997) used a group-based skills-oriented approach to teaching relaxation, cognitive restructuring, social skills, assertiveness, pleasant activity scheduling, and how to begin sexual adjustment. Subjects with high levels of depressed mood before treatment were significantly less depressed than were historical control subjects 1 year after treatment. At 2-year follow-up, those individuals who had received CBT had fewer hospital readmissions, used fewer drugs, and reported higher levels of adjustment compared with subjects in the control group (Craig et al. 1999). Kennedy et al. (2003) tested a "coping effectiveness training" approach that involves teaching cognitive appraisal and coping skills in small groups. Compared with matched historical control subjects, the treated subjects reported reduced depression and anxiety, although improvements were unrelated to changes in coping skills.

Group-based interventions provide unique opportunities to capitalize on the positive coping abilities modeled by participants with better adjustment. Therefore, group-based coping skills training is recommended for people with significant anxiety or depressive symptoms after SCI as an adjunct to or in lieu of individual psychotherapy.

Poor adjustment to disability and management of grief are also common reasons for referrals. As noted earlier, potentially harmful myths exist about the nature and course of grief. Empirically supported approaches to manage grief are lacking (Bonanno et al. 2002), but clinical experience provides guidance. Clinicians should resist the temptation to confront patients with their prognosis when they, for example, insist that they are going to walk again. It should be recognized that statements labeled as *denial* may simply reflect the common, understandable hope or wish for neurological recovery rather than psychopathology. Overly direct confrontation may damage defenses needed by patients, increase resistance, and risk eliciting excessive distress. We recommend tolerance of verbal denial and other adjustment patterns that do not interfere with rehabilitation progress for more than a day or so. For these patients, staff education about the range of normal adjustment may be the main intervention. When verbal denial is accompanied by behavioral denial (e.g., refusing to learn adaptive strategies such as wheelchair use and self-catheterization) or persistently interferes with rehabilitation progress, more directive interventions may be needed. In such cases, the psychiatrist may recommend that patients review information about the nature and extent of their injury (including radiographic evidence), prognosis for recovery, and current SCI research with the attending physician, possibly with the consultant present.

Given the action-oriented behavioral style of many patients with SCI, we believe that much adjustment is behaviorally mediated. That is, rather than verbally processing losses associated with SCI, patients accommodate to their impairments largely through physical and occupational therapy wherein they repeatedly experience their abilities and limitations through activities. To the extent that therapists can set attainable incremental goals and maximize the patients' sense of mastery, positive adjustment can be facilitated. Therapies also can be organized to help patients resume participation in their most meaningful, rewarding, and pleasant life activities. Prospective descriptive studies of bereavement (Bonanno et al. 2002) and the incipient empirical use of combined interpersonal therapy and CBT for "traumatic grief" (Shear et al. 2001) may lead to more valid approaches to treating adjustment to loss in SCI.

Nonadherence to treatment, and the associated conflicts with staff, often trigger psychiatric consultation. Causes of nonadherence are varied and include depression, amotivational states due to concomitant TBI, antisocial personality traits, ongoing substance abuse, and unrealistic staff expectations. Adherence is a function of the interaction among somatic, psychological, and environmental variables (Trieschmann 1988). Environmental factors may be particularly salient in cases of nonadherence. Once primary psychiatric disorders are ruled out, the consultant should examine how adherence to prescribed therapies may not be as rewarding for the patient as it should be, perhaps because of pain, withdrawal of social contact, or relinquishing a sense of control. In some cases, nonadherence may inadvertently be rewarded by engaging staff in negative social interactions, asserting independence, or avoiding unwanted responsibilities. One example is patients with dependent traits not improving toward independence because staff attention and expressions of support are contingent on dependent behavior. Behavioral principles such as rewarding successive approximations, ignoring disability-inappropriate behaviors, initiating behavioral activation, using quota systems, and explicitly linking progress in rehabilitation to desired outcomes (such as earlier discharge) may improve adherence to treatment (W.E. Fordyce 1976).

Conclusion

As society's attitudes toward disability continue to evolve and researchers work toward better understanding the potent effects of psychosocial factors in disability, psychiatrists will have an increasing role in the rehabilitation setting. To achieve comprehensive evaluation and treatment of persons with TBI and SCI, psychiatrists must appreciate and address the multiple complex facets of these conditions, from the acute neurological injury and attendant psychological trauma through the chronic neurological, medical, psychiatric, and social sequelae of the injury. The multidisciplinary rehabilitation setting affords an environment in which psychiatrists can utilize their pharmacological and psychotherapeutic skills in psychosomatic medicine to maximize the long-term functional potential of their patients.

References

Alexander MP: Mild traumatic brain injury: pathophysiology, natural history, and clinical management. Neurology 45:1253–1260, 1995

Alexander MP: Minor traumatic brain injury: a review of physiogenesis and psychogenesis. Semin Clin Neuropsychiatry 2:177–187, 1997

Allen CC, Ruff RM: Self-rating versus neuropsychological performance of moderate versus severe head-injured patients. Brain Inj 4:7–17, 1990

Alves WM, Colohan ART, O'Leary TJ, et al: Understanding posttraumatic symptoms after minor head injury. J Head Trauma Rehabil 1:1–12, 1986

Alves W, Macciocchi SN, Barth JT: Postconcussive symptoms after uncomplicated mild head injury. J Head Trauma Rehabil 8:48–59, 1993

Amador M, Lynne C, Brackett N: A Guide and Resource Directory to Male Fertility Following Spinal Cord Injury/Dysfunction: Miami Project to Cure Paralysis. Miami, FL, University of Miami, 2000

Amaducci LA, Fratiglioni L, Rocca WA, et al: Risk factors for clinically diagnosed Alzheimer's disease: a case-control study of an Italian population. Neurology 36:922–931, 1986

American Psychiatric Association: Diagnostic and Statistical Manual of Mental Disorders, 3rd Edition. Washington, DC, American Psychiatric Association, 1980

American Psychiatric Association: Diagnostic and Statistical Manual of Mental Disorders, 3rd Edition, Revised. Washington, DC, American Psychiatric Association, 1987

American Psychiatric Association: Diagnostic and Statistical Manual of Mental Disorders, 4th Edition. Washington, DC, American Psychiatric Association, 1994

American Psychiatric Association: Diagnostic and Statistical Manual of Mental Disorders, 4th Edition, Text Revision. Washington, DC, American Psychiatric Association, 2000

Anderson SW, Tranel D: Awareness of disease states following cerebral infarction, dementia, and head trauma: standardized assessment. Clin Neuropsychol 3:327–339, 1989

Anon J, Robinson C: Treatment of common male and female sexual concerns, in The Comprehensive Textbook of Behavioral Medicine. Edited by Ferguson J, Taylor C. New York, SP Medical & Scientific Books, 1980, pp 273–296

Ashman TA, Spielman LA, Hibbard MR, et al: Psychiatric challenges in the first 6 years after traumatic brain injury: cross-sequential analyses of Axis I disorders. Arch Phys Med Rehabil 85 (4 suppl 2):S36–S42, 2004

Auerbach SH: The pathophysiology of traumatic brain injury. Phys Med Rehabil 3:1–11, 1989

Azouvi P, Jokic C, Attal N, et al: Carbamazepine in agitation and aggressive behaviour following severe closed-head injury: results of an open trial. Brain Inj 13:797–804, 1999

Bakchine S, Lacomblez L, Benoit N, et al: Manic-like state after bilateral orbitofrontal and right temporoparietal injury: efficacy of clonidine. Neurology 39:777–781, 1989

Barncord SW, Wanlass RL: A correction procedure for the Minnesota Multiphasic Personality Inventory–2 for persons with spinal cord injury. Arch Phys Med Rehabil 81: 1185–1190, 2000

Battaglia J, Lindborg SR, Alaka K, et al: Calming versus sedative effects of intramuscular olanzapine in agitated patients. Am J Emerg Med 21:192–198, 2003

Bazarian JJ, Wong T, Harris M, et al: Epidemiology and predictors of post-concussive syndrome after minor head injury in an emergency population. Brain Inj 13:173–189, 1999

Ben-Yishay Y, Rattok J, Piasetsky EB, et al: Neuropsychologic rehabilitation: quest for a holistic approach. Semin Neurol 5:252–259, 1985

Beran RG, Gibson RJ: Aggressive behavior in intellectually challenged patients with epilepsy treated with lamotrigine. Epilepsia 39:280–282, 1998

Bergsneider M, Hovda DA, McArthur DL, et al: Metabolic recovery following human traumatic brain injury based on FDG-PET: time course and relationship to neurological disability. J Head Trauma Rehabil 16:135–148, 2001

Binder LM, Rohling ML: Money matters: meta-analytic review of the effects of financial incentives on recovery after closed head injury. Am J Psychiatry 153:7–10, 1996

Binder LM, Rohling ML, Larrabee GJ: A review of mild head trauma, part I: meta-analytic review of neuropsychological studies. J Clin Exp Neuropsychol 19:421–431, 1997

Bleiberg J, Garmoe W, Cederquist J, et al: Effects of dexedrine on performance consistency following brain injury: a double-blind placebo crossover case study. Neuropsychiatry Neuropsychol Behav Neurol 6:245–248, 1993

Boake C, Freeland JC, Ringholz GM, et al: Awareness of memory loss after severe closed-head injury. Brain Inj 9:273–283, 1995

Bogner J, Corrigan JD: Epidemiology of agitation following brain injury. Neurorehabilitation 5:293–297, 1995

Bohnen N, Jolles J, Twijnstra A: Neuropsychological deficits in patients with persistent symptoms six months after mild head injury. Neurosurgery 30:692–696, 1992

Bombardier CH: Alcohol and traumatic disability, in The Handbook of Rehabilitation Psychology. Edited by Frank R, Elliott T. Washington, DC, American Psychological Association Press, 2000, pp 399–416

Bombardier CH, Rimmele C: Alcohol use and readiness to change after spinal cord injury. Arch Phys Med Rehabil 79: 1110–1115, 1998

Bombardier CH, Kilmer J, Ehde D: Screening for alcoholism among persons with recent traumatic brain injury. Rehabil Psychol 42:259–271, 1997

Bombardier CH, Rimmele C, Zintel H: The magnitude and correlates of alcohol and drug use before traumatic brain injury. Arch Phys Med Rehabil 83:1765–1773, 2002

Bombardier CH, Temkin N, Machamer J, et al: The natural history of drinking and alcohol-related problems after traumatic brain injury. Arch Phys Med Rehabil 84:185–191, 2003

Bonanno G, Kaltman S: Toward an integrative perspective on bereavement. Psychol Bull 125:760–776, 1999

Bonanno GA, Wortman CB, Lehman DR, et al: Resilience to loss and chronic grief: a prospective study from preloss to 18-months postloss. J Pers Soc Psychol 83:1150–1164, 2002

Boyer B, Tollen L, Kafkalas C: A pilot study of posttraumatic stress disorder in children and adolescents with spinal cord injury. SCI Psychosocial Process 11:75–81, 1998

Brooke MM, Questad KA, Patterson PR, et al: Agitation and restlessness after closed head injury: a prospective study of 100 consecutive admissions. Arch Phys Med Rehabil 73:320–323, 1992a

Brooke MM, Patterson DR, Questad KA, et al: The treatment of agitation during initial hospitalization after traumatic brain injury. Arch Phys Med Rehabil 73:917–921, 1992b

Brown SJ, Fann JR, Grant I: Postconcussional disorder: time to acknowledge a common source of neurobehavioral morbidity. J Neuropsychiatry Clin Neurosci 6:15–22, 1994

Bryant RA, Harvey AG: Acute stress response: a comparison of head injured and non-head injured patients. Psychol Med 25:869–873, 1995

Bryant RA, Harvey AG: Relationship between acute stress disorder and posttraumatic stress disorder following mild traumatic brain injury. Am J Psychiatry 155:625–629, 1998

Bryant RA, Harvey AG: The influence of traumatic brain injury on acute stress disorder and posttraumatic stress disorder following motor vehicle accidents. Brain Inj 13:15–22, 1999

Bryant RA, Marosszeky JE, Crooks J, et al: Posttraumatic stress disorder following severe traumatic brain injury. Am J Psychiatry 157:629–631, 2000

Bullock MR, Lyeth BG, Muizelaar JP: Current status of neuroprotection trials for traumatic brain injury: lessons from animal models and clinical studies. Neurosurgery 45:207–220, 1999

Burnett DM, Kennedy RE, Cifu DX, et al: Using atypical neuroleptic drugs to treat agitation in patients with a brain injury: a review. Neurorehabilitation 13:165–172, 1999

Burns SP, Little JW, Hussey JD, et al: Sleep apnea syndrome in chronic spinal cord injury: associated factors and treatment. Arch Phys Med Rehabil 81:1334–1339, 2000

Caplan B: Staff and patient perception of patient mood. Rehabil Psychol 28:67–77, 1983

Capruso DX, Levin HS: Neurobehavioral outcome of head trauma, in Neurology and Trauma. Edited by Evans RW. Philadelphia, PA, WB Saunders, 1996, pp 201–221

Cardenas DD, McLean A, Farrell-Robers L, et al: Oral physostigmine and impaired memory in adults with brain injury. Brain Inj 8:579–587, 1994

Carter GM, Relles DA, Wynn BO, et al: Interim report on an inpatient rehabilitation facility prospective payment system. Rand Corp, DRU-2309-HCFA, July 2000

Cassidy JW: Fluoxetine: a new serotonergically active antidepressant. J Head Trauma Rehabil 4:67–69, 1989

Castriotta RJ, Lai JM: Sleep disorders associated with traumatic brain injury. Arch Phys Med Rehabil 82:1403–1406, 2001

Catsman-Berrevoets CE, Harskamp FV: Compulsive pre-sleep behavior and apathy due to bilateral thalamic stroke: response to bromocriptine. Neurology 38:647–649, 1988

Cavallo MM, Kay T, Ezrachi O: Problems and changes after traumatic brain injury: differing perceptions within and between families. Brain Inj 6:327–335, 1992

Caveness WF: Posttraumatic sequelae, in Head Injury Conference Proceedings. Edited by Caveness WF, Walker A. Philadelphia, PA, JB Lippincott, 1966, pp 209–219

Centers for Disease Control and Prevention, National Center for Injury Prevention and Control: Traumatic Brain Injury in the United States: A Report to Congress. Atlanta, GA, Centers for Disease Control and Prevention, 1999

Charlifue SW, Gerhart KA: Behavioral and demographic predictors of suicide after traumatic spinal cord injury. Arch Phys Med Rehabil 72:488–492, 1991

Chatham-Showalter PE: Carbamazepine for combativeness in acute traumatic brain injury. J Neuropsychiatry Clin Neurosci 8:96–99, 1996

Chatham-Showalter PE, Kimmel DN: Agitated symptom response to divalproex following acute brain injury. J Neuropsychiatry Clin Neurosci 12:395–397, 2000

Childers MK, Holland D: Psychomotor agitation following gabapentin use in brain injury. Brain Inj 11:537–540, 1997

Cicerone K, Dahlberg C, Kalmar K: Evidence-based cognitive rehabilitation: recommendations for clinical practice. Arch Phys Med Rehabil 81:1596–1615, 2000

Clark AF, Davison K: Mania following head injury: a report of two cases and a review of the literature. Br J Psychiatry 150:841–844, 1987

Clay DL, Hagglund KJ, Frank RG, et al: Enhancing the accuracy of depression diagnosis in patients with spinal cord injury using Bayesian analysis. Rehabil Psychol 40:171–180, 1995

Cohen SA, Ihrig K, Lott RS, et al: Risperidone for aggression and self-injurious behavior in adults with mental retardation. J Autism Dev Disord 28:229–233, 1998

Consortium for Spinal Cord Medicine: Depression Following Spinal Cord Injury: A Clinical Practice Guideline for Primary Care Physicians. Washington, DC, Paralyzed Veterans of America, 1998

Corrigan JD: Development of a scale for assessment of agitation following traumatic brain injury. J Clin Exp Neuropsychol 11:261–277, 1989

Corrigan JD: Substance abuse as a mediating factor in outcome from traumatic brain injury. Arch Phys Med Rehabil 76:302–309, 1995

Cowell LC, Cohen RF: Amantadine: a potential adjuvant therapy following traumatic brain injury. J Head Trauma Rehabil 10:91–94, 1995

Craig AR, Hancock KM, Dickson HG: A longitudinal investigation into anxiety and depression in the first 2 years following a spinal cord injury. Paraplegia 32:675–679, 1994

Craig AR, Hancock K, Dickson H, et al: Long-term psychological outcomes in spinal cord injured persons: results of a controlled trial using cognitive behavior therapy. Arch Phys Med Rehabil 78:33–38, 1997

Craig A, Hancock K, Dickson H: Improving the long-term adjustment of spinal cord injured persons. Spinal Cord 37:345–350, 1999

Crow S, Meller W, Christensen G, et al: Use of ECT after brain injury. Convuls Ther 12:113–116, 1996

Currier GW, Simpson GM: Risperidone liquid concentrate and oral lorazepam versus intramuscular haloperidol and intramuscular lorazepam for treatment of psychotic agitation. J Clin Psychiatry 62:153–157, 2001

Davidoff GN, Roth EJ, Richards JS: Cognitive deficits in spinal cord injury: epidemiology and outcome. Arch Phys Med Rehabil 73:275–284, 1992

Davidson J: Seizures and bupropion: a review. J Clin Psychiatry 50:256–261, 1989

Davison K, Bagley CR: Schizophrenia-like psychosis associated with organic disorders of the central nervous system. Br J Psychiatry 114:113–184, 1969

De Deyn PP, Rabheru K, Rasmussen A, et al: A randomized trial of risperidone, placebo, and haloperidol for behavioral symptoms of dementia. Neurology 53:946–955, 1999

Deb S, Lyons I, Koutzoukis C, et al: Rate of psychiatric illness 1 year after traumatic brain injury. Am J Psychiatry 156:374–378, 1999

DeLisa JA, Currie DM, Martin GM: Rehabilitation medicine: past, present, and future, in Rehabilitation Medicine: Principles and Practice, 3rd Edition. Philadelphia, PA, Lippincott Williams & Wilkins, 1998, pp 3–32

DeVivo MJ, Krause JS, Lammertse DP: Recent trends in mortality and causes of death among persons with spinal cord injury. Arch Phys Med Rehabil 80:1411–1419, 1999

Diamond S: Efficacy and safety profile of venlafaxine in chronic headache. Headache Quarterly 6:212–214, 1995

Dickel MJ, Renfrow SD, Moore PT, et al: Rapid eye movement sleep periodic leg movements in patients with spinal cord injury. Sleep 17:733–738, 1994

Dijkers M: Quality of life after spinal cord injury: a meta-analysis of the effects of disablement components. Spinal Cord 35:829–840, 1997

Dikmen SS, Temkin N, Armsden G: Neuropsychological recovery: relationship to psychosocial functioning and postconcussional complaints, in Mild Head Injury. Edited by Levin HS, Eisenberg HM, Benton AL. New York, Oxford University Press, 1989, pp 229–241

Dikmen S, Machamer JE, Winn HR, et al: Neuropsychological outcome at 1-year post head injury. Neuropsychology 9:80–90, 1995

Dikmen SS, Machamer JE, Winn HR, et al: Neuropsychological effects of valproate in traumatic brain injury: a randomized trial. Neurology 54:895–902, 2000

Dikmen S, Machamer J, Temkin N: Mild head injury: facts and artifacts. J Clin Exp Neuropsychol 23:729–738, 2001

Dinan TG, Mobayed M: Treatment resistance of depression after head injury: a preliminary study of amitriptyline response. Acta Psychiatr Scand 85:292–294, 1992

Doppenberg EMR, Bullock R: Clinical neuro-protection trials in severe traumatic brain injury: lessons from previous studies. J Neurotrauma 14:71–80, 1997

Duffy JD, Kant R: Clinical utility of clozapine in 16 patients with neurological disease. J Neuropsychiatry Clin Neurosci 8:92–96, 1996

Dunlop TW, Udvarhelyi GB, Stedem AFA, et al: Comparison of patients with and without emotional/behavioral deterioration during the first year after traumatic brain injury. J Neuropsychiatry Clin Neurosci 3:150–156, 1991

Eames P: The use of Sinemet and bromocriptine. Brain Inj 3:319–320, 1989

Eastwood EA, Hagglund KJ, Ragnarsson KT, et al: Medical rehabilitation length of stay and outcomes for persons with traumatic spinal cord injury: 1990–1997. Arch Phys Med Rehabil 80:1457–1463, 1999

Ellenberg JH, Levin HS, Saydjari C: Posttraumatic amnesia as a predictor of outcome after severe closed head injury. Arch Neurol 53:782–791, 1996

Elliott TR, Frank RG: Depression following spinal cord injury. Arch Phys Med Rehabil 77:816–823, 1996

Elliott T, Shewchuck R: Social support and leisure activities following severe physical disability: testing the mediating effects of depression. Basic Appl Soc Psychol 16:471–587, 1995

Elliott T, Umlauf R: Measurement of personality and psychopathology in acquired disability, in Psychological Assessment in Medical Rehabilitation Settings. Edited by Cushman L, Scherer M. Washington, DC, American Psychological Association, 1995, pp 325–358

Englander J, Hall K, Simpson T, et al: Mild traumatic brain injury in an insured population: subjective complaints and return to employment. Brain Inj 6:161–166, 1992

Ergh TC, Rapport LJ, Coleman RD, et al: Predictors of caregiver and family functioning following traumatic brain injury: social support moderates caregiver distress. J Head Trauma Rehabil 17:155–174, 2002

Ettinger AB, Weisbrot DM, Saracco J, et al: Positive and negative psychotropic effects of lamotrigine in patients with epilepsy and mental retardation. Epilepsia 39:874–877, 1998

Evans C, Sherer M, Nakase Thompson R, et al: Early impaired self-awareness, depression, and subjective well-being following TBI. J Int Neuropsychol Soc 9:253–254, 2003

Evans RW: The postconcussion syndrome and the sequelae of mild head injury, in Neurology and Trauma. Edited by Evans RW. Philadelphia, PA, WB Saunders, 1996, pp 91–116

Evans RW, Gualtieri CR, Patterson D: Treatment of chronic closed head injury with psychostimulant drugs: a controlled case study and an appropriate evaluation procedure. J Nerv Ment Dis 175:106–110, 1987

Fann JR: Neurological effects of psychopharmacological agents. Semin Clin Neuropsychiatry 7:196–206, 2002

Fann JR, Katon WJ, Uomoto JM, et al: Psychiatric disorders and functional disability in outpatients with traumatic brain injuries. Am J Psychiatry 152:1493–1499, 1995

Fann JR, Uomoto JM, Katon WJ: Sertraline in the treatment of major depression following mild traumatic brain injury. J Neuropsychiatry Clin Neurosci 12:226–232, 2000

Fann JR, Uomoto JM, Katon WJ: Cognitive improvement with treatment of depression following mild traumatic brain injury. Psychosomatics 42:48–54, 2001

Fann JR, Leonetti A, Jaffe K, et al: Psychiatric illness and subsequent traumatic brain injury: a case-control study. J Neurol Neurosurg Psychiatry 72:615–620, 2002

Fann JR, Burington B, Leonetti A, et al: Psychiatric illness following traumatic brain injury in an adult health maintenance organization population. Arch Gen Psychiatry 61:53–61, 2004

Federoff JP, Starkstein SE, Forrester AW, et al: Depression in patients with acute traumatic brain injury. Am J Psychiatry 149:918–923, 1992

Feeney DM, Gonzalez A, Law WA: Amphetamine, haloperidol, and experience interact to affect rate of recovery after motor cortex injury. Science 217:855–857, 1982

Fenton G, McClelland R, Montgomery A, et al: The postconcussional syndrome: social antecedents and psychological sequelae. Br J Psychiatry 162:493–497, 1993

Fichtenberg NL, Millis SR, Mann NR, et al: Factors associated with insomnia among post-acute traumatic brain injury survivors. Brain Inj 14:659–667, 2000

Fichtenberg NL, Putnam SH, Mann NR, et al: Insomnia screening in postacute traumatic brain injury: utility and validity of the Pittsburgh Sleep Quality Index. Am J Phys Med Rehabil 80:339–345, 2001

Fleminger S, Greenwood RJ, Oliver DL: Pharmacological management for agitation and aggression in people with acquired brain injury (Cochrane Review), in The Cochrane Library, Issue 1, Oxford, Update Software, 2003

Fordyce DJ, Roueche JR: Changes in perspectives of disability among patients, staff, and relatives during rehabilitation of brain injury. Rehabil Psychol 31:217–229, 1986

Fordyce WE: Behavioral Methods for Chronic Pain and Illness. St. Louis, MO, Mosby Year Book, 1976

Fox DD, Lees-Haley PR, Earnest K, et al: Post-concussive symptoms: base rates and etiology in psychiatric patients. Clin Neuropsychol 9:89–92, 1995

Frank RG, Chaney JM, Clay DL, et al: Dysphoria: a major symptom factor in persons with disability or chronic illness. Psychiatry Res 43:231–241, 1992

Fugate LP, Spacek LA, Kresty LA, et al: Measurement and treatment of agitation following traumatic brain injury, II: a survey of the Brain Injury Special Interest Group of the American Academy of Physical Medicine and Rehabilitation. Arch Phys Med Rehabil 78:924–928, 1997

Fuhrer M, Rintala D, Hart K, et al: Depressive symptomatology in persons with spinal cord injury who reside in the community. Arch Phys Med Rehabil 74:255–260, 1993

Fujii D, Ahmed I: Characteristics of psychotic disorder due to traumatic brain injury: an analysis of case studies in the literature. J Neuropsychiatry Clin Neurosci 14:130–140, 2002

Fullerton D, Harvey R, Klein M, et al: Psychiatric disorders in patients with spinal cord injury. Arch Gen Psychiatry 32:369–371, 1981

Galski T, Palasz J, Bruno RL, et al: Predicting physical and verbal aggression on a brain trauma unit. Arch Phys Med Rehabil 75:380–383, 1994

Gasquione PG: Affective state and awareness of sensory and cognitive effects after closed head injury. Neuropsychology 4:187–196, 1992

Gasquione PG, Gibbons TA: Lack of awareness of impairment in institutionalized, severely and chronically disabled survivors of traumatic brain injury: a preliminary investigation. J Head Trauma Rehabil 9:16–24, 1994

Gennarelli TA, Graham DI: Neuropathology of the head injuries. Semin Clin Neuropsychiatry 3:160–175, 1998

Gerhart KA, Koziol-McLain J, et al: Quality of life following spinal cord injury: knowledge and attitudes of emergency care providers. Ann Emerg Med 23:807–812, 1994

Go BK, DeVivo MJ, Richards JS: The epidemiology of spinal cord injury, in Spinal Cord Injury: Clinical Outcomes from the Model Systems. Edited by Stover S, DeLisa JA, Whiteneck GG. Gaithersburg, MD, Aspen, 1995, pp 21–55

Gosling J, Oddy M: Rearranged marriages: marital relationships after head injury. Brain Inj 13:785–796, 1999

Gouvier WD, Uddo-Crane M, Brown LM: Base rates of postconcussional symptoms. Arch Clin Neuropsychol 3:273–278, 1988

Gouvier WD, Cubic B, Jones G, et al: Postconcussion symptoms and daily stress in normal and head-injured college populations. Arch Clin Neuropsychol 7:193–211, 1992

Grant I, Alves W: Psychiatric and psychosocial disturbances in head injury, in Neurobehavioral Recovery from Head Injury. Edited by Levin HS, Grafman J, Eisenberg HM. New York, Oxford University Press, 1987, pp 234–235

Graves AB, White E, Koepsell TD, et al: The association between head trauma and Alzheimer's disease. Am J Epidemiol 131:491–501, 1990

Greendyke RM, Kanter DR: Therapeutic effects of pindolol on behavioral disturbances associated with organic brain disease: a double-blind study. J Clin Psychiatry 47:423–426, 1996

Greendyke RM, Kanter DR, Schuster DB, et al: Propranolol treatment of assaultive patients with organic brain disease: a double-blind, crossover, placebo-controlled study. J Nerv Ment Dis 174:290–294, 1996

Greve KW, Sherwin E, Stanford MW, et al: Personality and neurocognitive correlates of impulsive aggression in long-term survivors of severe traumatic brain injury. Brain Inj 15:255–262, 2001

Groom KN, Shaw TG, O'Connor ME, et al: Neurobehavioral symptoms and family functioning in traumatically brain-injured adults. Arch Clin Neuropsychol 13:695–711, 1998

Gualtieri CT: Buspirone for the behavior problems of patients with organic brain disorders. J Clin Psychopharmacol 11: 280–281, 1991

Gualtieri CT, Evans RW: Stimulant treatment for the neurobehavioural sequelae of traumatic brain injury. Brain Inj 2:273–290, 1988

Gualtieri T, Chandler M, Coons TB, et al: Amantadine: a new clinical profile for traumatic brain injury. Clin Neuropharmacol 12:258–270, 1989

Guilmette TJ, Rasile D: Sensitivity, specificity, and diagnostic accuracy of three verbal memory measures in the assessment of mild brain injury. Neuropsychology 9:338–344, 1995

Guerrero J, Thurman DJ, Sniezek JE: Emergency department visits associated with traumatic brain injury: United States, 1995–1996. Brain Inj 14:181–186, 2000

Gupta SR, Mlcoch AG: Bromocriptine treatment of nonfluent aphasia. Arch Phys Med Rehabil 73:373–376, 1992

Hall KM, Karzmark P, Stevens M, et al: Family stressors in traumatic brain injury: a two-year follow-up. Arch Phys Med Rehabil 75:876–884, 1994

Hamm RJ, Temple MD, Buck DL, et al: Cognitive recovery from traumatic brain injury: results of post-traumatic experimental interventions, in Neuroplasticity and Reorganization of Function After Brain Injury. Edited by Levin HS, Grafman J. New York, Oxford University Press, 2000, pp 49–67

Hanna-Pladdy B, Gouvier WD, Berry ZM: Postconcussional symptoms as predictors of neuropsychological deficits (abstract). Arch Clin Neuropsychol 12:329–330, 1997

Hanson R, Franklin M: Sexual loss in relation to other functional losses for spinal cord injured males. Arch Phys Med Rehabil 57:291–303, 1976

Hart T, Whyte J, Polansky M, et al: Concordance of patient and family report of neurobehavioral symptoms at 1 year after traumatic brain injury. Arch Phys Med Rehabil 84:204–213, 2003

Harvey AG, Bryant RA: Acute stress disorder following mild traumatic brain injury. J Nerv Ment Dis 186:333–337, 1998

Harvey AG, Bryant RA: A two-year prospective evaluation of the relationship between acute stress disorder and posttraumatic stress disorder following mild traumatic brain injury. Am J Psychiatry 157:626–628, 2000

Harvey AG, Brewin CR, Jones C, et al: Coexistence of posttraumatic stress disorder and traumatic brain injury: towards a resolution of the paradox. J Int Neuropsychol Soc 9:663–676, 2003

Hayes RL, Dixon CE: Neurochemical changes in mild head injury. Semin Neurol 14:25–31, 1994

Hayes RL, Jenkins LW, Lyeth BG: Neurotransmitter-mediated mechanisms of traumatic brain injury: acetylcholine and excitatory amino acids. J Neurotrauma 9 (suppl 1):173–187, 1992

Heaton RK, Pendleton MG: Use of neuropsychological test to predict adult patients' everyday functioning. J Consult Clin Psychol 49:807–821, 1981

Heilbronner RL, Roueche JR, Everson SA, et al: Comparing patient perspectives of disability and treatment effects with quality of participation in a post-acute brain injury rehabilitation programme. Brain Inj 3:387–389, 1989

Heinemann A, Keen M, Donohue R, et al: Alcohol use in persons with recent spinal cord injuries. Arch Phys Med Rehabil 69:619–624, 1988

Hendryx PM: Psychosocial changes perceived by closed-head-injured adults and their families. Arch Phys Med Rehabil 70:526–530, 1989

Hensley PL, Reeve A: A case of antidepressant-induced akathisia in a patient with traumatic brain injury. J Head Trauma Rehabil 16:302–305, 2001

Herrick S, Elliott T, Crow F: Social support and the prediction of health complications among persons with SCI. Rehabil Psychol 39:231–250, 1994

Hibbard MR, Grober SE, Stein PN, et al: Poststroke depression, in Comprehensive Casebook of Cognitive Therapy. Edited by Freeman A, Dattilio F. New York, Guilford, 1992, pp 303–310

Hibbard MR, Uysal S, Kepler K, et al: Axis I psychopathology in individuals with traumatic brain injury. J Head Trauma Rehabil 13:24–39, 1998

Hibbard MR, Gordon WA, Flanagan S, et al: Sexual dysfunction after traumatic brain injury. Neurorehabilitation 15:107–120, 2000a

Hibbard MR, Gordon WA, Kothera LM: Traumatic brain injury, in Cognitive-Behavioral Strategies in Crisis Intervention, 2nd Edition. Edited by Dattilio F, Freeman A. New York, Guilford, 2000b, pp 219–242

Hillbom E: After-effects of brain-injuries: research on the symptoms causing invalidism of persons in Finland having sustained brain-injuries during the wars of 1939–1940 and 1941–1944. Acta Psychiatr Scand 35 (suppl 142):1–95, 1960

Hiott DW, Labbate L: Anxiety disorders associated with traumatic brain injuries. Neurorehabilitation 17:345–355, 2002

Hornstein A, Seliger G: Cognitive side effects of lithium in closed head injury (letter). J Neuropsychiatry Clin Neurosci 1:446–447, 1989

Horton A, Howe N: Behavioral treatment of the traumatically brain injured: a case study. Percept Motor Skills 53:349–350, 1981

Iezzoni LI, Davis RB, Soukup J, et al: Quality dimensions that most concern people with physical and sensory disabilities. Arch Intern Med 163:2085–2092, 2003

Jennett B, Bond M: Assessment of outcome after severe brain damage. Lancet 1:480–484, 1975

Jorge R, Robinson RG: Mood disorders following traumatic brain injury. Neurorehabilitation 17:311–324, 2002

Jorge RE, Robinson RG, Arndt S: Are there symptoms that are specific for depressed mood in patients with traumatic brain injury? J Nerv Ment Dis 181:91–99, 1993a

Jorge RE, Robinson RG, Starkstein SE, et al: Depression and anxiety following traumatic brain injury. J Neuropsychiatry Clin Neurosci 5:369–374, 1993b

Jorge RE, Robinson RG, Starkstein SE, et al: Secondary mania following traumatic brain injury. Am J Psychiatry 150:916–921, 1993c

Jorge RE, Robinson RG, Moser D, et al: Major depression following traumatic brain injury. Arch Gen Psychiatry 61:42–50, 2004

Judd FK, Stone J, Webber JE, et al: Depression following spinal cord injury: a prospective in-patient study. Br J Psychiatry 154:668–671, 1989

Jung AC, Staiger T, Sullivan M: The efficacy of selective serotonin reuptake inhibitors for the management of chronic pain. J Gen Intern Med 12:384–389, 1997

Kaelin DL, Cifu DX, Matthies B: Methylphenidate effect on attention deficit in the acutely brain-injured adult. Arch Phys Med Rehabil 77:6–9, 1996

Kalisky Z, Morrison DP, Meyers CA, et al: Medical problems encountered during rehabilitation of patients with head injury. Arch Phys Med Rehabil 66:25–29, 1985

Kant R, Bogyi AM, Carosella NW, et al: ECT as a therapeutic option in severe brain injury. Convuls Ther 11:45–50, 1995

Kant R, Smith-Seemiller L, Zeiler D: Treatment of aggression and irritability after head injury. Brain Inj 12:661–666, 1998

Katz DI: Neuropathology and neurobehavioral recovery from closed head injury. J Head Trauma Rehabil 7:1–15, 1992

Katz IR, Jeste DV, Mintzer JE, et al: Comparison of risperidone and placebo for psychosis and behavioral disturbances associated with dementia: a randomized, double-blind trial. J Clin Psychiatry 60:107–115, 1999

Kay T, Cavallo MM: The family system: impact, assessment and intervention, in Neuropsychiatry of Traumatic Brain Injury. Edited by Hales RE. Washington, DC, American Psychiatric Press, 1994, pp 533–568

Kay T, Harrington DE, Adams R, et al: Definition of mild traumatic brain injury. J Head Trauma Rehabil 8:86–87, 1993

Kennedy P, Duff J: Post traumatic stress disorder and spinal cord injuries. Spinal Cord 39:1–10, 2001

Kennedy P, Evans MJ: Evaluation of post traumatic distress in the first 6 months following SCI. Spinal Cord 39:381–386, 2001

Kennedy P, Rogers BA: Anxiety and depression after spinal cord injury: a longitudinal analysis. Arch Phys Med Rehabil 81:932–937, 2000

Kennedy P, Duff J, Evans M, et al: Coping effectiveness training reduces depression and anxiety following traumatic spinal cord injuries. Br J Clin Psychol 42:41–52, 2003

Kim E: Agitation, aggression, and disinhibition syndromes after traumatic brain injury. Neurorehabilitation 17:297–310, 2002

King N: Mild head injury: neuropathology, sequelae, measurement and recovery. Br J Clin Psychol 36:161–184, 1997

King NS: Post-concussion syndrome: clarity amid the controversy? Br J Psychiatry 183:276–278, 2003

King NS, Crawford S, Wenden FJ, et al: The Rivermead Post Concussion Symptoms Questionnaire: a measure of symptoms commonly experienced after head injury and its reliability. J Neurol 242:587–592, 1995

Kishi Y, Robinson RG, Forrester AW: Prospective longitudinal study of depression following spinal cord injury. J Neuropsychiatry Clin Neurosci 6:237–244, 1994

Kishi Y, Robinson RG, Forrester AW: Comparison between acute and delayed onset major depression after spinal cord injury. J Nerv Ment Dis 183:286–292, 1995

Kiwerski J, Krauski M: Influence of alcohol intake on the course and consequences of spinal cord injury. Int J Rehab Res 15:240–245, 1992

Kolakowsky-Hayner SA, Gourley EV III, Kreutzer JS, et al: Pre-injury substance abuse among persons with brain injury and persons with spinal cord injury. Brain Inj 13:571–581, 1999

Kolakowsky-Hayner SA, Gourley EV III, Kreutzer JS, et al: Post-injury substance abuse among persons with brain injury and persons with spinal cord injury. Brain Inj 16:583–592, 2002

Koponen S, Taiminen T, Portin R, et al: Axis I and II psychiatric disorders after traumatic brain injury: a 30-year follow-up study. Am J Psychiatry 159:1315–1321, 2002

Kraus JF, McArthur DL: Incidence and prevalence of, and costs associated with, traumatic brain injury, in Rehabilitation of the Adult and Child with Traumatic Brain Injury, 3rd Edition. Edited by Rosenthal M, Kreutzer JS, Griffith ER, et al. Philadelphia, FA Davis, 1999, pp 3–18

Kraus MF, Maki PM: Effect of amantadine hydrochloride on symptoms of frontal lobe dysfunction in brain injury: case studies and review. J Neuropsychiatry Clin Neurosci 9:222–230, 1997

Krause J: Delivery of substance abuse services during spinal cord injury rehabilitation. Neurorehabilitation 2:45–51, 1992

Krause JS, Kewman D, DeVivo MJ, et al: Employment after spinal cord injury: an analysis of cases from the Model Spinal Cord Injury Systems. Arch Phys Med Rehabil 80:1492–1500, 1999

Kreutzer JS, Doherty KR, Harris JA, et al: Alcohol use among persons with traumatic brain injury. J Head Trauma Rehabil 5:9–20, 1990

Kreutzer JS, Wehman PH, Harris JA, et al: Substance abuse and crime patterns among persons with traumatic brain injury referred for supported employment. Brain Inj 5:177–187, 1991

Kreutzer JS, Gordon WA, Rosenthal M, et al: Neuropsychological characteristics of patients with brain injury: preliminary findings from a multicenter investigation. J Head Trauma Rehabil 8:47–59, 1993

Kreutzer JS, Gervasio AH, Camplair PS: Primary caregivers' psychological status and family functioning after traumatic brain injury. Brain Inj 8:197–210, 1994

Kreutzer JS, Marwitz JH, Witol AD: Interrelationship between crime, substance abuse, and aggressive behaviours among persons with traumatic brain injury. Brain Inj 9:757–768, 1995

Kreutzer JS, Witol AD, Marwitz JH: Alcohol and drug use among young persons with traumatic brain injury. J Learn Disabil 29:643–651, 1996

Kreutzer JS, Seel RT, Gourley E: The prevalence and symptom rates of depression after traumatic brain injury: a comprehensive examination. Brain Inj 15:563–576, 2001

Krieger D, Hansen K, McDermott C, et al: Loxapine versus olanzapine in the treatment of delirium following traumatic brain injury. Neurorehabilitation 18:205–208, 2003

Kwentus JA, Hart RP, Peck ET, et al: Psychiatric complications of closed head trauma. Psychosomatics 26:8–17, 1985

Lal S, Merbitz CP, Grip JC: Modification of function in head-injured patients with Sinemet. Brain Inj 2:225–233, 1988

Lang E, Hord AH, Denson D: Venlafaxine hydrochloride (Effexor) relieves thermal hyperalgesia in rats with an experimental mononeuropathy. Pain 68:151–155, 1996

Larrabee GJ: Neuropsychological outcome, post concussion symptoms and forensic considerations in mild closed head injury. Semin Clin Neuropsychiatry 2:196–206, 1997

Larrabee GJ: Current controversies in mild head injury, in The Evaluation and Treatment of Mild Traumatic Brain Injury. Edited by Varney NR, Roberts RJ. Mahwah, NJ, Lawrence Erlbaum Associates, 1999, pp 327–346

Lee MA, Leng MEF, Tierman EJJ: Risperidone: a useful adjunct for behavioural disturbance in primary cerebral tumours. Palliative Med 15:255–256, 2001

Leininger BE, Gramling SE, Farrell AD, et al: Neuropsychological deficits in symptomatic minor head injury patients after concussion and mild concussion. J Neurol Neurosurg Psychiatry 53:293–296, 1990

Leon-Carrion J: Dementia due to head trauma: an obscure name for a clear neurocognitive syndrome. Neurorehabilitation 17:115–122, 2002

Lesem MD, Zajecka JM, Swift RH, et al: Intramuscular ziprasidone, 2 mg versus 10 mg, in the short-term management of agitated psychotic patients. J Clin Psychiatry 62:12–18, 2001

Levin HS, O'Donnell VM, Grossman RG: The Galveston Orientation and Amnesia Test: a practical scale to assess cognition after head injury. J Nerv Ment Dis 167:675–684, 1979

Levin HS, Mattis S, Ruff RM, et al: Neurobehavioral outcome following minor head injury: a three-center study. J Neurosurg 66:234–243, 1987a

Levin HS, High WM, Goethe KE, et al: The Neurobehavioral Rating Scale: assessment of the behavioral sequelae of head injury by the clinician. J Neurol Neurosurg Psychiatry 50:183–193, 1987b

Levin HS, Brown SA, Song JX, et al: Depression and posttraumatic stress disorder at three months after mild to moderate traumatic brain injury. J Clin Exp Neuropsychol 23:754–769, 2001

Levitt P, Henry W, McHale D: Persistent movement disorder induced by buspirone. Mov Disord 8:331–334, 1993

Lewis L: A framework for developing a psychotherapy treatment plan with brain-injured patients. J Head Trauma Rehabil 6:22–29, 1991

Lindenmayer JP, Kotsaftis A: Use of sodium valproate in violent and aggressive behaviors: a critical review. J Clin Psychiatry 61:123–128, 2000

Livingston MG, Brooks DN, Bond MR: Patient outcome in the year following severe head injury and relatives' psychiatric and social functioning. J Neurol Neurosurg Psychiatry 48:876–881, 1985

MacDonald M, Nielson W, Cameron M: Depression and activity patterns of spinal cord injured persons living in the community. Arch Phys Med Rehabil 68:339–343, 1987

Malaspina D, Goetz RR, Friedman JH, et al: Traumatic brain injury and schizophrenia in members of schizophrenia and bipolar disorder pedigrees. Am J Psychiatry 158:440–446, 2001

Malec JF: Mild traumatic brain injury: scope of the problem, in The Evaluation and Treatment of Mild Traumatic Brain Injury. Edited by Varney NR, Roberts RJ. Mahwah, NJ, Lawrence Erlbaum Associates, 1999, pp 15–38

Malec J, Neimeyer R: Psychologic prediction of duration of inpatient spinal cord injury rehabilitation performance of self care. Arch Phys Med Rehabil 64:359–363, 1983

Marin RS: Apathy: a neuropsychiatric syndrome. J Neuropsychiatry Clin Neurosci 3:243–254, 1991

Marin RS, Fogel BS, Hawkins J, et al: Apathy: a treatable syndrome. J Neuropsychiatry Clin Neurosci 7:23–30, 1995

Marino RJ, Ditunno JF Jr, Donovan WH, et al: Neurologic recovery after traumatic spinal cord injury: data from the Model Spinal Cord Injury Systems. Arch Phys Med Rehabil 80:1391–1396, 1999

Martin R, Kuzniecky R, Ho S, et al: Cognitive effects of topiramate, gabapentin, and lamotrigine in healthy young adults. Neurology 52:321–327, 1999

Marwit SJ: Reliability of diagnosing complicated grief: a preliminary investigation. J Consult Clin Psychol 64:563–568, 1996

Maryniak O, Manchanda R, Velani A: Methotrimeprazine in the treatment of agitation in acquired brain injury patients. Brain Inj 15:167–174, 2001

Masand PS, Tesar GE: Use of stimulants in the medically ill. Psychiatr Clin North Am 19:515–547, 1996

Masel BE, Scheibel RS, Kimbark T, et al: Excessive daytime sleepiness in adults with brain injuries. Arch Phys Med Rehabil 82:1526–1532, 2001

Max W, MacKenzie EJ, Rice DP: Head injuries: costs and consequences. J Head Trauma Rehabil 6:76–91, 1991

Mayou R, Bryant B, Duthie R: Psychiatric consequences of road traffic accidents. BMJ 307:647–651, 1993

Mayou R, Black J, Bryant B: Unconsciousness, amnesia and psychiatric symptoms following road traffic accident injury. Br J Psychiatry 177:540–545, 2000

McAllister TW: Neuropsychiatric sequelae of head injuries. Psychiatr Clin North Am 15:395–413, 1992

McAllister TW, Ferrell RB: Evaluation and treatment of psychosis after traumatic brain injury. Neurorehabilitation 17:357–368, 2002

McCauley SR, Boake C, Levin HS, et al: Postconcussional disorder following mild to moderate traumatic brain injury: anxiety, depression, and social support as risk factors and comorbidities. J Clin Exp Neuropsychol 23:792–808, 2001

McClelland RJ, Fenton GW, Rutherford W: The postconcussional syndrome revisited. J R Soc Med 87:508–510, 1994

McDougle CJ, Holmes JP, Carlson DC, et al: A double-blind, placebo-controlled study of risperidone in adults with autistic disorder and other pervasive developmental disorders. Arch Gen Psychiatry 55:633–641, 1998

McElligott JM, Greenwald BD, Watanabe TK: Congenital and acquired brain injury. 4. New frontiers: neuroimaging, neuroprotective agents, cognitive-enhancing agents, new technology, and complementary medicine. Arch Phys Med Rehabil 84 (suppl 1):18–22, 2003

McGlynn SM, Schacter DL: Unawareness of deficits in neuropsychological syndromes. J Clin Exp Neuropsychol 11:143–205, 1989

McIntosh TK, Smith DH, Meaney DF, et al: Neuropathological sequelae of traumatic brain injury: relationship to neurochemical and biomechanical mechanisms. Lab Invest 74:315–342, 1996

McIntosh TK, Juhler M, Wieloch T: Novel pharmacological strategies in the treatment of experimental traumatic brain injury. J Neurotrauma 15:731–769, 1998

McKinlay WW, Brooks DN: Methodological problems in assessing psychosocial recovery following severe head injury. J Clin Neuropsychol 6:87–99, 1984

McKinlay WW, Brooks DN, Bond MR, et al: The short-term outcome of severe blunt head injury as reported by relatives of the injured persons. J Neurol Neurosurg Psychiatry 44:527–533, 1981

McKinley WO, Seel RT, Hardman JT: Nontraumatic spinal cord injury: incidence, epidemiology, and functional outcome. Arch Phys Med Rehabil 80:619–623, 1999

McLean A Jr, Temkin NR, Dikmen S, et al: The behavioral sequelae of head injury. J Clin Neuropsychol 5:361–376, 1983

McQuay HJ, Tramer M, Nye BA, et al: A systematic review of antidepressants in neuropathic pain. Pain 68:217–227, 1996

Meehan KM, Wang H, David SR, et al: Comparison of rapidly acting intramuscular olanzapine, lorazepam, and placebo: a double-blind, randomized study in acutely agitated patients with dementia. Neuropsychopharmacology 26:494–504, 2002

Meythaler JM, Peduzzi JD, Eleftheriou E, et al: Current concepts: diffuse axonal injury-associated traumatic brain injury. Arch Phys Med Rehabil 82:1461–1471, 2001

Meythaler JM, Brunner RC, Johnson A, et al: Amantadine to improve neurorecovery in traumatic brain injury-associated diffuse axonal injury: a pilot double-blind randomized trial. J Head Trauma Rehabil 17:300–313, 2002

Michals ML, Crismon ML, Robers S, et al: Clozapine response and adverse effects in nine brain-injured patients. J Clin Psychopharmacol 13:198–203, 1993

Middleboe T, Anderson HS, Birket-Smith M, et al: Minor head injury: impact on general health after one year. Acta Neurol Scand 85:5–9, 1992

Millis SR, Rosenthal M, Novack TA, et al: Long-term neuropsychological outcome after traumatic brain injury. J Head Trauma Rehabil 16:343–355, 2001

Mittenberg W, Strauman S: Diagnosis of mild head injury and the postconcussion syndrome. J Head Trauma Rehabil 15:783–791, 2000

Mittenberg W, Tremont G, Zielinski RE, et al: Cognitive-behavioral prevention of postconcussion syndrome. Arch Clin Neuropsychol 11:139–145, 1996

Mooney GF, Haas LJ: Effect of methylphenidate on brain injury-related anger. Arch Phys Med Rehabil 74:153–160, 1993

Moss NE, Crawford S, Wade DT: Postconcussion symptoms: is stress a mediating factor? Clin Rehabil 8:149–156, 1994

Muller U, Murai T, Bauer-Wittmund T, et al: Paroxetine versus citalopram treatment of pathological crying after brain injury. Brain Inj 13:805–811, 1999

Mysiw WJ, Jackson RD, Corrigan JD: Amitriptyline for post-traumatic agitation. Am J Phys Med Rehabil 67:29–33, 1988

Nahas Z, Arlinghaus KA, Kotrla KJ, et al: Rapid response of emotional incontinence to selective serotonin reuptake inhibitors. J Neuropsychiatry Clin Neurosci 10:453–455, 1998

National Institutes of Health Consensus Development Panel on Rehabilitation of Persons With Traumatic Brain Injury: Rehabilitation of persons with traumatic brain injury. JAMA 282:974–983, 1999

Newburn G, Edwards R, Thomas H, et al: Moclobemide in the treatment of major depressive disorder (DSM-3) following traumatic brain injury. Brain Inj 13:637–642, 1999

Nickels JL, Schneider WN, Dombovy ML, et al: Clinical use of amantadine in brain injury rehabilitation. Brain Inj 8:709–718, 1994

Niemcier JP, Burnett DM: No such thing as "uncomplicated bereavement" for patients in rehabilitation. Disabil Rehabil 23:645–653, 2001

Oddy M, Humphrey M, Uttley D: Stresses upon the relatives of head-injured patients. Br J Psychiatry 133:507–513, 1978a

Oddy M, Humphrey M, Uttley D: Subjective impairment and social recovery after closed head injury. J Neurol Neurosurg Psychiatry 41:611–616, 1978b

Ojemann LM, Baugh-Bookman C, Dudley DL: Effect of psychotropic medications on seizure control in patients with epilepsy. Neurology 37:1525–1527, 1987

Onghena P, Van Houdenhove B: Antidepressant-induced analgesia in chronic non-malignant pain: a meta-analysis of 39 placebo-controlled studies. Pain 49:205–219, 1992

Oyewumi LK, Lapierre YD: Efficacy of lithium in treating mood disorder occurring after brain stem injury. Am J Psychiatry 138:110–112, 1981

Pande AC, Davidson JR, Jefferson JW, et al: Treatment of social phobia with gabapentin: a placebo-controlled study. J Clin Psychopharmacol 19:341–348, 1999

Pande AC, Pollack MH, Crockatt J, et al: Placebo-controlled study of gabapentin treatment of panic disorder. J Clin Psychopharmacol 20:467–471, 2000

Paradiso S, Ohkubo T, Robinson RG: Vegetative and psychological symptoms associated with depressed mood over the first two years after stroke. Int J Psychiatry Med 27:137–157, 1997

Park NW, Ingles JL: Effectiveness of attention rehabilitation after an acquired brain injury: a meta-analysis. Neuropsychology 15:199–210, 2001

Parkes CM, Weiss RS: Recovery From Bereavement. New York, Basic Books, 1983

Perino C, Rago R, Cicolini A, et al: Mood and behavioural disorders following traumatic brain injury: clinical evaluation and pharmacological management. Brain Inj 15:139–148, 2001

Pinkston JB, Gouvier WD, Santa Maria MP: Mild head injury: differentiation of long-term differences on testing. Brain Cogn 44:74–78, 2000

Plenger PM, Dixon CE, Castillo RM, et al: Subacute methylphenidate treatment for moderate to moderately severe traumatic brain injury: a preliminary double-blind placebo-controlled study. Arch Phys Med Rehabil 77:536–540, 1996

Pope HG Jr, McElroy SL, Satlin A, et al: Head injury, bipolar disorder, and response to valproate. Compr Psychiatry 29:34–38, 1988

Povlishock JT: Pathophysiology of neural injury: therapeutic opportunities and challenges. Clin Neurosurg 46:113–126, 2000

Povlishock JT, Becker DP, Cheng CL, et al: Axonal change in minor head injury. J Neuropathol Exp Neurol 42:225–242, 1983

Prigatano GP: Personality and psychosocial consequences of brain injury, in Neuropsychological Rehabilitation After Brain Injury. Edited by Prigatano GP, Fordyce DJ, Zeiner HK, et al. Baltimore, MD, Johns Hopkins University Press, 1986, pp 29–50

Prigatano GP: Disordered mind, wounded soul: the emerging role of psychotherapy in rehabilitation after brain injury. J Head Trauma Rehabil 6:1–10, 1991

Prigatano GP: Behavioral limitations TBI patients tend to underestimate: a replication and extension to patients with lateralized cerebral dysfunction. Clin Neuropsychol 10:191–201, 1996

Prigatano GP: Principles of Neuropsychological Rehabilitation. New York, Oxford University Press, 1999

Prigatano GP, Altman IM: Impaired awareness of behavioral limitations after traumatic brain injury. Arch Phys Med Rehabil 71:1058–1064, 1990

Prigatano GP, Ben-Yishay Y: Psychotherapy and psychotherapeutic interventions in brain injury rehabilitation, in Rehabilitation of the Adult and Child With Traumatic Brain Injury. Edited by Rosenthal M, Griffith ER, Kreutzer JS, et al. Philadelphia, PA, FA Davis, 1999, pp 271–283

Prigatano GP, Fordyce DJ: Cognitive dysfunction and psychosocial adjustment after brain injury, in Neuropsychological Rehabilitation after Brain Injury. Edited by Prigatano GP, Fordyce DJ, Zeiner HK, et al. Baltimore, MD, Johns Hopkins University Press, 1986, pp 1–17

Prigatano GP, Altman IM, O'Brien KP: Behavioral limitations that brain injured patients tend to underestimate. Clin Neuropsychol 4:163–176, 1990

Radanov BP, di Stefano G, Schnidrig A, et al: Role of psychosocial stress in recovery from common whiplash. Lancet 338:712–715, 1991

Radnitz CL, Hsu L, Tirch DD, et al: A comparison of posttraumatic stress disorder in veterans with and without spinal cord injury. J Abnorm Psychol 107:676–680, 1998

Rammahan KW, Rosenberg JH, Pollak CP, et al: Modafinil: efficacy for the treatment of fatigue in patients with multiple sclerosis (abstract). Neurology 54 (suppl 3):24, 2000

Ranseen JD, Bohaska LA, Schmidt FA: An investigation of anosognosia following traumatic head injury. Int J Clin Neuropsychol 12:29–36, 1990

Rao V, Lyketsos C: Neuropsychiatric sequelae of traumatic brain injury. Psychosomatics 41:95–103, 2000

Rao V, Lyketsos CG: Psychiatric aspects of traumatic brain injury. Psychiatr Clin North Am 25:43–69, 2002

Richards JS: Psychologic adjustment to spinal cord injury during first postdischarge year. Arch Phys Med Rehabil 67:362–365, 1986

Rohe DE, Krause JS: Stability of interests after severe physical disability: an 11-year longitudinal study. J Vocat Behav 52:45–58, 1998

Rowland T, Mysiw WJ, Bogner J, et al: Trazodone for post traumatic agitation (abstract). Arch Phys Med Rehabil 73:963, 1992

Roy-Byrne P, Fann JR: Psychopharmacologic treatment for patients with neuropsychiatric disorders, in The American Psychiatric Press Textbook of Neuropsychiatry, 3rd Edition. Edited by Yudofsky SC, Hales RE. Washington, DC, American Psychiatric Press, 1997, pp 943–981

Ruff RM: Discipline-specific approach versus individual care, in The Evaluation and Treatment of Mild Traumatic Brain Injury. Edited by Varney NR, Roberts RJ. Mahwah, NJ, Lawrence Erlbaum Associates, 1999, pp 99–114

Ruff RM, Baser CA, Johnson JW, et al: Neuropsychological rehabilitation: an experimental study with head-injured patients. J Head Trauma Rehabil 4:20–36, 1989

Ruff RM, Marshall LF, Klauber MR, et al: Alcohol abuse and neurological outcome of the severely head injured. J Head Trauma Rehabil 5:21–31, 1990

Rutherford WH, Merrett JD, McDonald JR: Symptoms at one year following concussion from minor head injuries. Injury 10:225–230, 1979

Sachdev P, Smith JS, Cathcart S: Schizophrenia-like psychosis following traumatic brain injury: a chart-based descriptive and case-control study. Psychol Med 31:231–239, 2001

Sandel ME, Mysiw WJ: The agitated brain injured patient, part 1: definitions, differential diagnosis, and assessment. Arch Phys Med Rehabil 77:617–623, 1996

Sander AM, Kreutzer JS, Fernandez CC: Neurobehavioral functioning, substance abuse, and employment after brain injury: implications for vocational rehabilitation. J Head Trauma Rehabil 12:28–41, 1997

Santa Maria MP, Pinkston JB, Miller SR, et al: Stability of postconcussion symptomatology differs between high and low responders and by gender but not by mild head injury status. Arch Clin Neuropsychol 16:133–140, 2001

Saran AS: Depression after minor closed head injury: role of dexamethasone suppression test and antidepressants. J Clin Psychiatry 46:335–338, 1985

Sbordone RJ, Liter JC: Mild traumatic brain injury does not produce post-traumatic stress disorder. Brain Inj 9:405–412, 1995

Schiff HB, Sabin TD, Geller A, et al: Lithium in aggressive behavior. Am J Psychiatry 139:1346–1348, 1982

Schoenborn CA, Adams PF, Schiller JS: Summary health statistics for the U.S. population: National Health Interview Survey, 2000. National Center for Health Statistics. Vital Health Stat 10:214, 2003

Schreiber S, Backer MM, Pick CG: The antinociceptive effect of venlafaxine in mice is mediated through opioid and adrenergic mechanisms. Neurosci Lett 273:85–88, 1999

Schulz R, Decker S: Long-term adjustment to physical disability: the role of social support, perceived control, and self-blame. J Pers Soc Psychol 48:1162–1172, 1985

Seel RT, Kreutzer JS, Sander AM: Concordance of patients' and family members' ratings of neurobehavioral functioning after traumatic brain injury. Arch Phys Med Rehabil 78:1254–1259, 1997

Seel RT, Kreutzer JS, Rosenthal M, et al: Depression after traumatic brain injury: a National Institute on Disability and Rehabilitation Research Model Systems multicenter investigation. Arch Phys Med Rehabil 84:177–184, 2003

Shavelle RM, Strauss D, Whyte J, et al: Long-term causes of death after traumatic brain injury. Am J Phys Med Rehabil 80:510–516, 2001

Shear MK, Frank E, Foa E, et al: Traumatic grief treatment: a pilot study. Am J Psychiatry 158:1506–1508, 2001

Sherer M, Bergloff P, Boake C, et al: The Awareness Questionnaire: factor structure and internal consistency. Brain Inj 12:63–68, 1998a

Sherer M, Boake C, Levin E, et al: Characteristics of impaired awareness after traumatic brain injury. J Int Neuropsychol Soc 4:380–387, 1998b

Sherer M, Bergloff P, Levin E, et al: Impaired awareness and employment outcome after traumatic brain injury. J Head Trauma Rehabil 13:52–61, 1998c

Sherer M, Hart T, Nick TG, et al: Early impaired self-awareness after traumatic brain injury. Arch Phys Med Rehabil 84:168–176, 2003a

Sherer M, Nakase Thompson R, Nick T, et al: Patterns of neurobehavioral deficits in TBI patients at rehabilitation admission (abstract). J Int Neuropsychol Soc 9:251–252, 2003b

Shorvon SD: Safety of topiramate: adverse events and relationships to dosing. Epilepsia 37 (suppl 2):18–22, 1996

Shukla S, Cook BL, Mukherjee S, et al: Mania following head trauma. Am J Psychiatry 144:93–96, 1987

Silver JM, Yudofsky SC: Aggressive disorders, in Neuropsychiatry of Traumatic Brain Injury. Edited by Silver JM, Yudofsky SC, Hales RE. Washington, DC, American Psychiatric Press, 1994a, pp 313–353

Silver JM, Yudofsky SC: Psychopharmacology, in Neuropsychiatry of Traumatic Brain Injury. Edited by Silver JM, Yudofsky SC, Hales RE. Washington, DC, American Psychiatric Press, 1994b, pp 631–670

Silver JM, Hales RE, Yudofsky SC: Neuropsychiatric aspects of traumatic brain injury, in The American Psychiatric Publishing Textbook of Neuropsychiatry and Clinical Neurosciences, 4th Edition. Edited by Yudofsky SC, Hales RE. Washington, DC, American Psychiatric Publishing, 2002, pp 625–672

Sipski M, Alexander C: Sexual function in people with disabilities and chronic illness. Gaithersburg, MD, Aspen Publishers, 1997

Sipski ML, Alexander CJ, Rosen RC: Orgasm in women with spinal cord injuries: a laboratory-based assessment. Arch Phys Med Rehabil 76:1097–1102, 1995

Sloan RL, Brown KW, Pentland B: Fluoxetine as a treatment for emotional lability after brain injury. Brain Inj 6:315–319, 1992

Speech TJ, Rao SM, Osmon DC, et al: A double-blind controlled study of methylphenidate treatment in closed head injury. Brain Inj 7:333–338, 1993

Spitzer RL, Kroenke K, Williams JB: Validation and utility of a self-report version of PRIME-MD: the PHQ primary care study. Primary Care Evaluation of Mental Disorders. Patient Health Questionnaire. JAMA 282:1737–1744, 1999

Staas W, Formal C, Freedman M, et al: Spinal cord injury and spinal cord injury medicine, in Rehabilitation Medicine: Principles and Practice. Edited by DeLisa J, Gans BM. Philadelphia, PA, Lippincott-Raven Publishers, 1998, pp 1259–1291

Stanislav SW, Childs A: Evaluating the usage of droperidol in acutely agitated persons with brain injury. Brain Inj 14:261–265, 2000

Stanislav SW, Fabre T, Crismon ML, et al: Buspirone's efficacy in organic-induced aggression. J Clin Psychopharmacol 14:126–130, 1994

Stewart JT, Nemsath RH: Bipolar illness following traumatic brain injury: treatment with lithium and carbamazepine. J Clin Psychiatry 49:74–75, 1988

Stewart T, Shields CR: Grief in chronic illness: assessment and management. Arch Phys Med Rehabil 66:447–450, 1985

Stolp-Smith K, Wainberg K: Antidepressant exacerbation of spasticity. Arch Phys Med Rehabil 80:339–342, 1999

Street JS, Clark WS, Gannon KS, et al: Olanzapine treatment of psychotic and behavioral symptoms in patients with Alzheimer disease in nursing care facilities: a double-blind, randomized, placebo-controlled trial. The HGEU Study Group. Arch Gen Psychiatry 57:968–976, 2000

Stroebe MS, Hansson RO, Stroebe W, et al: Handbook of Bereavement Research. Washington, DC, American Psychological Association, 2001

Stuss DT, Binns MA, Carruth FG, et al: The acute period of recovery from traumatic brain injury: posttraumatic amnesia or posttraumatic confusional state? J Neurosurg 90:635–643, 1999

Suhr JA, Gunstad J: Postconcussive symptom report: the relative influence of head injury and depression. J Clin Exp Neuropsychol 24:981–993, 2002

Tate DG, Stiers W, Daugherty J, et al: The effects of insurance benefits coverage on functional and psychosocial outcomes after spinal cord injury. Arch Phys Med Rehabil 75:407–414, 1994

Tatum WO, French JA, Faught E, et al: Postmarketing experience with topiramate and cognition. Epilepsia 42:1134–1140, 2001

Taverni JP, Seliger G, Lichtman SW: Donepezil mediated memory improvement in traumatic brain injury during post acute rehabilitation. Brain Inj 12:77–80, 1998

Taylor LA, Kreutzer JS, Demm SR, et al: Traumatic brain injury and substance abuse: a review and analysis of the literature. Neuropsychological Rehabilitation 13:165–188, 2003

Teitelman E: Off-label uses of modafinil (letter). Am J Psychiatry 158:8, 2001

Tennant FS, Wild J: Naltrexone treatment for postconcussional syndrome. Am J Psychiatry 144:813–814, 1987

Terzoudi M, Gavrielidou P, Heilakos G, et al: Fatigue in multiple sclerosis: evaluation of a new pharmacological approach (abstract). Neurology 54 (suppl 3):A61–A62, 2000

Thompson RN, Sherer M, Yablon SA, et al: Confusion following TBI: inspection of indices of delirium and amnesia. J Int Neuropsychol Soc 7:177, 2001

Thomsen IV: Late outcome of very severe blunt head trauma: a 10–15 year second follow-up. J Neurol Neurosurg Psychiatry 47:260–268, 1984

Thurman D: The epidemiology and economics of head trauma, in Head Trauma: Basic, Preclinical, and Clinical Directions. Edited by Miller L, Hayes R. New York, Wiley, 2001, pp 327–348

Thurman DJ, Alverson C, Dunn KA, et al: Traumatic brain injury in the United States: a public health perspective. J Head Trauma Rehabil 14:602–615, 1999

Trahan DE, Ross CE, Trahan SL: Relationships among postconcussional-type symptoms, depression, and anxiety in neurologically normal young adults and victims of mild brain injury. Arch Clin Neuropsychol 16:435–445, 2001

Trieschmann RB: Spinal Cord Injuries: Psychological, Social and Vocational Rehabilitation. New York, Demos Publication, 1988

Trzepacz PT: Delirium, in Neuropsychiatry of Traumatic Brain Injury. Edited by Silver JM, Yudofsky SC, Hales RE. Washington, DC, American Psychiatric Press, 1994, pp 189–218

Trzepacz PT, Kennedy RE: Delirium and posttraumatic amnesia, in Textbook of Traumatic Brain Injury. Edited by Silver JM, McAllister TW, Yudofsky SC. Washington, DC, American Psychiatric Publishing, 2005, pp 175–200

Trzepacz PT, Baker RW, Greenhouse J: A symptom rating scale for delirium. Psychiatry Res 23:89–97, 1988

Tuohimaa P: Vestibular disturbances after acute mild head injury. Acta Otolaryngol Suppl 359:3–67, 1978

Turner AP, Bombardier CH, Rimmele CT: A typology of alcohol use patterns among persons with recent traumatic brain injury or spinal cord injury: implications for treatment matching. Arch Phys Med Rehabil 84:358–364, 2003

Umlauf R, Frank RG: A cluster-analytic description of patient subgroups in the rehabilitation setting. Rehabil Psychol 28:157–167, 1983

Uomoto J, Brockway J: Anger management training for brain injured patients and their family members. Arch Phys Med Rehabil 73:674–679, 1992

U.S. Department of Health and Human Services: Healthy People 2010: Understanding and Improving Health. Washington, DC, U.S. Department of Health and Human Services, 2001

Van der Naalt J, Van Zomeren AH, Sluiter WJ, et al: Acute behavioral disturbances related to imaging studies and outcome in mild-to-moderate head injury. Brain Inj 14:781–788, 1999

Van Reekum R, Cohen T, Wong J: Can traumatic brain injury cause psychiatric disorders? J Neuropsychiatry Clin Neurosci 12:316–327, 2000

Van Reekum R, Streiner DL, Conn DK: Applying Bradford Hill's criteria for causation to neuropsychiatry: challenges and opportunities. J Neuropsychiatry Clin Neurosci 13:318–325, 2001

van Workeom TC, Teelken AW, Minderhous JM: Difference in neurotransmitter metabolism in frontotemporal-lobe contusion and diffuse cerebral contusion. Lancet 1:812–813, 1977

Vargo JW: Some psychological effects of physical disability. Am J Occup Ther 32:31–34, 1978

Varney NR, Martzke JS, Roberts RJ: Major depression in patients with closed head injuries. Neuropsychology 1:7–9, 1987

Violon A, DeMol J: Psychological sequelae after head trauma in adults. Acta Neurochir (Wien) 85:96–102, 1987

Walker DE, Blankenship V, Ditty JA, et al: Prediction of recovery for closed-head-injured adults: an evaluation of the MMPI, the Adaptive Behavior Scale, and a "Quality of Life" Rating Scale. J Clin Psychol 43:699–707, 1987

Warden DL, Labbate LA, Salazar AM, et al: Posttraumatic stress disorder in patients with traumatic brain injury and amnesia for the event? J Neuropsychiatry Clin Neurosci 9:18–22, 1997

Webster G, Daisley A, King N: Relationship and family breakdown following acquired brain injury: the role of the rehabilitation team. Brain Inj 13:593–603, 1999

Westgren N, Levi R: Quality of life and traumatic spinal cord injury. Arch Phys Med Rehabil 79:1433–1439, 1998

Whelan FJ, Walker MS, Schultz SK: Donepezil in the treatment of cognitive dysfunction associated with traumatic brain injury. Ann Clin Psychiatry 12:131–135, 2000

Whitlock JA Jr: Brain injury, cognitive impairment and donepezil. J Head Trauma Rehabil 14:424–427, 1999

Whyte J, Hart T, Schuster K, et al: Effects of methylphenidate on attentional function after traumatic brain injury: a randomized placebo-controlled trial. Am J Phys Med Rehabil 76:440–450, 1997

Wilcox JH, Nasrallah HA: Childhood head trauma and psychosis. Psychiatry Res 21:303–306, 1987

Williams DH, Levin HS, Eisenberg HM: Mild head injury classification. Neurosurgery 27:422–428, 1990

Wilson JT, Teasdale GM, Hadley DM, et al: Posttraumatic amnesia: still a valuable yardstick. J Neurol Neurosurg Psychiatry 57:198–201, 1994

Witol AD, Sander AM, Seel RT, et al: Long-term neurobehavioral characteristics after brain injury: implications for vocational rehabilitation. J Voc Rehabil 7:159–167, 1996

World Health Organization: International Classification of Impairments, Disabilities and Handicaps: ICIDH. Geneva, Switzerland, World Health Organization, 1980

World Health Organization: International Statistical Classification of Diseases and Related Health Problems, 10th Revision. Geneva, Switzerland, World Health Organization, 1992

World Health Organization: International Classification of Functioning, Disability and Health: ICF. Geneva, Switzerland, World Health Organization, 2001

Wortman CB, Silver RC: The myths of coping with loss. J Consult Clin Psychol 57:349–357, 1989

Wroblewski BA, McColgan K, Smith K, et al: The incidence of seizures during tricyclic antidepressant drug treatment in a brain-injured population. J Clin Psychopharmacol 10:124–128, 1990

Wroblewski B, Glenn MB, Cornblatt R, et al: Protriptyline as an alternative stimulant medication in patients with brain injury: a series of case reports. Brain Inj 7:353–362, 1993

Wroblewski BA, Joseph AB, Cornblatt RR: Antidepressant pharmacotherapy and the treatment of depression in patients with severe traumatic brain injury: a controlled, prospective study. J Clin Psychiatry 57:582–587, 1996

Wroblewski BA, Joseph AB, Kupfer J, et al: Effectiveness of valproic acid on destructive and aggressive behaviors in patients with acquired brain injury. Brain Inj 11:37–47, 1997

Yoshino A, Hovda DA, Kawamata T, et al: Dynamic changes in local cerebral glucose utilization following cerebral concussion in rats: evidence of hyper- and subsequent hypometabolic state. Brain Res 561:106–119, 1991

Yudofsky SC, Silver JM, Jackson W, et al: The Overt Aggression Scale for the objective rating of verbal and physical aggression. Am J Psychiatry 143:35–39, 1986

Yudofsky SC, Silver JM, Schneider SE: Pharmacologic treatment of aggression. Psychiatr Ann 17:397–407, 1987

Yudofsky SC, Silver JM, Hales RE: Pharmacologic management of aggression in the elderly. J Clin Psychiatry 51:22–28, 1990

Yudofsky SC, Kopecky HJ, Kunik M, et al: The Overt Agitation Severity Scale for the objective rating of agitation. J Neuropsychiatry Clin Neurosci 9:541–548, 1997

Zafonte RD, Lexell J, Cullen N: Possible applications for dopaminergic agents following traumatic brain injury: part 2. J Head Trauma Rehabil 16:112–116, 2001

Zifko UA, Rupp M, Schwarz S, et al: Modafinil in treatment of fatigue in multiple sclerosis: results of an open-label study. J Neurol 249:983–987, 2002.

Zilbergeld B: Male Sexuality. New York, Bantam Books, 1978

36 Pain

Michael R. Clark, M.D., M.P.H.

Maciej P. Chodynicki, M.D.

IN THIS CHAPTER, we first review definitions, assessment, and epidemiology of pain. We then discuss selected specific acute and chronic pain syndromes, followed by the major psychiatric comorbidities of chronic pain, including somatization, substance use, depression, anxiety, and other emotional states. The chapter closes with a review of treatments, including medications, psychological therapies, and multidisciplinary programs. Some pain topics are covered elsewhere in this book, including arthritis (see Chapter 25, "Rheumatology"), fibromyalgia (see Chapter 26, "Chronic Fatigue and Fibromyalgia Syndromes"), postoperative pain (see Chapter 30, "Surgery"), headache (see Chapter 32, "Neurology and Neurosurgery"), pelvic pain and vulvodynia (see Chapter 33, "Obstetrics and Gynecology"), spinal cord injury (see Chapter 35, "Physical Medicine and Rehabilitation"), and palliative care (see Chapter 40, "Palliative Care").

Definition and Assessment

Pain has been defined by the International Association for the Study of Pain (IASP) as "an unpleasant sensory and emotional experience associated with actual or potential tissue damage, or described in terms of such damage" (Merskey et al. 1986, p. S217). Other terms relevant to pain are defined in Table 36–1. Pain is the most common reason a patient presents to a physician for evaluation (Kroenke 2003; Kroenke and Mangelsdorff 1989; Kroenke et al. 1990). If the patient suffers from chronic pain, defined as "pain without apparent biological value that has persisted beyond the normal tissue healing time (usually 3 months)," many specialists may be required in the successful care of the patient (Bonica 1990, p. 19). Most diseases associated with chronic pain, including

cancer, peripheral vascular disease, neuropathy, temporal arteritis, arthritis, and postherpetic neuralgia, are disproportionately represented in the elderly (Foley 1994; Gordon 1979). However, chronic pain and its consequences are now recognized complications of many illnesses, such as spinal cord injury, amputations, cerebral palsy, multiple sclerosis, HIV, Parkinson's disease, stroke, and neuromuscular diseases (Ehde et al. 2003).

Pain is a complex experience that varies demographically; is influenced by affective, cognitive, and behavioral factors; and has an extensive neurobiology (Meldrum 2003; Turk et al. 1983). Women are more sensitive to noxious stimuli and have higher risk for developing chronic pain (Fillingim 2000). African Americans with chronic pain report significantly higher levels of pain unpleasantness, avoidance, fearful thinking, and somatic complaints, that are not explained by their initially higher ratings of pain severity (McCracken et al. 2001; Riley et al. 2002). Elderly patients are often less likely to report pain or take opioids and other analgesics because of fears of addiction, tolerance that would limit pain relief in the future instance of disease progression, side effects, and a belief that pain is an indicator of disease that may distract the doctor from primary and possibly curative treatment (Ferrell 2004).

Pain is difficult to assess, especially in patients with terminal illness or cognitive impairment (Nikolaus 1997; Parmelee 1996). Patients' compliance with pain diaries is often poor, with only 11% actually following instructions, despite 90% of patients reporting compliance in one recent study (Stone et al. 2002). Pain rating scales attempt to measure the severity of pain. Many factors can influence these ratings, including contextual circumstances, disease states, mental disorders, distress, personality traits, memory of past experiences, and meaningful inter-

TABLE 36–1. Definitions relating to pain sensations

Allodynia	Pain from a stimulus that does not normally provoke pain
Deafferentation pain	Pain resulting from loss of sensory input into the central nervous system
Dysesthesia	An unpleasant, abnormal sensation that can be spontaneous or evoked
Hyperalgesia	An increased response to a stimulus that is normally painful
Hyperesthesia	Increased sensitivity to stimulation that excludes the special senses
Hyperpathia	Pain characterized by an increased reaction to a stimulus, especially a repetitive stimulus, and an increased threshold
Hypoesthesia	Diminished sensitivity to stimulation that excludes the special senses
Nociception	Detection of tissue damage by transducers in skin and deeper structures and the central propagation of this information via A delta and C fibers in the peripheral nerves
Paresthesia	An abnormal sensation, spontaneous or evoked, that is not unpleasant
Sensitization	Lowered threshold and prolonged/enhanced response to stimulation

Source. Adapted from Merskey et al. 1986.

pretations based on personal beliefs. Generally, there are poor correlations among pain reporting, tissue pathology, disability, and treatment response (Turk 1999). Drawings by patients of their pain distributions considered "nonorganic" were associated with significantly lower scores of psychological health (Dahl et al. 2001). Scores on simple numerical rating scales reflect the affective or emotional aspects of pain much more than the sensory intensity (Clark et al. 2002).

Even the simplest self-report measures used to record the presence of pain, such as a numeric rating scale or pain thermometer, cannot be effectively used by many individuals (Ferrell et al. 1995). Some patients have deficits in abstraction ability that make it difficult for them to rate pain using a visual analog scale (VAS) or a verbal descriptor scale (VDS). In a comparison study, the VDS was rated as the preferred, easiest, and best assessment tool for rating pain by the elderly (Herr and Mobily 1993). However, the ratings of pain intensity using these scales were poorly correlated with one another. The magnitude of a meaningful decrease on pain rating scales is difficult to define. Outcomes judged as clinically significant and referenced to a 7-point self-report global impression of change scale were associated with an approximately 30%

drop on a numerical rating (0–10) of pain intensity (Farrar et al. 2001). Alternative tools for evaluating pain, such as observations of pain behaviors, are limited by reliance on an outside observer to rate a patient's pain (Weiner et al. 1996, 1998).

A comprehensive evaluation should be performed for any patient who reports pain (Clark 2000a; Clark and Cox 2002). This evaluation should incorporate simple standardized tools for rating pain severity; observations of pain-related behaviors, including any problems with activities of daily living that would indicate the presence of pain; and a clinical examination to elicit evidence of pain and the signs of possible etiologies.

Epidemiology

The prevalence of chronic pain reported in the general population ranges from 10% to 55%, with an estimate of severe chronic pain of approximately 11% among adults (noting the lack of standard definitions for "chronic" or "severe") (Karlsten and Gordh 1997; Nickel and Raspe 2001; Ospina and Harstall 2002; Verhaak et al. 1998). In the most recent World Health Organization (WHO) review from multiple countries, the weighted mean prevalence of chronic pain was 31% in men, 40% in women, 25% in children up to age 18 years, and 50% in the elderly older than 65 years (Ospina and Harstall 2002). During a 2-week period, 13% of the U.S. workforce reported a loss in productivity due to a common pain condition such as headache, back pain, arthritis pain, or other musculoskeletal pain (Stewart et al. 2003).

An 8-year follow-up survey by the U.S. Center for Health Statistics found that 32.8% of the general population experienced chronic pain symptoms (Magni et al. 1993). In another WHO study of more than 25,000 primary care patients in 14 countries, 22% (17% in the United States) of patients suffered from pain that had been present for most of the time for at least 6 months (Gureje et al. 1998). In a study of 6,500 individuals aged 15–74 years in Finland, 14% experienced daily chronic pain that was independently associated with lower (odds ratio [OR]=11.8 for "poor") self-rated health (Mantyselka et al. 2003). A retrospective analysis of 14,000 primary care patients in Sweden reported that approximately 30% of patients seeking treatment had some kind of defined pain problem, with almost two-thirds diagnosed with musculoskeletal pain (Hasselstrom et al. 2002).

In a 24-year longitudinal study of chest, abdomen, and musculoskeletal pain, symptoms increased with age, and women reported more persistent and severe pain (Brattberg et al. 1997). In people 65 years or older, musculoskeletal pain is associated with three times the likelihood of significant difficulty performing three or more physical activities (Scudds and McD Robertson 1998). In persons older than 75 years, over two-thirds reported pain, almost half reported pain in multiple sites, and one-third rated pain as severe in at least one location (Brattberg et al. 1996).

Acute Pain

The Joint Commission on Accreditation of Healthcare Organizations has implemented pain management standards for all patient encounters (Phillips 2000). In the Veterans Affairs medical centers, pain intensity has been defined and tracked as the "5th vital sign." Acute pain is usually the result of trauma from a surgery, injury, or exacerbation of chronic disease, especially musculoskeletal conditions. Acute pain management will usually be successful with straightforward strategies such as relaxation, immobilization, analgesics (aspirin, acetaminophen, nonsteroidal anti-inflammatory drugs [NSAIDs], opioids), massage, and transcutaneous electrical nerve stimulation (TENS) (Acute Pain Management Guideline Panel 1992). Older adults are more likely to undergo surgery for degenerative problems, fractures, and cardiovascular disease (Ferrell 1996). The normal physiology of aging and the presence of chronic diseases must be taken into consideration when using pharmacotherapy for pain so as to avoid delirium, side effects, and toxicity.

In acute pain management, psychiatric consultation is requested when a patient requires more analgesia than expected or has a history of substance abuse. Patients with acute pain most frequently seek analgesic medications to alleviate pain. The absence of signs consistent with acute pain, such as elevated heart rate, blood pressure, and diaphoresis, does not rule out the presence of pain.

Acute pain management should be initiated as early as possible. If the management is focused on preventing occurrence and reemergence of pain, it may allow for lower total doses of analgesics. Analgesics, especially opioids, should be prescribed only for pain relief. Although analgesia may produce other benefits, other symptoms commonly coinciding with acute pain, such as insomnia and anxiety, should be managed separately from pain. Sleep deprivation and anxiety may intensify the sensation of pain and increase requests for more medication. Reducing anxiety and insomnia often reduces analgesic requirements.

Patients with active or recent history of opioid addiction, and those receiving methadone maintenance therapy, have increased tolerance to opioids and may require up to 50% higher doses of opioid analgesics than other

patients. Although it is important to carefully monitor opioid use in these patients, adequate treatment of acute pain is a priority. Inadequate dosing is significantly more common than abuse or diversion in these patients. Dosage should be carefully individualized, rather than based on preconceived expectations.

Selected Chronic Pain Conditions

Postherpetic Neuralgia

Postherpetic neuralgia is defined as pain persisting or recurring at the site of shingles at least 3 months after the onset of the acute varicella zoster viral rash (Bowsher 1997b). Postherpetic neuralgia occurs in about 10% of patients with acute herpes zoster. More than half of patients over 65 years of age with shingles develop postherpetic neuralgia, and it is more likely to occur in patients with cancer, diabetes mellitus, and immunosuppression. Other risk factors include greater acute pain and rash severity, sensory impairment, and psychological distress (Schmader 2002). Most cases gradually improve over time, with only about 25% of patients with postherpetic neuralgia experiencing pain at 1 year after diagnosis. Approximately 15% of referrals to pain clinics are for the treatment of postherpetic neuralgia.

Although degeneration and destruction of motor and sensory fibers of the mixed dorsal root ganglion characterize acute varicella zoster, other neurological damage may include inflammation of the spinal cord, myelin disruption, axonal damage, and decreases in the number of nerve endings from the affected skin. These injuries persist in postherpetic neuralgia patients, but the actual mechanism of pain is not well understood. Studies have suggested the role of both peripheral and central mechanisms resulting from the loss of large-caliber neurons and subsequent central sensitization or adrenergic receptor activation and alterations in C-fiber activity (Fields et al. 1998). Early treatment of varicella zoster with low-dose amitriptyline reduced the prevalence of pain at 6 months by 50% (Bowsher 1996, 1997a; Johnson 1997). Tricyclic antidepressants (TCAs), anticonvulsants, and opioids are the most common effective treatments for postherpetic neuralgia and may have potential for its prevention (Dworkin and Schmader 2003; Johnson and Dworkin 2003).

Peripheral Neuropathy Pain

Sensory neurons are damaged by many diseases, both directly and indirectly (Scadding 1994). Approximately 25% of patients with diabetes mellitus will experience painful diabetic neuropathy, with duration of illness and poor glycemic control contributing risk factors. If C-fiber input is preserved but large-fiber input is lost, paresthesias and pain are the predominant sensory experiences. The pain of a peripheral neuropathy can range from a constant burning to pain that is episodic, paroxysmal, and lancinating in quality (Mendell and Sahenk 2003). These phenomena are primarily the result of axonal degeneration and segmental demyelination. Sites of ectopic impulse generation can be found at any point along the peripheral nerve, including the dorsal root ganglion, regardless of where the nerve is actually damaged. Other changes can alter the magnitude and frequency of impulse generation, such as sensitivity to mechanical or neurochemical stimuli.

The paroxysms of pain that result from stimulation of hyperexcitable damaged neurons and subsequent recruitment of nearby undamaged sensory afferents may be explained by several forms of nonsynaptic (ephaptic) and prolonged (afterdischarge) impulse transmission described in models of peripheral neuropathic pain. Voltage-dependent sodium channels in the dorsal root ganglion undergo both up- and downregulation depending on the subpopulation (Rizzo 1997). When a peripheral nerve is damaged, central sensitization amplifies and sustains neuronal activity by a variety of mechanisms, such as reduced inhibition of dorsal horn cells.

Pharmacological treatments have been almost identical to those used for postherpetic neuralgia, but the new norepinephrine-serotonin reuptake inhibitor duloxetine has been the first agent to be approved by the U.S. Food and Drug Administration (FDA) for treatment of diabetic peripheral neuropathy pain.

Parkinson's Disease

Pain is the most common sensory manifestation of Parkinson's disease and reported by half of patients (Goetz et al. 1986; Koller 1984; Starkstein et al. 1991). The pain is typically described as cramping and aching, located in the lower back and extremities, but not associated with muscle contraction or spasm. These pains often decrease when the patient is treated with levodopa, which suggests a central origin. The loss of dopaminergic input could explain how pain is produced, perhaps through a loss of descending inhibition in the spinal cord (Burkey et al. 1996).

Central Poststroke Pain

Approximately 5% of patients who have suffered a stroke experience intractable pain in addition to other neurological deficits (Bowsher 1995). Patients typically have hemibody sensory deficits and pain associated with dysesthesias, allodynia, and hyperalgesia. Radiographic lesions are present in the thalamus, although other sites are often in-

volved. Excitatory amino acids may be involved in the development of this syndrome. Pharmacological treatment is usually not effective, and even ketamine, an N-methyl-D-aspartate (NMDA) receptor antagonist, reduced pain in less than 50% of patients (Yamamoto et al. 1997). Fluvoxamine significantly improved pain ratings but only in patients within 1 year after stroke (Shimodozono et al. 2002). In contrast, patients with spinal cord injury experienced reductions in continuous and evoked pain with ketamine and mu opioid receptor agonists, suggesting different mechanisms in different central pain states (Eide et al. 1995).

Migraine and Chronic Daily Headache

The International Headache Society has published guidelines for the classification of headache (Olesen 1988) (see also Chapter 32, "Neurology and Neurosurgery"). The peak incidence of migraine occurs between the third and sixth decades of life and then decreases with age. Over the life span, 18% of women and 6% of men will suffer from migraine (Lipton et al. 1997). Theories of pathogenesis include the involvement of the trigeminovascular system and plasma protein extravasation, antagonism of serotonin receptors, modulation of central aminergic control mechanisms, stabilizing effects on membranes through action at voltage-sensitive calcium channels, and involvement of substance P (Goadsby 1997; Solomon 1995). Common migraine is defined as a unilateral pulsatile headache, which may be associated with other symptoms such as nausea, vomiting, photophobia, and phonophobia (Szirmai 1997). The classic form of migraine adds visual prodromal symptoms such as scintillating scotomata. Complicated migraine includes focal neurological signs such as cranial nerve palsies and is often described by the name of the primary deficit (e.g., hemiplegic, vestibular, or basilar migraine).

Calcium channel blockers, beta-blockers, antidepressants, and anticonvulsants are the treatments with best-documented efficacy (Mathew 2001). A group-based multidisciplinary treatment consisting of stress management, supervised exercise, dietary education, and massage therapy significantly improved pain characteristics, functional status, quality of life, depression, and pain-related disability in patients with migraine (Lemstra et al. 2002).

Headache is the most common pain condition reported by the U.S. workforce as the reason for lost productive time (Stewart et al. 2003). Chronic daily headache affects about 5% of the population and is composed of constant (transformed) migraine, chronic tension-type headaches, new-onset daily persistent headache, and hemicrania continua (Lake and Saper 2002). Patients with chronic daily headache are more likely to overuse medication, leading to rebound headache; have psychiatric comorbidity such as depression and anxiety; report functional disability; and experience stress-related headache exacerbations (Lake 2001). Patients with transformed migraine have poor quality of life, having been found to have the worst SF-36 Health Survey profile compared with patients with episodic migraine or chronic tension-type headaches (Wang et al. 2001). Chronic tension-type headaches typically manifest as daily pain that is difficult to manage and unresponsive to many treatments.

A variety of medications have been recommended in addition to the traditional prophylactic agents and include serotonin agonists, serotonin antagonists, and alpha$_2$-adrenergic agonists. Olanzapine decreased headache severity and frequency in patients with refractory headaches who had undergone unsuccessful treatment with at least four preventive medications (Silberstein et al. 2002). Topiramate decreased migraine frequency, severity, number of headache days, and use of abortive medications in patients with both episodic and transformed migraine (Mathew et al. 2002). TCAs and stress management therapy significantly reduced headache activity, analgesic medication use, and headache-related disability (Holroyd et al. 2001). Combined medication and cognitive-behavioral psychotherapy are more effective than either treatment alone (Lake 2001; Lipchik and Nash 2002).

Low Back Pain

Low back pain (LBP) is one of the most common physical symptoms, and the most expensive condition when including lost productivity and health care costs (Stewart et al. 2003). Psychological factors are highly correlated with LBP; these factors include distress, depressed mood, and somatization, which predict the transition from acute to chronic LBP (Linton 2000; Pincus et al. 2002). A minority of patients with acute LBP will develop chronic LBP with disproportionate distress and disability. In one prospective cohort study of 1,246 patients with acute LBP who sought treatment, about 8% had chronic, continuous symptoms for 3 months, and less than 5% had unremitting pain for 22 months (T.S. Carey et al. 2000). Two-thirds of patients with chronic LBP at 3 months exhibited functional disability at 22 months. The most powerful predictor of chronicity was poor functional status 4 weeks after seeking treatment. In a study of secondary gain, both economic and social rewards were associated with higher levels of disability and depression in patients with chronic nonmalignant back pain (Ciccone et al. 1999). Depression has been identified as a presurgical risk factor associated with poor outcome in long-term follow-up of compen-

sated workers who underwent posterolateral lumbar fusion (DeBerard et al. 2001). Specifically, anxiety, depression, and occupational mental stress predicted lower rates of return to work in patients undergoing lumbar surgeries (Schade et al. 1999; Trief et al. 2000). Despite an extensive array of pain scales and functional instruments available to evaluate outcome, patient global assessment has been found a valid and responsive measure of overall treatment effect (Hagg et al. 2002).

The presence of a depressive disorder has been demonstrated to increase the risk of developing chronic musculoskeletal pain 3 years later (Leino and Magni 1993; Magni et al. 1993, 1994; Von Korff et al. 1993). In a 15-year prospective study of workers in an industrial setting, initial depression symptom scores were predictive of LBP and a positive clinical back examination in men but not women (Leino and Magni 1993). In a study of health care workers examined over 3 years with the Zung Depression Index, affective distress contributed to new-onset LBP (Adams et al. 1999). In a community-based sample, depression was associated with a nearly fourfold increase in the likelihood of seeking a consultation for the new complaint of back pain lasting greater than 3 months at follow-up (Waxman et al. 1998). In a 13-year follow-up study that examined the longitudinal relationship between LBP and depressive disorder, using lifetime reports of symptoms, and excluded other forms of affective distress such as demoralization, grief, and adjustment disorders, depressive disorder was a significant risk factor for incident LBP (Larson et al. 2004). While it is understandable that patients with LBP would experience reactive affective distress, a significant relationship between LBP and the subsequent onset of incident depressive disorder was not found. In another prospective analysis, participants who did not have current LBP were followed for 12 months (Croft et al. 1996). Patients with higher levels of distress at baseline were almost twice as likely to report a new episode of back pain. This study concluded that as much as 16% of LBP in the general population may be attributable to psychological distress.

The treatment of chronic LBP has been pursued with multiple modalities alone and in combination (Deyo and Weinstein 2001; Hildebrandt et al. 1996). Patients with chronic LBP exemplify the complexity of chronic pain treatment. Their symptoms may represent numerous diagnoses and require multimodal treatment plans. Although treatments often produce symptom reductions, there is conflicting evidence about their ability to improve functional status, particularly with respect to returning to work (Pfingsten et al. 1997; Saur et al. 1996; Staiger et al. 2003). Conservative interventions such as education, exercise, massage, and TENS produce inconsistent results (Furlan et al. 2002; Pengel et al. 2002). Studies of behavior therapies support their effectiveness in comparison with wait-list or no-treatment control conditions, but the efficacy data are less convincing for these therapies compared with usual treatment for chronic LBP (van Tulder et al. 2001). There is evidence that surgery may be effective for a carefully selected group of patients with chronic LBP (Fritzell et al. 2001). Multidisciplinary rehabilitation programs usually offer the best outcomes, but such programs are the most expensive approach, and high-quality randomized, controlled trials are still needed to document their efficacy (Huppe and Raspe 2003; Karjalainen et al. 2003; Lang et al. 2003). The patient's perception of disability is a critical factor that must be addressed for treatment to succeed.

Complex Regional Pain Syndrome (Causalgia and Reflex Sympathetic Dystrophy)

The term *complex regional pain syndrome* (CRPS)) now replaces reflex sympathetic dystrophy (CRPS type I) and causalgia (CRPS type II) (Stanton-Hicks et al. 1995). Type I involves ongoing spontaneous burning pain that is precipitated by a specific noxious trauma or cause of immobilization and is usually associated with hyperalgesia or allodynia to cutaneous stimuli. The symptoms are not limited to a single peripheral nerve, and there is often evidence of edema, blood flow abnormalities, or sudomotor dysfunction in the region of pain, usually an extremity. Motor changes such as tremor, weakness, and limitations in movement are common. If nerve injury is present, CRPS type II is appropriately diagnosed. Although the natural history varies, three clinical stages are classically described. Stage 1 (acute, early) is characterized by an inflammatory onset with constant aching or burning pain. Stage 2 (dystrophic, intermediate) is notable for cool, pale, and cyanotic skin. Stage 3 (atrophic, late) manifests as atrophy and wasting of multiple soft tissues, fixed joint contractures, and osteoporosis. When pain is relieved by blockade of the efferent sympathetic nervous system, the modifier, sympathetically maintained pain, is added (Wesselmann and Raja 1997). Patients with sympathetically maintained pain often report hyperalgesia to cold stimuli.

Patients with CRPS often exhibit emotional distress and psychological dysfunction. The reported prevalence of psychiatric disorders in patients with CRPS ranges from 18% to 64% (Bruehl and Carlson 1992). Examination using the Structured Clinical Interview for DSM-IV (SCID) demonstrated a high frequency of affective (46%), anxiety

(27%), and substance abuse disorders (14%) in patients with CRPS (Rommel et al. 2001). Some patients with CRPS may exhibit signs of conversion disorder, such as the normalization of hypoesthesia by nerve blocks. Nonanatomic and expansive areas of hypoesthesia or hyperalgesia with normal peripheral sensory nerve conduction or somatosensory evoked potentials in patients with CRPS type I are probably psychogenic in origin. Neurophysiological investigation suggests that certain positive motor signs (dystonia, tremors, spasms, irregular jerks) identified in patients with CRPS type I represent pseudoneurological illness (Verdugo and Ochoa 2000). A review of studies that used the Minnesota Multiphasic Personality Inventory (MMPI) concluded that patients with CRPS, like other patients with chronic pain, are somatically preoccupied, are depressed, and use repression as a psychological defense mechanism (Bruehl and Carlson 1992). However, there are no consistent differences in psychological characteristics or psychiatric diagnoses between CRPS and non-CRPS pain patients (Bruehl et al. 1996; Ciccone et al. 1997; DeGood et al. 1993; Fishbain 1999a; Geertzen et al. 1998; Monti et al. 1998; Nelson and Novy 1996; van der Laan et al. 1999; Zucchini et al. 1989).

Several literature reviews have examined whether psychological dysfunction was the cause or effect of CRPS (Bruehl and Carlson 1992; Haddox 1990; Lynch 1992). The majority of studies suffered flaws in methodology such as a lack of homogenous diagnostic groups, lack of control groups, and incorrect use of psychiatric or psychological terminology. Depression, anxiety, and fear of movement are common, but no unique personality traits or profile predisposes one to develop CRPS. In patients with CRPS, a recent study of daily diaries demonstrated that the prior day's depressed mood contributed to the present day's increased pain and that yesterday's pain also contributed to today's depression, anxiety, and anger (Feldman et al. 1999).

In summary, most authors have concluded that comorbid psychopathology in patients with CRPS is a consequence of the chronic pain rather than its cause. However, psychiatric conditions should be treated as primary barriers to functional rehabilitation. In addition, treatment for CRPS usually combines a variety of anesthetic blocks, typically regional sympathetic blocks, with oral sympatholytics, reactivating physical therapies, adjuvant analgesic medications, electrical stimulation, and possibly even surgical sympathectomy (Lee and Benzon 1999).

Orofacial Pain

Trigeminal neuralgia (tic douloureux) is a chronic pain syndrome with severe, paroxysmal, recurrent, lancinating pain in the distribution of cranial nerve V that is unilateral and most commonly involves the mandibular division (Elias and Burchiel 2002; Loeser 2001). Sensory or motor deficits are not usually present. Episodes of pain can be spontaneous or evoked by nonpainful stimuli to trigger zones, activities such as talking or chewing, or environmental conditions. Between episodes, patients are typically pain-free. Less common syndromes involving the intermedius branch of the facial nerve or the glossopharyngeal nerve present with pain that can involve the ear, posterior pharynx, tongue, or larynx (Zakrzewska 2002). Other related conditions include cluster headache, which occurs predominantly in men with an onset before age 25 and presents with pain that is episodic, unilaterally surrounding the eye, excruciating, lasts minutes to hours, and is associated with autonomic symptoms. Short-lasting, unilateral, neuralgiform pain with conjunctival injection and tearing (SUNCT) syndrome is a rare condition that more commonly affects older males. Tolosa-Hunt syndrome manifests as pain in the ocular area accompanied by ipsilateral paresis of oculomotor nerves and the first branch of the trigeminal nerve that is associated with compromise of ophthalmic venous circulation, and improves with steroids. The residual category of atypical facial pain is more commonly associated with psychopathology or other psychological factors that amplify the patient's pain, distress, and disability (Kapur et al. 2003).

The majority of patients with classical trigeminal neuralgia show evidence of trigeminal nerve root compression by blood vessels (85%), mass lesions, or other diseases that cause demyelination and hyperactivity of the trigeminal nucleus (multiple sclerosis, herpes zoster, postherpetic neuralgia) (Joffroy et al. 2001; Love and Coakham 2001). The ignition hypothesis postulates that afferent fibers become hyperexcitable as a result of injury and that paroxysms of pain are the manifestation of synchronized afterdischarge activity (Devor et al. 2002). Uncontrolled pain with frequent or severe prolonged attacks increases the risk of insomnia, weight loss, social withdrawal, anxiety, and depression, including suicide. Pharmacological treatment includes anticonvulsants, antidepressants, baclofen, mexiletine, lidocaine, and opioids (Cheshire 2002; Fisher et al. 2002; Sindrup and Jensen 2002). When pharmacological treatments fail, a variety of surgical procedures, such as microvascular decompression via suboccipital craniectomy, percutaneous gangliolysis, and stereotactic radiosurgery, may be undertaken.

Temporomandibular disorder (TMD) is a general term referring to complaints that involve the temporomandibular joint, muscles of mastication, and other orofacial musculoskeletal structures. Pain most commonly arises from the muscles of mastication and is precipitated by jaw function, such as opening the mouth or chewing. Associated symptoms include feelings of muscle fatigue, weakness, and tightness as well as changes in bite (malocclusion) or the ability to open/close the jaw. In contrast to the vague, diffuse pain of myalgia, temporomandibular joint dysfunction causes sharp, sudden, and intense pain with joint movement that is often localized to the preauricular area. Joint sounds such as clicking, popping, and crepitation are common. Patients may experience limitations in jaw movements, such as catching sensations or actual locking of the jaw. Joint problems are classified as relating to the condyle–disk complex, structural incompatibility of the articular surfaces, and inflammatory joint disorders.

Psychological distress is common in patients with TMD (McCreary et al. 1991). Patients with pain of muscular origin are usually more distressed and depressed, with greater levels of disability, than those with TM joint pain. These factors are responsive to treatment (Auerbach et al. 2001). Longitudinal data suggest that negative affect in patients with orofacial pain is more likely than pain to cause poor sleep quality (Riley et al. 2001). Patients with TMD classified as either "dysfunctional" or "interpersonally distressed" were at higher risk to develop chronic pain without treatment, suggesting a role for proactive prevention programs during the initial acute stages of illness or injury (Epker and Gatchel 2000). In treatment trials for patients with TMD, the dysfunctional group showed the best response to multidisciplinary treatment, with greater improvements in pain intensity, interference, catastrophizing, depression, and negative thoughts when compared with the other groups (Rudy et al. 1995; Sherman and Turk 2001). Patients with low levels of psychosocial dysfunction experienced significantly decreased pain, pain-related interference, numbers of painful muscles, and visits for TMD treatment when they received a less intensive self-care treatment program (Dworkin et al. 2002).

Burning mouth syndrome (BMS) is characterized as pain in oral and pharyngeal cavities, especially the tongue, often associated with dryness and taste alterations. Most cases are idiopathic, but BMS may coincide with a plethora of conditions such as bruxism, poorly fitting dentures, oral candidiasis, xerostomia, malnutrition, food allergies and contact dermatitis, gastroesophageal reflux disease, diabetes mellitus, hypothyroidism, neoplasia, menopause, and psychiatric conditions such as depression, anxiety, and somatoform disorders (Drage and Rogers 2003; Formaker and Frank 2000; Grushka et al. 2002). The condition mainly affects middle-aged and postmenopausal women, and the oral mucosa is usually normal. Psychological factors such as severe life events have been associated with the condition (Bergdahl and Bergdahl 1999; Bogetto et al. 1998).

Theories of etiology and pathogenesis include brain stem pathology, hyperactivity of sensory and motor components of the trigeminal nerve following loss of central inhibition that resulted from damage to the chorda tympani or glossopharyngeal nerves, disorders of the dopaminergic system, and small sensory fiber dysfunction (Forssell et al. 2002; Grushka et al. 2003; Scala et al. 2003). Potential underlying etiologies—such as depression/anxiety, nutritional deficiencies (iron, folate, B_{12}, and other B vitamins), maladaptive oral habits, and iatrogenic causes such as medications—should be identified and treated (Bogetto et al. 1998; Pinto et al. 2003). Treatment with TCAs or anticonvulsants has brought pain relief in some patients with BMS. Other treatments include benzodiazepines, topical analgesics, soft desensitizing oral appliances, serotonin reuptake inhibitors, vitamin and hormonal supplements, and habit awareness counseling (Formaker et al. 1998; Maina et al. 2002; Pinto et al. 2003; Zakrzewska et al. 2001).

Psychiatric Comorbidity

Patients' experiences of suffering, their language and behaviors, and the neurobiological conception of nociception all support a psychological component of pain (Hunt and Mantyh 2001; Price 2000). Cross-sectional studies have consistently found an association between chronic pain and psychological distress (Wilson et al. 2001). In a sample of more than 3,000 individuals, psychiatric disorder was a significant predictor of new-onset physical symptoms such as back, chest, and abdominal pain 7 years after evaluation (Hotopf et al. 1998). In a population-based case–control study, the prevalence of a mental disorder was more than three times higher in patients with chronic widespread pain than in those without such pain (Benjamin et al. 2000).

Pain Disorder and Somatization

Pain "caused" by emotional factors was first operationalized in DSM-II under psychophysiological disorders (American Psychiatric Association 1968). DSM-III introduced *psychogenic pain disorder*, in which pathophysiology was either absent or insufficient to explain the severity and duration of pain (American Psychiatric Association 1980). In DSM-III-R *somatoform pain disorder*, psychological factors were no longer required as an etiology of pain (American Psychiatric Association 1987). A preoccupation with pain, instead of the pain itself, was established as

the core criterion in conjunction with the absence of adequate physical findings. DSM-IV refined this diagnosis as *pain disorder* (American Psychiatric Association 1994; see also King and Strain 1992). The primary criteria require that pain be the chief complaint and that the pain cause significant distress or functional impairment. Psychological factors are recognized as having an important role in the pain. Unfortunately, the concept of psychological and physical dualism is still inherent in this diagnosis, undermining its validity and utility (Aronoff et al. 2000; King 2000; Sullivan 2000).

The lifetime prevalence of somatoform pain disorder (DSM-III-R) in the general population was 34% with a 6-month prevalence of 17% (Grabe et al. 2003). However, when the DSM-IV requirement of significant distress or psychosocial impairment was added to make the diagnosis, the lifetime prevalence was only 12% and the 6-month prevalence decreased to 5%, with the female:male ratio remaining 2:1. In a sample of more than 13,000 psychiatric consultations, a diagnosis of a somatoform pain disorder was made in 84% (Thomassen et al. 2003). Injured workers who developed somatoform pain disorder, compared with those injured workers who did not develop the condition, were characterized by more sites of pain, spread of pain beyond the area of the original injury, more opioid and benzodiazepine use, and greater involvement with compensation and with litigation (Streltzer et al. 2000).

Characterizing somatization as a psychophysiological process or a multidimensional construct such as somatic style rather than a categorical psychiatric diagnosis or a psychological trait is probably most appropriate (Barsky and Borus 1999; Mayou et al. 2003; Rief and Hiller 1999; Sullivan and Katon 1993). Symptoms, rather than specific diseases, are the most common reason for seeking medical care (Brown et al. 1971; Koch 1978; Kroenke 2003; Kroenke et al. 1990). Women report more severe, numerous, and frequent physical symptoms (including pain) than men (Barsky et al. 2001). Usually, a medical cause is never found for these "somatization" symptoms (Kroenke and Mangelsdorff 1989). As the number of medically unexplained symptoms increases, so does associated morbidity, such as functional disability, increased health care utilization, inappropriate treatment with medications, excessive evaluations, and higher rates of psychiatric disorders (Andersson et al. 1999; Katon et al. 1991; Kouyanou et al. 1998).

Although the actual diagnosis of somatization disorder is rare in patients with chronic pain, multiple pain complaints are present in somatization disorder by definition. Most patients with multiple unexplained symptoms have subsyndromal forms of somatization disorder, such as multisomatoform disorder, which has a prevalence in primary care of 4%–18% (Dickinson et al. 2003; Kroenke et al. 1997; Simon and Gureje 1999). Such patients are more likely to exhibit catastrophic thinking, believe the cause of their pain to be a mystery, have feelings of losing control, and think that physicians believe their pain is imaginary. Patients with chronic pain and medically unexplained symptoms also are at risk for iatrogenic consequences of excessive diagnostic tests, inappropriate medications, and unneeded surgery.

Substance Use

The prevalence of substance use disorders in patients with chronic pain is higher than in the general population (Dersh et al. 2002; Weaver and Schnoll 2002). In a study of primary care outpatients with chronic noncancer pain who received at least 6 months of opioid prescriptions during 1 year, behaviors consistent with opioid abuse were recorded in approximately 25% of patients (Reid et al. 2002). Almost 90% of patients attending a pain management clinic were taking medications and 70% were prescribed opioid analgesics (Kouyanou et al. 1997). In this population, 12% met DSM-III-R criteria for substance abuse or dependence. In another study of 414 chronic pain patients, 23% met criteria for active alcohol, opioid, or sedative misuse or dependence; 9% met criteria for a remission diagnosis; and current dependency was most common for opioid use (13%) (Hoffman et al. 1995). In reviews of substance dependence or addiction in patients with chronic pain, the prevalence ranges from 3% to 19% in high-quality studies (Fishbain et al. 1992; Nicholson 2003).

Recent efforts have attempted to standardize diagnostic criteria and definitions for problematic medication use behaviors and substance use disorders across professional disciplines (American Academy of Pain Medicine et al. 2001; Chabal et al. 1997; Greenwald et al. 1999; Savage 2003). The core criteria for a substance use disorder in patients with chronic pain include the loss of control in the use of the medication, excessive preoccupation with it despite adequate analgesia, and adverse consequences associated with its use (Compton et al. 1998). Items from the Prescription Drug Use Questionnaire that best predicted the presence of addiction in a sample of patients with problematic medication use were 1) the patient believing they were addicted, 2) increasing analgesic dose/frequency, and 3) a preferred route of administration. It must be emphasized that the presence of maladaptive behaviors must be demonstrated to diagnose addiction, because physical dependence and tolerance alone are normal physiological phenomena. In other words, dependence and tolerance are necessary but not sufficient for a diagnosis of addiction in the patient with chronic pain receiving treatment with opioids. Access to opioids may not be an issue because a physician has been prescribing them. If addiction is present, however, the patient may fear that opioid access will be limited and therefore try to conceal any problematic use of the medication.

Determining whether patients with chronic pain are abusing prescribed controlled substances is a routine but challenging issue in care (Compton et al. 1998; Miotto et al. 1996; Robinson et al. 2001; Savage 2002). In one survey of approximately 12,000 medical inpatients treated with opioids for a variety of conditions drawn from the Boston Collaborative Drug Surveillance Program, only four patients without a history of substance abuse were reported to have developed dependence on the medication (Porter and Jick 1980). While this report was based on a large sample and extensive medication database, the methods were not detailed and specifically did not describe the criteria for addiction or the extent of follow-up performed. Other studies of opioid therapy have found that patients who developed problems with their medication all had a history of substance abuse (Portenoy and Foley 1986; Taub 1982). However, inaccurate reporting and underreporting of medication use by patients complicate assessment (Fishbain et al. 1999b; Ready et al. 1982). Not infrequently, prior substance abuse history emerges only after current misuse has been identified, thus requiring physicians to be vigilant over the course of treatment. In patients with chronic pain who did develop new substance use disorders, the problem most commonly involved the medications prescribed by their physicians (Long et al. 1988; Maruta et al. 1979).

The causes and onset of substance use disorders have been difficult to characterize in relationship to chronic pain. During the first 5 years after the onset of chronic pain, patients are at increased risk for developing new substance use disorders and additional physical injuries (Brown et al. 1996; Savage 1993). This risk is highest in patients with a history of substance abuse or dependence, childhood physical or sexual abuse, and psychiatric comorbidity (Aronoff 2000; Fishbain et al. 1998; Miotto et al. 1996). In a study of chronic LBP patients, 34% had a substance use disorder, yet in 77% of cases the substance abuse was present before the onset of the chronic pain (Brown et al. 1996; Polatin et al. 1993). The mechanisms of relapse into substance abuse are not well understood and probably involve multiple factors. A cycle of pain followed by relief *after* taking medications is a classic example of operant reinforcement of *future* medication use that eventually becomes abuse (Fordyce et al. 1973). Research in patients with substance abuse has also demonstrated abnormalities in pain perception and tolerance. An increased sensitivity to pain and the reinforcing effects of relieving pain with substance use suggest a combined mechanism for the development of substance abuse in patients with chronic pain.

Careful monitoring of patients is essential to prevent this complication of the treatment of chronic pain. Increased function and opioid analgesia without side effects, not the avoidance of particular doses of opioids, are the goals of treatment (K.B. Carey et al. 2000; Hamilton 1999; Hathaway 2001; Marlatt 1996; Pappagallo and Heinberg 1997; Savage 1999). The evaluation of a patient suspected of misusing medications should be thorough and include an assessment of the pain syndrome as well as other medical disorders, patterns of medication use, social and family factors, patient and family history of substance abuse, and a psychiatric history (Miotto et al. 1996; Portenoy 1990). Reliance on medications that provide pain relief can result in a number of stereotyped patient behaviors that can either represent or be mistaken for addiction. Persistent pain can lead to increased focus on opioid medications. Patients may take extraordinary measures to ensure an adequate medication supply even in the absence of addiction. This may be manifested as requests for premature refills, higher doses, or extra quantities of medication or seeking medication from additional sources. Patients understandably fear the reemergence of pain and withdrawal symptoms if they run out of medication. Drug-seeking behavior may be the result of an anxious patient trying to maintain a previous level of pain control. In this situation, the patient's actions may represent pseudoaddiction that results from therapeutic dependence and current or potential undertreatment but not addiction (Kirsh et al. 2002; Weaver and Schnoll 2002). Since these behaviors occur in both pseudo- and true addiction, the distinction is based in part on whether the behaviors are infrequent and isolated vs. repetitive and persistent, and whether they abate with adequate opioid therapy. However, these are not distinct categories; overuse of analgesics occurs along a continuum.

In patients with higher risk of addiction, prevention should begin with a treatment contract to clarify the conditions under which opioids will be provided. The contract emphasizes a single physician being responsible for prescriptions, and explicitly describes all the conditions under which use of opioids will be considered inappropriate and may lead to discontinuation. Under optimal circumstances, opioid contracts attempt to improve compliance by distributing information and using a mutually agreed upon treatment plan that includes consequences for aberrant behaviors and incorporates the primary care physician to form a "trilateral" agreement with the patient

and pain specialist (Fishman et al. 1999, 2000, 2002). When there is concern that a patient will have difficulty taking medications as directed, a policy of prescribing small quantities, performing random pill counts, and not refilling lost supplies should be explicitly discussed and then followed. External sources of information such as urine toxicology testing, interviews with significant others, direct contact with pharmacists, data from prescription monitoring programs, and review of medical records can improve detection of substance use disorders. In one study, patients who denied using illicit substances that were detected on urine toxicology were more likely to be younger, receiving worker's compensation benefits, and have a previous diagnosis of polysubstance abuse (Katz and Fanciullo 2002).

The occurrence of any aberrant medication-related behaviors should prompt evaluation for addiction. Even when the diagnosis of a substance use disorder is suspected in patients taking opioids for chronic pain, behaviors such as stealing or forging prescriptions are relatively uncommon (Fishbain et al. 1992; Longo et al. 2000; Sees and Clark 1993). These more serious aberrant behaviors consistent with addiction also include selling medications, losing prescriptions, buying medications on the Internet, diverting medications from other patients, using oral medications intravenously, concurrently abusing alcohol or illicit drugs, repeatedly being noncompliant with the prescribed use of medications, and the patient's experiencing deterioration in the ability to function in family, social, or occupational roles. Concerns by family or friends about the patient's pattern of medication use, an appearance suggesting intoxication, or the patient's having other difficulties with functional abilities requires in-depth evaluation. Any unwillingness to discuss the possibility of addiction or changes in chronic opioid therapy is a red flag underlining the need for a full substance abuse evaluation.

Patients with substance use disorders have increased rates of chronic pain and are at the greatest risk for stigmatization and undertreatment with appropriate medications by health care practitioners (Gilson and Joranson 2002; Rosenblum et al. 2003). Ironically, this places them at additional risk of drug-seeking behaviors, including self-medication with illicit drugs. Almost one-quarter of patients admitted to inpatient residential substance abuse treatment and more than one-third of patients in methadone maintenance treatment programs reported severe chronic pain, with almost half of the inpatients and two-thirds of the methadone maintenance patients experiencing pain-related interference in functioning (Rosenblum et al. 2003). In another study of methadone maintenance therapy, patients with pain were more likely to overuse both prescribed and nonprescribed medications (Jamison et al. 2000). Patients with substance abuse and back pain were less likely to complete a substance abuse treatment program compared with those without pain (Stack et al. 2000). Ethical principles such as beneficence, quality of life, and autonomy can provide particularly useful guidance for the use of chronic opioid therapy (Cohen et al. 2002; Drug Enforcement Administration 2002; Nicholson 2003). Benefits of treatment should be optimized for each patient, recognizing a continuum of severity for both pain and addiction, within a context of risk management.

Depression and Distress

Pain in Patients With Depression

Physical symptoms are common in patients with major depression (Lipowski 1990). Approximately 60% of patients with depression report pain symptoms at the time of diagnosis (Magni et al. 1985; Von Knorring et al. 1983). In WHO data from 14 countries on five continents, 69% (range = 45%–95%) of patients with depression presented with only somatic symptoms, of which pain complaints were most common (Simon et al. 1999). Half the depressed patients reported multiple unexplained somatic symptoms, and 11% actively denied the psychological symptoms of depression. A survey of almost 19,000 Europeans found a fourfold increase in the prevalence of chronic painful conditions in respondents with major depression (Ohayon and Schatzberg 2003).

The presence of a depressive disorder has been demonstrated to increase the risk of developing chronic musculoskeletal pain, headache, and chest pain up to 3 years later (Leino and Magni 1993; Magni et al. 1993, 1994; Von Korff et al. 1993). Even after 8 years, the previously depressed patients remained twice as likely as the nondepressed subjects to develop chronic pain. In a 15-year prospective study of workers in an industrial setting, the presence of initial depression symptoms predicted LBP and a positive clinical back examination in men but not in women (Leino and Magni 1993). Five years later, self-assessed depression at baseline was a significant predictor in the 25% of at-risk women who developed fibromyalgia (Forseth et al. 1999).

Depression in Patients With Chronic Pain

In 1,016 health maintenance organization (HMO) members, the prevalence of depression was 12% in individuals with three or more pain complaints, compared with only 1% in those with one or no pain complaints (Dworkin et al. 1990). Depression was significantly more common in patients with rheumatoid arthritis, and the level of depression increased with greater levels of pain (Dickens et al. 2002). The Canadian National Population Health Survey found that the incidence of major depression was approximately doubled in subjects who reported a long-term medical condition such as back problems, migraine, and sinusitis (Patten 2001). In a community survey of people over age 65 who had activity limitations but no psychiatric morbidity, the incidence of depression three years later was highest in people with an acute illness and experienced pain (Livingston et al. 2000). In a similar study of late-onset depression in the elderly, joint pain was one of the most important predictors of incident depression 5 years later (Hein et al. 2003).

One-third to over half of patients presenting to clinics specializing in the evaluation of chronic pain have a current major depression (Dersh et al. 2002; Fishbain et al. 1997a; Reich et al. 1983; Smith 1992). In one study, 65% of patients hospitalized for rehabilitation for a musculoskeletal disease had a lifetime history of a psychiatric disorder (Harter et al. 2002). More than 30% of patients met criteria for a current mental disorder (11% major depression), with half having two or more psychiatric conditions. In groups of patients with medically unexplained symptoms such as back pain, orofacial pain, and dizziness, two-thirds of patients have a history of recurrent major depression, compared with less than 20% of medically ill control groups (Atkinson et al. 1991; Katon and Sullivan 1990; Sullivan and Katon 1993; Yap et al. 2002). Patients with higher levels of baseline affective distress on the General Health Questionnaire (GHQ) were 1.8 times more likely to seek consultation for a new episode of back pain 12 months later (Croft et al. 1996).

Affective Distress Versus Affective Disorder

The determination whether negative affect represents a diagnosis of major depression as opposed to psychological distress varies widely. Diagnostic criteria, structured interviews, and self-report questionnaires might lack validity or measure different concepts when applied to patients with chronic pain (Lebovits 2000). Self-report measures of depression are generally reliable and have predictive validity in patients with chronic pain (Turk and Okifuji 1994). Principal-components analyses of the responses of patients with chronic pain on the Beck Depression Inventory find three factors consistent with the core criteria of major depression: low mood, impaired self attitude, poor vital sense. One study described these factors as sadness, self-reproach, and somatic symptoms, and another described them in the similar terms of negative attitudes/suicide, physiological manifestations, and performance difficulty (Novy et al. 1995; Williams and Richardson 1993).

In a study comparing separate measures of affective distress, self-reported depressive symptoms, and major depression in patients with chronic pain at a pain clinic, the relationship between pain and depression remained significant even when the somatic items of depressive symptoms were excluded (Geisser et al. 2000). Self-reported depressive symptoms were also highly related to the evaluative or cognitive component of pain. In contrast, more general symptoms of affective distress were uniquely related to the sensory or emotional component of pain. Self-reported symptoms of affective distress and depressive symptoms were independently associated with increased pain, greater disability, and more negative thoughts about pain. A diagnosis of major depression was found only to make unique contributions to measures of negative thoughts about pain and self-reported disability. A diagnosis of major depression was determined to be a less sensitive indicator and less important predictor of the chronic pain experience than self-reported depressive symptoms. Therefore, practitioners should recognize the presence of depressive symptoms, even without the categorical diagnosis of major depression, as an important comorbidity for patients with chronic pain.

Consequences of Depression

The presence of depression has been shown to worsen other medical illnesses, interfere with their ongoing management, and amplify their detrimental effects on health-related quality of life (Cassano and Fava 2002; Gaynes et al. 2002). Depression in patients with chronic pain is associated with greater pain intensity, more pain persistence, less life control, more use of passive-avoidant coping strategies, noncompliance with treatment, application for early retirement, and greater interference from pain, including more pain behaviors observed by others (Hasenbring et al. 1994; Haythornthwaite et al. 1991; Kerns and Haythornthwaite 1988; Magni et al. 1985, 1993; Weickgenant et al. 1993). Primary care patients with musculoskeletal pain complicated by depression are significantly more likely than nondepressed patients with musculoskeletal pain to use medications daily, including sedative-hypnotics, and in combinations (Mantyselka et al. 2002). In a study of more than 15,000 employees who filed health claims, the cost of managing chronic conditions such as back problems was multiplied by 1.7 when comorbid depression was present (Druss et al. 2000). Depressed patients with chronic facial pain were more likely than nondepressed chronic facial pain patients to be noncompliant with medication changes, therapeutic injections, and splint therapy (Riley et al. 1999b).

Depression is a better predictor of disability than pain intensity and duration (Rudy et al. 1988). For example, fi-bromyalgia patients with depression compared with those without were significantly more likely to live alone, report functional disability, and describe maladaptive thoughts (Okifuji et al. 2000). A naturalistic follow-up study of patients with chronic pain who had substantial numbers of sick days found that a diagnosis of major depression predicted disability an average of 3.7 years later (Ericsson et al. 2002). The presence of depression in whiplash patients reduced the insurance claim closure rate by 37% (Cote et al. 2001). This rate was unaffected even after the insurance system eliminated compensation for pain and suffering. Preoperative major depression in patients undergoing surgery for thoracic outlet syndrome increased the rate of self-reported disability by over 15 times (Axelrod et al. 2001). The presence of preoperative depression in patients undergoing lumbar diskectomy predicted poorer surgical outcome at 1-year follow-up (Junge et al. 1995). In patients with rheumatoid arthritis, depressive symptoms were significantly associated with negative health and functional outcomes, as well as increased health services utilization (Katz and Yelin 1993). Depression consistently predicted level of functioning, pain severity, pain-related disability, less use of active coping, and more use of passive coping in patients on a university chronic pain inpatient unit (Fisher et al. 2001). In a clinical trial of 1,001 depressed patients older than 60 years with arthritis, antidepressants and/or problem-solving–oriented psychotherapy not only reduced depressive symptoms but also improved pain, functional status, and quality of life (Lin et al. 2003).

Patients suffering from chronic pain syndromes, including migraine, chronic abdominal pain, and orthopedic pain syndromes, report increased rates of suicidal ideation, suicide attempts, and suicide completion (Fishbain 1999b; Fishbain et al. 1991; Magni et al. 1998). In one study of patients who attempted suicide, 52% suffered from a chronic somatic disease and 21% were taking analgesics on a daily basis for pain (Stenager et al. 1994). Patients with chronic pain completed suicide at two to three times the rate in the general population (Fishbain et al. 1991). Cancer patients with pain and depression, but not pain alone, were significantly more likely to request assistance in committing suicide as well as actively to take steps to end their lives (Emanuel et al. 1996).

Relationship Between Pain and Depression

In addition to the epidemiology of pain and depression, as well as the effects of comorbidity on diagnosis, treatment, and outcome reviewed in the preceding subsections, the existing models of the relationship between pain and depression were recently detailed (Bair et al. 2003; Pincus and Williams 1999). Cognitive conceptualizations of depression have included the role of negative schemata, leading to processing biases, distorted perceptions, negative thoughts, and depressed mood; the role of learned helplessness in a context of having no control over adverse events; the focus on hopelessness that emerges as a result of the desired outcomes being improbable and undesired outcomes being inevitable; and a problem-solving mechanism that persuades others to interact with the ill person (Abramson et al. 1978, 1989; Beck 1976; Seligman 1974; Watson and Andrews 2002).

The rates of affective disorders in family members of patients with depression occurring after the onset of chronic pain are similar to those in the general population and significantly lower than those in family members of patients with major depression (Banks and Kerns 1996; Dworkin et al. 1999; Gallagher and Verma 1999). For example, major depression and depressive spectrum disorders were not more common in the first-degree relatives of patients with myofascial facial pain regardless of whether they had personal histories of early- or late-onset major depression (Dohrenwend et al. 1999). These results do not support the characterization of chronic nonmalignant pain as a variant of depression ("masked depression"), but they do support the hypothesis that depression emerges out of the stress of living with chronic pain.

In addition to depression as a consequence of chronic pain, there are mediating biopsychosocial factors in the interaction between depression and chronic pain (Banks and Kerns 1996; Fishbain et al. 1997a; Pincus and Williams 1999; Sheftell and Atlas 2002). The diathesis–stress model postulates an interaction between personal premorbid vulnerabilities activated and exacerbated by life stressors such as chronic pain and the subsequent outcome of depression or other psychopathology. In a study of patients with chronic LBP, regression models that included all cognitive-behavioral variables (self-control, cognitive distortion, interference with instrumental activities of daily living) produced the strongest association with self-reported depression (Maxwell et al. 1998). Without these cognitive factors, there was no significant association of pain and disability with depression—a finding consistent with the diathesis–stress model. Other intervening factors have also been identified. A study of nearly 4,000 twin pairs found that genetic factors accounted for 60% of the covariation in the best-fitting model for the association between back and neck pain and symptoms of depression and anxiety (Reichborn-Kjennerud et al. 2002).

More sophisticated models add the component of illness behaviors/disability, which functions both as a response of the vulnerable individual to a significant stressor and, later, as a stressor itself (Revenson and Felton 1989). The severity of depression has been found to be unaffected by pain intensity when pain-related disability is controlled for (Von Korff et al. 1992). If pain causes disability—such as loss of independence or mobility—that decreases an individual's participation in activities, the risk of depression is significantly increased (Williamson and Schulz 1992). In a clinical trial involving patients with chronic LBP, the association between pain and depression was found to be attributable to disability and illness attitudes (Dickens et al. 2000). A study of patients in primary care found that after a variety of factors, such as disability and perceived health, were controlled for, anxiety and depression were no longer associated with the diagnoses of headache, osteoarthritis, and abdominal pain (Wu et al. 2002).

The neurobiology of pain and depression overlap (Bair et al. 2003; Bolay and Moskowitz 2002; Hunt and Mantyh 2001; Price 2000; Riedel and Neeck 2001). In particular, the descending pathways of pain modulation in the central nervous system that utilize monoamine neurotransmitters in the limbic system, periaqueductal gray, rostral-ventromedial medulla, and dorsolateral pontine tegmentum influence aspects of affect and attention (Millan 2002). Pain can be decreased by descending inhibition as first postulated by the gate theory of Melzack and Wall (1965). Increased levels of serotonin and nephrine diminish peripheral nociceptive inputs and augment descending central inhibition. The functional deficiency of monoamine neurotransmitters or related neurochemical dysfunctions in affective disorder could partially explain the linkages between pain and depression. Similar associations between pain, depression, and sleep disturbance have been described (Moldofsky 2001). Reduced sleep quantity and quality have been correlated with pain, depression, and negative affectivity. Current models postulate that pain increases negative affect over time, with subsequent detrimental effects on sleep quality, although bidirectional relationships have also been proposed (McCracken and Iverson 2002; Riley et al. 2001). Physical functioning, duration of pain, and age have been implicated in mediation of the decreased sleep quality and latency in patients with chronic pain (Menefee et al. 2000).

Anxiety, Fear, Catastrophizing, and Anger

Patients with a variety of chronic pain syndromes, such as headache, LBP, neck pain after whiplash injury, and chronic pain from prostate cancer, have increased rates of both anxiety symptoms and current anxiety disorders (Dersh et al. 2002; Fishbain et al. 1986; Heim and Oei 1993; Juang et al. 2000; Lee et al. 1993; Polatin et al.

1993; Weissman and Merikangas 1986). Almost 50% of patients with chronic pain report anxiety symptoms, and up to 30% of patients have an anxiety disorder such as panic disorder and generalized anxiety disorder (Devlen 1994; Fishbain et al. 1998; Katon et al. 1985; Reich et al. 1983). One prospective study of 1,007 young adults found that a baseline history of migraine was significantly associated with an increased risk (OR=12.8) of first-incidence panic disorder (Breslau and Davis 1993). In a study of patients with fibromyalgia, more than half of the patients reported clinically relevant posttraumatic stress disorder (PTSD)–like symptoms that were significantly associated with greater levels of pain, emotional distress, interference, and disability (Sherman et al. 2000). Patients with chronic pain classified as Dysfunctional according to the Multidimensional Pain Inventory are almost twice as likely to complain of PTSD-like symptoms as patients classified as Interpersonally Distressed and more than three times as likely as Adaptive Copers (Asmundson et al. 2000, 2002).

Conversely, anxiety symptoms and disorders are associated with high levels of somatic preoccupation and physical symptoms. Pain intensity in rheumatoid arthritis patients was found to be significantly influenced by the presence of anxiety and depression even after disease activity had been controlled for (Smedstad et al. 1995). Men with high levels of anxiety were shown to experience greater pain severity, interference from pain, and limitations in daily activities (Edwards et al. 2000). Almost two-thirds of patients with panic disorder reported at least one current pain symptom, with chest pain and headache being the most common (Schmidt et al. 2002). Pain was related to higher levels of anxiety symptoms, panic frequency, and cognitive features of anxiety, but not to treatment response.

The fear–avoidance model and expectancy model of fear provide explanations for the initiation and maintenance of chronic pain disability, proposing that anxiety sensitivity amplifies reactions such as avoidance of specific activities (Greenberg and Burns 2003; Lethem et al. 1983; Reis 1991; Vlaeyen and Linton 2000). Anxiety sensitivity is a significant predictor of fear of, and anxiety about, pain (Zvolensky et al. 2001). Fear of pain, movement, reinjury, and other negative consequences that result in the avoidance of activities promote the transition to and sustaining of chronic pain and its associated disabilities such as muscular reactivity, deconditioning, and guarded movement (Asmundson et al. 1999). In one study, patients with chronic LBP who restricted their activities developed physiological changes (muscle atrophy, osteoporosis, weight gain) and functional deterioration attributed to deconditioning (Verbunt et al. 2003). This

process is reinforced by negative cognitions such as low self-efficacy, catastrophic interpretations, and increased expectations of failure regarding attempts to engage in rehabilitation. Higher levels of pain anxiety were shown to correlate with lower amounts of weight lifted and carried by men with chronic pain referred for work rehabilitation (Burns et al. 2000).

Fear–avoidance beliefs have been found to be one of the most significant predictors of failure to return to work in patients with chronic LBP (Waddell et al. 1993). Operant conditioning reinforces disability if the avoidance provides any short-term benefits, such as reducing anticipatory anxiety or relieving the individual of unwanted responsibilities. In a study of patients with chronic LBP, improvements in disability following physical therapy were associated with decreases in pain, psychological distress, and fear–avoidance beliefs but not in specific physical deficits (Mannion et al. 1999, 2001). Decreasing work-specific fears was a more important outcome than addressing general fears of physical activity in predicting improved physical capability for work among patients participating in an interdisciplinary treatment program (Vowles and Gross 2003).

Catastrophic thinking about pain has been attributed to the amplification of threatening information, and it interferes with the focus needed to facilitate patients' remaining involved with productive instead of pain-related activities (Crombez et al. 1998). Catastrophizing intensifies the experience of pain and increases emotional distress as well as self-perceived disability (Severeijns et al. 2001; Sullivan et al. 2001). This multidimensional construct includes elements of cognitive rumination, symptom magnification, and feelings of helplessness (Van Damme et al. 2002). Early treatment catastrophizing and helplessness of patients in a 4-week multidisciplinary pain program predicted late-treatment outcomes such as pain-related interference and activity level (Burns et al. 2003). These changes persisted despite changes in depression over the course of treatment being controlled for, supporting the model that changing negative cognitions improves treatment outcome.

Pain-related cognitions such as catastrophizing and fear–avoidance beliefs are considered some of the strongest psychological variables mediating the transition from acute to chronic pain and usually have more predictive power of poor adjustment to chronic pain than objective factors such as disease status, physical impairment, or occupational descriptions (Hasenbring et al. 2001). In a population-based study of individuals without LBP, high levels of catastrophizing and fear of injury prospectively predicted disability due to new-onset LBP 6 months later (Picavet et al. 2002). In a study of patients with pain after spinal cord injury, catastrophizing was the only form of coping significantly associated with poor adjustment (Turner et al. 2002).

Anger is characterized by a specific cognitive appraisal and action tendency (Fernandez and Turk 1995). This emotional state is distinguished from the trait of hostility and the goal-oriented behavior of aggression. In a sample of patients with chronic pain referred for comprehensive evaluation, 70% reported anger that was most commonly directed at themselves (74%) and health care professionals (62%) (Okifuji et al. 1999). Patients have different anger management styles that range from suppression (anger-in) to expression or engagement (anger-out). Women with chronic pain who were low in hostility and high on anger expression were more likely to report lower pain intensity and higher levels of activity (Burns et al. 1996). In contrast, patients who reported the highest levels of pain and associated interference were men with high hostility and suppression of anger. In men, anger suppression is associated with depression and limitations in performing general activities (Burns et al. 1998). In women with chronic headache, anger suppression was associated with depression, but expression was associated with anxiety (Venable et al. 2001).

Pharmacological Treatment

While medications are often prescribed for all types of chronic pain, research has consistently shown that several classes have proven efficacy for the treatment of neuropathic pain (Nitu et al. 2003). Ideally, pharmacotherapy of pain would be specifically selected on the basis of considerations of etiology (e.g., ischemic, neuropathic), pathophysiology (e.g., demyelination, central pain), and anatomy (e.g., C fibers, sympathetic nerves) (Woolf and Decosterd 1999; Woolf and Mannion 1999; Woolf et al. 1998). No experimental data exist to support or refute this clinical approach, and a number of drug classes have been found to improve many different kinds of pain. Unfortunately, medications are often underutilized and underdosed. In one study of patients with neuropathic pain, 73% complained of inadequate pain control, but 72% had never received anticonvulsants, 60% TCAs, or 41% opioids, and 25% had never received any of the above (Gilron et al. 2002). Physicians still attempt to alleviate pain with simple analgesics and fail to appreciate the subtleties of the "adjuvant" medications, which possess multiple pharmacological actions. These medications offer a sophisticated and multifaceted approach to antinociception that is usually required in the treatment of patients with chronic pain.

Opioids

Comprehensive reviews describe opioid pharmacology and opioid peptide systems (Ballantyne and Mao 2003; Bodnar and Hadjimarkou 2002; Drolet et al. 2001; Inturrisi 2002; Kieffer and Gaveriaux-Ruff 2002; O'Callaghan 2001; Przewlocki and Przewlocka 2001; Riedel and Neeck 2001; Vaccarino and Kastin 2001). The analgesic effects of opioids typically decrease the distressing affective component of pain more than the sensation of pain. This effect may be more pronounced in women who reported lower levels of affective distress despite higher levels of pain compared with men while being treated with opioids (Fillingim et al. 2003). The treatment of nonmalignant chronic pain with opioids remains a subject of considerable debate, with fears of regulatory pressure, medication abuse, and the development of tolerance creating reluctance to prescribe opioids (Chabal et al. 1992a; Maruta et al. 1979; Morgan 1985; Potter et al. 2001; Schug et al. 1991). Nevertheless, the prescription of long-term opioids for the treatment of chronic nonmalignant pain has increased (Clark 2002; Fanciullo et al. 2002; Moulin et al. 2002; Turk et al. 1994).

Opioids are effective in the treatment of chronic nonmalignant pain, as demonstrated in randomized, placebo-controlled trials, in reducing pain, pain-related disability, depression, insomnia, and physical dysfunction (Arkinstall et al. 1995; Caldwell et al. 2002; Maier et al. 2002; Moulin et al. 1996; Roth et al. 2000; Sittl et al. 2003). Studies of neuropathic pain show that opioids provide direct analgesic benefits and do not just counteract the unpleasantness of pain (Dellemijn and Vanneste 1997; Watt et al. 1996). Levorphanol reduced pain, affective distress, interference with function, and sleep difficulties in adults with neuropathic pain (Rowbotham et al. 2003). Continuous-release morphine decreased pain in patients with postherpetic neuralgia significantly more than did TCAs or placebo (Raja et al. 2002).

Successful treatment with opioids requires the assessment and documentation of improvements in function and analgesia without accompanying adverse side effects and aberrant behaviors (Mendelson and Mendelson 1991; Nedeljkovic et al. 2002; Passik and Weinreb 2000; Schug et al. 1991). The Federation of State Medical Boards, American Academy of Pain Medicine, American Pain Society, and American Geriatrics Society have all produced guidelines for the treatment of chronic pain (American Geriatrics Society Panel on Chronic Pain in Older Persons 1998). These efforts, combined with legislation to support these educational and governmental initiatives, are improving attitudes toward, acceptance of, and access to chronic opioid therapy (Gilson and Joranson 2001;

Joranson et al. 2002). If opioid therapy is unsuccessful, the medication should be gradually tapered and discontinued. Acute opioid withdrawal is not dangerous except in patients at risk from increased sympathetic tone, such as those with increased intracranial pressure or unstable angina. Intermittent discontinuation or tapering of opioids often results in exacerbation of the patient's pain (opioid-abstinence hyperalgesia, opioid-induced hyperalgesia), probably involving spinal sensitization (Li and Clark 2002; Li et al. 2001).

Generally, a constant rather than intermittent "as needed" schedule for pharmacotherapy should be followed, with the time between dosages and the individual dose amounts kept consistent. In particular, opioids with slow onset and longer duration of action are preferred so as to minimize the initial euphoria and interdose withdrawal symptoms of traditional short-acting opioids, which should be reserved for the treatment of breakthrough pain. Extended-release oral medications and transdermal routes of administration decrease these qualities of opioids that place patients at risk of inadequate treatment and abuse. In the United States, controlled-release formulations of morphine, oxycodone, fentanyl, and potentially hydromorphone and oxymorphone, as well as newer alternatives such as dihydroetorphine, transdermal buprenorphine, slow-release tramadol, and slow-release dihydrocodeine, are now available but still represent the minority of opioid prescriptions (Ohmori and Morimoto 2002; Portenoy et al. 2002; Tzschentke 2002; Wilder-Smith et al. 2001). Mixed agonist–antagonist opioids should be avoided because of their propensity to precipitate withdrawal symptoms in patients undergoing chronic opioid therapy.

Most long-acting opioids are expensive. Methadone offers a low-cost alternative with the unique advantage of suppressing withdrawal symptoms for more than 24 hours. Unfortunately, the analgesic properties of methadone are similar to those of immediate-release morphine, necessitating a 6-hour dosing schedule for the treatment of chronic pain. Generic formulations of continuous-release morphine and oxycodone offer affordable options. In a randomized, open-label, crossover trial in patients with chronic noncancer pain treated with opioids, transdermal fentanyl was preferred to sustained-release oral morphine (65% vs. 28%), with the greater preference attributed to better pain relief, an enhanced quality of life, and less constipation (Allan et al. 2001). Transdermal fentanyl produced significantly better cost–utility ratios than continuous-release formulations of morphine and oxycodone for each quality-adjusted life year gained despite higher costs of therapy (Neighbors et al. 2001).

The most common side effect of chronic opioid therapy is decreased gastrointestinal motility, potentially leading to constipation, vomiting, and abdominal pain. In some patients with chronic abdominal pain, the problem of "narcotic bowel" results from the vicious cycle of opioid treatment causing painful constipation, followed by the escalation of opioid dose, resulting in even more pain. This process is further complicated by rebound pain with attempts to taper the opioids, which leads to additional dose increases with no subsequent benefits, as well as the persistence of colonic dysmotility after opioid discontinuation. Oral opioids differ in their propensity to cause symptoms of gastrointestinal dysmotility (Heiskanen and Kalso 1997). Transdermal fentanyl is an effective analgesic with fewer gastrointestinal side effects than oral medications, with over 90% of patients choosing to continue the medication after completion of a study trial (Donner et al. 1996; Grond et al. 2000). Newer experimental opioid antagonists that do not cross the blood–brain barrier may offer relief of constipation without compromising analgesia or precipitating withdrawal (Kurz and Sessler 2003; Portenoy and Foley 1987).

Opioids induce centrally mediated hypogonadism with lower production of testosterone, manifested in fatigue, loss of libido, and impaired sexual function (Daniell 2002). Concerns about cognitive impairment are more often the reason opioids are not prescribed. Studies comparing patients taking opioids with those who are not or patients before and during treatment with opioids have not demonstrated deleterious effects on neuropsychological testing, computerized testing of performance, or electroencephalography (EEG), except in patients prescribed multiple medications, especially sedatives and hypnotics (Chapman et al. 2002; Hendler et al. 1980; Lomardo et al. 1976; McNairy et al. 1984; Sabatowski et al. 2003; Zielger 1994). Although no studies have examined the risk of delirium in chronic pain syndromes treated with opioids, meperidine poses a unique risk for causing an agitated hyperactive delirium.

Long-term administration of opioids predisposes one to tolerance, but chronic pain may actually facilitate its development (Christensen and Kayser 2000). While several physiological mechanisms have been described to explain this phenomenon, tolerance is uncommon in clinical practice (Borgland 2001; Cahill et al. 2001; Dogrul et al. 2002; France et al. 1984; Freye and Latasch 2003; Katz 2000; Mao et al. 2002; Portenoy 1990). The incidence of analgesic tolerance is lower with more potent opioids such as fentanyl, presumably because they are more receptor-specific and fewer receptors are needed to induce an analgesic effect. Although constipation is likely to persist, tolerance to most opioid side effects usually occurs.

The loss of preexisting analgesia can have many causes besides tolerance and should be carefully evaluated so as to determine its etiology. Disease progression or other changes in the patient's chronic pain condition should be considered before this loss is attributed to tolerance. A return of, or even an increase in, pain can be the result of new injury, worsening neurological damage, comorbid psychiatric disorders, or medication effects such as toxicity, withdrawal, or opioid-induced hyperalgesia (Liu and Anand 2001).

When tolerance to an analgesic agent develops, suggested strategies have included simultaneous administration of other agents (opioid agonists with differing receptor affinities; ultra-low-dose opioid antagonists; calcium channel blockers; alpha$_2$-adrenergic agonists; COX-2 inhibitors; NMDA receptor antagonists such as ketamine, dextromethorphan, memantine, and amantadine); opioid rotation to a more potent agonist; and intermittent cessation of certain agents (e.g., opioids, benzodiazepines) (Bolan et al. 2002; Pasternak 2001). Augmentation of analgesia may occur by using opioids that possess NMDA antagonist action, such as methadone, dextropropoxyphene, and ketobemidone, or those that inhibit monoamine reuptake, such as methadone, tramadol, and levorphanol (Rojas-Corrales et al. 2002; Sang 2000). Incomplete cross-tolerance of the analgesic effects of opioids probably accounts for the improved pain relief gained through rotating between different long-acting opioids or switching from short-acting to long-acting opioids (Quang-Cantagrel et al. 2000; Thomsen et al. 1999). Opioid rotation may also improve analgesia if morphine or hydromorphone is discontinued, because these agents' 3-glucuronide metabolites can accumulate within the cerebrospinal fluid and produce neuroexcitatory effects such as allodynia, myoclonus, delirium, and seizures (Forman 1996; Smith 2000).

Antidepressants

The neurobiology of pain suggests potential efficacy for all antidepressants in the treatment of chronic pain (Ansari 2000; Lynch 2001; Mattia et al. 2002). The analgesic effect of antidepressants is thought to be primarily mediated by the blockade of reuptake of nephrine and serotonin, increasing their levels to enhance the activation of descending inhibitory neurons (King 1981; Magni 1987; Ollat and Cesaro 1995). However, antidepressants may produce antinociceptive effects through a variety of other pharmacological mechanisms (Ansari 2000; Carter and Sullivan 2002; Feighner 1999; Kiefer et al. 1999). (See Chapter 37, "Psychopharmacology," for a discussion of the pharmacology of antidepressants.)

Tricyclic Antidepressants

The effectiveness of antidepressants for the treatment of major depression is well documented, but their analgesic properties are underappreciated (Barkin and Fawcett 2000). In 1960, the first report of imipramine use for trigeminal neuralgia was published (Paoli et al. 1960). Since then, antidepressants, particularly the TCAs, have been commonly prescribed for many chronic pain syndromes, including diabetic neuropathy, postherpetic neuralgia, central pain, poststroke pain, tension-type headache, migraine, and orofacial pain (Ansari 2000; Clark 2000b; Collins et al. 2000; Lynch 2001). TCAs have been most effective in relieving neuropathic pain and headache syndromes (Gruber et al. 1996; MacFarlane et al. 1997; Magni 1991; Max et al. 1987; McQuay et al. 1996; Volmink et al. 1996; Vrethem et al. 1997; Wesselmann and Reich 1996). A meta-analysis showed that TCAs were more effective than placebo for the treatment of chronic back pain in reducing pain severity but not functional disability (Salerno et al. 2002). Meta-analyses of randomized, controlled trials concluded that TCAs are the most effective agents for the treatment of postherpetic neuralgia and that nortriptyline is better tolerated than amitriptyline with equivalent efficacy (Dworkin and Schmader 2003; Lynch 2001; Roose et al 1981; Volmink et al. 1996; Watson et al. 1988). Protriptyline, compared with placebo, decreased chronic tension-type headache frequency by 86% in a study of women with this condition (Cohen 1997).

Only 25% of patients in one multidisciplinary pain center were prescribed TCAs, and 73% of treated patients were prescribed only the equivalent of 50 mg or less of amitriptyline, suggesting the potential for additional pain relief (Richeimer et al. 1997). The cost of TCAs for pain treatment is much lower (often less than $5.00/month) than the cost of other antidepressants and most analgesics (Adelman and Von Seggern 1995). A number of treatment studies of postherpetic neuralgia and painful diabetic peripheral neuropathy have used TCAs, with mean daily doses ranging from 100 to 250 mg (Max 1994; Onghena and Van Houdenhove 1992). Over 60% of patients reported improvement, usually beginning in the third week of treatment, with serum levels at the low end of the therapeutic range for the treatment of depression. Typically, the analgesic effects of antidepressants are independent of the presence of depression or improvement in mood. Analgesia usually occurs at lower doses and with earlier onset of action than expected for the treatment of depression. The results of investigations to determine drug concentrations needed for pain relief support higher serum levels but remain contradictory (Kishore-Kumar et al. 1990; Sindrup et al. 1989).

Noradrenergic activity is often associated with better analgesic effects than serotonergic activity alone. The relatively noradrenergic antidepressants (i.e., with a serotonin/norepinephrine ratio of less than 1.0) include amitriptyline, imipramine, doxepin, nortriptyline, desipramine, and maprotiline (Feighner 1999; Richelson 1994). Generally, the tertiary TCAs with balanced effects on serotonin and norepinephrine reuptake (imipramine, amitriptyline, doxepin) are considered more effective analgesic agents than the secondary TCAs with more selective norepinephrine reuptake inhibition (desipramine, nortriptyline, maprotiline). While tertiary amines have been used most commonly, the secondary amines have fewer side effects and are less likely to be discontinued. Randomized, controlled trials have not demonstrated consistent differences in efficacy between the TCAs (Bryson and Wilde 1996; Collins et al. 2000; Sindrup and Jensen 1999, 2000).

Selective Serotonin Reuptake Inhibitors

The selective serotonin reuptake inhibitors (SSRIs) produce weak antinociceptive effects in animal models of acute pain (Gatch et al. 1998; Paul and Hornby 1995; Schreiber et al. 1996). This antinociception is blocked by serotonin receptor antagonists and is enhanced by opioid receptor agonists. In human clinical trials, the efficacy of SSRIs in chronic pain syndromes has been variable and inconsistent (Belcheva et al. 1995; Jung et al. 1997; Tokunaga et al. 1998). In patients with chronic LBP without depression, nortriptyline or maprotiline, but not paroxetine, significantly reduced pain intensity (Atkinson et al. 1998, 1999). Desipramine was superior to fluoxetine in the treatment of painful diabetic peripheral neuropathy (Max et al. 1992). On the other hand, paroxetine and citalopram were beneficial in studies of patients with diabetic neuropathy (Sindrup et al. 1990, 1992). Fluoxetine significantly reduced pain in patients with rheumatoid arthritis and was comparable in efficacy to amitriptyline (Rani et al. 1996). A 12-week course of fluoxetine also improved outcome measures in women with fibromyalgia (Arnold et al. 2002). The SSRIs may be effective in the treatment of some headaches, especially migraine, and are well tolerated by patients (Bank 1994; Foster and Bafaloukos 1994; Saper et al. 1994). However, citalopram did not significantly reduce the duration of chronic tension headache, headache frequency, and the intake of analgesics (Bendtsen et al. 1996). In depressed patients with neuropathic pain, improvements in pain were dependent on improvements in depressive symptoms if patients were treated with fluoxetine but not fluvoxamine, which improved pain independently of antidepressant effects (Ciaramella et al. 2000).

Other Antidepressants

Venlafaxine and duloxetine inhibit the presynaptic reuptake of both serotonin and norepinephrine. Duloxetine more potently blocks serotonin and norepinephrine transporters both in vitro and in vivo when compared with venlafaxine (Bymaster et al. 2001). There is evidence of its analgesic efficacy in preclinical models and in clinical populations (Enggaard et al. 2001; Lang et al. 1996). Duloxetine is an effective treatment for major depression and significantly reduced pain complaints and time in pain while awake in these patients (Detke et al. 2002). Duloxetine has just been approved (September 2004) by the FDA for treatment of diabetic peripheral neuropathy pain. Controlled trials have shown duloxetine to be effective in fibromyalgia and diabetic neuropathy. A small controlled trial of venlafaxine in patients with neuropathic pain following treatment of breast cancer showed pain relief, with improved response at higher doses of venlafaxine that may be attributable to increased reuptake inhibition of norepinephrine (Tasmuth et al. 2002). In patients with neuropathic pain but without depression, bupropion decreased pain intensity and interference of pain with quality of life (Semenchuk et al. 2001). In a small open-label trial of diabetic neuropathy, nefazodone significantly reduced pain, paresthesias, and numbness (Goodnick et al. 2000). Monoamine oxidase inhibitors decrease the frequency and severity of migraine headaches (Merikangas and Merikangas 1995). Trazodone is commonly prescribed for insomnia, and several reports suggested efficacy for chronic pain. However, in higher-quality studies, trazodone was ineffective in decreasing pain in a double-blind, placebo-controlled study of patients with chronic LBP (Goodkin et al. 1990; Marek et al. 1992).

Comparing Relative Efficacy of Antidepressants and Other Agents

Comparing the relative efficacy of antidepressants and other pharmacological agents used in the treatment of pain can be calculated with the *number needed to treat* (NNT). NNT is defined as the number of patients who would need to receive the specific treatment for one patient to achieve at least 50% pain relief (Cook and Sackett 1995). Antidepressants, especially TCAs with optimized serum levels, are the most effective in the treatment of neuropathic pain, with the majority of clinical trials enrolling patients with postherpetic neuralgia and diabetic peripheral neuropathy (Collins et al. 2000; McQuay et al. 1996; Sindrup and Jensen 1999, 2000, 2002; Watson 2000). An NNT of 2.5 for TCAs, compared with an NNT of 6.7 for SSRIs, indicates that the difference in response between the active drug treatment and placebo is approximately 40%

versus only 15%, respectively. Subsequent meta-analyses of the treatment of functional gastrointestinal disorders, fibromyalgia, and chronic headache, including both migraine and tension headaches, found no differences in outcome between types of antidepressants with a pooled NNT of 3.2–4.0 (Jackson et al. 2000; O'Malley et al. 2000; Tomkins et al. 2001).

Anticonvulsants

Phenytoin was first reported as a successful treatment for trigeminal neuralgia in 1942 (Bergouignan 1942). Carbamazepine is the most widely studied anticonvulsant effective for neuropathic pain (Tanelian and Victory 1995). Anticonvulsants are effective for trigeminal neuralgia, diabetic neuropathy, postherpetic neuralgia, and migraine recurrence (McQuay et al. 1995; Tremont-Lukats et al. 2000; Wiffen et al. 2000). The NNT ranges from less than 2 to approximately 4 for anticonvulsants, with better compliance when compared with TCAs because of fewer adverse effects (Collins et al. 2000; Sindrup and Jensen 1999, 2000, 2002; Wiffen et al. 2000). Therapeutic serum levels have not been clearly established, but some evidence suggests lower levels than for seizures may be effective in decreasing pain (Moosa et al. 1993). (See Chapter 37, "Psychopharmacology," for a discussion of the anticonvulsants.)

Valproic acid is most commonly used in the prophylaxis of migraine but is also effective in the treatment of neuropathic pain (R. Jensen et al. 1994). Valproate was an effective prophylactic treatment in over two-thirds of patients with migraine and almost three-quarters of those with cluster headache (Gallagher et al. 2002; Mathew et al. 1995). Improvement occurred in frequency of headache, duration or headache days per month, intensity of headache, use of other medications for acute treatment of headache, the patient's opinion of treatment, and ratings of depression and anxiety (Kaniecki 1997; Klapper 1997; Rothrock 1997).

Gabapentin has been reported to reduce neuropathic pain in multiple sclerosis, migraine, postherpetic neuralgia, spinal cord injury, HIV-related neuropathy, and reflex sympathetic dystrophy (Houtchens et al. 1997; La Spina et al. 2001; To et al. 2002; Wetzel and Connelly 1997). Randomized, double-blind, placebo-controlled clinical trials have confirmed the efficacy of gabapentin in the treatment of diabetic peripheral neuropathy, postherpetic neuralgia, and postamputation phantom limb pain (Backonja et al. 1998; Bone et al. 2002; Mellegers et al. 2001; Rice et al. 2001; Rowbotham et al. 1998; Serpell 2002). A retrospective analysis found that patients were more likely to benefit from gabapentin if they had experienced allo-

dynia as a feature of their neuropathic pain (Gustorff et al. 2002). Gabapentin significantly decreased the pain associated with Guillain-Barré syndrome as well as the concomitant consumption of fentanyl (Pandey et al. 2002).

Lamotrigine may be effective in reducing the pain of phantom limbs, neuroma hypersensitivity, trigeminal neuralgia, causalgia, poststroke pain, and postherpetic neuralgia (Canavero and Bonicalzi 1996; Harbinson et al. 1997; T.S. Jensen 2002). Lamotrigine decreased the pain of diabetic neuropathy without associated improvements in mood or pain-related disability (Eisenberg et al. 2001). Lamotrigine produced analgesia that was correlated with serum drug concentrations and comparable to that obtained with phenytoin and dihydrocodeine (Webb and Kamali 1998).

Combinations of anticonvulsants with complementary mechanisms of action may increase effectiveness and decrease adverse effects of treatment. Patients with multiple sclerosis or trigeminal neuralgia who had failed treatment with carbamazepine or lamotrigine at therapeutic doses because of intolerable side effects were given gabapentin as an augmentation agent (Solaro et al. 2000). Gabapentin was titrated to pain relief, with no new side effects up to a maximum dosage of 1,200 mg/day, at which time either carbamazepine or lamotrigine was tapered until side effects were no longer present. Ten of 11 patients achieved pain control with no side effects.

Topiramate, tiagabine, pregabalin, vigabatrin, retigabine, levetiracetam, and zonisamide are new anticonvulsants with a spectrum of pharmacological actions and antinociceptive effects in animal models, but few clinical studies exist to support their use as a first-line therapy for patients with chronic pain (Cutrer 2001; Marson et al. 1997). Pregabalin is similar to gabapentin but with greater potency (Bryans and Wustrow 1999; Chen et al. 2001). Topiramate offers the advantages of low protein binding, minimal hepatic metabolism and unchanged renal excretion, few drug interactions, long half-life, and the unusual side effect of weight loss. A pilot study found that tiagabine improved pain symptoms and neuronal function assessed with quantitative sensory testing in patients with painful neuropathy (Novak et al. 2001).

Local Anesthetics

Topical lidocaine has been approved for the treatment of postherpetic neuralgia and does not produce significant serum levels (Argoff 2000). Oral mexiletine has been an effective treatment for neuropathic pain in painful diabetic neuropathy, peripheral nerve injury, alcoholic neuropathy, and phantom limb, but not cancer-related pain (Boulton 1993; Chabal et al. 1992b; Davis 1993; Kalso et al. 1998; Nishiyama and Sakuta 1995). Mexiletine not only decreased reports of pain but also the accompanying paresthesias and dysesthesias (Dejgard et al. 1988). Mexiletine also has been shown to decrease pain and sleep disturbances associated with painful diabetic neuropathy (Oskarsson et al. 1997). No significant correlations were found with plasma concentrations of mexiletine. Its effectiveness in widespread clinical use has been disappointing despite relatively few adverse effects.

Calcium Channel Blockers

Verapamil is the most commonly prescribed calcium channel blocker for chronic pain and has proven to be effective in the treatment of migraine and cluster headaches (Lewis and Solomon 1996; Markley 1991). The calcium channel blockers diltiazem and verapamil have also been found to potentiate morphine analgesia, but the results have been inconsistent (Hodoglugil et al. 1996; Taniguchi et al. 1995). Now in clinical trials, the experimental neuron-specific calcium channel blockers ziconotide and related omega-conopeptides possess potent analgesic, antihyperesthetic, and antiallodynic activity, as well as synergistic analgesic effects with morphine without producing tolerance (Bowersox et al. 1996; Brose et al. 1997; Jain 2000; M. T. Smith et al. 2002; Wang et al. 2000; Xiao and Bennett 1995).

Benzodiazepines

Benzodiazepines are commonly prescribed for insomnia and anxiety in patients with chronic pain (see Chapter 37, "Psychopharmacology"); however, there is little evidence of their utility for relief of pain, and they may even be counterproductive (Holister et al. 1981; King and Strain 1990). Only a limited number of chronic pain conditions, such as trigeminal neuralgia, tension headache, and temporomandibular disorder, were found to improve when treated with benzodiazepines (Dellemijn and Fields 1994). Clonazepam has been reported to provide long-term relief of the episodic lancinating variety of phantom limb pain (Bartusch et al. 1996). A recent extensive review failed to conclude that benzodiazepines significantly improve spasticity following spinal cord injury (Taricco et al. 2000).

Benzodiazepines also cause cognitive impairment (Buffett-Jerrott and Stewart 2002; Hendler et al. 1980). In patients with chronic pain, benzodiazepines, but not opioids, were associated with decreased activity levels, higher rates of health care visits, increased domestic instability, depression, and more disability days (Ciccone et al. 2000). Combining benzodiazepines with opioids may cause several problems. In methadone-related mortality, almost 75% of deaths were attributable to a combination of drug effects, and benzodiazepines were present in 74% of the deceased (Caplehorn and Drummer 2002; Ernst et al. 2002). Benzodiazepines have been associated with exacerbation of pain and interference with opioid analgesia (Nemmani and Mogil 2003; Sawynok 1985). They also increase the rate of developing tolerance to opioids (Freye and Latasch 2003).

Psychological Treatment

Patient Classifications

The biopsychosocial model of chronic pain recognizes the importance of a large number of factors, their interrelationships, and their contributions to ongoing suffering and eventually successful treatment (Keefe et al. 1996; Turk and Okifuji 2002). Controversy persists over which type of psychological treatment is most effective in the treatment of chronic pain. No differences were found between the treatment effects of cognitive versus behavioral therapies in patients mildly disabled by chronic LBP (Turner and Jensen 1993). Cognitive-behavioral therapy (CBT) provided as part of an individual therapy program offered no advantage over a group-based multidisciplinary program over 1 year (Turner-Stokes et al. 2003). Patients who are oriented toward self-management, with decreased perceptions of disability and less negative emotional responses to pain, are those most likely to improve (McCracken and Turk 2002). If treatment effects are to be optimized, more specific psychotherapies need to be designed for different types of pain patients.

Attempts to define more homogeneous subgroups of patients with chronic pain for the purpose of matching them with treatments have led to several empirical categorical or graded classifications based on different levels of psychosocial and functional impairment (Deardorff et al. 1993; Pfingsten et al. 2000; Riley et al. 1999a; Riley and Robinson 1998; Sanders and Brena 1993; Williams et al. 1995). Three groups have consistently been described across patient populations based on the Multidimensional Pain Inventory (Cook and Chastain 2001; Greco et al. 2003; Kerns et al. 1985; Turk and Rudy 1990; Weiner et al. 2001). The Dysfunctional group scores higher on pain severity, life interference due to pain, and psychological distress. This group also scores lower on perceptions of control and performance of daily activities. The Interpersonally Distressed group is characterized by the perception of poor support from others. The Adaptive Copers have lower ratings of pain severity, pain interference, affective distress, physical disability, and perceptions of being out of control. However, this subgroup classification did not predict the magnitude of positive treatment response for patients with chronic pain treated in a comprehensive interdisciplinary program (Gatchel et al. 2002). Tailoring psychological interventions to patient profiles based on psychosocial characteristics can result in greater and more prolonged improvement compared with usual care. In patients with early rheumatoid arthritis, tailoring or customizing CBT by assigning specific modules matched to patient priorities optimized the effectiveness of treatment (Evers et al. 2002).

Cognitive-Behavioral Therapy

Psychological treatment for chronic pain was pioneered by Fordyce, who used an operant conditioning behavioral model (Fordyce et al. 1973). The behavioral approach is based on an understanding of pain in a social context. The behaviors of the patient with chronic pain not only reinforce the behaviors of others but also are reinforced by others. Pain behaviors such as grimacing, guarding, and taking pain medication are indicators of perceived pain severity and functional disability, and such behaviors predict whether patients receive opioids (Chapman et al. 1985; Fordyce et al. 1984; Keefe et al. 1986; Romano et al. 1988; Turk and Matyas 1992; Turk and Okifuji 1997). In treatment, productive behaviors are targeted for reinforcement and pain behaviors are targeted for extinction. In practice, it remains unclear what type of patient benefits most from what type of behavioral treatment. For patients with chronic LBP, behavioral treatment decreased pain intensity and improved behavioral outcomes, including functional status, when compared with wait-listed control condition or no treatment, but not when it was added to usual treatment (van Tulder et al. 2001).

The cognitive-behavioral model of chronic pain assumes individual perceptions and evaluations of life experiences affect emotional and behavioral reactions to these experiences. If patients believe pain, depression, and disability are inevitable and uncontrollable, they will experience more negative affective responses, increased pain, and even more impaired physical and psychosocial functioning. The components of CBT, such as relaxation, cognitive restructuring, and coping self-statement training, interrupt this cycle of disability and enhance operant-behavioral treatment (Turner 1982a, 1982b; Turner and Chapman 1982). Patients are taught to become active participants in the management of their pain by using methods that minimize distressing thoughts and feelings.

Outcome studies of CBT in patients with syndromes ranging from specific painful diseases to vague functional somatoform symptoms have demonstrated significant improvements in pain intensity, pain behaviors, physical symptoms, affective distress, depression, coping, physical functioning, treatment-related and indirect socioeconomic costs, and return to work (Hiller et al. 2003; Keefe et al. 1990a; Kroenke and Swindle 2000; McCracken and Turk 2002; Turner 1982a; Turner and Romano 1990). The effectiveness of CBTs in adults with chronic pain has been documented in a meta-analysis across numerous outcome domains (Morley et al. 1999). The NNT was 2.3 in a meta-analysis of psychological treatment (relaxation, CBT) effectiveness for reducing the severity and frequency of chronic headache in children and adolescents (Eccleston et al. 2003). Pain reduction and improved physical function have been found to continue up to 12 months after the completion of active CBT (Gardea et al. 2001; Keefe et al. 1990b; Nielson and Weir 2001).

In a large HMO-based primary care study of back pain, a self-care intervention designed to provide education, reduce fear, promote attitudes favorable to self-management, and develop problem-solving skills to decrease pain and increase function significantly reduced back-related worry and fear–avoidance beliefs (Moore et al. 2000). Women, but not men, on sick leave for chronic spinal pain were at lower risk of taking early retirement at 18 months follow-up if they had been treated with physical therapy, CBT, or a combination of treatments compared with those in usual care (M.P. Jensen et al. 2001). Regardless of whether the women received CBT alone or in combination with physical therapy, CBT resulted in significant improvements in health-related quality of life. Elderly patients with chronic pain benefit more from CBT that presents information in concrete, well-organized, and brief formats (Kerns et al. 2001; Manetto and McPherson 1996; Middaugh and Pawlick 2002).

Patients on sick leave with nonspecific LBP treated with the addition of problem-solving therapy to behavioral graded activity had significantly fewer future sick leave days, higher rates of returning to work, and lower rates of receiving disability pensions (van den Hout et al. 2003). The risk for long-term sick absence of patients with spinal pain at risk for developing chronic pain was lowered by a factor of 9.3 at 1-year follow-up with a 6-session CBT group intervention (Linton and Andersson 2000). Pain-related fear and catastrophizing of patients were more likely to improve when the patients were exposed in vivo to individually tailored, fear-eliciting, and hierarchically ordered physical movements instead of following a general graded activity treatment program for back pain (Vlaeyen et al. 2002). A CBT program in a military population with nonmalignant chronic pain conditions reduced outpatient clinic visits by 87% in the first 3 months after treatment (Peters et al. 2000).

Mediators of Treatment Effects

The success of CBT has focused attention on many elements of the chronic pain experience to improve outcome. Adjustment is defined as the ability to carry out normal physical and psychosocial activities. The three dimensions of adjustment are social functioning (e.g., employment, functional ability), morale (e.g., depression, anxiety), and somatic health (e.g., pain intensity, medication use, health care utilization) (M.P. Jensen et al. 1991a; Lazarus and Folkman 1984). These concepts address resilience to the effects of chronic illness, the alleviation of suffering, and the development of a more positive concept of self or identity for the patient (Buchi et al. 2002).

Acceptance of chronic pain is a factor reported to influence patient adjustment. An analysis of patient accounts of their acceptance of chronic pain involved themes such as taking control, living day to day, acknowledging limitations, being empowered, accepting loss of self, believing that there is more to life than pain, not fighting battles that cannot be won, and relying on spiritual strength (Risdon et al. 2003). Therefore, acceptance is a realistic approach to living with pain that incorporates both disengagement from struggling against pain and engagement in productive everyday activities with achievable goals. Acceptance of pain is associated with reports of lower pain intensity, less pain-related anxiety and avoidance, less depression, less physical and psychosocial disability, more daily uptime, and better work status (McCracken 1998).

A *self-efficacy* expectancy is a belief about one's ability to perform a specific behavior, while an *outcome* expectancy is a belief about the consequences of performing a behavior. These variables have been derived from social learning theory and overlap with constructs such as locus of control and optimism (Anderson et al. 1995; Haugli et al. 2000; M.P. Jensen et al. 1991b; Keefe et al. 1992). Individuals are considered to be more likely to engage in coping efforts they believe are both within their capabilities and likely to result in a positive outcome. Patients with a variety of chronic pain syndromes who score higher on measures of self-efficacy or have an internal locus of control report lower levels of pain, higher pain thresholds, increased exercise performance, and more positive coping efforts (Asghari and Nicholas 2001; Barry et al. 2003; Berkke et al. 2001; Lackner and Carosella 1999). Evidence supports self-efficacy as a mediator of the relationship between pain intensity and disability (Arnstein 2000; Rudy et al. 2003).

The effectiveness of particular coping strategies is dependent on many aspects of a patient's experience. In a 6-month follow-up study of patients completing an inpatient pain program, improvement was associated with decreases in the use of passive coping strategies such as taking medications or hoping pain will decrease (M.P. Jensen et al. 1994). "Reinterpreting pain sensations as not being signs of ongoing injury" has been typically formulated as an active coping strategy. However, in a study of amputees with phantom limb pain, it was associated not with reduced pain levels but instead with greater psychosocial dysfunction. This coping strategy may not be appropriate for these patients because it requires greater amounts of time spent focusing on pain and disability, preventing them from engaging in social activities (Hill et al. 1995). Similarly, some types of emotion-focused coping are adaptive for some patients. For example, patients with myofascial pain were significantly more likely to report pain, impairment, and depression if they used passive coping strategies in contrast to emotion-focused coping, which was associated with significantly better adjustment (J.A. Smith et al. 2002). The coping strategies concept is consistent with the cognitive-behavioral model of chronic pain, although it still remains unclear how many unique coping strategies exist and whether changes in coping lead to or are the result of changes in patient adjustment (Hadjistavropoulos et al. 1999; M.P. Jensen et al. 1991a; Tan et al. 2001).

Placebo Response

Placebo effects are complex phenomena but similar to the effects of active treatments (Kleinman et al. 1994; Turner et al. 1994). The literature supporting the placebo effect has been criticized as flawed, misinterpreted, and overrated (Kienle and Kienle 1997). In a clinical setting it is difficult to separate "true" improvements from placebo responses to treatment as well as other factors such as regression to the mean and the natural history of the condition. Multiple patient and practitioner characteristics, such as expectancy, conditioning, and learning, affect the placebo response, and most are almost impossible to control for (Ploghaus et al. 2003; Price et al. 1999). Evidence supports a role of the endogenous opioid and sympathetic nervous systems in placebo-induced analgesia that can be reversed with opioid antagonists (Pollo et al. 2003; ter Riet et al. 1998).

Historically based on Beecher's original article, placebo interventions were a part of paternalistic medicine's treatment armamentarium (Kaptchuk 1998). In the era of randomized, controlled trials, placebos may be employed if cooperation of informed patients is secured. The magnitude of placebo analgesic effects was found to be significantly higher in studies that specifically investigated placebo analgesic mechanisms compared with those controlled trials that simply used a placebo for comparison

(Vase et al. 2002). However, there is controversy about the evidence of clinically important effects to justify the use of placebo interventions (Hrobjartsson and Gotzsche 2003). Using placebo to determine if the patient's pain is "real," or to "cure" a psychogenic condition by replacing an analgesic with a "neutral" substance, is dishonest, misleading, and counterproductive. A positive placebo response neither proves that the patient's pain is psychogenic nor shows that the patient would not benefit from an active treatment. Such an intervention can also result in loss of the patient's trust and render future treatment less effective.

Multidisciplinary Treatment

Methodology

Patients with chronic pain suffer dramatic reductions in physical, psychological, and social well-being with lower-rated health-related quality of life than those with almost all other medical conditions (Becker et al. 1997; Skevington 1998). The multidisciplinary pain center offers the full range of treatments for the most difficult pain syndromes in a setting that encourages patients to take an active role in improving their functional status and reinforces positive changes in behavior (Gibson et al. 1996; Helme et al. 1996). Specifically, interventions are designed to change maladaptive behavior such as inactivity and social withdrawal; alter maladaptive cognitions such as somatization, catastrophizing, and passive expectations of medical care; adopt active and positive coping skills; identify and stop operant conditioned behavior; and increase emotional control and stability while decreasing affective distress and depression.

Early failure of a single-modality treatment for chronic pain can have devastating consequences for future treatment attempts (Davies et al. 1997). A study of sequential trials of different treatment modalities found that the success of nerve blocks was diminished when used later in the treatment sequence.

A multidisciplinary approach starts with a serial evaluation by multiple specialists (Turk and Stieg 1987). Usually, this process implies a hierarchy of diagnostic importance. Psychiatry is often the last specialty to evaluate the patient, which may be perceived as signifying that psychological understanding is a low priority or that the other clinicians have decided the patient's pain is psychogenic. Even attempts at simultaneous evaluation by multiple specialists, including a psychiatrist or psychologist, can be misconstrued as trying to determine if symptoms are "real."

Interdisciplinary approaches combine areas of expertise to form a comprehensive formulation of chronic pain. The representatives of different fields of study recognize all symptoms can have a multiplicity of causes. These etiologies and diagnoses are all "real" and can be made by any number of specialists, if they are properly trained. When a specific diagnosis cannot be made, an etiology for the patient's symptoms has simply not yet been discovered. The patient no longer is stigmatized as having a "false" condition but instead is recognized as having a legitimate problem with understandable distress. The patient can remain in treatment to receive symptomatic interventions, functional rehabilitation, and the coordination of future evaluations.

Effectiveness

Multidisciplinary pain programs are often mistakenly equated with detoxification programs. It is true that most multidisciplinary programs pursue the goal of reducing inappropriate medication use. In one program, opioid use decreased from 83% to 58% of patients (Nissen et al. 2001). While reducing inappropriate medication use is necessary, it is almost never sufficient in achieving treatment goals. There is evidence that multidisciplinary pain programs improve patient functioning globally and in a number of specific areas, especially pain intensity, depression, disability, pain-related cognitions, and coping responses (Cutler et al. 1994; Fishbain et al. 1993; Flavell et al. 1996; M.P. Jensen et al. 2001). Multidisciplinary rehabilitation programs that include psychological and cognitive treatment are known to be effective for the treatment of chronic pain (Cutler et al. 1994; Fishbain et al. 1993; Flavell et al. 1996; Flor et al. 1992). Quality of life improves with multidisciplinary pain treatment, and good quality of life is associated with low levels of pain, distress, and interference with performing daily activities (Skevington et al. 2001). A meta-analysis of 65 studies evaluated the efficacy of treatments in patients who attended multidisciplinary pain clinics (Flor et al. 1992). Combination treatments were superior to unimodal treatments, treatment effects were maintained over a period of up to 7 years, and improvements were found not only on subjective but also on objective measures such as return to work and decreased health care utilization. Although more study is needed, the data support the conclusion that multidisciplinary pain clinic approaches are efficacious.

Ultimately, the goal of treating patients with chronic pain is to end disability and return them to work or other productive activities. Patients with chronic pain encounter many obstacles to returning to work, including their own negative perceptions and beliefs about work, such as poor self-efficacy and use of maladaptive coping strategies (Grossi et al. 1999; Marhold et al. 2002; Schult et al. 2000). In a longitudinal follow-up study of chronic back pain, patients who were not working and involved in litigation had the highest scores on measures of pain, depression, and disability (Suter 2002). One of the most important predictors is the patient's own intention of returning to work, which is less likely to be a function of pain than of job characteristics (Fishbain et al. 1997b). For example, job availability, satisfaction, dangerousness, physical demands, and litigation status are more likely to influence a patient's return to work (Fishbain et al. 1995, 1999a; Hildebrandt et al. 1997). In the longest follow-up study (13 years) of an inpatient pain management program, only half of the patients were unemployed, compared with almost 90% of the patients at the time of their admission (Maruta et al. 1998).

References

Abramson LY, Seligman MEP, Teasdale JD: Learned helplessness in humans: critique and reformulation. J Abnorm Psychol 87:49–74, 1978

Abramson LY, Alloy LB, Metalsky GI: Hopelessness depression: a theory-based subtype of depression. Psychol Rev 96:358–372, 1989

Acute Pain Management Guideline Panel: Acute Pain Management: Operative or Medical Procedures and Trauma. Clinical Practice Guideline. AHCPR Pub. No. 92–0032. Rockville, MD, Agency for Health Care Policy and Research, Public Health Service, U.S. Department of Health and Human Services, 1992

Adams MA, Mannion AF, Nolan P: Personal risk factors for first time low back pain. Spine 24:2497–2505, 1999

Adelman JU, Von Seggern R: Cost considerations in headache treatment, part 1: prophylactic migraine treatment. Headache 35:479–487, 1995

Allan L, Hays H, Jensen NH, et al: Randomised crossover trial of transdermal fentanyl and sustained release oral morphine for treating chronic non-cancer pain. BMJ 322:1154–1158, 2001

American Academy of Pain Medicine, the American Pain Society and the American Society of Addiction Medicine: Definitions related to the use of opioids for the treatment of pain. WMJ 100:28–29, 2001

American Geriatrics Society Panel on Chronic Pain in Older Persons: The management of chronic pain in older persons. J Am Geriatr Soc 46:635–651, 1998

American Psychiatric Association: Diagnostic and Statistical Manual of Mental Disorders, 2nd Edition. Washington, DC, American Psychiatric Press, 1968

American Psychiatric Association: Diagnostic and Statistical Manual of Mental Disorders, 3rd Edition. Washington, DC, American Psychiatric Press, 1980

American Psychiatric Association: Diagnostic and Statistical Manual of Mental Disorders, 3rd Edition, Revised. Washington, DC, American Psychiatric Press, 1987

American Psychiatric Association: Diagnostic and Statistical Manual of Mental Disorders, 4th Edition. Washington, DC, American Psychiatric Press, 1994

Anderson KO, Dowds BN, Pelletz RE, et al: Development and initial validation of a scale to measure self-efficacy beliefs in patients with chronic pain. Pain 63:77–84, 1995

Andersson HI, Ejlertsson G, Leden I, et al: Impact of chronic pain on health care seeking, self care, and medication: results from a population-based Swedish study. J Epidemiol Community Health 53:503–509, 1999

Ansari A: The efficacy of newer antidepressants in the treatment of chronic pain: a review of current literature. Harv Rev Psychiatry 7:257–277, 2000

Argoff CE: New analgesics for neuropathic pain: the lidocaine patch. Clin J Pain 16:S62–S66, 2000

Arkinstall W, Sandler A, Goughnour B, et al: Efficacy of controlled-release codeine in chronic non-malignant pain: a randomized, placebo-controlled clinical trial. Pain 62:169–178, 1995

Arnold LM, Hess EV, Hudson JI, et al: A randomized, placebo-controlled, double-blind, flexible-dose study of fluoxetine in the treatment of women with fibromyalgia. Am J Med 112:191–197, 2002

Arnstein P: The mediation of disability by self efficacy in different samples of chronic pain patients. Disabil Rehabil 22:794–801, 2000

Aronoff GM: Opioids in chronic pain management: is there a significant risk of addiction? Curr Rev Pain 4:112–121, 2000

Aronoff GM, Tota-Faucette M, Phillips L, et al: Are pain disorder and somatization disorder valid diagnostic entities? Curr Rev Pain 4:309–312, 2000

Asghari A, Nicholas MK: Pain self-efficacy beliefs and pain behaviour: a prospective study. Pain 94:85–100, 2001

Asmundson GJG, Norton PJ, Norton GR: Beyond pain: the role of fear and avoidance in chronicity. Clin Psychol Rev 19:97–119, 1999

Asmundson GJ, Bonin MF, Frombach IK, et al: Evidence of a disposition toward fearfulness and vulnerability to post-traumatic stress in dysfunctional pain patients. Behav Res Ther 38:801–812, 2000

Asmundson GJ, Coons MJ, Taylor S, et al: PTSD and the experience of pain: research and clinical implications of shared vulnerability and mutual maintenance models. Can J Psychiatry 47:930–937, 2002

Atkinson JH, Slater MA, Patterson TL, et al: Prevalence, onset and risk of psychiatric disorders in men with chronic low back pain: a controlled study. Pain 45:111–121, 1991

Atkinson JH, Slater MA, Williams RA, et al: A placebo-controlled randomized clinical trial of nortriptyline for chronic low back pain. Pain 76:287–296, 1998

Atkinson JH, Slater MA, Wahlgren DR, et al: Effects of noradrenergic and serotonergic antidepressants on chronic low back pain intensity. Pain 83:137–145, 1999

Auerbach SM, Laskin DM, Frantsve LM, et al: Depression, pain, exposure to stressful life events, and long-term outcomes in temporomandibular disorder patients. J Oral Maxillofac Surg 59:628–633, 2001

Axelrod DA, Proctor MC, Geisser ME, et al: Outcomes after surgery for thoracic outlet syndrome. J Vasc Surg 33:1220–1225, 2001

Backonja M, Beydoun A, Edwards KR, et al: Gabapentin for the symptomatic treatment of painful neuropathy in patients with diabetes mellitus: a randomized controlled trial. JAMA 280:1831–1836, 1998

Bair MJ, Robinson RL, Katon W, et al: Depression and pain comorbidity: a literature review. Arch Intern Med 163:2433–2445, 2003

Ballantyne JC, Mao J: Opioid therapy for chronic pain. N Engl J Med 349:1943–1953, 2003

Bank J: A comparative study of amitriptyline and fluvoxamine in migraine prophylaxis. Headache 34:476–478, 1994

Banks SM, Kerns RD: Explaining high rates of depression in chronic pain: a diathesis-stress framework. Psychol Bull 199:95–110, 1996

Barkin RL, Fawcett J: The management challenges of chronic pain: the role of antidepressants. Am J Ther 7:31–47, 2000

Barry LC, Guo Z, Kerns RD, et al: Functional self-efficacy and pain-related disability among older veterans with chronic pain in a primary care setting. Pain 104:131–137, 2003

Barsky AJ, Borus JF: Functional somatic syndromes. Ann Intern Med 130:910–921, 1999

Barsky AJ, Peekna HM, Borus JF: Somatic symptom reporting in women and men. J Gen Intern Med 16:266–275, 2001

Bartusch SL, Sanders BJ, D'Alessio JG, et al: Clonazepam for the treatment of lacinating phantom limb pain. Clin J Pain 12:59–62, 1996

Beck AT: Cognitive Therapy and the Emotional Disorders. London, Penguin, 1976

Becker N, Bondegaard Thomsen A, Olsen AK, et al: Pain epidemiology and health related quality of life in chronic non-malignant pain patients referred to a Danish multidisciplinary pain center. Pain 73:393–400, 1997

Belcheva S, Petkov VD, Konstantinova E, et al: Effects on nociception of the Ca2+ and 5-HT antagonist dotarizine and other 5-HT receptor agonists and antagonists. Acta Physiol Pharmacol Bulg 21:93–98, 1995

Bendtsen L, Jensen R, Olesen J: A non-selective (amitriptyline), but not a selective (citalopram) serotonin reuptake inhibitor is effective in the prophylactic treatment of chronic tension-type headache. J Neurol Neurosurg Psychiatry 61:285–290, 1996

Benjamin S, Morris S, McBeth J, et al: The association between chronic widespread pain and mental disorder: a population-based study. Arthritis Rheum 43:561–567, 2000

Bergdahl M, Bergdahl J: Burning mouth syndrome: prevalence and associated factors. J Oral Pathol Med 28:350–354, 1999

Bergouignan M: Cures heureuses de nevralgies faciales essentielles par le diphenyl-hydantoinate de soude. Rev Laryngol Otol Rhinol 63:34–41, 1942

Berkke M, Hjortdahl P, Kvien TK: Involvement and satisfaction: a Norwegian study of health care among 1,024 patients with rheumatoid arthritis and 1,509 patients with chronic noninflammatory musculoskeletal pain. Arthritis Rheum 45:8–15, 2001

Bodnar RJ, Hadjimarkou MM: Endogenous opiates and behavior: 2001. Peptides 23:2307–2365, 2002

Bogetto F, Maina G, Ferro G, et al: Psychiatric comorbidity in patients with burning mouth syndrome. Psychosom Med 60:378–385, 1998

Bolan EA, Tallarida RJ, Pasternak GW: Synergy between mu opioid ligands: evidence for functional interactions among mu opioid receptor subtypes. J Pharmacol Exp Ther 303:557–562, 2002

Bolay H, Moskowitz MA: Mechanisms of pain modulation in chronic syndromes. Neurology 59 (suppl 2):S2–S7, 2002

Bone M, Critchley P, Buggy DJ: Gabapentin in postamputation phantom limb pain: a randomized, double-blind, placebo-controlled, cross-over study. Reg Anesth Pain Med 27:481–516, 2002

Bonica JJ: Definitions and taxonomy of pain, in The Management of Pain. Edited by Bonica JJ. Philadelphia, PA, Lea & Febiger, 1990, pp 18–27

Borgland SL: Acute opioid receptor desensitization and tolerance: is there a link? Clin Exp Pharmacol Physiol 28:147–154, 2001

Boulton AJ: Causes of neuropathic pain. Diabet Med 10 (suppl 2): 87S–88S, 1993

Bowersox SS, Gadbois T, Singh T, et al: Selective N-type neuronal voltage-sensitive calcium channel blocker, SNX-111, produces spinal antinociception in rat models of acute, persistent and neuropathic pain. J Pharmacol Exp Ther 279:1243–1249, 1996

Bowsher D: The management of central post-stroke pain. Postgrad Med J 71:598–604, 1995

Bowsher D: Postherpetic neuralgia and its treatment: a retrospective survey of 191 patients. J Pain Symptom Manage 12:290–299, 1996

Bowsher D: The effects of pre-emptive treatment of postherpetic neuralgia with amitriptyline: a randomized, double-blind, placebo-controlled trial. J Pain Symptom Manage 13:327–331, 1997a

Bowsher D: The management of postherpetic neuralgia. Postgrad Med J 73:623–629, 1997b

Brattberg G, Parker MG, Thorslund M: The prevalence of pain among the oldest old in Sweden. Pain 67:29–34, 1996

Brattberg G, Parker MG, Thorslund M: A longitudinal study of pain: reported pain from middle age to old age. Clin J Pain 13:144–149, 1997

Breslau N, Davis GC: Migraine, physical health and psychiatric disorder: a prospective epidemiologic study in young adults. J Psychiatr Res 27:211–221, 1993

Brose WG, Gutlove DP, Luther RR, et al: Use of intrathecal SNX-111, a novel, N-type, voltage-sensitive, calcium channel blocker, in the management of intractable brachial plexus avulsion pain. Clin J Pain 13:256–259, 1997

Brown JW, Robertson LS, Kosa J, et al: A study of general practice in Massachusetts. JAMA 2216:301–306, 1971

Brown RL, Patterson JJ, Rounds LA, et al: Substance use among patients with chronic pain. J Fam Pract 43:152–160, 1996

Bruehl S, Carlson CR: Predisposing psychological factors in the development of reflex sympathetic dystrophy: a review of the empiric evidence. Clin J Pain 8:287–299, 1992

Bruehl S, Husfeldt B, Lubenow TR, et al: Psychological differences between reflex sympathetic dystrophy and non-RSD chronic pain patients. Pain 67:107–114, 1996

Bryans JS, Wustrow DJ: 3-substituted GABA analogs with central nervous system activity: a review. Med Res Rev 19:149–177, 1999

Bryson HM, Wilde MI: Amitriptyline: a review of its pharmacological properties and therapeutic use in chronic pain states. Drugs Aging 8:459–476, 1996

Buchi S, Buddeberg C, Klaghofer R, et al: Preliminary validation of PRISM (Pictorial Representation of Illness and Self Measure): a brief method to assess suffering. Psychother Psychosom 71:333–341, 2002

Buffett-Jerrott SE, Stewart SH: Cognitive and sedative effects of benzodiazepine use. Curr Pharm Des 8:45–58, 2002

Burkey AR, Carstens E, Wenniger JJ, et al: An opioidergic cortical antinociception triggering site in the agranular insular cortex of the rat that contributes to morphine antinociception. J Neurosci 16:6612–6623, 1996

Burns JW, Johnson BJ, Mahoney N, et al: Anger management style, hostility and spouse responses: gender differences in predictors of adjustment among chronic pain patients. Pain 64:445–453, 1996

Burns JW, Johnson BJ, Devine J, et al: Anger management style and the prediction of treatment outcome among male and female chronic pain patients. Behav Res Ther 36:1051–1062, 1998

Burns JW, Mullen JT, Higdon LJ, et al: Validity of the pain anxiety symptoms scale (PASS): prediction of physical capacity variables. Pain 84:247–252, 2000

Burns JW, Kubilus A, Bruehl S, et al: Do changes in cognitive factors influence outcome following multidisciplinary treatment for chronic pain? A cross-lagged panel analysis. J Consult Clin Psychol 71:81–91, 2003

Bymaster FP, Dreshfield-Ahmad LJ, Threlkeld PG, et al: Comparative affinity of duloxetine and venlafaxine for serotonin and norepinephrine transporters in vitro and in vivo, human serotonin receptor subtypes, and other neuronal receptors. Neuropsychopharmacology 25:871–880, 2001

Cahill CM, Morinville A, Lee MC, et al: Prolonged morphine treatment targets delta opioid receptors to neuronal plasma membranes and enhances delta-mediated antinociception. J Neurosci 21:7598–7607, 2001

Caldwell JR, Rapoport RJ, Davis JC, et al: Efficacy and safety of a once-daily morphine formulation in chronic, moderate-to-severe osteoarthritis pain: results from a randomized, placebo-controlled, double-blind trial and an open-label extension trial. J Pain Symptom Manage 23:278–291, 2002

Canavero S, Bonicalzi V: Lamotrigine control of central pain. Pain 68:179–181, 1996

Caplehorn JR, Drummer OH: Fatal methadone toxicity: signs and circumstances, and the role of benzodiazepines. Aust N Z J Public Health 26:358–362, 2002

Carey KB, Purnine DM, Maisto SA, et al: Treating substance abuse in the context of severe and persistent mental illness: clinicians' perspectives. J Subst Abuse Treat 19:189–198, 2000

Carey TS, Garrett JM, Jackman AM: Beyond the good prognosis: examination of an inception cohort of patients with chronic low back pain. Spine 25:115–120, 2000

Carter GT, Sullivan MD: Antidepressants in pain management. Curr Opin Invest Drugs 3:454–458, 2002

Cassano P, Fava M: Depression and public health: an overview. J Psychosom Res 53:849–857, 2002

Chabal C, Jacobson L, Chaney EF, et al: Narcotics for chronic pain: yes or no? A useless dichotomy. Am Pain Soc J 1:276–281, 1992a

Chabal C, Jacobson L, Mariano AJ, et al: The use of oral mexiletine for the treatment of pain after peripheral nerve injury. Anesthesiology 76:513–517, 1992b

Chabal C, Erjavec MK, Jacobson L, et al: Prescription opiate abuse in chronic pain patients: clinical criteria, incidence, and predictors. Clin J Pain 13:150–155, 1997

Chapman CR, Casey KL, Dubner R, et al: Pain measurement: an overview. Pain 22:1–31, 1985

Chapman SL, Byas-Smith MG, Reed BA: Effects of intermediate- and long-term use of opioids on cognition in patients with chronic pain. Clin J Pain 18:S83–S90, 2002

Chen SR, Xu Z, Pan HL: Stereospecific effect of pregabalin on ectopic afferent discharges and neuropathic pain induced by sciatic nerve ligation in rats. Anesthesiology 95:1473–1479, 2001

Cheshire WP: Defining the role for gabapentin in the treatment of trigeminal neuralgia: a retrospective study. J Pain 3:137–142, 2002

Christensen D, Kayser V: The development of pain-related behaviour and opioid tolerance after neuropathy-inducing surgery and sham surgery. Pain 88:231–238, 2000

Ciaramella A, Grosso S, Poli P: Fluoxetine versus fluvoxamine for treatment of chronic pain. Minerva Anestesiol 66:55–61, 2000

Ciccone DS, Bandilla EB, Wu W: Psychological dysfunction in patients with reflex sympathetic dystrophy. Pain 71:323–333, 1997

Ciccone DS, Just N, Bandilla EB: A comparison of economic and social reward in patients with chronic nonmalignant back pain. Psychosom Med 61:552–563, 1999

Ciccone DS, Just N, Bandilla EB, et al: Psychological correlates of opioid use in patients with chronic nonmalignant pain: a preliminary test of the downhill spiral hypothesis. J Pain Symptom Manage 20:180–192, 2000

Clark JD: Chronic pain prevalence and analgesic prescribing in a general medical population. J Pain Symptom Manage 23:131–137, 2002

Clark MR: Pain, in Textbook of Geriatric Neuropsychiatry. Edited by Coffey CE, Cummings JL. Washington, DC, American Psychiatric Press Inc., 2000a, pp 415–440

Clark MR: Pharmacological treatments for chronic nonmalignant pain. Int Rev Psychiatry 12:148–156, 2000b

Clark MR, Cox TS: Refractory Chronic Pain. Psychiatr Clin North Am 25:71–88, 2002

Clark WC, Yang JC, Tsui SL, et al: Unidimensional pain rating scales: a multidimensional affect and pain survey (MAPS) analysis of what they really measure. Pain 98:241–247, 2002

Cohen GL: Protriptyline, chronic tension-type headaches, and weight loss in women. Headache 37:433–436, 1997

Cohen MJ, Jasser S, Herron PD, et al: Ethical perspectives: opioid treatment of chronic pain in the context of addiction. Clin J Pain 18:S99–S107, 2002

Collins SL, Moore RA, McQuay HJ, et al: Antidepressants and anticonvulsants for diabetic neuropathy and postherpetic neuralgia: a quantitative systematic review. J Pain Symptom Manage 20:449–458, 2000

Compton P, Darakjian J, Miotto K: Screening for addiction in patients with chronic pain and "problematic" substance use: evaluation of a pilot assessment tool. J Pain Symptom Manage 16:355–363, 1998

Cook AJ, Chastain DC: The classification of patients with chronic pain: age and sex differences. Pain Res Manag 6:142–151, 2001

Cook RJ, Sackett DL: The number needed to treat: a clinically useful measure of treatment effect. BMJ 310:452–454, 1995

Cote P, Hogg-Johnson S, Cassidy JD, et al: The association between neck pain intensity, physical functioning, depressive symptomatology and time-to-claim-closure after whiplash. J Clin Epidemiol 54:275–286, 2001

Croft PR, Papageorgiou AC, Ferry S, et al: Psychological distress and low back pain: evidence from a prospective study in the general population. Spine 20:2731–2737, 1996

Crombez G, Eccleston C, Baeyens F, et al: When somatic information threatens, catastrophic thinking enhances attentional interference. Pain 75:187–198, 1998

Cutler BR, Fishbain DA, Rosomoff HL, et al: Does nonsurgical pain center treatment of chronic pain return patients to work? A review and meta-analysis of the literature. Spine 19:643–652, 1994

Cutrer FM: Antiepileptic drugs: how they work in headache. Headache 41:S3–S10, 2001

Dahl B, Gehrchen PM, Kiaer T, et al: Nonorganic pain drawings are associated with low psychological scores on the preoperative SF-36 questionnaire in patients with chronic low back pain. Eur Spine J 10:211–214, 2001

Daniell HW: Narcotic-induced hypogonadism during therapy for heroin addiction. J Addict Dis 21:47–53, 2002

Davies HT, Crombie IK, Brown JH, et al: Diminishing returns or appropriate treatment strategy? An analysis of short-term outcomes after pain clinic treatment. Pain 70:203–208, 1997

Davis RW: Successful treatment for phantom pain. Orthopaedics 16:691–695, 1993

Deardorff WW, Chino AF, Scott DW: Characteristics of chronic pain patients: factor analysis of the MMPI-2. Pain 54:153–158, 1993

DeBerard MS, Masters KS, Colledge AL, et al: Outcomes of posterolateral lumbar fusion in Utah patients receiving workers' compensation: a retrospective cohort study. Spine 26:738–746, 2001

DeGood DE, Cundiff GW, Adams LE, et al: A psychosocial and behavioral comparison of reflex sympathetic dystrophy, low back pain, and headache patients. Pain 54:317–322, 1993

Dejgard A, Petersen P, Kastrup J: Mexiletine for treatment of chronic painful diabetic neuropathy. Lancet 1:9–11, 1988

Dellemijn PL, Fields HL: Do benzodiazepines have a role in chronic pain management? Pain 57:137–152, 1994

Dellemijn PL, Vanneste JA: Randomised double-blind active-placebo-controlled crossover trial of intravenous fentanyl in neuropathic pain. Lancet 349:753–758, 1997

Dersh J, Polatin PB, Gatchel RJ: Chronic pain and psychopathology: research findings and theoretical considerations. Psychosom Med 64:773–786, 2002

Detke MJ, Lu Y, Goldstein DJ, et al: Duloxetine 60 mg once daily dosing versus placebo in the acute treatment of major depression. J Psychiatr Res 36:383–390, 2002

Devlen J: Anxiety and depression in migraine. J R Soc Med 87:338–341, 1994

Devor M, Amir R, Rappaport ZH: Pathophysiology of trigeminal neuralgia: the ignition hypothesis. Clin J Pain 18:4–13, 2002

Deyo RA, Weinstein JN: Low back pain. N Engl J Med 344:363–370, 2001

Dickens C, Jayson M, Sutton C, et al: The relationship between pain and depression in a trial using paroxetine in sufferers of chronic low back pain. Psychosomatics 41:490–499, 2000

Dickens C, McGowan L, Clark-Carter D, et al: Depression in rheumatoid arthritis: a systematic review of the literature with meta-analysis. Psychosom Med 64:52–60, 2002

Dickinson WP, Dickinson LM, deGruy FV, et al: The somatization in primary care study: a tale of three diagnoses. Gen Hosp Psychiatry 25:1–7, 2003

Dogrul A, Zagli U, Tulunay FC: The role of T-type calcium channels in morphine analgesia, development of antinociceptive tolerance and dependence to morphine, and morphine abstinence syndrome. Life Sci 71:725–734, 2002

Dohrenwend BP, Raphael KG, Marbach JJ, et al: Why is depression comorbid with chronic myofascial face pain? A family study of alternative hypotheses. Pain 83:183–192, 1999

Donner B, Zenz M, Tryba M, et al: Direct conversion from oral morphine to transdermal fentanyl: a multicenter study in patients with cancer pain. Pain 64:527–534, 1996

Drage LA, Rogers RS 3rd: Burning mouth syndrome. Dermatol Clin 21:135–145, 2003

Drolet G, Dumont EC, Gosselin I, et al: Role of endogenous opioid system in the regulation of the stress response. Prog Neuropsychopharmacol Biol Psychiatry 25:729–741, 2001

Drug Enforcement Administration: A joint statement from 21 health organizations and the Drug Enforcement Administration. Promoting pain relief and preventing abuse of pain medications: a critical balancing act. J Pain Symptom Manage 24:147, 2002

Druss BG, Rosenheck RA, Sledge WH: Health and disability costs of depressive illness in a major U.S. corporation. Am J Psychiatry 157:1274–1278, 2000

Dworkin RH, Schmader KE: Treatment and prevention of postherpetic neuralgia. Clin Infect Dis 36:877–882, 2003

Dworkin RH, Hetzel RD, Banks SM: Toward a model of the pathogenesis of chronic pain. Semin Clin Neuropsychiatry 4:176–185, 1999

Dworkin SF, Von Korff M, LeResche L: Multiple pains and psychiatric disturbance: an epidemiologic investigation. Arch Gen Psychiatry 47:239–244, 1990

Dworkin SF, Huggins KH, Wilson L, et al: A randomized clinical trial using research diagnostic criteria for temporomandibular disorders-axis II to target clinic cases for a tailored self-care TMD treatment program. J Orofac Pain 16:48–63, 2002

Eccleston C, Yorke L, Morley S, et al: Psychological therapies for the management of chronic and recurrent pain in children and adolescents. Cochrane Database Syst Rev 1: CD003968, 2003

Edwards R, Augustson EM, Fillingim R: Sex-specific effects of pain-related anxiety on adjustment to chronic pain. Clin J Pain 16:46–53, 2000

Ehde DM, Jensen MP, Engel JM, et al: Chronic pain secondary to disability: a review. Clin J Pain 19:3–17, 2003

Eide PK, Stubhaug A, Stenehjem AE: Central dysesthesia pain after traumatic spinal cord injury is dependent on N-methyl-D-aspartate receptor activation. Neurosurgery 37:1080–1087, 1995

Eisenberg E, Lurie Y, Braker C, et al: Lamotrigine reduces painful diabetic neuropathy: a randomized controlled study. Neurology 57:505–509, 2001

Elias WJ, Burchiel KJ: Trigeminal neuralgia and other neuropathic pain syndromes of the head and face. Curr Pain Headache Rep 6:115–124, 2002

Emanuel EJ, Fairclough DL, Daniels ER, et al: Euthanasia and physician-assisted suicide: attitudes and experiences of oncology patients, oncologists, and the public. Lancet 347:1805–1810, 1996

Enggaard TP, Klitgaard NA, Gram LF, et al: Specific effect of venlafaxine on single and repetitive experimental painful stimuli in humans. Clin Pharmacol Ther 69:245–251, 2001

Epker J, Gatchel RJ: Coping profile differences in the biopsychosocial functioning of patients with temporomandibular disorder. Psychosom Med 62:69–75, 2000

Ericsson M, Poston WS, Linder J, et al: Depression predicts disability in long-term chronic pain patients. Disabil Rehabil 24:334–340, 2002

Ernst E, Bartu A, Popescu A, et al: Methadone-related deaths in Western Australia 1993–99. Aust NZ J Public Health 26:364–370, 2002

Evers AW, Kraaimaat FW, van Riel PL, et al: Tailored cognitive-behavioral therapy in early rheumatoid arthritis for patients at risk: a randomized controlled trial. Pain 100:141–153, 2002

Fanciullo GJ, Ball PA, Girault G, et al: An observational study on the prevalence and pattern of opioid use in 25,479 patients with spine and radicular pain. Spine 27:201–205, 2002

Farrar JT, Young JP Jr, LaMoreaux L, et al: Clinical importance of changes in chronic pain intensity measured on an 11-point numerical pain rating scale. Pain 94:149–158, 2001

Feighner JP: Mechanism of action of antidepressant medications. J Clin Psychiatry 60 (suppl 4):4–11, 1999

Feldman SI, Downey G, Schaffer-Neitz R: Pain, negative mood, and perceived support in chronic pain patients: a daily diary study of people with reflex sympathetic dystrophy syndrome. J Consult Clin Psychol 67:776–785, 1999

Fernandez E, Turk DC: The scope and significance of anger in the experience of chronic pain. Pain 61:165–175, 1995

Ferrell BA: Overview of aging and pain, in Pain in the Elderly. Edited by Ferrell BR, Ferrell BA. Seattle, WA, IASP Press, 1996, pp 1–10

Ferrell BA: The management of pain in long-term care. Clin J Pain 20:240–243, 2004

Ferrell BA, Ferrell BR, Rivera L: Pain in cognitively impaired nursing home patients. J Pain Symptom Manage 10:591–598, 1995

Fields HL, Rowbotham M, Baron R: Postherpetic neuralgia: irritable nociceptors and deafferentation. Neurobiol Dis 5:209–227, 1998

Fillingim RB: Sex, gender, and pain: women and men really are different. Curr Rev Pain 4:24–30, 2000

Fillingim RB, Doleys DM, Edwards RR, et al: Clinical characteristics of chronic back pain as a function of gender and oral opioid use. Spine 28:143–150, 2003

Fishbain DA: Approaches to treatment decisions for psychiatric comorbidity in the management of the chronic pain patient. Med Clin North Am 83:737–760, 1999a

Fishbain DA: The association of chronic pain and suicide. Semin Clin Neuropsychiatry 4:221–227, 1999b

Fishbain DA, Goldberg M, Meagher BR, et al: Male and female chronic pain patients characterized by DSM-III diagnostic criteria. Pain 26:181–187, 1986

Fishbain DA, Goldberg M, Rosomoff RS, et al: Completed suicide in chronic pain. Clin J Pain 7:29–36, 1991

Fishbain DA, Rosomoff HL, Rosomoff RS: Drug abuse, dependence: addiction in chronic pain patients. Clin J Pain 8:77–85, 1992

Fishbain DA, Rosomoff HL, Goldberg M, et al: The prediction of return to the workplace after multidisciplinary pain center treatment. Clin J Pain 9:3–15, 1993

Fishbain DA, Rosomoff HL, Cutler RB, et al: Do chronic pain patients' perceptions about their preinjury jobs determine their intent to return to the same type of job post-pain facility treatment? Clin J Pain 11:267–278, 1995

Fishbain DA, Cutler R, Rosomoff HL, et al: Chronic pain-associated depression: antecedent or consequence of chronic pain? A review. Clin J Pain 13:116–137, 1997a

Fishbain DA, Cutler RB, Rosomoff HL, et al: Impact of chronic pain patients' job perception variables on actual return to work. Clin J Pain 13:197–206, 1997b

Fishbain D, Cutler R, Rosomoff H: Comorbid psychiatric disorders in chronic pain patients. Pain Clin 11:79–87, 1998

Fishbain DA, Cutler RB, Rosomoff HL, et al: Prediction of "intent," "discrepancy with intent," and "discrepancy with nonintent" for the patient with chronic pain to return to work after treatment at a pain facility. Clin J Pain 15:141–150, 1999a

Fishbain DA, Cutler RB, Rosomoff HL, et al: Validity of self-report drug use in chronic pain patients. Clin J Pain 15:184–191, 1999b

Fisher A, Zakrzewska JM, Patsalos PN: Trigeminal neuralgia: current treatments and future developments. Expert Opin Emerg Drugs 8:123–143, 2002

Fisher BJ, Haythornthwaite JA, Heinberg LJ, et al: Suicidal intent in patients with chronic pain. Pain 89:199–206, 2001

Fishman SM, Bandman TB, Edwards A, et al: The opioid contract in the management of chronic pain. J Pain Symptom Manage 18:27–37, 1999

Fishman SM, Wilsey B, Yang J, et al: Adherence monitoring and drug surveillance in chronic opioid therapy. J Pain Symptom Manage 20:293–307, 2000

Fishman SM, Mahajan G, Jung S, et al: The trilateral opioid contract: bridging the pain clinic and the primary care physician through the opioid contract. J Pain Symptom Manage 24:335–344, 2002

Flavell HA, Carrafa GP, Thomas CH, et al: Managing chronic back pain: impact of an interdisciplinary team approach. Med J Aust 165:253–255, 1996

Flor H, Fydrich T, Turk DC: Efficacy of multidisciplinary pain treatment centers: a meta-analytic review. Pain 49:221–230, 1992

Foley K: Pain in the elderly, in Principles of Geriatric Medicine and Gerontology. Edited by Hazzard WR, Bierman EL, Blass JP, et al. New York, McGraw-Hill, 1994, pp 317–331

Fordyce W, Fowler R, Lehmann J, et al: Operant conditioning in the treatment of chronic pain. Arch Phys Med Rehabil 54:399–408, 1973

Fordyce WE, Lansky D, Calsyn DA, et al: Pain measurement and pain behavior. Pain 18:53–69, 1984

Formaker BK, Frank ME: Taste function in patients with oral burning. Chem Senses 25:575–581, 2000

Formaker BK, Mott AE, Frank ME: The effects of topical anesthesia on oral burning in burning mouth syndrome. Ann N Y Acad Sci 855:776–780, 1998

Forman WB: Opioid analgesic drugs in the elderly. Clin Geriatr Med 12:489–500, 1996

Forseth KO, Husby G, Gran JT, et al: Prognostic factors for the development of fibromyalgia in women with self-reported musculoskeletal pain: a prospective study. J Rheumatol 26:2458–2467, 1999

Forssell H, Jaaskelainen S, Tenovuo O, et al: Sensory dysfunction in burning mouth syndrome. Pain 99:41–47, 2002

Foster CA, Bafaloukos J: Paroxetine in the treatment of chronic daily headache. Headache 34:587–589, 1994

France RD, Ruban BJ, Keefe FJ: Long-term use of narcotic analgesics in chronic pain. Soc Sci Med 19:1379–1382, 1984

Freye E, Latasch L: Development of opioid tolerance: molecular mechanisms and clinical consequences. Anasthesiol Intensivmed Notfallmed Schmerzther 38:14–26, 2003

Fritzell P, Hagg O, Wessberg P, et al: Lumbar fusion versus nonsurgical treatment for chronic low back pain: a multicenter randomized controlled trial from the Swedish Lumbar Spine Study Group. Spine 26:2521–2532, 2001

Furlan AD, Brosseau L, Imamura M, et al: Massage for low-back pain: a systematic review within the framework of the Cochrane Collaboration Back Review Group. Spine 27:1896–1910, 2002

Gallagher RM, Verma S: Managing pain and comorbid depression: a public health challenge. Semin Clin Neuropsychiatry 4:203–220, 1999

Gallagher RM, Mueller LL, Freitag FG: Divalproex sodium in the treatment of migraine and cluster headache. J Am Osteopath Assoc 102:92–94, 2002

Gardea MA, Gatchel RJ, Mishra KD: Long-term efficacy of biobehavioral treatment of temporomandibular disorders. J Behav Med 24:341–359, 2001

Gatch MB, Negus SS, Mello NK: Antinociceptive effects of monoamine reuptake inhibitors administered alone or in combination with mu opioid agonists in rhesus monkeys. Psychopharmacology 135:99–106, 1998

Gatchel RJ, Noe CE, Pulliam C, et al: A preliminary study of Multidimensional Pain Inventory profile differences in predicting treatment outcome in a heterogeneous cohort of patients with chronic pain. Clin J Pain 18:139–143, 2002

Gaynes BN, Burns BJ, Tweed DL, et al: Depression and health-related quality of life. J Nerv Ment Dis 190:799–806, 2002

Geertzen JH, de Bruijn-Kofman AT, de Bruijn HP, et al: Stressful life events and psychological dysfunction in complex regional pain syndrome type I. Clin J Pain 14:143–147, 1998

Geisser ME, Roth RS, Theisen ME, et al: Negative affect, self-report of depressive symptoms, and clinical depression: relation to the experience of chronic pain. Clin J Pain 16:110–120, 2000

Gibson SJ, Farrell MJ, Katz B, et al: Multidisciplinary management of chronic nonmalignant pain in older adults, in Pain in the Elderly. Edited by Ferrell BR, Ferrell BA. Seattle, WA, IASP Press, 1996, pp 91–99

Gilron I, Bailey J, Weaver DF, et al: Patients' attitudes and prior treatments in neuropathic pain: a pilot study. Pain Res Manag 7:199–203, 2002

Gilson AM, Joranson DE: Controlled substances and pain management: changes in knowledge and attitudes of state medical regulators. J Pain Symptom Manage 21:227–237, 2001

Gilson AM, Joranson DE: U.S. policies relevant to the prescribing of opioid analgesics for the treatment of pain in patients with addictive disease. Clin J Pain 18:S91–S98, 2002

Goadsby PJ: How do the currently used prophylactic agents work in migraine? Cephalalgia 17:85–92, 1997

Goetz CG, Tannen CM, Levy M, et al: Pain in Parkinson's disease. Mov Disord 10:541–549, 1986

Goodkin K, Gullion C, Agras WS: A randomized, double-blind, placebo-controlled trial of trazodone hydrochloride in chronic low back pain syndrome. J Clin Psychopharmacol 10:269–278, 1990

Goodnick PJ, Breakstone K, Kumar A, et al: Nefazodone in diabetic neuropathy: response and biology. Psychosom Med 62:599–600, 2000

Gordon RS: Pain in the elderly. JAMA 241:2191–2192, 1979

Grabe HJ, Meyer C, Hapke U, et al: Somatoform pain disorder in the general population. Psychother Psychosom 72:88–94, 2003

Greco CM, Rudy TE, Manzi S: Adaptation to chronic pain in systemic lupus erythematosus: applicability of the Multidimensional Pain Inventory. Pain Med 4:39–50, 2003

Greenberg J, Burns JW: Pain anxiety among chronic pain patients: specific phobia or manifestation of anxiety sensitivity? Behav Res Ther 41:223–240, 2003

Greenwald BD, Narcessian EJ, Pomeranz BA: Assessment of physiatrists' knowledge and perspectives on the use of opioids: review of basic concepts for managing chronic pain. Am J Phys Med Rehabil 78:408–415, 1999

Grond S, Radbruch L, Lehmann KA: Clinical pharmacokinetics of transdermal opioids: focus on transdermal fentanyl. Clin Pharmacokinet 38:59–89, 2000

Grossi G, Soares JJ, Angesleva J, et al: Psychosocial correlates of long-term sick-leave among patients with musculoskeletal pain. Pain 80:607–619, 1999

Gruber AJ, Hudson JI, Pope HG Jr: The management of treatment-resistant depression in disorders on the interface of psychiatry and medicine: fibromyalgia, chronic fatigue syndrome, migraine, irritable bowel syndrome, atypical facial pain, and premenstrual dysphoric disorder. Psychiatr Clin North Am 19:351–369, 1996

Grushka M, Epstein JB, Gorsky M: Burning mouth syndrome. Am Fam Physician 65:615–620, 622, 2002

Grushka M, Epstein JB, Gorsky M: Burning mouth syndrome and other oral sensory disorders: a unifying hypothesis. Pain Res Manag 8:133–135, 2003

Gureje O, Von Korff M, Simon GE, et al: Persistent pain and well-being: a World Health Organization study in primary care. JAMA 280:147–151, 1998

Gustorff B, Nahlik G, Spacek A, et al: Gabapentin in the treatment of chronic intractable pain. Schmerz 16:9–14, 2002

Haddox JD: Psychological aspects of reflex sympathetic dystrophy: pain and the sympathetic nervous system. Edited by Stanton-Hicks M. Boston, MA, Kluwer Academic, 1990, pp 207–224

Hadjistavropoulos HD, MacLeod FK, Asmundson GJ: Validation of the Chronic Pain Coping Inventory. Pain 80:471–481, 1999

Hagg O, Fritzell P, Oden A, et al: Simplifying outcome measurement: evaluation of instruments for measuring outcome after fusion surgery for chronic low back pain. Spine 27:1213–1222, 2002

Hamilton M: Researching harm reduction: care and contradictions. Subst Use Misuse 34:119–141, 1999

Harbinson J, Dennehy F, Keating D: Lamotrigine for pain with hyperalgesia. Ir Med J 90:56, 1997

Harter M, Reuter K, Weisser B, et al: A descriptive study of psychiatric disorders and psychosocial burden in rehabilitation patients with musculoskeletal diseases. Arch Phys Med Rehabil 83:461–468, 2002

Hasenbring M, Marienfeld G, Kuhlendahl D, et al: Risk factors of chronicity in lumbar disc patients: a prospective investigation of biologic, psychologic, and social predictors of therapy outcome. Spine 19:2759–2765, 1994

Hasenbring M, Hallner D, Klasen B: Psychological mechanisms in the transition from acute to chronic pain: over- or underrated? Schmerz 15:442–447, 2001

Hasselstrom J, Liu-Palmgren J, Rasjo-Wraak G: Prevalence of pain in general practice. Eur J Pain 6:375–385, 2002

Hathaway AD: Shortcomings of harm reduction: toward a morally invested drug reform strategy. Int J Drug Policy 12:125–137, 2001

Haugli L, Steen E, Laerum E, et al: Agency orientation and chronic musculoskeletal pain: effects of a group learning program based on the personal construct theory. Clin J Pain 16:281–289, 2000

Haythornthwaite JA, Sieber WJ, Kerns RD: Depression and the chronic pain experience. Pain 46:177–184, 1991

Heim HM, Oei TPS: Comparison of prostate cancer patients with and without pain. Pain 53:159–162, 1993

Hein S, Bonsignore M, Barkow K, et al: Lifetime depressive and somatic symptoms as preclinical markers of late-onset depression. Eur Arch Psychiatry Clin Neurosci 253:16–21, 2003

Heiskanen T, Kalso E: Controlled-release oxycodone and morphine in cancer related pain. Pain 73:37–45, 1997

Helme RD, Katz B, Gibson SJ, et al: Multidisciplinary pain clinics for older people: do they serve a role? Clin Geriatr Med 12:563–582, 1996

Hendler N, Cimini C, Ma T, et al: A comparison of cognitive impairment due to benzodiazepines and to narcotics. Am J Psychiatry 137:828–830, 1980

Herr KA, Mobily PR: Comparison of selected pain assessment tools for use with the elderly. Appl Nurs Res 6:39–46, 1993

Hildebrandt J, Pfingsten M, Franz C, et al: Mutltidisciplinary treatment program for chronic low back pain, part 1: overview. Schmerz 10:190–203, 1996

Hildebrandt J, Pfingsten M, Saur P, et al: Prediction of success from a multidisciplinary treatment program for chronic low back pain. Spine 22:990–1001, 1997

Hill A, Niven CA, Knussen C: The role of coping in adjustment to phantom limb pain. Pain 62:79–86, 1995

Hiller W, Fichter MM, Rief W: A controlled treatment study of somatoform disorders including analysis of healthcare utilization and cost-effectiveness. J Psychosom Res 54:369–380, 2003

Hodoglugil U, Guney HZ, Savran B, et al: Temporal variation in the interaction between calcium channel blockers and morphine-induced analgesia. Chronobiol Int 13:227–234, 1996

Hoffman NG, Olofsson O, Salen B, et al: Prevalence of abuse and dependency in chronic pain patients. Int J Addict 30:919–927, 1995

Holister LE, Conley FK, Britt R, et al: Long-term use of diazepam. JAMA 246:1568–1570, 1981

Holroyd KA, O'Donnell FJ, Stensland M, et al: Mangement of chronic tension-type headache with tricyclic antidepressant medication, stress management therapy, and their combination: a randomized controlled trial. JAMA 285:2208–2215, 2001

Hotopf M, Mayou R, Wadsworth M, et al: Temporal relationships between physical symptoms and psychiatric disorder: results from a national birth cohort. Br J Psychiatry 173:255–261, 1998

Houtchens MK, Richert JR, Sami A, et al: Open label gabapentin treatment for pain in multiple sclerosis. Mult Scler 3:250–253, 1997

Hrobjartsson A, Gotzsche PC: Placebo treatment versus no treatment. Cochrane Database Syst Rev 1:CD003974, 2003

Hunt SP, Mantyh PW: The molecular dynamics of pain control. Nat Rev Neurosci 2:83–91, 2001

Huppe A, Raspe H: Efficacy of inpatient rehabilitation for chronic back pain in Germany: a systematic review 1980–2001. Rehabilitation 42:143–154, 2003

Inturrisi CE: Clinical pharmacology of opioids for pain. Clin J Pain 18:S3–S13, 2002

Jackson JL, O'Malley PG, Tomkins G, et al: Treatment of functional gastrointestinal disorders with antidepressant medications: a meta-analysis. Am J Med 108:65–72, 2000

Jain KK: An evaluation of intrathecal ziconotide for the treatment of chronic pain. Expert Opin Investig Drugs 9:2403–2410, 2000

Jamison RN, Kauffman J, Katz NP: Characteristics of methadone maintenance patients with chronic pain. J Pain Symptom Manage 19:53–62, 2000

Jensen MP, Turner JA, Romano JM, et al: Coping with chronic pain: a critical review of the literature. Pain 47:249–283, 1991a

Jensen MP, Turner JA, Romano JM: Self-efficacy and outcome expectancies: relationship to chronic pain coping strategies and adjustment. Pain 44:263–269, 1991b

Jensen MP, Turner JA, Romano JM: Correlates of improvement in multidisciplinary treatment of chronic pain. J Consult Clin Psychol 62:172–179, 1994

Jensen MP, Turner JA, Romano JM: Changes in beliefs, catastrophizing, and coping are associated with improvement in multidisciplinary pain treatment. J Consult Clin Psychol 69:655–662, 2001

Jensen R, Brinck T, Olesen J: Sodium valproate has a prophylactic effect in migraine without aura: a triple-blind, placebo-controlled crossover study. Neurology 44:647–651, 1994

Jensen TS: Anticonvulsants in neuropathic pain: rationale and clinical evidence. Eur J Pain 6 (suppl A):61–68, 2002

Joffroy A, Levivier M, Massager N: Trigeminal neuralgia: pathophysiology and treatment. Acta Neurol Belg 101:20–25, 2001

Johnson RW: Herpes zoster and postherpetic neuralgia: optimal treatment. Drugs Aging 10:80–94, 1997

Johnson RW, Dworkin RH: Treatment of herpes zoster and postherpetic neuralgia. BMJ 326:748–750, 2003

Joranson DE, Gilson AM, Dahl JL, et al: Pain management, controlled substances, and state medical board policy: a decade of change. J Pain Symptom Manage 23:138–147, 2002

Juang KD, Wang SJ, Fuh JL, et al: Comorbidity of depressive and anxiety disorders in chronic daily headache and its subtypes. Headache 40:818–823, 2000

Jung AC, Staiger T, Sullivan M: The efficacy of selective serotonin reuptake inhibitors for the management of chronic pain. J Gen Intern Med 12:384–389, 1997

Junge A, Dvorak J, Ahrens S: Predictors of bad and good outcomes of lumbar disc surgery: a prospective clinical study with recommendations for screening to avoid bad outcomes. Spine 20:460–468, 1995

Kalso E, Tramer MR, McQuay HJ, et al: Systemic local-anaesthetic-type drugs in chronic pain: a systematic review. Eur J Pain 2:3–14, 1998

Kaniecki RG: A comparison of divalproex with propranolol and placebo for the prophylaxis of migraine without aura. Arch Neurol 54:1141–1145, 1997

Kaptchuk TJ: Powerful placebo: the dark side of the randomized controlled trial. Lancet 351:1722–1725, 1998

Kapur N, Kamel IR, Herlich A: Oral and craniofacial pain: diagnosis, pathophysiology, and treatment. Int Anesthesiol Clin 41:115–150, 2003

Karjalainen K, Malmivaara A, van Tulder M, et al: Multidisciplinary biopsychosocial rehabilitation for subacute low back pain among working age adults. Cochrane Database Syst Rev 1:CD002193, 2003

Karlsten R, Gordh T: How do drugs relieve neurogenic pain? Drugs Aging 11:398–412, 1997

Katon W, Sullivan M: Depression and a chronic medical illness. J Clin Psychiatry 150 (suppl):3–11, 1990

Katon W, Egan K, Miller D: Chronic pain: lifetime psychiatric diagnoses and family history. Am J Psychiatry 142:1156–1160, 1985

Katon W, Lin E, Von Korff M, et al: Somatization: a spectrum of severity. Am J Psychiatry 148:34–40, 1991

Katz NP: MorphiDex (MS:DM) double-blind, multiple-dose studies in chronic pain patients. J Pain Symptom Manage 19:S37–S41, 2000

Katz N, Fanciullo GJ: Role of urine toxicology testing in the management of chronic opioid therapy. Clin J Pain 18:S76–S82, 2002

Katz PP, Yelin EH: Prevalence and correlates of depressive symptoms among persons with rheumatoid arthritis. J Rheumatol 20:790–796, 1993

Keefe FJ, Crisson JE, Maltbie A, et al: Illness behavior as a predictor of pain and overt behavior patterns in chronic low back pain patients. J Psychosom Res 30:543–551, 1986

Keefe FJ, Caldwell DS, Williams DA, et al: Pain coping skills training in the management of osteoarthritic knee pain: a comparative study. Behav Ther 21:49–62, 1990a

Keefe FJ, Caldwell DS, Williams DA, et al: Pain coping skills training in the management of osteoarthritic knee pain, II: follow-up results. Behav Ther 21:435–447, 1990b

Keefe FJ, Dunsmore J, Burnett R: Behavioral and cognitive-behavioral approaches to chronic pain: recent advances and future directions. J Consult Clin Psychol 60:528–536, 1992

Keefe FJ, Beaupre PM, Weiner DK, et al: Pain in older adults: a cognitive-behavioral perspective, in Pain in the Elderly. Edited by Ferrell BR, Ferrell BA. Seattle, WA, IASP Press, 1996, pp 11–19

Kerns RD, Haythornthwaite JA: Depression among chronic pain patients: cognitive-behavioral analysis and effect on rehabilitation outcome. J Consult Clin Psychol 56:870–876, 1988

Kerns RD, Turk D, Rudy T: The West Haven–Yale Multidimensional Pain Inventory. Pain 23:345–356, 1985

Kerns RD, Otis JD, Marcus KS: Cognitive-behavioral therapy for chronic pain in the elderly. Clin Geriatr Med 17:503–523, 2001

Kiefer G, Fischer W, Feuerstein TJ: Effects of amitriptyline, amitriptylinoxide, doxepine, and clozapine on N-methyl-D-aspartate-evoked release of [3H]-acetylcholine in rat caudatoputamen. Arzneimittelforschung 49:820–823, 1999

Kieffer BL, Gaveriaux-Ruff C: Exploring the opioid system by gene knockout. Prog Neurobiol 66:285–306, 2002

Kienle GS, Kienle H: The powerful placebo effect: fact or fiction? J Clin Epidemiol 50:1311–1318, 1997

King RB: Neuropharmacology of depression, anxiety, and pain. Clin Neurosurg 28:116–136, 1981

King SA: The classification and assessment of pain. Int Rev Psychiatry 12:86–90, 2000

King SA, Strain JJ: Benzodiazepine use by chronic pain patients. Clin J Pain 6:143–147, 1990

King SA, Strain JJ: Revising the category of somatoform pain disorder. Hosp Community Psychiatry 43:217–219, 1992

Kirsh KL, Whitcomb LA, Donaghy K, et al: Abuse and addiction issues in medically ill patients with pain: attempts at clarification of terms and empirical study. Clin J Pain 18:S52–S60, 2002

Kishore-Kumar R, Max MB, Schafer SC, et al: Desipramine relieves post-herpetic neuralgia. Clin Pharm Ther 47:305–312, 1990

Klapper J: Divalproex sodium in migraine prophylaxis: a dose-controlled study. Cephalalgia 17:103–108, 1997

Kleinman I, Brown P, Librach L: Placebo pain medication: ethical and practical considerations. Arch Fam Med 3:453–457, 1994

Koch HK: The National Ambulatory Medical Care Survey: 1975 Summary (Publication No. PHS 78–1784). Hyattsville, MD, U.S. Department of Health, Education, and Welfare, 1978

Koller WC: Sensory symptoms in Parkinson's disease. Neurology 34:957–959, 1984

Kouyanou K, Pither CE, Wessely S: Medication misuse, abuse and dependence in chronic pain patients. J Psychosom Res 43:497–504, 1997

Kouyanou K, Pither CE, Rabe-Hesketh S, et al: A comparative study of iatrogenesis, medication abuse, and psychiatric morbidity in chronic pain patients with and without medically explained symptoms. Pain 76:417–426, 1998

Kroenke K: Patients presenting with somatic complaints: epidemiology, psychiatric comorbidity and management. Int J Methods Psychiatr Res 12:34–43, 2003

Kroenke K, Mangelsdorff A: Common symptoms in ambulatory care: incidence, evaluation, therapy, and outcome. Am J Med 86:262–266, 1989

Kroenke K, Swindle R: Cognitive-behavioral therapy for somatization and symptom syndromes: a critical review of controlled clinical trials. Psychother Psychosom 69:205–215, 2000

Kroenke K, Arrington ME, Mangelsdorff AD: The prevalence of symptoms in medical outpatients and the adequacy of therapy. Arch Intern Med 150:1685–1689, 1990

Kroenke K, Spitzer RL, deGruy FV, et al: Multisomatoform disorder: an alternative to undifferentiated somatoform disorder for the somatizing patient in primary care. Arch Gen Psychiatry 54:352–358, 1997

Kurz A, Sessler DI: Opioid-induced bowel dysfunction: pathophysiology and potential new therapies. Drugs 63:649–671, 2003

La Spina I, Porazzi D, Maggiolo F, et al: Gabapentin in painful HIV-related neuropathy: a report of 19 patients, preliminary observations. Eur J Neurol 8:71–75, 2001

Lackner JM, Carosella AM: The relative influence of perceived pain control, anxiety, and functional self efficacy on spinal function among patients with chronic low back pain. Spine 24:2254–2260, 1999

Lake AE 3rd: Behavioral and nonpharmacologic treatments of headache. Med Clin North Am 85:1055–1075, 2001

Lake AE 3rd, Saper JR: Chronic headache: new advances in treatment strategies. Neurology 59 (suppl 2):S8–S13, 2002

Lang E, Hord AH, Denson D: Venlafaxine hydrochloride (Effexor) relieves thermal hyperalgesia in rats with an experimental mononeuropathy. Pain 68:151–155, 1996

Lang E, Liebig K, Kastner S, et al: Multidisciplinary rehabilitation versus usual care for chronic low back pain in the community: effects on quality of life. Spine 3:270–276, 2003

Larson SL, Clark MR, Eaton WW: Depressive disorder as a long-term antecedent risk factor for incident back pain: a thirteen year follow-up study from the Baltimore Epidemiological Catchment Area sample. Psychol Med 34:1–9, 2004

Lazarus RA, Folkman S: Stress, Appraisal, and Coping. New York, Springer, 1984

Lebovits AH: The psychological assessment of patients with chronic pain. Curr Rev Pain 4:122–126, 2000

Lee DJ, Benzon HT: Anesthesiologic treatments for complex regional pain syndrome, in Essentials of Pain Medicine. Edited by Benzon HT, Raja SN. Philadelphia, Churchill-Livingstone, 1999, pp 255–258

Lee J, Giles K, Drummond PD: Psychological disturbances and an exaggerated response to pain in patients with whiplash injury. J Psychosom Res 37:105–110, 1993

Leino P, Magni G: Depressive and distress symptoms as predictors of low back pain, neck-shoulder pain, and other musculoskeletal morbidity: a 10 year follow-up of metal industry employees. Pain 53:89–94, 1993

Lemstra M, Stewart B, Olszynski WP: Effectiveness of multidisciplinary intervention in the treatment of migraine: a randomized clinical trial. Headache 42:845–854, 2002

Lethem J, Slade PD, Troup JDG, et al: Outline of fear-avoidance model of exaggerated pain perceptions. Behav Res Ther 21:401–408, 1983

Lewis TA, Solomon GD: Advances in cluster headache management. Cleve Clin J Med 63:237–244, 1996

Li X, Clark JD: Hyperalgesia during opioid abstinence: mediation by glutamate and substance P. Anesth Analg 95:979–984, 2002

Li X, Angst MS, Clark JD: A murine model of opioid-induced hyperalgesia. Brain Res Mol Brain Res 86:56–62, 2001

Lin EH, Katon W, Von Korff M, et al: Effect of improving depression care on pain and functional outcomes among older adults with arthritis: a randomized controlled trial. JAMA 290:2428–2439, 2003

Linton SJ: A review of psychological risk factors in back and neck pain. Spine 25:1148–1156, 2000

Linton SJ, Andersson T: Can chronic disability be prevented? A randomized trial of a cognitive-behavior intervention and two forms of information for patients with spinal pain. Spine 25:2825–2831, 2000

Lipchik GL, Nash JM: Cognitive-behavioral issues in the treatment and management of chronic daily headache. Curr Pain Headache Rep 6:473–479, 2002

Lipowski ZJ: Somatization and depression. Psychosomatics 31:13–21, 1990

Lipton RB, Stewart WF, von Korff M: Burden of migraine: societal costs and therapeutic opportunities. Neurology 48 (suppl 3):S4–S9, 1997

Liu JG, Anand KJ: Protein kinases modulate the cellular adaptations associated with opioid tolerance and dependence. Brain Res Brain Res Rev 38:1–19, 2001

Livingston G, Watkin V, Milne B, et al: Who becomes depressed? The Islington community study of old people. J Affect Disord 58:125–133, 2000

Loeser JD: Tic douloureux. Pain Res Manag 6:156–165, 2001

Lomardo WK, Lambardo B, Goldstein A: Cognitive functioning under moderate and low dosage methadone maintenance. Int J Addict 11:389–401, 1976

Long DM, Filtzer DL, BenDebba M, et al: Clinical features of the failed-back syndrome. J Neurosurg 69:61–71, 1988

Longo LP, Parran T Jr, Johnson B, et al: Addiction, part II: identification and management of the drug-seeking patient. Am Fam Physician 61:2401–2408, 2000

Love S, Coakham HB: Trigeminal neuralgia: pathology and pathogenesis. Brain 124:2347–2360, 2001

Lynch ME: Psychological aspects of reflex sympathetic dystrophy: a review of the adult and paediatric literature. Pain 49:337–347, 1992

Lynch ME: Antidepressants as analgesics: a review of randomized controlled trials. J Psychiatry Neurosci 26:30–36, 2001

MacFarlane BV, Wright A, O'Callaghan J, et al: Chronic neuropathic pain and its control by drugs. Pharmacol Ther 75:1–19, 1997

Magni G: On the relationship between chronic pain and depression when there is no organic lesion. Pain 31:1–21, 1987

Magni G: The use of antidepressants in the treatment of chronic pain: a review of the current evidence. Drugs 42:730–748, 1991

Magni G, Schifano F, DeLeo D: Pain as a symptom in elderly depressed patients: relationship to diagnostic subgroups. Eur Arch Psychiatry Neurol Sci 235:143–145, 1985

Magni G, Marchetti M, Moreschi C, et al: Chronic musculoskeletal pain and depressive symptoms in the National Health and Nutrition Examination, I: epidemiologic follow-up study. Pain 53:163–168, 1993

Magni G, Moreschi C, Rigatti-Luchini S, et al: Prospective study on the relationship between depressive symptoms and chronic musculoskeletal pain. Pain 56:289–297, 1994

Magni G, Rigatti-Luchini S, Fracca F, et al: Suicidality in chronic abdominal pain: an analysis of the Hispanic Health and Nutrition Examination Survey (HHANES). Pain 76:137–144, 1998

Maier C, Hildebrandt J, Klinger R, et al: Morphine responsiveness, efficacy and tolerability in patients with chronic nontumor associated pain: results of a double-blind placebo-controlled trial (MONTAS). Pain 97:223–233, 2002

Maina G, Vitalucci A, Gandolfo S, et al: Comparative efficacy of SSRIs and amisulpride in burning mouth syndrome: a single-blind study. J Clin Psychiatry 63:38–43, 2002

Manetto C, McPherson SE: The behavioral-cognitive model of pain. Clin Geriatr Med 12:461–471, 1996

Mannion AF, Muntener M, Taimela S, et al: A randomized clinical trial of three active therapies for chronic low back pain. Spine 24:2435–2448, 1999

Mannion AF, Junge A, Taimela S, et al: Active therapy for chronic low back pain, part 3: factors influencing self-rated disability and its change following therapy. Spine 26:920–929, 2001

Mantyselka P, Ahonen R, Viinamaki H, et al: Drug use by patients visiting primary care physicians due to nonacute musculoskeletal pain. Eur J Pharm Sci 17:210–216, 2002

Mantyselka PT, Turunen JH, Ahonen RS, et al: Chronic pain and poor self-rated health. JAMA 290:2435–2442, 2003

Mao J, Sung B, Ji RR, et al: Chronic morphine induces down-regulation of spinal glutamate transporters: implications in morphine tolerance and abnormal pain sensitivity. J Neurosci 22:8312–8323, 2002

Marek GJ, McDougle CJ, Price LH, et al: A comparison of trazodone and fluoxetine: implications for a serotonergic mechanism of antidepressant action. Psychopharmacology 109:2–11, 1992

Marhold C, Linton SJ, Melin L: Identification of obstacles for chronic pain patients to return to work: evaluation of a questionnaire. J Occup Rehabil 12:65–75, 2002

Markley HG: Verapamil and migraine prophylaxis: mechanisms and efficacy. Am J Med 90:48S–53S, 1991

Marlatt GA: Harm reduction: come as you are. Addict Behav 21:779–788, 1996

Marson AG, Kadir ZA, Hutton JL, et al: The new antiepileptic drugs: a systematic review of their efficacy and tolerability. Epilepsia 38:859–880, 1997

Maruta T, Swanson DW, Finlayson RE: Drug abuse and dependency in patients with chronic pain. Mayo Clin Proc 54:241–244, 1979

Maruta T, Malinchoc M, Offord KP, et al: Status of patients with chronic pain 13 years after treatment in a pain management center. Pain 74:199–204, 1998

Mathew NT: Antiepileptic drugs in migraine prevention. Headache 41 (suppl 1):S18–S24, 2001

Mathew NT, Saper JR, Silberstein SD, et al: Migraine prophylaxis with divalproex. Arch Neurol 52:281–286, 1995

Mathew NT, Kailasam J, Meadors L: Prophylaxis of migraine, transformed migraine, and cluster headache with topiramate. Headache 42:796–803, 2002

Mattia C, Paoletti F, Coluzzi F, et al: New antidepressants in the treatment of neuropathic pain: a review. Minerva Anestesiol 68:105–114, 2002

Max MB: Treatment of post-herpetic neuralgia: antidepressants. Ann Neurol 35:850–853, 1994

Max MB, Culnane M, Schafer SC, et al: Amitriptyline relieves diabetic neuropathy pain in patients with normal or depressed mood. Neurology 37:589–596, 1987

Max M, Lynch S, Muir J, et al: Effects of desipramine, amitriptyline and fluoxetine on pain in diabetic neuropathy. N Engl J Med 326:1250–1256, 1992

Maxwell TD, Gatchel RJ, Mayer TG: Cognitive predictors of depression in chronic low back pain: toward an inclusive model. J Behav Med 21:131–143, 1998

Mayou R, Levenson JL, Sharpe M: Somatoform disorders in DSM-V. Psychosomatics 44:449–451, 2003

McCracken LM: Learning to live with the pain: acceptance of pain predicts adjustment in persons with chronic pain. Pain 74:21–27, 1998

McCracken LM, Iverson GL: Disrupted sleep patterns and daily functioning in patients with chronic pain. Pain Res Manag 7:75–79, 2002

McCracken LM, Turk DC: Behavioral and cognitive-behavioral treatment for chronic pain: outcome, predictors of outcome, and treatment process. Spine 27:2564–2573, 2002

McCracken LM, Matthews AK, Tang TS, et al: A comparison of blacks and whites seeking treatment for chronic pain. Clin J Pain 17:249–255, 2001

McCreary CP, Clark GT, Merril RI, et al: Psychological distress and diagnostic subgroups of temporomandibular disorder patients. Pain 44:29–34, 1991

McNairy SI, Maruta T, Ivnik RJ, et al: Prescription medication dependence and neuropsychological function. Pain 18:169–177, 1984

McQuay H, Carroll D, Jadad AR, et al: Anticonvulsant drugs for management of pain: a systematic review. BMJ 311:1047–1052, 1995

McQuay HJ, Tramer M, Nye BA, et al: A systematic review of antidepressants in neuropathic pain. Pain 68:217–227, 1996

Meldrum ML: A capsule history of pain management. JAMA 290:2470–2475, 2003

Mellegers MA, Furlan AD, Mailis A: Gabapentin for neuropathic pain: systematic review of controlled and uncontrolled literature. Clin J Pain 17:284–295, 2001

Melzack R, Wall PD: Pain mechanisms: a new theory. Science 150:971–979, 1965

Mendell JR, Sahenk Z: Clinical practice: painful sensory neuropathy. N Engl J Med 348:1243–1255, 2003

Mendelson G, Mendelson D: Legal aspects of the management of chronic pain. Med J Aust 155:640–643, 1991

Menefee LA, Frank ED, Doghramji K, et al: Self-reported sleep quality and quality of life for individuals with chronic pain conditions. Clin J Pain 16:290–297, 2000

Merikangas KR, Merikangas JR: Combination monoamine oxidase inhibitor and beta-blocker treatment of migraine, with anxiety and depression. Biol Psychiatry 38:603–610, 1995

Merskey H, Lindblom U, Mumford JM, et al: Pain terms: a current list with definitions and notes on usage. Pain Suppl 3:S215–S221, 1986

Middaugh SJ, Pawlick K: Biofeedback and behavioral treatment of persistent pain in the older adult: a review and a study. Appl Psychophysiol Biofeedback 27:185–202, 2002

Millan MJ: Descending control of pain. Prog Neurobiol 66:355–474, 2002

Miotto K, Compton P, Ling W, et al: Diagnosing addictive disease in chronic pain patients. Psychosomatics 37:223–235, 1996

Moldofsky H: Sleep and pain. Sleep Med Rev 5:385–396, 2001

Monti DA, Herring CL, Schwartzman RJ, et al: Personality assessment of patients with complex regional pain syndrome type I. Clin J Pain 14:295–302, 1998

Moore JE, Von Korff M, Cherkin D, et al: A randomized trial of a cognitive-behavioral program for enhancing back pain self care in a primary care setting. Pain 88:145–153, 2000

Moosa RS, McFayden ML, Miller R, et al: Carbamazepine and its metabolites in neuralgias: concentration-effect relations. Eur J Clin Pharm 45:297–301, 1993

Morgan JP: American opiophobia: customary underutilization of opioid analgesics. Adv Alcohol Subst Abuse 5:163–173, 1985

Morley S, Eccleston C, Williams A: Systematic review and meta-analysis of randomized controlled trials of cognitive behaviour therapy and behaviour therapy for chronic pain in adults, excluding headache. Pain 80:1–13, 1999

Moulin DE, Iezzi A, Amireh R, et al: Randomised trial of oral morphine for chronic non-cancer pain. Lancet 347:143–147, 1996

Moulin DE, Clark AJ, Speechley M, et al: Chronic pain in Canada: prevalence, treatment, impact and the role of opioid analgesia. Pain Res Manag 7:179–184, 2002

Nedeljkovic SS, Wasan A, Jamison RN: Assessment of efficacy of long-term opioid therapy in pain patients with substance abuse potential. Clin J Pain 18:S39–S51, 2002

Neighbors DM, Bell TJ, Wilson J, et al: Economic evaluation of the fentanyl transdermal system for the treatment of chronic moderate to severe pain. J Pain Symptom Manage 21:129–143, 2001

Nelson DV, Novy DM: Psychological characteristics of reflex sympathetic dystrophy versus myofascial pain syndromes. Reg Anesth 21:202–208, 1996

Nemmani KV, Mogil JS: Serotonin-GABA interactions in the modulation of mu- and kappa-opioid analgesia. Neuropharmacology 44:304–310, 2003

Nicholson B: Responsible prescribing of opioids for the management of chronic pain. Drugs 63:17–32, 2003

Nickel R, Raspe HH: Chronic pain: epidemiology and health care utilization. Nervenarzt 72:897–906, 2001

Nielson WR, Weir R: Biopsychosocial approaches to the treatment of chronic pain. Clin J Pain 17 (suppl):S114–S127, 2001

Nikolaus T: Assessment of chronic pain in elderly patients. Ther Umsch 54:340–344, 1997

Nishiyama K, Sakuta M: Mexiletine for painful alcoholic neuropathy. Intern Med 34:577–579, 1995

Nissen LM, Tett SE, Cramond T, et al: Opioid analgesic prescribing and use: an audit of analgesic prescribing by general practitioners and The Multidisciplinary Pain Centre at Royal Brisbane Hospital. Br J Clin Pharmacol 52:693–698, 2001

Nitu AN, Wallihan R, Skljarevski V, et al: Emerging trends in the pharmacotherapy of chronic pain. Expert Opin Investig Drugs 12:549–559, 2003

Novak V, Kanard R, Kissel JT, et al: Treatment of painful sensory neuropathy with tiagabine: a pilot study. Clin Auton Res 11:357–361, 2001

Novy DM, Nelson DV, Berry LA, et al: What does the Beck Depression Inventory measure in chronic pain? A reappraisal. Pain 61:261–270, 1995

O'Callaghan JP: Evolution of a rational use of opioids in chronic pain. Eur J Pain 5 (suppl A):21–26, 2001

Ohayon MM, Schatzberg AF: Using chronic pain to predict depressive morbidity in the general population. Arch Gen Psychiatry 60:39–47, 2003

Ohmori S, Morimoto Y: Dihydroetorphine: a potent analgesic: pharmacology, toxicology, pharmacokinetics, and clinical effects. CNS Drug Rev 8:391–404, 2002

Okifuji A, Turk DC, Curran SL: Anger in chronic pain: investigations of anger targets and intensity. J Psychosom Res 47:1–12, 1999

Okifuji A, Turk DC, Sherman JJ: Evaluation of the relationship between depression and fibromyalgia syndrome: why aren't all patients depressed? J Rheumatol 27:212–219, 2000

Olesen J (ed): HIS classification and diagnostic criteria for headache disorders, cranial neuralgias and facial pain. Cephalalgia 8 (suppl 7):1–96, 1988

Ollat H, Cesaro P: Pharmacology of neuropathic pain. Clin Neuropharmacol 18:391–404, 1995

O'Malley PG, Balden E, Tomkins G, et al: Treatment of fibromyalgia with antidepressants: a meta-analysis. J Gen Intern Med 15:659–666, 2000

Onghena P, Van Houdenhove B: Antidepressant-induced analgesia in chronic non-malignant pain: a meta-analysis of 39 placebo-controlled studies. Pain 49:205–219, 1992

Oskarsson P, Ljunggren JG, Lins PE: Efficacy and safety of mexiletine in the treatment of painful diabetic neuropathy. Diabetes Care 20:1594–1597, 1997

Ospina M, Harstall C: Prevalence of Chronic Pain: An Overview (Report No. 28). Edmonton, Alberta, Alberta Heritage Foundation for Medical Research, Health Technology Assessment 2002

Pandey CK, Bose N, Garg G, et al: Gabapentin for the treatment of pain in Guillain-Barre syndrome: a double-blinded, placebo-controlled, crossover study. Anesth Analg 95:1719–1723, 2002

Paoli F, Darcourt G, Corsa P: Note preliminaire su l'action de l'impramine dans les etats douloureux. Revue de Neurologie 2:503–504, 1960

Pappagallo M, Heinberg LJ: Ethical issues in the management of chronic nonmalignant pain. Semin Neurol 17:203–211, 1997

Parmelee PA: Pain in cognitively impaired older persons. Clin Geriatr Med 12:473–487, 1996

Passik SD, Weinreb HJ: Managing chronic nonmalignant pain: overcoming obstacles to the use of opioids. Adv Ther 17:70–83, 2000

Pasternak GW: The pharmacology of mu analgesics: from patients to genes. Neuroscientist 7:220–231, 2001

Patten SB: Long-term medical conditions and major depression in a Canadian population study at waves 1 and 2. J Affect Disord 63:35–41, 2001

Paul D, Hornby PJ: Potentiation of intrathecal DAMGO antinociception, but not gastrointestinal transit inhibition, by 5-hydroxytryptamine and norepinephrine uptake blockade. Life Sci 56:PL83–PL87, 1995

Pengel HM, Maher CG, Refshauge KM: Systematic review of conservative interventions for subacute low back pain. Clin Rehabil 16:811–820, 2002

Peters L, Simon EP, Folen RA, et al: The COPE program: treatment efficacy and medical utilization outcome of a chronic pain management program at a major military hospital. Mil Med 165:954–960, 2000

Pfingsten M, Hildebrandt J, Saur P, et al: Multidisciplinary treatment program for chronic low back pain, part 4: prognosis of treatment outcomes and final conclusions. Schmerz 11:30–41, 1997

Pfingsten M, Schops P, Wille T, et al: Classification of chronic pain: quantification and grading with the Mainz Pain Staging System. Schmerz 14:10–17, 2000

Phillips DM: JCAHO pain management standards are unveiled. Joint Commission on Accreditation of Healthcare Organizations. JAMA 284:428–429, 2000

Picavet HS, Vlaeyen JW, Schouten JS: Pain catastrophizing and kinesiophobia: predictors of chronic low back pain. Am J Epidemiol 156:1028–1034, 2002

Pincus T, Williams A: Models and measurements of depression in chronic pain. J Psychosom Res 47:211–219, 1999

Pincus T, Burton AK, Vogel S, et al: A systematic review of psychological factors as predictors of chronicity/disability in prospective cohorts of low back pain. Spine 27:E109–E120, 2002

Pinto A, Sollecito TP, DeRossi SS: Burning mouth syndrome: a retrospective analysis of clinical characteristics and treatment outcomes. N Y State Dent J 69:18–24, 2003

Ploghaus A, Becerra L, Borras C, et al: Neural circuitry underlying pain modulation: expectation, hypnosis, placebo. Trends Cogn Sci 7:197–200, 2003

Polatin PB, Kinney RK, Gatchel RJ, et al: Psychiatric illness and chronic low back pain. Spine 18:66–71, 1993

Pollo A, Vighetti S, Rainero I, et al: Placebo analgesia and the heart. Pain 102:125–133, 2003

Portenoy RK: Chronic opioid therapy in non-malignant pain. J Pain Symptom Manage 5 (suppl 1):S46–S62, 1990

Portenoy RK, Foley KM: Chronic use of opioid analgesics in non-malignant pain: report of 38 cases. Pain 25:171–186, 1986

Portenoy RK, Foley KM: Constipation in the cancer patient. Med Clin North Am 71:303–312, 1987

Portenoy RK, Sciberras A, Eliot L, et al: Steady-state pharmacokinetics comparison of a new, extended-release, once-daily morphine formulation, Avinza, and a twice-daily controlled-release morphine formulation in patients with chronic moderate-to-severe pain. J Pain Symptom Manage 23:292–300, 2002

Porter J, Jick H: Addiction rare in patients treated with narcotics (letter). N Engl J Med 302:123, 1980

Potter M, Schafer S, Gonzalez-Mendez E, et al: Opioids for chronic nonmalignant pain: attitudes and practices of primary care physicians in the UCSF/Stanford Collaborative Research Network. University of California, San Francisco. J Fam Pract 50:145–151, 2001

Price DD: Psychological and neural mechanisms of the affective dimension of pain. Science 288:1769–1772, 2000

Price DD, Milling LS, Kirsch I, et al: An analysis of factors that contribute to the magnitude of placebo analgesia in an experimental paradigm. Pain 83:147–156, 1999

Przewlocki R, Przewlocka B: Opioids in chronic pain. Eur J Pharmacol 429:79–91, 2001

Quang-Cantagrel ND, Wallace MS, Magnuson SK: Opioid substitution to improve the effectiveness of chronic non-cancer pain control: a chart review. Anesth Analg 90:933–937, 2000

Raja SN, Haythornthwaite JA, Pappagallo M, et al: Opioids versus antidepressants in postherpetic neuralgia: a randomized, placebo-controlled trial. Neurology 59:1015–1021, 2002

Rani PU, Naidu MU, Prasad VB, et al: An evaluation of antidepressants in rheumatic pain conditions. Anesth Analg 83:371–375, 1996

Ready LB, Sarkis E, Turner JA: Self-reported vs. actual use of medications in chronic pain patients. Pain 12:285–294, 1982

Reich J, Tupin J, Abramowitz S: Psychiatric diagnosis in chronic pain patients. Am J Psychiatry 140:1495–1498, 1983

Reichborn-Kjennerud T, Stoltenberg C, Tambs K, et al: Back-neck pain and symptoms of anxiety and depression: a population-based twin study. Psychol Med 32:1009–1020, 2002

Reid MC, Engles-Horton LL, Weber MB, et al: Use of opioid medications for chronic noncancer pain syndromes in primary care. J Gen Intern Med 17:238–240, 2002

Reis S: Expectancy theory of fear, anxiety, and panic. Clin Psychol Rev 11:141–153, 1991

Revenson TA, Felton BT: Disability and coping as predictors of psychological adjustment to rheumatoid arthritis. J Consult Clin Psychol 57:344–348, 1989

Rice AS, Maton S, Postherpetic Neuralgia Study Group: Gabapentin in postherpetic neuralgia: a randomised, double blind, placebo controlled study. Pain 94:215–224, 2001

Richeimer SH, Bajwa ZH, Kahraman SS, et al: Utilization patterns of tricyclic antidepressants in a multidisciplinary pain clinic: a survey. Clin J Pain 13:324–329, 1997

Richelson E: Pharmacology of antidepressants: characteristics of the ideal drug. Mayo Clin Proc 69:1069–1081, 1994

Riedel W, Neeck G: Nociception, pain, and antinociception: current concepts. Z Rheumatol 60:404–415, 2001

Rief W, Hiller W: Toward empirically based criteria for the classification of somatoform disorders. J Psychosom Res 46:507–518, 1999

Riley JL 3rd, Robinson ME: Validity of MMPI-2 profiles in chronic back pain patients: differences in path models of coping and somatization. Clin J Pain 14:324–335, 1998

Riley JL 3rd, Robinson ME, Geisser ME: Empirical subgroups of the Coping Strategies Questionnaire–Revised: a multi-sample study. Clin J Pain 15:111–116, 1999a

Riley JL 3rd, Robinson ME, Wise EA, et al: Predicting treatment compliance following facial pain evaluation. Cranio 17:9–16, 1999b

Riley JL 3rd, Benson MB, Gremillion HA, et al: Sleep disturbance in orofacial pain patients: pain-related or emotional distress? Cranio 19:106–113, 2001

Riley JL 3rd, Wade JB, Myers CD, et al: Racial/ethnic differences in the experience of chronic pain. Pain 100:291–298, 2002

Risdon A, Eccleston C, Crombez G, et al: How can we learn to live with pain? A Q-methodological analysis of the diverse understandings of acceptance of chronic pain. Soc Sci Med 56:375–386, 2003

Rizzo MA: Successful treatment of painful traumatic mononeuropathy with carbamazepine: insights into a possible molecular pain mechanism. J Neurol Sci 152:103–106, 1997

Robinson RC, Gatchel RJ, Polatin P, et al: Screening for problematic prescription opioid use. Clin J Pain 17:220–228, 2001

Rojas-Corrales MO, Berrocoso E, Gibert-Rahola J, et al: Antidepressant-like effects of tramadol and other central analgesics with activity on monoamines reuptake, in helpless rats. Life Sci 72:143–152, 2002

Romano JM, Syrjala KL, Levy RL, et al: Overt pain behaviors: relationship to patient functioning and treatment outcome. Behav Ther 19:191–201, 1988

Rommel O, Malin JP, Zenz M, et al: Quantitative sensory testing, neurophysiological and psychological examination in patients with complex regional pain syndrome and hemisensory deficits. Pain 93:279–293, 2001

Roose SP, Glassman AH, Siris S: Comparison of imipramine and nortriptyline-induced orthostatic hypotension: a meaningful difference. J Clin Psychopharmacol 1:316–319, 1981

Rosenblum A, Joseph H, Fong C, et al: Prevalence and characteristics of chronic pain among chemically dependent patients in methadone maintenance and residential treatment facilities. JAMA 289:2370–2378, 2003

Roth SH, Fleischmann RM, Burch FX, et al: Around-the-clock, controlled-release oxycodone therapy for osteoarthritis-related pain: placebo-controlled trial and long-term evaluation. Arch Intern Med 160:853–860, 2000

Rothrock JF: Clinical studies of valproate for migraine prophylaxis. Cephalalgia 17:81–83, 1997

Rowbotham M, Harden N, Stacey B, et al: Gabapentin for the treatment of postherpetic neuralgia: a randomized controlled trial. JAMA 280:1837–1842, 1998

Rowbotham MC, Twilling L, Davies PS, et al: Oral opioid therapy for chronic peripheral and central neuropathic pain. N Engl J Med 348:1279–1281, 2003

Rudy TE, Kerns RD, Turk DC: Chronic pain and depression: toward a cognitive-behavioral mediation model. Pain 35:129–140, 1988

Rudy TE, Turk DC, Kubinski JA, et al: Differential treatment responses of TMD patients as a function of psychological characteristics. Pain 61:103–112, 1995

Rudy TE, Lieber SJ, Boston JR, et al: Psychosocial predictors of physical performance in disabled individuals with chronic pain. Clin J Pain 19:18–30, 2003

Sabatowski R, Schwalen S, Rettig K, et al: Driving ability under long-term treatment with transdermal fentanyl. J Pain Symptom Manage 25:38–47, 2003

Salerno SM, Browning R, Jackson JL: The effect of antidepressant treatment on chronic back pain: a meta-analysis. Arch Intern Med 162:19–24, 2002

Sanders SH, Brena SF: Empirically derived chronic pain patient subgroups: the utility of multidimensional clustering to identify differential treatment effects. Pain 54:51–56, 1993

Sang CN: NMDA-receptor antagonists in neuropathic pain: experimental methods to clinical trials. J Pain Symptom Manage 19 (suppl):S21–S25, 2000

Saper JR, Silberstein SD, Lake AE 3rd, et al: Double-blind trial of fluoxetine: chronic daily headache and migraine. Headache 34:497–502, 1994

Saur P, Hildebrandt J, Pfingsten M, et al: Multidisciplinary treatment program for chronic low back pain, part 2: somatic aspects. Schmerz 10:237–253, 1996

Savage SR: Addiction in the treatment of pain: significance, recognition and management. J Pain Symptom Manage 8:265–278, 1993

Savage SR: Opioid therapy of chronic pain: assessment of consequences. Acta Anaesthesiol Scand 43:909–917, 1999

Savage SR: Assessment for addiction in pain-treatment settings. Clin J Pain 18:S28–S38, 2002

Savage SR, Joranson DE, Covington EC, et al: Definitions related to the medical use of opioids: evolution towards universal agreement. J Pain Symptom Manage 26:655–667, 2003

Sawynok J: GABAergic mechanisms of analgesia: an update. Pharmacol Biochem Behav 26:463–474, 1985

Scadding FW: Peripheral neuropathies, in Textbook of Pain, 3rd Edition. Edited by Wall PD, Melzack R. Edinburgh, Churchill Livingstone, 1994, pp 667–683

Scala A, Checchi L, Montevecchi M, et al: Update on burning mouth syndrome: overview and patient management. Crit Rev Oral Biol Med 14:275–291, 2003

Schade V, Semmer N, Main CJ, et al: The impact of clinical, morphological, psychosocial and work-related factors on the outcome of lumbar diskectomy. Pain 80:239–249, 1999

Schmader KE: Epidemiology and impact on quality of life of postherpetic neuralgia and painful diabetic neuropathy. Clin J Pain 18:350–354, 2002

Schmidt NB, Santiago HT, Trakowski JH, et al: Pain in patients with panic disorder: relation to symptoms, cognitive characteristics and treatment outcome. Pain Res Manag 7:134–141, 2002

Schreiber S, Backer MM, Yanai J, et al: The antinociceptive effect of fluvoxamine. Eur Neuropsychopharmacol 6:281–284, 1996

Schug SA, Merry AF, Acland RH: Treatment principles for the use of opioids in pain of nonmalignant origin. Drugs 42:228–239, 1991

Schult ML, Soderback I, Jacobs K: Multidimensional aspects of work capability. Work 15:41–53, 2000

Scudds RJ, McD Robertson J: Empirical evidence of the association between the presence of musculoskeletal pain and physical disability in community-dwelling senior citizens. Pain 75:229–235, 1998

Sees KL, Clark HW: Opioid use in the treatment of chronic pain: assessment of addiction. J Pain Symptom Manage 8:257–264, 1993

Seligman MEP: Depression and learned helplessness, in The Psychology of Depression: Contemporary Theory and Research. Edited by Friedman RJ, Katz MM. Washington, DC, Hemisphere, 1974, pp 83–125

Semenchuk MR, Sherman S, Davis B: Double-blind, randomized trial of buproprion SR for the treatment of neuropathic pain. Neurology 57:1583–1588, 2001

Serpell MG: Neuropathic pain study group: gabapentin in neuropathic pain syndromes. A randomised, double-blind, placebo-controlled trial. Pain 99:557–566, 2002

Severeijns R, Vlaeyen JW, van den Hout MA, et al: Pain catastrophizing predicts pain intensity, disability, and psychological distress independent of the level of physical impairment. Clin J Pain 17:165–172, 2001

Sheftell FD, Atlas SJ: Migraine and psychiatric comorbidity: from theory and hypotheses to clinical application. Headache 42:934–944, 2002

Sherman JJ, Turk DC: Nonpharmacologic approaches to the management of myofascial temporomandibular disorders. Curr Pain Headache Rep 5:421–431, 2001

Sherman JJ, Turk DC, Okifuji A: Prevalence and impact of posttraumatic stress disorder-like symptoms on patients with fibromyalgia syndrome. Clin J Pain 16:127–134, 2000

Shimodozono M, Kawhira K, Kamishita T, et al: Reduction of central poststroke pain with the selective serotonin reuptake inhibitor fluvoxamine. Int J Neurosci 112:1173–1181, 2002

Silberstein SD, Peres MF, Hopkins MM, et al: Olanzapine in the treatment of refractory migraine and chronic daily headache. Headache 42:515–518, 2002

Simon GE, Gureje O: Stability of somatization disorder and somatization symptoms among primary care patients. Arch Gen Psychiatry 56:90–95, 1999

Simon GE, VonKorff M, Piccinelli M, et al: An international study of the relation between somatic symptoms and depression. N Engl J Med 341:1329–1335, 1999

Sindrup SH, Jensen TS: Efficacy of pharmacological treatments of neuropathic pain: an update and effect related to mechanism of drug action. Pain 83:389–400, 1999

Sindrup SH, Jensen TS: Pharmacologic treatment of pain in polyneuropathy. Neurology 55:915–920, 2000

Sindrup SH, Jensen TS: Pharmacotherapy of trigeminal neuralgia. Clin J Pain 18:22–27, 2002

Sindrup SH, Ejlertsen B, Froland A, et al: Imipramine treatment in diabetic neuropathy: relief of subjective symptoms without changes in peripheral and autonomic nerve function. Eur J Clin Pharmacol 37:151–153, 1989

Sindrup SH, Gram LF, Brosen K, et al: The SSRI paroxetine is effective in the treatment of diabetic neuropathy symptoms. Pain 42:135–144, 1990

Sindrup SH, Bjerre U, Dejaard A, et al: The SSRI citalopram relieves the symptoms of diabetic neuropathy. Clin Pharmacol Ther 52:547–552, 1992

Sittl R, Griessinger N, Likar R: Analgesic efficacy and tolerability of transdermal buprenorphine in patients with inadequately controlled chronic pain related to cancer and other disorders: a multicenter, randomized, double-blind, placebo-controlled trial. Clin Ther 25:150–168, 2003

Skevington SM: Investigating the relationship between pain and discomfort and quality of life, using the WHOQOL. Pain 76:395–406, 1998

Skevington SM, Carse MS, Williams AC: Validation of the WHOQOL-100: pain management improves quality of life for chronic pain patients. Clin J Pain 17:264–275, 2001

Smedstad LM, Vaglum P, Kvien TK, et al: The relationship between self-reported pain and sociodemographic variables, anxiety, and depressive symptoms in rheumatoid arthritis. J Rheumatol 22:514–520, 1995

Smith GR: The epidemiology and treatment of depression when it coexists with somatoform disorders, somatization, or pain. Gen Hosp Psychiatry 14:265–272, 1992

Smith JA, Lumley MA, Longo DJ: Contrasting emotional approach coping with passive coping for chronic myofascial pain. Ann Behav Med 24:326–335, 2002

Smith MT: Neuroexcitatory effects of morphine and hydromorphone: evidence implicating the 3-glucuronide metabolites. Clin Exp Pharmacol 27:524–528, 2000

Smith MT, Cabot PJ, Ross FB, et al: The novel N-type calcium channel blocker, AM336, produces potent dose-dependent antinociception after intrathecal dosing in rats and inhibits substance P release in rat spinal cord slices. Pain 96:119–127, 2002

Solaro C, Messmer Uccelli M, Uccelli A, et al: Low-dose gabapentin combined with either lamotrigine or carbamazepine can be useful therapies for trigeminal neuralgia in multiple sclerosis. Eur Neurol 44:45–48, 2000

Solomon GD: The pharmacology of medications used in treating headache. Semin Pediatr Neurol 2:165–177, 1995

Stack K, Cortina J, Samples C, et al: Race, age, and back pain as factors in completion of residential substance abuse treatment by veterans. Psychiatr Serv 51:1157–1161, 2000

Staiger TO, Gaster B, Sullivan MD, et al: Systematic review of antidepressants in the treatment of chronic low back pain. Spine 28:2540–2545, 2003

Stanton-Hicks M, Janig W, Hassenbusch S, et al: Reflex sympathetic dystrophy: changing concepts and taxonomy. Pain 63:127–133, 1995

Starkstein SE, Preziosi TJ, Robinson RG: Sleep disorders, pain, and depression in Parkinson's disease. Eur Neurol 31:352–355, 1991

Stenager EN, Stenager E, Jensen K: Attempted suicide, depression and physical diseases: a one-year follow-up study. Psychother Psychosom 61:65–73, 1994

Stewart WF, Ricci JA, Chee E, et al: Lost productive time and cost due to common pain conditions in the US workforce. JAMA 290:2443–2454, 2003

Stone AA, Shiffman S, Schwartz JE, et al: Patient non-compliance with paper diaries. BMJ 324:1193–1194, 2002

Streltzer J, Eliashof BA, Kline AE, et al: Chronic pain disorder following physical injury. Psychosomatics 41:227–234, 2000

Sullivan M: DSM-IV pain disorder: a case against the diagnosis. Int Rev Psychiatry 12:91–98, 2000

Sullivan M, Katon W: Somatization: the path between distress and somatic symptoms. Am Pain Soc J 2:141–149, 1993

Sullivan MJ, Thorn B, Haythornthwaite JA, et al: Theoretical perspectives on the relation between catastrophizing and pain. Clin J Pain 17:52–64, 2001

Suter PB: Employment and litigation: improved by work, assisted by verdict. Pain 100:249–257, 2002

Szirmai A: Vestibular disorders in patients with migraine. Eur Arch Otorhinolaryngol Suppl 1:S55–S57, 1997

Tan G, Jensen MP, Robinson-Whelen S, et al: Coping with chronic pain: a comparison of two measures. Pain 90:127–133, 2001

Tanelian DL, Victory RA: Sodium channel-blocking agents: their use in neuropathic pain conditions. Pain Forum 4:75–80, 1995

Taniguchi K, Miyagawa A, Mizutani A, et al: The effect of calcium channel antagonist administered by iontophoresis on the pain threshold. Acta Anaesthesiol Belg 46:69–73, 1995

Taricco M, Adone R, Pagliacci C, et al: Pharmacological interventions for spasticity following spinal cord injury. Cochrane Database Syst Rev 2:CD001131, 2000

Tasmuth T, Hartel B, Kalso E: Venlafaxine in neuropathic pain following treatment of breast cancer. Eur J Pain 6:17–24, 2002

Taub A: Opioid analgesics in the treatment of chronic intractable pain on non-neoplastic origin, in Narcotic Analgesics in Anesthesiology. Edited by Kitahata LM. Baltimore, MD, Williams & Wilkins, 1982, pp 199–208

ter Riet G, de Craen AJ, de Boer A, et al: Is placebo analgesia mediated by endogenous opioids? A systematic review. Pain 76:273–275, 1998

Thomassen R, van Hemert AM, Huyse FJ, et al: Somatoform disorders in consultation-liaison psychiatry: a comparison with other mental disorders. Gen Hosp Psychiatry 25:8–13, 2003

Thomsen AB, Becker N, Eriksen J: Opioid rotation in chronic non-malignant pain patients: a retrospective study. Acta Anaesthesiol Scand 43:918–923, 1999

To TP, Lim TC, Hill ST, et al: Gabapentin for neuropathic pain following spinal cord injury. Spinal Cord 40:282–285, 2002

Tokunaga A, Saika M, Senba E: 5-HT2A receptor subtype is involved in the thermal hyperalgesic mechanism of serotonin in the periphery. Pain 76:349–355, 1998

Tomkins GE, Jackson JL, O'Malley PG, et al: Treatment of chronic headache with antidepressants: a meta-analysis. Am J Med 111:54–63, 2001

Tremont-Lukats IW, Megeff C, Backonja MM: Anticonvulsants for neuropathic pain syndromes: mechanisms of action and place in therapy. Drugs 60:1029–1052, 2000

Trief PM, Grant W, Fredrickson B: A prospective study of psychological predictors of lumbar surgery outcome. Spine 25:2616–2621, 2000

Turk DC: The role of psychological factors in chronic pain. Acta Anaesthesiol Scand 43:885–888, 1999

Turk DC, Matyas TA: Pain-related behaviors: communication of pain. Am Pain Soc J 1:109–111, 1992

Turk DC, Okifuji A: Detecting depression in chronic pain patients: adequacy of self reports. Behav Res Ther 32:9–16, 1994

Turk DC, Okifuji A: What features affect physicians' decisions to prescribe opioids for chronic noncancer pain patients? Clin J Pain 13:330–336, 1997

Turk DC, Okifuji A: Psychological factors in chronic pain: evolution and revolution. J Consult Clin Psychol 70:678–690, 2002

Turk DC, Rudy TE: The robustness of an empirically derived taxonomy of chronic pain patients. Pain 42:27–35, 1990

Turk DC, Stieg RL: Chronic pain: the necessity of interdisciplinary communication. Clin J Pain 3:163–167, 1987

Turk DC, Brody MC, Okifuji EA: Physicians' attitudes and practices regarding the long-term prescribing of opioids for non-cancer pain. Pain 59:201–208, 1994

Turk DC, Meichenbaum D, Genest M (eds): Pain and Behavioral Medicine: A Cognitive-Behavioral Perspective. New York, Guilford, 1983

Turner JA: Comparison of group progressive-relaxation training and cognitive-behavioral group therapy for chronic low back pain. J Consult Clin Psychol 50:757–765, 1982a

Turner JA: Psychological interventions for chronic pain: a critical review, II: operant conditioning, hypnosis, and cognitive-behavioral therapy. Pain 12:23–46, 1982b

Turner JA, Chapman CR: Psychological interventions for chronic pain: a critical review, I: relaxation training and biofeedback. Pain 12:1–21, 1982

Turner JA, Jensen MP: Efficacy of cognitive therapy for chronic low back pain. Pain 52:169–177, 1993

Turner JA, Romano JM: Psychological and psychosocial techniques: cognitive-behavioral therapy, in The Management of Pain. Edited by Bonica JJ. Philadelphia, PA, Lea & Febiger, 1990, pp 1711–1720

Turner JA, Deyo RA, Loeser JD, et al: The importance of placebo effects in pain treatment and research. JAMA 271:1609–1614, 1994

Turner JA, Jensen MP, Warms CA, et al: Catastrophizing is associated with pain intensity, psychological distress, and pain-related disability among individuals with chronic pain after spinal cord injury. Pain 98:127–134, 2002

Turner-Stokes L, Erkeller-Yuksel F, Miles A, et al: Outpatient cognitive behavioral pain management programs: a randomized comparison of a group-based multidisciplinary versus an individual therapy model. Arch Phys Med Rehabil 84:781–788, 2003

Tzschentke TM: Behavioral pharmacology of buprenorphine, with a focus on preclinical models of reward and addiction. Psychopharmacology 161:1–16, 2002

Vaccarino AL, Kastin AJ: Endogenous opiates: 2000. Peptides 22:2257–2328, 2001

Van Damme S, Crombez G, Bijttebier P, et al: A confirmatory factor analysis of the Pain Catastrophizing Scale: invariant factor structure across clinical and non-clinical populations. Pain 96:319–324, 2002

Van den Hout JH, Vlaeyen JW, Heuts PH, et al: Secondary prevention of work-related disability in nonspecific low back pain: does problem-solving therapy help? A randomized clinical trial. Clin J Pain 19:87–96, 2003

van der Laan L, van Spaendonck K, Horstink MW, et al: The Symptom Checklist-90 Revised questionnaire: no psychological profiles in complex regional pain syndrome dystonia. J Pain Symptom Manage 17:357–362, 1999

Van Tulder MW, Ostelo R, Vlaeyen JW, et al: Behavioral treatment for chronic low back pain: a systematic review within the framework of the Cochrane Back Review Group. Spine 26:270–281, 2001

Vase L, Riley JL 3rd, Price DD: A comparison of placebo effects in clinical analgesic trials versus studies of placebo analgesia. Pain 99:443–452, 2002

Venable VL, Carlson CR, Wilson J: The role of anger and depression in recurrent headache. Headache 41:21–30, 2001

Verbunt JA, Seelen HA, Vlaeyen JW, et al: Disuse and deconditioning in chronic low back pain: concepts and hypotheses on contributing mechanisms. Eur J Pain 7:9–21, 2003

Verdugo RJ, Ochoa JL: Abnormal movements in complex regional pain syndrome: assessment of their nature. Muscle Nerve 23:198–205, 2000

Verhaak PF, Kerssens JJ, Dekker J, et al: Prevalence of chronic benign pain disorder among adults: a review of the literature. Pain 77:231–239, 1998

Vlaeyen JW, Linton SJ: Fear-avoidance and its consequences in chronic musculoskeletal pain: a state of the art. Pain 85:317–332, 2000

Vlaeyen JW, de Jong J, Geilen M, et al: The treatment of fear of movement/(re)injury in chronic low back pain: further evidence on the effectiveness of exposure in vivo. Clin J Pain 18:251–261, 2002

Volmink J, Lancaster T, Gray S, et al: Treatments for postherpetic neuralgia: a systematic review of randomized controlled trials. Fam Pract 13:84–91, 1996

Von Knorring L, Perris C, Eisemann M, et al: Pain as a symptom in depressive disorders, I: relationship to diagnostic subgroup and depressive symptomatology. Pain 15:19–26, 1983

Von Korff M, Ormel J, Katon W, et al: Disability and depression among high utilizers of health care: a longitudinal analysis. Arch Gen Psychiatry 49:91–100, 1992

Von Korff M, LeResche L, Dworkin SF: First onset of common pain symptoms: a prospective study of depression as a risk factor. Pain 55:251–258, 1993

Vowles KE, Gross RT: Work-related beliefs about injury and physical capability for work in individuals with chronic pain. Pain 101:291–298, 2003

Vrethem M, Boivie J, Arnqvist H, et al: A comparison of amitriptyline and maprotiline in the treatment of painful polyneuropathy in diabetics and nondiabetics. Clin J Pain 13:313–323, 1997

Waddell G, Newton M, Henderson I, et al: A fear-avoidance beliefs questionnaire (FABQ) and the role of fear-avoidance beliefs in chronic low back pain and disability. Pain 52:157–168, 1993

Wang SJ, Fuh JL, Lu SR, et al: Quality of life differs among headache diagnoses: analysis of SF-36 survey in 901 headache patients. Pain 89:285–292, 2001

Wang YX, Gao D, Pettus M, et al: Interactions of intrathecally administered ziconotide, a selective blocker of neuronal N-type voltage-sensitive calcium channels, with morphine on nociception in rats. Pain 84:271–281, 2000

Watson CP: The treatment of neuropathic pain: antidepressants and opioids. Clin J Pain 16 (suppl):S49–S55, 2000

Watson CP, Evans RJ, Watt VR, et al: Postherpetic neuralgia: 208 causes. Pain 35:289–298, 1988

Watson PJ, Andrews PW: Toward a revised evolutionary adaptationist analysis of depression: the social navigation hypothesis. J Affect Disord 72:1–14, 2002

Watt JW, Wiles JR, Bowsher DR: Epidural morphine for postherpetic neuralgia. Anaesthesia 51:647–651, 1996

Waxman R, Tennant A, Helliwell P: Community survey of factors associated with consultation for low back pain. BMJ 317:1564–1567, 1998

Weaver M, Schnoll S: Abuse liability in opioid therapy for pain treatment in patients with an addiction history. Clin J Pain 18:S61–S69, 2002

Webb J, Kamali F: Analgesic effects of lamotrigine and phenytoin on cold-induced pain: a crossover placebo-controlled study in healthy volunteers. Pain 76:357–363, 1998

Weickgenant AL, Slater MA, Patterson TL, et al: Coping activities in chronic low back pain: relationship with depression. Pain 53:95–103, 1993

Weiner D, Pieper C, McConnell E, et al: Pain measurement in elders with chronic low back pain: traditional and alternative approaches. Pain 67:461–467, 1996

Weiner D, Peterson B, Keefe F: Evaluating persistent pain in long term care residents: what role for pain maps? Pain 76:249–257, 1998

Weiner DK, Rudy TE, Gaur S: Are all older adults with persistent pain created equal? Preliminary evidence for a multiaxial taxonomy. Pain Res Manag 6:133–141, 2001

Weissman MM, Merikangas KR: The epidemiology of anxiety and panic disorders: an update. J Clin Psychiatry 47(suppl):11–17, 1986

Wesselmann U, Raja SN: Reflex sympathetic dystrophy/causalgia. Anesthesiol Clin North Am 15:407–427, 1997

Wesselmann U, Reich SG: The dynias. Semin Neurol 16:63–74, 1996

Wetzel CH, Connelly JF: Use of gabapentin in pain management. Ann Pharmacother 31:1082–1083, 1997

Wiffen P, Collins S, McQuay H, et al: Anticonvulsant drugs for acute and chronic pain. Cochrane Database Syst Rev 3:CD001133, 2000

Wilder-Smith CH, Hill L, Spargo K, et al: Treatment of severe pain from osteoarthritis with slow-release tramadol or dihydrocodeine in combination with NSAIDs: a randomised study comparing analgesia, antinociception and gastrointestinal effects. Pain 91:23–31, 2001

Williams AC de C, Richardson PH: What does the BDI measure in chronic pain? Pain 55:259–266, 1993

Williams DA, Urban B, Keefe FJ, et al: Cluster analyses of pain patients' responses to the SCL-90R. Pain 61:81–91, 1995

Williamson GM, Schulz R: Pain, activity restriction and symptoms of depression among community-residing elderly adults. J Gerontol 47:367–372, 1992

Wilson KG, Mikail SF, D'Eon JL, et al: Alternative diagnostic criteria for major depressive disorder in patients with chronic pain. Pain 91:227–234, 2001

Woolf CJ, Decosterd I: Implications of recent advances in the understanding of pain pathophysiology for the assessment of pain in patients. Pain Suppl 6:S141–S147, 1999

Woolf CJ, Mannion RJ: Neuropathic pain: aetiology, symptoms, mechanisms, and management. Lancet 353:1959–1964, 1999

Woolf CJ, Bennett GJ, Doherty M, et al: Towards a mechanism-based classification of pain. Pain 77:227–229, 1998

Wu LR, Parkerson GR Jr, Doraiswamy PM: Health perception, pain, and disability as correlates of anxiety and depression symptoms in primary care patients. J Am Board Fam Pract 15:183–190, 2002

Xiao WH, Bennett GJ: Synthetic omega-conopeptides applied to the site of nerve injury suppress neuropathic pains in rats. J Pharmacol Exp Ther 274:666–672, 1995

Yamamoto T, Katayama Y, Hirayama T, et al: Pharmacological classification of central post-stroke pain: comparison with the results of chronic motor cortex stimulation therapy. Pain 72:5–12, 1997

Yap AU, Tan KB, Chua EK, et al: Depression and somatization in patients with temporomandibular disorders. J Prosthet Dent 88:479–484, 2002

Zakrzewska JM: Diagnosis and differential diagnosis of trigeminal neuralgia. Clin J Pain 18:14–21, 2002

Zakrzewska JM, Glenny AM, Forssell H: Interventions for the treatment of burning mouth syndrome. Cochrane Database Syst Rev 3:CD002779, 2001

Zielger DK: Opiate and opioid use in patients with refractory headache. Cephalalgia 14:5–10, 1994

Zucchini M, Alberti G, Moretti MP: Algodystrophy and related psychological features. Funct Neurol 4:153–156, 1989

Zvolensky MJ, Goodie JL, McNeil DW, et al: Anxiety sensitivity in the prediction of pain-related fear and anxiety in a heterogeneous chronic pain population. Behav Res Ther 39:683–696, 2001

PART IV

Treatment

37 Psychopharmacology

Michael J. Robinson, M.D., F.R.C.P.C.

James A. Owen, Ph.D.

PSYCHOPHARMACOLOGICAL interventions are an essential part of the management of the medically ill; at least 35% of psychiatric consultations include recommendations for medication (Bronheim et al. 1998). Appropriate use of psychopharmacology in the medically ill requires careful consideration of the underlying medical illness, potential alterations to pharmacokinetics, drug–drug interactions, and contraindications. In this chapter, we review basic psychopharmacological concepts, including pharmacokinetics and pharmacodynamics in the medically ill, side effects, toxicity, drug interactions, and alternative routes of administration for each psychotropic drug class, as well as safety in pregnancy and lactation. Important considerations are critically examined for the use of psychotropic drugs in patients with major organ disorders. We also briefly review the use of complementary medicines, including herbal medicines and nonherbal dietary supplements.

Pharmacokinetics in the Medically Ill

Pharmacokinetics describes the absorption, distribution, metabolism, and excretion of drugs, whereas *pharmacodynamics* refers to the effects of drugs, primarily in the brain.

Absorption

Absorption of a drug is influenced by the characteristics of the absorption site and the physiochemical properties of a drug. Specific site properties that may affect absorption include surface area, ambient pH, mucosal integrity and function, and local blood flow. Orally administered drugs absorbed through the gastrointestinal tract may be extensively altered by "first-pass" hepatic metabolism before entering the systemic circulation. Sublingual and topical administration of drugs minimizes this first-pass effect, and rectal administration may reduce the first-pass effect by 50%. Drug formulation, drug interactions, gastric motility, and the characteristics of the absorptive surface all influence the *rate* of absorption, a key factor when rapid onset is desired. The *extent* of drug absorption, however, is more important with chronic administration. The *bioavailability* of a drug describes the rate and extent to which the drug ingredient is absorbed from the drug product and available for drug action. Intravenous drug delivery has 100% bioavailability.

Distribution

Systemic drug distribution is influenced by serum pH, blood flow, protein binding, lipid solubility, and the degree of ionization. Most drugs bind to proteins, either albumin or α_1 acid glycoprotein (AAGP), to a greater or lesser extent. Disease may alter the concentrations of serum proteins as well as binding affinities. For example, albumin binding is decreased in a number of illnesses (e.g., cirrhosis, bacterial pneumonia, acute pancreatitis, renal failure, surgery, and trauma), resulting in increased systemic toxicity with low therapeutic index drugs. In contrast, some disease states, such as hypothyroidism, may increase protein binding. AAGP concentrations may increase in Crohn's disease, myocardial infarction, stress, surgery, and trauma.

In general, acidic drugs (e.g., valproic acid, barbiturates) bind mostly to albumin, and more basic drugs (e.g., phenothiazines, tricyclic antidepressants [TCAs], amphetamines, most benzodiazepines) bind to globulins. In general, only free (unbound to plasma proteins) drug is pharmacologically active. Decreases in protein binding increase availability of the "free" drug to pharmacological action, metabolism, and excretion. When metabolic and excretory processes are unchanged by disease, changes to protein binding of a drug have little effect on steady-state plasma concentrations of pharmacologically active free drug. However, total plasma levels (free + bound drug) may be lowered; for this reason, clinical response to the drug, rather than laboratory-determined drug levels, should guide dosage. Most diseases that affect protein binding also affect metabolism and excretion. Therefore, disease-induced changes in free drug availability may have clinically significant consequences, especially for drugs with a low therapeutic index.

Volume of distribution is a function of a drug's lipid solubility and plasma- and tissue-binding properties. Most psychotropic drugs are lipophilic but are also extensively bound to plasma proteins. Volume of distribution is unpredictably altered by disease and is not useful is guiding dosage adjustments for medically ill patients.

Metabolism (or Biotransformation) and Elimination

Biotransformation occurs throughout the body, with the greatest activity in the liver and gut wall. Most psychotropic drugs are eliminated by hepatic metabolism and renal excretion. Hepatic biotransformation consists mostly of two types: phase I and phase II metabolism. Phase I metabolism consists of oxidation (i.e., cytochrome P450 monooxygenase system), reduction, or hydrolysis, which prepares medications for excretion or further metabolism by phase II pathways. The monoamine oxidases (MAOs) are also considered part of phase I. Phase II metabolism consists of many conjugation pathways, the most common being glucuronidation, acetylation, and sulfation. The hepatic clearance of drugs may be limited by either the rate of delivery (i.e., hepatic blood flow) of the drug to the hepatic metabolizing enzymes or the intrinsic capacity of the enzymes to metabolize the substrate. Clinically significant decreases in hepatic blood flow occur only in severe cirrhosis, and when possible, parenteral administration of drugs is preferred. Hepatic disease may preferentially affect anatomic regions of the liver, thereby altering specific metabolic processes. For example, oxidative metabolic reactions are more concentrated in the pericentral regions affected by acute viral hepatitis or alcoholic liver disease. Disease affecting the periportal regions, such as chronic hepatitis (in the absence of cirrhosis), may spare some hepatic oxidative function. In addition, acute and chronic liver diseases generally spare glucuronide conjugation reactions. Metabolic reactions altering the intrinsic capacity of the enzymes through inhibition and induction are discussed in the next section ("Drug–Drug Interactions").

The kidney's primary pharmacokinetic role is drug elimination. However, renal disease may affect absorption, distribution, and metabolism of drugs. Creatinine clearance is a more useful indicator of renal function than serum creatinine. Specific drugs and their use in renal failure are covered later in this chapter. In general, despite the complexity of pharmacokinetic changes in renal failure, few psychotropic agents other than lithium and gabapentin mandate dosage adjustment.

Disease processes, particularly those involving the gastrointestinal tract, liver, heart, and kidneys, can alter absorption, distribution, metabolism, and elimination. Table 37–1 summarizes how disease in these organ systems may alter the pharmacokinetics of psychotropic medications.

Drug–Drug Interactions

Drug–drug interactions are pharmacodynamic or pharmacokinetic in nature. Pharmacodynamic interactions involve alterations in the pharmacological response to a drug, which may be additive, synergistic or antagonistic. These interactions may occur directly, by altering the drug binding to the receptor site, or indirectly through other mechanisms. Pharmacokinetic interactions include altered absorption, distribution, metabolism, or excretion and can result in changing the drug concentration in tissues.

A *substrate* is an agent or a drug that is metabolized by an enzyme. An *inducer* is an agent or a drug that increases the activity of the metabolic enzyme, allowing for an increased rate of metabolism. Induction may lead to decreases in the amount of circulating parent drug and increases in the number and amount of metabolites produced. The clinical effect may be a loss or decrease in therapeutic efficacy or an increase in toxicity from metabolites. An *inhibitor* has the opposite effect, decreasing or blocking enzyme activity needed for the metabolism of other drugs. This results in increased levels of any drug dependent on that enzyme for biotransformation, thereby producing prolonged pharmacological effect or increased toxicity.

The hepatic cytochrome P450 enzyme system catalyzes phase I reactions and is responsible for most metabolic drug interactions. There are 11 cytochrome P450 enzyme families, of which 3 are important in humans: CYP1, CYP2, and CYP3. The families are divided into subfamilies that are identified by a capital letter (i.e., CYP3A). The subfamilies are further divided into isozymes based on the homology between the subfamily proteins and are denoted by a number following the capital letter (i.e., CYP3A4).

TABLE 37–1. Pharmacokinetics in the medically ill

Pharmacokinetic parameter	Potential factors	Clinical significance
Liver disease		
Absorption	Gastric acidity Gastric and intestinal motility Small intestine surface area (e.g., short gut) Enteric blood flow Reduced hepatic blood flow Portosystemic shunting	Minimize gastrointestinal side effects of psychotropics Liquid formulations may be better or more quickly absorbed than solid drug formulations Motility, secretory, and enteric blood flow changes in gastrointestinal disease usually do not require dosage change Consider parenteral administration

Distribution	Alterations in liver blood flow
	Changes in plasma proteins
	  Albumin may fall
	  AAGP may rise
	  Decreases in binding affinities
	Fluid shifts (e.g., ascites)
		Reduce dose
		Serum levels of drugs (bound + free) may be misleading

Metabolism and excretion	Reduced hepatic blood flow Intrinsic capacity of the enzymes	Clinically significant reductions only occur in severe cirrhosis
Renal disease		
Absorption	Ammonia buffering may raise gastric pH	Rarely clinically significant changes in pharmacokinetics Major exceptions—lithium and gabapentin
Distribution	Altered body water volume Reduced protein binding	Exact prediction of pharmacokinetic changes in the context of renal disease is impractical clinically Monitor drug levels more frequently but interpretation of blood levels difficult Serum levels of drugs (bound + free) may be misleading
Metabolism and excretion	Reduced renal blood flow Glomerular function	Creatinine clearance is a useful indicator of renal function to guide dose adjustments Serum creatinine may be confounded by some diseases that affect creatinine metabolism Dialysis alters pharmacokinetics
Cardiac disease		
Absorption	Decreased perfusion of drug absorption sites Intestinal wall edema may reduce absorption Changes in autonomic activity may affect GI motility and cause vasoconstriction	Congestive heart failure may decrease absorption of drugs through the gastrointestinal tract Intramuscular drug absorption may be decreased by vasoconstriction

Distribution	Changes in plasma proteins
	  AAGP may rise
	  Albumin may fall
	Volume of distribution is reduced
	Regional blood flow redistributions
		Acute doses should be reduced by approximately 50%
		Intravenous infusions should be given at a slower rate to avoid toxicity

Metabolism and excretion	Reduced renal and hepatic blood flow	A 50% reduction of dosage for chronic drug administration should be considered

Note. AAGP=alpha₁ acid glycoprotein; GI=gastrointestinal.

Cytochrome P450 enzymes exist in a variety of body tissues, including the gastrointestinal tract, liver, and brain. The most important cytochrome P450 enzymes in drug metabolism in humans are 1A2, 2C9, 2C19, 2D6, and 3A4. Because some of these enzymes exist in a polymorphic form, a small percentage of the population has one or more cytochrome P450 enzymes with significantly altered activity.

Phase II reactions are conjugation reactions in which water-soluble molecules are coupled to a drug to make it easily excreted. The most abundant phase II enzymes belong to the superfamily of uridine glucuronosyltransferases (UGTs). A classification system similar to the cytochrome P450 system has been developed to characterize the UGT superfamily of enzymes. There are two clinically significant UGT subfamilies: 1A and 2B. As with the cytochrome P450 system, there can be substrates, inhibitors, and inducers of UGT enzymes. For example, the benzodiazepines primarily metabolized by conjugation (oxazepam, lorazepam, and temazepam) are glucuronidated by UGT2B7. A number of nonsteroidal anti-inflammatory drugs (NSAIDs) are competitive inhibitors of UGT2B7. Phenobarbital, rifampin, and oral contraceptives appear to be inducers of UGT2B7. The role of UGTs in clinical pharmacology is being increasingly recognized.

Another system receiving increasing attention in clinical pharmacology is P-glycoproteins (P-gp). Human P-gps are divided into P-gp1 and P-gp3 (and they were renamed PGY1 and PGY3). PGY3 functions in phospholipid transport, whereas PGY1 (we use *P-gp* to refer to PGY1) is an efflux transporter. P-gps are present in the gut, liver and biliary systems, gonads, kidneys, brain, and other organs. They appear to be important for protecting the body from harmful substances and are involved in transporting certain hydrophobic substances into the gut, out of the brain, into urine, into bile, out of gonads, and out of other organs. They seem to play a large role in the distribution and elimination of many clinically important therapeutic substances.

As with the cytochrome P450 and UGT enzyme systems, there are substrates, inhibitors, and/or inducers of the P-gp transporters. Because intestinal P-gps are located in antecedent proximity to CYP3A4 and block absorption in the gut, they should be thought of as part of the first-pass effect, functioning as "gatekeepers" for later CYP3A4 actions. The effect of inhibiting P-gp is to "open the gates." For example, loperamide (an over-the-counter antidiarrheal) is a P-gp substrate and is normally transported out of the brain and therefore has no central opiate effects. When this drug is given with quinidine (a P-gp inhibitor), loperamide concentrations in the brain increase, and signs of respiratory depression can ensue (Sadeque et

al. 2000). Many factors can alter P-gp function and influence P-gp–based interactions; these include genetic differences, gender, herbal supplements, foods, and hormones (Cozza et al. 2003). Future understanding of the physiological regulation of these transporters may be key in designing and improving therapeutic actions of drugs.

General Principles

In medically ill patients, polypharmacy is usually the norm and requires vigilance regarding the many potential drug–drug interactions. To commit to memory all of the potential drug–drug interactions associated with psychotropic medications is practically impossible; these interactions are constantly changing as our knowledge increases and new medications are developed. Knowing the metabolic pathways of a drug and whether a drug to be combined has inhibitory or inductive effects on that enzyme provides a rough screen for predicting potential interactions. However, it should be remembered that drug concentration changes do not necessarily translate into clinically meaningful interactions. Cozza et al. (2003) advised that physicians prescribing in a polypharmacy environment should, whenever possible, avoid medications that significantly inhibit or induce cytochrome P450 enzymes and prefer those that are eliminated by multiple pathways and have a wide safety margin.

Identification of Potential Pharmacokinetic Interactions

Most pharmacokinetic drug–drug interactions involve the effects of an interacting drug on the cytochrome P450–mediated metabolism of a substrate drug. The interacting drug may be either an inhibitor or an inducer of the critical P450 isozymes involved in the substrate drug's metabolism. However, not all combinations of interacting drug with substrate will result in clinically significant drug–drug interactions. For these interactions to be clinically relevant, the substrate must have certain characteristics. A critical drug substrate is a drug with a narrow therapeutic index and one primary P450 isozyme mediating its elimination. For example, nifedipine, like all calcium-channel blockers, is primarily metabolized by the CYP3A4 isozyme. The addition of a drug that is a potent CYP3A4 inhibitor, such as fluvoxamine, will inhibit nifedipine's metabolism. Without a compensatory reduction in nifedipine dose, nifedipine levels will rise and toxicity may result. On the other hand, the addition of an inhibitor or inducer that interacts with a cytochrome P450 isozyme other than CYP3A4 will have no significant effect on nifedipine levels. Table 37–2 lists those drugs that are significant cytochrome P450 isozyme inhibitors, inducers, and critical substrates.

Metabolic drug interactions are most likely to occur in three situations: addition of an interacting drug (inhibitor or inducer) to an existing critical substrate drug; withdrawal of an interacting drug from a dosing regimen containing a substrate drug; or addition of a substrate drug to an existing regimen containing an interacting drug.

The addition of an interacting drug to a medication regimen containing a substrate drug at steady-state levels will dramatically alter the concentration of the substrate drug. If the interacting drug is an inhibitor, substrate drug concentrations will rise as its elimination is reduced. This rise in substrate levels may result in toxicity because of the drug's narrow therapeutic index. Conversely, addition of an enzyme inducer will increase elimination of the substrate, thereby lowering its concentration and therapeutic effect.

Withdrawal of an interacting drug from a drug regimen containing a critical substrate drug can also result in a drug interaction. The dosage of substrate drug will have been titrated, in the presence of the interacting drug, to optimize therapeutic effect and minimize adverse effects. Withdrawal of an enzyme inhibitor will allow metabolism to return (increase) to normal levels. This increased metabolism of the substrate drug will lower its levels and decrease therapeutic effect. In contrast, removal of an enzyme inducer will result in an increase in substrate drug levels and drug toxicity as metabolism of the substrate decreases to a normal rate.

The addition of a critical substrate drug to a drug regimen containing an interacting drug can result in a clinically significant interaction if the substrate is dosed according to established guidelines. Dosing guidelines do not account for the presence of a metabolic inhibitor or inducer and thus may lead to substrate concentrations that are, respectively, toxic or subtherapeutic.

Metabolic drug interactions can be minimized by avoiding drugs that are known critical substrates or potent inhibitors or inducers. Unfortunately, this is not always possible. However, by identifying medications that are critical substrates or potent inhibitors or inducers, making appropriate dosage adjustments, and monitoring drug levels (where possible), the adverse effects of these metabolic interactions will be reduced.

Drug interactions that affect renal drug elimination are clinically significant only if the parent drug or its active metabolite undergoes appreciable renal elimination. Changes in urine pH can modify the elimination of those compounds whose ratio of ionized/un-ionized forms is dramatically altered across the physiological range of urine pH (4.6 to 8.2) (i.e., the compound has a pKa within this pH range). Common drugs that alkalinize urine include antacids and carbonic anhydrase inhibitor diuretics. Un-ionized forms of drugs undergo greater glomerular resorption, whereas ionized drug forms are resorbed less and so have greater urinary excretion. For a basic drug such as amphetamine, alkalinization of urine increases the un-ionized fraction, enhancing resorption and so prolonging activity. Other basic psychotropic drugs, such as amitriptyline, imipramine, and meperidine, may be similarly affected (Cadwallader 1983).

Antidepressants

Antidepressant drugs are used to treat affective, anxiety, eating, and some somatoform disorders as well as insomnia, enuresis, incontinence, headaches, and chronic pain.

Side Effects and Toxicity

Selective Serotonin Reuptake Inhibitors and Novel/Mixed-Action Agents

Adverse effects of selective serotonin reuptake inhibitors (SSRIs) and novel/mixed-action agents are common, but they are usually mild, dose related, and abate over time. However, serotonergic agents, especially when used in combination, can induce the potentially fatal serotonin syndrome (see "Serotonin Syndrome" subsection later in this section).

Common short-term side effects with SSRIs and venlafaxine include nausea, vomiting, anxiety, headache, sedation, tremors, and anorexia. Common long-term side effects include sexual dysfunction, dry mouth, sweating, impaired sleep, and potential weight gain. Trazodone and nefazodone do not disrupt sexual function or sleep. Trazodone causes sedation in 20%–50% of patients and is often used for its sedating properties. It also infrequently causes priapism. Trazodone and nefazodone can cause orthostatic hypotension.

Frequent duloxetine side effects are nausea, dry mouth, fatigue, dizziness, constipation, somnolence, decreased appetite, and increased sweating (Nemeroff et al. 2002). Patients treated with reboxetine (used only in Europe) often report dry mouth, insomnia, constipation, sweating, and hypotension (Andreoli et al. 2002). Mirtazapine is associated with a high incidence of sedation, increased appetite, and weight gain (Nelson 1997). Common adverse effects of bupropion include agitation, insomnia, anxiety, dry mouth, constipation, postural hypotension, tachycardia, and cardiac arrhythmias. Nausea and vomiting are much less common with bupropion than with SSRIs (Vanderkooy et al. 2002).

TABLE 37–2. Drugs with clinically significant cytochrome P450 interactions

Drug	P450 isozyme[a]			
	1A2	**2C[c]**	**2D6**	**3A4**
Antiarrhythmics				
Amiodarone		X	X	S, X
Disopyramide				S
Encainide			S	
Flecainide			S	
Lidocaine				S
Mexiletine			S	
Propafenone			S, X	S
Quinidine			X	S
Anticoagulants/coagulation inhibitors				
Ticlopidine		X		
R-Warfarin	S	S		S
S-Warfarin		S		
Anticonvulsants/mood stabilizers				
Carbamazepine	I	I		S, I
Ethosuximide				S, I
Mephenytoin		S		
Phenytoin	I	S, I		I
Tiagabine		S	S	S
Valproate		I		
Antidepressants				
Amitriptyline	S	S	S	S
Bupropion			X	S
Clomipramine	S	S	S, X	S
Desipramine			S, X	
Doxepin			S	
Duloxetine	S		S, X	
Fluoxetine	X	X	S, X	S, X
Fluvoxamine	S, X	X		X
Gepirone				S
Imipramine	S	S	S	S
Maprotiline			S	
Moclobemide		S	X	
Nefazodone				S, X
Nortriptyline			S	
Paroxetine			S, X	
Tranylcypromine		X		
Trazodone			S	S
Trimipramine			S	
Venlafaxine			S	S

TABLE 37–2. Drugs with clinically significant cytochrome P450 interactions *(continued)*

Drug	P450 isozyme[a] 1A2	2C[c]	2D6	3A4
Antimicrobials				
Chloramphenicol		X		
Ciprofloxacin				X
Clarithromycin	X			S, X
Cotrimoxazole		X		
Enoxacin	X			
Erythromycin	X			S, X
Fluconazole		X		X
Griseofulvin	I			
Isoniazid	X			I
Itraconazole				S, X
Ketoconazole	X			S, X
Levofloxacin	X			
Metronidazole				X
Miconazole		S, X		S, X
Norfloxacin	X			X
Rifabutin				I
Rifampin	I	I		S, I
Roxithromycin				X
Sulfaphenazole		X		
Sulfonamides		X		
Troleandomycin	X			S, X
Antimigraine				
Ergotamine				S
Antineoplastic agents				
Tamoxifen	S	S		S
Antipsychotics				
Aripiprazole			S	S
Chlorpromazine	S		S	
Clozapine	S		S	S
Haloperidol	S		S, X	
Olanzapine	S		S	
Perphenazine			S	
Pimozide				S
Risperidone			S	
Thioridazine	S	S	S	
Antiretroviral agents				
Amprenavir				S
Atazanavir	X	X		S, X
Delavirdine		X		S, X
Efavirenz		X		S, X
Indinavir				S, X
Lopinavir				S
Lopinavir/ritonavir (Kaletra)	I	X	X	S, X
Nelfinavir				S, X
Nevirapine				S, I
Ritonavir	I	X	X	S, X
Saquinavir				S, X

TABLE 37–2.   Drugs with clinically significant cytochrome P450 interactions (*continued*)

Drug	P450 isozyme[a]			
	1A2	**2C**[c]	**2D6**	**3A4**
Anxiolytics/sedative-hypnotics				
Alprazolam				S
Bromazepam				S
Buspirone				S
Clonazepam				S
Diazepam		S		S
Hexobarbital		S		
Midazolam				S
Phenobarbital	I	I		I
Triazolam				S
Beta-blockers				
Alprenolol			S	
Bisoprolol			S	
Bufarolol			S	
Labetalol			S	
Metoprolol			S	
Pindolol			S	
Propranolol	S	S	S	
Timolol		S	S	
Bronchodilators				
Theophylline	S			S
Calcium channel blockers				
Amlodipine				S
Diltiazem				S, X
Felodipine				S
Isradipine				S
Nicardipine				S
Nifedipine				S
Nimodipine				S
Nisoldipine				S
Verapamil	S			S
Cognitive enhancers				
Tacrine	S			
Histamine H$_2$ antagonists				
Cimetidine	X	X	X	X
HMG-CoA reductase inhibitors				
Atorvastatin				S
Fluvastatin		X		S
Lovastatin		X		S
Pravastatin				S
Simvastatin		X		S
Immunosuppressive agents				
Cyclosporine				S, X
Rapamycin				S
Muscle relaxants				
Cyclobenzaprine	S		S	S
NSAIDs				
Phenylbutazone		S, X		

TABLE 37–2.   Drugs with clinically significant cytochrome P450 interactions (continued)

Drug	P450 isozyme[a]			
	1A2	2C[c]	2D6	3A4
Opiate analgesics				
Alfentanil				S
Hydrocodone			S	
Oxycodone			S	
Tramadol			S	
Oral hypoglycemics				
Chlorpropamide		S		
Glimepiride		S		
Glipizide		S		
Glyburide		S		
Tolbutamide		S, X		
Proton pump inhibitors				
Lansoprazole	I	S		
Omeprazole	I	S, X		S
Psychostimulants				
Atomoxetine			S, X	
Modafinil	I	X		S, I
Steroids				
Cortisol				S
Estradiol				S
Estrogen				S
Ethinylestradiol				S, X
Prednisolone				S
Prednisone				S
Progesterone				S
Testosterone				S
Uricosuric agents				
Sulfinpyrazone		X		
Miscellaneous agents				
Caffeine	S			S
Cannabinoids		S		S, X
Cruciferous vegetables[b]	I			
Grapefruit juice				X
Polyaromatic hydrocarbons	I			
St. John's wort				I
Smoking (tobacco, etc.)	I			

Note.   Drugs not present in this table generally do not have clinically significant cytochrome P450 interactions either as metabolic inhibitors or as critical substrates. NSAIDs=nonsteroidal anti-inflammatory drugs.

[a]Drug interactions with each cytochrome P450 isozyme: S=substrate; X=inhibitor; I=inducer. Only significant interactions are listed.

[b]Cruciferous vegetables include cabbage, cauliflower, broccoli, brussels sprouts, kale, etc.

[c]Combined properties on 2C9/10 and 2C19 cytochrome P450 isozymes.

Source.   Compiled, in part, from Alaka 2003; Bezchlibnyk and Jeffries 2000; Cozza et al. 2003; DeVane and Nemeroff 2002; Khachikian 2003; McEvoy 2003; Michalets 1998; Repchinsky 2003; USP DI Editorial Board 2003.

Central nervous system. An association between SSRI use and increased suicidal ideation was proposed by Teicher in 1990 on the basis of case reports (Teicher et al. 1990). Unfortunately, because of lack of definitive data, the existence of an association and the magnitude of effect remain unanswered. In a review of U.S. Food and Drug Administration (FDA) summary controlled clinical trial reports for nine modern antidepressants in 48,277 patients, Khan et al. (2003) concluded that there was no difference in suicide risk between antidepressant- and placebo-treated depressed patients or between treatment with SSRIs and with other antidepressants. In contrast, Healy (2003), from his review of randomized clinical trials, suggested that SSRIs possibly double the risk of suicide and suicide attempts in comparison with older antidepressants or no treatment. In June 2003, the United Kingdom Department of Health concluded that the rate of self-harm and potentially suicidal behavior is increased in children and adolescents receiving paroxetine for treatment of depression. Both the U.K. Department of Health and the FDA have issued recommendations that paroxetine not be used in this population. In March of 2004, the FDA asked manufacturers of antidepressant drugs (including fluoxetine, sertraline, paroxetine, fluvoxamine, citalopram, escitalopram, bupropion, venlafaxine, nefazodone, and mirtazapine) to include in their labeling a warning statement that recommends close observation of adult and pediatric patients treated with these agents for worsening depression or the emergence of suicidality. The FDA has not concluded that these drugs cause worsening depression or suicidality.

Bupropion causes a dose-related lowering of the seizure threshold and may precipitate seizures in susceptible patients receiving dosages above 450 mg/day. The incidence of seizure rises with increasing dosage, from 0.1% at 100–300 mg/day, through 0.4% at 300–450 mg/day, to 2.3% at dosages over 600 mg/day (McEvoy 2003). The seizure risk reported for other antidepressants ranges from 0.04% for mirtazapine to 15.6% ($n=32$) for maprotiline (Harden and Goldstein 2002; Jabbari et al. 1985). Given that the annual incidence of first unprovoked seizure is 0.06% in the general population, seizure risk for patients taking most antidepressants is not elevated. However, it is clear that certain antidepressants, including bupropion, clomipramine, and maprotiline, especially in higher doses, are associated with a greater seizure risk than are other antidepressants (Harden and Goldstein 2002).

Potential side effects of SSRIs include SSRI-induced extrapyramidal symptoms (EPS), likely resulting from serotonergic antagonism of dopaminergic pathways in the central nervous system (CNS). Akathisia, dystonia, parkinsonism, and tardive dyskinesia–like states have been reported, with akathisia being the most common effect and tardive dyskinesia–like states being the least common. Certain patients appear to be at increased risk, such as the elderly, patients with Parkinson's disease, and patients concurrently treated with dopamine antagonists (Leo 1996).

Serotonin syndrome. Serotonin syndrome is an uncommon but potentially life-threatening complication of treatment with serotonergic agents. Overall, there is considerable heterogeneity in the reported clinical features of serotonin syndrome (Table 37–3), likely reflecting the variation in the degree of severity of the syndrome. The incidence of the syndrome is unknown, partly due to the lack of uniform diagnostic criteria. Virtually all medications that potentiate serotonergic neurotransmission in the CNS have been reported in association with serotonin syndrome. The antidepressant combinations most commonly implicated have been monoamine oxidase inhibitors (MAOIs; reversible and irreversible) and TCAs, MAOIs and SSRIs, and MAOIs and venlafaxine. Table 37–4 lists selected other serotonergic drugs.

Currently there is no formal consensus regarding diagnostic criteria for serotonin syndrome. The first operationalized criteria were proposed in 1991 by Sternbach. Recently revised criteria are listed in Table 37–5 (Birmes et al. 2003; Keck and Arnold 2000). Laboratory findings have not been commonly reported in cases of serotonin syndrome, but some reports have noted leukocytosis, rhabdomyolysis with elevated creatine phosphokinase

TABLE 37–3. Clinical features of serotonin syndrome

Category	Clinical features
Mental status and behavioral	Delirium, confusion, agitation, anxiety, irritability, euphoria, dysphoria, restlessness
Neurological and motor	Ataxia/incoordination, tremor, muscle rigidity, myoclonus, hyperreflexia, clonus, seizures, trismus, teeth chattering
Gastrointestinal	Nausea, vomiting, diarrhea, incontinence
Autonomic nervous system	Hypertension, hypotension, tachycardia, diaphoresis, shivering, sialorrhea, mydriasis, tachypnea, pupillary dilation
Hyperthermia	

Source. Compiled in part from Keck and Arnold 2000.

TABLE 37–4. Drugs that potentiate serotonin in the central nervous system

Mechanism	Drug
Enhance serotonin synthesis	L-Tryptophan
Increase serotonin release	Cocaine
	Amphetamine
	Sibutramine
	Dextromethorphan, meperidine
	Methylene dioxymethamphetamine (MDMA, Ecstasy)
Serotonin agonist	Buspirone
	Lithium
	Triptans
	Ergots
	Trazodone, nefazodone
Inhibit serotonin catabolism	Antidepressant MAOIs
	Moclobemide
	Selegiline
Inhibit serotonin reuptake	SSRIs
	Mirtazapine
	Trazodone, nefazodone
	Venlafaxine, duloxetine
	Tricyclic antidepressants
	Dextromethorphan, meperidine
	Pethidine
	Tramadol

Note. MAOIs=monoamine oxidase inhibitors; SSRIs=selective serotonin reuptake inhibitors.

TABLE 37–5. Revised diagnostic criteria for serotonin syndrome

1. Addition of a serotonergic agent to an already established treatment (or increase in dosage) and manifestation of at least four major symptoms or three major symptoms plus two minor ones

   Mental (cognitive and behavioral) symptoms
   Major symptoms: confusion, elevated mood, coma, or semicoma
   Minor symptoms: agitation and nervousness, insomnia

   Autonomic symptoms
   Major symptoms: fever, hyperhidrosis
   Minor symptoms: tachycardia, tachypnea and dyspnea, diarrhea, low or high blood pressure

   Neurological symptoms
   Major symptoms: myoclonus, tremors, chills, rigidity, hyperreflexia
   Minor symptoms: impaired coordination, mydriasis, akathisia

2. These symptoms must not correspond to a psychiatric disorder, or its aggravation, that occurred before the patient took the serotonergic agent.
3. Infectious, metabolic, endocrine, or toxic causes must be excluded.
4. A neuroleptic treatment must not have been introduced, nor its dose increased, before the symptoms appeared.

Source. Adapted with permission from Birmes P, Coppin D, Schmitt L, et al.: "Serotonin Syndrome: A Brief Review." *CMAJ* 168:1439–1442, 2003.

(CPK), serum hepatic transaminase elevations, electrolyte abnormalities (hyponatremia, hypomagnesemia, hypercalcemia), and disseminated intravascular coagulopathy. The differential diagnosis includes other disorders producing cognitive and behavioral, neuromuscular, and autonomic nervous system dysfunction, with or without hyperthermia. Thus, the differential diagnosis for serotonin syndrome is similar to that for neuroleptic malignant syndrome (NMS) (see "Neuroleptic Malignant Syndrome" subsection later in the chapter). Differentiating serotonin syndrome from NMS can be very difficult in patients receiving both serotonergic and antipsychotic medications.

Serotonin syndrome is often self-limited and usually resolves quickly after discontinuation of serotonergic agents. Management includes the following basic principles: 1) provide necessary supportive care, 2) discontinue all serotonergic agents, 3) anticipate potential complications, 4) consider administering antiserotonergic agents, and 5) reassess the need for psychopharmacological ther-

apy before reinstituting drug therapy (Keck and Arnold 2000). Some patients will require admission to an intensive care unit, but most will show some improvement within 24 hours with supportive care alone. There are no specific antidotes available for the treatment of serotonin syndrome. The antihistamine cyproheptadine is the most consistently effective serotonin antagonist reported. The recommended adult dose is 4–8 mg and may be repeated every 1–4 hours up to a maximum daily dose of 32 mg. There is limited information on drug rechallenge in patients who have developed serotonin syndrome. General guidelines include reevaluating the necessity for drug therapy, considering a switch to a nonserotonergic medication, using single-drug therapy when serotonergic medications are required, and considering an extended (6-week) serotonin "drug-free" period before restarting a serotonergic agent (Mills 1997).

Autonomic and cardiovascular. The SSRIs and the novel/mixed-action antidepressants have a much safer cardiovascular profile than the TCAs and MAOIs. In general, the SSRIs have little effect on blood pressure or cardiac conduction (Glassman et al. 2002). Fluoxetine has been reported to rarely cause mild bradycardia in elderly patients with preexisting cardiac arrhythmias (Upward et al. 1988), and this may occur with other SSRIs as well.

The novel/mixed-action agents venlafaxine, duloxetine, bupropion, nefazodone, mirtazapine, and reboxetine have no effect on cardiac conduction but may affect blood pressure or heart rate (Khawaja and Feinstein 2003). Venlafaxine exhibits dose-related increases in heart rate (mean increase of 4 beats/minute over placebo) and blood pressure. Placebo-controlled clinical trials of venlafaxine observed an average diastolic pressure increase of 7 mm Hg at dosages of more than 300 mg/day and clinically significant diastolic pressure increases ($\geq$15 mm Hg) in 5.5% of patients taking the drug at dosages of more than 200 mg/day (Feighner 1995). Bupropion is reported to cause hypertension without affecting heart rate in some patients. In patients using transdermal nicotine, bupropion is associated with a 6.1% incidence of hypertension (Khawaja and Feinstein 2003). Reboxetine has also been associated with an increase in heart rate of 8–11 beats/minute (Fleishaker et al. 2001), but without any significant effect on electrocardiography (Andreoli et al. 2002). Trazodone lacks significant effects on cardiac conduction but in rare cases was reported to cause ventricular ectopy and ventricular tachycardia. The most frequent cardiovascular adverse effect of trazodone is postural hypotension, which may be associated with syncope. Nefazodone is structurally related to trazodone but has a lower incidence of postural hypotension (3%). Mirtazapine does not have significant effects on cardiac conduction, but because of its moderate alpha$_1$-antagonist activity, it has a 7% incidence of orthostatic hypotension (Khawaja and Feinstein 2003). Hypotension is observed in 10% of patients receiving reboxetine. Duloxetine appears to be without significant cardiovascular effects (Nemeroff et al. 2002).

Gastrointestinal.   Nausea is the most common adverse effect associated with the serotonergic antidepressants. Nausea is most likely to occur in patients receiving fluvoxamine (36%), venlafaxine (37%), and duloxetine at a starting dose of 60 mg qd (35%–40%) (Detke et al. 2002a, 2002b). Other serotonergic antidepressants have a lower incidence (20%–26%) of nausea, but these incidences are still much higher than those seen with placebo (9.3%–11.8%) (Nelson 1997; Repchinsky 2003). SSRIs and venlafaxine may also cause loose stools.

Although most adverse gastrointestinal effects of serotonergic antidepressants are dose related and generally decrease with continued treatment, sometimes severe side effects require antidepressant discontinuation. Potential

severe hepatotoxicity with nefazodone has led to its removal from the market in a number of countries, and it should not be used in patients with preexisting liver disease (Stewart 2002). Pancreatitis has also rarely been reported with mirtazapine (Lankisch and Werner 2003; Sommer et al. 2001).

Weight gain/loss.   Weight gain is a relatively common problem during both acute and long-term treatment with antidepressants. TCAs and MAOIs are more likely to cause weight gain than other antidepressants, with the exception of mirtazapine. Paroxetine may be more likely than other SSRIs to cause weight gain during long-term treatment. Bupropion rarely causes weight gain (Fava 2000).

Sexual dysfunction.   Please refer to Chapter 17, "Sexual Disorders," for a discussion of the sexual side effects of psychotropic medications.

Drug interactions.   Many SSRIs and novel/mixed-action antidepressants are potent inhibitors of cytochrome P450 isozymes and may significantly increase the blood levels, and the potential for toxic effects, of other co-administered narrow therapeutic index medications metabolized by these enzymes. See Table 37–2 for a listing of critical narrow therapeutic index drug substrates for these enzymes.

The use of multiple serotonergic drugs can induce serotonin syndrome (see "Serotonin Syndrome" subsection earlier in the chapter).

Abrupt discontinuation of SSRIs, especially those with short half-lives, may give rise to a discontinuation syndrome characterized by a wide variety of symptoms, including gastrointestinal, psychiatric, neurological, and flulike symptoms; sleep disturbances; and headache (Haddad 1998), usually resolving within 3 weeks. Antidepressants, like all psychoactive medications, should be gradually withdrawn. Discontinuation symptoms can cause misdiagnosis and inappropriate treatment, particularly in a patient with an active medical illness, as well as erode future compliance.

Tricyclic Antidepressants

TCAs are now viewed as second-line treatments for depression because their adverse effect profile is less benign than that of SSRIs. Death from TCA-induced cardiac conduction abnormalities was not uncommon in overdose.

Many adverse effects of TCAs are due not to their effects on serotonin (5-HT) or norepinephrine reuptake inhibition but rather to secondary pharmacological activities. TCAs are antagonists at histamine H_1, adrenergic alpha$_1$, and muscarinic receptors and have type-1A antiarrhythmic (quinidine-like) effects as a result of their blockade of voltage-dependent Na$^+$-channels. Adverse effects of the TCAs include sedation, anticholinergic effects (dry mouth, dry eyes, constipation, urinary retention, decreased sweating, confusion, memory impairment, tachycardia, blurred vision), and postural hypotension. Tolerance to these effects usually develops over time. TCAs at or just above therapeutic plasma levels frequently prolong PR, QRS, and QTc intervals, but rarely to a clinically significant degree in patients without preexisting cardiac disease or conduction defects (Glassman 1984). TCAs can cause heart block, arrhythmias, palpitations, tachycardia, syncope, and heart failure and should be used with caution in patients with preexisting cardiovascular disease or at risk of suicide. Following the discovery that class I antiarrhythmic drugs can increase mortality in patients with ischemic heart disease, it is prudent to assume that TCAs may carry the same risk in these patients (Cardiac Arrhythmia Suppression Trial [CAST] Investigators 1989; Glassman et al. 1993).

Drug interactions.   The combination of TCAs and other drugs with sedating, hypotensive, antiarrhythmic, or seizure threshold–lowering properties may lead to additive toxicity.

Concomitant use of TCAs and drugs with anticholinergic properties may cause an anticholinergic crisis characterized by delirium, hyperthermia (especially in hot environments), tachycardia, and paralytic ileus.

Coadministration of TCAs with direct-acting (e.g., isoproterenol, phenylephrine) or indirect-acting (MAOIs and other drugs with MAOI activity) sympathomimetics may precipitate a potentially fatal reaction, with symptoms of hyperpyrexia, sweating, confusion, myoclonus, seizures, hypertension, and tachycardia.

The combination of serotonergic effects from co-therapy with some TCAs and SSRIs may precipitate serotonin syndrome (see "Serotonin Syndrome" subsection earlier in this chapter).

TCAs are narrow therapeutic index drugs, each metabolized predominantly by either CYP2D6 or CYP3A4. Inhibitors of these enzymes can cause TCA toxicity by dramatically increasing TCA serum levels. Many agents, including several SSRIs and novel/mixed-action antidepressants, are potent inhibitors of these cytochromes (see Table 37–2). Plasma levels of TCAs should be monitored if they are coadministered with such inhibitors.

Toxicity/overdose.   TCA overdose carries a risk of death from cardiac conduction abnormalities that result in ma-

lignant ventricular arrhythmias. Initial symptoms of overdose involve CNS stimulation, in part due to anticholinergic effects, and include hyperpyrexia, delirium, hypertension, hallucinations, seizure, agitation, hyperreflexia, and parkinsonian symptoms. The initial stimulation phase is typically followed by CNS depression with drowsiness, areflexia, hypothermia, respiratory depression, severe hypotension, and coma. Risk of cardiotoxicity is high if the QRS interval is 100 msec or more (Boehnert and Lovejoy 1985) or if the total TCA plasma concentration is greater than 1,000 ng/mL; concentrations greater than 2,500 ng/mL are often fatal (Foulke and Albertson 1987).

Treatment for overdose includes removal of any unabsorbed medication from the stomach (gastric lavage or emesis with aspiration precautions and then activated charcoal to reduce absorption), followed by supportive therapy and close monitoring. Cardiac conduction abnormalities, arrhythmias, and hypotension may be treated with administration of intravenous sodium bicarbonate to produce a serum pH of 7.4–7.5. Life-threatening anticholinergic effects may be managed with physostigmine. Because of their large volumes of distribution and extensive protein binding, TCAs are not removed by dialysis.

Abrupt discontinuation of TCAs may give rise to a discontinuation syndrome characterized by dizziness, lethargy, headache, nightmares, and symptoms of anticholinergic rebound, including gastrointestinal upset, nausea, vomiting, diarrhea, excessive salivation, sweating, anxiety, restlessness, piloerection, and delirium (Dilsaver and Greden 1984). This syndrome can be avoided by gradual withdrawal.

Monoamine Oxidase Inhibitors

Monoamine oxidase inhibitors (MAOIs), with the possible exception of moclobemide (not available in the United States), are seen as third-line antidepressants because of their significant drug interactions and the dietary restrictions that accompany their use. Moclobemide, a short-half-life reversible inhibitor of monoamine oxidase type A (MAO-A), is less susceptible to dietary interactions providing it is taken after meals. Common adverse effects of MAOIs include orthostatic hypotension, dizziness, headache, sedation, insomnia or hypersomnia, tremor, and hyperreflexia. Interactions between MAOIs and direct- or indirect-acting sympathomimetics or dopaminergic agonists may cause a hypertensive crisis. MAOIs may trigger serotonin syndrome when combined with other medications (see "Serotonin Syndrome" subsection earlier in the chapter). Moclobemide shares the potential to cause hypertensive crises and serotonin syndrome with the irreversible agents. MAOIs may greatly potentiate the hypotensive effects of antihypertensive agents, including diuretics (British Medical Association 2003a).

Selegiline, a semiselective monoamine oxidase type B (MAO-B) inhibitor used to treat Parkinson's disease, may also contribute to serotonin syndrome. At dosages greater than 10 mg/day, selegiline also inhibits MAO-A and thus shares many of the adverse effects and drug/food interactions, including hypertensive crisis, of the antidepressant MAOIs.

Toxicity/overdose.   Symptoms of MAOI overdose are an extension of the normal adverse-effect profile. Treatment for overdose includes removal of any unabsorbed medication from the stomach and supportive measures.

Treatment for hypertensive crisis involves discontinuing the MAOI and slowly administering intravenous phentolamine (typical adult dose = 5 mg). *Beta-blockers should never be used*; beta-blockade allows unrestrained alpha-adrenergic stimulation, which further exacerbates the hypertension.

Mood Stabilizers

Mood stabilizers are used in the medically ill to treat primary and secondary mood disorders as well as for symptoms such as headache and chronic pain. Many but not all anticonvulsants appear to have mood-stabilizing properties. Valproic acid, carbamazepine, and oxcarbazepine are the most commonly used anticonvulsant mood stabilizers. Controlled studies do not support the use of gabapentin as a mood stabilizer (Evins 2003).

Side Effects and Toxicity

Lithium

Most patients using lithium experience some side effects, both acute (gastrointestinal distress and tremor) and long-term (polyuria and polydipsia, hypothyroidism, weight gain, impaired cognition, sedation, impaired coordination, edema, acne, and hair loss), most of which are mild and dose related (Peet and Pratt 1993). Adverse effects of lithium can be minimized by reducing the dose or decreasing the rate of absorption from the gut by administering the drug either in divided doses with meals or in a slow-release form.

Central nervous system.   Headache, fatigue, hand tremor, and mild cognitive impairment are reported by up to 50% of patients beginning lithium treatment. Hand tremor is usually a benign, fine, rapid intention tremor that resolves over time or can be managed by dose reduction or low-

dose beta-blockers. The tremor does not respond to antiparkinsonian drugs. Muscle weakness, fatigue, and ataxia are also common initial adverse effects that usually resolve (McEvoy 2003). Mild cognitive impairment may be experienced during the first 6–8 months of treatment; although rarely progressive, this impairment is the most common reason for noncompliance (Gitlin et al. 1989).

Autonomic and cardiovascular.   Lithium causes benign reversible repolarization electrocardiographic changes in 20%–30% of patients (Mitchell and Mackenzie 1982), including T-wave depression and inversion. Other cardiovascular effects of lithium include decreased heart rate and, rarely, cardiac conduction abnormalities and arrhythmias (Burggraf 1997).

Renal.   Lithium reduces renal response to antidiuretic hormone, resulting in polyuria and/or polydipsia initially in 30%–50% of patients and persisting in 10%–25%. Stopping lithium usually reverses this nephrogenic diabetes insipidus (McEvoy 2003). Apart from dry mouth, patients do not generally exhibit signs of dehydration. Management of polyuria may include changing to a single daily bedtime dose of lithium, decreasing dosage, and/or administering thiazide diuretics or amiloride. If thiazide diuretics are added, lithium dosage typically will have to be reduced by 50% to compensate for thiazide-induced reduction of lithium excretion (Jefferson et al. 1987). Use of amiloride does not require a reduction in lithium dosage (Bendz and Aurell 1999). Edema has been reported in patients with a high sodium intake (>170 mEq/day), responsive to reduction in sodium intake or spironolactone (Stancer and Kivi 1971).

Both functional and morphological changes of the kidneys have been reported in lithium-poisoned patients. Whether renal impairment is a direct effect of lithium on the kidneys or a secondary effect of systemic toxicicity is not resolved. Chronic use of lithium may result in altered kidney morphology in 10%–20% of patients, including interstitial fibrosis, tubular atrophy, urinary casts, and, occasionally, glomerular sclerosis (Bendz et al. 1996). These changes are not generally associated with impaired renal function. In 1979, the World Psychiatric Association convened a meeting in Copenhagen to discuss lithium and renal effects. The consensus was that the risk of lithium nephropathy in the absence of lithium toxicity is small. Most investigators continue to agree that the risk of renal dysfunction during chronic use is far less than the risk of psychiatric morbidity (Perry 1996).

Endocrine and metabolic.   The prevalence of overt hypothyroidism has been reported to be as high as 8%–19% for patients taking lithium, compared with a prevalence of 0.5%–1.8% in the general population. Subclinical hypothyroidism has been reported in up to 23% of patients receiving lithium therapy, compared with rates of up to 10.4% in the general population. Elevated thyroid-stimulating hormone is present in approximately 30% of patients taking lithium for 6 months or more, and progression to overt hypothyroidism (elevated thyroid-stimulating hormone and low free T_4) may occur in as many as 5%–10% of patients per year (Kleiner et al. 1999). Thyroid function should be assessed before lithium is started and periodically during therapy. Hypothyroidism can be treated with L-thyroxine and is not a contraindication to continuing lithium (Bauer and Whybrow 1990) (see also Chapter 23, "Endocrine and Metabolic Disorders").

Weight gain is the second most common reason cited by patients for lithium noncompliance (Gitlin et al. 1989). Weight gain is a consequence of increased caloric intake in part due to consumption of high-calorie fluids in response to increased thirst (McEvoy 2003).

Dermatological.   Dermatological adverse effects include dry skin and acne. Occurring in about 1% of patients taking lithium (Jefferson et al. 1987), these effects usually respond to standard treatment and rarely require lithium discontinuation. Alopecia and exacerbation of psoriasis occur less frequently (Chan et al. 2000) (see also Chapter 29, "Dermatology").

Drug interactions.   Lithium is almost entirely renally excreted, and most lithium filtered by the glomeruli is reabsorbed with sodium in the proximal tubule. Serum lithium levels are increased by thiazide diuretics, NSAIDs, angiotensin-converting enzyme inhibitors, sodium depletion, and dehydration (Dunner 2003). Verapamil, and possibly other calcium channel blockers, may also cause an increase in serum lithium levels (Wright and Jarrett 1991). For a more complete review, see the article by Thomsen and Schou (1999).

Lithium may potentiate the neurological adverse effects of other drugs, for example, EPS and tremor (Dunner 2000).

Toxicity/overdose.   Toxicity increases markedly as serum lithium levels exceed 1.5 mEq/L, and serum levels greater than 2.0 mEq/L are dangerous. However, some patients experience toxicity at "therapeutic" levels. Initial symptoms of toxicity include marked tremor, nausea, diarrhea, blurred vision, vertigo, confusion, and increased deep tendon reflexes, progressing to seizures, coma, cardiac arrhythmia, and possibly permanent neurological impairment as lithium levels increase.

Treatment for lithium toxicity includes gastric lavage or emesis followed by supportive measures. These measures include volume resuscitation with isotonic or one-half isotonic sodium chloride solution to enhance renal elimination of lithium in individuals with mild-to-moderate toxicity, or hemodialysis for patients with severe toxicity and/or lithium levels of 3.5 mEq/L or higher (Jaeger et al. 1993; Menghini and Albright 2000).

Anticonvulsants

Central nervous system.   The anticonvulsants valproate, carbamazepine, gabapentin, lamotrigine, oxcarbazepine, topiramate, tiagabine, zonisamide, and levetiracetam share a similar profile of CNS adverse effects. Sedation, ataxia, dizziness, muscle weakness, fatigue, and vision disturbances such as nystagmus and diplopia are common and often resolve with time, dosage reduction, or discontinuation. Studies of oxcarbazepine in epilepsy suggest a lower rate of adverse effects than carbamazepine (Dam et al. 1989). Psychotic symptoms are an infrequent adverse effect but reportedly occur more frequently with topiramate (Crawford 1998). Cognitive impairment is a common complication of anticonvulsant use. Among anticonvulsants used in psychiatry, the ranking of cognitive profile is (best to worst) gabapentin, lamotrigine, valproate and carbamazepine, and topiramate (Goldberg and Burdick 2001). There are insufficient data to rank oxcarbazepine and levetiracetam.

Gastrointestinal.   Symptoms of gastrointestinal distress, including nausea, vomiting, dyspepsia, diarrhea, and anorexia, are the most frequent adverse effects experienced with most anticonvulsants. These effects are often dose related and transient, and can be minimized by giving the drug in divided doses, with meals, or with slow titration.

Gastrointestinal effects appear less often with divalproex sodium than with valproic acid or sodium valproate. There are fewer gastrointestinal complaints with oxcarbazepine than with carbamazepine.

Hematological.   Carbamazepine is frequently associated with transient leukopenia and rarely may cause aplastic anemia. Carbamazepine should be discontinued in patients with white blood cell counts less than 3.0×10^9/L or neutrophil counts less than 1.0×10^9/L, and patients must be educated to report early signs of anemia, infection, or bleeding (Sobotka et al. 1990).

Mild, asymptomatic leukopenia and thrombocytopenia have been observed with valproate and are generally reversible with dosage reduction or discontinuation. More severe cases of thrombocytopenia and agranulocytosis have also been reported (Finsterer et al. 2001).

Renal. Carbamazepine and oxcarbazepine frequently cause the syndrome of inappropriate antidiuretic hormone secretion (SIADH), leading to hyponatremia and water intoxication. Carbamazepine-induced hyponatremia has been reported in as many as 6%–36% of patients, more commonly in the elderly (McEvoy 2003; van Amelsvoort et al. 1994). Hyponatremia may be more common with oxcarbazepine than with carbamazepine (Asconape 2002). (For a further discussion of SIADH, see "Antipsychotics" subsection later in this chapter.)

Endocrine and metabolic. Transient elevations in liver enzymes occur commonly with anticonvulsants. Significant changes in hepatic function are usually reversible with dosage reduction or discontinuation. However, fatal hepatotoxicity has been reported with valproate. The risk of hepatic failure may be increased by combination therapy and comorbid hepatic disorders (Konig et al. 1999).

Weight gain is a common factor in noncompliance (Mendlewicz et al. 1999). Weight gain is especially a problem with valproate, with 25% of patients gaining up to 20 kg (Pijl and Meinders 1996). Gabapentin is reported to result in about 10% gain of body weight in 25% of patients (DeToledo et al. 1997). Although carbamazepine is also reported to cause weight gain, the incidence is less than with valproate (Corman et al. 1997). Lamotrigine has little effect on weight, whereas topiramate causes a weight loss of about 3–5 kg (Chengappa et al. 1999; McElroy et al. 2000). Topiramate can cause hyperchloremic, non–anion gap metabolic acidosis; in clinical trials, persistent reductions in serum bicarbonate occurred in 23%–67% of patients, and levels were markedly low (<17 mEq/L) in 3%–11% (Ortho-McNeil, general letter, December 2003).

Polycystic ovarian syndrome occurs in women with epilepsy, with a prevalence 3.8 times greater than that in the general population. This increase has been variously attributed to either epilepsy (Joffe et al. 2001) or anticonvulsant medications, especially valproate. Whether valproate presents a similar risk when used as a mood stabilizer remains uncertain (see Chapter 23, "Endocrine and Metabolic Disorders").

Immune system. Benign skin rashes occur in 5%–20% of patients receiving anticonvulsants, including valproate, carbamazepine, and lamotrigine. However, serious and potentially fatal immune reactions to anticonvulsants are not uncommon. Anticonvulsant hypersensitivity syndrome has been observed in up to 1% of patients, with initial signs of rash, fever, malaise, and pharyngitis progressing to internal organ involvement. Severe and often fatal hypersensitivity cutaneous reactions include Stevens-Johnson syndrome and toxic epidermal necrolysis. Mortality occurs in about 5%–10% of patients with Stevens-Johnson syndrome and in up to 45% of those with toxic epidermal necrolysis. In comparison with general medical patients, the risk of developing Stevens-Johnson syndrome or toxic epidermal necrolysis during the first 2 months of anticonvulsant therapy is increased by 120-fold for carbamazepine, 25-fold for lamotrigine, and 24-fold for valproate (Rzany et al. 1999). Clinical trials suggest that 25% of patients with hypersensitivity reactions to carbamazepine will also cross-react to oxcarbazepine (USP DI Editorial Board 2003). The presence of an anticonvulsant-induced rash should prompt drug discontinuation (Hebert and Ralston 2001).

Drug interactions. Significant cytochrome P450 enzyme induction occurs with carbamazepine (CYP1A2, CYP2C, and CYP3A4), oxcarbazepine (CYP3A4), and valproate (CYP2C) (see Table 37–2). Because valproate is highly bound to plasma proteins, it can significantly displace other highly protein-bound drugs. Valproate can also compete for hepatic glucuronidation and so inhibit the elimination of drugs primarily using this route of metabolism, such as lamotrigine and morphine.

Toxicity/overdose. Symptoms of anticonvulsant overdose are often an extension of the normal adverse effects, including stupor, conduction disturbances, and hypotension. Treatment for overdose includes gastric lavage or emesis followed by supportive therapy. Hemodialysis is an effective means of enhancing drug elimination for valproate, gabapentin, topiramate, and levetiracetam.

Antipsychotics

Antipsychotic drugs are used in the medically ill to treat nearly all forms of psychosis, including psychosis secondary to general medical conditions, delirium, and dementia, and less frequently for nonspecific sedation and as analgesic adjuvants.

Side Effects and Toxicity

Central Nervous System

Acute extrapyramidal symptoms. Acute EPS—akathisia, akinesia, and dystonia—occur in as many as 50%–75% of patients who take typical antipsychotics (Collaborative Working Group on Clinical Trial Evaluations 1998). High-potency typical antipsychotics are associated with higher rates of EPS than are low-potency agents. Among the currently available atypical antipsychotics, the hierarchy of

EPS risk (greater to lesser) is risperidone > olanzapine = ziprasidone = aripiprazole (estimated) > quetiapine > clozapine (Tandon 2002).

Most akathisia and acute dystonic reactions in the medically ill are caused by phenothiazine antiemetics or metoclopramide, especially at high intravenous doses. When agitated medically ill patients are being treated with haloperidol, it can be very difficult to distinguish akathisia from the original target symptoms. It is also important to exclude other causes of restlessness that may mimic akathisia in medically ill patients, such as hypoglycemia, hypoxia, drug withdrawal, pain, electrolyte disturbances, iron deficiency, and restless legs syndrome. Severe dystonic reactions (e.g., opisthotonus) may be misdiagnosed in the medically ill as status epilepticus.

Chronic extrapyramidal symptoms.   Parkinsonian signs and tardive dyskinesia may result from chronic use of antipsychotics, phenothiazine antiemetics, or metoclopramide. Bradykinesia may easily be missed in the elderly or disabled medical patients. Tardive dyskinesias may be difficult to distinguish from other dyskinesias in elderly patients (e.g., "senile dyskinesias," ill-fitting dentures).

Seizures.   At higher doses, there appears to be an increased risk of seizures associated with antipsychotics. Various reports suggest a dose-dependent seizure risk with phenothiazines from 0.3%–1.2% compared with a rate of first unprovoked seizure in the general population of about 0.1%. Most of the early case reports were of seizures with chlorpromazine. Although there are no controlled comparative studies to allow an accurate assessment of relative seizure risk, it appears that high-potency typical antipsychotics and risperidone have the lowest rate of seizures; olanzapine, quetiapine, and low-potency typical antipsychotics have an intermediate risk; and clozapine has the highest risk (Alldredge 1999).

Sedation.   Sedation is the most common single side effect, especially with the low-potency typical antipsychotics. Among the atypical antipsychotics, the hierarchy of potential for sedation (greater to lesser) is clozapine > quetiapine > olanzapine > risperidone > ziprasidone = aripiprazole (estimated) (Tandon 2002). Sedation is most prominent in the early stages of therapy, with some degree of tolerance developing over time.

Thermoregulation.   Antipsychotics may interfere with temperature regulation, especially low-potency typical and anticholinergic atypical agents. Medically ill patients, especially elderly ones, are at particular risk because of other anticholinergic drugs and comorbidities impairing thermo-regulation (e.g., congestive heart failure, cerebrovascular disease). Depending on environmental exposure, either hyperthermia or hypothermia may result (Mann et al. 2003).

Neuroleptic malignant syndrome.   NMS is a rare, potentially fatal, idiosyncratic reaction to antipsychotics. NMS (or a similar syndrome) is also reported among patients with extrapyramidal disorders such as Wilson's disease, striatonigral degeneration, and Parkinson's disease who have received antipsychotics or dopamine-depleting agents or who have had dopamine agonists abruptly withdrawn (Friedman et al. 1985; Gibb 1988; Gibb and Griffith 1986; Kontaxakis et al. 1988). However, NMS is not specific to any neuropsychiatric diagnosis and has been reported in non–psychiatrically ill individuals who were treated with other dopamine antagonists such as metoclopramide and prochlorperazine (Nonino and Campomori 1999; Pesola and Quinto 1996). Estimates of the incidence of NMS have ranged from 0.02%–3.23%, reflecting differences in diagnostic criteria, survey techniques, patient populations, and treatment settings and practices (Lazarus et al. 1989). Malnutrition, dehydration, and iron deficiency all appear to increase risk for NMS.

NMS generally develops over a 1–3 day period and lasts for 5–10 days after a nondepot antipsychotic is discontinued. Mortality is high, often quoted at 20%–30% but probably lower now because of earlier recognition. The main clinical features of NMS include hyperthermia (>37°C), generalized muscle rigidity, mental status changes and autonomic instability. Temperature in hyperthermia is greater than 38°C in the majority of cases and can exceed 40°C, which predisposes the patient to severe complications, including irreversible CNS and other organ damage. Muscle rigidity is often heterogeneous and can be "lead-pipe" or cogwheeling. Autonomic dysfunction in NMS may include hypertension, orthostatic hypotension, labile blood pressure, tachycardia, tachypnea, sialorrhea, diaphoresis, skin pallor, and urinary incontinence. Neurological dysfunction may consist of tremor, myoclonus, focal dystonias, dysphagia, dysarthria, opisthotonus, oculogyric crisis, and dyskinesias. Altered level of consciousness may range from decreased awareness to coma. CPK levels are often elevated in NMS secondary to muscle necrosis from rigidity, hyperthermia, and ischemia. Elevated CPK levels are not proof of NMS, because they may result from agitation, use of physical restraints, and intramuscular injections. Extreme elevation of CPK (>100,000 U/L) constitutes rhabdomyolysis, which may be a consequence of NMS and/or other causes in the medically ill (e.g., sepsis, shock, alcohol). Serial CPK monitoring in NMS will typically show declining levels with the resolution of the syndrome. Leukocytosis with or without a left shift is common. Complications may include respiratory or renal failure, pulmonary embolus, electrolyte disturbances, and coagulopathy (Caroff and Mann 1993; Pelonero et al. 1998).

The differential diagnosis of NMS is large (Table 37–6). Although the vast majority of patients receiving antipsychotics who develop fever and rigidity will be found to have other conditions, the possibility of NMS should be considered because of the importance of promptly withholding antipsychotics. Basic and optional examinations for the clinical evaluation of possible NMS include those listed in Table 37–7.

The main interventions in NMS are early diagnosis, rapid cessation of the antipsychotic treatment, and intensive supportive care. Lithium, antipsychotics, and all other dopamine-blocking agents (including antiemetics and droperidol) should be discontinued. No specific therapy (e.g., dantrolene or bromocriptine) has been proven superior to other measures (for a detailed review, see Mann et al. 2003). Most cases of NMS require initial treatment in a medical intensive care unit and should be transferred back to a psychiatric service only after the patient is medically stable. Among patients who recover from NMS, there may be a 30% risk of recurrent episodes following subsequent antipsychotic rechallenge, but the majority of patients who require antipsychotic therapy can be cautiously re-treated.

TABLE 37–6. Differential diagnosis of neuroleptic malignant syndrome

Competing diagnosis	Distinguishing clinical features of the competing diagnosis
Malignant hyperthermia	Occurs after general anesthesia
Lethal catatonia	Similar symptoms before neuroleptic exposure
Heat stroke	Hot, dry skin; absence of rigidity; prior neuroleptic exposure may increase risk for heat stroke
Severe extrapyramidal symptoms or Parkinson's disease	Absence of fever, leukocytosis, autonomic changes
Central nervous system infection	Seizures more likely; significant abnormalities in cerebrospinal fluid
Allergic drug reaction	Rash, urticaria, wheezing, eosinophilia
Toxic encephalopathy, lithium toxicity	Absence of fever; low CPK
Anticholinergic delirium	Absence of rigidity; low CPK
Systemic infection plus severe EPS	May appear identical to neuroleptic malignant syndrome

Note. CPK = creatine phosphokinase; EPS = extrapyramidal symptoms.
Source. Adapted from Pelonero AL, Levenson JL, Pandurangi AK: "Neuroleptic Malignant Syndrome: A Review." *Psychiatric Services* 49:1163–1172, 1998. Used with permission.

TABLE 37–7. Examinations for possible neuroleptic malignant syndrome

Basic	Optional
Physical examination	Arterial blood gases
Electrolytes, including calcium and magnesium	Coagulation studies
	Blood cultures
Renal and hepatic function tests	Toxicology screen
Complete blood count	Lithium level
Serial tests of CPK levels	Iron deficiency test
Urinalysis	
Lumbar puncture	
CT or MRI of the head	

Note. CPK=creatine phosphokinase; CT=computed tomography; MRI=magnetic resonance imaging.
Source. Adapted from Pelonero AL, Levenson JL, Pandurangi AK: "Neuroleptic Malignant Syndrome: A Review." *Psychiatric Services* 49:1163–1172, 1998. Used with permission.

Autonomic and cardiovascular. Autonomic side effects result from cholinergic and alpha$_1$-adrenergic blockade, seen more frequently with low-potency typical antipsychotics. Among the atypical agents, the hierarchy for producing hypotension (from greatest risk to least risk) is clozapine > quetiapine > risperidone > olanzapine = ziprasidone = aripiprazole (estimated) (Tandon 2002).

QTc prolongation and torsades de pointes. A number of antipsychotics may be associated with QTc interval prolongation and risk for torsades de pointes. Sertindole was never marketed in the United States for this reason, but it is available in Europe with a restrictive label. Thioridazine, mesoridazine, and droperidol carry a "black box" warning regarding dose-related QTc prolongation and risk for sudden death. One study found that almost 30% of patients taking thioridazine had a change in QTc of 60 msec or more, followed by 21% for ziprasidone, 11% for quetiapine, and 4% each for risperidone, olanzapine, and haloperidol. A few subjects receiving thioridazine

(10%) and ziprasidone (3%) had a QTc prolongation of 75 msec or greater (Pfizer 2000). Case reports have also associated droperidol and pimozide with QTc prolongation. Controlled trials confirm QTc prolongation with droperidol (Carroll et al. 2002).

Other cardiac side effects.   Potentially fatal myocarditis, cardiomyopathy, and heart failure have been reported with clozapine. Estimated rates of clozapine-associated myocarditis range from 1 in 10,000 to 1 in 500. Eighty-five percent of these cases develop during the first 2 months of therapy and may be accompanied by eosinophilia. Clozapine-associated cardiomyopathy has most often occurred in patients under 50 years of age, with dilated cardiomyopathy accounting for two-thirds of the cases and one-third of the deaths. Withdrawal of the drug might result in improvement of the cardiomyopathy (Wooltorton 2002). Myocarditis and cardiomyopathy have also been reported in association with chlorpromazine, fluphenazine, risperidone, and haloperidol, but a causal link has not been demonstrated (Coulter et al. 2001).

Endocrinological and Metabolic

Glucose tolerance.   Pharmacoepidemiological studies and case reports reveal an association between the use of various atypical antipsychotics with hyperglycemia, new-onset type 2 diabetes, and occasional ketoacidosis. These effects are not fully understood and are not solely explained by weight gain; schizophrenia is itself a risk factor for type 2 diabetes regardless of treatment. New-onset diabetes has been reported more frequently with olanzapine and clozapine, but there have not been any systematic prospective studies. Current limited data report that hyperglycemia has been associated with all marketed atypical antipsychotics. To date, however, the only report of hyperglycemia associated with ziprasidone has been in the context of possible NMS with rhabdomyolysis and pancreatitis (Yang and McNeely 2002). Diabetic ketoacidosis has been reported in association with all atypical antipsychotics except for ziprasidone (see also Chapter 23, "Endocrine and Metabolic Disorders").

Lipids.   Phenothiazines, but not butyrophenones (Meyer 2001a), were long ago noted to elevate serum levels of cholesterol and triglycerides (Clark et al. 1967; Mefferd et al. 1958). More recent studies with atypical antipsychotics have demonstrated elevated serum triglyceride levels in patients taking clozapine, olanzapine, and quetiapine (Domon and Cargile 2002; Gaulin et al. 1999; Meyer 2001b), usually peaking in the first year of therapy.

Hyperprolactinemia.   Hyperprolactinemia is relatively common, especially with high-potency typical antipsychotics and risperidone, and can result in amenorrhea or irregular menses, galactorrhea, gynecomastia, sexual dysfunction, and osteoporosis.

Weight gain.   All currently marketed antipsychotics (with the possible exception of molindone, ziprasidone, and aripiprazole) are associated with weight gain, which may increase health risks (hypertension, atherosclerosis, type 2 diabetes, cardiovascular disease, and stroke), stigmatization, noncompliance, impairment in quality of life, and social withdrawal. The relative propensity to cause weight gain among the atypical antipsychotics (from greatest to least) is clozapine > olanzapine > risperidone = quetiapine = aripiprazole (estimated) > ziprasidone (Tandon 2002).

Syndrome of inappropriate antidiuretic hormone secretion.   SIADH can occur with typical as well as atypical antipsychotics (and some antidepressants and anticonvulsants). SIADH is characterized by a reduced ability to excrete water, resulting in extracellular dilution and hyponatremia. SIADH is distinguished from polydipsia (water intoxication) by urine osmolality, with relatively high urine osmolality in SIADH versus very low urine osmolality in polydipsia. Common symptoms include weakness, lethargy, headache, anorexia, and weight gain and may progress to confusion, convulsions, coma, and death.

Hematological.   Hematological side effects of antipsychotics include agranulocytosis, aplastic anemia, neutropenia, eosinophilia, and thrombocytopenia (for a full review, see Oyesanmi et al. 1999). Transient leukopenia and leukocytosis are not uncommon in the first few weeks of therapy and are usually not clinically significant. Agranulocytosis is the most common serious hematological side effect with typical antipsychotics (<0.1%) and occurs more frequently with low-potency agents. Clozapine-associated agranulocytosis occurs in about 1%–2% of patients, with highest risk in the first 6 months. A white blood count less than $2,000/mm^3$ or an absolute neutrophil count less than $1,000/mm^3$ is an indication for immediate cessation of clozapine.

Hepatic.   Liver function abnormalities during antipsychotic therapy have long been reported but seldom require drug discontinuation. Mild-to-moderate elevations in liver aminotransferases and alkaline phosphatase usually occur early in treatment and are unlikely to result in hepatic impairment. Cholestatic jaundice is an idiosyncratic reaction that occurs rarely with phenothiazines.

Allergic, dermatological, and ophthalmological. Dermatological adverse reactions include early allergic rashes, photosensitivity, and skin hyperpigmentation, especially with chlorpromazine. Pigmentary retinopathy occurred in patients taking more than 800 mg/day of thioridazine. Acute angle closure glaucoma may occur in patients with a physiologically narrow anterior chamber angle who take anticholinergic medications.

Sexual. Antipsychotics may cause sexual dysfunction (see Chapter 17, "Sexual Disorders," for detailed discussion).

Toxicity/overdose. Generally, antipsychotic overdose is associated with low morbidity and mortality. Most patients who have taken an antipsychotic overdose remain asymptomatic or develop mild sedation within 1–2 hours, but particular antipsychotics can cause serious cardiac effects (e.g., thioridazine-induced QTc prolongation) or neurotoxicity (e.g., clozapine-induced seizures), especially in medically vulnerable patients.

Drug interactions. Most antipsychotic drugs have sedating, hypotensive, anticholinergic, antiarrhythmic, and seizure threshold–lowering properties. Predictable drug interactions may occur when combining antipsychotics with other drugs also possessing these characteristics. For example, antipsychotics may strongly potentiate the sedative effects of other CNS depressants, and anticholinergic antipsychotics will have additive adverse effects with other anticholinergic drugs. Antipsychotics may greatly enhance the hypotensive effects of antihypertensive agents. Low-potency antipsychotics and ziprasidone should be avoided in patients receiving other drugs with quinidine-like properties.

Many antipsychotics, including aripiprazole, clozapine, olanzapine, and risperidone, are prone to pharmacokinetic drug interactions because of the limited number of cytochrome P450 isozymes involved in their metabolism (see Table 37–2).

Anxiolytics and Sedative-Hypnotics

Benzodiazepines have long been considered the cornerstone of pharmacotherapy for anxiety and insomnia. Alternatives include buspirone for anxiety and the nonbenzodiazepine hypnotics zolpidem, zopiclone, and zaleplon. These newer agents appear to have much less tolerance and abuse potential and fewer adverse effects than benzodiazepines. Chloral hydrate has been used as a sedative-hypnotic since 1869, but dependence occurs rapidly and withdrawal can be fatal.

Side Effects and Toxicity

Benzodiazepines

Benzodiazepines commonly cause dose-related CNS adverse effects but rarely affect organ systems other than the respiratory system.

Central nervous system. Acute adverse CNS effects, including sedation, fatigue and weakness, ataxia, slurred speech, confusion, and memory impairment, are common, especially in older individuals and the medically ill. When used for the treatment of insomnia, long-half-life benzodiazepines are more likely to cause daytime sedation and cognitive impairment than short-half-life drugs. The elderly and patients with brain injury are also susceptible to benzodiazepine-induced behavioral disinhibition resulting in excitement, aggression, and paradoxical rage (Kales et al. 1987).

Physical tolerance often develops with chronic use of benzodiazepines, and the therapeutic effects and adverse effects may diminish (Woods et al. 1992). A study of the cognitive effects of long-term benzodiazepine use in the elderly demonstrated that the impairment of memory, attention, and psychomotor speed evident with acute benzodiazepine use reverts to predrug levels over 6 months of therapy (McAndrews et al. 2003).

Respiratory. Benzodiazepines decrease the central respiratory response to hypoxia. Benzodiazepines differ in their ability to cause respiratory depression (Cohn 1983; Guilleminault 1990), with long-acting agents such as flurazepam (Dolly and Block 1982; Mendelson et al. 1981) and nitrazepam (Model 1973; Sanger and Zivkovic 1992) having the most pronounced effects. These drugs can cause apnea when used alone or in combination with other CNS depressants, most commonly alcohol (Guilleminault 1990; Mendelson et al. 1981). The respiratory depressant effects of benzodiazepines may become clinically significant in those with preexisting respiratory disorders, such as chronic obstructive pulmonary disease (COPD) (Clarke and Lyons 1977; Model 1973) or sleep apnea (Mendelson et al. 1981), or those with seizure disorders (which also can cause respiratory depression).

The incidence of respiratory depression associated with benzodiazepine treatment of seizure disorder ranges from 10.6% for lorazepam in adults (Alldredge et al. 2001) to 14% in children treated mainly with lorazepam (Stewart et al. 2002) and 9%–20% for children treated with diazepam (Appleton et al. 1995; Norris et al. 1999). Benzodiazepines should be used with caution in patients with compromised respiratory function or seizure disorders. Use in patients with obstructive sleep apnea is potentially fatal (Dolly and Block 1982) (see Chapter 16, "Sleep Disorders").

Drug interactions.   Additive CNS depressant effects, including respiratory depression, result from the combination of benzodiazepines and other CNS depressants, including alcohol.

Many benzodiazepines, including alprazolam, bromazepam, clonazepam, diazepam, midazolam, and triazolam, undergo hepatic and intestinal metabolism mediated by CYP3A4. Significant inhibitors of CYP3A4 may reduce the elimination of these benzodiazepines, whereas CYP3A4 inducers can increase their hepatic metabolism (see Table 37–2). Oxazepam, lorazepam, and temazepam are eliminated primarily by conjugation and renal excretion and so may be less problematic in patients with hepatic impairment.

Toxicity/overdose.   Benzodiazepines have a wide margin of safety; death from overdose is rare unless part of a polydrug overdose. Overdose may result in sedation, ataxia, slurred speech, confusion, seizures, respiratory depression, and coma. Treatment includes removal of any unabsorbed drug from the stomach (gastric lavage or emesis) followed by supportive therapy. The benzodiazepine antagonist flumazenil can also be used but may cause seizures.

Sudden discontinuation of benzodiazepines may result in severe withdrawal symptoms, including anxiety, agitation, dysphoria, anorexia, insomnia, sweating, vomiting, diarrhea, abdominal cramps, ataxia, psychosis, and seizures. The intensity of withdrawal symptoms is greater with higher doses, prolonged treatment, abrupt discontinuation, and short-half-life benzodiazepines. Patients should be gradually withdrawn from benzodiazepines; this is especially crucial for those with a history of seizure disorder. Withdrawal from short-half-life agents can be facilitated by switching to a long-half-life agent before tapering.

Nonbenzodiazepine Sedatives (Zolpidem, Zopiclone, and Zaleplon)

Zolpidem, zopiclone, and zaleplon are very well tolerated short-half-life hypnotics with very few dose-related adverse effects. Zolpidem's adverse effects include CNS (dizziness, drowsiness, and headache) and gastrointestinal effects (nausea and dyspepsia) (Hajak and Bandelow 1998). Zopiclone's adverse effects include bitter taste, dry mouth, difficulty arising in the morning, sleepiness, nausea, and nightmares (Allain et al. 1991). Clinical trials of zaleplon report adverse effects comparable to those seen with placebo. Tolerance to the hypnotic effects of these agents occurs less frequently than with benzodiazepines,

and they may be useful for treatment of rebound insomnia associated with benzodiazepine withdrawal (Pat-Horenczyk et al. 1998). Mild withdrawal symptoms have been reported in a small number of patients after discontinuation of zolpidem (Elie et al. 1999) and zopiclone (Bianchi and Musch 1990).

Respiratory.   Zolpidem has been reported to cause respiratory depression at high doses (Cirignotta et al. 1988). Zopiclone dose not appear to have significant effects on respiratory function. The respiratory effects of zaleplon are unknown.

Toxicity/overdose.   Although fatal overdose with zolpidem alone has been reported (Lichtenwalner and Tully 1997), it is rare. In a survey of 344 cases of intentional acute zolpidem overdose, death occurred in 6% of the cases but could not be directly linked to zolpidem because of multiple drug involvement (Garnier et al. 1994). Symptoms of intentional overdose of zolpidem include drowsiness, vomiting, coma, and respiratory failure. Treatment is generally limited to supportive measures and/or gastric lavage. Symptoms of toxicity rapidly subside in most cases (Garnier et al. 1994).

Fatal overdose with zopiclone has been reported but, as with zolpidem, appears rare (Boniface and Russell 1996; Bramness et al. 2001).

Chloral Hydrate

Chronic use and overdose of chloral hydrate have resulted in gastritis, gastric ulceration, hepatic and renal toxicity, and death (Graham et al. 1988). Chloral hydrate should be avoided in patients with severe renal, cardiac, or hepatic disease. Chloral hydrate is irritating to skin and mucous membranes and can cause dysgeusia, epigastric distress, nausea, and vomiting if taken on an empty stomach. Oral administration should be avoided in patients with esophagitis, gastritis, or peptic ulcer disease; rectal suppositories may be used instead. At high doses, chloral hydrate may cause hypotension and arrhythmias.

Drug interactions.   Chloral hydrate is highly bound to plasma proteins and may displace other highly bound drugs, such as warfarin. Chloral hydrate does potentiate warfarin's anticoagulant effect, but only to an extent too small to be clinically significant (Udall 1975; Wells et al. 1994).

Toxicity/overdose.   The average oral lethal dose of chloral hydrate in humans is 10 g; death has occurred with doses as low as 4 g. Symptoms of chloral hydrate overdose are similar to those of overdose with barbiturates and include hypotension, hypothermia, respiratory depression, arrhythmias, coma, and death. Hepatic and renal injury following overdose may result in jaundice and albuminuria. Treatment includes removal of any unabsorbed drug from the stomach (gastric lavage with endotracheal tube, with cuff inflated to prevent aspiration of gastric contents) followed by supportive therapy (Frankland and Robinson 2001).

Buspirone

Buspirone is a well-tolerated anxiolytic with no apparent effects on cognitive function or seizure threshold. Buspirone has little or no potential for physiological or psychological tolerance and so has no abuse liability or withdrawal syndrome on discontinuation. Dizziness, drowsiness, nervousness, nausea, and headache are the most frequent adverse affects and occur in about 5%–10% of patients. Adverse effects appear to be dose- and age-related and diminish with continued therapy. Unlike benzodiazepines, buspirone does not potentiate the effects of alcohol (Seppala et al. 1982) or suppress respiration (Garner et al. 1989). Buspirone does not exhibit cross-tolerance with benzodiazepines and so cannot be used to manage benzodiazepine withdrawal. Buspirone stimulates prolactin secretion in a dose-related manner, but the clinical significance of this effect is uncertain. Menstrual irregularities and galactorrhea have occasionally been reported, but their relation to buspirone is unclear.

Drug interactions.   Buspirone in combination with an MAOI has been associated with fatal serotonin syndrome as well as increased blood pressure (McEvoy 2003). Recent case reports also suggest that buspirone may very rarely precipitate serotonin syndrome when used in combination with St. John's wort (Dannawi 2002) or SSRIs (Manos 2000).

Buspirone undergoes hepatic and intestinal metabolism mediated by CYP3A4, so interactions are similar to those described earlier for benzodiazepines.

Toxicity/overdose.   No fatalities have been reported from buspirone overdose. Overdose symptoms include nausea, vomiting, drowsiness, miosis, and gastric distention. Treatment includes removal of any unabsorbed drug from the stomach (gastric lavage or emesis), followed by supportive therapy.

Psychostimulants

Psychostimulants are used in the treatment of attention-deficit/hyperactivity disorder (ADHD), narcolepsy, de-

pression, apathy, and analgesia augmentation in the medically ill. The well-established psychostimulant medications include methylphenidate, amphetamines (a mixture of amphetamine salts and dextroamphetamine), and pemoline.

Newer compounds include atomoxetine (a specific norepinephrine reuptake inhibitor) for ADHD (Kratochvil et al. 2003) and modafinil for narcolepsy. Modafinil also has demonstrated efficacy for fatigue accompanying multiple sclerosis (Rammohan et al. 2002) and excessive daytime sleepiness accompanying obstructive sleep apnea (Black 2003).

Side Effects and Toxicity

Methylphenidate, Amphetamines, and Pemoline

Common adverse effects include CNS (insomnia, headache, nervousness, and social withdrawal) and gastrointestinal (stomachache and anorexia) symptoms. Adverse effects are generally mild and diminish with continued treatment, adjustment of dose, or dose timing.

Chronic use of pemoline is associated with hepatotoxicity in 3% of patients, usually reversible on drug withdrawal, but potentially fatal hepatotoxicity may occur; concerns over the risk of fatal hepatotoxicity resulted in a "black box" warning for pemoline (Berkovitch et al. 1995). Pemoline may also decrease seizure threshold.

Although psychostimulants may suppress appetite, this does not tend to occur with the low doses used in medically ill patients (Masand et al. 1991). In healthy adults, methylphenidate (≤30 mg) and dextroamphetamine (≤15 mg) did not significantly alter heart rate or blood pressure (Martin et al. 1971). However, psychostimulants can cause elevated heart rate and blood pressure, palpitations, hypertension, hypotension, and cardiac arrhythmias when taken at doses higher than those routinely used in the medically ill. In a review of side effects associated with methylphenidate therapy in children with ADHD, methylphenidate increased heart rate by 3–10 beats/minute and blood pressure by 3.3–8 mm Hg systolic and 1.5–14 mm Hg diastolic (Rapport and Moffitt 2002).

Drug interactions.   Psychostimulants may interact with sympathomimetics and MAOIs (including selegiline), resulting in headache, arrhythmias, hypertensive crisis, and hyperpyrexia. Psychostimulants should not be administered with MAOIs or within 14 days of their discontinuation. Despite the paucity of empirical evidence regarding TCA–stimulant metabolic interactions, warning statements are included in many drug manuals. One review of the effects of stimulants on the pharmacokinetics of desipramine in children found no statistically or clinically significant interaction regardless of age, gender, or type of stimulant (Cohen et al. 1999). Several reports suggest that methylphenidate may interact pharmacodynamically with TCAs to cause increased anxiety, irritability, agitation, and aggression. Symptoms subsided on drug discontinuation (Grob and Coyle 1986; Gwirtsman et al. 1994; Markowitz and Patrick 2001).

Higher doses of psychostimulants may also reduce the therapeutic effectiveness of antihypertensive medications. When psychostimulants are used concurrently with beta-blockers, the excessive alpha-adrenergic activity may cause hypertension, reflex bradycardia, and possible heart block.

Toxicity/overdose. Symptoms of overdose include cardiovascular (flushing, palpitations, hypertension, arrhythmias, and tachycardia), CNS (delirium, euphoria, hyperreflexia, and psychosis), and autonomic (hyperpyrexia and sweating) effects. Treatment is primarily supportive. Any unabsorbed drug should be removed from the stomach (gastric lavage or emesis). A short-acting sedative may be needed in patients with severe intoxication.

Modafinil and Atomoxetine

Modafinil and atomoxetine have different adverse effect profiles than psychostimulants and do not have their same abuse potential. Modafinil's adverse effects include delayed sleep onset, nausea, and rhinitis (U.S. Modafinil in Narcolepsy Multicenter Study Group 2000). Palpitations, tachycardia, hypertension, excitation, and aggression have also been infrequently observed. Modafinil has been associated in rare cases with chest pain, palpitations, dyspnea, and transient ischemic T-wave changes in association with mitral valve prolapse or left ventricular hypertrophy. Modafinil does not cause appetite reduction (Rugino and Copley 2001).

Because of atomoxetine's recent introduction to the market (it received FDA approval in November 2002), experience with it is limited. Side effects in the clinical trials included insomnia, nausea, dry mouth, constipation, dizziness, decreased appetite, urinary hesitancy, sexual dysfunction, and palpitations (Alaka 2003).

Elimination of atomoxetine and modafinil is reduced in patients with hepatic impairment. Atomoxetine dose should be reduced by 50% in patients with moderate hepatic impairment and 75% in those with severe hepatic impairment (Alaka 2003). In patients with severe hepatic impairment, modafinil dose should be reduced by 50% (McEvoy 2003). Blood levels of modafinil acid, a modafinil metabolite, increase ninefold in patients with severe renal insufficiency, but its effects are unknown.

Drug interactions. Atomoxetine is a potent inhibitor of CYP2D6 and is primarily eliminated through metabolism by CYP2D6 (see Table 37–2). Atomoxetine may increase the toxicity of other coadministered narrow therapeutic index medications primarily metabolized by CYP2D6.

Drug interaction data for modafinil are limited. Clinical studies suggest that significant metabolic drug interactions are most likely with compounds, such as ethinylestradiol and triazolam, that undergo significant gastrointestinal CYP3A4-mediated first-pass metabolism (Robertson and Hellriegel 2003; Robertson et al. 2002). Modafinil–clozapine interactions have been the subject of two case reports, one showing an increase in clozapine level (Dequardo 2002) and the other showing a decrease in clozapine's therapeutic effect (Narendran et al. 2002).

Like other psychostimulants, atomoxetine and modafinil should not be administered to patients receiving MAOIs or within 14 days of MAOI withdrawal.

Cognitive Enhancers

The currently approved treatments for dementia of the Alzheimer's type are cholinesterase inhibitors, including tacrine, donepezil, rivastigmine, and galantamine. The NMDA receptor antagonist memantine has been approved in Germany for the treatment of dementia for more than 10 years (Reichman 2003) and in October 2003 was approved for use in the United States.

Side Effects and Toxicity

Cholinesterase Inhibitors

Tacrine is now rarely prescribed because of frequent reversible hepatotoxicity (Watkins et al. 1994). Other mainstream cholinesterase inhibitors are well tolerated; most of their adverse effects are mild, dose-related, and gastrointestinal in nature (nausea, vomiting, and diarrhea), as expected from procholinergic agents. Gastrointestinal side effects can be minimized by slow dose titration and administration with food. Adequate hydration reduces nausea.

Agent-specific side effects include muscle cramps and insomnia with donepezil and anorexia with rivastigmine and galantamine.

Overdose. Overdose of cholinesterase inhibitors can cause a potentially fatal cholinergic crisis, with bradycardia, hypotension, muscle weakness, nausea, vomiting, respiratory depression, sialorrhea, diaphoresis, and seizures. Treatment is with atropine (1–2 mg intravenously, repeat as required) and supportive care.

Drug interactions. Donepezil and galantamine are metabolized by CYP2D6 and CYP3A4 isozymes but are not associated with any clinically important cytochrome P450–mediated pharmacokinetic interactions (Tiseo et al. 1998a, 1998b, 1998c, 1998d, 1998e). Rivastigmine is metabolized primarily by esterase-mediated hydrolysis and has been shown not to interact with cytochrome P450 isozymes in vitro (Grossberg et al. 2000).

Cholinesterase inhibitors do, however, have the potential to exacerbate the effects of other cholinesterase inhibitors (e.g., physostigmine) or cholinomimetic agents (e.g., bethanechol). The neuromuscular blocking agents succinylcholine and mivacurium are metabolized by plasma cholinesterases, so cholinesterase inhibitors can prolong their effects and increase their toxicity.

Many prescription and nonprescription drugs possess anticholinergic activity that may impair cognitive function. In addition to those drug classes commonly recognized as having anticholinergic effects, such as antiparkinsonian agents, antispasmodics, tricyclic antidepressants, low-potency antipsychotics, and antihistamines, many individual drugs from unrelated drug classes also have these effects. Drugs with anticholinergic properties may decrease the effect of cognitive enhancers. The use of anticholinergic agents in a patient with compromised cognitive function should be minimized. A partial listing of drugs with significant CNS anticholinergic effects is presented in Table 37–8. Conversely, cholinesterase inhibitors may have a countertherapeutic effect in those patients receiving anticholinergic medication for medical conditions.

NMDA Receptor Antagonists

On the basis of limited data in small clinical trials (Forest Laboratories 2003), memantine appears well tolerated, with dizziness and constipation the most prominent side effects.

Drug interactions. The systematic evaluation of potential drug–drug interactions with memantine awaits more widespread use of the drug.

Alternative Routes of Administration

Some medically ill or surgical patients may not be able to take medication by mouth and therefore will require a parenteral route of administration. Parenteral routes of administration include sublingual, intravenous, intramuscular, intranasal, rectal, and topical or transdermal. The most common parenteral route of administration is intravenous. Some psychotropics are commonly available in parenteral forms, and customized formulations have been reported for a few of the others. Caution is indicated when using a medication for which adequate studies of safety and efficacy regarding parenteral administration are lacking.

The potential advantages of parenteral administration of psychotropics include guaranteeing compliance, providing options for those patients who cannot take oral medications, and potential pharmacokinetic advantages such as greater bioavailability, bypassing first-pass hepatic metabolism, potential reduction in toxic metabolites or adverse effects, and acceleration of achieving steady state plasma drug levels.

Antidepressants

Few antidepressants are available for parenteral administration. Intravenous clomipramine, imipramine, maprotiline, doxepin, dibenzepine, viloxazine, trazodone, and citalopram have been studied or widely used abroad, mainly in Europe. None are currently available in the United States. Recently, intravenous mirtazapine was found to be safe, efficacious, and well tolerated in 27 moderately to severely depressed inpatients (Konstantinidis et al. 2002). Citalopram is the only SSRI available for parenteral administration. To date, open and double-blind randomized, controlled clinical trials have shown that citalopram infusion followed by oral administration is an effective and well-tolerated treatment for severely depressed patients (Kasper and Muller-Spahn 2002). All the studies of intravenous antidepressants have been performed in medically healthy patients, leaving uncertain their safety and efficacy in the medically ill.

The rectal mucosa provides an alternative surface for drug absorption. The pharmacokinetics of rectal administration have been extensively reviewed by van Hoogdalem et al. (1991a, 1991b). No antidepressants are currently marketed in a rectal preparation. Rectal administration may be in the form of an enema, foam, semisolid suppository, and (to some extent) gelatin capsules. Independent or compounding pharmacies reportedly have made suppositories for amitriptyline, trazodone, imipramine, and clomipramine (Adams 1982; Chaumeil et al. 1988; Mirassou 1998). However, creating custom suppositories is a very labor-intensive process, and the bioavailability of rectal administration remains unpredictable.

Transdermal drug delivery offers several potential advantages, such as consistent drug levels, lack of peaks in plasma concentration, avoidance of first-pass metabolism, and convenience, with improvements in patient adherence. There has been one case report of transdermal amitriptyline gel in a depressed patient with chronic pain who

TABLE 37–8. Common drugs with significant anticholinergic effects

Antianginals Isosorbide dinitrate	**Antispasmodics** Atropine
Antiarrhythmics Disopyramide Procainamide Quinidine	Belladonna Clidinium Dicyclomine Glycopyrrolate
Antiasthmatics Theophylline	Homatropine Hyoscine
Anticoagulants Warfarin	Hyoscyamine Mepenzolate
Antidepressants Tricyclics Amoxapine Imipramine Maprotiline	Methscopolamine Oxybutynin Propantheline Scopolamine Tolterodine
Antidiarrheals Diphenoxylate	**Calcium channel blockers** Nifedipine
Antihistamines H_1 antagonists (e.g., diphenhydramine) H_2 antagonists (e.g., cimetidine)	**Cardiac glycosides** Digoxin
Antiparkinsonian agents Amantadine Benztropine Biperiden	**Diuretics** Furosemide
	Narcotic analgesics Codeine
Ethopropazine Orphenadrine	**Antiemetics** Prochlorperazine
Procyclidine Trihexyphenidyl	Promethazine
Antiplatelet agents Dipyridamole	**Skeletal muscle relaxants** Cyclobenzaprine
Antipsychotics Chlorpromazine Chlorprothixene Clozapine Loxapine Mesoridazine Olanzapine Pimozide Thioridazine	

Source. Compiled, in part, from Bezchlibnyk and Jeffries 2000; McEvoy 2003; Repchinsky 2003; Tune et al. 1992; USP DI Editorial Board 2003.

also had severe inflammatory bowel disease (Scott et al. 1999). The only potential transdermal antidepressant under development is selegiline (EmSam) (FDA approval letter February 2004) (Amsterdam 2003; Bodkin and Amsterdam 2002). The dose of oral selegiline needed for effective antidepressant treatment requires dietary tyramine restriction because of the clinically significant inhi-

bition of intestinal MAO-A. Transdermal administration of selegiline was developed to circumvent this problem. Transdermal selegiline has the following pharmacological advantages: 1) it limits intestinal MAO-A inhibition, leaving adequate intestinal MAO-A activity to digest tyramine; and 2) it circumvents first-pass metabolism, resulting in higher plasma concentrations and decreased metabolite formation. Double-blind, placebo-controlled studies found that transdermal selegiline was an effective and well-tolerated treatment for major depression (Amsterdam 2003; Bodkin and Amsterdam 2002). This agent may also be an option for the treatment of depression in medically ill patients and warrants further study.

Anxiolytics and Sedative-Hypnotics

Routes of administration available for some benzodiazepines include oral, sublingual, liquid, nasal, intramuscular, and intravenous. Intravenous formulations are available for midazolam, lorazepam, and diazepam. Intravenous benzodiazepines are commonly used to treat status epilepticus or to calm severely agitated patients. Intravenous lorazepam has the longest distribution half-life and therefore has the longest duration of effect after a single intravenous dose. Compared with diazepam, lorazepam pharmacokinetics after intravenous administration are more predictable. Because of its high lipid solubility, intravenous diazepam leads to rapid redistribution of the drug and a relatively rapid loss of clinical effect compared with lorazepam. Midazolam is a short-acting, water-soluble benzodiazepine frequently used in preoperative sedation, induction and maintenance of anesthesia, anxiolysis, and the treatment of status epilepticus. Midazolam's onset of action following intravenous administration is usually within 1–5 minutes, and the action lasts usually less than 2 hours. Intravenous flunitrazepam (Rohypnol), available in Europe, has been used in both the treatment and the prevention of alcohol withdrawal (Pycha et al. 1993; Spies et al. 1995). Intravenous benzodiazepine administration should always occur in a setting where there is ready access to personnel and equipment necessary for respiratory resuscitation.

Benzodiazepines that may be administered intramuscularly include lorazepam and midazolam. Lorazepam is usually chosen as the benzodiazepine for intramuscular administration because it is readily absorbed and has no active metabolites. Other benzodiazepines, such as diazepam, are not recommended for intramuscular use because they are erratically absorbed. Midazolam is also rapidly absorbed after intramuscular administration, with an onset of action between 5 and 15 minutes. When intravenous and intramuscular routes are not preferred or are unavailable, subcutaneous administration of some benzodiazepines, such as clonazepam, may be an option.

The pharmacokinetics of sublingual benzodiazepine administration has been studied by several groups. Several benzodiazepines, including lorazepam, alprazolam, triazolam, temazepam, prazepam, midazolam, clonazepam, and diazepam, have been administered sublingually,

using commercial nonsublingual formulations or custom preparations. The only benzodiazepines specifically marketed in a sublingual form are lorazepam in North America and temazepam in Europe (Russell et al. 1988). Although the sublingual form of lorazepam is more rapidly absorbed than the oral form, the pharmacokinetic profiles of sublingual and orally administered lorazepam are similar.

Rectal administration of benzodiazepines is routinely performed in the management of acute seizures in children. Diazepam can be administered rectally when venous access is not readily available. However, bioavailability seems to vary (Magnussen et al. 1979; Remy et al. 1992). Other benzodiazepines, such as triazolam, have been administered rectally but are not recommended for clinical use. In addition, since lorazepam may be given intravenously, intramuscularly, or sublingually, there is essentially no practical reason for rectal administration of benzodiazepines in adults.

Still other routes of administration for benzodiazepines include intrathecal and nasal midazolam. Intrathecal midazolam has been used principally for adjunctive pain management and has been found to be safe and effective in a variety of settings (Kim and Lee 2001; Sen et al. 2001; Serrao et al. 1992; Valentine et al. 1996). Intranasal administration via spray has been used effectively in a variety of settings, including acute seizure management in children, conscious sedation in children undergoing dental procedures, and management of claustrophobia in patients undergoing magnetic resonance imaging procedures (al Rakaf et al. 2001; Fisgin et al. 2002; Hollenhorst et al. 2001).

Antipsychotics

Haloperidol, droperidol, perphenazine, trifluoperazine, thiothixene, and triflupromazine are available in a form that may be administered by intravenous, intramuscular, or subcutaneous routes. Intravenous agents are usually reserved for acute agitation in which a rapid onset of effect is desirable. Droperidol is FDA approved for use as an intravenous anesthetic adjunct (but not for psychiatric conditions) but has been used for rapid tranquilization in the medical/surgical setting. Droperidol causes dose-dependent prolongation of the QTc interval and has been withdrawn from the United Kingdom and received a black-box warning in North America. Although haloperidol is not approved by the FDA for intravenous use, it is the antipsychotic most commonly administered intravenously in medical settings—usually in critical care units, in emergencies, or whenever there is a lack of oral access. High doses of haloperidol, up to 1,000 mg daily, in patients with severe delirium have been reported to have minimal effects on heart rate, respiratory rate, blood pressure, and pulmonary artery pressure, with minimal EPS (Levenson 1995; Stern 1985).

Many antipsychotics, including three atypical antipsychotics, ziprasidone, olanzapine, and risperidone, are available for intramuscular use. Intramuscular formulations can be subdivided into two categories on the basis of their pharmacokinetic features: short-acting preparations and long-acting depot preparations. Long-acting antipsychotics are typically used as antipsychotic maintenance treatment to ensure adherence and to eliminate bioavailability problems. Short-acting antipsychotics are usually used in acute management of delirium, psychosis, mania, or aggression (see Chapter 6, "Delirium"; Chapter 8, "Aggression and Violence"; and Chapter 11, "Mania, Catatonia, and Psychosis" for further discussion). Haloperidol is the most common (and least costly) intramuscularly administered antipsychotic in medical settings. However, acute parenteral administration of high-potency antipsychotics such as haloperidol is associated with more dystonia and other EPS. In patients who already have extrapyramidal disorders, an intramuscular antipsychotic other than haloperidol would be preferred. Parenteral administration of low-potency agents may cause more hypotension and lowered seizure threshold.

Intramuscular ziprasidone was launched in August 2002 and was recommended for the control of agitated behavior associated with schizophrenia. Peak plasma concentrations after an intramuscular dose of ziprasidone are achieved in 30–45 minutes. Unlike haloperidol, intramuscular ziprasidone cannot be mixed in the same syringe with a benzodiazepine. The magnitude of the QTc interval increase with intramuscular ziprasidone is comparable to that of the oral formulation. Ziprasidone is contraindicated in patients receiving other agents known to prolong the QTc interval and for patients with a known history of QTc prolongation, recent myocardial infarction, recent uncompensated heart failure, or a history of cardiac arrhythmias. Intramuscular ziprasidone has not been systematically studied in patients 65 years or older or in patients with significant hepatic or renal impairment. Intramuscular olanzapine is recommended for the management of agitation in patients with schizophrenia, bipolar mania, or dementia. At the time of this writing, there are no data on intramuscular ziprasidone or olanzapine in the management of agitation in medically ill patients without an underlying psychiatric condition, so caution is advised.

Subcutaneous administration is another route available for some antipsychotics. This route is more commonly used with haloperidol and methotrimeprazine (available

in Canada and Europe) in the management of terminal restlessness and for nausea/vomiting in palliative care patients. Loxapine has also been used subcutaneously in the palliative care setting.

Psychostimulants

There are no formulations of methylphenidate available for intravenous administration, and preparation of a solution from tablets is inadvisable. However, intravenous methylphenidate has been studied (Cantello et al. 1989; Janowsky et al. 1978; Lucas et al. 1987; Robinson et al. 1991), mostly in drug-induced provocation of psychotic symptoms. Dextroamphetamine has been administered intravenously to human subjects in research, but to date there are no reports of use of intravenous dextroamphetamine in clinical settings (Ernst and Goldberg 2002). There is one published case report of 5-mg dextroamphetamine suppositories compounded by a pharmacy for treating depressed mood in a woman with gastrointestinal obstruction (Holmes et al. 1994). Pemoline comes in a chewable tablet that was administered sublingually in four medically ill patients for the treatment of depression (Breitbart and Mermelstein 1992).

In summary, there are no systematic studies of safety and efficacy of psychostimulants given via non-enteral routes.

Mood Stabilizers

Mood stabilizers that have been administered intravenously include lithium carbonate and valproate. Published literature regarding parenteral administration of lithium salts is scarce. Because lithium is not subject to hepatic metabolism, the potential pharmacokinetic advantages of parenteral administration are much fewer than for other psychotropics. Parenteral lithium has rarely been used in the treatment of psychiatric disorders but has been used as a possible treatment in thyroid storm. Lithium was administered intraperitoneally in patients on continuous ambulatory peritoneal dialysis (Flynn et al. 1987). Lithium carbonate is not approved by the FDA for parenteral use, and there is not enough clinical experience or data to recommend its use by nonenteral routes.

Valproic acid has been available in parenteral form (Depacon) in Europe for over 18 years and was approved by the FDA in the United States in 1997. To date, there are no randomized, controlled trials documenting its safety and efficacy in psychiatric conditions, although case reports have been encouraging (Norton 2001; Norton and Quarles 2000; Regenold and Prasad 2001). The intravenous formulation of valproic acid can be given in dextrose, saline, or lactated Ringer's solution, prepared by adding 1 g to 500 mL of solution. The solution should not be infused at more than 20 mg/minute, with the dosage reduced in the elderly and in those with organic brain syndromes. The dosage varies between 1 and 3 g for most adults and one-half of this in the elderly. The infusion does not require cardiac monitoring and causes no significant risk of orthostatic hypotension (Norton 2001). Valproic acid is the only mood stabilizer available in an approved parenteral formulation supported by case reports of use in psychiatric conditions.

Cholinesterase Inhibitors

Currently, there have been no reports of non-enteral routes of administration for donepezil, galantamine, rivastigmine, or tacrine.

Complementary Medicines

An increasing number of patients are taking herbal medicines and nonherbal dietary supplements, often without disclosing their use. Many people assume that complementary medicines are "naturally" safe, and they combine complementary and conventional therapies, believing that the combination will be more effective (Eisenberg et al. 2001). This raises concerns about the appropriate therapeutic use, contraindications, adverse effects, and drug interactions of herbal and nonherbal drugs. Patients with chronic disease may be especially vulnerable to adverse effects from herbal medicines because of compromised organ function and polypharmacy with conventional agents.

The lack of government oversight and regulation further complicates attempts to assess the safety of herbal medicines. Manufacturers are not required to standardize the concentration of active ingredients or even to identify them (Chandler 2000; De Smet 2002). Herbal preparations may contain several plant species used under a single name (Chandler 2000) and may be adulterated with unlisted pharmacological agents, pesticides, and heavy metals, including cadmium, lead, mercury, or arsenic (Crone and Wise 1998). Drugs such as anti-inflammatory agents, steroids, diuretics, antihistamines, sildenafil-like compounds (Wooltorton 2003), and benzodiazepines may be intentionally added to the herbal product for therapeutic effect.

Contraindications, major adverse effects, and significant drug interactions for those herbal medicines and nonherbal dietary supplements commonly used for neuropsychiatric symptoms are summarized in the following subsections, derived from available reviews (Ang-Lee et al. 2001; Chandler 2000; Corns 2003; Crone and Wise 1998; Crone et al. 2001; De Smet 2002; Ernst 2002, 2003; Fugh-Berman 2000; Henney 2003; Izzo and Ernst 2001).

Selected Herbal Medicines

Black Cohosh

Purported use. Menopausal symptoms

Pharmacological effects and drug interactions. Black cohosh binds to estrogen receptors and lowers levels of luteinizing hormone. It is contraindicated in pregnancy and lactation and should be avoided by women with estrogen-dependent tumors.

Feverfew

Purported use. Migraine prophylaxis, anti-inflammatory

Pharmacological effects and drug interactions. Used as an abortifacient in animals, feverfew is contraindicated in pregnancy in humans. It inhibits platelet activation factor and may prolong bleeding time. Use caution with drugs known to increase bleeding times, such as anticoagulants, NSAIDs, and platelet inhibitors. Allergic reactions are common. Withdrawal syndrome (anxiety, fatigue, joint ache) may occur on sudden discontinuation.

Ginger

Purported use. Antispasmodic, antiemetic

Pharmacological effects and drug interactions. Ginger is a possible mutagen and abortifacient; avoid use in pregnancy. It inhibits thromboxane synthesis and thus may prolong bleeding time. Use caution with drugs known to increase bleeding times, such as anticoagulants, NSAIDs, and platelet inhibitors. These cautions do not apply to typical culinary doses.

Ginkgo Biloba

Purported use. Ginkgo biloba improves peripheral and CNS blood flow and is used as a treatment for ischemia associated with peripheral artery disease and vascular dementia.

Pharmacological effects and drug interactions. Ginkgo biloba inhibits platelet activation factor and prolongs bleeding time. It carries an increased risk for bleeding disorders when used with drugs known to increase bleeding times (anticoagulants, NSAIDs, platelet inhibitors). Intracerebral and intraocular hemorrhages have been reported, and it may cause palpitations. Seizures have been reported in children, and efficacy of anticonvulsants may be reduced. The ginkgo biloba fruit, including the seeds, is poisonous and very allergenic. Ingestion of the fruit has resulted in loss of consciousness, seizures, and death, with a mortality rate of 27%. Ingestion of fruit also causes contact dermatitis of mucous membranes. Discontinue use at least 2 days before surgery.

Ginseng

Purported use. Ginseng is promoted as a physical, mental, and sexual tonic, immunostimulant, and mood enhancer.

Pharmacological effects and drug interactions. Ginseng possesses estrogenic activity; it is contraindicated in patients with estrogen receptor–positive breast cancer. It may cause estrogen-related bleeding disorders (vaginal bleeding) and breast nodules. Sympathomimetic activity may cause tachycardia, hypertension, nervousness, agitation, mania, and headache. It also has hypoglycemic and anti–platelet aggregation properties. Ginseng may reduce the effects of loop diuretics (furosemide), antihypertensives, anxiolytics, antidepressants, mood stabilizers, and antiestrogens. It inhibits platelet activation factor and prolongs bleeding time. Ginseng increases the risk of bleeding disorders with drugs known to increase bleeding times (anticoagulants, NSAIDs, platelet inhibitors). Avoid use in patients with diabetes, hypertension, anxiety disorders, and bipolar disorder or those using estrogen therapy, antiestrogen therapy, or anticoagulants. Avoid long-term use, which may be associated with "ginseng abuse syndrome"; symptoms include hypertension, nervousness, insomnia, skin eruptions, diarrhea, and tremor. A withdrawal syndrome (hypotension, weakness, tremor) may occur on discontinuation. Discontinue at least 7 days before surgery.

Kava Kava

Purported use. Anxiolytic, sedative

Pharmacological effects and drug interactions. Kava kava is a possible dopamine antagonist; avoid use with antipsychotics and drugs used to treat Parkinson's disease. It potentiates the effects of CNS depressants, such as barbiturates, benzodiazepines, and alcohol. Dermopathy is common with heavy use. Antithrombotic action may prolong bleeding time. Use caution with drugs known to increase bleeding times. Kava kava is also hallucinogenic. Sale of kava has been banned in many jurisdictions because of

several incidents of fatal hepatotoxicity. Discontinue at least 24 hours before surgery.

Ma Huang (Ephedra)

Purported use. Weight loss, stimulant

Pharmacological effects and drug interactions. Ma huang is an indirect sympathomimetic; it contains ephedrine and pseudoephedrine, which cause release of epinephrine and norepinephrine. Excessive sympathetic stimulation can lead to dizziness, headache, decreased appetite, gastrointestinal distress, irregular heartbeat, tachycardia, hypertension, insomnia, flushing, seizures, stroke, and death. Drug interactions include increased risk of cardiac arrhythmia with cardiac glycosides and antiarrhythmics; reduced effects of antihypertensives, beta-blockers, sedative-hypnotics, and anesthetics; hypertensive crisis with MAOIs; and increased stimulant effects with theophylline and caffeine. Discontinue at least 24 hours before surgery.

St. John's Wort

Purported use. Antidepressant for mild to moderate depression, sedative

Pharmacological effects and drug interactions. St. John's wort increases serotonin and norepinephrine activity, which may cause sinus tachycardia and gastrointestinal distress and may exacerbate bipolar disorder, causing mania. It is a photosensitizer and may cause sun-induced skin rash, neuropathy, and possibly increased incidence of cataracts. It may exacerbate photosensitivity due to tetracycline, piroxicam, and phenothiazines. St. John's wort induces CYP3A4 and has the potential to interact with medications metabolized by this enzyme to lower drug levels and decrease therapeutic effect (see Table 37–2.) It induces renal P-gp drug transport systems, increasing renal elimination of several drugs, including digoxin and cyclosporine. St. John's wort may induce serotonin syndrome in combination with other serotonergic drugs. Discontinue at least 5 days before surgery.

Valerian

Purported use. Sedative, short-term treatment of insomnia, anxiolytic

Pharmacological effects and drug interactions. Tolerance to valerian may develop and lead to withdrawal effects if it is discontinued abruptly after prolonged usage. Withdrawal effects are similar to benzodiazepine withdrawal and can be managed with benzodiazepines. Valerian potentiates the sedative effects of CNS depressants.

Yohimbe, Yohimbine

Purported use.   Aphrodisiac, stimulant

Pharmacological effects and drug interactions.   Yohimbine, an alpha$_2$ antagonist, has indirect sympathomimetic activity. Adverse effects include insomnia, anxiety, panic attacks, hallucinations, hypertension, tachycardia, nausea, and vomiting. It should be avoided in patients with hypertension, sleep disorders, anxiety disorders, and psychosis. Yohimbine exacerbates the CNS and autonomic effects of stimulants and TCAs. Discontinue at least 2 days before surgery.

Selected Nonherbal Nutritional Supplements

DHEA (Dehydroepiandrosterone)

Purported use.   Depression, postmenopausal osteoporosis, systemic lupus erythematosus, erectile dysfunction, multiple sclerosis, dementia

Pharmacological effects and drug interactions.   DHEA is an endogenous anabolic steroid that may undergo conversion in vivo to testosterone or androstenedione followed by conversion to estriol, estrone, and estradiol. DHEA may cause weight gain, voice change, hirsutism, and menstrual irregularities in females and gynecomastia and prostatic hypertrophy in males. DHEA is contraindicated in patients who have liver dysfunction, prostate cancer, or hormone-dependent diseases such as estrogen-dependent breast cancer. DHEA may inhibit CYP3A4.

Gamma-Hydroxybutyrate (GHB), Gamma-Butyrolactone, and 1,4-Butanediol

Purported use.   Narcolepsy, recreational fast-acting hypnotic

Pharmacological effects and drug interactions.   GHB is a partial agonist at GABA$_B$ receptors with fast-onset hypnotic action. Gamma-butyrolactone and 1,4-butanediol are metabolized to GHB in vivo. Adverse effects include nystagmus, ataxia, apnea, sedation, dizziness, and respiratory depression. Coma, bradycardia, and death can result. Psychiatric side effects of GHB include hallucinations, delusions, agitation, confusion, and euphoria. A withdrawal syndrome (anxiety, insomnia, tremor, muscle cramps) has been observed. GHB is a banned drug in many jurisdictions, but its precursors, gamma-butyrolactone and 1,4-butanediol, are industrial solvents and are available as street drugs.

S-Adenosyl-L-Methionine (SAMe)

Purported use.   Depression, osteoarthritis, chronic liver disease

Pharmacological effects and drug interactions.   SAMe is the principal endogenous methyl donor for methylation reactions. Adverse effects include nausea, vomiting, and diarrhea. SAMe may increase anxiety and restlessness in patients with depression and mania and hypomania in patients with bipolar disorder. Serotonin syndrome has been reported. Use caution with SAMe in patients with bipolar disorder, patients with movement disorders, or patients taking serotonergic drugs.

Psychotropic Drug Use in the Medically Ill

Psychosomatic medicine specialists routinely prescribe and advise other physicians regarding the use of psychotropic medications in patients with multiple complex medical problems. This gives rise to many issues regarding changes in pharmacokinetics and pharmacodynamics as previously outlined in this chapter. This section outlines clinical recommendations for the use of psychotropic medications in specific medical/surgical populations.

Gastrointestinal Disease

Hepatic Disease

Alterations in psychopharmacology in patients with liver disease largely center on the changes in pharmacokinetics brought about by the disease (discussed earlier in this chapter). Acute hepatitis usually does not require dose alteration. The dosage of psychotropics in patients with chronic hepatitis may need to be modified depending on the severity of liver dysfunction. In patients with cirrhosis, drug dose will require significant modification. The severity of liver disease can be approximated using the Child-Pugh scoring system (see Chapter 21, "Gastrointestinal Disorders"). All plasma proteins are synthesized in the liver, so protein binding is altered in liver disease. The main clinical effect of chronically decreased protein binding is on the interpretation of blood levels (see discussion under "Distribution" subsection earlier in this chapter). When psychotropic medication is being prescribed for patients with impaired hepatic function, it is prudent to reduce the initial dose and titrate more slowly for any drug primarily metabolized by the liver, to carefully monitor for clinical response and side effects, and to choose drugs with a wide therapeutic index. Table 37–9 lists recommendations regarding dosing of psychotropics in patients with hepatic disease.

Antidepressants. Most antidepressants undergo extensive phase I hepatic oxidative metabolism and should be dosed according to the recommendations just described. Anticholinergic TCAs may exacerbate hepatic encephalopathy in susceptible individuals via intestinal stasis and central anticholinergic effects. The use of newer antidepressants in patients with hepatic disease has received very little study. Citalopram, paroxetine, sertraline, and fluoxetine have all been used safely in patients with hepatitis C, usually in the context of interferon-α treatment (Farah 2002; Gleason et al. 2002; Hauser et al. 2002; Kraus et al. 2002; Levenson and Fallon 1993; Sammut et al. 2002; Schramm et al. 2000).

Hepatotoxicity is a known rare side effect of many antidepressants, but nefazodone has a higher reported incidence than other current antidepressants and thus should be avoided in patients with preexisting hepatic disease (Carvajal et al. 2002; Stewart 2002). As a general guideline, minor elevations in transaminases are common and usually benign. Elevation of aspartate transaminase (AST) or alanine transaminase (ALT) levels of two to three times baseline or two times normal is significant, and any elevation of alkaline phosphatase (ALP) or bilirubin may be significant.

Antipsychotics. Although very little has been written about the use of antipsychotics in patients with liver failure, haloperidol remains the most commonly chosen antipsychotic for patients with hepatic disease. Chlorpromazine should be avoided because of its greater risk for hepatotoxicity. Low-potency typical antipsychotics, which are more anticholinergic than high-potency typicals, may precipitate hepatic encephalopathy in patients with cirrhosis (as described for TCAs). The atypical antipsychotics remain viable alternatives. Because they are extensively metabolized, their dosage should be reduced in patients with hepatic insufficiency.

Anxiolytics and sedative-hypnotics. Most benzodiazepines are metabolized by phase I processes, and liver disease affects phase I processes significantly more than phase II processes. For this reason, the preferred benzodiazepines for any patient with liver disease are lorazepam, oxazepam, and temazepam because they are principally metabolized by phase II processes. All benzodiazepines should be avoided in patients at risk for developing hepatic encephalopathy because they may precipitate its onset. When their use cannot be avoided (e.g., alcohol with-

drawal in a patient with cirrhosis), the benzodiazepines just mentioned are preferred, with vigilant monitoring of changes in mental status.

Mood stabilizers. Because of the risk of hepatotoxicity, carbamazepine and valproic acid are relatively contraindicated in patients with preexisting liver disease. If either of these agents is used, reduce dose and monitor liver function regularly, especially during the first 6 months of therapy. Gabapentin is renally excreted and does not require dosage adjustment in patients with hepatic disease. Lithium, although renally excreted, may require dose adjustment and close monitoring secondary to fluctuating fluid balance in patients with liver disease accompanied by ascites (secondary hyperaldosteronism). Oxcarbazepine's manufacturer states that no disease adjustment is needed for patients with mild to moderate hepatic insufficiency. Lamotrigine dose should be reduced according to the severity of hepatic impairment. There are no current dosing recommendations for topiramate.

Cholinesterase inhibitors. Donepezil clearance may be reduced in cirrhosis, but there are no specific dosing recommendations for hepatic insufficiency. Galantamine should be used with caution in patients with mild to moderate hepatic insufficiency, and its dose should not exceed 16 mg daily in patients with a Child-Pugh Score of 7–9 (see Chapter 21, "Gastrointestinal Disorders"). Rivastigmine clearance may be reduced by 60%–65% in patients with mild to moderate hepatic insufficiency, and dosing should be guided by monitoring efficacy and tolerability.

Psychostimulants. There are no specific dosing recommendations for methylphenidate. Modafinil clearance is reduced in hepatic insufficiency, and its dosage should be reduced by 50% in patients with severe hepatic insufficiency. For atomoxetine, initial doses should be reduced to 25% and 50% of the normal dose for patients with severe and moderate hepatic impairment, respectively (Chalon et al. 2003).

Gastrointestinal Bleeding

Antidepressants. Recent reports have raised concern regarding SSRIs and the risk of gastrointestinal bleeding (Dalton et al. 2003; de Abajo et al. 1999). Serotonin plays a role in hemostasis, and there have been cases of prolonged bleeding time, ecchymosis, purpura, and epistaxis, as well as gastrointestinal, genitourinary, and intracranial bleeding, in patients receiving SSRIs. Although the reports indicate an increase in the relative risk of gastrointestinal bleeding in patients taking SSRIs, the absolute effects are modest and about equivalent to low-dose

TABLE 37–9.   Selected psychotropic drugs in hepatic insufficiency (HI)

Antidepressants

MAOIs	Potentially hepatotoxic. No dosing guidelines.
SSRIs	Extensively metabolized. Decreased clearance and prolonged half-life. Initial dose should be reduced 50% and subsequent increments at longer intervals than usual. Target doses are typically substantially lower than usual.
TCAs	Extensively metabolized. Potentially serious hepatic effects. No dosing guidelines.
Bupropion	Extensively metabolized; decreased clearance. In even mild cirrhosis, use at reduced dose and/or frequency. In severe cirrhosis, dose should not exceed 75 mg daily for conventional tablets, or 100 mg daily for sustained-release formulations.
Duloxetine	Extensively metabolized; decreased metabolism and elimination. Do not use in patients with any hepatic insufficiency.
Mirtazapine	Extensively metabolized; decreased clearance. No dosing guidelines.
Nefazodone	May cause hepatic failure. Avoid use in patients with active liver disease.
Trazodone	Extensively metabolized. No dosing guidelines.
Venlafaxine	Decreased clearance and increased elimination half-life of venlafaxine and its active metabolite O-desmethylvenlafaxine. Dosage should be reduced by 50% in moderate HI.

Atypical antipsychotics

Clozapine	Extensively metabolized. Clozapine should be discontinued in patients with marked transaminase elevations or jaundice. No dosing guidelines.
Olanzapine	Extensively metabolized. Periodic assessment of transaminases is recommended. No dosage adjustment needed per manufacturer.
Quetiapine	Extensively metabolized; clearance decreased 30%. Start at 25 mg/day; increase by 25–50 mg daily.
Risperidone	Extensively metabolized; 35% increase in free fraction. Starting dosage and dose increments not to exceed 0.5 mg bid. Increases over 1.5 mg bid should be made at intervals of at least 1 week.
Ziprasidone	Extensively metabolized; increased half-life and serum level in mild to moderate HI. In spite of this, manufacturer recommends no dosage adjustment.

Conventional antipsychotics

Haloperidol et al.	All metabolized in the liver. No specific dosing recommendations.
	Phenothiazines (e.g., thioridazine and trifluoperazine) should be avoided. If nonphenothiazines are used, dosage should be reduced and titration should proceed more slowly than usual

Anxiolytic and sedative-hypnotic drugs

Alprazolam	Decreased metabolism and increased half-life. Dosage should be reduced by 50%–60%. Avoid use in patients with cirrhosis.
Buspirone	Extensively metabolized, half-life may be prolonged. Use at reduced dose. Do not use in patients with severe impairment.
Chlordiazepoxide	Extensively metabolized; reduced clearance and prolonged half-life in. Avoid use if possible.
Clonazepam	
Diazepam	
Flurazepam	
Triazolam	
Lorazepam	Metabolized by conjugation; clearance not affected. No dosage adjustment needed. Lorazepam preferred choice.
Oxazepam	
Temazepam	
Zaleplon	Metabolized in the liver. Reduced clearance. Usual ceiling dose is 5 mg.
Zolpidem	Not recommended in severe HI.

Mood stabilizers

Carbamazepine	Extensively metabolized. Perform baseline liver function tests and periodic evaluations during therapy. Discontinue for active liver disease or aggravation of liver dysfunction. No dosing guidelines.
Oxcarbazepine	Manufacturer states that no dosage adjustment is needed in mild to moderate HI.
Gabapentin	Renally excreted; not appreciably metabolized. No dosage adjustment needed.

TABLE 37–9. Selected psychotropic drugs in hepatic insufficiency (HI) *(continued)*

Mood stabilizers *(continued)*

Lamotrigine	Initial, escalation, and maintenance dosages should be reduced by 50% in moderate HI (Child-Pugh B) and by 75% in severe HI (Child-Pugh C).
Lithium	Renally excreted; not metabolized. Dosage adjustment depends on fluid status.
Topiramate	Reduced clearance. No dosing guidelines.
Valproate	Extensively metabolized; reduced clearance and increased half-life. Reduce dosage, monitor liver function tests frequently, especially in first 6 months of therapy. Avoid in patients with substantial hepatic dysfunction. Use with caution in patients with prior history of hepatic disease.

Cholinesterase inhibitors

Donepezil	Mildly reduced clearance in cirrhosis. No specific recommendations for dose adjustment.
Galantamine	Use with caution in mild to moderate HI. Dose should not exceed 16 mg daily in moderate HI (Child-Pugh 7–9). Use not recommended in severe HI (Child-Pugh 10–15).
Rivastigmine	Clearance reduced 60%–65% in mild to moderate HI, but dose adjustment may not be necessary.

Central nervous system stimulants

Methylphenidate	Unclear association with hepatotoxicity, particularly when co-administered with other adrenergic drugs. No dosing guidelines.
Modafinil	Decreased clearance. Reduce dose by 50% in severe HI.

Note. MAOI=monoamine oxidase inhibitor; SSRI=selective serotonin reuptake inhibitor; TCA=tricyclic antidepressant.
Source. Adapted from Jacobson S: "Psychopharmacology: Prescribing for Patients With Hepatic or Renal Dysfunction." *Psychiatric Times* 19, 2002. Used with permission.

ibuprofen. This relative risk is further increased by concurrent administration of NSAIDs and low-dose aspirin (Weinrieb et al. 2003).

Cholinesterase inhibitors. Increased cholinergic activity is expected to increase gastric acid secretion, thereby increasing risk of peptic ulcers. Therefore, caution is warranted when using cholinesterase inhibitors in patients who are at increased risk of developing ulcers or who are receiving NSAIDs.

Other Gastrointestinal Disorders

Many diseases can cause malabsorption. Depending on the type of malabsorption syndrome and the mechanism involved, varied effects on pharmacokinetics may be observed. In general, however, orally administered drugs may be poorly absorbed in the presence of malabsorption syndromes. In patients with delayed gastric emptying (due to diabetes mellitus, atrophic gastritis, gastric cancer, pyloric stenosis, pancreatitis, or gastric ulcer or drug induced), the pharmacokinetic effect may be to slow absorption rate and delay time to onset of the medication. The effects of gastric dysfunction, including reduced gastric acidity and reduced gastric emptying on drug absorption, are complex (see Gubbins and Bertch 1991; Parsons 1977). For non-enteric-coated preparations, increased gastric emptying is likely to increase the rate of drug absorption, and conversely, delayed gastric emptying will slow the rate of drug absorption. However, because of the large intestinal surface area, overall absorption is not likely to change significantly. Similarly, for most drugs, reduced gastric acidity is unlikely to significantly affect the extent of absorption. For enteric-coated preparations, however, reduced gastric acidity increases the rate of drug absorption because dissolution of the preparation will occur in the stomach. The rate and extent of absorption of drugs, such as clorazepate, that require gastric acid–induced hydrolysis for conversion to the active form (desmethyldiazepam in the case of clorazepate) are impaired by agents, and presumably disease states, that reduce gastric acidity (Greenblatt et al. 1978; Parsons 1977). Anticholinergic drugs should be avoided in patients with gastroparesis, constipation, or ulcerative colitis. SSRIs may be undesirable in patients with increased gastric motility or diarrhea.

Renal Disease

Although most psychotropic drugs do not depend on the kidney for excretion, a variety of factors may affect pharmacokinetics during renal failure, including changes in absorption, distribution, and protein binding (discussed earlier in this chapter). Despite the complexity of pharmacokinetic changes in renal failure, most psychotropics, other than lithium and gabapentin, do not require drastic dosage adjustment. However, many problems associated with use of psychotropics in patients with end-stage renal disease (ESRD) are related to comorbid illnesses rather than to the renal failure per se. Specific dosing guidelines based on creatinine clearance are not available for most psychotropics, but many clinicians use the rule of "two-thirds"—that is, for patients with renal insufficiency, use two-thirds of the dose (except for lithium and gabapentin) used for patients with normal renal function.

Because most psychotropics are lipophilic compounds with large volumes of distribution, they are not dialyzable. Only lithium, gabapentin, valproate, topiramate, and levetiracetam are removed by dialysis. Significant fluid shifts occur during and several hours after each hemodialysis treatment, making dialysis patients more prone to orthostasis. Hence, drugs that frequently cause orthostatic hypotension should ideally be avoided.

Table 37–10 provides recommendations for dosing psychotropics in patients with renal disease.

Antidepressants

Virtually all antidepressants may be used in patients with renal failure, although the greatest experience is with the TCAs. However, patients with ESRD tend to be more sensitive to the side effects of TCAs, including sedation, anticholinergic toxicity, and orthostatic hypotension. Hydroxylated metabolites have been shown to be markedly elevated in patients with ESRD and are hypothesized to be responsible for some TCA side effects. Nortriptyline is considered the preferred TCA because its blood levels correlate well with clinical effect, and the "therapeutic window" is the same in renal failure patients as in physically healthy patients. Limited data are available on the use of newer antidepressants in patients with renal failure. Some evidence suggests that dosage adjustments may not be needed for citalopram and fluoxetine in those with ESRD. However, the half-life of venlafaxine is prolonged in renal insufficiency; its clearance is reduced by over 50% in patients undergoing dialysis. Paroxetine clearance is also reduced in renal insufficiency. Because most antidepressants are metabolized by the liver and excreted by the kidney, initial dosage reduction of all antidepressants is reasonable as a way to reduce the possibility that potentially active metabolites will accumulate.

Antipsychotics

All antipsychotics may be used in patients with renal failure. Difficulties arise from the complications of renal failure and dialysis or from the chronic disease causing renal failure (e.g., diabetes). For example, patients with ESRD who also have diabetic autonomic neuropathy will be at higher risk for drug side effects, including postural hypotension and bladder, gastrointestinal, and sexual dysfunction.

Anxiolytics and Sedative-Hypnotics

Virtually all sedative-hypnotics can be used in patients with renal failure with the exception of barbiturates. Barbiturates should be avoided because they may increase osteomalacia and because of excessive sedation. Preferred benzodiazepines include those with inactive metabolites such as lorazepam and oxazepam. Even so, the half-lives of lorazepam and oxazepam may almost quadruple in patients with ESRD, and dosage reduction is required. Other benzodiazepines with inactive metabolites include clonazepam and temazepam, but less is known about changes in their half-lives in ESRD.

Mood Stabilizers

Lithium is almost entirely excreted by the kidneys. It is contraindicated in patients with acute renal failure, but not in those with chronic renal failure. For patients with stable partial renal insufficiency, dose conservatively and monitor renal function frequently. For patients on dialysis, lithium is completely dialyzed and may be given as a single oral dose (300–600 mg) following hemodialysis treatment. Lithium levels should not be checked until at least 2–3 hours after dialysis, because re-equilibration from tissue stores occurs in the immediate postdialytic period. For patients on peritoneal dialysis, lithium can be given in the dialysate. Dosage adjustment recommendations based on creatinine clearance are available for gabapentin, lithium, topiramate, and carbamazepine (Jacobson 2002).

Cholinesterase Inhibitors

It appears, from the limited data available, that dosage adjustment of donepezil is not required. As in patients without renal disease, rivastigmine dose should be titrated according to efficacy and individual tolerability. Galantamine should be used cautiously in patients with moderate renal insufficiency; according to the manufacturer, its use in patients with severe renal insufficiency is not recommended.

Psychostimulants

No specific dosing recommendations are currently available for psychostimulants.

Cardiovascular Disease

Potential adverse cardiovascular effects of psychotropics include orthostatic hypotension, conduction disturbances, and arrhythmias (see also Chapter 19, "Heart Disease"). Orthostatic hypotension can be a serious problem for many debilitated patients, aggravated by dehydration,

TABLE 37–10. Psychotropic drugs in renal insufficiency (RI)[a]

Antidepressants

MAOIs	May accumulate in RI.
Most SSRIs	Mild to moderate RI: no dosage adjustment needed.
	Severe RI: may need to reduce dosage or lengthen dosing interval.
Paroxetine	Mild RI: no dosage adjustment needed.
	Moderate RI: 50%–75% of usual dose.
	Severe RI: initial dosage of 10 mg/day; increase as needed by 10 mg at weekly intervals to a maximum dosage of 40 mg/day.
	Controlled-release formulation: initial dose of 12.5 mg/day; increase if needed by 12.5 mg at weekly intervals to a maximum dose of 50 mg/day.
TCAs	Water-soluble active metabolites may accumulate. No recommended dosage adjustments.
Bupropion	Water-soluble active metabolites may accumulate. Reduce initial dosage.
Duloxetine	Mild RI: population CPK analyses suggest no significant effect on apparent clearance.
	No data regarding use in moderate to severe RI.
	Not recommended for patients with end-stage renal disease.
Mirtazapine	Moderate RI: clearance decreased by 30%.
	Severe RI: clearance decreased by 50%.
Nefazodone	No dosage adjustment needed.
Trazodone	Mild RI: use with caution. No data regarding use in moderate to severe RI.
Venlafaxine	Moderate RI: 75% of usual dose.
	Severe RI: 50% of usual dose.
	Hemodialysis patients should be dosed after dialysis session.

Atypical antipsychotics

Clozapine, olanzapine, quetiapine	No dosage adjustment needed.
Risperidone	Clearance decreased in RI. Initiate therapy at 0.25–0.5 mg bid.
	Increase beyond 1.5 mg should be made at intervals of at least 7 days.
Ziprasidone	No recommendations made regarding dosage adjustment.

Conventional antipsychotics

Haloperidol et al.	No dosage adjustment needed.

Anxiolytics and sedative-hypnotics

Most benzodiazepines	No dosage adjustment needed.
Chlordiazepoxide	Severe RI: 50% of usual dose.
Buspirone	Use in severe RI not recommended.
Zaleplon	Mild to moderate RI: no dosage adjustment needed.
	Severe RI not adequately studied.
Zolpidem	Dosage adjustment may not be needed in RI.

Anticonvulsant/antimanic agents

Carbamazepine	Severe RI: 75% of usual dose.
Oxcarbazepine	Initiate therapy at 300 mg/day (50% of usual starting dose).
Gabapentin	Cl_{cr} <60 mL/min: 1,200 mg/day (400 mg tid).
	Cl_{cr} 30–60 mL/min: 600 mg/day (300 mg bid).
	Cl_{cr} 15–30 mL/min: 300 mg/day.
	Cl_{cr} <15 mL/min: 150 mg/day (300 mg every other day).
	Hemodialysis: 300–400 mg loading dose to patients who have never received gabapentin, then 200–300 mg after each dialysis session.
Lamotrigine	Reduced dose may be effective in significant RI.
Lithium	Moderate RI: 50%–75% of usual dose.
	Hemodialysis: usual dose 300 mg once after each dialysis session.

TABLE 37–10.   Psychotropic drugs in renal insufficiency (RI)[a] (continued)

Anticonvulsant/antimanic agents (continued)	
Topiramate	Mild RI: 100% of usual dosage.
	Moderate RI: 50% of usual dosage.
	Severe RI: 25% of usual dosage.
	Supplemental dose may be needed after hemodialysis.
Valproate	No dosage adjustment needed in RI, but valproate level measurements are misleading.
Cholinesterase inhibitors	
Donepezil	Limited data suggest no dosage adjustment needed.
Galantamine	Moderate RI: maximum dose 16 mg/day.
	Severe RI: use not recommended.
Rivastigmine	Dosage adjustment not recommended.
Central nervous system stimulants	
Methylphenidate	No dosage adjustment needed.
Modafinil	No dosage adjustment needed.
Antiparkinsonian agents	
Amantadine	Cl_{cr} 80 mL/min: 100 mg bid.
	Cl_{cr} 60 mL/min: 100 mg qd/bid on alternate days.
	Cl_{cr} 40 mL/min: 100 mg/day.
	Cl_{cr} 30 mL/min: 200 mg twice weekly.
	Cl_{cr} 20 mL/min: 100 mg three times weekly.
	Cl_{cr} 10 mL/min: 200 mg alternated with 100 mg every 7 days.

Note.   MAOIs=monoamine oxidase inhibitors; SSRIs=selective serotonin reuptake inhibitors; TCAs=tricyclic antidepressants.
[a]Mild RI is >50 mL/min; moderate RI is 10–50 mL/min; severe RI is <10 mL/min.
Source.   Adapted from Jacobson S: "Psychopharmacology: Prescribing for Patients With Hepatic or Renal Dysfunction." *Psychiatric Times* 19, 2002. Used with permission.

with increased morbidity resulting in patients with poor tissue perfusion and leading to injuries due to falls (fractures, subdural hematomas).

Antidepressants

For an extensive review of the safety of antidepressant drugs in patients with cardiac disease, please refer to the article by Alvarez and Pickworth (2003). In summary, patients most at risk for developing cardiac side effects include those with unstable coronary artery disease (especially recent myocardial infarction), conduction abnormalities, orthostatic hypotension, and congestive heart failure (Alvarez and Pickworth 2003). Although there are more studies of TCAs than other antidepressants in cardiac patients, the SSRIs have been studied in the largest number of patients.

Tricyclic antidepressants.   The TCAs have been shown to be relatively safe for short-term treatment of patients with stable ischemic heart disease, previous myocardial infarction, and congestive heart failure. Long-term safety has not been studied. In healthy individuals, the cardiovascular complications from TCAs administered at therapeutic levels are largely limited to orthostatic hypoten-

sion (Glassman 1984). In patients with heart disease, the cardiovascular risks become clinically significant. TCAs are more likely to cause orthostatic hypotension in patients with impairment in left ventricular function but are relatively safe to use in most patients with congestive heart failure. Caution is required if the patient has symptomatic orthostatic hypotension or markedly reduced cardiac ejection fraction. Nortriptyline is considered the safest TCA in patients with congestive heart failure because it is least likely to cause orthostasis (Roose et al. 1981) and has little to no effect on cardiac ejection fraction (Giardina et al. 1985; Roose et al. 1986).

All TCAs have quinidine-like antiarrhythmic properties that delay cardiac conduction and increase heart rate. In healthy individuals, this is usually not clinically significant. Patients with existing conduction delays (e.g., bundle branch block) may have clinically relevant deleterious effects on conduction time. In patients with bundle branch block (especially those with second-degree heart block), dissociative (third-degree) atrioventricular heart block may develop. Some calcium channel blockers (diltiazem and verapamil, but not nifedipine) may also slow atrioventricular conduction, making their combination with TCAs more dangerous.

Another potential quinidine-like effect of the TCAs is prolongation of the QTc interval, which may lead to the potentially fatal arrhythmia torsades de pointes. Those at particular risk include patients with a preexisting familial long QTc syndrome and those who develop undue QTc prolongation during treatment with TCAs (or other QTc-prolonging drugs). An electrocardiogram is indicated for patients treated with TCAs who have a personal or family history of sudden death or syncope or a personal history of angina, myocardial infarction, congestive heart failure, arrhythmias, hypokalemia, hypomagnesemia, or other significant cardiac risk factors (Vieweg 2002). If TCAs are absolutely necessary in patients with existing conduction disturbances, cardiology consultation should be sought prior to their use.

Wolff-Parkinson-White syndrome, or atrioventricular nodal reentrant tachycardia, affects approximately 0.15%–0.2% of the general population. Of these individuals, 60%–70% have no other evidence of heart disease. In some, more serious and potentially life-threatening abnormal rhythms may develop. The most common is atrial fibrillation. Quinidine-like drugs given to patients with atrial flutter-fibrillation may lead to ventricular tachycardia or fibrillation. All patients with Wolff-Parkinson-White syndrome should be evaluated by a cardiologist prior to considering TCA treatment.

Newer antidepressants.   SSRIs are currently considered the safest antidepressants in patients with cardiac disease. Paroxetine, sertraline, and fluoxetine have been studied, and citalopram is currently under study. In these studies, SSRIs have shown no orthostatic hypotension, minimal effects on conduction, and virtually no effects on ventricular function (Alvarez and Pickworth 2003). Trazodone and bupropion have been studied in small clinical trials. Trazodone is reportedly safe despite causing orthostatic hypotension. Bupropion has been used safely in patients with conduction disease and left ventricular dysfunction (Roose et al. 1991). Mirtazapine is currently being studied in patients following myocardial infarction (van den Brink et al. 2002).

Antipsychotics

Antipsychotics that cause orthostatic hypotension, including low-potency antipsychotics, clozapine, and perhaps quetiapine, should be avoided in patients with congestive heart failure. Orthostasis occurs far less frequently with high-potency typical antipsychotics such as haloperidol, which can usually be used safely even during acute unstable cardiac disease.

Patients with preexisting intraventricular conduction delays are at increased risk of heart block when given an-

tipsychotics with quinidine-like properties such as thioridazine. Although the cardiovascular risks with antipsychotics may vary, pimozide, thioridazine, mesoridazine, droperidol, sertindole, and ziprasidone carry the highest risk for prolonging the QTc interval and causing torsades de pointes. Other atypical antipsychotics and haloperidol appear to demonstrate the least risk for prolonging the QTc interval. Although haloperidol has caused QTc prolongation and torsades, especially when parenterally administered at a high dosage (>100 mg/day), it is generally accepted to be minimally cardiotoxic. An electrocardiogram is indicated in patients taking antipsychotic drugs with increased risk of QTc prolongation (droperidol, mesoridazine, thioridazine, pimozide, high intravenous dose haloperidol).

Anxiolytics and Sedative-Hypnotics

Generally, benzodiazepines are free of cardiovascular effects. Their safety has been documented even in the immediate post–myocardial infarction period (Risch et al. 1982). However, rapid intravenous administration may cause hypotension. Buspirone is essentially free of cardiovascular effects.

Mood Stabilizers

The cardiac effects of lithium at nontoxic levels are generally insignificant; there may be nonspecific electrocardiographic changes, which are usually benign. Lithium uncommonly causes sinus node dysfunction or first-degree atrioventricular block and should be used cautiously in patients at risk (Dasgupta and Jefferson 1990). For patients with congestive heart failure, reduced doses are required secondary to decreased lithium clearance. However, lithium is difficult to use in these patients because of salt restriction and diuretic therapy. Valproic acid is safe to use in patients with cardiovascular disease. Carbamazepine is more cardiotoxic and has been associated with the development of atrioventricular conduction disturbances. Before carbamazepine is prescribed, a baseline electrocardiogram should be obtained in patients at risk, and alternative therapy should be considered if there is evidence of heart block or atrioventricular conduction delay. Lamotrigine has been associated with clinically insignificant prolongation of the PR interval. Caution is warranted with other mood stabilizers because they have not been systematically studied in patients with cardiac disease.

Cholinesterase Inhibitors

Cholinesterase inhibitors may have vagotonic effects on the heart (e.g., bradycardia). This effect may be of particular concern in patients with "sick sinus syndrome" or other supraventricular conduction abnormalities. Cholinesterase inhibitors should be avoided in patients with most cardiac conduction abnormalities and those with unexplained syncopal episodes.

Psychostimulants

Methylphenidate and dextroamphetamine in low doses have no significant cardiovascular effects, including no effect on blood pressure or heart rate. Safe use has been described in many cardiac patients, including those with congestive heart failure, coronary artery disease, arrhythmias, and hypertension (Masand and Tesar 1996).

Central Nervous System Disease

Cerebrovascular Disease

The most common problems encountered when prescribing psychotropics to patients with cerebrovascular disease include lowered threshold for CNS side effects, orthostatic hypotension, and comorbid disorders (e.g., cardiac disease, diabetes).

Antidepressants.   Depression follows stroke in up to one-third of patients (see also Chapter 9, "Depression," and Chapter 32, "Neurology and Neurosurgery"). Treatment of poststroke depression has been most studied with nortriptyline, trazodone, fluoxetine, and citalopram, with favorable therapeutic effects in those patients able to tolerate these medications. Although more evidence is needed regarding the safety and efficacy of newer antidepressants in poststroke patients, they may be the drugs of choice given their favorable side-effect profile.

Antipsychotics.   In April 2003, Janssen Pharmaceutica, in conjunction with Health Canada, first reported a labeling change indicating that cerebrovascular events (stroke, transient ischemic attack), including fatalities, were reported in four placebo-controlled trials of risperidone in elderly patients ($N=1,230$; mean age, 85 years; range, 73–97) with dementia-related psychosis (Health Canada 2003). There was a significantly higher incidence of cerebrovascular adverse events in patients treated with risperidone than in those receiving placebo. Since then, Eli Lilly & Company has reported some data on cerebrovascular event rates in 5 placebo-controlled trials of olanzapine in elderly patients with dementia (including Alzheimer's, vascular, and mixed dementia). According to information supplied, the absolute increased risk for cerebrovascular accidents was 0.9% for patients taking olanzapine (Wooltorton 2004). These rates are similar to those reported for risperidone (Wooltorton 2002). Addi-

tionally, in placebo-controlled clinical trials of elderly patients with dementia-related psychosis, the incidence of death in olanzapine patients was significantly greater than that in placebo-treated patients (3.5% vs. 1.5%, respectively). Risk factors that may predispose this patient population to increased mortality when treated with olanzapine include age greater than 80 years, sedation, concomitant use of benzodiazepines or the presence of pulmonary conditions (e.g., pneumonia with or without aspiration) (Eli Lilly & Company 2004). In a retrospective analysis comparing mortality effects of haloperidol with those of atypical antipsychotics risperidone or olanzapine over a 2-year period in patients 65 years or older, the authors reported a statistically significant difference in mortality, with 21.4% (64 of 299) in the haloperidol group and 4.75% (61 of 1,254) in the atypical group (Nasrallah et al. 2004). It is difficult to know how to interpret this information, given the increased risk of stroke in the elderly and no reliable means to quantify the degree of vascular dementia (a marker for underlying cerebrovascular disease) in individual patients. It is unknown whether other antipsychotics pose elevated risk.

Psychostimulants.   Psychostimulants offer an alternative in treating poststroke depression, but poststroke patients may be more sensitive to their side effects. Hence, psychostimulants should be initiated at a very low dose and gradually increased as necessary (Masand and Tesar 1996).

Seizures

Psychotropics that may lower seizure threshold at normal doses primarily pose a risk in patients with untreated (or undertreated) seizure disorder.

Antidepressants.   Seizure disorder patients are frequently prescribed psychotropic medications, including antidepressants, because of high psychiatric comorbidity. How much risk for increased seizures do antidepressants cause in such patients? Studies to date are difficult to interpret because of methodological limitations and confounding factors. Clinical recommendations are based largely on observational studies and case reports. These include reports that assess risk for seizures after psychotropic drug overdose and during therapeutic use in patients with and without epilepsy (Alldredge 1999). Most antidepressants at therapeutic doses in nonepileptic patients exhibit a seizure risk close to that reported for the first spontaneous seizure in the general population (0.1%). Risk of seizures with bupropion SR (dosage of 450 mg/day) is comparable with that of SSRIs but elevated at dosages greater than 450 mg/day. The use of bupropion in patients with preexisting seizure disorder, or in patients who may be at higher risk for developing seizures, warrants caution. Although newer antidepressants are thought to have a decreased relative risk for seizures, identification of relative seizure risk is thwarted by lack of systematic prospective comparisons.

Antipsychotics. Low-potency typical antipsychotics, especially at high dosages (1,000 mg/day chlorpromazine), and clozapine have higher reported risk of seizures and ideally should be avoided in patients with existing seizure disorders. Seizures have been reported with most antipsychotics; however, haloperidol and atypical antipsychotics (other than clozapine) appear to have a much lower seizure risk (Alldredge 1999).

Cholinesterase inhibitors. Cholinomimetics may reduce the seizure threshold, and seizures have been reported during clinical trials with all cholinesterase inhibitors. However, seizure activity may also be a manifestation of Alzheimer's disease. Donepezil has been reported to increase seizure frequency in patients with epilepsy (Fisher et al. 2001). The risk–benefit ratio of cholinesterase treatment for patients with seizures must be carefully evaluated.

Psychostimulants. Many physicians believe that psychostimulants can lower seizure threshold, but evidence is lacking. One study of traumatic brain injury patients with posttraumatic seizures concluded that methylphenidate can be safely used even in those at high risk for seizures (Wroblewski et al. 1992). A small number of patients may experience an increase in seizure frequency when they are treated with psychostimulants. If seizure frequency rises, the drug should be discontinued. To our knowledge, seizures have not been reported during therapeutic use of atomoxetine.

Migraine Headache

Antidepressants. Many patients with migraine headaches take triptans, which are potent 5-HT$_{1B/1D}$ receptor agonists. Antidepressants are also frequently prescribed for migraine prophylaxis or comorbid depression. The two main concerns regarding the use of antidepressants in patients who use triptans are the risk for serotonin syndrome and the risk for pharmacokinetic interactions with the triptans. Serotonin syndrome as a complication of triptan use is quite rare, with only a few cases reported (Mathew et al. 1996; Putnam et al. 1999). Use of triptans does not contraindicate the use of serotonergic antidepressants. The pharmacokinetics of the triptans vary widely (Jhee et al. 2001). Some triptans, including rizatriptan and

sumatriptan, are metabolized by MAO and should not be used during MAOI therapy or within 2 weeks of MAOI discontinuation (McEvoy 2003). Almotriptan and naratriptan are eliminated primarily through metabolism by cytochrome P450 enzymes and/or renal elimination and thus can be more safely used in conjunction with MAOIs.

Parkinsonism

For additional discussion of use of medications in patients with Parkinson's disease, see Chapter 32, "Neurology and Neurosurgery."

Antidepressants. Double-blind studies of imipramine, nortriptyline, desipramine, and bupropion demonstrate antidepressant efficacy with no change in Parkinson's disease symptoms. The anticholinergic effects of TCAs may even be therapeutic for parkinsonism.

There is a theoretical concern that serotonergic antidepressants could worsen parkinsonism through inhibition of nigrostriatal dopamine release by serotonin—an effect that has been reported in a few cases (Hauser and Zesiewicz 1997). However, in open-label studies and case reports, sertraline, citalopram, reboxetine, paroxetine, and moclobemide have all been reported to be efficacious and well tolerated by patients with Parkinson's disease (Hauser and Zesiewicz 1997; Lemke 2002; Rampello et al. 2002; Steur and Ballering 1997; Tesei et al. 2000).

Early reports suggest that mirtazapine may reduce tremor (Gordon et al. 2002; Pact and Giduz 1999). Selegiline, a highly selective MAO-B inhibitor at doses used in the treatment of Parkinson's disease, is another antidepressant option, but it loses selectivity at the doses required for antidepressant efficacy and so requires standard MAOI precautions.

Antipsychotics. The major concern about using antipsychotics in treating patients with Parkinson's disease is that they all produce some degree of dopamine D$_2$ receptor blockade—especially high-potency typical antipsychotics—potentially aggravating the disease. Clozapine is the only atypical antipsychotic demonstrated in a controlled trial in patients with Parkinson's disease to be effective against psychosis without aggravating the disease, and it may even be beneficial in reducing tremor (Parkinson Study Group 1999). Initial case reports suggesting that olanzapine and risperidone were well tolerated were followed by other reports of deterioration in motor functioning. Case reports regarding quetiapine have been more positive.

To date, the limited case reports of the use of aripiprazole or ziprasidone in patients with Parkinson's disease have described mixed efficacy of these agents in reducing psychosis while not worsening parkinsonian symptoms (Connemann and Schonfeldt-Lecuona 2004; Fernandez et al. 2004; Schonfeldt-Lecuona and Connemann 2004).

Dementia With Lewy Bodies

Antipsychotics. Patients with dementia with Lewy bodies (see Chapter 7, "Dementia") typically present with extreme sensitivity to EPS of antipsychotics, a consideration that is especially important to remember when prescribing antipsychotics for the treatment of hallucinations, delusions, and/or agitation in patients with dementia. No randomized, controlled trials of antipsychotics in patients with dementia with Lewy bodies exist. Overall, atypical antipsychotics are probably safer than typical antipsychotics and should be used at very low dosages.

Endocrine Disease

Diabetes Mellitus

Antidepressants. An increase in catecholamine increases serum glucose levels while reducing both insulin release and insulin sensitivity. In contrast, increases in serotonergic function seem to increase sensitivity to insulin and reduce serum glucose. Thus, in theory, SSRIs may be preferred agents in patients with diabetes because of their minimal effects on glucose metabolism. However, in diabetic neuropathic pain, dual-action antidepressants appear more effective at lower doses than do specific serotonergic agents, perhaps because catecholamines and serotonin have both been implicated in pain pathways (Goodnick 2001).

Antipsychotics. An assessment of relative risks of particular antipsychotics in diabetes should include the risks of weight gain, glucose intolerance, and hyperlipidemia. Although there are insufficient data to define a first choice, it is generally agreed that clozapine and olanzapine should be avoided. There is no current consensus on when to monitor glucose and lipids when atypical antipsychotics are being prescribed.

Obesity

Antipsychotics.   Almost all antipsychotics can cause weight gain, but they vary in their propensity to cause this effect. There is some controversy as to who is more likely to gain weight on antipsychotics—those at normal weight to begin with or those who are already obese. Nevertheless, in patients who are already obese, weight-neutral antipsychotics such as molindone, ziprasidone, and aripiprazole are sensible as preferred agents.

Lipids

Antipsychotics. Phenothiazines, clozapine, olanzapine, and quetiapine are known to elevate serum triglyceride levels and thus should be avoided in patients who already have hypertriglyceridemia or hypercholesterolemia.

Respiratory Disease

For additional discussion of use of medications in patients with respiratory disease, see Chapter 20, "Lung Disease."

Antidepressants

Antidepressants generally do not cause problems in patients with respiratory disease. However, MAOIs are problematic in asthmatic patients because of their potential to interact with epinephrine and other sympathomimetic medications. Use of antidepressants with anticholinergic properties is of theoretical benefit because of their mild bronchodilator effect. Cyclic antidepressants, SSRIs, and other newer antidepressants have little to no effect on respiratory function.

Anxiolytics and Sedative-Hypnotics

The respiratory depressant effects of all benzodiazepines are well established; most of these agents can significantly reduce the ventilatory response to hypoxia. This may precipitate respiratory failure in a patient with marginal respiratory reserve. Patients with moderate-to-severe COPD are at risk for carbon dioxide retention with long-acting benzodiazepines, even at relatively low doses. However, benzodiazepines should not automatically be rejected for use in patients with COPD. Anxiety can often reduce respiratory efficiency, and benzodiazepines may actually improve respiratory status in some patients, especially those with asthma or emphysema ("pink puffers") (Mitchell-Heggs et al. 1980). Patients with severe bronchitis ("blue bloaters") or severe restrictive lung disease are the most vulnerable to the adverse effects of benzodiazepines. Intermediate-acting agents (oxazepam, temazepam, lorazepam) have fewer respiratory depressant effects and are the benzodiazepines of first choice for anxiolysis in patients with COPD. For patients with severe COPD, baseline assessment of blood gases and pulmonary consultation may be necessary in deciding whether benzodiazepines are appropriate for use. Oximetry is likely adequate for ongoing monitoring of the patient's clinical status during benzodiazepine use unless the patient is a known CO_2 retainer, in which case blood gases are more appropriate.

Controlled trials with short-acting hypnotics, including triazolam, zolpidem, and zaleplon, suggest that they may be safely used in selected patients who have mild to moderate COPD without daytime hypercapnia (George 2000). Zopiclone has been studied in patients with upper airway resistance syndrome and has no adverse effects on sleep architecture, respiratory parameters during sleep, and daytime sleepiness (Lofaso et al. 1997). Further study is needed to better define the risk–benefit ratio of hypnotics in patients with COPD. Benzodiazepines are currently contraindicated in individuals with sleep apnea.

Buspirone is potentially a safer anxiolytic in pulmonary patients because it does not depress respiration, at least in healthy volunteers ("Buspirone: Seven-Year Update" 1994). It also does not adversely affect sleep apnea (Mendelson et al. 1991). In the one open-label study of buspirone in subjects with severe lung disease, none of the subjects showed deterioration in respiratory function or increased carbon dioxide retention (Craven and Sutherland 1991). In patients with COPD, a double-blind study demonstrated no adverse effects on respiratory measures but also failed to show clinical benefit (Singh et al. 1993). Although buspirone does not adversely affect pulmonary function, its limitations are its potency and delayed therapeutic effect (Robinson and Levenson 2000).

Antipsychotics

Antipsychotics may be helpful in pulmonary patients who are incapacitated by extreme panic and dyspnea that mutually exacerbate each other. Most typical and atypical antipsychotics can be used in patients with chronic respiratory disease. Uncommon but serious concerns include the provocation of laryngeal dystonia and development of tardive dyskinesia affecting respiratory musculature. Low-potency typical antipsychotics may have some additional bronchodilatory effects. Clozapine has been associated with respiratory arrest and depression as well as allergic asthma (Lieberman and Safferman 1992; Stoppe et al. 1992).

Cholinesterase Inhibitors

Because acetylcholine is a potent mediator of bronchoconstriction, care must be taken in prescribing cholinesterase inhibitors to patients with asthma or COPD.

Cancer

For additional discussion of use of medications in patients with cancer, see Chapter 24, "Oncology."

Breast Cancer

Antidepressants. Recent case–control studies have reported an increased risk of developing breast cancer for patients taking some TCAs for longer than 10 years (Sharpe et al. 2002). Another case–control study concluded

that "paroxetine may be associated with a substantial increase in breast cancer risk" (Cotterchio et al. 2000, p. 779). These studies, and the resulting media attention, have caused considerable anxiety in women currently or previously taking antidepressants. A critical evaluation of these studies noted many methodological limitations and concluded that the current evidence does not merit changing depression treatment practice (Kurdyak et al. 2002; Sternbach 2003).

HIV/AIDS

See Chapter 28, "HIV/AIDS," and a review by Robinson and Qaqish (2002) for discussion of the use of psychotropics in patients with HIV/AIDS.

Psychotropic Drug Use During Pregnancy and Breast-Feeding

For additional discussion of the issues regarding medication use by pregnant or breast-feeding women, see Chapter 33, "Obstetrics and Gynecology."

Pregnancy

Fetal exposure to medications is common, especially during the first trimester. Because approximately 50%–65% of all pregnancies in the United States are unplanned (Koren et al. 1998; Rosenfeld and Everett 1996), the fetus may be exposed to a variety of drugs during the first trimester before the mother is aware of her pregnancy. Even during an established pregnancy, surveys estimate that 80% of women take prescription medications and 21%–33% are exposed to psychotropic drugs (Barki et al. 1998; Doering and Stewart 1978). For any woman of childbearing age, all drugs should be considered for their safety in pregnancy and breast-feeding.

Fetal risks associated with drug use during pregnancy include teratogenicity, direct toxicity, perinatal effects, and possible long-term effects on behavior and development. Known and possible risks of pharmacotherapy, however, must be balanced against the risks to the fetus from withholding therapy. Exacerbation of the mother's psychiatric illness may endanger the fetus in utero through maternal self-harm, suicide, malnutrition, lack of proper prenatal care, or excessive exposure to risks through impulsivity, delusions, disorientation, or denial of the pregnancy. Treatments for psychotic and bipolar disorders in severely ill patients should not be discontinued during pregnancy because of the fetal risks associated with the high incidence of relapse (Faedda et al. 1993).

Physiological changes associated with pregnancy alter drug pharmacokinetics and complicate therapy. In general, drug levels decline during pregnancy because of increases in renal elimination, volume of distribution, and cardiac output (Ward 1995, 1996). Over the course of the pregnancy, lithium clearance doubles (Schou et al. 1973) and TCA elimination increases 1.6 times (Wisner et al. 1993). Drug levels should be monitored during the pregnancy, and dosage should be adjusted to maintain a therapeutic response consistent with the lowest effective dose. During the early postpartum period, these physiological changes reverse. As maternal drug elimination returns to normal, any dosage adjustment required during pregnancy should be gradually reversed.

At parturition, the delivery of maternal drug to the neonate is discontinued and neonatal withdrawal symptoms may appear. Neonatal benzodiazepine withdrawal symptoms include irritability, tremor, diarrhea, vomiting, hypertonicity, and high-pitched crying (Rementeria and Bhatt 1977). Symptoms of TCA withdrawal in neonates include irritability, abdominal cramps, insomnia, tachycardia, tachypnea, and cyanosis. SSRIs have also been associated with a neonatal withdrawal syndrome (irritability, constant crying, shivering, increased tonus, eating and sleeping difficulties, and convulsions) (Nordeng et al. 2001). When possible, tapering and discontinuation of benzodiazepines and TCAs over a few weeks before delivery has been recommended to prevent neonatal withdrawal (Miller 1991, 1994), but this must be balanced against the risk of postpartum depression. Discontinued medications should be reinstated postpartum.

Neonates exposed to SSRIs and serotonin–norepinephrine reuptake inhibitors (SNRIs) late in the third trimester have developed complications requiring prolonged hospitalization, respiratory support, and tube feeding. Such complications can arise immediately upon delivery. Reported clinical findings have included respiratory distress, cyanosis, apnea, seizures, temperature instability, feeding difficulty, vomiting, hypoglycemia, hypotonia, hyperreflexia, tremor, jitteriness, irritability, and constant crying (Nordeng et al. 2001). These features are consistent with either a direct toxic effect of SSRIs and SNRIs or possibly a drug discontinuation syndrome. When treating a pregnant woman with an antidepressant during the third trimester, the physician should carefully consider the potential risks and benefits of treatment.

Breast-Feeding

During the postpartum period, women are at risk for the development of depression, mania, or psychosis. More than 60% of mothers breast-feed their infants (Llewellyn and Stowe 1998), and many will wish to do so while taking psychotropic medications. If informed that a medication is incompatible with breast-feeding, a mother may covertly breast-feed and discontinue her medication. Recurrence of the psychiatric disorder not only is dangerous for the mother but may place the infant at greater risk than that posed by breast-feeding while the mother is taking medication.

Unfortunately, case reports are the only source of adverse psychotropic effects during breast-feeding; there are no clinical trials of drug effects in breast-fed infants. With a few exceptions, psychotropic drugs seem to be relatively safe in breast-feeding. The American Academy of Pediatrics (2001) has classified medications according to the evidence supporting their safety in breast-feeding. Most psychotropic agents, however, are classified as "drugs for which the effect on nursing infants is unknown but may be of concern" (American Academy of Pediatrics 2001, p. 779) because of lack of clear data.

The use of medications during pregnancy and breast-feeding, including the risks, benefits, and treatment alternatives, must be discussed with the patient. Failure to fully inform may result in the patient discontinuing treatment because of excessive fear of risk to the fetus.

Increasing evidence suggests that most psychotropic medications are safe in pregnancy and breast-feeding. However, there are concerns about the anticonvulsant mood stabilizers, lithium, low-potency antipsychotics, and benzodiazepines. Concerns about psychotropic drug use in pregnancy and breast-feeding are listed below (compiled from American Academy of Pediatrics Committee on Drugs 2000; Burt et al. 2001; Ernst and Goldberg 2002; Gjere 2001; and Ward and Zamorski 2002).

Risks of Psychotropic Drug Use During Pregnancy and Breast-Feeding

Antipsychotics
- **Pregnancy:**
  - *Typical agents*—Not associated with any evidence of teratogenic, behavioral, emotional, or cognitive abnormalities.
  - *Low-potency drugs*—Can cause neonatal tachycardia, gastrointestinal dysfunction, sedation, and hypotension for a few days after birth. Best avoided so as to minimize anticholinergic, hypotensive, and antihistaminic effects.
  - *High-potency drugs*—Preferred despite the risk of fetal EPS. Incidence of fetal EPS (hyperactivity, hyperreflexia, abnormal movements, tremor, hand flapping, and crying that may persist for several months) is dose related.

– *Atypical agents*—Insufficient human data for recommendation.

– *Depot preparations*—Avoid because of long duration of action.

- **Breast-feeding:** Compatibility of antipsychotics with breast-feeding is unknown. Clozapine may be of concern because of possible agranulocytosis, sedation, and seizures (Iqbal et al. 2001). Sedating drugs such as chlorpromazine may produce drowsiness and lethargy in the infant. Monitor the neonate for antipsychotic side effects such as sedation, muscle rigidity, or tremor (Burt et al. 2001).

Antidepressants
- **Pregnancy:**
  – *TCAs*—Not associated with evidence of teratogenic effects. Avoid maprotiline because of increased maternal seizure risk. Neonatal TCA withdrawal symptoms include seizures, irritability, abdominal cramps, insomnia, tachycardia, tachypnea, and cyanosis.
  – *SSRIs*—Fluoxetine not associated with teratogenic effects. Other SSRIs do not appear to be teratogenic from limited human data.
  – *MAOIs*—Avoid because of hypotensive effects and potential for drug and food interactions.
- **Breast-feeding:** Compatibility with breast-feeding is unknown. Sedating drugs may cause neonatal lethargy. Limited case reports suggest that fluoxetine, paroxetine, and sertraline are relatively safe (Burt et al. 2001).

Antiparkinsonian Agents
- **Pregnancy:**
  – *Anticholinergics*—Not recommended for the treatment of EPS during pregnancy. Associated with increased risk of congenital anomalies, complications of pregnancy, and neonatal adverse effects (Gjere 2001). Akathisia can be treated during pregnancy with propranolol or atenolol.
- **Breast-feeding:** Anticholinergic drugs and amantadine are not classified.

Mood Stabilizers
- **Pregnancy:**
  – *Lithium*—Teratogenic potential is less than earlier thought. First-trimester exposure associated with a 10-fold increase in Ebstein anomaly, a rare (1 in 20,000) cardiovascular malformation. Cardiac ultrasonography at 18–20 weeks is recommended.
  – *Carbamazepine and valproate*—Associated with neural tube defects—carbamazepine (~1%) and valproate (~1% to 2%)—and fetal hydantoin syndrome (facial dysmorphism, cleft lip and palate, cardiac defects and digit hypoplasia). Screening for neural tube defects (amniocentesis and serum alpha-fetoprotein) before week 20 is advised. To minimize risk, all women of childbearing age should consume 0.4 mg folate daily. Women taking valproate or carbamazepine should supplement with 4 mg folate daily when planning to start pregnancy. Carbamazepine and valproate may cause transient vitamin K deficiency, resulting in neonatal clotting disorders. This risk can be minimized by supplementing with 20 mg oral vitamin K from week 36 to delivery, plus 1 mg intramuscularly to the newborn.
  – *Gabapentin, lamotrigine, topiramate:* Insufficient human data for recommendation. There is evidence of fetal toxicity (gabapentin) and teratogenicity (topiramate) in animal studies. Lamotrigine decreases folate in rats; consider folate supplementation (see previous item).
- **Breast-feeding:** Carbamazepine and valproate are compatible with breast-feeding; monitor for possible neonatal hepatotoxicity. Avoid breast-feeding if patient is taking lithium. High levels of lithium are present in breast milk, and therapeutic serum levels are found in breast-fed infants (Chaudron and Jefferson 2000), with reports of neonatal electrocardiographic changes and hypotonia (Ernst and Goldberg 2002). For lamotrigine, gabapentin, and topiramate, compatibility with breast-feeding is unknown. Lamotrigine may be of concern.

Anxiolytics and Sedative-Hypnotics
- **Pregnancy:**
  – *Benzodiazepines*—May be associated with a twofold increase in orofacial clefts. Neonatal benzodiazepine withdrawal (irritability, tremor, diarrhea, vomiting, hypertonicity, and high-pitched crying) may occur.
  – *Other anxiolytics/sedatives*—Insufficient data for recommendation.
- **Breast-feeding:** Compatibility with breast-feeding is unknown. Sedating drugs may cause neonatal lethargy.

General Guidelines for Psychotropic Drug Use in Pregnancy and Breast-Feeding

General guidelines for psychotropic drug use in pregnancy and breast-feeding (adapted from Fait et al. 2002; Newport et al. 2002; and Ward and Zamorski 2002) include the following:

1. For any woman of childbearing age, carefully select all drugs for their safety in pregnancy and breast-feeding.

2. Remember that the benefit of any medication to the mother must outweigh the risk to the fetus.

3. Discuss with the mother the risks and benefits of using psychotropic medications while pregnant or breast-feeding.

4. Avoid all drugs during pregnancy and breast-feeding if possible, including over-the-counter and herbal medicines.

5. Use the lowest effective dose of a short-half-life agent.

6. Prefer monotherapy to combination therapy.

7. Select established drugs with known effects in pregnancy and breast-feeding rather than agents with little supporting data.

8. Select medications for minimum teratogenic and behavioral toxicity.

9. Monitor clinical response and drug levels where possible during pregnancy. Adjust dosage as necessary to maintain therapeutic effect. At delivery, slowly return drug dose to prepregnancy levels.

10. Minimize drug exposure for the nursing infant by instructing the mother to take medication just after breast-feeding or before the infant is due for a long sleep (American Academy of Pediatrics 2001). SSRI levels peak in breast milk at 8–9 hours postdose. Infant exposure can be minimized if the milk during this period is "pumped and dumped" (Newport et al. 2002).

11. Consider electroconvulsive therapy for treatment of depression and especially for psychotic depression.

Conclusion

Rapid developments in medical care in general, and psychopharmacology in particular, challenge clinicians to remain current with new agents, new indications for established agents, and potential pharmacokinetic and pharmacodynamic interactions in a polypharmacy environment, which also includes over-the-counter and herbal preparations. In this chapter we have discussed the many key considerations relevant to the use of psychopharmacological agents in complex medically ill patients and during pregnancy and lactation. Detailed adverse effects, toxicities, drug interactions, and alternate administration routes for each major psychotherapeutic drug class have been described. We have endeavored to provide the most up-to-date information possible by making extensive use of Internet resources. Many of these Internet sources are cited in the reference section, and we encourage their general use as a means of following developments in this area.

References

Adams S: Amitriptyline suppositories (letter). N Engl J Med 306:996, 1982

al Rakaf H, Bello LL, Turkustani A, et al: Intra-nasal midazolam in conscious sedation of young paediatric dental patients. Int J Paediatr Dent 11:33–40, 2001

Alaka Y: Atomoxetine (Strattera) National PBM Drug Monograph. VHA Pharmacy Benefits Management Strategic Healthcare Group and Medical Advisory Panel 2003. Available at: www.vapbm.org/monograph/Atomoxetine.pdf. Accessed July 7, 2004

Allain H, Delahaye C, Le Coz F, et al: Postmarketing surveillance of zopiclone in insomnia: analysis of 20,513 cases. Sleep 14:408–413, 1991

Alldredge BK: Seizure risk associated with psychotropic drugs: clinical and pharmacokinetic considerations. Neurology 53:S68–S75, 1999

Alldredge BK, Gelb AM, Isaacs SM, et al: A comparison of lorazepam, diazepam, and placebo for the treatment of out-of-hospital status epilepticus. N Engl J Med 345:631–637, 2001

Alvarez W Jr, Pickworth KK: Safety of antidepressant drugs in the patient with cardiac disease: a review of the literature. Pharmacotherapy 23:754–771, 2003

American Academy of Pediatrics: Use of psychoactive medication during pregnancy and possible effects on the fetus and newborn. Committee on Drugs. Pediatrics 105(4 pt 1): 880–887, 2000

American Academy of Pediatrics: Transfer of drugs and other chemicals into human milk. Pediatrics 108:776–789, 2001

Amsterdam JD: A double-blind, placebo-controlled trial of the safety and efficacy of selegiline transdermal system without dietary restrictions in patients with major depressive disorder. J Clin Psychiatry 64:208–214, 2003

Andreoli V, Caillard V, Deo RS, et al: Reboxetine, a new noradrenaline selective antidepressant, is at least as effective as fluoxetine in the treatment of depression. J Clin Psychopharmacol 22:393–399, 2002

Ang-Lee MK, Moss J, Yuan C-S: Herbal medicines and perioperative care. JAMA 286:208–216, 2001

Appleton R, Sweeney A, Choonara I, et al: Lorazepam versus diazepam in the acute treatment of epileptic seizures and status epilepticus. Dev Med Child Neurol 37:682–688, 1995

Asconape JJ: Some common issues in the use of antiepileptic drugs. Semin Neurol 22:27–39, 2002

Barki ZHK, Kravitz HM, Berki TM: Psychotropic medications in pregnancy. Psychiatr Ann 28:486–500, 1998

Bauer MS, Whybrow PC: Rapid cycling bipolar affective disorder, II: treatment of refractory rapid cycling with high-dose levothyroxine: a preliminary study. Arch Gen Psychiatry 47:435–440, 1990

Bendz H, Aurell M: Drug-induced diabetes insipidus: incidence, prevention and management. Drug Saf 21:449–456, 1999

Bendz H, Sjodin I, Aurell M: Renal function on and off lithium in patients treated with lithium for 15 years or more: a controlled, prospective lithium-withdrawal study. Nephrol Dial Transplant 11:457–460, 1996

Berkovitch M, Pope E, Phillips J, et al: Pemoline-associated fulminant liver failure: testing the evidence for causation. Clin Pharmacol Ther 57:696–698, 1995

Bezchlibnyk KZ, Jeffries JJ: Clinical Handbook of Psychotropic Drugs. Toronto, ON, Hogrefe and Huber, 2000

Bianchi M, Musch B: Zopiclone discontinuation: review of 25 studies assessing withdrawal and rebound phenomena. Int Clin Psychopharmacol 5 (suppl 2):139–145, 1990

Birmes P, Coppin D, Schmitt L, et al: Serotonin syndrome: a brief review. CMAJ 168:1439–1442, 2003

Black J: Pro: modafinil has a role in management of sleep apnea. Am J Respir Crit Care Med 167:105–106, 2003

Bodkin JA, Amsterdam JD: Transdermal selegiline in major depression: a double-blind, placebo-controlled, parallel-group study in outpatients. Am J Psychiatry 159:1869–1875, 2002

Boehnert MT, Lovejoy FH Jr: Value of the QRS duration versus the serum drug level in predicting seizures and ventricular arrhythmias after an acute overdose of tricyclic antidepressants. N Engl J Med 313:474–479, 1985

Boniface PJ, Russell SG: Two cases of fatal zopiclone overdose. J Anal Toxicol 20:131–133, 1996

Bramness JG, Arnestad M, Karinen R, et al: Fatal overdose of zopiclone in an elderly woman with bronchogenic carcinoma. J Forensic Sci 46:1247–1249, 2001

Breitbart W, Mermelstein H: Pemoline: an alternative psychostimulant for the management of depressive disorders in cancer patients. Psychosomatics 33:352–356, 1992

British Medical Association, Royal Pharmaceutical Society of Great Britain: MAOIs. British National Formulary 47, 2004. Available at: http://bnf.org/bnf/bnf/current/doc/41001i257.htm. Accessed July 7, 2004

Bronheim HE, Fulop G, Kunkel EJ, et al: The Academy of Psychosomatic Medicine practice guidelines for psychiatric consultation in the general medical setting. The Academy of Psychosomatic Medicine. Psychosomatics 39:S8–S30, 1998

Burggraf GW: Are psychotropic drugs at therapeutic levels a concern for cardiologists? Can J Cardiol 13:75–80, 1997

Burt VK, Suri R, Altshuler L, et al: The use of psychotropic medications during breast-feeding. Am J Psychiatry 158:1001–1009, 2001

Buspirone: seven-year update. J Clin Psychiatry 55:222–229, 1994

Cadwallader DE: Biopharmaceutics and Drug Interactions. New York, Raven, 1983

Cantello R, Aguggia M, Gilli M, et al: Major depression in Parkinson's disease and the mood response to intravenous methylphenidate: possible role of the "hedonic" dopamine synapse. J Neurol Neurosurg Psychiatry 52:724–731, 1989

Cardiac Arrhythmia Suppression Trial (CAST) Investigators: Preliminary report: effect of encainide and flecainide on mortality in a randomized trial of arrhythmia suppression after myocardial infarction. N Engl J Med 321:406–412, 1989

Caroff SN, Mann SC: Neuroleptic malignant syndrome. Med Clin North Am 77:185–202, 1993

Carroll DH, Shyam R, Scahill L: Cardiac conduction and antipsychotic medication: a primer on electrocardiograms. J Child Adolesc Psychiatr Nurs 15:170–177, 2002

Carvajal GP, Garcia D, Sanchez SA, et al: Hepatotoxicity associated with the new antidepressants. J Clin Psychiatry 63:135–137, 2002

Chalon SA, Desager JP, Desante KA, et al: Effect of hepatic impairment on the pharmacokinetics of atomoxetine and its metabolites. Clin Pharmacol Ther 73:178–191, 2003

Chan HH, Wing Y, Su R, et al: A control study of the cutaneous side effects of chronic lithium therapy. J Affect Disord 57:107–113, 2000

Chandler F (ed): Herbs: Everyday Reference for Health Professionals. Ottawa, ON, Canadian Pharmacist Association and Canadian Medical Association, 2000

Chaudron LH, Jefferson JW: Mood stabilizers during breast-feeding: a review. J Clin Psychiatry 61:79–90, 2000

Chaumeil JC, Khoury JM, Zuber M, et al: Formulation of suppositories containing imipramine and clomipramine chlorhydrates. Drug Dev Ind Pharm 14:2225–2239, 1988

Chengappa KN, Rathore D, Levine J, et al: Topiramate as add-on treatment for patients with bipolar mania. Bipolar Disord 1:42–53, 1999

Cirignotta F, Mondini S, Zucconi M, et al: Zolpidem polysomnographic study of the effect of a new hypnotic drug in sleep apnea syndrome. Pharmacol Biochem Behav 29:807–809, 1988

Clark ML, Ray TS, Paredes A, et al: Chlorpromazine in women with chronic schizophrenia: the effect on cholesterol levels and cholesterol-behavior relationships. Psychosom Med 29:634–642, 1967

Clarke RS, Lyons SM: Diazepam and flunitrazepam as induction agents for cardiac surgical operations. Acta Anaesthesiol Scand 21:282–292, 1977

Cohen LG, Prince J, Biederman J, et al: Absence of effect of stimulants on the phamacokinetics of desipramine in children. Pharmacotherapy 19:746–752, 1999

Cohn MA: Hypnotics and the control of breathing: a review. Br J Clin Pharmacol 16 (suppl 2):245S–250S, 1983

Collaborative Working Group on Clinical Trial Evaluations: Assessment of EPS and tardive dyskinesia in clinical trials. J Clin Psychiatry 59 (suppl 12):23–27, 1998

Connemann BJ, Schonfeldt-Lecuona C: Ziprasidone in Parkinson's disease psychosis. Can J Psychiatry 49:73, 2004

Corman CL, Leung NM, Guberman AH: Weight gain in epileptic patients during treatment with valproic acid: a retrospective study. Can J Neurol Sci 24:240–244, 1997

Corns CM: Herbal remedies and clinical biochemistry. Ann Clin Biochem 40:489–507, 2003

Cotterchio M, Kreiger N, Darlington G, et al: Antidepressant medication use and breast cancer risk. Am J Epidemiol 151:951–957, 2000

Coulter DM, Bate A, Meyboom RH, et al: Antipsychotic drugs and heart muscle disorder in international pharmacovigilance: data mining study. BMJ 322:1207–1209, 2001

Cozza K, Armstrong S, Oesterheld JR: Concise Guide to Drug Interaction Principles for Medical Practice: Cytochrome P450s, UGTs, P-Glycoproteins, 2nd Edition. Washington, DC, American Psychiatric Publishing, 2003

Craven J, Sutherland A: Buspirone for anxiety disorders in patients with severe lung disease (letter). Lancet 338:249, 1991

Crawford P: An audit of topiramate use in a general neurology clinic. Seizure 7:207–211, 1998

Crone C, Wise T: Use of herbal medicines among consultation-liaison populations. Psychosomatics 39:3–13, 1998

Crone C, Gabriel G, Wise TN: Non-herbal nutritional supplements: the next wave. Psychosomatics 42:285–299, 2001

Dalton SO, Johansen C, Mellemkjaer L, et al: Use of selective serotonin reuptake inhibitors and risk of upper gastrointestinal tract bleeding: a population-based cohort study. Arch Intern Med 163:59–64, 2003

Dam M, Ekberg R, Loyning Y, et al: A double-blind study comparing oxcarbazepine and carbamazepine in patients with newly diagnosed, previously untreated epilepsy. Epilepsy Res 3:70–76, 1989

Dannawi M: Possible serotonin syndrome after combination of buspirone and St John's wort (letter). J Psychopharmacol 16:401, 2002

Dasgupta K, Jefferson JW: The use of lithium in the medically ill. Gen Hosp Psychiatry 12:83–97, 1990

de Abajo FJ, Rodriguez LA, Montero D: Association between selective serotonin reuptake inhibitors and upper gastrointestinal bleeding: population based case-control study. BMJ 319:1106–1109, 1999

De Smet PA: Herbal remedies. N Engl J Med 347:2046–2056, 2002

Dequardo JR: Modafinil-associated clozapine toxicity. Am J Psychiatry 159:1243–1244, 2002

Detke M, Lu Y, Goldstein DJ, et al: Duloxetine, 60 mg once daily, for major depressive disorder: a randomized double-blind placebo-controlled trial. J Clin Psychiatry 63:308–315, 2002

DeToledo JC, Toledo C, DeCerce J, et al: Changes in body weight with chronic, high-dose gabapentin therapy. Ther Drug Monit 19:394–396, 1997

DeVane CL, Nemeroff CB: 2002 Guide to Psychotropic Drug Interactions. Primary Psychiatry 9:28–57, 2002

Dilsaver SC, Greden JF: Antidepressant withdrawal phenomena. Biol Psychiatry 19:237–256, 1984

Doering PL, Stewart RB: The extent and character of drug consumption during pregnancy. JAMA 239:843–846, 1978

Dolly FR, Block AJ: Effect of flurazepam on sleep-disordered breathing and nocturnal oxygen desaturation in asymptomatic subjects. Am J Med 73:239–243, 1982

Domon SE, Cargile CS: Quetiapine-associated hyperglycemia and hypertriglyceridemia. J Am Acad Child Adolesc Psychiatry 41:495–496, 2002

Dunner DL: Optimizing lithium treatment. J Clin Psychiatry 61 (suppl 9):76–81, 2000

Dunner DL: Drug interactions of lithium and other antimanic/mood-stabilizing medications. J Clin Psychiatry 64 (suppl 5):38–43, 2003

Eisenberg DM, Kessler RC, Van Rompay MI, et al: Perceptions about complementary therapies relative to conventional therapies among adults who use both: results from a national survey. Ann Intern Med 135:344–351, 2001

Elie R, Ruther E, Farr I, et al: Sleep latency is shortened during 4 weeks of treatment with zaleplon, a novel nonbenzodiazepine hypnotic. Zaleplon Clinical Study Group. J Clin Psychiatry 60:536–544, 1999

Eli Lilly & Company: Zyprexa prescribing information. Available at: http://pi.lilly.com/us/zyprexa-pi.pdf. Accessed July 29, 2004

Ernst CL, Goldberg JF: The reproductive safety profile of mood stabilizers, atypical antipsychotics, and broad-spectrum psychotropics. J Clin Psychiatry 63 (suppl 4):42–55, 2002

Ernst E: The risk-benefit profile of commonly used herbal therapies: ginkgo, St John's wort, echinacea, saw palmetto, and kava. Ann Intern Med 136:42–53, 2002

Ernst E: Complementary medicine. Curr Opin Rheumatol 15:151–155, 2003

Evins AE: Efficacy of newer anticonvulsant medications in bipolar spectrum mood disorders. J Clin Psychiatry 64 (suppl 8):9–14, 2003

Faedda GL, Tondo L, Baldessarini RJ, et al: Outcome after rapid vs gradual discontinuation of lithium treatment in bipolar disorders. Arch Gen Psychiatry 50:448–455, 1993

Fait ML, Wise MG, Jachna JS, et al: Psychopharmacology, in American Psychiatric Publishing Textbook of Consultation-Liasion Psychiatry: Psychiatry in the Medically Ill, 2nd Edition. Edited by Wise MG, Rundell JR. Washington, DC, American Psychiatric Publishing, 2002, pp 939–987

Farah A: Interferon-induced depression treated with citalopram. J Clin Psychiatry 63:166–167, 2002

Fava M: Weight gain and antidepressants. J Clin Psychiatry 61 (suppl 11):37–41, 2000

Feighner JP: Cardiovascular safety in depressed patients: focus on venlafaxine. J Clin Psychiatry 56:574–579, 1995

Fernandez HH, Trieschmann ME, Friedman JH: Treatment of psychosis in Parkinson's disease: safety considerations. Drug Saf 26:643–659, 2003

Fernandez HH, Trieschmann ME, Friedman JH: Aripiprazole for drug-induced psychosis in Parkinson disease: preliminary experience. Clin Neuropharmacol 27:4–5, 2004

Finsterer J, Pelzl G, Hess B: Severe, isolated thrombocytopenia under polytherapy with carbamazepine and valproate. Psychiatry Clin Neurosci 55:423–426, 2001

Fisgin T, Gurer Y, Tezic T, et al: Effects of intranasal midazolam and rectal diazepam on acute convulsions in children: prospective randomized study. J Child Neurol 17:123–126, 2002

Fisher RS, Bortz JJ, Blum DE, et al: A pilot study of donepezil for memory problems in epilepsy. Epilepsy Behav 2:330–334, 2001

Fleishaker JC, Francom SF, Herman BD, et al: Lack of effect of reboxetine on cardiac repolarization. Clin Pharmacol Ther 70:261–269, 2001

Flynn CT, Chandran PK, Taylor MJ, et al: Intraperitoneal lithium administration for bipolar affective disorder in a patient on continuous ambulatory peritoneal dialysis. Int J Artif Organs 10:105–107, 1987

Forest Laboratories: Memantine HCl briefing document for FDA Peripheral and Central Nervous System Drug Advisory Committee Meeting, September 24, 2003. Available at: www.fda.gov/ohrms/dockets/ac/ 03/briefing/3979B1_01_ ForestLabs-Memantine.pdf. Accessed July 12, 2004.

Foulke GE, Albertson TE: QRS interval in tricyclic antidepressant overdosage: inaccuracy as a toxicity indicator in emergency settings. Ann Emerg Med 16:160–163, 1987

Frankland A, Robinson MJ: Fatal chloral hydrate overdoses: unnecessary tragedies. Can J Psychiatry 46:763–764, 2001

Friedman JH, Feinberg SS, Feldman RG: A neuroleptic malignant-like syndrome due to levodopa therapy withdrawal. JAMA 254:2792–2795, 1985

Fugh-Berman A: Herb-drug interactions. Lancet 355:134–138, 2000

Garner SJ, Eldridge FL, Wagner PG, et al: Buspirone, an anxiolytic drug that stimulates respiration. Am Rev Respir Dis 139:946–950, 1989

Garnier R, Guerault E, Muzard D, et al: Acute zolpidem poisoning: analysis of 344 cases. J Toxicol Clin Toxicol 32:391–404, 1994

Gaulin BD, Markowitz JS, Caley CF, et al: Clozapine-associated elevation in serum triglycerides. Am J Psychiatry 156:1270–1272, 1999

George CF: Perspectives on the management of insomnia in patients with chronic respiratory disorders. Sleep 23 (suppl 1):S31–S35, 2000

Giardina EG, Johnson LL, Vita J, et al: Effect of imipramine and nortriptyline on left ventricular function and blood pressure in patients treated for arrhythmias. Am Heart J 109:992–998, 1985

Gibb WR: Neuroleptic malignant syndrome in striatonigral degeneration. Br J Psychiatry 153:254–255, 1988

Gibb WR, Griffith DN: Levodopa withdrawal syndrome identical to neuroleptic malignant syndrome. Postgrad Med J 62:59–60, 1986

Gitlin MJ, Cochran SD, Jamison KR: Maintenance lithium treatment: side effects and compliance. J Clin Psychiatry 50:127–131, 1989

Gjere NA: Psychopharmacology in pregnancy. J Perinat Neonatal Nurs 14:12–25, 2001

Glassman AH: Cardiovascular effects of tricyclic antidepressants. Annu Rev Med 35:503–511, 1984

Glassman AH, Roose SP, Bigger JT Jr: The safety of tricyclic antidepressants in cardiac patients: risk-benefit reconsidered. JAMA 269:2673–2675, 1993

Glassman AH, O'Connor CM, Califf RM, et al: Sertraline treatment of major depression in patients with acute MI or unstable angina. JAMA 288:701–709, 2002

Gleason OC, Yates WR, Isbell MD, et al: An open-label trial of citalopram for major depression in patients with hepatitis C. J Clin Psychiatry 63:194–198, 2002

Goldberg JF, Burdick KE: Cognitive side effects of anticonvulsants. J Clin Psychiatry 62 (suppl 14):27–33, 2001

Goodnick PJ: Use of antidepressants in treatment of comorbid diabetes mellitus and depression as well as in diabetic neuropathy. Ann Clin Psychiatry 13:31–41, 2001

Gordon PH, Pullman SL, Louis ED, et al: Mirtazapine in Parkinsonian tremor. Parkinsonism Relat Disord 9:125–126, 2002

Graham SR, Day RO, Lee R, et al: Overdose with chloral hydrate: a pharmacological and therapeutic review. Med J Aust 149:686–688, 1988

Greenblatt DJ, Allen MD, MacLaughlin DS, et al: Diazepam absorption: effect of antacids and food. Clin Pharmacol Ther 24:600–609, 1978

Grob CS, Coyle JT: Suspected adverse methylphenidate-imipramine interactions in children. J Dev Behav Pediatr 7:265–267, 1986

Grossberg GT, Stahelin HB, Messina JC, et al: Lack of adverse pharmacodynamic drug interactions with rivastigmine and twenty-two classes of medications. Int J Geriatr Psychiatry 15:242–247, 2000

Gubbins PO, Bertch KE: Drug absorption in gastrointestinal disease and surgery: clinical pharmacokinetic and therapeutic implications. Clin Pharmacokinet 21:431–447, 1991

Guilleminault C: Benzodiazepines, breathing, and sleep. Am J Med 88:25S–28S, 1990

Gwirtsman HE, Szuba MP, Toren L, et al: The antidepressant response to tricyclics in major depressives is accelerated with adjunctive use of methylphenidate. Psychopharmacol Bull 30:157–164, 1994

Haddad P: The SSRI discontinuation syndrome. J Psychopharmacol 12:305–313, 1998

Hajak G, Bandelow B: Safety and tolerance of zolpidem in the treatment of disturbed sleep: a post-marketing surveillance of 16944 cases. Int Clin Psychopharmacol 13:157–167, 1998

Harden CL, Goldstein MA: Mood disorders in patients with epilepsy: epidemiology and management. CNS Drugs 16:291–302, 2002

Hauser P, Khosla J, Aurora H, et al: A prospective study of the incidence and open-label treatment of interferon-induced major depressive disorder in patients with hepatitis C. Mol Psychiatry 7:942–947, 2002

Hauser RA, Zesiewicz TA: Sertraline for the treatment of depression in Parkinson's disease. Mov Disord 12:756–759, 1997

Health Canada: Health Products and Food Branch, Important Drug Information Letter, 2003. Available at: http://www.hc-sc.gc.ca/hpfb-dgpsa/tpd-dpt/risperdal1_e.pdf. Accessed December 19, 2003

Healy D: Lines of evidence on the risks of suicide with selective serotonin reuptake inhibitors. Psychother Psychosom 72:71–79, 2003

Hebert AA, Ralston JP: Cutaneous reactions to anticonvulsant medications. J Clin Psychiatry 62 (suppl 14):22–26, 2001

Henney JE: Risk of drug interactions with St John's wort. JAMA 283:1679, 2003

Hollenhorst J, Munte S, Friedrich L, et al: Using intranasal midazolam spray to prevent claustrophobia induced by MR imaging. AJR Am J Roentgenol 176:865–868, 2001

Holmes TF, Sabaawi M, Fragala MR: Psychostimulant suppository treatment for depression in the gravely ill. J Clin Psychiatry 55:265–266, 1994

Iqbal MM, Gundlapalli SP, Ryan WG, et al: Effects of antimanic mood-stabilizing drugs on fetuses, neonates, and nursing infants. South Med J 94:304–322, 2001

Izzo AA, Ernst E: Interactions between herbal medicines and prescribed drugs: a systematic review. Drugs 61:2163–2175, 2001

Jabbari B, Bryan GE, Marsh EE, et al: Incidence of seizures with tricyclic and tetracyclic antidepressants. Arch Neurol 42:480–481, 1985

Jacobson S: Psychopharmacology: prescribing for patients with hepatic or renal dysfunction. Psychiatric Times 19(11), November 2002

Jaeger A, Sauder P, Kopferschmitt J, et al: When should dialysis be performed in lithium poisoning? A kinetic study in 14 cases of lithium poisoning. J Toxicol Clin Toxicol 31:429–447, 1993

Janowsky DS, Leichner P, Clopton P, et al: Comparison of oral and intravenous methylphenidate. Psychopharmacology (Berl) 59:75–78, 1978

Jefferson JW, Greist JH, Ackerman DL, et al: Lithium Encyclopedia for Clinical Practice, 2nd Edition. Washington, DC, American Psychiatric Press, 1987

Jhee SS, Shiovitz T, Crawford AW, et al: Pharmacokinetics and pharmacodynamics of the triptan antimigraine agents: a comparative review. Clin Pharmacokinet 40:189–205, 2001

Joffe H, Taylor AE, Hall JE: Polycystic ovarian syndrome: relationship to epilepsy and antiepileptic drug therapy. J Clin Endocrinol Metab 86:2946–2949, 2001

Kales A, Bixler EO, Vela-Bueno A, et al: Alprazolam: effects on sleep and withdrawal phenomena. J Clin Pharmacol 27:508–515, 1987

Kasper S, Muller-Spahn F: Intravenous antidepressant treatment: focus on citalopram. Eur Arch Psychiatry Clin Neurosci 252:105–109, 2002

Keck PEJ, Arnold LM: The serotonin syndrome. Psychiatr Ann 30:333–343, 2000

Khachikian D: Aripiprazole (Abilify) National PBM Drug Monograph. VHA Pharmacy Benefits Management Strategic Healthcare Group and Medical Advisory Panel 2003. Available at: www.vapbm.org/monograph/Aripiprazole.pdf. Accessed July 7, 2004.

Khan A, Khan S, Kolts R, et al: Suicide rates in clinical trials of SSRIs, other antidepressants, and placebo: analysis of FDA reports. Am J Psychiatry 160:790–792, 2003

Khawaja IS, Feinstein RE: Cardiovascular effects of selective serotonin reuptake inhibitors and other novel antidepressants. Heart Dis 5:153–160, 2003

Kim MH, Lee YM: Intrathecal midazolam increases the analgesic effects of spinal blockade with bupivacaine in patients undergoing haemorrhoidectomy. Br J Anaesth 86:77–79, 2001

Kleiner J, Altshuler L, Hendrick V, et al: Lithium-induced subclinical hypothyroidism: review of the literature and guidelines for treatment. J Clin Psychiatry 60:249–255, 1999

Konig SA, Schenk M, Sick C, et al: Fatal liver failure associated with valproate therapy in a patient with Friedreich's disease: review of valproate hepatotoxicity in adults. Epilepsia 40:1036–1040, 1999

Konstantinidis A, Stastny J, Ptak-Butta J, et al: Intravenous mirtazapine in the treatment of depressed inpatients. Eur Neuropsychopharmacol 12:57–60, 2002

Kontaxakis V, Stefanis C, Markidis M, et al: Neuroleptic malignant syndrome in a patient with Wilson's disease. J Neurol Neurosurg Psychiatry 51:1001–1002, 1988

Koren G, Pastuszak A, Ito S: Drugs in pregnancy. N Engl J Med 338:1128–1137, 1998

Kratochvil CJ, Vaughan BS, Harrington MJ, et al: Atomoxetine: a selective noradrenaline reuptake inhibitor for the treatment of attention-deficit/hyperactivity disorder. Exp Opin Pharmacother 4:1165–1174, 2003

Kraus MR, Schafer A, Faller H, et al: Paroxetine for the treatment of interferon-alpha-induced depression in chronic hepatitis C. Aliment Pharmacol Ther 16:1091–1099, 2002

Kurdyak PA, Gnam WH, Streiner DL: Antidepressants and the risk of breast cancer. Can J Psychiatry 47:966–970, 2002

Lankisch PG, Werner HM: Mirtazapine: another drug responsible for drug-induced acute pancreatitis? A letter of warning. Pancreas 26:211, 2003

Lazarus A, Mann SC, Caroff SN: The Neuroleptic Malignant Syndrome and Related Conditions. Washington, DC, American Psychiatric Press, 1989

Lemke MR: Effect of reboxetine on depression in Parkinson's disease patients. J Clin Psychiatry 63:300–304, 2002

Leo RJ: Movement disorders associated with the serotonin selective reuptake inhibitors. J Clin Psychiatry 57:449–454, 1996

Levenson JL: High-dose intravenous haloperidol for agitated delirium following lung transplantation. Psychosomatics 36:66–68, 1995

Levenson JL, Fallon HJ: Fluoxetine treatment of depression caused by interferon-alpha. Am J Gastroenterol 88:760–761, 1993

Lichtenwalner M, Tully R: A fatality involving zolpidem. J Anal Toxicol 21:567–569, 1997

Lieberman JA, Safferman AZ: Clinical profile of clozapine: adverse reactions and agranulocytosis. Psychiatr Q 63:51–70, 1992

Llewellyn A, Stowe ZN: Psychotropic medications in lactation. J Clin Psychiatry 59 (suppl 2):41–52, 1998

Lofaso F, Goldenberg F, Thebault C, et al: Effect of zopiclone on sleep, night-time ventilation, and daytime vigilance in upper airway resistance syndrome. Eur Respir J 10:2573–2577, 1997

Lucas PB, Gardner DL, Wolkowitz OM, et al: Dysphoria associated with methylphenidate infusion in borderline personality disorder. Am J Psychiatry 144:1577–1579, 1987

Magnussen I, Oxlund HR, Alsbirk KE, et al: Absorption of diazepam in man following rectal and parenteral administration. Acta Pharmacol Toxicol (Copenh) 45:87–90, 1979

Mann SC, Caroff SN, Keck PE Jr, et al: Neuroleptic Malignant Syndrome and Related Conditions, 2nd Edition. Washington, DC, American Psychiatric Publishing, 2003

Manos GH: Possible serotonin syndrome associated with buspirone added to fluoxetine. Ann Pharmacother 34:871–874, 2000

Markowitz JS, Patrick KS: Pharmacokinetic and pharmacodynamic drug interactions in the treatment of attention-deficit hyperactivity disorder. Clin Pharmacokinet 40:753–772, 2001

Martin WR, Sloan JW, Sapira JD, et al: Physiologic, subjective, and behavioral effects of amphetamine, methamphetamine, ephedrine, phenmetrazine, and methylphenidate in man. Clin Pharmacol Ther 12:245–258, 1971

Masand PS, Tesar GE: Use of stimulants in the medically ill. Psychiatr Clin North Am 19:515–547, 1996

Masand P, Pickett P, Murray GB: Psychostimulants for secondary depression in medical illness. Psychosomatics 32:203–208, 1991

Mathew NT, Tietjen GE, Lucker C: Serotonin syndrome complicating migraine pharmacotherapy. Cephalalgia 16:323–327, 1996

McAndrews MP, Weiss RT, Sandor P, et al: Cognitive effects of long-term benzodiazepine use in older adults. Hum Psychopharmacol 18:51–57, 2003

McElroy SL, Suppes T, Keck PE, et al: Open-label adjunctive topiramate in the treatment of bipolar disorders. Biol Psychiatry 47:1025–1033, 2000

McEvoy G (ed): American Hospital Formulary Service (AHFS) Drug Information 2003. Bethesda, MD, American Society of Health-System Pharmacists, 2003

Mefferd R, Labrose E, Gawienowski AM: Influence of chlorpromazine on certain biochemical variables of chronic male schizophrenics. J Nerv Ment Dis 127:167–179, 1958

Mendelson WB, Garnett D, Gillin JC: Flurazepam-induced sleep apnea syndrome in a patient with insomnia and mild sleep-related respiratory changes. J Nerv Ment Dis 169:261–264, 1981

Mendelson WB, Maczaj M, Holt J: Buspirone administration to sleep apnea patients. J Clin Psychopharmacol 11:71–72, 1991

Mendlewicz J, Souery D, Rivelli SK: Short-term and long-term treatment for bipolar patients: beyond the guidelines. J Affect Disord 55:79–85, 1999

Menghini VV, Albright RC Jr: Treatment of lithium intoxication with continuous venovenous hemodiafiltration. Am J Kidney Dis 36(3):E21, 2000

Meyer JM: Effects of atypical antipsychotics on weight and serum lipid levels. J Clin Psychiatry 62 (suppl 27):27–34, 2001a

Meyer JM: Novel antipsychotics and severe hyperlipidemia. J Clin Psychopharmacol 21:369–374, 2001b

Michalets E: Clinically significant cytochrome P450 drug interactions. Pharmacotherapy 18:84–112, 1998

Miller LJ: Clinical strategies for the use of psychotropic drugs during pregnancy. Psychiatr Med 9:275–298, 1991

Miller LJ: Psychiatric medication during pregnancy: understanding and minimizing risks. Psychiatr Ann 24:69–75, 1994

Mills KC: Serotonin syndrome: a clinical update. Crit Care Clin 13:763–783, 1997

Mirassou MM: Rectal antidepressant medication in the treatment of depression (letter). J Clin Psychiatry 59:29, 1998

Mitchell JE, Mackenzie TB: Cardiac effects of lithium therapy in man: a review. J Clin Psychiatry 43:47–51, 1982

Mitchell-Heggs P, Murphy K, Minty K, et al: Diazepam in the treatment of dyspnea in the "Pink Puffer" syndrome. Q J Med 49:9–20, 1980

Model DG: Nitrazepam induced respiratory depression in chronic obstructive lung disease. Br J Dis Chest 67:128–130, 1973

Narendran R, Young CM, Valenti AM, et al: Is psychosis exacerbated by modafinil? Arch Gen Psychiatry 59:292–293, 2002

Nasrallah HA, White T, Nasrallah AT: Lower mortality in geriatric patients receiving risperidone and olanzapine versus haloperidol: preliminary analysis of retrospective data. Am J Geriatr Psychiatry 12:437–439, 2004

Nelson JC: Safety and tolerability of the new antidepressants. J Clin Psychiatry 58 (suppl 6):26–31, 1997

Newport DJ, Hostetter A, Arnold A, et al: The treatment of postpartum depression: minimizing infant exposures. J Clin Psychiatry 63 (suppl 7):31–44, 2002

Nonino F, Campomori A: Neuroleptic malignant syndrome associated with metoclopramide. Ann Pharmacother 33:644–645, 1999

Nordeng H, Lindemann R, Perminov KV, et al: Neonatal withdrawal syndrome after in utero exposure to selective serotonin reuptake inhibitors. Acta Paediatr 90:288–291, 2001

Norris E, Marzouk O, Nunn A, et al: Respiratory depression in children receiving diazepam for acute seizures: a prospective study. Dev Med Child Neurol 41:340–343, 1999

Norton J: The use of intravenous valproate in psychiatry. Can J Psychiatry 46:371–372, 2001

Norton JW, Quarles E: Intravenous valproate in neuropsychiatry. Pharmacotherapy 20:88–92, 2000

Oyesanmi O, Kunkel EJ, Monti DA, et al: Hematologic side effects of psychotropics. Psychosomatics 40:414–421, 1999

Pact V, Giduz T: Mirtazapine treats resting tremor, essential tremor, and levodopa-induced dyskinesias. Neurology 53:1154, 1999

Parkinson Study Group: Low-dose clozapine for the treatment of drug-induced psychosis in Parkinson's disease. N Engl J Med 340:757–763, 1999

Parsons RL: Drug absorption in gastrointestinal disease with particular reference to malabsorption syndromes. Clin Pharmacokinet 2:45–60, 1977

Pat-Horenczyk R, Hacohen D, Herer P, et al: The effects of substituting zopiclone in withdrawal from chronic use of benzodiazepine hypnotics. Psychopharmacology (Berl) 140:450–457, 1998

Peet M, Pratt JP: Lithium: current status in psychiatric disorders. Drugs 46:7–17, 1993

Pelonero AL, Levenson JL, Pandurangi AK: Neuroleptic malignant syndrome: a review. Psychiatr Serv 49:1163–1172, 1998

Perry P: Lithium and renal effects. Clinical Psychopharmacology Seminar, 1996. Available at: http://www.vh.org/adult/provider/psychiatry/CPS/24.html. Accessed July 7, 2003

Pesola GR, Quinto C: Prochlorperazine-induced neuroleptic malignant syndrome. J Emerg Med 14:727–729, 1996

Pfizer: Food and Drug Administration Center for Drug Evaluation and Research, Briefing Information for Psychopharmacology Drug Advisory Committee, briefing document for Zeldox capsules (ziprasidone HCl), 2000. Available at: http://www.fda.gov/ohrms/dockets/ac/00/backgrd/3619b1a.pdf. Accessed July 7, 2003

Pijl H, Meinders AE: Body weight change as an adverse effect of drug treatment: mechanisms and management. Drug Saf 14:329–342, 1996

Putnam GP, O'Quinn S, Bolden-Watson CP, et al: Migraine polypharmacy and the tolerability of sumatriptan: a large-scale, prospective study. Cephalalgia 19:668–675, 1999

Pycha R, Miller C, Barnas C, et al: Intravenous flunitrazepam in the treatment of alcohol withdrawal delirium. Alcohol Clin Exp Res 17:753–757, 1993

Rammohan KW, Rosenberg JH, Lynn DJ, et al: Efficacy and safety of modafinil (Provigil) for the treatment of fatigue in multiple sclerosis: a two centre phase 2 study. J Neurol Neurosurg Psychiatry 72:179–183, 2002

Rampello L, Chiechio S, Raffaele R, et al: The SSRI citalopram improves bradykinesia in patients with Parkinson's disease treated with L-dopa. Clin Neuropharmacol 25:21–24, 2002

Rapport MD, Moffitt C: Attention deficit/hyperactivity disorder and methylphenidate: a review of height/weight, cardiovascular, and somatic complaint side effects. Clin Psychol Rev 22:1107–1131, 2002

Regenold WT, Prasad M: Uses of intravenous valproate in geriatric psychiatry. Am J Geriatr Psychiatry 9:306–308, 2001

Reichman WE: Current pharmacologic options for patients with Alzheimer's disease. Ann Gen Hosp Psychiatry 2:1, 2003

Rementeria JL, Bhatt K: Withdrawal symptoms in neonates from intrauterine exposure to diazepam. J Pediatr 90:123–126, 1977

Remy C, Jourdil N, Villemain D, et al: Intrarectal diazepam in epileptic adults. Epilepsia 33:353–358, 1992

Repchinsky C (ed): CPS 2003: Compendium of Pharmaceuticals and Specialties, the Canadian Drug Reference for Health Professionals. Ottawa, ON, Canadian Pharmacists Association, 2003

Risch SC, Groom GP, Janowsky DS: The effects of psychotropic drugs on the cardiovascular system. J Clin Psychiatry 43:16–31, 1982

Robertson P Jr, Hellriegel ET: Clinical pharmacokinetic profile of modafinil. Clin Pharmacokinet 42:123–137, 2003

Robertson P Jr, Hellriegel ET, Arora S, et al: Effect of modafinil on the pharmacokinetics of ethinyl estradiol and triazolam in healthy volunteers. Clin Pharmacol Ther 71:46–56, 2002

Robinson D, Mayerhoff D, Alvir J, et al: Mood responses of remitted schizophrenics to methylphenidate infusion. Psychopharmacology (Berl) 105:247–252, 1991

Robinson MJ, Levenson JL: The use of psychotropics in the medically ill. Curr Psychiatry Rep 2:247–255, 2000

Robinson MJ, Qaqish RB: Practical psychopharmacology in HIV-1 and acquired immunodeficiency syndrome. Psychiatr Clin North Am 25:149–175, 2002

Roose SP, Glassman AH, Siris SG, et al: Comparison of imipramine- and nortriptyline-induced orthostatic hypotension: a meaningful difference. J Clin Psychopharmacol 1:316–319, 1981

Roose SP, Glassman AH, Giardina EG, et al: Nortriptyline in depressed patients with left ventricular impairment. JAMA 256:3253–3257, 1986

Roose SP, Dalack GW, Glassman AH, et al: Cardiovascular effects of bupropion in depressed patients with heart disease. Am J Psychiatry 148:512–516, 1991

Rosenfeld JA, Everett KD: Factors related to planned and unplanned pregnancies. J Fam Pract 43:161–166, 1996

Rugino TA, Copley TC: Effects of modafinil in children with attention-deficit/hyperactivity disorder: an open-label study. J Am Acad Child Adolesc Psychiatry 40:230–235, 2001

Russell WJ, Badcock NR, Frewin DB, et al: Pharmacokinetics of a new sublingual formulation of temazepam. Eur J Clin Pharmacol 35:437–439, 1988

Rzany B, Correia O, Kelly JP, et al: Risk of Stevens-Johnson syndrome and toxic epidermal necrolysis during first weeks of antiepileptic therapy: a case-control study. Study Group of the International Case Control Study on Severe Cutaneous Adverse Reactions. Lancet 353:2190–2194, 1999

Sadeque AJ, Wandel C, He H, et al: Increased drug delivery to the brain by P-glycoprotein inhibition. Clin Pharmacol Ther 68:231–237, 2000

Sammut S, Bethus I, Goodall G, et al: Antidepressant reversal of interferon-alpha-induced anhedonia. Physiol Behav 75:765–772, 2002

Sanger DJ, Zivkovic B: Differential development of tolerance to the depressant effects of benzodiazepine and non-benzodiazepine agonists at the omega (benzodiazepine) modulatory sites of GABA$_A$ receptors. Neuropharmacology 31:693–700, 1992

Schonfeldt-Lecuona C, Connemann BJ: Aripiprazole and Parkinson's disease psychosis. Am J Psychiatry 161:373–374, 2004

Schou M, Amdisen A, Steenstrup OR: Lithium and pregnancy, II: hazards to women given lithium during pregnancy and delivery. BMJ 2:137–138, 1973

Schramm TM, Lawford BR, Macdonald GA, et al: Sertraline treatment of interferon-alfa-induced depressive disorder. Med J Aust 173:359–361, 2000

Scott MA, Letrent KJ, Hager KL, et al: Use of transdermal amitriptyline gel in a patient with chronic pain and depression. Pharmacotherapy 19:236–239, 1999

Sen A, Rudra A, Sarkar SK, et al: Intrathecal midazolam for postoperative pain relief in caesarean section delivery. J Indian Med Assoc 99:683–684, 686, 2001

Seppala T, Aranko K, Mattila MJ, et al: Effects of alcohol on buspirone and lorazepam actions. Clin Pharmacol Ther 32:201–207, 1982

Serrao JM, Marks RL, Morley SJ, et al: Intrathecal midazolam for the treatment of chronic mechanical low back pain: a controlled comparison with epidural steroid in a pilot study. Pain 48:5–12, 1992

Sharpe CR, Collet JP, Belzile E, et al: The effects of tricyclic antidepressants on breast cancer risk. Br J Cancer 86:92–97, 2002

Singh NP, Despars JA, Stansbury DW, et al: Effects of buspirone on anxiety levels and exercise tolerance in patients with chronic airflow obstruction and mild anxiety. Chest 103:800–804, 1993

Sobotka JL, Alexander B, Cook BL: A review of carbamazepine's hematologic reactions and monitoring recommendations. DICP 24:1214–1219, 1990

Sommer M, Dieterich A, Krause C, et al: Subclinical pancreatitis related to mirtazapine: a case report. Pharmacopsychiatry 34:158–159, 2001

Spies CD, Dubisz N, Funk W, et al: Prophylaxis of alcohol withdrawal syndrome in alcohol-dependent patients admitted to the intensive care unit after tumour resection. Br J Anaesth 75:734–739, 1995

Stancer HC, Kivi R: Lithium carbonate and oedema. Lancet 2(7731):985, 1971

Stern TA: The management of depression and anxiety following myocardial infarction. Mt Sinai J Med 52:623–633, 1985

Sternbach H: Are antidepressants carcinogenic? A review of preclinical and clinical studies. J Clin Psychiatry 64:1153-1162, 2003

Steur EN, Ballering LA: Moclobemide and selegeline in the treatment of depression in Parkinson's disease (letter). J Neurol Neurosurg Psychiatry 63:547, 1997

Stewart DE: Hepatic adverse reactions associated with nefazodone. Can J Psychiatry 47:375–377, 2002

Stewart WA, Harrison R, Dooley JM: Respiratory depression in the acute management of seizures. Arch Dis Child 87:225–226, 2002

Stoppe G, Muller P, Fuchs T, et al: Life-threatening allergic reaction to clozapine. Br J Psychiatry 161:259–261, 1992

Tandon R: Safety and tolerability: how do newer generation "atypical" antipsychotics compare? Psychiatr Q 73:297–311, 2002

Teicher MH, Glod C, Cole JO: Emergence of intense suicidal preoccupation during fluoxetine treatment. Am J Psychiatry 147:207–210, 1990

Tesei S, Antonini A, Canesi M, et al: Tolerability of paroxetine in Parkinson's disease: a prospective study. Mov Disord 15: 986–989, 2000

Thomsen K, Schou M: Avoidance of lithium intoxication: advice based on knowledge about the renal lithium clearance under various circumstances. Pharmacopsychiatry 32:83–86, 1999

Tiseo PJ, Perdomo CA, Friedhoff LT: Concurrent administration of donepezil HCl and cimetidine: assessment of pharmacokinetic changes following single and multiple doses. Br J Clin Pharmacol 46 (suppl 1):25–29, 1998a

Tiseo PJ, Perdomo CA, Friedhoff LT: Concurrent administration of donepezil HCl and digoxin: assessment of pharmacokinetic changes. Br J Clin Pharmacol 46 (suppl 1):40–44, 1998b

Tiseo PJ, Perdomo CA, Friedhoff LT: Concurrent administration of donepezil HCl and ketoconazole: assessment of pharmacokinetic changes following single and multiple doses. Br J Clin Pharmacol 46 (suppl 1):30–34, 1998c

Tiseo PJ, Foley K, Friedhoff LT: Concurrent administration of donepezil HCl and theophylline: assessment of pharmacokinetic changes following multiple-dose administration in healthy volunteers. Br J Clin Pharmacol 46 (suppl 1):35–39, 1998d

Tiseo PJ, Foley K, Friedhoff LT: The effect of multiple doses of donepezil HCl on the pharmacokinetic and pharmacodynamic profile of warfarin. Br J Clin Pharmacol. 46 (suppl 1): 45–50, 1998e

Tune L, Carr S, Hoag E, et al: Anticholinergic effects of drugs commonly prescribed for the elderly: potential means for assessing risk of delirium. Am J Psychiatry 149:1393–1394, 1992

Udall JA: Warfarin interactions with chloral hydrate and glutethimide. Curr Ther Res Clin Exp 17:67–74, 1975

Upward JW, Edwards JG, Goldie A, et al: Comparative effects of fluoxetine and amitriptyline on cardiac function. Br J Clin Pharmacol 26:399–402, 1988

U.S. Modafinil in Narcolepsy Multicenter Study Group: Randomized trial of modafinil as a treatment for the excessive daytime somnolence of narcolepsy. Neurology 54:1166–1175, 2000

USP DI Editorial Board (eds): USP Dispensing Information, Vol 1: Drug Information for the Health Care Professional. Greenwood Village, CO, MICROMEDEX Thompson Healthcare, 2003

Valentine JM, Lyons G, Bellamy MC: The effect of intrathecal midazolam on post-operative pain. Eur J Anaesthesiol 13:589–593, 1996

van Amelsvoort T, Bakshi R, Devaux CB, et al: Hyponatremia associated with carbamazepine and oxcarbazepine therapy: a review. Epilepsia 35:181–188, 1994

van den Brink RH, van Melle JP, Honig A, et al: Treatment of depression after myocardial infarction and the effects on cardiac prognosis and quality of life: rationale and outline of the Myocardial INfarction and Depression-Intervention Trial (MIND-IT). Am Heart J 144:219–225, 2002

van Hoogdalem E, de Boer AG, Breimer DD: Pharmacokinetics of rectal drug administration, part I: general considerations and clinical applications of centrally acting drugs. Clin Pharmacokinet 21:11–26, 1991a van Hoogdalem EJ, de Boer AG, Breimer DD: Pharmacokinetics of rectal drug administration, part II: clinical applications of peripherally acting drugs, and conclusions. Clin Pharmacokinet 21:110–128, 1991b

Vanderkooy JD, Kennedy SH, Bagby RM: Antidepressant side effects in depression patients treated in a naturalistic setting: a study of bupropion, moclobemide, paroxetine, sertraline, and venlafaxine. Can J Psychiatry 47:174–180, 2002

Vieweg W: Strategies to prevent fatal arrythmias in patients taking antipsychotics. Current Psychiatry Online 1(5), 2002

Ward RK, Zamorski MA: Benefits and risks of psychiatric medications during pregnancy. Am Fam Physician 66:629–636, 2002

Ward RM: Pharmacological treatment of the fetus: clinical pharmacokinetic considerations. Clin Pharmacokinet 28:343–350, 1995

Ward RM: Pharmacology of the maternal-placental-fetal-unit and fetal therapy. Prog Pediatr Cardiol 5:79–89, 1996

Watkins PB, Zimmerman HJ, Knapp MJ, et al: Hepatotoxic effects of tacrine administration in patients with Alzheimer's disease. JAMA 271:992–998, 1994

Weinrieb RM, Auriacombe M, Lynch KG, et al: A critical review of selective serotonin reuptake inhibitor–associated bleeding: balancing the risk of treating hepatitis C–infected patients. J Clin Psychiatry 64:1502–1510, 2003

Wells PS, Holbrook AM, Crowther NR, et al: Interactions of warfarin with drugs and food. Ann Intern Med 121:676–683, 1994

Wisner KL, Perel JM, Wheeler SB: Tricyclic dose requirements across pregnancy. Am J Psychiatry 150:1541–1542, 1993

Woods JH, Katz JL, Winger G: Benzodiazepines: use, abuse, and consequences. Pharmacol Rev 44:151–347, 1992

Wooltorton E: Antipsychotic clozapine (Clozaril): myocarditis and cardiovascular toxicity. CMAJ 166:1185–1186, 2002

Wooltorton E: Risperidone (Risperdal): increased rate of cerebrovascular events in dementia trials. CMAJ 167:1269–1270, 2002

Wooltorton E: Hua fo tablets tainted with sildenafil-like compound. CMAJ 166:1568, 2003

Wooltorton E: Olanzapine (Zyprexa): increased incidence of cerebrovascular events in dementia trials. CMAJ 170:1395, 2004

Wright BA, Jarrett DB: Lithium and calcium channel blockers: possible neurotoxicity. Biol Psychiatry 30:635–636, 1991

Wroblewski BA, Leary JM, Phelan AM, et al: Methylphenidate and seizure frequency in brain injured patients with seizure disorders. J Clin Psychiatry 53:86–89, 1992

Yang SH, McNeely MJ: Rhabdomyolysis, pancreatitis, and hyperglycemia with ziprasidone. Am J Psychiatry 159:1435, 2002

38 Psychosocial Treatments

Jennifer W. Kaupp, Ph.D.

Nathalie Rapoport-Hubschman, M.D.

David Spiegel, M.D.

WHEN DESCARTES UTTERED his famous dictum *"cogito ergo sum,"* separating mind from body, he did medicine a favor. At the time, the Church forbade autopsies because they were considered damaging to the soul. By declaring the soul distinct, Descartes freed doctors to examine the body and thereby helped to advance medical science. Now, however, the idea that mind and body are separate is holding medicine back from fully exploring the interactions among mind, brain, and body. It constrains our knowledge of how depression and anxiety complicate illnesses such as heart disease and cancer, and it obscures the obvious fact that medical treatment must encompass care as well as cure—involve the person with the illness and not just the disease in the body.

The psychosomatic medicine psychiatrist brings to the medical setting expertise in medicine, neurobiology, psychiatry, psychopharmacology, psychotherapy, and a working knowledge of psychosocial resources (Kaplan et al. 1994), as well as an appreciation of individual patients from a biopsychosocial perspective (Gabbard 1994; Gabbard and Kay 2001). Psychosocial interventions with the medically ill differ from standard psychotherapy in several important ways. Patients are generally referred by primary care physicians or specialists for distress associated with medical illness (Postone 1998), premorbid psychiatric disturbance (Hay and Passik 2000; Weitzner et al. 1999), or somatic symptoms with no medical foundation (Abramowitz et al. 2002; Ehlert et al. 1999; Hay and Passik 2000; Richter 1999). The methodology, timing, and goals of psychosocial interventions with the medically ill are determined by the interaction among disease factors (onset, etiology, course, prognosis, stigma) and medical treatment (disfiguring, painful, aversive, palliative,

complex) (Goodheart and Lansing 1997); the nature of emotional distress (anxiety, depression, disorientation, posttraumatic stress) (Andrykowski et al. 1998, 2000; Bauer and Whybrow 1999; Block 2000; Cordova et al. 2000; Guthrie 1996; Kaplan et al. 1994; Malt and Tjemsland 1999; Tjemsland et al. 1996a); availability of social support (Blechner 1997; Goodheart and Lansing 1997; Kaplan et al. 1994); psychological characteristics of the patient (premorbid psychopathology, personality traits, intelligence) (Blechner 1997; Gabbard 1994; Goodheart and Lansing 1997; Kaplan et al. 1994; McWilliams 1994); and response to the illness (usual coping skills, denial, hostility, dependency) (Andersen 2002; Diabetes Control and Complications Trial Research Group 1993; Fitzpatrick 1999; Gonder-Frederick et al. 2002; Goodheart and Lansing 1997).

In this chapter, we review the types of stress and distress that commonly affect patients with medical illness, psychological factors unique to these patients, and the psychotherapies that have been developed and evaluated to treat their symptoms and enhance their coping styles. There is growing evidence that a variety of psychotherapeutic strategies in individual and group formats are helpful in reducing distress, anxiety, and depression among the medically ill. Techniques employed include psychodynamic, supportive-expressive, and interpersonal psychotherapies, hypnosis, family therapy, cognitive-behavioral therapy (CBT), and psychoeducation. Psychotherapy is also discussed elsewhere in this book with respect to specific psychiatric disorders such as depression (Chapter 9, "Depression"), anxiety (Chapter 12, "Anxiety Disorders"), and somatoform disorders (Chapter 13, "Somatization and Somatoform Disorders"); in the specialty and subspecialty chapters; and in regard to its use in pain management (Chapter 36, "Pain") and palliative care (Chapter 40, "Palliative Care").

Stress and Distress Among the Medically Ill

Serious medical illnesses are often complicated by anxiety and depression, stress, adjustment disorder, interpersonal problems, and lack of social support for patients and their families (Andersen 2002; Holahan et al. 1995; Krumholz et al. 1998; Spiegel 1996; van Marle and Holmes 2002). Although these psychosocial factors appear to be outside the immediate realm of medicine, they have a profound impact on the patient's quality of life, symptom severity, disability level (Saravay 1996), and survival (Krumholz et al. 1998).

Psychosocial distress has been documented in almost all diseases studied, as reviewed in earlier chapters of this textbook (Kosslyn et al. 2000). Emotional disturbance, particularly anxiety and depression, may be an acute reaction to the diagnosis and treatment of catastrophic illness (Alter et al. 1996; Andrykowski and Cordova 1998; Andrykowski et al. 1998, 2000; Green et al. 1998; Guthrie 1996; Holahan et al. 1995; Smith et al. 1999; Spiegel 1996; Sutor et al. 1998; Tjemsland et al. 1996a, 1996b); a response to coping with a chronic medical disorder (Guthrie 1996; Kaplan et al. 1994); or an early indication of onset of diseases such as Parkinson's disease or pancreatic cancer (Maxmen and Ward 1995). Even for patients who do not develop Axis I psychiatric disorders, serious medical illness can be understood as a series of stressors that can elicit psychological and physiological stress responses (Koopman et al. 1998; Spiegel 2001).

Most individuals react to serious, life-threatening illness with a combination of emotions. Anxiety, experienced at somatic, cognitive, and emotional levels, is typically heightened during an illness (Guthrie 1996; Januzzi et al. 2000). Anxiety may be normal or pathological, acute or chronic, a state or a trait (Kaplan et al. 1994). Psychiatric consultation may be requested for critically ill or injured medical inpatients who are acutely highly anxious or in a regressed state (Kaplan et al. 1994). An intervention combining pharmacotherapy, emotional support, and reassurance from medical staff may be indicated (Kaplan et al. 1994). Chronic anxiety, on the other hand, can be a response to vague and unknown threats to the body, fear of separation or lack of support, shame and guilt, or helplessness (Abramowitz et al. 2002; Ehlert et al. 1999; Gottschalk 1978; Gottschalk and Gleser 1969; Kaplan et al. 1994; Richter 1999). Close collaboration between physician and psychiatrist, pharmacotherapy, and psycho-

therapy (CBT, brief or long-term psychodynamic) are recommended for the clinical management of these patients (Abramowitz et al. 2002). Does the medical patient have a history of childhood abuse or neglect underlying chronic anxiety? Supportive-expressive dynamic therapy that helps the patient examine reactions to medical illness, explore intrapsychic processes, and discuss and integrate abuse memories is suggested for long-term symptom reduction (Blechner 1997; Gabbard 1994; Goodheart and Lansing 1997; Herman 1992; Kaplan et al. 1994; McWilliams 1994, 1999; Postone 1998). Is chronic anxiety a function of a cancer patient's realistic concerns about recurrence, diminished functioning, or helplessness in the face of death? Educational and supportive interventions would be indicated. Interventions with the medically ill, regardless of the clinician's theoretical orientation, must be flexible enough to address illness-related problems as they arise during the course of the patient's illness (Blechner 1997; Goodheart and Lansing 1997; Postone 1998; Spiegel 1996; Spiegel and Classen 2000).

Treatment for comorbid depression, common in many chronic illnesses, will also vary as a function of disease factors and patient characteristics. For example, vegetative signs of depression, often attributed to the patient's medical illness and left untreated (Spiegel 1996; Spiegel and Giese-Davis 2003), can resolve with antidepressants (Block 2000; Nemeroff and Schatzberg 1998). Psychotherapy emphasizing social support, emotional expression, cognitive restructuring, and improved coping skills is effective in treating the psychosocial problems in depressed medically ill patients (Sutor et al. 1998).

Coping Skills Deficits

Medical patients are confronted with novel situations arising from the illness itself or from the demands of the treatment, including the need to preserve a reasonable emotional balance, maintain a sense of competence and mastery, sustain relationships with family and friends, and prepare for an uncertain future (Moos and Schaefer 1987). People with medical conditions may need help to improve existing coping skills or to learn new, more adaptive skills. Those who cannot adapt to the stresses of illness and medical care will have difficulty maintaining adequate levels of emotional, physical, and social functioning. The adaptive tasks needed to adjust to the illness may require new and unfamiliar ways of coping (e.g., learning to express emotions, mobilizing social support, increasing role flexibility) (Goodheart and Lansing 1997; Kaplan et al. 1994).

Adaptive coping has been divided into three types: information focused, emotion focused, and problem focused (Moos and Schaefer 1987; Valentiner et al. 1994). Problem-focused coping skills are important in helping the patient live with the illness and manage its treatment. Emotional adjustment to the illness is also essential. Research in the past decade suggests that medical patients are particularly inclined to use emotion-oriented strategies to reduce the high levels of distress caused by their illness, although many employ a wide range of strategies in stressful situations (Dunkel-Schetter and Westlake 1995; Newman et al. 1990). Some studies have shown that emotion-oriented and avoidant strategies may be less adaptive in the long run than task-oriented and approach strategies (De Ridder and Schreurs 2001). However, the impact of these coping strategies appears to depend on the specific constraints imposed by the circumstances of the illness. Recent studies suggest no specific coping strategy is more relevant than others in the context of medical illness (i.e., coping is situation-specific) (Folkman and Moskowitz 2000; Lazarus and Folkman 1984). A broad coping skills repertoire consisting of both problem- and emotion-focused strategies increases the probability of a constructive response to the particular demands of a stressful medical situation (Taylor 1999). This may explain the superior results of multicomponent psychosocial interventions that involve a broad repertoire of coping skills training, expanding patients' coping abilities in a flexible manner.

Timing of Intervention

Scheduling psychotherapeutic support at key moments during the course of an illness would seem extremely important. However, the literature specifically related to the timing of psychotherapeutic interventions is scarce. When is it appropriate to propose a psychological intervention to medical patients? Immediately following diagnosis, after acute medical treatment ends, just after relapse, during the chronic phase of the illness, during the terminal period, or when specific problems arise? What is the efficacy of early psychotherapeutic interventions? Obviously, the specific characteristics and course of various illnesses make it difficult to propose universally applicable answers.

The time of diagnosis is often overwhelming for the patient, who is also preoccupied with obtaining and assimilating diagnostic information and making treatment decisions. Because the patient's usual cognitive and emotional processes may be overwhelmed, this phase of intense distress is generally not an ideal time for proposing

psychological treatment, although crisis management can be beneficial for a newly diagnosed patient in an acute state of anxiety (Goodheart and Lansing 1997).

When the acute phase is completed, patients have more time to participate in treatment, may sometimes feel abandoned by the medical team that provided acute care, and/or may have postponed coming to grips with the meaning of the illness. Although illness-related issues may be one treatment focus, patients also present with psychosocial or interpersonal problems unrelated to illness, so it is important to avoid attributing all emotional symptoms to the medical illness (Blechner 1997; Goodheart and Lansing 1997; Postone 1998). Other issues come to the fore in the terminal stage of an illness. Depressive illness in a dying patient may be misunderstood as a normal reaction to imminent death; however, depressive symptoms can be relieved with antidepressants (Block 2000). A supportive dynamic intervention consisting of reviewing the life lived; addressing depression, anxiety, loneliness, loss, or fears about protracted and painful death; and preparing for death has been beneficial for many patients (e.g., late-stage AIDS patients) (Blechner 1997). Even some patients with AIDS-related dementia have responded favorably to supportive therapy (Blechner 1997).

Timing is also a consideration for patients undergoing acute medical interventions (e.g., surgery, cardiac catheterization). For example, when a chronic illness or malignancy necessitates amputation of a limb, a preoperative session with a psychiatrist may reduce the patient's distress following surgery (Fitzpatrick 1999). Postsurgical interventions are strongly recommended in the case of traumatic amputation (Fitzpatrick 1999). Psychosocial interventions immediately following surgery (Kuchler et al. 1999) and 2 months after diagnosis (McCorkle et al. 2000) have been beneficial in maintaining quality of life and increasing survival among cancer patients. In the case of diabetes, several researchers have suggested that family-based interventions may be scheduled early in the course of the disease to improve long-term metabolic control in pediatric patients (Anderson and Brackett 2000). Other studies suggest, however, that later intervention, even several years after diagnosis, is more efficacious when implemented at particular junctures during the course of the illness or when specific problems or complications arise (Grey et al. 1995; Kovacs et al. 1992).

Types of Interventions

Various psychotherapeutic treatments have been developed and evaluated for the broad array of psychiatric symptoms among the medically ill. Clearly, the appropriate treatment for depressive symptoms associated with cancer or heart disease will differ from psychotherapy for conversion disorder or early dementia in terms of therapeutic interventions and goals. Furthermore, variables unique to individual patients such as developmental history, stage in the life span and current roles, family history, extent and quality of emotional and social support, educational level, economic resources, cultural norms, and access to mental health services collectively shape psychosocial interventions (Blechner 1997; Goodheart and Lansing 1997; Kaplan et al. 1994). The efficacy of psychotherapeutic treatments for depression and anxiety in medically ill patients—particularly group therapy, supportive and interpersonal therapies grounded in psychodynamic theory, brief therapy, family therapy, behavioral and cognitive-behavioral methods, and psychoeducation—has been supported by numerous outcome studies (see Compas et al. 1998; Craighead et al. 1998; Niederehe and Schneider 1998).

Group Psychotherapy

Group intervention in a variety of forms has become an increasingly popular, effective, and efficient means of providing psychosocial support for the medically ill (Spiegel et al. 2000). Groups of different types reflect theoretical approaches that include the psychodynamic, existential, educational, and cognitive-behavioral, among others (Yalom 1995).

Clinical trials have demonstrated the benefits of group therapy for breast cancer patients (Andersen 2002; Classen et al. 2001; Fawzy et al. 2003; Goodwin et al. 2001), with notable reductions in pain and emotional distress and, in some cases, increased survival time (Kogon et al. 1997; Spiegel 2001; Spiegel et al. 1989), although not in others (Goodwin et al. 2001). Although group therapy has shown considerable success as an adjunctive treatment for cancer, HIV, heart disease, and other chronic illnesses (Allan and Scheidt 1998; Beresnevaite 2000; Classen et al. 2001; Kaplan et al. 1994; Spiegel 2001; Spiegel and Classen 2000; Stauffer 1998), some patients may not feel comfortable in a group setting. For example, patients treated for testicular cancer indicated a preference for individual rather than group psychotherapy (Moynihan et al. 1998). Group therapy may not be the treatment of choice for medically ill patients with severe psychopathology or brain damage (Levenson 1995; McWilliams 1999). Groups may be contraindicated for some patients with severe character pathology because their maladaptive interpersonal style can disrupt group process, alienating group members and therapists alike (Levenson 1995). In such

cases, the stress of serious medical illness would be compounded by removal from a support group. Although reactions to catastrophic illness may differ for individuals with preexisting psychopathology, such patients share with their emotionally healthy counterparts the need for support in dealing with diagnosis and treatment, changes wrought by disease, social isolation, and existential issues, whether offered individually or in a group.

Common elements of group intervention for the medically ill are described in the following subsections.

Social Support

Psychotherapy, especially in groups, can provide a new social network with the common bond of facing similar problems. At a time when the illness makes a person feel isolated, when many others withdraw out of awkwardness or fear, group psychotherapeutic support provides a new and important social connection. Indeed, the very thing that strains other social relationships is the ticket of admission to such groups, providing a surprising intensity of caring among members from the very beginning. Furthermore, members find that the process of giving help to others enhances their own sense of mastery of the patient role and increases their self-esteem, giving meaning to an otherwise meaningless tragedy.

Emotional Expression

The expression of emotion is important in reducing social isolation and improving coping, although it is an aspect of medical patient adjustment that is often overlooked or suppressed. A repressive coping strategy reduces expression of positive as well as negative emotion. Emotional suppression also reduces intimacy in families, limiting opportunities for direct expression of affection and concern. The use of the psychotherapeutic setting for dealing with painful affect also provides an organizing context for handling its intrusion. When unbidden thoughts involving fears of dying intrude, they can be better managed by patients who know that there is a time and a place during which such feelings can be expressed, acknowledged, and handled. Disease-related dysphoria is more intense when amplified by isolation, leaving the patient to feel that he or she is deservedly alone with the sense of anxiety, loss, and fear that he or she experiences. Being in a group in which many others express similar distress normalizes their reactions, making them less alien and overwhelming.

Detoxifying Dying: Processing Existential Concerns

Death anxiety in particular is intensified by isolation, in part because we often think of death in terms of separation from loved ones. There are powerful psychotherapeutic techniques that directly address such concerns (Yalom 1980). Yalom (1980) described the ultimate existential concerns as death, freedom, isolation, and meaninglessness. Rather than avoiding painful or anxiety-provoking topics in attempts to "stay positive," this form of group therapy addresses these concerns head-on with the intent of helping group members better use the time they have left. The goal is to help those facing the threat of death see it from a new point of view. When worked through, life-threatening problems can come to seem real but not overwhelming. Facing even life-threatening issues directly can help patients shift from emotion-focused to problem-focused coping. The process of dying is often more threatening than death itself. Direct discussion of death anxiety can help to divide the fear of death into a series of problems: loss of control over treatment decisions, fear of separation from loved ones, anxiety about pain, and so on. Discussion of these concerns can lead to addressing, if not completely resolving, each of these issues. Even the process of grieving can be reassuring at the same time that it is threatening. The experience of grieving others who have died of the same condition constitutes a deeply personal experience of the loss that will be experienced by others after one's own death.

Reorganizing Life Priorities and Living in the Present

Acceptance of the possibility of illness shortening one's life carries with it an opportunity for reevaluating life priorities. Facing the threat of death can aid in making the most of life. This attitude can help patients take control of those aspects of their lives they can influence, while grieving and relinquishing those they cannot. For cancer patients who are anticipating their imminent death and its impact on their loved ones, adjustment may be aided by a change from past- or future-focused orientation to a present-focused orientation more congruent with the reality of their foreshortened future. In addition, progress in reappraisal of life goals, reorganization of priorities, and perception of the benefits of the cancer experience may also mediate improvement in symptoms and enhance quality of life.

Enhancing Family Support

Group psychotherapeutic interventions can also be quite helpful in improving communication, identifying needs, increasing role flexibility, and adjusting to new medical, social, vocational, and financial realities confronting patients and their families. The group format is especially helpful for such tasks because problems expressing needs and wishes can be examined among group members as a model for clarifying communication in the family. For example, a patient who expresses dissatisfaction with support from her husband can be helped to clarify her requests for assistance and to deal with her ambivalence about needing help. Also, groups for family members of the medically ill have been conducted, helping them to manage their own emotional responses and develop active coping strategies for dealing with their family member's illness (Koopman et al. 1994; Spiegel and Classen 2000).

Improving Communication With Physicians

Support groups can be quite useful in facilitating better communication with physicians and other health care providers. Groups provide mutual encouragement to get questions answered, to participate actively in treatment decisions, and to consider alternatives carefully.

Symptom Control

Many group as well as individual psychotherapy programs teach specific coping skills designed to help patients reduce cancer-related symptoms such as anxiety, anticipatory nausea and vomiting, and pain. Techniques that can be employed in the group setting include specific self-regulation skills such as self-hypnosis, meditation, biofeedback, and progressive muscle relaxation. Hypnosis is widely used for pain and anxiety control in cancer to attenuate the experience of pain and suffering and to allow painful emotional material to be examined. Group sessions involving instruction in self-hypnosis provide an effective means of reducing pain and anxiety.

Implementation of Group Process Goals

Implementation of the themes discussed above can be facilitated by training group therapists to shift from a content to a process orientation, recognizing that their "patient" is the group itself and that group therapy is not merely a collection of individual therapeutic interactions. This means learning to keep the group's focus on the here and now, tracking the flow of emotion rather than pursuing completion of the content of discussions, maintaining an atmosphere in which all members feel that they are full participants with equal opportunities to share experience and maintain their points of view, and transforming shared problems into strategies for active coping.

Personalization. Leaders are taught to bring group discussions "into the room" by keeping the focus on interactions occurring among group members rather than directing discussion toward people and events outside the group. Thus, when one patient discusses how she feels that she is a burden to her husband, the discussion is better directed toward the questions "Do you feel like a burden to the group?" "Do other group members feel you are a burden?"

Affective expression. Leaders should "follow the affect" in the room rather than the content. If a silent group member shows signs of emotion, the leader should respectfully direct attention toward him or her: "You seem upset now—what are you feeling?" Expression of emotion produces vulnerability, and it is important to make sure that those who express feelings are heard and acknowledged.

Supportive group interactions. The leader is responsible for starting and ending the group on time and seeing that there are few interruptions of the group time. Each member should be made to feel that his or her problems are as important as anyone else's problems. It is necessary to inquire about missing members and to make sure that very silent members have a chance to talk. Also, it is critical to avoid scapegoating—allowing the group to fix on one patient as a displacement from dealing with their own problems. Leaders must remember that their "patient" is the group, not just a series of individuals.

Active coping. As problems are discussed, it is helpful for the leader to direct the group toward a means of responding to the problems rather than merely accumulating a series of unresolved difficulties or avoiding discussing them. Finding a means of addressing problems reduces the helplessness engendered by the problems.

Summary

Group therapy for the medically ill involves enhancing social support; encouraging emotional expression and processing; confronting existential concerns; improving relationships with family, friends, and physicians; and building coping skills. Such skills include taking a more active stance toward disease-related problems and learning techniques such as self-hypnosis for pain control. Group leaders emphasize the here and now, personalizing discussion by making the group interaction itself the focus of discussion. Thus, group relationships, feelings, and coping experiences intensify learning and solidarity.

Individual Psychodynamic Therapy

A large body of literature underscores the importance of human interaction in the lives of medically ill patients and their families. Lack of social support is predictive of psychiatric morbidity (Klausner and Alexopoulos 1999), dis-

ease course, treatment compliance (Christensen and Ehlers 2002; Gonder-Frederick et al. 2002), and increased mortality in the medically ill (Christensen and Ehlers 2002; House et al. 1988; Krumholz et al. 1998; Reynolds and Kaplan 1990; Reynolds et al. 1994; Smith and Ruiz 2002; Valentiner et al. 1994). Social isolation, perceived lack of social and emotional support, and interpersonal conflicts are risk factors for coronary disease and increased mortality in post–myocardial infarction (MI) patients (Berkman et al. 1992; Krumholz et al. 1998; Smith and Ruiz 2002). Lack of social support has also been implicated in anxiety and depression in caregivers of elderly and seriously medically ill loved ones (Donnelly et al. 2000; Gabbard 1994). Unfortunately, severe medical illness, especially when progressive or terminal, can lead to relationship problems with family and friends and loss of important sources of emotional and social support when most needed (Rolland 1989). Therefore, interventions based on theories that emphasize the innately human need for relationship—psychodynamic and object relations theories (Bemporad and Vasile 1990; Gabbard 1994; Kaplan et al. 1994; Maxmen and Ward 1995; McWilliams 1999) and interpersonal theories (Bemporad and Vasile 1990; Craighead et al. 1998; Donnelly et al. 2000; Gillies 2002; Guthrie 1996; Sullivan 1953)—are discussed in some detail (Compas et al. 1998; Gabbard 1994; Guthrie 1996; Kaplan et al. 1994; Levenson 1995; Milrod et al. 2000; Niederehe and Schneider 1998).

Clinical and empirical evidence support the benefits of psychodynamic psychotherapy for patients with cancer (Donnelly et al. 2000; Fitzpatrick 1999; Hay and Passik 2000; Postone 1998), HIV/AIDS (Blechner 1997), diabetes (Goodheart and Lansing 1997; Moran et al. 1991), irritable bowel syndrome (Guthrie 1996; Guthrie et al. 1991), rheumatoid arthritis (Alpay and Cassem 2000; Goodheart and Lansing 1997), and other chronic medical conditions (Goodheart and Lansing 1997). Patients with personality disorders, treatment-resistant somatic symptoms, and chronic medical illnesses may be good candidates for brief or long-term psychodynamic therapy (Compas et al. 1998; Gabbard 1994; Guthrie 1996; Kaplan et al. 1994; Levenson 1995; Milrod et al. 2000; Niederehe and Schneider 1998). Long-term supportive dynamic therapy is appropriate for patients with complex chronic medical illnesses because it improves patient management, service utilization, treatment compliance, anxiety management, and support for the patient and the family (van Marle and Holmes 2002). For example, a dynamic intervention with rheumatoid arthritis patients combining supportive techniques during an acute attack with interpretive, insight-oriented techniques in between has been effective in symptom management (Kaplan et al.

1994). Psychodynamic therapy has also been useful in treating anxiety and depression in medically ill elderly patients (Niederehe and Schneider 1998; Stern and Lovestone 2000; Thompson et al. 1987). Dynamic principles can inform interventions for patients with brain damage or early dementia by addressing the impaired self and altered object relationships (Gabbard 1994) and in terminal illness by easing a patient's loneliness and isolation (Blechner 1997; Donnelly et al. 2000).

Individual Supportive-Expressive Therapy

Supportive interventions are indicated for patients who are newly diagnosed with a life-threatening illness, acutely ill, terminal, cognitively impaired, seriously mentally ill, or lacking the ego strength and psychological-mindedness necessary for more expressive techniques (Bemporad and Vasile 1990; Gabbard 1994; Kaplan et al. 1994). The primary goal of supportive psychotherapy during an acute crisis is to return the patient to premorbid functioning by strengthening existing defenses, providing ego support and reality testing, and encouraging more adaptive object relationships (Gabbard 1994; Kaplan et al. 1994). Supportive interventions are designed to help the patient identify and express affect, cope with treatment demands, strengthen support systems, explore existential issues, and restore hope (Spiegel and Yalom 1978; Spiegel et al. 2000).

The unavoidable experiences of loss (of life, health, mobility, self-esteem, body parts, sense of the self as healthy), abandonment (because relationships often change when one becomes seriously ill), helplessness, and fear that accompany serious medical illness are major sources of distress (Spiegel and Yalom 1978; Spiegel et al. 2000). Supportive therapy provides a forum for medically ill patients to express anger and fear, grieve losses, and learn to live fully in spite of medical illness (McWilliams 1999; Spiegel and Yalom 1978; Spiegel et al. 2000).

Although transference and countertransference reactions, defensive operations, and resistances should be internally monitored throughout the sessions, these processes may never be interpreted in supportive interventions (Gabbard 1994; Kaplan et al. 1994; van Marle and Holmes 2002). However, even in a clearly supportive therapy it may be necessary to confront and interpret intrapsychic processes (e.g., resistance, defensive denial) that interfere with medical treatment and the well-being of the patient (Postone 1998).

Finally, therapists should be cautious about infantilizing medically ill patients with disproportionately supportive interventions. Unhealthy dependency can be avoided by terminating patients who are stable, using more expressive interventions as the acute phase passes, or offering brief or long-term psychodynamic therapy to patients who are interested in and able to benefit from insight (Kaplan et al. 1994; van Marle and Holmes 2002).

Individual Psychodynamic Treatment With Patients With Serious Medical Illness

This discussion is focused on psychodynamic interventions with cancer patients, although these principles are applicable to patients with a broad range of illnesses. Comorbid anxiety (Andrykowski and Cordova 1998; Andrykowski et al. 1998, 2000; Koopman et al. 2002; Malt and Tjemsland 1999; Tjemsland et al. 1996a) and depression (Derogatis et al. 1983; Evans et al. 1999; Spiegel 1996; Spiegel and Giese-Davis 2003; Spiegel et al. 1994; Van't Spijker et al. 1997) have been well documented in cancer patients, although diagnosis and treatment may also activate unconscious abandonment fears, dependency conflicts, control issues, and existential concerns (Postone 1998). Psychosocial treatments for cancer patients include crisis intervention during the acute stages of disease followed by supportive-expressive therapy, psychoeducation (Blechner 1997; Goodheart and Lansing 1997; Postone 1998; van Marle and Holmes 2002), and case management as needed (Blechner 1997; Donnelly et al. 2000; Postone 1998). Psychiatrists who move comfortably between illness-related concerns, supportive interventions, and in-depth explorations of psychological functioning are most effective (Blechner 1997; Postone 1998).

From the moment of diagnosis, cancer patients are faced with multiple losses. The stress of diagnosis and treatment activates a regressed state in most patients and old conflicts and primitive defenses in others (Postone 1998). Invasive or noxious medical treatments can evoke trauma memories, triggering flashbacks or dissociative states in patients who are survivors of childhood abuse (Hay and Passik 2000; Postone 1998). Clinical judgment will determine the appropriate balance between supportive and expressive interventions during the early phase of treatment.

Beyond the acute phase, treatment can shift to insight-oriented interventions for patients who are motivated, psychologically minded, and in reasonably stable emotional and physical health (Gabbard 1994; Kaplan et al. 1994; Postone 1998). Expressive therapy with the medically ill incorporates exploration of idiosyncratic meanings the patient has attached to the illness; interpretation of here-and-now experiences in the transference; clarification and interpretation of unconscious processes underlying current distress, maladaptive behaviors, and interpersonal problems; and supportive intervention at critical junctures during the course of illness (Gabbard 1994; Kaplan et al. 1994; Postone 1998) The real object relationship, vital because the psychiatrist has provided the patient with ego support, encouragement, and acceptance during crises, may overshadow the development of transference (Postone 1998). Positive or idealized transference is probable in cancer patients, although negative transference can develop if the psychiatrist is perceived as linked to the disease (Postone 1998). Countertransference issues to be aware of include rescue fantasies, feelings of helplessness and hopelessness, and personal conflicts about mortality (Postone 1998). The goal of therapy with cancer patients is to optimize quality of life, tend to unfinished business, strengthen important relationships, and deal with death, although the long-term goal of structural personality change is not unheard of for patients with a favorable prognosis (Postone 1998).

Individual Psychodynamic Intervention

Individual psychodynamic therapy is often the treatment of choice for individuals with personality disorders (Gabbard 1994). The present discussion focuses on a multi-component intervention for medically ill patients with borderline personality disorder. A diagnosis of a serious medical disorder such as cancer can be particularly disruptive for individuals with borderline personality disorder or other personality disorders (Hay and Passik 2000). For a patient with premorbid limitations to the observing ego, interpersonal deficits, abandonment fears, emotional dysregulation, and impulsivity (McWilliams 1994), the heightened anxiety associated with a frightening medical diagnosis can cause severe disequilibrium resulting in regressive defenses, diminished reality testing, intensified aggression and hostility, and aggravated interpersonal problems (Hay and Passik 2000). Coping with illness, hospitalization, and treatment is especially daunting for individuals who were in all probability raised in the context of chaos, neglect, and abuse (Hay and Passik 2000). Based on childhood history, these vulnerable patients expect to be abandoned, and the defenses against their intolerable anxiety and ambivalence and their splitting and other manipulative behaviors are highly disruptive in the medical setting (Hay and Passik 2000).

Psychiatrists can more effectively manage behaviors that typically disrupt treatment teams by working closely with both the patient and the medical staff (Hay and Passik 2000). Educating hospital staff about borderline pathology (etiology, abandonment fear, defenses); encouraging collaboration; providing a forum that supports the work of the treatment team and allows expression of frustration; choosing a single prescribing physician for analgesia; and encouraging staff to place strict limits on the patient's manipulative or aggressive behaviors, impulsivity, and boundary violations may forestall problems if implemented early (Hay and Passik 2000).

A multidimensional intervention that is highly structured and symptom focused is recommended (Clarkin et al. 1999; Gabbard 1994). The patient's physical and emotional well-being will be optimized by early treatment of comorbid psychiatric symptoms and pain and by tracking and intervening in the event of self-destructive acts (treatment sabotage, substance abuse, suicidal ideation, cutting), manipulativeness (demanding, rejecting, entitlement), defensive behaviors (splitting, good staff/bad staff), aggression, and impaired reality testing (medical noncompliance driven by denial) (Hay and Passik 2000). Therapy will be more supportive than expressive with this population, although judicious interpretation of idealized transference, self-destructive behavior, or denial will not necessarily upset the therapeutic alliance if offered empathically and skillfully (Clarkin et al. 1999; Gabbard 1994). Helping the patient understand the negative consequences of hostility in getting needs met, modeling effective communication, intervening with physicians and staff to facilitate or repair treatment relationships, and setting limits on boundary disturbances (interfering with other patients or staff) are useful additions to the psychiatrist's existing treatment protocol (Hay and Passik 2000).

Brief Psychodynamic Therapy

The supportive-expressive model presented earlier in this section can be effectively adapted to brief treatment, with similar goals and techniques depending on the nature of the presenting problem, dynamic formulation, and psychiatric and medical history (Gabbard 1994). The duration of brief dynamic therapy ranges from a single session to 1 year of weekly sessions (Gabbard 1994; Kaplan et al. 1994). There is a growing body of empirical evidence for the utility of brief dynamic therapy with medical patients (Donnelly et al. 2000; Guthrie et al. 1991). One randomized, controlled study investigating short-term dynamic psychotherapy with gastrointestinal clinic patients with irritable bowel syndrome demonstrated significant improvement in psychological and medical status posttreatment and at 1-year follow-up for patients in the treatment condition compared with those in the usual care condition (Guthrie et al. 1991). Furthermore, the psychological changes appeared to mediate the improvement in irritable bowel symptoms in anxious and depressed patients (Guthrie et al. 1991). Time-limited dynamic therapy (Levenson 1995) and interpersonal therapy (IPT) are brief dynamic interventions that have been effective in the medically ill.

Interpersonal Therapy

First developed as a brief therapy for depression, IPT has been beneficial in the treatment of anxiety, personality disorders, dysthymia, major depression, and subclinical psychiatric disturbances in medically ill patients (Alpay and Cassem 2000; Donnelly et al. 2000; Gillies 2002). Interpersonal therapy has also been useful for treating illness-related distress and interpersonal problems in patients with cancer (Donnelly et al. 2000), AIDS (Markowitz et al. 1998), rheumatoid arthritis (Alpay and Cassem 2000), and other chronic medical illnesses (Gillies 2002). Stressing the interactive nature of depression and interpersonal problems, IPT emphasizes symptom formation, relationships and social functioning, isolation, and (to a lesser degree) the developmental origins of personality traits in a flexible, short-term (16–20 weeks) intervention (Bemporad and Vasile 1990; Gillies 2002). The therapist plays the role of patient advocate and teacher, encourages affective expression, and helps patients identify relational difficulties (Alpay and Cassem 2000; Gillies 2002).

IPT with medically ill patients differs from that with nonpatients by addressing illness-related distress with or without depression, including loved ones in the treatment, facilitating interactions with medical personnel, being open to flexible scheduling (including phone sessions), and dispensing with the "sick role" called for in manualized IPT (Donnelly et al. 2000). The role transitions forced by illness can upset a patient's constant experience of self, with repercussions ranging from loss of self-esteem and self-worth, emotional distress, and social isolation to financial uncertainty (Donnelly et al. 2000). Treatment strategies include emotional support, strengthening adaptive defenses, improving coping methods, examining the physical and psychosocial impact of illness on the patient and the family, facilitating adaptive communication in all relationships, encouraging affective expression, and assisting the patient in gaining independence (Donnelly et al. 2000). Practical interventions include providing psychoeducation, increasing sources of social support, and helping the patient and family members cope with illness and treatment demands (Donnelly et al. 2000). The goal of treatment is reducing symptoms, improving interpersonal relationships, and optimizing medical and psychosocial care (Donnelly et al. 2000; Gillies 2002). Posttreatment booster sessions with IPT have been effective in relapse prevention (Frank et al. 1990, 1991) and are recommended for patients who are medically ill (Donnelly et al. 2000).

Summary

Psychodynamic theory informs psychosocial treatments specific to the medically ill. Interventions (Kuttner 1993) will differ as a function of current diagnosis, treatment, disease course, and prognosis as these factors interact with the psychological, genetic, environmental, social, and developmental aspects of the patient (Gabbard 1994; McWilliams 1994, 1999). Expressive-supportive dynamic theory may also incorporate cognitive and behavioral techniques, psychoeducation, and physician liaison, depending on the needs of the patient (Blechner 1997; Donnelly et al. 2000; Goodheart and Lansing 1997; Postone 1998). The goal is to help patients cope with current problems, alleviate symptoms, and facilitate adaptive decisions about health care (McWilliams 1999).

Hypnosis

Hypnosis is an altered state of consciousness that comprises heightened absorption in focal attention, dissociation of peripheral awareness, and enhanced responsiveness to social cues (Spiegel and Maldonado 1999).

Hypnosis has a long tradition of effectiveness in controlling somatic symptoms such as pain and anxiety (Faymonville et al. 1995; J. Holroyd 1996; Kuttner 1993). According to Patterson and Jensen (2003), in their recent authoritative review, "Randomized controlled studies with clinical populations indicate that hypnosis has a reliable and significant impact on acute procedural pain and chronic pain conditions" (p. 495).

Patients with the requisite hypnotic capacity can be taught to use self-hypnosis to reduce or eliminate pain and the tension that accompanies it (Maldonado and Spiegel 2000). Hypnotic analgesia seems to work via two mechanisms: physical relaxation and attention control. Patients in pain tend to splint the painful area instinctively, and yet this enhanced muscle tension around a painful area often increases pain. Most patients find that they can enhance their physical repose by focusing on a variety of images that connote physical relaxation, such as a sense of floating. Because hypnosis involves an intensification and narrowing of the focus of attention, it allows individuals to place pain at the periphery of their awareness by replacing it with some competing thought or sensation at the center of their attention. Thus, by focusing on a memory of dental anesthesia and spreading that numbness to the affected area, making the area warmer or cooler, substituting a sense of tingling or lightness, or focusing on sensation in some nonpainful part of the body, hypnotized individuals can diminish the amount of attention they pay to painful stimuli. Such hypnotic techniques have been shown to effectively reduce cancer pain in adults (Spiegel and Glafkides 1983) and procedural pain and other symptoms in children (Zeltzer and LeBaron 1982; Zeltzer et al. 1984). Hypnotic intervention actually alters perceptual processing in the brain, with reduced response to painful stimuli as measured by event-related potentials (Spiegel et al. 1989) and positron emission tomography (Rainville et al. 1999).

Because of its analgesic and anxiolytic properties, hypnosis is an effective tool in facilitating medical procedures. For example, Lang and colleagues (2000) demonstrated in a randomized prospective trial that the addition of training in self-hypnosis for individuals undergoing invasive radiological procedures resulted in significantly less pain and anxiety, fewer procedural complications, less use of analgesic medication, and saved an average of 17 minutes per procedure.

Hypnosis has also been effective in reducing symptoms in irritable bowel syndrome (Whorwell et al. 1984) and asthma (Morrison 1988) and in smoking control (Spiegel et al. 1993). Given the dissociative nature of many conversion symptoms, such as nonepileptic seizures (Bowman and Markand 1996), hypnosis is helpful in both their differential diagnosis and treatment (Barry and Sanborn 2001; Barry et al. 2000; Spiegel 2000). Thus, hypnosis is a particularly effective tool for symptoms among the medically ill because of its ability to help patients enhance control over mind/brain/body interactions (Greenberg et al. 1993; Kosslyn et al. 2000).

Family Therapy

The psychosocial impact of medical illness on families cannot be overestimated. The family is an integral force in personality development; a primary source for meeting basic human needs for relationship, self-expression, and meaning; and a complex, evolving system that strives for equilibrium (Foley 1989; Rolland 1989). It is not surprising that the psychosocial problems associated with medical illness extend to family members. In fact, from a family systems perspective, medical illness, especially if it is chronic, becomes part of the system (Rolland 1989). A diagnosis of major illness will always upset a family's equilibrium, but the impact on the family system differs by diagnosis, onset (acute or chronic), course (progressive or episodic), prognosis, level of incapacitation, and the idiomatic characteristics of the family (Rolland 1989). For example, the sudden onset of acute MI requires immediate attention to the existing family structure and role changes, whereas the progressive course of diabetes or multiple sclerosis enables a slow, gradual adjustment to these systemic processes (Rolland 1989). The diagnosis of catastrophic illness in a loved one can be overwhelming for any family, and healthier families tend to return to usual functioning with social and emotional support. Conversely, the presence of preexisting problems in communication, interpersonal conflicts, and abandonment issues are intensified by the stress of medical illness (Kaplan et al. 1994).

While the patient experiences illness-related stress and dependency fears, the family is affected by the burden of patient care, managing the household, and the existential fears associated with critical illness (Lehrer et al. 2002). Symptoms of anxiety and depression are common in family members caring for a loved one with cancer or other life-threatening disease (Donnelly et al. 2000; Kaplan et al. 1994; Marx et al. 2001). An illness with a progressive course requires constant adaptation and shifting roles as the illness advances, with little respite from symptoms (Rolland 1989). In recent years the field of psychooncology has been addressing emotional reactions, stress management, and caregiver burden in the family members of cancer patients (Holland 2002). A growing body of clinical and empirical evidence points to the utility of family therapy as a supportive intervention during the acute phase of medical illness, a preventive intervention for families at risk for psychiatric morbidity, and a therapeutic intervention for families with existing dysfunction (Bloch and Kissane 2000; Duff 2001; Goodheart and Lansing 1997; Kazak et al. 1999; Kissane et al. 1998; Lehrer et al. 2002; Radojevic et al. 1992; Shapiro 2002; Wysocki et al. 2001).

Family and couples therapies have been effective for patients and families living with cancer, asthma, cystic fibrosis, rheumatoid arthritis, type 2 diabetes, kidney disease, and somatoform disorders (Bloch and Kissane 2000; Donnelly et al. 2000; Duff 2001; Gonder-Frederick et al. 2002; Hener et al. 1996; Kazak et al. 1999; Keefe et al. 2002; Kissane et al. 1998; Kurnat and Murphy Moore 1999; Lehrer et al. 1992; Looper and Kirmayer 2002; Marchioro et al. 1996; Shapiro 2002; Wysocki et al. 2001). For example, an intervention with patients with rheumatoid arthritis treated with a combination of supportive family therapy and CBT resulted in improvements in joint swelling and pain at 2-month follow-up (Radojevic et al. 1992). A study comparing a supportive intervention, CBT, and a no-treatment control in dialysis patients and their partners found superior adjustment to home peritoneal kidney dialysis in both treatment groups (Hener et al. 1996).

Treatment Strategies

Family or couples therapy addresses the family interactions that may contribute to sickness (Looper and Kirmayer 2002), such as exacerbation of asthma (Lehrer et al. 1992, 2002) or poor control of diabetes (Wysocki et al. 2001). Family therapy with the medically ill is a time-limited, problem-focused, collaborative intervention informed by the psychiatrist's theoretical orientation; the diagnosis, treatment, and phase of illness; the patient's premorbid character, life cycle stage, and family role; the impact of illness, level of adaptive coping, and quality of family support; historical beliefs about disease and death;

the role of illness in the family system (e.g., illness behavior reinforced, overindulgence or isolation of the sick family member); and the premorbid and current state of family functioning (Foley 1989; Goodheart and Lansing 1997; Nichols and Schwartz 1991; Rolland 1989). A multimodal family intervention facilitating structural change in a dysfunctional system will help family members adapt to the changing needs of the patient while remaining uncontrolled by the disease (Goodheart and Lansing 1997). Adjunct interventions such as individual therapy, outside sources of support (support groups and self-help groups), and respite care also contribute to adaptive functioning of families (Goodheart and Lansing 1997).

Family Therapy With Seriously Ill Children

Serious chronic illnesses such as juvenile diabetes, some cancers, and childhood asthma tend to disrupt family systems, and family dysfunction can exacerbate the illness. Certain family dynamics have been implicated in acute asthma attacks in some children (Lehrer et al. 2002). Family dysfunction dominated by interpersonal problems, parental criticism, lack of affection, and parental psychopathology has been linked to poor treatment adherence and symptom exacerbation in asthmatic children, just as the stress of adapting to the needs of a family member with asthma can also lead to family disharmony (Lehrer et al. 2002). A child with life-threatening asthma may be overprotected by one or both parents, creating potential for secondary gain for the patient, possible exacerbation of symptoms, and sibling resentment (Rolland 1989). Fortunately, family therapy has been helpful in managing asthma in children (Duff 2001; Lehrer et al. 1992, 2002).

Serious illness interferes with normative developmental processes in children and adolescents (Goodheart and Lansing 1997). Frequent hospitalizations, restricted physical activity, and complex treatment protocols often leave sick children and adolescents feeling different from peers, particularly if the disease is visible (e.g., seizure disorders, certain cancers) (Duff 2001; Goodheart and Lansing 1997). Chronically ill children are vulnerable to developmental deficits, low self-esteem, interpersonal problems, isolation, and psychopathology (Duff 2001; Goodheart and Lansing 1997). Combined individual and family therapy addressing developmental, psychosocial, and behavioral problems in medically ill children is recommended (Duff 2001; Goodheart and Lansing 1997). Although behavioral and cognitive-behavioral techniques that focus on illness-related problems and parenting skills have been effective, a developmental approach utilizing expressive methods is more suitable for patients who are uncooperative with CBT or have severe depression and anxiety, developmental arrest, or enduring characterological problems (Duff 2001; Goodheart and Lansing 1997). Another family systems intervention shows clinical promise in the prevention and treatment of psychosocial problems associated with asthma and cystic fibrosis (Duff 2001). This multimodal intervention, which utilizes psychoeducation; open discussion about the interactive effect of feelings, thoughts, beliefs, and behaviors; communication skills training; and examination of strengths, relationships, expectations, and roles within the family is currently under investigation (Duff 2001). The goal of therapy with sick children is to allow them to experience as much normality as possible, given the circumstances of chronic disease, treatment, emergencies, and disability, in order to help them develop normally even in this context (Goodheart and Lansing 1997).

Summary

Important topics in family therapy with a medically ill member include current stressors, affective symptoms, grief and loss, communication patterns and dysfunctional interactions, and the role of the illness in the family system (e.g., illness behavior reinforced, overindulgence or isolation of the sick family member). The goal of family therapy is to establish constructive communication, improve interpersonal relationships among family members, and effect positive change in the structure of the system (Foley 1989).

Cognitive-Behavioral Therapy

Whereas the psychodynamic school sees the core structures of personality and psychopathology as unconscious and not easily accessible to the patient, the cognitive-behavioral view holds that these structures are largely in the realm of awareness and available for conscious examination (Freeman 1990; Hollon and Beck 1994). In Beck's cognitive model, previous social learning, developmental history, and significant experiences lead people to form a unique set of meanings and assumptions, or cognitive schemas, about themselves, the world, and the future (Beck and Weishaar 1989; Freeman 1990; Hollon and Beck 1994). These schemas are then used to organize perception and to govern and evaluate behavior (Hollon and Beck 1994). When specific schemas are activated, they directly influence the content of a person's perceptions, interpretations, associations, and memories from a given time (Beck and Weishaar 1989; Hollon and Beck 1994). Personality is understood as a set of cognitive schemas that predispose people to certain emotional disorders (Hollon and Beck 1994). For example, depression results from cognitions of sadness and loss, whereas anxiety is a function of an exaggerated sense of fear and danger—

important differences when defining the treatment focus (Hollon and Beck 1994). Assumptions that are extreme, dysfunctional, and resistant to change are thought to underlie and maintain some psychiatric disorders.

CBT was developed as a short-term (12–20 sessions) intervention for depression targeting patients' thoughts and their relation to behavior and affect (Hollon and Beck 1994). The efficacy of CBT as a treatment for depression is well established (Craighead et al. 1998), and cognitive, cognitive-behavioral, and behavioral interventions have been beneficial in addressing psychosocial problems associated with medical illness (Hollon and Beck 1994). Symptoms of major depression have been alleviated with CBT in patients with rheumatic diseases (e.g., rheumatoid arthritis, fibromyalgia), chronic fatigue syndrome (Alpay and Cassem 2000), type 2 diabetes (Lustman et al. 1998), and elderly medically ill patients (Niederehe and Schneider 1998). Cognitive-behavioral techniques have also been effective in the management of tension headache (K. A. Holroyd 2002), hypochondriasis (Simon et al. 2001), and a range of other somatoform disorders (Looper and Kirmayer 2002). Cognitive-behavioral interventions with patients who have osteoarthritis (Keefe et al. 2002) or rheumatoid arthritis (Keefe et al. 2002; Young 1992) have resulted in improved coping (e.g., stress management and pain management) and reduced anxiety and depression. A recent review concluded that CBT is efficacious for chronic pain management in rheumatic diseases, chronic pain syndrome, and low back pain and possibly efficacious for irritable bowel syndrome and some cancers (Compas et al. 1998). CBT has yielded substantial improvements in the disease course of a number of illnesses (Emmelkamp and van Oppen 1993).

Cognitive-Behavioral Therapy and Medical Illness

CBT for medically ill patients can be adapted to meet the patient's needs at a given time. Initially, the therapy may concentrate on alleviation of symptoms of distress, anxiety, and depression (Hollon and Beck 1994). For some patients, the treatment focus may be on psychosocial issues that act as barriers to optimal care, treatment adherence, and quality of life (Hollon and Beck 1994). In that case, enhancing self-care is an important goal that can be best attained through interventions developed on the basis of social learning and self-regulation theories (Glasgow et al. 1989; Tobin et al. 1986; Von Korff and Simon 1996; Von Korff et al. 1997). Cognitive and cognitive-behavioral techniques are indicated for patients who are adjusting to diagnosis, coping with unpleasant medical procedures or chemotherapy-induced nausea, in rehabilitation following brain injury, and for HIV prevention (Hollon and Beck 1994). Cognitive-behavioral interventions with

cancer patients generally include relaxation training and instruction in stress management and coping skills (Hollon and Beck 1994), although some address the issues of health education, communication, assertiveness, management of emotions, or psychosocial support in a group format (Compas et al. 1998). There is evidence for the need to incorporate medical management, such as treatment options and compliance, into the intervention in order to optimize the likelihood of treatment success (Lustman et al. 1998). For example, in treating a depressed patient with type 2 diabetes, it is especially important to integrate diabetes-related concerns into the therapy (Lustman et al. 1998). Treating a patient with a somatoform disorder may require repeatedly helping him or her question the evidence for maladaptive assumptions and cognitive distortions that underlie physical symptoms. For example, a hypochondriacal patient who is convinced he has a life-threatening disease will anxiously check his body repeatedly and perceive even normal body sensations as danger signals portending severe illness (Kaplan et al. 1994; Salkovskis 1989).

Summary

Cognitive, behavioral, and CBT techniques have demonstrated clinical utility in treating anxiety and depression, increasing treatment compliance, and coping with diagnosis and noxious treatments in the medically ill.

Psychoeducational Interventions

Group sessions that were held in the early 1900s for tuberculosis patients—interventions that involved educational as well as expressive components—educational interventions could be considered precursors to group psychotherapy for medically ill patients (Scheidlinger 1993). The provision of knowledge related to the illness has long been recognized as important, especially for information-focused coping. Psychoeducational interventions are designed to expand understanding of the mechanisms at work in the disease, improve treatment adherence, and enhance the sense of control and mastery a patient has over his or her disease. For example, interventions that reinforce information from the physician can be useful for patients navigating the difficult treatment regimen of diabetes or to reinforce safer-sex practices in HIV-positive patients. For noxious medical procedures, advanced information about the procedure, including what sensations to expect and why, may increase the coping abilities of the patient. Moreover, proposing cognitive or behavioral strategies to use during the procedure can further improve the patient's sense of control and adjustment (Taylor and Clark 1986). However, increased knowledge may have negative consequences, increasing stress and worry or inducing feelings of anxiety in particular individuals (Miller 1987) or circumstances (Burger 1989).

A variety of psychoeducational interventions have been proposed for people with medical illnesses. Many target psychosocial as well as medical factors in helping patients cope with the daily stresses of illness. Although they share some similarity across diseases, particular features are often quite disease specific in terms of goals and outcomes. Purely educational interventions have not always been sufficient for promoting adjustment to illness or improving quality of life and/or medical status (Kraimaat et al. 1995). Psychoeducational interventions for medical patients are usually more effective when they combine illness-specific knowledge and cues that will assist patients in the daily management of their disease (De Ridder and Schreurs 2001) or offer emotion-focused components that help them adjust to and live through the different phases of the illness. Problem-focused interventions may be particularly appropriate for diseases such as diabetes or asthma, in which the patient is responsible for essential aspects of treatment (Diabetes Control and Complications Trial Research Group 1993). Psychological interventions enable cognitive processing of medical information, support emotional adjustment to disease-related changes in daily life, and encourage the patient to take an active and collaborative role in his or her own care (e.g., performing daily tasks required by complex medical regimens, taking part in medical decision making, and communicating effectively with doctors and family).

Psychoeducational interventions often feature a combination of education and cognitive-behavioral techniques. These interventions are generally offered in a group format, and although they share some features with group psychotherapy (provision of social support, universality, helper-therapy principle), they tend to be more structured than psychotherapy per se. The goals of psychoeducational interventions may include modifying medical knowledge, health behaviors, and beliefs and improving treatment adherence, emotional adjustment, and communication. Depending on the type of intervention and on the illness, these interventions may focus on psychosocial variables (reducing anxiety and depression, enhancing self-efficacy or quality of life) or more directly on medical status and physiological factors (improving blood glucose control, respiratory capacity, or immunological status).

Psychosocial Treatment Outcomes

During the past two decades, several investigators have attempted to assess the efficacy of psychotherapy for the medically ill. Since the early studies evaluating the impact of group psychotherapy for cancer patients (Spiegel et al. 1989), interest in psychotherapeutic interventions for medical patients has been extended to a large number of other chronic illnesses. Many different types of psychosocial interventions are now available for the medically ill, although evaluation of psychotherapy outcomes has been hampered by enormous variability between studies. Psychosocial interventions appear to benefit patients with cancer (Andersen 1992; Andersen et al. 1994; Ashby et al. 1996; D.G. Cruess et al. 2000b; Devine and Westlake 1995; Fawzy et al. 1995; Greenberg et al. 1993; Kibby et al. 1998; Linden et al. 1996; Meyer and Mark 1995; Spiegel et al. 1981, 1989), heart disease (Dusseldorp et al. 1999; Ketterer 1993; Linden et al. 1996), diabetes (Delamater et al. 2001; Gonder-Frederick et al. 2002; Moran et al. 1991), arthritis (Astin et al. 2002; Bradley and Alberts 1999; Keefe et al. 2002; McCracken and Turk 2002; Parker et al. 1993), and HIV/AIDS (Antoni et al. 1991; Chesney et al. 1996; D.G. Cruess et al. 2000a, 2000c; S. Cruess et al. 2000; Esterling et al. 1992; Kelly et al. 1993; Lutgendorf et al. 1997). We review studies focusing on psychosocial interventions in primary care patients, cancer, heart disease, diabetes, arthritis, and HIV. Our goal is to present an overview of interventions that have the potential of leading to improved psychological or medical outcomes.

Primary Care

The need for psychosocial interventions in primary care is clear (Meredith et al. 1997; Saravay 1996; Sherbourne et al. 1996a, 1996b). Emotional distress has a negative impact on patients' medical symptoms, interferes with psychosocial functioning, and contributes to rising health care costs, yet psychiatric symptoms continue to be underdiagnosed and untreated by primary care providers (Coyne et al. 2002; Saravay 1996). A survey of depressed and anxious primary care patients found that a surprising 54.6%–72.9% receive no help from their physicians for personal or emotional problems (Evans et al. 1999). Yet negative treatment outcomes have been described in depressed primary care patients with asthma, diabetes, headache, and back pain (Koike et al. 2002). In one randomized, controlled study, depressed, chronically ill primary care patients were randomized into one of two treatment conditions (IPT or nortriptyline) or a control condition (usual physician care) (Coulehan et al. 1997). Remission of major depression was reported in 70% of the participants in both treatment conditions compared with 20% in the usual care condition at an 8-month follow-up (Coulehan et al. 1997).

Cancer

As treatments continue to improve, cancer is becoming more a chronic than a terminal illness. However, given the progressive nature of the disease, and the fact that approximately half of all people diagnosed with cancer will eventually die of it, the provision of effective psychosocial support is even more important. During the past 20 years, a growing number of research studies (summarized in Tables 38–1 and 38–2) assessing the benefit of psychosocial interventions for cancer patients have been conducted (Andersen 1992; Andersen et al. 1994; Ashby et al. 1996; Devine and Westlake 1995; Fawzy et al. 1995; Kibby et al. 1998; Linden et al. 1996; Meyer and Mark 1995). There is clear evidence that these interventions have a positive effect on psychological distress (Ferlic et al. 1979; Gustafson and Whitman 1978; Mulder et al. 1992; Spiegel and Bloom 1983; Spiegel et al. 1981; Wood et al. 1978), coping skills (Fawzy et al. 1993), and quality of life (Spiegel and Bloom 1983; Spiegel and Glafkides 1983). Psychoeducation and cognitive-behavioral interventions for cancer patients have led to improved treatment adherence (Richardson et al. 1990), stress reduction and enhanced psychological well-being (Allen et al. 2002; Elsesser et al. 1994; Helgeson et al. 1999; Larsson and Starrin 1992; McQuellon et al. 1998), and encouraging medical outcomes (Fawzy et al. 1993; Kuchler et al. 1999; McCorkle et al. 2000; Richardson et al. 1990).

Treatment Adherence

Despite the paucity of research on adherence to cancer treatment, it is an essential factor affecting disease outcome (Andersen et al. 1994). An early intervention study revealed that any one of three treatments (education, shaping of pill-taking behavior, or home visits) enhanced adherence to daily pill taking and follow-up visits (Richardson et al. 1987). Although patient knowledge was improved in each intervention group, the researchers pointed out that compliance was not directly affected by knowledge alone but rather by the behavioral components of the interventions (Richardson et al. 1987). Interventions designed to combat side effects of cancer treatment are important for improving treatment adherence (Fallowfield 1992). During the 1980s and 1990s, progressive muscle relaxation, with or without guided imagery, was considered efficacious in managing nausea and vomiting associated with chemotherapy (Carey and Burish 1988; Burish and Tope 1992). However, with newer antiemetic medications, the utility of psychological treatments in managing nausea and vomiting is less clear (Compas et al. 1998). For some patients, however, a combination of medication and behavioral techniques further reduces the noxious effects of cancer treatments, especially anticipatory nausea in chemotherapy patients (Compas et al. 1998).

Distress

A variety of psychosocial interventions have been helpful in reducing emotional distress in cancer patients (Allen et al. 2002; Elsesser et al. 1994; Larsson and Starrin 1992; McArdle et al. 1996). Even a minimal intervention such as a brief orientation tour led by a psychologist resulted in decreased anxiety, mood disturbance, and depressive symptoms in new medical oncology clinic patients (McQuellon et al. 1998). One study in which cancer patients received a minimal form of relaxation training resulted in significant improvement in mood and daily hassles and appraisal of radiation therapy as less threatening (Larsson and Starrin 1992). A recent randomized, controlled study of a cognitive-behavioral problem-solving intervention (an initial 2-hour in-person session followed by four telephone contacts, and a final 2-hour in-person session) for young women (age <50 years) with breast cancer resulted in improvements in mood, physical side effects, marital and sexual difficulties, and psychological problems at 4 months posttreatment (Allen et al. 2002). However, at the 8-month follow-up, treatment effects held only for women with moderate or good problem-solving ability, whereas women with high problem-solving skills received no benefit and women with low problem-solving skills were actually negatively affected by the intervention (Allen et al. 2002).

Finally, a program integrating psychoeducation, CBT, and family therapy for adolescent survivors of childhood cancer and their families has been positively received in early trials (Kazak et al. 1999). Families participate in a 1-day, 8-hour family group intervention focused on prevention of posttraumatic stress disorder, developmental deficits, and family dysfunction resulting from cancer (Kazak et al. 1999).

Coping

Helgeson and colleagues (1999) compared an eight-session education-based group providing informational support and relaxation training, a peer discussion–based group, and a combination of the two for women with breast cancer. The educational intervention facilitated initial adjustment in early-stage breast cancer patients, whereas the peer discussion group resulted in adverse effects. Education increased the patients' self-esteem, body image, perceived control, and reduced uncertainty about the illness. In another study, a multimodal cognitive-behavioral stress management (CBSM) group for women with breast cancer, combining 20 therapy hours of cognitive restructuring, relaxation, coping skills, assertiveness, anger man-

TABLE 38–1. Psychosocial interventions in cancer

Study	Participants	Diagnosis	Type of intervention	Results of intervention
Richardson et al. 1987	92 patients	Multiple myeloma, leukemia, lymphoma, or Hodgkin's disease	Compare combined education; shaping of pill-taking behavior; home visit	Improved adherence to daily pill-taking and follow-up visits in the three intervention groups
Richardson et al. 1990	94 patients	Hematological malignancies, newly diagnosed	Educational intervention: 1-hour session with nurse plus pill-taking procedure; home visit to organize "cueing" system for pill taking; or both, to increase treatment compliance	Low severity of disease and high compliance predicted increased survival for the three modalities
Larsson and Starrin 1992	64 patients	Breast cancer	Minimal form of relaxation training	Improvement in daily hassles, mood, appraise radiation as less threatening
Gruber et al. 1993	13 women	Stage I breast cancer	"Enhanced" relaxation, PMR/guided imagery exercises; electromyographic biofeedback	Positive endocrine/immune (higher cell counts, blastogenesis/lower cortisol); no differences in psychological measures
Fawzy et al. 1993	68 patients	Malignant melanoma	6- to 8-week CBSM group intervention shortly after surgery	Longer survival and recurrence times in treatment group
Elsesser et al. 1994	20 patients	Cancer, heterogeneous	6-week anxiety management training, PMR/cognitive restructuring	Significant reduction in anxiety (state and trait); no differences in depression, quality of life, or cell counts
McArdle et al. 1996	272 patients	Breast cancer surgery patients	Supportive nursing versus cancer patient volunteer support (pre- and postsurgery)	Improved self-report health and depressive symptoms in nursing condition
McQuellon et al. 1998	180 patients	Cancer, heterogeneous	Orientation tour for patients new to a medical oncology clinic	Reduction of state anxiety, mood disturbance, and depressive symptoms
Helgeson et al. 1999	312 women	Breast cancer	Educational/informational support group versus peer discussion group	Educational intervention increased self-esteem, body image, perceived control
Kuchler et al. 1999	271 patients	Gastrointestinal cancer, heterogeneous	Individual/inpatient psychotherapy (coping, support, and information on transition to recovery)	Increased survival (especially among women) in treatment group
Allen et al. 2002	164 women	Stages I–III A breast cancer; age <50 years	Individual cognitive-behavioral problem solving (a 2-hour one-on-one session, four phone contacts, and a final 2-hour one-on-one session)	Improved mood at 4 months in treatment group, no difference at 8 months Best with moderate level of problem-solving ability
D.G. Cruess et al. 2000b	34 women	Stage I or II breast cancer	See Antoni et al. 2001	Reduced cortisol levels in treatment group

TABLE 38–1. Psychosocial interventions in cancer (*continued*)

Study	Participants	Diagnosis	Type of intervention	Results of intervention
Larson et al. 2000	41 women	Breast cancer	Two presurgery support sessions, relaxation, information, problem solving	Lower declines in interferon-gamma production postsurgery in treatment group
McCorkle et al. 2000	375 patients	Solid cancers	Patient education, emotional and social support, and monitoring of physical and emotional activity provided during 4 weeks by nurses	No difference in survival with early stage patients versus improved survival in late stage patients
Antoni et al. 2001	136 patients	In situ disease or stage I or II breast cancer	CBSM group treatment, support, relaxation training, coping skills, cognitive restructuring, assertiveness and anger management training	No improvement in distress, self-reports of positive benefits, especially in patients low in optimism

Note. CBSM = cognitive-behavioral stress management; PMR = progressive muscle relaxation.

TABLE 38–2.   Randomized trials examining the hypothesis that psychosocial treatment affects cancer survival time

Study	Cancer type	Sample size	Psychotherapeutic intervention	Psychological outcome	Survival outcome
Linn et al. 1982	Lung, pancreatic, skin, sarcoma, leukemia, lymphoma	120	Individual existential psychotherapy	Improvement in depression, self-esteem, life satisfaction, alienation, locus of control	No difference
Spiegel et al. 1989	Metastatic breast	86	Supportive-expressive group therapy	Reduced anxiety and depression (POMS), improved coping, reduced pain	Hazard ratio for treatment = 0.51 (95% CI=0.31–0.82)
Richardson et al. 1990	Lymphoma, leukemia	94	Education, home visiting	Improved treatment adherence	RR = 0.39, independent of adherence
Fawzy et al. 1993	Malignant melanoma	66	Cognitive-behavioral group therapy emphasizing active coping skills training	Reduced anxiety and depression (POMS), improved coping	Improved at 4- and 10-year follow-up
Ilnyckyj et al. 1994	Breast, lymphoma, colon, ovarian	127	Heterogeneous group therapies, some leaderless	No benefit	No difference
Cunningham et al. 1998	Metastatic breast	66	Cognitive-behavioral therapy combined with supportive-expressive therapy	Increased anxious preoccupation and decreased helplessness in treatment group	No difference
Kuchler et al. 1999	Gastrointestinal	271	Individual psychotherapy at the time of diagnosis	Unreported	Hazard ratio for intervention group = 0.6 (95% CI= 0.45–0.84)
Edelman et al. 1999	Metastatic breast	124	Cognitive-behavioral therapy	Transient improvement in POMS	Interquartile range = 0.97 (0.59–1.46); no difference
McCorkle et al. 2000	Solid	375	Disease management and psychological support via three home visits and five telephone contacts	Unreported	RR of death for control subjects = 2.04 (95% CI= 1.33–3.12)
Goodwin et al. 2001	Metastatic breast	235	Supportive-expressive therapy	Improvement in distress on POMS but not EORTC; reduced pain	Hazard ratio for treatment = 1.06 (95% CI=0.78–1.45)

Note.   CI=confidence interval; EORTC=European Organisation for Research and Treatment of Cancer Quality-of-Life Measure; POMS=Profile of Mood States; RR=relative risk.

agement training, and social support, resulted in self-reported improvements in perceived benefits from their experience with cancer (e.g., enhanced sense of purpose and meaning, better family relationships, and altered life priorities), although no improvement in distress was noted. Women who scored low on an optimism scale at baseline reported the most benefit from the intervention (Antoni et al. 2001).

A pilot study for an intervention with IPT adapted for cancer patients has been helpful for patients and their partners in early trials (Donnelly et al. 2000). Female outpatients undergoing an aggressive treatment regimen for metastatic breast cancer ($n=14$) and their partners ($n=11$) participated in individual telephone IPT sessions coinciding with chemotherapy and continuing 4 weeks after treatment. Therapy focused on salient psychosocial issues (distress, family concerns, coping with illness and treatment demands, relationships with medical personnel), and overall the patients rated the intervention from good to excellent. Partners reported that the telephone contact was their only outlet to help them cope with role transitions, anticipated losses, depression and anxiety, and feelings of fear, anger, and frustration (Donnelly et al. 2000).

Family grief therapy, an empirically derived preventive intervention for families of cancer patients at risk for complicated bereavement, has also shown clinical promise in preliminary investigations (Bloch and Kissane 2000; Kissane et al. 1998). The treatment focused on current problems and concerns and family dynamics; beliefs about illness, death, and grief; and expression of negative affect, with the goal of improved coping, enhanced communication, increased cohesiveness, and more adaptive family functioning (Bloch and Kissane 2000; Kissane et al. 1998). Finally, a nonrandomized trial of an intervention for adolescent survivors of childhood cancer and their families received positive feedback from participants in a preliminary trial, who reported reduced anxiety and posttraumatic stress disorder symptoms at 6-month follow-up (Kazak et al. 1999).

Medical Effects

There is a small but surprising literature that raises the possibility that psychotherapeutic intervention may affect survival time as well as quality of life (Fawzy et al. 1993; Kuchler et al. 1999; McCorkle et al. 2000; Richardson et al. 1990; Spiegel et al. 1989). To date, 5 of 10 published randomized trials demonstrate such an effect (see Table 38–2) (Giese-Davis et al. 2002). To their initial surprise, Spiegel and colleagues (1989) found that 1 year (minimum) of supportive-expressive group psychotherapy resulted in a significant 18-month increase in survival time in metastatic breast cancer patients. In another study, a 6-

week cognitive-behavioral group intervention composed of education, stress management, coping skills training, and psychological support for malignant melanoma patients found significantly lower death rates at the 5–6 year follow-up in the treatment group (Fawzy et al. 1993). Interestingly, in this study, patients with higher baseline levels of distress seemed to experience lower rates of disease recurrence and death (Fawzy et al. 1993). An educational intervention aimed at increasing compliance with cancer treatment also had beneficial effects on survival in patients with newly diagnosed hematological cancer (Richardson et al. 1990). A recent study of individual psychotherapeutic support offered to a group of gastrointestinal cancer inpatients also yielded favorable results (Kuchler et al. 1999). In this study, standard care was supplemented with counseling (information on coping, transition to recovery, and emotional support) conducted at bedside by psychotherapists. At 2-year follow-up, the experimental group (especially female patients) experienced better survival than the control group (49% had died in the experimental group as opposed to 67% in the control group) (Kuchler et al. 1999). Finally, in a 4-week intervention consisting of patient education, psychological support, and implementation of a community-based network of support services, McCorkle and colleagues (2000) found improved survival in late-stage cancer patients, although no difference in survival time was found in patients with early-stage cancer.

Conversely, five other trials found no enhanced survival with psychosocial intervention. One excellent multicenter trial using supportive-expressive group psychotherapy with metastatic breast cancer patients showed reduced distress and pain but no survival advantage (Goodwin et al. 2001). However, the controversy over whether psychotherapy can increase survival should not obscure the finding that essentially every well-conducted study of psychotherapy in cancer patients—even studies showing no survival advantage—has found improved quality of life or reduced distress. Nevertheless, the potential benefits of psychotherapeutic support on cancer progression remains an important but unresolved research question (see also Chapter 24, "Oncology").

Heart Disease

Large prospective studies have shown an association among depressed affect, hopelessness, and ischemic heart disease (Anda et al. 1993) and among anxiety, phobic anxiety, and fatal coronary disease (Kawachi et al. 1994). Hostility has been linked to severity and progression of coronary artery disease as well as myocardial ischemia (Helmers et al. 1993; Julkunen et al. 1994; Suarez et al. 1998; Williams et al. 1985). There is now compelling evidence that psychosocial factors play an important role in the development and progression of heart disease. The addition of psychosocial treatment to standard cardiac care and rehabilitation has helped reduce morbidity and mortality, psychological distress, and some biological risk factors (Dusseldorp et al. 1999; Ketterer 1993; Linden et al. 1996).

Although studies published in the 1980s suggested that psychosocial interventions were valuable additions to usual medical care (Frasure-Smith and Prince 1985; Friedman et al. 1986), recent large, well-controlled trials have not yielded significant intervention effects (e.g., no reduction in cardiac deaths) (Frasure-Smith et al. 1997; Jones and West 1996). However, the exclusive focus on cardiac recurrences and mortality may underestimate intervention effects by overlooking positive psychological outcomes (Smith and Ruiz 2002). Despite some inconclusive results about the effects of psychological interventions on medical outcomes in heart disease, the literature supports the efficacy of psychosocial interventions in attenuating stress and enhancing quality of life (Dusseldorp et al. 1999; Linden 2000; Smith and Ruiz 2002). Studies in this area are summarized in Table 38–3. For example, an individual cognitive-behavioral intervention consisting of one or more sessions of relaxation training, stress management, behavioral risk reduction, treatment compliance, and cognitive interventions (e.g., identifying sources of distress) was provided for patients entering cardiac rehabilitation after hospitalization for angina, MI, angioplasty, or coronary artery bypass grafting (Black et al. 1998). The treatment was associated with decreased rehospitalization and depression (Black et al. 1998). A randomized, controlled trial of a brief hospital intervention (three sessions led by a psychologist) that emphasized cognitive restructuring of negative beliefs about post-MI consequences and preparation of a recovery action plan found significant changes in patients' perceptions of their MIs (e.g., length of illness and post-MI consequences on life) (Petrie et al. 2002). Patients in the intervention group returned to work sooner than those in the control group and had lower rates of angina symptoms at 3-month follow-up (Petrie et al. 2002). A nonrandomized clinical study comparing a cardiac rehabilitation program consisting of exercise, stress management, and counseling with a control group receiving standard medical care resulted in decreased negative affect over the 3-month intervention time and higher rates of survival over the following 9 years for the treatment group (Denollet and Brutsaert 2001).

Several studies of different types of multicomponent cognitive-behavioral interventions have yielded promising results in terms of functional or clinical outcomes. For example, a controlled pilot study of a stress management intervention for elderly patients with congestive heart failure resulted in significant improvement in perceived stress, emotional distress, depression, and exercise compliance (Luskin et al. 2002). A small study of patients with heart disease receiving eight 90-minute group therapy sessions that were focused on skills training to decrease antagonism (e.g., listening), cynicism (e.g., cognitive restructuring), and anger (e.g., problem-focused coping) was effective in reducing both hostility and blood pressure (Gidron et al. 1999). Blumenthal and colleagues (1997) compared the effects of a stress management intervention consisting of education, cognitive techniques, and relaxation training with those of an exercise condition in a group of patients with coronary artery disease and symptoms of ambulatory or mental stress–induced ischemia. The stress management intervention (sixteen 90-minute group sessions) was associated with a significant reduction in clinical coronary artery disease events at 2- and 5-year follow-up (Blumenthal et al. 1997). The multicomponent program developed by Ornish includes psychological interventions as one of multiple components targeting the risk factors for heart disease (stress management, aerobic exercise, very-low-fat diet, and group support) (Ornish et al. 1998). This intervention has produced a clear reduction in recurrent cardiac events and in severity of coronary artery disease, as well as evidence of improved coronary circulation, compared with standard medical care (Ornish et al. 1998). This intriguing finding is limited by the fact that patients were informed as to which arm of the study they would be entering prior to randomization. In this study, it also remains unclear which components of the multimodal program were the most influential in producing positive outcomes—the psychological components or others directly targeting risk factors for coronary artery disease such as diet or exercise (Ornish et al. 1998; see also Chapter 19, "Heart Disease").

Diabetes

The past decade has seen a growing awareness of the importance of psychosocial factors in diabetes. The goals of treatment for diabetes have undergone radical changes resulting from the findings of the Diabetes Control and Complications Trial Research Group, which presented strong evidence that diabetes complications could be delayed or prevented should patients maintain tight control of their blood glucose levels (Diabetes Control and Complications Trial Research Group 1993; Gonder-Frederick et al. 2002). These treatment recommendations and their psychological implications have had an enormous impact on the study of psychosocial factors in diabetes (see Table

TABLE 38–3. Psychosocial interventions in heart disease

Study	Participants	Diagnosis	Type of intervention	Results of intervention
Ornish et al. 1998	48 patients	Coronary artery disease	Stress management, exercise, very-low-fat diet, group support	Reduced recurrent cardiac events, CAD severity, improved coronary circulation
Black et al. 1998	60 cardiac rehabilitation patients	Post–angina, MI, angioplasty, bypass grafting	One-on-one CBT, relaxation training, stress management for risk factor reduction and improved treatment compliance	Reduced depression in treatment groups; 35% versus 48% rehospitalized
Gidron et al. 1999	22 patients	Coronary heart disease and high level of hostility	Group CBT to modify hostility: listening, cognitive restructuring, and problem-focused coping	Reduction in hostility and blood pressure
Denollet and Brutsaert 2001	150 patients	Coronary heart disease	Multicomponent cardiac rehabilitation: exercise, stress management, and counseling	Less negative affect during 3-month treatment; improved survival for following 9 years
Luskin et al. 2002	14 patients	Congestive heart failure	One-on-one stress management intervention for elderly patients	Improvement in perceived stress, emotional distress, depression, exercise
Petrie et al. 2002	65 patients	First MI	Brief hospital intervention, cognitive restructuring and preparation of a recovery action plan	Significant changes in patient perceptions of their MI; treatment group returned to work faster; lower rate of angina at 3-month follow-up
Blumenthal et al. 1997	107 patients	CAD and ischemia during mental stress testing	Group intervention with stress management training, cognitive techniques, and relaxation training versus exercise	Reduction in clinical CAD events over 2 years of follow-up and after 5 years in group treatment condition

Note. CAD=coronary artery disease; CBT=cognitive-behavioral therapy; MI=myocardial infarction.

38–4 for a summary of these studies). Psychosocial factors are relevant to nearly every aspect of diabetes management (Ciechanowski et al. 2001; Fosbury et al. 1997; Glasgow and Eakin 1998; Gonder-Frederick et al. 2002; Grey et al. 1998; Lustman et al. 1998; Moran et al. 1991; Rubin et al. 1989; Van der Ven et al. 2000; Zettler et al. 1995). It is now clear that psychological interventions can have a positive impact on emotional and physical well-being (Gonder-Frederick et al. 2002), regimen adherence (Ciechanowski et al. 2001), and glycemic control in people living with diabetes (Delamater et al. 2001; Fosbury et al. 1997; Gonder-Frederick et al. 2002; Grey et al. 1998; Lustman et al. 1998; Moran et al. 1991; Rubin et al. 1989; Van der Ven et al. 2000; Zettler et al. 1995).

CBT has proved to be an effective treatment for comorbid depression in diabetes patients (Fosbury et al. 1997; Gonder-Frederick et al. 2002; Grey et al. 1998; Lustman et al. 1998; Rubin et al. 1989; Van der Ven et al. 2000; Zettler et al. 1995). A randomized, controlled trial comparing 10 weeks of individual CBT plus diabetes education with diabetes education alone in depressed patients with type 2 diabetes resulted in greater remission of major depression in the CBT group posttreatment and at 6-month follow-up (Lustman et al. 1998). Other investigators have shown that brief, group-based CBT targeting diabetes-specific issues (e.g., anxiety about complications, relationship problems, beliefs about diabetes that represent barriers to self-care) has shown decreased diabetes-related distress and improved emotional well-being and metabolic control (Van der Ven et al. 2000). Another cognitive approach, cognitive-analytic therapy, has been tested in patients with poorly controlled type 1 diabetes (Fosbury et al. 1997). The intervention, which addressed psychosocial difficulties contributing to self-management problems, resulted in improved interpersonal relationships and glycemic status (Fosbury et al. 1997).

Coping skills training and stress management for adolescents with diabetes have been successful in reducing diabetes-related stress, enhancing social interactions and quality of life, and improving metabolic control (Grey et al. 1998). Similarly, coping skills training in adults effectively decreases diabetes-related anxiety and avoidance behaviors, enhances coping ability and emotional well-being, and improves self-care and glycemic control (Rubin et al. 1989; Zettler et al. 1995). Nonetheless, Gonder-Frederick and colleagues (2002) noted in their recent review that the long-term impact of CBSM on lifestyle factors crucial to the management of the diabetes regimen (such as diet and exercise) has been minimal thus far. Inconsistencies in the effectiveness of psychosocial interventions studied may be due to limited scope, level of competence of the clinicians, and factors specific to the

patients. Brief, goal-directed therapy may not be adequate for overwhelmed chronic medically ill patients.

Long-standing psychosocial problems, dysfunctional interpersonal style, and maladaptive personality traits can interfere with medical management of illness (Ciechanowski et al. 2001; Goodheart and Lansing 1997; Moran et al. 1991). For example, diabetic patients who have an insecure attachment style, particularly a dismissing style, are more likely than patients with secure attachment to be treatment noncompliant, have a poor relationship with medical personnel, and have poor glycemic control (Ciechanowski et al. 2001). The impact of emotional problems, environmental stressors, and intrapsychic processes on medical management of illness has been studied in a small, controlled treatment trial with hospitalized child and adolescent brittle diabetes patients (Moran et al. 1991). Intensive psychoanalytic psychotherapy (three to five sessions per week for 15 weeks) and medical management, compared with medical management alone, was found to produce a notable improvement in glycemic control at posttreatment and 1-year follow-up (Moran et al. 1991). The psychoanalytic treatment protocol was based on the individual participants' medical and psychological assessment, social factors (family, education), and intrapsychic and interpersonal conflicts thought to underlie poor treatment compliance (Moran et al. 1991). The authors concluded that abnormal blood glucose control interfered with daily living, and that multimodal inpatient treatment (psychoanalytic therapy, dynamically informed parental and staff support, and close collaboration with the physician) led to long-term change in this brittle diabetes population (Moran et al. 1991; see also Chapter 23, "Endocrine and Metabolic Disorders").

Arthritis

A number of studies, summarized in Table 38–5, have demonstrated the importance of psychosocial interventions for arthritis patients (Alpay and Cassem 2000; Astin et al. 2002; Bradley and Alberts 1999; Keefe et al. 2002; Leibing et al. 1999; Lorig et al. 1985; McCracken 1991; Mullen et al. 1987; Parker et al. 1993; Sharpe et al. 2001). Although the early studies focused mainly on arthritis pain (Bradley and Alberts 1999; McCracken 1991; Parker et al. 1993), emphasis has recently shifted toward a broader range of arthritis-related problems. Psychosocial interventions currently address issues such as psychological disturbance, interpersonal distress, and physical functioning (Alpay and Cassem 2000; Keefe et al. 2002). Psychoeducation and cognitive-behavioral interventions have led to substantial benefits in the management of arthritis (Lorig et al. 1985; Mullen et al. 1987), resulting in dimin-

TABLE 38–4. Psychosocial interventions in diabetes

Study	Participants	Diagnosis	Type of intervention	Results of intervention
Lane et al. 1993	38 patients	Type 2 diabetes	Biofeedback assisted relaxation training	Improved glycosylated hemoglobin level, no improvement in glucose tolerance
Zettler et al. 1995	17 patients	Diabetes	Group CBT (exposure, relaxation and cognitive restructuring)	Reduced fear of long-term complications, improved acceptance of diabetes and metabolic control
Aikens et al. 1997	22 patients	Type 2 diabetes	Relaxation training (PMR/imagery)	No difference
Fosbury et al. 1997	26 patients	Type 1 diabetes, poorly controlled	Cognitive analytic therapy versus diabetes education	Improved interpersonal problems and glycemic control in treatment group, maintained at 9-month follow-up
Grey et al. 1998	65 adolescents	Type 1 diabetes	Intensive insulin therapy with coping skills training versus insulin treatment	Improved glycemic control, diabetes self-efficacy, quality of life in treatment group
Lustman et al. 1998	51 patients	Type 2 diabetes with major depression	One-on-one CBT	Remission of depression greater (85% in CBT group, 27.3% in control group); improved glycemic control with treatment
Snoek et al. 2001	24 patients	Type 1 diabetes, poorly controlled	Group CBT	Improved glycemic control
Surwit et al. 2002	108 patients	Type 2 diabetes	Group diabetes education program with or without stress management training	Significant reduction in glycosylated hemoglobin level at 1-year follow-up in the stress management group

Note. CBT=cognitive-behavioral therapy; PMR=progressive muscle relaxation.

TABLE 38–5. Psychosocial interventions in arthritis

Study	Participants	Diagnosis	Type of intervention	Results of intervention
Lorig et al. 1989	707 patients	Osteoarthritis and rheumatoid arthritis	Psychoeducation, lay-leaders: illness and treatment, nutrition and exercise, training in relaxation, problem-solving, communication	Improved knowledge, increased adaptive behaviors, and reduced pain
Kelley et al. 1997	70 patients	Rheumatoid arthritis	Oral emotional disclosure: 15 minutes on 4 consecutive days	Immediate increase in negative mood, better physical functioning, decreased affective disturbance at 3 months
Leibing et al. 1999	55 patients	Rheumatoid arthritis	12 weekly sessions of CBT	Reduction in passive, emotion-focused coping; helplessness, depression; anxiety; affective pain; and fluctuation of pain
Sharpe et al. 2001	53 patients	Rheumatoid arthritis (onset <2 years)	CBT intervention	Reduced depressive symptoms posttreatment and at follow-up; reduced C-reactive protein levels; improved joint involvement
Smyth et al. 1999	112 patients	Rheumatoid arthritis	Written exercise of emotional disclosure	Reduced disease severity

Note. CBT=cognitive-behavioral therapy.

ished psychological distress, improved marital adjustment, and reduced disease-related symptomatology (e.g., joint swelling and fatigue) (Astin et al. 2002; Keefe et al. 2002). Interpersonal therapy has been effective in treating major depression in patients with rheumatological diseases (Alpay and Cassem 2000).

Several studies have shown that CBT is more effective in managing some disease-related symptoms of rheumatoid arthritis than some standard treatments such as physical or occupational therapy (Leibing et al. 1999; Radojevic et al. 1992; Sharpe et al. 2001). A recent randomized, controlled study of patients with rheumatoid arthritis found improvements in pain fluctuation, affect, coping, and emotional stability as well as a slower progression of disease course in the treatment group (12 weekly sessions of CBT) (Leibing et al. 1999). In a blind, randomized, controlled study with early stage rheumatoid arthritis patients (less than 2 years post-diagnosis), a multicomponent CBT intervention consisting of education, relaxation training, attention diversion, goal setting, pacing, problem solving, cognitive restructuring, assertiveness and communication, and management of high-risk situations was compared with a control group receiving standard care (Sharpe et al. 2001). The treatment produced significant reduction in depressive symptoms and improvement in joint involvement at 6-month follow-up (Sharpe et al. 2001). A reduction in C-reactive protein levels (a sensitive measure of disease activity in rheumatoid arthritis) was found in the intervention group posttreatment, although this disappeared at follow-up (Sharpe et al. 2001).

A different type of stress management approach has shown interesting results in arthritis patients. Emotional disclosure, a model in which individuals write or talk privately about a stressful life event, disclosing their intimate thoughts and feelings, led to decreased physiological activity and better self-reported health in healthy people (Pennebaker and Beall 1986; Pennebaker et al. 1988). A recent quantitative review indicated that emotional disclosure is associated with significant improvement in physical health, psychological well-being, and physiological and general functioning (Kelley et al. 1997; Smyth 1998; Smyth et al. 1999; Spiegel 1999). A study of oral emotional disclosure for persons with rheumatoid arthritis found significantly less physical dysfunction and affective disturbance in participants in the disclosure condition compared with control participants at 3-month follow-up (Kelley et al. 1997). In this case, however, the intervention did not lead to any group differences in pain or joint condition. Immediate increases in negative mood were experienced by disclosure patients following the intervention, although participants with more negative mood at baseline experienced the best long-term improvement in

joint condition (Kelley et al. 1997). This paradigm has also been applied to written emotional disclosure exercises with arthritis patients (Smyth 1998; Smyth et al. 1999).

Despite the promising results of these interventions, a recent literature review failed to confirm the superior efficacy of cognitive-behavioral interventions over other interventions (Astin et al. 2002). For arthritis-related outcomes such as pain and disability, long-term effects of the interventions seemed difficult to maintain, whereas depression and joint tenderness may further improve over time (Astin et al. 2002). Identifying the mechanisms of action of psychosocial interventions is obviously complex. In arthritis, however, it appears that patients' enhanced self-efficacy may be a pivotal factor in achieving and maintaining important treatment gains (Lorig et al. 1989; see also Chapter 25, "Rheumatology").

HIV/AIDS

Psychosocial interventions have been used as an adjunct to medical treatment and have benefited emotional health as well as physiological parameters in people with HIV/AIDS (Antoni et al. 2000a, 2000b, 2001; Chesney et al. 1996; D.G. Cruess et al. 2000a, 2000c; Kalichman et al. 1995; Kelly 1998; Kelly et al. 1993; Lutgendorf et al. 1997, 1998; Mulder et al. 1994; Spiegel and Classen 2000; Spiegel et al. 1981; Treisman et al. 2001).

Interventions designed to decrease distress, improve coping mechanisms, influence disease progression (Chesney et al. 1996), increase self-efficacy, and decrease perceived anxiety, depressed mood, hostility, anger, and somatization (Antoni et al. 1991; Antoni et al. 2001; Chesney et al. 1996; S. Cruess et al. 2000; Kelly et al. 1993; Lutgendorf et al. 1997, 1998; Mulder et al. 1994) have met with success (see Table 38–6 for a summary of relevant studies). These studies frequently have employed cognitive and/or behavioral approaches, CBSM, and IPT. The interventions described, using an individual or group format, include relaxation skills training and practice, cognitive restructuring, instruction in self-monitoring of environmental stressors, social skills training, and interpersonal psychotherapy.

Two studies compared different psychotherapy approaches for individuals with HIV (Kelly et al. 1993; Mulder et al. 1994). Kelly et al. (1993) compared eight sessions of group-based CBSM, supportive-expressive group therapy (Spiegel and Classen 2000; Spiegel et al. 1981), and a control group (individual counseling on demand) in depressed men with HIV/AIDS. The authors (Kelly et al. 1993) found that both the CBSM and the supportive-expressive groups had reduced depressed mood, hostility,

TABLE 38–6. Psychosocial interventions in HIV

Study	Participants	Diagnosis	Type of intervention	Results of intervention
Antoni et al. 1991	47 healthy gay men	Asymptomatic	CBSM intervention, anticipating HIV test results for 5 weeks; adjust to HIV status, lifestyle needs during following 5 weeks	Treatment group had less anxiety or depression after notification; decreased CD4 and NK cell counts in response to the HIV-positive diagnosis in control group
Kelly et al. 1993	68 men	HIV/AIDS; moderate depression	Group CBSM versus socially supportive group therapy	Reduced depressed mood, hostility, somatization in CBSM and socially supportive groups; reduced psychiatric symptoms and anxiety in socially supportive group; reduced illicit drug use in CBSM group; socially supportive group therapy superior to CBSM in reducing psychological distress at 3 months
Mulder et al. 1994	39 men	Asymptomatic HIV-positive	Group CBSM, group experiential therapy, or wait-list control	CBSM and experiential therapy decreased POMS-defined total mood disturbance and Beck Depression Inventory scores
Chesney et al. 1996	149 gay men	HIV-positive	Coping effectiveness training (problem-focused or emotion-focused), HIV education group, or wait-list control	Increased self-efficacy and decreased perceived stress with coping effectiveness training; no differences among conditions in changes in CD4 count or symptoms
Lutgendorf et al. 1997	40 men	Symptomatic HIV-positive	Group CBSM	Decreased dysphoria, anxiety, total distress, and HSV-2 antibody titers in CBSM group; no difference in CD4 count
Antoni et al. 2000a	73 gay men	HIV-positive	10-week CBSM intervention	CBSM decreased anxiety, anger, total mood disturbance, perceived stress; decreased urinary norepinephrine predicted a slower decline in CD8 count at 6- to 12-month follow-up in CBSM group
Antoni et al. 2000b	59 gay men	HIV-positive	CBSM intervention	Decreased depressed mood paralleled by reductions in urinary free cortisol
D. G. Cruess et al. 2000c	30 gay men	HIV-positive	Weekly relaxation training sessions in a 10-week group-based CBSM intervention	Decreases in mood disturbance and anxiety related to reductions in pre-session salivary cortisol levels; reduced cortisol levels in early sessions associated with more frequent relaxation practice
D. G. Cruess et al. 2000a	65 gay men	Symptomatic HIV-positive	Group CBSM	Increased urinary free testosterone levels associated with reduced distress

Note. CBSM = cognitive-behavioral stress management; HSV-2 = herpes simplex virus type 2; POMS = Profile of Mood States.

and somatization. Whereas the CBSM group had reduced illicit drug use, the social support group experienced a reduction in overall psychiatric symptoms and anxiety. The social support group was superior to the CBSM group in reducing psychological distress and maintaining treatment gains at 3-month follow-up (Kelly et al. 1993). Mulder and colleagues (1994) compared group-based CBSM with experiential therapy (17 sessions over 15 weeks) for HIV-positive men. Men in both conditions experienced decreased distress, although no differences were noted between the two treatments with regard to coping, social support, or emotional expression (Mulder et al. 1994).

In a 3-month coping effectiveness training intervention based on Lazarus and Folkman's (1984) stress and coping theory, a group of HIV-positive homosexual men were taught to match coping strategies to stressors (e.g., emotion-focused strategies for uncontrollable stressors and problem-focused coping strategies for controllable stressors) (Chesney et al. 1996). Men in the coping effectiveness training condition reported less perceived stress, reduced emotional distress, and improved self-efficacy (Chesney et al. 1996). A recent study using the National Institute of Mental Health Treatment of Depression Collaborative Research Program four-group design (IPT, CBT, support with imipramine, support only) with depressed HIV-positive patients found that patients in both the IPT and the support with imipramine conditions had more symptom reduction than did those in the CBT and support-only conditions (Markowitz et al. 1998).

Several studies suggest that psychological interventions have the potential to improve not only psychological well-being but also biological parameters for people with HIV/AIDS (Antoni et al. 2000a, 2000b; D.G. Cruess et al. 2000a, 2000c; S. Cruess et al. 2000). Interventions characterized by a strong emphasis on relaxation (CBSM, relaxation techniques, and cognitive-behavioral packages) have been demonstrated to have positive psychosocial effects while effecting modulations in biological variables in HIV-positive patients, including reduction in cortisol levels, increase in urinary free testosterone levels, reduction in 24-hour urinary norepinephrine output, reduction in herpes simplex virus type-2 antibody titers, and changes in CD8 counts. Such neuroendocrine and immunological changes are currently considered positive biological system markers of HIV status (Antoni et al. 2000a, 2000b; D.G. Cruess et al. 2000a, 2000c; S. Cruess et al. 2000; Lutgendorf et al. 1997; Schneiderman et al. 2001).

One randomized, controlled study of a 10-week CBSM intervention targeting homosexual and bisexual men awaiting notification of HIV status focused on anticipation of HIV test results for the first 5 weeks and on ad-

justing to HIV status and lifestyle needs during the following 5 weeks (Antoni et al. 1991). The intervention group had increased CD4 (T-helper) cell counts and CD56 (natural killer) cells (Antoni et al. 1991). Another randomized, controlled study investigated a CBSM intervention that included 10 sessions of education about stress and the benefits of relaxation, cognitive restructuring, coping skills and assertiveness training, anger management, and identification of social supports for symptomatic HIV-positive men (Lutgendorf et al. 1998). The CBSM group had significant improvement in cognitive coping strategies (positive reframing and acceptance of the illness) and social supports (attachment and alliance formation). Men in the intervention group also had significant decreases in self-reported dysphoria, anxiety, and total distress. Although neither group showed changes in CD4 counts, the intervention group had decreases in herpes simplex virus type 2 antibody titers, a parameter that may be a marker of immunocompetence (Lutgendorf et al. 1998). Two other studies using the same model of CBSM showed decreases in depressed mood that were closely paralleled by reductions in urinary free cortisol (Antoni et al. 2000b; D.G. Cruess et al. 2000c). In the study by Cruess and colleagues (2000c), greater reductions in cortisol during early sessions were associated with more frequent relaxation practice at home.

Consultation psychiatry is integral in the treatment of patients with HIV/AIDS who have chronic mental illness, personality disorders, and addiction. Difficulties include risky sexual practices, continued drug abuse and needle sharing, limited access to treatment, treatment noncompliance, and a range of psychosocial problems associated with living on the fringes of society (poverty, homelessness, isolation) (Clark and Everall 1997; Kalichman et al. 1995; Treisman et al. 2001; see Chapter 28, "HIV/AIDS").

Conclusion

There is considerable evidence that a variety of psychotherapeutic interventions provide substantial benefits for people in various stages of coping with medical illness (Compas et al. 1998). Techniques ranging from intensive individual psychotherapies to group, psychoeducational, and family approaches can enhance coping, reduce distress, improve adherence to medical treatment, diminish pain, and facilitate optimal functioning. Furthermore, better adjustment to illness may translate into a reduction of the cost of care (reduction in utilization of medical services, reduction in medication needs) (Lang and Rosen 2002; Sobel 1995). Further research should enable a better identification of the most efficient interventions and allow researchers to identify which components of these interventions are the most promising with respect to the type and stage of illness and the specific needs of patients. More study is needed to better understand psychophysiological mechanisms affected by psychotherapeutic interventions. However, it is clear that psychotherapeutic techniques are effective complements to modern biotechnological medical treatment, particularly in improving quality of life.

References

Abramowitz JS, Schwartz SA, Whiteside SP: A contemporary conceptual model of hypochondriasis. Mayo Clin Proc 77:1323–1330, 2002

Aikens JE, Kiolbasa TA, Sobel R: Psychological predictors of glycemic change with relaxation training in non-insulin-dependent diabetes mellitus. Psychother Psychosom 66:302–306, 1997

Allan R, Scheidt S: Group psychotherapy for patients with coronary heart disease. Int J Group Psychother 48:187–214, 1998

Allen SM, Shah AC, Nezu AM, et al: A problem-solving approach to stress reduction among younger women with breast cancer: a randomized controlled trial. Cancer 94:3089–3100, 2002

Alpay M, Cassem EH: Diagnosis and treatment of mood disorders in patients with rheumatic disease. Ann Rheum Dis 59:2–4, 2000

Alter CL, Pelcovitz D, Axelrod A, et al: Identification of PTSD in cancer survivors. Psychosomatics 37:137–143, 1996

Anda R, Williamson DF, Jones D, et al: Depressed affect, hopelessness, and the risks of ischaemic heart disease in a cohort of U.S. adults. Epidemiology 4:285–294, 1993

Andersen BL: Psychological interventions for cancer patients to enhance the quality of life. J Consult Clin Psychol 60:552–568, 1992

Andersen BL: Biobehavioral outcomes following psychological interventions for cancer patients. J Consult Clin Psychol 70:590–610, 2002

Andersen BL, Kiecolt-Glaser JK, Glaser R, et al: A biobehavioral model of cancer stress and disease course. Am Psychol 49:389–404, 1994

Anderson BJ, Brackett J: Diabetes during childhood, in Psychology in Diabetes Care. Edited by Snoek FJ, Skinner C. London, Wiley, 2000, pp 1–24

Andrykowski MA, Cordova MJ: Factors associated with PTSD symptoms following treatment for breast cancer: test of the Anderson model. J Trauma Stress 11:189–203, 1998

Andrykowski MA, Cordova MJ, Studts JL, et al: Posttraumatic stress disorder after treatment for breast cancer: prevalence of diagnosis and the use of the PTSD Checklist—Civilian Version (PCL-C) as a screening instrument. J Consult Clin Psychol 66:586–590, 1998

Andrykowski MA, Cordova MJ, McGrath PC, et al: Stability and change in posttraumatic stress disorder symptoms following breast cancer treatment: a 1-year follow-up. Psycho-Oncology 9:69–78, 2000

Antoni MH, Baggett L, Ironson G, et al: Cognitive-behavioral stress management intervention buffers distress responses and immunologic changes following notification of HIV-1 seropositivity. J Consult Clin Psychol 59:906–915, 1991

Antoni MH, Cruess DG, Cruess S, et al: Cognitive-behavioral stress management intervention effects on anxiety, 24-hr urinary norepinephrine output, and T-cytotoxic/suppressor cells over time among symptomatic HIV-infected gay men. J Consult Clin Psychol 68:31–45, 2000a

Antoni MH, Cruess S, Cruess DG, et al: Cognitive-behavioral stress management reduces distress and 24-hour urinary free cortisol output among symptomatic HIV-infected gay men. Ann Behav Med 22:29–37, 2000b

Antoni MH, Lehman JM, Kilbourn KM, et al: Cognitive-behavioral stress management intervention decreases the prevalence of depression and enhances the benefit finding among women under treatment for early stage breast cancer. Health Psychol 20:20–32, 2001

Ashby MA, Kissane DW, Beadle GF, et al: Psychosocial support, treatment of metastatic disease and palliative care. Med J Aust 164:43–49, 1996

Astin JA, Beckner W, Soeken K, et al: Psychological interventions for rheumatoid arthritis: a meta-analysis of randomized controlled trials. Arthritis Rheum 47:291–302, 2002

Barry JJ, Sanborn K: Etiology, diagnosis, and treatment of nonepileptic seizures. Curr Neurol Neurosci Rep 1:381–389, 2001

Barry JJ, Atzman O, Morrell MJ: Discriminating between epileptic and nonepileptic events: the utility of hypnotic seizure induction. Epilepsia 41:81–84, 2000

Bauer M, Whybrow PC: Depression and other psychiatric illnesses associated with medical conditions. Curr Opin Psychiatry 12:325–329, 1999

Beck AT, Weishaar ME: Cognitive therapy, in Current Psychotherapies, 4th Edition. Edited by Corsini RJ, Wedding D. Itasca, IL, F.E. Peacock, 1989, pp 285–320

Bemporad JR, Vasile RG: Psychotherapy. New York, Wiley, 1990

Beresnevaite M: Exploring the benefits of group psychotherapy in reducing alexithymia in coronary heart disease patients: a preliminary study. Psychother Psychosom 69:117–122, 2000

Berkman LF, Leo-Summers L, Horwitz RI: Emotional support and survival after myocardial infarction: a prospective, population-based study of the elderly. Ann Intern Med 117:1003–1009, 1992

Black JL, Allison TG, Williams DE, et al: Effect of intervention for psychological distress on rehospitalization rates in cardiac rehabilitation patients. Psychosomatics 39:134–143, 1998

Blechner ML: Psychodynamic Approaches to AIDS and HIV. Mahwah, NJ, Analytic Press, 1997

Bloch S, Kissane D: Psychotherapies in psycho-oncology. An exciting new challenge. Br J Psychiatry 177:112–116, 2000

Block SD: Assessing and managing depression in the terminally ill patient. ACP-ASIM End-of-Life Care Consensus Panel. American College of Physicians–American Society of Internal Medicine. Ann Intern Med 132:209–218, 2000

Blumenthal JA, Jiang W, Babyak MA, et al: Stress management and exercise training in cardiac patients with myocardial ischemia: effects on prognosis and evaluation of mechanisms. Arch Intern Med 157:2213–2223, 1997

Bowman ES, Markand ON: Psychodynamics and psychiatric diagnoses of pseudoseizure subjects. Am J Psychiatry 153:57–63, 1996

Bradley LA, Alberts KR: Psychological and behavioral approaches to pain management for patients with rheumatic disease. Rheum Dis Clin North Am 25:215–232, viii, 1999

Burger JM: Negative reactions to increases in perceived personal control. J Pers Soc Psychol 56:246–256, 1989

Burish TG, Tope DM: Psychological techniques for controlling the adverse side effects of cancer chemotherapy: findings from a decade of research. J Pain Symptom Manage 7:287–301, 1992

Carey MP, Burish TG: Etiology and treatment of the psychological side effects associated with cancer chemotherapy: a critical review and discussion. Psychol Bull 104:307–325, 1988

Chesney M, Folkman S, Chambers D: Coping effectiveness training for men living with HIV: preliminary findings. Int J STD AIDS 7 (suppl 2):75–82, 1996

Christensen AJ, Ehlers SL: Psychological factors in end-stage renal disease: an emerging context for behavioral medicine research. J Consult Clin Psychol 70:712–724, 2002

Ciechanowski PS, Katon WJ, Russo JE, et al: A patient–provider relationship: attachment theory and adherence to treatment in diabetes. Am J Psychiatry 158:29–35, 2001

Clark BR, Everall IP: What is the role of the HIV liaison psychiatrist? Genitourin Med 73:568–570, 1997

Clarkin JF, Yeomans FE, Kernberg OF: Psychotherapy for Borderline Personality. New York, Wiley, 1999

Classen C, Butler LD, Koopman C, et al: Supportive-expressive group therapy and distress in patients with metastatic breast cancer: a randomized clinical intervention trial. Arch Gen Psychiatry 58:494–501, 2001

Compas BE, Haaga DA, Keefe FJ, et al: Sampling of empirically supported psychological treatments from health psychology: smoking, chronic pain, cancer, and bulimia nervosa. J Consult Clin Psychol 66:89–112, 1998

Cordova MJ, Studts JL, Hann DM, et al: Symptom structure of PTSD following breast cancer. J Trauma Stress 13:301–319, 2000

Coulehan JL, Schulberg HC, Block MR, et al: Treating depressed primary care patients improves their physical, mental, and social functioning. Arch Intern Med 157:1113–1120, 1997

Coyne JC, Thompson R, Klinkman MS, et al: Emotional disorders in primary care. J Consult Clin Psychol 70:798–809, 2002

Craighead WE, Wilcoxon Craighead L, Ilardi SS, et al: Psychosocial treatments for major depressive disorder, in A Guide to Treatments that Work. Edited by Nathan PE, Gorman JM. New York, Oxford University Press, 1998, pp 226–239

Cruess DG, Antoni MH, Schneiderman N, et al: Cognitive-behavioral stress management increases free testosterone and decreases psychological distress in HIV-seropositive men. Health Psychol 19:12–20, 2000a

Cruess DG, Antoni MH, McGregor BA, et al: Cognitive-behavioral stress management reduces serum cortisol by enhancing benefit finding among women being treated for early stage breast cancer. Psychosom Med 62:304–308, 2000b

Cruess DG, Antoni MH, Kumar M, et al: Reductions in salivary cortisol are associated with mood improvement during relaxation training among HIV-seropositive men. J Behav Med 23:107–122, 2000c

Cruess S, Antoni M, Cruess D, et al: Reductions in herpes simplex virus type 2 antibody titers after cognitive behavioral stress management and relationships with neuroendocrine function, relaxation skills, and social support in HIV-positive men. Psychosom Med 62:828–837, 2000

Cunningham AJ, Edmonds CV, Jenkins GP, et al: A randomized controlled trial of the effects of group psychological therapy on survival in women with metastatic breast cancer. Psychooncology 7:508–517, 1998

De Ridder D, Schreurs K: Developing interventions for chronically ill patients: is coping a helpful concept? Clin Psychol Rev 21:205–240, 2001

Delamater AM, Jacobson AM, Anderson B, et al: Psychosocial therapies in diabetes: report of the Psychosocial Therapies Working Group. Diabetes Care 24:1286–1292, 2001

Denollet J, Brutsaert DL: Reducing emotional distress improves prognosis in coronary heart disease: 9-year mortality in a clinical trial of rehabilitation. Circulation 104:2018–2023, 2001

Derogatis LR, Morrow GR, Fetting J, et al: The prevalence of psychiatric disorders among cancer patients. JAMA 249:751–757, 1983

Devine EC, Westlake SK: The effects of psychoeducational care provided to adults with cancer: meta-analysis of 116 studies. Oncol Nurs Forum 22:1369–1381, 1995

Diabetes Control and Complications Trial Research Group: The effect of intensive treatment of diabetes on the development and progression of long-term complications in insulin-dependent diabetes mellitus. N Engl J Med 329:977–986, 1993

Donnelly J, Kornblith AB, Fleishman S, et al: A pilot study of interpersonal psychotherapy by telephone with cancer patients and their partners. Psycho-Oncology 9:44–56, 2000

Duff AJA: Psychological interventions in cystic fibrosis and asthma. Paediatr Respir Rev 2:350–357, 2001

Dunkel-Schetter EC, Westlake SK: The effects of psychoeducational care provided to adults with cancer: meta-analysis of 116 studies. Oncol Nurs Forum 22:1369–1381, 1995

Dusseldorp E, van Elderen T, Maes S, et al: A meta-analysis of psychoeduational programs for coronary heart disease patients. Health Psychol 18:506–519, 1999

Edelman S, Lemon J, Bell DR, et al: Effects of group CBT on the survival time of patients with metastatic breast cancer. Psychooncology 8:474–481, 1999

Ehlert U, Wagner D, Lupke U: Consultation-liaison service in the general hospital: effects of cognitive-behavioral therapy in patients with physical nonspecific symptoms. J Psychosom Res 47:411–417, 1999

Elsesser K, van Berkel M, Sartory G, et al: The effects of anxiety management training on psychological variables and immune parameters in cancer patients: a pilot study. Behavioral and Cognitive Psychotherapy 22:13–23, 1994

Emmelkamp PM, van Oppen P: Cognitive interventions in behavioral medicine. Psychother Psychosom 59:116–130, 1993

Esterling BA, Antoni MH, Schneiderman N, et al: Psychosocial modulation of antibody to Epstein-Barr viral capsid antigen and human herpesvirus type-6 in HIV-1-infected and at-risk gay men. Psychosom Med 54:354–371, 1992

Evans DL, Staab JP, Petitto JM, et al: Depression in the medical setting: biopsychological interactions and treatment considerations. J Clin Psychiatry 60:40–55, 1999

Fallowfield LJ: Behavioural interventions and psychological aspects of care during chemotherapy. Eur J Cancer 28 (suppl 1): S39–S41, 1992

Fawzy FI, Fawzy NW, Hyun CS, et al: Malignant melanoma: effects of an early structured psychiatric intervention, coping, and affective state on recurrence and survival 6 years later. Arch Gen Psychiatry 50:681–689, 1993

Fawzy FI, Fawzy NW, Arndt LA, et al: Critical review of psychosocial interventions in cancer care. Arch Gen Psychiatry 52:100–113, 1995

Fawzy FI, Canada AL, Fawzy NW, et al: Malignant melanoma: effects of a brief, structured psychiatric intervention on survival and recurrence at 10-year follow-up. Arch Gen Psychiatry 60:100–103, 2003

Faymonville ME, Fissette J, Mambourg PH, et al: Hypnosis as adjunct therapy in conscious sedation for plastic surgery. Reg Anesth 20:145–151, 1995

Ferlic M, Goldman A, Kennedy BJ: Group counseling in adult patients with advanced cancer. Cancer 43:760–766, 1979

Fitzpatrick MC: The psychologic assessment and psychosocial recovery of the patient with an amputation. Clin Orthop 361:98–107, 1999

Foley VD: Family therapy, in Current Psychotherapies, 4th Edition. Edited by Corsini RJ, Wedding D. Itasca, IL, FE Peacock, 1989, pp 455–500

Folkman S, Moskowitz JT: Positive affect and the other side of coping. Am Psychol 55:647–654, 2000

Fosbury JA, Bosley CM, Ryle A, et al: A trial of cognitive analytic therapy in poorly controlled type I patients. Diabetes Care 20:959–964, 1997

Frank E, Kupfer DJ, Perel JM, et al: Three-year outcomes for maintenance therapies in recurrent depression: contributing factors. Arch Gen Psychiatry 47:1093–1099, 1990

Frank E, Kupfer DJ, Wagner EF, et al: Efficacy of interpersonal psychotherapy as a maintenance treatment of recurrent depression. Arch Gen Psychiatry 48:1053–1059, 1991

Frasure-Smith N, Prince R: The ischemic heart disease life stress monitoring program: impact on mortality. Psychosom Med 47:431–445, 1985

Frasure-Smith N, Lesperance F, Prince RH, et al: Randomised trial of home-based psychosocial nursing intervention for patients recovering from myocardial infarction. Lancet 350:473–479, 1997

Freeman A: Cognitive therapy, in Handbook of Comparative Treatments for Adult Disorders. Edited by Bellack AS, Hersen M. New York, Wiley, 1990, pp 64–87

Friedman M, Thoreson CE, Gill JJ, et al: Alteration of type-A behavior and its effects on cardiac recurrences in post-myocardial infarction in patients: summary results of the Recurrent Coronary Prevention Project. Am Heart J 112: 653–665, 1986

Gabbard G: Psychodynamic Psychiatry in Clinical Practice. Washington, DC, American Psychiatric Press Inc, 1994

Gabbard G, Kay J: The fate of integrated treatment: whatever happened to the biopsychosocial psychiatrist? Am J Psychiatry 158:1956–1963, 2001

Gidron Y, Davidson K, Bata I: The short-term effects of a hostility-reduction intervention on male coronary heart disease patients. Health Psychol 18:416–420, 1999

Giese-Davis J, Koopman C, Butler LD, et al: Change in emotion-regulation strategy for women with metastatic breast cancer following supportive-expressive group therapy. J Consult Clin Psychol 70:916–925, 2002

Gillies L: Interpersonal Therapy. New York, Oxford University Press, 2002

Glasgow RE, Eakin EG: Issues in diabetes self-management, in The Handbook of Health Behavior Change. Edited by Shumaker SA, Schron EB, Ockene J, et al. New York, Springer, 1998, pp 435–461

Glasgow RE, Toobert DJ, Riddle M, et al: Diabetes-specific social learning variables and self-care behaviors among persons with type II diabetes. Health Psychol 8:285–303, 1989

Gonder-Frederick LA, Cox DJ, Ritterband LM: Diabetes and behavioral medicine: the second decade. J Consult Clin Psychol 70:611–625, 2002

Goodheart CD, Lansing MH: Treating People With Chronic Disease: A Psychological Guide. Washington, DC, American Psychological Association, 1997

Goodwin PJ, Leszcz M, Ennis M, et al: The effect of group psychosocial support on survival in metastatic breast cancer. N Engl J Med 345:1719–1726, 2001

Gottschalk LA: Content analysis of speech in psychiatric research. Compr Psychiatry 19:387–392, 1978

Gottschalk LA, Gleser GC: The Measurement of Psychological States Through the Content Analysis of Verbal Behavior. Berkeley, CA, University of California Press, 1969

Green BL, Rowland JH, Krupnick JL, et al: Prevalence of post-traumatic stress disorder in women with breast cancer. Psychosomatics 39:102–111, 1998

Greenberg LS, Ford CL, Alden LS, et al: In-session change in emotionally focused therapy. J Consult Clin Psychol 61: 78–84, 1993

Grey M, Cameron ME, Lipman TH, et al: Psychosocial status of children with diabetes in the first 2 years after diagnosis. Diabetes Care 18:1330–1336, 1995

Grey M, Boland EA, Davidson M, et al: Short-term effects of coping skills training as adjunct to intensive therapy in adolescents. Diabetes Care 21:902–908, 1998

Gruber BL, Hersh SP, Hall NR, et al: Immunological responses of breast cancer patients to behavioral interventions. Biofeedback Self Regul 18:1–22, 1993

Gustafson J, Whitman H: Towards a balanced social environment on the oncology service. Soc Psychiatry 13:147–152, 1978

Guthrie E: Emotional disorder in chronic illness: psychotherapeutic interventions. Br J Psychiatry 168:265–285, 1996

Guthrie EA, Creed FH, Dawson D, et al: A controlled trial of psychological treatment for the irritable bowel syndrome. Gastroenterology 100:450–457, 1991

Hay J, Passik SD: The cancer patient with borderline personality disorder: suggestions for symptom-focused management in the medical setting. Psycho-Oncology 9:91–100, 2000

Helgeson VS, Cohen S, Schulz R, et al: Education and peer discussion group interventions and adjustment to breast cancer. Arch Gen Psychiatry 56:340–347, 1999

Helmers KF, Krantz DS, Howell RH, et al: Hostility and myocardial ischemia in coronary artery disease patients: evaluation by gender and ischemic index. Psychosom Med 55:29–36, 1993

Hener T, Weisenberg M, Har-Even D: Supportive versus cognitive-behavioral intervention programs in achieving adjustment to home peritoneal kidney dialysis. J Consult Clin Psychol 64:731–741, 1996

Herman JL: Trauma and Recovery. New York, Basic Books, 1992

Holahan CJ, Moos RH, Holahan CK, et al: Social support, coping, and depressive symptoms in a late-middle-aged sample of patients reporting cardiac illness. Health Psychol 14:152–163, 1995

Holland JC: History of psycho-oncology: overcoming attitudinal and conceptual barriers. Psychosom Med 64:206–221, 2002

Hollon SD, Beck AT: Cognitive and cognitive-behavioral therapies, in Handbook of Psychotherapy and Behavior Change. Edited by Bergin AE, Garfield SL. New York, Wiley, 1994, pp 428–466

Holroyd J: Hypnosis treatment of clinical pain: understanding why hypnosis is useful. Int J Clin Exp Hypn 44:33–51, 1996

Holroyd KA: Assessment and psychological management of recurrent headache disorders. J Consult Clin Psychol 70:656–677, 2002

House JS, Landis KR, Umberson D: Social relationships and health. Science 241:540–545, 1988

Ilnyckyj A, Farber J, Cheang MC, et al: A randomized controlled trial of psychotherapeutic intervention in cancer patients. Ann R Coll Physicians Surg Can 27:93–96, 1994

Januzzi JL, Stern TA, Pasternack RC, et al: The influence of anxiety and depression on outcomes of patients with coronary artery disease. Arch Intern Med 160:1913–1921, 2000

Jones DA, West RR: Psychological rehabilitation after myocardial infarction: a multicenter randomized controlled trial. BMJ 313:1515–1521, 1996

Julkunen J, Salonen R, Kaplan GA, et al: Hostility and the progression of carotid atherosclerosis. Psychosom Med 56:519–525, 1994

Kalichman SC, Sikkema KJ, Kelly JA, et al: Use of a brief behavioral skills intervention to prevent HIV infection among chronic mentally ill adults. Psychiatr Serv 46:275–280, 1995

Kaplan HI, Sadock BJ, Gregg JA, et al: Synopsis of Psychiatry. Baltimore, MD, Williams & Wilkins, 1994

Kawachi I, Colditz GA, Ascherio A, et al: Prospective study of phobic anxiety and risk of coronary heart disease in men. Circulation 89:1992–1997, 1994

Kazak AE, Simms S, Barakat L, et al: Surviving Cancer Competently Intervention Program (SCCIP): a cognitive-behavioral and family therapy intervention for adolescent survivors of childhood cancer and their families. Fam Process 38:175–190, 1999

Keefe FJ, Smith SJ, Buffington AL, et al: Recent advances and future directions in the biopsychosocial assessment and treatment of arthritis. J Consult Clin Psychol 70:640–655, 2002

Kelley JE, Lumley MA, Leisen JC: Health effects of emotional disclosure in rheumatoid arthritis patients. Health Psychol 16:331–340, 1997

Kelly JA: Group psychotherapy for persons with HIV and AIDS-related illnesses. Int J Group Psychother 48:143–162, 1998

Kelly JA, Murphy DA, Bahr GR, et al: Outcome of cognitive-behavioral and support group brief therapies for depressed, HIV-infected persons. Am J Psychiatry 150:1679–1686, 1993

Ketterer MW: Secondary prevention of ischemic heart disease. Psychosomatics 34:478–484, 1993

Kibby MY, Tyc VL, Mulhern RK, et al: Effectiveness of psychological intervention for children and adolescents with chronic medical illness: a meta-analysis. Clin Psychol Rev 18:103–117, 1998

Kissane DW, Bloch S, McKenzie M, et al: Family grief therapy: a preliminary account of a new model to promote healthy family functioning during palliative care and bereavement. Psycho-Oncology 7:14–25, 1998

Klausner EJ, Alexopoulos GA: The future of psychosocial treatments for elderly patients. Psychiatr Serv 50:1198–1204, 1999

Kogon MM, Biswas A, Pearl D, et al: Effects of medical and psychotherapeutic treatment on the survival of women with metastatic breast carcinoma. Cancer 80:225–230, 1997

Koike AK, Unutzer J, Wells KB: Improving the care for depression in patients with comorbid medical illness. Am J Psychiatry 159:1738–1745, 2002

Koopman C, Classen C, Speigel D: Predictors of posttraumatic stress symptoms among survivors of the Oakland/Berkeley, Calif, firestorm. Am J Psychiatry 151:888–894, 1994

Koopman C, Hermanson K, Diamond S, et al: Social support, life stress, pain and emotional adjustment to advanced breast cancer. Psycho-Oncology 7:101–111, 1998

Koopman C, Butler L, Classen C, et al: Traumatic stress symptoms among women with recently diagnosed primary breast cancer. J Trauma Stress 15:277–287, 2002

Kosslyn SM, Thompson WL, Costantini-Ferrando MF, et al: Hypnotic visual illusion alters color processing in the brain. Am J Psychiatry 157:1279–1284, 2000

Kovacs M, Goldston D, Obrosky DS, et al: Prevalence and predictors of pervasive noncompliance with medical treatment among youths with insulin-dependent diabetes mellitus. J Am Acad Child Adolesc Psychiatry 31:1112–1119, 1992

Kraimaat FW, Brons MR, Geenen R, et al: The effect of cognitive behavior therapy in patients with rheumatoid arthritis. Behav Res Ther 33:487–495, 1995

Krumholz HM, Butler J, Miller J, et al: Prognostic importance of emotional support for elderly patients hospitalized with heart failure. Circulation 97:958–964, 1998

Kuchler T, Henne-Bruns D, Rappat S, et al: Impact of psychotherapeutic support on gastrointestinal cancer patients undergoing surgery: survival results of a trial. Hepatogastroenterology 46:322–335, 1999

Kurnat EL, Murphy Moore C: The impact of a chronic condition on the families of children with asthma. Pediatr Nurs 25:288–302, 1999

Kuttner L: Managing pain in children. Changing treatment of headaches. Can Fam Physician 39:563–568, 1993

Lane JD, McCaskill CC, Ross SL, et al: Relaxation training for NIDDM. Predicting who may benefit. Diabetes Care 16:1087–1094, 1993

Lang EV, Rosen MP: Cost analysis of adjunct hypnosis with sedation during outpatient interventional radiologic procedures. Radiology 222:375–382, 2002

Lang EV, Benotsch EG, Fick LJ, et al: Adjunctive nonpharmacological analgesia for invasive medical procedures: a randomised trial. Lancet 355:1486–1490, 2000

Larson MR, Duberstein PR, Talbot NL, et al: A presurgical psychosocial intervention for breast cancer patients: psychological distress and the immune response. J Psychosom Res 48:187–194, 2000

Larsson G, Starrin B: Relaxation training as an integral part of caring activities for cancer patients: effects on well-being. Scand J Caring Sci 6:179–185, 1992

Lazarus A, Folkman S: Stress, Appraisal, and Coping. New York, Springer, 1984

Lehrer PM, Sargunaraj D, Hochron S: Psychological approaches to the treatment of asthma. J Consult Clin Psychol 60:639–643, 1992

Lehrer PM, Feldman J, Giardino N, et al: Psychological aspects of asthma. J Consult Clin Psychol 70:691–711, 2002

Leibing E, Pfingsten M, Bartmann U, et al: Cognitive-behavioral treatment in unselected rheumatoid arthritis outpatients. Clin J Pain 15:58–66, 1999

Levenson H: Time-Limited Dynamic Psychotherapy: A Guide to Clinical Practice. New York, Basic Books, 1995

Linden W: Psychological treatments in cardiac rehabilitation: review of rationales and outcomes. J Psychosom Res 48:443–454, 2000

Linden W, Stossel C, Maurice J: Psychosocial interventions for patients with coronary artery disease: a meta-analysis. Arch Intern Med 156:745–752, 1996

Linn MW, Linn BS, Harris R: Effects of counseling for late stage cancer patients. Cancer 49:1048–1055, 1982

Looper KJ, Kirmayer LJ: Behavioral medicine approaches to somatoform disorders. J Consult Clin Psychol 70:810–827, 2002

Lorig K, Lubeck D, Kraines RG, et al: Outcomes of self-help education for patients with arthritis. Arthritis Rheum 28:680–685, 1985

Lorig K, Seleznick M, Lubeck D, et al: The beneficial outcomes of the arthritis self-management course are not adequately explained by behavior change. Arthritis Rheum 32:91–95, 1989

Luskin F, Reitz M, Newell K, et al: A controlled pilot study of stress management training of elderly patients with congestive heart failure. Prev Cardiol 5:168–172, 2002

Lustman PJ, Griffith LS, Freedland KE, et al: Cognitive behavior therapy for depression in type 2 diabetes mellitus: a randomized, controlled trial. Ann Intern Med 129:613–621, 1998

Lutgendorf SK, Antoni MH, Ironson G, et al: Cognitive-behavioral stress management decreases dysphoric mood and herpes simplex virus-type 2 antibody titers in symptomatic HIV-seropositive gay men. J Consult Clin Psychol 65:31–43, 1997

Lutgendorf SK, Antoni MH, Ironson G, et al: Changes in cognitive coping skills and social support during cognitive behavioral stress management intervention and distress outcomes in symptomatic human immunodeficiency virus (HIV)-seropositive gay men. Psychosom Med 60:204–214, 1998

Maldonado J, Spiegel D: Medical hypnosis, in Psychiatric Care of the Medical Patient. Edited by Stoudemire A, Fogel B, Greenberg D. New York, Oxford University Press, 2000

Malt UF, Tjemsland L: PTSD in women with breast cancer. Psychosomatics 40:89–89, 1999

Marchioro G, Azzarello G, Checchin F, et al: The impact of a psychological intervention on quality of life in non-metastatic breast cancer. Eur J Cancer 32A:1612–1615, 1996

Markowitz JC, Kocsis JH, Fishman B, et al: Treatment of depressive symptoms in human immunodeficiency virus–positive patients. Arch Gen Psychiatry 55:452–457, 1998

Marx A, Bollmann A, Dunbar SB, et al: Psychological reactions among family members of patients with implantable defibrillators. Int J Psychiatry Med 31:375–387, 2001

Maxmen JS, Ward NG: Essential Psychopathology and Its Treatment, 2nd Edition, Revised for DSM-IV. New York, WW Norton, 1995

McArdle JM, George WD, McArdle CS, et al: Psychological support for patients undergoing breast cancer surgery: a randomised study. BMJ 312:813–816, 1996

McCorkle R, Strumpf NE, Nuamah IF, et al: A specialized home care intervention improves survival among older post-surgical cancer patients. J Am Geriatr Soc 48:1707–1713, 2000

McCracken LM: Cognitive behavioral treatment of rheumatoid arthritis: a preliminary review of efficacy and methodology. Ann Behav Med 13:57–65, 1991

McCracken LM, Turk DC: Behavioral and cognitive-behavioral treatment for chronic pain: outcome, predictors of outcome, and treatment process. Spine 27:2564–2573, 2002

McQuellon RP, Wells M, Hoffman S, et al: Reducing distress in cancer patients with an orientation program. Psycho-Oncology 7:207–217, 1998

McWilliams N: Psychoanalytic Diagnosis: Understanding Personality Structure in the Clinical Process. New York, Guilford, 1994

McWilliams N: Psychoanalytic Case Formulation. New York, Guilford, 1999

Meredith L, Sherbourne CD, Jackson CA, et al: Treatment typically provided for comorbid anxiety disorders. Arch Fam Med 6:231–237, 1997

Meyer TJ, Mark MM: Effects of psychosocial interventions with adult cancer patients: a meta-analysis of randomized experiments. Health Psychol 14:101–108, 1995

Miller SM: Monitoring and blunting: validation of a questionnaire to assess styles of information seeking under threat. J Pers Soc Psychol 52:345–353, 1987

Milrod B, Busch F, Leon AC, et al: Open trial of psychodynamic psychotherapy for panic disorder: a pilot study. Am J Psychiatry 157:1878–1880, 2000

Moos RH, Schaefer JA: The crisis of physical illness: an overview and conceptual approach, in Coping With Physical Illness: New Perspectives. Edited by Moos RH. New York, Plenum, 1987, pp 3–25

Moran G, Fonagy P, Kurtz A, et al: A controlled study of the psychoanalytic treatment of brittle diabetes. J Am Acad Child Adolesc Psychiatry 30:926–935, 1991

Morrison JB: Chronic asthma and improvement with relaxation induced by hypnotherapy. J R Soc Med 81:701–704, 1988

Moynihan C, Bliss JM, Davidson J, et al: Evaluation of adjuvant psychological therapy in patients with testicular cancer: randomised controlled trial. BMJ 316:429–435, 1998

Mulder C, Van der Pompe G, Spiegel D, et al: Do psychosocial factors influence the course of breast cancer? A review of recent literature methodological problems and future directions. Psycho-Oncology 1:155–167, 1992

Mulder CL, Emmelkamp PM, Antoni MH, et al: Cognitive-behavioral and experiential group psychotherapy for HIV-infected homosexual men: a comparative study. Psychosom Med 56:423–431, 1994

Mullen PD, Laville EA, Biddle AK, et al: Efficacy of psycho-educational interventions on pain, depression, and disability in people with arthritis: a meta-analysis. J Rheumatol 14 (suppl 15):33–39, 1987

Nemeroff CB, Schatzberg AF: Pharmacological Treatment of Unipolar Depression. New York, Oxford University Press, 1998

Newman SP, Fitzpatrick MC, Lamb R, et al: Patterns of coping in rheumatoid arthritis. Psychol Health 4:187–200, 1990

Nichols MP, Schwartz RC: Family Therapy, Concepts and Methods. Boston, MA, Allyn and Bacon, 1991

Niederehe G, Schneider LS: Treatments for Depression and Anxiety in the Aged. New York, Oxford University Press, 1998

Ornish D, Scherwitz LW, Billings JH, et al: Intensive lifestyle changes for reversal of coronary heart disease. JAMA 280:2001–2007, 1998

Parker JC, Iverson GL, Smarr KL, et al: Cognitive-behavioral approaches to pain management in rheumatoid arthritis. Arthritis Care Res 6:207–212, 1993

Patterson DR, Jensen MP: Hypnosis and clinical pain. Psychol Bull 129:495–521, 2003

Pennebaker JW, Beall SK: Confronting a traumatic event: toward an understanding of inhibition and disease. J Abnorm Psychol 95:274–281, 1986

Pennebaker JW, Kiecolt-Glaser JK, Glaser R: Disclosure of traumas and immune function: health implications for psychotherapy. J Consult Clin Psychol 56:239–245, 1988

Petrie KJ, Cameron LD, Ellis CJ, et al: Changing illness perceptions after myocardial infarction: an early intervention randomized controlled trial. Psychosom Med 64:580–586, 2002

Postone N: Psychotherapy with cancer patients. Am J Psychother 52:412–424, 1998

Radojevic V, Nicassio PM, Weisman MH, et al: Behavioral intervention with and without family support for rheumatoid arthritis. Behav Ther 23:13–30, 1992

Rainville P, Hofbauer RK, Paus T, et al: Cerebral mechanisms of hypnotic induction and suggestion. J Cogn Neurosci 11:110–125, 1999

Reynolds P, Kaplan GA: Social connections and risk for cancer: prospective evidence from the Alameda County Study. Behav Med 16:101–110, 1990

Reynolds P, Boyd PT, Blacklow RS, et al: The relationship between social ties and survival among black and white breast cancer patients. National Cancer Institute Black/White Cancer Survival Study Group. Cancer Epidemiol Biomarkers Prev 3:253–259, 1994

Richardson JL, Marks G, Johnson CA, et al: Path model of multidimensional compliance with cancer therapy. Health Psychol 6:183–207, 1987

Richardson JL, Shelton DR, Krailo M, et al: The effect of compliance with treatment on survival among patients with hematologic malignancies. J Clin Oncol 8:356–364, 1990

Richter EL: Managing somatic preoccupation. Am Fam Physician 59:3113–3120, 1999

Rolland JS: Chronic illness and the family life cycle, in The Changing Family Life Cycle. Edited by Carter B, McGoldrick M. Boston, MA, Allyn and Bacon, 1989, pp 433–456

Rubin RR, Peyrot M, Saudek CD: Effect of diabetes education on self-care, metabolic control, and emotional well-being. Diabetes Care 12:673–679, 1989

Salkovskis PM: Somatic problems, in Cognitive Behaviour Therapy for Psychiatric Problems: A Practical Guide. Edited by Hawton K. Oxford, UK, Oxford University Press, 1989, pp 235–276

Saravay SM: Psychiatric interventions in the medically ill. Psychiatr Clin North Am 19:467–479, 1996

Scheidlinger S: History of group psychotherapy, in Comprehensive Group Psychotherapy, 3rd Edition. Edited by Kaplan HI, Sadock BJ. Baltimore, MD, Williams & Wilkins, 1993, pp 2–9

Schneiderman N, Antoni MH, Saab PG, et al: Health psychology: psychosocial and biobehavioral aspects of chronic disease management. Annu Rev Psychol 52:555–580, 2001

Shapiro ER: Chronic illness as a family process: a social-developmental approach to promoting resilience. Psychother Pract 58:1375–1384, 2002

Sharpe L, Sensky T, Timberlake N, et al: A blind, randomized, controlled trial of cognitive-behavioural intervention for patients with recent onset rheumatoid arthritis: preventing psychological and physical morbidity. Pain 89:275–283, 2001

Sherbourne CD, Wells KB, Meredith LS, et al: Comorbid anxiety disorder and the functioning and well-being of chronically ill patients of general medical providers. Arch Gen Psychiatry 53:889–895, 1996a

Sherbourne CD, Jackson CA, Meredith LS, et al: Prevalence of comorbid anxiety disorders in primary care outpatients. Arch Fam Med 5:27–35, 1996b

Simon GE, Manning WG, Katzelnick DJ, et al: Cost-effectiveness of systematic depression treatment for high utilizers of general medical care. Arch Gen Psychiatry 58:181–187, 2001

Smith MY, Redd W, DuHamel K, et al: Validation of the PTSD Checklist–Civilian Version in survivors of bone marrow transplantation. J Trauma Stress 12:485–499, 1999

Smith TW, Ruiz JM: Psychosocial influences on the development and course of coronary heart disease: current status and implications for research and practice. J Consult Clin Psychol 70:548–568, 2002

Smyth JM: Written emotional expression: effect sizes, outcome types, and moderating variables. J Consult Clin Psychol 66:174–184, 1998

Smyth JM, Stone AA, Hurewitz A, et al: Effects of writing about stressful experiences on symptom reduction in patients with asthma or rheumatoid arthritis: a randomized trial. JAMA 281:1304–1309, 1999

Snoek FJ, van der Ven NC, Lubach CH, et al: Effects of cognitive behavioural group training (CBGT) in adult patients with poorly controlled insulin-dependent (type 1) diabetes: a pilot study. Patient Educ Couns 45:143–148, 2001

Sobel DS: Rethinking medicine: improving health outcomes with cost-effective psychosocial interventions. Psychosom Med 57:234–244, 1995

Spiegel D: Cancer and depression. Br J Psychiatry 168:109–116, 1996

Spiegel D: Healing words: emotional expression and disease outcome. JAMA 281:1328–1329, 1999

Spiegel D: Efficacy and cost-effectiveness of group psychotherapy for patients with cancer. ONE (Oncology Economics) 1(5):53–58, 2000

Spiegel D: Mind matters: group therapy and survival in breast cancer. N Engl J Med 345:1767–1768, 2001

Spiegel D, Bloom FR: Pain in metastatic breast cancer. Cancer 52:341–345, 1983

Spiegel D, Classen C: Group Therapy for Cancer Patients. New York, Basic Books, 2000

Spiegel D, Giese-Davis J: Depression and cancer: mechanisms and disease progression. Biol Psychiatry 54:269–282, 2003

Spiegel D, Glafkides MC: Effects of group confrontation with death and dying. Int J Group Psychother 33:433–447, 1983

Spiegel D, Maldonado J: Hypnosis, in The American Psychiatric Press Textbook of Clinical Psychiatry, 3rd Edition. Edited by Hales RE, Yudofsky SC, Talbot JA. Washington, DC, American Psychiatric Press Inc, 1999, pp 1243–1274

Spiegel D, Yalom ID: A support group for dying patients. Int J Group Psychother 28:233–245, 1978

Spiegel D, Bloom JR, Yalom I, et al: Group support for patients with metastatic cancer: a randomized outcome study. Arch Gen Psychiatry 38:527–533, 1981

Spiegel D, Bloom JR, Kraemer HC, et al: Effect of psychosocial treatment on survival of patients with metastatic breast cancer. Lancet 2:888–901, 1989

Spiegel D, Frischholz EJ, Fleiss JL, et al: Predictors of smoking abstinence following a single-session restructuring intervention with self-hypnosis. Am J Psychiatry 150:1090–1097, 1993

Spiegel D, Sands S, Koopman C: Pain and depression in patients with cancer. Cancer 74:2570–2578, 1994

Spiegel H, Greenleaf M, Spiegel D: Hypnosis, in Kaplan and Sadock's Comprehensive Textbook of Psychiatry, 7th Edition, Vol 2. Edited by Sadock BJ, Sadock VA. Philadelphia, PA, Lippincott Williams & Wilkins, 2000, pp 2128–2146

Stauffer MH: A long-term psychotherapy group for children with chronic medical illness. Bull Menninger Clin 62:15–32, 1998

Stern JM, Lovestone S: Therapy with the elderly: introducing psychodynamic psychotherapy to the multi-disciplinary team. Int J Geriatr Psychiatry 15:500–505, 2000

Suarez EC, Kuhn CM, Schanberg SM, et al: Neuroendocrine, cardiovascular, and emotional responses of hostile men: the role of interpersonal challenge. Psychosom Med 60:78–88, 1998

Sullivan HS: The Interpersonal Theory of Psychiatry. New York, WW Norton, 1953

Surwit RS, van Tilburg MA, Zucker N, et al: Stress management improves long-term glycemic control in type 2 diabetes. Diabetes Care 25:30–34, 2002

Sutor B, Rummans TA, Jowsey SG, et al: Major depression in medically ill patients. Mayo Clin Proc 73:329–337, 1998

Taylor SE: Health Psychology. Boston, MA, McGraw-Hill, 1999

Taylor SE, Clark LF (eds): Does Information Improve Adjustment to Noxious Events? Advances in Applied Social Psychology. Hillsdale, NJ, Erlbaum, 1986

Thompson LW, Gallagher D, Breckenridge JS: Comparative effectiveness of psychotherapies for depressed elders. J Consult Clin Psychol 55:385–390, 1987

Tjemsland L, Soreide JA, Malt UF, et al: Traumatic distress symptoms in early breast cancer, I: acute response to diagnosis. Psycho-Oncology 5:1–8, 1996a

Tjemsland L, Soreide JA, Malt UF, et al: Traumatic distress symptoms in early breast cancer, II: outcome six weeks postsurgery. Psycho-Oncology 5:295–303, 1996b

Tobin DL, Reynolds RV, Holroyd KA, et al: Self-management and social learning theory, in Self-Management of Chronic Disease: Handbook of Clinical Interventions and Research. Edited by Holroyd KA, Creer TL. Orlando, FL, Academic Press, 1986

Treisman GJ, Angelino AF, Hutton HE: Psychiatric issues in the management of patients with HIV infection. JAMA 286:2857–2864, 2001

Valentiner DP, Holahan CJ, Moos RH, et al: Social support, appraisals of event controllability, and coping: an integrative model. J Pers Soc Psychol 66:1094–1102, 1994

Van der Ven M, Chatrou M, Snoek FJ, et al: Cognitive behavioral group training (CBGT), in Psychology in Diabetes Care. Edited by Snoek FJ, Skinner TC. London, Wiley, 2000, pp 207–233

van Marle S, Holmes J: Supportive Psychotherapy As an Integrative Psychotherapy. New York, Oxford University Press, 2002

Van't Spijker A, Trijsburg RW, Duivenvoorden HJ: Psychological sequelae of cancer diagnosis: a meta-analytical review of 58 studies after 1980. Psychosom Med 59:280–293, 1997

Von Korff M, Simon G: The prevalence and impact of psychological disorders in primary care: HMO research needed to improve care. HMO Pract 10:150–155, 1996

Von Korff M, Gruman J, Schaefer J, et al: Collaborative management of chronic illness. Ann Intern Med 127:1097–1102, 1997

Weitzner MA, Lehininger F, Sullivan D, et al: Borderline personality disorder and bone marrow transplantation: ethical considerations and review. Psycho-Oncology 8:46–54, 1999

Whorwell PJ, Prior A, Faragher EB: Controlled trial of hypnotherapy in the treatment of severe refractory irritable bowel syndrome. Lancet 2:1232–1234, 1984

Williams RB, Barefoot JC, Shekelle R, et al: The health consequences of hostility, in Anger and Hostility in Cardiovascular and Behavioral Disorders. Edited by Chesney M, Rosenman RH. New York, Hemisphere, 1985, pp 173–185

Wood PE, Milligan M, Christ D, et al: Group counseling for cancer patients in a community hospital. Psychosomatics 19:555–561, 1978

Wysocki T, Greco P, Harris MA, et al: Behavior therapy for families of adolescents with diabetes: maintenance of treatment effects. Diabetes Care 24:441–446, 2001

Yalom ID: Existential Psychotherapy. New York, Basic Books, 1980

Yalom ID: The Theory and Practice of Group Psychotherapy. New York, Basic Books, 1995

Young L: Psychological factors in rheumatoid arthritis. J Consult Clin Psychol 60:619–627, 1992

Zeltzer L, LeBaron S: Hypnosis and nonhypnotic techniques for reduction of pain and anxiety during painful procedures in children and adolescents with cancer. J Pediatr 101:1032–1035, 1982

Zeltzer L, LeBaron S, Zeltzer PM: The effectiveness of behavioral intervention for reduction of nausea and vomiting in children and adolescents receiving chemotherapy. J Clin Oncol 2:683–690, 1984

Zettler A, Duran G, Waadt S, et al: Coping with fear of long-term complications in diabetes mellitus: a model clinical program. Psychother Psychosom 64:178–184, 1995

39 Electroconvulsive Therapy

Keith G. Rasmussen, M.D.

Teresa A. Rummans, M.D.

Teresa S.M. Tsang, M.D.

Roxann D. Barnes, M.D.

THE CORNERSTONES IN the management of medically ill patients receiving electroconvulsive therapy (ECT) include the following: 1) careful pretreatment identification, assessment, and stabilization of medical comorbidity; 2) proper treatment technique (anesthesia, muscle paralysis, continuous oxygenation, electrocardiographic monitoring, and rational use of cardioprotective agents); 3) vigilant assessment of the patient's medical status between treatments; and 4) identification and management of treatment-emergent medical complications.

In this chapter, we focus on the first two of these cornerstones. Management of ECT-induced medical complications, whether in the ECT suite or between treatments, is beyond the scope of this chapter. The importance of careful management is illustrated in a 1968 case report (Hussar and Pachter 1968) in which an elderly man with known heart disease received ECT without cardiac assessment or electrocardiographic monitoring, resulting in myocardial infarction (MI), cardiac arrest, and death. In the modern era, with sophisticated cardiac imaging techniques and better treatments (both before and during ECT), along with continuous electrocardiography and pulse oximetry during the treatment, the outcome likely would have been quite different.

ECT has been a core component of the psychiatrist's treatment armamentarium for more than 60 years. ECT is an extremely safe procedure; average death rates due to treatment are estimated to be approximately 1 per 10,000 patients treated (American Psychiatric Association 2001). Nonetheless, medical comorbidity in ECT patients is so common that the ECT clinician should be familiar with strategies to prevent morbidity and mortality.

Ideally, prospective controlled trials would establish the safety and efficacy of ECT in patients with a given medical disorder, but such trials are impractical and unlikely. However, a substantial number of case reports and series, combined with extensive clinical experience, allow for rational and prudent risk-reduction strategies in ECT practice. In this chapter, we treat organ systems separately; for more extensive reviews of other aspects of ECT practice (e.g., electrode placement, stimulus intensity), the reader is referred to recent ECT texts and practice guidelines (Abrams 2002; American Psychiatric Association 2001). The *Journal of ECT* (formerly *Convulsive Therapy*) contains many case reports of the use of ECT in literally dozens of illnesses. In this chapter, we assume the reader is generally familiar with ECT practice, including the indications for ECT, aspects of modern ECT technique, and the routine pre-ECT workup (which includes a comprehensive medical and psychiatric history, physical examination, basic laboratory screen, and electrocardiogram). We provide recommendations for additional investigations and interventions for patients with various medical conditions.

Cardiovascular Disorders

The potent effects of ECT on cardiovascular physiology have been well characterized for several decades. Unfortunately, the same cannot be said for risk-reduction strategies in such patients. In this section, we review the available literature and provide prudent recommendations. We first review ECT's cardiovascular effects, which are relevant to the care of the cardiac patient receiving ECT. Following that, we outline specific considerations for patients with particular cardiac conditions. For most patients with known or suspected cardiovascular illness, pretreatment consultation with a cardiologist is recommended.

Cardiac Physiology of ECT

Hemodynamic Effects

Anesthetic medications can cause a decrease or increase in cardiac output, depending on the type of agent selected. Typically in ECT, a barbiturate anesthetic is used, with an approximately 25% increase in pulse rate and a 13% decrease in cardiac output immediately after anesthesia (Wells and Davies 1987). After the electrical stimulus, there is a vagally (i.e., parasympathetically) mediated short-lived bradycardia, occasionally with asystole of several seconds (Rasmussen et al. 1999). If the electrical stimulus is suprathreshold (i.e., strong enough to cause a seizure), this initial parasympathetic phase is rapidly replaced by a sympathetically mediated tachycardia and rise in blood pressure during the seizure (Rasmussen et al. 1999). Accordingly, there is also a transient sharp rise in plasma catecholamine levels (Gravenstein et al. 1965). During the seizure, the rate pressure product (the product of heart rate and systolic blood pressure, a measure of myocardial workload) often increases severalfold (Huang et al. 1989; Rasmussen et al. 1999; Rumi et al. 2002), and cardiac output increases by 81% (Wells and Davies 1987). These effects generally subside within a few minutes to an hour. In the immediate postictal phase, if no antimuscarinic premedication (e.g., glycopyrrolate or atropine) has been given, there is often transient bradycardia, followed again by a smaller increase in heart rate that typically reverts to prestimulus levels within a few minutes. A mild increase in heart rate may persist over the preanesthesia baseline depending on the half-life of the antimuscarinic premedication if given. Thus, from a hemodynamic standpoint, the factor that is most relevant to cardiac patients is the sympathetically mediated sharp increase in myocardial workload, which may pose significant risk for patients with coronary artery disease (CAD), dysrhythmias, or congestive heart failure (CHF).

If the electrical stimulus is not of sufficient intensity to cause a seizure (referred to in ECT practice as a subconvulsive, or subthreshold, stimulus), then the initial parasympathetically mediated bradycardia/asystole will not be replaced by the sympathetically mediated phase; there have been rare reports of prolonged asystole requiring resuscitative efforts, especially in patients who have not been given antimuscarinic premedication or who have been given beta-blockers (Burd and Kettl 1998; Decina et al. 1984; Tang and Ungvari 2001; Wells et al. 1988). This is especially important in patients with cardiac disease who may not tolerate several-second asystoles well (Zielinski et al. 1993). Thus, the use of antimuscarinic premedication is encouraged in ECT, especially if the patient has received beta-blockade or when a stimulus titration procedure is to be used to determine seizure threshold, in which case subconvulsive stimuli are expected (Abrams 2002; American Psychiatric Association 2001).

Electrocardiographic Effects

Several studies have examined electrocardiographic changes associated with ECT. Troup et al. (1978) performed 12-hour Holter monitoring in ECT before and after treatment in young, cardiovascularly healthy patients. A slight increase in QTc interval occurred just postictally in some patients, but a return to baseline was noted a few minutes later. The authors found no increase in ventricular or atrial premature contractions in the 12-hour post-ECT period. Kitamura and Page (1984) also performed Holter monitoring 12 hours before and after ECT in 13 patients with a mean age of just more than 50 years. No malignant ventricular dysrhythmias were noted. However, rate-dependent ST-segment depressions were observed which subsided by 1 hour post-ECT. The increase in heart rate caused by the seizure returned to prestimulus levels (i.e., postanesthesia, which included use of atropine) within 4 minutes. Hejtmancik et al. (1949) found a mean decrease in QTc interval of 38 milliseconds just after the seizure. Deliyiannis et al. (1962) performed continuous electrocardiographic monitoring in ECT patients before, during, and for 2 minutes after the seizure. During the seizure itself, ST-segment depression of 1–4 mm was seen in 15 of 20 patients; increased T-wave amplitude, premature atrial complexes (PACs), and premature ventricular complexes (PVCs) were also common. Postictally, there was immediate bradycardia with frequent PACs and PVCs, varying degrees of atrioventricular block or nodal rhythms, and ST-segment depression, all of which resolved within a few minutes. These findings are consistent with sympathetic stimulation during the seizure, followed by vagal response immediately after. Guttmacher and Greenlund (1990) performed 24-hour Holter monitoring on eight elderly subjects with stable cardiac disease (the majority with past histories of MI or heart block) who were receiving ECT. Other than the expected seizure-induced tachycardia and hypertension, which rapidly resolved, no significant electrocardiographic changes were seen.

Zvara et al. (1997) performed Holter monitoring on 19 elderly patients for at least 2 hours after two of their

ECT treatments. For each patient, there was one study with, and one without, preanesthetic administration of the ultra-short-acting beta-blocker esmolol. The purpose of the study was to determine whether pretreatment with a beta-blocker reduced electrocardiographic evidence of myocardial ischemia during and after ECT. Eleven of 19 patients showed at least some ST-segment change (mostly depression) in the postictal period. Interestingly, although esmolol did potently blunt the seizure-induced tachycardia and hypertension, it had no effect on ST-segment ischemic changes. Dysrhythmias, mostly PVCs, were equally common in the postictal period with or without esmolol pretreatment.

Rumi et al. (2002) performed 24-hour ambulatory blood pressure and Holter monitoring on 47 young, healthy patients (mean age=30.3 years; range=18–40 years) without cardiac disease. Three patients (ages 23, 33, and 36 years) showed ST-segment depression of at least 1 mm before, during, and after ECT. All were demonstrated to have normal coronary arteries on subsequent angiography. Other than occasional PACs or PVCs, the Holter results were normal. Hemodynamic responses returned to baseline within 1 hour following the seizure.

Huuhka et al. (2003) performed 24-hour Holter monitoring before and after ECT in 26 elderly patients. Although there was a slight increase in bigeminy/trigeminy in the 24 hours post-ECT, there was no significant increase in the total number of PVCs. Supraventricular tachycardia increased slightly, but supraventricular extrasystoles did not, in the 24 hours post-ECT; none of the significant changes were seen in the 1-hour period post-ECT as compared with the 1-hour period pre-ECT. Nine of the patients also showed ST-segment depression of at least 1 mm in the post-ECT period, although the data on the precise timing and recovery of the ST-segments were not provided. McCully et al. (2003) performed 12-lead electrocardiograms on a series of 53 ECT patients at baseline before ECT and again after the first, fourth, and final treatments. Transient ECG changes, mostly T-wave amplitude changes, were seen in approximately one-third of the patients. Rasmussen et al. (2004) performed 3-hour Holter monitoring on 11 ECT patients (mean age 45 years) before the first treatment and after the last treatment in an ECT series. No significant changes were seen in frequency of dysrhythmias or in the ST segments.

The dysrhythmic changes described in the paragraphs above can be divided into those that are sympathetically mediated (e.g., PVCs in the context of tachycardia) and those that are parasympathetically mediated (e.g., ventricular ectopy during periods of bradycardia, nodal rhythms). In general, it is not uncommon, even in young, healthy patients, to see a variety of brief, rapidly resolving electro-

cardiographic changes during and shortly after the seizure in P-R, QTc, and ST-T wave as well as PACs, PVCs, paroxysmal supraventricular tachycardia (PSVT), and short, nonhemodynamically significant runs of ventricular tachycardia. In the immediate postictal time period, with the relative parasympathetic predominance, it is not uncommon to see vagally mediated changes such as junctional rhythms and PVCs in the face of bradycardia. These latter phenomena are less intense when antimuscarinic premedication is used.

Transient, benign T-wave inversions are also occasionally seen in ECT and can occur in the absence of myocardial compromise (Cockey and Conti 1995; Gould et al. 1983). Khoury and Benedetti (1989) found that 23% of ECT patients showed increased T-wave amplitude lasting an average of 6 minutes during and after the seizure. There has been some controversy as to whether these common, transient ECG changes in ECT represent benign, neurally mediated phenomena or myocardial ischemia. Most ECG changes are felt to be neurally mediated and probably benign (Deliyiannis et al. 1962), requiring no specific intervention. Close attention to proper pretreatment ventilation can largely abate many of these changes (McKenna et al. 1970). Changes in myocardiospecific enzymes suggesting ischemia generally do not occur with ECT (Dec et al. 1985). Some echocardiographic findings (reviewed later in the chapter), however, suggest that myocardial ischemia can occur with ECT. Obviously, if serious atrial or ventricular dysrhythmias occur, or if there is evidence of hemodynamic compromise, immediate treatment is important.

Echocardiographic Effects

There are at least eight reports in which transthoracic echocardiographic assessment was performed in the periictal period in ECT. Mensah et al. (1990) reported two cases in which pretreatment echocardiogram revealed left ventricular intracardiac thrombi. There were no apparent complications with full courses of ECT in either case. However, no post-ECT echocardiographic assessment was undertaken.

Messina et al. (1992) performed baseline and immediate postictal echocardiograms on 11 patients. All baseline studies were normal. Immediately postictally, 5 of the patients had transient new regional wall motion abnormalities (all hypokinesis; no akinesis or dyskinesis). Of these 5 patients, 3 had electrocardiographic evidence of 1 mm downsloping or horizontal ST-segment depressions associated with the presence of regional wall motion abnormalities; 1 had peaked T-waves; and 1 had normal electrocardiographic results during hypokinesis. The other 6 patients had normal postictal electrocardiograms. As the echocardiographic and electrocardiographic changes occurred with doubling of the rate–pressure product, the authors interpreted them as ischemic in nature. All the measures that had changed returned to baseline within a few minutes postictally, and no patient complained of angina or had an MI.

Zhu et al. (1992) treated a 77-year-old woman without known heart disease with ECT. Postictally, the electrocardiogram revealed 1–2 mm ST-segment elevations. Immediate echocardiography showed an ejection fraction of 35% with inferior wall akinesis and anteroseptal and anterior wall hypokinesis. Coronary angiogram demonstrated relatively mild atherosclerosis. During the next 2 days post-ECT, giant T-wave inversions developed in the absence of increased myocardial enzymes. Electrocardiography and echocardiography results normalized 4 days posttreatment, and no further ECT treatments were given at that time. During a depressive relapse 6 months later, ECT was again undertaken. Nitrates and diltiazem were given before the first treatment, but electrocardiography 24 hours later showed return of the giant T-wave inversions and echocardiographic abnormalities. Before each of the remaining six ECT treatments, 15 mg labetalol was given, and no electrocardiographic or echocardiographic abnormalities recurred. The authors attributed the findings to myocardial stunning; electrocardiographic ST-segment changes, T inversions, and U waves have all been associated with acute central nervous system (CNS) events (Perron and Brady 2000). The electrocardiographic changes probably reflected ischemia from marked sympathetic stimulation.

Ruwitch et al. (1994) performed two-dimensional (2-D) echocardiography immediately before and 1 minute postictally in 10 ECT patients with known CAD. Additionally, technetium Tc 99m sestamibi was injected 45 seconds after the end of the seizure, and scans were completed within 3 hours and compared with baseline thallous chloride Tl 201 stress scintigraphy in five patients in whom such a study was available. On 2-D echocardiogram, postictal wall motion abnormalities were identified in six patients (segmental in three and global in three). One patient did not have the postictal echocardiogram performed for technical reasons. Of the remaining three patients, no new abnormalities were identified. The Tc 99m sestamibi scans showed reversible (two complete, three partial) or fixed (two) defects; in the five patients with baseline scintigraphic studies, the findings were concordant in all cases. The authors concluded that myocardial ischemia is common in ECT patients with CAD and may be predictable with scintigraphy.

Eitzman et al. (1994) performed echocardiography 30 minutes postictally on a 76-year-old woman with 1-mm ST-segment elevation 15 minutes post-ECT. The echocardiogram revealed distal septal and apical akinesis. Intravenous nitroglycerin promptly resolved the ST-segment elevation. Adenosine thallium imaging 3 days later was entirely normal. Coronary artery spasm was presumed to be the etiology of the ECT effects. Repeat echocardiogram 6 days post-ECT was normal, but transient akinesis was replicated after hyperventilation, and this was felt to support a diagnosis of coronary artery spasm. Repeat hyperventilation echocardiogram 2 days later, while the patient was taking nifedipine (a common treatment for coronary artery spasm), was normal. The patient subsequently underwent a full course of ECT treatments without electrocardiographic changes while continuing to take the nifedipine.

O'Connor et al. (1996) performed echocardiography on 13 ECT patients at baseline, after anesthetic administration, 1 minute postictally, and 15 minutes later. For each patient, one study was done with, and one without, concomitant esmolol before anesthesia. Of the 26 seizures thus monitored with echocardiography, new regional wall motion abnormalities were seen in only one (and that was with esmolol pretreatment). In contrast to the sample of Messina et al. (1992), 31% of the patients had baseline regional wall motion abnormalities (4 with inferior hypokinesis and 1 with inferior akinesis). Concomitant electrocardiography showed nonspecific ST changes, PACs, PVCs, and one three-beat run of ventricular tachycardia, none associated with wall motion abnormalities. Thus, O'Connor et al. (1996) concluded that in their sample, in contrast to the sample of Messina et al. (1992), new regional wall motion abnormalities are rare in ECT, and the common electrocardiographic changes seen postictally do not generally occur with echocardiographic evidence of ischemia. Of note, in both the O'Connor et al. (1996) and Zvara et al. (1997) studies, pretreatment with the beta-blocker esmolol was not associated with a reduction of ECT effects on echocardiogram or electrocardiogram.

Fuenmayor and colleagues (1997) performed baseline, 20-minute post-ECT, and 6-hour post-ECT echocardiography on 11 patients without cardiac disease and focused their analysis on left ventricular pump function. The mean age of the patients was 23 years. End systolic area was increased, and ejection fraction decreased 20 minutes postictally but returned to normal at the 6 hour study. No change in diastolic function was observed. The authors concluded that ECT temporarily reduces left ventricular systolic function.

Kadoi et al. (2001) performed echocardiography with an automated border detection system that allowed continuous monitoring of systolic function in nine ECT patients with American Society of Anesthesiologists (ASA) status of I or II, starting from just prior to anesthesia induction until 10 minutes postictally. Mean age was 51 years. Immediately postictally, there was a significant reduction in fractional area change of the left ventricle, indicating higher end-systolic area, suggesting impaired overall left ventricular function. However, no regional wall motion abnormalities were seen, nor were there any ST-segment changes on electrocardiography. All measures of systolic function that had changed returned to baseline within a few minutes postictally.

In the most recent study, McCully et al. (2003) performed echocardiography at baseline and approximately 20–30 minutes after the first, fourth, and final ECT treatments. Changes were transient and included new left ventricular systolic dysfunction in 15 of the sample of 53 patients. In 7 of these 15 patients, the systolic dysfunction was global. In the other 8 patients, dysfunction was regional and included the ventricular septum and anterior wall in 5; ventricular septal and inferior wall hypokinesis in 2; and isolated ventricular septal hypokinesis in 1 patient. No baseline clinical characteristics, such as medical history, age, or gender, differentiated these patients from those who did not show echocardiographic changes during ECT. Furthermore, there was no difference between the two groups in peak rate–pressure product or electrocardiographic changes during ECT. In two of the patients showing echocardiographic changes, there was nonsustained ventricular tachycardia and moderate global left ventricular dysfunction (ejection fractions of 30% and 40%). None of the patients showing echocardiographic changes suffered any cardiac events during or up to 1 month after ECT. One patient, an 84-year-old woman with preexisting left ventricular systolic function that did not change during ECT, suffered a stroke 3 days after the last treatment and subsequently died. She had no mural thrombus on the echocardiograms.

In summary, the echocardiographic studies of ECT show transiently reduced left ventricular systolic function. Although the literature is mixed, in some patients, especially those with CAD, temporary new regional hypokinesis may be induced.

Summary

ECT produces temporary parasympathetic and sympathetic nervous system stimulation with expected alterations in heart rate, blood pressure, and rate–pressure product, with a brief, but substantial, increase in myocardial workload. Transient electrocardiographic and echocardiographic changes, some of which are probably ischemic and some likely neurally mediated, also occur. Echocardiographic studies of small sample sizes have shown

brief reductions in left ventricular function. Thus, for the prospective ECT patient with cardiac disease, physicians should be vigilant with regard to stabilizing and monitoring any pathological cardiovascular responses or complications.

In the following section, we turn our attention to assessment and management of ECT patients with specific cardiac conditions.

Congestive Heart Failure

Special attention should be given to patients with CHF. These patients are particularly vulnerable to the stress of hyperdynamic states, such as that associated with strong sympathetic stimulation from ECT, resulting in an increase in myocardial demand and possibly transient ischemia (Fuenmayor et al. 1997; Kadoi et al. 2001). Zielinski et al. (1993) reported on a series of 40 ECT patients with a variety of cardiac diagnoses who were compared with a similarly treated age- and sex-matched group of noncardiac ECT patients. Twelve of the 40 cardiac patients had CHF (mean ejection fraction, 34.6%; range, 22%–47%), and many had other cardiac diagnoses, including conduction defects, ischemic heart disease, and rhythm disturbances. Cardiac complications were classified as major (prolonged ischemic changes on electrocardiogram, MI, prolonged dysrhythmias, or symptoms of coronary ischemia) or minor (transient dysrhythmias or ST-T wave changes without hemodynamic compromise that occurred during or shortly after the seizure). One cardiac patient in the series had an MI, but the authors did not report on whether this patient had CHF. No patient in the series died. Of the 12 patients with CHF, 3 had "major" complications: 2 had (unspecified) ischemic changes on electrocardiography, and 1 had dysrhythmias. Seven of the CHF patients had minor cardiac complications, consisting usually of transient dysrhythmias (atrial or ventricular). Finally, 2 of the CHF patients underwent ECT without cardiac complications. The authors found that in patients who were not initially pretreated with antimuscarinic medication, bradycardia and brief periods of asystole were common and preventable with subsequent atropine. The group of noncardiac patients had no major complications and a significantly lower rate of minor complications with ECT. No specific recommendations were proffered to aid in the management of CHF patients in ECT.

Unfortunately, in this and another commonly cited series (Rice et al. 1994), cardiac illnesses were treated as a homogeneous group without specific considerations for CHF, so no useful information can be gleaned from these studies with regard to management of CHF patients during ECT.

Stern et al. (1997) reported on three patients with CHF, aged 59–78 years and with ejection fractions of 20%–25%, who received ECT without any cardiac complications. The authors used nitroglycerin patch, sublingual nifedipine, and intravenous labetalol pre-ECT to lower the risk of decompensation of heart failure during the procedure. Goldberg and Badger (1993) reported on two patients with CHF and implantable cardioverter defibrillators (ICDs). The first, a 54-year-old man (unspecified ejection fraction), tolerated eight ECT treatments without consequence except for dramatic relief from depression. The second, a 65-year-old man with dilated cardiomyopathy and pre-ECT ejection fraction of 20%, had a total of four treatments. Upon recovery from the first and third treatments, he had respiratory difficulties and bouts of hypotension that responded to an intravenous pressor (ephedrine). After the fourth treatment, he developed a wide complex tachycardia without palpable pulse and was resuscitated. No further ECT was administered, but he suffered a hypotensive episode 5 days later that ultimately led to his death from progressive heart failure several days thereafter.

Gerring and Shields (1982) provided detailed outcome data on four patients with CHF who were treated with ECT for depressive illness. A 60-year-old woman with mitral stenosis received ECT without complication. A 58-year-old woman, also with mitral stenosis in addition to CHF, suffered atrial fibrillation leading to severe decompensation of the CHF after the second treatment; upon stabilization, she went on to receive another course of ECT without complication. A 71-year-old woman with a history of MI in addition to CHF had a cardiopulmonary arrest 45 minutes after her fifth treatment and died. Finally, a 69-year-old woman showed transient ventricular and atrial dysrhythmias after several of her ECT treatments, which she otherwise tolerated well.

Petrides and Fink (1996), in a series of ECT patients with atrial fibrillation, reported that one 89-year-old woman with CHF converted to sinus rhythm after receiving a course of ECT. The other case of interest in their series of CHF patients was a 76-year-old woman in atrial fibrillation who received a course of seven ECT treatments, during which she fluctuated between atrial fibrillation and sinus rhythm. The CHF did not seem to worsen.

As shown in the case series cited above, patients with CHF need to be closely monitored before and during ECT and are particularly sensitive to sympathetic stimulation. In the case of compromised left ventricular function, an increase in sympathetic stimulation with an associated increase in myocardial workload may aggravate CHF. Because of the failing heart's decreased ability to increase its contractile function, it is more sensitive than the normal heart to increases in afterload such as those caused by the sympathetic stimulation with ECT. If the underlying pathology is ischemic heart disease, sympathetic stimulation may induce ishemia with worsening of CHF.

CHF should be optimally treated and stabilized prior to ECT treatments. Once the patient is scheduled for ECT, cardiac medications should be administered in the morning before the treatment with a small amount of water, with enough time to ensure absorption. Recent practice guidelines caution against administration of diuretic agents the morning of ECT to avoid bladder rupture or incontinence during the seizure (American Psychiatric Association 2001). However, we generally recommend administering patients' usual stable medications, including diuretics, to avoid any abrupt changes in their medical regimen. The full bladder problem can be managed simply by having the patient void just before the treatment or, if necessary, by making transient use of a urinary catheter.

The most important principles in the management of CHF patients during actual ECT include vigilance in monitoring hemodynamic status, cardiac rhythm, oxygenation, and ventilation and prompt intervention. Beta receptors are downregulated in CHF, leading to a significantly decreased ability of the patient to respond to exogenously administered catecholamines should resuscitation be required. Patients with CHF are particularly prone to malignant ventricular dysrhythmias, which are also less responsive to conventional therapy. Zielinsky et al. (1993) noted that the presence of ventricular dysrhythmias at baseline predicted post-ECT dysrhythmias, so anesthesia providers should pay particular attention to rhythm disturbances and be aware that they may be more difficult to treat in the patient with CHF. In patients with right ventricular heart failure (especially those with increased pulmonary vascular resistance from hypoxic pulmonary vasoconstriction or hypercapnia and associated respiratory acidosis), an increase in pulmonary vascular resistance can quickly increase right ventricular afterload and precipitate right ventricular failure.

Whether to use an antimuscarinic agent in the patient with CHF must be decided on a case-by-case basis. The potential for such medication to increase myocardial workload through added tachycardia and hypertension is established (Rasmussen et al. 1999). On the other hand, as discussed previously, if a patient receives a subconvulsive electrical stimulus, especially if he or she is also receiving beta-blocking medication, the risk of unopposed parasympathetic stimulation and resultant prolonged asystole is real (Burd and Kettl 1998; Decina et al. 1984; Tang and Ungvari 2001; Wells et al. 1988).

The attending anesthesiologist may elect to use other cardioprotective agents when ECT is being administered to the patient with CHF. For example, a beta-blocker such as esmolol or labetalol may dampen the seizure-induced sympathetic stimulation. The rationale for either agent's use is that the sympathetic stimulation worsens arterial compliance and increases vascular resistance. Because cardiac function is already borderline, even small increases in the impedance of the arterial vasculature can acutely drop cardiac output. Lessening the tachycardia with a beta-blocker reduces myocardial oxygen demand, increases diastolic filling time, and optimizes preload. On the other hand, with an intermediate-duration agent such as labetalol, or long-acting agents such as metoprolol or propranolol, effects lingering after the treatment may predispose to undesirable hypotension. Other strategies include preload reduction (e.g., nitrates), peripheral vasodilators (e.g., hydralazine), and calcium channel blockade (e.g., verapamil or diltiazem).

Finally, intertreatment assessment in patients with CHF is especially important, as demonstrated by the case report of a patient who died of congestive decompensation that began several days after the last ECT treatment (Goldberg and Badger 1993). Daily rounds should include not only assessment of mood and cognitive status but inquiries about symptoms of CHF (e.g., shortness of breath, orthopnea) and physical examination for signs of CHF (e.g., gallops, jugular venous distension, peripheral edema, pulmonary crackles). Any new or worsening findings should prompt careful evaluation and, if necessary, halting of ECT (even if temporarily) to stabilize the patient. Deterioration of left ventricular function over time may also occur without obvious symptoms, and thus patients with CHF should be periodically assessed by a cardiologist.

Coronary Artery Disease/ Post–Myocardial Infarction

In case series cited earlier (Gerring and Shields 1982; Petrides and Fink 1996; Rice et al. 1994; Zielinski et al. 1993), numerous patients with CAD—some with remote history of MI—underwent ECT without major complications. Unfortunately, there are few reports in which patients with precisely defined severity of CAD were prospectively followed for any effects of ECT. In the echocardiographic/sestamibi study by Ruwitch et al. (1994), ECT did not cause any clinical complications (e.g., angina, MI, clinically significant depression of ventricular dysfunction). Nonetheless, the electrocardiographic and echocardiographic studies mentioned previously showed that in patients undergoing ECT, especially those with preexisting CAD, ischemic changes were often noted on electrocardiogram and/or echocardiogram. Thus,

although the risks of significant morbidity in ECT are probably small, caution is advised in the treatment of patients with CAD. Pre-ECT cardiac testing may be necessary depending on the initial assessment.

Applegate (1997) reviewed the evaluation of patients with ischemic heart disease scheduled to undergo ECT, with emphasis on the 1996 American College of Cardiology/American Heart Association Task Force guidelines, including optimization of the patient's anti-ischemic regimen. Other than the small study by Ruwitch et al. (1994), in which baseline scintigraphy correlated with ECT-induced sestamibi findings, no particular studies inform the ECT clinician whether cardiac imaging has predictive value for ECT complications. Whether to perform cardiac imaging in patients with CAD prior to ECT would depend on the time since the patient's last imaging study and the severity and status of their cardiac disease.

After the prospective ECT patient with CAD has had the appropriate pretreatment evaluation and stabilization, there are measures that may further reduce cardiac risk. Many studies have shown that pretreatment with a variety of antihypertensive agents (e.g., beta-blockers, calcium channel blockers, other vasodilators, or nitrates) lowers the seizure-induced rise in heart rate or blood pressure (Abrams 2002). Whether this reliably translates into actual protection against cardiac complications is unknown. In fact, Zvara et al. (1997) found no difference in electrocardiographic evidence of ischemia during and after ECT with the use of esmolol, in spite of reductions in the elevation in rate–pressure product. Castelli et al. (1995) also found that neither labetalol nor esmolol affected postictal ST-segment changes, even though both drugs blunted the heart rate and blood pressure elevations during ECT. Additionally, in one echocardiographic study, the use of esmolol did not appear to affect changes associated with ECT treatment (O'Connor et al. 1996), although the incidence of patients in that study with underlying CAD is unknown. Furthermore, given its small size (16 patients, 26 sessions) and the low incidence of new regional wall motion abnormalities (4%), it is unlikely that this study can provide much guidance with respect to the use of esmolol. However, it is interesting to compare the peak heart rate after esmolol treatment in relation to incidence of new regional wall motion abnormalities between studies. In the O'Connor et al. (1996) study, peak heart rate post-esmolol (1 mg/kg) was 77 (±17) beats/minute, with an incidence of 4% new regional wall motion abnormalities. In the Messina et al. (1992) study, in which no esmolol was used, the heart rate post-ECT was 127 beats/minute with a new regional wall motion abnormality incidence of 45%. Thus, it remains uncertain whether beta-blocker pretreatment reduces morbidity associated with ECT. Given the well-documented salutary effects of such drugs in patients with ischemic heart disease, it seems reasonable to use them in selected cases either before, during, or shortly after the treatment depending on the patient's hemodynamic status, after carefully weighing the risks and potential benefits of such treatment.

A final issue regarding ECT in the patient with CAD concerns the frequently asked question "How soon after an MI can ECT be safely performed?" Severe depression is common in the post-MI period. When the patient sinks into a state of suicidal despair, profound psychomotor retardation, or psychosis, ECT may be the preferred treatment of choice. De Silva and Bachman (1995) consider the first 3 months post-MI to be a particularly high-risk time period for ECT. However, there is no strict rule as to how soon one can perform ECT in a post-MI patient, because it depends on the severity of CAD and whether the patient is considered revascularized or stabilized. A cardiologist should be consulted. Treatment with nitrates or beta-blockade during ECT in a patient with a recent MI would seem prudent, along with the provision for longer-than-usual monitoring in the recovery room to check for late-occurring ischemic changes on electrocardiography or symptoms suggestive of myocardial ischemia or impaired ventricular function. It would not be advisable to perform ECT in a patient in the first few weeks after coronary stenting, although one must weigh the risks of ECT against those of the illness requiring ECT on a case-by-case basis.

Dysrhythmias, Pacemakers, and Implantable Defibrillators

It is not uncommon for patients with known cardiac dysrhythmia or with a pacemaker or ICD to be referred for ECT. The most common dysrhythmia is atrial fibrillation. There are several reports of patients in atrial fibrillation who safely received ECT and who remained in atrial fibrillation (Geretsegger and Rochowanski 1987; Gerring and Shields 1982; Kitamura and Page 1984; Petrides and Fink 1996; Regestein and Reich 1985; Tancer and Evans 1989). There are also reports of patients in atrial fibrillation who converted to sinus rhythm, sometimes transiently, during ECT (Harsch 1991; Ottoway 2002; Petrides and Fink 1996). Ottoway (2002) reported on a 78-year-old man who had had four-vessel coronary artery bypass grafting 1 month prior to receiving ECT and who had rate-controlled atrial fibrillation. The first two treatments proceeded uneventfully. Electrical cardioversion was attempted just prior to the third treatment and converted the patient to sinus rhythm only for 30 seconds, whereupon he reverted back to atrial fibrillation,

and the third ECT treatment was then administered. The patient converted to sinus rhythm during the resultant seizure and remained there for the rest of his subsequent three treatments, and the depression resolved. Harsch (1991) described a patient in atrial fibrillation who converted to sinus rhythm twice during a course of ECT. Petrides and Fink (1996) reported on three patients who also converted from atrial fibrillation to sinus rhythm during ECT (albeit transiently in one case). ECT has been given after successful cardioversion for atrial fibrillation. Moriarty (1972) reported on a 62-year-old man with depression and chronic atrial fibrillation who received his first ECT session immediately after failed electrical cardioversion attempts. However, just prior to his second treatment, cardioversion was successful, and the patient went on to receive five more treatments without complication or return of atrial fibrillation. On follow-up 8 months later, he remained in sinus rhythm while taking quinidine.

Two cases of apparently new-onset atrial fibrillation occurring during ECT have also been described (O'Melia 1970; Petrides and Fink 1996). O'Melia (1970) described a previously healthy 57-year-old woman who was found to be in atrial fibrillation after her second ECT treatment. She reverted back to sinus rhythm 36 hours later, but further ECT treatments were not given. In the Petrides and Fink (1996) series, a patient with a past history of atrial flutter converted from sinus rhythm to atrial fibrillation after her sixth ECT treatment. She was then converted to sinus rhythm with medication but received no more ECT.

Atrial fibrillation newly identified before ECT should be assessed by a cardiologist for optimal management. The decision to choose rate control versus cardioversion depends on a number of factors and should be made by the cardiologist. Management of chronic atrial fibrillation would be the same whether the patient is receiving ECT or not. There are several considerations when performing ECT in a patient with chronic atrial fibrillation. First, in the appropriate patient without contraindications, therapeutic anticoagulation should be maintained throughout the course of ECT (American Psychiatric Association 2001). For the patient who is not receiving chronic anticoagulation, consideration should be given to short-term anticoagulation (e.g., with heparin) during the ECT course. Second, consideration should be given to performing a transesophageal echocardiogram to check if an atrial clot is present. Third, the patient's heart rate should remain well controlled. Fourth, any associated cardiovascular comorbidities, such as CAD, CHF, or valvular disease, must be taken into account. Fifth, consideration should probably be given to premedication with a beta-blocker before inducing the seizure to lessen sympathetic stimulation. Sixth, and perhaps most important, close and meticulous monitoring of the patient's hemodynamic status, oxygenation, and electrocardiographic changes in response to treatment is critically important during ECT. Electrocardiographic rhythm should be inspected prior to each treatment. As the cases cited above demonstrate, conversion from atrial fibrillation to sinus rhythm is possible during ECT, thus reinforcing the need for anticoagulation. If the patient in atrial fibrillation does convert to sinus rhythm, the attending cardiologist should be notified. Finally, the patient without history of atrial fibrillation who develops this rhythm during ECT obviously should have a cardiac workup before treatment is resumed.

Atrial fibrillation is the most common, but not the only, cardiac dysrhythmia in patients referred for ECT. Because cardiac patients are predisposed to a variety of atrial or ventricular dysrhythmias, it is important to ensure that electrolytes (especially sodium, potassium, calcium, and magnesium) are normal. Electrolyte abnormalities and other metabolic perturbations (e.g., thyroid dysfunction) can be even more pro-dysrhythmic along with medications that may prolong the QT interval, including some psychotropics.

A related issue concerns the prospective ECT patient with a cardiac pacemaker or an ICD. There have been numerous case reports of patients with pacemakers who have undergone successful and uncomplicated ECT (Abiuso et al. 1978; Alexopoulos and Frances 1980; Alexopoulos et al. 1984; Ballenger 1973; Blitt and Kirschvink 1976; Dolenc et al., in press; Gibson et al. 1973; Jauhar et al. 1979; Youmans et al. 1972), as well as a few reports of patients with ICDs (Dolenc et al., in press; Goldberg and Badger 1993; Lapid et al. 2001; Pornnoppadol and Isenberg 1998). In the case by Goldberg and Badger (1993) described earlier, a man with an ICD and CHF underwent ECT and died of what appeared to be decompensated CHF. It was unlikely that the ICD contributed to the fatal outcome. In fact, with modern pacemakers and ICDs, there is no risk of electrical damage to the device during ECT, assuming proper grounding of the patient (Abrams 2002).

Pre-ECT device assessment to ensure normal functioning is advisable. It is particularly important for the ECT clinicians to know what type of pacemaker a patient has. Patients who are pacemaker-dependent should have their pacemaker assessed and programmed to an appropriate mode where necessary. Those patients with an activity-driven sensor generally will not need to have the rate response programmed off for ECT, because variation in rate between the programmed upper and lower rates should be tolerated. Furthermore, if the activity sensor does respond to either the electrical stimulus or the seizure, patient safety will not be compromised. Pacemaker

patients with minute ventilation devices will need the rate response turned off before ECT. Some practitioners have used a magnet placed on the chest above the device to convert a demand mode pacemaker to fixed mode during ECT in order to avoid spurious discharge of the device, which theoretically could occur as the result of muscle electrical activity; however, there is no evidence to support this practice (Abrams 2002).

ICDs should be turned off prior to each ECT treatment while the patient is on an electrocardiographic monitor, the latter being continued until the ICD is turned back on. All patients with ICDs or pacemakers that have been reprogrammed prior to ECT should have device assessment after the procedure. In summary, presence of a pacemaker or defibrillator does not constitute a contraindication to ECT, but cardiology consultation for appropriate assessment and management of the underlying cardiac disease and device interrogation/adjustment is required.

Vascular Disease

A number of case reports cite safe and effective use of ECT in patients with a variety of aortic aneurysms, some after surgical correction (Abramczuk and Rose 1979; Attar-Levy et al. 1995; Chapman 1961; Devanand et al. 1990; Dowling and Francis 1993; Goumeniouk et al. 1990; Greenbank 1958; Monke 1952; Moore 1960; Pomeranze et al. 1968; Rosenfeld et al. 1988; Weatherly and Villien 1958; Wolford 1957). Assuming that there are no preexisting conditions or surgical complications, there is no specific reason to assume that patients who have had an aneurysm repair are at increased risk during ECT.

The chief concern in patients with aneurysms is the potential risk of rupture or leakage caused by the rapid rise in blood pressure during ECT. If a patient is known to have an aortic aneurysm, evaluation of the size (e.g., by ultrasound) should be undertaken prior to ECT. Consultation with a vascular surgeon would be prudent to evaluate the stability of the aneurysm and strategies for risk reduction. Pretreatment with antihypertensives before ECT anesthesia can optimize control of blood pressure and reduce arterial wall stress. Labetalol would seem to be ideal for this purpose, as it has both alpha- and beta-blockade and thus can reduce peripheral vascular resistance and attenuate the rise in blood pressure during and shortly after the seizure (McCall et al. 1991). Repetitive imaging may be necessary during the course of ECT treatments if there is any concern with respect to the stability of the aneurysm.

Hypertension is probably the most common cardiovascular condition in patients receiving ECT. Although it seems intuitively obvious that good control of blood pressure is ideal before ECT, undue delays while waiting for complete normalization are unwarranted. In the 65-year history of ECT, reports of intracerebral hemorrhage during treatment are exceedingly rare; in fact, we are aware of only two reports, both in patients without known prior vascular instability (Rikher et al. 1997; Weisberg et al. 1991). Swartz and Inglis (1990) found that blood pressure actually went down after a course of ECT. Prudic et al. (1987) and Webb et al. (1990) both found that patients with the highest blood pressures pre-ECT had the lowest rise in blood pressure and rate–pressure product during and after the seizure. Finally, with the availability of short-acting antihypertensive agents (e.g., esmolol), high blood pressure can generally be managed rapidly and effectively during the treatments.

Miscellaneous Cardiac Conditions

Numerous reports exist of safe use of ECT in patients with various valvular abnormalities with or without prior surgical correction (Hardman and Morse 1972; Levin et al. 2000; Rasmussen 1997). If a patient has had mechanical valve replacement and has received appropriate anticoagulation, the risk of ECT treatment should not be significantly increased (assuming that no other cardiac dysfunction, such as impaired ventricular function or dysrhythmia, is present). However, if a patient has a valvular abnormality that has not been optimally treated or is newly identified, then echocardiography should be obtained.

Heart transplant patients are rarely encountered in ECT practice. There are three published cases of uncomplicated ECT in heart transplant recipients (Kellner et al. 1991a; Lee et al. 2001; Pargger et al. 1995). Because the transplanted heart is denervated, theoretically there is less risk of vagally mediated bradydysrhythmias during ECT (Lee et al. 2001). Although sympathetic innervation is also lacking, the acute seizure-induced rise in plasma catecholamines still occurs, which causes increases in pulse and blood pressure (Gravenstein et al. 1965), as was seen in the cases just referenced. One must also remember that if bradycardia is encountered during ECT in such a patient, the heart rate will not change in response to antimuscarinic medication. If resuscitation is necessary, the drugs of choice are epinephrine or isoproterenol. Pre-ECT echocardiographic evaluation is recommended, and use of intratreatment medications such as beta-blockers or nitrates can reduce unfavorable cardiac stress. Obviously, one should only undertake ECT in a cardiac transplant patient in close consultation with the patient's cardiologist.

Anticoagulation

There are several common indications for anticoagulation in ECT patients, including atrial fibrillation, deep venous thrombosis, and valvular replacement. Many reports exist of patients receiving therapeutic anticoagulation who underwent ECT without complications (Bleich et al. 2000; Hay 1989; Loo et al. 1985). One theoretical concern about maintaining anticoagulation during ECT is the risk of spontaneous hemorrhage during the blood pressure surge in the peri-ictal period. However, to our knowledge no cases have been reported of hemorrhage during ECT in patients receiving anticoagulation, so therapeutic anticoagulation should be continued throughout ECT. Indices of anticoagulation (i.e., the international normalized ratio for coumadin or the partial thromboplastin time for heparin) may fluctuate, especially in patients with acute illnesses or medication changes, and should be carefully monitored. The blood pressure cuff used to block the effects of muscle paralysis in assessing the motor seizure duration should not be placed on the affected limb in patients with deep venous thrombosis (e.g., a forearm should be cuffed rather than the calf).

Neurological Disorders

In considering the medical risks of ECT in patients with neurological disorders, there are four main differences between the neurological and cardiovascular aspects of ECT: 1) the effects of ECT on CNS function are not as well characterized; 2) there are essentially no functional tests to assess degree of risk in a neurological patient before ECT; 3) there are no neuroprotective strategies of note, as there are in the context of cardiac disease (i.e., availability of various cardioprotective agents to blunt the cardiac effects of ECT); and 4) ECT may actually improve the underlying neurological disorder for some conditions (as discussed later in this section). One similarity with the cardiac literature is that there are virtually no controlled data informing the ECT clinician. Fortunately, a large body of case series and reports, as well as accumulated clinical experience, does provide confidence that the majority of patients with various neurological disorders can safely and effectively be treated with ECT. The few areas of probable high neurological risk are well characterized and represent a very small percentage of patients referred for ECT.

Although neurodiagnostic tests (e.g., computed tomography, magnetic resonance imaging [MRI], electroencephalography, single photon emission computed tomography, positron emission tomography) may be helpful in diagnosing suspected neurological disease, none of these tests is routinely indicated prior to ECT (American Psychiatric Association 2001), nor do any lead to a confident ability to predict risk level with ECT. In patients with known neurological disease, the best pre-ECT assessment consists of a careful neurological exam and diagnostic tests for particular indications. In this section, before considering the various neurological disorders encountered in ECT practice, we review some of the neurophysiological effects of ECT.

Neurophysiological Effects of ECT

A great deal of research has been conducted on the electroencephalographic, cerebral blood flow, neurometabolic, and neurohormonal effects of electrically induced seizures both in animals and humans (reviewed in Abrams 2002). The purpose of this research is to elucidate the mechanism of action of ECT as well as the underlying neurobiology of psychiatric illnesses and is beyond the scope of this chapter. Furthermore, other than perhaps the blood flow effects, none of these findings is relevant to assessing degree of risk in the prospective ECT patient with comorbid neurological disease.

The most well-characterized clinical effect of ECT on the brain is that on memory function (reviewed in Abrams 2002), which is also beyond the scope of this chapter. No laboratory tests reliably predict extent of cognitive dysfunction with ECT in neurological patients, nor are any nootropic agents available to prevent these effects.

There is a dramatic increase in cerebral blood flow during the seizure in ECT (Nobler et al. 1994), which leads to a transient increase in intracranial pressure. Thus, it would be expected that conditions already causing increased intracranial pressure would represent high-risk situations (American Psychiatric Association 2001).

Dementia

Numerous reports indicate that ECT can be efficacious for depressive symptoms in depressed dementia patients without causing undue or long-lasting increases in memory disturbance (Rao and Lyketsos 2000). Most of these reports do not establish a dementia diagnosis separate from the cognitive dysfunction related to depression (Rasmussen et al. 2002). In fact, in routine clinical circumstances, it is often difficult to determine whether the patient with coexisting severe depression and cognitive dysfunction has a separate dementing illness or depression-related cognitive dysfunction (Stoudemire et al. 1995). A further problem with this literature is the lack of long-term cognitive follow-up in most reports.

Reynolds et al. (1987) prospectively followed depression ratings in three depressed dementia patients receiving ECT. Two of the patients enjoyed an excellent antidepressant response to ECT without cognitive worsening, whereas one patient suffered acute cognitive worsening as assessed with the Mini-Mental State Examination (MMSE) (Folstein et al. 1975) and had no antidepressant response. Gaspar and Samarasinghe (1982) treated three patients with ECT who carried diagnoses of primary dementia and depression. As with the Reynolds et al. (1987) series, two of the three patients experienced a good antidepressant effect with ECT; none of the patients seemed to have long-lasting cognitive impairment, although no systematic follow up was reported.

Nelson and Rosenberg (1991) treated 21 depressed dementia patients with ECT. Antidepressant efficacy ratings based on chart review were similar to those of a depressed ECT comparison group without dementia. Post-ECT confusion was believed to be greater in the dementia patients, although no efficacy or cognitive follow-up data were presented.

In the largest series to date, Rao and Lyketsos (2000) administered ECT in 31 depressed dementia patients: 16 with vascular dementia, 4 with Alzheimer's dementia, and 11 with dementia of uncertain cause. No outcome data were presented separately for the different dementia groups. Half of the patients experienced delirium (criteria not specified) with ECT. Two-thirds had a good antidepressant response to treatment. The MMSE score actually increased an average of 1.62 points during ECT, indicating the beneficial effect of ECT on attention after clearing of the acute posttreatment confusion. One patient had tardive seizures in the recovery room after ECT.

McDonald and Thompson (2001) reported on three dementia patients with medication-refractory mania who showed excellent benefits with index and maintenance courses of right unilateral ECT and who seemed to tolerate the treatments well from a cognitive standpoint. Grant and Mohan (2001) described four dementia patients whose agitation and aggression were reduced with ECT.

In the most recent ECT series in patients with dementia, Rasmussen et al. (2003) treated seven patients with probable Lewy body dementia. All seven experienced acute antidepressant effects with ECT, which were sustained in three patients for several months to 2 years with maintenance ECT. Acute confusional states were common in this series.

In summary, several dozen cases of patients with dementia have been reported in the ECT literature, with approximately two-thirds showing antidepressant (or antimanic) benefit, and about half showing greater-than-usual cognitive impairment. If the patient's dementia syndrome etiology is well characterized, there is no need to perform neurodiagnostic testing in preparation for ECT. If, however, there is still diagnostic uncertainty about the dementia etiology, further workup may be indicated.

The frequency with which elderly, cognitively impaired patients are referred for ECT points to the need for a large, prospective trial in patients whose dementia severity and subtype are well characterized, with long-term follow up of cognitive and psychopathological outcome. In the meantime, the ECT clinician treating such patients would be well advised to consider right unilateral or bifrontal electrode placement with twice-weekly treatment frequency. There is no evidence from the available literature that the number of treatments to achieve efficacy is different from that for patients without dementia, although the treatments may need to be halted if excessive cognitive dysfunction occurs.

Another common technical issue in treating dementia patients with ECT is whether to have the patients continue taking a cholinesterase inhibitor such as donepezil, galantamine, or rivastigmine. Such medications are commonly used in treating patients with dementia, but there has been concern over a possible interaction of such drugs with succinylcholine, which is metabolized by plasma cholinesterases (Folk et al. 2000). Theoretically, such drugs may prolong the action of succinylcholine, and practitioners have been cautioned either to discontinue such therapy before anesthesia or at least to proceed with caution (Folk et al. 2000; Heath 1997, 2003; Walker and Perks 2002). Rasmussen et al. (2003) reported that patients taking donepezil for dementia symptoms were safely treated with ECT. A further practical problem is that the half-life of the most commonly used cholinesterase inhibitor, donepezil, is so long (i.e., about 50 hours) that a complete washout would take about a week and a half, a period that is prohibitively long in treating a typical patient severely ill enough to warrant ECT treatment. A prudent approach, in our opinion, would be to continue the cholinesterase inhibitor if there has been benefit with it and proceed with ECT but remain mindful of a possible prolongation of succinylcholine action.

Movement Disorders

In this section, we discuss the most commonly encountered movement disorders in ECT practice: Parkinson's disease and neuroleptic-induced movement disorders. The scarce literature on rare conditions such as Huntington's disease, Wilson's disease, progressive supranuclear palsy, and multiple system atrophy is also briefly reviewed.

Parkinson's Disease

Several case reports, case series, and one placebo (sham-ECT)–controlled trial indicate that ECT is effective for treating depression in patients with Parkinson's disease (Rasmussen et al. 2002). An intriguing finding in this literature is that ECT may also improve motor function (Moellentine et al. 1998; Rasmussen and Abrams 1991). Common side effects of ECT in patients with Parkinson's disease include delirium and treatment-emergent dyskinesia, which probably indicate a dopaminomimetic effect (Douyon et al. 1989). The duration of ECT-related antiparkinsonian effects has been variable. Fall et al. (1995) followed 16 nondemented, nondepressed patients with Parkinson's disease before, immediately after, and for up to 1.5 years after courses of mostly unilateral ECT. Fifteen had measurable (occasionally dramatic) improvement in the motor symptoms of Parkinson's disease. Although maintenance ECT was not used, 8 patients had sustained improvement for 3–18 months after ECT. Five patients developed severe confusional states, the duration of which was up to 2 weeks. Four of these 5 patients went on to have long-lasting (i.e., at least several months) motor improvement.

Pridmore et al. (1995) treated seven nondepressed Parkinson's disease patients with four unilateral ECT treatments. Immediate post-ECT and 2-week post-ECT ratings in all spheres of motor function indicated improvements. Four patients developed severe, although temporary, confusion. One patient developed dyskinesia, which responded to lowering of the levodopa dose. In a follow-up report on these and several other such patients who had been given index (but not maintenance) ECT, three of nine initial ECT responders had improvements lasting 2–10 weeks, whereas six of nine had improvements lasting 10–35 months (Pridmore and Pollard 1996).

There are several case reports of patients with Parkinson's disease given maintenance ECT to extend the initial motoric improvement of index courses of treatment (Aarsland et al. 1997; Fall and Granerus 1999; Hoflich et al. 1995; Serby et al. 1994; Wengel et al. 1998; Zervas and Fink 1991). Maintenance ECT seemed to prevent relapses. The frequency of such treatments was quite variable depending on the period of improvement each patient sustained. Cognitive impairment was noticeable in some cases.

In summary, ECT seems to be effective for the depression commonly encountered in patients with Parkinson's disease and may even improve the motoric signs. The duration of such benefits is unpredictable and may be extended with maintenance ECT, although the benefits need to be balanced against cognitive impairment. Acute confusional states and dyskinesias are common during ECT and may be reduced with cautious lowering of dopamine agonist dosage. As with demented patients, we recommend that the ECT clinician consider twice, versus thrice, weekly treatment frequency and the use of electrode placements that may cause less cognitive impairment (i.e., right unilateral or bifrontal).

Neuroleptic-Induced Movement Disorders

A few case series and case reports indicate variable results in patients with tardive dyskinesia (Besson and Palin 1991; Flaherty et al. 1984; Holcomb et al. 1983; Price and Levin 1978; Yassa et al. 1990). In one case, dyskinesias were induced in a Wilson's disease patient (DeQuardo et al. 1992). It is not surprising that some cases of tardive dyskinesia worsen with ECT, considering the known propensity of ECT to increase levodopa-induced dyskinesias in patients with Parkinson's disease (Douyon et al. 1989). Several cases of improvement in tardive dystonia with ECT have been reported (Kaplan et al. 1991; Kwentus et al. 1984; Postalache et al. 1995), although one case without improvement has been reported (Hanin et al. 1995).

Numerous series have documented that ECT represents a life-saving option for patients with neuroleptic-induced malignant catatonia (also known as neuroleptic malignant syndrome) who do not respond to more conservative measures (Davis et al. 1991; Mann et al. 1990; Nisijima and Ishiguro 1999; Philbrick and Rummans 1994; Scheftner and Shulman 1992; Troller and Sachdev 1999). Typically, ECT should be reserved for patients who fail to respond to withdrawal of neuroleptic medication and institution of supportive measures, such as muscle relaxants and benzodiazepines; additionally, ECT can treat both the signs of neuroleptic-induced malignant catatonia as well as catatonia, psychosis, or mood disorder as part of the underlying psychopathological condition, which are sometimes difficult to distinguish (Mann et al. 2003).

There is no particular reason to believe that ECT is unsafe in patients who have these neuroleptic-induced movement disorders, although the clinician should monitor the effects ECT may have on the movements as well as on cognitive function.

Cerebrovascular Disease

Several isolated reports of safe use of ECT in patients poststroke have been published (DeQuardo and Tandon 1988; Weintraub and Lippmann 2000). In a large series of such patients given ECT (Currier et al. 1992; Murray et al. 1986), 32 of 34 attained an antidepressant response, and none of the patients deteriorated neurologically. Nei-

ther location nor time since stroke was associated with clinical outcome. Five of six patients showed improvement in preexisting cognitive impairment with treatment, again reflecting the enhancement in sustained attention with the antidepressant benefit of ECT.

Martin et al. (1992) treated 14 poststroke patients with ECT and compared their outcomes with those of 14 age- and sex-matched control ECT patients. They found a similar incidence of 4 of 14 in each group developing interictal delirium. All four of the poststroke patients developing delirium had caudate strokes, supporting the investigators' contention that basal ganglia lesions predispose to ECT-related delirium. The poststroke ECT patients had a good clinical response without worsening in noncognitive neurological functions. Of note, the more ECT treatments given after the delirium became apparent, the longer the delirium lasted.

In addition to patients with a history of stroke, those with known intracerebral aneurysms or vascular malformations might be expected to have a higher than average risk of complications with ECT. At least two cases of patients safely administered ECT after cerebral aneurysm repair have been reported (Farah et al. 1996; Husum et al. 1983), and numerous cases of patients with known aneurysms that have not been surgically corrected pre-ECT have been reported; in none of those did a bleed occur (Bader et al. 1995; Drop et al. 1988; Gardner and Kellner 1998; Hunt and Kaplan 1998; Kolano et al. 1997; Najjar and Guttmacher 1998; Salaris et al. 2000; Viguera et al. 1998). Two cases of ECT-associated intracerebral hemorrhages have been reported (Rikher et al. 1997; Weisberg et al. 1991), both in patients without known pre-ECT cerebrovascular disease. Most investigators reporting on ECT in patients with known aneurysms used antihypertensive treatments to dampen the ECT-related increase in blood pressure. Drop et al. (2000) considered intracerebral aneurysms at high risk for rupture during ECT and recommended that appropriate antihypertensive measures (e.g., beta-blockade, sodium nitroprusside) and monitoring should be undertaken during ECT in such patients.

In summary, the literature on ECT in patients with histories of stroke or intracerebral aneurysm contains numerous reports of safe ECT administration. This should provide some confidence to the clinician, but caution is still warranted. Patients with hemorrhagic strokes probably present a greater risk than those with ischemic ones. Measures to control excessive blood pressure increases that do not cause a later drop in blood pressure should be considered, given stroke patients' common impairment in cerebral autoregulation of blood pressure (Drop et al. 2000). Thus, relatively short-acting antihypertensives, such as esmolol, probably provide safer hemodynamic control than longer-acting compounds.

Epilepsy

ECT has anticonvulsant activity, as indicated by a progressive increase in seizure threshold and decrease in seizure length during the course of treatments (Sackeim et al. 1983). In the pre-anticonvulsant era, and sporadically in the modern era, ECT has been used successfully to treat intractable epilepsy (Caplan 1946; Griesemer et al. 1997; Regenold et al. 1998; Sackeim et al. 1983; Schnur et al. 1989; Taylor 1946; Viparelli and Viparelli 1992; Wolff 1956) and even status epilepticus (Lisanby et al. 2001). These effects are short-lived, however, and the use of ECT to treat epilepsy is largely only of historical interest, with current treatments including anticonvulsant medications, surgery, and vagal nerve stimulation.

Occasional reports document that status epilepticus can occur, fortunately rarely, after ECT, even in nonepileptic patients given ECT for a mood, psychotic, or behavioral dyscontrol disorder (Grogan et al. 1995; Hansen-Grant et al. 1995; Rao et al. 1993). There are two reports of status epilepticus following ECT in epileptic patients: one patient had been administered multiple monitored ECT (Maletzky 1981), a technique no longer recommended for routine use (American Psychiatric Association 2001); the other had previously unrecognized seizures and was not receiving anticonvulsant medication during ECT (Moss-Herjanic 1967). At present, there is no evidence that spontaneous seizure frequency increases with ECT in epileptic patients. However, no large series have been published. Furthermore, it does not appear that the incidence of chronic epilepsy is increased in nonepileptic patients who receive ECT (Blackwood et al. 1980).

The more common clinical challenge is how to treat the epileptic patient whose psychopathological features indicate ECT. Surprisingly few reports describe ECT for psychiatric indications in epileptic patients (Hsiao et al. 1987). There are two cases of successful and safe ECT in depressed patients after neurosurgery for a seizure disorder (Kaufman et al. 1996; Krahn et al. 1993). In assessing risk with ECT, one must consider the etiology of the seizure disorder: a patient with seizures secondary to a brain tumor would obviously be at higher risk of complications from ECT than a patient with idiopathic epilepsy, a normal head MRI, and no focal neurological findings. Before undertaking a course of ECT in a patient with epilepsy, consultation with the patient's neurologist is advised. Pretreatment head imaging or electroencephalography is not needed unless such testing is indicated as part of the patient's neurological care.

The most common technical problem in ECT with epileptic patients is elicitation of therapeutic seizures in the face of concomitant treatment with anticonvulsant medications. We have personally treated numerous epileptic patients successfully with ECT without having to alter the patient's anticonvulsant regimen; however, occasionally patients either do not obtain seizures or have extremely short ones. In such a scenario, strategies include hyperventilation before the electrical stimulus, use of non-anticonvulsant anesthetic agents such as etomidate or ketamine, pretreatment with intravenous caffeine before anesthesia, and cautious lowering of the patient's anticonvulsant medication dosages (American Psychiatric Association 2001). The latter method brings the risk of spontaneous seizures and should be undertaken with the aid of a neurologist. At present, it is not known whether various anticonvulsant agents differentially affect seizure threshold and duration in ECT.

Intracranial Tumors

Two early reports of dire outcomes in ECT patients found to have brain tumors following treatment led to the common belief that intracranial masses represent an absolute contraindication to ECT (Maltbie et al. 1980; Shapiro and Goldberg 1957). Mattingly et al. (1991), however, reviewed 10 cases in which presence of the tumor was known in advance of ECT (eight with meningiomas and two with metastatic breast cancer). None of the patients had focal neurological findings, increased intracranial pressure, or papilledema before treatment, nor did any of them die or experience neurological deterioration with ECT up to 1 month afterward. Several other cases of successful and neurologically uncomplicated administration of ECT to patients with meningiomas have been described (Kellner and Rames 1990; Kellner et al. 1991b; McKinney et al. 1998; Starkstein and Migliorelli 1993). Recently, a patient with increased intracranial pressure associated with a brain tumor was reported to enjoy a good therapeutic response without neurological deterioration (Patkar et al. 2000). The investigators used dexamethasone, furosemide, and beta-blockade before treatment to decrease brain edema and to blunt the increase in intracranial pressure associated with ECT. Most recently, Kohler and Burock (2001) reported a 35-year-old woman with intractable depression after two resections and radiation therapy for recurrent left frontal neurocytoma. Pretreatment MRI revealed a complex mass in the left lateral ventricle and left frontal encephalomalacia. She had mild right-sided weakness and mild transcortical expressive dysphasia. After three ECT treatments and on follow-up several months later, she was much better and without any neurological worsening.

Whether intracranial pressure was elevated pretreatment was not reported.

Presence of any CNS tumor may present an increased risk for neurological complications caused by ECT. In the absence of focal neurological signs, brain edema, mass effect, or papilledema, the risks likely are relatively small. In the presence of such findings, the increased risk may be quite high, and ECT should be considered only when no other reasonable option exists and only after consultation with a neurosurgeon or neurologist.

Other Neurological Disorders

As discussed previously, ECT may be lifesaving in some cases of refractory neuroleptic-induced malignant catatonia (neuroleptic malignant syndrome). There have also been several reports that ECT may be effective in a variety of other states falling under the rubric of "delirium" (Stromgren 1997). However, most of the reports involve patients who would be described in the United States as having catatonic features as part of a mood or psychotic disorder (American Psychiatric Association 1999; Stromgren 1997). We agree with recent practice guidelines that ECT should not be considered effective against delirium as a global phenomenon (American Psychiatric Association 1999). However, there may be specific types of delirium in which ECT may play a role. For example, there are some reports of a beneficial effect of ECT in delirium tremens (Dudley and Williams 1972; Kramp and Bolwig 1981), although this is probably only of historical interest. Additionally, there are reports of patients with protracted delirium after traumatic brain injury who responded to ECT (Kant et al. 1995; Silverman 1964). A prudent summary statement on this issue would be that although ECT is not a primary treatment for delirium, it sometimes may be dramatically effective in cases in which, in spite of intense medical and neurological assessment and management, a patient persists with severe agitation, psychosis, or catatonic features.

Several cases have been reported of patients with multiple sclerosis receiving ECT for psychopathological states (Mattingly et al. 1992; Savitsky and Karliner 1951), with the suggestion that gadolinium-enhancing lesions on MRI before treatment may indicate a high risk for neurological deterioration (Mattingly et al. 1992). Isolated case reports and small series also describe, with greatly varying levels of detail on outcome, the safe use of ECT for psychopathological states in patients with a diversity of other neurological conditions such as cerebral palsy (Rasmussen et al. 1993), hydrocephalus with shunt (Levy and Levy 1987), spinocerebellar ataxia (Folkerts et al. 1998), Huntington's disease (Beale et al. 1997; Broth-

ers and Meadows 1955; Evans et al. 1987; Folstein et al. 1983; Heathfield 1967; Lewis et al. 1996; McHugh and Folstein 1975; Ranen et al. 1994), progressive supranuclear palsy (Barclay et al. 1996), Friedreich's ataxia (Singh et al. 2001), and multiple system atrophy (Hooten et al. 1998; Roane et al. 2000). Of course, these do not prove ECT has the same risk profile as for patients without these conditions. A prudent approach in such patients is to be cautious for signs of neurological worsening and especially for excessive cognitive side effects.

Miscellaneous Medical Disorders

The heart and brain bear most of the physiological effects of ECT. Fortunately, most of the other organ systems are not substantially affected by ECT, nor do their diseases generally cause much concern for greater risk of complications during ECT. We do, however, cover some additional considerations in the following discussion.

Pulmonary

With the obvious paralyzing effect of anesthetic medications on respiration, careful attention to airway management is of the highest importance in ECT practice, and patients with pulmonary disorders should receive special attention. For example, bronchospasm is a risk in patients with chronic obstructive pulmonary disease or asthma (Taylor 1968). Patients who are using inhalers should do so in the morning shortly before treatment. Theophylline has been associated with a risk of prolonged seizures and status epilepticus in ECT (Abrams 1997; Devanand et al. 1988; Peters et al. 1984), and discontinuation before ECT if medically safe has been recommended (American Psychiatric Association 2001), although Rasmussen and Zorumski (1993) described seven patients with therapeutic theophylline levels during ECT, none of whom developed status epilepticus. If discontinuing theophylline is medically contraindicated, then the lowest therapeutic blood level should be maintained, caffeine augmentation should be avoided, and there should be ready access to rapidly acting anticonvulsant medication (e.g., intravenous diazepam).

Pregnancy

The two most common adverse events in pregnant women during ECT are aspiration and those related to premature labor, uterine contractions, and vaginal bleeding, although ECT can be delivered safely during pregnancy (American Psychiatric Association 2001; Ishikawa et al. 2001; Miller

1994; Walker and Swartz 1994). Safety measures to prevent aspiration include tracheal intubation and alkalinizing intragastric pH with a nonparticulate antacid. Pretreatment obstetrical assessment, preferably to include fetal ultrasound, can identify high-risk pregnancies. Noninvasive monitoring of fetal heart tones before and after the seizure can document that no fetal distress occurred. Finally, probably the most important aspect of safe ECT in pregnant women is ready availability of obstetrical intervention in case of untoward events (American Psychiatric Association 2001).

Diabetes Mellitus

A recent large series describing patients with insulin-dependent type 2 diabetes mellitus concluded that clinically significant changes in glucose levels are rare during ECT (Netzel et al. 2002). Diabetic patients should have blood glucose levels monitored closely during the ECT course, including fingerstick checks just before treatment and probably during recovery and shortly thereafter. Typically, insulin-dependent diabetics are administered half their morning insulin doses and are treated with ECT promptly. They are then fed breakfast and given the remaining half of their insulin dose. Intravenous access should be maintained well into recovery in case glucose needs to be administered for hypoglycemic episodes in brittle patients.

Other Considerations

Electrolyte abnormalities can lead to cardiac dysrhythmias and should be corrected. Histamine$_2$ antagonists or antacids may decrease gastric acid secretion and the risk of aspiration in patients with gastroesophageal reflux disease, gastroparesis, or obesity (as well as pregnancy, as discussed above). Patients at severe risk for aspiration may require intubation. Urinary retention from antimuscarinic agents given during ECT is quite uncomfortable for patients and can predispose to urinary tract infections and even bladder rupture if not monitored. In those patients who do experience significant urinary retention after treatments, antimuscarinics can be avoided, recognizing that the vagal effect of the electrical stimulus is not blocked and prolonged asystole can occur. Patients with severe osteoporosis or recent fractures require careful titration of muscle relaxant dosing; the adequacy of paralysis can be tested with a peripheral nerve stimulator. Extra care should be exercised in ventilating the patient with unstable cervical spine disease to avoid spinal cord injury. With the brief increase in intraocular pressure lasting a few minutes after the seizures (Edwards et al. 1990; Good et al. 2004; Saad

et al. 2000), glaucoma patients should receive their medications in the mornings before treatment, an exception being anthicholinesterase drugs, which theoretically could prolong the action of succinylcholine (American Psychiatric Association 2001; Saad et al. 2000).

Conclusion

ECT represents a remarkably safe and effective treatment option for depressed, manic, or psychotic patients with concomitant medical illnesses. With proper attention to pretreatment medical evaluation, rational use of cardioprotective medications during the treatments, and ongoing monitoring of medical status in between treatments, virtually all patients requiring ECT can be safely treated.

References

Aarsland D, Larsen JP, Oyvind W, et al: Maintenance electroconvulsive therapy for Parkinson's disease. Convuls Ther 13:274–277, 1997

Abiuso P, Dunkelman R, Proper M: Electroconvulsive therapy in patients with pacemakers. JAMA 240:2459–2460, 1978

Abramczuk JA, Rose NM: Pre-anesthetic assessment and the prevention of post-ECT morbidity. Br J Psychiatry 134: 582–587, 1979

Abrams R: Electroconvulsive Therapy, 3rd Edition. New York, Oxford University Press, 1997

Abrams R: Electroconvulsive Therapy, 4th Edition. New York, Oxford University Press, 2002

Alexopoulos GS, Frances RJ: ECT and cardiac patients with pacemakers. Am J Psychiatry 137:1111–1112, 1980

Alexopoulos GS, Shamoian CJ, Lucas J, et al: Medical problems of geriatric psychiatric patients and younger controls during electroconvulsive therapy. J Am Geriatr Soc 32:651–654, 1984

American Psychiatric Association, Committee on Electroconvulsive Therapy: The Practice of Electroconvulsive Therapy, 2nd Edition. Edited by Weiner RD. Washington, DC, American Psychiatric Association, 2001

American Psychiatric Association, Task Force on Delirium: Practice Guidelines for the Treatment of Patients with Delirium. Am J Psychiatry 156 (suppl):1–20, 1999

Applegate RJ: Diagnosis and management of ischemic heart disease in the patient scheduled to undergo electroconvulsive therapy. Convuls Ther 13:128–144, 1997

Attar-Levy D, Fidelle G, Bochier P, et al: Electroconvulsive therapy and aortic aneurysm: apropos of a case. Encephale 21:473–476, 1995

Bader GM, Silk KR, DeQuardo JR, et al: Electroconvulsive therapy and intracranial aneurysm. Convuls Ther 11:139–143, 1995

Ballenger JC: Electroconvulsive therapy and cardiac pacemakers. Psychosomatics 14:233–234, 1973

Barclay CL, Duff J, Sandor P, et al: Limited usefulness of electroconvulsive therapy in progressive supranuclear palsy. Neurology 46:1284–1286, 1996

Beale MD, Kellner CH, Gurecki P, et al: ECT for the treatment of Huntington's disease: a case study. Convuls Ther 13:108–112, 1997

Besson JAO, Palin AN: Tardive dyskinesia, depression, and ECT (letter). Br J Psychiatry 159:446, 1991

Blackwood DHR, Cull RE, Freeman CPL, et al: A study of the incidence of epilepsy following ECT. J Neurol Neurosurg Psychiatry 43:1098–1102, 1980

Bleich S, Degner D, Scheschonka A, et al: Electroconvulsive therapy and anticoagulation. Can J Psychiatry 45:87–88, 2000

Blitt CD, Kirschvink LJ: Electroconvulsive therapy with a cardiac pacemaker (letter). Anesthesiology 45:580, 1976

Brothers CRD, Meadows AW: An investigation of Huntington's chorea in Victoria. J Ment Sci 101:548–563, 1955

Burd J, Kettl P: Incidence of asystole in electroconvulsive therapy in elderly patients. Am J Geriatr Psychiatry 6:203–211, 1998

Caplan G: Electrical convulsion therapy in the treatment of epilepsy. J Ment Sci 92:784–793, 1946

Castelli I, Steiner LA, Kaufman MA, et al: Comparative effects of esmolol and labetolol to attenuate hyperdynamic states after electroconvulsive therapy. Anesth Analg 80:557–561, 1995

Chapman AH: Aortic dacron graft surgery and electroshock: report of a case. Am J Psychiatry 117:937–938, 1961

Cockey GH, Conti CR: Electroconvulsive therapy-induced transient T-wave inversions on ECG. Clin Cardiol 18:418–420, 1995

Currier MB, Murray GB, Welch CC: Electroconvulsive therapy for post-stroke depressed geriatric patients. J Neuropsychiatry Clin Neurosci 4:140–144, 1992

Davis JM, Janicak PJ, Sakkar P, et al: Electroconvulsive therapy in the treatment of the neuroleptic malignant syndrome. Convuls Ther 7:111–120, 1991

Dec GW, Stern TA, Welch C: The effects of electroconvulsive therapy on serial electrocardiograms and serum cardiac enzyme values: a prospective study of depressed hospitalized inpatients. JAMA 253:2525–2529, 1985

Decina P, Malitz S, Sackeim HA, et al: Cardiac arrest during ECT modified by β-adrenergic blockade. Am J Psychiatry 141:298–300, 1984

Deliyiannis S, Eliahim M, Bellet S: The electrocardiogram during electroconvulsive therapy as studied by radioelectrocardiography. Am J Cardiol 10:187–194, 1962

DeQuardo JR, Tandon R: ECT in post-stroke major depression. Convuls Ther 4:221–224, 1988

DeQuardo JR, Liberzon I, Tandon R: Recurrent post-ECT dyskinesias (letter). Convuls Ther 8:42–43, 1992

De Silva RA, Bachman WR: Cardiac consultation in patients with neuropsychiatric problems. Cardiol Clin 13:225–239, 1995

Devanand DP, Malitz S, Sackeim HA: ECT in a patient with aortic aneurysm. J Clin Psychiatry 51:255–256, 1990

Devanand DP, Sackeim HA, Decina P, et al: Status epilepticus following ECT in a patient taking theophylline (letter). J Clin Psychopharmacol 8:153, 1988

Dolenc TJ, Barnes RD, Hayes DL, et al: Electroconvulsive therapy in patients with pacemakers and ICDs. Pacing Clin Electrophysiol (in press)

Douyon R, Serby M, Klutchko B, et al: ECT and Parkinson's disease revisited: a "naturalistic" study. Am J Psychiatry 146:1451–1455, 1989

Dowling FG, Francis A: Aortic aneurysm and electroconvulsive therapy. Convuls Ther 9:121–127, 1993

Drop LJ, Bouckoms AJ, Welch CA: Arterial hypertension and multiple cerebral aneurysms in a patient treated with electroconvulsive therapy. J Clin Psychiatry 49:280–282, 1988

Drop LJ, Viguera A, Welch CA: ECT in patients with intracranial aneurysm (letter). J ECT 16:71–72, 2000

Dudley WHC, Williams JG: Electroconvulsive therapy in delirium tremens. Compr Psychiatry 13:357–360, 1972

Edwards RM, Stoudemire A, Vela MA, et al: Intraocular pressure changes in nonglaucomatous patients undergoing electroconvulsive therapy. Convuls Ther 6:209–213, 1990

Eitzman DT, Bach DS, Rubenfire M: Management of myocardial stunning associated with electroconvulsive therapy guided by hyperventilation echocardiography. Am Heart J 127:928–929, 1994

Evans DL, Pederson CA, Tancer ME: ECT in the treatment of organic psychosis in Huntington's disease. Convuls Ther 3:145–150, 1987

Fall P-A, Granerus A-K: Maintenance ECT in Parkinson's disease. J Neural Transm 106:737–741, 1999

Fall P-A, Ekman R, Granerus A-K, et al: ECT in Parkinson's disease: changes in motor symptoms, monoamine metabolites and neuropeptides. J Neural Transm 10:129–140, 1995

Farah A, McCall WV, Amundson RH: ECT after cerebral aneurysm repair. Convuls Therapy 12:165–170, 1996

Flaherty JA, Naidu J, Dysken M: Emergent dyskinesia and depression. Am J Psychiatry 141:808–809, 1984

Folk JW, Kellner CH, Beale MD, et al: Anesthesia for electroconvulsive therapy: a review. J ECT 16:157–170, 2000

Folkerts HE, Stadtland C, Reker T: ECT for organic catatonia due to hereditary cerebellar ataxia. J ECT 14:53–55, 1998

Folstein MF, Folstein SE, McHugh PR: "Mini-Mental State": a practical method for grading the cognitive status of patients for the clinician. J Psychiatr Res 12:189–198, 1975

Folstein SE, Abbott MH, Chase GA, et al: The association of affective disorder with Huntington's disease in a case series and in families. Psychol Med 13:537–542, 1983

Fuenmayor AJ, el Fakih Y, Moreno J, et al: Effects of electroconvulsive therapy on cardiac function in patients without heart disease. Cardiology 88:254–257, 1997

Gardner MW, Kellner CH: Safe use of ECT with an intracranial aneurysm (letter). J ECT 14:290–292, 1998

Gaspar D, Samarasinghe LA: ECT in psychogeriatric practice: a study of risk factors, indications and outcome. Compr Psychiatry 23:170–175, 1982

Geretsegger C, Rochowanski E: Electroconvulsive therapy in acute life-threatening catatonia with associated cardiac and respiratory decompensation. Convuls Ther 3:291–295, 1987

Gerring JP, Shields HM: The identification and management of patients with a high risk for cardiac arrythmias during modified ECT. J Clin Psychiatry 43:140–143, 1982

Gibson TC, Leaman DM, Devors J, et al: Pacemaker function in relation to electroconvulsive therapy. Chest 63:1025–1027, 1973

Goldberg RK, Badger JM: Major depressive disorder in patients with the implantable cardioverter defibrillator: two cases treated with ECT. Psychosomatics 34:273–277, 1993

Good MS, Dolenc TJ, Rasmussen KG: Electroconvulsive therapy in a patient with glaucoma. J ECT 20:48–49, 2004

Gould L, Gopalaswamy C, Chandy F, et al: Electroconvulsive therapy-induced ECG changes simulating a myocardial infarction. Arch Intern Med 143:1786–1787, 1983

Goumeniouk AD, Fry PD, Zis AP: Abdominal aortic aneurysm and ECT administration. Convuls Ther 6:55–57, 1990

Grant JE, Mohan SN: Treatment of agitation and aggression in four demented patients using ECT. J ECT 17:205–209, 2001

Gravenstein JS, Anton AH, Weiner SM, et al: Catecholamine and cardiovascular response to electroconvulsive therapy in man. Compr Psychiatry 37:833–839, 1965

Greenbank RK: Aortic homograft surgery and electroshock. Am J Psychiatry 115:469, 1958

Griesemer DA, Kellner CH, Beale MD, et al: Electroconvulsive therapy for treatment of intractable seizures: initial findings in two children. Neurology 49:1389–1392, 1997

Grogan R, Wagner DR, Sullivan T, et al: Generalized nonconvulsive status epilepticus after electroconvulsive therapy. Convuls Ther 11:51–56, 1995

Guttmacher LB, Greenlund P: Effects of electroconvulsive therapy on the electrocardiogram in geriatric patients with stable cardiovascular diseases. Convuls Ther 6:5–12, 1990

Hanin B, Lerner Y, Srour N: An unusual effect of ECT on drug-induced parkinsonism and tardive dystonia. Convuls Ther 11:271–274, 1995

Hansen-Grant S, Tandon R, Maixner D, et al: Subclinical status epilepticus following ECT. Convuls Ther 11:139–143, 1995

Hardman JB, Morse RM: Early electroconvulsive treatment of a patient who had artificial aortic and mitral valves. Am J Psychiatry 128:895–897, 1972

Harsch HH: Atrial fibrillation, cardioversion and electroconvulsive therapy. Convuls Ther 7:139–142, 1991

Hay D: ECT in the medically ill elderly. Convuls Ther 5:8–16, 1989

Heath ML: Donepezil, Alzheimer's disease, and suxamethonium (letter). Anaesthesia 52:1018, 1997

Heath ML: Donepezil and succinylcholine (letter). Anaesthesia 58:202, 2003

Heathfield KWG: Huntington's chorea. Brain 90:203–232, 1967

Hejtmancik MR, Bankhead AJ, Herrmann GR: Electrocardiographic changes following electroshock therapy in curarized patients. Am Heart J 37:790–805, 1949

Hoflich G, Kasper S, Burghof K-W, et al: Maintenance ECT for treatment of therapy-resistant paranoid schizophrenia and Parkinson's disease. Biol Psychiatry 37:892–894, 1995

Holcomb HH, Sternberg DE, Heninger GR: Effects of electroconvulsive therapy on mood, parkinsonism, and tardive dyskinesia in a depressed patient: ECT and dopamine systems. Biol Psychiatry 18:865–873, 1983

Hooten WM, Melin G, Richardson JR: Response of the parkinsonian symptoms of multiple system atrophy to ECT (letter). Am J Psychiatry 155:1628, 1998

Hsiao J, Messenheimer J, Evans DL: ECT and neurological disorders. Convuls Ther 3:121–136, 1987

Huang KC, Lucas LF, Tsueda K, et al: Age-related changes in cardiovascular function associated with electroconvulsive therapy. Convuls Ther 5:17–25, 1989

Hunt SA, Kaplan E: ECT in the presence of a cerebral aneurysm (letter). J ECT 14:123–124, 1998

Hussar AE, Pachter M: Myocardial infarction and fatal coronary insufficiency during electroconvulsive therapy. JAMA 204:1004–1007, 1968

Husum B, Vester-Andersen T, Buchmann G, et al: Electroconvulsive therapy and intracranial aneurysm: prevention of blood pressure elevation in a normotensive patient by hydralazine and propranolol. Anaesthesia 38:1205–1207, 1983

Huuhka MJ, Seinela L, Reinikainen P, et al: Cardiac arrhythmias induced by ECT in elderly psychiatric patients: experience with 48-hour Holter monitoring. J ECT 19:22–25, 2003

Ishikawa T, Kawahara S, Saito T, et al: Anesthesia for electroconvulsive therapy during pregnancy: a case report. Masui 50:991–997, 2001

Jauhar P, Weller M, Hirsch SR: Electroconvulsive therapy for patient with cardiac pacemaker. BMJ 1:901, 1979

Kadoi Y, Saito S, Seki S, et al: Electroconvulsive therapy impairs systolic performance of the left ventricle. Can J Anaesth 48:405–408, 2001

Kant R, Bogyi A, Carasella N, et al: ECT as a therapeutic option in severe brain injury. Convuls Ther 11:45–50, 1995

Kaplan Z, Benjamin J, Zohar J: Remission of tardive dystonia with ECT. Convuls Ther 7:280–283, 1991

Kaufman KR, Saucedo C, Schaeffer J, et al: Electroconvulsive therapy (ECT) for intractable depression following epilepsy neurosurgery. Seizure 5:307–312, 1996

Kellner CH, Rames L: Dexamethasone pretreatment for ECT in a patient with meningioma. Clin Gerontol 10:67–72, 1990

Kellner CH, Monroe RR, Burns C, et al: Electroconvulsive therapy in a patient with a heart transplant (letter). N Engl J Med 325:663, 1991a

Kellner CH, Burns CM, Bernstein HJ, et al: Safe administration of ECT in a patient with a calcified frontal mass (letter). J Neuropsychiatry Clin Neurosci 3:353–354, 1991b

Khoury GF, Benedetti C: T-wave changes associated with electroconvulsive therapy. Anesth Analg 69:677–679, 1989

Kitamura T, Page AJF: Electrocardiographic changes following electroconvulsive therapy. Eur Arch Psychiatry Neurol Sci 234:147–148, 1984

Kohler CG, Burock M: ECT for psychotic depression associated with a brain tumor (letter). Am J Psychiatry 158:2089, 2001

Kolano JE, Chibber A, Calalang CC: Use of esmolol to control bleeding and heart rate during electroconvulsive therapy in a patient with an intracranial aneurysm. J Clin Anesth 9:493–495, 1997

Krahn LE, Rummans TA, Peterson GC, et al: Electroconvulsive therapy for depression after temporal lobectomy for epilepsy. Convuls Ther 9:217–219, 1993

Kramp P, Bolwig TG: Electroconvulsive therapy in acute delirious states. Compr Psychiatry 22:368–371, 1981

Kwentus JA, Schulz SC, Hart RP: Tardive dystonia, catatonia, and electroconvulsive therapy. J Nerv Ment Dis 172:171–173, 1984

Lapid MI, Rummans TA, Hofmann VE, et al: ECT and automatic internal cardioverter-defibrillator. J ECT 17:146–148, 2001

Lee HB, Jayaram G, Teitelbaum ML: Electroconvulsive therapy for depression in a cardiac transplant patient. Psychosomatics 42:362–364, 2001

Levin L, Wambold D, Viguera A, et al: Hemodynamic responses to ECT in a patient with critical aortic stenosis. J ECT 16:52–61, 2000

Levy SD, Levy SB: Electroconvulsive therapy in two former neurosurgical patients: skull prosthesis and ventricular shunt. Convuls Ther 3:46–48, 1987

Lewis CF, DeQuardo JR, Tandon R: ECT in genetically confirmed Huntington's disease. J Neuropsychiatry Clin Neurosci 8:209–210, 1996

Lisanby SH, Bazil CW, Resor SR, et al: ECT in the treatment of status epilepticus. J ECT 17:210–215, 2001

Loo H, Kuche H, Benkelfat C: Electroconvulsive therapy during anticoagulant therapy. Convuls Ther 1:258–262, 1985

Maletzky BM: Multiple Monitored Electroconvulsive Therapy. Boca Raton, FL, CRR Press, 1981

Maltbie AA, Wingfield MS, Volow MR, et al: Electroconvulsive therapy in the presence of brain tumor: case reports and an evaluation of risk. J Nerv Ment Dis 168:400–405, 1980

Mann SC, Caroff SN, Bleier H, et al: Electroconvulsive therapy of the lethal catatonia syndrome. Convuls Ther 6:239–247, 1990

Mann SC, Caroff SN, Keck PE Jr, et al: Neuroleptic Malignant Syndrome and Related Conditions, 2nd Edition. Washington, DC, American Psychiatric Publishing, 2003

Martin M, Figiel GS, Mattingly G, et al: ECT-induced interictal delirium in patients with a history of CVA. J Geriatr Psychiatry and Neurology 5:149–155, 1992

Mattingly G, Figiel GS, Jarvis MR, et al: Prospective uses of ECT in the presence of intracranial tumors (letter). J Neuropsychiatry Clin Neurosci 3:459–463, 1991

Mattingly G, Baker K, Zorumski CF, et al: Multiple sclerosis and ECT: possible value of gadolinium-enhanced magnetic resonance scans for identifying high-risk patients. J Neuropsychiatry Clin Neurosci 4:145–151, 1992

McCall WV, Shelp FE, Weiner RD, et al: Effects of labetolol on hemodynamics and seizure duration during ECT. Convuls Ther 7:5–14, 1991

McCully RB, Karon BL, Rummans TA, et al: Frequency of left ventricular dysfunction after electroconvulsive therapy. Am J Cardiol 91:1147–1150, 2003

McDonald WM, Thompson TR: Treatment of mania in dementia with electroconvulsive therapy. Psychopharmacol Bull 35:72–82, 2001

McHugh PR, Folstein MF: Psychiatric syndromes of Huntington's chorea: a clinical and phenomenologic study, in Psychiatric Aspects of Neurological Disease. Edited by Benson DF, Blumer D. Orlando, FL, Grune & Stratton, 1975, pp 267–286

McKenna G, Engle RP, Brooks H, et al: Cardiac arrhythmias during electroshock therapy: significance, prevention, and treatment. Am J Psychiatry 127:172–175, 1970

McKinney PA, Beale MD, Kellner CH: Electroconvulsive therapy in a patient with a cerebellar meningioma. J ECT 14:49–52, 1998

Mensah GA, Shoen RE, Devereaux RB: Intracardiac thrombi in patients undergoing electroconvulsive therapy. Am Heart J 119:684–685, 1990

Messina AG, Paranicas M, Katz B, et al: Effect of electroconvulsive therapy on the electrocardiogram and echocardiogram. Anesth Analg 75:511–514, 1992

Miller L: Use of electroconvulsive therapy during pregnancy. Hosp Community Psychiatry 45:444–450, 1994

Moellentine C, Rummans TA, Ahlskog JE, et al: ECT and Parkinson's disease. J Neuropsychiatry Clin Neurosci 10:187–193, 1998

Monke JV: Electroconvulsive therapy following surgical correction of aortic coarctation by implantation of an aortic isograft: a case history. Am J Psychiatry 109:378–379, 1952

Moore MB: Electroconvulsive therapy and the aorta. CMAJ 83:1258–1259, 1960

Moriarty JD: Combined cardioversion and ECT in chronic auricular fibrillation. Psychosomatics 13:388–389, 1972

Moss-Herjanic B: Prolonged unconsciousness following electroconvulsive therapy. Am J Psychiatry 124:112–114, 1967

Murray GB, Shea V, Conn DK: Electroconvulsive therapy for poststroke depression. J Clin Psychiatry 47:258–260, 1986

Najjar F, Guttmacher LB: ECT in the presence of intracranial aneurysm (letter). J ECT 14:266–271, 1998

Nelson JP, Rosenberg DR: ECT treatment of demented elderly patients with major depression: a retrospective study of efficacy and safety. Convuls Ther 7:157–165, 1991

Netzel PJ, Mueller PS, Rummans TA, et al: Safety, efficacy, and effects on glycemic control of electroconvulsive therapy in insulin-requiring type 2 diabetic patients. J ECT 18:16–21, 2002

Nisijima K, Ishiguro T: Electroconvulsive therapy for the treatment of neuroleptic malignant syndrome with psychotic symptoms: a report of 5 cases. J ECT 15:158–163, 1999

Nobler MS, Sackeim HA, Prohovnik I, et al: Regional cerebral blood flow in mood disorders, III: treatment and clinical response. Arch Gen Psychiatry 51:884–897, 1994

O'Connor CJ, Rothenberg DM, Soble JS, et al: The effect of esmolol pretreatment on the incidence of regional wall motion abnormalities during electroconvulsive therapy. Anesth Analg 82:143–147, 1996

O'Melia J: A case of auricular fibrillation following the use of suxamethonium during ECT (letter). Br J Psychiatry 117: 718, 1970

Ottoway A: Atrial fibrillation, failed cardioversion, and electroconvulsive therapy. Anaesth Intensive Care 30:215–218, 2002

Pargger H, Kaufmann MA, Schouten R, et al: Hemodynamic responses to electroconvulsive therapy in a patient 5 years after cardiac transplantation. Anesthesiology 83:625–627, 1995

Patkar AA, Hill KP, Weinstein SP, et al: ECT in the presence of brain tumor and increased intracranial pressure: evaluation and reduction of risk. J ECT 16:189–197, 2000

Perron AD, Brady WJ: Electrocardiographic manifestations of CNS events (comment). Am J Emerg Med 18:715–720, 2000

Peters S, Wochos D, Peterson G: Status epilepticus as a complication of concurrent electroconvulsive and theophylline therapy. Mayo Clin Proc 59:568–579, 1984

Petrides G, Fink M: Atrial fibrillation, anticoagulation, and electroconvulsive therapy. Convuls Ther 12:91–98, 1996

Philbrick KL, Rummans TA: Malignant catatonia. J Neuropsychiatry Clin Neurosci 6:1–13, 1994

Pomeranze JP, Karliner W, Triebel WA, et al: Electroshock therapy in presence of serious organic disease: depression and aortic aneurysm. Geriatrics 23:122–124, 1968

Pornnoppadol C, Isenberg K: ECT with implantable cardioverter defibrillator. J ECT 14:124–126, 1998

Postalache TT, Londono JH, Halem RG, et al: Electroconvulsive therapy in tardive dystonia. Convuls Ther 11:275–279, 1995

Price TRP, Levin R: The effects of ECT on tardive dyskinesia. Am J Psychiatry 135:991–993, 1978

Pridmore S, Pollard C: Electroconvulsive therapy in Parkinson's disease: 30 month follow up (letter). J Neurol Neurosurg Psychiatry 61:693, 1996

Pridmore S, Yeo PT, Pasha MI: Electroconvulsive therapy for the physical signs of Parkinson's disease without depressive disorder (letter). J Neurol Neurosurg Psychiatry 58:641–642, 1995

Prudic J, Sackeim HA, Decina P, et al: Acute effects of ECT on cardiovascular functioning: relations to patient and treatment variables. Acta Psychiatr Scand 75:344–351, 1987

Ranen NG, Peyser CE, Fostein SE: ECT as a treatment for depression in Huntington's disease. J Neuropsychiatry Clin Neurosci 6:154–159, 1994

Rao KMJ, Gangadhar BN, Janakiramiah N: Nonconvulsive status epilepticus after the ninth electroconvulsive therapy. Convuls Ther 9:128–134, 1993

Rao V, Lyketsos CG: The benefits and risks of ECT for patients with primary dementia who also suffer from depression. Int J Geriatr Psychiatry 15:729–735, 2000

Rasmussen KG: Electroconvulsive therapy in patients with aortic stenosis. Convuls Ther 13:196–199, 1997

Rasmussen K, Abrams R: Treatment of Parkinson's disease with electroconvulsive therapy. Psychiatr Clin North Am 14: 925–933, 1991

Rasmussen KG, Zorumski CF: Electroconvulsive therapy in patients taking theophylline. J Clin Psychiatry 54:427–431, 1993

Rasmussen KG, Zorumski CF, Jarvis MR: ECT in patients with cerebral palsy. Convuls Ther 9:205–208, 1993

Rasmussen KG, Jarvis MR, Zorumski CF, et al: Low-dose atropine in electroconvulsive therapy. J ECT 15:213–221, 1999

Rasmussen KG, Rummans TA, Richardson JR: Electroconvulsive therapy in the medically ill. Psychiatr Clin North Am 25:177–194, 2002

Rasmussen KG, Russell JC, Kung S, et al: Electroconvulsive therapy for patients with major depression and probable Lewy body dementia. J ECT 19:103–109, 2003

Rasmussen KG, Karpyak VM, Hammill SC: Lack of effect of ECT on Holter monitor recordings before and after treatment. J ECT 20:45–47, 2004

Regenold WT, Weintraub D, Taller A: Electroconvulsive therapy for epilepsy and major depression. Am J Geriatr Psychiatry 6:180–183, 1998

Regestein QR, Reich P: Electroconvulsive therapy in patients at high risk for physical complications. Convuls Ther 1:101–114, 1985

Reynolds CF, Perel JM, Kupfer DJ, et al: Open-trial response to antidepressant treatment in elderly patients with mixed depression and cognitive impairment. Psychiatry Res 21:111–122, 1987

Rice EH, Sombrotto LB, Markowitz JC, et al: Cardiovascular morbidity in high-risk patients during ECT. Am J Psychiatry 151:1637–1641, 1994

Rikher KV, Johnson R, Kamal M: Cortical blindness after electroconvulsive therapy. J Am Board Fam Pract 10:141–143, 1997

Roane DM, Rogers JD, Helew L, et al: Electroconvulsive therapy for elderly patients with multiple system atrophy: a case series. Am J Geriatr Psychiatry 8:171–174, 2000

Rosenfeld JE, Glassberg S, Sherrid M: Administration of ECT four years after aortic aneurysm dissection. Am J Psychiatry 145:128–129, 1988

Rumi DO, Solimene MC, Takada JY, et al: Electrocardiographic and blood pressure alterations during electroconvulsive therapy in young adults. Arq Bras Cardiol 79:149–160, 2002

Ruwitch JF, Perez JE, Miller TR, et al: Myocardial ischemia induced by electroconvulsive therapy (abstract 2034). Circulation 90 (suppl 4, pt 2):I379, 1994

Saad D, Black J, Krahn L, et al: ECT post eye surgery: two cases and a review of the literature. J ECT 16:409–414, 2000

Sackeim HA, Decina P, Prohovnik I, et al: Anticonvulsant and antidepressant properties of electroconvulsive therapy: a proposed mechanism of action. Biol Psychiatry 18:1301–1310, 1983

Salaris S, Szuba MP, Traber K: ECT and intracranial vascular masses. J ECT 16:198–203, 2000

Savitsky N, Karliner W: Electroshock therapy and multiple sclerosis. New York State Journal of Medical Science 51: 788, 1951

Scheftner WA, Shulman RB: Treatment choice in neuroleptic malignant syndrome. Convuls Ther 8:267–279, 1992

Schnur DD, Mukherjee S, Silver J, et al: Electroconvulsive therapy in the treatment of episodic aggressive dyscontrol in psychotic patients. Convuls Ther 5:353–361, 1989

Serby M, Moros D, Rowan J, et al: Maintenance ECT as adjunctive treatment to dopaminergic drugs in Parkinson's disease (abstract). Biol Psychiatry 35:654, 1994

Shapiro MF, Goldberg HH: Electroconvulsive therapy in patients with structural diseases of the central nervous system. Am J Med Sci 233:186–195, 1957

Silverman M: Organic stupor subsequent to severe head injury treated with ECT. Br J Psychiatry 110:648–650, 1964

Singh G, Binstadt BA, Black DF, et al: Electroconvulsive therapy and Friedreich's ataxia. J ECT 17:53–54, 2001

Starkstein SE, Migliorelli R: ECT in a patient with a frontal craniotomy and residual meningioma. J Neuropsychiatry Clin Neurosci 5:428–430, 1993

Stern L, Hirschmann S, Grunhaus L: ECT in patients with major depressive disorder and low cardiac output. Convuls Ther 13:68–73, 1997

Stoudemire A, Hill CD, Morris R, et al: Improvement in depression-related cognitive dysfunction following ECT. J Neuropsychiatry Clin Neurosci 7:31–34, 1995

Stromgren LS: ECT in acute delirium and related clinical states. Convuls Ther 13:10–17, 1997

Swartz CM, Inglis AE: Blood pressure reduction with ECT response. J Clin Psychiatry 51:414–416, 1990

Tancer ME, Evans DL: Electroconvulsive therapy in geriatric patients undergoing anticoagulation therapy. Convuls Ther 5:102–109, 1989

Tang W-K, Ungvari GS: Asystole during electroconvulsive therapy: a case report. Aust N Z J Psychiatry 35:382–385, 2001

Taylor G: Electroshock therapy in the asthmatic patient. Can Psychiatr Assoc J 13:187–188, 1968

Taylor JH: Control of grand mal epilepsy with electro-shock. Dis Nerv Syst 7:284–285, 1946

Troller JN, Sachdev PS: Electroconvulsive treatment of neuroleptic malignant syndrome: a review and report of cases. Aust N Z J Psychiatry 33:650–659, 1999

Troup PJ, Small JG, Milstein V, et al: Effect of electroconvulsive therapy on cardiac rhythm, conduction, and repolarization. Pacing Clin Electrophysiol 1:172–177, 1978

Viguera A, Rordorf G, Schouten R, et al: Intracranial haemodynamics during attenuated responses to electroconvulsive therapy in the presence of an intracerebral aneurysm. J Neurol Neurosurg Psychiatry 64:802–805, 1998

Viparelli U, Viparelli G: ECT and grand mal epilepsy (letter). Convuls Ther 8:39–42, 1992

Walker C, Perks D: Do you know about donepezil and succinylcholine? (letter). Anaesthesia 57:1041, 2002

Walker R, Swartz C: Electroconvulsive therapy during high-risk pregnancy. Gen Hosp Psychiatry 16:348–353, 1994

Weatherly MD, Villien LM: Treatment of psychotic depression complicated by aortic homograft replacement. Am J Psychiatry 114:1120, 1958

Webb MC, Coffey CE, Saunders WR, et al: Cardiovascular response to unilateral electroconvulsive therapy. Biol Psychiatry 28:758–766, 1990

Weintraub D, Lippmann S: Electroconvulsive therapy in the acute poststroke period. J ECT 16:415–418, 2000

Weisberg LA, Elliott D, Mielke D: Intracerebral hemorrhage following electroconvulsive therapy (letter). Neurology 41:1849, 1991

Wells DG, Davies GG: Hemodynamic changes associated with electroconvulsive therapy. Anesth Analg 66:1193–1195, 1987

Wells DG, Zelcer J, Treadrae C: ECT-induced asystole from a sub-convulsive shock. Anaesth Intensive Care 16:368–373, 1988

Wengel SP, Burke WJ, Pfeiffer RF, et al: Maintenance electroconvulsive therapy for intractable Parkinson's disease. Am J Geriatr Psychiatry 6:263–269, 1998

Wolff GE: Electro-convulsive treatment: a help for epileptics. Am Pract Dig Treat 7:1791–1793, 1956

Wolford JA: Electroshock therapy and aortic aneurysm. Am J Psychiatry 113:656, 1957

Yassa R, Hoffman H, Carakis M: The effect of electroconvulsive therapy on tardive dyskinesia: a prospective study. Convuls Ther 6:194–198, 1990

Youmans CR Jr, Bourianoff G, Allensworth DC, et al: Cardiovascular alterations during electroconvulsive therapy in patients with cardiac pacemakers. South Med J 65:361–365, 1972

Zervas IM, Fink M: ECT for refractory Parkinson's disease (letter). Convuls Ther 7:222–223, 1991

Zhu W-X, Olson DE, Karon BL, et al: Myocardial stunning after electroconvulsive therapy. Ann Intern Med 117:914–915, 1992

Zielinski RJ, Roose SP, Devanand DP, et al: Cardiovascular complications of ECT in depressed patients with cardiac disease. Am J Psychiatry 150:904–909, 1993

Zvara DA, Brooker RF, McCall WV, et al: The effect of esmolol on ST-segment depression and arrhythmias after electroconvulsive therapy. Convuls Ther 13:165–174, 1997

40 Palliative Care

William Breitbart, M.D.

Christopher Gibson, Ph.D.

Harvey Max Chochinov, M.D., Ph.D., F.R.C.P.C.

ONE OF THE most challenging roles for the psychosomatic medicine psychiatrist is to help guide terminally ill patients physically, psychologically, and spiritually through the dying process. Patients with advanced cancer, AIDS, and other life-threatening medical illnesses are at increased risk for developing major psychiatric complications and have an enormous burden of both physical as well as psychological symptoms (Breitbart et al. 2004a). In fact, surveys suggest that psychological symptoms such as depression, anxiety, and hopelessness are as frequent, if not more so, than pain and other physical symptoms (Portenoy et al. 1994; Vogl et al. 1999).

In 1999 the Academy of Psychosomatic Medicine published its position statement titled "Psychiatric Aspects of Excellent End-of-Life Care" (Shuster et al. 1999), which stressed the importance of psychiatric issues in palliative care and the need for competent psychiatric care to be an integral component of palliative care. Major textbooks provide comprehensive reviews of the interface of psychiatry and palliative medicine (Chochinov and Breitbart 2000; Lloyd-Williams 2003), and a new international journal with that focus has recently been started (Breitbart 2003b).

The importance of the psychiatric, psychosocial, and spiritual aspects of palliative care has also been recognized in reports from the American Board of Internal Medicine (Subcommittee on Psychiatric Aspects of Life-Sustaining Technology 1996), the Institute of Medicine (Field and Cassel 1997; Foley and Helband 2001), the National Comprehensive Cancer Network (Levy et al. 2003), and the U.S. Health Resources and Services Administration (O'Neill et al. 2003). Several major national and international palliative care organizations also exist, and more

than 10 national and international palliative care scientific journals have been published (Stjernsward and Clark 2004).

This chapter prepares the psychosomatic medicine practitioner to become an effective psychiatric clinician involved in the care of patients with advanced, life-threatening medical illnesses, either as a consultant to or a part of the palliative care team. In this chapter, we review basic concepts and the role of the psychiatrist in palliative care, including assessment and management of common psychiatric disorders in the terminally ill, with special attention to suicide and desire for hastened death. We describe the psychotherapies developed for use in palliative care settings and then discuss spirituality, cultural sensitivity, communication, grief and bereavement, and control of common physical symptoms.

Related topics are discussed elsewhere in this book, including advance directives and end-of-life decisions (see Chapter 4, "Ethical Issues," and Chapter 5, "Psychological Responses to Illness"), physician-assisted suicide (see Chapter 10, "Suicidality"), terminal sedation (see Chapter 20, "Lung Disease"), dialysis discontinuation (see Chapter 22, "Renal Disease"), and pain management (see Chapter 36, "Pain").

Palliative Care

Historical Perspectives

The term *palliation* is derived from the Latin root word *palliare*, which means "to cloak" or "to conceal." *Pallium* also refers to the cloth that covers or cloaks burial caskets.

These root words suggest that the dying patient, although not amenable to cure, can be "cloaked" or "embraced" in the comforting arms of the caregiver. What cannot be cured can always be comforted. The nature and focus of palliative care has evolved over the past century, expanding beyond just comfort for the dying to include palliative care and symptom control that begins with the onset of a life-threatening illness and proceeds past death to include bereavement interventions for family and others.

Modern palliative care is an outgrowth of the hospice movement that began in the 1840s with Calvaires in Lyon, France, and progressed through 1900 and the establishment of the St. Joseph's Hospice in London, finally culminating with the progenitor of all modern hospices, St. Christopher's Hospice, established in 1967. By 1975 a large number of independent hospices had been developed in the United Kingdom, Canada, and Australia. The first hospice in the United States was established in 1974 in Connecticut. Soon after, the U.S. government established limited Medicare coverage for hospice benefits. This period also saw the establishment of the first "palliative care" program at Royal Victoria Hospital in Montreal, founded by Balfour Mount and his colleagues. This period of evolution from the traditional stand-alone, home-based hospice also saw the development of hospital-based pain and palliative care consultation services such as the pain service established in 1978 by Kathleen Foley at the Memorial Sloan-Kettering Cancer Center. Modern palliative care thus evolved from the hospice movement into a mixture of academic and nonacademic clinical care delivery systems that had components of home care and hospital-based services (Stjernsward and Papallona 1998).

Defining Palliative Care

The Palliative Care Foundation (1981) defined *palliative care* as "active compassionate care of the terminally ill at a time that their disease is no longer responsive to traditional treatment aimed at cure or prolongation of life, and when the control of symptoms is paramount" (p. 10). According to this definition, palliative care applies primarily at the end of life. In 1990, the World Health Organization (WHO) defined *palliative care* as

> the active total care of patients whose disease is not responsive to curative treatment. Control of pain, of other symptoms, and of psychological, social and spiritual problems, is paramount. The goal of palliative care is achievement of the best quality of life for patients and their families. Many aspects of palliative care are also applicable earlier in the course of the illness in conjunction with anti-cancer treatment. (p. 2)

This definition is the first to suggest applicability even at stages of disease that precede the end of life.

In 1995, the Canadian Palliative Care Association published its definition of *palliative care*:

> Palliative care, as a philosophy of care, is the combination of active and compassionate therapies, intended to comfort and support individuals and families who are living with a life-threatening illness. During periods of illness and bereavement, palliative care strives to meet physical, psychological, social and spiritual expectations and needs, while remaining sensitive to personal, cultural and religious values, beliefs and practices. Palliative care may be combined with therapies aimed at reducing or curing illness, or it may be the total focus of care. (p. 3)

This definition is perhaps the most expansive to date. It suggests not only that palliative care is applicable at all stages of life-threatening disease (intensifying once cure is no longer possible) but that psychological, social, spiritual, and cultural issues are elements of palliative care as important as the control of pain and other physical symptoms. According to the WHO, palliative care 1) affirms life and regards dying as a normal process; 2) views the dying process as a valuable experience; 3) neither hastens nor postpones death; 4) provides relief from pain and other symptoms; 5) integrates psychological and spiritual care; 6) offers a support system to help patients live as actively as possible until death; 7) helps family cope with illness and bereavement; and 8) is multidisciplinary, including physicians, nurses, mental health professionals, clergy, and volunteers (World Health Organization 1990, 1997, 1998).

Palliative Care Programs/ Models of Care Delivery

Fully developed model palliative care programs ideally include all of the following components: 1) a home care program (e.g., hospice program); 2) a hospital-based palliative care consultation service; 3) a day care program or ambulatory care clinic; 4) a palliative care inpatient unit (or dedicated palliative care beds in hospital); 5) a bereavement program; 6) training and research programs; and 7) Internet-based services. It is estimated that there are currently more than 3,000 hospices in the United States and over 300 hospital-based pain and palliative care services. In addition, there are 4 academic medical school–affiliated departments of palliative medicine, and 10 pain and palliative medicine fellowship training programs in the United States.

Death in America

To understand and treat psychiatric issues in the dying patient today, one must have an appreciation of why, when, where, and how Americans now die.

Where and How Do Americans Die?

Although two Gallup polls, conducted in 1992 and 1996, found that 9 of 10 terminally ill patients with less than 6 months to live would prefer to die at home (Foreman 1996; National Hospice Organization 1996; Seidlitz et al. 1995), today most Americans die in institutions, surrounded by medical caregivers.

The SUPPORT clinical trial (Study to Understand Prognoses and Preferences for Outcomes and Risks of Treatments) (SUPPORT Principal Investigators 1995) and other studies have suggested that a technological imperative characterizes Western medical practice, including care of the dying. SUPPORT found substantial shortcomings in the care of seriously ill hospitalized patients—including poor communication between physicians and dying patients and implementation of overly aggressive treatment, often against patients' wishes. The findings of this study emphasized the need for greater skills and education in end-of-life issues as well as increased communication with and support of dying patients. Perhaps the most perturbing conclusion from this study is that in general, Americans are dying not good deaths but bad deaths, characterized by needless suffering and disregard for patients' or families' wishes or values.

The concept of death trajectories (see Figure 40–1) has been used to describe the unique as well as relatively predictable patterns of approaching death (Field and Cassel 1997). Some people die suddenly and unexpectedly, as shown in Figure 40–1A (e.g., cardiac arrest). Among those with forewarning of death, many have a steady and relatively predictable decline, as shown in Figure 40–1B (e.g., advanced cancer). There is a third pattern (Figure 40–1C) of long periods of chronic illness punctuated by crises, any of which may result in death (e.g., AIDS, congestive heart failure, or chronic obstructive pulmonary disease). Each type of death trajectory brings with it a unique set of problems and illustrates the challenges of determining prognoses for patients with life-threatening illnesses.

What Is a "Good" Death?

A meaningful dying process is one throughout which the patient is physically, psychologically, spiritually, and emotionally supported by his or her family, friends, and care-givers. Weisman (1972) described four criteria for what he called an "appropriate death": 1) internal conflicts, such as fears about loss of control, should be reduced as much as possible; 2) the individual's personal sense of identity should be sustained; 3) critical relationships should be enhanced or at least maintained, and conflicts should be resolved, if possible; and 4) the person should be encouraged to set and attempt to reach meaningful goals, even though limited, such as attending a graduation, a wedding, or the birth of a child, as a way to provide a sense of continuity into the future.

Role of the Psychiatrist

The traditional role of the psychiatrist is broadened in several ways in the care of the dying patient. Psychosomatic medicine psychiatrists can provide expert care and teaching about the management of depression, anxiety, delirium, and pain in terminally ill patients (Breitbart and Holland 1993; Chochinov and Breitbart 2000). Psychiatrists can also play an important role in the management of social, psychological, ethical, legal, and spiritual issues that complicate the care of dying patients. The psychiatrist can provide assistance in dealing with the existential crisis posed by a terminal diagnosis. Through discussions with the primary care physician, the patient and family may have begun to confront the reality that the disease is no longer curable or controllable. The psychiatrist can help the patient deal with the prognosis and explore treatment options, including palliative care. The psychiatrist's unique expertise in the care of the dying patient is to diagnose and treat comorbid psychiatric disorders that may complicate the course of illness as well as evaluate and intervene regarding suicide risk.

The psychiatrist helps resolve conflicts among patient, family, and staff by opening lines of communication and helping families to deal with the strong emotions that surround the imminent death of a loved one. Conflicts with the physician and staff are common because the clinicians are also stressed; resolution of these conflicts is a critical intervention for the patient's physical and psychological well-being.

Psychotherapeutic interventions for patients and families who are experiencing anticipatory grief are also important. During the bereavement period, the family may turn to the psychiatrist who participated in the patient's care and who shares memories of the patient for continuing support.

The psychiatrist also has an ethical role in encouraging discussion of end-of-life decisions regarding treatment, withholding resuscitation, and life support. The ca-

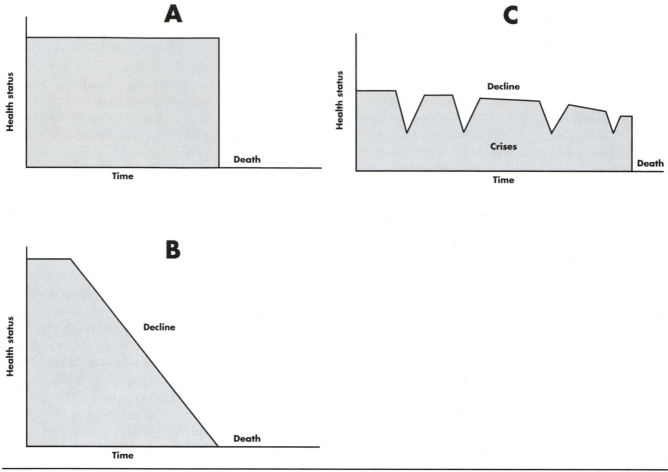

FIGURE 40–1.   Prototypical death trajectories.

(A) Sudden death from an unexpected cause. **(B)** Steady decline from a progressive disease with a "terminal" phase. **(C)** Advanced illness marked by slow decline with periodic crises and "sudden" death.

pacity of the patient to make rational judgments and the proxy's ability to make an appropriate decision for the patient may require psychiatric evaluation. The decision to withdraw life support is highly emotional and may require psychiatric consultation (Subcommittee on Psychiatric Aspects of Life-Sustaining Technology 1996).The psychiatrist's role can include teaching the medical staff about the psychological issues involved in care of dying patients, including how to deliver bad news and discuss do-not-resuscitate (DNR) orders and other treatment preferences with the patient or with family when the patient is unable to make such decisions (Misbin et al. 1993).

Psychiatric Disorders in the Palliative Care Setting

Patients with advanced disease, such as advanced cancer, are particularly vulnerable to psychiatric disorders and

complications (Breitbart et al. 1993, 1995, 2004a; Minagawa et al. 1996). The incidence of specific psychiatric disorders in advanced diseases is discussed in earlier chapters in this volume, for example, cancer (Chapter 24, "Oncology"), heart failure (Chapter 19, "Heart Disease"), chronic obstructive pulmonary disease (Chapter 20, "Lung Disease"), end-stage renal disease (Chapter 22, "Renal Disease"), and AIDS (Chapter 28, "HIV/AIDS").

Anxiety Disorders

The terminally ill patient presents with a complex mixture of physical and psychological symptoms in the context of a frightening reality, making the identification of anxious symptoms requiring treatment challenging (see also Chapter 12, "Anxiety Disorders"). Patients with anxiety complain of tension or restlessness, or they exhibit jitteriness, autonomic hyperactivity, vigilance, insomnia, distractibility, shortness of breath, numbness, apprehension, worry, or rumination. Often the physical or somatic manifestations of anxiety overshadow the psychological or cognitive ones and are the symptoms that the patient most often presents (Holland 1989). The consultant must use these symptoms as a cue to inquire about the patient's psychological state, which is commonly one of fear, worry, or apprehension.

The assumption that a high level of anxiety is inevitably encountered during the terminal phase of illness is neither helpful nor accurate. In deciding whether to treat anxiety during the terminal phase of illness, the clinician should consider the patient's subjective level of distress as the primary impetus for the initiation of treatment. Other considerations include problematic patient behavior such as noncompliance due to anxiety, family and staff reactions to the patient's distress, and the balancing of the risks and benefits of treatment (Payne and Massie 2000).

Prevalence

Prevalence of anxiety disorders among terminally ill cancer and AIDS patients ranges from 15% to 28% (Kerrihard et al. 1999). Prevalence studies of anxiety, primarily in cancer populations, report a higher prevalence of mixed anxiety and depressive symptoms rather than anxiety alone (Payne and Massie 2000). Prevalence of anxiety increases with advancing disease and decline in the patient's physical status (Rabkin et al. 1997). Brandberg et al. (1995) reported that 28% of advanced melanoma patients were anxious compared with 15% of control subjects. The prevalence of anxiety disorders in HIV/AIDS has been reported to range from 0% to 39% (Kerrihard et al. 1999). As disease progresses, patients' anxiety may include fears about the disease process, the clinical course, possible treatment outcomes, and death. In addition, anxiety may result from fear of increasing social stigma as the medical illness becomes more evident as well as from fear of the increasing financial consequences of treatments.

As outlined in Table 40–1, anxiety can occur in terminally ill patients as an adjustment disorder, a disease- or treatment-related condition, or an exacerbation of a pre-existing anxiety disorder (Kerrihard et al. 1999; Massie 1989). Adjustment disorder with anxiety is related to adjusting to the existential crisis and the uncertainty of the prognosis and the future (Holland 1989). When faced with terminal illness, patients with preexisting anxiety disorders are at risk for reactivation of symptoms. A generalized anxiety disorder or panic disorder is apt to recur, especially in the presence of dyspnea or pain. Persons with phobias will have an especially difficult time if the disease or treatment confronts them with their fears (e.g., claustrophobia, fear of needles, fear of isolation). Posttraumatic stress disorder (PTSD) may be activated in dying patients as they relate their situation to some prior near-death experience, such as the Holocaust, a combat experience, or a cardiac arrest, and the terror associated with that experience.

Assessment

As noted in Table 40–1, symptoms of anxiety in the terminally ill patient may arise from a medical complication of the illness or treatment (Breitbart et al. 1993, 1995; Holland 1989; Payne and Massie 2000). Hypoxia, sepsis, poorly controlled pain, drug reactions such as akathisia, and withdrawal states often present as anxiety. In the dying patient, anxiety can represent impending cardiac or respiratory arrest, pulmonary embolism, sepsis, electrolyte imbalance, or dehydration (Strain et al. 1981).

During the terminal phase of illness, when patients become less alert, there is a tendency to minimize the use of sedating medications. It is important to consider the need to slowly taper benzodiazepines and opioids, which may have been sustained at high doses for extended relief of anxiety or pain, in order to prevent acute withdrawal states. Withdrawal states in terminally ill patients often manifest first as agitation or anxiety and become clinically evident days later than might be expected in younger, healthier patients due to impaired metabolism.

Despite the fact that anxiety in terminal illness commonly results from medical complications, it is important to consider psychological factors that may play a role, particularly in patients who are alert and not confused (Holland 1989; Payne and Massie 2000). Patients frequently fear the isolation and separation of death. Claustrophobic patients may fear the idea of being confined and buried in a coffin. These issues can be disconcerting to consultants, who may find themselves at a loss for words that are consoling to the patient.

Pharmacological Treatment

The pharmacotherapy of anxiety in terminal illness has been extensively reviewed (Breitbart et al. 1993, 1995; Holland 1989; Payne and Massie 2000) and is similar in most respects to its treatment in the medically ill in general (see Chapter 12, "Anxiety Disorders," and Chapter 37, "Psychopharmacology"). In this subsection, we note selected aspects specific to the terminally ill.

Dying patients can be administered diazepam rectally when no other route is available, with dosages equivalent to those used in oral regimens. Rectal diazepam (Twycross and Lack 1984) has been used widely in palliative care to control anxiety, restlessness, and agitation associated with the final days of life. Neuroleptics are perhaps the safest class of anxiolytics in patients for whom there is legitimate concern regarding respiratory depression or compromise. The utility of antidepressants for anxiety disor-

TABLE 40–1.   Anxiety in terminally ill patients

Types of anxiety	Causes
Reactive anxiety/adjustment disorder	Awareness of terminal condition Fears and uncertainty about death Conflicts with family or staff Do-not-resuscitate order discussion

Disease- and treatment-related anxiety	Poor pain control
	 Related metabolic disturbances
	      Hypoxia
	      Hypoglycemia
	      Electrolyte imbalance
	 Delirium
	 Sepsis
	 Bleeding
	 Pulmonary embolus

Substance-induced anxiety	Anxiety-producing drugs
	 Corticosteroids
	 Antiemetics
	      Metoclopramide
	      Prochlorperazine
	 Bronchodilators
	 Withdrawal
	      Opioids
	      Benzodiazepines
	      Alcohol

Preexisting anxiety disorders
    General anxiety disorder
    Panic
    Phobias
    Posttraumatic stress disorder
	Exacerbation of symptoms related to fears and distressing medical symptoms

ders is often limited in the dying patient because these agents require weeks to achieve therapeutic effect.

Opioid drugs such as the narcotic analgesics are primarily indicated for the control of pain but are also effective in the relief of dyspnea and associated anxiety (Bruera et al. 1990). Continuous intravenous infusions of morphine or other narcotic analgesics allow for careful titration and control of respiratory distress, anxiety, pain, and agitation (Portenoy et al. 1989). Occasionally one must maintain the patient in a state of unresponsiveness in order to maximize comfort. When respiratory distress is not a major problem, it is preferable to use the opioid drugs solely for analgesia and to add more specific anxiolytics to control concomitant anxiety.

Nonpharmacological Treatment

Nonpharmacological interventions for anxiety and distress include supportive psychotherapy and behavioral interventions that are used alone or in combination (see discussion later in this chapter and in Chapter 12, "Anxiety Disorders," and Chapter 38, "Psychosocial Treatments"). Brief supportive psychotherapy is often useful in dealing with both crises and existential issues confronted by the terminally ill (Massie et al. 1989). Inclusion of the family in psychotherapeutic interventions should be considered, particularly as the patient with advanced illness becomes increasingly debilitated and less able to interact.

Relaxation, guided imagery, and hypnosis may help reduce anxiety and thereby increase the patient's sense of control. Many patients with advanced illness are still appropriate candidates for the use of behavioral techniques despite physical debilitation. The utility of such interventions for a terminally ill patient is limited by the degree of mental clarity of the patient (Breitbart et al. 1995). In some cases, techniques can be modified so as to include even mildly cognitively impaired patients. This involves the therapist taking a more active role by orienting the patient, creating a safe and secure environment, and evoking a conditioned response to his or her voice or presence. A typical behavioral intervention for anxiety in a terminally ill patient would include a relaxation exercise combined with some distraction or imagery technique. The patient is first taught to relax using passive breathing accompanied by either passive or active muscle relaxation. When in a relaxed state, the patient is taught a pleasant, distracting imagery exercise. In a randomized study comparing a relaxation technique with alprazolam in the treatment of anxiety and distress in non–terminally ill cancer patients, both treatments were demonstrated to be quite effective for mild to moderate degrees of anxiety or distress. Alprazolam was more effective for greater levels of distress or anxiety and had more rapid onset of beneficial effect (Holland et al. 1987). Of course, relaxation techniques can be prescribed concurrently with anxiolytic medications in highly anxious terminal patients.

Depression

See also Chapter 9, "Depression," for additional information.

Prevalence

Two recent studies of the prevalence of major depression in terminally ill cancer patients in palliative care units suggest that the prevalence of depression in patients during the last weeks to months of life ranges from 9% to 18% (Breitbart et al. 2000; Wilson et al. 2000). Family history of depression and history of previous depressive episodes further increase the patient's risk of developing a depressive episode. Recent reports suggest that loss of meaning and low scores on measures of spiritual well-being are associated with higher levels of depressive symptoms, suggesting that the relationship between existential distress and depression in terminal illness warrants further investigation (Nelson et al. 2002). Many studies have also found a correlation between depression, pain, and functional status (Breitbart 1989b). In addition, evaluation of depression must also include an examination of treatments and physical conditions that may be the cause of depression. Corticosteroids (Stiefel et al. 1989), chemotherapeutic agents (vincristine, vinblastine, asparaginase, intrathecal methotrexate, interferon, interleukin) (Adams et al. 1984; Denicoff et al. 1987; Holland et al. 1974; Young 1982), amphotericin (Weddington 1982), whole brain radiation (DeAngelis et al. 1989), central nervous system (CNS) metabolic–endocrine complications (Breitbart 1989a), and paraneoplastic syndromes (Patchell and Posner 1989; Posner 1988) can all cause depressive symptoms.

Assessment

Depressed mood and sadness can be appropriate responses as the terminally ill patient faces death. These emotions can be manifestations of anticipatory grief over the impending loss of one's life, health, loved ones, and autonomy. Despite this, major depression is common in the palliative care setting, where it has been underdiagnosed and undertreated. Minimization of depressive symptoms as "normal reactions" by clinicians and the difficulties of accurately diagnosing depression in the terminally ill both contribute to the underdiagnosis of depression, and undertreatment is due in part to the concern that severely medically ill patients will not be able to tolerate the side effects of antidepressants (Block 2000). Strategies for accurately diagnosing depression in seriously medically ill patients are reviewed in Chapter 9, "Depression." Their application in terminally ill patients in a palliative care facility is exemplified by Chochinov et al. (1994).

The diagnosis of a major depressive syndrome in a terminally ill patient, as in medically ill patients in general, often relies more on the psychological or cognitive symptoms of major depression than the neurovegetative symptoms. The strategy of relying on the psychological symptoms of depression for diagnostic specificity is itself not without problems. How is the clinician to interpret feelings of hopelessness in the dying patient when there is no hope for cure or recovery? Feelings of hopelessness, worthlessness, or suicidal ideation must be explored in detail. Although many dying patients lose hope for a cure, they are able to maintain hope for better symptom control. For many patients hope is contingent on the ability to find continued meaning in their day-to-day existence. Hopelessness that is pervasive and accompanied by a sense of despair or despondency is more likely to represent a symptom of a depressive disorder. Such patients often state that they feel they are burdening their families unfairly, causing them great pain and inconvenience. Those beliefs are less likely to represent a symptom of depression than if the patient feels that his or her life has never had any worth or that the illness is punishment for evil things he or she has done. Even mild and passive forms of suicidal ideation are very often indicative of significant degrees of depression in terminally ill patients (Breitbart 1987, 1990).

Chochinov et al. (1997) studied brief screening instruments to measure depression in the terminally ill, including a single-item interview assessing depressed mood ("Have you been depressed most of the time for the past 2 weeks?"), a two-item interview assessing depressed mood and loss of interest in activities, a visual analogue scale for depressed mood, and the Beck Depression Inventory. Semistructured diagnostic interviews served as the standard against which the screening performance of the four brief screening methods was assessed. Most noteworthy, the single-item question correctly identified the diagnosis of every patient, substantially outperforming the questionnaire and visual analogue measures.

Passik and colleagues demonstrated that the Zung Depression Rating Scale could be used effectively by oncologists and nurses as a rapid screening tool for depression in patients with advanced cancer and that oncologists could be trained to diagnose and initiate further evaluation and treatment of clinical depression (Dugan et al. 1998; McDonald et al. 1999; Passik et al. 1998, 2000, 2001).

Pharmacological Treatment

Antidepressant medications are the mainstay of management for gravely ill patients meeting diagnostic criteria for major depression (Block 2000; Wilson et al. 2000) and have established efficacy (Massie and Popkin 1998; Wilson et al. 2000). Pharmacotherapy of depression in the medically ill is reviewed in detail in Chapter 9, "Depression," and Chapter 37, "Psychopharmacology," and in this discussion we note specific aspects relevant to palliative care. Factors such as prognosis and the time frame for treatment may play an important role in determining the type of pharmacotherapy for depression in the terminally ill. A depressed patient with several months of life expectancy can afford to wait the 2–4 weeks it may take to respond to a standard antidepressant. The depressed dying patient with less than 3 weeks to live may do best with a rapid-acting psychostimulant (Block 2000; Homsi et al. 2001; Tremblay and Breitbart 2001). Patients who are within hours to days of death and in distress are likely to benefit most from the use of sedatives or narcotic analgesic infusions. For the terminally ill, antidepressants are usually initiated at approximately half the usual starting dose because of the patients' sensitivity to adverse effects.

Psychostimulants are particularly helpful in the treatment of depression in the terminally ill because they have a rapid onset of action and energizing effects and typically do not cause anorexia, weight loss, or insomnia at therapeutic doses. In fact, at low doses, stimulants may actually increase appetite (see also Chapter 9, "Depression," and Chapter 37, "Psychopharmacology"). Abuse is almost always an irrelevant concern in the terminally ill, and stimulants should not be withheld on the basis of a patient's prior history of substance abuse. Occasionally, treatment with a selective serotonin reuptake inhibitor (SSRI) and a psychostimulant may be initiated concurrently so that depressed patients may receive the immediate benefits of the psychostimulant drug while waiting the necessary weeks for the SSRI to work. At that point the psychostimulant may be withdrawn. Methylphenidate and dextroamphetamine are usually initiated at low doses (2.5–5 mg in the morning and at noon). The benefits can be assessed

during the first 1–2 days of treatment and the dose gradually titrated (usually to no greater than 30 mg/day total). An additional benefit of stimulants is that they have been shown to reduce sedation secondary to opioid analgesics and provide adjuvant analgesic effects (Bruera et al. 1987). Pemoline comes in a chewable tablet form that can be absorbed through the buccal mucosa and thus can be used by patients who have difficulty swallowing or have intestinal obstruction, and it appears to be as effective as methylphenidate or dextroamphetamine in the treatment of depressive symptoms in terminally ill cancer patients (Breitbart and Mermelstein 1992). Pemoline can be started at a dose of 18.75 mg in the morning and at noon and increased gradually over a period of days. Patients typically require 75 mg/day or less. Pemoline should be used with caution in patients with liver impairment.

Nonpharmacological Treatment

Depression in cancer patients with advanced disease is optimally managed with a combination of supportive psychotherapy, cognitive-behavioral techniques, and antidepressant medications (Wilson et al. 2000). Psychotherapeutic interventions, in the form of either individual or group counseling, have been shown to effectively reduce psychological distress and depressive symptoms in advanced-stage cancer patients (Massie et al. 1989; Spiegel and Bloom 1983; Spiegel et al. 1981). Cognitive-behavioral interventions such as relaxation and distraction with pleasant imagery also have been shown to decrease depressive symptoms in patients with mild to moderate levels of depression (Holland et al. 1987).

Supportive psychotherapy for the dying patient consists of active listening with supportive verbal interventions and the occasional interpretation (Peck et al. 1983). Despite the seriousness of the patient's plight, it is not necessary for the psychiatrist or psychologist to appear overly solemn or emotionally restrained. Often the psychotherapist is the only person among all of the patient's caregivers who is comfortable enough to converse lightheartedly and to allow the patient to talk about his or her life and experiences rather than focus solely on impending death. The dying patient who wishes to talk or ask questions about death should be encouraged to do so freely, with the therapist maintaining an interested, interactive stance.

Psychotherapies other than supportive psychotherapy have been described as potentially useful in the treatment of depressive symptoms and distress in palliative care patients. Chochinov and Breitbart (2000) extensively reviewed interpersonal, existential, life narrative, and group psychotherapies in palliative care. Recently, several novel psychotherapies have been developed and are being tested in the treatment of depression, hopelessness, loss of meaning, and demoralization; these new modalities include meaning-centered psychotherapy (Breitbart 2002) and dignity-conserving care (Chochinov 2002), both of which are described later in this chapter.

Suicide, Assisted Suicide, and Desire for Hastened Death

Suicide, suicidal ideation, and desire for hastened death are all important and serious consequences of unrecognized and inadequately treated clinical depression (see also Chapter 10, "Suicidality"). Although clinical depression has been demonstrated to be a critically important factor in desire for hastened death (through suicide or other means), understanding more fully why some patients with a terminal illness wish or seek to hasten their death remains an important element in the practice of palliative care. Despite the continued legal prohibitions against assisted suicide in the United States (except Oregon), a substantial number of patients think about and discuss those alternatives with their physicians, family, and friends (Rosenfeld 2000).

Suicide

Factors associated with increased risk of suicide in patients with serious medical illnesses are reviewed in Chapter 10, "Suicidality," and elsewhere (Breitbart 1987, 1990).

Cancer patients commit suicide most frequently in the advanced stages of disease (Bolund 1985; Farberow et al. 1963; Fox et al. 1982; Louhivuori and Hakama 1979). With advancing disease the incidence of significant pain increases, and uncontrolled pain is a dramatically important risk factor for suicide (Bolund 1985; Farberow et al. 1971).

Hopelessness is a key variable linking depression and suicide in the terminally ill. Chochinov et al. (1998) demonstrated that hopelessness was correlated more highly with suicidal ideation in terminally ill cancer patients than was level of depression. In Scandinavia, the highest incidence of suicide was found in cancer patients who were offered no further treatment and no further contact with the health care system (Bolund 1985; Louhivuori and Hakama 1979). Being left to face illness alone creates a sense of isolation and abandonment that is critical to the development of hopelessness.

The prevalence of organic mental disorders reaches as high as 85% during the terminal stages of illness (Massie et al. 1983). Although early work suggested that delirium was a protective factor in regard to suicide among cancer patients (Farberow et al. 1963), clinical experience has found confusional states to be a major contributing factor in impulsive suicide attempts, especially in the hospital setting (see Chapter 10, "Suicidality").

Loss of control and a sense of helplessness in the face of terminal illness are important factors in suicide vulnerability. *Control* refers to the helplessness induced by symptoms, deficits due to the illness or its treatments, and the excessive need on the part of some patients to be in control of all aspects of living or dying. Farberow et al. (1971) noted that patients who were accepting and adaptable were much less likely to commit suicide than those who exhibited a need to be in control of even the most minute details of their care. However, it is not uncommon for terminal illness to induce a great sense of helplessness even in those who are not typically controlling individuals, for example through loss of mobility, paraplegia, loss of bowel and bladder function, amputation, aphonia, sensory loss, and inability to eat or swallow. Most distressing to patients is the sense that they are losing control of their minds, especially when they are confused or sedated by medications. The risk of suicide is increased with such impairments, especially when accompanied by psychological distress and disturbed interpersonal relationships (Farberow et al. 1971).

Fatigue in the form of emotional, spiritual, financial, familial, communal, and other resource exhaustion increases risk of suicide in patients with terminal illness (Breitbart 1987). Increased survival in cancer, AIDS, chronic obstructive pulmonary disease, congestive heart failure, and other diseases is accompanied by increased numbers of hospitalizations, complications, and expenses. Symptom control thus becomes a prolonged process with frequent advances and setbacks. The dying process also can become extremely long and arduous for all concerned. It is not uncommon for both family members and health care providers to withdraw prematurely from the patient under these circumstances. A suicidal patient can thus feel even more isolated and abandoned. The presence of a strong support system for the patient that may act as an external control of suicidal behavior reduces risk of suicide significantly.

Suicidal Ideation

It is widely held that most terminally ill patients experience occasional thoughts of suicide as a means of escaping the threat of being overwhelmed by their illness ("If it gets too bad, I always have a way out") and will reveal this to a sensitive interviewer. However, some studies suggest that suicidal ideation is relatively infrequent and is limited to those who are significantly depressed (Achte and Vanhkouen 1971; Brown et al. 1986; Silberfarb et al. 1980). Among a cohort of cancer patients with pain, suicidal ideation was found in just 17% (Breitbart 1987). The actual prevalence of suicidal ideation may be considerably higher, because patients may be less likely to disclose these thoughts to a research interviewer than in a well-established doctor–patient relationship.

Assessment and Management of the Suicidal Terminally Ill Patient

Assessment and management of suicidal ideation in the medically ill are discussed in Chapter 10, "Suicidality." Some physicians, nurses, and other caregivers fail to intervene for suicidal ideation in the terminally ill, either because they think it is rational ("I would feel that way too") or because they think that intervention is futile ("He's going to die anyway"). This is a serious error for several reasons. Suicide can be very traumatic to family and health care givers, even in the terminally ill. Patients often reconsider and reject the idea of suicide after they have an opportunity to express underlying issues to an attentive physician, particularly fears of loss of control over aspects of their death. Suicidal ideation is often driven by unbearable symptoms that may not have been recognized and should become the focus of palliative care

Psychiatric hospitalization can sometimes be helpful but is usually not desirable in the terminally ill patient. Thus, the medical hospital or home is the setting in which management most often takes place. Although it is appropriate to intervene when medical or psychiatric factors are clearly the driving force in a cancer patient's suicide, there are circumstances when usurping control from the patient and family with overly aggressive intervention may be contraindicated. This is most evident in those with advanced illness for whom comfort and symptom control are the primary concerns.

Ultimately, palliative care clinicians are not able to prevent all suicides in terminally ill patients for whom they provide care. Intervention should emphasize an aggressive attempt to prevent suicide that is driven by the desperation of physical and psychological symptoms, such as uncontrolled pain and unrecognized or untreated delirium or depression. Prolonged suffering caused by poorly controlled symptoms can lead to such desperation, and it is the appropriate role of the palliative care team to provide effective management of physical and psychological symptoms as an alternative to desire for death, suicide, or request for assisted suicide by patients. (Requests for assisted suicide are covered in Chapter 10, "Suicidality.")

Desire for Hastened Death

Desire for hastened death may be thought of as a unifying construct underlying requests for assisted suicide or euthanasia, as well as suicidal thoughts in general. Several studies have demonstrated that depression plays a significant role in the terminally ill patient's desire for hastened

death. Chochinov et al. (1995) found that 45% of terminally ill patients in a palliative care facility acknowledged at least a fleeting desire to die, but these episodes were mostly brief and did not reflect a sustained or committed desire to die. However, 9% reported an unequivocal desire for death to come soon and indicated that they held this desire consistently over time. Among this group, 59% received a diagnosis of depression, compared with a prevalence of 8% in patients who did not endorse a genuine, consistent desire for death. Patients with depression were approximately six to seven times more likely to have a desire for hastened death than patients without depression. Patients with a desire for death were also found to have significantly more pain and less social support than those patients without a desire for death.

Breitbart et al. (2000) studied the relationships among depression, hopelessness, and desire for death in terminally ill cancer patients. Seventeen percent of the patients were classified as having a high desire for death (; Rosenfeld et al. 1999, 2000), and 16% met criteria for a current major depressive episode. Of the patients who met criteria for major depressive episode, 47% were classified as having a high desire for hastened death; only 12% of those without a desire for death met criteria for depression. Thus, patients with major depression were four times more likely to have a high desire for hastened death. In addition, Breitbart et al. (2000) found that both depression and hopelessness, characterized as a pessimistic cognitive style rather than an assessment of one's poor prognosis, appear to be synergistic determinants of desire for hastened death. No significant association with the presence or the intensity of pain was found.

Desire for hastened death also appears to be a function of psychological distress and social factors such as social support, spiritual well-being, quality of life, and perception of oneself as a burden to others. Recent data suggest that among dying patients the "will to live," as measured with a visual analogue scale, tends to fluctuate rapidly over time and is correlated with anxiety, depression, and shortness of breath as death approaches (Chochinov et al. 1999).

Treatment of depression can reduce the wish for hastened death and also increase desire for life-sustaining medical therapies (Ganzini et al. 1994). When it is practical to do so, in severely depressed patients—particularly those who are hopeless—decisions about withdrawal of treatment should be discouraged until after treatment of their depression.

Interventions for Despair at the End of Life

The response of a clinician to despair at the end of life as manifest by a patient's expression of desire for death or request for assisted suicide has important and obvious implications for all aspects of care and affects patients, family, and staff (Breitbart et al. 2004a). These issues must be addressed both rapidly and thoughtfully, offering the patient a nonjudgmental willingness to discuss the factors contributing to the kind of suffering and despondency that leads to such a desire for death. Such despair has been variably described as "spiritual" suffering, "demoralization," loss of "dignity," and "loss of meaning" (Breitbart 2002; Cherny 2004; Chochinov et al. 2002b; Greenstein and Breitbart 2000; Kissane et al. 2001; Rousseau 2000). Specific therapeutic approaches for despair at the end of life are described in detail in the section on "Psychotherapy Interventions in Palliative Care" later in the chapter.

Most palliative care clinicians believe that aggressive management of physical and psychological distress will prevent wishes for hastened death or requests for assisted suicide. For example, there is a general consensus that major depression can be effectively treated in the context of terminal illness. However, no research has yet addressed whether such treatment for depression directly influences desire for hastened death. There are currently two large trials in cancer and AIDS populations examining this specific question (Breitbart et al. 2000). Because depression and hopelessness are not identical constructs (although highly correlated), it is important to empirically test clinical interventions.

Delirium

Delirium is discussed in detail in Chapter 6, "Delirium"; in this discussion we focus on aspects most relevant to palliative care. In addition to its own adverse effects, delirium can interfere dramatically with the recognition and control of other physical and psychological symptoms such as pain in later stages of illness (Breitbart and Sparrow 1998; Bruera et al. 1992; Coyle et al. 1994; Fainsinger et al. 1991).

Prevalence

Delirium is the most common and serious neuropsychiatric complication in patients with advanced illnesses such as cancer and AIDS, particularly in the last weeks of life, with prevalence rates ranging from 25% to 85% (Breitbart 2001; Breitbart et al. 1996a; Bruera et al. 1992; Fainsinger et al. 1991; Levine et al. 1978; Massie et al. 1983; Murray 1987). Pereira et al. (1997) found the prevalence of cognitive impairment in cancer inpatients to be 44%, and just prior to death, the prevalence rose to 62%. Lawlor et al. (2000a) reported that whereas 42% of advanced cancer patients had delirium upon admission to their pal-

liative care unit, terminal delirium occurred in 88% of patients before their deaths.

In a recent study of terminally ill cancer patients, Breitbart et al. (2002) found that 54% of patients recalled their delirium experience after recovery from delirium. Factors predicting delirium recall included the degree of short-term memory impairment, delirium severity, and the presence of perceptual disturbances (the more severe, the less likely recall). Patients, spouses or other caregivers, and nurses each rated distress related to the episode of delirium. The most significant factor predicting distress for patients was the presence of delusions. Patients with hypoactive delirium were just as distressed as patients with hyperactive delirium. Spouse distress was predicted by the patients' Karnofsky Performance Status (the lower the Karnofsky score, the worse the spouse distress), and nurse distress was predicted by delirium severity and perceptual disturbances.

Assessment

Delirium, in contrast with dementia, is classically conceptualized as a reversible process. Reversibility of delirium is often possible even in the patient with advanced illness, but it may not be reversible in the last 24–48 hours of life, with the outcome probably attributable to irreversible processes such as multiple organ failure occurring in the final hours of life. In the palliative care literature, delirium occurring in the last days of life is often referred to as "terminal restlessness" or "terminal agitation." Unfortunately, delirium is often underrecognized or misdiagnosed and inappropriately treated or untreated in terminally ill patients.

Instruments available for diagnosing and monitoring severity of delirium are described in Chapter 6, "Delirium." Of those, the Memorial Delirium Assessment Scale (MDAS) is one specifically validated in hospitalized inpatients with advanced cancer and AIDS (Breitbart et al. 1997). The MDAS is a 10-item tool useful both for diagnostic screening and for assessing delirium severity among patients with advanced disease. Lawlor and colleagues (2000b) found that a cutoff score of 7 out of 30 yielded the highest sensitivity (98%) and specificity (76%) for a delirium diagnosis in advanced cancer patients in a palliative care unit.

Reversible Versus Irreversible Delirium

The standard approach to managing delirium outlined in Chapter 6, "Delirium," remains relevant in the terminally ill, including a search for underlying causes, correction of those factors, and management of the symptoms of delirium (Breitbart 2001; Breitbart et al. 2000). The ideal and often achievable outcome is a patient who is awake, alert, calm, cognitively intact, not psychotic, and communicating coherently with family and staff. In the terminally ill patient who develops delirium in the last days of life (terminal delirium), the management differs, presenting a number of dilemmas, and the desired clinical outcome may be significantly altered by the dying process.

Delirium can have multiple potential etiologies (see Table 40–2). In patients with advanced cancer, for instance, delirium can be due to the direct effects of cancer on the CNS, indirect CNS effects of the disease or treatments (medications, electrolyte imbalance, failure of a vital organ, infection, vascular complications), and/or preexisting CNS disease (e.g., dementia) (Bruera et al. 1992; Lawlor et al. 2000a). Given the large numbers of drugs cancer patients require and the fragile state of their physiological functioning, even routinely ordered hypnotic agents may be enough to tip patients over into delirium. Narcotic analgesics, especially meperidine, are common causes of confusional states, particularly in the elderly and terminally ill.

In confronting delirium in the terminally ill or dying patient, a differential diagnosis should always be formulated as to the likely etiology. However, there is an ongoing debate as to the appropriate extent of diagnostic evaluation that should be pursued in a dying patient with a terminal delirium (Breitbart 2001). Most palliative care clinicians would undertake diagnostic studies only when a clinically suspected etiology can be identified easily, with minimal use of invasive procedures, and treated effectively with simple interventions that carry minimal burden or risk of causing further distress. Diagnostic workup in pursuit of an etiology for delirium may be limited by either practical constraints such as the setting (home, hospice) or the focus on patient comfort, so that unpleasant or painful diagnostics may be avoided. Most often, however, the etiology of terminal delirium is multifactorial or may not be determined. Bruera et al. (1992) reported that an etiology is discovered in less than 50% of terminally ill patients with delirium. When a distinct cause is found for delirium in the terminally ill, it may be irreversible or difficult to treat. Studies in patients with earlier stages of advanced cancer have demonstrated the potential utility of a thorough diagnostic assessment (Bruera et al. 1992; Coyle et al. 1994). When such diagnostic information is available, specific therapy may be able to reverse delirium. One study found that 68% of delirious cancer patients could be improved, despite a 30-day mortality of 31% (Lawlor et al. 2000a). Another study found a cause in 43% of the patients evaluated, and of these, one-third of the episodes of cognitive failure improved (Bruera et al. 1992).

TABLE 40–2. Causes of delirium in patients with advanced disease

Direct central nervous system (CNS) causes
Primary brain tumor
Metastatic spread to CNS
Seizures
CNS infection

Indirect causes
Hyperthermia
Organ failure
  Uremia
  Hepatic encephalopathy
  Congestive heart failure
  Pulmonary failure
    Pulmonary edema
    Pulmonary emboli
Electrolyte imbalance
Treatment side effects from
  Chemotherapeutic agents
  Steroids
  Radiation
  Narcotics
  Anticholinergics
  Antiemetics
  Antivirals
Infection
  Sepsis
  Opportunistic infections
Hematological abnormalities
  Severe anemia
  Disseminated intravascular coagulopathy (DIC) and other hypercoagulable states
Nutritional deficiencies
Paraneoplastic syndromes

A recent prospective study of delirium in patients on a palliative care unit found that the etiology of delirium was multifactorial in the great majority of cases (Lawlor et al. 2000a). Although delirium occurred in 88% of dying patients in the last week of life, delirium was reversible in approximately 50% of episodes. Causes of delirium that were most associated with reversibility included dehydration and psychoactive or opioid medications. Hypoxic and metabolic encephalopathies were less likely to be reversible in terminal delirium.

Therefore, even in terminal delirium a diagnostic workup should include basic assessment of potentially reversible causes of delirium while minimizing any investigation that would be burdensome for the patient. A full physical examination should be conducted to assess for evidence of sepsis, dehydration, or major organ failure. Medications that could contribute to delirium should be reviewed. Oximetry can rule out hypoxia, and one set of blood draws can screen for metabolic disturbances (e.g., hypercalcemia) and hematological abnormalities (e.g., anemia, leukocytosis). Imaging studies of the brain and assessment of the cerebrospinal fluid may be appropriate in some instances if they have the potential to identify lesions amenable to palliative treatment (e.g., radiosensitive CNS metastases).

Interventions

Pharmacological

Pharmacotherapy of delirium is reviewed in detail in Chapter 6, "Delirium." Low doses of neuroleptic medication are usually sufficient in treating delirium in the terminally ill, but high doses have sometimes been required (Fernandez et al. 1989). Haloperidol remains the drug of first choice and may be given orally or parenterally. Delivery of haloperidol by the subcutaneous route is utilized by many palliative care practitioners (Bruera et al. 1992; Twycross and Lack 1983).

Many palliative care clinicians are using low dosages of risperidone (e.g., 0.5–1.0 mg bid) or olanzapine (2.5–20 mg/day in divided doses) in the management of delirium in terminally ill patients, particularly in those who have demonstrated intolerance to the extrapyramidal side effects of the classic neuroleptics (Breitbart 2001). However, there is less experience with (and few data on) using atypical antipsychotics for delirium, and most are unavailable for parenteral administration. Breitbart and colleagues (2002b) recently published a large open trial of olanzapine for the treatment of delirium in hospitalized patients with advanced cancer. Olanzapine was highly effective, resolving delirium in 76% of patients with no extrapyramidal side effects. Poorer response to treatment occurred in those with age over 70, history of dementia, and hypoactive delirium. Sedation was the most common side effect.

Although neuroleptic drugs are generally very beneficial in reducing agitation, anxiety, and confusion in delirium, this is not always possible in terminal delirium. A significant group (at least 10%–20%) of terminally ill patients experience delirium that can only be controlled by sedation to the point of a significantly decreased level of consciousness (Fainsinger et al. 1991; Ventafridda et al. 1990). The goal of treatment in those cases is quiet sedation only. Midazolam, given by subcutaneous or intravenous infusion in doses ranging from 30 to 100 mg per 24 hours, can be used to control agitated terminal delirium (Bottomley and Hanks 1990; De Sousa and Jepson 1988). Propofol, a short-acting anesthetic agent, has also begun to be used for this purpose, given in, for example, an in-travenous loading dose of 20 mg followed by a continuous infusion with initial doses of 10–70 mg/hour titrated up to as high as 400 mg/hour in severely agitated patients (Mercadante et al. 1995; Moyle 1995). Propofol's level of sedation may be more easily controlled, with more rapid recovery upon decreasing the rate of infusion than with midazolam (Mercadante et al. 1995).

Nonpharmacological

In addition to seeking out and potentially correcting underlying causes for delirium, environmental and supportive interventions are important, as described in Chapter 6, "Delirium." In fact, in the dying patient these may be the only steps taken. The presence of family, frequent reorientation, correction of hearing and visual impairment, reversal of dehydration, and a quiet well-lit room with familiar objects all are helpful in reducing the severity and impact of delirium in seriously ill patients. However, these interventions are less applicable in the last days of life, and there is little likelihood that they would prevent terminal delirium.

Controversies in the Management of Terminal Delirium

Several aspects of the use of neuroleptics and other pharmacological agents in the management of delirium in the dying patient remain controversial in some circles. Some view delirium as a natural part of the dying process that should not be altered and argue that pharmacological interventions are inappropriate in the dying patient. In particular, some who care for the dying view hallucinations and delusions in which dead relatives communicate with dying patients or welcome them to heaven as important elements in the transition from life to death. There are some patients who experience hallucinations during delirium that are pleasant and even comforting, and many clinicians question the appropriateness of intervening pharmacologically in such instances.

Another concern often raised is that these patients are so close to death that aggressive treatment is unnecessary. Parenteral neuroleptics or sedatives may be mistakenly avoided because of exaggerated fears that they might hasten death through hypotension or respiratory depression. There is the possibility that sedation may worsen confusion in delirium. Many clinicians are unnecessarily pessimistic about the possible results of neuroleptic treatment for delirium. They argue that since the underlying pathophysiological process (such as hepatic or renal failure) often continues unabated, no improvement can be expected in the patient's mental status.

Clinical experience in managing delirium in dying patients suggests that the use of neuroleptics in the management of agitation, paranoia, hallucinations, and altered sensorium is safe, effective, and often quite appropriate (Breitbart 2001). Management of delirium on a case-by-case basis seems wisest. The agitated, delirious dying patient should usually have a trial of neuroleptics to help restore calm. A "wait and see" approach prior to using neuroleptics may be appropriate with some patients who have a lethargic, somnolent presentation of delirium or those who are having frankly pleasant or comforting hallucinations. Such an approach must be tempered by the knowledge that a lethargic delirium may very quickly and unexpectedly become an agitated delirium that can threaten the serenity and safety of the patient, family, and staff. An additional rationale for intervening pharmacologically with patients who have "hypoactive" delirium is evidence that neuroleptics are effective in controlling the symptoms of delirium in both hyperactive as well as hypoactive subtypes of delirium (Breitbart et al. 1996a).

Finally, a very challenging clinical problem is management of terminal delirium that is unresponsive to standard neuroleptics and for which symptoms can only be controlled by sedation to the point of significantly decreased consciousness. Before undertaking interventions such as midazolam or propofol infusions, in which the aim is a calm, comfortable, but sedated and unresponsive patient, the clinician should discuss with the family (and the patient if he or she has lucid moments) the concerns and wishes for the type of care that can best honor the patient's and family's values. Family members should be informed that the goal of sedation is to provide comfort and symptom control and not to hasten death. Terminal sedation intended to maximize the patient's comfort is not euthanasia. After the patient receives this degree of sedation, the family may experience a premature sense of loss, and they may feel their loved one is in some sort of limbo state, not yet dead but yet no longer alive in the vital sense. The distress and confusion that family members can experience during such a period can be ameliorated by including them in the decision making and emphasizing the shared goals of care. Sedation in such patients is not always complete or irreversible; some patients have periods of wakefulness despite sedation, and many clinicians will periodically lighten sedation to reassess the patient's condition.

Psychotherapy Interventions in Palliative Care

The potential benefits of psychotherapy for seriously medically ill patients are frequently underestimated by clinicians (Rodin and Gillies 2000). This bias against psychotherapeutic interventions tends to be even more pronounced in patients who are months away from death. However, psychotherapeutic interventions have been demonstrated to be useful and effective for patients struggling with advanced life-threatening medical illness. This section briefly describes different psychotherapeutic interventions and their relative applicability and efficacy for patients near the end of life. Psychotherapy in the medically ill is reviewed in detail in Chapter 38, "Psychosocial Treatment."

Individual Psychotherapy

Traditional insight-oriented psychotherapy has had limited application among dying patients. Insight-oriented psychotherapy is based on the development of a trusting relationship between the psychotherapist and the patient and an exploration of various unconscious conflicts and issues (Rodin and Gillies 2000). Resolution of conflicts, through a process involving interpretation, catharsis, and enhanced insight, requires time, energy, and commitment. This approach may be too demanding for most patients nearing death, but elements of psychodynamic therapy have an important role in all palliative psychotherapies. Cognitive-behavioral and interpersonal therapies have been widely studied in the medically ill. In full extended form they too may not be practical in imminently dying patients, but there are important cognitive and interpersonal elements in the specific psychotherapies as described in the following sections.

Existential Therapies

Existential therapies explore ways in which suffering can be experienced from a more positive and meaningful perspective. *Logotherapy* is one approach with the primary tenet that one always has control over one's attitude or outlook, no matter the enormity of the adversity. The goal is to decrease patients' suffering and encourage them to live life to its fullest by engaging in activities that bring the greatest amount of meaning and purpose to their lives (Frankl 1959/1992). The focus is on goals to achieve, tasks to fulfill, and responsibilities toward others. Rather than covering up patients' distress, logotherapy acknowledges and fully explores patients' suffering (Spira 2000). Although it was not designed for patients who were imminently dying, Zuehlke and Watkins (1975) explored the use of logotherapy with six dying patients and reported them to have a greater sense of freedom to change their attitudes and to see themselves and their lives as meaningful and worthwhile.

Another form of existential therapy useful with dying patients is the *life narrative*. This treatment explores the meaning of the physical illness in the context of the patient's life trajectory. It is designed to create a new perspective of dealing with the illness, emphasize past strengths, increase self-esteem, and support effective past coping strategies. The therapist emphatically summarizes the patient's life history and response to the illness to convey a sense that the therapist understands the patient over time (Viederman 2000; Viederman and Perry 1980). Life narrative can bolster patients' psychological and physical well-being. One study by Pennebaker and Seagal (1999) demonstrated that when patients wrote about important personal experiences in an emotional way for 15 minutes over 3 days, improvements in mental and physical health occurred. Life narrative has traditionally been used for treating depressed patients whose depression is a response to physical illness. However, the written form of this approach can be too demanding for patients at the end stage of their illness.

A similar method of intervention is the *life review*, which provides patients with the opportunity to identify and reexamine past experiences and achievements to find meaning, resolve old conflicts and make amends, or resolve unfinished business (Byock 1996; Heiney 1995; Lichter et al. 1993). The process of life review can be achieved through written or taped autobiographies, by reminiscing, through storytelling about past experiences or discussion of the patient's career or life work, and by creating family trees (Lewis and Butler 1974). Examples of other life review activities include going on pilgrimages, artistic expression (e.g., creating a collage or drawings, writing poetry), and journal writing (Pickrel 1989). Life review has traditionally been used in the elderly as a means of conflict resolution and to facilitate a dignified acceptance of death (Butler 1963). For dying patients, their stories have a special meaning. In negotiating one's way through serious illness and its treatment, the telling of one's own story takes on a renewed urgency. This approach has not, however, been widely utilized in palliative care settings.

Group Psychotherapy

Group interventions may offer benefits less available in individual therapies, such as a sense of universality, sharing a common experience and identity, a feeling of helping oneself by helping others, hopefulness fostered by seeing how others have coped successfully, and a sense of belonging to a larger group (self-transcendence, meaning, common purpose). However, patients in advanced stages of terminal illness are often too sick to participate in group therapy. Group psychotherapeutic interventions for medically ill patients are reviewed in detail in Chapter 38, "Psychosocial Treatment."

Emerging Psychotherapeutic Interventions in the Terminally Ill

Spiritual Suffering

Palliative care practitioners have recognized the importance of spiritual suffering in their patients and have begun to design interventions to address it (Puchalski and Romer 2000; Rousseau 2000). Rousseau (2000) has developed an approach for the treatment of spiritual suffering that centers on facilitating religious expression while also controlling physical symptoms; providing a supportive presence; encouraging life review to assist in recognizing purpose, value, and meaning; exploring guilt, remorse, forgiveness, and reconciliation; reframing goals; and encouraging meditative practices. Although this approach blends basic principles common to many psychotherapies, it should be noted that this intervention contains a heavy emphasis on facilitating religious expression and confession and thus, although very useful to many patients, is not applicable to all and is not an intervention that all clinicians feel comfortable providing.

Meaning-Centered Psychotherapy

Breitbart and colleagues (Breitbart 2002; Breitbart and Heller 2003; Gibson CA, Breitbart W: "Individual Meaning-Centered Psychotherapy Treatment Manual," unpublished, 2004; Greenstein and Breitbart 2002) have applied Viktor Frankl's (1955, 1963, 1969, 1988, 1992, 1997) concepts of meaning-based psychotherapy (logotherapy) to address spiritual suffering in dying patients. This "Meaning-Centered Group Psychotherapy" (Greenstein and Breitbart 2000) utilizes a mixture of didactics, discussion, and experiential exercises that focus on particular themes related to meaning and advanced cancer. It is designed to help patients with advanced cancer sustain or enhance a sense of meaning, peace, and purpose in their lives even as they approach the end of life. Gibson and Breitbart ("Individual Meaning-Centered Psychotherapy Treatment Manual," unpublished, 2004) have manualized an individual form of this therapy and are currently conducting outcome studies to determine the feasibility and efficacy of both the group and individual forms of this therapy.

Demoralization

Kissane and colleagues (2001) described a syndrome of "demoralization" in the terminally ill that they propose is distinct from depression and consists of a triad of hopelessness, loss of meaning, and existential distress expressed as a desire for death. It is associated with life-threatening medical illness, disability, bodily disfigurement, fear, loss of dignity, social isolation, and feelings of being a burden. Because of the sense of impotence and hopelessness, those with the syndrome predictably progress to a desire to die or commit suicide. The authors (Kissane et al. 2001) formulated a treatment approach for demoralization syndrome that emphasizes a multidisciplinary, multimodal approach consisting of 1) ensuring continuity of care and active symptom management; 2) ensuring dignity in the dying process; 3) using various types of psychotherapy to help sustain a sense of meaning, limit cognitive distortions, and maintain family relationships (i.e., meaning-based, cognitive-behavioral, interpersonal, and family psychotherapy interventions); 4) using life review and narrative and attention to spiritual issues; and 5) administering pharmacotherapy for comorbid anxiety, depression, and delirium.

Dignity-Conserving Care

Ensuring dignity in the dying process is a critical goal of palliative care. Despite use of the term *dignity* in arguments for and against a patient's self-governance in matters pertaining to death, there is little empirical research on how this term has been used by patients who are nearing death. Chochinov et al. (2002a, 2002b) examined how dying patients understand and define *dignity* in order to develop a model of dignity in the terminally ill (see Figure 40–2). A semistructured interview was designed to explore how patients cope with their illness and their perceptions of dignity. Three major categories emerged, which included illness-related concerns (concerns related to the illness itself that threaten or impinge on the patient's sense of dignity), dignity-conserving repertoire (internally held qualities or personal approaches that patients use to maintain their sense of dignity), and social dignity inventory (social concerns or relationship dynamics that enhance or detract from a patient's sense of dignity). These broad categories and their carefully defined themes and subthemes form the foundation for an emerging model of dignity among the dying. The concept of dignity and the notion of dignity-conserving care offer a way of understanding how patients face advancing terminal illness and present an approach that clinicians can use to explicitly target the maintenance of dignity as a therapeutic objective.

Accordingly, Chochinov (2002) has developed a short-term dignity-conserving care intervention for palliative care patients that incorporates various facets from this model most likely to bolster the dying patient's will to live, lessen their desire for death or overall level of distress, and improve their quality of life. The dignity model establishes

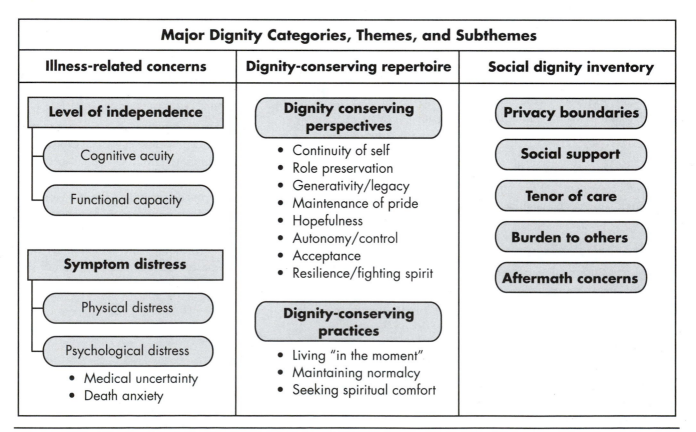

FIGURE 40–2.   Model of dignity for the terminally ill.

the importance of generativity as a significant dignity theme. As such, the sessions are taped, transcribed, and edited, and the transcription is returned to the patient within 1–2 days. The creation of a tangible product that will live beyond the patient acknowledges the importance of generativity as a salient dignity issue. The immediacy of the returned transcript is intended to bolster the patient's sense of purpose, meaning, and worth while giving them the tangible experience that their thoughts and words continue to be valued. In most instances, these transcripts will be left for family or loved ones and form part of a personal legacy that the patient will have actively participated in creating and shaping.

Spirituality in Palliative Care

Addressing spirituality as an essential element of quality palliative care has been identified as a priority by medical professionals as well as by patients (Field and Cassel 1997; Moadel et al. 1999; Singer et al. 1999). Spirituality encompasses concepts of faith and/or meaning (Karasu 1999; Puchalski and Romer 2000). Viewing spirituality as a construct composed of faith and meaning is reflected in the FACIT Spiritual Well-Being Scale (Brady et al. 1999; Peterman et al. 1996). This scale generates a total score as well as two subscale scores; one corresponding to "Faith" and a second corresponding to "Meaning/Peace." Other measures that are commonly used to gauge aspects of spirituality include the Daily Spiritual Experiences Scale (Underwood and Teresi 2002) and the Spiritual Beliefs Inventory (Baider et al. 2001).

Spirituality and Life-Threatening Medical Illness

There has been great interest in spirituality, faith, and religious beliefs and their impact on health outcomes and their role in palliative care (Baider et al. 1999; Holland et al. 1999; Koenig et al. 1992, 1998; McCullough and Larson 1999; Sloan et al. 1999). Sloan and colleagues (1999) concluded in their review of the literature that evidence of an association between religion and health was weak and inconsistent and that it was premature to promote faith and religion as adjunctive treatments. Elderly men who use religious beliefs or practices as a means of coping with physical illness appear to be less depressed than their nonreligious peers (Koenig et al. 1992). Researchers theorize that religious beliefs may help patients construct meaning from the suffering inherent in illness, which may in turn facilitate acceptance (Koenig et al. 1998). Recent studies have found that religion and spirituality generally play a

positive role in patients' coping with illnesses such as cancer or HIV (Baider et al. 1999; Nelson et al. 2002; Peterman et al. 1996).

Several recent studies (Breitbart et al. 2000; McClain et al. 2003; Nelson et al. 2002) have demonstrated a central role for spiritual well-being and meaning as a buffering agent against depression, hopelessness, and desire for hastened death among advanced cancer patients. Although spiritual well-being (per the FACIT Spiritual Well-Being Scale) has a generally positive influence on the incidence of depression, hopelessness, and desire for death, it is the score on the Meaning/Peace subscale that has the most significant effect. These findings are significant in the face of what we have come to learn about the consequences of depression and hopelessness in palliative care patients. Depression and hopelessness are associated with poorer survival in cancer patients (Watson et al. 1999) and dramatically higher rates of suicide, suicidal ideation, desire for hastened death, and interest in physician-assisted suicide (Breitbart et al. 1996b, 2000; Chochinov et al. 1994, 1995, 1998). Such findings point to the need for interventions in terminal patients that address depression, hopelessness, and loss of meaning and impact on desire for death.

Communicating About Spiritual Issues

Several factors may inhibit effective communication with patients about spirituality in a palliative care setting (Clayton 2000; Ellis et al. 1999; Post et al. 2000; Sloan et al. 1999). Promoting religion, faith, or specific religious beliefs or rituals (e.g., prayer, belief in an afterlife) in an effort to deal with patients' spiritual concerns or suffering at the end of life has limited acceptance among health care providers and is not universally applicable to all patients. Maugans and Wadland (1991) suggested that there is often a great discrepancy between physicians and patients on such issues as belief in God, belief in an afterlife, regular prayer, and feeling close to God, with physicians endorsing such beliefs or practices less than half as often as patients (none greater than 40%).

Additional barriers include lack of time on the part of the provider, lack of training, fear of projecting one's own beliefs onto the patient, and concerns about patient autonomy (Ellis et al. 1999). Finally, providers may feel that these discussions are inappropriate because they are outside of their area of expertise or intrusive to the patient's privacy (Ellis et al. 1999; Post et al. 2000; Sloan et al. 1999). However, the majority of studies have demonstrated that patients welcome these discussions (Anderson et al. 1993; King and Bushwick 1994; Maugans 1996).

Communicating effectively with patients about spirituality requires comfort in several domains. These include 1) a basic knowledge of common spiritual concerns and sources of spiritual pain for patients; 2) the principles and beliefs of the major religions common to the patient populations one treats; 3) basic clinical communication skills, such as active and empathetic listening, with an ability to identify and highlight spiritually relevant issues; and 4) the ability to remain present while patients struggle with spiritual issues in light of their mortality (Storey and Knight 2001). This final domain is often the most trying, especially for clinicians early in their career.

The American Academy of Hospice and Palliative Medicine offers the following guidelines for clinicians when communicating about spiritual issues (Doyle 1992; Hay 1996; Storey and Knight 2001). First, it is important to recognize that every patient is an individual and has a unique belief system that should be honored and respected. A patient's spiritual views may or may not incorporate religious beliefs, as *spirituality* is considered the more inclusive category. Therefore, initial discussions should focus on broad spiritual issues and then, when appropriate, on more specific religious beliefs. Caregivers should maintain appropriate boundaries and avoid discussions of their own religious beliefs because they are usually not relevant. Finally, fostering hope and integrating meaning into a patient's life is a more important aspect of providing spiritual healing than adherence to a particular belief system or religious affiliation. Methods for taking a spiritual history are reviewed elsewhere (Puchalski and Romer 2000). Formal assessment tools are also available (Kuhn 1988; Maugans 1996).

Psychosomatic medicine clinicians should be aware of the importance of spirituality and the value of pastoral care services not only for the patient but also for the family coping with a terminal illness. Referrals to chaplains are as important as referrals to any other specialist and an essential part of comprehensive care (Thiel and Robinson 1997).

Cross-Cultural Issues in Care of the Dying

Ethnicity and culture strongly influence attitudes toward death and dying. A full discussion of cultural and ethnic differences in the face of life-threatening illness is beyond the scope of this chapter, but some illustrative points should be noted. Although fears of cancer and other debilitating diseases are universal (Butow et al. 1997), it appears that individuals from mainstream Western cultures generally use different coping strategies than those used in non-Western cultures (Barg and Gullatte 2001). Wide differences also exist within countries.

Blackhall et al. (1995) studied ethnic attitudes in the United States toward patient autonomy regarding disclosure of the diagnosis and prognosis of a terminal illness and toward end-of-life decision making. They found that different cultures have distinct opinions about how much information physicians should provide concerning diagnoses and prognoses. The investigators determined that African Americans (88%) and European Americans (87%) are significantly more likely than Mexican Americans (65%) or Korean Americans (47%) to believe that a patient should always be informed of a diagnosis of metastatic cancer. They also found that African Americans (63%) and European Americans (69%) are more likely than Korean Americans (35%) and Mexican Americans (48%) to believe a patient should be informed of a terminal prognosis and be actively involved in decisions concerning use of life-sustaining technology. They concluded that physicians should ask their patients whether they wish to be informed of their diagnoses and prognoses and to be involved in treatment decisions or prefer to let family members or caregivers handle such matters.

A similar study of Navajo Indian beliefs concerning autonomy in patient diagnosis and prognosis found that in the Navajo culture, physicians and patients must speak in only a positive way, avoiding any negative thought or speech (Carrese and Rhodes 1995). Because Navajos believe that language can "shape reality and control events," informing patients of a negative diagnosis or prognosis is considered disrespectful and physically and emotionally dangerous (Carrese and Rhodes 1995). As these two studies show, physicians must be careful to respect their patients' cultural beliefs in disclosing the diagnosis and prognosis of a terminal illness. Important differences between cultures include those that exist in the roles of religion (Musick et al. 1998a, 1998b), family, alternative healing traditions and folk healers (Canive and Castillo 1997; Chan et al. 2001), attitudes toward pain and suffering (Gordon 2002), beliefs about afterlife, and customs regarding the deceased's body and burial preparations (Parkes et al. 1997). At the same time, one should beware of cultural stereotypes and not assume that every member of a particular ethnic or cultural group holds identical shared values.

Doctor–Patient Communication

Doctor–patient communication is an essential component in caring for a dying patient (Baile and Beale 2001; Buckman 1993, 1998; Fallowfield 2004; Parker et al. 2001; Smith 2000). A study of cancer patients' predictions regarding outcome and the treatments they chose revealed that inadequate communication between cancer patients and their physicians resulted in overestimation of survival by patients and a resulting tendency to choose more aggressive treatment (Weeks et al. 1996).

In a study of oncologists' communication skills (Fallowfield et al. 1998), less than 35% reported having received any previous communication training, but most desired to learn better communication techniques. Psychosomatic medicine specialists can help improve communication skills in physicians and other health care professionals caring for dying patients. Intensive training programs in doctor–patient communication that use a variety of teaching methods, including role playing, videotaped feedback, experiential exercises, and didactics, have been demonstrated to have both short-term as well as long-term efficacy in improving communication skills among physicians (Fallowfield 2004; Maguire 1999).

One critical aspect of doctor–patient communication is how to break bad news. A useful six-step protocol for breaking bad news includes 1) getting the physical context right, 2) finding out how much the patient knows, 3) finding out how much the patient wants to know, 4) sharing information (aligning and educating), 5) responding to the patient's feelings, and 6) planning and following through (Baile and Beale 2001; Buckman 1998).

Bereavement

Bereavement care is an integral dimension of palliative care, particularly for the 20% of bereaved individuals who develop complicated grief, for which effective therapies are available (Kissane 2004). Normal grief is an inevitable dimension of humanity, an adaptive adjustment process, and one that, with support, can be approached with courage.

Although words such as *grief*, *mourning*, and *bereavement* are commonly used interchangeably, the following definitions may be helpful:

- *Bereavement* is the state of loss resulting from death (Parkes 1998).
- *Grief* is the emotional response associated with loss (Stroebe et al. 1993).
- *Mourning* is the process of adaptation, including the cultural and social rituals prescribed as accompaniments (Raphael 1983).
- *Anticipatory grief* precedes the death and results from the expectation of that event (Raphael 1983).
- *Complicated grief* represents a pathological outcome involving psychological, social, or physical morbidity (Rando 1983).

- *Disenfranchised grief* represents the hidden sorrow of the marginalized patient, for whom there is less social permission to express many dimensions of loss (Doka 2000).

The Nature of Normal Grief

The expression of normal grief is evident through its emotional, cognitive, physical, and behavioral features (Parkes 1998). In Lindemann's classic (1944) study of people who lost a relative in Boston's Coconut Grove Nightclub fire, he identified key features of grief including somatic distress with numbness, preoccupation with sad memories of the deceased, guilt, anger, loss of regular patterns of conduct, and identification with the deceased.

Emotional distress occurs in waves with unavoidable crying and a range of associated affects including sadness, anger, despair, anxiety, and guilt. Cognitive processes become dominated by memories, reflected in storytelling, reminiscences, and conversations about the deceased. Physical responses include numbness, restlessness, tension, tremors, sleep disturbance, anorexia, weight loss, fatigue, and painful symptoms. Finally, behavioral aspects are variously reflected in social withdrawal, wandering, searching, and seeking company and consolation.

A number of physiological changes have been identified in grief in neuroendocrine functioning (Jacobs et al. 1997), immune indices (Esterling et al. 1996), and sleep efficiency (Hall et al. 1998).

Clinical Presentations of Grief

As the patient and family journey through palliative care, the clinical phases of grief progress from anticipatory grief through to the immediate news of the death, to the stages of acute grief, and potentially for some, to the complications of bereavement.

Anticipatory Grief

Anticipatory grief generally draws the supportive family closer. In contrast, for some families difficulties emerge as they express their anticipatory grief. Impaired coping is exhibited through protective avoidance, denial of the seriousness of the threat, anger, or withdrawal from involvement. Sometimes family dysfunction is glaring. More commonly, however, subthreshold or mild depressive or anxiety disorders develop gradually as individuals struggle to adapt to unwelcome changes. Although anticipatory grief was historically suggested to reduce postmortem grief (Parkes 1975), intense distress is now well recognized as a marker of risk for complicated grief. During this phase of anticipatory grief, families that are capable of effective communication should be encouraged to openly share their feelings as they go about the care of their dying family member or friend. Saying goodbye needs to be recognized as a process that evolves over time, with opportunities for reminiscence, celebration of the life and contribution of the dying person, expressions of gratitude, and completion of any unfinished business (Meares 1981). These tasks have the potential to generate creative and positive emotional aspects of what is otherwise a sad time for all.

Sometimes staff will have concerns about the emotional response of the bereaved. If there is uncertainty about its cultural appropriateness, consultation with an informed cultural intermediary may prove helpful.

Caution is needed in those settings where grief could be marginalized, well exemplified by ageism (see Doka 2000). If a death is normalized because it appears in step with the life cycle, family members may receive less support and reduced permission to express many aspects of their loss.

Acute Grief and Time Course of Bereavement

The sequence or phases through which the bereaved move over time are not rigidly demarcated but merge gradually one into the other (Parkes 1998; Raphael 1983). Starting with 1) initial numbness and sense of unreality, 2) waves of distress begin to occur as the bereaved experience intense pining and yearning for their lost one. Memories of the deceased trigger these acute pangs of grief. Then, as the pain of separation grows, 3) a phase of disorganization emerges as loneliness resulting from the loss sets in. Hofer (1984) described this phase aptly as a constant background disturbance of restlessness, inattention, sadness, and despair with social withdrawal that can last for several months. Eventually 4) a phase of reorganization and recovery develops as nostalgia replaces sadness, morale improves, and an altered world view is constructed.

The time course of mourning is proportional to the strength of attachment to the lost person and also varies with cultural expression, there being no sharply defined end point to grief. Just as a mother's grief following sudden infant death syndrome usually lasts longer than grief following a neonatal death, so too with adult loss—the mourning that follows many years of marriage is generally longer than that in brief relationships. Some, including older widows and widowers, may continue to display their grief for several years (Zisook and Schucter 1985). This may represent a continuing relationship with the deceased that, for some, is their choice and leads to a prolonged period of bereavement that may be quite appropriate and within the normal range of grief experience. The clinical task is then to differentiate those that remain

within the spectrum of normality from those that cross the threshold of complicated grief.

Complicated Grief

Normal and abnormal responses to bereavement span a spectrum in which intensity of reaction, presence of a range of related grief behaviors, and time course determine the differentiation. Psychiatric disorders commonly complicating grief include clinical depression, anxiety disorders, alcohol abuse or other substance abuse, and psychotic disorders. When frank psychiatric disorders complicate bereavement, they are more likely to be recognized and treated than subthreshold states. Studies of the bereaved identify clusters of intense grief symptoms distinct from uncomplicated grief (Parkes 1983; Prigerson et al. 1995a, 1995b). Their recognition calls for an experienced clinical judgment that does not normalize the distress as understandable.

Inhibited or Delayed Grief

Although avoidance may serve some as a temporary coping mechanism, its persistence is usually associated with relationship or other difficulties. Cultural and individual variation significantly influences grief expression; a placid external emotional response cannot be equated with internal avoidance. Empirical studies have generally identified avoidant forms of complicated grief in up to 5% of the bereaved—the grief may not always present clinically but may reappear in later years as an unresolved issue.

Chronic Grief

A common form of complicated grief, chronic grief is particularly associated with overly dependent relationships in which a sense of abandonment is avoided by perpetuation of the relationship through memorialization of the deceased and maintenance of continuing bonds. Social withdrawal and depression are common. A fantasy of reunion with the deceased can cause suicide to be an increasingly attractive option. Active treatment using antidepressants and cognitive-behavioral therapy to reality test the loss and promote socialization (via activity scheduling) is often appropriate for chronic grief (keeping in mind that not all persistent grief is pathological).

Traumatic Grief

When death has been unexpected or its nature in some way shocking—traumatic, violent, stigmatized, or perceived as undignified—its integration and acceptance may be interfered with by the arousal and increased distress that memories can trigger. Intensive recollections including flashbacks, nightmares, and recurrent intrusive memories cause hyperarousal, disbelief, insomnia, irritability, and disturbed concentration that distort normal grieving (Prigerson and Jacobs 2001). The shock of the death can precipitate mistrust, anger, detachment, and an unwillingness to accept its reality. These reactions at a subthreshold level are on a continuum with the full features of acute and posttraumatic stress disorders, but subthreshold states have been observed to persist for years and contribute substantial morbidity. Palliative care deaths involving profound breakdown of bodily surfaces, gross disfigurement due to head and neck cancers, or other changes eliciting fear, disgust, or mortification may generate traumatic memories in the bereaved. Schut and colleagues (1997) found that PTSD was often correlated with the perceived inadequacy of the goodbye and suggested that rituals to complete this be incorporated into related grief therapies.

Psychiatric Disorders in Bereavement

Rates of major depression in the bereaved have varied between 16% and 50%, peaking during the first 2 months (Clayton 1990; Zisook and Schuchter 1991) and gradually decreasing to 15% across the next 2 years (Harlow et al. 1991; Zisook et al. 1994). The features of any major depressive episode following bereavement resemble major depression at other points of the life cycle (Karam 1994). There is a tendency toward chronicity, considerable social morbidity, and risk of inadequate treatment.

Anxiety disorders take the form of adjustment disorders, generalized anxiety disorder, acute and posttraumatic stress disorders, and phobias and occur in up to 30% of the bereaved (Jacobs 1993).

Individuals predisposed to alcohol or other substance use disorders are at higher risk for relapse during grief (Jacobs 1993), as are those with psychotic disorders. The latter should not be confused with the "normal" hallucinations that can occur in grief, typically limited to the voice, sight, and/or sense of presence of the deceased.

Risk factors that, when present, can aid recognition of those at greater risk of complicated grief are summarized in Table 40–3.

Grief Therapies

The most basic model is a supportive/expressive intervention in which the person is invited to share his or her feelings about the loss to a health professional who will listen and seek to understand the other's distress in a comforting manner. The key therapeutic aspects of this encounter are the sharing of distress and, through the relational understanding that is acknowledged, some shift in cognitive appraisal of the reality that has been forever altered. There are multiple possible formal interventions for bereaved people, but the first question is whether an intervention is actually warranted. For most, although bereavement is painful, personal resilience will ensure normal adaptation. There can therefore be no justification for routine intervention, because grief is not a disease. Early intervention should be considered for those at risk of maladaptive outcomes and those who later develop complicated bereavement need active treatments.

The spectrum of interventions spans individual-, group-, and family-oriented therapies and encompasses all schools of psychotherapy as well as appropriately indicated pharmacotherapy. A typical intervention entails six to eight sessions over several months. In this sense, grief therapy is focused and time limited, but multimodal therapies are common. Table 40–4 lists commonly used forms of grief therapy (Kissane 2004).

TABLE 40–3. Risk factors for complicated grief	
Category	**Range of circumstances**
Nature of the death	Untimely within the life cycle (e.g., death of a child)
	Sudden and unexpected
	Traumatic/shocking
	Stigmatized
Strengths and vulnerabilities of the caregiver/bereaved	Past history of psychiatric disorder
	Personality and coping style
	Cumulative experience of losses
Nature of the relationship with the deceased	Overly dependent
	Ambivalent
Family and support network	Dysfunctional family
	Isolated
	Alienated

TABLE 40–4.   Models of grief therapy

Model	Potential focus for application	Clinical issues when indicated
Supportive/expressive therapy (guided grief work, crisis intervention)	Individual and/or group	Avoidance of emotional expression Inhibited or delayed grief Isolated and needing support Established psychiatric disorders including depression
Interpersonal or psychodynamic therapy	Individual and/or group	Relational issues dominate Role transition difficulties
Cognitive-behavioral therapy	Individual and/or group	Chronic grief with "stuck" behaviors Traumatic grief Posttraumatic stress disorder
Family-focused grief therapy	Family	Family either at risk or clearly dysfunctional in its relating Adolescents or children at risk
Combined pharmacotherapies with any of the psychotherapeutic models	Individual	Depressive disorders Anxiety disorders Sleep disorders

Pharmacotherapy is widely used to support the bereaved, but prescribing should be judicious. Benzodiazepines allay anxiety and assist sleep, but excessive use may interfere with adaptive mourning. Antidepressants are indicated when bereavement is complicated by major depression or panic disorder (Jacobs et al. 1987; Pasternak et al. 1991; Zisook et al. 2001).

Palliation of Selected Physical Symptoms

Although the diagnosis and treatment of psychiatric disorders in the patient with advanced illness is important, pain and other distressing physical symptoms must also be aggressively treated to enhance the patient's quality of life (Foley 1985; Foley and Helband 2001). Some key points are noted in this discussion, but a comprehensive review of pharmacological and nonpharmacological interventions for common physical symptoms encountered in the terminally ill can be found in a curriculum published by the American Society of Clinical Oncology (2001) and in major palliative care texts (Chochinov and Breitbart 2000; Doyle et al. 2003).

Pain

The Agency for Health Care Policy and Research (1994) published a practice guideline for management of cancer pain in the early 1990s, with more recent guidelines from the National Comprehensive Cancer Network (Benedetti et al. 2000). Breitbart et al. (2004b) provided an up-to-date detailed discussion of the use of behavioral, psychotherapeutic, and psychopharmacological interventions for pain control in palliative care (see also Chapter 36, "Pain"). After adequate medical treatment, mild to moderate levels of residual pain can be effectively managed with behavioral techniques that are quite similar to those used for anxiety, phobias, and anticipatory nausea and vomiting. Relaxation techniques, imagery, hypnosis, biofeedback, and multicomponent cognitive-behavioral interventions have been used to provide comfort and minimize pain in adults, children, and adolescents.

Anorexia and Weight Loss

Whereas physiological changes associated with terminal illness account for most of the anorexia and cachexia in the terminally ill, with additional contributions from adverse effects of treatments, psychological and psychiatric factors, including anxiety, depression, and conditioned food aversions, may also play a role (Lesko 1989). The treatment of anorexia and weight loss begins with the identification and correction of reversible causes (e.g., opioid-induced nausea, stomatitis from chemotherapy, or thrush). Progestational drugs (medroxyprogesterone or megesterol acetate) are often tried for nonspecific cachexia. Appetite-stimulating antidepressants (e.g., tricyclic antidepressants, mirtazapine, trazodone) should be prescribed when the cause is major depression, but depression should never be diagnosed solely on the basis of unexplained anorexia and weight loss. Treatment of conditioned nausea and vomiting is discussed later.

Asthenia/Fatigue

Asthenia and fatigue are extremely common in patients with advanced cancer, AIDS, and organ failure as a result of deconditioning, catabolism, malnutrition, infection, profound anemia, metabolic abnormalities, or adverse effects of treatment, but a reversible cause often cannot be identified. As with unexplained weight loss in advanced disease, there is a tendency to overdiagnose depression in the terminally ill patient with extreme fatigue.

The literature in support of the pharmacotherapy of fatigue in cancer patients is largely anecdotal, but practice guidelines are available (Mock et al. 2000). Identifiable causes should be specifically treated when possible, for example, erythropoietin for anemia. Some patients respond to corticosteroids, but the benefits tend to be fleeting and prolonged use can cause proximal myopathy. Psychostimulants have been used in the treatment of asthenia with good results (Breitbart et al. 2001; see also Chapter 28, "HIV/AIDS"). Low doses of stimulants do not appear to cause appetite suppression or weight loss and may actually improve energy and appetite in fatigued terminally ill patients.

Nausea and Vomiting

Common causes of nausea and vomiting in cancer patients include radiation, medications, toxins, metabolic derangements, obstruction of the gastrointestinal tract, and chemotherapy. Conditioned by the experience of profound nausea and vomiting secondary to highly emetic chemotherapy agents, some patients report being nauseated in anticipation of treatment. Anticipatory nausea and vomiting used to be very frequent but has become less so with current antiemetic therapy.

Antiemetic drugs are the mainstay of managing chemotherapy-induced nausea and vomiting in patients with advanced disease. Several antiemetics (e.g., metoclopramide, prochlorperazine, promethazine) have dopamine-blocking properties and so can cause the same extrapyramidal side effects as neuroleptics, with acute akathisia and dystonia common. Extrapyramidal side effects are not a problem with newer antiemetics like ondansetron. Rapid-onset, short-acting benzodiazepines are also helpful in controlling anticipatory nausea and vomiting once they have developed (Greenberg et al. 1987). Behavioral control of anticipatory nausea and vomiting was shown to be highly effective (Barnes 1988) but has largely been replaced by antiemetic drugs.

Conclusion

The psychosomatic medicine practitioner can play an important role in the care of patients with advanced, life-threatening medical illnesses. Palliative care for terminally ill patients must include not only control of pain and physical symptoms but also assessment and management of psychiatric and psychosocial complications. The psychosomatic medicine practitioner working in the palliative care setting must be knowledgeable in the assessment and management of major psychiatric complications such as anxiety, depression, and delirium, and also must be adept in dealing with issues of existential despair and spiritual suffering. Cultural issues, communication issues, ethical issues, and issues of bereavement are all areas requiring attention and awareness. As part of a multidisciplinary team, the psychosomatic medicine practitioner can play an important role in the provision of comprehensive palliative care.

References

Achte KA, Vanhkouen ML: Cancer and the psyche. Omega 2:46–56, 1971

Adams F, Quesada JR, Gutterman JU: Neuropsychiatric manifestations of human leukocyte interferon therapy in patients with cancer. JAMA 252:938–941, 1984

Agency for Health Care Policy and Research: Management of cancer pain: adults. Clin Pract Guidel Quick Ref Guide Clin 9:1–29, 1994

American Society of Clinical Oncology: Optimizing Cancer Cure: The Importance of Symptom Management. Alexandria, VA, American Society of Clinical Oncology Publishing, 2001

Anderson JM, Anderson LJ, Felsenthal G: Pastoral needs for support within an inpatient rehabilitation unit. Arch Phys Med Rehabil 74:574–578, 1993

Baider L, Russak SM, Perry S, et al: The role of religious and spiritual beliefs in coping with malignant melanoma: an Israeli sample. Psychooncology 8:27–35, 1999

Baider L, Holland JC, Russak SM, et al: The System of Belief Inventory–15 (SBI-15). Psycho-Oncology 10:534–540, 2001

Baile W, Beale E: Giving bad news to cancer patients: matching process and content. J Clin Oncol 19:2575–2577, 2001

Barg FK, Gullatte MM: Cancer support groups: meeting the needs of African Americans with cancer. Semin Oncol Nurs 17:171–178, 2001

Barnes M: Nausea and vomiting in the patient with advanced cancer. J Pain Symptom Manage 3:81–85, 1988

Benedetti C, Brock C, Cleeland C, et al: NCCN Practice Guidelines for Cancer Pain. Oncology (Huntingt) 14:135–150, 2000

Blackhall LJ, Murphy ST, Frank G, et al: Ethnicity and attitudes toward patient autonomy. JAMA 274:820–825, 1995

Block SD: Assessing and managing depression in the terminally ill patient. Ann Intern Med 132:209–218, 2000

Bolund C: Suicide and cancer, II: medical and care factors in suicide by cancer patients in Sweden. Journal of Psychosocial Oncology 3:17–30, 1985

Bottomley DM, Hanks GW: Subcutaneous midazolam infusion in palliative care. J Pain Symptom Manage 5:259–261, 1990

Brady MJ, Peterman AH, Fitchett G, et al: A case for including spirituality in quality of life measurement in oncology. Psycho-Oncology 8:417–428, 1999

Brandberg Y, Mansson-Brahme E, Ringborg U, et al: Psychological reactions in patients with malignant melanoma. Eur J Cancer 31A:157–162, 1995

Breitbart W: Suicide in cancer patients. Oncology (Huntingt) 1:49–55, 1987

Breitbart W: Endocrine-related psychiatric disorders, in Handbook of Psychooncology: Psychological Care of the Patient With Cancer. Edited by Holland JC, Rowland JH. New York, Oxford University Press, 1989a, pp 356–368

Breitbart W: Psychiatric management of cancer pain. Cancer 63:2336–2342, 1989b

Breitbart W: Cancer pain and suicide, in Advances in Pain Research and Therapy, Vol 16. Edited by Foley K, Bonica JJ, Ventafridda V, et al. New York, Raven, 1990, pp 399–412

Breitbart W: Diagnosis and management of delirium in the terminally ill, in Topics in Palliative Care, Vol 5. Edited by Bruera E, Portenoy R. New York, Oxford University Press, 2001, pp 303–321

Breitbart W: Spirituality and meaning in supportive care: spirituality- and meaning-centered group psychotherapy interventions in advanced cancer. Support Care Cancer 10:272–280, 2002

Breitbart W: Palliative and Supportive Care: introducing a new international journal; the "care" journal of palliative medicine. Palliative and Supportive Care 1:1–2, 2003

Breitbart W, Heller KS: Reframing hope: meaning-centered care for patients near the end of life. J Palliat Med 6:979–988, 2003

Breitbart W, Holland JC (eds): Psychiatric Aspects of Symptom Management in Cancer Patients. Washington, DC, American Psychiatric Press, 1993

Breitbart W, Mermelstein H: Pemoline: an alternative psychostimulant for the management of depressive disorders in cancer patients. Psychosomatics 33:352–356, 1992

Breitbart W, Sparrow B: Management of delirium in the terminally ill. Progress in Palliative Care 6:107–113, 1998

Breitbart W, Levenson JA, Passik SD: Terminally ill patients, in Psychiatric Aspects of Symptom Management in Cancer Patients. Edited by Breitbart W, Holland JC. Washington, DC, American Psychiatric Press, 1993, pp 173–230

Breitbart W, Bruera E, Chochinov H, et al: Neuropsychiatric syndromes and psychological symptoms in patients with advanced cancer. J Pain Symptom Manage 10:131–141, 1995

Breitbart W, Marotta R, Platt MM, et al: A double-blind comparison trial of haloperidol, chlorpromazine, and lorazepam in the treatment of delirium in hospitalized AIDS patients. Am J Psychiatry 153:231–237, 1996a

Breitbart W, Rosenfeld BD, Passik SD: Interest in physician-assisted suicide among ambulatory HIV-infected patients. Am J Psychiatry 153:238–242, 1996b

Breitbart W, Rosenfeld B, Roth A, et al: The Memorial Delirium Assessment Scale. J Pain Symptom Manage 13:128–137, 1997

Breitbart W, Rosenfeld B, Pessin H, et al: Depression, hopelessness, and desire for death in terminally ill patients with cancer. JAMA 284:2907–2911, 2000

Breitbart W, Rosenfeld B, Kaim M, et al: A randomized, double-blind, placebo-controlled trial of psychostimulants for the treatment of fatigue in ambulatory patients with human immunodeficiency virus disease. Arch Intern Med 161:411–420, 2001

Breitbart W, Gibson C, Tremblay A: The delirium experience: delirium recall and delirium-related distress in hospitalized patients with cancer, their spouses/caregivers, and their nurses. Psychosomatics 43:183–194, 2002a

Breitbart W, Tremblay A, Gibson C: An open trial of olanzapine for the treatment of delirium in hospitalized cancer patients. Psychosomatics 43:175–182, 2002b

Breitbart W, Chochinov H, Passik S: Psychiatric symptoms in palliative medicine, in Oxford Textbook of Palliative Medicine, 3rd Edition. Edited by Doyle D, Hanks G, Cherny N, et al. New York, Oxford University Press, 2004a, pp 746–771

Breitbart W, Payne D, Passik S: Psychological and psychiatric interventions in pain control, in Oxford Textbook of Palliative Medicine, 3rd Edition. Edited by Doyle D, Hanks G, Cherny N, et al. New York, Oxford University Press, 2004b, pp 424–438

Brown JH, Henteleff P, Barakat S, et al: Is it normal for terminally ill patients to desire death? Am J Psychiatry 143:208–211, 1986

Bruera E, Chadwick S, Brenneis C, et al: Methylphenidate associated with narcotics for the treatment of cancer pain. Cancer Treat Rep 71:67–70, 1987

Bruera E, Macmillan K, Pither J, et al: Effects of morphine on the dyspnea of terminal cancer patients. J Pain Symptom Manage 5:341–344, 1990

Bruera E, Miller L, McCallion J, et al: Cognitive failure in patients with terminal cancer: a prospective study. J Pain Symptom Manage 7:192–195, 1992

Buckman R: How to Break Bad News: A Guide for Healthcare Professionals. London, Macmillan Medical, 1993

Buckman R: Communication in palliative care: a practical guide, in Oxford Textbook of Palliative Medicine, 2nd Edition. Edited by Doyle D, Hanks GWC, MacDonald N. New York, Oxford University Press, 1998, pp 141–156

Butler RN: The life review: an interpretation of reminiscence in the aged. Psychiatry 26:65–75, 1963

Butow P, Tattersall M, Goldstein D: Communication with cancer patients in culturally diverse societies. Ann N Y Acad Sci 809:317–329, 1997

Byock IR: The nature of suffering and the nature of opportunity at the end of life. Clin Geriatr Med 12:237–252, 1996

Canadian Palliative Care Association: Palliative Care: Towards a Consensus in Standardized Principles of Practice. Ottawa, ON, Canadian Palliative Care Association, 1995

Canive JM, Castillo D: Hispanic veterans diagnosed with PTSD: assessment and treatment issues. NCP Clinical Quarterly 7(1), Winter 1997

Carrese J, Rhodes L: Western bioethics on the Navajo reservation. JAMA 274:826–829, 1995

Chan C, Ho P, Chow E: A body-mind-spirit model in health: an Eastern approach. Social Work Health and Mental Care 34:261–282, 2001

Cherny N: The problem of suffering, in Oxford Textbook of Palliative Medicine, 3rd Edition. Edited by Doyle D, Hanks G, Cherny N, et al. New York, Oxford University Press, 2004, pp 7–13

Chochinov HM: Dignity-conserving care—a new model for palliative care: helping the patient feel valued. JAMA 287: 2253–2260, 2002

Chochinov HM, Breitbart W (eds): Handbook of Psychiatry in Palliative Medicine. New York, Oxford University Press, 2000

Chochinov HM, Wilson KG, Enns M, et al: Prevalence of depression in the terminally ill: effects of diagnostic criteria and symptom threshold judgments. Am J Psychiatry 151: 537–540, 1994

Chochinov HM, Wilson KG, Enns M, et al: Desire for death in the terminally ill. Am J Psychiatry 152:1185–1191, 1995

Chochinov H, Wilson K, Enns M, et al: "Are You Depressed?" screening for depression in the terminally ill. Am J Psychiatry 154:674–676, 1997

Chochinov H, Wilson K, Enns M, et al: Depression, hopelessness, and suicidal ideation in the terminally ill. Psychosomatics 39:366–370, 1998

Chochinov HM, Tataryn D, Clinch JJ, et al: Will to live in the terminally ill. Lancet 354:816–819, 1999

Chochinov HM, Hack T, Hassard T, et al: Dignity in the terminally ill: a cross-sectional, cohort study. Lancet 360:2026–2030, 2002a

Chochinov HM, Hack T, McClement S, et al: Dignity in the terminally ill: an empirical model. Soc Sci Med 54:433–443, 2002b

Clayton CL: Barriers, boundaries, and blessings: ethical issues in physicians' spiritual involvement with patients. Medical Humanities Report 21:234–256, 2000

Clayton P: Bereavement and depression. J Clin Psychiatry 51: 34–38, 1990

Coyle N, Breitbart W, Weaver S, et al: Delirium as a contributing factor to "crescendo" pain: three case reports. J Pain Symptom Manage 9:44–47, 1994

DeAngelis LM, Delattre J, Posner JB: Radiation-induced dementia in patients cured of brain metastases. Neurology 39:789–796, 1989

Denicoff KD, Rubinow DR, Papa MZ, et al: The neuropsychiatric effects of treatment with interleukin-2 and lymphokine activated killer cells. Ann Intern Med 107:293–300, 1987

DeSousa E, Jepson A: Midazolam in terminal care (letter). Lancet 1(8577):67–68, 1988

Doka K: Disenfranchised grief, in Disenfranchised Grief: Recognizing Hidden Sorrow. Edited by Doka K. Lexington, MA, Lexington Books, 2000, pp 3–11

Doyle D: Have we looked beyond the physical and psychosocial? J Pain Symptom Manage 7:302–311, 1992

Doyle D, Hanks GWC, Cherny N, et al (eds): Oxford Textbook of Palliative Medicine, 3rd Edition. New York, NY, Oxford University Press, 2003

Dugan W, McDonald MV, Passik SD, et al: Use of the Zung Self-Rating Depression Scale in cancer patients: feasibility as a screening tool. Psychooncology 7:483–493, 1998

Ellis M, Vinson D, Ewigman B: Addressing spiritual concerns of patients: family physicians' attitudes and practices. J Fam Pract 48:105–109, 1999

Esterling B, Kiecolt-Glaser J, Glaser R: Psychosocial modulation of cytokine-induced natural killer cell activity in older adults. Psychosomatics 38:529–534, 1996

Fainsinger R, Miller MJ, Bruera E, et al: Symptom control during the last week of life in a palliative care unit. J Palliat Care 7:5–11, 1991

Fallowfield L: Communication and palliative medicine, in Oxford Textbook of Palliative Medicine, 3rd Edition. Edited by Doyle D, Hanks G, Cherny N, et al. New York, NY, Oxford University Press, 2004, pp 101–107

Fallowfield L, Lipkin M, Hall A: Teaching senior oncologists communication skills: results from phase I of a comprehensive longitudinal program in the United Kingdom. J Clin Oncol 16:1961–1968, 1998

Farberow NL, Schneidman ES, Leonard CV: Suicide Among General Medical and Surgical Hospital Patients With Malignant Neoplasms (Medical Bulletin 9). Washington, DC, U.S. Veterans Administration, 1963

Farberow NL, Ganzler S, Cutter F, et al: An eight-year survey of hospital suicides. Suicide Life Threat Behav 1:984–201, 1971

Fernandez F, Levy JK, Mansell PWA: Management of delirium in terminally ill AIDS patients. Int J Psychiatry Med 19: 165–172, 1989

Field M, Cassel C (eds): Approaching Death: Improving Care at the End of Life. Washington, DC, National Academy Press, 1997

Foley KM: The treatment of cancer pain. N Engl J Med 313:84–95, 1985

Foley KM, Helband H (eds): Improving Palliative Care for Cancer. National Cancer Policy Board, Institute of Medicine and National Research Council. Washington, DC, National Academy Press, 2001

Foreman J: 70% would pick hospice, poll finds. Boston Globe, October 4, 1996, p A3

Fox BH, Stanek EJ, Boyd SC, et al: Suicide rates among cancer patients in Connecticut. J Chronic Dis 35:89–100, 1982

Frankl V: Man's Search for Meaning. New York, Washington Square Press, 1963

Frankl VF: The Doctor and the Soul (1955). New York, Random House, 1986

Frankl VF: The Will to Meaning: Foundations and Applications of Logotherapy, Expanded Edition (1969). New York, Penguin Books, 1988

Frankl VF: Man's Search for Meaning, 4th Edition (1959). Massachusetts, Beacon Press, 1992

Frankl VF: Man's Search for Ultimate Meaning (1975). New York, Plenum Press, 1997

Ganzini L, Lee MA, Heintz RT, et al: The effect of depression treatment on elderly patients' preferences for life-sustaining medical therapy. Am J Psychiatry 151:1631–1636, 1994

Gordon JS: Asian spiritual traditions and their usefulness to practitioners and patients facing life and death. J Altern Complement Med 5:603–608, 2002

Greenberg DB, Surman OS, Clarke J, et al: Alprazolam for phobic nausea and vomiting related to cancer chemotherapy. Cancer Treat Rep 71:549–550, 1987

Greenstein M, Breitbart W: Cancer and the experience of meaning: a group psychotherapy program for people with cancer. Am J Psychother 54:486–500, 2000

Hall M, Baum A, Buysse D, et al: Sleep as a mediator of the stress-immune relationship. Psychosom Med 60:48–51, 1998

Harlow S, Goldberg E, Comstock G: A longitudinal study of the prevalence of depressive symptomatology in elderly widowed and married women. Arch Gen Psychiatry 48:1065–1068, 1991

Hay MW: Developing guidelines for spiritual caregivers in hospice: principles for spiritual assessment. Presented at the National Hospice Organization Annual Symposium and Exposition, Chicago, IL, November 1996

Heiney PS: The healing power of story. Oncol Nurs Forum 6:899–904, 1995

Hofer M: Relationships as regulators: a psychobiologic perspective on bereavement. Psychosom Med 46:183–197, 1984

Holland JC: Anxiety and cancer: the patient and the family. J Clin Psychiatry 50 (suppl):20–25, 1989

Holland JC, Fasanello S, Ohnuma T: Psychiatric symptoms associated with L-asparaginase administration. J Psychiatr Res 10:105–113, 1974

Holland JC, Morrow G, Schmale A, et al: Reduction of anxiety and depression in cancer patients by alprazolam or by a behavioral technique (abstract). Proceedings of the American Society of Clinical Oncology 6:258, 1987

Holland JC, Passik S, Kash KM, et al: The role of religious and spiritual beliefs in coping with malignant melanoma. Psycho-Oncology 8:14–26, 1999

Homsi J, Nelson KA, Sarhill N, et al: A phase II study of methylphenidate for depression in advanced cancer. Am J Hosp Palliat Care 18:403–407, 2001

Jacobs S: Pathological Grief. Washington, DC, American Psychiatric Press, 1993

Jacobs S, Nelson J, Zisook S: Treating depressions of bereavement with antidepressants: a pilot study. Psychiatr Clin North Am 10:501–510, 1987

Jacobs S, Bruce M, Kim K: Adrenal function predicts demoralisation after losses. Psychosomatics 38:529–534, 1997

Karam E: The nosological status of bereavement-related depressions. Br J Psychiatry 165:48–52, 1994

Karasu BT: Spiritual psychotherapy. Am J Psychother 53:143–162, 1999

Kerrihard T, Breitbart W, Dent K, et al: Anxiety in patients with cancer and human immunodeficiency virus. Semin Clin Neuropsychiatry 4:114–132, 1999

King DE, Bushwick B: Beliefs and attitudes of hospital inpatients about faith healing and prayer. J Fam Pract 39:349–352, 1994

Kissane DW: Bereavement, in The Oxford Textbook of Palliative Medicine, 3rd Edition. Edited by Doyle D, Hanks G, Cherny N, et al. Oxford, UK, Oxford University Press, 2004, pp 1135–1154

Kissane D, Clarke DM, Street AF: Demoralization syndrome: a relevant psychiatric diagnosis for palliative care. J Palliat Care 17:12–21, 2001

Koenig HG, Cohen HJ, Blazer DG, et al: Religious coping and depression among elderly, hospitalized medically ill men. Am J Psychiatry 149:1693–1700, 1992

Koenig HG, George, LK, Peterson BL: Religiosity and remission of depression in medically ill older patients. Am J Psychiatry 155:536–542, 1998

Kuhn CC: A spiritual inventory of the medically ill patient. Psychiatr Med 6:87–100, 1988

Lawlor PG, Gagnon B, Mancini IL, et al: Occurrence, causes, and outcome of delirium in patients with advanced cancer: a prospective study. Arch Intern Med 160:786–794, 2000a

Lawlor PG, Nekolaichuk C, Gagnon B, et al: Clinical utility, factor analysis, and further validation of the memorial delirium assessment scale in patients with advanced cancer: Assessing delirium in advanced cancer. Cancer 88:2859–2867, 2000b

Lesko L: Anorexia, in Handbook of Psychooncology: Psychological Care of the Patient with Cancer. Edited by Holland JC, Rowland JH. New York, Oxford University Press, 1989, pp 434–443

Levine PM, Silberfarb PM, Lipowski ZJ: Mental disorders in cancer patients: a study of 100 psychiatric referrals. Cancer 42:1385–1391, 1978

Levy MH, NCCN Palliative Care Panel Members: Palliative care. Journal of the National Comprehensive Cancer Network 1:394–420, 2003

Lewis MI, Butler R: Life review therapy: putting memories to work in individual and group psychotherapy. Geriatrics 29:165–169, 1974

Lichter I, Mooney J, Boyd M: Biography as therapy. Palliative Medicine 7:133–137, 1993

Lindemann E: Symptomatology and management of acute grief. Am J Psychiatry 101:141–148, 1944

Lloyd-Williams M (ed): Psychosocial Issues in Palliative Care. New York, Oxford University Press, 2003

Louhivuori KA, Hakama J: Risk of suicide among cancer patients. Am J Epidemiol 109:59–65, 1979

Maguire P: Improving communication with cancer patients. Eur J Cancer 35:2058–2065, 1999

Massie MJ: Anxiety, panic, phobias, in Handbook of Psycho-oncology: Psychological Care of the Patient With Cancer. Edited by Holland JC, Rowland JH. New York, Oxford University Press, 1989, pp 300–309

Massie MJ, Popkin MK: Depressive disorders, in Psycho-Oncology. Edited by Holland JC. New York, Oxford University Press, 1998, pp 518–540

Massie MJ, Holland JC, Glass E: Delirium in terminally ill cancer patients. Am J Psychiatry 140:1048–1050, 1983

Massie MJ, Holland JC, Straker N: Psychotherapeutic interventions, in Handbook of Psychooncology: Psychological Care of the Patient with Cancer. Edited by Holland JC, Rowland JH. New York, Oxford University Press, 1989, pp 455–469

Maugans TA: The SPIRITual history. Arch Fam Med 5:11–16, 1996

Maugans TA, Wadland WC: Religion and family medicine: a survey of physicians and patients. J Fam Pract 32:210–213, 1991

McClain CS, Rosenfeld B, Breitbart W: Effect of spiritual well-being on end-of-life despair in terminally ill cancer patients. Lancet 361:1603–1607, 2003

McCullough ME, Larson DB: Religion and depression: a review of the literature. Twin Research 2:126–136, 1999

McDonald MV, Passik SD, Dugan W, et al: Nurses' recognition of depression in their patients with cancer. Oncol Nurs Forum 26:593–599, 1999

Meares R: On saying goodbye before death. JAMA 246:1227–1229, 1981

Mercadante S, De Conno F, Ripamonti C: Propofol in terminal care. J Pain Symptom Manage 10:639–642, 1995

Minagawa H, Uchitomi Y, Yamawaki S, et al: Psychiatric morbidity in terminally ill cancer patients. Cancer 78:1131–1137, 1996

Misbin RI, O'Hare D, Lederberg MS, et al: Compliance with New York State's do-not-resuscitate law at Memorial Sloan-Kettering Cancer Center: a review of patient deaths. N Y State J Med 93:165–168, 1993

Moadel A, Morgan C, Fatone A, et al: Seeking meaning and hope: self-reported spiritual and existential needs among an ethnically diverse cancer patient population. Psycho-Oncology 8:1428–1431, 1999

Mock V, Atkinson A, Barsevick A, et al: NCCN practice guidelines for cancer-related fatigue. Oncology (Huntingt) 14:151–161, 2000

Moyle J: The use of propofol in palliative medicine. J Pain Symptom Manage 10:643–646, 1995

Murray GB: Confusion, delirium, and dementia, in Massachusetts General Hospital Handbook of General Hospital Psychiatry, 2nd Edition. Edited by Hackett TP, Cassem NH. Littleton, MA, PSG Publishing, 1987, pp 84–115

Musick M, Koenig H, Larson D: Religion and spiritual beliefs, in Psycho-Oncology. Edited by Holland JC. New York, Oxford University Press, 1998a, pp 780–789

Musick MA, Koenig HG, Hays JC, et al: Religious activity and depression among community-dwelling elderly persons with cancer: the moderating effect of race. Journal of Gerontology: Social Sciences 53B:S218–S227, 1998b

National Hospice Organization: New findings address escalating end-of-life debate (press release). Arlington, VA, National Hospice Organization, October 3, 1996

Nelson CJ, Rosenfeld B, Breitbart W, et al: Spirituality, religion, and depression in the terminally ill. Psychosomatics 43:213–220, 2002

O'Neill JF, Selwyn PA, Schietinger H (eds): A Clinical Guide to Supportive and Palliative Care for HIV/AIDS. Washington, DC, U.S. Department of Health and Human Services, Health Resources and Services Administration, HIV/AIDS Bureau, 2003

Palliative Care Foundation: Palliative Care Services in Hospitals, Guidelines. Report of the Working Group on Special Services in Hospitals, Ottawa, Ontario. Toronto, Canada, National Health and Welfare, Palliative Care Foundation, 1981

Parker B, Baile W, deMoor C, et al: Breaking bad news about cancer: patients' preferences for communication. J Clin Oncol 19:2049–2056, 2001

Parkes C: Determinants of outcome following bereavement. Omega 6:303–323, 1975

Parkes C: Bereavement: Studies of Grief in Adult Life, 3rd Edition. Madison, CT, International Universities Press, 1998

Parkes C, Weiss R: Recovery from Bereavement. New York, Basic Books, 1983

Parkes C, Laungani P, Young B (ed): Death and bereavement across cultures. London, Routledge, 1997

Passik SD, Dugan W, McDonald MV, et al: Oncologists' recognition of depression in their patients with cancer. J Clin Oncol 16:1594–1600, 1998

Passik SD, Donaghy KB, Theobald DE, et al: Oncology staff recognition of depressive symptoms on videotaped interviews of depressed cancer patients: implications for designing a training program. J Pain Symptom Manage 19:329–338, 2000

Passik SD, Kirsh KL, Donaghy KB, et al: An attempt to employ the Zung Self-Rating Depression Scale as a "lab test" to trigger follow-up in ambulatory oncology clinics: criterion validity and detection. J Pain Symptom Manage 21:273–281, 2001

Pasternak R, Reynolds C, Schlernitzauer M: Acute open-trial nortriptyline therapy of bereavement-related depression in late life. J Clin Psychiatry 52:307–310, 1991

Patchell RA, Posner JB: Cancer and the nervous system, in Handbook of Psychooncology: Psychological Care of the Patient With Cancer. Edited by Holland JC, Rowland JH. New York, Oxford University Press, 1989, pp 327–341

Payne DK, Massie MJ: Anxiety in palliative care, in Handbook of Psychiatry in Palliative medicine. Edited by Chochinov HM, Breitbart W. New York, Oxford University Press, 2000, pp 63–74

Peck AW, Stern WC, Watkinson C: Incidence of seizures during treatment with tricyclic antidepressant drugs and bupropion. J Clin Psychiatry 44:197–201, 1983

Pennebaker JW, Seagal JD: Forming a story: the health benefits of narrative. J Clin Psychol 55:1243–1254, 1999

Pereira J, Hanson J, Bruera E: The frequency and clinical course of cognitive impairment in patients with terminal cancer. Cancer 79:835–842, 1997

Peterman AH, Fitchett G, Cella DF: Modeling the relationship between quality of life dimensions and an overall sense of well-being. Paper presented at the Third World Congress of Psycho-Oncology, New York, October 3–6, 1996

Pickrel J: "Tell me your story": using life review in counseling the terminally ill. Death Studies 13:127–135, 1989

Portenoy R[K], Foley KM: Management of cancer pain, in Handbook of Psychooncology: Psychological Care of the Patient With Cancer. Edited by Holland JC, Rowland JH. New York, Oxford University Press, 1989, pp 369–382

Portenoy RK, Thaler HT, Kornblith AB, et al: The Memorial Symptom Assessment Scale: an instrument for the evaluation of symptom prevalence, characteristics, and distress. Eur J Cancer 30A:1326–1336, 1994

Posner JB: Nonmetastatic effects of cancer on the nervous system, in Cecil's Textbook of Medicine, 8th Edition. Edited by Wyngaarden JB, Smith LH. Philadelphia, PA, WB Saunders, 1988, pp 1104–1107

Post SG, Puchalski CM, Larson DB: Physicians and patient spirituality: professional boundaries, competency, and ethics. Ann Intern Med 132:578–583, 2000

Prigerson H, Jacobs S: Traumatic grief as a distinct disorder: a rationale, consensus criteria, and a preliminary empirical test, in Handbook of Bereavement Research: Consequences, Coping, and Care. Edited by Stroebe M, Hansson R, Stroebe W, et al. Washington, DC, American Psychological Association, 2001, pp 613–637

Prigerson H, Frand E, Kasl S: Complicated grief and bereavement-related depression as distinct disorders: preliminary empirical validation in elderly bereaved spouses. Am J Psychiatry 152:22–30, 1995a

Prigerson H, Maciejewski P, Newson J, et al: Inventory of complicated grief. Psychiatry Res 59:65–79, 1995b

Puchalski C, Romer AL: Taking a spiritual history allows clinicians to understand patients more fully. Journal of Palliative Medicine 3:129–137, 2000

Rabkin JG, Goetz RR, Remien RH, et al: Stability of mood despite HIV illness progression in a group of homosexual men. Am J Psychiatry 154:231–238, 1997

Rando T: Treatment of Complicated Mourning. Champaign, IL, Research Press, 1983

Raphael B: The Anatomy of Bereavement. London, Hutchinson, 1983

Rodin G, Gillies LA: Individual psychotherapy for the patient with advanced disease, in Handbook of Psychiatry in Palliative Medicine. Edited by Chochinov HM, Breitbart W. New York, Oxford University Press, 2000

Rosenfeld B: Assisted suicide, depression, and the right to die. Psychol Public Policy Law 6:467–488, 2000

Rosenfeld B, Breitbart W, Stein K, et al: Measuring desire for death among patients with HIV/AIDS: the schedule of attitudes toward hastened death. Am J Psychiatry 156:94–100, 1999

Rosenfeld B, Breitbart W, Galietta M, et al: The schedule of attitudes toward hastened death: Measuring desire for death in terminally ill cancer patients. Cancer 88:2868–2875, 2000

Rousseau P: Spirituality and the dying patient. J Clin Oncol 18:2000–2002, 2000

Schut H, Stroebe M, de Keijser J, et al: Intervention for the bereaved: gender differences in the efficacy of two counseling programmes. Br J Clin Psychol 36:63–72, 1997

Seidlitz L, Duberstein PR, Cox C, et al: Attitudes of older people toward suicide and assisted suicide: an analysis of Gallup poll findings. J Am Geriatr Soc 43:993–998, 1995

Shuster JL, Breitbart W, Chochinov HM: Psychiatric aspects of excellent end-of-life care: position statement of the Academy of Psychosomatic Medicine. Psychosomatics 40:1–3, 1999

Silberfarb PM, Maurer LH, Crouthamel CS: Psychosocial aspects of neoplastic disease, I: functional status of breast cancer patients during different treatment regimens. Am J Psychiatry 137:450–455, 1980

Singer P, Martin DK, Kelner M: Domains of quality end-of-life care from the patient perspective. JAMA 281:163–168, 1999

Sloan RP, Bagiella E, Powell T: Religion, spirituality, and medicine. Lancet 353:664–667, 1999

Smith TJ: Tell it like it is. J Clin Oncol 18:3441–3445, 2000

Spiegel D, Bloom JR: Group therapy and hypnosis reduce metastatic breast carcinoma pain. Psychosom Med 4:333–339, 1983

Spiegel D, Bloom JR, Yalom ID: Group support for patients with metastatic cancer: a randomized prospective outcome study. Arch Gen Psychiatry 38:527–533, 1981

Spira J: Existential psychotherapy in palliative care, in Handbook of Psychiatry in Palliative Medicine. Edited by Chochinov H, Breitbart W. New York, Oxford University Press, 2000, pp 197–214

Stiefel FC, Breitbart W, Holland JC: Corticosteroids in cancer: neuropsychiatric complications. Cancer Invest 7:479–491, 1989

Stjernsward J, Clark D: Palliative medicine: a global perspective, in Oxford Textbook of Palliative Medicine, 3rd Edition. Edited by Doyle D, Hanks GWC, Cherny N, et al. New York, Oxford University Press, 2004, pp 1197–1224

Stjernsward J, Papallona S: Palliative medicine: a global perspective, in Oxford Textbook of Palliative Medicine, 2nd Edition. Edited by Doyle D, Hanks GWC, MacDonald N. New York, Oxford University Press, 1998, pp 1227–1245

Storey P, Knight C: UNIPAC Two: Alleviating Psychological and Spiritual Pain in the Terminally Ill, American Academy of Hospice and Palliative Medicine. Larchmont, NY, Mary Ann Liebert, Inc, 2001

Strain JJ, Liebowitz MR, Klein DF: Anxiety and panic attacks in the medically ill. Psychiatr Clin North Am 4:333–350, 1981

Stroebe M, Stroebe W, Hansson R (ed): Handbook of Bereavement. Cambridge, United Kingdom, Cambridge University Press, 1993

Subcommittee on Psychiatric Aspects of Life-Sustaining Technology: The role of the psychiatrist in end-of-life treatment decisions, in Caring for the Dying: Identification and Promotion of Physician Competency (Educational Resource Document). Philadelphia, PA, American Board of Internal Medicine, 1996, pp 61–67

SUPPORT Principal Investigators: A controlled trial to improve care for seriously ill hospitalized patients: the study to understand prognoses and preferences for outcomes and risks of treatments (SUPPORT). JAMA 274:1591–1598, 1995

Thiel MM, Robinson MR: Physicians' collaboration with chaplains: difficulties and benefits. J Clin Ethics 8:94–103, 1997

Tremblay A, Breitbart W: Psychiatric dimensions of palliative care. Neurol Clin 19:949–967, 2001

Twycross RG, Lack SA: Symptom Control in Far Advanced Cancer: Pain Relief. London, Pitman, 1983

Twycross RG, Lack SA: Therapeutics in Terminal Disease. London, Pitman, 1984, pp 99–103

Underwood LG, Teresi JA: The daily spiritual experience scale. Ann Behav Med 24:22–33, 2002

Ventafridda V, Ripamonti C, De Conno F, et al: Symptom prevalence and control during cancer patients' last days of life. J Palliat Care 6:7–11, 1990

Viederman M: The supportive relationship, the psychodynamic life narrative, and the dying patient, in Handbook of Psychiatry in Palliative Medicine. Edited by Chochinov HM, Breitbart W. New York, Oxford University Press, 2000, pp 215–223

Viederman M, Perry SW: Use of a psychodynamic life narrative in the treatment of depression in the physically ill. Gen Hosp Psychiatry 3:177–185, 1980

Vogl D, Rosenfeld B, Breitbart W, et al: Symptom prevalence, characteristics and distress in AIDS outpatients. J Pain Symptom Manage 18:253–262, 1999

Watson M, Haviland JJ, Greer S, et al: Influence of psychological response on survival in breast cancer population-based cohort study. Lancet 354:1331–1336, 1999

Weddington WW: Delirium and depression associated with amphotericin B. Psychosomatics 23:1076–1078, 1982

Weeks JC, Cook EF, O'Day SJ, et al: Relationship between cancer patients' predictions of prognosis and their treatment preferences. JAMA 279:1709–1714, 1996

Weisman AD: On Dying and Denying: A Psychiatric Study of Terminality. New York, Behavioral Publications, 1972

Wilson KG, Chochinov HM, de Faye BJ, et al: Diagnosis and management of depression in palliative care, in Handbook of Psychiatry in Palliative Medicine. Edited by Chochinov HM, Breitbart W. New York, Oxford University Press, 2000, pp 25–49

World Health Organization: Cancer Pain Relief and Palliative Care: Report of a WHO Expert Committee (Technical Bulletin 804). Geneva, Switzerland, World Health Organization, 1990

World Health Organization: Cancer Pain Relief and Palliative Care: Report of a WHO Expert Committee (Technical Bulletin 804). Geneva, Switzerland, World Health Organization, 1997

World Health Organization: Symptom Relief in Terminal Illness. Geneva, Switzerland, World Health Organization, 1998

Young DF: Neurological complications of cancer chemotherapy, in Neurological Complications of Therapy: Selected Topics. Edited by Silverstein A. New York, Futura, 1982, pp 57–113

Zisook S, Schuchter S: The first four years of widowhood. Psychiatr Ann 16:288–294, 1985

Zisook S, Schuchter S: Depression through the first year after the death of a spouse. Am J Psychiatry 148:1346–1352, 1991

Zisook S, Schuchter S, Sledge P: The spectrum of depressive phenomena after spousal bereavement. J Clin Psychiatry 55 (suppl 4):29–36, 1994

Zisook S, Shuchter SR, Pedrelli P, et al: Bupropion sustained release for bereavement: results of an open trial. J Clin Psychiatry 62:227–230, 2001

Zuehlke TE, Watkins JT: The use of psychotherapy with dying patients: an exploratory study. J Clin Psychol 31:729–732, 1975

Index

*Page numbers printed in **boldface** type refer to tables or figures.*

Stress Profile, 27
Stroke, 701–705
  behavioral changes after, 703–705
    affective dysprosodia, 703
    anosognosia, 703
    anxiety, 259, 704
    apathy, 703
    aphasia, 703
    catastrophic reactions, 705
    depression, 195, 203, 703–704
      antidepressants for, 203, 205, 704
      brain lesions associated with, 203
      cognitive-behavioral therapy for, 704
      electroconvulsive therapy for, 203, 207
      etiology of, 704
      prevalence of, 203
      psychostimulants for, 207
    emotional lability, 704–705
    executive dysfunction, 705
    inhibition dyscontrol, 705
    loss of empathy, 705
    mania, 237
    obsessive-compulsive disorder, 705
    psychosis, 705
    sexual dysfunction, 369–370, **370,** 705
  catatonia and, 240
  clinical features of, 702
  cocaine abuse and, 406
  cognitive impairment and delirium due to, 702–703
  due to infarction, 702
  electroconvulsive therapy after, 969–970
  epidemiology of, 702
  hemorrhagic, 702
  interpreting Minnesota Multiphasic Personality Inventory in patients with, 23
  mechanisms of, 702
  mortality from, 702
  neuroimaging of, 702
  neuropsychological evaluation after, 19–20, 29–30
  pain after, 830
  psychotropic drug use in, 908
  rheumatoid arthritis and, 538
  risk factors for, **135**
  sickle cell anemia and, 774
  vascular dementia and, 142, 702
  vertebrobasilar, 702

Structured Clinical Interview for DSM-IV (SCID), 791, 832
Structured Interview of Reported Symptoms, 30
Study to Understand Prognoses and Preferences for Outcomes and Risks of Treatments (SUPPORT), 981
Stupor
  in catatonia, 240
  vs. hypoactive delirium, 91
Subacute sclerosing panencephalitis (SSPE), 713
Subarachnoid hemorrhage, 20, 723
  headache due to, 719, 723
  vs. migraine, 719
Subcortical arteriosclerotic encephalopathy, 142
Subcutaneous drug administration
  of antipsychotics, 897
  of benzodiazepines, 896
Subdural hematoma, 177, 722–723
  acute vs. chronic, 722
  clinical features of, 722–723
  investigation and differential diagnosis of, 723
  management of, 723
  pathology of, 723
Sublimation, **79**
Sublingual drug administration
  of benzodiazepines, 896
  of psychostimulants, 897
Substance-induced disorders, 387–388
  anxiety, 256, **257–258**
  delirium, 100, 112, **114**
  dementia, **133,** 143
  depression, 204–205, **205**
  mania, 236, **237**
  psychosis, 243, **245**
  sexual dysfunction, 370–375, **372–374**
  sleep disturbances, 348–353, **350–352**
  withdrawal syndromes (See Withdrawal)
Substance P
  in alopecia areata, 632
  fibromyalgia and, 564
Substance use disorders (SUDs), 387–411
  abuse in, 388
  acute assessment of, 389, **389**
  addiction in, 388
  aggressive behavior and, 171, 172, **178,** 180
  among inpatients, 174

  victims of domestic violence, 183
  alcohol-related disorders, 391–400
  amphetamine-related disorders, 407
  cannabis-related disorders, 409–410
  club drugs and hallucinogens, 408–409
  cocaine-related disorders, 405–406
  definitions related to, 338
  dependence in, 338
  DSM-IV-TR substance-related disorders, 387–388
  heritability of, 389
  high index of suspicion for, 388–389
  inhalant-related disorders, 411
  maternal competency and, 46–47
  medical illness and
    burn trauma, 657–659
    chronic hepatitis C infection, 473
    high-risk sexual behaviors and HIV transmission, 366
    HIV infection, 612
    renal failure, 485
    spinal cord injury, 391, 804
    traumatic brain injury, 21, 795–796
  negative reactions to patients with, 388, 389
  nicotine-related disorders, 410–411
  opioid-related disorders, 401–404
  in patients with chronic pain, 835–837
  phencyclidine-related disorders, 407–408
  in pregnancy, 743, 778
  psychiatric comorbidity with
    antisocial personality disorder, 614
    body dysmorphic disorder, 286
    dementia, **133,** 134, 143
    eating disorders, 313
    schizophrenia/psychosis, 7, 243, 244
    somatization, 273–275, 281
    suicidality, 221–222
  roles of psychiatrists in medical settings regarding, 387
  sedative-, hypnotic-, and anxiolytic-related disorders, 400–401
  social network of patients with, 388
  tolerance in, 338
  toxicology screening for, 10, 389
  transplant surgery for patients with, 679, 683–685
  treatment of, 389–391
    aftercare, 389–390
    barriers to, 388